PEDIATRIC ACUTE CARE

A Guide for Interprofessional Practice

Edited by

KARIN REUTER-RICE, PhD, NP, FCCM

Assistant Professor
School of Nursing
School of Medicine, Department of Pediatrics
Duke University
Durham, North Carolina

BETH NACHTSHEIM BOLICK, DNP, NP

Associate Professor
Department of Women, Children, & Family Nursing
College of Nursing
Rush University
Chicago, Illinois

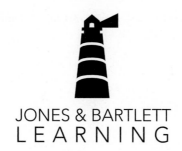

JONES & BARTLETT
LEARNING

World Headquarters

Jones & Bartlett Learning
5 Wall Street
Burlington, MA 01803
978-443-5000
info@jblearning.com
www.jblearning.com

Jones & Bartlett Learning
Canada
6339 Ormindale Way
Mississauga, Ontario L5V 1J2
Canada

Jones & Bartlett Learning
International
Barb House, Barb Mews
London W6 7PA
United Kingdom

Jones & Bartlett Learning books and products are available through most bookstores and online booksellers. To contact Jones & Bartlett Learning directly, call 800-832-0034, fax 978-443-8000, or visit our website, www.jblearning.com.

Substantial discounts on bulk quantities of Jones & Bartlett Learning publications are available to corporations, professional associations, and other qualified organizations. For details and specific discount information, contact the special sales department at Jones & Bartlett Learning via the above contact information or send an email to specialsales@jblearning.com.

The authors, editors, and publisher have made every effort to provide accurate information. However, they are not responsible for errors, omissions, or for any outcomes related to the use of the contents of this book and take no responsibility for the use of the products and procedures described. Treatments and side effects described in this book may not be applicable to all people; likewise, some people may require a dose or experience a side effect that is not described herein. Drugs and medical devices are discussed that may have limited availability controlled by the Food and Drug Administration (FDA) for use only in a research study or clinical trial. Research, clinical practice, and government regulations often change the accepted standard in this field. When consideration is being given to use of any drug in the clinical setting, the health care provider or reader is responsible for determining FDA status of the drug, reading the package insert, and reviewing prescribing information for the most up-to-date recommendations on dose, precautions, and contraindications, and determining the appropriate usage for the product. This is especially important in the case of drugs that are new or seldom used.

Production Credits
Publisher: Kevin Sullivan
Acquisitions Editor: Amanda Harvey
Editorial Assistant: Sara Bempkins
Production Editor: Amanda Clerkin
Associate Marketing Manager: Katie Hennessy
Permissions and Photo Researcher: Amy Mendosa
V.P., Manufacturing and Inventory Control: Therese Connell
Composition: diacriTech, Chennai, India
Cover Design: Scott Moden
Cover Image: © Prudkov/ShutterStock, Inc.
Printing and Binding: Courier Kendallville
Cover Printing: Courier Kendallville

Library of Congress Cataloging-in-Publication Data
Pediatric acute care : a guide for interprofessional practice/edited
by Karin Reuter-Rice, Beth Bolick.
  p. ; cm.
  Includes bibliographical references and index.
  ISBN 978-0-7637-7971-9 (alk. paper)
  1. Pediatric emergencies. 2. Pediatric intensive care. 3. Pediatric nursing. I. Reuter-Rice, Karin. II. Bolick, Beth.
  [DNLM: 1. Critical Illness—nursing. 2. Acute Disease—nursing. 3. Child. 4. Critical Care—methods. 5. Infant. 6. Nurse Practitioners. WY 159]
RJ370.P382 2012
618.92'0025—dc22
                    2010040548

6048

Printed in the United States of America
15 14 13 12 11 10 9 8 7 6 5 4 3 2 1

Dedication

We dedicate this book to the members of the pediatric interprofessional
team. Your commitment, passion, and expertise improve the lives
of pediatric patients and their families.
We thank the contributors and reviewers for your time, enthusiasm, wisdom,
and guidance. We also would like to extend our thanks to our many colleagues
who stood steadfast with us in this project and supported our efforts.
We sincerely appreciate the counsel and detailed direction we received
from the Jones & Bartlett Learning editorial staff that
allowed us to complete the first edition of this work.
Last and certainly not least, without the patience, encouragement,
support, and love of our husbands, children, families, and dogs this
huge undertaking would not have been possible.

Karin and Beth

Contents

The catalog page for this text, found at the publisher's website, contains the following additional online resources for students, professionals, and instructors. The URL for the catalog page is: http://www.jblearning.com/catalog/9780763779719. You can also visit the publisher's main website at http://www.jblearning.com and search for either of the lead editor's last names.

Instructional Materials
These are complete chapters on patient simulation and the role of assessment in teaching and learning that supplement the chapters found in the book.

Prepared Lectures
A selection of PowerPoint lectures, developed from the text material, has been provided for your use. Please feel free to adapt the lectures to your setting or use the lecture template to create new lectures of your own from the text material.

Prepared Simulation Scenarios
A selection of simulation scenarios, developed from text material, has been provided for your use. Please feel free to adapt the scenarios to your setting or use the simulation template in the preceding chapter to create new scenarios of your own from the text material.

Sample Simulation Scenario Videos
Several recorded simulations have been provided for your viewing. They are meant to offer you ideas for implementing your own simulations. These are examples only.

Foreword

There is an ongoing explosion of scientific knowledge and technological advances in pediatrics. To provide care in this dynamic field, health care professionals need to constantly reassess and revise their approach to pediatric patients and their families. Effective patient- and family-centered care requires a commitment to care on a 24 hours a day, 365 days a year basis. Consequently, it takes a large team of competent professionals from many disciplines to promote the best outcomes in this challenging environment. The complexity of today's health care system and the increasing acuity of our patients demand smart, motivated, and dedicated team members.

Pediatric Acute Care: A Guide for Interprofessional Practice, edited by Drs. Karin Reuter-Rice and Beth Bolick, reaches out to the entire interprofessional team. It provides insights into care, safety, systems, and regulations across the pediatric spectrum. *Pediatric Acute Care* is intended as a reference for practice and as a resource for training health care professionals who care for pediatric patients in a variety of settings, such as emergency, transport, inpatient, and critical care. Reuter-Rice and Bolick's book uniquely exemplifies the interprofessional movement in pediatrics. More than 200 professionals from diverse disciplines such as child life, education, epidemiology, law, medicine, military, nursing, nutrition, oriental medicine, pharmacy, public health, psychology, regulatory agencies, and research came together to provide you with their expertise and an evidence-based approach to practice.

Our hope is that this book will serve as a valuable resource to you throughout your personal journey. Reuter-Rice and Bolick's *Pediatric Acute Care* has the depth and diversity needed to address today's complex and dynamic health care environment and to ensure optimal outcomes for patients and their families.

William R. Hayden, MD
Section Chief, Pediatric
Critical Care
John H. Stroger, Jr. Hospital
of Cook County/Rush
University Medical Center
Rush Children's Hospital
Chicago, Illinois

Judy Verger, PhD, NP
Director, Pediatric Critical
Care and Neonatal Nurse
Practitioner Programs
School of Nursing
University of Pennsylvania
Philadelphia, Pennsylvania
Nurse Practitioner, Pediatric
Critical Care
Children's Hospital of
Philadelphia

Foreword

Reviewers

Donna L. Agan, EdD
Nursing Data Analyst
Scripps Mercy Hospital
San Diego, California

John W. Berkenbosch, MD, FRCPC, FAAP, FCCM
Professor of Pediatrics, Pediatric Critical Care
Director, University Children's Sedation Services
University of Louisville
Attending Physician, "Just For Kids" Critical Care Center
Kosair Children's Hospital
Louisville, Kentucky

Cindy Etzler Budek, MS, NP
Nurse Practitioner, Pulmonary Habilitation
Children's Memorial Hospital
Chicago, Illinois

Edward E. Conway, Jr., MD, MS, FCCM, FAAP
Professor of Clinical Pediatrics
Albert Einstein College of Medicine
Chairman, Milton and Bernice Stern Department of
    Pediatrics
Chief, Pediatric Critical Care
Beth Israel Medical Center
New York, New York

Edmundo Cortez, MD
Assistant Professor, Department of Pediatrics
Rush Medical College
Director, Pediatric Critical Care
Rush University Medical Center, Rush Children's
    Hospital
Chicago, Illinois

Donna Miles Curry, PhD, CNS
Associate Professor, Associate Dean for Graduate
    Programs
College of Nursing & Health
Wright State University
Dayton, Ohio

Gretchen Delametter, MSN, NP
Nurse Practitioner, Pediatric Neurosurgery
University of North Carolina Hospitals and Clinics
Chapel Hill, North Carolina

Valarie Eichler, MSN, NP
Adjunct Clinical Faculty
University of Texas, Arlington/University of Alabama,
    Birmingham
Nurse Practitioner, Pediatric Critical Care
Children's Medical Center Dallas
Dallas, Texas

Sarah Gutknecht, DNP, NP
Affiliate Faculty
University of Minnesota School of Nursing
Nurse Practitioner
Gillette Children's Hospital
St. Paul, Minnesota
Shriners Hospital for Children
Minneapolis, Minnesota

Patricia Kunz Howard, RN, PhD, FAEN
Adjunct Faculty
University of Kentucky College of Nursing
Operations Manager, Emergency and Trauma
    Services
University of Kentucky Chandler Hospital
Lexington, Kentucky

Sara E. Jandeska, MD
Assistant Professor, Department of Pediatrics
Rush Medical College
Attending Physician, Pediatric Nephrology
Director, Pediatric Dialysis
Rush University Medical Center, Rush Children's
    Hospital
Attending Physician, Pediatric Nephrology
John H. Stroger, Jr. Hospital of Cook County
Chicago, Illinois

Christine Kennelly, MS, CNS
Clinical Nurse Coordinator, Pediatric Critical Care
Rush University Medical Center, Rush Children's
    Hospital
Chicago, Illinois

Richard A. Levy, MD
Assistant Professor, Medicine and Pediatrics
Rush University
Physician, Pediatric Endocrinology
Rush University Medical Center, Rush Children's
    Hospital
Chicago, Illinois

Maureen A. Madden, MSN, NP, FCCM
Assistant Professor, Department of Pediatrics
UMDNJ, Robert Wood Johnson Medical School
Nurse Practitioner, Pediatric Critical Care
Bristol-Myers Squibb Children's Hospital at
    Robert Wood Johnson University Hospital
New Brunswick, New Jersey

Barry P. Markovitz, MD, MPH
Professor of Clinical Anesthesiology and Pediatrics
University of Southern California Keck School of
    Medicine
Director, Pediatric Critical Care
Children's Hospital of Los Angeles
Los Angeles, California

Lisa M. Milonovich, MSN, NP
Nurse Practitioner, Pediatric Critical Care
Children's Medical Center Dallas
Dallas, Texas

Lynn D. Mohr, MS, CNS
Instructor, Department of Women, Children, and
    Family Nursing
Rush University College of Nursing
Chicago, Illinois

Jeffrey M. Pearl, MD
Director, Pediatric Cardiovascular Surgery
Phoenix Children's Hospital
Phoenix, Arizona

Amy Phipps, MSN, NP
Nurse Practitioner, Pediatric Bariatric Surgery
University of Illinois Medical Center
Chicago, Illinois

John W. Polley, MD
Chairman, Craniomaxillofacial Surgery, Aesthetic and
    Pediatric Plastic Surgery

John W. Curtin Chair
Professor and Chairman
Department of Plastic and Reconstructive Surgery
Co-director, Rush Craniofacial Center
Rush University Medical Center
Chicago, Illinois

Faisal G. Qureshi, MD
Assistant Professor of Surgery and Critical Care
George Washington University School of Medicine
    and Public Health
Director, Surgical Care Unit
Children's National Medical Center
Washington, DC

Tom B. Rice, MD, FAAP, FCCP
Professor of Pediatrics
Chief, Division of Pediatric Critical Care
Medical College of Wisconsin
Director, Pediatric Critical Care Services
Children's Hospital of Wisconsin
Milwaukee, Wisconsin

Beth Shields, PharmD
Rush Medical College
Clinical Specialist Pediatrics
Specialty Operations Supervisor
Rush University Medical Center, Rush Children's
    Hospital
Chicago, Illinois

Emily Siffermann, MD, FAAP
Attending Physician, Child Protective Services
John H. Stroger, Jr. Hospital of Cook County
Chicago, Illinois

Erin R. Stucky, MD, FAAP, SFHM
Clinical Professor, Division of Pediatrics and
    Hospital Medicine
Vice-Chair for Clinical Affairs
Associate Program Director, Pediatric Residency
    Program
Director, Pediatric Hospital Medicine Fellowship
Director, Graduate Medical Education
Director, Quality and Patient Safety
University of California, San Diego
Attending Physician, Hospitalist
Rady Children's Hospital San Diego
San Diego, California

Mary P. White, MSN, NP
United States Navy Nurse Corps
Naval Branch Health Clinic Kings Bay Georgia
St. Mary's, Georgia

Contributors

Mary Ruth Abelt, MSN, NP
Assistant Professor, Department of Pediatrics, Section of
    Critical Care
Baylor College of Medicine
Director of Advanced Level Practitioners, Pediatric
    Critical Care
Texas Children's Hospital
Houston, Texas

Sherri Adams, MSN, NP
Lecturer
University of Toronto
Nurse Practitioner, Paediatric Medicine Complex Care
    Program
The Hospital for Sick Children
Toronto, Ontario

Christine Agee, MSN, NP
Nurse Practitioner, Pediatric Electrophysiology/Cardiology
Pediatric Critical Care
Duke University Children's Hospital
Durham, North Carolina

Maryann Alexander, RN, PhD
Chief Officer, Nursing Regulation
National Council of State Boards of Nursing
Chicago, Illinois

Joseph J. Amato, MD, MJ
Professor, Cardiovascular and Thoracic Surgery
Professor, Pediatrics
Rush College of Medicine
Rush University Medical Center
Chicago, Illinois

Amy S. Babuich, MD
Instructor, Department of Ophthalmology
Attending Physician, Ophthalmology
Bascom Palmer Eye Institute
Miami, Florida

David Barnett, PhD
Associate Director, University Assessment and Student
    Learning
Rush University
Chicago, Illinois

Dean Barone, MPAS, PA
Physician Assistant, Pediatric Critical Care
Bristol-Myers Squibb Children's Hospital at
    Robert Wood Johnson University Hospital
New Brunswick, New Jersey

Jennifer Bevacqua, MSN, NP
Nurse Practitioner, Pediatric Emergency Medicine
Doernbecher Children's Hospital, Oregon Health and
    Sciences University
Portland, Oregon

Abigail R. Blackmore, RN
Trauma Nurse Registrar
St. Anthony Central Hospital
Denver, Colorado

Pamela W. Bourg, RN, MS
Director Trauma Program
St. Anthony Central Hospital
Denver, Colorado

Rosemary Briars, ND, NP
Adjunct Faculty, Rush University College of
    Nursing and
University of Illinois Chicago College of Nursing
Co-director, Chicago Children's Diabetes Center
La Rabida Children's Hospital
Chicago, Illinois

Lori Broderick, MD, PhD
Physician, Pediatric Allergy and Immunology
Rady Children's Hospital San Diego
San Diego, California

Richard Brown, MSN, JD, NP, FAANP
Instructor Graduate Studies
University of Alabama Birmingham
Nurse Practitioner
Children's Hospital of Alabama
Birmingham, Alabama

Cindy Etzler Budek, MS, NP
Nurse Practitioner, Pulmonary Habilitation
Children's Memorial Hospital
Chicago, Illinois

Anthony M. Burda, BS, PharmD, ABAT
Assistant Professor, Department of Pharmacology
Rush University Medical Center
Chief Specialist in Poison Information
Illinois Poison Center
Chicago, Illinois

Ruth Bush, PhD, MPH
Adjunct Professor, Allied Health
San Diego Mesa College
Epidemiologist
Rady Children's Hospital San Diego
San Diego, California

Marianne Buzby, MSN, NP
Lecturer
University of Pennsylvania
Nurse Practitioner, Diabetes Center for Children
Children's Hospital of Philadelphia
Philadelphia, Pennsylvania

Jennifer Chaikin, RN, MSN, MHA
Clinical Nurse Educator, Pediatric Acute and Critical Care
Georgetown University Hospital
Washington, DC

Johanna Chang, MD, FAAP
Department of Pediatrics, Division of Rheumatology
Stanford University School of Medicine
Physician, Pediatric Rheumatology
Lucile Salter Packard Children's Hospital at Stanford
Stanford, California

Samantha Chinderle, MSN, NP
Nurse Practitioner, Pediatric Critical Care
Medical College of Wisconsin, Children's Hospital of Wisconsin
Milwaukee, Wisconsin

Nancy Chornick, RN, PhD
Director of Nursing Regulation
National Council of State Boards of Nursing
Chicago, Illinois

Dana Connolly, PhD, NP
Nurse Practitioner/Research Scientist, Pediatric Cardiology and Cardiothoracic Surgery
Heart Institute at Rady Children's Hospital San Diego
San Diego, California

Kathleen Corcoran, MS, BBA, NP
Nurse Practitioner, Pediatric Trauma
Children's Medical Center
Dallas, Texas

Karen Corlett, MSN, NP
Nurse Practitioner, Pediatric Cardiac Intensivists of North Texas
Congenital Heart Surgery Unit
Medical City Children's Hospital
Dallas, Texas

Edmundo Cortez, MD
Assistant Professor, Department of Pediatrics
Rush Medical College
Director, Pediatric Critical Care
Rush University Medical Center, Rush Children's Hospital
Chicago, Illinois

Paula Costanzo, MSN, NP
Nurse Practitioner, Pediatric Pulmonary
Rady Children's Hospital San Diego
San Diego, California

Vicki L. Craig, MD
Assistant Professor, Department of Pediatrics
UMDNJ, Robert Wood Johnson Medical School
Attending Physician, Pediatric Critical Care
Bristol-Myers Squibb Children's Hospital at Robert Wood Johnson University Hospital
New Brunswick, New Jersey

Marguerite Degenhardt, DNP, NP
Assistant Professor, Department of Women, Children, and Family Nursing
Rush University College of Nursing
Chicago, Illinois

Sylvia del Castillo, MD
Assistant Professor of Pediatrics, Department of Anesthesia Critical Care Medicine
Associate Fellowship Director, Pediatric Critical Care Medicine Fellowship Program
University of Southern California Keck School of Medicine
Attending Physician, Pediatric Critical Care
Children's Hospital Los Angeles
Los Angeles, California

Jessica L. Diver, MSN, NP
Nurse Practitioner, Pediatric Bone Marrow Transplant
Children's Hospital of Michigan
Detroit, Michigan

Sharron L. Docherty, PhD, NP
Associate Professor
Duke University School of Nursing
Nurse Practitioner, Valvano Day Hospital, Children's
    Health Center
Duke University Children's Hospital
Durham, North Carolina

Valerie Ebert, DO, FAAP
Assistant Professor Clinical Pediatrics
Department of Pediatrics, Section of Hospital Medicine
University of Arizona
Tucson, Arizona

Julie Edwards, RN, MSN
Clinical Faculty
St. Francis Medical Center College of Nursing
Peoria, Illinois

Darcy Egging, MS, NP
Affiliate Faculty
Loyola University School of Nursing
Maywood, Illinois
Nurse Practitioner, Valley Emergency Care Inc.
Delnor Hospital
Geneva, Illinois

Valarie Eichler, MSN, NP
Adjunct Clinical Faculty
University of Texas, Arlington/University of
    Alabama, Birmingham
Nurse Practitioner, Pediatric Critical Care
Children's Medical Center Dallas
Dallas, Texas

Elizabeth P. Elliott, MS, BA, PA
Instructor, Department of Pediatrics
Clinical Adjunct Instructor, Physician Assistant Program
Baylor College of Medicine
Physician Assistant, Pediatric Critical Care
Texas Children's Hospital
Houston, Texas

Sandra L. Elvik, MS, NP
Associate Professor, Pediatrics
UCLA School of Medicine
Assistant Medical Director, Child Abuse Crisis Center
Harbor, UCLA Medical Center
Torrance, California

Kathy Enright, MS, CCLS
Child Life Specialist, Pediatric Critical Care
Rady Children's Hospital San Diego
San Diego, California

Daniel B. Fagbuyi, MD, FAAP
Assistant Professor of Pediatrics and Emergency
    Medicine
George Washington University School of Medicine and
    Public Health
Director, Disaster Preparedness and Emergency
    Management
Attending Physician, Pediatric Emergency Medicine
Children's National Medical Center
Washington, DC

Elizabeth Farrington, PharmD, FCCP, FCCM, BCPS
Clinical Assistant Professor of Pharmacotherapy
University of North Carolina Eschelam School of
    Pharmacy
Clinical Specialist, Pediatrics
University of North Carolina Hospitals and Clinics
Chapel Hill, North Carolina

Ann Marie Felauer, MSN, NP
Nurse Practitioner, Pediatric Critical Care
Medical College of Wisconsin, Children's Hospital of
    Wisconsin
Milwaukee, Wisconsin

**Ronald M. Ferdman, MD, MEd, FAAP, FAAAAI,
    FACAAI**
Assistant Professor Clinical Pediatrics, Department of
    Pediatrics
University of Southern California
Attending Physician, Clinical Immunology and Allergy
Children's Hospital of Los Angeles
Los Angeles, California

Kelly Finkbeiner, MSN, NP
Nurse Practitioner, Pediatric Surgery
Children's Memorial Hospital
Chicago, Illinois

Corey B. Fritz, MS, NP
Nurse Practitioner, Pediatric Trauma
Children's Medical Center Dallas
Dallas, Texas

Sammé Fuches, RD, CNSC
Clinical Dietitian, Pediatric Critical Care
Rady Children's Hospital San Diego
San Diego, California

Jennifer Lorayne Fuller, MD
Pediatrician
Physician, General Anesthesiology
The Johns Hopkins Hospital
Baltimore, Maryland

Katheryn Gambetta, MD
Physician, Heart Failure and Heart Transplant
Children's Memorial Hospital
Chicago, Illinois

Rani Ganesan, MD
Assistant Professor
Rush Medical College
Attending Physician, Pediatric Critical Care
Rush University Medical Center, Rush Children's
    Hospital/John H. Stroger, Jr. Hospital of Cook County
Chicago, Illinois

Ann E. Gerhart, MSN, NP
Nurse Practitioner, Emergency Department
Naval Medical Center San Diego
Rady Children's Hospital San Diego
San Diego, California

Terea Giannetta, MSN, NP
Lecturer, Pediatric Nurse Practitioner Program
    Coordinator
California State University
Fresno, California
Nurse Practitioner, Pediatric Hematology/Oncology
Children's Hospital Central California
Madera, California

Samuel B. Goldfarb, MD
Assistant Professor, Department of Pediatrics, Division of
    Pulmonary Medicine
University of Pennsylvania
Director, Lung and Heart/Lung Transplant Programs
Children's Hospital of Philadelphia
Philadelphia, Pennsylvania

Mary Astor Gomez, MSN, NP
Advanced Practice Nurse, Educator, Pediatric
    Transport Team
Children's Memorial Hospital
Chicago, Illinois

Catherine J. Goodhue, MN, NP
Research Program Administrator, Pediatric Surgery
Children's Hospital Los Angeles
Los Angeles, California

Daniel J. Goodman, PhD
Psychologist, Eating Disorders Program

Rush University Medical Center, Rush Children's
    Hospital
Chicago, Illinois

Prasad Gourineni, MD
Assistant Professor, Department of Pediatrics
University of Illinois Chicago
Chicago, Illinois
Director, Pediatric Orthopedic Surgery
Advocate Hope Children's Hospital
Oak Lawn, Illinois

Gerald J. Gracia, MD
Physician, Pediatric Surgical Critical Care
Children's Hospital of Los Angeles
Los Angeles, California

Michele Grimason, MSN, NP
Nurse Practitioner, Pediatric Neuro-Critical Care
Children's Memorial Hospital
Chicago, Illinois

Justin Thames Hamrick, MD
Pediatrician
Physician, General Anesthesiology
The Johns Hopkins Hospital
Baltimore, Maryland

Brian D. Hanna, MDCM, PhD
Clinical Professor Pediatrics
University of Pennsylvania School of Medicine
Director, Section of Pulmonary Hypertension
Division of Cardiology
Children's Hospital of Philadelphia
Philadelphia, Pennsylvania

Keli Hansen, MN, NP
Nurse Practitioner, Pediatric Gastroenterology and
    Transplant
Seattle Children's Hospital
Seattle, Washington

Cathy M. Haut, DNP, NP
Assistant Professor
Specialty Director, Pediatric Acute Care Nurse
    Practitioner Program
University of Maryland School of Nursing
Nurse Practitioner, Pediatric Critical Care
Herman and Walter Samuelson Children's Hospital
    at Sinai
Baltimore, Maryland

Harriet S. Hawkins, RN, FAEN
Resuscitation Education Coordinator
Children's Memorial Hospital
Chicago, Illinois

Pamela A. Herendeen, DNP, NP
Associate Professor
Director, Care of Children's and Families Program
University of Rochester School of Nursing
Senior Pediatric Nurse Practitioner
Golisano Children's Hospital at Strong
Rochester, New York

Peter Heydemann, MD
Section Chief, Pediatric Neurology
Rush University Medical Center, Rush Children's
    Hospital
Chicago, Illinois

Judie Holleman, MSN, NP
Nurse Practitioner, Pediatric Neurosurgery
University of Chicago, Comer Children's Hospital
Chicago, Illinois

Renée Semonin Holleran, RN, PhD, FAEN
Staff Nurse, Emergency Department
Intermountain Medical Center
Salt Lake City, Utah

Emily Hopper, MSN, NP
Nurse Practitioner, Pediatric Trauma
Dell Children's Medical Center of Central Texas
Austin, Texas

Gail Hornor, MS, NP
Nurse Practitioner, Child Abuse and Neglect
Nationwide Children's Hospital
Columbus, Ohio

Karen Sue Hoyt, PhD, NP, FAEN, FAANP
Nurse Practitioner, Emergency Medicine
St. Mary Medical Center
Long Beach, California

Joyce Hsu, MD
Clinical Assistant Professor in Pediatric Rheumatology
Stanford University
Palo Alto, California
Attending Physician, Pediatric Rheumatology
Lucile Salter Packard Children's Hospital at Stanford
Stanford, California

Jean B. Ivey, DSN, NP
Associate Professor, Coordinator Pediatric Graduate
    Options
University of Alabama at Birmingham
Birmingham, Alabama

Phillip Jacobson, MD
Attending Physician, Pediatric Critical Care
John H. Stroger, Jr. Hospital of Cook County
Rush University Medical Center, Rush Children's
    Hospital
Chicago, Illinois

Sara E. Jandeska, MD
Assistant Professor, Department of Pediatrics
Rush Medical College
Attending Physician, Pediatric Nephrology
Director, Pediatric Dialysis
Rush University Medical Center, Rush Children's
    Hospital
Attending Physician, Pediatric Nephrology
John H. Stroger, Jr. Hospital of Cook County
Chicago, Illinois

Amanda Johnson, MSN, NP
Nurse Practitioner, Pediatric Neurosurgery
University of Chicago, Comer Children's Hospital
Chicago, Illinois

Angela M. Johnson, MSTOM, MPH, Dipl OM
Assistant Professor, Department of Adult Health and
    Gerontologic Nursing
Rush University College of Nursing
Practitioner of Oriental Medicine
Cancer Integrative Medicine Center
Rush University Medical Center
Chicago, Illinois

Jason M. Kane, MD, MS, FAAP
Assistant Professor, Department of Pediatrics
Rush Medical College
Attending Physician, Pediatric Critical Care
Rush University Medical Center, Rush Children's
    Hospital
Chicago, Illinois

Lindsey Katzmark, MSN, NP
Nurse Practitioner, Adult Congenital Heart Disease
    Program
Children's Hospital of Wisconsin, Froedtert Hospital
Milwaukee, Wisconsin

Yasir Kazmi, MD
Physician, Pediatrics
Rush University Medical Center
Chicago, Illinois

Paul M. Kent, MD
Assistant Professor, Department of Pediatrics

Attending Physician, Pediatric Hematology/Oncology
Rush University Medical Center, Rush Children's
 Hospital/University of Illinois, Chicago
Chicago, Illinois

Cindy L. Kerr, MSN, NP
Nurse Practitioner, Interventional Radiology
Children's Hospital Boston
Boston, Massachusetts

Anita Kewalramani, MD
Assistant Professor, Department of Pediatrics
Rush College of Medicine
Attending Physician, Pediatrics
Rush University Medical Center, Rush Children's
 Hospital
Chicago, Illinois

Bonnie Kitchen, MNSc, NP
Nurse Practitioner, General Pediatrics
Arkansas Children's Hospital
Little Rock, Arkansas

Ruth Kleinpell, PhD, NP, FAAN, FCCM
Director, Center for Clinical Research and Scholarship
Rush University Medical Center
Professor, Department of Adult Health and
 Gerontological Nursing
Rush University College of Nursing
Nurse Practitioner, Emergency Medicine
Our Lady of the Resurrection Medical Center
Chicago, Illinois

Andrea M. Kline, MS, NP, FCCM
Nurse Practitioner, Pediatric Pulmonary, Critical Care,
 and Allergy
Riley Hospital for Children
Indianapolis, Indiana

Jane E. Kramer, MD, FAAP
Associate Professor, Department of Pediatrics
Rush Medical College
Director, Pediatric Residency Program
Attending Physician, Pediatrics and Emergency Medicine
Rush University Medical Center, Rush Children's Hospital
Chicago, Illinois

Arthur Kubic, PharmD
Specialist in Poison Information
Illinois Poison Center
Chicago, Illinois

Susan C. Kuehn, MSN, NP
Nurse Practitioner, Neonatal Intensive Care

Children's Medical Center Dallas
Dallas, Texas

Julie Kuzin, MSN, NP
Nurse Practitioner, Pediatric Cardiology
Texas Children's Hospital
Houston, Texas

Anne K. Lam, MSN, NP
Instructor, Department of Pediatric Critical Care Medicine
Baylor College of Medicine
Nurse Practitioner, Pediatric Critical Care
Texas Children's Hospital
Houston, Texas

Elaine R. Lamb, MSN, NP
Nurse Practitioner, Pediatric Trauma and Burn Service
Children's National Medical Center
Washington, DC

Patricia R. Lawrence, MSN, NP
Nurse Practitioner, Pediatric Cardiovascular Surgery
Children's Hospital Boston
Boston, Massachusetts

John A. D. Leake, MD, MPH
Associate Professor, Department of Pediatrics, Division of
 Pediatric Infectious Diseases
University of California, San Diego
Attending Physician, Pediatric Infectious Diseases
Rady Children's Hospital San Diego
San Diego, California

Karen LeRoy, MSN, NP
Clinical Faculty
Touro University
Nurse Practitioner, Children's Acute Care Hospitalist Service
Summerlin Hospital and Medical Center
Las Vegas, Nevada

Daniel Lesser, MD
Assistant Professor, Department of Pediatrics
University of California, San Diego
Attending Physician, Pediatric Respiratory Medicine
Rady Children's Hospital San Diego
San Diego, California

Richard A. Levy, MD
Assistant Professor, Medicine and Pediatrics
Rush University
Physician, Pediatric Endocrinology
Rush University Medical Center, Rush Children's
 Hospital
Chicago, Illinois

Rose Linsler, BSN, RN
Flight Nurse, Pediatric Practice Coordinator
Intermountain Healthcare Pediatric Life Flight
Salt Lake City, Utah

Jeffrey F. Linzer, Sr., MD, FAAP, FACEP
Associate Professor, Pediatrics and Emergency Medicine
Emory University School of Medicine
Co-director, Children's Sedation Service
Associate Medical Director, Compliance and Business
    Affairs,
Emergency Pediatric Group, Division of Pediatric
    Emergency Medicine
Children's Healthcare of Atlanta at Egleston and Hughes
    Spalding
Atlanta, Georgia

Jeanne M. Little, MS, NP
Instructor, Department of Women, Children, and Family
    Nursing
Rush University College of Nursing
Chicago, Illinois

Barbara Lockart, MSN, NP
Nurse Practitioner, Pediatric Oncology
Children's Memorial Hospital
Chicago, Illinois

Grace Macek, MSN, NP
Nurse Practitioner, Pediatric Cardiothoracic Surgery
University of Chicago, Comer Children's Hospital
Chicago, Illinois

Tracy Lynn Mackie, MN, NP
Sessional Instructor, Department of Pediatrics
University of Calgary
Nurse Practitioner, Unit 31 (Pediatrics)
Peter Lougheed Center
Calgary, Alberta

Jennifer R. Madden, MSN, NP
Assistant Professor, Pediatrics
University of Colorado
Nurse Practitioner, Pediatric Neuro-oncology
The Children's Hospital
Aurora, Colorado

Maureen A. Madden, MSN, NP, FCCM
Assistant Professor, Department of Pediatrics
UMDNJ, Robert Wood Johnson Medical School
Nurse Practitioner, Pediatric Critical Care
Bristol-Myers Squibb Children's Hospital at Robert
    Wood Johnson University Hospital
New Brunswick, New Jersey

Sanjay Mahant, MD, FRCPC
Assistant Professor, Department of Pediatrics
University of Toronto
Attending Physician, Pediatric Medicine
Hospital for Sick Children
Toronto, Ontario

Kelly Keefe Marcoux, MSN, NP
Clinical Assistant Professor of Pediatrics
UMDNJ, Robert Wood Johnson Medical School
Director of Advanced Practice Nursing
Nurse Practitioner, Pediatric Critical Care
Bristol-Myers Squibb Children's Hospital at Robert Wood
    Johnson University Hospital
New Brunswick, New Jersey

Jill Marks, MSN, NP
Nurse Practitioner, Pediatric Emergency Medicine
Children's Memorial Hospital
Chicago, Illinois

Minnette Markus-Rodden, MSN, NP
Clinical Instructor, Department of Pediatrics
UMDNJ, Robert Wood Johnson Medical School
Nurse Practitioner, Pediatric Critical Care and
    Transport
Bristol-Myers Squibb Children's Hospital at
    Robert Wood Johnson University Hospital
New Brunswick, New Jersey

Sarah A. Martin, MS, NP
Nurse Practitioner, Pediatric Surgery
Children's Memorial Hospital
Chicago, Illinois

Samuel M. Maurice, MD
Physician, Pediatric Plastic Surgery
Children's Healthcare of Atlanta at Egleston and
    Hughes Spalding
Atlanta, Georgia

Riza V. Mauricio, MSN, NP
Nurse Practitioner, Pediatric Critical Care
Children's Hospital of M. D. Anderson Cancer
    Center
Houston, Texas

Randolph A. McConnie, MD
Director, Clinical Services
Pediatric Gastroenterology
Rush University Medical Center
Chicago, Illinois

Mary E. McCulley, MS, NP
Assistant Clinical Professor, Department of Family
    Health Nursing
University of California San Francisco School of Nursing
San Francisco, California
Nurse Practitioner, Pediatric Cardiothoracic Surgery
Children's Hospital Los Angeles
Los Angeles, California

Steven A. McDonald, MSN, NP
Nurse Practitioner, Pediatric Acute Care
University of Minnesota Amplatz Children's Hospital
Minneapolis, Minnesota

John D. Mead, PhD
Psychologist, Eating Disorders Program
Rush University Medical Center
Chicago, Illinois

Milton W. Meadows, MD
Physician, Pediatric Critical Care
Rady Children's Hospital San Diego
San Diego, California

Cheryl Mele, MSN, NP
Assistant Professor, Department of Nursing
Drexel University
Philadelphia, Pennsylvania
Nurse Practitioner, Neonatology
Alfred I. du Pont Children's Hospital
Wilmington, Delaware

Jon N. Meliones, MD
Professor of Pediatrics
Duke University School of Medicine
Director, PCICU
Director, Performance Improvement Children's Services
Duke University Children's Hospital
Durham, North Carolina

Theresa A. Mikhailov, MD, FAAP
Associate Professor, Division of Pediatric Critical Care
Director, Pediatric Critical Care Nurse Practitioner and
    Pediatric Critical Care Nutrition Program
Medical College of Wisconsin
Associate Director, Pediatric Critical Care
Children's Hospital of Wisconsin
Milwaukee, Wisconsin

Lisa M. Milonovich, MSN, NP
Nurse Practitioner, Pediatric Critical Care
Children's Medical Center Dallas
Dallas, Texas

Jennifer A. Misasi, MSN, NP
Nurse Practitioner, Pediatric Hematology/Oncology/
    Palliative Care
Rush University Medical Center, Rush Children's Hospital
Chicago, Illinois

David Mittelman, MD, FAAO
Associate Professor, Department of Ophthalmology
Rush Medical College
Attending Physician, Ophthalmology
Rush University Medical Center
Chicago, Illinois

Jeffrey M. Mjaanes, MD
Assistant Professor, Departments of Pediatrics and
    Orthopedic Surgery
Team Physician, DePaul University
Team Physician, Trinity International University
Attending Physician, Midwest Orthopedics at Rush
Adult and Pediatric Sports Medicine
Chicago, Illinois

Lynn D. Mohr, MS, CNS
Instructor, Department of Women, Children, and
    Family Nursing
Rush University College of Nursing
Chicago, Illinois

Regina Mosier, MSN, NP
Nurse Practitioner, Pediatric Cardiothoracic Intensive Care
Nationwide Children's Hospital
Columbus, Ohio

Laurette E. Mouat, MSN, NP
Nurse Practitioner, Pediatric Gastroenterology,
    Hepatology, and Nutrition
Rady Children's Hospital San Diego
San Diego, California

David Nathalang, DO, FAAP
Assistant Professor of Clinical Pediatrics, Section of
    Pediatric Critical Care
University of Arizona College of Medicine
Attending Physician, Pediatric Critical Care
University of Arizona Medical Center, Diamond
    Children's Medical Center
Tucson, Arizona

Amy Newman, MSN, NP
Nurse Practitioner, Pediatric Oncology
Medical College of Wisconsin, Children's Hospital of
    Wisconsin
Milwaukee, Wisconsin

Nicole Fortier O'Brien, MD
Assistant Professor, Clinical Pediatrics
The Ohio State University

Attending Physician, Pediatric Critical Care
Nationwide Children's Hospital
Columbus, Ohio

Catherine O'Keefe, DNP, NP
Assistant Professor
Creighton University School of Nursing
Nurse Practitioner, Pediatric Infectious Diseases
Creighton University School of Medicine
Omaha, Nebraska

Kristen L. Osborn, MSN, NP
Instructor
University of Alabama School of Nursing
Nurse Practitioner, Pediatric Hematology/Oncology
Birmingham, Alabama

Dana Palermo, RD
Clinical Dietitian
Rady Children's Hospital San Diego
San Diego, California

Andrea Lynne Parker, MSN, BA, NP
Nurse Practitioner, Pediatric Surgery
Children's Hospital of Los Angeles
Los Angeles, California

Holly S. Parker, MSN, NP
Consulting Associate Faculty
Duke University School of Nursing
Durham, North Carolina

Asha Soyini Payne, MD, MPH, FAAP
Adjunct Instructor
George Washington University School of Medicine
    and Public Health
Physician, Pediatric Emergency Medicine
Children's National Medical Center
Washington, DC

James Pierce, MD
Pediatrician and Surgeon
Children's Hospital of Los Angeles
Los Angeles, California

Sarah Pihl, MSN, NP
Nurse Practitioner, Pediatric Intensive Care
The Children's Hospital
Aurora, Colorado

Megan Pike, MS, CCLS
Child Life Specialist
Rady Children's Hospital San Diego
San Diego, California

Kathleen Piotrowski-Walters, MSN, CNS
Clinical Faculty, Department of Women, Children, and
    Family Nursing
Rush University College of Nursing
Staff Nurse, Pediatric Critical Care
Rush University Medical Center
Chicago, Illinois

John W. Polley, MD
Chairman, Craniomaxillofacial Surgery, Aesthetic and
    Pediatric Plastic Surgery
John W. Curtin Chair
Professor and Chairman
Department of Plastic and Reconstructive Surgery
Co-director, Rush Craniofacial Center
Rush University Medical Center
Chicago, Illinois

Alice Pong, MD
Associate Clinical Professor
University of California San Diego
Attending Physician, Pediatric Infectious Diseases
Rady Children's Hospital San Diego
San Diego, California

Stephen G. Pophal, MD
Chief, Pediatric Cardiology
St. Joseph's Hospital and Medical Center
Director, Pediatric Cardiology
Scott and Laura Eller Congenital Heart Center
Phoenix, Arizona

Elizabeth M. Preze, MSN, NP
Director, Cardiac Nursing
Children's Memorial Hospital
Chicago, Illinois

Kenneth Quinto, MD
Physician, Allergy and Immunology
University of California San Diego
La Jolla, California

Alyssa Rake, MD, FAAP
Clinical Instructor in Pediatrics
University of Southern California Keck School of Medicine
Attending Physician, Pediatric Critical Care
Children's Hospital Los Angeles
Los Angeles, California

Thomas H. Rand, MD, PhD, FAAP
Clinical Associate Professor of Pediatrics
University of Washington
Seattle, Washington

Attending Physician, Pediatric Infectious Diseases
St. Luke's Children's Hospital
Boise, Idaho

Natalie B. Ratz, MS, RD
Instructor
Rush University College of Health Sciences
Clinical Dietitian
Rush University Medical Center
Chicago, Illinois

Brenda Reid, MN, CNS
Lecturer, Faculty of Nursing
University of Toronto
Clinical Nurse Specialist, Immunology and Allergy
The Hospital for Sick Children
Toronto, Ontario

Melissa Reider-Demer, NP
Nurse Practitioner, Pediatric Neurology
Children's Hospital Los Angeles
Los Angeles, California

Mark Riccioni, MSN, NP
Instructor, Department of Pediatrics, Section of
    Critical Care
Baylor College of Medicine
Nurse Practitioner, Pediatric Critical Care
Texas Children's Hospital
Houston, Texas

Tom B. Rice, MD, FAAP, FCCP
Professor of Pediatrics
Chief, Division of Pediatric Critical Care
Medical College of Wisconsin
Director, Pediatric Critical Care Services
Children's Hospital of Wisconsin
Milwaukee, Wisconsin

Christopher C. Rich, MD
Assistant Clinical Professor, Department of Psychiatry
University of California, San Diego
Director, Child and Adolescent Psychiatric Services
University of California San Diego Medical Center
San Diego, California

Courtney Robinson, MSN, CNS, NP
Nurse Practitioner, Pediatric Emergency Medicine
Texas Children's Hospital
Houston, Texas

Karen A. Rodriguez, MN, NP
Nurse Practitioner, Pediatric Trauma
Children's Hospital Los Angeles
Los Angeles, California

Nancy A. Rodriguez, PhD, NP
Assistant Professor, Department of Women, Children,
    and Family Health
Rush University College of Nursing
Chicago, Illinois
Nurse Practitioner, Neonatal Intensive Care
Evanston Hospital, North Shore University Health System
Evanston, Illinois

Mary R. Rodts, DNP, NP, FAAN
Associate Professor, Department of Women,
    Children, and Family Nursing
Rush University College of Nursing
Nurse Practitioner, Orthopedic Surgery
Midwest Orthopedics at Rush
Chicago, Illinois

Jodie Roth, MSN, NP
Nurse Practitioner, Pediatric Trauma
Dell Children's Medical Center of Central Texas
Austin, Texas

Pamela A. Ruppel, MSN, NP
Nurse Practitioner, Pediatric Gastroenterology
Peyton Manning Children's Hospital
Indianapolis, Indiana

Randall Ruppel, MD
Attending Physician, Pediatric Critical Care
Peyton Manning Children's Hospital
Indianapolis, Indiana

Terri Russell, DNP, NP
Assistant Professor, Department of Women,
    Children, and Family Nursing
Coordinator Neonatal Nurse Practitioner
    Program
Rush University College of Nursing
Nurse Practitioner, Neonatal Intensive Care
University of Chicago, Comer Children's Hospital
Chicago, Illinois

Gina M. Sanchez, MSN, NP
Instructor
Baylor College of Medicine
Nurse Practitioner, Pediatric Critical Care
Texas Children's Hospital
Houston, Texas

Lisa G. Sansalone, MSN, NP
Clinical Instructor, Pediatric Surgery
University of Texas Health Science Center
Nurse Practitioner, Pediatric Trauma

Children's Memorial Hermann Hospital
Houston, Texas

Jennifer Schoonover, MSN, NP
Nurse Practitioner, Pediatric Anesthesia
Kosair Children's Hospital
Louisville, Kentucky

Paul N. Severin, MD, FAAP
Associate Professor, Department of Pediatrics
Rush Medical College
Chairman, Division of Pediatric Critical Care Medicine
Director, Pediatric Intensive Care Unit
John H. Stroger, Jr. Hospital of Cook County
Director, PICU Transport
John H. Stroger, Jr. Hospital of Cook County, Rush
    University Medical Center, Rush Children's Hospital
Chicago, Illinois

Katherine K. Shannon, MS, NP
Adjunct Faculty
University of Illinois at Chicago College of Nursing
Nurse Practitioner, Pediatric Orthopedic Surgery
Children's Memorial Hospital
Chicago, Illinois

Emily Siffermann, MD, FAAP
Attending Physician, Child Protective Services
John H. Stroger, Jr. Hospital of Cook County
Chicago, Illinois

Jill M. Siegrist, MSN, NP
Nurse Practitioner, Pediatric Critical Care
University of Maryland Medical System
Baltimore, Maryland

Shari Simone, DNP, NP, FCCM
Associate Faculty, Pediatric Acute Care Nurse
    Practitioner Program
University of Maryland School of Nursing
Lead Nurse Practitioner, Women's & Children's Services
Nurse Practitioner, Pediatric Critical Care
University of Maryland Medical Center
Baltimore, Maryland

Adam B. Smith, MD
Physician, Plastic Surgery
Rush University Medical Center
Chicago, Illinois

Lauren R. Sorce, MSN, NP, FCCM
Nurse Practitioner, Pediatric Critical Care
Children's Memorial Hospital
Chicago, Illinois

Bonnie J. Stojadinovic, DNP, NP
Nurse Practitioner, Pediatric Critical Care
Medical College of Wisconsin/Children's Hospital of
    Wisconsin
Milwaukee, Wisconsin

Gary R. Strokosch, MD
Director, Eating Disorders Program
Rush University Medical Center
Chicago, Illinois

Rosemarie Suhayda, PhD, NP, LANP
Associate Professor, Department of Women, Children,
    and Family Nursing
Director, Evaluation
Rush University College of Nursing
Director, University Assessment and Student Learning
Rush University
Chicago, Illinois

Kristen T. Sullivan, MSN, NP
Adjunct Faculty, Department of Women, Children, and
    Family Nursing
Rush University College of Nursing
Chicago, Illinois
Nurse Practitioner, Pediatric Cardiovascular Surgery
Phoenix Children's Hospital
Phoenix, Arizona

Audrey C. Taylor, MSN, NP
Nurse Practitioner, Pediatric Hematology
Rush University Medical Center, Rush Children's Hospital
Chicago, Illinois

Bradley Tilford, MD
Assistant Professor of Clinical Pediatrics, Section of
    Pediatric Pulmonology, Critical Care, and Allergy
Indiana University School of Medicine
Attending Physician, Pediatric Critical Care
Riley Hospital for Children
Indianapolis, Indiana

Tara Trimarchi, MSN, NP
Lecturer
University of Pennsylvania School of Nursing
Senior Solutions Consultant
Children's Hospital of Philadelphia
Philadelphia, Pennsylvania

Dawn Tucker, MSN, NP
Nurse Practitioner, Cardiothoracic Surgery
Children's Mercy Hospitals and Clinics
Kansas City, Missouri

Jamie Tumulty, MS, NP, CNS
Nurse Practitioner/Clinical Nurse Specialist, Pediatric
    Acute Care
University of Maryland Medical Center
Baltimore, Maryland

Jeffrey S. Upperman, MD
Associate Professor of Surgery
University of Southern California Keck School of
    Medicine
Director, Pediatric Trauma Program
Children's Hospital Los Angeles
Los Angeles, California

Leonard A. Valentino, MD
Associate Professor of Pediatrics, Assistant Professor
    of Internal Medicine and Immunology/
    Microbiology
Rush University
Director, Pediatric Hematology/Oncology
Rush University Medical Center
Chicago, Illinois

Michael Wahl, MD, FACEP, FACMT
Clinical Instructor, Division of Emergency
    Medicine
University of Chicago
Director, Illinois Poison Center
Chicago, Illinois
Attending Physician, Emergency Medicine
Evanston Hospital, North Shore University
    Health System
Evanston, Illinois

Elizabeth Murphy Waibel, MSN, NP
Pediatric Trauma and Burn Nurse Practitioner
Children's National Medical Center
Washington, DC

Mark S. Wainwright, MD. PhD
Associate Professor
Northwestern University Feinberg School of
    Medicine
Attending Physician, Pediatric Neurology and
    Critical Care
Children's Memorial Hospital
Chicago, Illinois

Brittany N. Wall, MSN, NP
Nurse Practitioner, Neonatal Intensive Care
Children's Medical Center Dallas
Dallas, Texas

Deborah Walter, MSN, NP
Nurse Practitioner, Pediatric Cardiology/Cardiac
    Surgery
Rady Children's Hospital San Diego
San Diego, California

Summer Watkins, MSN, NP
Adjunct Faculty, Department of Women,
    Children, & Family Nursing
Rush University College of Nursing
Chicago, Illinois
Nurse Practitioner, Orthopedic Surgery
Advocate Hope Children's Hospital
Oak Lawn, Illinois

Mark D. Weber, MSN, NP
Nurse Practitioner, Pediatric Critical Care
Duke University Children's Hospital
Durham, North Carolina

Barbara Weintraub, MSN, MPH, NP, FAEN
Director, Adult and Pediatric Emergency and
    Trauma Services
Northwest Community Hospital
Arlington Heights, Illinois

John J. Whitcomb, PhD, RN
Assistant Professor, School of Nursing
College of Health, Education, and Human
    Development
Clemson University
Clemson, South Carolina

Laurie Beth Williams, MSN, NP
Nurse Practitioner, Cardiovascular Intensive Care
Children's Hospital of Orange County
Orange, California

Sarah A. Wilson, MSN, NP
Nurse Practitioner, Pediatric Trauma
Children's Medical Center Dallas
Dallas, Texas

Barbara V. Wise, PhD, NP
Nurse Practitioner, Pediatric Oncology
National Cancer Institute
Bethesda, Maryland

Michael Worthen, MD
Physician, Pediatric Anesthesia and Critical Care
Rady Children's Hospital San Diego
San Diego, California

Elizabeth Louise Yu, MD
Physician, Pediatric Gastroenterology and Hepatology
Rady Children's Hospital San Diego
San Diego, California

Tamara Zagustin, MD
Assistant Professor, Pediatrics
University of California, San Diego School
    of Medicine
Director, Pediatric Rehabilitation Medicine
Rady Children's Hospital San Diego
San Diego, California

Paula Zakrzewski, MSN, NP
Nurse Practitioner, Pediatric Neurosurgery
University of Chicago, Comer Children's Hospital
Chicago, Illinois

Christine A. Zawistowski, MD, FAAP
Assistant Professor of Pediatrics
Mount Sinai School of Medicine
Attending Physician, Pediatric Critical Care, Pain Team,
    and Palliative Care
Mount Sinai Kravis Children's Hospital
New York, New York

Tresa E. Zielinski, MS, NP
Nurse Practitioner, Pediatric Kidney Transplant
Children's Memorial Hospital
Chicago, Illinois

PART I

Interprofessional Patient Care

Theresa Mikhailov and Tom Rice

The Interprofessional Team

- Team Members
- Roles and Functions of Team Members
- Best Practice for Successful Teams
- References

TEAM MEMBERS

Interprofessional patient care is an integrated approach in which members of a clinical team actively coordinate care and services across disciplines (Ray, 1998). A health care discipline is an area of clinical knowledge and related research that is pertinent to patient care (Ray). For the care of a given patient, a team of professionals is selected from the multitude of health care disciplines. These disciplines can be categorized into medicine, nursing, allied health professions, and administration. Moreover, many subcategories exist within each of these categories.

The discipline of medicine includes physicians and surgeons, physicians-in-training, medical students, and physician assistants (PA). The discipline of nursing includes advanced practice registered nurses—a category that can be subdivided into nurse practitioners, nurse anesthetists, and clinical nurse specialists—as well as staff nurses and nursing students. The discipline of the allied health professions includes many separate disciplines, such as pharmacists, respiratory care practitioners, dietitians, therapists (occupational, physical, speech), social workers, chaplains, child life specialists, case managers, paramedics, and emergency personnel. The discipline of administration includes medical directors, nurse managers, supervisors, and health unit coordinators.

ROLES AND FUNCTIONS OF TEAM MEMBERS

The role of each team member depends on the patient, the setting, the desired outcome, and the composition of the team.

Attending physicians are health care professionals (HCP) who counsel patients on diet, hygiene, and preventive health care and who diagnose illnesses and prescribe and administer treatment for patients suffering from disease or injury (American Medical Association [AMA], n.d. [h]). Individuals who want to become physicians must complete 4 years of training at an accredited medical school, including 2 years of didactic training and 2 years of clinical training under the supervision of experienced physicians. Students may attend an allopathic medical school and become a medical doctor (MD) or an osteopathic medical school and become a doctor of osteopathic medicine (DO). After completion of medical school, students become physicians-in-training, first as residents in an area of general practice such as pediatrics or surgery, and then in some cases, as fellows in an area of specialized practice such as endocrinology or cardiothoracic surgery. Physicians must take national examinations to become board certified in their specialty and subspecialty area of practice. Both allopathic and osteopathic boards design and administer these examinations.

A physician assistant is an HCP who is academically and clinically prepared to practice medicine under the direction and supervision of a physician. A physician assistant makes clinical decisions and provides a broad range of diagnostic, therapeutic, preventive, and health maintenance services (AMA, n.d. [g]).

Advanced practice registered nurses (APRN) have additional graduate-level didactic and clinical training in a particular population, which may be further divided into acute or primary care. APRN programs typically require a bachelor of science degree in nursing and clinical nursing experience for entry; they award a master of science degree in nursing. The recommendation from the American Association of Colleges of Nursing (2009) is to transition to award the doctor of nursing practice (DNP) with additional education by 2015. Four types of APRNs are distinguished: nurse practitioners (NP), certified nurse–midwives (CNM), clinical nurse specialists (CNS), and certified registered nurse anesthetists (CRNA).

Nurse practitioners deliver primary and/or acute care in a variety of clinical settings; they diagnose and treat common acute illnesses and injuries, perform physical examinations, and manage chronic health conditions. Pediatric nurse practitioners can be trained as primary care or acute care nurse practitioners. Primary care pediatric nurse practitioners (PNP) provide health maintenance and well-child examinations, developmental screenings, school physicals, immunizations, anticipatory guidance, and diagnosis and treatment of common childhood illnesses (National Association of Pediatric Nurse Practitioners [NAPNAP], 2009). Acute care pediatric nurse practitioners (AC PNP) are trained to meet the specialized physiologic and psychological needs of children with complex acute, critical, and chronic health care needs (NAPNAP, 2005). Neonatal nurse practitioners (NNP) are acute care practitioners whose formal education and clinical competencies focus on the care of infants (through 2 years of age) with complex acute, critical, and chronic conditions (National Association of Neonatal Nurses, 2009).

Certified nurse–midwives provide prenatal and gynecological care to healthy women, deliver babies, and provide postpartum care. Clinical nurse specialists are expert clinicians who provide care to an identified population, offer consultation to staff nurses, and implement improvements in health care delivery systems (National Association of Clinical Nurse Specialists, 2009). Certified registered nurse anesthetists specialize in anesthetic care of patients (American Association of Nurse Anesthetists, 2009).

Nurses are HCPs who perform a variety of health care services, including recording patients' medical histories and symptoms, performing diagnostic testing, administering treatments and medication, helping patients with follow-up care and rehabilitation, and teaching patients and families (AMA, n.d. [c]). Individuals who want to become nurses must complete nursing education through one of two pathways: a bachelor of science degree in nursing or an associate degree in nursing. All nursing education requires both classroom instruction and supervised clinical instruction in hospitals and other health care facilities.

A wide range of allied health professionals participate in the care of patients across the spectrum of health care.

- Pharmacists distribute medications prescribed by other providers, inform patients about medications, and advise practitioners on selection, dosages, interactions, and side effects of medications (AMA, n.d. [e]).
- Respiratory therapists evaluate and treat patients of all ages with respiratory illnesses and other cardiopulmonary conditions (AMA, n.d. [i]).
- Dietitians integrate and apply the principles derived from the sciences of food, nutrition, biochemistry, physiology, food management, and behavior to achieve and maintain health status of patients in a variety of clinical settings (AMA, n.d. [a]).
- Occupational therapists promote health and wellness to those persons who have or are at risk for developing an illness, injury, disease, disorder, condition, impairment, disability, activity limitation, or participation restriction. Occupational therapy addresses the physical, cognitive, psychosocial, sensory, and other aspects of performance in a variety of contexts to support engagement in everyday life activities that affect health, well-being, and quality of life (AMA, n.d. [d]).
- Physical therapists provide services to patients who are recovering from accidents or illness and to people with disabilities. They help improve patients' strength and mobility, relieve pain, and prevent or limit permanent physical disabilities (AMA, n.d. [f]).
- Speech therapists evaluate, diagnose, and treat speech, language, and swallowing disorders in individuals of all ages, from infants to the elderly (AMA, n.d. [j]).
- Social workers assist individuals, groups, or communities to restore or enhance their capacity for social functioning, while creating societal conditions favorable to their goals. They help prevent and mitigate crises and counsel individuals, families, and communities to cope more effectively with the stresses of everyday life (National Association of Social Workers, 2009).
- Chaplains help people in health care settings cope with life-changing medical situations (Health Care Chaplaincy, 2009).
- Child life specialists are trained professionals with expertise in helping children and their families overcome life's most challenging events. They promote effective coping through play, preparation, education, and self-expression activities; provide emotional support for families; and encourage optimal development

of children facing a broad range of challenging experiences, particularly those related to health care and hospitalization (Child Life Council, 2009).
- Case managers are professionals who help patients understand their current health status, what they can do about it, and why those treatments are important. Case managers guide patients and provide cohesion to other professionals in the health care delivery team (Case Management Society of America, 2009).
- Emergency medical technicians (EMT) and paramedics are trained to provide emergency care to people who have suffered from an illness or an injury outside of the hospital setting. EMTs and paramedics work under protocols to recognize, assess, and manage medical emergencies and transport patients to facilities where they can obtain definitive medical care. EMTs provide basic life support, and paramedics provide advanced life support (AMA, n.d. [b]).

Administration and leadership are also important aspects of health care.

- A medical director is a physician who provides administrative and clinical leadership for a clinical area, such as an inpatient unit, an outpatient clinic, or a clinical program.
- A nurse manager is a nurse who provides administrative and clinical leadership for a clinical area, such as an inpatient unit, an outpatient clinic, or a clinical program.
- Nursing supervisors are nurses who are responsible for clinical and administrative oversight of a given clinical area during a designated period of time.
- Health unit coordinators are administrative professionals who help maintain a health care facility's service and performance by preparing documents, transcribing medical orders, maintaining patient charts and records, coordinating patient activities for the unit, ordering supplies, and communicating with the other clinical departments (Health Careers Center, 2009).

BEST PRACTICE FOR SUCCESSFUL TEAMS

Health care teams are ubiquitous in both inpatient and outpatient health care (Chen & Yang, 2008; Darling & Ogg, 1984; Kuziemsky et al., 2009; Lingard et al., 2004; Pavilanis, 2005; Penson et al., 2006; Wilson, 2008). These teams always include HCPs from at least two disciplines and provide a framework for members to work together to achieve better patient outcomes.

The structure and composition of health care teams depend on the setting and the purpose of the team. Some teams remain intact over a prolonged period so as to provide care to patients with chronic health care needs (Pavilanis, 2005; Penson et al., 2006; Wilson, 2008). The composition of these teams may remain consistent for weeks, months, or even longer. Other teams assemble quickly to meet the needs of a given patient, only to disband just as quickly once the purpose of the team has been achieved. The composition of these teams may vary with respect to the individual participants, but generally includes providers from specified disciplines. Still other teams exist that provide care to a given patient or group of patients on a short-term basis. These teams may be more fluid in composition, as team members come and go based on the needs of the patients or the dynamics of the health care team (Chen & Yang, 2008; Lingard et al., 2004). The model of teams may also vary from the most basic parallel model, in which providers work independently in the same setting, to the most complex model, in which providers work in a nonhierarchical, interprofessional manner and decision making occurs by consensus (Boon et al., 2004).

Regardless of the structure, composition, or model of the health care team, members must agree in advance on the role of each team member and must respect one another's roles. Individual team members must be competent within their discipline and accountable to other members (Odegard et al., 2009). Additionally, members require training in teamwork skills to function effectively within the team (Burke et al., 2004; Fernandez et al., 2007; Hamman, 2004; Ray, 1998). Interprofessional education may be a key factor in achieving success among interprofessional health care teams (Bellack et al., 1997; Headrick & Khaleel, 2008; Headrick et al., 1996). It is essential that interprofessional teams have a shared mission, purpose, or goal (Patterson et al., 2002). Other keys to successful teamwork include integrated scheduling, physical proximity of team members, strong interpersonal communication skills, regular opportunities for communication, a shared language for communication, a lack of therapeutic territorialism, and a commitment to the interprofessional process (Chen & Yang, 2008; Darling & Ogg, 1984).

Team process can be characterized into the "12 C's of teamwork":

1. Communication (the *sine qua non* of teamwork)
2. Cooperation (empowerment of team members)
3. Cohesiveness (the team sticks together)
4. Commitment (investing in the team process)
5. Collaboration (equality in the team)
6. Confronts problems directly
7. Coordination of efforts (ensuring actions support a common plan)
8. Conflict management
9. Consensus decision making
10. Caring (patient-centered outcomes)
11. Consistency (with one another and the environment)
12. Contribution (feeling this is being made)

A modern interprofessional team is a consistent grouping of people from relevant clinical disciplines, ideally inclusive of the patient, who interact guided by these 12 processes to achieve team-defined favorable patient outcomes (Wiecha & Pollard, 2004).

The goals of the health care team in pediatric acute care vary with the setting and with the patient or type of patients for whom the team is providing care. For example, a pediatric trauma team is designed to rapidly assess a patient and intervene promptly. This team requires rapid assembly of a team of providers who are skilled in both their individual areas of patient care expertise and their ability to function as a team. The leader of this team is generally a physician who receives immediate consultation from the other HCPs on the team but who is responsible for making critical decisions regarding the plan of care. Another example is a pediatric oncology team, which is designed to diagnose and treat children with oncological conditions. This team includes physicians, APRNs, staff nurses, and many different providers such as pharmacists, dietitians, social workers, case managers, and chaplains. It may function in a more interprofessional manner, with all members of the team contributing to the individual patient's care and meeting as a group to discuss the patient's needs. While the physician may still be viewed as the leader for such a team, this may differ from the trauma or transport team leader role, in that decisions may be made through group consensus. Teams can be led by providers other than physicians, but team leaders serve an essential role in teams as they facilitate decision making and exchange of information (Kuziemsky et al., 2009).

The trauma team and the oncology team are very different models of health care teams, yet both depend on cohesive teamwork to be successful. Both require effective team communication. Health care teams such as these solve complex patient problems on an ongoing basis. Thus they require critical information, infrastructure to access information, and a process to facilitate communication (Kuziemsky et al., 2009; Reddy & Spence, 2006). Open communication allows team members to share concerns about safety or quality of patient care and to ask questions in an attempt to improve understanding of patient care. This open communication between interprofessional team members is vital to successful teamwork (McCauley & Irwin, 2006; Reader et al., 2007). Interprofessional rounds can also provide an opportunity for this open communication and collaboration between team members to occur (Blough, C., & Walrath, J. (2007); O'Mahony et al., 2007; Vazirani et al., 2005).

Team debriefing is another essential feature of successful teamwork. Team debriefings allow team members to review team performance, identify errors and evaluate them in relation to team function, and provide and receive constructive feedback to improve team performance (Hunt et al., 2007; Odegard et al., 2009). Teamwork has been demonstrated to result in better communication and collaboration between HCPs, higher job and career satisfaction, less burnout, and, paradoxically, an increased sense of autonomy (Rafferty et al., 2001; Vazirani et al., 2005). Objectively, teamwork has resulted in shorter lengths of stay and improved quality of care as measured by quality core measure performance (Friedman & Berger, 2004; O'Mahony et al., 2007).

REFERENCES

1. American Association of Colleges of Nursing. (2009). The doctor of nursing practice fact sheet. Retrieved from http://www.aacn.nche.edu/Media/FactSheets/dnp.htm

2. American Association of Nurse Anesthetists. (2009). Retrieved from http://www.aana.com/Default.aspx

3. American Medical Association (AMA). (n.d. [a]). Dietitian health care careers directory 2009–2010. Retrieved from http://www.ama-assn.org/ama1/pub/upload/mm/40/diet01-dietitian.pdf

4. American Medical Association (AMA). (n.d. [b]). Emergency medical technician–paramedic 2009–2010. Retrieved from http://www.ama-assn.org/ama1/pub/upload/mm/40/ah06-emerg-med-tech-para.pdf

5. American Medical Association (AMA). (n.d. [c]). Nurse health care careers directory 2009–2010. Retrieved from http://www.ama-assn.org/ama1/pub/upload/mm/40/nurse.pdf

6. American Medical Association (AMA). (n.d. [d]). Occupational therapist health care careers directory 2009–2010. Retrieved from http://www.ama-assn.org/ama1/pub/upload/mm/40/tr01-occup-ther.pdf

7. American Medical Association (AMA). (n.d. [e]). Pharmacist health care careers directory 2009–2010. Retrieved from http://www.ama-assn.org/ama1/pub/upload/mm/40/pharm01-pharmacist.pdf

8. American Medical Association (AMA). (n.d. [f]). Physical therapist health care careers directory 2009–2010. Retrieved from http://www.ama-assn.org/ama1/pub/upload/mm/40/tr03-phys-ther.pdf

9. American Medical Association (AMA). (n.d. [g]). Physician assistant health care careers directory 2009–2010. Retrieved from http://www.ama-assn.org/ama1/pub/upload/mm/40/physician-asst.pdf

10. American Medical Association (AMA). (n.d. [h]). Physician health care careers directory 2009–2010. Retrieved from http://www.ama-assn.org/ama1/pub/upload/mm/40/physician.pdf

11. American Medical Association (AMA). (n.d. [i]). Respiratory therapist health care careers directory 2009–2010. Retrieved from http://www.ama-assn.org/ama1/pub/upload/mm/40/ah14-respira-ther.pdf

12. American Medical Association (AMA). (n.d. [j]). Speech-language pathologist health care careers directory 2009–2010. Retrieved from http://www.ama-assn.org/ama1/pub/upload/mm/40/comm02-speech-lang-path.pdf

13. Bellack, J., Gerrity, P., Moore, S., Novotny, J., Quinn, D., Norman, L., & Harper, D. (1997). Taking aim at interdisciplinary education for continuous improvement in health care. *Nursing and Health Care Perspectives, 18*(6), 308–315.

14. Blough, C., & Walrath, J. (2007). Improving patient safety and communication through care rounds in a pediatric oncology outpatient clinic. *Journal of Nursing Care Quality, 22*(2), 159–163. doi:10.1097/01.NCQ.0000263106.15720.9f

15. Boon, H., Verhoef, M., O'Hara, D., & Findlay, B. (2004). From parallel practice to integrative health care: A conceptual framework. *BMC Health Services Research, 4*(1), 15. doi:10.1186/1472-6963-4-15

16. Burke, C., Salas, E., Wilson-Donnelly, K., & Priest, H. (2004). How to turn a team of experts into an expert medical team: Guidance from the aviation and military communities. *Quality & Safety in Health Care, 13*(suppl 1), i96–i104. doi:10.1136/qhc.13.suppl_1.i96

17. Case Management Society of America. (2009). Retrieved from http://www.cmsa.org/

18. Chen, J., & Yang, R. (2008). A look inside an interdisciplinary spine center at an academic medical center. *Iowa Orthopaedic Journal, 28*, 98–101.

19. Child Life Council. (2009). The child life profession. Retrieved from http://www.childlife.org/The%20Child%20Life%20Profession/

20. Darling, L., & Ogg, H. (1984). Basic requirements for initiating an interdisciplinary process. *Physical Therapy, 64*(11), 1684–1686.

21. Fernandez, R., Parker, D., Kalus, J., Miller, D., & Compton, S. (2007). Using a human patient simulation mannequin to teach interdisciplinary team skills to pharmacy students. *American Journal of Pharmaceutical Education, 71*(3), 51.

22. Friedman, D., & Berger, D. (2004). Improving team structure and communication: A key to hospital efficiency. *Archives of Surgery, 139*(11), 1194–1198. doi:10.1001/archsurg.139.11.1194

23. Hamman, W. (2004). The complexity of team training: What we have learned from aviation and its applications to medicine. *Quality & Safety in Health Care, 13*(suppl 1), i72–i79. doi:10.1136/qhc.13.suppl_1.i72

24. Headrick, L., & Khaleel, N. (2008). Getting it right: Educating professionals to work together in improving health and health care. *Journal of Interprofessional Care, 22*(4), 364–374. doi:10.1080/13561820802227871

25. Headrick, L., Knapp, M., Neuhauser, D., Gelmon, S., Norman, L., Quinn, D., & Baker, R. (1996). Working from upstream to improve health care: The IHI interdisciplinary professional education collaborative. *The Joint Commission Journal on Quality Improvement, 22*(3), 149–164.

26. Health Care Chaplaincy. (2009). Finding meaning: Bringing comfort. Retrieved from http://www.healthcarechaplaincy.org/about-us/finding-meaning-bringing-comfort.html

27. Health Careers Center. (2009). Health unit coordinator. Retrieved from http://www.mshealthcareers.com/careers/healthunitcoord.htm

28. Hunt, E., Heine, M., Hohenhaus, S., Luo, X., & Frush, K. (2007). Simulated pediatric trauma team management: Assessment of an educational intervention. *Pediatric Emergency Care, 23*(11), 796–804. doi:10.1097/PEC.0b013e31815a0653

29. Kuziemsky, C., Borycki, E., Purkis, M., Black, F., Boyle, M., Cloutier-Fisher, D., et al. (2009). An interdisciplinary team communication framework and its application to healthcare "e-teams" systems design. *BMC Medical Informatics and Decision Making, 9*, 43. doi:10.1186/1472-6947-9-43

30. Lingard, L., Espin, S., Evans, C., & Hawryluck, L. (2004). The rules of the game: Interprofessional collaboration on the intensive care unit team. *Critical Care (London, England), 8*(6), R403–R408. doi:10.1186/cc2958

31. McCauley, K., & Irwin, R. (2006). Changing the work environment in ICUs to achieve patient-focused care: The time has come. *Chest, 130*(5), 1571–1578. doi:10.1378/chest.130.5.1571

32. National Association of Neonatal Nurses. (2009). Retrieved from http://www.nann.org/pdf/09_requirements_neonatal_nursing_practice.pdf

33. National Association of Clinical Nurse Specialists. (2009). Retrieved from http://www.nacns.org/AboutNACNS/FAQs/tabid/109/Default.aspx

34. National Association of Pediatric Nurse Practitioners (NAPNAP). (2005). The acute care pediatric nurse practitioner. *Journal of Pediatric Health Care, 19*(5), A38–A39. doi:10.1016/j.pedhc.2005.07.005

35. National Association of Pediatric Nurse Practitioners (NAPNAP). (2009). Retrieved from http://www.nAPRNap.org/PNPResources/PatientInformation/WhatIsPNP.aspx

36. National Association of Social Workers. (2009). Retrieved from http://www.naswdc.org/pressroom/features/general/profession.asp

37. Odegard, P., Robins, L., Murphy, N., Belza, B., Brock, D., Gallagher, T., et al. (2009). Interprofessional initiatives at the University of Washington. *American Journal of Pharmaceutical Education, 73*(4), 63.

38. O'Mahony, S., Mazur, E., Charney, P., Wang, Y., & Fine, J. (2007). Use of multidisciplinary rounds to simultaneously improve quality outcomes, enhance resident education, and shorten length of stay. *Journal of General Internal Medicine, 22*(8), 1073–1079. doi:10.1007/s11606-007-0225-1

39. Patterson, K., Grenny, J., McMillan, B., & Switzer, A. (2002). In N. Hancock (Ed.), *Crucial conversations: Tools for talking when stakes are high.* New York: McGraw-Hill.

40. Pavilanis, A. (2005). Interdisciplinary collaborative care: Face of the future. *Canadian Family Physician (Medecin de Famille Canadien), 51,* 779–781.

41. Penson, R., Kyriakou, H., Zuckerman, D., Chabner, B., & Lynch, T. Jr. (2006). Teams: Communication in multidisciplinary care. *The Oncologist, 11*(5), 520–526. doi:10.1634/theoncologist.11-5-520

42. Rafferty, A., Ball, J., & Aiken, L. (2001). Are teamwork and professional autonomy compatible, and do they result in improved hospital care? *Quality in Health Care, 10*(suppl 2), ii32–ii37.

43. Ray, M. (1998). Shared borders: Achieving the goals of interdisciplinary patient care. *American Journal of Health-System Pharmacy, 55*(13), 1369–1374.

44. Reader, T., Flin, R., Mearns, K., & Cuthbertson, B. (2007). Interdisciplinary communication in the intensive care unit. *British Journal of Anaesthesia, 98*(3), 347–352. doi:10.1093/bja/ael372

45. Reddy, M., & Spence, P. (2006). Finding answers: Information needs of a multidisciplinary patient care team in an emergency department. *AMIA Symposium,* 649–653.

46. Vazirani, S., Hays, R., Shapiro, M., & Cowan, M. (2005). Effect of a multidisciplinary intervention on communication and collaboration among physicians and nurses. *American Journal of Critical Care, 14*(1), 71–77.

47. Wiecha, J., & Pollard, T. (2004). The interdisciplinary eHealth team: Chronic care for the future. *Journal of Medical Internet Research, 6*(3), e22. doi:102196/jmir.6.3.e22. http://www.jmir.org/2004/3/e22/

48. Wilson, C. (2008). Dream-team for optimal care. *Canadian Family Physician (Medecin de Famille Canadien), 54*(2), 317–318.

Research, Evidence-Based Practice, and Clinical Decision Making

Promoting research in clinical practice is an essential component in ensuring best practices and promoting positive outcomes for patients. Unfortunately, it is often difficult for those in clinical practice to devote time to research activities, as the daily demands of practice often take precedence. Of equal importance is the use and integration of evidence-based practice (EBP) to improve pediatric care outcomes. This chapter reviews key strategies for implementing EBP and research in pediatric clinical practice. Examples of clinical EBP and research related to pediatric care are used to showcase the processes involved and to highlight strategies for implementing EBP and clinically focused research initiatives.

RESEARCH AS A BASIS FOR CLINICAL PRACTICE

Research indicates that patients who receive care based on evidence from well-designed studies experience better care and better outcomes (Melynk & Fineout-Overholt, 2005). Clinical research provides a mechanism for assessing aspects of health care so as to advance the science of clinical care (Burns & Grove, 2005; Hulley et al., 2006; Polit & Beck, 2006). In addition, using and conducting research helps to ensure that clinical care is relevant and effective (Burns & Grove, 2005). In acute and critical care pediatric settings, research is especially important for evaluating the impact of health care interventions on patient outcomes, including recovery from critical illness and prevention of complications during acute illness states.

The U.S. Department of Health and Human Services (HHS) Office of Extramural Research (2010) has defined research as a systematic investigation designed to develop new knowledge about disease and health care. Separate definitions allow for the protection and inclusion of children and adolescents in the HHS regulations. The National Institutes of Health (NIH, 1998) defines children as an individual younger than the age of 21 years. Special oversight of research studies involving children is often required to protect the well-being of young subjects, but addresses concerns that treatment modalities are otherwise based on adult-only research.

Research forms the basis for clinical practice, yet many health care interventions stem from limited investigation. Clinicians may also lack the time needed to gather and evaluate research literature. However, identifying opportunities for conducting research is important to advancing the practice of pediatric acute care.

Clinical Research Example

A pediatric intensive care unit (PICU) had a policy related to family presence during resuscitation; however, it did not have a policy related to family presence during invasive procedures. As a result, a clinical team formed to review the research literature related to family presence during invasive procedures and assessed options for better informing clinical practice. In conducting the search, several national organizations supporting family presence programs were identified and position statements on the topic were considered (Emergency Nurses Association, 2007). A literature search revealed a synthesis on parental presence during resuscitation and invasive procedures (Dingeman et al., 2007) as well as a practice alert highlighting the benefits of family presence (American Association of Critical Care Nurses, 2004).

Based on this information, the clinical team determined that a descriptive study assessing family members' perceptions and clinical staff attitudes of family presence during invasive procedures would be beneficial to better inform the clinical team about options for standardizing care processes and contribute to the research literature. They proceeded to prepare a research proposal, submitted it to the institutional review board (IRB) for approval, and conducted a descriptive study with a convenience sample of staff and family members. The results of the study helped to inform the PICU clinical team that, while some staff members were resistant to allowing family presence, family members unanimously preferred the option of being present during invasive procedures. The PICU implemented a 6-month pilot and established that both staff and family found it beneficial. The clinical team then began preparing a manuscript of study results for submission to a clinical journal.

This example highlights the basic processes involved in implementing clinical research, including a literature review, research plan formulation, proposal development, IRB submission, research implementation, results evaluation, clinical practice application, and results dissemination to inform practice.

While once perceived as a rigorous, time-intensive activity, conducting research is now recognized to be a professional responsibility. As highlighted in the preceding example, pursuing a clinical research project is feasible when the venture is championed by a clinical team. Conducting research and integrating findings in clinical practice both improves care for pediatric patients and their family members and ensures best outcomes for the health care team.

EVIDENCE-BASED PRACTICE

EBP uses research to promote best outcomes, is characterized by using the best proven information when making clinical decisions, and is considered the new standard in health care (Melynk & Fineout-Overhold, 2005; Sackett et al., 2000). EBP, which is defined as an approach to practicing health care, emphasizes that the clinician must be aware of the evidence in support of clinical practice and evaluate the strength of that evidence (Evidence-Based Medicine Working Group, 1992). This process involves searching for the evidence via literature reviews, critically appraising the evidence for validity and clinical usefulness, and applying the results in clinical practice (Sackett et al., 2000).

The EBP movement began with Archie Cochrane (1999), a British epidemiologist. In 1972, Cochrane wrote a landmark book that criticized the medical profession for not conducting rigorous reviews of health care evidence. His promotion of the strength of randomized controlled trial evidence led to the development of the Cochrane Library, a database of systematic reviews; the Cochrane Centre in Oxford, United Kingdom; and the International Cochrane Collaboration, a group of more than 10,000 volunteers in more than 90 countries who review the effects of health care interventions tested in clinical research (Cochrane Collaboration, 2010).

EBP and research is evaluated based on the amount and quality of existing evidence. As shown in Figure 2-1, the evidence pyramid depicts the most clinically relevant evidence at the top and the least clinically relevant at the bottom. The most clinically relevant evidence comes from meta-analyses and systematic reviews, followed by randomized clinical trial evidence. Research designs such as cohort studies and case-control studies provide the next strongest level of evidence, followed by case reports and expert opinion. Evidence such as that gleaned from animal-based laboratory studies are the least clinically relevant, but can be useful as a background resource.

Locating the best evidence involves several approaches, including conducting a literature review, examining the existing research, and critiquing the evidence. Evaluating the evidence requires analyzing both the quantity of research on a certain topic or aspect of clinical care and the quality of the research methods, including the study design, sample size, overall results, validity, and generalizability of the research (Polit & Beck, 2006). The growing number of powerful search engines available has greatly eased the task of identifying research evidence relevant to a clinical practice. Various resources in locating EBP and research include databases such as the Cochrane Library and medical search engines such as PubMed, MedlinePlus, and Ovid (Table 2-1). As a starting point, the essential steps in investigating the literature in EBP and research evidence include identifying a clinical question or area of interest, determining the appropriate database to employ, and using suitable key search terms to narrow the literature search to the specific area of interest. Selected publications are then reviewed to identify useful resources and evaluate the available evidence (Table 2-2).

Clinical EBP Example

A subacute unit identified that providing support to parents of chronically, critically ill children with repeat hospitalizations was a clinical challenge. The unit's recently established

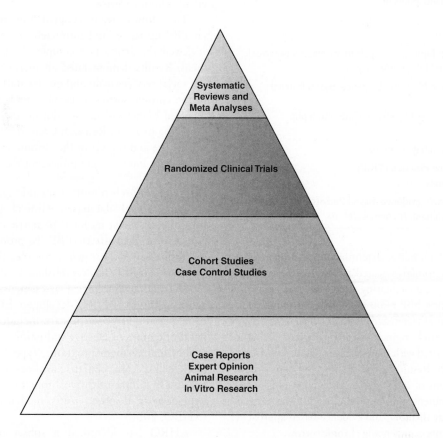

FIGURE 2-1

Evidence Pyramid.

Source: Adapted from Sackett et al., 2000.

TABLE 2-1

Evidence-Based Practice and Research Resources

Agency for Healthcare Research and Quality
http://www.ahrq.gov

American Academy of Pediatrics
http://www.aap.org

American Pediatric Society/Society for Pediatric Research
http://www.aps-spr.org

Canadian Pediatric Society
http://www.cps.ca

Cochrane Collaborative
http://www.cochrane.org

Collaborative Pediatric Critical Care Research Network
http://www.nichd.nih.gov/research/supported/cpccrn.cfm

Database of Abstracts of Reviews of Effectiveness (DARE)
http://www.york.ac.uk/inst/crd/crddatabases.htm

Joanna Briggs Institute
http://www.joannabriggs.edu.au/about/home.php

MedlinePlus
http://medlineplus.gov/

National Guideline Clearinghouse (AHRQ)
http://www.guideline.gov

National Association of Children's Hospitals and Related Institutions
http://www.childrenshospitals.net

Ovid
http://www.ovid.com

Pediatric Acute Lung Injury and Sepsis Investigators Network
http://pedsccm.org/PALISI_network.php

Pediatric Critical Care Medicine Evidence-Based Journal Reviews
http://www.pedsccm.org/EBJournal_Club_intro.php

PubMed
http://www.ncbi.nlm.nih.gov/entrez

Turning Research into Practice (TRIP)
http://www.tripdatabase.com

University of Michigan's Evidence-Based Pediatric Website
http://www.med.umich.edu/pediatrics/ebm/

TABLE 2-2

Essential Steps in Conducting a Literature Search	
Step 1	Identify a clinical question or query. *Example:* What is the evidence for family presence during pediatric invasive procedures?
Step 2	Determine the type of database that is appropriate to search for literature related to the clinical question. *Example:* PubMed
Step 3	Enter key search terms in the subject heading.
Step 4	Combine search terms to find relevant evidence/research.
Step 5	Review the search findings to identify useful resources and evaluate available evidence.

Source: Adapted from Melynk & Fineout-Overholt, 2005.

article were made available to staff in the break rooms. As an incentive, continuing education credit was offered to those completing a post-review competency assessment. This review highlighted that chronic sorrow can be part of the normal grief response and that, although parents might experience symptoms of depression, chronic sorrow is not the same thing as clinical depression. In addition, Gordon's (2009) article discussed the use of a framework to identify parents experiencing chronic sorrow.

The clinical team adopted this theoretical model as an EBP initiative, and ultimately 95% of the clinical staff reviewed the article and completed the competency assessment. Results demonstrated an increase in consultations to the social services team and greater staff satisfaction with use of the chronic sorrow assessment tool; in addition, families reported higher satisfaction during their child's hospitalization. The EBP and Research Committee continued to monitor the use and impact of the chronic sorrow assessment tool as a quality improvement project for the unit.

EBP and research resources include general and pediatric-specific clinical databases, clinical practice guidelines, information about national pediatric organizations, and a consortium for pediatric EBP. To promote the use of EBP in clinical care, the Agency for Healthcare Research and Quality (AHRQ) has established EBP centers to generate reports and technological assessments on relevant clinical care topics. AHRQ-developed EBP reviews relevant to neonatal and pediatric care include maternal and neonatal outcomes of elective induction, child and adolescent weight management programs, type 1 diabetes education, sickle cell disease, pediatric anthrax and bioterrorism preparedness, failure-to-thrive, bronchiolitis, attention-deficit/hyperactivity disorder, otitis media, and acute sinusitis (AHRQ, 2006).

AHRQ has identified a subset of pediatric quality indicators (PQIs) based on a retrospective medical record review of patients discharged from the National Association

EBP and Research Committee determined that implementing a clinically relevant initiative geared toward assisting parents in managing sorrow and facilitating effective coping strategies would entail searching EBP resources. The team sought assistance from the hospital's reference librarian to help identify key terms and medical search engines for a comprehensive literature review. The team started with the Cochrane database, followed by a Medline search. Results included stress and coping management, descriptions of tools (e.g., a parental coping scale), strategies for assessment and interventions for the targeted population (e.g., play therapy), and evidence-based approaches for supporting parents experiencing chronic sorrow.

After careful review, the committee identified one EBP article (Gordon, 2009) as a useful resource; copies of this of Children's Hospitals and Related Institutions (NACHRI; see Scanlon et al., 2008). These indicators, which are listed in Table 2-3, can be useful in developing specific EBP and research initiatives. As an example, targeting best practices for the prevention of decubitus ulcers or the early identification of sepsis based on the PQI indicators could promote adoption of EBP and provide a means of formally tracking the effect of interventions on improved performance.

To promote interprofessional EBP and collaborative research, leaders from 18 children's hospitals and universities formed the National Consortium for Pediatric and Adolescent EBP. In addition to hosting an EBP Leadership Summit, this consortium promotes the use of EBP and research for improving child and adolescent health (Melnyk et al., 2007). Other pediatric-specific resources are outlined in Table 2-1.

USING EBP AND RESEARCH FOR CLINICAL DECISION MAKING

Evaluating research for use in clinical practice involves reviewing studies for their merits and strengths as well as for their limitations, then making a determination of whether the findings are applicable to clinical care. A research

critique goes beyond a review or summary of a study: It reflects an objective assessment of a study's validity and significance as evaluated based on its component parts, after thoroughly examining all aspects of the research design, results, and conclusions. Table 2-4 outlines some common questions to guide a research critique.

Despite the acknowledged benefits of research, many barriers to clinical research have been identified, including lack of knowledge about research techniques, lack of institutional support, research findings limited to a specific clinical setting lacking generalizability, and negative attitudes about clinical research (Ahrens, 2005; Carroll et al., 2009; Chulay, 2005).

A number of strategies can be employed to promote research in clinical settings (Table 2-5), including increased awareness of the importance of research to clinical practice. Supporting and mentoring investigations help to inform clinicians about research processes and promote improvements in clinical practice. Identifying and encouraging active research projects can range from being the responsibility of a formal research committee to being an agenda item on routine staff meetings. Designating teams or unit-based clinical champions can also encourage the use of EBP and research.

Journal clubs promote peer review and a critique of research through periodic meetings, providing a forum for a collective effort to upgrade knowledge and hone skills consistent with the latest developments and findings (Dwarakanath & Khan, 2000; Sidorov, 1995). Advantages of participating in a journal club include exposure to new knowledge, enhancing awareness of current nursing research findings, learning to critique and appraise research, becoming familiar with the best current clinical research, reinforcing best practices, and encouraging research utilization. Table 2-6 demonstrates how to organize a journal club and facilitate discussion of EBP and research in the clinical setting.

Clinical Journal Club Example

Clinical staff at one institution questioned the reliability of blood pressure measurements in a 12-year-old patient who weighed 155 pounds, as the measurements were taken using both pediatric and adult blood pressure cuffs. Two staff members volunteered to search the literature for relevant evidence. They located an EBP article that focused on noninvasive blood pressure measurement in children and organized a journal club session to facilitate discussion of the article as well as application to the current patient situation. The evidence-based research article noted that selection of a proper-sized cuff was considered one of the most important factors when measuring blood pressure.

During the journal club discussion, one of the clinical residents cited evidence from the National High Blood Pressure Education Program Working Group on High Blood Pressure in Children and Adolescents (2004), which suggested that

TABLE 2-3

Pediatric Quality Indicators

Provider-Level Pediatric Quality Indicators

- Accidental Puncture or Laceration (PDI 1)
- Decubitus Ulcer (PDI 2)
- Foreign Body Left During Procedure (PDI 3)
- Iatrogenic Pneumothorax in Neonates at Risk (PDI 4)
- Iatrogenic Pneumothorax in Non-neonates (PDI 5)
- Pediatric Heart Surgery Mortality (PDI 6)
- Pediatric Heart Surgery Volume (PDI 7)
- Postoperative Hemorrhage or Hematoma (PDI 8)
- Postoperative Respiratory Failure (PDI 9)
- Postoperative Sepsis (PDI 10)
- Postoperative Wound Dehiscence (PDI 11)
- Selected Infections Due to Medical Care (PDI 12)
- Transfusion Reaction (PDI 13)

Area-Level Pediatric Quality Indicators

- Asthma Admission Rate (PDI 14)
- Diabetes Short-Term Complication Rate (PDI 15)
- Gastroenteritis Admission Rate (PDI 16)
- Perforated Appendix Admission Rate (PDI 17)
- Urinary Tract Infection Admission Rate (PDI 18)

Source: Agency for Healthcare Research and Quality, 2006.

TABLE 2-4

Questions to Guide a Research Critique	
A. Description of the study	What was the purpose of the research? Does the problem have significance to clinical care? Why is the problem significant/important? What are the research questions, objectives, or hypotheses?
B. Literature evaluation	Is this a thorough review of the literature? Do the citations include recent literature? Does the content of the review relate directly to the research problem? Does the research cited in the literature review support the need for this study?
C. Conceptual framework	Does the research report use a theoretical or conceptual model for the study? Does the model guide the research and seem appropriate? How did the model contribute to the design and execution of the study? Are the findings linked back to the model or framework?
D. Sample	Who were the subjects? What were the inclusion/exclusion criteria? How were subjects recruited? Are the size and key characteristics of the sample described? How representative is the sample?
E. Methods and design	Which methodology was employed? How were the data collected? Are the data collection instruments clearly described? Were the instruments appropriate measures of the variables? If so, what were the validity and reliability of the instrument? Would the same results be expected in subsequent testing?
F. Analysis	How were the data analyzed? Do the selected statistical tests appear appropriate? Is a rationale provided for the use of selected statistical tests? Were the results significant?
G. Results	What were the research findings? Are the results clear and understandable? Are the interpretations consistent with the results? Were the conclusions accurate and relevant to the problem? Were the authors' recommendations appropriate? Are study limitations addressed?
H. Clinical significance	How does the study contribute to the body of knowledge? What are the implications to practice/education/research? Which additional questions does the study raise?

Sources: Frank-Stromborg & Olsen, 2004; Polit & Beck, 2006; Whitley, 2002.

TABLE 2-5

Strategies for Promoting Research in Clinical Practice
Foster awareness of the important of research to clinical practice:
• Use of journal clubs
• Formulation of a research committee
• Use of clinicians to champion research projects
Identify current quality-based or best practice initiatives that can be formulated into research projects.
Develop research projects that target established indicators.
Consider nursing interest areas for additional research projects.
Showcase research projects to promote interest in conducting additional projects:
• Grand rounds
• Formal programs/continuing education forums
• Institutional newsletter updates
• Poster presentations
• Participation in institutional research day forums
Garner administrative support to allocate clinician time for research activities.
Identify research resources (access to online databases, librarian-assisted literature searchers, toolkits, practice guidelines).
Create formal project protocols and submit them for institutional review board approval.
Designate project leaders and unit-based champions.
Seek funding for clinical pilot studies.
Establish partnerships between academic researchers and health care institutions.
Assess the availability of research consultants.
Link participation in research to incentives (e.g., clinical ladder advancement/promotion).
Publish and present research projects.

Source: Adapted with permission from Kleinpell R, (2008). Promoting research in clinical practice: strategies for implementing research initiatives. *AACN Advanced Critical Care, 19*(2), 155–161.

the degree of overestimation with a small cuff was greater than the degree of underestimation with a large cuff. Additionally, despite the labeling of blood pressure cuffs (e.g., infant, child, small adult), the specific cuff size might differ from one manufacturer to another. In reviewing the journal club article, the clinical team identified that the accurate cuff should be selected by arm circumference (Schell et al., 2006). Based on the literature, the 12-year-old patient required use of an adult-sized blood pressure cuff. From this journal club session, the clinical team identified that monthly journal clubs would be valuable in reviewing and discussing clinically relevant research and improving clinical practice.

The use of EBP and research promote best practices for pediatric acute care. While busy clinicians face time constraints in searching EBP and research literature, the benefits of integrating these elements and conducting research

TABLE 2-6

Steps to Organizing a Journal Club to Facilitate Discussion of Evidence-Based Practice and Research in the Clinical Setting

1. Select a relevant research article that would be of interest to the clinical staff or that addresses a recent clinical issue.

2. Post and distribute copies of the research article and the journal club discussion questions.

3. Establish a convenient meeting time and location (e.g., monthly).

4. Identify a facilitator for the meeting. Initially, this could be a health care professional or other clinical leader. Once the group is well established, journal club members could alternate in leading subsequent sessions.

5. Encourage active participation of those attending through discussion questions and prompts.

6. Assess the journal club experience at the end of the session (e.g., evaluation forms).

7. Solicit improvements to both journal club meeting structure and dissemination of information (e.g., how to increase participation, variable or multiple meeting times for the convenience of all shifts, video or audio tape session for those unable to attend).

argue for their ongoing integration into clinical practice as a means to promote the best outcomes for pediatric patients and their family members.

Critical Thinking

Strategies for implementing EBP and research in pediatric clinical practice include fostering awareness of the importance of research to clinical practice, using journal clubs to promote review and critique of research, forming a research committee to identify and promote active research projects, and designating unit-based clinical champions for promoting the use of EBP and research.

REFERENCES

1. Agency for Healthcare Research and Quality. (2006). Pediatric quality indicators overview. Retrieved from http://www.qualityindicators.ahrq.gov/pdi_overview.htm

2. Ahrens, T. (2005). Evidenced-based practice: Priorities and implementation strategies. *AACN Clinical Issues, 16*(1), 36–42.

3. American Association of Critical Care Nurses. (2004). AACN practice alert: Family presence during CPR and invasive procedures. Retrieved from http://www.aacn.org/WD/Practice/Docs/PracticeAlerts/Family_Presence_During_CPR_11-2004.pdf

4. Burns, N., & Grove, S. (2005). *The practice of nursing research: Conduct, critique, and utilization* (5th ed.). St. Louis: Elsevier Saunders.

5. Carroll, D., Greenwood, R., Lynch, K., Sullivan, J., Ready, C., & Fitzmaurice, J. (1997). Barriers and facilitators to the utilization of nursing research. *Clinical Nurse Specialist, 11*(5), 207–212.

6. Chulay, M. (2006). Good research ideas for clinicians. *AACN Advanced Critical Care, 17*(3), 253–265.

7. Cochrane, A. (1999). *Effectiveness and efficiency: Random reflections of health services* (2nd ed.). London: Royal Society of Medicine Press.

8. Cochrane Collaboration. (2010). Archie Cochrane: The name behind The Cochrane Collaboration. Retrieved from http://www.cochrane.org/about-us/history/archie-cochrane#Bio

9. Dingeman, R., Mitchell, E., Meyer, E., & Curley, M. (2007). Parent presence during complex invasive procedures and cardiopulmonary resuscitation: A systematic review of the literature. *Pediatrics, 120,* 842–854.

10. Dwarakanath, L., & Khan, K. (2000). Modernizing the journal club. *Hospital Medicine, 61,* 425–427.

11. Emergency Nurses Association. (2007). *Presenting the option for family presence.* Des Plaines, IL: Author.

12. Evidence-Based Medicine Working Group. (1992). Evidence-based medicine: A new approach to teaching the practice of medicine. *Journal of the American Medical Association, 268,* 2420–2425.

13. Frank-Stromborg, M., & Olsen, S. (2004). *Instruments for clinical health care research.* Sudbury, MA: Jones and Bartlett.

14. Gordon, J. (2009). An evidence-based approach for supporting parents experiencing chronic sorrow. *Pediatric Nursing, 35,* 115–119.

15. Hulley, S., Cummings, S., Browner, W., Grady, D., & Newman, T. (Eds.). (2006). *Designing clinical research: An epidemiologic approach* (3rd ed.). Philadelphia: Lippincott Williams & Wilkins.

16. Kleinpell, R. (2008). Promoting research in clinical practice: Strategies for implementing research initiatives. *AACN Advanced Critical Care, 19,* 155–163.

17. Melynk, B., & Fineout-Overholt, E. (2005). *Evidence-based practice in nursing and healthcare.* Philadelphia: Lippincott Williams & Wilkins.

18. Melynk, B., Fineout-Overholt, E., Hockenberry, M. et al. (2007). Improving healthcare and outcomes for high-risk children and teens: Formation of the National Consortium for Pediatric and Adolescent Evidence-Based Practice. *Pediatric Nursing, 33,* 525–529.

19. National High Blood Pressure Education Program Working Group on High Blood Pressure in Children and Adolescents. (2004). The fourth report on the diagnosis, evaluation, and treatment of high blood pressure in children and adolescents. *Pediatrics, 114,* 555–576.

20. National Institutes of Health (NIH). (1998). NIH policy and guidelines on the inclusion of children as participants in research involving human subjects. Retrieved from http://grants.nih.gov/grants/guide/notice-files/not98-024.html

21. Polit, D., & Beck, C. (2006). *Essentials of nursing research: Methods, appraisal, and utilization* (6th ed.). Philadelphia: Lippincott Williams & Wilkins.

22. Sackett, D., Straus, S., Richardson, W., Rosenberg, W., & Haynes, R. (2000). *Evidence-based medicine: How to practice and teach EBM* (2nd ed.). Edinburgh: Churchill Livingstone.

23. Scanlon, M., Harris, M., Levy, F., & Sedman, A. (2008). Evaluation of the Agency for Healthcare Research and Quality pediatric quality indicators. *Pediatrics, 121,* e1723–e1731.

24. Schell, K., Lyons, D., Bradley, E. et al. (2006). Clinical comparison of automatic, noninvasive measurements of blood pressure in the forearm and upper arm with the patient supine or with the head of the bed raised 45 degrees: A follow-up study. *American Journal of Critical Care, 15*(2), 196–205.

25. Sidorov, J. (1995). How are internal medicine residency journal clubs organized, and what makes them successful? *Archives in Internal Medicine, 155,* 1193–1197.

26. U.S. Department of Health and Human Services Office of Extramural Research. (2010). Glossary & acronym list. Retrieved from http://grants.nih.gov/grants/glossary.htm

27. Whitley, B. (2002). *Principles of research in behavioral science.* Boston: McGraw-Hill.

Certification, Licensure, and Credentialing/Privileging for the Health Care Professional

- Certification
- Licensure
- Credentialing and Privileging
- Health Care Professionals in Pediatric Acute Care

- Regulatory Issues for Health Care Professionals in Pediatric Acute Care
- References

Ensuring that an individual is qualified and competent to practice is a fundamental step and crucial factor in the safe delivery of care to children. Certification, licensure, and credentialing/privileging are different processes that share a common purpose: Individuals are required to demonstrate that they have met the qualifications and professional standards to safely practice within a health care profession. The administration of a certification, license, or credentialing/privileging is the responsibility of various entities, which include professional organizations (certification), state governments' regulatory boards or agencies (licensure), and employers (credentialing/privileging).

This chapter provides an overview of the pediatric health care disciplines and outlines the regulatory and professional requirements to practice in this field. In addition, it outlines some of the most pertinent regulatory issues facing health care professionals (HCPs) in the twenty-first century.

CERTIFICATION

Certification indicates qualification; however, it often represents more than minimum competency. Certification is administered by a professional organization and serves as an indicator that an individual has achieved an advanced level of expertise in a specialized area or population. Requirements for certification may include a specific level of education, clinical hrs of practice or training in a given population, and passage of an examination. Depending on the profession and the state, certification may or may not be a requirement to legally practice in the state. While it is often left to the discretion of the HCP to decide whether he or she will pursue professional certification, for many professionals, certification may be required by the employer. In addition, for members of some professions such as advanced practice nurses, certification is a prerequisite for licensure. Certification requirements can be found on the certifying body's website.

LICENSURE

Licensure is granted by state boards (or other government agencies) to individuals deemed qualified and competent to practice a profession. A license is required by law when the role, activities, and procedures performed by members of that profession are considered to carry a high risk to the public. State practice acts, rules, and regulations outline the requirements for licensure and grant authority to a specific governing body, such as a state board of nursing or medicine, or other state agency, to issue licenses and have regulatory authority over the profession. Each state sets different requirements for licensure; these requirements also vary according to the profession.

To achieve licensure within a health care profession, the individual must prove he or she has met the minimum requirements and standards to practice safely. Licensure requirements generally include a specified level of education from an accredited program and passage of a required examination. Requirements may include clinical practice hrs and/or certification. Individual states may impose additional obligations, such as criminal background checks and licensure fees.

CREDENTIALING AND PRIVILEGING

Credentialing and privileging are the processes used by health care institutions to verify HCPs' credentials and define the services they will provide to patients in that facility or organization.

Credentialing is the assessment and evaluation of the credentials of the HCP. It includes confirmation of the applicant's education, certification, and licensure. The credentialing process also verifies professional references, examines past claims history, and scrutinizes disciplinary actions. It is the responsibility of the institution credentialing the HCP to determine if the individual's credentials match the scope of practice for the role sought at that facility.

Privileging is the authorization to provide specific services and perform certain procedures within an institution. It is determined by the institution that hires the HCP. Health care institutions are mandated by law to establish a governing body whose role it is to ensure that every practitioner providing care or performing surgical procedures within that institution has the requisite knowledge, skills, and competencies necessary to safely carry out that role (Centers for Medicare and Medicaid Services [CMS], 2004; Health Resources and Services Administration [HRSA], 2006).

The institution's governing body, in accordance with state law, determines which categories of practitioners must be privileged. These may include, but are not limited to, physicians, dentists, advanced practice nurses, and physician assistants. The institution also determines the duties, scope, and extent (e.g., active, temporary, honorary) of those privileges. Advanced practice registered nurses (APRN), for example, are subject to state laws that specify the level of independence and prescriptive authority they are granted. Institutional clinical privileges granted to the APRN must be in accordance with the nurse practice act and regulations as well as the institution's bylaws.

Privileging is also influenced by federal laws (CMS; Federal Tort Claims Act [FTCA]) and the institution's accreditation agency, such as The Joint Commission (TJC). Some years ago, privileging was a process exclusively applied to physicians. In 1983, however, The Joint Commission revised its medical staff standards to allow for nonphysician practitioners to be privileged and adopted standards that allowed licensed HCPs who were not physicians to independently provide patient care as long as that practice was permitted by both state law and the institution's bylaws.

Within a given health care organization, the HCP may apply for both clinical and admitting privileges. Clinical privileges refer to the tasks, procedures, and activities that a practitioner is granted by the governing body of the institution. These are assigned in accordance with the institution's bylaws, state laws authorizing scope of practice, and the individual's qualifications and competencies. Clinical privileges may or may not include admitting privileges. The ability to admit a patient to an institution is also determined by the institution's governing body and based on the institution's bylaws, state laws, and standards set by the accreditation agency. Once granted, these privileges must be available for referencing throughout the institution.

Since the change in The Joint Commission standards regarding who is considered medical staff, institutions have created another category to describe nonphysician medical staff. Based on the institutional bylaws, these individuals may have voting rights and serve on the medical staff committees. Nonphysicians may be called "affiliates" or a similar term denoting that the individual does not have full privileges. Very often, "affiliates" have specific circumstances under which they can practice and specific functions they can perform. The institution may require supervision by a physician for admitting and discharging patients. Persons who are classified into the "affiliate" staff category often may not vote or be members on institutional committees regarding matters related to policy governing the medical staff. Requirements for obtaining credentialing and privileging are outlined in an institution's bylaws.

HEALTH CARE PROFESSIONALS IN PEDIATRIC ACUTE CARE

PHYSICIANS

Licensure

Physicians (MD: medical doctor; DO: doctor of osteopathy) are licensed under state boards of medicine. Some states have separate medical boards licensing MDs and DOs; other state boards license both. Although the criteria for licensure vary among states, all state boards of medicine require passing a national examination, either U.S. Medical Licensing Examination (USML) for MDs or the Comprehensive Osteopathic Medical Licensing Examination (COMLEX) for DOs. Other criteria include an accredited educational program and 1 to 3 years of postgraduate training.

Certification and recertification

Physicians certify in a specialty area after becoming a licensed physician. For physicians, certification is voluntary.

Standards are set by the profession. Requirements vary among the specialties. In the United States, three organizations certify MDs and DOs in approximately 26 specialties: the American Boards of Medical Specialties, the American Osteopathic Association Bureau of Osteopathic Specialties, and the American Board of Physician Specialties. Recertification is required by these organizations, with the time varying between 7 and 10 years depending on the specialty.

PHYSICIAN ASSISTANTS

Certification and recertification

After successful completion of an accredited educational program, a physician assistant (PA) is eligible to take the Physician Assistant National Certifying Examination. This multiple-choice examination consists of basic medical and surgical knowledge. The PA must complete 100 hrs of Category II continuing medical education (CME) every 2 years, and must pass a recertification examination every 6 years. Category II credits must be related to patient care, medicine, and professional issues. For recertification, three versions of the certification exam are now available, covering primary care, adult medicine, and surgery (began 2009). PAs have a choice of taking whichever examination most closely fits their area of practice.

Licensure

PAs are licensed under the state boards of medicine. To be eligible for licensure, they must have graduated from an accredited program and successfully passed the national certification examination. In practice, they are supervised by physicians. When applying to the state boards of medicine for licensure, the PA candidate must simultaneously submit an application for his or her supervising physician. State laws generally identify the responsibilities and duties of the supervising physician, including the number of PAs they are allowed to supervise. The scope of practice of the PA includes the medical services deemed to be within the education and experience of the PA, which are delegated by the supervising physician. In summary, the supervising physician delegates the medical tasks to the PA, after determining which are appropriate to the PA's level of competence (American Association of Physician Assistants, n.d.).

ADVANCED PRACTICE REGISTERED NURSES

Certification and recertification

Certification for APRNs occurs after completion of an accredited educational program. Certification for nurse practitioners (NPs) and clinical nurse specialists (CNSs) requires graduation from an accredited program with a focus on the role and population the individual for which the nurse seeks to be certified. It also requires passage of a certification examination that tests the knowledge and skills related to the role and population the individual has studied and wishes to address in the nurse's practice. For example, pediatric nurse practitioners must have graduated from an accredited pediatric NP program, either primary or acute care, and passed the state-approved certification examination for that specialty.

Each state determines which APRN certification examinations are acceptable for legal recognition to practice as an APRN. The National Council of State Boards of Nursing (NCSBN) has identified criteria for legally defensible examinations that include the following characteristics: national in scope; meets acceptable testing standards; tests entry-level practice; and represents knowledge, skills, and abilities needed for safe APRN practice. Several major certification programs develop APRN certification examinations: American Academy of Nurse Practitioners, American Association of Critical Care Nurses, American Nurses Credentialing Center, National Certification Corporation, Pediatric Nursing Certification Board, American Midwifery Certification Board, and Council on Certification of Nurse Anesthetists. All of these major APRN certification organizations have recertification programs that include continuing education units (CEUs) and practice requirements.

Licensure

An APRN license, in addition to an RN license, is the national recommended standard for granting legal recognition to advanced practice registered nurses. Not all states issue licenses; however, APRNs in most jurisdictions are required to obtain some form of legal recognition and must meet specific requirements prior to being granted the authority to practice. APRNs are required by law to graduate from an accredited graduate-level educational program. There is a recommendation to transition to the doctor of nursing practice (DNP) as entry to practice by 2015 (American Association of Colleges of Nursing, 2009). APRNs must also successfully pass a certification examination in their advanced practice specialty.

REGISTERED NURSES

Education, licensure, and certification

Registered nurse (RN) licensure is based on graduation from a state-approved school of nursing, which is accredited by either the National League for Nursing Accrediting Commission (NLNAC) or the Commission on Collegiate Nursing Education (CCNE). Nursing education is provided

by four-year baccalaureate and two-year associate degree programs. However, the American Association of Colleges of Nursing (2000) recommends transition to baccalaureate education as the standard entry to professional nursing practice.

Upon graduation from either degree program, an individual must pass a licensing exam, the National Council Licensure Examination for Registered Nurses (NCLEX-RN), in order to practice as an RN. Each state has a board of nursing which regulates nursing practice. Furthermore, state boards of nursing govern and set continuing education or competency requirements for licensure renewal (American Nurses Association, 2004).

Licensure encompasses the minimum requirements for practice as a professional registered nurse. Certification recognizes an individual as having attained a higher level of expertise or degree of proficiency with a specific population in a defined area of clinical practice. Certification is optional for practice as an RN. There are numerous population specific certification examinations available for pediatric RNs. These include certified pediatric nurse (CPN), certified pediatric emergency nurse (CPEN), certified pediatric oncology nurse (CPON), and certification as a pediatric critical care nurse (CCRN) (American Nurses Association, 2004).

RESPIRATORY THERAPISTS

Respiratory therapists (RTs) provide care for pediatric patients who range from premature infants being ventilated to adolescents with lung disease or respiratory problems. RTs take histories, assess patients while focusing on the respiratory system, perform diagnostic tests, and treat patients under the orders of a physician, physician assistant, or advanced practice registered nurse. These HCPs also provide education for the patient and family on procedures such as chest physiotherapy or caring for the child on a ventilator in the home setting.

Education, certification, and licensure

The minimum education requirement for an RT is an associate degree, although potential students are encouraged to pursue a bachelor's or master's degree. RT programs are offered through universities, colleges, and vocational schools and are accredited through the Commission on Accreditation of Allied Health Programs (CAAHC) or the Committee on Accreditation for Respiratory Care (CoARC). Graduates are eligible to sit for the certification examination from the National Board for Respiratory Care (NBRC).

Forty-eight states and the District of Columbia require RTs to be licensed; Hawaii and Alaska do not (American Association for Respiratory Care [AARC], 2010).

Licensure is based on graduation from an accredited program and passage of the NBRC examination. Certified RTs who graduated from advanced level programs and passed two separate exams are eligible for becoming registered respiratory technicians (RRTs). These individuals are then qualified to fill supervisory positions and to work in intensive care units (U.S. Bureau of Labor Statistics, 2010a).

The NBRC also offers specialty exams. For example, RTs can specialize in pediatric care and become certified in this area by taking the Neonatal/Pediatric Respiratory Care Specialist examination. The individual is then certified as a CRT-NPS or RRT-NPS.

OCCUPATIONAL THERAPISTS

Occupational therapists (OTs) work with children to develop and improve fine and gross motor skills. In particular, these HCPs may work with children who have fine and gross motor delays or children with severe disabilities such as cerebral palsy, muscular dystrophy, or brain injuries. OTs work in both hospitals and outpatient settings.

Education, certification, and licensure

A master's degree from an accredited program is the minimal education requirement for OTs. Programs are accredited through the Accreditation Council for Occupational Therapy Education. Graduation qualifies the individual to sit for the national certifying examination.

OTs are regulated in all states. Forty-seven states issue licenses to individuals who meet the qualifications required. Three states (Colorado, Hawaii, and Michigan) have established registration laws for OTs (American Occupational Therapy Association, 2008).

PHYSICAL THERAPISTS

Physical therapists provide assessment and treatment of children who have musculoskeletal, movement, and functional disorders due to disease process, disability, or injury.

Education, certification, and licensure

A post-baccalaureate degree from an accredited physical therapy program is required for licensure as a physical therapist. While some programs offer a master's degree, most offer the doctor of physical therapy degree. Also required for licensure is successful passage of the National Physical Therapy Examination. Some states also require candidates for PT licensure to pass a jurisprudence exam (Federation of State Boards of Physical Therapy, 2010).

AUDIOLOGISTS

Audiologists screen and evaluate children for hearing, balance, and related sensory and neural disorders. They administer hearing tests, assess hearing loss, and use various procedures for diagnosing disorders. The role of the audiologist includes fitting the hearing-impaired child with amplification devices and providing aural rehabilitation to decrease the impact of hearing loss on communication and learning (All Allied Health Schools, 2010).

Education, licensure, and certification

Audiology students must complete a two-year master's or a four-year doctoral (AuD) program in audiology. According to the American Speech-Language-Hearing Association (ASHA), as of the year 2012, audiologists will have to earn a doctoral degree to be certified (ASHA, 2010b). In 2009, 18 states required a doctoral degree or its equivalent for licensure of new applicants.

Audiologists are regulated through licensure in all 50 states. Some states regulate the dispensing of hearing aids separately, by requiring an additional Hearing Aid Dispenser license. Although state requirements vary, in addition to graduate education in audiology, requirements for licensure may include clinical experience, passage of an examination or certification, and supervised postgraduate paid professional experience (ASHA, 2010b).

Certification of audiologists is voluntary. The Certificate of Clinical Competence in Audiology (CCC-A), which is granted by ASHA, is a nationally recognized professional credential. this certification goes beyond the minimal requirements for licensure to require a master's or doctoral degree from an accredited academic program, clinical experience supervised by an ASHA-certified professional, and a passing score on the national examination (ASHA, 2010c). Audiologists may also be credentialed through the American Board of Audiology. Professional credentialing may satisfy some or all of the requirements for state licensure.

SPEECH AND LANGUAGE PATHOLOGISTS

Speech-language pathologists, sometimes called *speech therapists*, assess, diagnose, and treat children who cannot vocalize sounds, are unable to clearly pronounce words, or have speech rhythm problems, such as stuttering or problems with swallowing.

Education, certification, and certification

Most states require a speech-language pathologist to be licensed. Requirements for licensure include at least a master's degree from an accredited program, a passing score on the national examination on speech-language pathology,

300 to 375 hours of supervised clinical experience, and 9 months of postgraduate professional clinical experience. Regulations may differ for speech-language pathologists who plan to work in a school setting.

The Certificate of Clinical Competence in Speech-Language Pathology (CCC-SLP) credential offered by the ASHA is obtained on a voluntary basis. The certification process requires a graduate degree from a program accredited by the Council on Academic Accreditation in Audiology and Speech-Language Pathology (CAA) of the ASHA. The candidate must have completed a 36-week full-time postgraduate clinical fellowship and must pass the Praxis Series examination in speech-language pathology (ASHA, 2009; U.S. Bureau of Labor Statistics, 2010b). In addition, a minimum of 400 clock hours of supervised clinical experience is required (ASHA, 2009).

CHILD LIFE THERAPISTS

Child life therapists use play, educational strategies, and self-expression to optimize a child's development and provide emotional support during illness. As part of their roles, they offer support, information, and guidance during procedures and hospitalizations to children and their families and work as part of an interprofessional team to optimize health outcomes (Child Life Council, 2010a).

Education and certification

Licensure is not required for child life therapists. Certification, however, is recommended and often required for employment. Qualifications for certification includes a bachelor's degree or higher. Ten college-level courses in child life or a related subject and a minimum of 480 hours of child life clinical experience under the direct supervision of a Certified Child Life Specialist are also required. Certification is obtained through the Child Life Council (Child Life Council, 2010b).

REGULATORY ISSUES FOR HEALTH CARE PROFESSIONALS IN PEDIATRIC ACUTE CARE

Regulatory issues in today's complex healthcare environment have resulted, in part, from a variety of economic, social, and technologic influences. These factors include mobility across jurisdictions, continued competence, and the redefining of scopes of practice among HCPs.

MOBILITY OF HEALTH CARE PROFESSIONALS

Telehealth and other technological advances have now made it possible for HCPs to deliver health care across state lines and even across international borders from one remote location. While technology has increased access to care and opened new avenues for health care delivery, differing state laws and regulations in the United States have complicated this practice for HCPs. For physicians, APRNs, and many of the allied health professions, a license may be required in every state the HCP practices. The state in which the practitioner is practicing is determined by the location of the *patient.* Thus it does not matter whether the patient receives care on-site or from a remote location: The HCP may be required to be licensed in the state where the patient is located if he or she wants to provide care. In addition, the HCP is subject to that state's laws and regulations.

Individuals who wish to practice telehealth and care for patients in multiple states may find the process of obtaining multiple licenses cumbersome and potentially prohibitive to practice if they do not meet another state's differing licensure requirements. A mélange of diverse licensure requirements, the expense involved in obtaining multiple licenses, differing practice acts, and other regulations can make practice in multiple states complex and burdensome (American Medical Association, 2010).

In addition to the complexities required for delivering care via telehealth, HCPs themselves are increasingly becoming more mobile. Personal preferences, economic issues, and the growing need for HCPs in underserved areas or during times of disasters are all reasons for HCPs to have the privilege of mobility and gain access to practice across state lines. Uniformity of state laws would greatly enhance the portability of HCPs' practice and may provide additional relief to states that are experiencing clinician shortages.

One method for addressing these issues in nursing is the Nurse Licensure Compact (NLC). Under the NLC, which is based on a model of mutual recognition, registered nurses are granted a license in their state of residence and are authorized to practice in any other state that is part of the compact. Nurses working in NLC-covered states are required to follow the laws and regulations of the state in which they are working. However, not all states belong to the NLC. The states that do not use the single-state model require nurses who wish to practice in that state to apply for a license.

An increasing number of states have enacted laws and regulations to address the issue of practicing medicine across state lines. These states require a physician to obtain a special license to engage in such practice or to obtain a full unrestricted state medical license (AMA, 2010). State boards, for their part, are recognizing the growing need for uniformity in practice requirements and are taking steps to promote uniform licensure requirements in the form of Model Practice Acts that set standards and provide legislative language for state professional boards.

MAINTAINING PROFESSIONAL COMPETENCE

Continued competence is a critical regulatory issue. As early as 1970, the U.S. Health Service called upon certifiers and regulators to develop better methods of evaluations for relicensure and recertification. In *Crossing the Quality Chasm: A New Health System for the 21st Century* (2001), the Institute of Medicine stated that "There are no consistent methods for ensuring the continued competence of health professionals within the current state licensing functions or other processes" (p. 215). Professions and regulatory boards alike are challenged to provide assurance to the public that individuals are qualified to practice throughout their careers.

Many questions exist regarding continued competence:

- Who is responsible for assuring competence? Should it be the profession or the licensing boards that set standards and are responsible for ongoing competence requirements of HCPs?
- Which standards should be used to evaluate continued competence?
- Should the standard be based on a generalist's competencies or focus on the HCP's specialty practice?

Currently, the continued competence method required by most states for license renewal is continuing education. Studies have shown, however, that this method is not optimal for ensuring the ongoing competency of a licensed practitioner. It often does not fill gaps in knowledge and does not provide assurance that the practitioner's knowledge is current and competent to care for patients.

Other continued competence requirements in state practice acts and regulations include maintaining a minimum number of practice hrs, maintaining a professional portfolio, self-reflection (in which the individual reflects on his or her own practice knowledge and gaps in knowledge), and certification. Hard evidence is not available to support the contention that these methods help HCPs maintain the ongoing knowledge, skills, and abilities necessary to practice competently throughout their careers. Many of the professional state licensure boards are currently addressing this gap by examining methods and collecting data to ensure the that individuals practicing within the profession are competent to practice.

REDEFINING SCOPES OF PRACTICE

Until the end of the twentieth century, physicians were the exclusive patient care providers who managed pediatric patients. This position was fortified by regulations that prevented alternative providers from serving these patients, as laws dictated their scope of practice and prevented others from practicing independently. In the 1990s, this exclusive position was eroded by an explosion in the supply of nonphysician clinicians and a demand for providers to underserved populations (Rosenbaum, 2008). Today, nonphysician providers are providing increasing amounts of health care in these environments. For APRNs, state legislative activity in this area has been significant. In particular, the Balanced Budget Act of 1997 removed the need for physician supervision and extended direct Medicare reimbursement to nurse practitioners in nonhospital settings. In 2008 alone, 24 states introduced bills to widen the scope of practice for APRNs (Croasdale, 2008).

The literature is peppered with articles discussing whether this overlapping scope of practice is collaborative or competitive in nature. A long-term study reporting 1987 to 1997 data concluded that it is a collaborative relationship and suggested that physicians are increasingly collaborating with nonphysician providers as a means to extend their practice (Druss et al., 2003). Another example of collaboration is the use of APRNs in providing care to underserved populations. However, there is a fine line between collaboration and competition. Changes in policies by federal, state, or large health care organizations could easily change the definition of roles in the direction of competition between physicians and APRNs. The challenge is to continue to develop new models of care delivery that provide safe care without creating conflict within the health care system.

REFERENCES

1. All Allied Health Schools. (2010). Becoming an audiologist. Retrieved from http://www.allalliedhealthschools.com/faqs/audiology
2. American Association of Colleges of Nursing. (2000). The baccalaureate degree in nursing as minimal preparation for professional practice. Retrieved from http://www.aacn.nche.edu/Publications/positions/baccmin.htm
3. American Association of Colleges of Nursing. (2009). The doctor of nursing practice fact sheet. Retrieved from http://www.aacn.nche.edu/Media/FactSheets/dnp.htm
4. American Association of Physician Assistants. (n.d.). Becoming a physician's assistant. Retrieved from www.aapa.org
5. American Association for Respiratory Care. (2010). Licensure matrix. Retrieved from http://www.aarc.org/advocacy/state/2000_licensure_matrix.html#matrix
6. American Medical Association. (2010). Physician licensure: An update of trends. Retrieved from http://www.ama-assn.org/ama/pub/about-ama/our-people/member-groups-sections/young-physicians-section/advocacy-resources/physician-licensure-an-update-trends.shtml
7. American Nurses Association. (2004). *Nursing: Scope and standards of practice.* Washington, DC: Author.
8. American Occupational Therapy Association. (2008). Jurisdictions regulating occupational therapists (OTs). Retrieved from http://www.aota.org/Practitioners/Licensure/StateRegs/OTRegs/36459.aspx
9. American Speech-Language-Hearing Association. (2009). 2005 standards and implementation procedures for the Certificate of Clinical Competence in Speech-Language Pathology: Revised March 2009. Retrieved from http://www.asha.org/certification/slp_standards.htm#Std_IImpl
10. American Speech-Language-Hearing Association. (2010a). ASHA state-by-state. Retrieved from http://www.asha.org/advocacy/state/default.htm

11. American Speech-Language-Hearing Association. (2010b). Fact sheet. Retrieved from http://www.asaha.org/careers/professions/audiology.htm

12. American Speech-Language-Hearing Association. (2010c). 2010 state licensure trends. Retrieved from http://www.asha.org/uploadedFiles/StateLicensureTrends.pdf

13. Centers for Medicare and Medicaid Services (CMS). (2004). Requirements for hospital medical staff privileging. Retrieved from http://www.cms.gov/SurveyCertificationGenInfo/downloads/SCLetter05-04.pdf

14. Child Life Council. (2010a). The child life profession. Retrieved from http://www.childlife.org/The%20Child%20Life%20Profession/

15. Child Life Council. (2010b). Certification for the child life profession. Retrieved from http://www.childlife.org/Certification/

16. Croasdale, M. (2008). Advanced practice nurses seek wider scope in 24 states. *AMNews*. Retrieved from www.ama-assn.org/amednews/2008/04/21/prl20421.htm

17. Druss, B., et al. (2003). Trends in care by nonphysician clinicians in the United States. *New England Journal of Medicine, 348*, 130–137.

18. Federation of State Boards of Physical Therapy. (2010). For candidates and licensees. Retrieved from https://www.fsbpt.org/ForCandidatesAndLicensees/index.asp

19. Health Resources and Services Administration (HRSA). (2006). Policy Information Notice 01-16: Credentialing and privileging of health center practitioners. Retrieved from http://www.bphc.hrsa.gov/policy/pin0116.htm

20. Institute of Medicine. (2001). Crossing the quality chasm: A new health system for the 21st century. Retrieved from http://www.iom.edu/Reports/2001/Crossing-the-Quality-Chasm-A-New-Health-System-for-the-21st-Century.aspx

21. Rosenbaum, S. (2008). The impact of United States law on medicine as a profession. *Journal of the American Medical Association, 289*, 1546–1556.

22. U.S. Bureau of Labor Statistics. (2010a). Respiratory therapists. Retrieved from http://data.bls.gov/cgi-bin/print.pl/oco/ocos321.htm

23. U.S. Bureau of Labor Statistics. (2010b). Speech and language pathologists. Retrieved from http://www.bls.gov/oco/ocos099.htm

Jeffrey F. Linzer, Sr.

Documentation and Coding

- Reimbursement for Professional Services
- Documentation Guidelines and Rules
- Basic Evaluation and Management Documentation
- Basic Diagnosis Coding
- References

Medicolegal documentation is the record of patient events and management. It provides information to evaluate and therapeutically manage the patient. With certain exceptions, information is recorded by the physician, advanced practice nurse, physician assistant, or other nonphysician practitioners (NPP) operating within their state-defined scope of practice.

Appropriate documentation describes the following aspects of care:

- What was heard (history)
- What was seen (exam)
- What was thought (medical decision making)

The medical record is like a short story that should easily lead the "reader" from the complaint to the findings. The health care professional (HCP) should record the source of information, particularly if someone other than the patient or the primary caregiver is providing the details of the complaint or events. This point may be especially important if the historian fails to give important information (such as a medication allergy) that has the potential to lead to an adverse outcome and the information was not otherwise obtainable (such as by the review of old records).

The use of direct quotes whenever possible aids in the "retelling" of events and may be supportive in situations that have potential for legal action. For example, in an assault exam, a pediatric patient may have a pet name for a specific body area in question. In this situation, write the pet name in quotes and then indicate with which area the child associated the word. The HCP should also avoid accusatory statements and list the history exactly as it is provided by the patient and/or caregiver.

Caregivers often use poorly defined medical words in their description of the child. Avoiding potentially inflammatory words in patient descriptions is essential to document an objective description. For example, the caregiver may say the pediatric patient has been "lethargic." Ask the person to define what he or she means, and include this definition with the history. It is also important that the description uses clearly understood language such as "sleepy but wakes easily to voice."

A lengthy summary of the history, physical examination, and orders is not required to document the HCP's thought process. However, for conditions that are not straightforward or that may require a particularly extensive work-up, it is valuable to indicate the differential diagnoses and reasons for the choice of laboratory or radiographic tests ordered. Also, the HCP should note why an expected test or procedure is deferred. For example, there is an expectation that a gynecologic examination should be performed in an adolescent female with lower back pain, fever, and vaginal discharge. If this exam was not performed, the reason should be clearly noted in the record—for instance, "patient refused gynecologic examination." It is also important to record any changes (or lack thereof) after a therapy or therapeutic management strategy has been implemented. For example, the HCP might document "No change in the patient's blood pressure following a normal saline (20 mL/kg) fluid bolus" or "Pain after morphine decreased to 2/10 on the pain scale."

Separate documentation should occur for each performed procedure (such as lumbar puncture and laceration repair). Documentation formats used for this purpose may include a written note in the progress note, a stand-alone procedure form, a computer-generated form, or a fully electronic medical record template. The documentation should include the following details: the time and date when the procedure was performed; the type of procedure and the associated indication; the name of the consenting/assenting patient and/or caregiver; the name of the person primarily responsible for performing the procedure and any assistants; a "time out" universal protocol statement (identification of the correct procedure, on the correct patient, in the correct location); a narrative of the procedure itself; and details of any complications that may have occurred. A statement regarding the condition of the patient at the end of the procedure should complete the note.

REIMBURSEMENT FOR PROFESSIONAL SERVICES

Two types of professional health care services are distinguished: *evaluation and management* (E/M), or "thinking" work, and *procedures*, or "hands on" work. Professional services are also referred to as *physician work* by the Center for Medicare and Medicaid Services (CMS). Identifier codes for these services are listed in the Current Procedural Terminology (CPT) developed by the American Medical Association. New codes are published annually and become effective on January 1 of each year.

Traditionally services have been reimbursed based on local or regional "usual, customary, and reasonable" fee schedules. In this case, third-party payers may set reimbursement fees based on factors that may not be clear to either the patient or the provider. This type of reimbursement is most common with providers who do not have a contract with the payer.

A large percentage of payers provide reimbursement based on the *Resource-Based Relative Value Scale* (*RBRVS*), especially for contracted services. The RBRVS was developed as a way to balance reimbursement for different types of professional services. A "relative value unit" (RVU) is set for a professional service through the Relative Value Update Committee (RUC). The RUC, which includes members from a variety of medical professional societies, acts as an expert panel and makes recommendations to CMS, which may then accept, reject, or modify its RVU recommendations. CMS publishes the accepted values annually in the *Federal Register*. While primarily intended for use in Medicare-billed services, almost all professional services utilize these published RVUs, which have become the de facto standard payment scale used by third-party payers.

Each RVU consists of three components: physician work, practice expense, and malpractice costs. These values may be modified based on geographic differences. Due to the differences in practice expenses, RVUs for the same service will be slightly different for services performed in a facility (hospital) versus a nonfacility outpatient site (office or clinic). This variation is attributed to coverage of practice expenses in the nonfacility setting, ranging from turning on the lights to paying for staff services. In contrast, in a facility setting, these costs may be separately billed.

The RVU is multiplied by a "conversion factor" (CF) to determine the payment for services. The Medicare CF is published annually along with the RVU values in the *Federal Register* (Table 4-1). Medicaid systems in many states set reimbursement as a percentage of the Medicare value. The CF between private payers and the provider is set as part of their contract.

An E/M service may be billed on the same day as a procedure is performed provided it is a "significant and separately identifiable service." When this occurs, a –25 modifier is added to the E/M CPT code. For example, a patient presenting with a forehead laceration after a fall would be examined for signs of additional injury before the laceration is repaired. In this situation, both the E/M service and the procedure may be billed. The level of billing is based on medical necessity, rather than on how much is written in the patient's record. In other words, it is based on whether the care provided reflects the presenting or primary problem.

TABLE 4-1

2009 Medicare Reimbursement Calculation for Comprehensive Established Patient Office

99215 (Outpatient Office/Clinic, Established)	
Facility (hospital)	Nonfacility (office)
• Work = 2.00	• Work = 2.00
• Practice = 0.65	• Practice = 1.38
• Malpractice = 0.08	• Malpractice = 0.08
• Total = 2.73	• Total = 3.46
2.73 × 36.07 (CF) = $98.46	3.46 × 36.07 (CF) = $124.79

Note: The Medicare conversion factor (CF) for 2009 was $36.0666.

Sources: Centers for Medicare and Medicaid Services. (2008, November 19). 73 *Federal Register;* CPT code copyright 2009 by American Medical Association.

DOCUMENTATION GUIDELINES AND RULES

The first documentation guidelines were listed in CPT when the E/M codes were first published. They are subjective and, therefore, open to varied interpretation. To facilitate chart auditing for payment purposes, the Health Care Finance Administration (now CMS) published the first Medicare documentation guidelines in 1995, with a revision subsequently occurring in 1999. Providers have a choice as to which set of guidelines they prefer to use. These guidelines are now the standard used by most third-party payers in determining the level of physician work. The guidelines define how much history, physical examination, and medical decision making need to be documented to support coding for a specific level of E/M service.

Diagnosis coding rules derive from *International Classification of Diseases, Ninth Edition, Clinical Modification* (ICD-9; to be replaced by ICD-10-CM in 2013) and *Coding Guidelines*, published quarterly by the American Hospital Association. New codes are published annually and become effective on October 1 of each year. The codes and associated rules that come with CPT and ICD-9 are considered part of the Health Insurance Portability and Accountability Act (HIPAA) transaction code sets that must be used by all users who practice within HIPAA guidelines. Additional coding rules may come from state Medicaid agencies, Medicare Administrative Contractors, and third-party payer contracts.

BASIC EVALUATION AND MANAGEMENT DOCUMENTATION

Three key elements exist in basic E/M documentation: history, physical examination, and medical decision making (MDM). Four types of history and physical examination include: problem focused, expanded problem focused, detailed, and comprehensive. The type of history and physical examination is based on the amount of detail documented (Tables 4-2 and 4-3).

The history consists of the chief complaint (CC), history of the present illness (HPI), review of systems (ROS), and past, family, and social histories (PFSH). A chief complaint is always required. The documentation should concisely indicate the nature of the presenting or primary problem. While the CC may reflect the presenting problem, occasionally other more significant issues may be identified as the primary problem. For example, the caregiver may bring the child to the primary care provider's office with a complaint of an upper respiratory infection (URI), but the examiner may find that the child is actually wheezing and in acute respiratory distress. While the chief complaint and presenting problem in this patient would be the URI, the primary problem addressed would be the respiratory distress.

TABLE 4-2

Levels of History: Based on 1995 and 1997 CMS Documentation Guidelines							
Level of History	Chief Compliant (CC)	History of the Present Illness (HPI)		Review of Systems (ROS)		Past, Family, and Social History (PFSH)	
		CPT	CMS (Medicare)	CPT	CMS (Medicare)	CPT	CMS (Medicare)
Problem focused	Required	Brief	1–3 elements	Not required		Not required	
Expanded problem focused	Required	Brief	1–3 elements	Problem pertinent	1 system	Not required	
Detailed	Required	Extended	≥ 4 elements OR ≥ 3 chronic or inactive conditions	Extended	2–9 systems	Pertinent	1 item
Comprehensive	Required	Extended	≥ 4 elements OR ≥ 3 chronic or inactive conditions	Complete	≥ 10 systems	Complete	2 or 3 items

Note: Current Procedural Terminology (CPT).

Source: Data from Centers for Medicare & Medicaid Services.

TABLE 4-3

Levels of Exam: Based on 1995 and 1997 CMS Documentation Guidelines			
Level of Physical Exam	CPT Definitions	CMS (Medicare) Documentation Guidelines	
		1995 Guidelines	1997 Guidelines
Problem focused	Limited exam of affected body area	1 body area or organ system	1–5 bullets in one or more areas/systems
Expanded problem focused	Limited exam of affected body area + other symptomatic or related organ systems	Limited exam of affected body area + other symptomatic or related organ systems (usually 2–4 body areas/organ systems including affected area)	6 or more bullets in one or more areas/systems
Detailed	Extended exam of affected body area + other symptomatic or related organ systems	Extended exam of affected body area + other symptomatic or related organ systems (usually 5–7 body areas/organ systems including affected area)	12 or more bullets in 2 or more areas/systems OR at least 2 bullets from 6 or more areas/systems
Comprehensive	General multisystem exam or complete examination of a single organ system	8 or more organ systems	At least 2 bullets from 9 or more areas/systems

Note: Current Procedural Terminology (CPT).

Source: Data from Centers for Medicare & Medicaid Services.

Immediately following the CC is the HPI, which consists of eight elements: location, quality, severity, duration, timing, context, modifying factors, and associated signs and symptoms. A brief HPI consists of one to three elements; an extended HPI includes four or more elements or the status of at least three chronic or inactive conditions.

Fourteen systems are covered in the ROS: constitutional (such as fever), eyes, ears/nose/mouth/throat, cardiovascular, respiratory, gastrointestinal, genitourinary, musculoskeletal, integumentary, neurological, psychiatric, endocrine, hematologic/lymphatic, and allergic/immunologic. Pertinent positives and negatives should be recorded for each of these systems. The HCP should not redocument the CC in the ROS. A *problem pertinent* ROS relates the system(s) directly to the HPI. An *extended* ROS would also include a limited number of additional systems (total of 2 to 9 systems). A *complete* ROS documents at least 10 of the 14 systems.

Two types of PFSH are included: pertinent and complete. A *pertinent* PFSH is one specific item from any area. For example, "no known allergies" would give credit for past medical history and "attends daycare program" would count for social history. The number of areas needed to be documented for a *complete* PFSH depends on the patient setting. For patients seen in the emergency department or established patients seen in any outpatient venue (e.g., office, clinic), two of the three areas must be documented. For all other patients (e.g., new patient seen in any outpatient venue, consultation, initial inpatient interview, observational care), all three areas must be documented.

The HPI must be personally recorded by the physician or NPP. An intake history obtained by any other type of HCP cannot be used as the HPI, even if a note is attached stating that it was reviewed and accepted by a licensed physician. In contrast, the ROS and PFSH may be written by any HCP, student, patient, or caregiver provided that the physician or NPP indicate that they reviewed the information and made appropriate modifications. If there have been no interval changes between visits, a notation to that fact combined with the date of the last ROS/PFSH is sufficient for the current visit.

The physical examination always includes a general description of the patient. The body is separated into body areas and organ systems. The detail required in the physical examination depends on whether the 1995 or 1999 guidelines are used (Table 4-4). The 1995 guidelines are thought to favor nonspecialty general medical exams.

MDM is the most important key element in documentation. The amount of detail written for the history and physical examination must support the level of MDM. As with the history and physical examination, four types of MDM are possible: straightforward, low complexity, moderate complexity, and high complexity. MDM is made up of three components:

- The number of diagnostic and/or therapeutic management options that need to be considered
- The amount and/or complexity of data that must be obtained and analyzed
- The risk involved in either the presenting or primary problem, the diagnostic testing for the problem, and the management of the problem

At least two of these components must be included to determine the level of decision making. The level of MDM may be calculated in various ways: The simplest option is to use the risk table provided by CMS (Table 4-5). Once the level of risk is substantiated, the HCP must then support the overall level of MDM.

Generally, all three of the key elements (history, physical examination, medical decision making) must be present to determine the CPT level of E/M service. Services such as an established office visit require only two of the three key elements; however, MDM should always be one of the elements to support the medical necessity of the service. Some E/M services have an associated time component. If counseling and coordination of care exceed 50% of the visit

TABLE 4-4

Exam Body Areas and Organ Systems: Based on 1995 and 1997 CMS Documentation Guidelines		
CMS (Medicare)		
1995 Guidelines		**1997 Guidelines**
Body Areas	**Organ Systems**	**General Multisystem Exam Systems and Areas**
• Head (face) • Neck • Chest (breasts and axillae) • Abdomen • Genitalia, groin, buttocks • Back (spine) • Each extremity	• Constitutional • Eyes • Ears, nose, mouth, and throat • Cardiovascular • Respiratory • Gastrointestinal • Genitourinary • Musculoskeletal • Skin • Neurologic • Psychiatric • Hematologic, lymphatic, immunologic	• Constitutional • Eyes • Ears, nose, mouth, and throat • Neck • Respiratory • Cardiovascular • Chest (breasts) • Gastrointestinal (abdomen) • Genitourinary • Lymphatic • Musculoskeletal • Skin • Neurological • Psychiatric

Source: Data from Centers for Medicare & Medicaid Services.

TABLE 4-5

Table of Risk: Based on 1995 and 1997 CMS Documentation Guidelines			
Level of Risk	**Presenting Problem(s)**	**Diagnostic Procedure(s) Ordered**	**Management Options Selected**
Minimal	• One self-limited or minor problem (e.g., cold, insect bite, tinea corporis)	• Laboratory tests requiring venipuncture • CXR • ECG/EEG • Urinalysis • Ultrasound (e.g., echocardiography) • KOH prep	• Rest • Gargles • Elastic bandages • Superficial dressings
Low	• Two or more self-limited or minor problems • One stable chronic illness (e.g., well-controlled hypertension, non-insulin-dependent diabetes, cataract, BPH) • Acute uncomplicated illness or injury (e.g., cystitis, allergic rhinitis, simple sprain)	• Physiologic tests not under stress (e.g., pulmonary function tests) • Noncardiovascular imaging studies with contrast (e.g., barium enema) • Superficial needle biopsies • Clinical laboratory tests requiring arterial puncture • Skin biopsies	• Over-the-counter drugs • Minor surgery with no identified risk factors • Physical therapy • Occupational therapy • IV fluids without additives
Moderate	• One or more chronic illnesses with mild exacerbation, progression, or side effects of treatment • Two or more stable chronic illnesses • Undiagnosed new problem with uncertain prognosis (e.g., lump in breast) • Acute illness with systemic symptoms (e.g., pyelonephritis, pneumonitis, colitis) • Acute complicated injury (e.g., head injury with brief loss of consciousness)	• Physiologic tests under stress (e.g., cardiac stress test, fetal contraction stress test) • Diagnostic endoscopies with no identified risk factors • Deep needle or incisional biopsy • Cardiovascular imaging studies with contrast and no identified risk factors (e.g., arteriogram, cardiac catheterization) • Obtain fluid from body cavity (e.g., lumbar puncture, thoracentesis, culdocentesis)	• Minor surgery with identified risk factors • Elective major surgery (open, percutaneous, or endoscopic) with no identified risk factors • Prescription drug management • Therapeutic nuclear medicine • IV fluids with additives • Closed treatment of fracture or dislocation without manipulation
High	• One or more chronic illnesses with severe exacerbation, progression, or side effects of treatment • Acute or chronic illnesses or injuries that pose a threat to life or bodily function (e.g., multiple trauma, acute MI, pulmonary embolus, severe respiratory distress, progressive severe rheumatoid arthritis, psychiatric illness with potential threat to self or others, peritonitis, acute renal failure) • An abrupt change in neurologic status (e.g., seizure, TIA, weakness, sensory loss)	• Cardiovascular imaging studies with contrast with identified risk factors • Cardiac electrophysiological tests • Diagnostic endoscopies with identified risk factors • Discography	• Elective major surgery (open, percutaneous, or endoscopic) with identified risk factors • Emergency major surgery (open, percutaneous, or endoscopic) • Parenteral controlled substances • Drug therapy requiring intensive monitoring for toxicity • Decision not to resuscitate or to de-escalate care because of poor prognosis

Notes: Center for Medicare and Medicaid Services (CMS), chest radiograph (CXR), electrocardiograph (ECG), electroencephalograph (EEG), intravenous (IV), benign prostatic hyperplasia (BPH), myocardial infarct (MI), transient ischemic attack (TIA).

Source: Data from Centers for Medicare & Medicaid Services.

time, then time may be used in determining the level of service. A very limited number of services, such as critical care, are based on time only.

It is important to remember that these documentation guidelines relate solely to reimbursement issues. At all times the medical record is first and foremost a medicolegal document and, therefore, should include any and all notations needed to accurately reflect the events and plans associated with the patient's episode of care.

BASIC DIAGNOSIS CODING

The World Health Organization (WHO) provides the foundation for the *International Classification of Diseases* for epidemiological tracking of illness and injury. Unlike the CPT, the WHO information is available in the public domain. In the United States, the ICD clinical modification is managed by four cooperating parties: CMS, National Center for Health Statistics/U.S. Centers for Disease Control and Prevention, American Hospital Association, and American Health Information Management Association. The current version, ICD-9-CM, is divided into three parts: diseases and injuries (001–999), supplementary factors (V01–V89), and external factors (E000–E999).

In choosing a diagnosis, the code that best explains the reason or significant finding for the encounter should be used. Any contributing diagnosis is listed as a secondary code; diagnoses that do not affect the visit are not listed. Next, a diagnosis code that reflects the highest level of clinical certainty should be selected. It is appropriate to use clinical judgment even in absence of laboratory or radiographic confirmation to make this determination. If the condition is unclear, then the diagnosis code for the presenting symptoms and/or complaints should be selected. A "final" diagnosis is not needed. Indeterminist terms, unless specifically in the code title, such as "rule out," "possible," or "probable," and descriptors such as "mild," "slight," or "moderate" are not appropriate. *These descriptors are part of the patient assessment, not the diagnosis.*

The assessment is the HCP's overall evaluation of the patient encounter. The diagnosis should reflect the specific terminology found in ICD-9. For example, a patient with a swollen ankle after a fall may have a Salter-Harris type I fracture that is not yet visible on radiograph. The assessment would be "possible SH-I ankle fracture," while the diagnosis—"ankle injury"—would reflect the highest level of clinical certainty.

Presenting problems or findings that are inherent to a condition should not be separately coded. For example, fever and ear pain (otalgia) are a part of acute otitis media and should not be coded individually. However, conditions that explain the reason for a diagnostic study should be coded separately. This separation of codes is especially helpful if the code is not later justified by the final diagnosis.

Use specific diagnosis codes for neonates younger than 29 days of age, or for conditions that began in the neonatal period and still affect the patient.

Writing diagnoses such as "ROM (right-sided otitis media)," "RAD (reactive airway disease)," or "AGE (acute gastroenteritis)" can lead to down-coding of the E/M level and/or denial of service by a third-party payer. In these examples, the diagnoses would translate into the codes for "unspecified otitis media," "asthma (stable)," and "other and unspecified noninfectious gastroenteritis," respectively. By comparison, the use of specific terminology would include "acute suppurative otitis media," "acute bronchospasm," and "presumed infectious acute gastroenteritis" (a diagnosis with the indeterminate term included in the code title).

Supplementary or "V-codes" may reflect either the primary reason or a contributing factor for the encounter. V-codes are used to describe the following circumstances:

- Patient allergy to certain medications
- Infection with a resistant organism
- Medical apparatus, such as a tracheostomy
- Procedure, such as suture removal
- Sequential vaccination, such as rabies vaccination
- End-of-treatment evaluation
- A concern or possible exposure when there are no actual findings

For example, for an encounter with a pediatric patient who was involved in a motor vehicle crash where the patient has no complaints, symptoms, or physical findings would be V-coded as "exam after motor vehicle crash."

External condition or "E-codes" are always secondary codes. They denote factors that contribute to an injury. In the previous example, an E-code might be used to indicate the patient's status as a passenger in a motor vehicle collision.

REFERENCES

1. American Medical Association (AMA). (2009). *Current procedural terminology (CPT®)*. Chicago, IL: Author.
2. Center for Medicare and Medicaid Services (CMS). (1995). 1995 documentation guidelines for evaluation & management services. Retrieved from http://www.cms.hhs.gov/MLNProducts/Downloads/1995dg.pdf
3. Center for Medicare and Medicaid Services (CMS). (1997). 1997 documentation guidelines for evaluation & management services. Retrieved from http://www.cms.hhs.gov/MLNProducts/Downloads/MASTER1.pdf
4. Center for Medicare and Medicaid Services (CMS) & the National Center for Health Statistics (NCHS). ICD-9-CM official guidelines for coding and reporting. Retrieved from http://www.cdc.gov/nchs/data/icd9/icdguide09.pdf
5. U.S. Department of Health and Human Services, Centers for Medicare and Medicaid Services (CMS). (2008, November 19). Medicare program: Payment policies under the physician fee schedule and other revisions to Part B for CY 2009 (short title). 73 Fed Reg 69725–70238.

Structures of Communication within Organizations

- **Communication**
- **Committees and Task Forces**

- **Shared Governance**
- **References**

COMMUNICATION

In 2001, the American Association of Critical Care Nurses (AACN) made a commitment to actively promote the creation of healthy work environments that support and foster excellence in patient care wherever acute and critical care nurses practice. The six standards deemed necessary to achieve this goal consist of skilled communication, true collaboration, effective decision making, appropriate staffing, meaningful recognition, and authentic leadership (AACN, 2005). Although they were determined by a nursing organization, these standards apply to all health care professionals (HCPs). The Joint Commission singles out the breakdown of one of these elements—skilled communication—as a frequent problem in sentinel events (unexpected events leading to death or serious injury) and has included improving communication in the 2010 National Patient Safety Goals (2009, 2010).

In skilled communication, the communicators invite and hear all relevant perspectives and listen with respect. They demonstrate congruence between words and actions, and they hold others accountable for doing the same. Health care organizations committed to skilled communication establish formal structures and processes that ensure effective information sharing among patients, families, and the health care team and require individuals and teams to formally evaluate the impact of communication on clinical, financial, and work environment outcomes. Maxfield (2007) provides an excellent metaphor demonstrating the critical need for skilled communication:

> Jet fighters landing on carriers at sea and squads of firefighters parachuting into forest fires provide the best models for the communication skills required in hospitals. What they share are frequent unexpected emergencies. In predictable environments, success depends on planning and controlling the future. But on aircraft carriers, in firefighting teams, and in many parts of a hospital, the best don't look at the future beyond about 4 hours. Instead, they focus on managing the complexity of the present—the three planes landing, the explosion or flames, or [the] multiple complexities of an operating room. Juggling these multiple inputs and outputs in real-time requires a much higher and better level of communication. (p. 16)

Effective communication has at least one sender, one receiver, and one message. It can be verbal, nonverbal, or written; in today's world, it can also be an electronic "instant message." Both internal and external factors may affect how the message is delivered or received. Internal factors are intrinsic to the communicators, such as culture, gender, language, generation, or level of understanding. For instance, Rudan (2003) found that gender is a significant factor in organizational communication simply because men and women use verbal and nonverbal language differently. He found that when conducting business meetings, the males were more business-like whereas the females were more socially oriented. External factors include the size of the organization and whether the communication is formal or informal. Ultimately, the key question is this: Does the message reach those it is intended to reach and convey what it is intended to convey and does it do so in a timely manner?

To ensure the message is clear and understood, several organizational strategies can be implemented:

- Keep information concise, regardless of the format or purpose. Provide a context to the information so that the receiver understands the message.
- Seek feedback from the receiver to ensure that the message was received accurately, on time, and as intended. This approach is often referred to as "closed-loop" communication.
- Use multiple modes of delivery when possible. This strategy works especially well for messages dealing with policy, new practice, or emergency.
- Use direct eye contact if the message is delivered in person.

Information within an organization does not just flow between two people or within a small group of people, as happens on a clinical unit. It also flows in multiple directions within an organization's structure—upward, downward, horizontal, diagonal, and in an informal way often referred to as "the grapevine." The modes or media in which communication takes place also vary. Traditional modes such as email, face-to-face contact, telephone/voicemail, and pager remain in use; however, savvy organizations are now incorporating social networks and text messaging in their communication plans as well, recognizing that their younger staff will more quickly retrieve communications from these sources than the more traditional ones. Even so, despite the evolving technology, chance face-to-face meetings are still regularly used to communicate important information. This form of communication can be highly interruptive to the work environment and increases the potential for misunderstood or forgotten messages (Parker & Coiera, 2000). Regardless of the setting or mode, communication is an important skill to master as part of the effort to provide a healthy work environment and reduce medical errors.

COMMITTEES AND TASK FORCES

Health care is a business. As such, certain work needs to be accomplished to meet the mission of caring for patients. Committees and task forces are important methods to accomplish this work.

Committees function by engaging in group activity across traditional lines or departments. They are prescribed within the organizational structure and report to a particular officer within the structure. These ongoing groups are organized around a specific function such as quality improvement, disaster preparedness, or strategic planning and can be formed at the unit, department, or senior administrative level. The advantages of committees include that multiple stakeholders with investment in the final output or work product come together to complete tasks and make decisions. The committee members may come to decisions through either vote or consensus. The major disadvantage of committees is that decision making can be slowed due to the need for consensus building and meeting schedules. There is also the risk that quieter voices may go unheard. Committees usually have a leader or chairperson and maintain a formal structure of agendas, minutes, and reports. Meetings are often scheduled at regular, predetermined intervals.

Task forces, by comparison, are temporary groups that are formed to work on very specific projects or tasks. These short-lived groups have defined dates for task completion. Examples of task forces include those devoted to construction design and specific protocol development. In fact, search committees are actually task forces that are commonly mislabeled as committees. Task forces have the same advantages and disadvantages as committees. They may not have the same depth of structure as committees, such as regular, predetermined meetings, but they often do have a chairperson, an agenda, minutes, and a final report.

The outcomes for both committees and task forces can often be measured through a practice or policy change result, such as a reduction in patient falls or medication errors. Commitment to either committee or task force work can be difficult given the constraints of patient care. Nevertheless, these groups are a means by which HCPs in the organization as a whole can have a lasting impact.

To be effective within a committee or task force, one needs to understand group dynamics. Tuckman and Jensen (1977) identified four stages of small group development: forming, storming, norming, and performing.

- *Forming* occurs when the members introduce themselves to the group. The introduction will often delineate their basis as a stakeholder and explain what they have to offer the group in expertise. The goals for the group are reviewed and plans made. This stage is a good time for most groups, as members are usually excited about the task and enthusiastic to reach project completion.
- *Storming* occurs as individuals establish their identity within the group and a level of trust develops. A level of competition may also develop. Most groups will have some differing of opinions. Although these different perspectives are what make group decisions stronger when reached, they can also make consensus building a long and difficult process. Group leaders need to make

sure that all group members are respected and that even quiet members are heard.
- *Norming* is seen when roles are established and work is identified.
- *Performing* is the stage in which the work is actually under way and the members work independently and efficiently to complete their tasks within the larger group.

As a group forms, specific tasks and roles are identified, such as information seeker, coordinator, evaluator, and recorder. During the storming and norming stages, an element of group building occurs and a level of sustainment emerges that needs to be maintained. Examples of group-building roles include encourager, harmonizer, compromiser, gatekeeper, standard setter, group commentator, and follower. Within the group-building roles, individual roles are likely to develop based on individual members' strengths and weaknesses. Group leaders need to be cognizant of each member's roles so that group progress is not inhibited by someone who becomes an aggressor or recognition seeker. As Marquis and Huston (2006) state, "Managers must be well grounded in group dynamics and group roles because of the need to facilitate group communication and productivity within the organization" (p. 487). They further state, "Dynamic leaders inspire followers toward participative management by how they work and communicate in groups. Leaders keep group members on course, draw out the shy, politely cut out the garrulous, and protect the weak" (p. 487).

SHARED GOVERNANCE

Shared governance was developed in the early 1980s as an alternative to the traditional bureaucratic, top-down organizational structure. The aim of shared governance is to empower groups within a system to make change and have control over their own practice. This model is interpreted and implemented differently within each organization and can be implemented at the unit, department, or organizational level. For instance, it may be exemplified by councils (groups designated to govern), committees, or task forces. Research suggests that using a shared governance model results in a constructive hospital culture, HCP retention, work satisfaction, and positive patient outcomes (Upenieks, 2000). At the same time, shared governance requires a sustained and long-term commitment on the part of the HCPs and the organization to maintain these effects.

REFERENCES

1. American Association of Critical Care Nurses. (2005). *AACN standards for establishing and sustaining healthy work environments.* Aliso Viejo, CA: Author. Retrieved from http://www.aacn.org/WD/HWE/Docs/HWEStandards.pdf

2. The Joint Commission. (2009). Sentinel events. Retrieved from http://www.jointcommission.org/SentinelEvents/

3. The Joint Commission. (2010). National safety goals.Retrieved from http://www.jointcommission.org/PatientSafety/NationalPatient SafetyGoals/

4. Marquis, B., & Huston, C. (2006). *Leadership roles and management functions in nursing: Theory and application* (5th ed.). Philadelphia: Lippincott Williams and Wilkins.

5. Maxfield, D. (2007). Creating healthy work environments: Skilled communication. *American College of Chest Physicians, 2*(2), 16.

6. Parker, J., & Coiera, E. (2000). Improving clinical communication: A view from psychology. *Journal of the American Medical Informatics Association, 7*(5), 453–461.

7. Rudan, V. (2003). The best of both worlds: A consideration of gender in team building. *Journal of Nursing Administration, 33*(3), 179–186.

8. Tuckman, B., & Jensen, M. (1977). Stages of small group development revisited. *Group and Organization Studies, 2*(4), 419.

9. Upenieks, V. (2000). The relationship of nursing practice models and job satisfaction outcomes. *Journal of Nursing Administration, 30*(6), 330–335.

Patient Safety

Despite the expertise and dedication of pediatric health care professionals (HCP), pediatric patients are frequently harmed or killed during the delivery of care that is intended to make them well (Kohn et al., 1999; Leape & Berwick, 2005). Inadvertent harm to pediatric patients may occur as a result of an *adverse event* in which injury is caused by medical management rather than by a patient's underlying disease or by a medical error. A *medical error* is the failure of a planned intervention to be carried out as intended, the inappropriate use of an intervention, or the failure to enact a necessary intervention (Garbutt et al., 2007; Kohn et al.; Woods & Johnson, 2005). Table 6-1 lists additional definitions of adverse events and medical errors. Although harm from adverse events can be minimized through monitoring and planned mitigation strategies, adverse events cannot be prevented in all circumstances. The development of a harmful side effect to an appropriately prescribed and administered medication is an example of an adverse event. In contrast to adverse events, medical errors, such as miscalculating the dose of a medication, are nearly always preventable.

In 1999, an Institute of Medicine (IOM) report, titled *To Err Is Human: Building a Safer Health System,* documented that approximately 100,000 people died every year in the United States as the result of medical errors made by HCPs (Kohn et al., 1999). The report ranked errors as the eighth leading cause of death, attributed 7,000 of these deaths to medication errors, and estimated that the annual cost incurred by the errors is as high as $29 billion (American Hospital Association [AHA], 1999; Brennan et al., 1991; Centers for Disease Control and Prevention [CDC], 2002; Kohn et al.; Leape et al., 1991). More startlingly, subsequent research indicates that the *To Err Is Human* report may have actually underestimated the magnitude of inadvertent harm inflicted on patients. For example, CDC data suggest that nosocomial bloodstream infections alone may account for as many as 90,000 patient deaths every year (CDC, 2000; Leape & Berwick, 2005) and that deaths due to medical errors outpace deaths due to pneumonia, influenza, or diabetes (CDC, 2004; Health Grades, 2004). Furthermore, Leape and Berwick (2005) have reported that since the

publication of *To Err Is Human,* there has been little reduction in the rate of errors and adverse events that harm patients in the United States.

The discipline of patient safety, which focuses on the prevention of accidental injury due to adverse events or medical errors—collectively referred to as *patient safety events*—has emerged in response to the IOM report and related research. The annual rate of patient safety events in hospitalized patients younger than age 18 years is 1–2.9 events per 100 admissions. It has been estimated that 60% of pediatric patient safety events are preventable. In keeping with a national average of 7 million pediatric hospital admissions per year, this rate equates to at least 70,000 children experiencing adverse events annually, more than one-half of which could be prevented through the use of patient safety interventions (McDonald et al., 2007; Woods et al., 2005). To administer high-quality care, it is imperative that pediatric HCPs understand the principles of patient safety and are able to identify and implement strategies to prevent patient safety events.

THEORETICAL FOUNDATION FOR PATIENT SAFETY

THEORIES OF HUMAN ERROR AND PERFORMANCE RELIABILITY

An understanding of human error and performance reliability of human systems provides a theoretic foundation for the discipline of patient safety. Much of what is known about human error and performance reliability has been generated by industries such as manufacturing, nuclear power, and aviation. Studies of such industries have identified that people process information using *skill-, rule-,* and *knowledge-based* modes of behavior (Rasmussen et al., 1994). The *generic error modeling system (GEMS;* see Table 6-2) associates a specific propensity for error with each behavior mode. According to the GEMS, decision making that relies on knowledge, judgment, and memory results in the highest rate of error. This theory illustrates that in addition

TABLE 6-1

Patient Safety Event Definitions	
Adverse event	An injury that was caused by medical management rather than by a patient's underlying disease
Medical error	The failure of a planned action to be completed as intended or to achieve its intended goal, the use of the wrong action to achieve a goal, or negligence to carry out a necessary action Minor error: A medical error that causes harm that is neither permanent nor life threatening Serious error: A medical error that causes permanent injury or transient, but life-threatening harm
Near miss	An adverse event or medical error that would have caused harm to a patient, but did not because of timely intervention or chance
Sentinel event	An adverse event or medical error that results in death or serious physical or psychological injury

Source: Corrigan et al., 1999.

TABLE 6-2

Generic Error Modeling System	
Behavior Mode	**Propensity for Error**
Skill Based	
Performance of highly practiced actions in a familiar situation *Example*: HCP prescribes a drug that she has used to treat patients on a daily basis for many years	1 error per 1,000 actions
Rule Based	
Following preestablished rules to perform an action that has not been highly practiced or to perform in an unfamiliar situation *Example*: When writing a prescription for an unfamiliar medication, the HCP refers to the hospital's formulary to review the medication's indications and contraindications for use and to select a dose	1 error per 100 actions
Knowledge Based	
Use of judgment to perform an action that has not been highly practiced or to perform in an unfamiliar situation *Example*: When writing a prescription for an unfamiliar medication, the HCP uses her knowledge of other drugs in the same class to determine that a drug is appropriate for a patient and to select a dose	3 errors per 10 actions

Source: Reason, 1990.

to education and practical experience, people need decision support tools, such as reminders, written instructions, and checklists, to reliably perform activities (Reason, 1990, 1997, 2000). Furthermore, industrial theories of *quality control* demonstrate that performance reliability improves with standardization of practices and with strict control for variation from standards (Evans, 2005).

ERROR-PROOFING SYSTEMS

The causes of patient safety events can be categorized as either *active failures,* which are unsafe behaviors enacted by people, or *latent conditions,* which are flaws in the design of systems in which people work. For a system to be safe, it must possess layers of defense that prevent or trap both active failures and latent conditions before they cause harm (Marx, 1999; Medvedev, 1991). The term *Swiss cheese model* (Figure 6-1) has been coined to represent the need for layers of defense in systems. The Swiss cheese model illustrates the possibility for holes in safeguards to line up and allow an error to pass through a system and cause harm to a patient. This model demonstrates that to maximally reduce the risk of failure, multiple and redundant defense layers must be built into systems (Reason, 1990, 1997, 2000).

CREW RESOURCE MANAGEMENT

Studies of nuclear power and aviation accidents have noted that in addition to stemming from inadequate defense barriers, over-reliance on human memory, and lack of

procedural standardization, system failures are commonly associated with authoritative behavior, ineffective communication, stress, and fatigue among people functioning within the system (Ciavarelli et al., 1999; Helmriech et al., 1999; Tamuz & Harrison, 2006; Weiner et al., 1993). By error-proofing systems and by employing *crew resource management (CRM),* industries have significantly improved the safety of their services. CRM entails the use of tools and training that enhance the interpersonal and communication skills, as well as the technical skills, among members of a team. Tools such as structured briefings and training via simulation are common features of CRM. In health care, this model is often applied to emergency management teams such as trauma, rapid response, and resuscitation teams. It is equally important as part of effective "time-outs" (universal protocol), which confirm the correctness of the patient, site, and procedure before invasive interventions; for routine care planning during daily rounds; and for hand-off communication between HCPs (Eppich et al., 2008).

More than 50% of patient safety events are attributed to communication failures (Hunt et al., 2007; Kohn et al., 1999). The use of structured templates for communicating patient information is an example of CRM that is known to improve the completeness and clarity of knowledge exchange in health care (Hunter, 2007; Norton, 2007; Sandlin, 2007). Most importantly, effective communication can prevent failure to rescue. *Failure to rescue* is an event in which a patient dies or incurs considerable morbidity due to a complication of care or because of a condition other than the reason for admission that is acquired during the hospitalization (Bobay et al., 2008; Clarke & Aiken, 2003).

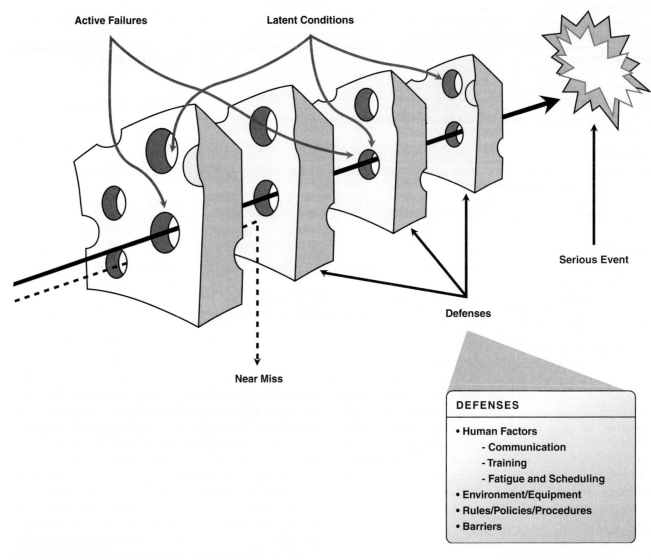

Active Failures

Latent Conditions

Serious Event

Defenses

Near Miss

DEFENSES

- **Human Factors**
  - **- Communication**
  - **- Training**
  - **- Fatigue and Scheduling**
- **Environment/Equipment**
- **Rules/Policies/Procedures**
- **Barriers**

FIGURE 6-1

Swiss Cheese Model of System Defenses and Patient Safety Events.

Source: Used with permission Reason, J. (1990). Human Error. New York: Cambridge University Press.

In addition to vigilant physiologic surveillance, elements of CRM—including effective communication of patient data and needs between HCPs, and highly practiced rapid response and resuscitation teams—can prevent failure to rescue events (Clarke & Aiken, 2003; France et al., 2008; Nishisaki et al., 2007; Sharek et al., 2007; Van Voorhis & Willis, 2009).

HIGH-RELIABILITY ORGANIZATIONS

The combination of standardization, layers of defense, and CRM allows organizations to produce desired outcomes, despite error-prone activities, with a very low rate of failure. Organizations that achieve low failure rates are designated as *high-reliability organizations* (HROs). Regardless of the type of industry, HROs share the following characteristics:

- Preoccupation with error prevention
- Appreciation of the complexity of errors and reluctance to simplify the causes or the strategies to prevent errors
- A focus on system failures rather than individual performance, including nonpunitive approaches to addressing errors
- Ability to learn from errors and continually improve
- A flat organization hierarchy in which staff of any level can call out safety concerns and make recommendations for improvement (Oriol, 2006; Tamuz & Harrison, 2006)

CULTURE OF SAFETY

To be an HRO, a health care system must possess a *culture of safety*. Fundamental elements of a culture of safety (Table 6-3) include cohesive teamwork, unyielding leadership support for patient safety goals, nonpunitive approaches to errors that are reported, and transparency regarding patient safety events for the purposes of learning and preventing recurrence (Hinshaw, 2008; Milstead, 2005; Nance, 2004; Oriol, 2006; Singer et al., 2007). In addition, elements of *ideal work environments* are necessary for a safety culture. Ideal work environments possess the following attributes:

- Highly educated staff
- Work hr restrictions
- Appropriate staffing ratios and workload distribution
- Ergonomically sound physical workspace
- Decision support aids at the point of care
- Teamwork and collaboration (Hinshaw, 2008; Holden, 2006)

A determination of whether the characteristics of a HRO, including elements of a safety culture and an ideal work environment exist, can be made by examining Table 6-4.

METHODS FOR IMPROVING SAFETY

Preoccupation with error prevention and performance improvement is inherent within a culture of safety. Three analysis tools commonly used to manage patient safety

TABLE 6-3

Characteristics of a Culture of Safety

- Leadership support for patient safety goals
- Widespread preoccupation with error prevention and safety-proofing systems
- Nonpunitive responses to errors and adverse events
- Transparency regarding errors and adverse events for the purpose of continual learning
- Work hour restrictions and appropriate staffing ratios and workload distribution
- Ergonomically sound physical workspaces
- Decision support aids readily available at the point of care and reduced staff reliance on use of memory
- Standardization of practices and staff adherence to established policies and procedures
- Cohesive teamwork and communication
- A flat organization hierarchy in which staff of any level are empowered to escalate safety concerns and make recommendations for improvement

TABLE 6-4

Does a Culture of Safety Exist?

The following questions, which are adapted from the Agency for Healthcare Research and Quality (AHRQ) Hospital Survey Questions on Patient Safety Culture, can be used to determine if a culture of safety is present in a pediatric acute care setting

Teamwork and Collaboration

- Do people support one another in this unit?
- When a lot of work needs to be done quickly, do we work together as a team to get the work done?
- In this unit, do people treat one another with respect?
- Are staff members afraid to ask questions when something does not seem right?
- Do staff feel free to question the decisions or actions of those with more authority?
- Are shift changes problematic for patients in this unit or in the hospital?
- When one area in this unit gets really busy, do others help out?
- Is there good cooperation among hospital units that need to work together?
- Do hospital units work well together to provide the best care for patients?
- Is it often unpleasant to work with staff from other hospital units?
- Do hospital units coordinate well with one another?
- Do things "fall between the cracks" when transferring patients from one unit to another?
- Is important patient care information often lost during shift changes?
- Do problems often occur in the exchange of information across hospital units?

(Continued)

TABLE 6-4

Does a Culture of Safety Exist? *(Continued)*

Staffing, Work Hours, and Workload

- Do we have enough staff to handle the workload?
- Do we work in "crisis mode" trying to do too much, too quickly?
- Is patient safety ever sacrificed to get more work done?
- Do staff in this unit work longer hours than is best for patient care?
- Do we use more agency/temporary staff than is best for patient care?
- Are staff appropriately educated and trained to do their jobs?

Leadership Support

- Do the actions of hospital management show that patient safety is a top priority?
- Does hospital management seem interested in patient safety only after an adverse event happens?
- Does hospital management provide a work climate that promotes patient safety?
- Does my supervisor/manager overlook patient safety problems that happen repeatedly?
- Does my supervisor/manager say a good word when he or she sees a job done according to established patient safety procedures?
- Does my supervisor/manager seriously consider staff suggestions for improving patient safety?
- Whenever pressure builds up, does my supervisor/manager wants us to work faster, even if it means taking shortcuts?

Transparency and Nonpunitive Approaches to Patient Safety Events

- Do staff members feel like their mistakes are held against them?
- When an event is reported, does it feels like the *person* is being written up, not the *problem*?
- Do staff worry that mistakes they make are documented and maintained in their personnel file?
- Will staff freely speak up if they see something that may negatively affect patient care?
- Are we are informed about errors that happen in this unit?
- Are we are given feedback about changes put into place based on event reports?

Preoccupation with Error Prevention

- Is it just by chance that more serious mistakes don't happen around here?
- In this unit, do we discuss ways to prevent errors from happening again?
- Are we are actively doing things to improve patient safety?
- Do mistakes lead to positive changes here?
- After we make changes to improve patient safety, do we evaluate their effectiveness?
- When a mistake is made, but is caught and corrected before affecting the patient, how often is it reported?
- When a mistake is made, but has no potential to harm the patient, how often is it reported?
- When a mistake is made that could harm the patient, but does not, how often is it reported?

Application of Human Error and Performance Reliability Theory

- Are our procedures and systems are good at preventing errors from happening?
- Do we implement multiple layers of interventions to trap errors from occurring?
- Are procedures and processes standardized?
- Do staff adhere to policies and procedures?
- Are decision support aids immediately available at the bedside?
- Do we focus on system failures rather than individual performance?

Ergonomics of the Physical Workspace

- Is the layout of physical workspace conducive to carrying out patient care?
- Can I easily access all necessary supplies and equipment while caring for patients?
- Are calls for assistance immediately heard and acknowledged?
- Is the unit noisy?
- Do staff on the unit become desensitized to sounding alarms?
- Am I frequently distracted while carrying out complex clinical tasks?

Source: Adapted from AHRQ Hospital Survey on Patient Safety Culture, http://www.ahrq.gov/qual/hospculture/

TABLE 6-5

Patient Safety Analysis Tools	
Tool	**Purpose**
Failure mode effects analysis	A prospective analysis used to identify and assign a risk priority to system vulnerabilities, called *failure modes*, so that the organization can implement safeguards before errors occur
Incident report	A qualitative narrative of an adverse event, near miss, or medical error that is constructed by staff directly involved in the incident at the time of discovery
Root cause analysis	A retrospective analysis of a serious medical error or sentinel event that has occurred so as to identify contributing factors: <ul><li>Human factors such as problems with communication, training, fatigue, or scheduling</li><li>Environment or equipment defects</li><li>Absence of or deviation from policies and procedures</li><li>Failure or absence of defense barriers in systems</li></ul>

Sources: Duwe et al., 2005; Garbutt et al., 2007; Iedema et al., 2006; Kunac & Reith, 2005; Le Duff et al., 2005; Robinson et al., 2006; Sheridan-Leos et al., 2006; Veterans Administration National Center for Patient Safety, 2008; Wald & Shojanian, 2001; Wetterneck et al., 2006.

TABLE 6-6

Model for Improvement Applied to Patient Safety

Step 1: Identify care delivery that is unsafe.

Step 2: Select interventions that will improve the safety of care.

Step 3: Determine how improvement in safety will be evaluated.

Step 4: Run the following plan–do–study–act (PDSA) cycles for the safety improvement interventions:

- **Plan:** Plan the improvement intervention.
- **Do:** Implement the improvement intervention.
- **Study:** Evaluate the effectiveness of the improvement intervention.
- **Act:** Determine the next steps based on the evaluation.

Repeat these cycles for each improvement interventions.

Source: Langley et al., 1996.

are *failure mode effects analysis, incident reporting,* and *root cause analysis.* Table 6-5 describes each of these analysis tools. The ultimate goal of these endeavors is to identify the variables that might lead to system failure, so that the organization can design and implement safeguards to improve patient safety (Apostolakis & Barach, 2004; Duwe et al., 2005; Garbutt et al., 2007; Iedema et al., 2006; Le Duff et al., 2004). Once identified, the *model for improvement* (Table 6-6) can be used to implement and evaluate the effectiveness of patient safety improvement efforts.

PATIENT SAFETY: APPLICATION TO PEDIATRIC ACUTE CARE

To Err Is Human, as well as subsequent reports that spawned the discipline of patient safety, primarily focused on adult medical care. Moreover, quality and patient safety indicators, such as those developed by the U.S. Agency for Healthcare Research and Quality (AHRQ) to evaluate the safety of hospital services are primarily based on adult safety events. Studies that have specifically examined the quality of children's health care have found that pediatric patient safety events occur less frequently than adult events, but are of equal severity (as measured by their impact on length of stay, cost, and risk of mortality) and are more often preventable. Pediatric patient safety events also have different defining characteristics than events encountered in adult health care (McDonald et al., 2007; Woods et al., 2005).

MEDICATION SAFETY

Perhaps the most important age-based difference in patient safety events is the fact that pediatric patients—particularly infants and toddlers—are three times more likely than adults to experience medication errors or adverse drug events (ADEs) (Holdsworth et al., 2003; Kaushal et al., 2001;

TABLE 6-7

Strategies for Pediatric Medication Safety and Application to Phases of the Medication Use Process			
Medication Ordering	**Medication Preparation and Dispensing**	**Medication Administration**	**Medication Monitoring**
• Use of computerized provider order entry	• Immediate access to patient history, allergies, and relevant laboratory data	• Documentation of medication administration in an electronic medical record	• Use of standardized monitoring protocols (for physiologic monitoring or drug-level monitoring)
• Use of verbal orders only in urgent or emergent situations	• Checking of all medication orders by a pharmacist	• Immediate access to patient history, allergies, and relevant laboratory data	• Vigilant monitoring for patients receiving high-risk medications, particularly analgesics and sedatives
• Immediate access to patient history, allergies, and relevant laboratory data	• Standardization of drug concentrations	• Collaboration with unit-based pharmacists	• Collaboration with unit-based pharmacists
• Collaboration with unit-based pharmacists	• Unit-dosed dispensing	• Restricted access to drugs until orders are checked by pharmacists	
• Medication reconciliation during times of transition in patient care	• Storage of medications in patient-specific storage bins	• Identification and special management of high-risk medications	
• Identification and special management of high-risk medications	• Identification and special management of high-risk medications, including dispensing by a pharmacist only	• Absence of concentrated electrolytes on nursing units	
• Prohibition of the use of error-prone medication abbreviations	• Use of tall-man letters to identify look-a-like or sound-a-like medications	• Use of two patient identifiers and potentially bar-code identification before every drug administration	
• Prohibition of the use of trailing zeros in medication doses	• Separate storage of look-a-like or sound-a-like medications	• Use of tall-man letters to identify look-a-like or sound-a-like medications	
• Use of leading zeros in medication doses			
• Use of tall-man letters to identify look-a-like or sound-a-like medications and separately storing look-a-like or sound-a-like medications			

Sources: Hicks et al., 2006; Holdsworth et al., 2003; Kaushal et al., 2001.

Leape & Berwick, 2005. Medication errors and ADEs are more likely to occur in pediatric patients because growth and physiologic maturation issues require complex dose calculations, frequent dose modifications, and narrower therapeutic-to-lethal dose ranges. Dosing complexity is further compounded by the lack of available pediatric pharmacokinetics and pharmacodynamics data. Furthermore, the inability of pediatric patients to question the appropriateness of a medication or to report side effects prevents them from serving as a layer of protection against errors and ADEs (Hicks et al., 2003; Kaushal et al., 2001; Kaushal et al., 2004; Takata et al., 2008). Table 6-7 presents strategies for ensuring pediatric medication safety, and Table 6-8 lists the medication most commonly ordered in error in pediatrics.

TABLE 6-8

Medications Commonly Associated with Errors in Pediatrics
• Analgesics and sedatives
• Anticoagulants
• Antimicrobials
• Antineoplastic agents
• Corticosteroids
• Electrolytes and fluids
• Insulin
• Vasoactive drugs

Sources: Hicks et al., 2006; Holdsworth et al., 2003; Kaushal et al., 2001.

DIAGNOSTIC-RELATED ADVERSE EVENTS

Like medication safety events, *diagnostic-related adverse events* occur more often in pediatric patients than in adults for two reasons: (1) disease presentations often vary across pediatric age-groups and (2) pediatric patients are less capable of reporting symptoms and participating in history taking. Diagnostic-related adverse events include incorrect diagnosis, due to the misuse or misinterpretation of clinical assessments, and study results (Woods et al., 2005). Diagnostic-related adverse events cause harm via neglect or delay to enact necessary treatment of patients, including delays in admissions and transfers to intensive care units. Premature transfer of a patient to a less acute level of care or premature discharge of a patient is also categorized as a diagnostic-related adverse event (Scanlon et al., 2007; Woods).

PEDIATRIC PATIENT SAFETY INDICATORS: IDENTIFICATION OF PRIORITY SAFETY ISSUES

The uniqueness of pediatric patient safety risks requires adaptation of standard, adult-based patient safety indicators and improvement efforts. Accordingly, the AHRQ, in conjunction with pediatric organizations such as the American Academy of Pediatrics (AAP), the National Association of Children's Hospitals and Related institutions (NACHRI), and the Child Health Corporation of America (CHCA), has developed pediatric-specific patient safety priorities and related quality indicators. Indicators of safe care were identified by meta-analysis of clinical outcomes research that investigated the epidemiology of adverse events and errors during acute care. Table 6-9 illustrates the AHRQ's standard patient safety indicators and the pediatric-specific quality indicators. There is overlap between the AHRQ's general, adult-based

TABLE 6-9

U.S. Agency for Healthcare Research and Quality Patient Safety Indicators and Pediatric Quality Indicators	
Patient Safety Indicators (Adult Based)	**Pediatric Quality Indicators**
• Complications of anesthesia	• Accidental puncture or laceration*
• Death in low-mortality DRGs	• Decubitus ulcer*
• Decubitus ulcer*	• Foreign body left during procedure*
• Failure to rescue	• Iatrogenic pneumothorax in neonates at risk*
• Foreign body left in during procedure*	• Iatrogenic pneumothorax in non-neonates*
• Iatrogenic pneumothorax*	• Pediatric heart surgery mortality
• Selected infections due to medical care	• Pediatric heart surgery volume
• Postoperative hip fracture	• Postoperative hemorrhage or hematoma*
• Postoperative hemorrhage or hematoma*	• Postoperative respiratory failure*
• Postoperative physiologic and metabolic derangements	• Postoperative sepsis*
• Postoperative respiratory failure*	• Postoperative wound dehiscence*
• Postoperative pulmonary embolism or deep vein thrombosis	• Selected infections due to medical care
• Postoperative sepsis*	• Transfusion reaction*
• Postoperative wound dehiscence in abdominopelvic surgical patients*	• Asthma admission rate
• Accidental puncture and laceration*	• Diabetes short-term complication rate
• Transfusion reaction*	• Gastroenteritis admission rate
• Birth trauma—injury to neonate	• Perforated appendix admission rate
• Obstetric trauma—vaginal delivery with instrument	• Urinary tract infection admission rate
• Obstetric trauma—vaginal delivery without instrument	
• Obstetric trauma—cesarean delivery	
• Selected infections due to medical care	

* Indicates overlap in indicators.

DRG: diagnostic related groups.

Source: Pediatric quality indicators overview. (2006). In *AHRQ quality indicators.* Rockville, MD: Agency for Healthcare Research and Quality.

patient safety indicators and pediatric quality indicators for the following phenomena:

- Accidental puncture or laceration
- Decubitus ulcer
- Foreign body left during procedure
- Iatrogenic pneumothorax
- Postoperative hemorrhage or hematoma, respiratory failure, sepsis, and wound dehiscence
- Transfusion reaction

AHRQ indicators that are unique to pediatrics include the following:

- Pediatric heart surgery mortality
- Diabetes short-term complication rates
- Admission rates for gastroenteritis, perforated appendix, and urinary tract infection (as indications of inaccurate diagnosis or ineffective initial management of signs and symptoms)

Additional opportunities for preventing harm to patients in pediatric acute care settings include the following concerns:

- Fall prevention
- Deep vein thrombosis (DVT) prophylaxis
- Pain assessment and management
- Prevention of unplanned readmissions due to premature discharge from the hospital
- Hand hygiene

Indicators can be used to prioritize issues for patient safety improvement initiatives and to track performance trends in care delivery. Nevertheless, improvement efforts should not be limited to the phenomenon included in these lists. Health care organizations should also target improvement efforts at the causes of patient safety events identified internally via incident reports, root cause analysis (RCAs), and failure mode and effect analysis (FMEAs) (Scanlon et al., 2008; Scanlon et al., 2007).

HEALTH CARE–ASSOCIATED INFECTIONS

In addition to the quality and safety indicators previously listed, prevention of health care–associated infections is an important focus for maximizing pediatric patient safety. Variables that predispose hospitalized pediatric patients to infection include age less than one year, immunosuppression, antibiotic use, chronic disease, need for critical care, and the presence of invasive devices (Cavalcante et al., 2006; National Nosocomial Infections Surveillance System (NNIS), 2004; Stockwell, 2007; Urrea et al., 2003). Surgical site infections, hospital-acquired pneumonia (particularly in pediatric patients who are mechanically ventilated), and urinary tract infections associated with indwelling bladder catheters are also encountered all too frequently in pediatrics. Bloodstream infections, however, are the most common health care–associated infections in pediatric patients (NNIS, 2004; Stockwell, 2007; Urrea et al., 2003). Indeed, the NNIS and the CDC report that more than 90% of bloodstream infection in hospitalized children and adolescents are associated with central venous catheters and, therefore, are adverse events that can be prevented (Leape & Berwick, 2005; NNIS, 2004; Stockwell, 2007; Wachter & Pronovost, 2006).

TABLE 6-10

Strategies for the Prevention of Central Line–Associated Bloodstream Infections

Hand Hygiene
- Perform hand hygiene:
  - Before and after inserting a catheter and handling a catheter insertion site
  - Before and after inserting, replacing, accessing, repairing, or dressing a wound

Maximal Barrier Precautions During Insertion
- Use maximal barrier precautions, including a cap, mask, sterile gown, and sterile gloves as well as a sterile drape

Chlorhexidine Skin Antisepsis
- Prep skin for line insertion with a solution of 2% chlorhexidine / 70% isopropyl alcohol

Optimal Catheter Site Selection
- The subclavian vein is the preferred site; however, in children or in individuals with a high risk for bleeding, the femoral vein may be used

Daily Review of Line Necessity
- Promptly remove unnecessary lines

Source: Institute for Healthcare Improvement, 2007.

Central line–associated bloodstream infections (CLABSI) increase morbidity and mortality and hospital length of stay (NNIS, 2004; Stockwell, 2007). The Joint Commission (2008), the Institute for Health Care Improvement, the National Initiative for Children's Health Care Quality (NICHQ), and CHCA all sponsor programs for the reduction of CLABSI. Table 6-10 describes strategies commonly included in programs to reduce the incidence of CLABSI.

In addition to implementing strategies to prevent CLABSI, comprehensive infection prevention and control programs are paramount to patient safety. Attention to hand hygiene; isolation and cohorting of patients with transmittable diseases, and particularly infections with multidrug-resistant organisms; and adherence to sterile and aseptic technique when required are all necessary to prevent harm to hospitalized pediatric patients. For more information on health care–associated infections, see Chapter 30.

Prevention of harm to acutely ill pediatric patients during the delivery of care that is intended to make them well is a fundamental responsibility of all pediatric-focused HCPs. Through the application of human error and the performance reliability theory, HCPs can minimize or prevent medical errors and adverse events in this vulnerable population. A number of patient safety priorities have been published by governmental and professional organizations dedicated to health care improvement. Together with internal evaluations of a hospital's performance, national priorities can be used by HCPs to identify the elements of care delivery that are most vulnerable to patient safety events and to implement strategies to prevent patient safety events. At the same time, successful implementation of patient safety interventions depends on an existing culture of safety within a health care organization. In keeping with this point, it is equally important that pediatric HCPs can identify and promote elements of a safety culture, such as the attributes of a high-reliability organizations and ideal work environments.

REFERENCES

1. Agency for Healthcare Research and Quality (AHRQ). (2006). Patient safety indicators overview. In *AHRQ quality indicators.* Rockville, MD: Author. Retrieved from http://www.qualityindicators.ahrq.gov/psi_overview.htm

2. American Hospital Association. (1999). *Hospital statistics.* Chicago: Author.

3. Apostolakis, G., & Barach, P. (2004). Reporting and preventing medical mishaps: Safety lessons learned from nuclear power. In B. Youngberg & M. Hatlie (Eds.), *The patient safety handbook.* (pp. 205–224). Sudbury, MA: Jones and Bartlett.

4. Bobay, K., Fiorelli, K., & Anderson, A. (2008). Failure to rescue: A preliminary study of patient-level factors. *Journal of Nursing Care Quality, 23*(3), 211–215.

5. Brennan, T., Leape, L., Laird, N., Hebert, L., Localio, A., Lawthers, A., et al. (1991). Incidence of adverse events and negligence in hospitalized patients: Results of the Harvard Medical Practice Study I. *New England Journal of Medicine, 324*(6), 370–376.

6. Cavalcante, S., Mota, E., Silva, L., Teixeira, L., & Cavalcante, L. (2006). Risk factors for developing nosocomial infections among pediatric patients. *Pediatric Infectious Disease Journal, 25*(5), 438–445.

7. Centers for Disease Control and Prevention (CDC). (2000). Monitoring hospital acquired infections to promote patient safety—United States, 1990–1999. *Morbidity & Mortality Weekly Report, 49,* 149–153.

8. Centers for Disease Control and Prevention (CDC). (2004). Death: Preliminary data for 2002. *National Vital Statistics Report, 52*(13), 4.

9. Ciavarelli, A., Figlock, R., & Sengupta, K. (1999). Organizational factors in aviation accidents. *Naval Postgraduate School Research 9,* 40–43.

10. Clarke, S., & Aiken, L. (2003). Failure to rescue. *American Journal of Nursing, 103*(1), 42– 47.

11. Corrigan, J. M., Donaldson, M. D. (1999). *To err is human: Building a safer health system.* Washington, DC: National Academy Press.

12. Duwe, B., Fuchs, B., & Hansen-Flaschen, J. (2005). Failure mode and effects analysis application to critical medicine. *Critical Care Clinics, 21*(1), 21–30.

13. Eppich, W., Brannen, M., & Hunt, E. (2008). Team training: Implications for emergency and critical care pediatrics. *Current Opinion in Pediatrics, 20*(3), 255–260.

14. Evans, J. (2005). *Total quality: Management, organization and strategy* (4th ed.). Cleveland: Thompson South Western.

15. France, D., Leming-Lee, S., Jackson, T., Feistritzer, N., & Higgins, M. (2008). An observational analysis of surgical team compliance with perioperative safety practices after crew resource management training. *American Journal of Surgery, 195*(4), 546–553.

16. Garbutt, J., Brownstein, D., Klein, E., Waterman, A., Krauss, M., Marcuse, E., et al. (2007). Reporting and disclosing medical errors: Pediatricians' attitudes and behaviors. *Archives of Pediatrics & Adolescent Medicine, 161*(2), 179–185.

17. Health Grades, Inc. (2004). *Patient safety in American hospitals.* Retrieved from http://www.healthgrades.com/media/english/pdf/HG_Patient_Safety_Study_Final.pdf

18. Helmreich, R., Merritt, A., & Wilhelm, J. (1999). The evolution of crew resource management training in commercial aviation. *International Journal of Aviation Psychology, 9*(1), 19–32.

19. Hicks, R., Becker, S., & Cousins, D. (2006). Harmful medication errors in children: A 5-year analysis of data from the USP's MEDMARX program. *Journal of Pediatric Nursing, 21*(4), 290–298.

20. Hinshaw, A. (2008). Navigating the perfect storm: Balancing a culture of safety with workforce challenges. *Nursing Research. 57*(1 suppl), S4–S10.

21. Holden, J. (2006). How can we improve the nursing work? *Maternal Child Nursing, 1*(31), 34–38.

22. Holdsworth, M., Fichtl, R., Behta, M., Raisch, D., Mendez-Rico, E., Adams, A., et al. (2003). Incidence and impact of adverse drug events in pediatric inpatients. *Archives of Pediatrics & Adolescent Medicine, 157*(1), 60–65.

23. Hunt, E., Shilkofski, N., Stavroudis, T., & Nelson, K. (2007) Simulation: Translation to improved team performance. *Anesthesiology Clinics, 25*(2), 301–319.

24. Hunter, J. (2007). Extend the universal protocol, not just the surgical time out. *Journal of the American College of Surgeons, 205*(4), e4–e5.

25. Iedema, R., Flabouris, A., Grant, S., & Jorm, C. (2006). Narrativizing errors of care: Critical incident reporting in clinical practice. *Social Science & Medicine, 62*(1), 134–144.

26. Institute for Healthcare Improvement. (2007). 5 Million Lives campaign: How-to guide: Prevent central line infections. Retrieved from http://www.ihi.org/NR/rdonlyres/0AD706AA-0E76-457B-A4B0-78C31A5172D8/0/CentralLineInfectionsHowtoGuide.doc

27. The Joint Commission. (2008). Sentinel events. Retrieved from http://www.jointcommission.org/SentinelEvents

28. Kaushal, R., Bates, D., Landrigan, C., McKenna, K., Clapp, M., Federico, F., et al. (2001). Medication errors and adverse drug events in pediatric inpatients. *Journal of the American Medical Association, 285*(16), 2114–2120.

29. Kohn, K., Corrigan, J., & Donaldson, M. (1999). *To err is human: Building a safer healthcare system.* Washington, DC: National Academy Press.

30. Kunac, D., & Reith, D. (2005). Identification of priorities for medication safety in neonatal intensive care. *Drug Safety, 28*(3), 251–261.

31. Langley, G., Nolan, K., Nolan, T., Norman, C., & Provost, L. (1996). *The ImprovementGuide.* San Francisco: Jossey-Bass.

32. Leape, L., & Berwick, D. (2005). Five years after *To Err Is Human*: What have we learned? *Journal of the American Medical Association, 19*(293), 2384–2390.

33. Leape, L., Brennan, T., Laird, N., Lawthers, A., Localio, A., Barnes, B., et al. (1991). The nature of adverse events in hospitalized patients: Results of the Harvard Medical Practice Study II. *New England Journal of Medicine, 324*(6), 377–384.

34. Le Duff, F., Daniel, S., Kamendje, B., Le Beux, P., & Duvauferrier, R. (2005). Monitoring incident report in the healthcare process to improve quality in hospitals. *International Journal of Medical Informatics, 74*(2–4), 111–117.

35. Marx, D. (1999). *Maintenance error causation.* Washington, DC: Federal Aviation Authority Office of Aviation Medicine.

36. McDonald, K., Davies, S., Haberland, C., & Geppert, J. (2007). Preliminary assessment of pediatric health care quality and patient safety in the United States using readily available administrative data. *Pediatrics, 122*, e416–e425.

37. Medvedev, G. (1991). *The truth about Chernobyl.* New York: Basic Book.

38. Milstead, J. (2005). The culture of safety. *Policy, Politics & Nursing Practice, 6*(1), 51–54.

39. Nance, J. (2004). Admitting imperfection: Revelations from the cockpit for the world of medicine. In B. Youngberg & M. Hatlie (Eds.), *The patient safety handbook* (pp. 187–203). Sudbury, MA: Jones and Bartlett.

40. National Nosocomial Infections Surveillance System (NNIS). (2004). National Nosocomial Infections Surveillance (NNIS) system report, data summary from January 1992 through June 2004, issued October 2004. *American Journal of Infection Control, 32*(8), 470–485.

41. Nishisaki, A., Keren, R., & Nadkarni V. (2007). Does simulation improve patient safety? Self- efficacy, competence, operational performance, and patient safety. *Anesthesiology Clinics, 25*(2), 225–236.

42. Norton, E. (2007). Implementing the universal protocol hospital-wide. *AORN Journal, 85*(6), 1187–1197.

43. Oriol, M. (2006). Crew resource management: Applications in healthcare organizations. *Journal of Nursing Administration, 36*(9), 402–406.

44. Rasmussen, J., Pejtersen, A., & Goodstein, L. (1994). *Cognitive systems engineering.* New York: Wiley.

45. Reason, J. (1990). *Human error.* New York: Cambridge University Press.

46. Reason, J. (1997). *Managing the risks of organizational accidents.* Hampshire, UK: Ashgate.

47. Reason, J. (2000). Human error: Models and management. *British Medical Journal, 320*, 768–770.

48. Robinson, D., Heigham, M., & Clark, J. (2006). Using failure mode and effects analysis for safe administration of chemotherapy to hospitalized children with cancer. *Joint Commission Journal on Quality & Patient Safety, 32*(3), 161–166.

49. Sandlin, D. (2007). Improving patient safety by implementing a standardized and consistent approach to hand-off communication. *Journal of PeriAnesthesia Nursing, 22*(4), 289–292.

50. Scanlon, M., Harris, J., Levy, F., & Sedman, A. (2008). Evaluation of the Agency for Healthcare Research and Quality pediatric quality indicators. *Pediatrics, 121*, e1723–e1731.

51. Scanlon, M., Mistry, K., & Jeffries, H. (2007). Determining pediatric intensive care unit quality indicators for measuring pediatric intensive care unit safety. *Pediatric Critical Care Medicine, 8*(2), S3–S10.

52. Sharek, P., Parast, L., Leong, K., Coombs, J., Earnest, K., Sullivan, J., et al. (2007). Effect of a rapid response team on hospital-wide mortality and code rates outside the ICU in a children's hospital. *Journal of the American Medical Association, 298*(19), 2267–2274.

53. Sheridan-Leos, N., Schulmeister, L., & Hartranft, S. (2006). Failure mode and effect analysis: A technique to prevent chemotherapy errors. *Clinical Journal of Oncology Nursing, 10*(3), 393–398.

54. Singer, S., Meterko, M., Baker, L., Gaba, D., Falwell, A., & Rosen, A. (2007). Workforce perceptions of hospital safety culture: Development and validation of the Patient Safety Climate in Healthcare Organizations survey. *Health Services Research, 42*(5), 1999–2021.

55. Stockwell, J. (2007). Nosocomial infections in the pediatric intensive care unit: Affecting the impact on safety and outcome. *Pediatric Critical Care Medicine, 8*(2 suppl), S21–S37.

56. Takata, G., Taketomo, C., & Waite, S. (2008). Characteristics of medication errors and adverse drug events in hospitals participating in the California pediatric patient safety initiative. *American Journal of Health-Systems Pharmacists, 65*(1), 2036–2044.

57. Tamuz, M., & Harrison, M. (2006). Improving patient safety in hospitals: Contributions of high- reliability theory and normal accident theory. *Health Services Research, 41*(4 pt 2), 1654–1676.

58. Urrea, M., Pons, M., Serra, M., Latorre, C., & Palomeque, A. (2003). Prospective incidence study of nosocomial infections in a pediatric intensive care unit. *Pediatric Infectious Disease Journal, 22*(6), 490–494.

59. Van Voorhis, K., & Willis, T. (2009). Implementing a pediatric rapid response system to improve quality and patient safety. *Pediatric Clinics of North America, 56*(4), 919–933.

60. Veterans Administration National Center for Patient Safety. (2008). Root cause analysis. Retrieved from http://www.va.gov/NCPS/CogAids/Triage/index.html?8

61. Wachter, R., & Pronovost, P. (2006). The 100,000 Lives campaign: A scientific and policy review. *Joint Commission Journal on Quality & Patient Safety, 32*(11), 621–627.

62. Wald, H., & Shojania, K. (2001). Incident reporting. In Agency for Health Care Research and Quality, *Making health care safer: A critical analysis of patient safety practices* (pp. 41–51). Rockville, MD: Agency for Health Care Research and Quality.

63. Weiner, E., Kanki, B., & Helmreich, R. (1993). *Cockpit resource management.* San Diego: Harcourt, Brace.

64. Wetterneck, T., Skibinski, K., Roberts, T., Kleppin, S., Schroeder, M., Enloe, M., et al. (2006). Using failure mode and effects analysis to plan implementation of smart i.v. pump technology. *American Journal of Health-System Pharmacy, 63*(16), 1528–1538.

65. Woods, D., Johnson, J., Holl, J., Mehra, M., Thomas, E., Ogata, E., & Lannon, C. (2005). Anatomy of a patient safety event: A pediatric safety taxonomy. *Quality & Safety in Health Care, 14*, 422–427.

66. Woods, D., Thomas, E., Holl, J., Altman, S., & Brennan, T. (2005). Adverse events and preventable adverse events in children. *Pediatrics, 115*(1), 155–160.

PART II

Approach to the Pediatric Patient and Family

Megan Pike and Kathy Enright

CHAPTER

7

Child Life: Developmental Considerations

"I have the right to be viewed first as a child, then as patient."

—Canadian Institute of Child Health, 1980

All children need to feel safe, to express themselves, and to make sense of their world. Children in the hospital experience these same needs, often with a greater sense of urgency and intensity. Hospitalization, serious illness, and life-threatening injury all have the potential to create emotional stress and even psychological trauma (Bronner et al., 2008). However, careful attention to the psychosocial needs of individual pediatric patients will help minimize developmental vulnerabilities and maximize each patient's ability to cope. This chapter provides health care professionals (HCPs) with the information they need to engage in developmentally appropriate interactions that will increase a pediatric patient's ability to cope with the stress of hospitalization.

CHILD LIFE SPECIALISTS

Concern for the psychosocial and developmental well-being of pediatric patients and their families is the primary focus of the child life profession. Certified Child Life Specialists (CCLS) are HCPs who promote effective coping through play, preparation, education, and self-expression activities (Child Life Council, 2009). Child life specialists attempt to ensure that pediatric patients' opportunities for growth and development continue despite the stresses of hospitalization. Health care institutions now employ child life specialists in a variety of care areas, including inpatient units, emergency departments (ED), ambulatory care clinics, and inpatient adult units (for work with young family members). While CCLSs provide specialized psychosocial interventions, pediatric patients benefit most when all members of the health care team are also educated in promoting patients' psychosocial wellness.

STRESSORS IN THE HEALTH CARE SETTING

How and why a child is admitted to the hospital will greatly influence the pediatric patient's perception of the experience. Admissions due to trauma or acute illness will be experienced differently than those that are planned. Even transitions within the hospital can cause stress. For example, patients who are transferred to a pediatric intensive care unit (PICU) from another care area will encounter different surroundings, greater restrictions on movement and visitation, different routines, heightened emotion in family and caregivers, and perhaps new or more frequent medical tests and procedures.

Regardless of the reason for admission, pediatric patients consistently face certain psychosocial stressors. Developing an awareness of these factors will help HCPs alter the environment and tailor their approach to meet a patient's specific needs. These common stressors include physical pain; separation from caregivers; frequent, new, or invasive medical tests and procedures; unfamiliar staff (i.e., "strangers"); strange noises; bright lights; disturbing smells; uncomfortable temperatures; changes in routines (e.g., the child who had begun toilet training but must now wear diapers); fast pace and the lack of time to process new information; and limited ability to comprehend what is happening due to young age, developmental delay, or disease process.

The effects that any of these stressors have on a pediatric patient are highly individual. Even so, studies have consistently shown that children who are most severely ill, who stay in the hospital longer, and who have more invasive procedures demonstrate more psychological disturbances for a longer period of time after their hospitalization (Rennick et al., 2002). This relationship is important to note, as it is often these children whose need for information and play are overlooked due to their extreme medical needs.

Hospitals seeking to alleviate some of these stressors are increasingly providing access to multiple healing modalities. Licensed therapists trained in the use of art, music, and animals have the potential to help children and families cope with the stressors of hospitalization and illness. These therapies can help children find new ways to express feelings and find a distraction from pain. Access to these types of specialized services, along with daily opportunities for play and developmentally supportive interactions, can help hospitalized children cope with the myriad of stressors present in their lives.

STRESS AND COPING IN PEDIATRIC PATIENTS

All individuals engage in a daily balancing act of stress and coping. Lazarus and Folkman (1984) proposed that stress is not just an emotion, but rather a reaction to the judgments we all make about the happenings in our environment. According to this model, the hospitalized child will make two separate judgments about the world around him or her; Lazarus and Folkman termed these judgments "appraisals." First, the child will appraise whether the situation is threatening. Then, the child will decide which course of action is appropriate (coping). For example, when a HCP first walks into the patient's room, the child may make the primary appraisal of "I don't know what you're going to do to me." According to Lazarus and Folkman, once a situation has been deemed a threat, individuals make a secondary appraisal, or an assessment of the available options. In this case, the pediatric patient may try to cope with this perceived threat by crying, by hiding, or even by being overly compliant.

Children and adolescents in the hospital will attempt to utilize coping behaviors that have helped them in the past.

Unfortunately, they may not find continued success with these behaviors in the face of new, more intense traumatic situations. Caregivers and HCPs may be caught off guard by extremes in a child's behavior as the individual tries to find new ways of coping with the situation. For example, hiding under the covers or refusing to come out of the bathroom may be how the child reacts to the multitude of "strangers" who come and go. The child life specialist will try to understand the cause of the behavior so as to help the child develop more appropriate coping strategies.

All HCPs can help encourage positive coping behaviors in their pediatric patients. Clearly, the multitude of stressors that exist in the health care setting can be overwhelming. Therefore, removing even one stressor can simplify the situation and make it easier for the child (Brenner, 1997). In the previous example, HCPs may assign primary nurses and attempt to reduce the number of students and ancillary personnel who enter the patient's room. In addition, HCPs can support the pediatric patient's need for information. When pediatric patients perceive the hospital environment as predictable, their initial reactions to potentially stressful situations may change.

There is no one-size-fits-all method for helping children and adolescents learn to cope. Prior experiences with the health care environment will play a significant role in the pediatric patient's ability to cope with these stressors. In addition, patients' developmental level will especially influence the way in which they respond to these perceived threats. It is vital for HCPs to understand the basic cognitive and psychosocial abilities typical for each developmental stage of childhood and adolescence.

HOSPITALIZATION AND PSYCHOSOCIAL DEVELOPMENT

According to Erikson (1963), all people advance through life in specific psychosocial stages. These stages are defined by a primary crisis, or a conflict that the individual must learn to resolve to successfully integrate that stage of life into his or her personality. These stages follow a consistent and predictable sequence and occur whenever an individual is most ready to meet them. Therefore, when major stressors occur, including hospitalization and illness, children may be at risk for missing out on key psychosocial advances. Even so, steps may be taken to minimize these threats to development (Table 7-1).

EFFECTIVE COMMUNICATION WITH PEDIATRIC PATIENTS

Preparing children for health care experiences is a key role of the child life specialist, yet all HCPs can benefit from learning what to say and what not to say to a child preparing for an interview, test, or procedure. The child life specialist's goal in preparing a child for health care experiences is to *help make an otherwise unknown situation seem familiar and predictable* (Goldberger et al., 2009). Communication with children should be honest, but gentle. Health care professionals must

TABLE 7-1

Erikson's Stages of Development and HCP Approaches	
Infancy	
Trust versus mistrust "Is the world a good place?"	*Developmental Considerations* • Encourage caregiver involvement as much as possible and limit unnecessary separations • Maintain routines • Provide soothing stimulation in the environment (mobiles, quiet music, soft lights) • Maintain day/night lighting • Provide swaddling and contain limbs close to the body during periods of stress • Consider use of sucrose-plus-pacifier to help soothe during painful procedures *Play* • Face-to-face interactions with trusted caregivers (singing, talking, holding, reading) • Items that respond to the infant's actions (cause and effect) • Toys with a variety of textures, colors, and shapes • Items that can be mouthed/sucked on • Beware toys with small parts and choking hazards • Limit television exposure and attempt to eliminate TV watching for children younger than two years of age (American Academy of Pediatrics, Committee on Public Education, 2001)
Toddlerhood	
Autonomy versus shame and doubt "I will do it myself."	*Developmental Considerations* • Encourage caregiver presence as much as possible and limit unnecessary separations • Maintain routines • Provide normalization through play and interaction with the environment • Create a "safe zone" by utilizing treatment rooms and avoiding procedures in the crib or bed

(Continued)

TABLE 7-1

Erikson's Stages of Development and HCP Approaches (Continued)

	Play
	• Continued exploration of cause-and-effect relationships
	• Gross motor opportunities to stretch, walk, and crawl
	• Fine motor skill-building that includes shape sorting, block stacking, and similar activities
	• Beginning of art exploration through scribbling and painting
	• Beware toys with small parts and choking hazards
Preschool	
Initiative versus guilt "I need to try new things."	*Developmental Considerations*
	• Maintain home routines as much as possible
	• Provide appropriate choices
	• Encourage caregiver presence as much as possible and limit unnecessary separations
	• Give ample opportunities for control
	• Allow for expressive play opportunities
	• Praise a job well-done to encourage independence and positive self-concept
	• Ensure age-appropriate understanding; avoid causing misconceptions with confusing language
	• Magical thinking can contribute to misconceptions and guilt about causes of illness and injury
	Play
	• Dolls, animals, cars, and play medical equipment to allow for role-playing and expression
	• Creative art such as drawing, painting, and cutting and pasting
	• Fine motor activities such as simple puzzles and large construction blocks
	• Beware toys with small parts and choking hazards
School Age	
Industry versus inferiority "What am I good at?"	*Developmental Considerations*
	• Provide age-appropriate explanations
	• Maintain connections with friends and school
	• Provide opportunities to feel successful and competent
	• Give choices and involve in care as much as possible to increase sense of control and self-efficacy
	Play
	• Creative expression through art
	• Will enjoy toys and games that can be mastered or in which there can be order and rules
	• Allow opportunities for socialization as appropriate
Adolescence	
Identity versus role confusion "Who am I?"	*Developmental Considerations*
	• Maintain privacy
	• Encourage peer interaction/socialization
	• Include in decision making
	• Provide opportunities for self-expression
	• Avoid talking down to adolescent patients, but also avoid treating adolescents as adults
	• Maintain professional boundaries in relationships and conversations, as adolescent patients may seek to deal with their isolation by trying to make personal connections with trusted HCPs
	Play
	• Expression through art or journaling
	• Socializing with peers
	• Maintaining friendships through the Internet or by phone
	• Participating in child life–sponsored "teen nights" with other patients

Source: Adapted from CHILDHOOD AND SOCIETY by Erik H. Erikson. Copyright 1950, © 1963 by W. W. Norton and Company, Inc., renewed © 1978, 1991 by Erik H. Erikson. Used by permission of W. W. Norton & Company, Inc.

accurately communicate a sequence of events, while leaving out things that the child will not directly experience. In doing so, they should avoid the use of confusing words and explain any medical terms (Table 7-2).

These points are important to keep in mind even when you are talking in front of the pediatric patient and not directly to him or her. In one example, a 7-year-old patient in the pediatric emergency department, who appeared to be intently watching cartoons, overheard a HCP discussing the anesthesia consent/permission form with her caregivers. When the patient became extremely fearful about her procedure, the child life specialist was called in. The child

TABLE 7-2

Communicating with Pediatric Patients

Use minimally threatening language. Use softened and more descriptive words.	The word HURT is emotionally loaded and not very descriptive. Use "*pinch*," "*sting*," or "*pressure*." Instead of CUT or HOLE, use "*make a small opening*." Instead of BURN, use "*stinging*" or "*very warm*." Instead of TAKE OUT, use "*remove*." Instead of SHOT, use "*poke*" or "*needle*.
Avoid confusing words. Avoid words with double meanings.	Consider these common terms from a child's perspective: STOOL, FLUSH, PICU ("pick-you"), DRAW Blood, CAT SCAN, DYE, DRESSING Change, Take a NAP. ("Nap" implies a sleep wherein children control whether they fall asleep and then wake up if they choose. When talking of anesthesia, more explanation is required.)
Avoid too much detail.	Limit explanations to aspects that children will see, hear, taste, smell, and feel. Avoid discussion of things that they will not experience.
Always explain potentially confusing terms.	When using medical terms, explain them using concrete examples that the child can understand. For example, the term "IV" may be meaningless to a child until someone explains to him or her that "The small tube in your hand that helps you get medicine is called an 'IV.'"
Reflect the child's natural language.	Ask how things felt and looked to children to help clarify their experiences. Use the child's own words and phrases as appropriate.
Use pronouns appropriately.	For example, use "I will help you get ready to take a bath now" instead of "We're going to take a bath now."
Give choices only when a choice exists.	Consider the difference between "Do you want to take your medicine?" and "Would you like to take your medicine now or in 10 minutes?" Be aware of adding "Okay?" at the end of a statement, as it implies a choice. "We are going to take your X-ray now . . . Okay?"
Allow the child to express emotion and maintain integrity.	Avoid the following phrases: • "Don't cry." • "Why are you crying?" • "You didn't cry!" Crying is a natural response to stress and should be an accepted expression of emotion. If the child feels that something hurts, validate that experience, rather than belittling it ("It's just tape that I'm taking off!"). • "Be brave." • "You were so brave!" A typical response to this statement is "I don't feel brave!" Try instead: "That seemed really hard, can you tell me what it was like?" • "Be a big boy/girl." Being unable to hold still for an IV start should not make the child feel she has lost status as a "big girl."

Source: Gaynard et al., 1990.

life specialist learned from the girl that she had heard she would be "put to sleep," a phrase she associated with the death of a family pet.

While language is, indeed, important in preparing children for health care experiences, studies have shown that modeling and rehearsal are more helpful preparation techniques than didactic, verbal explanations (Hatava et al., 2000). For this reason, child life specialists will include a variety of age-appropriate preparatory materials (e.g., books, dolls, model medical equipment) that will help pediatric patients prepare for the entire sensory experience. Preparation for any medical encounter should focus on what the child will directly experience and what will be expected of the child. What will the child see, hear, taste, smell, feel, and do? Finally, the child life specialist will work with the pediatric patient to help him or her develop a plan to cope with the stressful parts of the experience. This plan may include relaxation exercises, choosing a support person to accompany him or her, and utilizing alternative focus techniques.

SUPPORTING CHILDREN DURING HEALTH CARE EXPERIENCES

As described previously, the child life specialist will not only prepare the patient for the experience, but will also help him or her develop an appropriate coping strategy.

During the test or procedure, the HCP can continue to support the patient's plan for coping and contribute to a child-friendly environment. Deciding on a *single* person to be the patient's coach during a stressful event is a helpful technique to reduce anxiety and increase compliance. The "one voice" approach minimizes confusion and helps the patient stay focused on the planned coping strategy (Goldberger et al., 2009). In addition, the use of comfort or upright positioning can greatly reduce anxiety in pediatric patients during painful procedures (Sparks et al., 2007).

Family-centered care promotes caregiver presence during examinations and procedures. Caregivers are trusted allies of the child and should remain at the bedside for support. Child life specialists may work with caregivers to help them find their role during the procedure (e.g., providing comfort, being a coping-strategy "coach"). *Caregivers should not be used to help restrain an uncooperative patient.* If the caregiver holds the patient during the test or procedure, positioning for comfort is the best technique. It allows the caregiver to gently restrain the child if needed, while maintaining a sense of comfort. In developmentally appropriate patients, providing them with coping strategies prepares them for future examinations or procedures (Spagrud et al., 2008). Regardless of the patient's level of compliance during the test or procedure, all patients should be reassured and praised for things they did well.

SIBLINGS AND FAMILIES

For most people, the hospital is filled with firsts. For families facing an inpatient hospitalization for a new diagnosis, these firsts are many and scary. Child life specialists attempt to prepare children and families for new experiences. Armed with knowledge and a sense of empowerment, patients, siblings, and caregivers alike can learn to navigate unfamiliar situations. Caregivers need to understand what the typical psychosocial responses to hospitalization are and what they may expect from their young patient as well as from their well children at home. Child life specialists may explain new diagnoses and complicated treatments to siblings and patients in ways the children can understand. Siblings visiting the hospital for the first time may meet with a child life specialist to prepare them to see unfamiliar medical equipment or to visit a patient who looks much different than he or she did at home. All HCPs may support siblings by encouraging visitation and family togetherness at the bedside, learning the names of siblings who are present and speaking to them directly, and reporting any concerns about the psychosocial well-being of siblings to the child life specialist.

PLAY IN THE HOSPITAL SETTING

To comprehend and cope with their health care experiences, pediatric patients must be given the opportunity to play. Play allows children to assimilate and solidify new information with existing knowledge (Piaget, 1962). It enables children to prepare for adult life and to understand the world around them (Montessori, 1965). Play is necessary in the hospital setting not only to process and understand information, but also to comfort, to engage, to cope, and to express feelings. "Play is often the only place of comfort that children are able to bring with them into health care settings, and keep with them on a continual basis" (Jessee & Gaynard, 2009, p. 150). In play, the pediatric patient is allowed to make choices and take control.

Child life specialists use therapeutic play in the health care setting on the premise that all children have within themselves the ability to create great psychological resilience (Axline, 1969). Play is most productive and therapeutic for pediatric patients when a knowledgeable adult is present to help facilitate it. In examining the play behaviors of pediatric patients in an intensive care unit, researchers found that the presence of a child life specialist greatly increased the patients' positive affect and interaction with play materials, as opposed to just being given toys without a child life specialist in attendance (Cataldo et al., 1979).

Play in the health care setting may happen in the patient's room, in waiting areas, or in hospital playrooms. Having established the value of play opportunities, HCPs should respect any child at play as much as possible. Scheduling medical examinations and procedures so that the child can have frequent, uninterrupted playtimes helps create a daily routine and allows the child to become completely immersed in the activity. Hospital playrooms should be safe places that are free of medical procedures, examinations, and conversations. A child at play in the child life playroom is working on the serious tasks of assimilating traumatic experiences, interacting with other children, and regaining a sense of normalcy. Unnecessary interruptions should be limited.

The play of hospitalized children may be more emotionally intense than the play that HCPs are accustomed to witnessing. Three key principles should guide play interactions between HCPs and pediatric patients:

- *Play belongs to the child.* Anything within reason should be allowed. All feelings and expressions should be received without judgment. Adults will often say, "Do you really mean that?" or "Why are you acting so . . . [angry, loud, quiet, and so on]?" Instead of taking this approach, HCPs can try asking children to tell them more about the actions or simply observing and allowing the play to continue as long as it is safe.
- *Play is meant to be enjoyable.* Adults will sometimes try to guide children toward play that the adult feels is

beneficial, educational, or fun. The child should take the lead and choose what is enjoyable.

- *Any child can play.* HCPs should support any patient who has a desire to engage in play. Pediatric patients in the ICU who are alert but unable to move or speak can still communicate with either their caregiver or child life specialist, who can be directed to string beads, build with blocks, or to play for the patient in the way he or she chooses.

DEATH AND GRIEF IN THE HEALTH CARE SETTING

Hospitals are intended to be places of healing—somewhere people go to get better. Therefore, when a death occurs on a pediatric unit, staff and families may feel at a loss to help young children cope with the grief. Similarly, resources to help a pediatric patient who is facing end-of-life issues can be scarce, and families may shy away from even discussing the subject. Health care professionals can work with child life specialists to ensure that the concepts of death and dying are presented to patients and siblings in developmentally appropriate ways.

THE PEDIATRIC PATIENT AT THE END-OF-LIFE

Death in a pediatric setting can happen quickly; alternatively, it may be a long-anticipated event. When it becomes clear that a pediatric patient is going to die, the most powerful tool available to HCPs and families is communication. As with all other aspects of hospitalization, children crave honesty. When adults try to shield children from information, children are left with an incomplete understanding and may come to believe that adults are not to be trusted to tell the truth. Pediatric patients at the end of their lives frequently have questions and fears regarding being alone, suffering pain, leaving a legacy, and saying goodbye. If no open communication exists, then neither does an avenue for exploring or ameliorating these fears.

Even within the most trusting and open families, some pediatric patients may choose not to discuss their fears of death and dying with caregivers. In an attempt to shelter their loved ones, or because it is less emotionally taxing, pediatric patients may turn to trusted HCPs. Adolescents, especially, may seek out trusted HCPs in an attempt to express their feelings. Health care professionals can support pediatric patients in these interactions by listening and asking questions. Sharing personal beliefs or making judgments should be avoided. Children and adolescents may ask questions about another's beliefs on death, but rarely need to hear a particular person's response. Often at the heart of these questions is the desire to express feelings. This interaction should be taken as an opportunity to help the child

or adolescent figure out what he or she believes. The child life specialist and health care team should work together to identify psychosocial needs and provide appropriate therapeutic interventions. No single clinician can effectively address all of the needs of the dying adolescent. Through an interprofessional team approach, the adolescent patient's need to understand, to find meaning, to express feelings, to make decisions, and to exert control can be met (Freyer et al., 2006).

Not all pediatric patients at the end of their lives will engage in conversations about death and dying issues. Child life specialists will work with these patients to help them express feelings in a variety of ways. Through therapeutic relationship development, art, writing, reading, being with friends, or participating in support groups, children and adolescents can discover developmentally appropriate ways of coping with complex situations.

GRIEVING CHILDREN AND FAMILIES

Understanding the natural grief process is critical for all HCPs working in a pediatric setting. Most professionals are familiar with the widely accepted five stages of grief: denial, anger, bargaining, depression, and acceptance (Kübler-Ross, 1969). However, Kübler-Ross's research in this area applied to adults at the end of their lives; it was not intended for grieving family members or pediatric grief.

More recent research in the field of bereavement proposes a task-oriented model, characterized by six basic tasks of grieving:

- Acknowledging the reality of the death and understanding what happened
- "Feeling the feelings" of the loss
- Keeping the loved one's memory alive
- Adjusting to a life without the presence of the loved one
- Finding meaning or context to the experience
- Moving on with life, but not forgetting (Brown, 2009)

The work of grieving begins as soon as the child learns of the death and continues throughout life. In an inpatient setting, child life specialists and other HCPs are uniquely placed to help grieving children cope with the first three tasks of the natural grief process. As soon as possible after the death, the child life specialist can help caregivers explain the death to the surviving children and prepare them for any future events. Knowing what to expect and being supported by a child life specialist will help children cope with such situations as viewing the body, saying goodbye, or attending a funeral. The child life specialist will attempt to address any misconceptions or confusion that may lead to anxiety or guilt.

To aid with the second task of "feeling the feelings," the child life specialist will create a supportive, trusting environment. Grieving children should be given the opportunity to talk, express feelings, or even play if they wish. The child life specialist will make sure that both children and caregivers understand that a wide variety of feelings are natural and accepted and that their feelings will change over time.

In the hospital, surviving children may choose to take part in memory-making activities about their loved one, thereby beginning work on the third task. Most pediatric hospitals offer mementos to families after their child's death, such as a handprint, lock of hair, memory quilt, or photo album. The child life specialist may help surviving children and trusted caregivers to participate in the creation of these items. Some family members, or even some HCPs, may feel that it is detrimental for a child to see a deceased loved one. Others may strongly believe that it is a vital part of saying goodbye. Understanding that all children are different, the child life specialist will assess and support the individual needs of each child and family. Notably, no child should be either forced to view the body or be kept away if it is against the child's and family's wishes.

The HCP's approach to working with pediatric patients must include an appreciation for the fact that children and adolescents comprehend information and express emotions differently than adults. This is especially true when dealing with the concepts of death and grief. A complete understanding of death consists of five separate components (Speece & Brent, 1996). To realize a complete understanding of death, children must learn that death is universal, that it is irreversible, that a dead person's body is completely nonfunctional, and that there are specific physical causes of death (rather than magical or fantastical ones). The fifth component is understanding noncorporeal continuation, which refers to the belief that some part of a person's being continues beyond his or her physical death (Speece & Brent).

Death must be explained to children at their level, addressing any potential for confusion. For example, very young children may have an incomplete understanding of the nonfunctionality of death and worry that their dead loved one will be cold without a blanket. Others may wonder if their own negative thoughts or bad behaviors caused the death. Older children may worry that other people they care about will also die soon.

The feelings and reactions of children will differ greatly from those expressed by adults. Children are not equipped to experience prolonged sadness, nor should they be expected to outwardly or directly express their grief. There is no doubt that grieving children experience intense emotions, yet these feelings will be intermittent, occurring between periods of normalcy. Playing, laughing, and wanting to return to school or other routines are all natural behaviors of grieving children. Conversely, playing less, not wanting to go back to school, and desiring to stay close to surviving loved ones are also natural reactions to extreme loss and should be respected.

While adjusting to their loss and in response to the emotional turmoil surrounding them, grieving children may display new or intensified behaviors. Some children may regress to earlier stages of development—backsliding in toilet training or refusing to sleep in their own bed, for example. Other children may exhibit new fears, such as a fear of the dark or of being left alone. Still others may cope with their family's sense of loss by taking on characteristics of their deceased loved one—for example, by eating their brother's favorite foods or partaking in their sister's favorite games or activities. Grieving adolescents may begin to feel disconnected from their life before the loss. Friends and activities that they previously enjoyed may not hold the same appeal.

All grieving children deserve to be treated as individuals; certainly, no one-size-fits-all approach exists. Thus an approach that may be helpful for one family may not be appropriate for another. To support a healthy grief process, caregivers and HCPs can use the following suggestions to communicate with children about death.

Use the word "dead." Children understand language in absolute terms. Phrases such as "passed on," "asleep," and "no longer with us" are confusing. Many adults are afraid of saying the words "dead," "death," or "dying," but children do not necessarily fear these words. These words, more than any euphemisms, convey accurate meanings.

Avoid references to religion. While adults may find comfort in spiritual or religious phrases, they have the potential to be confusing to children. Consider the double meanings inherent in "Your brother is in heaven" and "God took your dad last night."

Take your cues from the child. Every child will react differently. Take the time to ask questions and listen. Allow the child to dictate the course of the interaction. The grieving child is the only expert on his or her needs. Assessing these needs in each moment involves listening and paying careful attention. The needs of a grieving child change quickly and drastically within the walls of the hospital.

Allow families to grieve together. Many hospitals have family rooms or grief rooms where family members can remain with the body of a deceased loved one for as long as needed. Whether in this setting or in the patient's room, children should be allowed join in this process with their family members. An alternative area should also exist to support children who do not wish to stay in the room or who wish to leave before other family members are ready. Often, caregivers of deceased children are too distraught to fully address all the needs of the surviving siblings. Health care professionals can encourage families to identify a trusted person to take responsibility for the support of the children while in the hospital. This person can be a comfort to the surviving children when grieving caregivers are unable to fully attend to them.

For families who experience the death of a child in the hospital, the work of bereavement is long and difficult. For their part, child life specialists and HCPs in an inpatient setting are uniquely placed to help surviving children and families on a path toward healthy grieving and remembering.

DEVELOPMENTAL CONSIDERATIONS IN THE ACUTE CARE SETTING

With the right information and careful attention to the developmental needs of each patient, all HCPs can help children reduce stress and maximize coping in the hospital. Suffering a traumatic injury, receiving a life-altering diagnosis, or being admitted to the hospital will be less likely to cause psychological distress if all HCPs work together to create a child-friendly environment. Providers who communicate openly with pediatric patients and choose their words carefully will see a difference in their patients' ability to understand and cope. Families and children who receive compassionate, but honest care during or after a death will feel more empowered. Child life specialists and HCPs should work together to ensure that all pediatric patients are recognized as individuals who have to right to understand what is happening, to play, and to express themselves.

REFERENCES

1. American Academy of Pediatrics, Committee on Public Education. (2001). Policy statement: Children, adolescents and televison. *Pediatrics,107*(2), 423–426.
2. Axline, V. (1969). *Play therapy.* New York: Ballantine.
3. Brenner, A. (1997). *Helping children cope with stress.* Lexington, MA: Jossey-Bass.
4. Bronner, M., Knoester, H., Bos, A., Last, A., & Grootenhuis, M. (2008). Posttraumatic stress disorder (PTSD) in children after paediatric intensive care treatment compared to children who survived a major fire disaster. *Child and Adolescent Psychiatry and Mental Health, 2*(1–9).
5. Brown, C. (2009). Working with grieving children and families. In R. Thompson (Ed.), *The handbook of child life: A guide for pediatric psychosocial care* (pp. 238–256). Springfield, IL: Charles C. Thomas.
6. Canadian Institute of Child Health. (1980). The rights of a child. Canadian Institute of Child Health, Resources and Publications. Retrieved from http://www.cich.ca/Publications_Voice.html
7. Cataldo, M., Bessman, C., Parker, L., Pearson, J., & Rogers, M. (1979). Behavioral assessment for pediatric intensive care units. *Journal of Applied Behavioral Analysis, 12,* 83–97.
8. Child Life Council. (2009). The child life profession. Retrieved from http://www.childlife.org
9. Erikson, E. (1963). *Childhood and society.* New York: W. W. Norton.
10. Freyer, D., Aura, K., Sterken, D., Pastyrnak, S., Hudson, D., & Rishards, T. (2006). Multidisciplinary care of the dying adolescent. *Pediatric Palliative Medicine, 15*(3), 694–715.
11. Gaynard, L., Wolfer, J., Goldberger, J., Thompson, R., Redburn, L., & Laidley, L. (1990). *Psychosocial care of children in hospitals: A clinical practice manual for the ACCH Child Life Research Project.* Bethesda, MD: Association for the Care of Children's Health.
12. Goldberger, J., Luebering Mohl, A., & Thompson, R. (2009). Psychological preparation and coping. In R. H. Thompson (Ed.), *The handbook of child life: A guide for pediatric psychosocial care* (pp. 160–198). Springfield, IL: Charles C. Thomas.
13. Hatava, P., Olsson, G., & Lagerkranser, M. (2000). Preoperative psychological preparation for children undergoing ENT operations: A comparison of two methods. *Paediatric Anaesthesia, 10*(5), 477–486.
14. Jessee, P., & Gaynard, L. (2009). Paradigms of play. In R. H. Thompson (Ed.), *The handbook of child life: A guide for pediatric psychosocial care* (pp. 136–159). Springfield, IL: Charles C. Thomas.
15. Kübler-Ross, E. (1969). *On death and dying.* New York: Macmillan.
16. Lazarus, R., & Folkman, S. (1984). *Stress, appraisal and coping.* New York: Springer.
17. Montessori, M. (1965). *Dr. Montessori's own handbook.* New York: Schocken.
18. Piaget, J. (1962). *Play, dreams and imitation in childhood.* New York: Norton.
19. Rennick, J., Johnston, C., Dougherty, G., Platt, R., & Ritchie, J. (2002). Children's psychological responses after critical illness and exposure to invasive technology. *Journal of Developmental and Behavioral Pediatrics, 23,* 133–144.
20. Spagrud, L., von Baeyer, C., Kaiser, A., Mpofu, C., Fennell, L., Friesen, K., et al. (2008). Pain, distress, and adult–child interaction during venipuncture in pediatric oncology: An examination of three types of venous access. *Journal of Pain and Symptom Management, 36*(2), 173–184.
21. Sparks, L., Setlik, J., & Luhman, J. (2007). Parental holding and positioning to decrease IV distress in young children: A randomized controlled trial. *Journal of Pediatric Nursing, 22*(6), 440–447.
22. Speece, M., & Brent, S. (1996). The development of children's understanding of death. In C. A. Corr (Ed.), *Helping Children Cope with Death and Bereavement.* New York: Springer Publishing Company, Inc.

Terea Giannetta and Lynn Mohr

Patient- and Family-Centered Care

Family-centered care is primary health care that recognizes the family as the constant in the child's life; it includes an assessment of the health of the entire family, the identification of actual or potential factors that might influence family members, and the implementation of interventions to maintain or improve the health of the family members. The term "family-centered care" was first used in relation to maternity nursing in the 1960s (Beach Center on Families and Disability, 1996; Wiedenbach, 1967). More recently, family-centered care has focused on the family–professional relationship and models for patient/caregiver/health care professional collaboration.

The Institute for Family Centered Care, founded in 1992, serves as a central repository for information for patients, families, and health care professionals (HCPs) in the promotion of family-centered care. Initially, the institute worked on behalf of only pediatric patients and their families; soon, however, its scope moved beyond childhood to encompass the patient throughout the life span. In tandem, the term used to describe such care evolved to "patient- and family-centered care" (PFCC).

Patient- and family-centered care is supported and promoted by a growing body of research and by many organizations, such as the Institute for Medicine (IOM), the American Academy of Pediatrics (AAP), American Association of Critical Care Nurses (AACN), National Association of Pediatric Nurse Practitioners (NAPNAP), Child Life Council, Children's Hospice International, Collaborative Family Healthcare Association, Emergency Nurses Association (ENA), Society of Critical Care Medicine (SCCM), and Society of Pediatric Nurses (SPN). The last organization, in conjunction with the American Nurses Association, published *The SPN/ANA Guide to Family Centered Care* (Lewandowski & Tesler, 2003).

One of the benefits of PFCC is that stronger partnerships are created with the family in promoting the child's health and development. Another benefit is the improvement of patient and family outcomes. Evidence cited in the literature supports the contention that family presence during health care procedures decreases anxiety for both children and their caregivers (Blesch & Fisher, 1996; LaRosa-Nash & Murphy, 1997). In a study reported by Fina et al. (1997), when parents were present and helped with their child's pain assessment and management, the child cried less, was less restless, and required less medicine.

Family-to-family support has also been reported to benefit the mental health of mothers of children with chronic illness (Ireys et al., 2001). A multisite evaluation of parent-to-parent support demonstrated that one-to-one support of parents boosted their confidence and problem-solving capacity (Ainbinde et al., 1998; Singer et al., 1999).

In addition, increased hospital staff satisfaction has been shown when PFCC has been instituted. Hemmelgarn and

Dukes (2001) reported that when PFCC is incorporated in the pediatric emergency department, staff members have more positive feelings about their work. This leads to improved job performance and decreased staff turnover, resulting in decreased costs for the sponsoring organization.

CORE PRINCIPLES OF PATIENT- AND FAMILY-CENTERED CARE

The foundation for PFCC is the partnership between families and HCP at all levels in planning the delivery and evaluation of health care. The partnerships are guided by four core principles: dignity and respect, information sharing, participation, and collaboration (Institute of Family Centered Care, 2009).

The first core principle, *dignity and respect*, is evident when the HCP listens to, and honors, patient and family perspectives and choices. This includes knowledge of the patient's and family's values, beliefs, and cultural background.

Many theories and models for cultural assessment stress the importance of understanding how a person is influenced by communication, time orientation, spirituality, and nutrition—for example, the culture care theory (Leininger, 2006), the model for cultural competence (Purnell & Paulanka, 2005), the transcultural assessment model (Giger & Davidhizar, 1991), and the HEALTH traditions model (Spector, 2009). Using the transcultural assessment model with a Mexican American client, for example, requires the development of a trusting relationship built on awareness and understanding of the cultural phenomena of social organization and environmental control. Using the HEALTH traditions model, one would recognize that an individual may use traditional foods and wear clothing that was proven successful within that person's culture.

To meet the cultural needs of the patient and family, a cultural assessment must be performed in a language that is common to both the HCP and the child and family. If a common language is not available, then an interpreter should be employed. Careful observation to identify cultural influences on health beliefs is necessary when asking about the family's understanding and perceptions of the cause of the illness/condition, the impact and severity of illness/condition, the length of the illness/condition, preferred treatments the child and family might have, the child's and family's expectations of the preferred treatments, and any concerns the child and family have about the illness/condition.

Several resources are available to assist the HCP in the provision of culturally competent care. The U.S. Department of Health and Human Services' (HHS) Cultural Competence and Health Literacy website offers numerous resources for

HCPs, including assessment tools, specific language and culture information, specific disease information, health professional education, research, information regarding special populations, and web-based educational offerings. The Office of Minority Health (www.hhs.gov) offers online educational programs for both the physician and the nurse to improve skills that facilitate effective nurse–physician interactions and to enhance the quality of care for diverse populations. The National Center for Cultural Competence (NCCC) (2004) offers online resources that are available to both individual practitioners and health care organizations, which can be used to promote and improve cultural and linguistic competence. The National Prevention Information Network (NPIN) is the U.S. reference and referral service for information and resources related to human immuno-deficiency virus/acquired immune deficiency syndrome (HIV/AIDS), viral hepatitis, sexually transmitted infections (STIs), and tuberculosis (TB) (U.S. Department of Health and Human Services, Office of Minority Health, 2007). Cultural competence is listed under the subheading of "communities at risk," and the NPIN offers the HCP specific information as to how cultural competence applies to these medical conditions. Several books are also available to guide the HCP in the provision of culturally competent care, such as *The Health Care Professional's Guide to Clinical Cultural Competence* (Srivastava, 2006) and Mosby's *Pocket Guide to Cultural Assessment* (D'Avanzo, 2007).

The second core principle in PFCC is *information sharing*. Information should be communicated in a timely manner, and should be shared completely and without bias with patients and families. On occasion, differences in style of communication between patients, families, and HCPs may lead to discomfort and miscommunication. Miscommunication may include both verbal and nonverbal behaviors such as eye contact, touch, and personal space. Evidence clearly links HCP–patient communication to levels of patient satisfaction, adherence to therapeutic plans, and health outcomes; thus this principle is a key consideration in acute care practices (Betancourt & Green, 2009; MacKean et al., 2005).

When patients and families have established open communication and developed trusting relationships, litigation is also less likely to occur. Risk management literature contains ample evidence that patients and families are less likely to sue even when mistakes are made provided open communication and trusting relationships have been the norm (Beckman et al.,1994; Levinson, 1997).

The third core principle is that patients and families are encouraged to *participate* in health care decision making and should be supported in the decisions that are made at any level of participation the family chooses. Some families do not wish to be involved simply because they may feel too overwhelmed or inadequate to make decisions. For these families, greater reliance is placed upon the HCP

for decision making. When partnerships between families and HCPs are strong, better clinical decisions can be made because communication is open and honest (AAP, 2003).

The fourth core principle is *collaboration* between patients, families, HCPs, and the health care system. This collaboration includes all aspects of care planning, from policy to program development to facility arrangements.

DEFINITION OF FAMILY

According to Shelton and Sepanek (1994), the first step in the provision of PFCC is to understand what constitutes "family" and who the child considers as family members. The definition of family varies according to the source and the reason for the definition. The field of biology defines the family based on the biological function of the continuation of the species, while the field of psychology emphasizes the interpersonal aspects of family responsibility placed on the individual's personality development within the family. Economists view the family as a productive unit responsible for the provision of material needs, whereas sociologists regard the family as a social unit which reacts to a larger society.

Family can also mean those persons in a direct household or may encompass all members linked by relationships, both direct and indirect, within the family. The U.S. Census Bureau (2006) defines a family unit by household, which includes all the people who occupy a housing unit as their usual place of residence and a person, or one of the people, in whose name the unit is owned, being purchased, or. Two types of householders are distinguished by the Census Bureau: a family householder and a nonfamily householder. A family householder is a householder living with one or more people who are related to him or her by birth, marriage, or adoption. The householder and all people in the household related to him or her are family members. In contrast, a nonfamily householder is a householder living alone or with nonrelatives only. The U.S. Census Bureau (2006) identifies caregivers with a foster child and domestic partners as two examples of nonfamilies.

According to Bozett (1987) and Patterson (1995), an even broader definition of family exists in which the family is seen as including anyone whom the patient says it does. Under this definition, family members may include spouses, domestic partners, same-sex parent, step-parents, others serving as parents, and any other persons operating in the caregiver role.

The traditional nuclear family, a blended family, an extended family, a binuclear family, and a gay or lesbian family are several of the family types that exist in contemporary society. Crawford (1999) identifies society's definition of family as one that includes single parents, biracial couples, blended families, unrelated individuals living cooperatively, and homosexual couples.

While most experts in the field have concluded that there is no single correct definition of what constitutes family (Fine, 1993), approaches taken to define the family have ranged in meaning from specific to broad, from theoretical to practical, and from culturally specific to culturally diverse. Even though family definitions may vary, HCPs must still identify who the family members are and what their roles in the household are to promote optimal patient and family-centered care.

ASSESSING FAMILIES

Once the family members have been identified, a family assessment guides the HCP in determining which interventions may be helpful for the family. The *Friedman family assessment model* and the *Calgary family assessment model* are available to facilitate this process.

The Friedman family assessment model incorporates elements of general system theory, developmental theory, structural–functional theory, and cross-cultural theory in an effort to provide a macroscopic view of families. This model views the family as an open system, such that attention is directed to the family structure, functions, and interplay with social systems (Friedman et al., 2003).

The Calgary family assessment model consists of three categories of information that are collected to help assess the family's strengths and problems (Wright & Leahey, 2005):

- *Structural* family data include information regarding family composition, extended family, and social aspects such as ethnicity and spirituality.
- *Developmental* family data include information about the stages of the family's life cycle.
- *Functional* family data include routines of daily living as well as roles and interactions involved in usual family activities.

Health care professionals can focus on those specific data that match family challenges, ranging from acute illness to hospitalization.

Both of these models require the use of genograms or ecomaps to aid in family assessment and promotion of collaborative family–HCP relationships. A genogram is a graphic way to organize the family information gathered during an assessment and to look for patterns within the family that may need a targeted intervention (McGoldrick et al., 2008). The family ecomap provides a visual picture of the family's social network and an understanding of the family functioning by portraying the family connections to larger systems. These systems may involve social networks, community services, churches, agencies, and workplaces, for example.

EXAMPLES OF PATIENT- AND FAMILY-CENTERED CARE

The hospitalization of a child disrupts a family's usual routines, and the parental roles change when the child's care is provided by others (Sarajarvi et al., 2006). Initially, it is common for HCPs to perform and provide all of the daily care. Nevertheless, care is optimal when HCPs work with the family to determine which care is best provided by the HCP and which by the family. Working together, they then can plan to either continue care or resume usual home routines upon discharge.

Delivery of care through short-stay, surgical, and ambulatory units providing minor procedures, diagnostic testing, and radiologic studies is the least disruptive to family life. Care in these settings requires a concerted effort to compress all the information and teaching needed into a very short time frame, however; thus a variety of teaching modalities—such as written materials, videos, pamphlets, and repeat demonstrations—may be used. Working with families to determine their preferred learning styles and knowledge deficits is central to educating patients and families appropriately in such brief encounters.

Emergency care places an extraordinarily high level of stress on families, as the need for unexpected, rapid decision making and the fast pace of treating an emergent condition may be very unfamiliar and uncomfortable for caregivers. When care is provided out of sight, anxiety and stress increase even further. Additional stress may occur when families have other children requiring care outside the emergency department, which divides the caregivers' attention and loyalties as they struggle to be in multiple places at one time. Patient- and family-centered care provides opportunities for patients and families to be present during procedures and resuscitation.

Intensive care units, both pediatric and neonatal, are highly specialized units for patients with prematurity, congenital anomalies, and life-threatening injury and illness. Some hospitals add to this burden by limiting visitation time and the number of visitors to patients in these units. These limitations may cause frustration and disruption of communication with the HCPs. Neonatal units have the greatest burden in this regard, which may be exacerbated by fears that the initial separation of mother and child will impair attachment (Griffin, 2006). Patient- and family-centered care provides opportunities for open visitation, caregivers working as coaches, or support persons for other caregivers. Not all hospitals are equipped to care for critically ill pediatric patients, however, and the need to transfer the patient to another facility may add to the already high level of family stress.

Isolation units require special instructions for the family. The HCP must ensure that the family understands the need for the special precautions and the proper use of protective equipment and procedures. Visitation may be limited when the patient is confined to such a unit, so encouraging contact with all family members via available forms—such as telephone or computer—is important.

Rehabilitation units provide an opportunity for pediatric patients to reach their full potential following significant illness or injury. These stays can be lengthy and may require caregivers to cohabit so that they can learn special techniques for care of their child. This demand may put extra stress on families as they work to adapt to the changes in lifestyle, finances, and family dynamics that occur with such responsibilities.

Caring for siblings also represents a significant stressor for the family when a child is acutely ill. The developmental age of the sibling may help determine the concerns that need to be addressed. Younger children may not tolerate the separation from the caregiver or may fear they contributed to the illness in some way. Helping to orient siblings to the sights, sounds, smells, and rules of the hospital is important when they come to see the patient. Older siblings may feel separated and in the way. Family-centered care encourages siblings to visit often, although some seasonal variations regarding sibling visitation (e.g., respiratory infections) might require using alternative methods to help the siblings know how the hospitalized child is doing, such as phone calls, video messages, and exchanges of cards or letters. Child life therapists can be very helpful in working with siblings before they visit critically ill or injured family members as well as in finding strategies for communication that work for the family.

EMPOWERING THE FAMILY IN CARE GOALS

The health care environment has a culture of its own, and the art of negotiating in that culture is an important skill for HCPs to possess. Negotiation is not about trying to convince the patient and family to do what we want them to do; rather, it focuses on being open to learning the patient's and family's perspective, explaining the health care perspective, acknowledging the differences and similarities between the two to create a common ground, and then agreeing to a mutually acceptable plan (Block, 2009). Patient- and family-centered care is acknowledging that the patient and family have the ultimate decision-making power in regard to their health care and that the HCP is there to provide expert support and guidance to them as they make this journey.

REFERENCES

1. Ainbinde, J., Blanchard, L., Singer, G., Sullivan, M., Powers, L., Marquis, J., et al. (1998). A qualitative study of parent to parent support for parents of children with special needs. *Journal Pediatric Psychology, 23,* 99–109.

2. Beach Center on Families and Disability. (1996). *What research says: Family centered service delivery.* Lawrence, KS: University of Kansas.

3. Beckman, H., Markakis, K., Suchman, A., & Frankel, R. (1994). The doctor–patient relationship and malpractice. *Archives of Internal Medicine, 154,*1365–1370.

4. Betancourt, J., & Green, A. (Eds.). (2009). Cross-cultural care and communication. Retrieved from http://www.utdol.com

5. Blesch, P., & Fisher, M. (1996). The impact of parental presence on parental anxiety and satisfaction. *AORN Journal, 63,* 761–768.

6. Block, S. (2009). Grief and bereavement. Retrieved from http://www.utdol.com

7. Bozett, F. (1987). Family nursing and life-threatening illness. In M. Leahey & L. Wright (Eds.), *Families and life threatening illness.* Springhouse, PA: Springhouse.

8. Crawford, J. (1999). Co-parent adoptions by same-sex couples: From loophole to law. *Families in Society: The Journal of Contemporary Human Services, 80,* 271–278.

9. D'Avanzo, C. (2007). *Mosby's pocket guide to cultural assessment.* Philadelphia, PA: Elsevier.

10. Fina, D., Lopas, L., Stagnone, J., & Santucci, P. (1997). Parent participation in the postanesthesia care unit: Fourteen years of progress at one hospital. *Journal of Perianesthia Nursing, 12,* 152–162.

11. Fine, M. (1993). Current approaches to understanding family diversity: An overview of the special issue. *Family Relations, 42,* 235–237.

12. Friedman, M., Bowden, V., & Jones, E. (2003). *Family nursing: Research, theory and practice* (5th ed.). Upper Saddle River, NJ: Prentice Hall.

13. Giger, J., & Davidhizar, R. (1991). The Giger & Davidhizar transcultural model: A roadmap for addressing cultural factors in health care. Retrieved from http://www.aannet.org/files/public/Giger_template.pdf

14. Griffin, T. (2006). Family-centered care in the NICU. *Journal of Perinatal and Neonatal Nursing, 20,* 98–102.

15. Hemmelgarn, A., & Dukes, D. (2001). Emergency room culture and the emotional support component of family-centered care. *Child Health Care, 30,* 93–110.

16. Institute of Family Centered Care. (2009). Changing the concepts of families as visitors: Family presence and participation bibliography. Retrieved from www.familycenteredcare.org

17. Ireys, H., Chernoff, R., DeVet, K., & Kim, Y. (2001). Maternal outcomes of a randomized controlled trial of a community-based support program for families of children with chronic illnesses. *Archives of Pediatric & Adolescent Medicine, 155,* 771–777.

18. LaRosa-Nash, P., & Murphy, J. (1997). An approach to pediatric perioperative care: Parent- present induction. *Nursing Clinics of North America, 32,* 183–199.

19. Leininger, M. (2006). Culture care diversity and universality theory and evolution of the ethno-nursing method. In M. Leininger & M. McFarland (Eds.), *Culture care diversity and universality: A worldwide nursing theory.* (2nd ed., pp. 1–41). Sudbury, MA: Jones and Bartlett.

20. Levinson, W. (1997). Doctor–patient communication and medical malpractice: Implications for pediatricians. *Pediatric Annals, 26,* 186–193.

21. Lewandowski, L., & Tesler, M. (2003). Family-centered care: Putting it into action. In *The SPN/ANA guide to family-centered care.* Washington, DC: American Nurses Association.

22. MacKean, G., Thurston, W., & Scott, C. (2005). Bridging the divide between families' and health professionals' perspectives on family centered care. *Health Expect, 8,* 74–85.

23. McGoldrick, M., Gerson, R., & Petry, S. (2008). *Genograms: Assessment and intervention* (3rd ed.). New York: W. W. Norton.

24. Patterson, J. (1995). Promoting resilience in families experiencing stress. *Pediatric Clinics of North America, 42,* 47–63.

25. Purnell, L., & Paulanka, B. (2005). *Guide to culturally competent health care.* Philadelphia: F. A. Davis.

26. Sarajarvi, A., Haapamaki, M., & Paavilainen, E. (2006). Emotional and information support for families during their child's illness. *International Nursing Review, 53*, 205–210.

27. Shelton, T., & Sepanek, J. (1994). *Family centered care for children needing specialized health and developmental services*. Bethesda, MD: Association for the Care of Children's Health.

28. Singer, G., Marquis, J., Powers, L., Blanchard, L., DiVenere, N., Santelli, B., et al. (1999). A multi-site evaluation of parent to parent programs for parents of children with disabilities. *Journal of Early Intervention, 22*, 217–229.

29. Spector, R. (2009). *Cultural diversity in health and illness* (7th ed.). Upper Saddle River, NJ: Pearson Prentice Hall.

30. Srivastava, R. (2006). *The health care professional's guide to clinical cultural competence*. Philadelphia: Elsevier.

31. U.S. Census Bureau. (2006). Definition: Household and family. Retrieved from http://ask.census.gov

32. U.S. Department of Health and Human Services, Office of Minority Health. (2007). National standards for culturally and linguistically appropriate services in health care. Retrieved from http://www.hhs.gov

33. Wiedenbach, E. (1967). *Family centered maternity nursing*. New York: Putnam.

34. Wright, L., & Leahy, M. (2005). *Nurses and families: A guide to family assessment and intervention* (4th ed.). Philadelphia: F. A. Davis.

Christine A. Zawistowski

Communicating Bad News

- **Steps to Communicating Bad News**
- **References**

Bad news is any information that produces a negative alteration to a person's expectations about his or her present and future. The information conveyed may or may not pertain to a terminal diagnosis to be considered bad news. For example, a new diagnosis of insulin-dependent diabetes, a 10-day-old neonate requiring a lumbar puncture, or reporting a medication error to a family can all be considered "bad news." There are gradations to what constitutes bad news; the determination is ultimately subjective and dependent on the recipient's life experiences, personality, spiritual beliefs, philosophical standpoint, perceived social supports, and emotional hardiness.

The SPIKES protocol is one of the more common frameworks to use when delivering bad news. It is divided into six steps: **S**etting, **P**atient perception, **I**nvitation, **K**nowledge, **E**xploring/empathy, and **S**trategy/summary (Baile et al., 2000). Other models are available (Levetown et al., 2008), but all include variations of the following steps.

STEPS TO COMMUNICATING BAD NEWS

STEP 1

When setting up the interview, a health care professional (HCP) familiar to the patient and family should be the one who delivers the news. Check the accuracy of facts and plan to answer common questions. Determine with the family who should be present. If this is the first meeting and the pediatric patient is of the age of assent, determine whether the patient is to attend the meeting. At least one supportive individual (e.g., family member, social worker, child life specialist, psychologist, clergy) should be requested to accompany the recipient(s) to provide emotional support. Information about the recipient's background and beliefs should be obtained prior to the discussion.

Whenever possible, the information should be delivered in person, and not via telephone. Those persons who will participate in the conversation should turn off, or set to vibrate, telephones and pagers. Ask colleagues for privacy and to avoid interruptions during the meeting. A private room with facial tissues and adequate seating should be used. The HCP delivering the news should be seated and calm. All persons present should introduce themselves.

STEP 2

Explore the patient's and family's understanding of the disease or injury process, symptoms, findings, care to date, and reason for the meeting. Ask how much information the patient and family want to know. If they do not desire to have the information at that time, offer to talk again in the future or have them designate a family member with whom the information can be shared.

STEP 3

Once the patient and family have established that they want to receive the information, the HCP needs to deliver it in a simple and empathetic manner. A warning statement such as "I have some bad news to give you about your son's/daughter's condition" should be issued. At this point, pause for a moment. The initial information is then delivered using simple words understandable to laypersons. Communicate the information in small parcels. Continue to pause frequently.

STEP 4

Acknowledge the emotions of the patient and family and allow for silence and tears. After delivering the initial information, the HCP should stop talking and listen to what the patient and family have to say without interruption.

STEP 5

Summarize what is said by the patient or family. Notice and validate feelings, and then expand on further information as necessary. Depending on the news, patients and families may have a limited ability to comprehend more detail. Further meetings may be needed.

STEP 6

The interview will then come to a close with the use of a final summary and plan for the next course of action. Asking the family to summarize what they understand aids with misconceptions and allows for correction and the opportunity to repeat key information. In the plan, provide clear direction for what comes next. Discuss therapeutic options. Telephone numbers and referrals should be ready and given to the patient and family at the meeting.

If the first meeting was with caregivers, then often the plan includes a follow-up meeting to inform the pediatric patient. Discuss who should be at the next meeting. If the caregivers are concerned about how to tell the pediatric patient, child life specialists may be employed to assist them in this effort, as they are uniquely prepared to communicate with pediatric patients at their developmental level.

The HCP should close the discussion with a brief summary of the next plan of action. Document the conference in the chart and contact the primary care provider (PCP) or pertinent subspecialist to inform this HCP of the conference and the information shared. Be prepared to repeat what occurred during each meeting at subsequent meetings. Families under stress often need repetition to enhance memory.

REFERENCES

1. Baile, W. F., Buckman, R., Lenzi, R., Glober, G., Beale, E. A., & Kudelka, A. P. (2000). SPIKES: A six-step protocol for delivering bad news: Application to the patient with cancer. *Oncologist, 5*(4), 2–11.
2. Levetown, M., Diekeman, D. S., Antommaria, A. H., Fallat, M. E., Holzman, I. R., Leuthner S. R., et al. (2008). Communicating with pediatric patients and families: From everyday interactions to skill in conveying distressing information. *Pediatrics, 121*(5), e1441–e1460.

Ethical Considerations

Medical ethics is primarily a field of applied ethics—that is, the study of moral values and judgments as they apply to medicine. Four major principles of medical ethics have been defined (Table 10-1).

Many of the ethical issues that arise in medicine involve some component of decision making. Two major decision standards are applied in this forum: substituted judgment and best interests. *Substituted judgment* is a judgment made on behalf of a noncompetent patient based on what that person would have decided had he or she been competent.

The *best interest* standard has its origins in family law and has become the prevailing standard used to judge the adequacy of medical decision making on behalf of pediatric patients. The surrogate decision maker must determine the highest net balance among available options, weighing the positives against the negatives. The best interest standard incorporates the total well-being of the individual rather than just his or her medical well-being. This standard can be difficult to apply, as it can be challenging to define the best interest in a medical setting. Values and the nature of the various interests can be complex; therefore, it is not entirely clear that "best interest" should be the sole consideration when making a medical decision on behalf of a pediatric patient.

ETHICAL APPROACH TO CONSENT

Informed consent is a process that involves a competent individual voluntarily receiving and understanding information and then making a decision. Implied within this concept is the notion that the individual involved has the ability to understand and communicate, reason and deliberate. It is assumed that the individual is also able to analyze conflicting elements and use personal values to come to a decision. The age at which a person possesses these characteristics varies from state to state and may be limited to specific medical conditions.

Pediatric patients are legally presumed by these statutes to be incompetent and are not allowed to provide their own consent for medical treatment. Technically, legal guardians cannot truly give consent for medical treatment on behalf of their pediatric patient, as the person for whom the treatment is planned is the only one who can give informed consent. Rather, *parental permission* is the more correct term when legal guardians give permission for medical treatment on behalf of their child or adolescent. Parental permission

implies shared decision making between legal guardians and health care professionals (HCPs). Legal guardians are granted wide discretion in these decisions as long as the intervention will not harm the pediatric patient, it will not significantly harm others, and potential benefit from the intervention is possible. In situations involving the potential for substantial harm, the focus shifts to what is best for the pediatric patient.

Pediatric patients should not be excluded from the process of obtaining permission for a medical treatment or intervention. The concept of *assent* was developed in the 1980s to address decision making by adolescents with cancer. Pediatric patients should participate in the decision-making process commensurate with their developmental level. Their assent to medical care should be sought whenever reasonable, and caregivers and HCPs should not exclude them without persuasive reasons (American Academy of Pediatrics Committee on Bioethics, 1995). Assent includes four components:

- Helping the pediatric patient achieve developmentally appropriate awareness of the condition
- Telling the pediatric patient what to expect with clinical management
- Assessing understanding and factors influencing response
- Soliciting expression of the pediatric patient's willingness to accept the proposed treatment

ADVANCE DIRECTIVES

An advance directive (AD) allows patients and/or surrogates to designate desired medical interventions under applicable circumstances. The federal Patient Self-Determination Act requires health care institutions to ask anyone older than the age of 18 years whether he or she has completed one, and if not, to inform the patient of his or her right to do so. Advance directives dealing with resuscitation status have, in the past, been termed "do not resuscitate" orders; the negative connotations associated with this terminology have since led to the adoption of the terms "do not attempt resuscitation" (DNR) and "allow natural death" (AND) for such directives. When discussing a resuscitative issue with patients and families, using the terminology "allow natural death" is better received, has a more positive connotation, and states what will be done rather than what will not be done for the patient.

TABLE 10-1

Four Principles of Medical Ethics
Beneficence: provide care that benefits the patient
Nonmaleficence: avoid harming the patient
Autonomy: individuals should decide what constitutes their own best interest
Justice: provide services fairly without bias from factors irrelevant to the medical situation

REFUSAL OF CARE

Refusal of care can occur in all health care settings and at any stage of treatment—from diagnostic studies such as newborn metabolic screening and sepsis work-up, to preventive care such as immunizations, and to life-saving treatments such as blood transfusions and chemotherapy. The refusal can come from the pediatric patient, the caregiver, or both; in some cases, there may be conflict between the two parties. Not all refusals of care are the same, however; there is variability in the degree of harm, likelihood of harm, and role of the pediatric patient.

Many times, refusals of care are a result of communication problems. An approach to discerning the cause behind the refusal is as follows:

- Ensure good communication.
  - Make use of interpreter services when necessary.
  - Enlist other professionals such as social workers and clergy.
  - Make use of caregiver support groups.
  - Offer to include additional family members.
- Consider accommodating the family's preference.
- Share management with alternative or complementary medicine providers when safe to do so.
- Ensure that the pediatric patient's voice is heard and determine the patient's level of decision-making capacity.
- Reassess the seriousness of the consequences of various options for the pediatric patient's current and future well-being.
- Consider obtaining a second opinion.
- Consider whether certain features of the pediatric patient's situation, including family views and practical matters, may mean that a medically less preferable treatment regimen is overall better for the patient.

If, after addressing issues with communication, the situation remains unresolved, then an ethics consult should be obtained. If the ethics consult does not resolve the situation, then seeking legal counsel may be the next required step. Depending on the urgency and seriousness of the patient's illness, the court system may be required to determine the patient's next best therapeutic plan. This option is most often used as a last resort.

INAPPROPRIATE CARE/FUTILE CARE

Just as caregivers sometimes refuse seemingly appropriate care, so they may also request inappropriate or futile care. *Futile* or *inappropriate care* refers to medical interventions that are unlikely to produce any significant benefit to the patient. Therapeutic plans can be quantitatively futile, where the likelihood that the plan will benefit the patient is very poor, or qualitatively poor, where the quality of benefit the treatment will produce is very poor. HCPs have a moral duty to refuse to provide a therapeutic option that may harm a patient and a social duty to conserve resources.

The motivation behind requests for inappropriate or futile care may be guilt, denial, mistrust, or any combination of the three. Most often, they result from miscommunication and inadequate understanding of the issues involved in care of the patient. Requests for futile or inappropriate treatment are best handled in a similar manner to refusals of care.

ISSUES IN DEATH AND DYING

The current prevailing view is that no moral distinction exists between withholding or withdrawing life-sustaining therapies. However, because there is always uncertainty in predicting a patient's response to treatment, withdrawing treatment based on a failure to respond may be morally preferable to withholding that same treatment. Withholding treatment out of the concern that withdrawing it in the future would be more difficult, risks undertreating a patient who might respond to that treatment.

Euthanasia, or physician-assisted suicide, is a deliberate intervention undertaken with the intention of ending a life to relieve intractable suffering. Laws in most U.S. states and countries around the world prohibit this practice. The concern regarding this practice is the "slippery slope" effect—that is, the idea that lowering the barrier against killing will make it easier for HCPs to kill others, that boundaries will become less distinct, and that individuals with severe physical or mental disabilities will be at risk for involuntary euthanasia.

The American Academy of Pediatrics does not support physician-assisted suicide. The provision of adequate sedation and analgesia to a patient, even if it hastens his or her death, however, is not considered euthanasia because of the *doctrine of double effect* (DDE). The DDE is a set of ethical criteria for evaluating the permissibility of acting when one's otherwise legitimate act will also cause a negative effect that one would normally be obliged to avoid. The set of criteria states the following:

- An action having foreseen harmful effects practically inseparable from the good effect is justifiable upon satisfaction of the following—the nature of the act is itself good, or at least morally neutral.
- The agent intends the good effect and not the bad effect, either as a means to the good or as an end itself.
- The good effect outweighs the bad effect in circumstances sufficiently grave to justify causing the bad effect and the agent exercises due diligence to minimize the harm.

One of the more psychologically distressing issues in withholding or withdrawing life-sustaining care relates to artificial nutrition and hydration. When administered through a feeding tube or intravenously, it is considered a form of life-sustaining treatment. Under appropriate circumstances, it is ethically defensible to forgo or withdraw this form of therapy (Diekema & Botkin, 2009).

CONFIDENTIALITY

Confidentiality is the HCP's obligation to prevent unauthorized access to information about a patient. It is based on the fiduciary relationship between the HCP and the patient. Exceptions may be made in certain instances because of competing values:

- When necessary to promote public health and safety (e.g., in cases involving pediatric patient neglect and abuse or communicable diseases)
- When public interest demands disclosure (e.g., in cases involving dangerousness to self or others or gunshot wounds)

RESEARCH

Research is a systematic investigation designed to develop or contribute to general knowledge. The risks of research should be minimized and reasonable with respect to the anticipated benefits of the subjects and importance of the knowledge gained. Further restrictions are placed on research involving pediatric patients because children cannot give informed consent. Generally, it is permissible to involve pediatric patients in research that poses "minimal risk"—in other words, risk equivalent to those risks encountered in daily life or during performance of routine physical or psychological exams or tests. It is controversial as to whether pediatric patients should be allowed to participate in nontherapeutic research.

For pediatric patients to participate in research, a few requirements should be met. First, the pediatric patient's legal guardians need to give permission. Second, assent of the patient should be obtained (if age appropriate); while this is not an absolute requirement, depending on the developmental level of the pediatric patient, the opportunity to dissent, especially for nontherapeutic research, should be made available. Third, as with all research, institutional review board (IRB) approval must be granted for the study to be conducted.

REFERENCES

1. American Academy of Pediatrics Committee on Bioethics. (1995). Informed consent, parental permission, and assent in pediatric practice. *Pediatrics, 95*(2), 314–317.
2. Diekema, D., & Botkin, J. (2009). American Academy of Pediatrics Committee on Bioethics. Clinical report: Forgoing medically provided nutrition and hydration in children. *Pediatrics, 124*(2), 813–822.

Care of the Minor and Legal Implications

Pediatric health care is complex and often unpredictable. Health care professional (HCPs) face unique legal and ethical challenges, which compound the complexity of the medical care, especially when conflicts arise between the wishes of the child and the wishes of the child's parents or guardians. For the purposes of this chapter, the pediatric patient, either child or adolescent, will be referred to as *child,* as that is the term most commonly used in state statutes.

WHO IS A MINOR?

A *minor* is a person who is younger than the age of legal competence. *Majority* is the legal age at which a person is no longer a minor. Majority is generally accepted to be the age at which, by law, a person is capable of being legally responsible for all of his or her acts (e.g., contractual obligations) and is entitled to the management of his or her own affairs and enjoyment of civic rights (e.g., the right to vote). The age of majority varies from state to state, and adult rights and responsibilities are gradually attained. For example, state laws may still prohibit certain

acts, such as alcohol consumption, until a person reaches a greater age.

STATE STATUTES

All states and the District of Columbia have positions on the age of majority, with most identifying 18 years as the age. Alabama and Nebraska have set the age of majority at 19 years; in Colorado and Mississippi, this age is 21 years. Other states have provisions that the individual must graduate from high school to attain majority status. In addition, states often have statutes dealing with emancipation, consent for medical procedures, and the ability to sue, enter into contracts, and other matters that vary by state (Table 11-1). Persons who have reached the age of majority may not, however, be considered competent to make their own health care decisions; this is especially true in the health care setting. HCPs are expected to be able to assess the competency and maturity of their patients. This issue can often be challenging in the face of serious or chronic illness or injury when the patient is already experiencing physical or psychological stress.

TABLE 11-1

Age of Majority, Age for Emancipation, and Age to Consent to Medical Treatment, Including Applicable Statute		
State	**Age of Majority (Years)**	**Age of Emancipation**	**Age to Consent to Medical Treatment**
Alabama	19 (§26-1-1)	18 years (§26-13-1)	14 years (§22-8-4)
Alaska	18 (§25.20.010)	16 years (§09.55.590)	If living apart from parents or if parent of child, minor may give own consent (§25.20.025)
Arizona	18 (§1-215)	Not specified	If homeless, marries, or emancipated (§44-132 et seq.)
Arkansas	18 (§9-25-101)	16 (§9-26-104)	Any minor who is married, emancipated, incarcerated, or sufficiently intelligent to understand consequences of consent (§20-9-602)
California	18 (Fam. §6500)	14 years (Fam. §7120), or if married or in military (Fam. §7002)	Minor may consent if 15 years or older, living apart from parents, and managing own finances (§6922)
Colorado	21 (2-4-401(6))	Occurs upon attainment of majority; *Koltay v. Koltay* 667 P.2d 1374 (Colo. 1983)	18 years (§13-22-101(1)[d]), or 15 years if living apart from parents and paying own expenses (§13-22-103[1])
Connecticut	18 (§1-1d)	16 (§46b-150)	18 years or upon emancipation (§46b-150d)
Delaware	18 (1 §701)	Not specified	Not specified
District of Columbia	18 (§46-101)	Not specified	If connected to pregnancy, substance abuse, psychological disturbance, or sexually transmitted disease (22 DCMR §600.7)
Florida	18 (§743.07)	If legal marriage occurs (§743.01); upon petition if 16 or older (§743.015)	If emergency (§743.064)

(Continued)

TABLE 11-1

Age of Majority, Age for Emancipation, and Age to Consent to Medical Treatment, Including Applicable Statute *(Continued)*

State	Age of Majority (Years)	Age of Emancipation	Age to Consent to Medical Treatment
Georgia	18 (§39-1-1)	Not specified	18 years for treatment in general (§31-9-2); if treatment is for venereal disease, minor may consent; female minor has valid consent for treatment in connection with pregnancy
Hawaii	18 (§577-1)	Legal marriage (§577-25)	For counseling services for alcohol or drug abuse (§577-26); if for pregnancy, venereal disease, or family planning services (§577A-2)
Idaho	18 (§32-101)	Marriage (§32-101)	14 years; treatment of infectious, contagious, or communicable diseases (§39-3801)
Illinois	18; common law	Minors between 16 and 18 years may apply if no parental objection (§§750 ILCS 30/1 et seq.)	Consent by minor if married, parent, or victim of sexual assault (410 ILCS 210/1 et seq.)
Indiana	18; common law	Not specified	Minors may consent if emancipated, 14 years or older and living apart from parents, married, or in military service (16-36-1-3)
Iowa	18 (§599.1)	Marriage (§599.1)	Not specified
Kansas	18; 16 if married (§38-101)	At discretion of the court (§38-109)	Unmarried pregnant minor may consent to hospital, medical, and surgical care (§38-123); or any minor older than 16 (§38-123b)
Kentucky	18 (§2.015)	Not specified	Minors of any age may consent to emergency care or treatment for pregnancy, drug/alcohol abuse, or venereal disease. Minors 16 years or older may consent to mental health treatment. Emancipated minors may consent to any treatment (§222.441).
Louisiana	18 (CC §29)	Through notarial act by parent at age 15 years (CC §366); through judicial consent at age 16 years (CC §385); marriage (CC §379)	May consent without parental consent (R.S.40 §1095 et seq.)
Maine	18 (1§72(11))	Not specified	Minors may consent to any treatment if married, emancipated, in the military, or living apart from parents. Otherwise, minors may consent to substance abuse or mental health treatment (22 §1502 et seq.).
Maryland	18 (Art. 1, §24)	Married minor may buy or sell property and to join in deed, mortgage, lease, or notes if spouse is of age (Est. & Tr. Art. 13 §503[a]); age 15 years regarding insurance and cannot repudiate on basis of minority (Est. & Tr. Art. 13 §503[c]); or if in military, can enter into real estate transactions (Est. & Tr. Art. 13 §503 [b])	If married or a parent or seeking help with drug use, alcoholism, venereal disease, sexual assault, pregnancy, or contraception, or if seeking consent would be life threatening (Health- Gen. Art. 20 §102); minor 16 years or older can consent to treatment for emotional disorder (Health- Gen. Art. 20 §104)

(Continued)

TABLE 11-1

Age of Majority, Age for Emancipation, and Age to Consent to Medical Treatment, Including Applicable Statute *(Continued)*			
State	**Age of Majority (Years)**	**Age of Emancipation**	**Age to Consent to Medical Treatment**
Massachusetts	18 (Ch. 231 §85P)	Not specified	If 12 years or older and certified to be drug dependent, may consent to appropriate medical care (Ch. 112 §12E); minor may also consent to emergency care when married, widowed, or divorced; a parent; a member of the armed forces; living separately from parents and managing own financial affairs; has come into contact with dangerous public health disease; or pregnant (Ch. 112 §12F)
Michigan	18 (722.1(a))	Through marriage, military service, or by judicial petition at age 16 (722.4 et seq.)	If pregnant (§333.9132); human immunodeficiency virus or venereal disease treatment (§333.5127); substance abuse treatment (§333.6121)
Minnesota	18 (§645.45[4])	Not specified	Minor may consent if living apart from parents and managing own financial affairs, if married or parent, or for pregnancy, venereal disease, or substance abuse (§144.341 et seq.)
Mississippi	21 (§1-3-27)	By petition; no minimum age specified (§93-19-3)	Not specified
Missouri	18 (common law)	If married, minor may convey or encumber real estate if spouse is of age (§442.040)	Minor may consent if married; treatment is for pregnancy, excluding abortion; venereal disease; or drug or substance abuse
Montana	18 (§41-1-101)	Occurs upon marriage (§40-6-234) or by judicial petition after reaching age 16 years (§41-1-501)	Yes, if emancipated; separated from parents and self-supporting; pregnant; has a communicable disease; addicted to alcohol or drugs; has had a child or graduated from high school; needs emergency care (§41-1-402)
Nebraska	19 (§43-2101)	Marriage (§43-2101); common law (209 Neb. 94[1981])	Not specified
Nevada	18 (§129.010)	16 years by court order (§129.080)	If emancipated (§129.130); or if living apart from parents, married, has a child, or has a health hazard (§129.030); or under the influence of drugs (§129.050); or has a sexually transmitted disease (§129.060)
New Hampshire	18 (§21-B:1)	Not specified	12 years or older may consent to drug treatment (§318-B:12-a)
New Jersey	18 (9:17B-3)	Not specified	If married or pregnant (9:17A-1.9)
New Mexico	18 (§32A-1-4[B])	Through marriage, death, adoption, or majority of minor (32A-21-1 et seq.)	If married or emancipated (§24-10-1)
New York	18 (Dom. Rel. §2)	Not specified	If married, parent, pregnant, or in an emergency (Pub. He. §2504)

(Continued)

TABLE 11-1

Age of Majority, Age for Emancipation, and Age to Consent to Medical Treatment, Including Applicable Statute *(Continued)*			
State	**Age of Majority (Years)**	**Age of Emancipation**	**Age to Consent to Medical Treatment**
North Carolina	18 (48A-2)	Upon marriage or becoming 18 years; may petition court if 16 years or older (§7B-3500 et seq.)	Venereal disease, pregnancy, drug abuse, or emotional disturbance; any emancipated minor may consent to medical, dental, or health treatment for himself or herself or the minor's child (§90-21.5)
North Dakota	18 (§14-10-01)	Marriage (§14-09-20)	Any minor may consent to emergency medical care (§14-10-17.1); minors 14 years or older may consent to treatment for venereal disease or substance abuse (§14-10-17)
Ohio	18 (§§3109.01)	Not specified	Not specified
Oklahoma	18 (15§13)	Through court order; upon marriage (10 §10; 10 §91 et seq.)	Minors may consent if married, a parent, emancipated, or for emergencies, substance abuse, communicable diseases, or pregnancy (63 §2602)
Oregon	18(§109.510)	By marriage or court decree (109.520; 419B.552)	15 years or older may consent to any treatment; 14 years or older may consent to mental health or substance abuse treatment; any age may consent to venereal disease treatment (109.610 et seq.)
Pennsylvania	18 (23§5101)	Not specified	Not specified
Rhode Island	18 (§15-12-1)	Common law applies, *Pardey v. American Ship Windlass Co.* 34 A. 737 (1896)	If married or 16 years, may consent to any treatment (§23-4.6-1)
South Carolina	18 (§15-1-320)	Not specified	Married minor or his or her spouse may consent to diagnostic, therapeutic, or postmortem care (§20-7-270); or may consent if older than 16 (20-7-280)
South Dakota	18 (§26-1-1)	Upon marriage or age of majority; by express agreement if no longer dependent for support or active military duty (25-5-19; 25-5-24)	Minors of any age may consent to treatment for venereal disease (§34-23-16)
Tennessee	18 (§1-3-105[1])	By judicial petition, no minimum age specified (§29-31-101 et seq.)	Minors may receive contraceptives if pregnant, parent, or married (§68 34-107)
Texas	18 (Civ. Prac. & Rem. §129.001)	If resident and 17 or 16 years if living apart from guardian or parents and is self-supporting or by marriage (Fam. §31.001 et seq.)	Minors may consent to any treatment if in military or 16 years old and living apart from parents; any minors may consent to treatment for pregnancy, substance abuse, or infectious diseases (Fam. §32.003)
Utah	18 (§15-2-1)	Marriage (15-2-1)	Any female in connection with pregnancy or childbirth (78-14-5)
Vermont	18 (1§173)	Not specified	Minors 12 years or older may consent to treatment for venereal disease or substance abuse (18§4226).

(Continued)

TABLE 11-1

Age of Majority, Age for Emancipation, and Age to Consent to Medical Treatment, Including Applicable Statute *(Continued)*

State	Age of Majority (Years)	Age of Emancipation	Age to Consent to Medical Treatment
Virginia	18 (§1-13.42)	By judicial petition at age 16 years (§16.1-331 et seq.)	Minors may consent to treatment for venereal disease, pregnancy, substance abuse, or mental illness; married minors may consent to any treatment (§54.1-2969 [E])
Washington	18 (§26.28.010 et seq.)	By judicial petition at age 16 years (§13.64.010 et seq.)	Not specified
West Virginia	18 (§2-2-10[aa])	By marriage, if younger than 16 years; if older than 16 years and unmarried, may apply to court; must show ability to support oneself and make decisions (§49-7-27)	Not specified
Wisconsin	18 (§990.01[3])	By marriage, unless incompetent (880.04[1])	Not specified
Wyoming	18 (§14-1-101)	Through marriage, military service, or at age 17 years if living separate, apart from parents; parents consent to living arrangement; minor deemed capable of handling financial affairs; and income is lawfully derived (14-1-201 et seq.)	Yes if married, military, guardian cannot be located, or living apart and self-supporting or is emancipated (14-1-101)

Abbreviations: Civil Practice and Remedies (Civ. Prac. & Rem.), Colorado (Colo.), civil court (CC), domestic relations (Dom. Rel.), District of Columbia Municipal Regulations (DCMR), Estate and Trust Articles (Es. & Tr Art), et sequentes, Latin for "the following ones" (et seq.), family (Fam), Health-General Article (Health Gen. Art), public health (Pub He), Nebraska (Neb), versus (v), sections (§).

PARENTAL RIGHTS

Traditionally, the law recognized the fundamental right of parents to make decisions about the health care of their minor children (*Meyer v. Nebraska,* 1923; *Parham v. J.R.,* 1979; *Pierce v. Society of Sisters,* 1925; *Prince v. Massachusetts,* 1944; *Troxel v. Granville,* 2000). This concept arises from the *parental liberty doctrine,* which recognizes, as a matter of civil liberty, the parent's right to make decisions regarding a child's education, health care, lifestyle, regimen, religious observance, and discipline. In contrast, minors are not typically afforded the same rights to make decisions about these kinds of matters even if their will differs from their parents'. Parental authority is usually considered to outrank the child's wishes, but that control gradually diminishes as the child's capacity to make reasonable decisions increases.

The right of parents to make decisions regarding the health care of their minor children is not unlimited, however. Limitations are placed on parents' rights when their behavior is deemed to not be in the best interest of the child. Under the common law doctrine of *parens patriae* (Latin for "parent of the nation"), the state may intervene against a child's natural parent or legal guardian and act as the parent of any child or individual who is in need of protection (*Troxel v. Granville,* 2000; *West Virginia v. Chas. Pfizer & Co.,* 1971). This intervention may extend to the appointment of a guardian to act on behalf of the child and, in some cases, includes prosecution of parents for neglecting their child's health or welfare (*State v. Norman,* 1991); however, the state will have the burden of proving that it has not unjustifiably interfered with the parental liberty doctrine.

EMANCIPATED MINOR AND MATURE MINOR

Parents' rights are also limited when minors are deemed to have the capacity to make their own decisions. Two classes of minors—the emancipated minor and the mature minor—may be granted decision-making authority regarding their own health care.

An *emancipated minor* is defined as a minor who has been made free of parental control. Minors are usually automatically emancipated when they become pregnant or have children of their own, regardless of their age. Some states have a legal process whereby a minor, or a guardian for the minor, may petition the court to emancipate the minor and grant him or her some or all of the rights of legal adulthood.

The *mature minor* doctrine allows a minor to demonstrate requisite capacity and maturity to make independent decisions with regard to health care. This doctrine takes into consideration the age of the minor, the nature of the situation, the ability of the minor to understand the medical procedure in question, and, the laws of the state in which the minor resides. Not all states have adopted the mature minor doctrine.

In some cases, minors are given the right to refuse treatment, just as they are sometimes given the right to consent to treatment. The right to refuse treatment may be granted even if the minor's decision to refuse the treatment conflicts with the wishes of the parents or goes against the advice of the HCP. The right to refuse treatment is generally based on a determination of the minor's capacity to make health care decisions, just as in the case of the right to consent to treatment.

IMMATURE MINOR

The presumption under U.S. law is that a minor who is younger than 18 years of age is immature and, therefore, may not make his or her own decisions regarding health care. Under several conditions, however, a minor may be determined to be mature enough to make those decisions. Regardless of the maturity level, it is well accepted that even the most immature minor is owed an opportunity to participate in his or her health care decisions unless the family and HCP determine that giving the child the information needed for assent (described later in this chapter) would be detrimental to the child's psychological or physical condition. The parent or guardian and HCP make the determination what is in the immature minor's best interest.

RECENT RULINGS

ABRAHAM'S LAW

In August 2005, Starchild Abraham Cherrix of Virginia was diagnosed with Hodgkin's disease at the age of 15 years. Abraham, as he preferred to be called, received a first course of chemotherapy. He was set to receive a second course, followed by radiation, when he and his parents elected to discontinue conventional therapy and begin an herbal treatment plan known as the Hoxsey method. There was no evidence base supporting the Hoxsey method as effective, but Abraham and his family believed that it would be less toxic than his first course of chemotherapy. Subsequently,

Abraham's parents were charged with medical neglect and a county social services agency sought a court order to force Abraham to receive the recommended chemotherapy and radiation. After months of court challenges, Abraham's parents were ultimately cleared of all charges and the family was allowed to pursue alternative treatments.

As a result of this case, in March 2007, the Virginia legislature amended its child abuse statute. The new statute, called Abraham's Law, allows parents and children 14 years or older to refuse medical treatment for a life-threatening condition. It also prevents parents from being charged with medical neglect if the decision to refuse such treatment is made jointly, and in good faith, by the parents and the child who is 14 years or older. The child must be sufficiently mature to have an informed opinion on the subject of his or her medical treatment. The adoption of Abraham's Law has since compelled many states to explore the concept of the mature minor doctrine.

PARKER JENSEN CANCER CASE

In 2003, a 12-year old Utah boy named Parker Jensen was diagnosed with Ewing's sarcoma. His oncologist recommended treatment with chemotherapy. His parents resisted the therapy and requested second opinions and an option to pursue alternative therapies. His oncologist filed a complaint with the Utah Department of Child and Family Services (DCFS). When the DCFS moved to take custody of Parker, the parents fled the state with their son to avoid losing their parental rights. The parents were subsequently charged with kidnapping by the state of Utah. After many legal proceedings, the Jensens pleaded guilty to a misdemeanor charge of custodial interference, which was eventually removed from their records. The state of Utah ultimately abandoned its efforts to force Parker to receive chemotherapy. The family has since filed multiple suits alleging that the state of Utah and others violated and interfered with their constitutional and parental rights. At last report, Parker was alive with no evidence of cancer.

Courts are usually unsympathetic when parents refuse treatment based on religious beliefs for their minor children with serious medical conditions (*Schmidt v. Mutual Hosp. Svcs.*, 2005; *State v. Norman*, 1991). The courts weigh the seriousness of the condition and risks to the patient of proceeding in either direction when making their decisions. The question in such cases is whether the state's interest is superior to the parents' desire for religious autonomy in a particular situation. For example, courts will often allow a parent to refuse immunizations for their children based on religious beliefs because the state's interest is secondary to the interests of the family for a primary care issue (*Diana H. v. Rubin*, 2007).

Outcomes in cases where parents or minor children refuse treatment recommended by HCPs vary depending on the circumstances in each case and the state law for the particular jurisdiction. The general trend, however, is to allow parents and children to have autonomy regarding decisions related to medical treatment, even if their decisions contradict conventional wisdom. If parents can demonstrate that they are advocating for their position based on reasonable information and a plan for treatment that they truly feel is in the best interest of the child, courts will often side with the parent (*In re Nikolas E.,* 1998). In some cases, the courts must make a determination as to whether the parents are capable of making a rational and informed decision regarding the best interests of their child (*A.D.H. v. State Dep't of Human Resources,* 1994). Courts will often side with children even if their decisions conflict with those of the parent under the mature minor doctrine if the court finds that the child is sufficiently informed about the diagnosis and treatment alternatives and reasonably understands the consequences of the decision (*In re Conner,* 2006; *H.L. v. Matheson,* 1981; *Hodgson v. Minnesota,* 1990).

CONSENT, PERMISSION, AND ASSENT

In 1989, the United Nations Children's Fund (UNICEF) held the Convention on the Rights of the Child (CRC). At this meeting, 193 ratifying parties agreed to protect the rights of children to be actively involved in decisions and actions that concern them, to express their opinions, and to have those opinions weighed and considered in medical decision making (UNICEF, 2005).

Despite the CRC, U.S. state statutes vary widely regarding the rights of children and parents and health care decisions. In some states, the age of consent is unspecified or differs depending on the circumstances. For example, in one state, the age of consent for health care is 14 years, and the age for sexual consent is 16 years; however, once a person is married, regardless of age, he or she becomes an adult and is granted the ability to consent. Adolescent mothers may give legal consent for decisions pertaining to their children. In some cases, poor decision making may lead to removal of the child and/or formal supervision by adult family members or social service agencies. Other regulations may apply to children with substance abuse or other specific conditions and problems.

CONSENT

The American Academy of Pediatrics (AAP) Committee on Bioethics has outlined the parameters for informed consent, parental consent/permission, and child assent (Mercurio et al., 2008). Informed consent is based on the assumption that a person of the age of majority has the full and accurate information needed to make a decision. It is further assumed that the decision maker has the mental capacity and ability to recognize the probable consequences of the decision. Consent is decision making for oneself; as such, it is not a term that commonly applies to children except as previously described.

PERMISSION

Informed permission is obtained from the parent or guardian for a minor child. Generally the parent/guardian is fully informed of the purpose, benefits, and risks for the child and is asked for permission to perform the procedure or enroll the child in the research study. In the case of the older child, the parental permission form may be abbreviated or even waived if there is minimal risk. U.S. federal regulations (Code of Federal Regulations, 1991; U.S. Department of Health and Human Services [USDHHS], 1983) and U.S. Food and Drug Administration guidelines (FDA, 2001) specify accepted rules in these cases.

ASSENT

Article 12 of the Children's Act (United Nations, 1989) is the basis for the concept of *self-determination*, which requires that the child be allowed to hold and express his or her own views if capable of doing so and that the child's perspective be considered. Assent is the process of self-determination by which a child, having been fully informed or informed to the limits of his or her ability to understand the aspects of the decision, participates in decision making. Participation may be a simple expression of opinion, or it may entail a thorough and involved discussion of all aspects of an issue. The AAP recommends that all efforts should be made to inform the child and seek assent when possible and applicable. Further recommendations include the following:

- Involve children in health care discussions, even when their assent is not being sought.
- Help them achieve developmentally appropriate awareness of their condition when possible.
- Provide information regarding what to expect during tests and treatment.
- Evaluate their understanding and factors that influence their response.
- Solicit, when possible, the child's willingness to accept the proposed care.
- Do not ask a child for an opinion if it is not to be taken seriously.
- Do not seek assent if the medical care is essential and there is no choice (Mercurio et al., 2008, p. e1).

Assent may be waived if the child is mentally or physically unable to participate in decision making. However, this situation is becoming rarer as more innovative and creative means of communication have been devised for those with communication disorders. Communication boards, sign language, and speech adjuncts, for example, are now more common in health care settings.

Institutional research review boards recognize the variability of maturity and competency of minors and the importance of minors either giving their assent to participate in clinical trials or having their assent waived by their parent or guardian. Assent, therefore, follows parental permission. In many situations, children who are old enough to write their name, and are assessed by the family and HCP to be mature enough to understand decisions regarding trial participation, are routinely asked to provide assent. This provision applies to children as young as 6 to 7 years of age. Alternatively, the parents or guardians may waive the minor's assent for reasons such as age, maturity, or psychological state if they believe it is not in the minor's best interest to provide assent. For routine medical care such as examinations, vaccinations, noninvasive testing, or minor procedures, it is well accepted that reviewing the procedure, including risks and benefits, with an immature minor is done for the purpose of achieving the child's cooperation with the procedure, not for obtaining the child's assent.

There is a growing body of literature concerning the right of self-determination for children who have disabilities and receive their care in outpatient settings and/or the medical home (Alderson et al., 2006; Foederer, 2007). In the case of disabled or chronically ill children, the seriousness and continuing nature of their health problem(s) frequently mean that the parents are more involved and are required to participate in activities of daily living (toileting, dressing, feeding) well past the age at which these activities become independent functions for other children. Consequently, such children are less likely to develop other independent functions or make decisions, particularly if there is a communication or cognition problem.

CONFIDENTIALITY

Communication between HCPs and children and their families frequently involves the principle of *confidentiality*. This principle holds that HCPs must not share confidences between themselves and a patient or parent with others without the patient's or parent's express permission. There are specific exceptions to the principle. First, if the HCP believes that the patient is in danger of self-harm or harm to another, then the information must be shared appropriately to prevent such injuries. Second, the HCP must report disclosures of illegal activity.

Lyren et al. (2006) reported that minors and parents understood the principle of confidentiality differently. Parents assumed that HCP would inform them of high-risk behaviors that their children confided to the professionals, whereas

minors expected the HCP to keep the information private. What is actually protected varies state to state. HCPs should be specific when explaining confidentiality; one method may involve the use of examples of types of information that may and may not be shared without the patient's consent.

RESEARCH AND CLINICAL PRACTICE DEFINITIONS

Institutional research review boards are charged with supervision and evaluation of research protocols to assure that the rights of patients are respected and that ethical principles are used in the conduct of research. Obtaining informed parental consent or parental permission for participation in research, without undue influence or coercion, is the responsibility of the study investigator. The nature of the study; whether it is experimental or invasive; whether there is a potential for physical, emotional, or psychological harm; and possible alternatives to the study design must be reviewed with the family. It is the HCP's responsibility, in the role of patient and family advocate, to verify that consent is legitimately obtained and that consent protocols are followed. The HCP may not advise or direct the decision to participate. If the HCP has any interest in the research protocol or study, he or she should exclude himself or herself from the consent process.

EMERGENCY PROCEDURES

Hospitals that provide care for children should have written policies and procedures that define their process for obtaining emergency consent/permission and for waiving the informed consent/permission process in certain circumstances while still providing emergency care. When the parent or guardian is not present but is available by telephone or other video medium, a procedure for obtaining consent/permission must include a third-party "auditory witness." This witness must be able to hear the entire conversation and consent/permission. When a parent or guardian is unavailable and the minor child is awake and alert, the HCP may make a determination that the child is mature enough and able to understand his or her condition and make decisions as a mature minor, thereby giving consent in the absence of the parent or guardian. In emergent situations where the patient, regardless of age, is unconscious or unable to communicate his or her wishes, most hospitals have a procedure in place where two licensed medical professionals (often two licensed physicians) may make a declaration that life-saving or emergency care is needed and that a delay in delivery of that care to obtain consent/permission would be deleterious. These declarations should be committed to writing in the patient's medical record.

ORGAN DONATION

According to the AAP (2002), approximately 3% of all transplantations occur in children younger than 17 years of age. Concerns regarding organ transplantation include the source of the organ (i.e., from a live donor versus a cadaver), the health status of the donor, and the presence of communicable disease or damage to the transplanted organ. Cadaver donors are matched by height, weight, ABO (blood type), and serology status according to the organ or organs requested. Ethical issues are less problematic for cadaver organs due to the strict protocols and policies for organ distribution; however, how families are advised that their child is unlikely to survive and asked to consider organ donation has serious implications (Bellali et al., 2007; Rodrigue et al., 2008).

Live donor transplantation raises several additional concerns. First, the identification of potential live donors is particularly important when a child is a recipient. A sibling has a 1:4 chance of being a perfect match and an identical twin is the best match. Families may latch on to those "chances" without thinking about the implications for the child they want to donate the organ (AAP, 2010). The emotional cost to the child for choosing to donate, or guilt if he or she does not, may be high. The child might feel that the sibling is more important to the family, or that he or she did not receive adequate attention for making the sacrifice (Fleck, 2004). The child who receives the organ will know that he or she owes his or her recovery to the donor child. This could result in overt or covert pressure to "pay back" the sibling and lead to problematic issues between the siblings or family members in the future. It is, therefore, preferred that a related adult donor or an unrelated donor be used. This practice avoids the complicated dynamic of the parent having to decide that one child's suffering is more significant than the other child's. It also avoids producing guilt in the sibling if he or she is not willing to donate the organ (Fleck).

REPRODUCTIVE DECISION MAKING

In emergency departments, minors may be seen for sexually related health disorders, diseases such as sexually transmitted infections (STIs), and pregnancy tests. In some instances, minors may seek information regarding birth control, pregnancy termination, and prevention of infection with human immunodeficiency virus (HIV) and other STIs. In addition, parents with chronically ill children or children who are developmentally delayed or cognitively impaired may seek pregnancy prevention strategies to protect them from sexual abuse and STIs.

Some states require parental permission to provide any kind of education related to sexuality or birth control. Other states have laws that allow children of a particular age—for example, 14 years or 16 years—to consent to

their own health care, including sexual education and birth control (Harty-Golder, 2008). Married adolescents generally can consent to their own health care and that of their children. Consent laws for pregnancy termination also vary from state to state.

When the parents' insurance policy is used for payment of service by the child, it is difficult to manage and protect confidentiality (when permitted by law) without the parents' awareness. Unless there is reason not to, the HCP should suggest open discussion of options and plans between the parent and the child.

In the case of chronically ill, developmentally delayed, and cognitively impaired children, state laws also vary widely. In some states, parents may have total responsibility for decision making regarding sexual education, birth control, pregnancy termination, and sterilization.

SPERM BANKING, OVARIAN TISSUE PRESERVATION, AND OTHER PROTECTIVE REPRODUCTIVE STRATEGIES

Some medical conditions in children warrant consideration of future reproductive ability, especially in cases where prognosis for survival is good and risk of treatment-related infertility is high. HCPs should be aware of which options are available and empower patients and families to make informed decisions about pursuing fertility preservation techniques (Reebals et al., 2006; Zakak, 2009). Currently, the only established option for male fertility preservation is cryopreservation of spermatozoa; for female fertility preservation, options include cryopreservation of oocytes, cryopreservation of embryos, and ovarian transposition before treatment with radiation therapy (Zakak).

Fertility preservation has significant ethical and legal issues associated with it. Minors must provide consent for the procedures and storage of reproductive tissue. The female preservation options are invasive, and their risks and benefits must be considered. There are also financial concerns, because most medical insurance plans do not provide coverage for storage of reproductive tissue. Another very serious ethical and legal dilemma that may be encountered is posthumous use of stored reproductive tissue. HCPs should obtain written instructions from the tissue donor indicating what he or she would like to happen to the reproductive tissue if the person should die, including whether it should be destroyed, used, or not used in the event of the individual's death.

GENETIC TESTING

The science of genetics has rapidly expanded and continues to do so. In some cases, children may be tested for adult-onset familial cancers when they are not yet able to understand the ramifications of the results (Gilbar, 2009). While genetic experts have developed guidelines for counseling families and individuals about testing, there are still many settings that lack such guidelines. Recently, the ethics of performing genetic screening of children being considered for adoption has been explored, including the potential for adoption rejection based on the results (Newson & Leonard, 2009).

It is important that HCPs and the interprofessional team discuss and develop policies, and patient/family education materials to assist with explaining legal and ethical questions when genetic testing is considered. Most hospitals that provide genetic testing also have genetic counselors who provide genetic counseling before and after all such testing. A variety of issues—such as who should receive the information, what responsibility patients and families have to inform other family members, and what long-term ramifications the outcome may have for the child or family member—must be addressed.

THE HEALTH CARE PROFESSIONAL AND CARE OF THE MINOR

The legal implications of caring for children and families are complex and further complicated by varying state statutes. Written policies that are state and setting specific are invaluable references for HCPs who work with children in acute care. Health care professionals must be aware of the conflicting viewpoints and potential for litigation when assisting parents and minors with informed decision making. In situations where there is overt conflict or where parents appear to be having difficulty making decisions, the atmosphere may become highly charged and stressful; therefore, support and advocacy for the patient and family members is crucial. In such cases, HCPs may consider seeking a formal ethics committee consultation where available.

REFERENCES

1. *A.D.H. v. State Dep't of Human Resources*, 640 So.2d 969 (Ala. Civ. App. 1994).
2. Alderson, P., Sutcliffe, K., & Curtis, K. (2006). Children's competence to consent to medical treatment. *Hastings Center Report, 36*(6), 25–34.
3. American Academy of Pediatrics (AAP), Committee on Hospital Care and Section on Surgery. (2010). Pediatric organ donation and transplantation. *Pediatrics, 125*(4), 822–828.
4. Bellali, T., Papazogulou, I., & Papadatou, D. (2007). Empirically based recommendations to support parents facing the dilemma of paediatric cadaver organ donation. *Intensive and Critical Care Nursing, 23*, 216–225.
5. Code of Federal Regulations. (1991). Federal policy for the protection of human subjects (Subpart A). Washington, DC: United States Department of Health and Human Services, 5CFR (46), 116–117.
6. *Diana H. v. Rubin*, 171 P.3d 200 (Ariz. Ct. App. 2007).
7. Food and Drug Administration, US Department of Health and Human Services. (2001). Additional safeguards for children in clinical investigations of FDA regulated products. *Federal Regist, 21*CFR, (50,56, 66), 20589–20600.
8. Fleck, L. (2004). Children and organ donation: Some cautionary remarks. *Cambridge Quarterly of Healthcare Ethics, 13*(2), 161–166.
9. Foederer, A. (2007). Who will decide for Angel: A child's fight to receive adequate health care. *Journal of Nursing Law, 11*(3), 129–140.
10. Gilbar, R. (2009, July 17). Genetic testing of children for familial cancers: A comparative legal perspective on consent, communication of information and confidentiality. *Familial Cancer.* doi: 10.1/1007/s10689-009-0268-2
11. Harty-Golder, B. (2008). Defining minors under the law. *Medical Laboratory Observer, 40*(11), 40.
12. *H.L. v. Matheson,* 450 U.S. 398 (1981). *In re Conner,* 140 P.3d 1167 (Or. Ct. App. 2006).
13. *Hodgson v. Minnesota,* 497 U.S. 417 (1990). *In re Nikolas E.,* 720 A.2d 562 (Me. 1998).
14. Lyren, A., Kodish, E., Lazebnik, R., & O'Riordan, M. (2006). Understanding confidentiality: Perspectives of African American adolescents and their parents. *Journal of Adolescent Health, 39*, 261–265.
15. Mercurio, M., Adam, M., Forman, E., Ladd, E., Ross, L., & Silber, T. (2008). American Academy of Pediatrics policy statements on bioethics. *Pediatrics in Review, 29,* e1–e8. doi: 10.1542/10.1542/pir.29-1-e1. Retrieved from http://pedsinreview.aappublications.org/cgi/content/extract/29/1/e1
16. *Meyer v. Nebraska,* 262 U.S. 390 (1923).
17. Newson, A., & Leonard, S. (2009). Childhood genetic testing for familial cancer: Should adoption make a difference. *Familial Cancer,* published online ahead of print June 25, 2009. doi: 10.1007/s10689-009-9262-8
18. *Parham v. J.R.,* 442 U.S. 584 (1979).
19. *Pierce v. Society of Sisters,* 268 U.S. 510 (1925).
20. *Prince v. Massachusetts,* 321 U.S. 158 (1944).
21. Reebals, J. F., Brown, R., & Buckner, E. B. (2006). Nurse practice issues regarding sperm banking in adolescent male cancer patients. *Journal of Pediatric Oncology Nursing, 23*, 182–188.
22. Rodrigue, J., Cornell, D., & Howard, R. J. (2008). Pediatric organ donation: What factors most influence parents' donation decisions? *Pediatric Critical Care, 9*(2), 180–185.
23. *Schmidt v. Mutual Hosp. Svcs., Inc.,* 832 N.E.2d 977 (Ind. Ct. App. 2005).
24. *State v. Norman,* 808 P.2d 1159 (Wash. Ct. App. 1991).
25. *Troxel v. Granville,* 530 U.S. 57 (2000).
26. United Nations Children's Fund (UNICEF). (2005). Path to the Convention on the Rights of the Child. Retrieved from http://www.unicef.org/crc/index_30197.html
27. United Nations General Assembly. (1989). Convention on the Rights of the Child. *Resolution 25* session 44.
28. US Department of Health and Human Services. (1983). 45 CFR Part 46: additional protections for children involved as subjects in research (hereafter "subpart D"). *Federal Regist.* 48, 9814–9820.
29. *West Virginia v. Chas. Pfizer & Co.,* 440 F.2d 1079 (2d Cir. 1971).
30. Zakak, N. (2009). Fertility issues of childhood cancer survivors: The role of the pediatric nurse practitioner in fertility preservation. *Journal of Pediatric Oncology Nursing, 26*, 48–59.

Lindsey Katzmark

Transition to Adulthood

The number of pediatric patients with chronic medical conditions has increased in the past 20 years, and advances in pharmacological, surgical, and technological methods have resulted in many pediatric patients with chronic illnesses surviving well into adulthood (American Academy of Pediatrics [AAP], 2002). Ninety percent of all children with disabilities now live beyond 20 years of age (Blum, 1995). Therefore, large cohorts of young people requiring complex, interprofessional care must make the transition to adult services (Blum et al., 2003).

DEFINITION OF HEALTH CARE TRANSITION

In general, transitions are a part of normal, healthy life. A medical transition is defined by Blum (1995) as "the purposeful, planned movement of adolescents and young adults with chronic physical and medical conditions from child-centered to adult-oriented health care systems" (p. 3). The definition of "transition" is very different from the concept of "transfer." A transition is an anticipated and coordinated effort, whereas a transfer is only one component of a transition (Blum, 1995). Transition from the pediatric health care professional (HCP) to the adult HCP should transmit a positive message that pediatric patients can survive to adulthood; like their peers without chronic illness, they can become adults with independent, productive futures (Callahan et al., 2001; Kennedy & Sawyer, 2008).

Transition should occur for all pediatric patients with chronic illness who are expected to live beyond adolescence. In the same way that pediatric HCPs are specially trained to meet the family-centered needs of the pediatric patient; adult HCPs are specifically trained in the patient-centered care of their target population (Rosen, 1995). Patient and family needs for transition vary. For some patients, it may mean transitioning from a pediatric hematologist to an adult hematologist for care of sickle cell disease. For other patients, it may mean transition from an entire team of HCPs who provided care for a wide range of problems such as developmental delay, gastroesophageal reflux, and seizures (Rosen, 1994; Society for Adolescent Medicine, 2003; Werner, 2009).

Regardless of the complexity of the transition, it is important to recognize that transition for those with chronic medical conditions from pediatric to adult care can be extremely challenging and stressful not only for the pediatric patient but also for the caregiver and HCP. Relationships in such cases are often strong and trust implicit.

NATIONAL POLICIES AND STATEMENTS

In 2002, the AAP, in concert with the American Academy of Family Physicians and the American Society of Internal Medicine, produced a consensus statement regarding the transition of young people with special health care needs. This document not only outlines the challenge of transition for pediatric patients with complex illness, but also suggests a process for taking the critical first steps for successful transition (AAP, 2002):

- Identifying a specialized HCP who attends to the unique challenges of transition to adulthood
- Identifying the knowledge and skills needed to care for young people with special health care needs and making this a part of health care training
- Preparing up-to-date medical summaries for the transition
- Starting to develop a written transition plan by at least age 14 years
- Recognizing that young people with special health care needs may require more resources during their transition to adulthood
- Ensuring affordable, continuous health insurance coverage for all young people with special health care needs throughout adolescence and into adulthood

An objective for *Healthy People 2020* specifically addresses increasing the proportion of youth with disabilities (aged 12 to 17 years) who have transition plans for pediatric to adult health care. This objective supports the goal that all young people with special health care needs receive the services needed to make necessary transitions to all aspects of adult life, including health care, work, and independent living (U.S. Department of Health and Human Service, 2010).

ROLE OF THE HEALTH CARE TEAM

The transition health care team includes not only the pediatric primary care provider (PCP), but also pertinent specialists, the adult PCP, and the family. Communication is essential to the process of transition. Regular discussions with patients, caregivers, and the transition health care team should occur to assure that when young people view transition not as a sudden change, but rather as an anticipated, coordinated, comfortable, and trusted transfer of services (Flume, 2009).

TIMING OF TRANSITION

Specifying a defined time of transition is a critical step in ensuring a successful transition (Flume, 2009). Whether this time is dictated by milestones or individualized by patient readiness, it should be established early in the transition process and be chronicled in a written document. The idea that there will be a transition plan in the future should begin early in life. Chronic illness care can often focus on bleak outcomes, so it is important to convey a message that outcomes are continually improving and that children with special health care needs often survive well into adulthood (Flume, 2009).

GOALS FOR TRANSITION

Guiding principles for the transition should include ensuring a gradual and individual process, involving the entire family, setting goals for independence and self-care, and recognizing the young person's need for empowerment and the caregivers' simultaneous need for support (McCurdy et al., 2006).

PLANNING FOR TRANSITION

To achieve the goal that all young people with special needs receive services necessary to make the transition to adult life, including independent living and health care, there should be a plan for transition education. As the patient becomes older, a program can be developed to encourage responsibility and independent decision making.

Regardless of the barriers for a specific individual, optimal health care is achieved when the chronically ill patient is ensured primary medical care that is accessible and medically and developmentally appropriate from those specifically trained to provide it.

REFERENCES

1. American Academy of Pediatrics. (2002). Health care transitions: destinations unknown. *Pediatrics, 110*(6), 1307–1314.
2. Blum, R. (1995). Transition to adult care: Setting the stage. *Journal Adolescent Health, 17,* 3–5.
3. Blum, R., Garell, D., Hodgman, C., et al. (2003). Transition to adult healthcare for adolescents and young adults with chronic conditions. *Journal of Adolescent Health, 33,* 309–311.
4. Callahan, S., Feinstein-Winitzer, R., & Keenan, P. (2001). Transition from pediatric to adult-oriented health care: A challenge for patients with chronic disease. *Current Opinion in Pediatrics, 13,* 310–316.
5. Flume, P. (2009). Smoothing the transition from pediatric to adult care: Lessons learned. *Current Opinion in Pulmonary Medicine, 15,* 611–614.
6. Kennedy, A., & Sawyer, S. (2008). Transition from pediatric to adult services: Are we getting it right? *Current Opinion in Pediatrics, 20,* 403–409.
7. McCurdy, C., DiCenso, A., Boblin, S., Ludwin, D., Bryant-Lukosius, D., & Bosompra, K. (2006). There to here: Young adult patients' perceptions of the process of transition from pediatric to adult transplant care. *Progress in Transplantation, 16*(6), 309–316.
8. Rosen, D. (1994). Transition from pediatric to adult-oriented health care for the adolescent with chronic disease or disability. *Adolescent Medicine: State of the Art Reviews, 5,* 241–248.
9. Rosen, D. (1995). Between two worlds: Bridging the cultures of child health and adult medicine. *Journal Adolescent Health, 17,* 10–16.
10. Society for Adolescent Medicine. (2003). Transition to adult health care for adolescents and young adults with chronic conditions. *Journal of Adolescent Health, 33,* 309–311.
11. U.S. Department of Health and Human Services. (2010). *Developing healthy people 2020: Disability and secondary conditions* (DSC HP2020–15). Retrieved from http://www.healthypeople.gov/hp2020/Objectives
12. Werner, R. (2009). Crossing the bridge to adult care: Transitioning youth from pediatric to adult care. *ACNN Currents, 2*(3), 1–5.

Sharron L. Docherty

Care of the Medically Fragile

TERMS AND CLASSIFICATIONS

Children with special health care needs (CSHCN) are defined by the U.S. Maternal and Child Health Bureau as a group of pediatric patients who have, or are at increased risk for, a chronic physical, developmental, behavioral, or emotional condition that requires health and related services of a type or amount beyond that required by other children (McPherson et al., 1998). A growing subset of CSHCN who are of particular concern to acute care health care professionals (HCPs) is that set of children and adolescents described as *medically fragile*. These pediatric patients have complex chronic conditions involving several organ systems and require multiple specialists, technological supports, and community services to assist them to function to their healthiest potential. The medical complexity of their conditions, the high level of skill required to meet their daily health care needs, and the continuous nature and potential volatility of the conditions set this group apart from the broader population of CSHCN (Harrigan et al., 2002; Rehm & Bradley, 2005).

A variety of terms, such as "medically complex," "technology dependent," and "multiply handicapped," have been used to describe this vulnerable population of CSHCN (Carnevale et al., 2008; Cohen et al., 2008; Gordon et al., 2007; Harrigan et al., 2002; Miles et al., 1999; O'Brien & Wegner, 2002; Watson et al., 2002). Frequent and prolonged hospitalizations, complex and multisystem health

and developmental needs, and reliance upon technology and care across hospital, clinic, and home settings are the key characteristics that all of these terms seek to signify about the pediatric patients whom they are used to represent (Harrigan et al., 2002). However, the multiplicity of terms used by researchers and HCPs has contributed to the challenges in understanding the prevalence of such patients and synthesizing best practices and policies for this vulnerable group of patients. For the purposes of this chapter, they will be described as *medically fragile* pediatric patients.

The nature and severity of conditions that render children medically fragile is quite diverse. Table 13-1 is a nonexhaustive sampling of conditions, organized by specialty, that commonly contribute to the medical fragility of a pediatric patient. Nevertheless, it is the health and developmental consequences of these diagnoses—such as ongoing functional impairment, neurodevelopmental disability, dependence on medical technology, and need for ongoing skilled and supportive care from HCPs and family members—that unite these children into an especially vulnerable subpopulation of CSHCN. It is truly the care needs that define medically fragile pediatric patients. These needs are usually extensive, with patients often relying on medical equipment to compensate for the loss of vital body functioning and requiring continual, comprehensive care for the prevention of further disability and death (Office of Technology Assessment, 1987).

TABLE 13-1

Conditions Commonly Associated with Medically Fragile Pediatric Patients		
System	**Diagnoses**	**Possible Technology**
Neurology	Cerebral palsy; ataxia teleangiectasia; muscular dystrophy; seizure disorder; spina bifida; traumatic brain injury	Shunts; oropharyngeal/nasopharyngeal suctioning; urinary bladder catheterization; cardiorespiratory monitoring
Cardiology	Complex congenital heart lesion	Cardiorespiratory monitoring; oxygen
Pulmonology	Chronic lung disease; cystic fibrosis; congenital diaphragmatic hernia	Cardiorespiratory monitoring; oxygen; tracheostomy; mechanical ventilation; percussion therapy
Gastroenterology	Intestinal failure; biliary atresia; failure-to-thrive; bowel disease	Parenteral or enteral nutrition
Hematology	Sickle cell anemia; Fanconi's anemia	Vascular access catheter; chronic blood product need
Oncology	Brain tumor	Shunts; vascular access catheter
Rheumatology	Systemic lupus erythematosus; dermatomyositis	
Immunology	Immune deficiency; HIV	
Transplants	Bone marrow; stem cell; solid organ	
Urology/nephrology	Prune belly syndrome; kidney disease	Veno/peritoneal dialysis

HIV: Human immunodeficiency virus.

EPIDEMIOLOGY

The 2005–2006 National Survey of Children with Special Health Care Needs reported that 13.9% of children younger than 18 years of age have a special health care need (U.S. Health Resources Service Administration [HRSA], 2008). While many authors have described the increase in prevalence of medically fragile pediatric patients as resulting from advances in medical care (Cohen et al., 2008; Council on Children with Disabilities, 2005; Haffner & Schurman, 2001; Mentro, 2003), accurate estimates of the size of this population are rare (Carnevale et al., 2008). The last systematic estimation of the numbers of medically fragile pediatric patients was conducted in 1987 by the now defunct congressional U.S. Office of Technology Assessment (OTA). This agency estimated that there were between 11,000 and 68,000 children in the United States who were medically fragile and dependent on technology (OTA, 1987). The OTA categorized children into four groups based on health care needs: ventilator dependence, intravenous medication or nutritional support, other device-based respiratory or nutritional support, and medical devices that compensate for vital bodily functions.

Advances in medical and nursing care, such as the increasing viability of extremely preterm infants, advances in the portability of life-sustaining technology (e.g., parenteral nutrition, ventilatory support), and life-extending treatments for children with conditions that previously would have led to an early death (e.g., malignancies, genetic conditions) (Feudtner et al., 2001), have led to an exponential rise in the prevalence of medically fragile pediatric patients. As survival rates have increased, a concomitant rise in morbidity has occurred (Mahon & Kibirige, 2004).

Epidemiological trends describing health care utilization by medically fragile pediatric patients help to illustrate the profound needs that exact a high physical, emotional, social, and economic toll on the child, family, health care system, and society. Estimates suggest that this population accounts for the majority of nontraumatic hospitalizations for children, with this proportion more than doubling over the past four decades (Mahon & Kibirige, 2004; Wise, 2004). Medically fragile patients are hospitalized at least four times more often and spend up to seven times as many days in hospital as compared to nonmedically fragile patients; the increased length of stay has been attributed to technology dependence and the requirement for medical devices on discharge. Moreover, the likelihood of multiple admissions in a given year is substantially higher for medically fragile patients than for their short-stay counterparts (Marcin et al., 2001; Wise). Lastly, it is known that these children account for more than half of childhood deaths (Brandon et al., 2007; Feudtner et al., 2002). Thus, although medically fragile pediatric patients make up a relatively small subset of CSHCN, their vulnerabilities and disproportionate impact on health expenditures and resources make them an important group for targeted interventions (Newacheck & Halfon, 1998).

HIGH DEPENDENCY CARE NEEDS

While the nature and severity of conditions that render children medically fragile vary widely, certain key therapeutic and technologic management needs are common to many conditions. The list of needs presented in this section serves to acquaint the HCP with possible management requirements for medically fragile pediatric patients. The reader is encouraged to consult a prescriptive source for detailed instruction on the application of these interventions.

PHYSIOLOGIC MONITORING

Many medically fragile children require the use of technology to transmit objective data on physiologic variables that may require immediate interventions. These technologies perform either episodic or continuous monitoring of vital signs and physiologic status and have been used across care settings, from inpatient and outpatient environments to home care. Variables that are typically monitored include electrical activity of the heart, respiratory rate, blood pressure, body temperature, cardiac output, and amount of oxygen and carbon dioxide in the blood. A pulse oximeter monitors the arterial hemoglobin oxygen saturation through use of a sensor clipped over the finger or toe. An apnea monitor continuously monitors breathing via electrodes or sensors placed on the patient.

RESPIRATORY ASSISTANCE

The use of supplemental oxygen is a common management need for medically fragile pediatric patients with conditions such as chronic lung disease, end-stage cystic fibrosis, pulmonary hypertension, obstructive sleep apnea, neuromuscular conditions, and disorders of the chest wall, and those in whom palliative care for symptom relief is indicated (Balfour-Lynn et al., 2005; Haffner & Schurman, 2001). The advent of liquid oxygen has made home discharge a more realistic goal in such cases. Although liquid oxygen has many advantages over the gas form, it is more expensive; thus it may be difficult to gain approval for use of this technology from many third-party payers. Conditions for home discharge of a child on oxygen should include that the oxygen requirement remains relatively stable with a mean SaO_2 of 93% or higher without frequent episodes of desaturation. The SaO_2 should not fall below 90% for more than 5% of any recording period and the child should be able to cope with short periods in room air without rapid deterioration (Balfour-Lynn et al., 2005).

A variety of clinical situations can result in a medically fragile patient requiring tracheostomy placement. One recent study identified the principal indications for tracheostomy use with children as airway control (37%), airway obstruction (25%), chronic lung disease (23%), central hypoventilation (9%), and neuromuscular disease (6%) (Graf et al., 2008).

Children who depend on mechanical ventilation for oxygenation are often the most complex of patients. Conditions that may require long-term mechanical ventilation include neuromuscular disorders, chest wall deformities, and primary pulmonary disorders (Kingston, 2007). Types of ventilatory support range from noninvasive positive-pressure ventilation for those patients requiring intermittent assistance to multiple positive-pressure ventilators (Haffner & Schurman, 2001).

FLUID AND NUTRITION ASSISTANCE

One of the success stories in long-term management strategies for medically fragile pediatric patients has occurred in the area of enteral and parenteral nutrition. Enteral nutrition involves the nonvolitional delivery of nutrients by a tube to the gastrointestinal (GI) tract (Haffner & Schurman, 2001). A wide range of conditions associated with medically fragile pediatric patients may require the use of enteral nutrition, such as, neurologic impairment, cancer, human immunodeficiency virus (HIV) infection, and cystic fibrosis. When the child does not have an intact GI tract that supports the absorption of nutrients, then parenteral nutrition must be employed. Conditions such as intestinal failure (e.g., short gut syndrome), biliary atresia, and organ and stem cell transplant are often associated with the need for mid- to long-term parental nutrition. This nutrition is administered through a central venous catheter, which may comprise a percutaneous, tunneled, or implanted device.

PAIN AND SEDATION ISSUES

Children with medically fragile conditions experience pain or discomfort along a continuum that ranges from episodic bouts of discomfort through continuous severe pain that impacts the child's affect and interferes with quality of life and sleeping patterns. The emotional toll on caregivers of children experiencing chronic pain can be profound and requires close attention by the HCP.

BEHAVIORAL AND ADJUSTMENT ISSUES

Research has supported the contention that most children with chronic illness will experience the same level of psychologic and behavioral problems as other children their age. Behavioral and adjustment problems are more likely to occur when the onset of the illness occurs earlier in life, and particularly if it emerges in infancy. The risk of psychologic and behavioral problems does not appear to be associated with the severity of the chronic illness. The effects can be seen across all diagnoses, but are more profound with disorders that affect the central nervous system, including cerebral palsy, traumatic brain injury, and treatment-related complications that involve the brain, such as chemotherapy for cancer (Wise, 2004).

MODELS OF CARE

THE MEDICAL HOME

The medical home is a conceptual model that describes holistic care as "accessible, continuous, comprehensive, compassionate, coordinated, family-centered, and culturally effective" (American Academy of Pediatrics [AAP], 1992, p. 774). The AAP further characterizes the medical home as an approach to providing continuous and comprehensive primary pediatric care from infancy through young adulthood, with availability 24 hours a day, 7 days a week, from a physician whom the family trusts (AAP, 2004). Studies of potential enhanced continuity of care proposed by the medical home model have predicted overall cost savings with adoption of this concept (McBurney et al., 2004).

Despite efforts to apply the medical home concept to the care of medically fragile pediatric patients, most applications persist in assuming the provision of primary care, defined as the point of access to the health care system for all new needs and problems (Trivedi et al., 2010). Results from a large survey of children with special health care needs over the 2005–2006 period demonstrated that approximately 50% of CSHCN did not have access to all aspects of a medical home, including access to needed referrals, care coordination, and family-centered care (Strickland et al., 2009). Additionally, these researchers found significant disparities in regard to poverty, race, and ethnicity when it came to applying the concept of the medical home. The proportion of CSHCN without a medical home increased significantly as family income decreased. Those patients with the most severe limitations in activities of daily living were at highest risk of not having a medical home.

ACUTE CARE HOSPITALS

The traditional model of the acute care hospital has assumed that this facility provides acute or definitive management of illness rather than engaging in chronic care. Much has been written about the benefits of home and community care for patients who require ongoing health services (Koop, 1987). Home- and community-focused care recognizes that the family is the constant in the medically fragile child's life and facilitates caregiver–provider collaboration in all aspects of care (Garwick et al., 1998). Despite persistent efforts to transfer chronic care to community and home settings, recent surveys have suggested that pediatric patients with chronic conditions make up only 55% to 60% of all hospital discharges (Neff & Valentine, 2002; Wise, 2004). Indeed, over the past two decades, children's hospitals and mixed-population acute care hospitals have continued to serve as the medical home for the majority of medically fragile pediatric patients.

Several recent authors (Cohen et al., 2008; Roesler et al., 2002) have posited a number of potential benefits to increasing the care coordination role of children's hospitals in regard to medically fragile pediatric patients. A survey of families of children with chronic conditions revealed that they prefer "one-stop shopping" for health care in the location where the majority of their care is provided (Garwick et al., 1998). Hospital-based HCPs have the expertise, comfort, and resources to manage the complex and multisystem needs; by comparison, HCPs in primary care settings are often overburdened and under-trained to shoulder the enormous administrative responsibilities of care coordination for medically complex children (Cohen et al.). The financial disincentives often faced by individual practitioners in providing holistic care to medically fragile pediatric patients may be offset by the organizational savings on a hospital level from improved efficiency of care coordination for this population (Matlow et al., 2006).

Cohen et al. (2008) described two current hospital-based models. In the *specialist model,* hospitals have multidisciplinary programs for well-defined conditions that are relatively common among the medically fragile population (e.g., cancer, cystic fibrosis, spina bifida, sickle cell disease). Teams of specialist HCPs (including specialist physicians, nurses, therapists, nutritionists, and social workers) efficiently coordinate care for these populations of children. Although few controlled studies have been conducted, the literature seems to support the development of these programs when outcomes such as lower mortality or resource utilization are primary goals (Homer et al., 2008).

An alternative model, the *generalist model,* organizes care that is not condition focused, but rather encompasses a broader range of childhood conditions using, when necessary, specialist consultations (Cohen et al., 2008). Because medically fragile pediatric patients suffer from conditions that affect relatively small groups of children, and because many of these conditions have multisystem impacts, organizing care around groups of conditions that share common care needs can be more efficient and cost-effective. Proponents of the generalist model suggest that this organization of care tends to allow for more of a focus on the needs of the child and family.

HOME CARE

The benefits of home care in enhancing normal growth and development for medically fragile pediatric patients have been well described in the literature since the 1990s and early 2000s (Ahmann & Bond, 1992; Fields et al., 1991). Moreover, cost-comparison studies done during this period purported to find that home-based versus acute care management of medically fragile pediatric patients resulted in fewer hospitalization days and significantly decreased financial costs associated with the delivery of home care (Fields et al.; Miller et al., 1998).

More recently, Carnevale and colleagues (2008) have suggested that researchers have not accurately assessed the social, health, and financial costs incurred by families who are attempting to provide acute and chronic care in the home setting. Studies comparing living contexts, caregiving arrangements, and pediatric patients' preferences for places and providers of care have yet to be done. Irrespective of their individual circumstances, many caregivers feel as though they have little choice except to care for their children, despite a lack of support in communities that are characterized by significant physical, social, and policy barriers (Carnevale et al., 2008). Although some exceptional home care programs providing coordinated and comprehensive health and social services do exist, many families continue to cite poor access to health care services as an ongoing problem (Newachek et al., 2009).

IMPACT ON FAMILIES

A large number of studies have documented the impact on parents and families of having a child with a medically fragile condition (Aite et al., 2003; Black et al., 2009; Carnevale et al., 2006; Docherty et al., 2002). These burdens have been described as multidimensional and interconnected (Ratliffe et al., 2002), such that any particular event can have a major effect on the family system. The challenge of parenting in a context of constant uncertainty has been described in detail (Anderson et al., 2010; Ray, 2002; Rempel & Harrison, 2007) and modeled through the use of concepts such as extraordinary parenting, which involves a constant awareness and anticipation of needs and gaps for the child. For example, Rempel and Harrison (2007) examined this concept through a study of parenting a child with a life-threatening heart condition; they highlighted the efforts to safeguard the survival of the child through extensive assessment and problem solving such as ensuring weight gain and protecting the child from infection. This complex provision of care occurs as caregivers work diligently to maintain critical relationships that would minimize the consequences of their child's condition.

THE MEDICALLY FRAGILE PATIENT AND THE HEALTH CARE TEAM

The historical shift in the distribution of pediatric hospitalization and mortality reflects not only the increased prevalence of childhood chronic illness, but also a markedly reduced incidence of serious acute pediatric illness (Wise, 2004). To begin to address the issues that families face and to redress the inequities that they experience, strong interprofessional bridges must be built among clinicians, health scientists, social scientists, and humanists—linking childhood, disability, gender, housing, and science and technology studies scholars together with critical geographers, architects, ethicists, economists, educators, and health professionals. New insights are needed to spur new lines of scholarship that will lead to innovative practices and policies, thereby ensuring that caregiving responsibilities and costs are distributed fairly and that medically fragile children enjoy the rights of citizenship and the entitlements of contemporary childhood (Carnevale et al., 2008).

REFERENCES

1. Ahmann, E., & Bond, N. J. (1992). Promoting normal development in school-age children and adolescents who are technology dependent: A family centered model. *Pediatric Nursing, 18*(4), 399–405.
2. Aite, L., Trucchi, A., Nahom, A., Zaccara, A., Casaccia, G., & Bagolan, P. (2003). A challenging intervention with maternal anxiety: Babies requiring surgical correction of a congenital anomaly after missed prenatal diagnosis. *Infant Mental Health Journal, 24,* 571–579.
3. American Academy of Pediatrics (AAP). (1992). The medical home. *Pediatrics, 90,* 774.
4. American Academy of Pediatrics (AAP), Medical Home Initiatives for Children with Special Needs Project Advisory Committee. (2004). Policy statement: Organizational principles to guide and define the child health care system and/or improve the health of all children. *Pediatrics, 113*(suppl), 1545–1547.
5. Anderson, L., Riesch, S., Pridham, K., Lutz, K., & Becker, P. (2010). Furthering the understanding of parent–child relationships: A nursing scholarship review series. Part 4: Parent–child relationships at risk. *Journal for Specialists in Pediatric Nursing, 15*(2), 111–134.
6. Balfour-Lynn, I., Primhak, R., & Shaw, B. (2005). Home oxygen for children: Who, how and when? *Thorax, 60*(1), 76–81.
7. Black, B., Holditch-Davis, D., & Miles, M., (2009). Life course theory as a framework to examine becoming a mother of a medically fragile preterm infant. *Research in Nursing and Health, 32*(1), 38–49.
8. Brandon, D., Docherty, S., & Thorpe, J. (2007). Infant and child deaths in acute care settings: Implications for palliative care. *Journal of Palliative Medicine, 10*(4), 910–918.
9. Carnevale, F., Alexander, E., Davis, M., Rennick, J., & Troini, R. (2006). Daily living with distress and enrichment: The moral experience of families with ventilator assisted children at home. *Pediatrics, 117*(1), e48–e60.
10. Carnevale, F., Rehm, R., Kirk, S., & McKeever, P. (2008). What we know (and don't know) about raising children with complex continuing care needs. *Journal of Child Health Care, 12,* 4–6.
11. Cohen, E., Friedman, J., Nicholas, D., Adams, S., & Rosenbaum, P. (2008). A home for medically complex children: The role of hospital programs. *Journal of Health Care Quality, 30*(3), 7–15.
12. Council on Children with Disabilities. (2005). Care coordination in the medical home: Integrating health and related systems of care for children with special health care needs. *Pediatrics, 116*(5), 1238–1244.
13. Docherty, S., Miles, M., & Holditch-Davis, D. (2002). Worry about child health in mothers of hospitalized medically fragile infants. *Advances in Neonatal Care, 2*(2), 84–92.
14. Feudtner, C., Hays, R., Haynes, G., Geyer, J., Neff, J., & Koepsell, T. (2001). Deaths attributed to pediatric complex chronic conditions: National trends and implications for supportive care services. *Pediatrics, 107*(6), E99.
15. Feudtner, C., Silveira, M., & Christakis, D. (2002). Where do children with complex chronic conditions die? Patterns in Washington state, 1980–1998. *Pediatrics, 109*(4), 656–660.
16. Fields, A., Coble, D., Pollack, M., & Kaufman, J. (1991). Outcome of home care for technology-dependent, community-based case management model. *Pediatric Pulmonology, 11*(4), 310–317.
17. Garwick, A., Kohrman, C., Wolman, C., & Blum, R. W. (1998). Families' recommendations for improving services for children with chronic conditions. *Archives of Pediatrics and Adolescent Medicine, 152*(4), 440–448.
18. Gilgoff, R., & Gilgoff, I. (2003). Long term follow up of home mechanical ventilation in young children with spinal cord injuries and neuromuscular conditions. *Journal of Pediatrics, 142,* 476–480.
19. Gordon, J., Colby, H., Bartelt, T., Jablonski, D., Krauthoefer, M., & Havens, P. (2007). A tertiary care–primary care partnership model for medically complex and fragile children and youth with special health care needs. *Archives of Pediatric and Adolescent Medicine, 161*(10), 937–944.
20. Graf, J., Montagnino, B., Hueckel, R., & McPherson, M. (2008). Pediatric tracheostomies: A recent experience from one academic center. *Pediatric Critical Care Medicine, 9*(1), 96–100.
21. Haffner, J., & Schurman, S. (2001). The technology dependent child. *Pediatric Clinics of North American, 48,* 751–764.
22. Harrigan, R., Ratliffe, C., Patrinos, M., & Tse, A. (2002). Medically fragile pediatric patients: An integrative review of the literature and recommendations for future research. *Issues in Comprehensive Pediatric Nursing, 25,* 1–20.
23. Health Resources and Services Administration, Maternal and Child Health Bureau. (2008). *The National Survey of Children with Special Health Care Needs chartbook 2005–2006.* Rockville, MD: Author.
24. Homer, C., et al. (2008). A review of the evidence for the medical home for children with special health care needs. *Pediatrics, 122*(4), e922–e937.
25. Kingston, R. (2007). Home care of the ventilator dependent child. *Home Health Care Management & Practice, 19*(6), 436–441.
26. Kirk, S., Glendinning, C., & Callery, P. (2005). Parent or nurse? The experience of being the parent of a technology-dependent child. *Journal of Advanced Nursing, 51*(5), 456–464.
27. Koop, C. (1987). *Surgeon General's report: Children with special health care needs—Campaign 87—Commitment to family-centered, coordinated care for children with special health care needs.* Washington, DC: U.S. Department of Health and Human Services.
28. Mahon, M., & Kibirige, M. (2004). Patterns of admission for children with special needs to the paediatric assessment unit. *Archives of Disease in Childhood, 89*(2), 165–169.
29. Marcin, J., Slonim, A. D., Pollock, M. M., & Ruttimann, U. E. (2001). Long-stay patients in the pediatric intensive care unit. *Critical Care Medicine, 29,* 652–657.
30. Matlow, A., Wright, J., Zimmerman, B., Thomson, K., & Valente, M. (2006). How can the principles of complexity science be applied to improve the coordination of care for complex pediatric patients? *Quality and Safety in Health Care, 15*(2), 85–88.
31. McBurney, P., Simpson, K., & Darden, P. (2004). Potential cost savings of decreased emergency department visits through increased continuity in a pediatric medical home. *Ambulatory Pediatrics, 4*(3), 204–208.

32. McPherson M., et al. (1998). A new definition of children with special health care needs. *Pediatrics, 102*(1), 137–140.

33. Mentro, A. (2003). Health care policy for medically fragile pediatric patients. *Journal of Pediatric Nursing, 18*(4), 22.

34. Miles, M., Holditch-Davis, D., Burchinal, M., & Nelson, D. (1999). Distress and growth outcomes in mothers of medically fragile infants. *Nursing Research, 48*, 129–140.

35. Miller, V., Rice, J., DeVoe, M., & Fos, P. (1998). An analysis of program and family costs of case managed care for technology-dependent infants with bronchopulmonary dysplasia. *Journal of Pediatric Nursing, 13*(4), 244–251.

36. Neff, J., & Valentine, J. (2002). Trends in pediatric hospitalization by hospital type and chronic condition status: Washington state 1987–1998. *Academy Health Annual Research Conference.*

37. Newacheck, P., & Halfon, N. (1998). Prevalence and impact of disabling chronic conditions in childhood. *American Journal of Public Health, 88*(4), 610–617.

38. Newacheck, P., Houtrow, A., Romm, D., Kuhlthau, K., Bloom, S., Van Cleave, J., et al. (2009). The future of health insurance for children with special health care needs. *Pediatrics, 123*(5), e940–e947.

39. O'Brien, M., & Wegner, C. (2002). Rearing the child who is technology dependent: Perceptions of parents and home care nurses. *Journal for Specialists in Pediatric Nursing, 7*(1), 7–15.

40. Office of Technology Assessment (OTA). (1987). *Technology-dependent children: Home care vs. home care. A technical memorandum.* Washington, DC: U.S. Congress.

41. Ratliffe, C., Harrigan, R., Haley, J., Tse, A., & Olson, T. (2002). Stress in families with medically fragile children. *Issues in Comprehensive Pediatric Nursing, 25*(3), 167–188.

42. Ray, L. (2002). Parenting and childhood chronicity: Making visible the invisible work. *Journal of Pediatric Nursing, 17*(6), 424–438.

43. Rehm, R., & Bradley, J. (2005). Normalization in families raising a child who is medically fragile/technology dependent and developmentally delayed. *Qualitative Health Research, 15*(6), 808–820.

44. Rempel, G. R., & Harrison, M. J. (2007). Safeguarding precarious survival: Parenting children who have life-threatening heart disease. *Qualitative Health Research, 17*(6), 824–837.

45. Roesler, T., Rickerby, M., Nassau, J., & High, P. (2002). Treating a high risk population: A collaboration of child psychiatry and pediatrics. *Medicine & Health, Rhode Island, 85*(9), 265–268.

46. Trivedi, H., Pattison, N., & Baptista Neto, L. (2010). Pediatric medical home: Foundations, challenges, and future directions. *Child & Adolescent Psychiatric Clinics of North America, 19*(2), 183–197.

47. Watson, D., Townsley, R., & Abbott, D. (2002). Exploring multi-agency working in services to disabled children with complex health care needs and their families. *Journal of Clinical Nursing, 11*, 367–375.

48. Wise, P. (2004). Chronic illness in childhood. In R. Kliegman, R. Behrman, H. Jenson, & B. Stanton (Eds.), *Nelson textbook of pediatrics* (18th ed., pp. 188–191). St. Louis: Saunders.

Management in the Emergency Setting

U.S. emergency departments (ED) reported more than 28 million pediatric patient visits in 2005 (Merrill et al., 2005). The most common reasons for visits among patients aged 15 years and younger were fever, cough, vomiting, earache, and unspecified injury to the head, neck, or face (Pitts et al., 2008; Studdert et al., 2005). Infants younger than 12 months of age were the highest per capita ED population, with a rate of 84.5 visits per 100 infants per year, representing approximately 3.5 million ED visits annually. While 75% of these visits were to general EDs, 9.2% were to pediatric EDs within general hospitals and 14.3% to EDs in pediatric hospitals (Pitts et al.). Taking into account all ambulatory care visits for children 15 years and younger, 75% of these visits were to primary care provider (PCP) offices and 14% to EDs (Studdert et al.).

LEVELS OF CARE

Hospital-based emergency care is provided in a variety of settings with an array of names—emergency room (ER), emergency ward, emergency care, emergency department—reflecting the changes over the last few decades in the depth and breadth of care provided in this arena. Levels of care in an emergency setting can be difficult to define, as there are no generally agreed-upon guidelines.

One widely utilized means of defining levels of care is that of triage. The term "triage" comes from the Old French verb *trier*; it was originally used to refer to the sorting of injured and allocation of resources to battle and disaster victims (Merriam-Webster, 2009). It is used today to refer to the sorting of patients in an emergency department according to the urgency of their need for medical care.

Just as there are no general guidelines for levels of care, so there are no generally agreed-upon definitions of individual levels of triage acuity or the optimal flow within triage. Triage systems are most commonly divided into three, four, or five levels, based on factors such as presenting chief complaint, time to physician evaluation, and resources needed to treat. In 2004, the Emergency Nurses Association (ENA) and the American College of Emergency Physicians (ACEP) issued a joint position statement recommending that triage be based on a valid five-level scale (ENA, 2004b). While a number of five-level triage scales are currently used (e.g., Manchester, Emergency Severity Index, Canadian Triage Acuity Scale), there is no universal agreement on any one triage scale that meets these criteria and there is limited evidence of such a scale's validity with children.

HISTORY

Obtaining an accurate and timely history in the midst of the stress and chaos that are common in the emergency department presents its own unique challenges.

One difficulty is establishing a therapeutic relationship in such a setting. Trust and comfort with the health care professional (HCP) often supports more open and honest communication; the forging of this relationship must be accomplished quickly, as the health history provides 85% of the information an HCP needs to make a diagnosis (Kaufmann, 2009).

The ED health history should focus on the chief complaint, rather than the full, comprehensive history usually obtained in primary care or inpatient settings. Treat the caregiver's concerns as valid, regardless of their nature; assess and treat the patient's pain in a timely manner; refer to the patient by name and not as "him," "her," "them," "your child," or another generic term; and speak directly to the child as appropriate. These strategies will build trust with the caregiver and initiate the therapeutic relationship. Maintaining open, two-way communication while asking the caregiver questions and giving voice to your findings during the examination also help establish trust and elicit the most accurate history possible.

The components of a pediatric history in the emergency department may be organized using any of a number of methods. One that is easy to remember uses the mnemonic CIAMPEDS (Table 14-1) (ENA, 2004a). Another mnemonic that is commonly used is AMPLE, which stands for allergies, medications, past medical history, last meal, event.

Certain situations require a special approach to obtain needed components of the ED health history. One common situation is the need to obtain information from non-English-speaking families. Access to trained translators is essential in these circumstances, as utilization of family members and friends may lead to misunderstanding—either intentional or unintentional—of medical terms. Emergency departments employ numerous means of accessing translation services, including in-house translators, technologic formats such as a Cyracom and the AT&T language line, and a "language bank" of bilingual employees.

Trauma is another situation requiring a unique approach to history taking. In patients with severe traumatic injuries, resuscitation will take priority over the acquisition of the standard ED health history. Concurrent to care, however, an injury-focused health history needs to be completed so that those attending the resuscitation have the information they need for care. A simple mnemonic that can be used is MIVT (see Chapter 38):

M = Mechanism of injury
I = Injuries suspected
V = Vital signs assessment
T = Treatment initiated prior to arrival in the ED (ENA, 2004a)

Children with special health care needs (CSHCN) are another group whose distinctive concerns must be addressed in the acquisition of an ED health history. Such patients will

TABLE 14-1

CIAMPEDS Mnemonic for Obtaining a Pediatric Health History	
Historical Information	**Components and Rationale**
Chief complaint	Reason for the current ED visit.
Immunizations	Patient's immunization status.
Isolation	Recent exposures to communicable diseases and need for isolation.
Allergies	Allergies to food and environmental allergens, including reactions.
Medications	All medications, including prescribed, over-the-counter, herbal, or dietary supplements, including the name, dosage, route, frequency, duration, and most recent dose. Elicit the reason the medication is being given.
Past medical history	Include a birth history for children younger than 2 years of age and children with disabilities.
Parent's impression of child's health	What prompted the ED visit? What is it that the caregiver is most concerned about?
Events surrounding illness or injury	Onset, duration, and progression of symptoms, and any treatments given prior to arrival.
Diet	Time of last oral intake. How has the patient been eating and drinking?
Diapers	Last urine output; last stool if pertinent.
Symptoms associated with illness/injury	Description of the symptoms and any aggravating and alleviating factors.

ED: Emergency department.

have a different baseline than their healthy counterparts. Consequently, it is important to review both their medical record and the perceptions of their caregivers to complete the history. One useful adjunct in the emergency care of CSHCN is the *Emergency Information Form* (available at http://www.aap.org/advocacy/emergprep.htm), which was developed by the American Academy of Pediatrics (AAP) and is supported by many other organizations. This form is designed to be shared with all HCPs the child encounters, and specifies health information particular to the patient's previous medical and surgical history.

Another population requiring a modified approach to history taking is the patient in whom maltreatment is suspected. In these patients, it is often necessary to separate the patient from the caregiver and obtain two independent histories (see Chapter 36).

PHYSICAL EXAMINATION

Conducting a pediatric physical examination in the ED requires altering both the goal and the process normally employed. The goal of the ED physical examination is to accomplish a focused exam of those areas related or potentially related to the chief complaint. A complete exam is not indicated; indeed, it may add unnecessary delay and cost to the visit. In the ED setting, the most important point is to determine whether the condition is *serious versus not serious* and whether the patient *needs treatment versus doesn't need treatment.*

In addition, the usual order of the exam is altered in the ED. Whereas the customary physical examination follows a sequence from head to toe, exams in the ED are best conducted from least invasive to most invasive or painful (invasive as perceived by the pediatric patient). For example, the HCP might observe the patient's breathing pattern, listen to breath sounds, take an oral temperature measurement, and examine the tympanic membranes.

Reassessment is another key component of the physical exam in the ED. In the primary care or inpatient setting, HCPs typically have an established relationship with the pediatric patient and caregivers and a baseline to which the illness state may be compared. In contrast, the only baseline available in the emergency department is the arrival state. Thus frequent reassessment provides the opportunity to compare the patient only to his or her own earlier baseline.

DIFFERENTIAL DIAGNOSIS

Differential diagnoses are most commonly formulated by first considering the statistically most probable conditions, and then narrowing the possibilities down from there. In emergency departments, this entire process is condensed into a brief, intense interval with minimal information and high stakes. A definitive diagnosis is not always possible, or even necessary, in this setting (Garmel, 2005). Sometimes, ruling out any urgent or emergent conditions and determining appropriate disposition provides the best outcome possible for the situation. Thus ED generated differential diagnoses are usually formed on a bifurcated path, with one path being the typical versus the rare, and the other being the "Are there any life threats, and am I missing anything?" path. In general, ED differentials proceed from answering the following questions (Rosen, 1996):

- What is the life threat?
- Does the patient need admission?
- Can the diagnosis be supported by the evidence available?

- What is the most serious diagnosis possible?
- What is the appropriate disposition for the patient?

PLAN OF CARE

Laboratory testing, radiologic testing, and other diagnostic studies such as electrocardiographs (ECGs) are performed to evaluate for the considered diagnoses. Diagnostic studies are also used to determine the disposition for a patient. For instance, while a complete blood count (CBC) revealing a hemoglobin value below the normal range does not provide a definitive diagnosis, it may point to the need for admission and further work-up. The following questions are typically asked when ordering a diagnostic study:

- Will the results of this study change my management?
- Will the results of this study change the disposition of the case?
- Have I done a brief cost–risk–benefit analysis of this study?

Two concerns common to the ED warrant review. The first is "defensive medicine"—that is, the practice of ordering diagnostic studies, therapeutic interventions, or a higher level of care than is warranted in evidence-based practice in an attempt to reduce the incidence of malpractice claims. If a claim is made, defensive medicine is also used to demonstrate to the courts that a high standard of care has been met (Studdert et al., 2005). Answering the three questions previously noted will help the HCP determine whether the reason for the test is diagnostic or defensive. Unfortunately, in today's litigious society, some HCPs feel the need to "prove" that the patient does not have a condition that has already has been negated through a focused history and physical examination. Research has demonstrated, however, that a strong HCP–caregiver therapeutic relationship is a more effective deterrent to expressed intent to file malpractice claims—even more important than extra studies, interventions, or hospital admission ("Bad Rapport with Patients to Blame for Most Malpractice Suits," 1997; Martin, 2008).

The second concern is that of "parental or caregiver request." In one survey, 24% of pediatricians stated that they had changed prescribing habits due to parental request (Kuzujanakis et al., 2003). Out of concern for their child, caregivers may seek or receive medical advice from numerous and often conflicting sources, including extended family, television, and the Internet. This may result in families' self-diagnosing conditions, having unrealistic expectations, and voicing distrust of the HCP if the provider's recommended plan differs from the other advice. While it may be frustrating and time-consuming to clarify with families why a certain request may not be in their child's best interest, remembering that sometimes the care that needs to be provided is education and reassurance, rather than antibiotics, may make these interactions proceed more smoothly.

In the United States, emergency departments must perform screening exams on everyone who presents for treatment, regardless of insurance or specialty fit, under the federal Emergency Medical Treatment and Labor Act (EMTALA). Consequently, pediatric emergency HCPs must have basic educational preparation or continuing education that allows them to treat a myriad number of problems and diverse populations. Seeing a wide variety of problems may result in the need to consult subspecialty services. These consultations do not always need to occur during the ED visit. Some consults, such as the reduction of a fractured extremity, clearly must occur prior to discharge; others, such as follow-up care for a corneal abrasion, may be arranged at a set time after discharge.

PATIENT AND FAMILY TEACHING

Education must be provided to both the pediatric patient and his or her caregivers. Critical components of this education include—at a minimum—knowledge of the disorder for which they sought treatment, the therapeutic management goals, and the risks and benefits of following or not following the management plan. Perhaps the most important aspect of ED discharge instructions is writing them at the appropriate literacy level. In one study, the mean reading ability of discharged patients was found to be at the sixth-grade level, while the average set of printed discharge instructions were actually written at the eleventh-grade level. Physicians also consistently overestimated their patients' understanding of the written instructions (Wei & Camargo, 2000).

Numerous prepackaged ED discharge instruction programs are available to provide materials at the appropriate reading level, such as Logicare and *Emergency Department Patient Discharge Manual* by Beard, Berman, and Somes (2002). Some products are also available in several languages, such as ExitCare. Each of these commercially available discharge instruction products should be reviewed by the HCP to ensure that the discharge teaching is congruent with his or her own practice. Many of these products can be tailored to specific practice patterns.

DISPOSITION AND DISCHARGE PLANNING

Regardless of disposition type, communication with the patient's primary care provider is critical in ensuring appropriate follow-up at the conclusion of the illness episode. Patients admitted to the hospital or transferred to other hospitals may be cared for by providers other than their own; thus a call from the emergency provider to the primary care provider is pivotal. SBAR (Situation–Background–Assessment–Recommendation) is a useful tool for organizing all such communication (Institute for Healthcare Improvement, n.d.).

Follow-up should be planned and not dictated. Telling a family that they need to call a consulting service for a follow-up appointment in 3 weeks does not always result in the intended action. Some families will have good intentions of arranging the follow-up, yet forget to do so; others will find legitimate barriers to such follow-up. Emergency departments may want to investigate and implement strategies that support follow-up for their discharged patients. These strategies may include telephone follow-up calls, a follow-up clinic, or staff who arrange the follow-up visits for the families.

REFERENCES

1. Bad rapport with patients to blame for most malpractice suits. (1997). *University of Chicago Chronicle, 16*(11).

2. Beard, S., Berman, A., & Somes, J. (Eds.). (2002). *Emergency department patient discharge manual.* New York: Aspen Law and Publishing.

3. Emergency Nurses Association (ENA). (2004a). *Emergency nursing pediatric course.* Des Plaines: Author.

4. Emergency Nurses Association (ENA). (2004b). Standardized ED triage scale and acuity categorization: Joint ENA/ACEP statement. Retrieved from http://www.ena.org/SiteCollectionDocuments/Position%20Statements/Standardized_ED_Triage_Scale_and_Acuity_Categorization_-_ENAACEP.pdf

5. Garmel, G. (2005). Approach to the emergency patient. In S. Mahadevan & G. Garmel (Eds.), *An introduction to clinical emergency medicine: Guide for practitioners in the emergency department* (pp. 3–18). New York: Cambridge University Press.

6. Institute for Healthcare Improvement. (n.d.). SBAR technique for communication: A situational briefing model. Retrieved from http://www.ihi.org/IHI/Topics/PatientSafety/SafetyGeneral/Tools/SBARTechniqueforCommunicationASituationalBriefingModel.htm

7. Kaufmann, J. (2009). Health history and physical assessment. In D. Thomas & L. Bernardo, *Core curriculum for pediatric emergency nursing* (pp. 55–70). Des Plaines: Emergency Nurses Association.

8. Kuzujanakis, M., Kleinman, K., Rifas-Shiman, S., & Finkelstein, J. (2003). Correlates of parental antibiotic knowledge, demand, and reported use. *Ambulatory Pediatrics, 3*(4), 203–210.

9. Martin, J. (2008). Physicians practicing defensive medicine to avoid malpractice. Retrieved from www.bidmc.org/YourHealth/HealthResearch Journals.aspx?ChunkIK=93884

10. Merriam-Webster. (2009). *Merriam-Webster online dictionary.*

11. Merrill, C., Owens, P., & Stocks, C. (2005). Pediatric emergency department visits in community hospitals from selected states, 2005. Retrieved from Healthcare Cost and Utilization Project (HCUP): www.hcup-us.ahrq.gov/reports/statbriefs/sb52.jsp

12. Pitts, S., Niska, R., Xu, J., & Burt, C. (2008). *National Hospital Ambulatory Medical Care survey: 2006 emergency department summary.* Retrieved from National Center for Health Statistics: http://www.cdc.gov/nchs/data/nhsr/nhsr007.pdf

13. Rosen, P. (1996). General approach to the emergency patient. In D. Rund, R. Barkin, P. Rosen, & G. Sternbach (Eds.), *Essentials of emergency medicine* (2nd ed., pp. 7–15). St. Louis: Mosby.

14. Studdert, D., Mello, M., Sage, W., DesRoches, C., Peugh, J., Zapert, K., et al. (2005). Defensive medicine among high-risk specialist physicians in a volatile malpractice environment. *Journal of the American Medical Association, 293*(21), 2609–2617.

15. Wei, H., & Camargo, C. (2000). Patient education in the emergency department. *Academic Emergency Medicine, 7*(6), 710–717.

Management in the Inpatient Setting

- Levels of Care
- Pediatric Intensive Care Admission Criteria
- Level I and II Units
- Pediatric Risk of Mortality (PRISM)
- History
- Physical Examination
- Problem Lists

- Differential Diagnosis
- Plan of Care
- Communication Among HCPs
- Presenting During Hospital Rounds
- Transfer or Discharge of the Hospitalized Pediatric Patient
- References

LEVELS OF CARE

Health care professionals (HCPs) in pediatric hospital settings decide on a daily basis whether a child is to be admitted to a medical–surgical unit or a pediatric intensive care unit (PICU). HCPs rely on essential assessment skills to determine the appropriate level of care. The American Academy of Pediatrics (AAP) and the Society of Critical Care Medicine (SCCM) have developed guidelines for admission and discharge criteria for the PICU to help direct these critical decisions (AAP & SCCM, 1999). Changes to the guidelines are made by each institution based on its available resources. For example, some general pediatric oncology units will accept patients who are on low-dose dopamine infusions because nurse-to-patient ratios support their level of care. Other institutions may not have the same capabilities to care for an oncology patient on vasopressor therapy on a general medical–surgical unit and the patient will require admission to a unit that provides higher-acuity care. When possible, adding physiologic parameters (e.g., blood potassium of > 6.0 mEq, fraction of inspired oxygen of 0.5 L/min or greater) provides an objective means of determining the severity of illness and guides the appropriate admission setting for a pediatric patient.

PEDIATRIC INTENSIVE CARE ADMISSION CRITERIA

The guidelines for admission to a PICU are organized by organ system (Table 15-1). Any patient with a condition that is considered life-threatening, potentially life-threatening, or unstable *must* be admitted to the PICU. A patient with a condition that requires special technologic needs, invasive or intense monitoring (e.g., intracranial, arterial,

TABLE 15-1

Summary of the American Academy of Pediatrics and Society of Critical Care Medicine Admission Criteria for the Pediatric Intensive Care Unit	
Respiratory system	Endotracheal intubation or at high risk for potential intubation; progressive upper or lower airway disease with probable respiratory failure; high oxygen requirement (FIO_2 > 0.5); new tracheostomy; acute barotrauma affecting the upper/lower airway; frequent or continuous inhaled medications
Cardiovascular system	Shock; postcardiopulmonary resuscitation; life-threatening arrhythmias; unstable congestive heart failure; congenital heart disease with unstable cardiorespiratory status; following high-risk cardiovascular (CV) procedures; need for arterial, central venous, or pulmonary artery monitoring; temporary cardiac pacing
Neurologic	Seizures unresponsive to therapy or requiring continuous infusion of anti-epileptics; acute or severe alteration in mental status; preoperative neurosurgical conditions with neurological compromise; following neurosurgical procedures requiring invasive monitoring or frequent neurovascular checks; acute meningitis with altered mental status; head trauma with increased intracranial pressure; progressive neuromuscular dysfunction; spinal cord compression; placement of external ventricular drainage device
Hematology/oncology	Exchange transfusions; plasmapheresis; severe coagulopathy; severe anemia leading to cardiorespiratory compromise; severe complications of sickle cell disease; anticipated tumor lysis syndrome; masses threatening the airway, organs, or vital vessels
Endocrine/metabolice	Severe diabetic ketoacidosis; severe electrolyte abnormalities; inborn errors of metabolism with acute deterioration
Gastrointestinal	Significant gastrointestinal bleeding; following foreign body removal via endoscopy; acute hepatic failure
Surgical	Following CV, thoracic, neurologic, otolaryngologic, craniofacial, orthopedic/spine, and organ transplant surgeries; general surgery with cardiorespiratory compromise; multiple trauma; or any surgery with major blood loss
Renal system	Renal failure; unstable patient requiring dialysis or renal replacement therapies; acute rhabdomyolysis
Multisystem and other	Toxic ingestions; multiple-organ dysfunction syndrome; malignant hyperthermia; electrical injury; burns covering >10% of body surface
Special intensive technologic needs	Any condition that requires technologic needs or interventions that exceed a general care unit's abilities

Source: Adapted from Academy of Pediatrics Committee on Hospital Care and Section on Critical Care and Society of Critical Care Medicine Pediatric Section Admission Criteria Task Force, 1999, reaffirmed 2008.

pulmonary artery, central venous pressure monitoring), or therapies that exceed individual patient care unit policies must be admitted to the PICU (AAP & SCCM, 1999). For example, a patient with a newly placed tracheostomy, with or without mechanical ventilation, should be admitted to the PICU; in contrast, a patient with a mature and stable tracheostomy, requiring baseline mechanical ventilation, could be admitted to a lower-acuity unit. The lower-acuity unit may be what was formerly considered an intermediate care unit. Billing for an intermediate care unit and PICU are no longer differentiated, so the distinction of intermediate care unit is becoming extinct.

LEVEL I AND II UNITS

Critical care experts have also created guidelines to distinguish between pediatric critical care services provided by level I and level II units. Level I pediatric intensive care units are equipped to care for the most severely ill patients. These units must have the ability to provide interprofessional care for a wide range of complex illnesses and are often located in a major medical center or within a children's hospital (Rosenberg & Moss, 2004). Level II critical care units may need to temporarily manage severely ill patients until they are stabilized and arrangements are made to transfer them to a level I facility. Well-established relationships with a level I unit are necessary for safe functioning of a level II unit (Rosenburg & Moss). Level II units can care for patients with less complexity or lower patient acuity.

The main differences between level I and level II units relate to staff availability, existence of subspecialties, and in-house presence of physicians. Level II units may not have a full complement of subspecialists and their availability may be limited. Quality of care standards are expected to be the same for both levels of care (Rosenburg & Moss, 2004).

PEDIATRIC RISK OF MORTALITY (PRISM)

The application of pediatric scoring systems has increased over the past 20 years because their use has proven beneficial for those involved with quality improvement (Marcin & Pollack, 2007). Acuity scoring systems measure illness severity, morbidity and mortality, cost of care, and length of stay. One scoring system that is frequently used to predict pediatric mortality is the Pediatric Risk of Mortality (PRISM III) (Marcin & Pollack; Pollack et al., 1996). The PRISM III provides an objective way to assist pediatric critical care professionals with identifying physiologic variables that predict mortality. The PRISM III variables with the greatest predictive value of mortality are low systolic blood pressure, abnormal pupillary reflexes, and altered mental status (Pollack et al.).

HISTORY

A thorough history and physical examination are the foundation of effective clinical decisions. The main goal of gathering a patient history is to obtain accurate and complete information that will guide patient diagnosis and management. Skilled interviewers are efficient and establish a professional and trusting relationship with both the pediatric patient and the caregiver.

A private and quiet environment is ideal for conducting such an interview, but is often unrealistic in the acute care setting. It helps to start with open-ended questions, such as "What made you decide to bring your child into the emergency department (ED) today?" Follow with questions that will elicit more precise and measurable details. Meeting the caregiver's level of understanding, not speaking too fast, avoiding looking at your watch, actively listening, and maintaining the same eye level as the caregiver or patient are helpful tips for ensuring a successful interview. Furthermore, avoid using a surrogate term such as "Mom"; it is more respectful to take the time to learn the caregiver's preferred name (Seidel et al., 2003). A more complete history may be gathered from an adolescent if the patient and the HCP are alone for part of the interview.

Obtaining a thorough health history follows a process that has been widely accepted by health professionals for many years. The history components include the chief complaint, history of present illness, past medical history, medications, allergies, immunizations, travel and contagion exposure, family history, psychosocial history, and spiritual and cultural assessment, and review of systems (Table 15-2). The history-taking process does not need to be rigid and orderly, as long as all the components are covered. Older children and adolescents should have questions directed at them as often as appropriate. It is important to

TABLE 15-2

Health History Components
Chief complaint
History of present illness
Past medical history
Medications
Allergies
Immunizations
Exposures: travel and contagion
Family history
Psychosocial history
Spiritual and cultural assessment
Review of systems

document the relationship of the person who provides the history, as the historian may not be a parent.

CHIEF COMPLAINT

The chief complaint (CC) is a brief statement indicating the reason for seeking health care; it also includes the duration of illness. Directly quoting the patient or caregiver is helpful. The history of present illness is a very detailed evaluation of the circumstances surrounding the chief complaint, including problem onset, duration, severity, effect on daily functioning, exacerbating or relieving factors, and attempted home, alternative, and/or medical therapies.

PAST MEDICAL HISTORY

The patient's past medical history (PMH) elicits information regarding past medical problems, chronic illness, special health care needs, surgical procedures, hospitalizations (including length of stay and level of care received), ED visits, and neonatal/birth history. Collecting a thorough and accurate past medical history might be challenging if the pediatric patient has received care at multiple institutions.

MEDICATION

Soliciting information regarding current and past medication use, integrative medicine and therapies, over-the-counter medications, vitamin/herb use, and prescription therapies allows the HCP to explore attempted therapies that were beneficial or had untoward side effects. Medication dosing, frequency, last time of administration, and length of use should be documented to help determine whether and when the medication may be administered during hospitalization. Often caregivers know only the volume amount and frequency prescribed for a medication; if necessary, the patient's pharmacy can be contacted to obtain further details.

ALLERGIES, IMMUNIZATIONS, AND EXPOSURES

A description of allergies to medications, environmental allergens, and foods, along with the type and severity of a reaction, should also be documented. In addition, immunization status and any adverse reactions require documentation. The HCP will find that patients and caregivers often do not recall exact immunization dates, so this aspect of the history might require further investigation by contacting the primary care provider (PCP).

Every patient should be screened for exposure to contagions and recent travel. If a contagious exposure is suspected, notification of the institution's infectious control department/policies can guide isolation procedures.

FAMILY HEALTH HISTORY

Family health history includes details of the maternal gestational history, the mother's health during pregnancies, the health status of siblings and parents, and death information on closely related relatives. A review of at least two generations is preferable. A genogram, or family pedigree, is a great graphic representation of a family's medical history and can help detect risk for disease inheritance.

PSYCHOSOCIAL HISTORY

The personal and psychosocial history for the pediatric patient explores areas such as school or daycare attendance, developmental milestones, and details about the home environment (e.g., primary caregiver, smokers, pets, stairs, guns, smoke detectors, window guards, violence). Health habits to be discussed include nutrition, exercise, helmet/seat belt use, sunscreen use, elimination patterns, sleep schedules, breast and testicular self-examinations, and dental care. The assessment tool known by the acronym HEADSSS can be useful when gathering an adolescent's pyschosocial history:

- Home environment
- Education and employment history
- Activity involvement
- Drug, alcohol, and tobacco use
- Sexuality and sexual abuse
- Safety issues (including violence and gang involvement)
- Suicide and depression (Duderstadt & Shapiro, 2006)

SPIRITUAL AND CULTURAL ASSESSMENT

Illness may lead to feelings of vulnerability and even thoughts of death in patients and their families. HCP awareness of spirituality and cultural influences helps assure compassionate and holistic care. Inquiring about spiritual, religious, cultural heritage, and/or involvement in a spiritual or religious community can help the HCP understand a patient's background and possible decision-making process. Although spirituality and cultural values can be a great source of strength for patients and their families, the degree of importance varies from patient to patient. The HCP can ask the patient and family how they would like these issues addressed during hospitalization.

REVIEW OF SYSTEMS

The review of systems (ROS) is a detailed review of possible complaints specific to each body system. Areas of inquiry may differ depending on the age of the child. The ROS questions may prompt the patient and caregiver to provide details they might have felt were insignificant, but actually assist with diagnosis. The HCP may discover seemingly unrelated symptoms that did not surface during the rest of the history. In essence, the ROS is a time for investigation. Before concluding with the history, ask the patient and/or caregiver if there is anything else they want to share.

PHYSICAL EXAMINATION

Performing the examination with a young child in the caregiver's lap may decrease anxiety, especially beginning at 6 months of age (Duderstadt, 2006). For their part, school-age and older children will have decreased anxiety if you talk them through every step of the examination. Remember not to offer a choice to the child when there is no choice. For example, do not ask the child if it is okay for you to listen to the lungs, as this is a task that must be completed. Experienced professionals approach the physical examination of a pediatric patient using the quiet to active approach (Duderstadt). Begin the assessment with techniques that require minimal child participation and allow the child to remain quiet. In other words, try to avoid beginning the examination with more invasive procedures that will likely agitate the child. The most practiced order followed is inspection, auscultation, palpation, and percussion. However, flexibility in varying the order of the examination is essential when caring for young children because their activity and anxiety levels are unpredictable.

The sequence of the physical examination is not as important as using a systematic approach that is followed each time the exam is performed. Omitting parts of the assessment for convenience is not in the best interest of the pediatric patient and may lead to misdiagnosis. It is crucial to recognize that in settings such as the ED, the physical examination may be abbreviated to address life-threatening problems. The focus in the ED might be to stabilize a child who is critically ill and transfer him or her safely to the PICU. Hence, the physical examination done in the inpatient unit must be extremely detailed, as an abnormality that may not be obvious in the ED may become more apparent over time. The physical examination approach for a trauma patient is reviewed in detail in Chapter 38.

INSPECTION

Valuable information can be gathered by careful observation or inspection of the patient. For example, a child observed sleeping can appear very comfortable, but may exhibit significantly increased work of breathing when awake and upset. Inspecting a patient thoroughly requires that all body parts are visible at some point during the examination, including a full review of the skin. Adequate light is important when examining a patient to ensure that subtle findings are not overlooked.

AUSCULTATION

Auscultation of heart tones, respiratory sounds, and abdominal sounds is usually minimally disturbing to the child. The best time to hear these sounds is often when the pediatric patient is sleeping. An essential skill for an HCP to acquire is the ability to screen out adventitious sounds. Notably, the close proximity of organs in children leads to sounds from different areas of the chest being heard simultaneously during auscultation (Duderstadt, 2006). Breath sounds, especially if noisy, can mask heart tones. Conversely, a loud and transmittable heart murmur might make it difficult to accurately assess lung sounds.

The bell of the stethoscope can be used to more effectively isolate heart sounds in small children (Duderstadt, 2006). Stethoscopes and any other equipment shared among patients should be thoroughly washed with soap and water or sanitizer between patients. Cloth covers for stethoscopes, although helpful in distracting young children, should be avoided, as they pose a significant risk for infection transmission.

PALPATION

Palpation is a technique used to gather information using the sense of touch. With this assessment method, the HCP uses his or her fingertips to explore various body parts (e.g., lymph nodes, muscles, tissues, body organs, masses) to detect and discriminate temperature, vibration/pulsation, location, size, mobility, and sensitivity or tenderness (Duderstadt, 2006). The examiner begins with light touch and move toward firm pressure.

PERCUSSION

Percussion is an evaluation method that uses the examiner's hand to produce body sounds. The HCP's finger is used to strike the middle finger of the opposite hand, which is in contact with the patient's skin surface. Percussion deciphers the density of body parts, helps define organ borders, and assists with mass and tumor identification. The stomach and intestines are the least dense and generate a resonance sound, while bone produces a very dense, dull sound (Duderstadt, 2006).

ADDITIONAL COMPONENTS OF A PHYSICAL EXAMINATION

The cranial nerve evaluation can be done toward the end of the examination, as it often requires patient cooperation. In addition, cranial nerves II through XII can be grossly assessed by simply observing patients during the interview process. If a cranial nerve appears to be abnormal, then a full, detailed evaluation of all the nerves is necessary. Of course, a patient who sought health care due to a neurological illness requires thorough cranial nerve testing.

Consider a brief genital inspection on every patient at each health care visit, especially to look for any signs of sexual maltreatment (see Chapter 36). The oral and ear examinations are often left to the end of the examination because these assessments are more invasive.

Weight, height, and head circumference should also be plotted for all children on a growth chart. Body surface area (BSA) can be calculated on the pediatric patient by taking the square root of the product of the patient's weight in kilograms times the patient's height in centimeters divided by 3,600 (Table 15-3) (Mosteller, 1987). The BSA is valuable in that it is used to calculate tests such as glomerular function and cardiac index. Many chemotherapy agents and other pharmacotherapies require the BSA for medication dosing.

PROBLEM LISTS

A comprehensive history and physical examination will serve as concrete building blocks for the creation of complete problem lists and differential diagnoses. The most familiar approach to medical decision making stems from the problem-oriented medical record introduced by Dr. Lawrence Weed in 1965 (Schneiderman, 1994). The database (history, background information, physical examination, laboratory findings) directs the formulation of a complete problem list (Schneiderman). Problems can be medical, psychiatric, psychosocial, and educational, and each problem can be rendered active, inactive, or resolved (Schneiderman).

It is helpful if the problem list is numbered and coherent. The listing of problems can begin with birth, such as Down syndrome or prematurity at 30 weeks, to help with organization. Health maintenance should always be included in the problem list. Furthermore, any medication a patient is taking needs to correspond with a problem on the list.

TABLE 15-3

Calculation of Body Surface Area
Body surface area (m²) = ([Height (cm) × Weight (kg)] / 3,600)

Source: Mosteller, 1987.

If a medication does not match a problem on the list, you are either missing a problem or the medication needs to be re-evaluated.

The more complex the patient's illness or injury, the more important it is to maintain an up-to-date problem list. The problem list is an important communication tool for the interprofessional team. A diagnosis may have several minor symptoms that can be grouped as a problem, while major symptoms can be listed separately to promote a sound management plan (Schneiderman, 1994). For example:

1. *Streptococcus pneumoniae* pneumonia with fever and leukocytosis
2. Respiratory failure secondary to problem 1

DIFFERENTIAL DIAGNOSIS

Often the HCP is formulating differential diagnoses the minute the chief complaint is heard (Oski & Oski, 2006). This line of thinking leads to detailed questions throughout the interview geared at those potential diagnoses. A common pitfall for the novice HCP is to have tunnel vision, that is, to focus on only one possible diagnosis. Formulating several potential diagnoses that relate to the chief complaint and physical examination findings avoids missing a diagnosis (Oski & Oski).

At the same time, it is crucial to remember Fulginiti's principle: "Common diseases and conditions occur commonly" (Oski & Oski, 2006, p. 43). Diagnostic decision making can be difficult because a common disease may present with symptoms that are not typical for that particular illness. "A single disorder can produce a wide spectrum of signs and symptoms, and many disorders can produce similar signs and symptoms" (Berman, 2003, p. 2). Consider the most common differential diagnosis first, but do not exclude more rare diagnoses.

Misdiagnosis due to tunnel vision can delay treatment and cause harm to the patient (Oski & Oski, 2006). It is human nature to want to discredit evidence that does not support the most prevalent differential diagnosis, as doing so requires forming new potential diagnoses. Practicing in this mindset will limit diagnostic success. Moreover, a patient's complaints may be due to more than one diagnosis, although a single disease can usually explain most symptoms (Oski & Oski).

An overall statement following the patient's problem list and differential diagnoses addresses the HCP's impression or assessment of the patient's condition. This impression statement includes a brief summary of the patient's significant health history, the active problems and reason for hospitalization, and the most likely etiology for these problems. It also includes whether the pediatric patient's health condition is improving, deteriorating, or stable. An impression is often included during patient care rounds to summarize the presented findings and to help guide the discussion for therapeutic management.

PLAN OF CARE

DIAGNOSTIC STUDIES

A thorough problem list guides initial planning efforts, with a corresponding plan to be developed for each problem (Schneiderman, 1994). Plans are generally categorized as diagnostic, therapeutic, and patient/family education (Schneiderman).

Initial *diagnostic studies* should be directed at the most probable diagnoses. HCPs should be conscientious of the cost of care and do their best to optimize the use of limited resources. When ordering a diagnostic study, consider how the results will influence the plan of care. Will the study (also referred to as a test) confirm a diagnosis, offer prognostic information, or better guide the health care team to the best therapeutic management plan? If the purpose of an ordered study is not specific or does not correlate with the problem list, the necessity of the test should be re-evaluated. It is also important to carefully consider the risks associated with each test (Oski & Oski, 2006).

Even the most skilled HCPs will encounter clinical situations where the appropriate plan of care is uncertain. Thorough evaluation of current literature that relates to the patient's diagnosis can help guide the correct course of therapeutic management.

THERAPEUTIC MANAGEMENT

Be specific when describing each plan so that other members of the health care team will understand the rational for the plan. Often plans have several components, and organizing these elements by type assists with comprehensive management (Schneiderman, 1994). For example, in a seven-year-old patient with suspected pneumonia, the plan might look like this:

Diagnostic: chest radiograph, white blood cell count, respiratory viral screen

Therapeutic management: oxygen via nasal cannula to maintain oxygen saturation at greater than 92%, encourage coughing, deep breathing, and incentive spirometry, cefuroxime IV for 7 days

Educational: provide the family with antibiotic information, teach the patient and family how to use an incentive spirometer, encourage ambulation as able

CONSULTATIONS

"The consultant is expected to offer greater experience and wider perspective in the area of concern" (Lake, 1994, p. 48).

Obtaining consults from subspecialty services may be obvious based on the patient diagnosis and, therefore, the consult may be directed at assisting with therapeutic management. Alternatively, the referring HCP might request a consult to help establish a diagnosis. Consultants also serve to lessen the stress and anxiety of the patient and family when a diagnosis is unknown or uncommon.

It is helpful if the referring HCP formulates specific questions or concerns for the consultant. The HCP also is responsible for preparing the pediatric patient and caregiver for the consultation so the purpose and expectations of the consult are understood (Lake, 1994).

COMMUNICATION AMONG HCPs

Effective communication among HCPs is central to providing the highest level of patient care. Clear and concise communication during an admission or a transport between or within a facility facilitates safe patient care. The pediatric patient's bedside nurse should be an integral part of the discussions involving diagnosis and therapeutic management plans. Improved communication occurs when the transport team caring for the pediatric patient between facilities stays with the patient until the HCP responsible for admitting the patient has evaluated the patient and all questions have been answered. The acronym SBAR describes a commonly used format to communicate crucial patient information during transfer of care:

- Situation
- Background information
- Assessment of the illness and possible etiologies
- Recommendation for further care

Some institutions have added an "I" before SBAR as a reminder to HCPs to introduce themselves to the receiving provider before communicating patient information.

Effective communication with the PCP may prevent health information gaps. Ideally, the PCP should be notified at the time of admission, updated with any changes in patient status, and kept well informed of the hospitalization course prior to discharge.

PRESENTING DURING HOSPITAL ROUNDS

Hospital rounds may be informal or have a structured, organized, interprofessional health care team approach. Regardless, hospital rounds serve as a critical communication tool. During rounds, patient data (e.g., vital signs, laboratory results, physical examination findings) are reviewed, the problem list and impression statement are presented, and a detailed therapeutic plan addressing the problem list is discussed. The plans decided on during rounds guide the patient goals for that day, and sometimes for the week. Despite the acuity of the patient, the goals of returning home and achieving prehospitalization health or better are to be considered during every hospital day. As unexpected changes in patient status occur, the HCP and team consistently re-evaluate the therapeutic plans and goals throughout the patient's hospital stay.

PROFESSIONALISM

An HCP's dress and hygiene will go a long way toward establishing positive first impressions and respectful relationships with patients, caregivers, and other members of the health care team. Clothing and lab coats should be nonrevealing, clean, and unwrinkled. Most positions within hospitals require close-toed shoes for safety reasons. Avoiding gum chewing, visible body piercing and tattoos, and overdone make-up promotes a professional appearance. Dangling or large earrings pose an injury risk for the HCP. Pulling longer hair back and keeping natural fingernails short, clean, and unpolished protects patients from infection risks. Body sprays and perfumes should be avoided, especially when caring for patients with respiratory ailments.

Nametags are visible best on the upper chest. Lanyards hang nametags near the lower abdomen and are difficult to read. They may also hang into patient care spaces, posing a risk for infectious transmission.

Body language that is uninviting, such as arms crossed in front of the chest, slouching, or hands on the hips, can make the HCP appear unapproachable. Additionally, inflammatory statements of any kind hinder effective communication among the health care team members. Opinions must always be expressed in a respectful manner.

The AAP Committee on Bioethics (2007) has developed a statement of principles to guide medical professional behavior when caring for children. The following key points from this statement deserve emphasis:

- Be honest with patients and caregivers at all times.
- Admit when an error has happened.
- Be accountable for your actions.
- Acknowledge your limits and know when to ask for help.
- Always place the patient's well-being first.
- Make a commitment to continued education.

PICU TRANSFER/DISCHARGE CRITERIA AND FOLLOW-UP

There are generally four destination options for a patient who is transferred or discharged from the PICU: a designated medical–surgical care unit, a rehabilitative facility,

a long-term care facility, or home. The AAP and SCCM (1999) guidelines require reversal of the unstable condition that necessitated PICU admission before a patient leaves this unit. A patient is generally ready to transfer out of the PICU when certain criteria are met: stable hemodynamics and respiratory status for several hours; minimal oxygen requirement; no intravenous vasopressor, vasodilator, or antiarrhythmic infusions; hemodynamic catheters and intracranial devices for monitoring are removed; cardiac arrhythmias and seizures are well controlled; chronically ventilated patients have reversal of the unstable physiologic condition and have returned to baseline ventilation; tracheostomies are mature with minimal to moderate suctioning requirements; and dialysis needs are routine (AAP & SCCM, 1999). Patients who were intubated generally need to remain in the PICU 12 to 24 hours following extubation. Overall, the patient interventions required must not exceed the capabilities of the accepting unit or facility (AAP & SCCM). These guidelines are adjusted depending on the facility, as levels of care vary at each institution.

TRANSFER OR DISCHARGE OF THE HOSPITALIZED PEDIATRIC PATIENT

The SBAR tool and a thorough discharge or transfer summary will assist with patient transfer of care and prevent gaps in communication. All patient problems—inactive and active—are to be included in the discharge/transfer summary, along with a detailed plan for future care and follow-up for each problem (Schneiderman, 1994). Follow-up information includes therapeutic management plans and goals, medication instructions including start and completion dates, anticipated future tests, and necessary appointments with the PCP or subspecialists.

REFERENCES

1. American Academy of Pediatrics (AAP), Committee on Hospital Care and Section on Critical Care, & Society of Critical Care Medicine (SCCM), Pediatric Section Admission Criteria Task Force. (1999). Guidelines for developing admission and discharge policies for the pediatric intensive care unit. *Pediatrics, 103*(4), 840–842.
2. American Academy of Pediatrics (AAP) Committee on Bioethics. (2007). Professionalism in pediatrics: Statement of principles. *Pediatrics, 120*(4), 895–897.
3. Berman, S. (2003). Clinical decision making. In *Pediatric decision making* (4th ed., pp. 2–4). Philadelphia: Mosby.
4. Duderstadt, K. G. (2006). Approach to child and adolescent assessment. In *Pediatric physical examination* (pp. 3–10). St. Louis: Mosby.
5. Duderstadt, K. G., & Shapiro, N. A. (2006). Comprehensive information gathering. In K. Duderstadt (Ed.), *Pediatric physical examination* (pp. 33–45). St. Louis: Mosby.
6. Lake, A. M. (1994). The consultation. In F. Oski, C. DeAngelis, R. Feigin, J. McMillan, & J. Warshaw (Eds.), *Principles and practice of pediatrics* (2nd ed., pp. 48–51). Philadelphia: J. B. Lippincott.

7. Marcin, J. P., & Pollack, M. M. (2007). Review of the acuity scoring systems for the pediatric intensive care unit and their use in quality improvement. *Journal of Intensive Care Medicine, 22*(3), 131–140.

8. Mosteller, R. D. (1987). Simplified calculation of body surface area. *New England Journal of Medicine, 317*(17), 1098.

9. Oski, F. A., & Oski, J. A. (2006). Diagnostic process. In J. McMillan, R. Feigin, C. DeAngelis, & D. Jones, Jr. (Eds.), *Oski's pediatrics: Principles and practice* (4th ed., pp. 41–44). Philadelphia: Lippincott Williams & Wilkins.

10. Pollack, M. M., Patel, K. M., & Ruttimann, U.E. (1996). PRISM III: An updated pediatric risk of mortality score. *Critical Care Medicine, 24*(5), 743–752.

11. Rosenberg, D. I., & Moss, M. M., Section on Critical Care and Committee on Hospital Care. (2004). American Academy of Pediatrics and Society of Critical Care Medicine clinical report: Guidelines and levels of care for pediatric intensive care units. *Pediatrics, 114*(4), 1114–1125.

12. Schneiderman, H. (1994). The problem oriented medical record. In F. Oski, C. DeAngelis, R. Feigin, J. McMillan, & J. Warshaw (Eds.), *Principles and practice of pediatrics* (2nd ed., pp. 45–48). Philadelphia: J. B. Lippincott.

13. Seidel, H. M., Ball, J. W., Dains, J. E., & Benedict, G. W. (2003). The history and interviewing process. In *Mosby's guide to physical examination* (5th ed., pp. 1–37). St. Louis: Mosby.

Susan Kuehn and Brittany N. Wall

Management of the Premature Infant in the Pediatric Acute Care Setting

- The Premature Infant
- History and Physical Examination Findings Specific to the Newborn
- Environment of Care

- Selected Problems in the Newborn or Premature Infant
- Planning for Home
- References

THE PREMATURE INFANT

The preterm or premature infant is any infant born prior to 37 weeks' gestational age. Every year, more than 500,00 preterm births occur in the United States, accounting for 12.8% of all live births in this country. Premature birth rates rose by more than 16% between 1996 and 2006 (March of Dimes, 2006). Advances in neonatal care and research continue to markedly improved the survival rates of preterm infants to 97.4% in 2005 (National Center for Health Statistics, 2009). With increasing survival rates, however, have come preterm infants who experience many immediate- and long-term sequelae.

HISTORY AND PHYSICAL EXAMINATION FINDINGS SPECIFIC TO THE NEWBORN

GESTATIONAL AGE

The American Academy of Pediatrics (AAP) recommends that newborns be classified by both gestational age and birth weight (Gomella et al., 2004). The infant's estimated gestational age (EGA) provides insight into expected developmental characteristics, growth patterns, and health risks.

Basic measurements to classify infants are length, weight, and head circumference. Length is measured from crown to heel; normal values are based on gestational age and should be plotted on a standard growth chart (Colson, 2005). Once the infant is plotted on the growth chart, one may determine if the infant is small, appropriate, or large for gestational age.

Regardless of the gestational age of the infant, the preterm neonate may fall into any one of the growth evaluation categories (Table 16-1). Each category is associated with its own set of risk factors and health problems. For example, within the category SGA, there are two subcategories.

The first subcategory, *asymmetrical* SGA, refers to infants whose weight falls below the 10th percentile and who are average in length and head circumference. This set of criteria is also known as "head-sparing" SGA due to the infant's head circumference remaining average for gestational age. Asymmetrical SGA can be caused by bleeding from placental abruption or previa, placental insufficiency, or pregnancy induced hypertension. The second subcategory is *symmetrical* SGA, in which the infant is noted to be uniformly small. Typically, this small size is due to the infant experiencing some type of chronic stressor. Examples of such stressors are chromosomal defects, maternal chronic hypertension, and congenital viral infections.

Conversely, a large for gestational age (LGA) infant is one whose weight is above the 90th percentile for age. Large for gestational age infants are frequently associated with diabetic mothers. Appropriate for gestational age (AGA) infants are those who are at the expected weight, head circumference, and length for their age (Charsha, 1997).

Three methods of determining postnatal gestational age (listed in order of accuracy and usefulness) by physical examination are the following: New Ballard Score (Table 16-2), rapid delivery room assessment, and direct visualization of the anterior vascular capsule of the lens by ophthalmoscope (Gomella et al., 2004).

CORRECTED AGE

Serial evaluation of the premature infant postnatally should use the "corrected age." Corrected age is calculated by subtracting the number of weeks of prematurity from the infant's chronological age. Thus an infant born at 31 weeks would have 9 weeks of prematurity. If the child presents at age 3 months (12 weeks), the corrected age would be 3 weeks. There is no consensus as to when health care

TABLE 16-1

Terms Related to Prematurity Regarding Age and Size

Preterm or premature infant: An infant born prior to 37 weeks of estimated gestational age

Low birth weight (LBW): Birth weight < 2,500 gm (5 lb, 8 oz)

Very low birth weight (VLBW): Birth weight < 1,500 gm (3 lb, 5 oz)

Extremely low birth weight (ELBW): Birth weight < 1,000 gm (2 lb, 3 oz)

Chronologic or birth age: Time since birth

Estimated gestational age (EGA): Approximate time since conception

Corrected gestational age (CGA): Age adjusted to reflect current gestational age from date of birth to present

Postconceptual age (PCA): Weeks gestation + weeks of life

TABLE 16-2

New Ballard Score: Assessment of Gestational Age

NEUROMUSCULAR MATURITY							
SCORE	**-1**	**0**	**1**	**2**	**3**	**4**	**5**
POSTURE							
SQUARE WINDOW (WRIST)	> 90°	90°	60°	45°	30°	0°	
ARM RECOIL		180°	140° - 180°	110° - 140°	90° - 110°	< 90°	
POPLITEAL ANGLE	180°	160°	140°	120°	100°	90°	< 90°
SCARF SIGN							
HEEL TO EAR							

PHYSICAL MATURITY							
SKIN	Sticky, friable transparent	Gelatinous, red translucent	Smooth, pink; visible veins	Superficial peeling and/or rash; few veins	Cracking, pale areas; rare veins	Parchment, deep cracking; no vessels	Leathery, cracked, wrinkled
LANUGO	None	Sparse	Abundant	Thinning	Bald areas	Mostly bald	**MATURITY RATING**
PLANTAR SURFACE	Heel - toe 40-50mm -1 < 40 mm: -2	> 50mm, no crease	Faint red marks	Anterior transverse crease only	Creases anterior 2/3	Creases over entire sole	Score / Weeks: -10 / 20; -5 / 22
BREAST	Imperceptible	Barely perceptible	Flat areola, no bud	Stippled areola, 1-2mm bud	Raised areola, 3-4 mm bud	Full areola, 5-10mm bud	0 / 24; 5 / 26; 10 / 28
EYE/EAR	Lids fused loosely: -1 tightly: -2	Lids open; pinna flat; stays folded	Slightly curved pinns; soft; slow recoil	Well curved pinna; soft but ready recoil	Formed and firm, instant recoil	thick cartilage; ear stiff	15 / 30; 20 / 32; 25 / 34
GENITALS (MALE)	Scrotum flat, smooth	Scrotum empty, faint rugae	Testes in upper canal, rare rugae	Testes descending, few rugae	Testes down, good rugae	Testes pendulous, deep rugae	30 / 36; 35 / 38; 40 / 40
GENITALS (FEMALE)	Clitoris prominent, labia flat	Clitoris prominent, small labia minora	Clitoris prominent, enlarging minora	Majora and minora equally prominent	Majora large, minora small	Majora cover clitoris and minors	45 / 42; 50 / 44

MATURITY RATING

Score	Weeks
-10	20
-5	22
0	24
5	26
10	28
15	30
20	32
25	34
30	36
35	38
40	40
45	42
50	44

Dilation and tortuosity of the veins and arterioles; may be present at any stage of ROP. Associated with Rapid progression and unfavorable outcomes.

Source: Ballard, J., Khoury, J., & Wedig, K., et al: New Ballard score, expanded to include extremely premature infants. The Journal of Pediatrics, 119(3), 417–423, 1991; Used with permission by Elsevier Limited.

professionals (HCPs) should stop using the corrected age, but many continue to adjust the child's age until the patient is 2 years old.

HISTORY

Historical information should include maternal/obstetric data (e.g., gravida, para, spontaneous and therapeutic abortions, maternal infections, sexually transmitted infections, any therapies, medications, acute/chronic disorders, mental health) and labor and delivery data (e.g., APGAR scores, infant resuscitation, therapies, medications). The past medical, family, and psychosocial history includes information as to genetic or prevalent diseases within the family.

PHYSICAL EXAMINATION

Vital signs

Temperature. No single environmental temperature is appropriate for all sizes, gestational ages, and conditions of preterm infants. However, the optimal temperature range should be between 36.5 and 37.5°C (97.7–99.5°F) (World Health Organization [WHO], 1997).

The WHO defines three categories of hypothermia and two categories of hyperthermia:

Hypothermia:

- *Cold stress* of 36.0–36.4°C (96.8–97.5°F) is cause for concern. Warm the infant and identify the cause(s); check equipment and temperature probe function.
- *Moderate hypothermia* of 32.0–35.9°C (89.6–96.6°F) requires immediate rewarming of the infant.
- *Severe hypothermia* < 32.0°C (< 89.6°F) requires urgent resuscitation; the prognosis is grim (WHO, 1997).

Hyperthermia:

- *Hyperthermia* > 37.5°C (99.5°F) is cause for concern. Identify the cause(s); suspect and assess for infection; check equipment and temperature probe function.
- *Severe Hyperthermia* > 40°C (104°F) requires a tepid water bath (the water temperature should be 2°C [3.6°F] cooler than infant's body temperature); maintain hydration.

To prevent hypothermia or hyperthermia, the infant's skin and axillary temperatures should be monitored continuously. The premature infant usually gains the ability to regulate his or her own body temperature at around 34 weeks' gestation.

Heart rate. Typically, the resting heart rate is in the range of 100–170 beats/min. The infant's rate varies with changes in activity as well as chronologic age. Average heart rate at birth is 141 beats/min at birth, 171 beats/min at 2 months of age, and approximately 142 beats/min at 1 year of age (Trachtenberg & Golemon, 1998). The cardiac rhythm should be regular, with the exception of an occasional premature atrial or ventricular contraction, which is not uncommon.

Respiratory rate. Normal respiratory rate is in the range of 40–60 breaths/min. Infants are primarily nose breathers whose breathing pattern is *normally* irregular and periodic. For example, the preterm infant may have a regular rate for a minute or so and then a period of time (5–10 seconds) where no respirations occur. However, if the infant experiences a drop in the heart rate and any cyanotic color changes with a pause in respiration for more than 15–20 seconds, this condition is abnormal and is known as apnea of prematurity (AOP). AOP is related to immaturity of the central respiratory center and most often occurs in preterm infants born before 34 weeks' gestation (Balaraman, 2003). AOP is treated with methylxanthines; caffeine and theophylline are the most commonly used medications. If the infant has several episodes of apnea, new apneic episodes, or apnea with clinical deterioration, consider sepsis in the differential diagnosis. Signs of respiratory distress other than AOP include tachypnea, grunting, nasal flaring, retractions, and increased oxygen requirements.

Blood pressure. As many as 50% of all very low birth weight (VLBW) neonates receive treatment for low blood pressure; however, there is no consensus regarding the actual definition of hypotension in the neonate. A point of reference accepted by some clinicians is the recommendation by the Joint Working Group of the British Association of Perinatal Medicine, which states that the mean arterial blood pressure (MBP) should be maintained at a level (in mmHg) equal to or greater than the gestational age (in weeks) of the infant during the first day of life (Taeusch, 2005). For example, a mean blood pressure of 28 mmHg or greater would correlate with a 28-week infant. Birth weight, gestational age, and postconceptional age are significant determinants in blood pressure of the LBW infant (Zubrow et al., 1995). Blood pressure typically increases with increasing gestational age, weight, and postnatal age during the first week of life (Leflore et al., 2000).

The normal physiologic blood pressure range that ensures adequate organ perfusion is unknown (Short et al., 2006). Therefore, include hypotension as a differential diagnosis when any of the following clinical features are evident in a neonate in conjunction with a questionable adequate blood pressure: tachypnea, tachycardia, bradycardia, mottling of the skin, prolonged capillary refill time, cool extremities, or decreased urine output. Factors that may affect the blood pressure include blood loss, route of delivery (vaginal or cesarean section), asphyxia, patent ductus arteriosus (PDA), and apnea (Engle, 2001). There is great variation in the approach to treatment of hypotension. For example, management may include observation, blood products, colloid or crystalloid fluid replacements, inotropic support, or corticosteroids (Engle).

Hypertension, or a higher than expected blood pressure, occurs in the neonate when the systolic or diastolic blood pressure is sustained more than two standard deviations above the mean values (95% or greater). However, this definition is more frequently applied to the term infant than to the preterm infant. Etiologies of hypertension in neonates include congenital or acquired renovascular disease or volume overload; this condition may be seen in as many as 3% of all neonatal intensive care admissions. Infants may be asymptomatic or symptomatic, depending on the severity of the blood pressure increase. Signs of hypertension include feeding difficulties, unexplained tachypnea, irritability, and hematuria. Management may include observation, fluid restriction, beta blockers, angiotensin-converting enzyme inhibitors, calcium-channel blockers, and diuretics (Fanaroff & Fanaroff, 2006).

The optimal method of blood pressure measurement for the premature infant is via an umbilical or peripheral arterial catheter. This is a direct invasive measurement, which provides for continuous monitoring. The HCP can also measure blood pressure noninvasively by using oscillometric techniques with an appropriate-size cuff that is placed around the infant's arm or leg (Engle, 2001). If possible, it is desirable to obtain four extremity blood pressures within the first 24 hours of life to assess for aortic obstruction. If there is a 15–20 mmHg differential between the upper and lower extremities, coarctation of the aorta should be suspected.

Environment

Take care to keep the infant warm during assessment. Use radiant heat or an incubator with skin probes to maintain constant body temperature as previously described. Expose only parts of the infant's body needed for assessment to reduce cold stress. Prevent direct light from shining in the infant's face, minimize stimulation as much as possible, and perform assessment tasks in order from least to most invasive.

Central nervous system

Early in gestation, the infant's resting posture is hypotonic. Flexion and hip adduction increases with increasing gestational age. However, a frog-leg position noted after 36 weeks' gestation is abnormal (Verklan & Walden, 2003).

Most spontaneous movements occur during active sleep and are very primitive in nature. Due to the immaturity of the nervous system, one may observe jerky, irregular, tremulous activity of the premature neonate. In the awake state, the preterm infant may exhibit random stretching movements, which may be bilateral or asynchronous. Deep tendon reflexes are present, but less active in preterm infants (Pursley & Henry, 2008).

Skin

Transparency of the skin and visibility of the veins increase with decreasing gestational age. The 26-week gestation infant has –three to six layers of skin, as compared to the 16 layers of skin observed in the term infant. Note the presence of lanugo (fine, downy hair) and vernix caseosa (white, "cheese-like" matter from sebaceous gland secretions and skin cells), as it will be more abundant with decreasing gestational age. Plantar creases first appear on the anterior portion of the foot between 28 and 30 weeks' gestation and extend toward the heel as gestational age progresses. Note any signs of jaundice: This condition occurs in as many as 80% of preterm infants, progresses cephalocaudally, and peaks at days 5–6 of life; its presence within the first 24 hours after birth is abnormal (Verklan & Walden, 2003). Total and direct serum bilirubin levels should be monitored carefully within the first 2 weeks of life (see Chapter 26).

Head

Palpate sutures and the anterior/posterior fontanel (overriding sutures may be present for more than 1 week in the extremely low birth weight [ELBW] infant). Evaluate for fused eyelids, which normally open spontaneously between 26 and 30 weeks' gestation. Assess ear formation and the amount of pinna cartilage. Prior to 34 weeks' gestation, little cartilage exists, and the ear has a tendency to stay folded on itself. At 36 weeks' gestation, some cartilage is present and the pinna rebounds when folded and released. Inward curving of the upper pinna usually begins by 34 weeks (Verklan & Walden, 2003). Evaluate the mouth and note the development of the suck and swallow reflex, which is usually complete between 32 and 34 weeks. The rooting reflex is well established by 32 weeks. At 34 weeks' gestation, the infant may have the ability to tolerate full oral feedings (Pursley & Henry, 2008).

Chest/thorax

The preterm infant's rib margins will likely be apparent due to the thinner layers of muscle and decreased subcutaneous fat noted in such neonates compared to term infants (Verklan & Walden, 2003). Evaluate the breasts; breast buds will be imperceptible in the extremely premature infant and will be more noticeable with advancing gestational age. Full-term infants have a stippled or raised areola with bud measuring 1 to 4 mm (Ballard et al., 1991).

Abdomen and genitalia

Inspect the umbilical cord, which normally contains two arteries and one vein. In more than 20% of those infants with a single artery, associated congenital anomalies are present (Thummula et al., 1998). In females, the clitoris is prominent, with small, widely separated labia. The testes of the male preterm infant begin to descend at 28 weeks' gestation and can be palpated high in the scrotum at 37 weeks' gestation (Verklan & Walden, 2003).

ENVIRONMENT OF CARE

THERMOREGULATION

In the womb, the fetus prepares for its arrival to the outside world by storing glycogen, producing catecholamines, and depositing brown adipose fat in the third trimester. "Brown fat" is highly vascular and appears only in infants. This type of fat, which is first noted between 26 and 30 weeks' gestation, is metabolized for heat production. The immature, preterm infant has little time to prepare prior to delivery and does not fully complete these processes.

At birth, rapid environmental cooling ensues, with the infant's body temperature decreasing at a rate of 0.2–1.0°C per minute. If there is a 20°C (36°F) difference between the intrauterine and extrauterine environment, the failure rate for a preterm infant to successfully adapt from the fetal state of warmth to the outside environment without intervention is high (Aylott, 2006). When the rate of heat loss exceeds the rate of heat production and heat retention is at a minimum, the neonate's body temperature falls. To compensate for this condition, the infant tries to minimize heat loss by peripheral vasoconstriction and encourage heat production by increasing metabolism and the oxidation of brown fat—a process known as nonshivering thermogenesis. If the infant is not successful, hypothermia occurs. The signs and symptoms vary according to the level of severity, but the infant typically exhibits acrocyanosis, cool extremities, decreased peripheral perfusion, apnea, bradycardia, lethargy, irritability, poor feeding, hypoglycemia, metabolic acidosis, decreased cardiac output, and increased oxygen requirements. The preterm infant is at a greater risk of hypothermia due to low birth weight, SGA status, immature skin and central nervous system function, greater body water content, a large surface area-to-body mass ratio, decreased brown fat, and primitive and insufficient metabolic response to thermal stress (Aylott, 2006; Hawdon, 2006; Short, 2008).

Although it is less common, hyperthermia can occur just as easily as hypothermia and is just as dangerous. Its clinical presentation may include increased oxygen consumption (secondary to increased metabolic rate), tachycardia, tachypnea, irritability, dehydration, acidosis, and lethargy (WHO, 1997). Initially, the HCP should determine whether the cause of the infant's elevated body temperature is due to excessive environmental temperature or increased endogenous heat production, such as is noted with infection. To verify environmental temperature, note the temperature reading and mode of the incubator or radiant warmer, and ensure that there are no loose or nonfunctioning temperature probes. If the infant has a "true fever" due to infection, one would expect a low incubator air temperature as well as the child's extremities being cool to touch secondary to peripheral vasoconstriction. In all cases of hyperthermia, the HCP should examine the infant for infection. Other interventions include hydration (with intravenous or oral fluids), removal of some layers of clothing or blankets, a tepid bath, or the administration of acetaminophen (Gomella et al., 2004).

The ultimate goal of thermoregulation is to maintain the infant in a neutral thermal environment (NTE). NTE is defined as one in which the infant can maintain the peripheral and core body temperature with minimal changes in oxygen consumption and metabolic need. In addition, this environment facilitates growth and development (White, 2000). Four basic mechanisms of heat exchange with the environment exist: conduction, convection, radiation, and evaporation (Figure 16-1). For the neonate, much heat is lost during physical examinations, bathing, and weighing. To counteract this possibility, use radiant heat sources, keep port holes closed on incubators, warm scales, and keep infants dry to reduce heat loss.

ELBW infants born at 25 weeks' gestation lose 15 times more water through their skin from insensible loss than term infants, due to immaturity of the preterm infant's skin. Use of an incubator with a humidity level of 50% or greater will minimize the insensible or transepidermal water loss. Body temperature is critical to regulating cellular function; thus successfully maintaining the preterm infant in a NTE will improve clinical outcomes, ultimately increasing the infant's likelihood of survival (Soll, 2008).

PERCEPTION OF PAIN

Until the late 1980s, the health care community had a long history of denying that the infant—and especially the preterm infant—was able to perceive pain because of the immaturity of the central nervous system (Walden & Carrier, 2009). Other myths associated with neonates suggested that they had no memory of pain, objective assessment of pain was impossible, analgesia could not be administered safely,

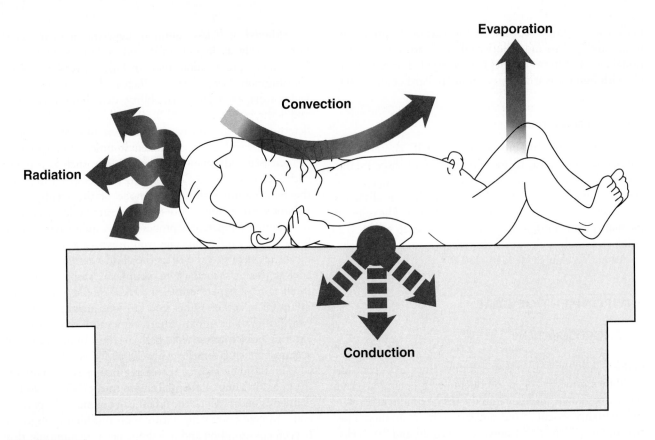

FIGURE 16-1

Four Ways a Newborn May Lose Heat to the Environment.

Source: Used with permission. Courtesy of World Health Organization. (1997). Thermal Protection of the Newborn: A Practical Guide.

and the infant experiencing it could not communicate pain. Pain is formally defined as "an unplanned sensory and emotional experience associated with actual or potential tissue damage, or described in terms of such damage" (Merskey & Bagduk, 1994). With admission to an intensive care unit, an infant experiences many medically necessary diagnostic and therapeutic procedures that are painful—on average, 14 procedures per day (Walden & Gibbins, 2008).

The neonate's nervous system begins to develop early in gestation and continues to mature after delivery. Although differences in pain responses are observed related to gestational age and development of the cortex, even the very premature infant shows behavioral and physiological reactions and hormonal stress responses to painful stimuli. Behavioral indicators of pain include facial expression (e.g., brow bulge, eye squeeze, nasolabila furrow, open mouth), body movement (posture and tone), cry, behavioral state, consolability, and skin color. Physiologic indicators include variation in heart rate, blood pressure, respiratory rate, oxygen saturation, skin color, and palmar sweating.

Since 1992, at least 16 pain tools have been introduced as means to assess and guide pain management in the neonatal population. The most frequently used of these instruments

are the Neonatal Infant Pain Scale (NIPS), the Premature Infant Pain Profile (PIPP), the Crying, Requires oxygen, Increased vital signs, Expressions, Sleepless (CRIES) tool, and the Neonatal Pain, Agitation, and Sedation Scale (NPASS). These tools typically incorporate a combination of behavioral and physiologic indicators to assess pain.

Regardless of the tool used for assessment, education and a consistent interprofessional team approach to pain management of neonates is important. Pain experienced in the intensive care unit can be viewed as acute procedural pain, acute prolonged pain, or chronic pain; these forms may occur either separately or simultaneously.

Both pharmacologic and nonpharmacologic methods of pain management should be utilized in the intensive care unit, with the most appropriate approach depending on the situation. Nonpharmacologic interventions should be used to minimize an infant's pain and stress and increase the child's coping and regulatory abilities; pharmacologic interventions should be used to treat moderate to severe pain. Nonpharmacologic methods of pain management include swaddling, positioning for self-comforting behavior (hand to mouth), modifying the environment (decreasing light and noise), containment, non-nutritive sucking, facilitated tucking, skin-to-skin contact (kangaroo care), and breastfeeding. Pharmacologic interventions include the use of anesthetic agents (EMLA cream, lidocaine), nonsteroidal anti-inflammatory drugs (acetaminophen, ibuprofen), and opioid analgesics (morphine, fentanyl). Oral sucrose is an inexpensive intervention that is thought to modulate transmission or processing of nociception by mediating the release of endogenous opioids. The safety and efficacy of oral sucrose in infants of less than 27 weeks' gestation has not been established, however, and its administration should be considered on a case-by-case basis.

Both short-term pain and long-term pain have consequences for the neonate. Short-term consequences include decreased oxygen saturation, increased heart rate, increased intracranial pressure (increasing the risk of intraventricular hemorrhage), and depression of the immune system (increasing the risk of infection). Long-term effects include failure to activate or delay in the stress response, elevated basal cortisol levels, and altered tactile sensation.

Parents naturally have concerns and fears about their infants experiencing pain. Education should focus on teaching them which cues their infant displays when stressed or in pain, which medications are being given and why, and why pain management for their infant is important. Involving caregivers in the care of their infants fosters the parent–infant relationship. Allowing parents to voices their concerns is vital, and recognition of cultural and religious needs will also help to promote their comfort with caregivers.

DEVELOPMENTAL CARE

Developmental care of the preterm infant is a philosophy that takes into consideration the environment required to provide optimal intensive care as well as fulfillment of the mental and physical needs of the infant. The goal of developmental care is to assist growth and foster development of the infant as a whole being without promoting instability or signals of stress.

Positioning

Compared to term newborns, preterm infants have immature physiologic flexion of the extremities, trunk, and pelvis. Therefore, extension of the limbs dominates unless the infant is provided with external support to maintain a developmentally appropriate flexed posture. Supportive devices and techniques include nesting, bumpers, containment devices, and swaddling. Without the necessary positioning support, preterm infants are at risk for developing an abnormal head shape, increased neck extension, scapular adduction, shoulder retraction, external hip rotation and abduction, and eversion of the ankles and feet. Goals of proper positioning include maintaining neutral alignment of the head and trunk and providing a variety of positions in response to the infant's current behavioral state. Consultation with a physical therapist, if available, is encouraged to help facilitate these positions.

Clustering of care

Ensuring prolonged periods of minimal stimulation and providing undisturbed rest and sleep is essential for the preterm infant. Infants and children between 28 weeks' gestation and 3 to 4 years of age rely on preservation of sleep cycles to build sensory systems and preserve brain plasticity, which is the preservation of the capacity to change, adapt, and learn in response to environmental experiences and new needs.

REM sleep—which has been referred to as "a period of maximal brain activity"—is a critical component of the sleep cycle for the neonate. Sensory systems that require REM sleep for normal development include somatesthetic (touch), kinesthetic (motion), proprioception (position), chemosensory (smell and taste), auditory (hearing), vision, limbic, social learning, and hippocampal (memory). The hippocampus processes learned behaviors, information, and creates long-term memories throughout an entire sleep cycle. In the absence of a complete sleep cycle, such as occurs with sleep deprivation, the sensory experiences remain in short-term memory, most of which is ultimately lost.

The ultimate goal, then, is the coordination or "clustering" of care by the interprofessional team in conjunction with the family to provide the infant with a comfortable, protective environment that allows for organized sleep patterns and facilitates development of the brain and sensory systems.

Modification of external stimuli

In keeping with the desire to promote organized sleep patterns, HCPs should monitor the infant's cues in response to the surrounding environment. Premature infants are able to communicate signs of stability and stress via the autonomic, motor, and state-related systems (Engle, 2006). Physiologic stress cues include changes in heart rate, respiratory rate, apnea, grunting, gasping, cyanosis, and decreased blood oxygen level. Behavioral cues that indicate stress in the premature infant include hiccupping, gaze aversion, finger splaying, vomiting, crying, fussing, tongue protrusion, yawning, and facial grimace. The neonate may also demonstrate a variety of self-consoling behaviors, which facilitate the coping response to stress. These behaviors include sucking, bringing the hands to the face, grasping of linens or the child's own body parts, and hand or foot bracing.

The presence of these cues warrant investigation by HCPs and steps to assess and modulate the environment. Examples of environmental measures to ensure a nurturing atmosphere include use of isolette covers, dim lighting, cycled lighting, and background noise level of 50 dB or less. Everyone in the infant's environment should keep the voice level down at the bedside, abstain from writing and placing equipment on top of isolettes, and take care in opening and closing port holes and trashcans. Developmentally appropriate tactile and sensory stimulation improves short-term growth outcomes and results in a shorter length of hospital.

SELECTED PROBLEMS IN THE NEWBORN OR PREMATURE INFANT

INTRAVENTRICULAR HEMORRHAGE

Pathophysiology

In premature infants, intraventricular hemorrhage (IVH) occurs first in the subependymal germinal matrix at the head of the caudate nucleus near the foramen of Monro. Immature and fragile blood vessels in the premature infant's brain begin to hemorrhage, with bleeding potentially continuing through the ependymal lining and into the lateral ventricle. Such hemorrhages are termed periventricular–intraventricular hemorrhages (PIVH). PIVH is classified by the location and severity of the hemorrhage:

Grade I: Isolated germinal matrix hemorrhage
Grade II: Intraventricular hemorrhage without ventricular dilation
Grade III: Intraventricular hemorrhage with ventricular dilation
Grade IV: Intraventricular hemorrhage with ventricular dilation and hemorrhage into the parenchyma of the brain

Epidemiology and etiology

Any perinatal or neonatal event that results in hypoxia, an alteration in cerebral blood flow, or an alteration in intravascular pressure increases the risk for PIVH. Some examples are occipital pressure, crying, hypoxia, and hypercapnia. Approximately 50% of hemorrhages in premature infants occur within the first 24 hours of life. and 90% of infants with IVH bleed within the first 72 hours after birth. Overall, the incidence of IVH ranges from 15% to 20% in premature infants weighing less than 1,500 grams at birth.

Presentation

Manifestations of IVH are often nonspecific and subtle. The clinical signs that are most closely correlated with evidence of IVH by CT scan include changes in activity level or tone, a full anterior fontanel, a decreased hematocrit level, and the inability of the hematocrit to rise following a blood transfusion. The diagnosis of PIVH is often made by cranial ultrasonography.

It is imperative that preterm infants be monitored closely for IVH. Serial cranial ultrasounds are essential for accurate and reliable detection of ischemia, hemorrhage, or brain damage. By performing serial screenings, the HCP can identify not only the evolution of present lesions, but also determine the times when they occurred. Many acute care units have established specific guidelines regarding when to obtain serial ultrasounds for premature infants: For example, the first head ultrasound may be performed within the first 24 hours of life; the second ultrasound may be performed on the third day of life; and a third ultrasound is performed on the seventh day of life. Almost all hemorrhages will be detected, and their maximum extent identified, during this time. If a lesion or hemorrhage is identified, sequential ultrasounds are necessary throughout the neonatal period to assess evolution and resolution over an extended period.

Plan of care

Extension of a hemorrhage occurs in 20% to 40% of cases; posthemorrhagic hydrocephalus occurs in 10% to 15% of all preterm infants with PIVH. The type of treatment depends on the ventricular size, intracranial pressure, and rate of progression. If hydrocephalus progresses, a ventriculoperitoneal shunt is often placed. However, because of the high risk of infection and the high rate of failure when a shunt is placed too early, temporizing measures are often employed first, until the infant is deemed ready for shunt placement. These measures can range from use of medications that decrease the production of cerebrospinal fluid (CSF), to serial lumbar punctures to drain CSF, to placement of an external ventricular drain.

Risk prevention

The morbidity and mortality rates with IVH correlate most directly with the degree of parenchymal damage the infant has endured. Prevention is the best treatment. Many types of stresses to premature infants put them at higher risk for PIVH. Therefore, the interprofessional team must work together to minimize risks. Measures to reduce the risk of PIVH include the following:

- Maintain temperature within a neutral thermal environment.
- Avoid rapid fluid infusions. If sodium bicarbonate is necessary, give a dilute solution slowly.
- Monitor blood pressure closely—any fluctuating pattern of arterial pressure could be cause for concern.
- Minimize suctioning, which can increase cerebral blood flow velocity and reduce oxygenation.

RETINOPATHY OF PREMATURITY

Pathophysiology

Blood vessels in the retina begin to develop at approximately 14 to 16 weeks' gestation and complete development at approximately 40 to 44 weeks gestation. When the infant is premature, the development or vascularization of the blood vessels in the retina is incomplete (Askin & Diehl-Jones, 2009). Vascular growth will continue, however, in the retinal bed after the infant's birth. Abnormal vascular growth in the retinal bed of a premature infant is known as retinopathy of prematurity (ROP). If the infant is not screened and treated quickly, he or she will likely have visual impairment and/or vision loss.

Epidemiology and etiology

The risk of developing ROP is inversely proportional to the gestational age of the infant at birth; thus, the more premature the infant, the higher the risk for ROP. Of infants who weigh less than 1,251 grams at birth, 66% to 68% go on to develop ROP. By comparison, 90% to 93% of infants who weigh less than 750 grams at birth develop this condition.

Since the 1950s, there has been an increasing awareness of the association between exposure to high concentrations of oxygen and the development of ROP. Normally, when the infant is in the womb, PaO_2 averages 30 mmHg with a saturation level of 70%. This hypoxic environment *stimulates* the production of two growth factors: vascular endothelial growth factor (VEGF) and insulin-like growth factor 1 (IGF-1). VEGF has been found in the retinal bed of the eye where new blood vessels are growing. These vessels grow more slowly without IGF-1. When the infant is born, it transitions from an environment of hypoxia to hyperoxia (in room air, PaO_2 is in the range of 60–100 mmHg), which in turn *suppresses* the secretion of VEGF. This effect leads to cessation of normal vessel growth, vasoconstriction of immature retinal vessels, and the demise of newly developed capillaries. VEGF levels remain low until further growth in the retinal bed results in a localized area of hypoxia, thereby increasing the levels of growth factor (Askin & Diehl-Jones, 2009; Pollan, 2009).

Although the results of research studies have helped to explain the pathogenesis of ROP, many questions related to this condition remain unanswered. The single greatest risk factor for the development of ROP is prematurity. The list of associated risk factors for ROP is ever changing, but includes growth restriction, varied levels of carbon dioxide, surfactant therapy, postnatal steroid use, blood transfusions, IVH, sepsis, dopamine administration, birth weight, and severity of illness (Askin & Diehl-Jones, 2009).

Presentation

In 2006, the AAP, in conjunction with the Academy of Ophthalmology (AO) and the American Association for Pediatric Ophthalmology and Strabismus (AAPOS), released screening guidelines for ROP. All examinations should be performed by an ophthalmologist, with timing of the initial exam based on the infant's gestational age at birth and postnatal age:

- All infants with birth weight of less than 1,500 grams or less than 32 weeks' gestational age
- Infants with a birth weight in the range of 1,500–2,000 grams with a history of unstable clinical course and deemed to be "high risk" by the HCP

Indirect ophthalmoscopy or digital images are most often used to perform this assessment; these techniques require dilation of the pupils. The presence of ROP is graded based on three zones of disease and five stages of abnormal vascular development (Figure 16-2). Zone I involvement is most concerning, owing to a greater chance of retinal detachment occurring secondary to the presence of extensive scar tissue in this location. The specific area affected in the identified zone is described by how many clock hours of the eye's circumference are affected. Stages of ROP are described in varying degrees of severity (Table 16-3), with 1 being the least severe and 5 being the most severe (Askin & Diehl-Jones, 2009; International Committee for the Classification of Retinopathy of Prematurity, 2005).

ROP may regress gradually without any need for surgical intervention. The AAP, AO, and AAPOS (2006) guidelines recommend intervention when ROP meets the following criteria: zone I ROP at any stage when plus disease is present, stage 3 ROP in zone I in the absence of plus disease, or stage 2 or 3 ROP in zone II with plus disease.

Plan of care

For many years, the cornerstone surgical treatment for ROP was cryotherapy, which uses a liquid nitrogen probe to destroy the avascular "scar" tissue. More recently, it has been noted that cryotherapy causes more inflammation and discomfort than laser surgery; consequently, laser surgery is now the first-line surgical procedure for ROP (Askin & Diehl-Jones, 2009). If the retina has detached, however, laser therapy is ineffective and a vitrectomy or a scleral buckle (SB) must be performed. A vitrectomy involves removal of the scar tissue, which allows the retina to reconnect with the back of the eye. The lens of the eye may or may not be removed, depending on the amount and location of scar tissue. With SB, the globe is not instrumented; instead, a silicone band is placed around the globe, which modifies the shape of the eye and pushes the retina back toward the posterior wall, where it may reattach.

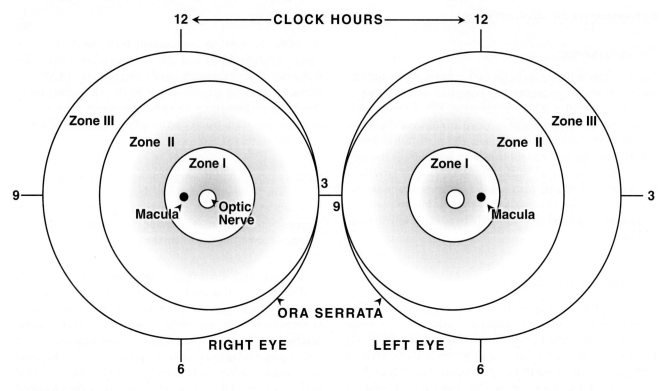

FIGURE 16-2

Retinopathy of Prematurity Zones.

Source: © Crown copyright [2000–2007] Auckland District Health Board www.adhb.govt.nz/newborn/Guidelines/Developmental/ROP.htm

Disposition and discharge planning

All treatments for ROP have a limited degree of success, with more than 10% of affected infants considered to be legally blind (vision worse than 20/200), despite the best efforts of HCPs (Repka, 2005, 2006).

Follow-up is individualized and depends on whether management is for observation or surgery. Ophthalmologic examinations may be performed every 1 to 3 weeks depending on patient response and continue until the retinal vessels are mature.

CHRONIC LUNG DISEASE

Chronic lung disease (CLD) is the most common issue that affects the preterm infant and is a sequela of respiratory distress syndrome (RDS). RDS is caused by a deficiency or dysfunction of pulmonary surfactant (Seger & Soll, 2009). The incidence of RDS is 10% for all premature infants, but increases to 50% for the 26 to 28 weeks' gestational age infant. Refer to Chapter 35 for detailed information on this disease.

ANEMIA OF PREMATURITY

Pathophysiology

All newborn infants, whether term or preterm, experience a gradual decrease in the level of hemoglobin over the first 3 months of life related to physiological changes. This low point is referred to as the "physiologic nadir." The physiologic changes associated with hematopoiesis include transition from hepatic to bone marrow production of the red blood cells (RBCs) and from liver to kidney production of erythropoietin (EPO). In the preterm neonate, EPO production continues to occur primarily in the liver for a longer period of time than in the term infant; the complete transition to kidney-based production does not occur until 4 to 6 weeks after delivery in such children. Liver EPO is less sensitive to hypoxia; consequently, the preterm neonate has a higher risk of developing anemia.

Epidemiology and etiology

In the healthy term infant, symptoms of anemia are rare when the infant reaches the physiologic nadir (9 gm/dL).

TABLE 16-3

Stages of Retinopathy of Prematurity

STAGE 1	**Demarcation line**—a sharp, white clear-cut demarcation between vascularized and avascular retina (normal retina has a tenuous, nonlinear, feathery border).
STAGE 2	**Elevated ridge**—ridge of scar tissue present within the region of white demarcation line.
STAGE 3	**Neovascularization**—"new vessel growth" from posterior aspect of ridge; further divided into mild, moderate, severe dependent upon amount of growth present.
STAGE 4	**Retinal detachment**—scar tissue hardens and retracts, transforming the retina.
	4A—partial detachment of retina, affecting the outermost (peripheral) retina.
	4B—subtotal or total detachment of retina, with a "fold" evident extending through all zones.
STAGE 5	**Total retinal detachment**—retina "funnel-shaped"; extends from optic nerve to front of the eye.
PLUS DISEASE	Dilation and tortuosity of the veins and arterioles; may be present at any stage of ROP. Associated with Rapid progression and unfavorable outcomes.
	PrePlus Disease—dilated and tortuous veins and arterioles noted; abnormal but not severe enough to be classified as "Plus disease"; may be present at any stage ROP.
	Aggressive Posterior ROP (AP-ROP)—rapid in progression; dilated and tortuous veins/arterioles in posterior portion, zone 1 most common. May not sequentially advance through Stage 1 to 3 but often rapidly advances to stage 4 or 5.

Source: © Crown copyright [2000–2007] Auckland District Health Board
www.adhb.govt.nz/newborn/Guidelines/Developmental/ROP.htm

By comparison, in the preterm infant, the physiologic nadir (8 gm/dL for infants weighing 1–1.5 kg; 7 gm/dL for infants weighing less than 1kg) is reached more quickly, is lower, and is exacerbated by a neonatal intensive care admission, frequent blood sampling, shortened life of the RBCs, and rapid growth. The nadir for the preterm infant is inversely related to gestational age. Neonatal anemia is defined as a hemoglobin or hematocrit concentration that is more than two standard deviations below the mean for postnatal age.

Presentation

Anemia of prematurity (AOP) is similar to neonatal anemia, except that there may be more rapid development of clinical signs and symptoms such as tachypnea, apnea, increased oxygen requirement, bradycardia, poor weight gain, decreased activity, and pallor. This anemia may also be a normal physiologic response, though in these infants it occurs sooner after delivery and lasts through the infant's first 3 to 5 months of life. AOP becomes pathologic when the clinical signs and symptoms require intervention.

Differential diagnosis

Anemia of prematurity should be clinically differentiated from other types of anemia to determine the appropriate therapeutic management.

Plan of care

Strategies for the treatment of AOP include limiting the amount of blood lost through phlebotomy procedures, providing appropriate nutritional support, and RBC transfusion. As many as 80% of infants weighing less than 1,000 grams receive one transfusion prior to discharge home. Prior to the 1990s, transfusions were given liberally and the criteria for transfusion were not standardized. When EPO became available, guidelines for restrictive use of RBC transfusions were developed. These criteria have helped to decrease the frequency of RBC transfusion in the ELBW population.

The use of EPO in the preterm population remains controversial. Early use of EPO therapy (started before the neonate reaches 8 days of age) is not recommended due to the increased risk of retinopathy of prematurity associated with this treatment. EPO administration must be accompanied by appropriate nutritional support.

Disposition and discharge planning

There remains some controversy related to neurological outcomes with the use of restrictive RBC transfusion guidelines. Regardless, many neonatal intensive care units have adopted such guidelines, resulting in decreased use of this therapy.

The AAP recommends that all preterm infants receive iron supplementation. Iron supplementation should begin as early as 2 weeks of age. Administer 2–4 mg/kg elemental iron to the breastfed preterm infant and administer 1 mg/kg to the formula-fed infant.

PATENT DUCTUS ARTERIOSUS

Patent ductus arteriosus (PDA) is a common condition in preterm infants, occurring in as many as 45% of infants weighing less than 1,750 grams at birth, and as many as 80% of ELBW infants weighing less than 1,000 grams (DiMenna et al., 2006). Refer to Chapter 22 for detailed information on this condition.

NECROTIZING ENTEROCOLITIS

Pathophysiology

The pathophysiology of necrotizing enterocolitis (NEC) is still unknown but is believed to be multifactorial. Immaturity of the gastrointestinal (GI) system related to motility, digestive ability, circulatory regulation, barrier function, and immune defense predisposes the preterm infant to intestinal injury. This intestinal injury then leads to an abnormal and uncontrolled inflammatory response that produces NEC. Abnormal bacterial colonization and genetic predisposition are other contributing factors in the development of this condition.

Epidemiology and etiology

Necrotizing enterocolitis bowel is the most common GI disease process to affect neonatal acute care patients, with the preterm infant being at the highest at risk. The overall incidence of NEC is approximately 1 to 3 per 1,000 live births. In the preterm population, the incidence of NEC ranges from 2% to 13%. Overall mortality rates for NEC are 25%, with a range from 9% to 50%. Gestational age (less than 28 weeks) and, most importantly, birth weight (less than 1,500 grams) are the strongest indicators of mortality, with decreasing age and size resulting in increased incidence and mortality.

Numerous risk factors are associated with the development of NEC, though prematurity is the most common. Maternal risk factors associated with NEC include placental insufficiency, pregnancy-induced hypertension, suspected or known drug use or abuse, antenatal steroids, and chorioamnionitis. Neonatal risk factors include gestation, low birth weight, type and onset of enteral feedings, hypoxic

events with associated GI ischemia, exchange transfusions, PDA, and infections. While the term infant is at risk for developing NEC within the first week of life, the preterm infant faces this risk for several weeks.

Presentation

The clinical presentation of NEC varies, with symptoms ranging from mild to life-threatening. GI symptoms may include feeding intolerance, abdominal distention, gastric residuals, vomiting, blood in stool (gross or occult), and abdominal tenderness. Other generalized signs and symptoms may include lethargy, apnea, respiratory distress, bradycardia, temperature instability, and shock.

Plan of care

Abdominal radiographs (anterior–posterior and left lateral decubitus films) may reveal findings such as ileus, dilated loops of bowel, pneumatosis intestinalis, ascites, intrahepatic portal venous air, and persistent sentinel loops of bowel (Figures 16-3 and 16-4). Laboratory findings commonly reveal early metabolic acidosis, thrombocytopenia, neutropenia, coagulopathies, and electrolyte imbalances.

Management of NEC should focus on halting progression of the disease. Initial care is nothing-by-mouth (NPO) status and decompression of the GI tract. An evaluation for infection related to other causes (e.g., blood, urine, CSF) should be completed and broad spectrum antibiotic therapy started. Treatment of hypotension, metabolic acidosis, hyponatremia, and other signs and symptoms of shock is essential. The infant with NEC typically experiences a

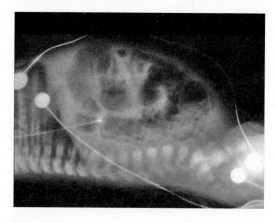

FIGURE 16-3

Necrotizing Enterocolitis.

Source: Courtesy of Sam Alaish, M.D., 2005, Baltimore, Maryland.

prolonged period of parenteral nutrition and bowel rest; consequently, central venous catheter access must be available.

Surgical treatment is indicated when there is evidence of bowel perforation or bowel gangrene, or when the patient experiences continued clinical deterioration (tender abdominal wall mass, abdominal erythema, increased abdominal tenderness and distention, persistent sentinel loop of bowel on radiograph, portal venous air, persistent thrombocytopenia, and/or acidosis) despite adequate medical management. Surgical interventions can range from placement of a peritoneal drain to an exploratory laparotomy. Peritoneal drains (PDs) are usually inserted on those infants who are too sick for surgery but require immediate intervention. A large percentage of infants with PD go on to require a laparotomy. The exploratory laparotomy is done to remove diseased segments of bowel, to preserve as much viable bowel as possible, and to exteriorize the loop of functioning bowel with creation of a stoma (Hughes et al., 2009). Infants will require additional surgery for reversal of the enterostomy, though the exact timing depends on the location of the ostomy and the overall health status of the infant.

Morbidity related to NEC includes significantly prolonged hospital stays and long-term neurodevelopmental impairment. Prolonged hospital stays are related to not only existing comorbidities (i.e., bronchopulmonary dysplasia), but also the infant's poor nutritional status owing to the loss of bowel and the length of time needed for reversal of the stoma. Infants who have NEC are at increased risk for cerebral palsy and neurodevelopmental, visual, cognitive, and psychomotor impairment as compared to infants of similar age and gestation without NEC.

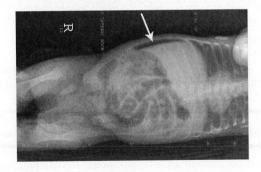

FIGURE 16-4

Necrotizing Enterocolitis.

Source: Courtesy of Sam Alaish, M.D., 2005, Baltimore, Maryland.

Disposition and discharge planning

Discharge of the infant with NEC requires planning and monitoring. The infant who has made an adequate recovery and is being discharged home remains at high risk for failure-to-thrive. Care must be directed toward maintaining adequate caloric intake and monitoring overall growth. These infants frequently have feeding aversions that require placement of gastrostomy tubes for management of feedings at discharge. For those infants who lost large segments of bowel with resulting intestinal failure (short-gut syndrome), home parenteral nutrition and future small bowel transplant may be warranted.

Follow-up is coordinated with both the primary care provider and gastroenterologist to ensure that the child maintains adequate growth and development and to address any ongoing GI issues that occur as a long-term consequence of NEC. Referral is also necessary to specialists in developmental care, nutrition, physical therapy, occupational therapy, and speech therapy. Parental education and support are vital in transitioning the infant to a home environment and meeting the developmental needs of the baby.

SEPSIS IN THE PREMATURE INFANT

Pathophysiology

Preterm birth interrupts the maturation process of the immune system, leaving the premature infant at risk for infection in a pathogen-rich environment. Most elements of the immune system are present in premature infants; however, their number and function may be insufficient. For example, the neutrophil proliferating pool (NPP) and the neutrophil storage pool (NSP) account for as much as 90% of all neutrophils in the body. During an inflammatory process, such as sepsis, neutrophils are released from the NSP. Once these stores are exhausted, immature cells are mobilized from the NPP. The size of the NPP of a premature infant is only one-tenth the size (per kilogram of body weight) of the NPP of the adult (Chandra et al., 2007). Phagocytic cells, T and B lymphocytes, and humoral mediators such as complement factors, fibronectin, and cytokines are all similarly affected by prematurity (Kemp & Campbell, 1996).

Epidemiology and etiology

The incidence of sepsis among preterm infants is inversely proportional to birth weight and gestational age. Ten percent of those infants who weigh 1,000 to 1,500 grams at birth, 35% of those who weigh less than 1,000 grams, and as many of 50% of those who weigh less than 750 grams experience a serious systemic infection (Kaufman & Fairchild, 2004).

Several factors increase the risk for sepsis in the preterm infant. The first is the immature and thin epidermal and epithelial skin barrier (described earlier in this chapter). This already minimized barrier is made more so by injury from adhesives; intravenous, arterial, and heelstick punctures; and aggressive handling. A second factor is the immaturity of the GI mucosa. In the preterm infant, reduced immunoglobulin A (IgA), mucin, and acid production allow for bacterial and fungal overgrowth. Mucosal surfaces are similarly affected, as skin barriers and microbial invasion can occur in the nasopharynx or oropharynx through erosion from the gastric and endotracheal tubes. Third, administration of certain medications may increase risk for infection. For example, indomethicin may affect neutrophil function; H_2 antagonists may lower gastric pH, thereby supporting microbial overgrowth; and the extensive use of antibiotics may further alter the intestinal flora and allow fungal proliferation (Kaufman & Fairchild, 2004).

Early-onset sepsis

The researchers conducting the Neonatal Early Onset Sepsis Study (National Institute of Child Health and Human Development [NICHD], 2009) have defined early-onset sepsis (EOS) as a positive blood or CSF culture drawn within the first 72 hours of life. The organisms most commonly implicated in EOS are *Escherichia coli* (*E. coli*) and Group B *Streptococcus* (GBS). *E. coli* infections in VLBW infants have become more common, increasing from 3.2 cases per 1,000 live births in the period 1991–1993 to 7 cases per 1,000 live births in 2002–2003 (Puopolo, 2008). Gram negative bacteria account for 41% of infections in infants with EOS (Kaufman & Fairchild, 2004). At the same time, infections from GBS are decreasing. This trend is thought to reflect the prophylactic use of intrapartum antibiotics instituted in 1996. Prior to that time, GBS sepsis occurred in 78% of all preterm infants with EOS as opposed to only 47% of preterm infants from 2003 to 2006 (Hoogen et al., 2010). Gram negative sepsis is associated with the highest mortality rates.

EOS can appear as bacteremia, meningitis, pneumonia, or infection of the urinary tract. It is typically acquired via ascent of organisms from the birth canal to the amniotic fluid. Maternal risk factors for EOS (other than premature delivery) include lack of prenatal care, premature or prolonged rupture of membranes, chorioamnionitis, and history of or current urinary tract infection. Clinical signs and symptoms may include respiratory distress, temperature instability, hypotonia, irritability, poor feeding, early-onset jaundice, apnea, poor perfusion, tachycardia, and seizures.

The AAP recommends that all neonates younger than 35 weeks of age with a history or physical examination concerning for EOS have a complete blood count with differential and blood culture drawn and empiric administration

of intravenous antibiotics started. The inclusion of a CSF sample depends on the clinical presentation of the infant, the facility, and physician preference. Ampicillin and gentamicin are the drugs of choice for treating EOS.

Late-onset sepsis

Late-onset sepsis (LOS) is defined by NICHD as a positive blood culture, obtained in the presence of clinical signs of sepsis, occurring after 72 hours of life (Short, 2004) (Table 16-4). This disease is strongly associated with decreasing birth weight and gestational age and has been reported to occur in as many as 20% of VLBW infants. The Neonatal Research Network reported that 43% of infants with birth weights in the range of 401–750 grams had at least one episode of LOS, compared to 7% of infants with birth weights in the range of 1,251–1,500 grams. Similarly, 46% of infants born after less than 25 weeks' gestation developed LOS, compared to only 2% in infants born after 32 weeks' gestation (Stoll et al., 2002).

The clinical presentation of LOS is nonspecific. Signs and symptoms exhibited by the affected neonate may include temperature instability, increased apnea/bradycardia, feeding intolerance (abdominal distention, emesis, residuals, increased frequency of stools), hematochezia, increased oxygen requirements and support, hypotonia, and lethargy (Karlowicz & Buescher, 2008). LOS is responsible for the majority of nosocomial infections, including bloodstream infections from central venous catheters (CVCs).

Pathogens causing LOS include coagulase-negative *Staphylococcus* (CONS), *Staphylococcus aureus* (including methicillin-resistant *S. aureus* [MRSA]), *Klebsiella*, *Pseudomonas aeruginosa*, *Candida* species, and GBS. Gram negative bacteria are responsible for 36% of the LOS infections in VLBW infants (Kaufman & Fairchild, 2004). Peak occurrence of *Candida* infections occurs between postnatal days 11 and 20; the species most commonly implicated are *C. albicans* and *C. parapsilosis*. *Enterococcus* is an emerging pathogen that has been noted in LOS (Cohen-Wolkowiez et al., 2009; Karlowicz & Buescher, 2008).

Evaluation of LOS consists of a complete blood count with manual differential, blood cultures (central and peripheral if possible), urine culture (suprapubic tap or catheter), and CSF sample (lumbar puncture or ventricular tap) (Table 16-5). In addition, obtaining a fungal culture should be considered in the infant who is deemed at high risk for fungal infection. Factors increasing the rise of LOS include presence of a CVC, parenteral nutrition, history of NEC, and previous use of broad spectrum antibiotics, postnatal steroids, or H_2 antagonists.

Initial empiric therapy for LOS consists ampicillin and gentamicin, unless the suspected infectious process is *S. aureus* infection or a skin, soft-tissue, bone, or joint infection; in the latter cases, vancomycin is used instead of ampicillin to cover for resistant organisms.

TABLE 16-4

Timing of Bacterial and Fungal Sepsis in Very Low Birth Weight Infants

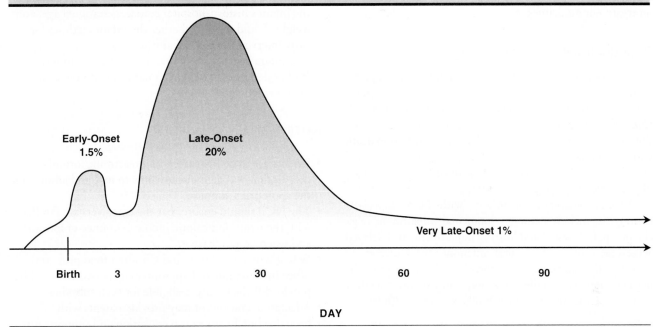

Source: Percentages indicate the approximate number of very low birth weight (VLBW) infants with septicemia. Late onset sepsis (LOS) occurs with vertical and horizontal spread of organisms. While the vast majority of cases of sepsis in VLBW infants occur in the first 30 days of life, VLBW infants requiring prolonged intensive care are at risk for VLOS beyond 2 months of age.
Reprinted with permission of American Society for Microbiology; from Kaufman, Fairchild, K. (2004). Clinical Microbiology of Bacterial and Fungal Sepsis in Very-Low-Birth-Weight-Infants. Clinical Microbiology Reviews 17(3), p. 638–680.

TABLE 16-5

A Comparison of Cerebrospinal Fluid Ranges in Low Birth Weight Infants			
	Sarff et al. (1976)	**Rodriguez et al. (1990)**	**Rodriguez et al. (1990)**
Birth weight	970–2,500 gm	≤ 1,000 gm	1,001–1,500 gm
White blood cells per mm3 blood	0–29	0–14	0–44
Glucose (mg/dL)	24–63	29–217	31–109
Protein (mg/dL)	65–150	76–370	45–227

Source: Adapted from Rodriguez et al., 1990; Sarff et al., 1976.

The U.S. Centers for Disease Prevention and Control (CDC) recommends against global empiric prescription of vancomycin due to the risk of fostering vancomycin-resistant *Enterococcus* species. Some centers have a protocol to start vancomycin and gentamicin empirically for the first 48 hours after the initial LOS evaluation. Then, when the organism is identified and susceptibilities are available, the therapy can be tailored as appropriate. Vancomycin prophylaxis decreases both CONS and overall sepsis, but does not reduce mortality or duration of hospitalization.

For meningitis, cefotaxime is added to the ampicillin and gentamicin regimen to provide broader spectrum coverage against pathogens that might cross the blood–brain barrier. When the infectious process is suspected to originate from the gastrointestinal system, clindamycin may be added as an adjunct to improve therapy coverage for anaerobic pathogens. In the presence of fungal sepsis, amphotericin B is generally preferred as a first-line agent. Fluconazole has been used for fungal prophylaxis with inconclusive results (Kaufman & Fairchild, 2004). Therefore, its use for LOS is limited.

Ultimately, there is always variation in the LOS pathogens by geographic area and individual facility. The most recent edition of the *Red Book* (AAP) provides information on treatment guidelines.

Disposition and discharge planning

Each episode of LOS lengthens the hospital stay by approximately 19 days. Sepsis is the leading cause of death in infants older than 2 weeks of age. Infection with Gram negative rods (*Enterobacter, Pseudomonas, Bordetalla, Klebsiella*) is responsible for the most fulminant infections and may lead to death within 48 hours of onset. The highest fatality rate is associated with *Pseudomonas* infection (40%) (Cohen-Wolkowiez et al., 2009; Karlowicz & Buescher, 2008).

Adverse outcomes for infants with EOS, especially meningitis, include neurodevelopmental impairment (e.g., cerebral palsy), visual and hearing impairment, and delayed achievement of developmental milestones (McGuire et al., 2004). Although therapy for sepsis is evolving, most of the newer therapies have failed to demonstrate a significant effect on neonatal outcomes (Cohen-Wolkowiez et al., 2009).

PLANNING FOR HOME

Many premature infants have prolonged hospital stays that require various levels of care. Consequently, HCPs in all areas of the acute care setting need to be knowledgeable about the home care requirements and follow-up for the premature (or formerly premature) infant.

According to the AAP, routine discharge planning for high-risk infants incorporates a detailed assessment, evaluation, and plan for the following aspects of care (AAP, 2008; CHOP, 2010):

- Physical, developmental, and neurological exam
- Nutritional counseling
- Safety
- Caregiver support
- Preventive health (newborn screening, hearing screening, immunizations)
- Continuing care needs

PHYSICAL, DEVELOPMENTAL, AND NEUROLOGICAL EXAMINATION

- The HCP should ensure that the infant has a documened consistent weight gain of 15 to 30 grams per day.
- Medical or surgical problems that require care in an acute care unit should be resolved.
- Feedings must be successful, without any distress.

- The infant must demonstrate the ability to maintain a stable temperature in an open crib for several days.
- Results of the physical examination and consideration of the infant's history, hospital course, gestational age, and weight should dictate whether the infant qualifies for early intervention referral at discharge.
- The infant must have no documented arrhythmias (unless determined benign in nature) and no recent documented apneic events.

NUTRITIONAL COUNSELING

- Parents are to be instructed on breastmilk/formula preparation and demonstrate how to mix and administer the appropriate amount.
- The HCP should ensure that the caregivers are familiar with the name and caloric intake per ounce of formula and where to purchase it.
- WIC (Women, Infants, and Children food program) office information and appropriate paperwork should be provided if the family is eligible for such subsidies.
- A lactation consultant may provide parents with breastfeeding breast pump education and support. An appropriate latch should be demonstrated by the infant prior to discharge.

SAFETY

- Infant cardiopulmonary resuscitation (CPR) training should be completed.
- Safe sleep positions should be reviewed. Supine positioning—"back to sleep"—should be recommended unless another position is medically necessary and advised (Engle, 2006).
- Basic baby care should be reviewed (e.g., instruction on safe bath-water temperature, how to properly take an infant's temperature, bulb suction technique).
- Review when to call the primary care provider or take the infant to the emergency department.
- Provide for appropriate administration and/or demonstration of medications.
- Review the use and care of special medical devices, dressings, or equipment; this includes care of catheters and ostomies, apnea monitors, and durable medical equipment.
- Make sure that the caregivers have a car seat that meets safety standards, and that the infant has completed and passed a car seat test.

PARENT/CAREGIVER SUPPORT

- All questions should be answered and appropriate literature provided.

- Caregivers should be offered the opportunity to stay overnight in a "rooming in" room with the infant. This provides for security of the caregiving routine and allows the caregivers to assume total care and responsibility while being supervised by the health care team.
- Review symptoms of illness and distress; ensure that the caregivers know when to call the HCP or take the infant to the hospital.
- Review the discharge instructions/summary with the parents.

PREVENTIVE HEALTH

- Ensure that the primary care provider is identified and a follow-up appointment scheduled.
- Immunizations should be up-to-date.
- Vision and hearing screens should be complete.
- Newborn screens should be completed.

CONTINUING CARE NEEDS

- Make sure that follow-up clinic and therapy appointments are scheduled.
- Confirm that durable medical equipment and supplies have been ordered for home use and will be available on home arrival.
- Schedule home health visits if needed.

REFERENCES

1. American Academy of Pediatrics (AO) Section on Ophthalmology, American Academy of Ophthalmology (AO), & American Association for Pediatric Ophthalmology and Strabismus (AAPOS). (2006). Screening examination of premature infants for retinopathy of prematurity [Policy statement]. *Pediatrics, 117*, 572–576.
2. American Academy of Pediatrics Committee on the Fetus and Newborn. (2008). Hospital discharge of the high-risk neonate. *Pediatrics, 122*(5), 1119–1126.
3. Askin, D., & Diehl-Jones, W. (2009). Retinopathy of prematurity. *Critical Care Nursing Clinics of North America, 21*, 213–233.
4. Aylott, M. (2006). The neonatal energy triangle. Part 1: Metabolic adaptation. *Paediatric Nursing, 18*(6), 38–42.
5. Balaraman, V. (2003). Common problems of the premature infant. Retrieved from http://www.hawaii.edu/medicine/pediatrics/pedtext/s03c05.html
6. Ballard, J. L., Khoury, J., Wedig, K., Wang, L., Eilers-Walsman, B., & Lipp, R. (1991). New Ballard Score expanded to include extremely premature infants. *Journal of Pediatrics, 119*(3), 417–423.
7. Chandra, S., Haines, H., Michie, C., & Maheshwari, A. (2007). Developmental defects in neutrophils from preterm infants. *NeoReviews, 8*(9), e368–e376.
8. Charsha, D. (1997). *Neonatal physical assessment: Gestational age and growth evaluation.* St. Louis: Mosby Year-Book.
9. The Children's Hospital of Philadelphia. (2010). Health Information: Taking Your Baby Home. Retrieved from http://www.chop.edu/healthinfo/taking-your-baby-home.html

10. Cohen-Wolkowiez, M., Moran, C., Benjamin, D., Cotten, C., Clark, R., Benjamin, Jr., D., et al. (2009). Early and late onset sepsis in late preterm infants. *Pediatric Infectious Disease Journal, 28*(12), 1052–1056.
11. Colson, E. (2005). Evaluation and care of the normal neonate. Retrieved from http://www.merck.com/mmpe/print/sec19/ch266/ch266b.html
12. DiMenna, L. et al. (2006). Management of the neonate with patent ductus arteriosus. *Journal of Perinatal and Neonatal Nursing, 20*(4), 333–340.
13. Engle, W. (2001). Blood pressure in the very low birth weight neonate. *Early Human Development, 62*, 97–130.
14. Engle, W., Wyckoff, M., and Rosenfeld, C. (2006). Developmental issues in prematurity. House Staff Nursery Manual, Division of Neonatal-Perinatal Medicine Department of Pediatrics, The University of Texas Southwestern Medical Center at Dallas.
15. Fallat, et al. (1998). Central venous catheter bloodstream infections in the neonatal intensive care unit. *Journal of Pediatric Surgery, 33*, 1383–1387.
16. Fanaroff, A., & Fanaroff, J. (2006). Blood pressure disorders in the neonate: Hypotension and hypertension. *Seminars in Fetal & Neonatal Medicine, 11*, 174–181.
17. Gomella, T., et al. (2004). Assessment of gestational age. In *Neonatology: Management, procedures, on-call problems, diseases, drugs* (5th ed.). Stamford, CT: Appleton & Lange.
18. Hawdon, J. (2006). Thermal regulation and effects on nutrient substrate metabolism. In Neonatal nutrition and metabolism (2nd ed.). New York: Cambridge University Press.
19. Hoogen, A., et al. (2010). Long-term trends in the epidemiology of neonatal sepsis and antibiotic susceptibility of causative agents. *Neonatology, 97*, 22–28.
20. Hughes, B., Baez, L., and McGrath, J. M. (2009). Necrotizing enterocolitis: Past tends and current concerns. *Newborn & Infant Nursing Reviews, 9*(3), 156–162.
21. International Committee for the Classification of Retinopathy of Prematurity. (2005). The international classification of retinopathy of prematurity revisited. *Archives of Ophthalmology, 123*, 991–999.
22. Karlowicz, G., & Buescher, S. (2008). Nosocomial infections in the neonate lung. In *Principles and practice of pediatric infectious diseases* (3rd ed.). Churchill Livingstone. Retrieved from http: www.mdconsult.com
23. Kaufman, D., & Fairchild, K. (2004). Clinical microbiology of bacterial and fungal sepsis in very-low-birth-weight infants. *Clinical Microbiology Reviews, 17*(3), 638–680.
24. Kemp, A., & Campbell, D. (1996). The neonatal immune system. *Seminars in Neonatology, 1*(2), 67–75.
25. Leflore, J. L., et al. (2000). Determinants of blood pressure in very low birth weight neonates: Lack of effect of antenatal steroids. *Early Human Development, 59*, 37–50.
26. March of Dimes. (2006). Perinatal Data Center PeriStats, 2006. Retrieved from http://www.marchofdimes.com/peristats/alldata.aspx?reg=99&dv=es
27. McGuire, W., et al. (2004). ABC of preterm birth: Infection in the preterm infant. *British Medical Journal, 329*, 1277–1280.
28. Merskey, H., Bogduk, N. (1994). Part III: Pain Terms, A Current List with Definitions and Notes on Usage. Classification of Chronic Pain, (2nd ed)., IASP Task Force on Taxonomy, Seattle: IASP Press: 209–214,
29. National Center for Health Statistics. (2009). Number and percentage of infant deaths by gestational age U.S., 1995 and 2005. Prepared by March of Dimes Perinatal Data Center.
30. National Institute of Child Health and Human Development (NICHD). (2009). NICHD Neonatal Research Network: Early-onset sepsis: An NICHD/CDC surveillance study. Retrieved from https://neonatal.rti.org/pdf/StudySummary/summ_EOS.pdf
31. Pollan, C. (2009). Retinopathy of prematurity: An eye toward better outcomes. *Neonatal Network 28*(2), 93–101.

32. Puopolo, K. (2008). Epidemiology of neonatal early-onset sepsis. *NeoReviews, 19*(12), e571–e579.

33. Pursley, D., & Henry, A. (2008). Developmental characteristics of preterm infants. *Pediatrics in Review, 29*, 67–68.

34. Repka, M. & Stavroudis, T. (2005). Retinopathy of prematurity. *Johns Hopkins: eNeonatal Review Newsletter, 3*(2).

35. Repka, M. X., Tung, B., Good, W. V., Shapiro, M., Capone, A., Baker, J. D., et al. (2006). Outcome of eyes developing retinal detachment during the early treatment for retinopathy of prematurity study (ETROP). *Archives of Ophthalmology, 124*(1), 24–30.

36. Rodriguez, A.F., et al. (1990). Cerebrospinal fluid values in the very low birth weight infant. *The Journal of Pediatrics, 116*, 971.

37. Sarff, L.D., Platt, L.H. & McCracken, G.H. (1976). Cerebrospinal fluid evaluation in neonates: Comparison of high-risk infants with and without meningitis. *The Journal of Pediatrics, 883*, 473–477.

38. Seger, N. and Soll, R. (2009). Animal derived surfactant extract for treatment of respiratory distress syndrome (Review). The Cochrane Collaboration. John Wiley & Sons.

39. Short, B. L., Van Meurs, K., Evans, J. R., & the Cardiology Group. (2006, March). Summary proceedings from the Cardiology Group on Cardiovascular Instability in Preterm Infants. *Pediatrics, 117*, S34–S39.

40. Short, M. (2008). Keeping infants warm: Challenges in hypothermia. *Advances in Neonatal Care, 8*(1), 6–12.

41. Soll, R. F. (2008). Heat loss prevention in neonates. *Journal of Perinatology, 28*, 557–559.

42. Stoll, B., Hansen, N., et al. (2002). Late-onset sepsis in very low birth weight neonates: The experience of the NICHD Neonatal Research Network. *Pediatrics, 110*(2), 285–291.

43. Taeusch, H. W. (2005). Avery's diseases of the newborn (8th ed.). Philadelphia: Elsevier Saunders: 1328.

44. Thummula, M., Raju, T., & Langenberg, P. (1998). Isolated single umbilical artery anomaly and the risk for congenital malformations: A meta-analysis. *Journal of Pediatric Surgery, 4*(33), 580–585.

45. Trachtenbarg, D., & Golemon, T. (1998). Care of the premature infant: Part 1. Monitoring growth and development. Retrieved from http:www.aafp.org/afp/AFPprinter/980501ap/trachten.html?print=yes

46. Walden, M. & Carrier, C. (2009). The ten commandments of pain assessment and management in preterm neonates. *Critical Care Nursing Clinics of North America, 21*(2), 235–52.

47. Walden, M. & Gibbins, S. (2008). *Pain assessment and management: Guideline for practice.* Glenview, IL: National Association of Neonatal Nurses.

48. White, L. (2000). Foundations of nursing: caring for the whole person. (1st ed.)., New York: Delmar Cengage Learning: 1358–1359.

49. Verklan, M., & Walden, M. (2003). Core curriculum for neonatal intensive care nursing (3rd ed.). St. Louis: Elsevier Saunders: 135–172.

50. World Health Organization (WHO). (1997). *Thermal control of the newborn: A practical guide.* Geneva, Switzerland: Maternal and Safe Motherhood Program, Division of Family Health.

51. Zubrow, A.B., et al. (1995). Determinants of blood pressure in neonates admitted to neonatal intensive care units: a prospective multicenter study. *Journal of Perinatology, 15*, 470–479.

Reneé S. Holleran and Rose Linsler

Transport

- Goal of Transport
- Indications for Pediatric Transport
- Transport Team Crew Composition
- Communication
- Air Transport
- Ground Transport
- Safety

- Physiologic Stressors of Transport
- Equipment
- Preparation for Transport
- Families
- Outreach Education and Follow-up
- References

In 1985, legislation was passed and funding provided to ensure that states would develop systems to improve the care of ill or injured pediatric patients in the prehospital and emergency settings. In addition, the American Academy of Pediatrics, the American College of Emergency Physicians, the National Association of EMS Physicians, and the National Association of Emergency Medical Technicians undertook similar initiatives (Tunik & Foltin, 2008). Today, as a result of these efforts, both ground and air services are available throughout the United States to transport pediatric patients.

GOAL OF TRANSPORT

The primary goal for any type of transport is to get the right patient to the right level of care, in the right amount of time, and in the safest manner possible (Stroud et al., 2008).

INDICATIONS FOR PEDIATRIC TRANSPORT

Many factors influence the decision to transport a pediatric patient. These include the scope of practice for the referring agent, the comfort level of the referring staff, the available onsite resources, and the need for a higher level of care (Holleran, 2010; Holleran & Linsler, 2006; Orr et al., 2006).

TRANSPORT TEAM CREW COMPOSITION

The composition of transport teams varies. For example, teams may be composed of free-standing generalists who care for patients across the lifespan, or they can be dedicated to pediatrics. One of the criticisms of using a generalist team is that members may lack pediatric clinical experience and the ability to recognize pertinent differences between ill or injured adult and pediatric patients (Orr et al., 2009). Such experience and knowledge are most important for advanced airway management and initial resuscitation.

Another transport team model utilizes staff from neonatal or pediatric intensive care units. This kind of team typically provides care directed by a physician and functions as an extension of the intensive care unit. With the unit-based model, the major advantage is that staff members are highly trained in treating the pediatric population. However, a disadvantage is that the team members may feel pressure to complete the transport too quickly so as to return to a staff position (Aijzian & Nakagawa, 2007).

Regardless of whether the team is generalist, pediatric, or unit based, the team members themselves may be drawn from various roles. Members may include registered nurses, nurse practitioners, physicians/assistant, pediatric residents, respiratory care practitioners, or paramedics and emergency medical technicians (EMT's) (Horowitz & Rozenfeld, 2007). Teams may be composed of these members in any combination, with some teams determining composition on a case-by-case basis and using standardized guidelines to meet patient needs. The overall goal is to match the team composition with the needs of the patient during transport (Holleran & Linsler, 2006; Horowitz & Rozenfeld; Orr et al., 2009).

All teams must have a method for ensuring that the personnel selected as members acquire and maintain the skills required to serve the needs of the ill or injured neonate and pediatric patient. These skills include pediatric advance life support with advanced airway management, chest drainage, vascular access, and appropriate medication selection (Fenton & Leslie, 2009; Ratnavel, 2009).

COMMUNICATION

In the event of a scene transport, the information provided to the team may be as brief as a street address, geographical reference, or latitude/longitude position. In many rotor-wing programs, as a safety precaution, the pilot is "blinded" to patient information; thus the flight crew may or may not know the patient's age or mechanism of injury.

In interfacility transfers, more information is typically available. The referring facility contacts the accepting facility; the accepting facility then must confirm the availability of a bed for the patient and its willingness to accept the transfer. Information is shared regarding the current illness or injury, past medical history, treatment given, and needs for further specialized treatment (Table 17-1). This information allows the team to determine the personnel and equipment required for safe transport. Stabilization begins at the time of the referral, and the transport team provides additional advice as needed to stabilize the patient while the team is en route (Slota, 2006).

Permission for transport from the patient's parents or guardians (including a review of the risks associated with the transport) and copies of radiographic images, diagnostic results, and the medical record must be prepared by the referring facility so as to be ready to accompany the patient back to the receiving facility (Orr et al., 2006). At the scene or referring facility, the transport team communicates back to the accepting facility an update on the patient's condition, any interventions performed, and an estimated time of arrival to the receiving facility. Additional interventions to be initiated prior to transport are discussed as well. The treatments and procedures provided to the patient at the referring facility are based on how urgent the patient's condition is, what is needed to provide safe transport without undue deterioration, and what can be accomplished quickly at the receiving facility based on the length of transport. A plan of care (POC) is developed, and the patient is transported following the accepting program's guidelines and standing orders.

TABLE 17-1

Transport Communication Information: Initial Call

Information Obtained

- History of present illness or injury
  - Current condition
  - Treatment rendered
- Pertinent past medical history, allergies, weight
- Vital signs
- Level of consciousness and Glasgow Coma Scale score
- Laboratory data
- Radiographic studies

Information Provided

- Treatment recommendations
  - Airway placement: type and size
  - Ventilator management
  - Fluid resuscitation
  - Medications: selections, doses, routes
- Transport team estimated time of arrival

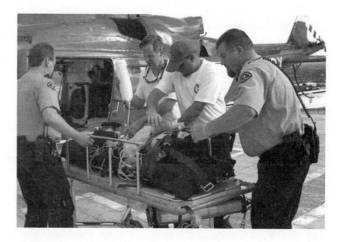

FIGURE 17-1

Transport Team and Receiving Facility Safely Unloading a Pediatric Patient from a Helicopter.

Source: Courtesy of Reneé Holleran and Rose Linsler.

Upon arrival at the accepting facility, an updated verbal report, including information on any changes in assessment findings and the patient's response to interventions, is given to the medical team. This face-to-face exchange of information is augmented by delivery of the transport team's written documentation.

AIR TRANSPORT

Transport by air can be accomplished by both rotor and fixed-wing aircraft. Team compositions for air transport vary (Figure 17-1). The advantages of air medical transport include timeliness and speed of transport (AAP, 2007). Disadvantages include the limited cabin size, weight and balance concerns, access to air medical transport, weather considerations, cost, and landing zone requirements (AAP).

GROUND TRANSPORT

There are both advantages and disadvantages to transferring and transporting the pediatric patient by ground, just with air medical transport. The primary advantage with the use of a ground vehicle is the ability to bring the necessary equipment and personnel to manage the patient. Weight and balance are generally not issues in the ground vehicle. Other advantages of this method of transport include its ready availability, the door-to-door service, a lower cost than with air transport, the ability to operate in weather conditions that would restrict air medical transport, the ability

to carry more than one patient without difficulty, and the ability to pull over and move out of traffic to undertake care interventions such as intubation (AAP, 2007).

Disadvantages of ground transport include the length of transport time, speed limitations due to traffic and road access, a rough ride because of the vehicle suspension (which may cause patient harm), and the greater risk of complications because of the length of time the child is outside of the hospital setting. If the ground vehicle is staffed by paramedics or EMTs, there may be an additional risk that the level of care is insufficient for patient needs. Also, during transport, the vehicle is lost to the community it serves (AAP, 2007).

SAFETY

The decision to use either air or ground transport should always be based first and foremost on transport team and patient safety. There is some level of risk associated with all modes of transport. For example, just because a ground vehicle may be able to travel in weather that has grounded an air medical vehicle, it does not mean that the vehicle *should* go. A snowstorm with ice and fog may impede travel for either method of transportation (Worley, 2010).

Each patient transport requires both mission planning and risk assessment. Factors that should be taken into account during in these preparatory steps include the type of vehicle available and the safety equipment on board, current and future weather conditions, fatigue of the transport team (how many transports have they accomplished as well as attempted), time of day (night versus daytime) of the transport, the type of transport (interfacility or scene), and transport team experience (Worley, 2010).

There should be no consequences if the transport team decides to decline or halt a transport. A procedure should be in place to review each transport, especially those declined or terminated. The program philosophy for safe transport should follow the idiom, "Three to say go and one to say no" (Worley, 2010).

In addition to patient care skill training, transports teams need to receive basic and continuing education regarding survival training. Each vehicle and person should carry survival gear. Every transport environment presents unique challenges, and all team members should be prepared for emergencies. In addition, all personnel who interact with the transport team must receive education and training so they can work competently with the team members and efficiently support their practice. Safety should always be the number one priority of pediatric transport.

PHYSIOLOGIC STRESSORS OF TRANSPORT

Whether the patient is transported by air or ground, additional physiologic stressors come into play that may affect transport. These stressors may result in, for example, cyanosis, hypotension, tachycardia, or cardiac arrest. Dislodgement of endotracheal tubes, loss of power, and lack of light are only some of the many undesirable events that may occur during transport (Holleran & Treadwell, 2010; Kanter & Tompkins, 1989). Other stressors associated with transport include hypoxia, barometric pressure changes, thermal changes, decreased humidity, noise, vibration, gravitational forces, spatial disorientation, flicker vertigo, and fuel vapors (Figures 17-2 through Figure 17-8). Many of these stressors are possible with air and ground transport, but especially hypoxia, vibration, noise, thermal

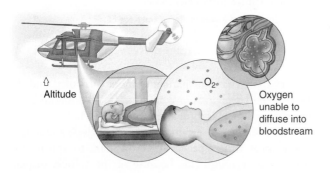

FIGURE 17-2

Hypoxic hypoxia results from a lack of oxygen or an inability of oxygen to diffuse into the bloodstream.

Source: From American Academy of Orthopaedic Surgeons (AAOS) and the American College of Emergency Physicians (ACEP), Pollak, A. (Ed.) (2011). Critical Care Transport, Sudbury. MA: Jones and Bartlett Publishers.

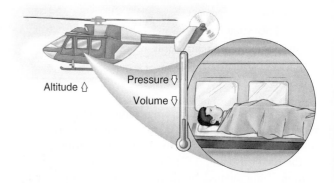

FIGURE 17-4

Charles' law. The volume of a gas is directly proportional to the temperature, with the pressure remaining constant.

Source: From American Academy of Orthopaedic Surgeons (AAOS) and the American College of Emergency Physicians (ACEP), Pollak, A. (Ed.) (2011). Critical Care Transport, Sudbury. MA: Jones and Bartlett Publishers.

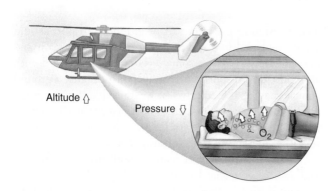

FIGURE 17-3

Boyle's law. As altitude increases, atmospheric pressure decreases, and gases inside the body expand.

Source: From American Academy of Orthopaedic Surgeons (AAOS) and the American College of Emergency Physicians (ACEP), Pollak, A. (Ed.) (2011). Critical Care Transport, Sudbury. MA: Jones and Bartlett Publishers.

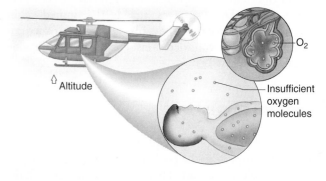

FIGURE 17-5

Dalton's law. The total pressure of a gas mixture is the sum of the individual pressures. Insufficient oxygen molecules can lead to hypoxia.

Source: From American Academy of Orthopaedic Surgeons (AAOS) and the American College of Emergency Physicians (ACEP), Pollak, A. (Ed.) (2011). Critical Care Transport, Sudbury. MA: Jones and Bartlett Publishers.

changes, flicker vertigo, and fuel vapors. Stresses specific to air medical transport include gravitational forces, spatial disorientation, and barometric pressure changes.

EQUIPMENT

The transport team provides advanced critical care management for patients at remote sites and during transport; consequently, dedicated, readily available, and self-sufficient equipment is purchased with the team, patient, and environment in mind. The selected equipment must be compatible with seasonal temperature fluctuations, vehicle vibrations, altitude changes, and spatial limitations, while producing no electromagnetic interference with vehicle performance (Figure 17-9).

Broken and missing equipment must be replaced, expiration dates checked, and battery life determined prior to every shift and after every use. Due to the nature of the transport environment and the daily abuse the equipment receives, there is always a chance that primary equipment may fail and gases may become depleted. The team needs to anticipate these events and have the backup equipment in serviceable condition and readily available.

Basic monitoring for all patients includes continuous electrocardiograph (ECG) and oxygen saturation readings;

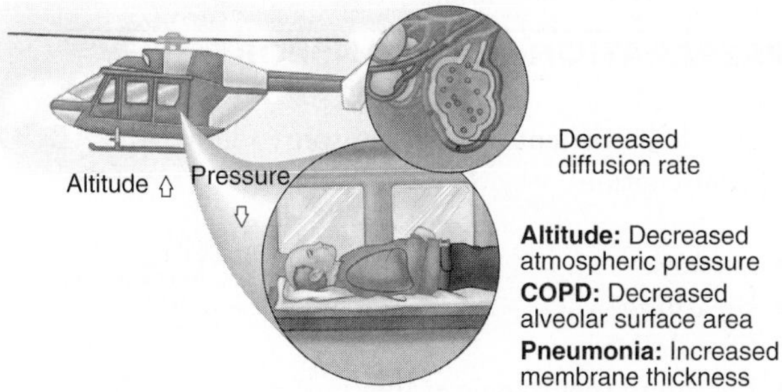

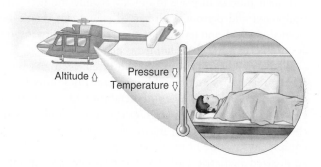

FIGURE 17-6

Fick's law. The diffusion rate of a gas is affected by atmospheric pressures, the surface area of the membrane, and the thickness of the membrane. A patient with COPD and pneumonia will have decreased gas exchange.

Source: From American Academy of Orthopaedic Surgeons (AAOS) and the American College of Emergency Physicians (ACEP), Pollak, A. (Ed.) (2011). Critical Care Transport, Sudbury. MA: Jones and Bartlett Publishers.

FIGURE 17-8

Gay-Lussac's law. As pressure decreases, temperature decreases. Remember to keep your patients warm.

Source: From American Academy of Orthopaedic Surgeons (AAOS) and the American College of Emergency Physicians (ACEP), Pollak, A. (Ed.) (2011). Critical Care Transport, Sudbury. MA: Jones and Bartlett Publishers.

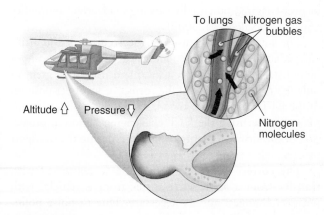

FIGURE 17-7

Henry's law. As the pressure of gas over a liquid decreases, the amount of gas dissolved in the liquid will also decrease. In decompression sickness, nitrogen saturates the tissues, then forms gas bubbles that travel to the lungs.

Source: From American Academy of Orthopaedic Surgeons (AAOS) and the American College of Emergency Physicians (ACEP), Pollak, A. (Ed.) (2011). Critical Care Transport, Sudbury. MA: Jones and Bartlett Publishers.

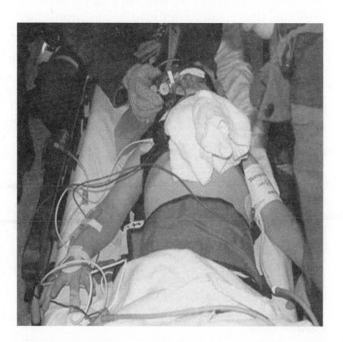

FIGURE 17-9

Equipment Used During Pediatric Transport.

with intubated patients, continuous $ETCO_2$ is needed as well. The hypothermic or hyperthermic patient requires continuous core temperature monitoring, which may be performed via a urinary catheter with a temperature probe or a thermometer.

The ability to obtain and run basic laboratory studies such blood gases, hematocrit, and glucose contributes to delivery of a higher level of care in the transport setting. Bedside testing devices are useful tools during transport.

Additional equipment and personnel may occasionally be required to deliver care including extracorporeal life support, nitric oxide administration, high-frequency ventilation, use of an incubator, or invasive hemodynamic and intracranial pressure monitoring. The transport team should have an expedient process in place to quickly acquire the necessary equipment and personnel. Borrowed equipment should be cleaned, tracked, and returned to the referring facility as soon as possible, as it may have limited pediatric resources.

Pediatric transports involve children aged newborn through 17 years and weighing several kilograms to an excess of 100 kg. The unpredictability of the patient characteristics, owing to large range of ages and sizes in the pediatric population, means that appropriately sized equipment must be immediately available for neonates to adult-sized pediatric patients. For example, size-specific equipment includes $ETCO_2$ adapters, pulse oximeter probes, blood pressure cuffs, advanced airway equipment, safety restraints, cervical collars and backboards, defibrillators, intravenous (IV) pumps, chest tubes, and venous access catheters. A transport ventilator capable of providing appropriate flow and settings to compensate for the large range of pediatric sizes is imperative. Adjustable trigger sensitivity, an oxygen blender, and multiple modes of ventilation (i.e., pressure ventilation, volume ventilation, pressure support) are desirable as well (Figure 17-10).

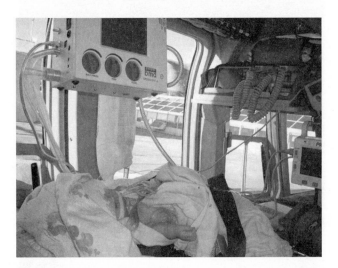

FIGURE 17-10

Transport Ventilator.

Source: © Jones & Bartlett Learning. Courtesy of MIEMSS.

Knowledge of pharmacotherapy for the ill or injured pediatric patient is required of all team members. Transport personnel regularly intubate young patients using rapid-sequence induction and manage patients requiring analgesia and sedation during transport (Ajizian & Nakagawa, 2007). Commonly used pharmacological agents in the transport environment include opiates, sedative/hypnotics, neuromuscular blocking agents, anticonvulsants, and vasoactive agents. Due to the large variance in pediatric weights, the ability to calculate and administer the correct volume of medication requires small-volume syringes and IV pumps capable of delivering medications in 0.1 mL/h increments.

PREPARATION FOR TRANSPORT

Care of the patient during transport follows the ABCDE of resuscitation:

- Airway
- Breathing
- Circulation
- Disability (neurologic evaluation)
- Exposure

AIRWAY

The preponderance of respiratory emergencies in children requires the transport team members to be experts in rapid and efficient assessment of the respiratory system. Team members should position themselves in a way so that they can efficiently manage the patient's airway. Inaccurate assessment may result in delay to definitive care or over-triaging, potentially causing inadvertent morbidity (Ajizian & Nakagawa, 2007).

The importance of ensuring the security of the artificial pediatric airway (i.e., endotracheal tube [ETT]) cannot be overstated. For instance, a head and neck movement of only 0.5 cm can determine the correct or incorrect position of the ETT in an infant. Blood, secretions, and facial burns may make securing the ETT challenging; however, protection of the airway is a primary concern during the transport process.

The correct position of the ETT is reassessed with transfer from a stretcher, transfer from a vehicle, with position changes, and as necessary. Due to noise pollution and inability to auscultate breath sounds in transport, especially in a helicopter, proper positioning and integrity of the artificial airway requires close attention. Correct positioning is monitored by chest rise, continuous $ETCO_2$ monitoring, visualization of the known depth indicator of the airway, and vigilant observation of proper ventilator function with absence of alarms. If there is any doubt, correct ETT placement is confirmed via direct laryngoscopy.

BREATHING

Assessment of breathing evaluates the quality and quantity of the patient's spontaneous respiratory rate (tachypnea—can be nonspecific; bradypnea and apnea—more ominous), amount of chest rise (tidal volume), absence or presence and equality of breath sounds, and work of breathing (e.g., retractions, nasal flaring, grunting, use of accessory muscles). Continuous visual assessment of the patient's respiratory status and the ability to provide emergent airway and breathing interventions must be accounted for within the spatial limitations of the transport environment (Figure 17-11).

Ventilator management and strategies to maintain oxygenation and ventilation are developed and discussed in the POC for each individual patient by health care professionals (HCPs) who routinely manage pediatric mechanical ventilation. Potential risks based on patient pathophysiology are planned for as needed (Ajizian & Nakagawa, 2007; Rhoades & Linsler, 2010).

CIRCULATION

Assessment of cardiovascular function includes evaluation of the presence or absence of pulses—distal and central—and their quality and rate. Heart rhythm, blood pressure, end-organ function (e.g., mental status, urine output), capillary refill time, and skin color and temperature are all indicators of circulatory function. In a cool environment, peripheral vasoconstriction occurs, affecting capillary refill time and skin color and temperature, and potentially altering the physical assessment despite normal cardiovascular function.

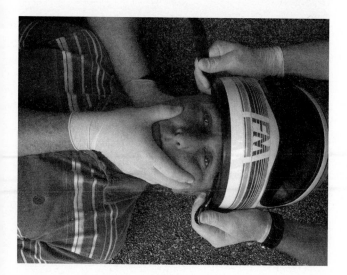

FIGURE 17-11

Stabilization.

Source: Courtesy of Mark Woolcock.

The cardiorespiratory monitor should be located in a secure position that is readily observable throughout the transport. The monitor provides a variety of visual (waveforms) and numerical data, including ECG, heart rate, respiratory rate, oxygen saturation, and, for the intubated patient, $ETCO_2$.

Establishment of vascular access is a common and often challenging problem in infants and smaller children (Ajizian & Nakagawa, 2007). This difficulty is more pronounced in the moving transport environment. Generally, at least one peripheral vein or intraosseous access is obtained prior to transport; additional access can be obtained en route.

Hypotension is supported with the administration of IV fluids, blood and blood products, and/or ionotropic agents. Active bleeding is controlled with direct pressure or indirect pressure (pelvic fracture). During a prolonged transport, serial hematocrit readings are valuable to guide treatment of ongoing blood loss.

DISABILITY

An abnormal level of consciousness (LOC) may result from a non-neurologic cause (such as shock and hypoxia) or from a primary neurologic disorder (such as traumatic brain injury). The LOC provides an important indication of brain perfusion. It can be quickly categorized using the AVPU scale:

A: alert
V: responds to verbal commands
P: responds to painful stimuli
U: unresponsive

The Pediatric Glasgow Coma Scale score (see Chapter 33) provides assessment of the patient's LOC and motor function. A GCS change of at least 2 points indicates a clinically important change in the patient's neurologic status.

Pupillary response is an indicator of brain stem function. Medications administered to the patient may also affect papillary responses; therefore, monitoring should occur throughout the transport as warranted by the patient condition or treatment strategies.

Prior to departure, cervical and spinal precautions are taken with trauma victims. Sensation and motor function are noted prior to and following such placement. Skeletal deformities are splinted in the position of comfort of function, with frequent neurovascular reassessments occurring throughout transport.

EXPOSURE

The initial examination requires that as much of the patient's body as possible be exposed. Children, however, are highly sensitive to environmental temperature conditions. Care should be taken during their exposure, and during transport, to prevent iatrogenic hypothermia. To help eliminate inadvertent hypothermia, HCPs may increase ambient room or vehicle temperature, adjust the neonatal transport incubator, examine the patient under a radiant warmer, administer warmed IV fluids or blood, shield the patient from rotor wash, apply chemical heat packs, cover the patient with warm blankets and a hat, and, if possible, provide warm and humidified oxygen (Figures 17-12 and 17-13). Devices to assess patient temperature should be available as standard equipment for pediatric transports.

Findings such as mottled skin, a distended abdomen, and traumatic injuries are more readily observed upon full exposure. Also, the team is better able to observe the patency and accessibility of existing intravascular devices and chest tubes, and to determine correct skeletal alignment with traction devices, when full exposure is available.

FAMILIES

Health care professionals cannot assume that the concerned persons they meet at the bedside are part of the child's nuclear family and therefore, the patient's legal guardians. Adopted children, blended families, biological parents, and legal guardians are examples of the diverse, family constellations that the transport team will encounter during their brief time at the child's bedside. Regardless of who the identified family members are, they are recognized as an integral part of the transport process, and an extension of the patient. They are generally the experts on the patient's well-being. Due to the nature of the environment and its inherent limitations, the transport team may have limited interaction with the family. The referring personnel's expectations of the transport team include approaching the family with an unbiased, respectful, and nonjudgmental attitude (Funk & Farber, 2009).

The unplanned, emergent transport is a new and frightening process for the caregivers and family members. This unfamiliar environment may provoke anxiety related to multiple variables such as loss of control, feelings of helplessness, and fear of the unfamiliar environment. Added to this mix are the stressors associated with the patient's injury or illness, physical separation from the patient, and the risk that the patient may die en route before he or she arrives at the accepting facility. To minimize these stressors, the transport team members should make every effort to speak with a family member before departing. As part of this communication, they should obtain a history and subjective information from the family, discuss a brief POC, answer questions, and ascertain the family's plan to arrive at the referring location. When possible, the family is encouraged to escort the team to the transport vehicle. If the family is not accompanying the patient, a good-bye show of affection is recommended before departing the referral facility. The

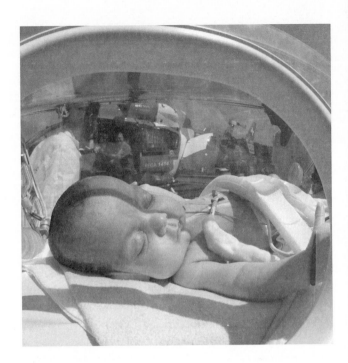

FIGURE 17-12

Neonatal Transport Incubator.

Source: Courtesy of Rega, Swiss Air-Rescue.

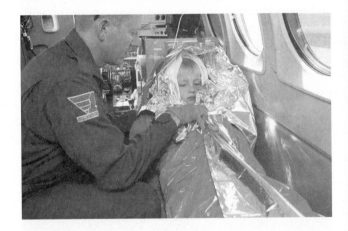

FIGURE 17-13

To manage a hypothermic pediatric patient, remove wet clothing, place him or her under a heat lamp, and provide warm blankets and liquids.

Source: © Jones & Bartlett Learning. Courtesy of MIEMSS.

team's competence, compassion, and empathy will help to alleviate caregiver anxieties and promote confidence in the transport process.

Transport programs should have established guidelines defining when or if a caregiver or family member may accompany a child in the transport vehicle. Every situation is different and must be handled accordingly. Safe completion of the transport is always the primary factor governing the decision to accept a family member in the vehicle. If safety is at risk, any member of the transport team has the right to veto a caregiver's traveling with the child (Funk & Farber, 2009). Examples of such concerns include, but are not limited to, impairment from substance abuse, inability to fit in the safety restraint, inappropriate level of anxiety related to the form of travel, and concerns expressed by the referring facility regarding the emotional stability of the identified family member. Other factors to consider include the spatial and weight limitations of the vehicle (often seen with rotor-wing flights); the existence of marginal weather; the length of transport time; liability concerns; an unstable patient requiring extensive care, reducing the team's ability to support the parent; concerns of occult injuries in the family member acquired in the same accident as the patient; and concern for caregiver interference with patient care.

In the prehospital urban setting, rotor-wing transport of a family member is less likely; however, in a rural backcountry setting, consideration may be made owing to the geographical distance to the referring facility. The family member must satisfy all requirements to allow safe completion of the transport.

OUTREACH EDUCATION AND FOLLOW-UP

Referring hospital staff and prehospital providers commonly desire education focusing on pediatric management until the transport team arrives. Nonpediatric care providers admit to feelings of increased stress related to caring for the critically ill or injured pediatric patient. Patient follow-up and outreach education allow the transport team to share their expertise in a nonacute, low-stress learning environment. They also provide an opportunity for referring staff to meet and interact with the transport team, develop confidence in the program, and recognize competence in the team members (AAP, 2007).

Pediatric outreach education may be proactive, such as addressing topics common to stabilization of the ill or injured patient and when to call for transport, or reactive, such as when a team member witnesses a knowledge deficit during the transfer process. The information provided is usually the current, evidence-based practice from the accepting facility, thereby supporting the referring facility's ability to initiate care prior to the transport team's arrival.

Follow-up information provides valuable feedback to the referring facility or HCPs and encourages the exchange of educational opportunities. This information must comply with Health Insurance Portability and Accountability Act (HIPAA) regulations and meet the guidelines set by both the transport program and the accepting facility. A telephone call, immediately following the transport, informs the referring facility that the patient and team arrived safely to their destination. A patient care update is relayed and questions answered. Verbal feedback is encouraged and provided, and future educational opportunities are identified. If permitted by the transport service, a confidential follow-up letter provides additional information including an update of the patient's hospital course and outcome. Follow-up may also include stress debriefing—immediately following the death and possibly at a later time, in a more formal environment—with staff members who are emotionally distraught over the tragic, sudden death of a pediatric patient.

REFERENCES

1. Ajizian, S., & Nakagawa, T. (2007). Interfacility transport of the critically ill pediatric patient. *Chest, 132,* 1361–1367.
2. American Academy of Pediatrics (AAP). (2007). *Guidelines for air and ground transport of neonatal and pediatric patients* (3rd ed.). Elk Grove Village, IL: Author.
3. Fenton, A., & Leslie, A. (2009). Who should staff neonatal transport teams? *Early Human Development, 85,* 487–490.
4. Funk, R., & Farber, J. (2009). Partners in care: Implementing a policy on family member passengers. *Air Medical Journal, 28,* 31–36.
5. Holleran, R. (2010). *ASTNA patient transport: Principles and practice* (4th ed.). St. Louis: Mosby/Elsevier.
6. Holleran, R., & Linsler, R. (2006). Pediatric transport team: Intermountain life flight. *Pediatric Emergency Care, 22,* 1–5.
7. Holleran, R., & Treadwell, D. (2010). Patient assessment and preparation for transport. In R. Holleran (Ed.), *ASTNA patient transport: Principles and practice* (pp. 138–180). St. Louis: Mosby/Elsevier.
8. Horowitz, R., & Rozenfeld, R. (2007). Pediatric critical care interfacility transport. *Clinical Pediatric Emergency Medicine, 8,* 190–202.
9. Kanter, R., & Tompkins, J. (1989). Adverse events during interhospital transport: Physiologic deterioration associated with pretransport severity of illness. *Pediatrics, 84,* 43–48.
10. Orr, R. A., Felmet, K., Han, Y., McCloskey, K., Dragotta, M., Bills, D., et al. (2009). Pediatric specialized transport teams are associated with improved outcomes. *Pediatrics, 124,* 40–48.
11. Orr, R., Han, Y., & Roth, K. (2006). Pediatric transport: Shifting the paradigm to improve patient outcomes. In B. Furhman & J. Zimmerman (Eds.), *Pediatric critical care* (3rd ed., pp. 141–150). St. Louis: Elsevier.
12. Ratnavel, N. (2009). Safety and governance issues for neonatal transport services. *Early Human Development, 85,* 483–486.
13. Rhoades, C., & Linsler, R. (2010). Mechanical ventilation. In R. Holleran (Ed.), *Air and surface patient transport: Principles and practice,* (4th ed., pp. 234–254). St. Louis: Mosby/Elsevier.
14. Slota, M. (2006). *Core curriculum for pediatric critical care nursing* (2nd ed.). Philadelphia: Saunders: 792–819.
15. Stroud, M., Prodhan, P., Moss, M., & Anand, K. (2008). Redefining the golden hour in pediatric transport. *Pediatric Critical Care Medicine, 9,* 435–437.
16. Tunik, G., & Foltin, G. (2008). Emergency medical services and transport. In J. Baren, S. Rothrock, & L. Brown (Eds.), *Pediatric emergency medicine* (pp. 1035–1042). St. Louis: Elsevier.
17. Worley, G. (2010). Safety and survival. In R. Holleran (Ed.), *ASTNA patient transport: Principles and practice* (4th ed., pp. 106–139). St. Louis: Mosby/Elsevier.

Angela M. Johnson

Integrative Medicine

In recent decades, the use of complementary and alternative medicine (CAM) in the United States has grown steadily. A major reason for the increased popularity of CAM is that it provides the opportunity to maintain a degree of control over one's care and offers hope for symptom management, and even cure (Sencer & Kelly, 2007). The National Center for Complementary and Alternative Medicine (NCCAM, 2007) defines CAM as a group of diverse medical and health care systems, practices, and products that are not generally considered part of conventional medicine. An important distinction to note is that the term "complementary" medicine denotes therapies used "in conjunction with" conventional medicine—for example, acupuncture used in conjunction with analgesics to help better manage pain. In contrast, the term "alternative" medicine denotes therapies used "as a replacement for" conventional medicine—for example, the use of herbs to treat depression) (Kemper et al., 2008). More recently, the term "integrative medicine" has emerged to describe complementary therapies. For the purposes of this chapter, the term *integrative medicine* (IM) will be used.

IM involves using evidence-based CAM therapies in conjunction with conventional medicine. Kemper and Shannon (2007) suggest that IM encompasses four core concepts:

- Patient-centered care (individualized, consistent with patient values and goals)
- Sustainable, healing environment
- Comprehensive approaches to therapies
- Health promotion and wellness; promotion of the innate healing potential

One integrative medicine care model that has been widely accepted in the field of pediatrics is the Kemper Model of Holistic Care (Table 18-1). This paradigm integrates conventional and complementary therapies into a coherent construct of treatment options (Kemper et al., 2008).

A second, also frequently referenced model has been developed NCCAM (2009). This model groups individual therapies into five main domains:

- Whole medical systems (e.g., traditional Chinese medicine, Ayurveda, naturopathic, and homeopathic medicine) are built upon complete systems of theory and practice.
- Mind–body medicine (e.g., meditation, visualization, and prayer) comprises a combination of techniques used to enhance the mind's ability to positively affect physical and mental functioning.
- Biologically based practices include vitamins, minerals, fatty acids, dietary supplements, animal-derived extracts, probiotics, prebiotics, whole diets, functional foods, and herbal products.
- Manipulative and body-based practices involve the manipulation or movement of one or more body part; examples include chiropracty and massage.
- Energy medicine (e.g., qi gong, reiki, and therapeutic touch) involves the use of manipulating energy fields that purportedly surround and penetrate the body.

PREVALENCE OF USE

In 2008, NCCAM and National Center for Health Statistics released findings on adult and pediatric use of IM. The reports from more than 32,000 people revealed IM use among 38.3% and 11.8% of U.S. adults and pediatrics, respectively. Among healthy pediatric patients seen in outpatient settings, the American Academy of Pediatrics (AAP) has estimated current levels of utilization of IM

TABLE 18-1

Kemper Model of Holistic Care			
Biochemical	**Lifestyle**	**Biomechanical**	**Bioenergetic**
Medications	Nutrition	Massage and bodywork	Acupuncture
Dietary supplements	Exercise/rest	Chiropractic and osteopathic adjustments	Radiation therapy
Vitamins	Environmental therapies (heat, ice, music, vibration, light)	Surgery	Magnets
Minerals	Mind–body therapies (behavior management, meditation, hypnosis, biofeedback, counseling)		Reiki
Herbal remedies			Healing touch Qi gong Therapeutic touch Homeopathy

Source: Kemper et al., 2008.

to range between 20% and 40%. Among patients with chronic, recurrent, or incurable illnesses such as asthma, juvenile rheumatoid arthritis, and cancer, the rate of IM use is as high as 72% (Jean & Cyr, 2007).

Factors influencing IM use among pediatric patients include word-of-mouth, fear of side effects from traditional drugs, chronic medical problems, dissatisfaction with conventional medicine, and more personalized attention from IM providers (Pitetti et al., 2001). Additionally, studies find that when a person actively participates in his or her own care, it provides a sense of autonomy (Gardiner & Wornham, 2000), which often increases compliance, leads to a feeling of empowerment and, in adult studies, has been found to be therapeutically beneficial (Sencer & Kelly, 2007).

EVIDENCE-BASED IM IN PEDIATRIC CARE

When counseling pediatric patients and their caregivers about IM, it is the health care professional's (HCP's) ethical responsibility to seek information and evaluate the scientific merits of specific modalities. While a number of reviews have focused on the use of IM in the pediatric population, detailed information about the safety and efficacy of many IM therapies used in pediatrics is limited or has yet to be compiled.

Guidelines outlined by the AAP recommend that practitioners apply common sense to balancing the risks and benefits when making therapeutic decisions. The following factors should be considered in the decision-making process:

- Severity and acuteness of illness
- Curability with conventional care
- Degree of invasiveness
- Toxicities and adverse effects of conventional treatment
- Quality of evidence for efficacy and safety of the complementary therapy
- The family's understanding of the risks and benefits of IM treatment, voluntary acceptance of those risks, and persistence of the family's intention to use IM therapy (Kemper et al., 2008)

After gathering evidence-based information, the decision-making process and plan should be conducted in a collaborative manner in which the patient and caregiver are given unbiased information so that they can make informed decisions together with the HCP.

EXAMPLES OF EVIDENCE-BASED IM IN PEDIATRIC CARE

Some of the most popular forms of IM among the pediatric population include chiropracty, herbal supplements, and acupuncture. Examples of other forms of IM used by pediatrics include massage therapy and mind–body medicine (i.e., breathing, visualization, biofeedback).

CHIROPRACTY

One of the most common IM modalities used among pediatrics is chiropractic medicine. An estimated 14% of all visits to chiropractors involve pediatric patients (Kemper et al., 2008). Most patients seek out chiropractors for help with conditions ranging from musculoskeletal pain and otitis media to allergies and attention-deficit/hyperactivity disorder (ADHD). NCCAM describes chiropractic care as a health care approach that focuses on the relationship between the body's structure—mainly the spine and its functioning. While few randomized controlled trials have demonstrated clinical benefit from chiropractic care, data on pediatric safety are lacking (Vohra et al., 2007). According to Kemper et al. (2008), anecdotal evidence suggests severe complications are possible with chiropractic treatment of the pediatric patient, although such outcomes seem to be rare. Lin et al. (2005) suggest that pediatric chiropractic care is often not consistent with recommended medical guidelines, and national guidelines are needed to assess safety, efficacy, and cost of chiropractic care for children.

NONPHARMACEUTICAL HERBS, DIETARY SUPPLEMENTS, HOMEOPATHY, AND VITAMINS

Biologically based practices, such as use of nonpharmaceutical herbs, dietary supplements, homeopathy, and vitamins, are another popular form of IM among pediatrics. An estimated 20% to 40% of young children and adolescents in the United States take dietary supplements (Gardiner & Riley, 2007). Other surveys of older pediatric patients suggest that as many as 75% use of herbal supplements (Kemper et al., 2008). The increased use of herbal products among older pediatric patients may be correlated with anabolic steroid use, which studies have shown to be on the rise in as early as eighth grade.

Trends suggest that pediatrics with medical conditions, such as ADHD, asthma, cancer, allergic rhinitis, headache, and inflammatory bowel disease, are more likely to take dietary supplements. Some of the more commonly used herbs in pediatrics include Echinacea, German chamomile (*Matricaria recuita*), ginger, lemon balm (*Melissa officinalis*), and valarian (*Valarian officinalis*). Gardiner and Riley (2007) suggest that scientific studies support use of these herbs for some uses (i.e., calming effects of chamomile), but note that all have been found to have either potential side effects or contraindications.

While a number of review articles have addressed the use of herbal products (i.e., efficacy, toxicity, and drug–herb interactions), most supplements are not subject to government regulation, suffer from a lack of standardization, and have not undergone rigorous trials. To help potential users, their caregivers, and HCPs navigate through the decision-making process, Woolf (2003) makes two points:

- Peer-reviewed studies on the efficacy of herbal remedies should be critically reviewed and the HCP should form his or her own conclusions.
- The limited information regarding IM available for pediatric use suggests that these products may extend hospitalization or interfere with successful diagnosis and therapies.

Some reputable websites and other resources related to these products are summarized in Table 18-2.

ACUPUNCTURE

Another IM modality commonly used among pediatric patients is acupuncture. Of all IM modalities, acupuncture has been reported as among the most frequently recommended by HCPs; it is currently practiced in more than 140 hospitals in the United States (Gold et al., 2008). Despite conventional thought that pediatric patients are afraid of

needles, most studies reveal that they find acupuncture helpful and highly acceptable (Zeltzer et al., 2002).

Originating in China, acupuncture has been practiced for more than 2,000 years. It is part of the medical system called traditional Chinese medicine (TCM). From a TCM perspective, energy or *qi* (pronounced "chee") is distributed throughout the body via meridians. Along these meridians lie approximately 2,000 acupuncture points with specific functions to help restore obstructed qi, which is suggested to contribute to pain, illness, and disease. From a Western medical perspective, an agreed-upon physiological basis for acupuncture's clinical effects remains unclear. Pain studies suggest acupuncture "releases endogenous opioid peptides, such as beta-endorphin, and perhaps other neurotransmitters and neurohormones in the brain" (Wu et al., 2009).

One of the most common ways a practitioner accesses qi is through acupuncture. This technique involves the gentle insertion of hair-thin, solid, single-use, stainless-steel needles into the skin at various acupoints along the meridians. When performed by trained professionals, acupuncture is generally considered safe. While there have been case reports of some fatalities from acupuncture-related complications (i.e., pneumothorax, cardiac tamponade, serious infection), Kemper et al. (2000) suggest that the

TABLE 18-2

Resources

Internet Resources

Academy for Guided Imagery
American Holistic Medical Association

AMSA Foundation EDCAM Curriculum Resource Materials

CAMLAW blog (Michael H. Cohen)
Cancer.gov CAM Resources
Center for Mind–Body Medicine
Center for Mindfulness at University of Massachusetts
Children's Complementary Therapy Network (CCTN), United Kingdom
Children's Hospitals and Clinics of Minnesota Integrative Medicine Program
Consumer Labs Reviews

FDA Dietary Supplements Page

Canadian Pediatric Complementary and Alternative Medicine Network (PedCAM)
HerbMed Index
International Bibliographic Information on Dietary Supplements (IBIDS)
Longwood Herbal Task Force
MedlinePlus—Alternative Medicine
Medscape
Mind–Body Medical Institute at Harvard University
National Center for Complementary and Alternative Medicine (NCCAM/NIH)
Native American Ethnobotany (University of Michigan–Dearborn)
Natural Medicines Comprehensive Database
Natural Standard
Office of Dietary Supplements

(Continued)

TABLE 18-2

Resources (Continued)
Books

The American Holistic Medical Association Guide to Holistic Health (Trivieri), 2001
Aromatherapy for the Healthy Child (Worwood), 2000
Creating the Peaceable Classroom (Bothmer), 2003
Everyday Blessings: The Inner Work of Mindful Parenting (Kabat-Zinn), 1998
Guided Imagery for Healing Children and Teens (Curran), 2001
Healing Images for Children: Teaching Relaxation and Guided Imagery to Children Facing Cancer and Other Serious Illnesses (Klein), 2001
Healthy Child, Whole Child: Integrating the Best of Conventional and Alternative Medicine to Keep Your Kids Healthy (Ditchek and Greenfield), 2001
The Holistic Pediatrician, second edition (Kemper), 2002
Hypnosis and Hypnotherapy with Children (Olness and Kohen), 1996
Integrative Medicine (Rakel), 2003
Integrative Medicine: Principles for Practice (Kligler and Lee), 2004
Itsy Bitsy Yoga (Garabedian), 2004
Nature Cures: The History of Alternative Medicine in America (Whorton), 2002
Pediatric Acupuncture (Loo), 2002
Raising Healthy Children in a Toxic World (Landrigan), 2001
Smart Medicine for a Healthier Child: A Practical A-to-Z Reference to Natural and Conventional Treatments for Infants and Children, second edition (Zand), 2003
The Whole Food Market Cookbook (Petusevsky), 2002
Yoga for the Special Child (Sumar), 1998

Source: Courtesy of Lawrence D. Rosen, MD, The Whole Child Center.

incidence of serious side effects from acupuncture is in the range of 1:10,000 to 1:100,000—about the same risk as for a serious adverse event from taking penicillin. In a review of pediatric adverse events, Jindal et al. (2008) labeled acupuncture as low risk (i.e., 1.55 adverse events occurring in 100 treatments).

In pediatric populations, researchers have found some efficacy to support the use of acupuncture for conditions such as postoperative nausea and vomiting, seasonal allergic rhinitis, recurrent headaches, and nocturnal enuresis (Jindal et al., 2008; Kemper et al., 2008; Libonate et al., 2008). Additionally, in combination with hypnosis, acupuncture has been found to be feasible and acceptable for chronic pediatric pain (Zeltzer et al., 2002). As suggested by many authors, there is an ongoing need for continued randomized controlled studies of all IM modalities for various medical conditions in pediatric populations.

COMMUNICATION AND COLLABORATION

Today's pediatric patients and caregivers have a great desire to be involved in decisions about their own health care. This is especially the case for caregivers with chronically ill children, who will often search for every means possible to help alleviate their children's pain and suffering. IM offers a unique opportunity to address pain and suffering in a patient-centered, holistic, collaborate manner. Communication is essential in promoting this collaboration. Unfortunately, communication between the patient and family and the HCP is often lacking. In fact, some studies show that as many as 50% of families who use IM do not reveal this fact to their HCP (Sawni et al., 2007; Woolf, 2003). The most cited reason for nondisclosure: The HCP did not ask. Other reasons include that the caregiver or patient did not believe the IM modality was relevant and that the family sensed disinterest or disapproval from their HCP regarding IM (Sibinga et al., 2004).

Experts in the field recommend HCPs routinely ask patients about IM use in an open and nonjudgmental manner. To help gather as much information as possible, HCPs are encouraged to ask specifically if the patient is using any herbs, supplements, home remedies, massage, acupuncture, or other services to enhance health. Additionally, when making referrals to IM practitioners, encourage the patient and caregiver to become familiar with IM practitioners' credentials (i.e., education, training, licensing, credentialing, areas of expertise), and include the IM provider in your overall care-coordinating activities.

Interest in and use of integrative medicine among pediatric patients is steadily increasing. Depending on the available evidence, a HCP should encourage communication and support use when appropriate. Having thoughtful conversations that provide knowledgeable guidance about therapeutic options may bridge gaps in beliefs about wellness and disease, further strengthen the patient–practitioner relationship, and, most importantly, promote improved heath of the pediatric patient.

REFERENCES

1. Gardiner, P., & Riley, D. (2007). Herbs to homeopathy: Medicinal products for children. *Pediatric Clinics of North America, 54*, 859–874.

2. Gardiner, P., & Wornham, W. (2000). Recent review of complementary and alternative medicine used by adolescents. *Current Opinion in Pediatrics, 12*, 298–302.

3. Gold, J., Nicolaou, C., Belmont, K., Katz, A., Benaron, D., & Yu, W. (2008). Pediatric acupuncture: A review of clinical research. Retrieved from http://ecam.oxfordjournals.org/cgi/reprint/6/4/429

4. Jean, D., & Cyr, C. (2007). Use of complementary and alternative medicine in a general pediatric clinic. *Pediatrics, 120,* e148–e141.

5. Jindal, V., Ge, A., & Mansky, P. (2008). Safety and efficacy of acupuncture: A review of the evidence. *Journal of Pediatric Hematology Oncology, 30*(6), 431–442.

6. Kemper, K., Sarah, R., Silver-Highfield, E., Xiarhos, E., Barnes, L., & Berde, C. (2000). On pins and needles? Pediatric pain patients' experience with acupuncture. *Pediatrics, 105*(4), 941–947.

7. Kemper, K., & Shannon, S. (2007). Complementary and alternative medicine therapies to promote healthy moods. *Pediatric Clinics of North America, 54*, 901–926.

8. Kemper, K., Vohra, S., & Walls, R. (2008). The use of complementary and alternative medicine in pediatrics. *Pediatrics, 122*, 1374–1386.

9. Libonate, J., Evans, S., & Tsao, J. (2008). Efficacy of acupuncture for health conditions in children: A review. *Scientific World Journal, 8*, 670–682.

10. Lin, Y., Lee, A., Kemper, K., & Berde C. (2005). Use of complementary and alternative medicine in pediatric pain service: A survey. *Pain Management, 6*(6), 452–458.

11. National Center for Complementary and Alternative Medicine (NCCAM). (2007). The use of complementary and alternative medicine in the united states. Retrieved from http://nccam.nih.gov/news/camstats/2007/camsurvey_fs1.htm

12. National Center for Complementary and Alternative Medicine (NCCAM). (2009). What is CAM? Retrieved from http://nccam.nih.gov/health/whatiscam/overview.htm

13. Pitetti, R., Singh, S., Hornyak, D., Garcia, S., & Herr, S. (2001). Complementary and alternative medicine use in children. *Pediatric Emergency Care, 54*(3), 165–169.

14. Sawni, A., Ragothaman, R., Thomas, R., & Mahajan, P. (2007). The use of complementary/alternative therapies among children attending an urban pediatric emergency department, *Clinical Pediatrics, 46*(7), 36–41.

15. Sencer, S., & Kelly, K. (2007). Complementary and alternative therapies in pediatric oncology. *Pediatric Clinics of North America, 54*, 1043–1060.

16. Sibinga, E., Ottonlini, M., Duggan, M., & Wilson, M. (2004). Parent–pediatrician communication about complementary and alternative medicine use for children. *Clinical Pediatrics, 43*(4), 367–373.

17. Vohra, S., Johnston, B., Cramer, K., & Humphreys, K. (2007). Adverse events associated with pediatric spinal manipulation: A systemic review. *Pediatrics, 119*(1), e275–e283.

18. Woolf, A. (2003). Herbal remedies and children: Do they work? Are they harmful? *Pediatrics, 112*(1): 240–246.

19. Wu, S., Sapru, A., Stewart, M., Millet, M., Hudes, M., Livermore, L., & Flori, H. (2009). Using acupuncture for acute pain in hospitalized children. *Pediatric Critical Care, 10*(3), 291–296.

20. Zeltzer, L., Tsao, J., Stelling, C., Powers, M., Levy, S., & Waterhouse, M. (2002). A phase I study of the feasibility and acceptability of an acupuncture/hypnosis intervention for chronic pediatric pain. *Journal of Pain and Symptom Management, 24*(4), 437–446.

Rehabilitation

- Prolonged Immobility
- Oromotor Dysfunction
- Stimulation Therapy
- Circadian Rhythm Aids

- Seizures
- Spasticity
- References

Rehabilitation health care professionals (HCPs) identify patient strengths and deficits after illness or injury so as to facilitate patients' function in mobility, cognition, swallowing, communication, and independence in the activities of daily living. Early consultation with the rehabilitation team optimizes therapeutic interventions, management goals, and communication between the rehabilitation HCPs and pediatric patients and their caregivers, thereby enabling a smoother transition to the acute inpatient rehabilitation service with eventual reintegration of the patient back home, in school, and in the community.

Rehabilitation should be initiated early during the intensive care stay, as this approach will shorten both the overall hospital and inpatient rehabilitation stays. Early transfer to the inpatient rehabilitation unit is appropriate once the pediatric patient is medically stable enough to leave the intensive care unit.

The attending physiatrist, physical therapist, occupational therapist, speech therapist, and other subspecialists (e.g., psychologist, orthotist) are but a few of the many members of the interprofessional team of rehabilitation HCPs who are involved in the acute care of pediatric patients in the intensive care setting.

PROLONGED IMMOBILITY

Prolonged immobility predisposes a patient to develop pressure ulcers, muscle contractures with loss of range of motion, heterotopic ossification (most commonly in the hip and knee), and peripheral mononeuropathies secondary to compression of body parts (Hurvitz et al., 1992). The rehabilitation team works to ameliorate the effects of immobility through medical management, therapeutic exercises and activities, equipment (e.g., wheelchairs, tilt tables, standers), and orthotics. The occupational therapist initiates activities of daily living to facilitate hygiene and general care of the patient with patient-specific adaptive equipment that can facilitate this task. These HCPs also focus on designing upper extremity splints for positioning and function. Use of orthotics and splints, especially in the sedated pediatric patient, requires strict skin vigilance and on/off schedules to optimize the benefits of these devices and prevent complications from their use.

OROMOTOR DYSFUNCTION

The speech pathologist and the occupational therapist work together in facilitating communication and oromotor skills, especially once the patient is extubated. The pediatric patient with a tracheostomy and on a ventilator, for example, can eat by mouth. A feeding trial is performed at the bedside. If concerns for aspiration exist, an instrumental or radiological evaluation of swallowing skill may

be performed to evaluate for dysphagia. Once dysphagia has been identified, therapists may trial different maneuvers, diet textures or consistencies, and ways of presenting and offering the food (e.g., quantities, bottles, frequencies) to improve feeding. Thin, liquid consistencies are the hardest and least safe to manage orally in those patients with acquired brain injury (ABI) and delayed oral motor response. Conversely, patients who fatigue easily and have significant deconditioning are more likely to have difficulty with chewing of solids.

STIMULATION THERAPY

Stimulation therapy is useful in the acute period for those patients with low-level consciousness. Its use, however, must be considered in relationship to ongoing medical problems such as increased intracranial pressure. Stimulation therapy is usually initiated as a structured stimulus that is brief and of low intensity. Its intensity and duration are then increased as tolerated. Stimulation therapy may include environmental modification, multisensory stimulation, or the use of technology and pharmacological interventions. During this early intervention phase of rehabilitation within the intensive care setting, clear communication with the critical care service is important so that contraindications to rehabilitation therapies are understood.

Pharmacologic neurostimulation is a standard therapeutic approach for both pediatric and adult patients with ABI. The pharmacological agents used vary depending on the targeted signs or symptoms (Patrick et al., 2003; Williams, 2007). Amantadine, a dopamine agonist, is a well-tolerated neurostimulant in children. The dosage of amantadine in the pediatric patient with ABI is usually higher than that used for prophylaxis and treatment of parainfluenza. Amantadine may also be of use for the management of agitation; however, beta blockers such as propranolol are generally considered more effective than amantadine, valproic acid, carbamazepine, or methylphenidate (Fleminger et al., 2003; Vargus-Adams et al., 2010). Other medications used as neurostimulants in the pediatric population include bromocriptine, levo/carbodopa, and methylphenidate; however, their long-term effects are unknown (Williams et al., 1998).

CIRCADIAN RHYTHM AIDS

An early goal is to reestablish the sleep–wake circadian rhythm, which is commonly lost in the intensive care setting. Trazodone, an antidepressant, is commonly administered to help with night sleep, which is important during the recovery phase (Lombard & Zafonte, 2005).

Melatonin (*N*-acetyl-5-methoxytryptamine) is a chronobiotic—that is, a neurohormone involved in the regulation of the sleep–wake cycle. Produced in the pineal gland through the conversion of tryptophan, it is normally secreted during darkness, in response to the release of norepinephrine from retinal photoreceptors and the resulting activation of the retino-hypothalamic-pineal system. Levels are highest in children, but and decline as individuals age. Levels begin to rise at nightfall and peak in adults at 2 to 4 A.M.; therefore minimal secretion occurs during daylight hours. Exogenous melatonin is sold as an over-the-counter (OTC) dietary supplement in the United States. It is synthesized from the amino acid tryptophan, which occurs naturally in certain foods, such as turkey, seeds, and nuts. Melatonin's use has not been FDA reviewed for safety, efficacy, or purity; thus this agent is used to only a limited extent in children. Melatonin has been studied in pediatrics to promote circadian rhythm and administered in the evening as a natural sleep aid (Owens et al., 2003). Dosage is based on weight and age and institutional protocol. Side effects at higher adult dosing have been associated with seizures.

One of the scales commonly used to assess cognitive function and rate of disability is the Rancho Los Amigos Scale of Cognitive Levels (Hagen et al., 1972). In addition, tools are available to evaluate stimulus therapy or intervention, such as the Coma/Near Coma Scale (Rappaport et al., 1992) and the Glasgow Outcome Scale (Jennett et al., 1981). Other scales used in the inpatient rehabilitation setting that are probably not as applicable to the intensive care setting are the Functional Independence Measures for Children (WeeFIM), the Pediatric Evaluation of Disability Inventory (PEDI), the Functional Rehabilitation Evaluation of Sensori-Neurologic Outcomes (FRESNO), and the Barthel Index (Golomb et al., 2004; Mahoney & Barthel, 1965; Roberts et al., 1999). The Coma/Near Coma Scale is useful in evaluating small and reproducible changes in states of low-level consciousness in both pediatric and adult patients who are being challenged with a structured yet brief stimulus for which one anticipates a response.

SEIZURES

Prophylactic antiepileptic drugs (AEDs) are not recommended to prevent the development of late seizures (Adelson et al., 2003; Young et al., 1983); however, they may be considered as a treatment to prevent early seizures (between 24 hours and 7 days) in high-risk pediatric patients. For children, having early seizures after a traumatic brain injury does not correlate with the development of late seizures as it does in the adult (Annegers et al., 1980) yet the incidence of post-traumatic seizures is greater in children than in adults, especially in children younger than 1 year of age at the time of injury (Raimondi & Hirschauer, 1984). There is concern that the use of AEDs in young children

may interfere with the developing brain; therefore, these agents should be used only when clinically required and at the lowest clinically effective dose to facilitate maximum cognitive recovery (Ikonomidou & Turski, 2010). More studies are needed to establish clear guidelines in the use of AEDs, including the newer-generation forms, in children.

SPASTICITY

Spasticity, posturing, and movement disorders in the patient with ABI can be a challenge to control. Initial therapies include conservative management with range of motion exercises, slow stretching, functional electrical stimulation, casting, and splinting. If these interventions fail, then pharmacological interventions may be considered.

Diazepam is a long-acting benzodiazepine that acts at the gamma-aminobutyric acid (GABA) A receptor. It is effective in controlling spasticity; however, due to its sedation side effects and propensity to exacerbate cognitive deficits, this medication's use for spasticity of cerebral origin may be limited (Watanabe, 2009). Dependence and withdrawal are additional concerns with the use of the benzodiazepines for spasticity management. Diazepam may be best used for pediatric patients with significant spasticity and seizure disorders.

Baclofen is a GABA B agonist that may have beneficial effects on spasticity but also may have significant side effects such as confusion, sedation, dizziness, nausea, and constipation. Abrupt withdrawal from this agent is life-threatening and produces effects similar to neuroleptic malignant syndrome. Oral baclofen may be effective for generalized spasticity and dystonia, either alone or in combination with other medications.

Intrathecal baclofen (ITB) therapy is very effective in the patient with ABI and significant spasticity, posturing, and severe autonomic dysfunction (Albright & Ferson, 2006). It may also be effective in secondary dystonia, an involuntary sustained or intermittent muscle contraction with variable repetitive movements and posturing, although it has not yet been approved for this use by the U.S. Food and Drug Administration. ITB therapy is delivered via a programmable infusion pump whose implantation requires a surgical procedure, but that results in fewer side effects (Albright & Ferson, 2006; Turner, 2003). ITB has proven effective for treating spasticity caused by cerebral palsy, multiple sclerosis, brain injury, spinal cord injury, strokes, and secondary dystonia in acute and chronic stages of therapy (Francisco et al., 2005; 2007).

Dantrolene may be effective in managing spasticity by blocking calcium release from the sarcoplasmic reticulum of skeletal muscle (it works peripherally). Side effects associated with this medication include fatigue, lethargy, and possibly weakness in the nonaffected limbs with decreased postural control. Dantrolene is hepatotoxic; therefore, its use requires close monitoring of liver function over time and with each dose adjustment (Watanabe, 2009).

Other medications used for treatment of spasticity include clonidine, tizanidine, cyproheptadine, gabapentin, pregabalin, cannabinoids, and 4-aminopyridine (Watanabe, 2009). These medications, however, may decrease spasticity with variable results and their side effects may limit their effectiveness. There is no good evidence of functional improvement with the use of these medications.

When spasticity is localized within a specific group of muscles, chemodenervation and neurolysis are techniques that may be utilized to control the spasticity without having the potential sedating side effects of the previously described medications (Elovic et al., 2009). Common agents for chemodenervation are botulism neurotoxin (BoNT), phenol, and alcohol.

Botulism neurotoxin (BoNT), in the form of BoNT type A (Botox and Dysport) and BoNT type B may be used for spasticity management in localized muscles. It is given by intramuscular injection, so it is easy to administer (anesthesia not required); in addition, this agent easy to titrate. The disadvantages are that it is very costly, only a limited amount of BoNT can be injected into any one muscle, the drug has a longer onset of action (delayed benefit), and it can be reinjected only every 3 months (Elovic et al., 2009). Caution should be used when BoNT is administered to very ill patients with acute respiratory problems due to the possible systemic effects of dysphagia, dyspnea, and visual problems (the subject of a FDA "black box" warning on BoNT's label).

Phenol and alcohol may be used for neurolysis with a perineural injection or as a motor-point block injection (Elovic et al., 2009). Both of these agents have an immediate onset of action, are potent, are inexpensive, and may be reinjected within 1 week if necessary. The disadvantages are that patients need to be sedated for injection, there is a risk of dysesthesias, fibrosis can develop in the soft tissue, and injection is technically more difficult than for botulism toxins. Phenol and alcohol are good options whenever the use of botulism toxin is contraindicated or when there is an increased risk of systemic effects and complications from the botulism toxins.

REFERENCES

1. Adelson, P., Bratton, S., & Carney, N. (2003). Guidelines for the acute medical management of severe traumatic brain injury in infants, children, and adolescents: The role of antiseizure prophylaxis following severe pediatric traumatic brain injury. *Pediatric Critical Care Medicine, 4*(3 suppl), S72–S75.

2. Albright, A., & Ferson, S. (2006). Intrathecal baclofen therapy in children. *Neurosurgery Focus, 21*(2), 1–6.

3. Annegers, J., Grabow, R., Laws, E. Jr., Elveback, L., & Kurland, L. (1980). Seizures after head trauma: A population study. *Neurology, 30*(7 Pt 1), 683–689.

4. Elovic, E., Esquenazi, A., Alter, K., Lin, J., Alfaro, A., & Kaelin, D. (2009). Chemodenervation and nerve blocks in the diagnosis and management of spasticity and muscle overactivity. *PM & R; The Journal of Injury, Function, and Rehabilitation, 1*(9), 842–851.

5. Fleminger, S., Greenwood, R., & Oliver, D. (2003). Pharmacological management for agitation and aggression in people with acquired brain injury. *Cochrane Database of Systematic Reviews, 1*, Art. No.: CD003299. doi: 10.1002/14651858.CD003299

6. Francisco, G., Hu, M., Boake, C., & Ivanhoe, C. (2005). Efficacy of early use of intrathecal baclofen therapy for treating spastic hypertonia due to acquired brain injury. *Brain Injury, 19*(5), 359–364.

7. Francisco, G., Latorre, J., & Ivanhoe, C. (2007). Intrathecal baclofen therapy for spastic hypertonia in chronic traumatic brain injury. *Brain Injury, 21*(3), 335–338.

8. Golomb, M., Garg, B., & Williams, L. (2004). Measuring gross motor recovery in young children with early brain injury. *Pediatric Neurology, 31*(5), 311–317.

9. Hagen, C., Malkmus, D., & Durham, P. (1972). *Levels of cognitive functioning*. Downey, CA: Rancho Los Amigos Hospital.

10. Hurvitz, E., Mandac, B., Davidoff, G., Johnson, J., & Nelson, V. (1992). Risk factors for heterotopic ossification in children and adolescents with severe traumatic brain injury. *Archives of Physical Medicine and Rehabilitation, 73*, 459–462.

11. Ikonomidou, C., & Turski, L. (2010). Antiepileptic drugs and brain development. *Epilepsy Research, 88*(1), 11–22.

12. Jennett, B., Snoek, J., Bond, M., & Brooks, N. (1981). Disability after severe head injury: Observations on the use of the Glasgow Outcome Scale. *Journal of Neurology, Neurosurgery & Psychiatry, 44*(4), 285–293.

13. Lombard, L., & Zafonte, R. (2005). Agitation after traumatic brain injury. *American Journal of Physical Medicine and Rehabilitation, 84*, 797–812.

14. Mahoney, F., & Barthel, D. (1965). Functional evaluation: The Barthel Index. *Mississippi State Medical Journal, 14*, 61–65.

15. Owens, J., Rosen, C., & Mindell, J. (2003). Medication use in the treatment of pediatric insomnia: Results of a survey of community-based pediatricians. *Pediatrics, 111*(5), 628–635.

16. Patrick, P., Buck, M., Conway, M., & Blackman, J. (2003). The use of dopamine enhancing medications with children in low response states following brain injury. *Brain Injury, 17*, 497–506.

17. Raimondi, A., & Hirschauer, J. (1984). Head injury in the infant and toddler: Coma scoring and outcome scale. *Child's Brain, 11*(1), 12–35.

18. Rappaport, M., Dougherty, A., & Kelting, D. (1992). Evaluation of coma and vegetative states. *Archives of Physical Medicine and Rehabilitation, 73*(7), 628–634.

19. Roberts, S., Wells, R., Brown, I., et al. (1999). The FRESNO: A pediatric functional outcome measurement system. *Journal of Rehabilitation Outcomes and Measures, 3*(1), 11–19.

20. Turner, M. (2003). Early use of intrathecal baclofen in brain injury in pediatric patients. *Acta Neurochirurgica (Wien), 87*, 81–83.

21. Vargus-Adams, J., McMahon, M., Michaud, L., Bean, J., & Vinks, A. (2010). Pharmacokinetics of amantadine in children with impaired consciousness due to acquired brain injury: Preliminary findings using a sparse-sampling technique. *PM & R Journal, 2*, 37–42.

22. Watanabe, T. (2009). Role of oral medications in spasticity management. *PM & R Journal, 1*, 839–841.

23. Williams, S. (2007). Amantadine treatment following traumatic brain injury in children. *Brain Injury, 21*, 885–889.

24. Williams, S., Ris, M., Ayyangar, R., Schefft, B., & Berch, D. (1998). Recovery in pediatric brain injury: Is psychostimulant medication beneficial? *Journal of Head Trauma Rehabilitation, 13*, 73–81.

25. Young, B., Rapp, R., Norton, J., Haack, D., & Walsh, J. (1983). Failure of prophylactically administered phenytoin to prevent post-traumatic seizures in children. *Child's Brain, 10*(3), 185–192.

Christine A. Zawistowski

Palliative Care

Palliative care is care provided to patients with life-limiting or life-threatening conditions that seeks to prevent and relieve suffering while supporting the best quality of life for patients and their families (National Consensus Project for Quality Palliative Care [NCP], 2009). Palliative care enhances quality of life in the face of an ultimately terminal condition. When such care is delivered, the overall goal is to add life to the pediatric patient's years, *not* years to the patient's life. The focus of care shifts more to symptom relief than purely curative measures, and seeks to strike a balance between the two. Good palliative care follows the family after the patient's death and ensures that bereaved families remain functional and intact. Most importantly, palliative care is an interprofessional approach that requires the skills and talents of every member of the health care team.

Palliative care is sometimes confused with hospice care, although some important differences separate the two. Hospice care is a subset of palliative care and most often takes place in a patient's home; in contrast, palliative care is provided wherever the patient is cared for. To be eligible to receive hospice care, a patient must be deemed "terminal," with a life expectancy of no more than 6 months. Palliative care, however, begins with the initial diagnosis of a life-limiting illness and continues throughout its course. The focus of hospice care is comfort rather than disease abatement, whereas palliative care addresses both comfort care and life-prolonging therapies.

THE NEED FOR PEDIATRIC PALLIATIVE CARE

Approximately 55,000 pediatric patients in the United States die every year from trauma, lethal congenital conditions, extreme prematurity, heritable disorders, or acquired illnesses. Of this number, one-half die in the first year of life; of those deaths, two-thirds occur in the neonatal period (Martin et al., 2008). In addition, 1 million pediatric patients are currently coping with chronic life-limiting or life-threatening conditions; although the incidence of death in these pediatric patients is decreasing, the population requiring care is steadily increasing. One-fourth of all pediatric patient deaths result from complex chronic conditions (Feudtner et al., 2001).

PRINCIPLES OF PALLIATIVE CARE

In August 2000, the American Academy of Pediatrics (AAP) Committees on Bioethics and Hospital Care published a position paper titled "Palliative Care for Pediatric Children" (Nelson et al., 2000). Contained within this document are principles that serve as the foundation for a sound and integrated model of palliative care:

- Respect for the dignity of patients and families. This includes respecting the patient's and family's wishes and incorporating their goals into the plan of care.

- Access to competent and compassionate palliative care. This includes not only caring for the physical needs of the patient, but also providing for his or her psychosocial and spiritual needs. Incorporating therapies that improve the patient's and family's quality of life—such as education, music and art therapy, integrative medicine (Chapter 18), child life interventions (Chapter 7), support for parents and siblings, and respite care—is a necessary and essential part of good integrated palliative care.

- Support for the caregivers. Health care professionals (HCPs) support the patients and families in the dying process and death. Support for the HCPs, in turn, may include counseling, remembrance services, and allowing them to take time away from the bedside to attend funerals.

- Improved professional and social support for pediatric palliative care. Many barriers prevent families from accessing palliative care services (e.g., regulatory, financial, educational). Professional and public education is necessary to demonstrate the need for and value of these services.

- Continued improvement of pediatric palliative care through research and education.

From these principles, the AAP generated a list of recommendations. The most important of these guidelines states that *all HCPs who care for pediatric patients need to be familiar with, and comfortable providing, palliative care to pediatric patients.*

CHALLENGES ASSOCIATED WITH PEDIATRIC PALLIATIVE CARE

Providing good palliative for any patient can be difficult, but the pediatric population poses some unique challenges. These challenges are identified in Table 20-1.

ESSENTIAL ELEMENTS IN THE APPROACH TO PEDIATRIC PALLIATIVE CARE

The NCP clinical practice guidelines for quality palliative care apply to both pediatric and adult patients but do not fully address the unique aspects of the pediatric population. To remedy this omission, four domains have been described to provide a specific pediatric perspective (Himelstein et al., 2004).

PHYSICAL

It is necessary to identify pain and other troubling symptoms that the patient may be experiencing. A plan for both pharmacologic and nonpharmacologic treatment of these symptoms must be created and disseminated among all HCPs providing care to the patient. The family should have pain medications safeguard in the home at all times to prevent accidental ingestion. When the HCP for the patient is no longer comfortable or able to address the patient's

TABLE 20-1

Challenges Associated with Pediatric Palliative Care
Determining which pediatric patients will benefit most from services
Difficulty in predicting time to death in patients with rare diseases; disease processes that are different from those in adults
The success of technology, which leads families and HCP to think that death can always be averted
Attitudes of families and HCPs; perception of death as a therapeutic misadventure rather than a natural process
HCPs who do not have experience discussing death and dying with patients and families
Coordination of care; pediatric patients with complex medical conditions who have multiple HCPs, so that it is not clear who should be in charge of the care
Lack of pediatric-specific palliative care and hospice services in the community
Few reliable, validated, developmentally appropriate tools to measure the efficacy of symptom control
Eligibility and reimbursement for services that are currently based on adult hospice criteria

symptomatic needs, referral to a pain and/or palliative care specialist is appropriate.

PSYCHOLOGICAL AND SOCIAL

Patients and families may not always be able or willing to express their psychosocial concerns. Both the pediatric patient's and the family's fears and concerns must be identified. It is helpful to learn about the pediatric patient's coping and communication styles. Eliciting the family's previous experience with traumatic life or chronic illness events is important as well. Therefore, the family's resources in terms of support systems during the illness and in the bereavement period should be assessed early on.

SPIRITUAL

Both the pediatric patient as an individual and the family as a whole should undergo a spiritual assessment. This entails reviewing the pediatric patient's hopes, dreams, and values, as well as those of the family. The meaning of life should be explored. It is important to understand the role of prayer and ritual, in addition to beliefs related to death.

CULTURAL

Attempts should be made to the meet the needs of the pediatric patient and their family in a manner that is culturally sensitive. The culturally based desires and concerns of the patient and family need to be explored and addressed. Communication should occur in a way that is understandable to the pediatric patient and family. Acquisition of interpreter services, if appropriate, is an important part of allowing for accurate communication. Respect for truth telling, disclosure, and decision making are key components of maintaining a culturally sensitive environment.

CARE OF THE IMMINENTLY DYING PATIENT

The family should be educated about signs and symptoms of impending death. The patient's care during this phase should occur in a location the family is comfortable with, whether that be the home or the hospital. It is essential to determine the best location to have this discussion before death is imminent (see Chapter 9). After death, the family should be assisted with making arrangements for a funeral, memorial, and burial. Bereavement follow-up and support should be established.

PRACTICAL ASPECTS OF CARE

Advance care planning is a process that is revisited as the trajectory of the patient's illness changes over time. Decision makers should be identified early on; this determination is especially important for patients who are close to the age of 18 years. The trajectory of the illness is important to discuss with the patient and family, as goals of care should be elucidated initially and then change over time. Issues regarding care or concerns near the end-of-life are best discussed prior to the imminent-death phase. Modes of communication and coordination with the health care team need to be established. In addition, the HCP caring for the pediatric patient should become familiar with the patient's home and school environment so that the child's current and future functional status can be appropriately addressed.

INTRODUCING PALLIATIVE CARE TO THE PEDIATRIC PATIENT AND FAMILY

Introducing the concept of palliative care to a pediatric patient and his or her family is a process that occurs over time. It should never be a discrete single conversation. After the possibility that the pediatric patient may die from the disease process is introduced, it is then helpful to elicit the desirable goals of care from both the pediatric patient and the family. This exploration leads to the topic of palliation, so that palliative care may be tailored to meet the goals and needs of the pediatric patient and family. Depending on the developmental stage of the pediatric patient, the child may be included in these conversations and the information should be presented in an age-appropriate manner. In many instances, a child life specialist can aid with these conversations.

REFERENCES

1. Feudtner, C., Hays, R. M., Haynes, G., Geyer, J. R., Neff, J. M., & Koepsell, T. D. (2001). Deaths attributed to pediatric complex chronic conditions: National trends and implications for supportive care services. *Pediatrics, 107*(6), e99–103.

2. Himelstein, B. P., Hilden, J. M., Boldt, A. M., & Weissman, D. (2004). Pediatric palliative care. *New England Journal of Medicine, 350*, 1752–1762.

3. Martin, J. A., Hsiang-Ching, K., Mathews, T. J., Hoyert, D. L., Strobino, D. M., Guyer, B., et al. (2008). Annual summary of vital statistics 2006. *Pediatrics, 121*(4), 788–801.

4. National Consensus Project for Quality Palliative Care (NCP). (2009). Clinical practice guidelines for quality palliative care (2nd ed.). Retrieved from http://www.nationalconsensusproject.org

5. Nelson, R. M., Botkin, J. R., Kodish, E. D., Levetown, M., Truman, J. T., & Wilfond, B. S. (2000). American Academy of Pediatrics Committee on Bioethics and Committee on Hospital Care: Palliative care for pediatric patients. *Pediatrics, 106*(2), 351–357; AAP publications retired or reaffirmed, October 2006. American Academy of Pediatrics. (2007). *Pediatrics, 119*(2), 405.

PART III

Selected Disorders and Their Management

Shari Simone and Lauren Sorce

Analgesia, Paralytics, Sedation, and Withdrawal

Managing anxiety and pain in children who require diagnostic or therapeutic procedures or maintaining comfort and safety in mechanically ventilated pediatric patients can be challenging. Ensuring safe and optimal sedation and pain management necessitates recognition of the unique considerations in pediatric patients. A comprehensive assessment of the pediatric patient includes the acute medical condition, emotional and cognitive capabilities, anatomical and physiologic state related to chronic medical conditions, and age. Health care professionals (HCPs) must also use knowledge of pain physiology to interpret assessment data and to prescribe the most appropriate agents that will minimize pain and anxiety for the individual patient while limiting side effects.

CLASSIFICATION OF PAIN

The International Association for the Study of Pain (IASP, 2007) defines pain as an unpleasant, subjective, sensory, and emotional experience associated with actual or potential tissue damage. Pain is recognized as a complex multidimensional phenomenon that is an individual experience. Pain is classified as nociceptive, neuropathic, or functional based on the inferred pathophysiologic condition.

- *Nociceptive* or acute pain is defined as either somatic (arising from skin, bone, joint, muscle, or connective tissue) or visceral (arising from internal organs).
- *Neuropathic* pain is pain due to nerve damage. In pediatric patients, it is more commonly related to trauma (e.g., localized nerve or spinal cord injury), surgery (post amputation), and chemotherapy (peripheral neuropathy).
- *Functional* pain (fibromyalgia, irritable bowel syndrome) refers to the abnormal presence of, or inappropriate activation of, abnormal pain pathways within the nervous system. Pain circuits may rewire themselves and produce spontaneous nerve stimulation.

Pain is further classified as acute or chronic. *Acute pain* is short lived and occurs with injury or near injury to the tissue due to an adverse chemical, thermal, or mechanical stimulus. *Chronic pain* can be nociceptive, neuropathic, or functional; it is defined as pain lasting longer than one month (ISAP, 2007). Chronic pain in pediatric patients is less common than in adults but may be experienced with medical conditions such as cancer, rheumatologic disorders, and sickle cell disease.

ANXIETY AND AGITATION

Anxiety is a state of apprehension that develops in response to stress and includes behavioral, emotional, and physiologic responses. In contrast, agitation is an exaggerated state involving excessive, often nonpurposeful motor activity. Nonpurposeful activity is associated with physiological responses that may be accompanied by anxiety, panic, depression, delusions, hallucinations, or delirium.

The hospital environment is a significant source of anxiety for both younger children and adolescents. In the younger child, anxiety may be intensified by being separated from the caregivers. The HCP must be able to identify the child who is anxious as a result of environmental factors versus the child who is agitated as a result of a pathological condition. For example, agitation in pediatric patients may be the result of intolerable levels of pain and anxiety or the result of hypoxia, bronchospasm, or inadequate ventilatory support.

PHYSIOLOGY OF PAIN

Nociception refers to a complex series of physiological events resulting in the sensation of pain. Nociception consists of four primary processes: transduction, transmission, modulation, and perception.

Transduction refers to the pain initiation phase. During this process, noxious stimuli activate free nerve endings known as primary afferent nociceptors at the site of tissue damage and transmit these impulses to the spinal cord (Figure 21-1). Nociceptors located in the periphery are contained within somatic and visceral structures and may be activated by mechanical, thermal, and chemical factors. Two types of nociceptor fibers exist: A-delta and C fibers. A-delta fibers are thinly myelinated, rapidly conducting fibers that are primarily responsible for sensations characterized as sharp, stabbing, well-localized pain. A-delta fibers have a high threshold for firing in response to mechanical or thermal stimuli. Once activated, they dramatically increase their rate of firing as the stimulus intensity increases. C fibers are unmyelinated fibers that respond to noxious mechanical, thermal, and chemical stimuli, conduct impulses at a slower rate, and tend to induce pain more characterized as dull, aching, and poorly localized (Cohen, 2004; Fitzgerald & Howard, 2003).

Tissue injury causes the production and release of a variety of substances that stimulate or sensitize nociceptors, including bradykinins, serotonin, histamine, potassium ions, norepinephrine, prostaglandins, leukotrienes, and substance P. Both A-delta and C fiber nociceptors have the property of sensitization, which results in the receptors becoming more sensitive and more reactive with repeated stimuli. This process results in a decreased pain threshold and produces an enhanced response to subsequent painful stimuli. The use of presurgical regional nerve blocks and analgesics has increased in popularity as a method to reduce hypersensitization and disrupt the chain of events leading to acute pain in anticipation of postoperative pain (Brislin & Rose, 2005).

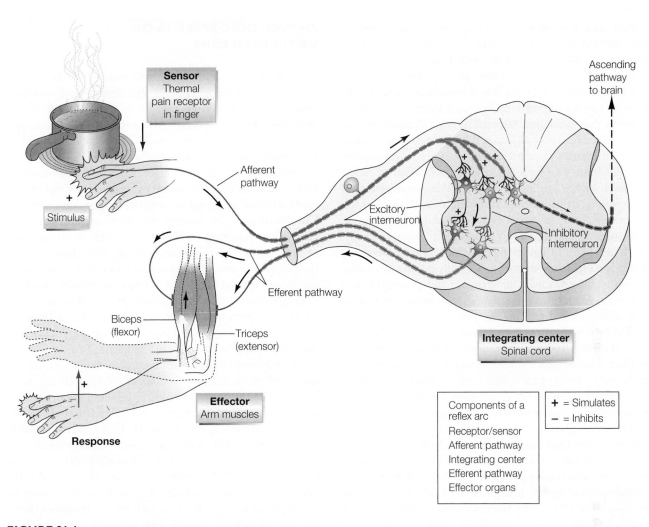

FIGURE 21-1

Transmission of Pain Impulse from Periphery to Spinal Cord.

Source: From Chiras, D. (2008). Human Biology. Sudbury, MA: Jones and Bartlett Publishers.

In addition to the release of chemical substances as a result of tissue injury, cellular damage causes the release of phospholipids and other substances from the cell's lipid membrane into the intracellular space. The release of phospholipids initiates the arachidonic acid cascade. The arachidonic acid cascade activates 5-lipo-oxygenase and cyclo-oxygenase (COX), resulting in the synthesis of leukotrienes and prostaglandins. Leukotrienes and prostaglandins sensitize the nociceptors so that they may be activated by weaker stimuli that normally would not induce pain signals. Inhibition of leukotriene and prostaglandin synthesis may improve pain control when tissue damage is known or suspected. The nonsteroidal anti-inflammatory drugs (NSAIDs) decrease the synthesis of these leukotrienes, thereby decreasing pain, swelling, and edema in the peripheral tissues. Several NSAIDs also appear to be potent inhibitors of prostaglandin synthesis. Those that are more lipophilic (e.g., ibuprofen) penetrate better in the

central nervous system (CNS) and inhibit synthesis of both peripheral and central prostaglandins, whereas acetaminophen blocks only prostaglandin synthesis in the CNS.

Following transduction, the afferent (i.e., incoming) signals must be transmitted to the CNS before the body perceives the stimulus as pain. *Transmission*, the second process of nociception, comprises the propagation of the impulses through the sensory nervous system by primary afferent neurons that synapse in the dorsal horn of the spinal cord and then ascend to the brain stem, thalamus, limbic system, and areas in the cerebral cortex. Although multiple pathways are assumed to affect the pain signals, the dorsal horn of the spinal cord is the primary coordinating site and is largely affected by descending stimulating and inhibitory signals from the brain.

Modulation is the third step in the nociception process and refers to the alteration of pain sensation by endogenous mechanisms. Modulation may result in either attenuation or amplification (also termed "wind-up") of the pain intensity and duration. The most important site where these effects occur is the dorsal horn of the spinal cord. Amplification or pain wind-up refers to the slow, prolonged depolarization and hyperexcitability by the dorsal horn neurons seen with repeated painful stimulation. This mechanism is thought to be partly due to the slow response of NMDA receptors and the sustained release of substance P. Several neuronal changes occur during this hyperexcitability state. First, subsequent painful stimuli evoke a longer and intense period of action potential firing, leading to hyperalgesia (increased pain sensitivity to damaged tissues). In addition, the size of the receptive fields increase, leading to a secondary hyperalgesia (increased pain sensitivity to surrounding tissues). Finally, the threshold for firing action potentials is lowered, resulting in allodynia (pain in response to normally minimally painful stimuli). This propensity for increased and prolonged pain as a result of this mechanism is a rationale for implementing early treatment and ensuring that pain is well controlled.

Modulation occurs between interneurons and by pathways of descending inhibition originating in the thalamus and brain stem, which inhibit synaptic pain transmission at the dorsal horn of the spinal cord. In addition, neurons within these pathways release inhibitory neurotransmitters, including norepinephrine, serotonin, gamma-aminobutyric acid (GABA), glycine, and enkephalin. The inhibitory neurotransmitters then block the release of substance P, glutamine, and other excitatory neurotransmitters. Opioids mimic this descending pain inhibitory system by binding to endorphin receptors throughout the CNS. Another class of drugs that affects this system includes alpha$_2$ agonists (e.g., clonidine, dexmedetomidine). Alpha$_2$ agonists act both before and after synapses at alpha$_2$ receptors in the dorsal horns of the spinal cord to hyperpolarize cell membranes and inhibit generation of the action potential.

The endogenous opiate system is another mechanism responsible for modulating pain impulses. This system consists of neurotransmitters such as enkephalins, dynorphins, and beta endorphins that are found throughout the CNS and bind to specific opioid receptors. The three main types of opioid receptors are designated as mu, delta, and kappa, each of which has its own subtypes. All three receptors induce membrane hyperpolarization, which inhibits generation of an action potential, thereby modulating the transmission of pain impulses.

Finally, the brain processes the nociceptive input as perceived pain. Pain is perceived as a multidimensional sensory and emotional experience to which the body mounts both physical and behavioral responses. Expression of pain clearly is different in pediatric patients when compared to adults, and is affected by a number of factors including developmental age and medical condition. In nonverbal children, the HCP must rely on the pediatric patient's behavioral and physiologic responses as well as information provided by the caregiver on the child's usual response to pain.

PHYSIOLOGIC EFFECTS OF UNTREATED PAIN

Inadequate treatment of pain and anxiety in the pediatric patient can significantly—and detrimentally—affect patient outcomes. Acute pain leads to activation of the physiologic stress response and significant adverse changes in multiple organ systems, including the cardiovascular, respiratory, metabolic, kidney, hemostasis, and immune systems. Physiologic responses to acute pain include tachycardia, hyperventilation, hypertension, diaphoresis, mydriasis, and increased myocardial oxygen consumption. Unrelieved pain and anxiety may also lead to inadequate ventilation, resulting in hypoxia, as well as stimulation of neuroendocrine responses, causing the release of corticosteroids, growth hormone, and catecholamines, plus decreased insulin secretion. These responses produce hyperglycemia and a breakdown in carbohydrates and fat stores, which may lead to metabolic acidosis from an increase in blood levels of lactate, pyruvate, ketone bodies, and fatty acids.

In addition to the adverse physiologic effects of untreated pain, other psychologic adverse effects have been well described in neonates, children in the perioperative setting, and children with cancer (Kain et al., 1999; Rennick et al., 2004; Weisman et al., 1998). When Rennick and Rashotte (2009) performed a systematic review of psychologic outcomes in children following pediatric intensive care unit (PICU) hospitalization, they found that negative psychologic sequelae may manifest for as long as 1 year post discharge. Reported adverse psychologic effects include behavioral changes such as avoidance behaviors, interrupted sleep patterns, irritability, outbursts of anger, and depression (Rennick & Rashotte, 2009).

In addition, an emerging literature has described post-traumatic stress disorder (PTSD) and acute stress disorder (ASD) in hospitalized children with injury-related traumatic events and illness-related traumatic events (Ward-Begnoche, 2007). Criteria for PTSD involve three main categories of symptoms: (1) the patient re-experiences the traumatic event (e.g., nightmares); (2) the patient shows avoidance behaviors toward trauma-related stimuli (e.g., avoids conversations, people, or places); and (3) the patient experiences a heightened arousal state (e.g., sleep disturbances). Symptoms must be present for at least 1 month to support a diagnosis of PTSD. Some reported predictors for PTSD include uncontrolled pain, parental stress, preexisting psychiatric disorders, and previous hospitalizations (Ward-Begnoche, 2007); refer to Chapter 38 for more information on PTSD.

Hospitalized pediatric patients should be monitored carefully for potential signs of PTSD or ASD both during the hospital stay and following discharge. Attempts to minimize or prevent negative psychologic sequelae are necessary and should include maximizing pain management, enhancing parental involvement and communication, and providing supportive counseling services during the hospitalization and following discharge for the patient and family. In addition, child life services are instrumental in facilitating coping and adjustment of patients and their families in both inpatient and outpatient settings. The American Academy of Pediatrics' (AAP, 2006) policy statement on child life services describes an effective child life program as one that provides pediatric patients with developmentally appropriate play and communication, engages in psychologic preparation before and during procedures, establishes therapeutic relationships, and provides support to family members for all pediatric patients.

DEVELOPMENTAL CONSIDERATIONS

Although there are fundamental developmental differences in pain perception in infants and children, the neurological structures required to perceive pain are fully developed by 26 weeks' gestation (Brislin & Rose, 2005). In the neonate, neural transmission in peripheral nerves is slower as myelination is incomplete at birth; however, both unmyelinated C fibers and the thinly myelinated A-delta fibers are developed (Rose & Logan, 2004), making the neonate capable of perceiving pain. Research demonstrates that, similar to the case for the older child or adult, repeated stimulation of these nociceptive fibers decreases the infant's excitatory thresholds, resulting in peripheral sensitization and increased responsiveness to repeated stimuli (Fitzgerald & Howard, 2003). Therefore, neonates can also experience the same types of pain as are seen in the older child.

In addition, pharmacokinetic differences in pediatric patients have implications for analgesic and sedation medication dosages and intervals. Important principles include the following (Berde & Sethna, 2002):

- Neonates have delayed maturation of the cytochrome P450 hepatic enzyme system involved in drug metabolism, resulting in a reduced clearance of drugs, particularly opioids and amino-amide local anesthetics. In general, maturation of these enzyme functions occurs by 6 months of age.
- The relatively higher body water content in neonates and infants results in a larger volume of distribution of water-soluble drugs and the potential for a longer duration of medication action.
- The relatively smaller fat and muscle stores in neonates result in higher plasma concentrations of drugs because fewer active sites for drug binding or uptake are available; this factor leads to increased risk of toxicity and adverse effects.
- Protein binding of drugs is reduced in neonates compared with older children due to lower plasma levels of albumin; this factor may cause a greater medication effect or increased plasma free drug concentration.
- Renal excretion of medications depends on renal blood flow, glomerular filtration rate, and tubular secretory function, all of which are decreased in infants. These variations may require adjustments in drug dosages and intervals to prevent adverse effects.
- Neonates have decreased ventilatory responses to hypoxemia and hypercarbia. These ventilatory responses can be further impaired by CNS depressant medications such as opioids and benzodiazepines.

PAIN AND SEDATION ASSESSMENT

Assessment is critical to the management of pain and agitation in the acutely ill patient. While a variety of assessment tools exist, careful selection of the appropriate tool is paramount to proper assessment. Assessment tools include self-report, observational, and physiologic-based instruments. A combination of these tools may also be used.

Selection of the appropriate self-report pain tool is predicated upon the patient's age and developmental level. Historically, the *FACES* scale has been widely used for patients as young as 3 years of age (Wong & Baker, 1988). This scale uses pictures of faces with varying expression of pain; the patient is asked to select the face that accurately reflects his or her pain. The faces in the scale are depicted with tears or smiles during pain; however, if the patient is in pain but not smiling or crying, he or she may have difficulty adequately scoring the pain level, as the scale lacks the appropriate face to select. Children with different ethnic backgrounds who do not express facial signs of pain may also have trouble selecting a face to represent their level of pain. Additionally, the numeric scores associated with the selected face do not correspond to scores on a numeric rating scale.

In an effort to improve the application of the FACES scale, Bieri et al. (1990) created and validated the *Faces Pain Scale*. This scale has seven face pictures and a numeric rating between 0 and 6 to correspond with various levels of pain. In 2001, Hicks and colleagues published the revised version of the Faces Pain Scale. The *Faces Pain Scale—Revised* (*FPS-R*) has six faces with a 0 to 5 or 0 to 10 metric application. This scale has been validated in patients aged 4 years and older and was created to align with the numeric rating scale metric. Stanford et al. (2006) examined hypothetical vignettes of pain and the use of the FPS-R in patients aged 3 to 6 years. Their study demonstrated that patients between the ages of 5 and 6 years were significantly more accurate in their use of the FPS-R than those aged 3 and 4 years. This finding suggests that care should be taken in applying any single tool in the evaluation of pediatric pain.

The *numeric rating scale* (*NRS*) is a self-reporting pain scale that is widely used in pediatric and adult patients. Variants of the scale include the NRS-11, which includes

11 items that are scored from 0 to 10, and the NRS-101, which includes items that are scored from 0 to 100. The use of this tool in pediatrics depends on the individual child's understanding of numeracy. With recent interest in validating this tool in pediatrics, Miro et al. (2009) performed two separate studies comparing the NRS-11 to the FPS-R in pediatric patients aged 6 to 16 years and 8 to 12 years, respectively. The results of these studies demonstrated validity of the NRS as compared to the FPS-R; however, the subjects, in both studies, preferred to use the FPS-R. Additional validation of the NRS-11 is supported by three data sets described by von Baeyer and colleagues (2009), which advocate the use of the NRS-11 for patients 8 years of age or older, with recommendations for continued study in younger patients.

Self-report tools have been demonstrated as valid and reliable in the literature. However, a variety of situations may affect the child's actual reporting of pain, such as family culture, ethnic culture, prior pain experiences, and societal norms. Careful evaluation should be done when a child is demonstrating pain behaviors but not verbalizing it.

The *faces, legs, activity, cry and consolability behavioral scale* (*FLACC*) is an observational scale to evaluate pain in patients aged 2 months through 7 years (Merkel et al., 1997). It is designed to rate the patient's pain by assessing five behavioral items and obtaining a total score between 0 and 10. Recently, the FLACC scale was validated in patients younger than 16 years of age who were able to self-report pain (Nilsson et al., 2008; Willis et al., 2003). A revised version of the FLACC scale has also been validated as a means to measure pain in the cognitively impaired patient (Malviya et al., 2005; Voepel-Lewis et al., 2008).

Agitation assessment scales can be used to evaluate the level of sedation; however, few scales have been validated in the pediatric population. In 1970, Dr. J. Antonio Aldrete created a recovery assessment tool to evaluate postanesthesia recovery and discharge criteria in adult patients. The *Aldrete Recovery* scale was modeled after the *Neonatal APGAR* scale and has since been modified for use in pediatrics (Soliman et al., 1988). This tool scores the pediatric patient in the categories of motor activity, respirations, blood pressure, consciousness, and color. Although it is helpful in evaluating pediatric patients, simultaneous oxygen saturation and vital sign monitoring are imperative to accurately assess recovery.

The *Ramsay Sedation Scale* (*RSS*), created by Ramsay, Savage, Simpson, and Goodwin in 1974, is a subjective tool with a scoring range from 1 (anxious and agitated) to 6 (unresponsive to light touch/loud noise). Limited reliability and validity studies of this scale have been conducted in adults; the RSS has not been validated in children (Sessler et al., 2008).

The *COMFORT* scale, developed by Ambuel et al. in 1992, evaluates the efficacy of therapies aimed at reducing distress in critically ill children who are receiving invasive and noninvasive respiratory support. The scale includes eight dimensions: alertness, calmness, respiratory response, movement, mean arterial blood pressure, heart rate, muscle tone, and facial expression. Each dimension is scored 1 through 5 to create a total COMFORT score. As this tool contains constructs of both pain and sedation, the decision to treat pain versus agitation may be unclear. Psychometric testing of the original COMFORT scale revealed poor inter-rater reliability when determining the physiologic domains other than heart rate and mean arterial blood pressure, which demonstrated good overall inter-rater reliability. As some of the physiologic measurements may be affected by disease state and/or medication, the reliability and validity of the entire tool has come into question. Further testing of the COMFORT scale to evaluate its usefulness (without the physiologic parameters) determined that removal of the physiologic indexes allowed for a reliable alternative to the scale (Itsa, 2005). However, the revised COMFORT tool has not yet been studied for validity.

The *State Behavioral Scale* (*SBS*) measures sedation in patients who are being supported by mechanical ventilation (Curley et al., 2006). The tool comprises seven dimensions on the sedation to agitation continuum. The scores range from –3 (unresponsive) to +2 (agitated). While the SBS tool has been determined to be reliable and valid in mechanically ventilated pediatric patients, its application to other pediatric acute care settings has not been tested.

SEDATION AGENTS

The acutely ill patient often requires sedation for a variety of reasons. As such, ensuring safe and effective pharmacologic treatment is critical to this vulnerable population. Table 21-1 provides a comprehensive list of sedation agents that are commonly used in pediatric patients.

Sedative agents belong to different drug classes and, as a result, work somewhat differently in the body. Barbiturates, for example, act by binding to the GABA receptor and enhance its activity, subsequently reducing firing of the neuron. Benzodiazepines act similarly to barbiturates, but also include some antagonists (flumazenil) and reverse agonists that increase neuron firing and may stimulate seizures. Each barbiturate and benzodiazepine has a different length of activity; as such, the agent should be selected based on the specific clinical situation. Anesthetics are also used for sedation and affect GABA activity. Other sedatives—specifically chloral hydrate—act as CNS depressants but have an unknown mechanism of action. Dexmedetomidine, the newest sedating agent, is currently classified as an anesthetic that works as a selective alpha$_2$-adrenoceptor agonist, resulting in inhibition of norepinephrine release (www.online.lexi.com).

Sedatives used in the pediatric population include midazolam and lorazepam. These medications are benzodiazepine, hypnotic drugs. They are commonly used for short-term sedation for diagnostic imaging, therapeutic interventions (intravascular line placement), and diagnostic procedures (lumbar puncture). When using these medications as sedation prior to painful procedures, an analgesic should also be administered—these medications have no analgesic properties.

Midazolam may be administered a variety of routes, including enterally, parenterally, intramuscularly, and intranasally. However, this medication is not palatable; as such, its administration may be difficult without a mixing vehicle, particularly in the patient designated as nothing by mouth (NPO) status. While the intranasal route is not routinely used, it may be the route of choice for a patient who is NPO status and has no intravenous (IV) access. The dose of intranasal midazolam is specified as 0.2 mg/kg body weight, with a range of 0.2 to 0.3 mg/kg per dose. This dose may be repeated in 15 minutes if the patient is not sedated adequately. Midazolam may also be used for continuous infusion in critically ill pediatric patients. When using this medication in critically ill patients, dose titration to effect is an important consideration, as patients with hepatic and renal insufficiency or failure may require lower doses because of the medication's active metabolite (Table 21-1).

Lorazepam is longer acting than midazolam; thus it may be a better option for procedures requiring a longer time frame. This agent can be administered enterally, parenterally, and intramuscularly. Although it may be used in critically ill patients, it does not lend itself to continuous infusion because of its long half-life (Table 21-1).

Other sedation medications used in pediatrics include diazepam, chloral hydrate, etomidate, pentobarbital, methohexital, thiopental, propofol, and dexmedetomidine. While these medications are used, no standards for their use in pediatric patients have been developed. Some are used routinely for diagnostic imaging sedation or sleep diagnostic studies (e.g., chloral hydrate, pentobarbital); others are used for diagnostic procedures requiring no movement on the patient's part (e.g., propofol). Adrenal suppression and myoclonus may occur after one dose of etomidate (www .online.lexi.com). As such, careful consideration is required prior to the selection of this medication. Dexmedetomidine is the newest of these sedation agents. While some literature describes its use in pediatric patients, this medication is currently not FDA approved for use in patients younger than 18 years of age.

Propofol was initially regarded as an excellent choice for PICU sedation secondary to its pharmacokinetics and rapid reversibility. However, continuous infusion of this medication for days has resulted in propofol infusion syndrome (PRIS) in some pediatric patients. Symptoms of PRIS include bradycardia, metabolic acidosis, rhabdomyolysis, enlarged or fatty liver, hyperlipidemia, cardiac failure, and, in some cases, death (Parke et al., 1992). As a

consequence, propofol's labeling now carries a warning against continuous infusion administration in pediatric critical care (www.online.lexi.com). However, short-term administration of this agent is feasible in pediatric patients. As with all the medications mentioned in this chapter, hospital/unit policies will dictate medication protocols and routines for use (Table 21-1).

ANALGESIC AGENTS

A variety of pain-relieving medications can be used in pediatric patients, ranging from over-the-counter (OTC) to prescription medications. As with the sedation agents, it is necessary to match the clinical condition of the patient with the need for the analgesic medication to achieve adequate pain relief. For a complete listing of opioid and alpha adrenergic analgesic agents used in pediatric patients, refer to Table 21-1.

Opioids act as previously described, by mimicking the descending pain inhibitory system and binding to endorphin receptors in the CNS. Additionally, they bind to specific opiate receptors, including mu, delta, and kappa receptors and their subtypes, and modulate the transmission of pain impulses. Commonly used opioids include morphine, hydromorphone, fentanyl, and methadone.

Morphine is a narcotic analgesic that works by binding to mu receptors, thereby producing both analgesia and sedation. Its secondary effects may include anxiolysis and euphoria. This medication is used frequently in critically ill pediatric patients; however, it is on the list of "high alert" medications set forth by the Institute for Safe Medication Practice (ISMP). As a result, careful consideration should be undertaken with using morphine in young patients. The dose of morphine varies depending on the route of administration (Table 21-1). This medication is metabolized in the liver through glucuronidation and results in active and inactive metabolites. The active metabolite (morphine-6-gucuronide) may contribute to the analgesic effects after the first dose of morphine and, when used on a long-term basis, may supersede morphine's analgesic effects (Heard & Fletcher, 2006). Morphine is excreted by the kidneys almost completely within 24 hours. Its administration causes histamine release, which may result in erythema at the infusion site or bronchospasm in children with asthma.

Adverse responses to morphine include CNS depression, which may lead to unconsciousness. Respiratory rate may decrease, resulting in decreased minute ventilation. The patient also may have a decreased response to hypercarbia. In some patients, morphine's effects on respiratory drive may only be secondary to its hypoxic stimulation of the carotid chemoreceptors. All of these effects may occur at analgesic doses, so careful dosing and monitoring are required if morphine is used. Other side effects of

TABLE 21-1

Pharmacologic Agents, Dosing, and Actions

Medication	Pharmacology	Pharmacokinetics/dynamics	Indications	Dosing	Significant Side Effects
Benzodiazepines					
Midazolam	CNS depressant, hypnotic	Onset of action: IV: 1–5 min PO: 10–20 min IM: 5 min Duration: IV: 20–30 min IM: 2–6 hr Protein binding: ~97% to albumin Metabolism: Liver via cytochrome P450 Active primary metabolite Half-life: IV: 2.9–4.5 hr PO: 2.2–6.8 hr Elimination: ~80% in urine ~10% in feces	Sedation, anxiolysis, ventilatory synchrony	**Anxiolysis or amnesia:** IV: 0.25–0.5 mg/kg *Adult:* IM 0.07–0.08 mg/kg IV: 0.02–0.04 mg/kg **Procedural sedation:** IM: 0.1–0.15 mg/kg IV: 0.025–0.1 mg/kg Intranasal: 0.2–0.3 mg/kg *Adult:* IV 0.5–2 mg IV **Mechanical ventilation:** IV continuous infusion: Load with 0.05–0.2 mg/kg Infusion: 0.06–0.12 mg/kg/hr *Adult:* 0.04–0.2 mg/kg/hr *All doses should be titrated to goal level of sedation*	Respiratory depression or arrest, cardiac arrest, hypotension, bradycardia.
Lorazepam	CNS depressant, hypnotic	Onset of action: IV: 15–30 min PO: 60 min IM: 30–60 min Duration: 8–12 hr Protein binding: 85% bound Metabolism: Glucuronide conjugation in the liver to inactive metabolite Half-life: 6–17 hr Elimination: Urine	Sedation, anxiolysis	**Sedation:** IV/PO: 0.02–0.1 mg/kg every 4–8 hr *Adult:* PO 1–10 mg/day divided in 2–3 doses Preoperative: IV 0.044 mg/kg, maximum dose 2 mg IM: 0.05 mg/kg, maximum dose 4 mg **Procedural sedation:** PO/IV/IM: 0.02–0.09 mg/kg **Mechanical ventilation:** IV/PO: 0.02–0.1 mg/kg every 4–8 hr Infusion: 0.025–0.2 mg/kg/hr (Tobias, 1995) *All doses should be titrated to goal level of sedation*	Significant respiratory depression, apnea, bradycardia, circulatory collapse. Parenteral formulation mixed with polyethylene glycol, which may result in toxicity (kidney failure, lactic acidosis, osmolar gap) with high doses or long-term therapy.

| Diazepam | CNS depressant, hypnotic | Sedation, anxiolysis, | **Procedural Sedation:**
PO: 0.2–0.3 mg/kg
IV: 0.05–0.1 mg/kg
Sedation/anxiolysis:
PO: 0.12–0.8 mg/kg/day divided Q6–8 hr
IV/IM: 0.04–0.3 mg/kg/dose to maximum 0.6 mg/kg within 8 hr
Adolescent sedation:
PO: 10 mg
IV: 5 mg, may repeat 2.5 mg
Adult sedation:
PO: 2–10 mg/day 3–4 times per day
IV: 0.03–0.1mg/kg every 30 min–6 hr | Onset of action:
IV: 1–3 min
Rectal: 2–10 min
Duration: 15–30 min
Protein binding: ~85% in neonates
Metabolism: Liver, active metabolite*
Half-life:
Child 1 month–2 years: 40–50 hr
Child 2–12 years: 15–21 hr
Child 12–16 years: 18–20 hr
Elimination: Urine
*Adult data | Rapid IV push may cause sudden hypotension, cardiac arrest, apnea, or respiratory depression. Laryngospasm. Injection and rectal gel contain benzoic acid, benzyl alcohol and sodium benzoate; use with caution in neonates. |

Other Agents

| Chloral hydrate | Hypnotic, sedative | Short-term sedation or hypnosis, nonpainful procedures | **Sedation:**
25–50 mg/kg/day divided every 6–8 hr maximum 500 mg/dose
Procedural sedation:
50–75 mg/kg/dose; may repeat to maximum 120 mg/kg or 1 gm total in infants, 2 gm total in child
Hypnotic:
50 mg/kg/dose;
1 gm total/day in infants, 2 gm total/day in child
Adult sedation:
PO/PR: 250 mg 3 times/day | Onset of action: 10–20 min
Duration: 4–8 hr
Protein binding: 35–94% (metabolite specific)*
Metabolism: Liver by alcohol dehydrogenase, some kidney metabolism*
Half-life:
Infant: 1 hr
Metabolite in neonates: 8.5–66 hr
Mean half-life:
Child: 10 hours
Elimination: Urine and small amount in bile*
*Adult data | Death and permanent neurological injury secondary to respiratory compromise, respiratory depression when combination therapy used, paradoxical excitement. |

(Continued)

TABLE 21-1

Pharmacologic Agents, Dosing, and Actions (Continued)

Medication	Pharmacology	Pharmacokinetics/dynamics	Indications	Dosing	Significant Side Effects
Other Agents					
Etomidate	General anesthetic	Onset of action: IV: 30–60 sec Duration: IV: 2–10 min (dose dependent) Protein binding: 76% Metabolism: Hepatic and plasma esterase Half-life, terminal: 2.6–3.5 hr Elimination: 75% in urine over 24 hr	Procedural sedation, anesthesia induction	**Procedural sedation:** 0.1–0.3 mg/kg (limited data in children) *Adult:* IV: 0.2–0.6 mg/kg for anesthesia induction	Single dose may impact stress-induced increase in cortisol production for up to 24 hours in certain people. Bradycardia, apnea, hypertension, hypotension, laryngospasm, myoclonus.
Barbiturates					
Pentobarbital	General anesthetic, hypnotic, sedative	Onset of action: IV: ≤ 1 min IM: 10–15 min Duration: IV: 15 min Protein binding: 35–55% Metabolism: Liver via hydroxylation and oxidation pathways Half-life, terminal: Child: 25 hr Elimination: < 1% unchanged renally	Procedural sedation, hypnosis, failed sedation in intubated children	**Procedural sedation:** Child: IV 2 mg/kg, repeat 1–2 mg/kg every 5–10 min until desired state, to maximum 6 mg/kg Infant: IV 1–3 mg/kg, to maximum of 100 mg until asleep **Hypnotic:** Child: IM 2–6 mg/kg *Adult:* IV 100 mg every 1–3 min (total dose 500 mg) IM: 150–200 mg **Failed sedation in intubated patient:** 1–2 mg/kg/hr continuous infusion	Arrhythmias, bradycardia, hypotension, laryngospasm, apnea, respiratory depression.
Methohexital	General anesthetic, sedative	Onset of action: IV: 1 min IM: 2–10 min PR: 5–15 min	Procedural sedation,	**Procedural sedation:** ≥ 1 month to child: IM: 6.6–10 mg/kg 5% solution	"Black box" warning: only administer in a facility where continuous monitoring and resuscitation/intubation

Drug	Classification	Pharmacokinetics	Indications	Dosing	Adverse Effects
		Duration: IV: 7–10 min, IM/PR: 1–1.5 hr; Metabolism: Liver via demethylation and oxidation*; Elimination: Kidney*; *Adult data		IV: 0.5 mg/kg 1% solution, titrate by 0.5 mg/kg; *Adult anesthesia induction:* IV: 1–1.5 mg/kg; maintenance: 50–120 mcg/kg/min	equipment is available (hospital, ambulatory care site). Hypotension, circulatory depression, peripheral vascular collapse, cardiorespiratory arrest, apnea, laryngospasm, bronchospasm. *No analgesic properties.*
Thiopental	General anesthetic, sedative, hypnotic	Onset of action: IV: 30–60 sec; Duration: IV: 5–30 min; Protein binding: 72–86%*; Metabolism: Liver to inactive metabolites; also forms pentobarbital*; Half-life: 3–11.5 hr in adults (less in children); Elimination: ~80% in urine ~10% in feces	Adjunct for intubation in head injury; induction of anesthesia; sedation	**Anesthesia induction:** Infants: IV 3–4 mg/kg; Children: IV 5–6 mg/kg; Adult: 3–5 mg/kg; **Increased intracranial pressure:** IV 1.5–5 mg/kg/doses, repeat as needed; *Adult: same dosing;* **Sedation:** Children: rectal 5–10 mg/kg/dose	Decreased cardiac output, hypotension, laryngospasm, bronchospasm, respiratory depression, apnea, anaphylaxis.

Analgesics

Drug	Classification	Pharmacokinetics	Indications	Dosing	Adverse Effects
Morphine	Narcotic analgesic	Peak action: IV: 20 min, PO: 1 hr, IM: 30–60 min, SQ: 50–90 min; Duration: IV/IM/SQ: 3–5 hr, PO: 3–5 hr; Protein binding: < 20% in neonates	Pain management, adjunct for sedation management	**Pain management:** PO: 0.2–0.5 mg/kg/dose every 4–6 h PRN; *Adults:* 10–30 mg Q 4 hr PRN; IV/IM/SQ: 0.1–0.2 mg/kg/dose every 2–4 hr as needed; *Adult:* 2.5–20 mg/dose Q 4 hr PRN; Continuous infusion: 0.02 mg/kg/hr; titrate as needed; *Adult:* 0.8–10 mg/hr	CNS depression, respiratory depression, severe hypotension, syncope, increased intracranial pressure peripheral vasodilation, orthostatic hypotension, noncardiogenic pulmonary edema. Histamine release.

(Continued)

TABLE 21-1

Pharmacologic Agents, Dosing, and Actions (Continued)

Medication	Pharmacology	Pharmacokinetics/dynamics	Indications	Dosing	Significant Side Effects
		Metabolism: Liver via glucuronide conjugation to active and inactive metabolites Half-life: Infants: 5–10 hr Child: 1–8 hr Elimination: Unchanged in the urine		Epidural: 0.03–0.05 mg/kg; maximum 5 mg/24 hr *Adult:* 2–4 mg/24 hr; maximum dose 10 mg/24 hr **Sedation:** IV: 0.05–0.1 mg/kg/dose *Adolescent/Adult:* IV: 3–4 mg	
Analgesics					
Hydromorphone	Narcotic analgesic	Onset of action: IV: within 5 min PO: 15–30 min Duration: IV/PO: 4–5 hr Protein binding: 8–19% Metabolism: Liver via glucuronide conjugation to inactive metabolites Half-life: 1–3 hr Elimination: Urine	Pain management	Young children: PO: 0.03–0.08 mg/kg/dose every 3–4 hr as needed; maximum 5 mg/dose IV: 0.015 mg/kg/dose every 3–6 hr as needed Older children and adults: PO: 1–2 mg/dose every 3–4 hr as needed; may titrate dose to effect IV/IM/SC: 0.2–0.6 mg/dose every 2–4 hr as needed; may titrate to effect	Significant respiratory depression, especially in patients with preexisting respiratory conditions. Hypotension exaggerated in patients with hypovolemia. Orthostatic hypotension, peripheral vasodilation, CNS depression, increased intracranial pressure, histamine release.
Fentanyl	Synthetic narcotic analgesic	Onset of action: IV: nearly immediate IM: 7–15 min Duration: IV: 30–60 min IM: 1–2 hr Protein binding: 80–85% Metabolism: Liver via cytochrome P450	Pain management, sedation	Neonates and young infants: Sedation/analgesia: IV: 1–4 mcg/kg/dose, may repeat every 2–4 hr Continuous sedation/analgesia: 0.5–1 mcg/kg/hr; titrate to effect Children: Sedation/analgesia: IV: 1–2 mcg/kg/dose Continuous sedation/analgesia: IV: 1–3 mcg/kg/hr; titrate to effect	May cause life-threatening hypotension, respiratory depression. Orthostatic hypotension, chest wall rigidity, arrhythmia, syncope, bradycardia, CNS depression. Fentanyl is 50–100 times more potent than morphine.

Drug	Classification	Pharmacokinetics	Dosing	Adverse Effects/Comments
(continued)		Half-life: Infant to 4.5 years: mean 2.4 hr Child: 11–36 hr Elimination: Urine	Adolescents and adults: Sedation/analgesia: IV: 0.5–1 mcg/kg/dose, may repeat at 30–60 min or 25–50 mcg may repeat 4–5 times with 25 mcg Postoperative pain: Adolescents and adults: IV/IM: 50–100 mcg/dose	Prolonged QT interval or torsades de pointes, death, life-threatening respiratory depression, cardiac arrhythmias. Increased intracranial pressure, histamine release.
Methadone	Narcotic analgesic	Onset of action: IV: 10–20 min PO: 30–60 min Duration: IV: maximum effect 1–2 hr PO: 6–8 hr Protein binding: 85–90% Metabolism: Liver via *N*-demethylation to an inactive metabolite Half-life: 4–62 hr Elimination: Urine	Pain management, iatrogenic narcotic dependency Pain management: Children: IV: 0.1 mg/kg/dose every 4 hr for 2–3 doses; titrate every 6–12 hr as needed; dose decrement may be required with long-term therapy due to tissue accumulation PO/IM/SQ: 0.1 mg/kg/dose every 4 hr for 2–3 doses; titrate every 6–12 hr as needed Maximum dose: 10 mg/dose *Adult:* PO: 5–10 mg, interval range Q 4–12 hr IV/IM/SQ: 2.5–10 mg Q 8–12 hr Iatrogenic narcotic dependency: dosing must be individualized to the patient	

Alpha₂ Adrenergic Agents

Drug	Classification	Pharmacokinetics	Dosing	Adverse Effects/Comments
Dexmedetomidine	Sedative	Onset of action: IV: near immediate Protein binding:* ~94% Metabolism: Liver via *N*-glucuronidation, *N*-methylation, CYP2A6 Half-life:* Distribution: 6 min Terminal: 2 hr	Continuous sedation in intubated patients Child: IV load: 0.5–1 mcg/kg Continuous infusion: 0.2–0.7 mcg/kg/hr No studies currently available to support therapy > 24 hr in children *Adult:* ICU sedation: 1 mcg/kg load over 10 min with infusion 0.2–0.7 mcg/kg/hr	Bradycardia, sinus arrest, hypotension, hypertension, pulmonary edema, respiratory acidosis.

(Continued)

TABLE 21-1

Pharmacologic Agents, Dosing, and Actions (Continued)

Medication	Pharmacology	Pharmacokinetics/dynamics	Indications	Dosing	Significant Side Effects
	Elimination:* 95% in urine 4% in feces *Adult data			Procedural sedation: 0.5–1 mcg/kg load with 0.2–1 mcg/kg/hr during procedure	

Alpha₂ Adrenergic Agents

Medication	Pharmacology	Pharmacokinetics/dynamics	Indications	Dosing	Significant Side Effects
Clonidine	Non-narcotic analgesic	Onset of action: Transdermal: ~2 days Duration: Transdermal: 7 days Protein binding: 20–40% Metabolism: Liver to inactive metabolites Half-life: Child: 8–12 hr Elimination: 65% in urine 22% in feces	Pain and sedation management Withdrawal management	Child: PO: 2 mcg/kg/dose every 4–6 hr; increase over days as needed to range 2–4 mcg/kg/dose Epidural: 0.5 mcg/kg/hr; titrate to effect Transdermal: Convert oral dosing to patch Adult: PO: 0.1–0.2 mg 3 times/day (Malchow & Black, 2008)	Sudden death or serious cardiovascular events when combined with stimulant medications, hypotension, CHF, sedation.

General Anesthetics

Medication	Pharmacology	Pharmacokinetics/dynamics	Indications	Dosing	Significant Side Effects
Ketamine	General anesthetic	Onset of action: IV: 30 sec PO: within 30 min IM: 3–4 min Duration: IV: 5–10 min IM: 12–30 min Protein binding: ~97% to albumin Metabolism: Liver via N-dealkylation, hydroxylation, glucuronide conjugation Half-life: Terminal 2.5 hr	Procedural sedation Continuous sedation in intubated patients	PO: 6–10 mg/kg 30 min preprocedure IM: 3–7 mg/kg IV: 0.5–2 mg/kg Continuous sedation: 5–20 mcg/kg/min; titrate to effect Adult: IM: 3–8 mg/kg IV: 1–4.5 mg/kg	Hypersalivation, respiratory depression, postanesthetic delirium, hypertension, tachycardia, hypotension, increased cerebral blood flow, laryngospasm.

Drug	Classification	Indication	Dosing	Pharmacokinetics	Comments
Propofol	General anesthetic	Procedural sedation	Sedation: IV: 1–1.5 mg/kg over 20–30 sec, then 0.5–1 mg/kg PRN for goal effect. Anesthesia: IV 2.5–0.5 mg/kg over 20–30 sec, then 125–150 mcg/kg/min for 10–15 min; decrease to goal level of sedation (usual dose is 125–150 mcg/kg/min). Adult ICU sedation: IV: 100–150 mcg/kg/min or 0.5 mg/kg, then continuous infusion 0.3–3 mg/kg/hr	Onset of action: IV: 9–51 sec. Duration: 3–10 min. Protein binding: 97–99%. Metabolism:* Liver via glucuronide and sulfate conjugation. Half-life:* Alpha: 2–8 min, Terminal 300–700 min. Elimination:* Urine and feces. *Adult data	Not currently recommended for continuous sedation of PICU patient secondary to propofol infusion syndrome (severe metabolic acidosis, hyperkalemia, lipemia, rhabdomyolysis, hepatomegaly, cardiac and kidney failure). Significant hypotension, bradycardia, hypothermia and respiratory depression in the patient without an artificial airway.

Neuromuscular Blocking Agents

Drug	Classification	Indication	Dosing	Pharmacokinetics	Comments
Succinylcholine	Depolarizing NMBA, Fast-acting NMBA	Rapid-sequence endotracheal intubation	IM: 3–4 mg/kg. Infant: IV: 2 mg/kg. Child: IV: 1 mg/kg. Adult: IM/IV: 0.6 mg/kg with maintenance 0.04–0.07 mg/kg every 5–10 min PRN. Continuous infusion: 2.5 mg/min (range 0.5–10 mg/min)	Onset of action: IV: 30–60 sec, IM: 2–3 min. Duration: IV: 4–6 min, IM: 10–30 min. Metabolism:* Plasma pseudocholinesterase. *Adult data	Malignant hyperthermia may be triggered. Rhabdomyolysis when used in a patient with undiagnosed myopathy; thus caution is warranted before use in male infants < 3 months of age (may have undiagnosed Duchenne muscular dystrophy). Asystole, hypotension, arrhythmias, myoglobinuria, apnea.
Cisatracurium	Nondepolarizing NBMA, Intermediate-acting NMBA	Muscle blockade	Children 2–12 years: IV: 0.1 mg/kg. Children more than 12 years: IV: 0.15–0.2 mg/kg. Continuous infusion: 1–4 mcg/kg/min. Adults: IV: 1–3 mcg/kg/min (range 0.06–0.18 mg/kg/hr)	Onset of action: IV: 2–3 min. Maximum effect: 3–5 min. Duration: IV: 35–45 min. Metabolism:* Hofmann elimination. Half-life:* 22–31 min. Elimination:* < 10% in urine. *Adult data	Must be prepared for airway management when dosing. Potentiating effects: severe hypokalemia, hypocalcemia, hyponatemia, hypermagnesemia, acidosis, acute intermittent porphyria, renal/hepatic failure. Antagonizing effects: alkalosis, hypercalcemia, demyelinating lesions, peripheral neuropathies, diabetes mellitus.

(Continued)

TABLE 21-1

Pharmacologic Agents, Dosing, and Actions (Continued)

Medication	Pharmacology	Pharmacokinetics/dynamics	Indications	Dosing	Significant Side Effects
		Neuromuscular Blocking Agents			
Pancuronium	Nondepolarizing NMBA Long-acting NMBA	Onset of action: Maximum effect: within 2–3 min Duration: IV: 40–60 min Protein binding:* 87% Metabolism:* 30–40% in liver Half-life:* 110 min Elimination:* 60% unchanged in urine 40% in bile *Adult data	Muscle blockade	Neonates and infants: IV: 0.1 mg/kg Continuous infusion: 0.4–0.6 mcg/kg/min Children: IV 0.15 mg/kg Continuous infusion: 0.5–1.7 mcg/kg/min Adolescents and adults: IV: 0.15 mg/kg every 30–60 min PRN Continuous infusion: 0.02/0.04 mg/kg/hr	Pancuronium: tachycardia. Use with caution in patients with baseline tachycardia or at risk for tachyarrhythmias.
Rocuronium	Nondepolarizing NMBA Fast-acting NMBA	Onset of action: Child maximum effect: 30–60 sec Duration: Infants: 40 min Child: 26–30 min Protein binding:* 30% Metabolism:* Liver Half-life: 0.5–1.8 hr Hepatic dysfunction: 4.3 hr Kidney dysfunction: 2.4 hr Elimination: 70% in bile 30% unchanged in liver *Adult data	Muscle blockade; may be considered for use for rapid- sequence intubation	Rapid-sequence intubation: IV: 0.6–1.2 mg/kg Continuous infusion: 7–12 mcg/kg/min Adult: Same	

Drug	Class	Indication	Dosing	Pharmacokinetics	Comments
Vecuronium	Nondepolarizing NMBA Intermediate-acting NMBA	Muscle blockade	Neonate: 0.1 mg/kg Infant: 0.1 mg/kg Continuous infusion: 1–1.5 mcg/kg/min Child: 0.1 mg/kg Continuous infusion: 1.5–2.5 mcg/kg/min Adult: 0.1 mg/kg/dose Continuous infusion: 1.5–2 mcg/kg/min	Onset of action: IV: 1–3 min Duration: 30–40 min Protein binding:* 60–80% Metabolism:* Liver Half-life (elimination): Infant: 65 min Child: 41 min Hepatic dysfunction: 4.3 hr Kidney dysfunction: 2.4 hr Elimination:* 50% in feces via bile 25% in urine *Adult data	

Reversal Agents

Drug	Class	Indication	Dosing	Pharmacokinetics	Comments
Flumazenil	Benzodiazepine antidote	Reversal of sedation	Initial dose: 0.01 mg/kg over 15 sec, may repeat 0.01 mg/kg after 45 sec, then every minute for maximum cumulative dose of 0.05 mg/kg or 1 mg Adult: 0.2 mg over 15 sec, repeat 0.2 mg after 45 sec, then every 60 sec up to total 1 mg; maximum dose 3 mg in 1 hr	Onset of action: IV: 1–3 min Maximum effect: 6 min Duration: <1 hr Protein binding: 50% primarily to albumin Metabolism: Liver Half-life: 20–75 min Elimination: 99% hepatic 1% unchanged in urine	May result in seizures in patients dependent on medication. Resedation after duration has worn off.

(Continued)

TABLE 21-1

Pharmacologic Agents, Dosing, and Actions (Continued)

Medication	Pharmacology	Pharmacokinetics/dynamics	Indications	Dosing	Significant Side Effects
			Reversal Agents		
Naloxone	Antidote narcotic agonists	Onset of action: IV: within 2 min ET/IM/SQ: within 2–5 min Duration: 20–60 min Metabolism: Liver via glucuronidation Half-life: Neonate: 0.5–1.5 hr Elimination: Urine	Narcotic oversedation	**Total reversal of narcotic effect:** Infant, child ≤ 5 years 0.1 mg/kg Child > 5 years 2 mg/dose PALS guidelines recommend 2–10 times the IV dose via IM, SQ, or ET route **Post anesthetic narcotic reversal:** 0.01 mg/kg, repeat every 2–3 min as needed *Adult:* 0.005–0.01 mg/dose every 2–3 min	May precipitate withdrawal. Hypertension, hypotension, ventricular arrhythmias, cardiac arrest.
Neostigmine	Antidote to nondepolarizing NMBA	Onset of action: IV: 1–20 min IM: within 20–30 min Duration: IV: 1–2 hr IM: 2–4 hr Metabolism:* Liver Half-life:* 0.5–2.1 hr Elimination:* 50% unchanged in urine *Adult data	Reversal of nondepolarizing NMBA	Infant: IV: 0.025–0.1 mg/kg Child: IV: 0.025–0.8 mg/kg *Adult:* 0.5–2.5 mg; total dose not to exceed 5 mg	Administer with atropine or glycopyrrolate to limit salivation/ Bradycardia, asystole, AV block, agitation, seizures, bronchoconstriction, laryngospasm, dyspnea, respiratory arrest, salivation.

NMBA: neuromuscular blocking agent; IV intravenous; PO: by mouth; IM: intramuscular; SQ: subcutaneous; PR: by rectum; ET: endotracheal; PRN: as needed; CNS: central nervous system; AV: atrioventricular; CHF: congestive heart failure; TID: thrice daily; PAL: Pediatric Advanced Life Support.

Source: Tobias, J. (1995). Lorazepam versus midazolam for sedation. *Critical Care Medicine, 23*(6), 1151; Malchow, R., & Black, I. (2008). The evolution of pain management in the critically ill trauma patient: Emerging concepts from the global war on terrorism. *Critical Care Medicine, 36*(1), s346–s357; http://online.lexi.com

morphine include hypotension, peripheral vasodilation, pupillary constriction, and constipation. Constipation may be mediated by the use of oral or continuous infusion naloxone (Tofil et al., 2006).

Hydromorphone is another mu-agonist narcotic analgesic and is a hydrogenated ketone of morphine (Heard & Fletcher, 2006). This medication is approximately five to seven times stronger than morphine; it is also on the ISMP list of "high alert" medications. The dosage of hydromorphone varies with the route of delivery (Table 21-1). This agent is metabolized by the liver through glucuronidation to mostly inactive metabolites and is excreted in the urine. Its adverse response profile is similar to that of morphine. Specifically, hydromorphone's label carries a "black box" warning for respiratory depression (www.online.lexi.com).

Fentanyl is a synthetic narcotic analgesic (and mu agonist) that is 100 times more potent than morphine. Its dosage on the route of administration (Table 21-1). In areas where both morphine and fentanyl are used, careful dosing is essential, as these medications are not dosed in the same units of measurement. Fentanyl is highly lipophilic; as a result, it has a rapid onset of action and an equally rapid cessation of effects. Fentanyl is metabolized by the liver through the cytochrome P450 system into inactive metabolites.

A well-known, often feared, and real adverse response to fentanyl is chest wall rigidity. This idiopathic response to the medication usually occurs after large doses are administered. In this condition, the chest wall becomes rigid and air entry into the lungs is restricted. To alleviate the rigidity, a neuromuscular blocking agent or naloxone may be used. Unlike morphine, fentanyl does not cause hypotension and does not stimulate histamine release. However, respiratory depression is also listed as a "black box" warning on fentanyl's label (www.online.lexi.com).

Methadone is a long-acting narcotic analgesic that is commonly used for the prevention of withdrawal syndromes; however, it may also be used as an adjunct medication as part of pain management. Methadone works by binding to the opiate receptors in the CNS and inhibiting ascending pain pathways. It is metabolized in the liver into inactive metabolites. Methadone builds up in the body tissues, which prolongs its narcotic effect. The benefit of methadone is that it is long acting and, as such, can be administered every 8 to 12 hours.

Methadone's label carries a boxed warning focusing on the potential for respiratory depression, as the effect of the medication persists longer than the peak analgesic effect. Additionally, there is a boxed warning for the risk of prolongation of the QTc interval or torsades de pointes. Adult data recommend careful evaluation of the patient, including known risk factors (electrolyte abnormalities, diuretic therapy, cardiac hypertrophy), to decrease the risk of life-threatening arrhythmias (Krantz et al., 2009).

Antipyretic and OTC medications are also used in acutely ill pediatric patients to control pain. Acetaminophen is a commonly used antipyretic and analgesic in pediatrics. In general, it is safe to use. The dose range is 10 to 15 mg/kg, not to exceed 5 doses in 24 hours or 90 mg/kg in 24 hours. Rectal dosing may go up to 20 mg/kg; however, the medication should be titrated to effect. Acetaminophen may be given orally or rectally, as it is available in a variety of dosage forms. This medication is metabolized by the liver, then conjugated with glutathione and inactivated. When excessive amounts are taken, glutathione stores can become depleted, leading to increased levels of the active metabolite *N*-acetyl-imidoquinone, which may produce hepatic cellular necrosis (www.online.lexi.com). As such, this medication should be used with extreme caution in pediatric patients with hepatic insufficiency or failure.

Ibuprofen is an NSAID used as an antipyretic and analgesic in pediatrics. Specifically, its mechanism of action is the inhibition of prostaglandin biosynthesis through blocking cyclo-oxygenase (Patzer, 2008). The dose range is 4 to 10 mg/kg, given every 6 to 8 hours. Currently, only enteral dosage forms are available for pediatric analgesic use. An injectable form of ibuprofen is available, but is not FDA approved for children younger than 17 years of age. Because ibuprofen is oxidized in the liver, it should be used with caution in patients with hepatic insufficiency or failure. Additionally, ibuprofen inhibits platelet aggregation, resulting in increased bleeding time. Patients with thrombocytopenia, coagulation disorders, or bleeding problems should not be prescribed this medication. Significant side effects of ibuprofen include nausea, vomiting, gastrointestinal bleed, Stevens-Johnson syndrome (SJS), and toxic epidermal necrosis (www.online.lexi.com).

Naproxen is an NSAID used as an analgesic and antipyretic medication. The usual dose in children is 5 to 7 mg/kg, given every 8 to 12 hours orally. Naproxen is metabolized in the liver and excreted in the urine. Its significant side effects are similar to those for the other NSAIDs; thus naproxen should not be used in patients with thrombocytopenia, coagulation disorders, or bleeding problems.

Ketorolac is another NSAID used as an antipyretic and analgesic agent in the pediatric population. Its dose range is 0.5 mg/kg intravenously or 1 mg/kg intramuscularly. This medication is approved only for single-dose administration—not ongoing use—in patients 2 to 16 years of age. The literature, however, describes clinical experiences with dosing every 6 hours for pain management. Ketorolac is metabolized by the liver via hydroxylation and glucuronide conjugation and primarily excreted by the kidneys. Its significant side effects include gastrointestinal bleeding, ulceration, and perforation of the stomach or intestines. Like ibuprofen, ketorolac is contraindicated in patients with thrombocytopenia, coagulation disorders, or bleeding problems; gastrointestinal prophylaxis is recommended.

The previously described NSAIDs carry a "black box" warning for patients who have advanced kidney disease. In addition, kidney toxicity may develop in patients with dehydration, cardiac failure, liver dysfunction, and in patients receiving other potentially nephrotoxic medications (Patzer, 2008).

OTHER AGENTS

Additional agents that are useful in controlling pain and agitation in pediatric patients include alpha adrenergic agents (e.g., clonidine, dexmedetomidine) and anesthetics (e.g., ketamine, propofol). For example, dexmedetomidine may be chosen for the pediatric patient who is difficult to sedate, and ketamine is a good alternative for a short painful procedure. Table 21-1 provides a comprehensive list of these medications and information on dosing and side effects.

LOCAL ANESTHETICS

A variety of topical agents exist to limit pain during procedures. Topical creams containing lidocaine are therapeutic for minor painful procedures such as IV line placement or venous port access (EMLA, LMX). These topical agents are placed on the skin in a "dollop" and covered with an occlusive dressing. The cream begins to work within 30 to 60 minutes, depending on the product. Once the ingredient is active, the occlusive dressing is removed and the cream is wiped off the skin. The procedure should proceed as usual with cleansing of the skin. Blanching of the skin may occur in the area of penetration. The topical agent penetrates the skin and provides a local anesthesia whose effects last less than 4 hours. Systemic absorption may occur if the cream is used over a significant surface area of the body; in particular, lidocaine toxicity may occur. Side effects of lidocaine toxicity include CNS effects (seizures), cardiac arrhythmias, and increased risk for methemoglobinemia. Topical anesthetic creams should never be applied to broken skin, as their absorption will be affected (www.online.lexi.com).

Intradermal injection of lidocaine-containing solutions may also be used to anesthetize areas for minor procedures such as IV access or lumbar puncture. The amount to be injected depends on the vascularity of the tissues and the procedure being performed. For example, IV access requires a very small area of analgesia compared to an incision and drainage or suture placement, both of which require a larger area of analgesia. The dose of lidocaine used should not exceed 4.5 mg/kg.

Buffered lidocaine 1% in a jet injector, commonly known as J-Tip (National Medical Products Inc, Irvine, California), is the newest addition to topical anesthetics. J-Tip is a needle-free injection system containing buffered lidocaine 1% that is delivered using a high-pressure carbon dioxide gas cartridge. The medication penetrates the skin 5 to 8 millimeters in 0.2 second, allowing for rapid onset of anesthetic and subsequent insertion of an intravenous catheter (Jimenez et al., 2006). In comparison studies with topical lidocaine-containing cream anesthetics, J-Tip worked faster and relieved pain better during intravenous catheter placement (Jimenez et al.; Spanos et al., 2008).

NEUROMUSCULAR BLOCKING AGENTS

The use of neuromuscular blocking agents (NMBAs) in the pediatric population is generally reserved for critically ill children. These medications are used to facilitate diagnostic and therapeutic procedures, promote mechanical ventilation synchrony, reduce metabolic demands, and facilitate muscle control (shivering). These medications are not without side effects and complications, however; thus the decision to integrate them into the therapeutic profile should be made only after thorough consideration of the risks and benefits. Furthermore, these medications possess no sedating or analgesic properties, and their use limits HCPs' ability to perform neurologic examination. For all these reasons, the pediatric patient must be adequately sedated and pain free prior to the use of an NMBA.

To fully comprehend the mechanisms of action of NMBAs, one must understand muscle physiology. Muscle contractions are initiated when the action potential travels through the CNS to the nerve terminal (Figure 21-2). At the nerve terminal, an influx of calcium ions causes the release of acetylcholine. Acetylcholine then crosses the synaptic cleft, binds with its receptors on the motor end plate, and facilitates opening of the sodium channels. When an adequate number of acetylcholine receptors have been engaged, the membrane potential decreases, the voltage-dependent sodium channels are activated, and an action potential results. Subsequently, the action potential is propagated and a muscle contraction occurs (Martin et al., 1999).

NMBAs are classified as depolarizing (agonist) or nondepolarizing (antagonist). Depolarizing NMBAs bind to acetylcholine receptors in the synaptic cleft and produce muscle paralysis. Succinylcholine is the only depolarizing NMBA currently available in the United States (Table 21-1). This agent has the quickest onset of the available NMBAs. As such, rapid-sequence intubation is the primary indication for using this medication. Succinylcholine is contraindicated in pediatric patients who have malignant hyperthermia or who have a family history of malignant hyperthermia. Additionally, in children with neuromuscular diseases, there have been reports of rhabdomyolysis, hyperkalemia, and death with administration of succinylcholine. In a systematic analysis, Gurnaney et al. (2009) identified that patients with muscular dystrophies who receive succinylcholine are at risk for the development of

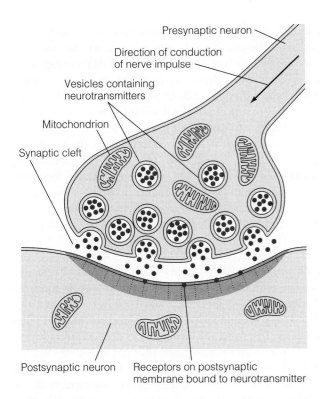

Presynaptic neuron

Direction of conduction
of nerve impulse

Vesicles containing
neurotransmitters

Mitochondrion

Synaptic cleft

Postsynaptic neuron

Receptors on postsynaptic
membrane bound to neurotransmitter

FIGURE 21-2

Neuromuscular Junction.

Source: From Chiras, D. (2008). Human Biology. Sudbury, MA: Jones
and Bartlett Publishers.

life-threatening hyperkalemia and, as such, should not
receive this agent. In light of this finding, children should
be screened for the presence of a neuromuscular disorder
prior to administration of this medication.

Nondepolarizing NMBAs act by competitively binding
at acetylcholine receptor sites without creating depolarization. A variety of nondepolarizing NMBAs are available that
are classified based on their chemical structure—namely,
as either benzylisoquinolinium derivatives or aminosteroid
compounds. Agents commonly used in pediatrics include the
aminosteroid NMBAs such as pancuronium, vecuronium,
and rocuronium (Table 21-1). These agents differ in their
duration of action; therefore, agent selection will depend on
the desired duration of activity and rationale for paralysis. For
example, a short-acting agent (rocuronium) is often selected
for intubation, whereas a longer-acting agent (vecuronium) is
used to facilitate mechanical ventilation. Most of the nonde-
ploarizing NBMAs are metabolized by the liver or excreted
unchanged in the urine. Cisatracurium is a unique agent
in that it is eliminated through several pathways, including
spontaneous degradation in plasma (Hofmann elimination);
this medication may be used for patients with renal or hepatic
dysfunction (Taketomo et al., 2010).

The use of NMBAs may complicate care, as several
medications can potentiate or antagonize the action of

NMBAs. Medications known to potentiate the activity
of NMBAs include steroids, aminoglycosides, antiarrhythmics, calcium-channel blockers, diuretics, beta adrenergic
blockers, and inhalation anesthetics. Medications known to
antagonize the effects of NMBA include phenytoin, theophylline, and sympathomimetic medications. Furthermore,
prolonged neuromuscular blockade and disuse atrophy are
well-known complications associated with NMBAs.

MONITORING

Continuous monitoring is essential for pediatric patients
receiving sedation, analgesia, and neuromuscular blockade
to ensure safe care. Monitoring pediatric patients who are
receiving NMBAs is critical, as these patients are at risk
for excessive NMBA dosing, which may prolong mechanical ventilation and hospitalization and compromise patient
safety. The current pediatric guideline from the United
Kingdom Paediatric Intensive Care Society recommends
evaluating level of neuromuscular blockade at least once
every 24 hours using *train-of-four* (*TOF*) testing (Playfor
et al., 2007). This clinical guideline is consistent with the
adult guideline, which recommends assessing the patient
clinically and implementing TOF monitoring to direct
titration of NMBA (Murray et al., 2002).

Currently, limited methods are available for monitoring
pediatric patients on NBMAs. The easiest method to monitor
the depth of neuromuscular blockade is to assess the patient
for muscle movement during a noxious stimulus (suctioning).
During the stimulus, if the patient is not maximally muscle
blocked, the observer will note muscle movement with
coughing. However, this method is considered unreliable:
The muscle contraction may be so small that it is not
apparent to the observer. Thus clinical monitoring alone is
inadequate.

TOF monitoring is an evaluation of the depth of neuromuscular blockade used in pediatric and adult patients
receiving NMBAs. Monitoring TOF is performed with
a *peripheral nerve stimulator* (*PNS*). The PNS is a device
that delivers four rapid-sequence electrical stimuli via
electrodes applied over a nerve. The most commonly
used peripheral nerves are the ulnar or facial nerve. The
number of responses noted in the thumb (ulnar) or eyelid
(facial) are counted and scored as zero to four twitches
of the four stimuli. Each number of twitches is considered to correlate with a percentage of depth of neuromuscular blockade. For example, zero out of four twitches
means the patient is 100% blocked, whereas four out of
four twitches corresponds with no blockade. Adequate
blockade is achieved when the patient has at least one
twitch. Two pediatric studies have compared clinical
observation and TOF in the evaluation of muscle movement in patients receiving NMBAs. Both studies found
poor correlation between observation and TOF testing,

supporting the need to develop a more objective method when evaluating a patient receiving NMBAs (Corso, 2008; Pena et al., 2000).

A daily "drug holiday" is another option for monitoring NMBA effects in pediatrics. This method stops the NMBA being administered and monitors the patient until movement is observed (Shapiro et al., 1995). The time it takes the patient to move is compared with the duration of the particular NMBA being used. For example, the effects of a medication lasting 60 minutes in duration should be absent after 60 minutes off the medication. However, concomitant therapies may potentiate the medication's actions; thus a time range should be allowed to first movement. If the patient does not demonstrate any movement for many hours, the HCP can safely titrate the medication to a lower dose, as the patient appears to be receiving more medication than needed. Provided the patient is meeting the goals of therapy (e.g., ventilatory synchrony), the dose of NMBA should be adjusted to the minimum effective dose. Continuous monitoring of the pediatric patient during NMBA titration is critical to ensure safe use and limit complications.

Bispectral index (*BIS*) monitoring is an electroencephalographic method to evaluate the hypnotic state of the sedation effect on the brain (Aneja et al., 2003). This monitoring device uses a quadruple electrode placed on the forehead of the patient and results in a single number reading from 0 to 100. Scores less than 40 are associated with deep hypnosis, whereas scores greater than 80 are associated with recall (Aneja et al.). This technology potentially lends itself nicely to the evaluation of sedation in critically ill pediatric patients and those receiving NMBAs.

Berkenbosch et al. (2002) studied sedated, mechanically ventilated pediatric patients and compared sedation scoring with a modified RSS to BIS scoring. These researchers found that BIS scoring was correlated, independent of prescribed medication, with inadequate and adequate sedation but was less sensitive in identifying excessive sedation.

In another study, BIS values in infants 6 months of age or younger were identified as lower at each sedation level as compared with older children using the University of Michigan Sedation Scale. Additionally, it was noted that BIS values were high in the face of limited patient responsiveness when ketamine and opioids were used as part of patient management (Malviya et al., 2007).

Several studies have compared sedation scoring with the COMFORT scale and BIS monitoring in critically ill, mechanically ventilated children. BIS monitoring has been found to correlate well with COMFORT scores overall (Twite et al., 2005). The BIS monitoring also correlates with light and moderate sedation (Froom et al., 2008) and deep sedation when low electroencephalograph (EEG) impedance is used (Triltsch et al., 2005).

BIS monitoring has been studied in pediatric patients receiving NMBAs. Trope et al. (2005) found BIS scoring did not correlate with autonomic variable changes in the pediatric patient. That is, increased heart rate or blood pressure did not correlate with increased BIS scoring; hence the HCP was not alerted to the patient being less sedated. Tobias and Grindstaff (2005) found similar results. Given these findings, it is unclear if reliance on autonomic variables is sufficient to determine level of sedation in pediatric patients, although it has historically been the method of choice; they are flawed in the face of an EEG monitoring device. BIS monitoring has also been evaluated for procedural sedation in pediatric patients. BIS data correlate well with RSS measurements in children receiving propofol (Powers et al., 2005) or midazolam, fentanyl, and pentobarbital (Agrawal et al., 2004). However, a study by Mason and colleagues (2006) examined patients receiving sedation with pentobarbital and found that the BIS monitoring did not correlate well with the RSS findings during moderate to deep sedation. Overall, it has been demonstrated that BIS data correlate with increasing levels of sedation: The lower the BIS score, the more sedated the patient. However, it has not been demonstrated that the BIS data correlate well with specific sedation goals such as mild, moderate, or deep sedation. As such, multifactorial assessments should be done to maximize the safety of patients using BIS monitoring technology.

REVERSAL AGENTS

Reversing sedation, analgesia, and NMBAs may be required under certain circumstances, such as in pediatric patients experiencing over-sedation, respiratory depression, and prolonged neuromuscular blockade. Reversal agents include flumazenil, naloxone, and neostigmine (Table 21-1). Reversing sedation with benzodiazepines can be accomplished using flumazenil. However, rapid reversal of a benzodiazepine may result in abrupt withdrawal symptoms, including seizures, in patients with physiologic dependence or those who are receiving benzodiazepines for seizure management. Flumazenil antagonizes the benzodiazepine effect at the GABA/benzodiazepine receptor complex (www.online.lexi.com). The activity of flumazenil is short acting, thus repeat dosing is often needed because the patient may become resedated when the action has worn off.

In a study by Shannon et al. (1997), incremental doses of flumazenil (0.01 mg/kg [maximum dosage 0.2 mg] given every minute up to a cumulative total dose of 0.05 mg/kg) partially or completely reversed conscious sedation from midazolam therapy in 96% of the patients within 10 minutes. The authors recommend monitoring for resedation for as long as 2 hours after the final flumazenil dose. These data support the contention that titration of flumazenil is important to achieve the desired effect of reversal of the sedating agent.

Naloxone reverses the narcotic effect by replacing the drug at the receptor site. Like flumazenil, naloxone often requires repeat dosing, as it has a shorter duration of action than the narcotic and should be titrated to effect. Continuous infusion of naloxone has been used not only for patients with overdose, but also to combat tolerance in patients receiving long-term opioid infusions (Darnell et al., 2008). It is imperative to recognize that a dose of naloxone may reverse not only the adverse event that being treated, but also reverse the pain relief activity of the narcotic. Patients may subsequently experience acute pain. In patients who require reversal of opioids due to respiratory suppression, a partial dose of naloxone (usual dose of 0.1 mg/kg for life-threatening toxicity) every 2 to 3 minutes can be given in attempt to maintain the analgesic effect of the medication while reversing the respiratory depression (Perry & Shannon, 1996). Repeat dosing or continuous infusion may continue until the desired effect is achieved and the patient is no longer at risk for resedation (Dahan et al., 2010).

Naloxone may also be used to treat opioid-induced pruritus and constipation (Table 21-1). Studies support the use of low-dose naloxone (0.25 mcg/kg/hr) to decrease opioid-induced side effects without reversing the analgesic effect (Maxwell et al., 2005).

Neostigmine is the reversal agent for nondepolarizing NMBAs. It is not effective for the depolarizing NMBA succinylcholine. Neostigmine is often used to reverse the NMBA effects following an operative procedure. For the pediatric patient with prolonged muscle paralysis following NMBA use, neostigmine may be given to determine if the paralysis is secondary to the NMBA or another different pathology (Table 21-1).

PROCEDURAL SEDATION STRATEGIES

Procedural sedation has evolved into a distinct skill set and is provided by many different practitioners in various practice settings (Cravero et al., 2006; Krauss & Green, 2006; Meyer et al., 2007). In response to the rapid evolution in sedation practices, recent national safety initiatives and sedation guidelines promulgated by the American Association of Anesthesiologists (ASA), the American Academy of Pediatrics (AAP), and the American Academy of Pediatric Dentistry have resulted in increased state regulation surrounding procedural sedation practices (Hertzog & Havidich, 2007; Joint Commission on Accreditation of HealthCare Organizations [JCAHO], 2006). HCPs must be aware of these specific state regulations as well as credentialing and competency requirements within institutions, and ensure their individual compliance with the standards set by regulatory bodies and national organizations.

Procedural sedation and analgesia for pediatric patients entails the use of sedative, analgesic, and dissociative medications to provide anxiolysis, amnesia, analgesia, sedation, and motor control during painful or unpleasant diagnostic and therapeutic procedures (Cote & Wilson, 2006; Kraus & Green, 2006). The progression from mild sedation to general anesthesia is not perceived as a series of discrete levels, but rather constitutes a continuum. Professional organizations such as American College of Emergency Physicians (ACEP), AAP, and ASA have defined four states of procedural sedation and analgesia:

- *Minimal sedation*: a medically controlled state of depressed consciousness that (1) allows protective reflexes to be maintained; (2) retains the patient's ability to maintain a patent airway independently and continuously; and (3) permits appropriate response by the patient to physical stimulation or verbal command.
- *Moderate sedation/analgesia*: a drug-induced depression of consciousness during which pediatric patients respond purposefully to verbal commands, either alone or accompanied by light tactile stimulation. No assistance is required to maintain a patent airway.
- *Deep sedation*: a medically controlled state of depressed consciousness or unconsciousness from which the patient is not easily aroused. It may be accompanied by a partial or complete loss of protective reflexes, and includes the inability to maintain a patent airway independently and respond purposefully to physical stimulation or verbal command.
- *General anesthesia*: a drug-induced loss of consciousness during which patients are not arousable, even by painful stimulation. The ability to independently maintain ventilatory function is often impaired.

The AAP (2002), ASA (2002), and ACEP (2005) have set guidelines for procedural sedation. Although these guidelines are nonbinding in nature, they are relevant to all locations and to all HCPs who provide care for pediatric patients. Any procedure requiring sedation requires a presedation assessment and should address factors associated with the procedure, patient, and personnel requirements.

Factors related to the procedure include the following:

- *Duration of procedure*: Influences the choice of short-acting versus long-acting medication.
- *Painful versus nonpainful procedure*: Sedation regimens differ based on type of procedure. For example, a sedative and analgesic agent should be chosen for a painful procedure, whereas an agent that achieves anxiolysis or sedation alone may be sufficient for a nonpainful procedure (diagnostic procedure).
- *Location of procedure*: The availability of rescue resources influences the choice of agents and the number of doses administered to minimize risk of deep sedation.

Factors related to the patient are as follows:

- *Past experience*: Elicit a sedation/anesthetic history that includes positive and negative experiences and drugs received.
- *Allergies*: Determine the type of reaction that occurred with the drug and whether symptoms included urticaria or respiratory distress, suggesting the possibility of anaphylaxis and requiring avoidance of this agent.
- *Aspiration risk*: Determine the time of last oral intake. Fasting guidelines (NPO status) are based on anesthesia recommendations, as the exact depth of sedation achieved in pediatric patients is difficult to predict following a dose of a sedative; therefore it should be assumed that airway reflexes may be lost with sedation and steps to minimize risk should be taken. Although no national guidelines for fasting prior to sedation exist, generally accepted guidelines endorsed by the AAP and ASA are presented in Table 21-2. Currently, there is no evidence suggesting a correlation between fasting, emesis, and pulmonary aspiration in healthy pediatric patients undergoing procedural sedation (Mace et al., 2008). However, if the HCP elicits a history of gastroesophageal reflux disease and severity, that factor may prompt referral to an anesthesiologist with or without elective intubation.

TABLE 21-2

Preprocedure Fasting Guidelines	
Diet	**Minimal Fasting Period**
Clear liquids	2 hours
Human breastmilk	4 hours
Infant formula or milk	6 hours
Solid food	8 hours

Source: American Society of Anesthesiologists.

- *General health*: Includes health history (the focus should include any history of stridor, snoring, sleep apnea, neuromuscular disease, cardiovascular disease, or chromosomal abnormalities); physical examination including body habitus (significant obesity) and the airway, cardiovascular and respiratory systems; and age and weight. The ASA classification system (Table 21-3) categorizes patients based on general health to determine their suitability for sedation. Consultation with an anesthesia specialist is recommended if significant risk factors are identified or the patient qualifies as having an ASA classification of 3 or greater. More recently, however, a greater emphasis has been placed on airway evaluation, as agreement on the value of the rating system varies (Burgoyne et al., 2007).
- *Current medication*: Including dosage, time, and route.
- *Airway issues*: Abnormalities of the head, neck, face, jaw, and airway should be noted. Any pediatric patient with dysmorphic facial features requires close inspection to determine the potential for difficulty in maintaining a patent airway. A small mandible or large tongue is often associated with difficult spontaneous ventilation as well as difficult assisted ventilation. It is also important to inspect the teeth for potentially loose teeth. The modified Mallampati classification may be helpful as part of the presedation airway assessment (Langeron et al., 2006; Mallampati et al., 1985; Mashour & Sandberg, 2006). This examination classifies the size of the tongue by opening the patient's mouth as wide as possible, visualizing the oropharynx, and determining the degree of visualization of the uvula and tonsillar pillars (Figure 21-3). Determination that the patient belongs in Class III or IV, in which only the soft or hard palate is visualized, should prompt consultation with an anesthesiologist. A recent systematic review and meta-analysis found the original and modified Mallampati tests have limited accuracy for predicting a difficult airway when used alone for airway screening (Lee et al., 2006). Although no

TABLE 21-3

ASA Physical Status Classification System		
ASA Class	**Description**	**Suitability for Sedation**
P1	Normal healthy patient	Excellent
P2	Patient with mild systemic disease	Generally good
P3	Patient with severe systemic disease	Intermediate to poor; consider benefits to relative risks
P4	Patient with severe systemic disease that is a constant threat to life	Poor; benefits rarely outweigh risks
P5	Moribund patient who is not expected to survive without the operation	Extremely poor

Source: American Association of Anesthesiologists (ASA), http://www.asahq.org/clinical/physicalstatus.htm

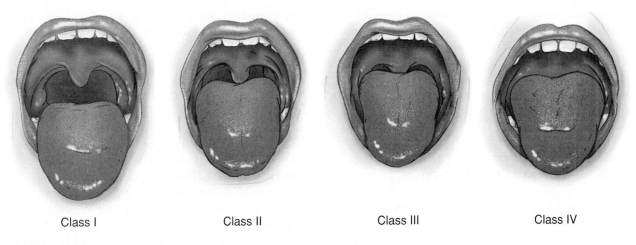

| Class I | Class II | Class III | Class IV |

FIGURE 21-3

Mallampati Airway Classification.

Source: From American Academy of Orthopaedic Surgeons (AAOS) and the American College of Emergency Physicians (ACEP), Pollak, A. (Ed.) (2011). Critical Care Transport, Sudbury. MA: Jones and Bartlett Publishers.

pediatric studies were included in this analysis, the Mallampati test is still considered a useful adjunct in evaluating the pediatric airway (ASA, 2003).

- *Developmental issues*: Requirements for sedation will change based on the patient's neurodevelopmental status, the level of cooperation needed for the procedure, and the pediatric patient's anxiety associated with the procedure.

The major history assessment parameters may be remembered by using the mnemonic "AMPLE": allergies, medications, past medical history, last meal, and events leading up to scenario (why sedation is required).

Factors related to the personnel requirements include the following:

- *Regulatory requirements*: Some states mandate the presence of a licensed independent practitioner and an experienced nurse.
- *HCP's sedation skills*: The HCP must be able to rapidly identify and treat respiratory and hemodynamic complications, knowledgeable about medications, and capable of responding to these complications, including maintaining or establishing a patent airway and initiating assisted ventilation.

The 2006 recommendation from JCAHO (now called The Joint Commission [TJC]) states that a licensed independent provider administering sedation medications must be trained to manage or "rescue" a patient from one level of sedation "deeper" than that which is intended. The provider must be immediately available to intervene in the event of complications associated with sedation administration. Adverse events associated with procedural

sedation include decreased respiratory drive, inability to maintain a patent airway, inability to maintain airway protective reflexes (cough and gag), and hemodynamic compromise. TJC also mandates that the standard of care for procedural sedation is the same regardless of the setting in which care is delivered. General guidelines are outlined here, but the HCP must recognize that specific details for procedural sedation will vary between institutions.

PREPARATION

- Maintain the patient on NPO status.
- Obtain informed consent/permission for the procedure and sedation and assent if appropriate. The consent form should include potential risks associated with medications and/or the underlying disease condition(s) present.
- Complete appropriate presedation assessment documentation.
- Obtain all necessary equipment. Use the mnemonic "SOAPME": suction, oxygen, airway (self-inflating bag, appropriate-size mask, advanced airway equipment), pharmaceuticals (sedation agents, reversal agents, intravenous fluids), monitors (cardiorespiratory monitor, pulse oximeter, capnography, noninvasive blood pressure), equipment (other needed for procedure and available resuscitative equipment)
- Even with the most careful titration of sedation medications, the HCP must be prepared for potential respiratory depression or airway obstruction and the need for resuscitative measures.
- The sedation team includes a licensed independent practitioner not performing the procedure and a skilled

nurse whose responsibility is to monitor appropriate physiologic parameters, administer care, and assist with any supportive or resuscitation measures as needed.

- The presence of child life and/or caregiver involvement to provide comfort measures and use of nonpharmacologic methods such as distraction, guided imagery, and relaxation are essential to decrease anxiety and minimize pain.

CONSIDERATIONS IN CHOOSING AGENTS

There are several key points to consider when selecting drugs for procedural sedation. As previously noted, the potential for pain with the procedure, the patient's prior experience with drugs, the duration of the procedure, and the patient's medical condition should all be determined as part of the presedation assessment. In addition, it is important to consider the following:

- *Mechanism of action of the drug*: Does it have primarily sedative or analgesic properties?
- *Pharmacokinetics of the drug*, including duration and route of administration: The intravenous route is usually the preferred route, as the HCP can more easily titrate the medication to the desired effect. In addition, combinations of medications should be administered with caution, as they may be more potent than an individual medication.
- *Dose response*: It is important to avoid repeated administration of medications before the peak effect of a previous dose has been reached. Repeat dosing can result in an excessive total drug effect over time and potentiates the effect of the drugs. The HCP must also recognize the risks associated with the use of combinations of medications. For example, the use of both an opioid and a benzodiazepine increases the risk of respiratory depression above that seen when either type of medication is used exclusively.

SEDATION AGENTS

Agents used for moderate sedation in pediatric patients are listed in Table 21-4. In addition to these agents, local (lidocaine) and topical (EMLA, LMX cream) anesthetics can successfully decrease pain perception and are used as adjunct measures for invasive procedures. Oral sucrose has been shown to be safe and effective in reducing signs of distress associated with minor, painful procedures in neonates and is moderately effective in infants up to 6 months of age (Mace et al., 2008). Single agents are often used for diagnostic procedures; however, moderate sedation for therapeutic procedures is often best achieved with a combination of a benzodiazepine and an opioid (e.g., midazolam and fentanyl).

PROCEDURE

- Completion of any presedation institutional documentation.
- Cardiorespiratory monitors applied to the patient.
- Equipment checked by sedation nurse and HCP: includes, but is not limited to, oxygen, bag-mask ventilation, suction, immediate access to airway adjuncts, advance airway support, and resuscitation equipment.
- "Time out" (universal protocol) performed by sedation nurse and HCP.
- Monitoring: includes vital signs (heart rate, respiratory rate, blood pressure), oxygen saturation, level of consciousness, and pain and sedation scores before and at regular intervals during the procedure, including before and after all sedation is administered. In addition, capnography should be considered for lengthier procedures or for those during which access to the patient is limited (e.g., magnetic resonance imaging [MRI]).
- Documentation: includes record of vital signs, medications with doses and times, supportive measures, and any significant events.

DISCHARGE CRITERIA

Pediatric patients are at continued risk for complications after the completion of sedation for a procedure; thus they require monitoring until they are fully recovered and the risks no longer exist. The recovery area must be equipped with suction, oxygen, and advanced airway equipment. Monitoring equipment includes a cardiorespiratory monitor, a pulse oximeter, and a blood pressure monitor. Vital signs are recorded at regular intervals until the child is back to his or her neurological baseline.

Currently, there is no universally applicable evidence-based set of clinical indicators for safe discharge following procedural sedation (Mace et al., 2008). General criteria used to make this decision include (1) stable vital signs, (2) good control of pain, (3) return to baseline level of consciousness, (4) good control of nausea and/or vomiting, and (5) adequate tolerance of oral intake to maintain hydration. Discharge must be approved by the HCP, with appropriate documentation. Sedation records must include the patient's status at time of discharge. Finally, specific instructions should be given to the caregiver regarding appropriate diet, medications, level of activity, and situations in which to notify the HCP (e.g., sudden unexpected problems).

TABLE 21-4

Commonly Used Sedation and Analgesic Agents

Indication	Drug	Route	Dose	Onset	Recommended Use
Sedation	Chloral hydrate	Oral or rectal	50–75 mg/kg (maximum: infants 1 gm, child 2 gm)	15–30 min	Noninvasive diagnostic procedure (age < 3 years)
	Midazolam	Oral or rectal	0.25–0.5 mg/kg	15–30 min	Noninvasive diagnostic procedure or minor invasive procedure
		Nasal	0.2–0.5 mg/kg	10–15 min	Same as oral or rectal but unable to take oral route
		IM	0.1–0.15 mg/kg	10–20 min	Same as oral or rectal but unable to take oral route
		IV	Initial dosage 0.025–0.1 mg/kg, titrate to desired effect	3 min	Diagnostic or therapeutic procedures, in combination with analgesic for painful procedures
	Pentobarbital	IV	Initial dosage 1–2 mg/kg, repeat in 1 mg/kg increments to desired effect; maximum 4 mg/kg	10–15 min	Diagnostic procedures requiring cooperation for a prolonged period of time
	Etomidate	IV	0.1–0.3 mg/kg	1–2 min	Patients ≥ 12 years to assist with procedures requiring maximal cooperation
	Propofol	IV	2.5–3.5 mg/kg bolus, then continuous infusion	1 min	Painful procedures, regulated medication
Analgesia	Fentanyl Oralet (sweetened lozenge on a plastic stick)	Oral transmucosal fentanyl citrate (OTFC)	10–15 mcg/kg	10–20 min	Patients without an IV for minor painful procedure
	Fentanyl	IV	1 mcg/kg	2–4 min	Painful procedures
	Ketamine	IM	3–7 mg/kg	3–5 min	Sedate the "out of control" patient without an IV or for a moderately painful procedure
		IV	0.5 – 2 mg/kg	1–2 min	Painful procedures

IV: intravenous; IM: intramuscular.

Source: Taketomo, C., Hodding, J., & Kraus, D. (2010). *Pediatric dosage handbook* (17th ed.). Hudson, OH: Lexi-Comp.

OUTCOME

In 2009, the Consensus Panel on Sedation Research of Pediatric Emergency Research Canada (PERC) and the Pediatric Emergency Care Applied Research Network (PECARN) published recommendations for standardizing terminology and reporting adverse events for procedural sedation in children, with the ultimate goal being the creation of a uniform reporting mechanism to enhance future research. The overall estimated incidence of serious adverse outcomes associated with procedural sedation is less than 1 per 10,000 (Cravero et al., 2006; Meyer et al., 2007). Cote and colleagues (2000) reported that the rate of adverse effects was related to three factors: (1) the number of sedative agents administered, but particularly if two or more agents were given; (2) inadequate monitoring; and (3) poor rescue system. Adverse events were found to occur irrespective of physician type, but were rather associated with the skill of the practitioner (Cote et al., 2000). A large prospective pediatric study of 1,367 pediatric patients found that the highest risk of serious adverse events occurred within 25 minutes of receiving the last dose of intravenous sedative (Newman et al., 2003). Instituting sedation practices based on current national guidelines and best evidence is necessary to ensure safe sedation practices.

PATIENT-, CAREGIVER-, AND NURSE-CONTROLLED ANALGESIA

Patient-controlled analgesia (PCA) comprises a preprogrammed delivery system that administers comparatively small preset doses of an analgesic medication (usually an opioid) intravenously when a patient activates the pump by depressing an attached button. A lockout period between doses, typically lasting 6 to 10 minutes, prevents administration of repeated doses within short periods of time, thereby decreasing the potential for toxicity. PCA benefits include more consistent and sustained analgesia, lower total doses of opioid use, and opioid dosing titration for individualized variations in pain. PCA opioid administration offers some advantages over continuous intravenous infusion in terms of ease of dose titration and the management of incident pain such as with dressing changes and physical therapy. PCA devices may administer a basal or continuous infusion along with intermittent bolus doses.

PCA protocols and standardized order sets for pediatric patients are becoming widely used. Data demonstrate that improved monitoring of pediatric patients and increased identification of potential adverse events occur with the use of standardized PCA order sets (Wrona et al., 2007).

Intravenous PCA has been shown to provide optimal pain management for pediatric patients with postoperative pain, sickle cell pain crisis, or cancer. It has also been used for those in palliative care (Anghelescu et al., 2008;

Greco & Berde, 2005; Melzer-Lange et al., 2004; Shin et al., 2001). The most commonly prescribed opioids for PCA infusions are morphine, hydromorphone, and fentanyl (Table 21-5). Hydromorphone is often reserved for patients experiencing complications such as significant pruritus and nausea associated with morphine infusion.

PCA has been shown to be safe and effective in children 7 years of age or older (Greco & Berde, 2005). Although selected younger children may be suitable candidates for PCA, monitoring the patient's understanding of pushing the device button to receive pain relief is critical, as a higher frequency of failed analgesia has been found in children younger than 7 years of age (Greco & Berde). Other considerations with PCA use include the child's physical ability to push the device button (adequate strength, unrestrained) and willingness to push the button when experiencing pain.

"PCA-by-proxy" allows a person authorized or designated by the institution—the registered nurse or caregiver, for example—to activate the analgesic infusion pump in lieu of the patient doing so. In general, nurse-controlled analgesia (NCA) may be used in patients who are cognitively or physically unable to push the button. Evidence suggests that NCA is an efficient and safe method to control pain in the hospital setting (Birmingham et al., 2009; Monitto et al., 2000; Peters et al., 1999; Pillitteri & Clark, 1998). The value of caregiver-controlled analgesia has also been well established for children with advanced cancer or in palliative care (Anghelescu et al., 2005; Monitto et al.), but remains controversial for other patient populations (Greco & Berde, 2005). In 2004, TJC issued a sentinel event alert to inform hospitals and medical personnel of the risks associated with *unauthorized* PCA-by-proxy and has charged pediatric institutions with developing clear defined policies and procedures that specifically outline patient selection criteria, education, and appropriate monitoring of these patients.

Epidural analgesic infusions may also be useful in patients for postoperative pain management and may decrease requirements for other pain medications. Epidural infusions commonly involve combinations of local

TABLE 21-5

Patient-Controlled Analgesic Dosing			
	Fentanyl	Hydromorphine	Morphine
Basal rate (mcg/kg/hr)	0.5–1	3–5	10–30
Bolus dose (mcg/kg)	0.5–10	3–5	10–30
Lockout period (min)	6–10	6–10	6–10
Bolus limit (per hour)	2–3	4–6	4–6

anesthetics with opioids, such as bupivicaine with fentanyl, hydromorphone, or morphine. Studies have confirmed the safety and efficacy of epidural infusion use in infants and children (Greco & Berde, 2005; Kost-Byerly, 2002; Saudan et al., 2007; Tobias, 2004) and have compared the use of epidural infusions to PCA (Anghelescu et al., 2008; Gauger et al., 2009). In all patients, the potential for age-related differences in hepatic degradation and clearance of local anesthetics and opioids should be considered. Also, dosages

TABLE 21-6

Patient-Controlled Analgesia and Epidural Infusion Adverse Effects and Management Adverse Effect	
Adverse Effect	**Treatment**
Respiratory depression	Decrease PCA dosing Increase the lockout interval Decrease/discontinue the basal rate if present Consider adding an NSAID Consider low-dose naloxone 2–10 mcg/kg IV
Apnea	Stop the infusion Assist ventilation as needed Reverse the opioid with naloxone 0.1 mg/kg/dose (maximum 2 mg)
Pruritis	Diphenhydramine 1 mg/kg/dose IV every 6 hours (maximum 50 mg/dose) Consider low-dose naloxone Consider decreasing the opioid dosage or changing the opioid Consider adding an NSAID
Nausea and vomiting	Treat with antiemetics such as ondansetron: in patients weighing less than 10 kg, 0.1 mg/kg/dose every 4–6 hours; in patients weighing 10 kg or more, 1 mg/dose IV every 4–6 hours Consider decreasing the opioid dosage or changing the opioid Consider adding an NSAID
Constipation	Ducosate 10–40 mg PO daily Bisacodyl (Dulcolax) 5 mg PO/PR daily
Urinary retention	More common with intrathecal-administered opioid Consider decreasing the opioid dosage Bladder catheterization

PCA: patient-controlled analgesia; NSAID: nonsteroidal anti-inflammatory drug; IV: intravenous; PO: by mouth; PR: by rectum.

of opioids and amide local anesthetics should be reduced in infants younger than 6 months of age (Kost-Byerly, 2002). Adverse events are similar for PCA and epidural infusions (Table 21-6).

Patients are typically transitioned from PCA or epidural infusions when able to tolerate oral medications. If the pediatric patient is being treated for chronic pain, the total daily PCA dose (basal rate plus boluses) received is calculated and converted to the oral equivalent based on drug potency. For example, the conversion of IV morphine to oral morphine is approximately 3:1 potency. Thus, if the pediatric patient received a total of 40 mg IV morphine, the oral equivalency is $40 \times 3 = 120$ mg in divided doses (30 mg every 6 hours). For treatment of acute pain, patients typically remain on PCA until the acute process is resolved and the transition to an oral analgesic agent such as oxycodone or morphine has been tolerated.

SEDATION STRATEGIES FOR MECHANICALLY VENTILATED CHILDREN

Multiple factors need to be considered in sedating critically ill pediatric patients. Specifically, the degree of illness, therapeutic goal, and concomitant pharmacotherapy will affect the choice of intermittent or continuous infusion medications. For example, a patient with a critical airway would likely require continuous infusions to maintain a steady therapeutic medication state, thereby minimizing the risk of agitation and possible inadvertent extubation. A patient with respiratory distress requiring noninvasive positive-pressure ventilation may require minimal "as needed" dosing to tolerate the ventilation equipment while avoiding the risk of exacerbating the respiratory compromise. These two examples demonstrate the spectrum of analgesic and sedation needs in the intensive care unit and highlight the difficulty in standardizing an approach to analgesia and sedation for critically ill children (Table 21-1; Table 21-7). The HCP must recognize that the infusion rate will need to be titrated based on the patient's response (Hartman et al., 2009).

Dexmedetomidine, a relatively new alpha$_2$ adrenergic agonist, has shown promise as a sedation agent in the adult population but has not been approved by the FDA for use in pediatric patients. Preliminary research suggests that there may be a role for dexmedetomidine as an alternative sedation agent or as a means to reduce the need for other sedation medications (Czaja & Zimmerman, 2009; Tobias, 2002; Tobias & Berkenbosch, 2003, 2004)

Some adult sedation practices are also drawing the attention of pediatric-focused HCPs. In 2000, Kress and colleagues evaluated the effectiveness of daily interruption of continuous infusion agents in adult critically ill patients. Each day, the sedation infusions were stopped until the

TABLE 21-7

Commonly Used Continuous Infusions for Sedation and Analgesia in the Pediatric Intensive Care Unit		
Agent	**Dosing**	**Comments**
Fentanyl	1–3 mcg/kg/hr	Approximately 100 times the analgesic potency of morphine. Relatively long elimination half-life. Substantial clinical experience in infants and children following surgery for congenital heart disease.
Morphine	10–30 mcg/kg/hr	Longer duration of action than fentanyl, possibly providing improved analgesia. Delayed onset of tolerance and potentially less withdrawal when compared to fentanyl. Use with caution in asthmatic patients due to potential histamine release.
Midazolam	0.05–0.2 mg/kg/hr	Abundant clinical experience with its use as a continuous agent. Problems with tolerance and withdrawal syndrome. Reduced efficacy in infants.
Ketamine	1–2 mg/kg/hr	Limited pediatric research describing use as continuous infusion. Suggested use in patients with status asthmaticus and burns and as an adjunct agent in mechanically ventilated children who are difficult to sedation.

Source: Playfor, S., Jenkins, I., Boyles, C., et al. (2006). Consensus guidelines on sedation and analgesia in critically ill children. *Intensive Care Medicine, 32*(10), 1125–1136; Tobias, J. (2005). Sedation and analgesia in the pediatric intensive care unit. *Pediatric Annals, 34*(8), 636–645.

adult could respond, and then were resumed at a decremented dose. The medications were titrated to a goal level of sedation. The authors surmised that a daily interruption in sedation medications led to decreases in both the number of mechanical ventilation days and the number of intensive care unit (ICU) days (Kress et al., 2000). In another study, Schweickert and colleagues (2004) demonstrated that a sedation protocol based on daily interruptions of continuous infusions decreased complications associated with critical illness. Patients managed by the daily interruption protocol had a sedation-associated complication incidence of 2.6% versus 6.2% for patients managed without such a protocol (Schweickert et al., 2004). Mechanical ventilation

complications evaluated included ventilator-associated pneumonia, upper gastrointestinal hemorrhage, bacteremia, barotrauma, deep venous thrombosis, cholestasis, and sinusitis requiring surgical intervention. Kress and colleagues (2003) also evaluated the impact of daily sedation interruption on psychological outcomes. When these investigators compared patients managed with a daily sedation interruption versus patients managed without a protocol, they found that the adults in the daily interruption group had a tendency toward improved psychological outcomes and lower incidence of PTSD (Kress et al., 2003). Although the daily sedation interruption strategy has shown success in reducing the length of mechanical ventilation in adults, this strategy is less feasible in pediatric patients, primarily because children's developmental and cognitive immaturity requires deeper sedation to ensure safety, cooperation, and adequate mechanical ventilation.

Another novel approach to adult sedation management has been the creation of a nurse-driven sedation protocol. Brook and colleagues (1999) studied the application of a nurse-driven sedation protocol in the care of critically ill adults on mechanical ventilation. In their study, adults in the protocol arm had significant decreases in duration of mechanical ventilation, ICU and hospital stay, overall sedation requirements, and need for tracheostomy (Brook et al., 1999). In contrast to these findings, a recent study duplicating the Brook et al. work found no statistical significance in duration of mechanical ventilation or ICU or hospital stay (Bucknall et al., 2008). Currently, no published data support the concept that either of these sedation management strategies would be effective in pediatrics; however, a multicenter, controlled clinical trial is under way to evaluate the effectiveness of a nurse-managed sedation protocol in pediatric critically ill children.

WEANING NARCOTICS AND SEDATIVES

The most frequently used medications to minimize pain and anxiety in critically ill pediatric patients are opioids and benzodiazepines (Ista et al., 2007). Unfortunately, continuous use of sedative and analgesic agents for several days increases the risk of tolerance, dependence, and withdrawal (Cunliffe et al., 2004; Suresh & Anand, 1998).

- *Tolerance* is defined as a decrease in a drug's effect over time or the need to increase the dose to achieve the same effect (Ista et al., 2007; Tobias, 2000).
- *Dependence* refers to the continued need for the drugs administration to prevent withdrawal.
- *Withdrawal* is a constellation of physical symptoms that occurs when an opioid or benzodiazepine is abruptly discontinued in a patient who has developed tolerance (Ista et al., 2007; Tobias, 2000). The symptoms of withdrawal vary among patients and may be affected

by the agent and the patient's age, cognitive state, and associated medical conditions (Ista et al., 2007; Tobias, 2000). The predominant manifestations include central nervous system effects, sympathetic hyperactivity, and gastrointestinal disturbances (Ista et al.).

Researchers first described opioid dependency and withdrawal in neonates and infants in the 1970s in infants of drug-addicted mothers (Finnegan et al., 1975). However, dependency and opioid withdrawal syndrome were not recognized as a problem in PICU patients until 1990 (Arnold et al., 1990). A 1993 survey found that 62% of PICU patients experienced withdrawal symptoms; however, only 24% of PICUs routinely tapered sedatives to prevent withdrawal (Marx et al., 1993). Opiates were typically tapered only after withdrawal symptoms occurred, with the duration of tapering lasting as long as 6 weeks. Several reports describe opioid and benzodiazepine withdrawal characteristics in critically ill pediatric patients (Dominguez et al., 2006; Franck et al., 2004; Franck et al., 1998; Hughes et al., 1994; Katz et al., 1994; Lugo et al., 2001).

Today, a mounting body of evidence suggests that critically ill pediatric patients who receive benzodiazepines and/or opioids for 5 days or longer are at risk for experiencing withdrawal, with clinical manifestations typically occurring 8 to 48 hours after discontinuation of these medications (Cunliffe et al., 2004; Lugo et al., 2001; Robertson et al., 2000; Siddappa et al., 2003). In addition, some reports indicate that cumulative drug dosage is another predictor of withdrawal risk. A cumulative dose of midazolam greater than 60 mg/kg and a cumulative dose of fentanyl greater than 2,500 mcg/kg were associated with withdrawal syndrome in children (Fonsmark et al., 1999; Katz et al., 1994).

Despite increasing evidence of withdrawal syndrome in pediatric patients, few policies exist addressing the management or prevention of withdrawal syndrome. The AAP developed neonatal withdrawal syndrome guidelines in 1983 and updated these guidelines in 1998. Recent Cochrane reviews have examined treatment of opioid withdrawal in neonates (Osborn et al., 2005a, 2005b). However, consensus regarding optimal agents, route, or dosing of opioids or sedatives currently does not exist in pediatrics. The United Kingdom Paediatric Intensive Care Society published recommendations in 2006 regarding analgesia and sedation in critically ill children, but none of these guidelines were based on randomized control trials or addressed the issue of drug withdrawal (Jenkins et al., 2007).

Methods to assess benzodiazepine and opioid withdrawal vary among studies. Four tools currently exist to assess neonates after prolonged use of opioids or newborns of drug-addicted mothers (Ista et al., 2007). The most frequently used assessment scale that captures withdrawal behaviors in children of all ages is the *neonatal abstinence score* (*NAS*), although it has not been validated in the pediatric population.

Three tools have been developed to measure withdrawal symptoms in children. The Sedation Withdrawal Score developed by Cunliffe et al. (2004) included 12 symptoms of withdrawal, each scored subjectively on a three-point scale. The Sophia Observation Withdrawal Symptoms Scale was designed to measure opioid and benzodiazepine withdrawal in ventilated pediatric patients aged 0 to 18 years (Ista et al., 2008). Although these tools appear to be clinically useful, psychometric evaluations of their sensitivity, validity, and reliability are currently under way. In 2008, Franck and colleagues developed the *withdrawal assessment tool-version 1 (WAT-1)*—a pediatric-specific tool containing 11 items and 12 possible points. This tool was tested in 83 children between the ages of 7 months and 10 years with acute respiratory failure who were being weaned from continuous infusion or around-the-clock opioids and benzodiazepines. The WAT-1 demonstrated excellent psychometric performance for the study population but requires further testing in other "at-risk" groups.

Emerging evidence supports the use of novel sedation strategies during mechanical ventilation to reduce tolerance and withdrawal in both adult and pediatric critically ill patients. The data suggest that use of nurse-led sedation protocols during mechanical ventilation, daily interruptions in sedation infusions, and sequential rotations of different classes of opioids and benzodiazepines may all decrease incidence of tolerance and withdrawal, duration of mechanical ventilation, duration of sedation, and ICU stay (Alexander et al., 2002; Parran & Pederson, 2002; Quenot et al., 2007).

Despite a growing body of evidence documenting significant withdrawal effects in critically ill children, there remains great variation in sedation weaning practices. Clinicians often rely on their knowledge of opioids and benzodiazepines, intuition, and previous clinical experiences to guide decisions regarding the agent, dosage, rate of taper, and assessment and treatment of withdrawal symptoms. Although the use of an evidence-based, standardized method for weaning patients off of sedation may improve patient outcomes and reduce inconsistencies associated with weaning agents too rapidly or too slowly, evidence demonstrating reduced withdrawal symptoms in children following mechanical ventilation with the use of a standardized sedation weaning protocol is limited and may not be practical.

The use of methadone for opioid withdrawal is supported by the largest body of evidence, although the data obtained from such studies are primarily retrospective and observational. These findings suggest the use of methadone to prevent opioid withdrawal is safe and effective in critically ill pediatric patients (Berens et al., 2006; Ducharme et al., 2005; Lugo et al., 2001; Meyer & Berens, 2001; Robertson et al., 2000; Siddappa et al., 2003). Pharmacokinetic data show that methadone has the longest half-life of the commonly available opiates and good oral bioavailability, thus allowing for conversion from the intravenous to oral route of administration and extended dosing intervals (Yaster et al., 1996). At the same time, evidence pertaining to the optimal methadone starting dosage and duration of wean remains limited. Conversion from one opioid or benzodiazepine to another requires equianalgesic dosing. To prevent underdosing or overdosing when converting from one drug to another, recommendations include taking a conservative approach and utilizing dose titration to achieve the desired effect (Robertson et al., 2000; Tobias, 2000).

Recent reports examining methadone taper protocols indicate that these plans have successfully reduced opioid withdrawal symptoms in critically ill children but used larger starting doses of methadone than previously reported (Berens et al., 2006; Lugo et al., 2001; Meyer & Berens, 2001; Robertson et al., 2000). Despite the larger starting dose, the duration of weaning was reduced without increased incidence of withdrawal. The concurrent use of lorazepam in these studies raises the question as to whether the simultaneous use alleviated withdrawal symptoms and potentially expedited methadone weaning.

Fewer studies have examined the occurrence of benzodiazepine withdrawal and optimal weaning strategies (Dominguez et al., 2006; Ducharme et al., 2005; Franck et al., 2004). The findings of these studies suggest that concurrent use of benzodiazepine and opioid weaning requires a longer titration; however, further investigation is needed to determine whether agents should be weaned sequentially or concurrently.

PREVENTION OF WITHDRAWAL

Ideally sedation and analgesic agents should be weaned as soon as deemed possible based on the patient's improving status. According to current evidence, pediatric patients receiving less than a 5-day course of sedation agents can be weaned from these agents fairly rapidly (Anand et al., 2010). By comparison, patients receiving sedation and analgesic agents for 5 days or longer are at risk for withdrawal and require a slower weaning process.

Katz and colleagues (1994) found that opioid withdrawal occurred in 100% of pediatric patients receiving fentanyl for 9 days or longer. In addition, several studies have demonstrated that withdrawal symptoms often occur 8 to 48 hours after discontinuation of opioid agents (Cunliffe et al., 2004; Katz et al., 1994; Robertson et al., 2000; Siddappa et al., 2003).

Few reports exist in the literature describing opioid tapering (Berens et al., 2006; Franck et al., 2004; Meyer & Berens, 2001; Robertson et al., 2000) and benzodiazepine tapering (Ducharme et al., 2004; Ista et al., 2009) as pediatric weaning strategies. Sedation weaning strategies should consider the following factors:

- Single versus multiple drug tolerance
- Equipotent conversion of intravenous to oral medications
- Total infusion days
- Method of assessment
- Treatment of breakthrough withdrawal
- Tapering adjustments for repeated withdrawal symptoms or symptoms consistent with oversedation

Although limited evidence exists to support tapering strategies, many providers advocate for weaning the agent(s) over a time equal to the duration of the infusion. In many cases, however, patients who have received sedation and analgesic agents for more than 2 weeks may require a prolonged weaning process, occurring over several weeks. The importance of frequent assessment and aggressive treatment of withdrawal symptoms using pharmacologic, environmental, and nursing care approaches is critical to promote optimal outcomes.

MEDICATION CONVERSION

Pediatric patients who have received opioids or other sedative agents for 5 or more days typically benefit from switching from IV agents to long-acting oral agents. The most common conversions of IV to oral agents are fentanyl to methadone and midazolam to lorazepam.

He conversion between these medications must take into account differences in these drugs' potency, half-life, and bioavailability. For example, fentanyl is 100 times more potent than methadone; however, the half-life of methadone is 75 to 100 times as long as that of fentanyl. The difference in potency (fentanyl to methadone 100:1) is offset by the difference in half-life (fentanyl to methadone 1:100); therefore, the total daily dose of methadone equals the total daily dose of fentanyl (Table 21-8). Although the bioavailability of oral methadone (75–80%) is less than that of fentanyl, it is generally not necessary to increase the dose to compensate for this difference.

The starting total daily dose of methadone is equivalent to the total daily IV dose of fentanyl (in milligrams). The enteral methadone dose is divided into an every 12-hour dosing regimen. The fentanyl infusion is decreased by 50% after the second dose, decreased by 50% after the third dose, and discontinued after the fourth dose. If symptoms of withdrawal are observed during the weaning process, an intravenous dose of rescue morphine (0.05–0.1 mg/kg) should be administered; in this instance, the total morphine requirement over a 24-hour period is calculated and added to the next day's methadone dose. Once the fentanyl infusion is discontinued, the methadone dose should not be changed for approximately 48 to 72 hours to allow the patient to achieve a steady-state serum concentration. If however, the patient appears excessively sedated, a dose of

TABLE 21-8

Conversion of Intravenous Fentanyl to Enteral Methadone

Conversion Factors

Potency (fentanyl to methadone) 100:1
Half-life (fentanyl to methadone) 1:75–100
Oral bioavailability (methadone) 75–80%

Conversion Factors

- A 10-kg patient is receiving a fentanyl infusion of 5 mcg/kg/hr
- The total daily fentanyl dose is 1.2 mg
- An equivalent enteral methadone total dose is started in divided doses and the fentanyl infusion weaned over 24–48 hours

Conversion Factors

1. The starting dose of methadone is 1.2 mg daily divided every 12 hours
2. After the second dose of methadone, the fentanyl infusion is decreased by 50% (e.g., 2.5 mcg/kg/hr)
3. After the third dose of methadone, the fentanyl infusion is decreased by 50% (e.g., 1.3 mcg/kg/hr)
4. After the fourth dose of methadone, the fentanyl infusion is discontinued

Source: Tobias, J. (2003). Pain management for the critically ill child in the pediatric intensive care unit. In N. Schechter, C. Berde, & M. Yaster (Eds.), *Pain in infants, children, and adolescents* (2nd ed., pp. 807–840). Philadelphia: Lippincott Williams & Wilkins.

methadone may be held and the subsequent dose decreased by 10% to 20%.

Other strategies advocate for a higher starting dose and include giving 2.5 times the total daily fentanyl dose divided every 8 hours (Siddappa et al., 2003). Another regimen calls for 4 times the total daily fentanyl dose divided every 6 hours (Robertson et al., 2000). Tapering begins 24 to 48 hours after conversion.

As with the opioids, longer-acting oral agents are available within the benzodiazepine class, yet limited conversion information is available for these agents. The conversion of midazolam to lorazepam should also account for their differences in potency (1:2–3) and half-life (1:3–6) as well as the decrease in bioavailability (60–70%) with oral administration of lorazepam. Lugo and colleagues (1999) reported a potency ratio of 1:6 when switching from IV midazolam to oral lorazepam; thus, in their calculation conversion, one-sixth of the total daily dose of IV midazolam was given as enteral lorazepam. The starting total daily dose of enteral lorazepam is then divided every 4 to 6 hours; the infusion is decreased by 50% after the second and all subsequent doses of enteral lorazepam until the infusion is discontinued (fourth dose). If symptoms

of withdrawal are observed, an intravenous rescue dose of lorazepam (0.05–0.1 mg/kg) should be administered and the infusion titration slowed.

Reported weaning enteral sedation (methadone and/or lorazepam) strategies vary significantly. In general, medication titration should not be started until steady-state levels of the enteral agents have been achieved (48–72 hours). Research examining methadone weaning strategies in patients exposed to opioids for more than 7 days demonstrated success by weaning patients from these agents over 5 to 10 days and by decreasing the dose by 10% to 20% per day (Berens et al., 2006; Meyer & Berens, 2001; Robertson et al., 2000). Robertson and colleagues (2000) found that patients who had prolonged opioid exposure (more than 14 days) were successfully weaned by decreasing the daily dose of methadone by 10%. Those with fewer than 14 days' exposure were successfully weaned by decreasing the dose by 20% each day. Patients who received prolonged benzodiazepine exposure in addition to opioids were found to require a longer taper if both agents were being weaned concurrently (Ducharme et al., 2005; Franck et al., 2004; Meyer & Berens). Strategies for weaning patients from two-agent regimens include weaning each agent by 10% to 20% every other day or weaning methadone first followed by a lorazepam taper (Durcharme et al.; Franck et al.; Meyer & Berens; Robertson et al.).

Adjunctive therapy to enhance sedation titration and minimize withdrawal has been explored. The agent most commonly used is clonidine, which is administered to prevent opioid and benzodiazepine withdrawal (Arenas-Lopez et al., 2004; Playfor et al., 2006). Clonidine is an alpha$_2$ adrenergic medication that partially mediates its pharmacologic action in a fashion similar to opioids. It is available in an oral form and as a transdermal patch. Starting doses range from 3 to 5 mcg/kg/day (Arenas-Lopez et al.). The transdermal patch is available in 100 mcg and 200 mcg concentrations. The peak effect of the transdermal patch is achieved within 72 hours, and the medication remains potent for a total of 7 days, at which time the patch is replaced. Adverse effects include sedation, bradycardia, and hypotension.

SUMMARY

Weaning pediatric patients from sedation regimens can pose significant challenges to the health care team. The weaning strategies presented here are based on the current evidence and are intended to assist the HCP in the initiation and titration of commonly administered medications. However, the HCP must recognize that due to the diversity of patients and clinical scenarios, designing specific weaning protocols may be difficult. In all cases, an understanding of medication principles and close monitoring of the pediatric patient for observed symptoms of withdrawal are crucial for optimal management.

REFERENCES

1. Agrawal, D., Feldman, H., Krauss, B., & Waltzman, M. (2004). Bispectral Index monitoring quantifies depth of sedation during emergency department procedural sedation and analgesia in children. *Annals of Emergency Medicine, 43*(2), 247–255.

2. Aldrete, J., & Kroulik, D. (1970). A postanesthetic recovery score. *Anesthesia and analgesia, 49*(6), 924–933.

3. Alexander, E., Carnevale, F., & Razack, S. (2002). Evaluation of a sedation protocol for intubated critically ill children. *Intensive and Critical Care Nursing, 18*(5), 292–301.

4. Ambuel, B., Hamlett, K., Marx, C., & Blumer, J. (1992). Assessing distress in pediatric intensive care environments: The COMFORT scale. *Journal of Pediatric Psychology, 17*(1), 95–109.

5. American Academy of Pediatrics (AAP). (2002). Guidelines for monitoring and management of pediatric patients during and after sedation for diagnostic and therapeutic procedures: Addendum. *Pediatrics, 110*(4), 836–838.

6. American Academy of Pediatrics (AAP). (2006). Child life services: Policy statement. *Pediatrics, 118*(4), 1757–1763.

7. American Academy of Pediatrics (AAP), Committee on Drugs. (1998). Neonatal drug withdrawal. *Pediatrics, 101*(6), 1079–1088.

8. American College of Emergency Physicians (ACEP). (2005). Clinical policy: Procedural sedation and analgesia in the emergency department. *Annuals of Emergency Medicine, 45*(4), 177–196.

9. American Society of Anesthesiologists (ASA), Task Force on Management of the Difficult Airway. (2003). *Anesthesiology, 98*(4), 1269–1276.

10. American Society of Anesthesiologists (ASA), Task Force on Sedation and Analgesia by Non-Anesthesiologists. (2002). Practice guidelines for sedation and analgesia by non-anesthesiologists. *Anesthesiology, 96*(2), 1004–1017.

11. Anand, K., Wilson, D., Berger, J., Harrison, R., Meert, K., Zimmerman, J., et al. (2010). Tolerance and withdrawal from prolonged opioid use in critically ill children. *Pediatrics, 125*, e1208–e1225.

12. Aneja, R., Heard, A., Fletcher, J., & Heard, C. (2003). Sedation monitoring of children by the bispectral index in the pediatric intensive care unit. *Pediatric Critical Care Medicine, 4*(1), 60–64.

13. Anghelescu, D., Burgoyne, L., Oakes, L., & Wallace, D. (2005). The safety of patient-controlled analgesia by proxy in pediatric oncology patients. *Anesthesia & Analgesia, 101*(6), 1623–1627.

14. Anghelescu, D., Ross, C., Oakes, L., & Burgoyne, L. (2008). The safety of concurrent administration of opioids via epidural and intravenous routes for postoperative pain in pediatric oncology patients. *Journal of Pain and Symptom Management, 35*(4), 412–419.

15. Arenas-Lopez, S., Riphagen, S., Tibby, S., Durward, A., Tomlin, S., Davies, G., et al. (2004). Use of oral clonidine for sedation in ventilated pediatric intensive care patients. *Intensive Care Medicine, 30*(10), 1625–1629.

16. Arnold, J., Truog, R., Orav, E., Scavone, J., & Hershenson, M. (1990). Tolerance and dependence in neonates sedated with fentanyl during extracorporeal membrane oxygenation. *Anesthesiology, 73*(6), 1136–1140.

17. Berde, C., & Sethna, N. (2002). Analgesics for the treatment of pain in children. *New England Journal of Medicine, 347*(14), 1094–1103.

18. Berens, R., Meyer, M., Mikhailov, T., Colpaert, K., Czarnecki, M., Ghanayem, N., et al. (2006). A prospective evaluation of opioid weaning in opioid-dependent pediatric critical care patients. *Pediatric Anesthesia, 102*(1), 1045–1050.

19. Berkenbosch, J., Fichter, C., & Tobias, J. (2002). The correlation of the bispectral index monitor with clinical sedation scores during mechanical ventilation in the pediatric intensive care unit. *Anesthesia and Analgesia, 94*(3), 506–511.

20. Bieri, D., Reeve, R., Champion, G., Addicoat, L., & Ziegler, J. (1990). The Faces Pain Scale for the self-assessment of the severity of pain experienced by children: Development, initial validation, and preliminary investigation for ratio scale properties. *Pain, 4*(2), 139–150.

21. Birmingham, P., Suresh, S., Ambrosy, A., & Porfyris, S. (2009). Parent-assisted or nurse-assisted epidural analgesia: Is this feasible in pediatric patients? *Paediatric Anaesthesia, 19*(11), 1084–1099.

22. Brislin, R., & Rose, J. (2005). Pediatric acute pain management. *Anesthesiology Clinics of North America, 23*(4), 789–814.

23. Brook, U., Mendelberg, A., Galili, A., Priel, I., & Bujanover, Y. (1999). Effect of a nurse-implemented sedation protocol on the duration of mechanical ventilation. *Patient Education and Counseling, 37*(1), 49–53.

24. Bucknall, T. K., Manias, E., & Presneill, J. J. (2008). A randomized trial of protocol-driven sedation management for mechanical ventilation in an Australian Intensive Care Unit. *Critical Care Medicine, 36*(5), 1444–1450.

25. Burgoyne, L., Smeltzer, M., Pereiras, M., Norris, L., Armendi, A., & De, A. (2007). How well do pediatric anesthesiologists agree when assigning ASA physical status classifications to their patients? *Pediatric Anaesthesia, 17*(10), 956–962.

26. Cohen, S. (2004). Pathophysiology of pain. In C. Warfield & Z. Bajun (Eds.), *Principles and practice of pain medicine* (2nd ed., pp. 35–44). New York: McGraw-Hill.

27. Corso, L. (2008). Train-of-four results and observed muscle movement in children during continuous neuromuscular blockade. *Critical Care Nurse, 28*(3), 30–38.

28. Cote, C., Karl, H., Notterman, D., Weinberg, J., & McCloskey, C. (2000). Adverse sedation events in pediatrics: A critical incident analysis of contributing factors. *Pediatrics, 105*(4), 805–814.

29. Cote, C. J., & Wilson, S. (2006). Guidelines for monitoring and management of pediatric patients during and after sedation for diagnostic and therapeutic procedures: An update. American Academy of Pediatrics, American Academy of Pediatric Dentistry. *Pediatrics, 118*(6), 2587–2602.

30. Cravero, J., Blike, G., Beach, M., Gallagher, S., Hertzog, J., Havidich, J., et al. (2006). Incidence and nature of adverse events during pediatric sedation/anesthesia for procedures outside the operating room: Report from the Pediatric Sedation Research Consortium. *Pediatrics, 118*(3), 1087–1096.

31. Cunliffe, M., McArthur, L., & Dooley, F. (2004). Managing sedation withdrawal in children who undergo prolonged PICU admission after discharge to the ward. *Pediatric Anesthesia, 14*(1), 293–298.

32. Curley, M., Harris, S., Fraser, K., Johnson, R., & Arnold, J. (2006). State Behavioral Scale: A sedation assessment instrument for infants and children supported on mechanical ventilation. *Pediatric Critical Care Medicine, 7*(2), 107–114.

33. Czaja, A., & Zimmerman, J. (2009). The use of dexmedetomidine in critically ill children. *Pediatric Critical Care Medicine, 10*(3), 381–386.

34. Dahan, A., Aarts, L., & Smith, T. (2010). Incidence, reversal, and prevention of opioid-induced respiratory depression. *Anesthesiology, 112*(1), 226–238.

35. Darnell, C., Thompson, J., Stromberg, D., Roy, L., & Sheeran, P. (2008). Effect of low-dose naloxone infusion on fentanyl requirements in critically ill children. *Pediatrics, 121*(5), e1363–e1371.

36. Dominguez, K., Crowley, M., Coleman, D., Katz, R., Wilkins, D., & Kelly, H. (2006). Withdrawal from lorazepam in critically ill children. *Annals of Pharmacotherapy, 40*(6), 1035–1039.

37. Ducharme, C., Carnevale, F., Clermont, M., & Shea, S. (2005). A prospective study of adverse reactions to the weaning of opioids and benzodiazepines among critically ill children. *Intensive & Critical Care Nursing: The Official Journal of the British Association of Critical Care Nurses, 21*(3), 179–186.

38. Finnegan, L., Connaughton, J., Kron, R., & Emich, J. (1975). Neonatal abstinence syndrome: Assessment and management. *Addiction Diseases, 2*(1–2), 141–158.

39. Fitzgerald M., & Howard, R. (2003). The neurobiologic basis of pediatric pain. In N. L. Schechter, C. B. Berde, & M. Yaster (Eds.), *Pain in infants, children and adolescents* (2nd ed., pp. 19–42). Baltimore: Lippincott Williams & Wilkins.

40. Fonsmark, L., Rasmussen, Y., & Carl, P. (1999). Occurrence of withdrawal in critically ill sedated children. *Critical Care Medicine, 27*(1), 196–199.

41. Franck, L., Harris, S., Soentenga, D., Amling, J., & Curley, M. (2008). The Withdrawal Assessment Tool-1 (WAT-1): An assessment instrument for monitoring opioid and benzodiazepine withdrawal symptoms in pediatric patients. *Pediatric Critical Care Medicine, 9*(6), 573–580.

42. Franck, L., Naughton, I., & Winter, I. (2004). Opioid and benzodiazepine withdrawal symptoms in paediatric intensive care patients. *Intensive and Critical Care Nursing, 20*(1), 344–351.

43. Franck, L., Vilardi, J., Durand, D., & Powers, R. (1998). Opioid withdrawal in neonates after continuous infusions of morphine or fentanyl during extracorporeal membrane oxygenation. *American Journal of Critical Care: An Official Publication, American Association of Critical-Care Nurses, 7*(5), 364–369.

44. Froom, S., Malan, C., Mecklenburgh, J., Price, M., Chawathe, M., Hall, J., et al. (2008). Bispectral index asymmetry and COMFORT score in paediatric intensive care patients. *British Journal of Anaesthesia, 100*(5), 690–696.

45. Gauger, V., Voepel-Lewis, T., Burke, C., Kostrzewa, A., Caird, M., Wagner, D., et al. (2009). Epidural analgesia compared with intravenous analgesia after pediatric posterior spinal fusion. *Journal of Pediatric Orthopedics, 29*(6), 588–593.

46. Greco, C. & Berde, C. (2005). Pain management for the hospitalized pediatric patient. *Pediatric Clinics of North America, 52*(4), 995–1027.

47. Gurnaney, H., Brown, A., & Litman, R. S. (2009). Malignant hyperthermia and muscular dystrophies. *Pediatric Anesthesiology, 109*(4), 1043–1048.

48. Hartman, M., McCrory, D., & Schulman, S. (2009). Efficacy of sedation regimens to facilitate mechanical ventilation in the pediatric intensive care unit: A systematic review. *Pediatric Critical Care Medicine, 10*(2), 246–254.

49. Heard, C., & Fletcher, J. (2006). Sedation and analgesia. In B. P. Fuhrman & J. Zimmerman (Eds.), *Pediatric critical care* (3rd ed., pp. 1748–1779). Philadelphia: Mosby.

50. Hertzog, J. H., & Havidich, J. E. (2007). Non-anesthesiologist-provided pediatric procedural sedation: An update. *Current Opinions in Anesthesiology, 20*(4), 365–372.

51. Hicks, C., von Baeyer, C., Spafford, P., van Korlaar, I., & Goodenough, B. (2001). The Faces Pain Scale—Revised: Toward a common metric in pediatric pain measurement. *Pain, 93*(2), 173–183.

52. Hughes, J., Gill, A., Leach, H., Nunn, A., Billingham, I., Ratcliffe, J., et al. (1994). A prospective study of the adverse effects of midazolam on withdrawal in critically ill children. *Acta Paediatrica (Oslo, Norway: 1992), 83*(11), 1194–1199.

53. International Association of the Study of Pain (IASP). (2007). Pain terminology. Retrieved from http://www.iasp-pain.org

54. Itsa, E., vanDijk, M., Tibboel, D., & de Hoog, M. (2005). Assessment of sedation levels in pediatric intensive care patients can be improved by using the comfort "behavior" scale. *Pediatric Critical Care Medicine, 6*(1), 58–63.

55. Ista, E., van Dijk, M., Gamel, C., Tibboel, D., & de Hoog, M. (2007). Withdrawal symptoms in children after long-term administration of sedatives and/or analgesics: A literature review: "Assessment remains troublesome." *Intensive Care Medicine, 33*(1), 1396–1406.

56. Ista, E., van Dijk, M., Gamel, C., Tibboel, D., & de Hoog, M. (2008). Withdrawal symptoms in critically ill children after long-term administration of sedatives and/or analgesics: A first evaluation. *Critical Care Medicine, 36*(8), 2427–2432.

57. Jenkins, I., Playfor, S., Bevan, C., Davies, G., & Wolf, A. (2007). Current United Kingdom sedation practice in pediatric intensive care. *Paediatric Anaesthesia, 17*(7), 675–683.

58. Jimenez, N., Bradford, H., Seidel, K., Sousa, M., & Lynn, A. (2006). A comparison of a needle-free injection system for local anesthesia versus EMLA® for intravenous catheter insertion in the pediatric patient. *Anesthesia and Analgesia, 102*(2), 411–414.

59. Joint Commission on Accreditation of Healthcare Organizations. (2006). *Comprehensive accreditation manual for hospitals (CAMH): The official handbook.* Oakbrook Terrace, IL: Author: PC41–PC43.

60. Kain, Z., Mayes, L., Wang, S., & Hofstadter, M. (1999). Postoperative behavioral outcomes in children: Effects of sedative medications. *Anesthesiology, 90*(37), 758–765.

61. Katz, R., Kelly, H., & Hsi, A. (1994). Prospective study on the occurrence of withdrawal in critically ill children who receive fentanyl by continuous infusion. *Critical Care Medicine, 4*(1), 763–767.

62. Kost-Byerly, S. (2002). New concepts in acute and extended postoperative pain management in children. *Anesthesiology Clinics of North America, 20*(1), 115–135.

63. Krantz, M., Martin, J., Stimmel, B., Mehta, D., & Haigney, M. (2009). QTc interval screening in methadone treatment. *Annals of Internal Medicine, 150*(6), 387–395.

64. Krauss, B., & Green, S. (2006). Procedural sedation and analgesia in children. *Lancet, 367*(4), 766–780.

65. Kress, J. P., Pohlman, A. S., O'Connor, M. F., & Hall J. B. (2000). Daily interruption of sedative infusions in critically ill patients undergoing mechanical ventilation. *New England Journal of Medicine, 342*(20), 1471–1477.

66. Kress, J. P., Gehlbach, B., Lacy, M., Pilskin, N., Pohlman, A. S., & Hall, J. B. (2003). The long term psychological effects of daily sedative interruptions on critically ill patiens. *American Journal of Respiratory Critical Care Medicine, 168*(12), 1457–1561.

67. Langeron, O., Amour, J., Vivien, B., & Aubrun, F. (2006). Clinical review: Management of difficult airways. *Critical Care, 10*(6), 243–248.

68. Lee, A., Fan, L. T., Gin, T., Karmakar, M. K., & Ngan Kee, W. D. (2006). A systematic review (meta-analysis) of the accuracy of the mallampati tests to predict the difficult airway. *Anesthesia and Analgesia, 102*(6), 1867–1878.

69. Lexi-Drug book. (2009). Retrieved from http://www.online.lexi.com

70. Lugo, R. A., Chester, E. A., Cash, J., Grant, M. J., & Vernon, D. D. (1999). A cost analysis of enterally administered lorazepam in the pediatric intensive care unit. *Critical Care Medicine, 27*(2), 417–421.

71. Lugo, R., MacLaren, R., Cash, J., Pribble, C., & Vernon, D. (2001). Enteral methadone to expedite fentanyl discontinuation and prevent opioid abstinence syndrome in the PICU. *Pharmacotherapy, 21*(12), 1566–1573.

72. Mace, S., Brown, L., Francis, L., Godwin, S., Han, S., Howard, P., et al. (2008). Clinical policy: Critical issues in the sedation of pediatric patients in the emergency department. *Journal of Emergency Nursing, 34*(3), e33–e107.

73. Mallampati, S., Gatt, S., Gugino, L., Desai, S., Waraksa, B., Freiberger, D., et al. (1985). A clinical sign to predict difficult tracheal intubation: A prospective study. *Canadian Journal of Anaesthesia, 32*(4), 429–434.

74. Malviya, S., Voepel-Lewis, T., Burke, C., Merkel, S., & Tait, A. (2005). The revised FLACC observational pain tool: Improved reliability and validity for pain assessment in children with cognitive impairment. *Pediatric Anesthesia, 16*(3), 258–265.

75. Malviya, S., Voepel-Lewis, T., Tait, A., Watcha, M., Sadhasivam, S., & Friesen, R. (2007). Effect of age and sedative agent on the accuracy of bispectral index in detecting depth of sedation in children. *Pediatrics, 120*(3), e461–470.

76. Martin, L., Bratton, S., & O'Rourke, P. (1999). Clinical uses and controversies of neuromuscular blocking agents in infants and children. *Critical Care Medicine, 27*(7), 1358–1368.

77. Marx, C., Rosenberg, D., Ambuel, B., Hamlet, K., & Blumer, J. (1993). Pediatric intensive care sedation: Survey of fellowship training programs. *Pediatrics, 91*(1), 369–378.

78. Mashour, G., & Sandberg, W. (2006). Craniocervical extension improves the specificity and predictive value of the Mallampati airway evaluation. *International Anesthesia Research Society, 103*(5), 1256–1259.

79. Mason, K. P., Michna, W., Zurakowski, D., Burrows, P., Pirich, M., Carrier M., et al. (2006). Value of bispectral index monitor in differentiating between moderate and deep Ramsay Sedation Scores in children. *Pediatric Anesthesia, 16*(12), 1226–1231.

80. Maxwell, L., Kaufmann, S., Bitzer, S., Jackson E., McGready, J., Kost-Byerly, S., et al. (2005). The effects of a small-dose naloxone infusion on opioid-induced side effects and analgesia in children and adolescents treated with intravenous patient-controlled analgesia: A double-blind, prospective, randomized controlled study. *Anesthesia and Analgesia, 100*(4), 953–958.

81. Melzer-Lange, M., Walsh-Kelly, C., Lea, G., Hillery, C., & Scott, J. (2004). Patient-controlled analgesia for sickle cell pain crisis in a pediatric emergency department. *Pediatric Emergency Care, 20*(1), 2–4.

82. Merkel, S., Voepel-Lewis, T., Shayevitz, J., & Malviya, S. (1997). The FLACC: A behavioral scale for scoring postoperative pain in young children. *Pediatric Nursing, 23*(3), 293–297.

83. Meyer, M., & Berens, R. (2001). Efficacy of an enteral 10-day methadone wean to prevent opioid withdrawal in fentanyl-tolerant pediatric intensive care unit patients. *Pediatric Critical Care Medicine, 2*(4), 329–333.

84. Meyer, S., Grundmann, U., Gottschling, S., Kleinschmidt, S., & Gortner, L. (2007). Sedation and analgesia for brief diagnostic and therapeutic procedures in children. *European Journal of Pediatrics, 166*(10), 291–302.

85. Miro, J., Castarlenas, E., & Huguet, A. (2009). Evidence for the use of a numerical rating scale to assess the intensity of pediatric pain. *European Journal of Pain, 13*(10), 1089–1095.

86. Monitto, C., Greenberg, R., & Kost-Byerly, S. (2000). The safety and efficacy of parent-/nurse-controlled analgesia in patients less than six years of age. *Anesthesia Analgesia, 91*(3), 573–579.

87. Murray, M. J., Cowen, J., DeBlock, H., Erstad, B., Gray, A. W. Jr., Tescher, A. N., et al. (2002). Clinical practice guidelines for sustained neuromuscular in the adult critically ill patient. Task Force of American College of Critical Care Medicine (ACCM) of the Society of Critical Care Medicine (SCCM), American Society of Health-System Pharmacists, American College of Chest Physicians. *Critical Care Medicine, 30*(1), 142–156.

88. Newman, D., Azer, M., Pitetti, R., & Singh, S. (2003). When is a patient safe for discharge after procedural sedation? The timing of adverse events in 1367 pediatric procedural sedations. *Annuals of Emergency Medicine, 42*(5), 627–635.

89. Nilsson, S., Finnstrom, B., & Kokinsky, E. (2008). The FLACC behavioral scale for procedural pain assessment in children aged 5–16 years. *Pediatric Anesthesia, 18*(8), 767–774.

90. Osborn, D., Jeffery, H., & Cole, M. (2005a). Opiate treatment for opiate withdrawal in newborn infants. *Cochrane Database Systematic Review, 20*(3), CD002059.

91. Osborn, D., Jeffery, H., & Cole, M. (2005b). Sedatives for opiate withdrawal in newborn infants. *Cochrane Database Systematic Review, 20*(3), CD002053.

92. Parke, T., Rice, A., Greenaway, C., Bray, R., Smith, P., Waldmann, C. S., et al. (1992). Metabolic acidosis and fatal myocardial failure after propofol infusion in children: Five case reports. *British Medical Journal, 305*(6854), 613–616.

93. Parran, L., & Pederson, C. (2002). Effects of an opioid taper algorithm in hematopoietic progenitor cell transplant recipients. *Oncology Nursing Forum, 29*(1), 41–50.

94. Patzer, L. (2008). Nephrotoxicity as a cause of acute kidney injury in children. *Pediatric Nephrology, 23*(12), 2159–2173.

95. Pena, O., Prestjohn, S., & Guzzetta, C. (2000). Agreement between muscle movement and peripheral nerve stimulation in critically ill pediatric patients receiving neuromuscular blocking agents. *Heart & Lung, 29*(5), 309–318.

96. Perry, H., & Shannon, M. (1996). Diagnosis and management of opioid- and benzodiazepine-induced comatose overdose in children. *Current Opinion in Pediatrics, 8*(3), 243–247.

97. Peters, J., Bandell Hoekstra, I., Huijer Abu-Saad, H., Bouwmeester, J., Meursing, A., & Tibboel, D. (1999). Patient controlled analgesia in children and adolescents: A randomized controlled trial. *Pediatric Anaesthesia, 9*(3), 235–241.

98. Pillitteri, L., & Clark, R. (1998). Comparison of a patient-controlled analgesia system with continuous infusion for administration of diamorphine for mucositis. *Transplantation, 22*(5), 495–498.

99. Playfor, S., Jenkins, I., Boyles, C., Choonara, I., Davies, G., Haywood, T., et al. (2007). Consensus guidelines on sedation and analgesia in critically ill children. *Intensive Care Medicine, 32*(8), 1125–1136.

100. Powers, K., Nazarian, E., Tapyrik, S., Kohli, S., Yin, H., van der Jagt, E., et al. (2005). Bispectral index as a guide for titration of propofol during procedural sedation among children. *Pediatrics, 115*(6), 1666–1674.

101. Quenot, J., Ladoire, S., Devoucoux, F., Doise, J., Cailliod, R., Cunin, N., et al. (2007). Effect of a nurse-implemented sedation protocol on the incidence of ventilator-associated pneumonia. *Critical Care Medicine, 35*(9), 2031–2036.

102. Ramsay, M., Savage, T., Simpson, B., & Goodwin, R. (1974). Controlled sedation with alphaxalone-alphadolone. *British Medical Journal, 2*(5920), 656–659.

103. Rennick, J., Morin, I., Kim, D., Johnston, C., Dougherty, G., & Platt, R. (2004). Identifying children at high risk for psychological sequelae after pediatric intensive care unit hospitalization. *Pediatric Critical Care Medicine, 5*(4), 358–363.

104. Rennick, J., & Rashotte, J. (2009). Psychological outcomes in children following pediatric intensive care unit hospitalization: A systematic review of the research. *Journal of Child Health Care, 13*(2), 128–149.

105. Robertson, R., Darsey, E., Fortenberry, J., Pettignano, R., & Hartley, G. (2000). Evaluation of an opiate-weaning protocol using methadone in pediatric intensive care unit patients. *Pediatric Critical Care Medicine, 1*(2), 119–123.

106. Rose, J., & Logan, D. (2004). Pediatric pain assessment. In: R. S. Litman (Ed.), *Pediatric anesthesia: The requisites in anesthesiology* (pp. 191–195). Philadelphia: Mosby.

107. Saudan, S., Habre, W., Ceroni, D., Meyer, P., Greeberg, R., Kaelin, A., et al. (2007). Safety and efficacy of patient controlled epidural analgesia following pediatric spinal surgery. *Pediatric Anesthesia, 18*(2), 132–139.

108. Schweickert, W., Gehlbach, B., Pohlman, A., Hall, J., & Kress, J. (2004). Daily interruption of sedative infusions and complications of critical illness in mechanically ventilated patients. *Critical Care Medicine, 32*(6), 1272–1276.

109. Sessler, C., Grap, M., & Ramsay, M. (2008). Evaluating and monitoring analgesia and sedation in the intensive care unit. *Critical Care, 12*(suppl 3), S2.

110. Shannon, M., Albers, G., Burkhart, K., Liebelt, E., Kelley, M., McCubbin, M., et al. (1997). Safety and efficacy of flumazenil in the reversal of benzodiazepine-induced conscious sedation. *Journal of Pediatrics, 131*(4), 582–586.

111. Shapiro, B., Warren, J., Egol, A., Geenbaum, D., Jacobi, J., Nasraway, S., et al. (1995). Practice parameters for sustained neuromuscular blockade in the adult critically ill patient: An executive summary. *Critical Care Medicine, 23*(9), 1601–1605.

112. Shin, D., Kim, S., Kim, C., & Kim, H. (2001). Postoperative pain management using intravenous patient-controlled analgesia for pediatric patients. *Journal of Craniofacial Surgery, 12*(2), 129–133.

113. Siddappa, R., Fletcher, J., Heard, A., Kielma, D., Cimino, M., & Heard C. (2003). Methadone dosage for prevention of opioid withdrawal in children. *Pediatric Anesthesia, 13*(1), 805–810.

114. Soliman, I., Patel R., Ehrenpreis, M., & Hannallah, R. (1988). Recovery scores do not correlate with postoperative hypoxemia in children. *Anesthesia and Analgesia, 67*(1), 53–56.

115. Spanos, S., Booth, R., Koenig, H., Sikes, K., Graceley, E., & Kim, I. (2008). Jet injection of 1% buffered lidocaine versus topical

ELA-Max for anesthesia before peripheral intravenous catheterization in children: A randomized controlled trial. *Pediatric Emergency Care, 24*(8), 511–515.

116. Stanford, E., Chambers, C., & Craig, K. (2006). The role of developmental factors in predicting young children's use of a self-report scale for pain. *Pain, 120*(1–2), 16–23.

117. Suresh, S., & Anand, K. (1998). Opioid tolerance in neonates: Mechanisms, diagnosis, assessment, and management. *Seminars in Perinatology, 22*(5), 425–433.

118. Taketomo, C., Hodding, J., & Kraus, D. (2010). *Pediatric dosage handbook*. Hudson, OH: Lexi-Comp.

119. Tobias, J. (1995). Lorazepam versus midazolam for sedation. *Critical Care Medicine, 23*(6), 1151.

120. Tobias, J. (2000). Tolerance, withdrawal, and physical dependency after long-term sedation and analgesia of children in the pediatric intensive care unit. *Critical Care Medicine, 28*(6), 2122–2132.

121. Tobias, J. D. (2002). Therapeutic application of regional anaesthesia in paediatric-aged patients. *Paediatric Anaesthesia, 12*(3), 272–277.

122. Tobias J. D. & Berkenbosch, J. W. (2003). Developemnt of bradycardia during sedation with dexmedetomidine in infant concurrently receiving digoxin. *Pedaitric Critical Care Medicine, 4*(2), 203–205.

123. Tobias, J. (2004). A review of intrathecal and epidural analgesia after spinal surgery in children. *Anesthesia & Analgesia, 98*(2), 956–965.

124. Tobias, J., & Berkenbosch, J. (2004). Sedation during mechanical ventilation in infants and children: Dexmedetomidine versus midazolam. *South Medicine Journal, 97*(5), 451–455.

125. Tobias, J., & Grindstaff, R. (2005). Bispectral index monitoring during the administration of neuromuscular blocking agents in the pediatric intensive care unit. *Journal of Intensive Care Medicine, 20*(4), 233–237.

126. Tofil, N., Benner, K., Faro, S., & Winkler, M. (2006). The use of enteral naloxone to treat opioid-induced constipation in a pediatric intensive care unit. *Pediatric Critical Care Medicine, 7*(3), 252–254.

127. Triltsch, A., Nestmann, G., Orawa, H., Moshirzadeh, M., Sander, S., GroBe, J., et al. (2005). Bispectral index versus COMFORT score to determine the level of sedation in paediatric intensive care unit patients: A prospective study. *Critical Care, 9*(1), R9–R17.

128. Trope, R., Silver, R., & Sagy, M. (2005). Concomitant assessment of depth of sedation by changes in bispectral index and changes in autonomic variables (heart rate and/or BP) in pediatric critically ill patients receiving neuromuscular blockade. *Chest, 128*(1), 303–307.

129. Twite, M., Zuk, J., Gralla, J., & Friesen, R. (2005). Correlation of the bispectral index monitor with the COMFORT scale in the pediatric intensive care unit. *Pediatric Critical Care Medicine, 6*(6), 648–653.

130. Voepel-Lewis, T., Malviya, S., Tait, A., Merkel, S., Foster, R., & Krane, E. (2008). A comparison of the clinical utility of pain assessment tools for children with cognitive impairment. *Pediatric Anesthesiology, 106*(1), 72–78.

131. Von Baeyer, C.L., Spagrud, L.J., McCormick, J.C., Choo, E., Neville, K, Connolly, M. A. (2009). Three new datasets supporting use of the numerical rating scale (NRS-II) for children's self-reports of pain intensity. *Pain, 143*(3), 223–227.

132. Ward-Begnoche, W. (2007). Posttraumatic stress symptoms in the pediatric intensive care unit. *Journal of Specialty Pediatrics, 12*(2), 84–92.

133. Weisman, S. L., Bernstein, B., & Schechter, N. (1998). Consequences of inadequate analgesia during painful procedures in children. *Archives in Pediatric Adolescent Medicine, 152*(2), 147–149.

134. Willis, M. H., Mekel, S. I, Voepel-Lewis, T. & Malviya, S. (2003). FLACC Behavioral Pain Assessment Scale: A comparison with the child's self report. *Pediatric Nursing, 29*(3), 195–198.

135. Wong, D., & Baker, C. (1988). Pain in children: Comparison of assessment scales. *Pediatric Nursing, 149*(1), 9–17.

136. Wrona, S., Chisolm, D., Powers, M., & Miler, V. (2007). Improving processes of care in patient-controlled analgesia: The impact of computerized order sets and acute pain service patient management. *Pediatric Anesthesia, 17*(11), 1083–1089.

137. Yaster, M., Kost-Byerly, S., Berde, C., & Billet, C. (1996). The management of opioid and benzodiazepine dependence in infants, children, and adolescents. *Pediatrics, 98*(1), 135–140.

Cardiac Disorders

- Physiology and Diagnostics
- Advanced Life Support Education
- Arrhythmias and Pacemakers
- Cardiac Transplantation
- Cardiomyopathy
- Cardiogenic Shock
- Cardiovascular Agents
- Carditis
- Chylothorax
- Congenital Heart Lesions
- Congestive Heart Failure
- Extracorporeal Life Support
- Postpericardiotomy Syndrome
- Pulmonary Hypertension
- Rheumatic Fever
- Syncope
- References

PHYSIOLOGY AND DIAGNOSTICS

Brian D. Hanna

PHYSIOLOGY

Normal and pathologic cardiovascular function in pediatrics is continually colored by the developmental changes associated with growth from birth to adulthood. In the first years of life, the human myocardium increases both the number and size of myocytes and changes the collagen in the interstitum from stiff type 1 to the more compliant type 2. In addition, the neonate's myocytes do not have a developed t-tubular system to handle intracellular calcium for excitation–contraction coupling; thus the neonatal heart is more heavily dependent on extracellular calcium than the adult heart. In these ways, the infant myocardium resembles a failing adult heart, where function has been degraded by loss of myocytes, degradation of intracellular signaling pathways and calcium handling, and activation of fetal genes leading to myofibrosis with collagen type 1.

Cardiac function

Mammalian cardiac function is defined by the concepts of preload, afterload, contractility, automaticity, and rhythmicity (Lakatta & Maughan, 1990).

Preload, afterload, and contractility. Figure 22-1 and Table 22-1 describe the relationships between preload, afterload, and contractility. In classical experiments, *preload* was defined in terms of the stretch of the sarcomere before contraction. In clinical practice, it is defined as the intramyocardial pressure at end diastole and is approximated by the ventricular end-diastolic pressure.

The absolute definition of ventricular *afterload* has evaded clinicians for decades. It is understood that afterload must be defined in terms of the intramyocardial tension at the beginning of ejection (in keeping with the *Laplace* equation, tension is a function of the ventricular internal pressure and the wall radius and thickness) and the arterial input impedance (a characterization of the properties of blood and the vascular tree that limit forward motion of blood; calculated by *Fourier analysis* of the instantaneous pressure-flow relationship). Clinically, it is common practice to designate the early systolic arterial pressure as the ventricular afterload.

Contractility can be defined as the pressure/volume ratio at end systole. A boundary line exists that defines the lower limit of ventricular volume where the sarcomere cannot shorten further (Figure 22-1). This line identifies the inotropic state of the ventricle; the instantaneous slope is contractility. Heart failure and infancy move this line downward and to the right, signaling lower contractility; inotropic agents move it upward and to the left, signaling higher contractility.

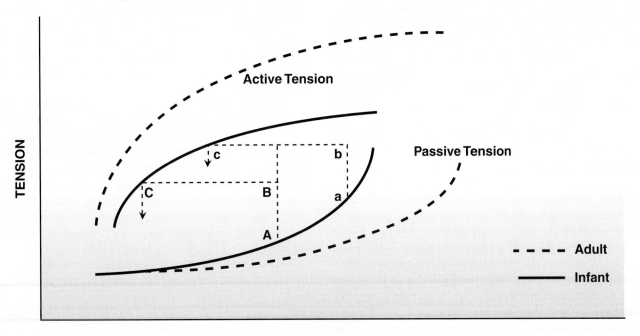

FIGURE 22-1

The Effects of Load on Stroke Volume at Different Ages. The graphic representation of the Frank-Starling relationship of tension versus length applies to all mammalian muscle. Applying this relationship to the clinical setting, although approximated, tension corresponds to ventricular pressure and length to the ventricular diameter. The infant heart has more passive tension (stiffer) and lower active tension (less contractility) when compared to the adult. Consequently, in the infant, passive tension increases more for an increase in length, but active tension increases less with increasing length.

TABLE 22-1

Descriptions of Preload, Stroke Volume, Afterload, and Contractility

Preload: The tension at the time that the ventricle starts to contract. The increase in preload for an infant is seen as the difference between point *A* and point *a*.

Stroke volume: In this representation, the length of either line *B-C* or line *b-c*.

Afterload: The afterload seen by the ventricle is the tension seen at either point *B* or *x*. Graphically it is easy to see that dropping the afterload from *x* to *B* dramatically increases the stroke volume. Although it is possible to increase the stroke volume by increasing preload, the symptoms of heart failure are more obvious with high preload rather than lower afterload.

Contractility: In this figure, the instantaneous slope of the active tension curve at the end of systole (points *C* and *c*). In clinical medicine, it is difficult to move either the infant heart or the heart experiencing chronic heart failure back toward the adult active tension curve because there are few myocytes and less effective calcium handling.

There is an important interdependence between right and left ventricle function. The intraventricular septum is normally a left ventricular structure. When the preload and afterload conditions are normal for both ventricles, right ventricular ejection is highly dependent on septal contraction. In patients with high right ventricular preload (as in large atrial-level left-to-right shunts) or high right ventricular afterload (as in a nonrestrictive ventricular septal defect, right ventricular outflow obstruction, or severe pulmonary hypertension), or in patients with abnormal ventricular sizes (as seen in some congenital heart diseases), the septal position and contraction are abnormal, with degradation being noted in biventricular diastolic and systolic function.

Cardiac rate (automaticity, overdrive suppression, and impulse conduction).   *Automaticity* is a property of all myocardial cells; however, the ionic mechanisms are different for the Purkinji fibers, atrial cells, and ventricular cells compared to the pacemaker cells of the sinoatrial and atrioventricular nodes. Nonpacemaker cells respond to a change in the resting membrane potential with a rapid increase in intracellular sodium and, therefore, membrane potential. This fast response does not exist in pacemaker cells, where the action potential results from changes in the relatively slow-acting calcium and sodium channels.

The *rhythmicity* (regularity) of pacemaker activity is the result of slow depolarization of the action potential during phase 4 (the resting membrane potential). In nonpacemaker cells, it appears to follow from a slow reduction in the outward potassium current; by comparison, in pacemaker cells,

a steady inward calcium current is involved. Cardiac rate is determined by the cell with the fastest intrinsic rate, usually the sinoatrial nodal cell; all slower cells have their rates suppressed, known as *overdrive suppression.*

Impulse conduction is an important characteristic that determines cardiac rate and rhythm. The atrioventricular grove does not conduct impulses; only the atrioventricular node conducts atrial impulses to the ventricle. In addition, Purkinji cells have a faster conduction velocity than the surrounding myocardium, determining the timing of ventricular activation: intraventricular septum and papillary muscles first, then the apical and central endocardium, and finally the ventricular base.

Neural and hormonal control of the heart

First principles in the control of the heart dictate the presence and maturity of the receptor and intracellular signaling, the afferent (sensing) and efferent (effector) neuronal connections, and the central neuronal processing. This is true for both normal physiologic reflexes and the response to pharmacologic agents (e.g., inotropic drugs).

The autonomic nervous system, which consists of both the vagal and sympathetic neuronal systems, is responsible for reflex neuronal control of the heart. In general, the sinoatrial and atrioventricular nodes are innervated by postganglionic fibers. This results in the vagus system slowing the heart rate and conduction and depressing ventricular contractility, and the sympathetic system increasing this rate and conduction and enhancing ventricular contractility. Considerable interplay between the vagal and sympathetic systems occurs both at the ganglia on the heart and at the level of the myocytes.

Central nervous system (CNS)–mediated reflexes rely on afferent information on atrial volume (*Bainbridge reflex*), arterial blood pressure (*baroreceptor reflex*), and blood or cerebrospinal fluid (CSF) levels of carbon dioxide, pH, or oxygen (*chemoreceptor reflexes*). These reflexes control cardiac rate and contractility, resulting in homeostasis of the aforementioned parameters. The afferent information for the peripheral reflexes travels in the vagi, where both efferent vagal and sympathetic nerves are involved in the ensuing effects.

Humeral control over the heart is predominantly exerted by adrenal gland secretion of adrenaline and noradrenaline, both of which increase cardiac rate and contractility. In addition, adrenocortical steroid hormones, thyroid hormones, and glucagon are potent inotropic agents. The importance of recognizing these other hormonal inotropic agents becomes clear when treatment of heart failure is attempted.

Cardiorespiratory interactions

Respiratory-induced alterations in heart rate are neuronally stimulated; respiratory rate and volume information is determined by the firing pattern of both the vagus nerves and the sympathetic innervation of the heart. In addition, the change in preload and afterload caused by the inspiration–expiration cycle affects both cardiac rate and stroke volume, with a concomitant cyclical change being observed in the arterial blood pressure.

Pathophysiologic changes in this interaction may be seen in several clinical situations (Healy et al., 2010). Profound alteration in lung function caused by left ventricular failure and high left atrial pressures, and right ventricular failure caused by pathologic pulmonary vascular hypertension, are extreme examples.

Vascular physiology

Fluid dynamics and lymphatic flow. The important concepts that determine flow through the capillary bed include the control of the number of open capillaries and the transmural pressure, oncotic pressure, and permeability of the capillary membrane.

The control of the number of open capillaries is tissue specific. Metabolically active tissues, such as those found in the myocardium, have both a higher capillary density and more capillaries open at any one time compared to, for example, adipose tissue. The control of capillary flow occurs at the precapillary sphincter, which is under the control of the local transmural pressure, the autonomic nervous system, hormonal influences, and local metabolic mediators. Physiologic states that have high cardiac output, such as those that occur with epinephrine therapy, do not necessarily have high capillary flow rates in all tissues, as all tissues have arteriovenous connections that can shunt blood past the capillary bed when the metabolic needs are reduced.

Adequate flow across capillary membranes into the tissues is necessary to meet the metabolic demands of the body's tissues. This flow occurs as a balance of the hydrostatic (blood pressure) and oncotic (protein concentration) pressures between the capillary and the tissue. The *capillary hydrostatic pressure* is the difference between the pressures at the arterial and venous ends, estimated at 32 and 15 mmHg, respectively, for most tissues. The *tissue hydrostatic pressure* is usually zero. The oncotic pressure averages 25 mmHg in the capillary and less than 5 mmHg in the tissue. Because each tissue has a different permeability of the capillary membrane to proteins, the tissue oncotic pressure in highly permeable tissues (e.g., in the liver) increases toward the venous end of a capillary.

Hydrostatic forces push fluid out into the tissue and oncotic forces pull it back; thus more fluid is filtered at the arterial end than is reabsorbed at the venous end. The result is lymphatic flow. The volume of this flow, in a 24-hour period, approximates the total body plasma volume. It contains between one-fourth and one-half of the body's total plasma protein. Lymphatic flow, therefore, is increased when plasma proteins are low, capillary permeability is high, or hydrostatic pressure across the capillary increases. Edema states occur when the total lymphatic flow exceeds the capability of the lymphatic system, when lymphatic obstructions are present, or when central venous pressures are high (because the thoracic duct must drain back into the supracardiac venous system).

Vascular resistance, capacitance, and capacity. The concepts of vascular resistance, capacitance, and capacity are central to most of clinical cardiology. Unfortunately, the formulas that we use are based on assumptions not met in the body, which is a pulsatile, nonlaminar system with distensible tubes that is filled with blood, a non-Newtonian fluid with varying viscosity. However, despite these limitations, day-to-day clinical care is based on these formulas.

Poiseuille's law states the relationship of flow ($\mathbf{Q}$) and pressure ($\mathbf{P}$) to resistance ($\mathbf{R}$):

$$\mathbf{Q} = \frac{\pi(\mathbf{P}_{in} - \mathbf{P}_{out})\mathbf{r}^4}{8\eta l}, \ \mathbf{r} = \text{radius}; \ \eta = \text{viscosity}; \ \mathbf{l} = \text{length};$$
$$\text{and } \pi/\mathbf{8} = \text{a constant}$$

or

$$\mathbf{R} = (\mathbf{P}_{in} - \mathbf{P}_{out})/\mathbf{Q} = 8\eta l/\pi \mathbf{r}^4$$

Therefore, if Poiseuille's law is applicable, the *resistance* to flow is determined only by the radius and length of the vessel and the viscosity of the blood. In tissue, the radius, length, and blood viscosity vary throughout the vascular bed; the major resistance factor is the precapillary arterioles. The arterioles are able to constrict and relax to a great degree (because R is proportional to r^4); thus the major changes in resistance to meet physiologic needs occur at this level.

Capacitance is the term used to describe the dispensability of blood vessels. When the left ventricle ejects its full stroke volume into the ascending aorta, the blood does not rush down the vascular tree, but rather first distends the ascending aorta and then is transferred more distally over the rest of the cardiac cycle. Without the capacitance of the ascending aorta, the heart would need to eject blood directly against the total distal resistance, increasing both the systolic blood pressure and the afterload on the ventricle. This phenomenon is observed, for example, in patients who have had late repairs of coarctation of the aorta or who have had conduits placed between the right ventricle and the pulmonary branches.

Capacity comprises the ability of the distal vascular bed to accept flow. This concept is probably most relevant to the pulmonary circuit, where the vascular bed is the only one in the body that must take the full cardiac stroke volume with every beat. Cardiac output can be as much as six times higher than the average rate in trained athletes; thus the vascular bed must have sufficient capacity to increase the available capillaries to accommodate the flow. In the lung, this flexibility is accomplished through a system of supranumary blood vessels; in the systemic circuit, it is accomplished through the vascular bed of the skin and abdominal organs. This vast ability for over-capacity in the pulmonary circuit means that over a wide range of blood flows, the pressure does not increase; therefore, the resistance decreases with increased flow—clearly not following Poiseuille's law. Pathologic loss of this capacity, as in the disease of pulmonary hypertension, results in increased pressure and right ventricular afterload with increased blood flow.

Neural and hormonal control of the vasculature. Neural control of blood pressure, flow, and vascular capacitance involve complex CNS-mediated reflexes similar to the reflexes that control cardiac function. These reflexes respond to perturbations of daily living from postural changes to exercise and from anxiety owing to the fight-or-flight response. However, all of this CNS activity flows through the autonomic nervous system, its neurotransmitters, and receptors. Development, disease, and trauma can alter this fine balance, leading to pathologic changes in regional blood pressure, flow, and capacitance.

All vessels except true capillaries are innervated to some extent by postganglionic sympathetic neurons that release noradrenaline, resulting in vasoconstriction. In addition, a basal activity occurs in vasoconstrictor sympathetic nerves such that the affected vessels are somewhat constricted at rest. Vasoconstriction of arterioles and precapillary arteriolar sphincters will decrease capillary flow, increase the vascular resistance of that bed, and shunt blood away from that organ. At the same time, vasoconstriction of postcapillary venules is associated with a decrease in vascular capacitance and, if widespread, will increase venous return to the heart, effectively increasing preload.

Neurally mediated vasodilation occurs either by a decrease in the resting sympathetic vasoconstrictor activity or by activation of β_2-adrenergic receptors that are present in some tissues. In addition, the parasympathetic vagal system selectively innervates specialized tissues. When this system is activated, it produces vasoconstriction (e.g., in coronary, respiratory epithelial, and salivary gland vessels).

Humeral control of vascular resistance, flow, and capacitance is intimately tied to both local metabolic mediators and the neural control systems. Co-release of the neuropeptide Y from sympathetic nerves increases vasoconstriction and modulates release of vasoactive hormones, whereas co-release of kallikrein from vagal nerves is a potent vasodilator agent. Reflex control of the autonomic nervous system also affects release of humeral agents in well-described responses to behavior, blood loss, or changes in metabolic demands. Notably, humeral responses tend to be more global and less involved in regional vascular responses.

Several vasoactive molecules are locally released and have limited activity past their immediate environment. Endothelin (a potent vasoconstrictor) and prostacyclin (a potent vasodilator) are examples of substances whose release into the local environment causes release and profound changes in local blood flow. In addition, thyroid, parathyroid, adrenal, and sex hormones are involved in modulating reflex control of electrolyte and water handling, vascular resistance, and capacitance; thus the release of these substances affects overall (systemic) blood pressure.

Specific reflex mechanisms that involve humeral modulation of vascular tone include the vasoconstrictor effects on the renin–angiotensin system and the arginine vasopressin hypothalamic osmoreceptor system; the natriuretic, vasodilation effects produced by atrial natriuretic peptide; and the ventricle-derived, brain-type natriuretic peptide.

DIAGNOSTICS

History

A past history of prolonged neonatal hospitalization, poor growth, injury associated with syncopy, shortness of breath, chest pain at rest, and/or poor school performance are nonspecific and important considerations when pediatric cardiac conditions are suspected. Therefore, the health care professional (HCP) should obtain a detailed, comprehensive health history and review of systems that will identify key signs that the patient or family may not necessarily equate with the heart or a heart problem.

Physical examination

Inspection, cardiac auscultation, and palpation are crucial components in the pediatric cardiac examination; resulting in a wealth of diagnostic information (Table 22-2). A comprehensive cardiac examination requires that patients be fully disrobed and the entire body examined. Additional pearls are summarized here:

- The right ventricular impulse is under the xiphoid sternum 99% of the time. If it is more prominent than the left apical impulse after 12 hours of age, this finding is considered abnormal and requires evaluation.
- At fast heart rates, it is difficult to tell which is the A_2 sound and which is the P_2 sound; A_2 is always loudest at the lower left sternal border.
- All high-frequency murmurs at the apex occur in systole.
- Coarctation of the aorta may be missed in infancy when an HCP misidentifies the femoral pulse while an infant is crying. If there are pedal pulses, then there are femoral pulses.

Electrocardiograph

An electrocardiograph (ECG/EKG) may be the most often performed cardiac test in any patient's life, yet its sensitivity and specificity for congenital and acquired heart disease, outside of arrhythmia detection, is suspect. Some very rational cardiologists advocate that all neonates have an ECG prior to discharge from the hospital and believe that this screening will decrease the risk of sudden death associated with structural heart disease and fatal arrhythmias, as in congenital long QT syndromes. Unfortunately, because a long QT interval is frequently normal in neonates, this may not be the right test at the right time. Preathletic screening with an ECG is also recommended and has better characteristics as a screening test than the same test performed in infancy.

ECG findings vary with age (Table 22-3), such that what is considered grossly abnormal in an adult is quite normal in a child—for example, a prominent R wave in lead V_1. Voltage versus lead and age data have been validated and are widely available (Davignon, 1980). Recognition of abnormal ECG patterns should be the goal for new HCPs. For instance, a qR pattern in lead V_1 denotes right ventricular hypertrophy (RVH) (Table 22-4), but when it is absent in lead V_6 it is highly associated with hypoplastic left heart syndrome.

Radiograph

The sensitivity and specificity of chest radiographs (CXR) as screening tests are not high; however, when interpreted by a pediatric radiologist with cardiovascular training,

TABLE 22-2

Age-Based Estimates for Vital Signs and Weight (Blood Pressure Mean ± 2 Standard Deviations)					
Age	Weight (kg)	Heart Rate	Respiratory Rate	Systolic BP	Diastolic BP
Premature	1	145/min	~40	42 ± 10	21 ± 8
Premature	1–2	135	~40	50 ± 10	28 ± 8
Newborn	2–3	125	~40	60 ± 10	37 ± 8
1 month	4	120	24–35	80 ± 16	46 ± 16
6 month	7	130	24–35	89 ± 29	60 ± 10
1 year	10	120	20–30	96 ± 30	66 ± 25
2–3 years	12–14	115	20–30	99 ± 25	64 ± 25
4–5 years	16–18	100	20–30	99 ± 20	65 ± 20
6–8 years	20–26	100	12–25	100 ± 15	60 ± 10
10–12 yr	32–42	75	12–25	110 ± 17	60 ± 10
>14 yr	>50	70	12–18	118 ± 20	60 ± 10

Source: Rothrock, S. (2007). *Tarascon pediatric emergency pocketbook* (5th ed.). Loma Linda, CA: Tarascon Publishing.

TABLE 22-3

Normal Electrocardiograph Values				
Age	P–R Interval[a]	QRS Interval[a]	QRS Axis (mean)	QTc[b]
0–7 days	0.08–0.12	0.04–0.08	80–160 (125)	0.34–0.54
1–4 weeks	0.08–0.12	0.04–0.07	60–160 (110)	0.30–0.50
1–3 months	0.08–0.12	0.04–0.08	40–120 (80)	0.32–0.47
3–6 months	0.08–0.12	0.04–0.08	20–80 (65)	0.35–0.46
6–12 months	0.09–0.13	0.04–0.08	0–100 (65)	0.31–0.49
1–3 years	0.10–0.14	0.04–0.08	20–100 (55)	0.34–0.49
3–8 years	0.11–0.16	0.05–0.09	40–80 (60)	< 0.45
8–16 years	0.12–0.17	0.05–0.09	20–80 (65)	< 0.45

a. Seconds.

b. QTc = QT interval/(square root of RR interval).

Source: Rothrock, S. (2007). *Tarascon pediatric emergency pocketbook* (5th ed.). Loma Linda, Ca Tarascon Publishing.

TABLE 22-4

ECG Diagnosis of Chamber Enlargement

Right ventricular hypertrophy/RVH

- R in V_1 > 20 mm (> 25 mm < 1 month)
- S in V_6 > 6 mm (> 12 mm < 1 month)
- Upright T in V_3R, R in V_1 after 5 days
- QR pattern in V_3R, V_1

Left ventricular hypertrophy/LVH

- R in V_6 > 25 mm (> 21 mm < 1 year)
- S in V_1 > 30 mm (> 20 mm <1 year)
- R in V_6 + S in V_1 > 60 mm (use V_5 if R in V_5 > R in V_6)
- Abnormal R/S ratio
- S in V_1 > 2 × R in V_5

Biventricular hypertrophy

- RVH and (S in V_1 or R in V_6) exceeding mean for age
- LVH and (R in V_1 or S in V_6) exceeding mean for age

Right atrial hypertrophy

- Peak P value > 3 mm (< 6 months), > 2.5 mm (≥ 6 months)

Left atrial hypertrophy

- P in II > 0.09 second
- P in V_1 with late negative deflection > 0.04 second and > 1 mm deep

Source: Rothrock, S. (2007). *Tarascon pediatric emergency pocketbook* (5th ed.). Loma Linda, CA Tarascon Publishing.

they can be an excellent tool. For example, when the situs of the heart is in question, the lower hemidiaphragm denotes the position of the cardiac apex, independent of the situs of the abdominal viscera.

Imaging studies

Cardiac computed tomography. The ready availability of cardiac computed tomography (CT) has made it a useful tool in the diagnosis of cardiovascular structures. Most chest CTs are not ECG gated, however, so data on chamber volumes, shunt lesions, and systolic function are not reliable. Chest CT angiograms, by comparison, provide excellent data about systemic and pulmonary venous anatomy, proximal pulmonary artery anatomy, and the relationships of the great arteries and arch abnormalities.

Many questions arise regarding the radiation dose children receive with CT. Current studies suggest that an infant is exposed to an average of 0.28 millisevert during this type of study, or the same amount of radiation received during approximately five to eight CXRs. The rapidity with which excellent images are obtained, often without sedation, make this a very valid imaging modality.

Cardiac magnetic resonance imaging. Although cardiac magnetic resonance imaging (MRI) studies are long, are technically complicated, and require either procedural sedation or general anesthesia, the anatomical, functional, volumetric, and hemodynamic data via this technique are obtained without radiation exposure or invasive catheterization. In addition to the obvious lesions where ECG-gated imaging is helpful, gadolinium-based assessments of myocardial scar, viability, and edema have great potential to assist in diagnosis and treatment of cardiac rejection

post-transplant, myocarditis, and chronic cardiomyopathy. Flow quantification is used to estimate pulmonary-to-systemic flow ratios, the regurgitant fraction even in the face of both atrioventricular and semilunar valve regurgitation, and the contribution of aortopulmonary connections to total pulmonary flow in caval–pulmonary connections. In the future, MRI-derived estimates of vascular impedance and capacitance are expected to significantly improve our understanding of ventricular loading conditions and cardiac failure.

Echocardiograph. Echocardiograph interrogation of the heart and great vessels, using two-dimensional imaging, Doppler flow interrogation, and color flow mapping, has become the standard imaging modality in pediatric cardiology (Lai et al., 2009). Whereas several years ago a child would not undergo a cardiac surgical procedure without a cardiac catheterization, today most diagnoses no longer require preoperative catheterization if the echocardiograph evaluation is diagnostic.

There are a few diagnoses for which an echocardiograph may not give a definitive diagnosis: anomalous left coronary from the pulmonary artery, complex aortic arch abnormalities, and complex pulmonary artery or pulmonary vein abnormalities. In addition, echocardiograph-derived hemodynamic evaluations may be inaccurate. Assessment of aortic valve stenosis may be misleading; the same is true with pulmonary outflow tract stenosis when it occurs at several levels. Most pediatric echocardiograph laboratories do not perform load-independent measures of ventricular function, as in velocity of circumferential fiber shortening (Vcf) or end-systolic wall stress (WS), but instead rely on shortening fraction (SF) and fixed-geometric estimates of ejection fraction (EF). Likewise, echocardiograph-based estimates of pulmonary vascular obstruction do not include an accurate pulmonary blood flow, or venous pressure estimate, thus making the assessment difficult to interpret.

The following equations apply when using an echocardiogram:

- Simplified *Bernoulli Equation*: the relationship between pressure and velocity

$$\Delta P = 4(v_2^2 - v_1^2)$$

ΔP = change in pressure across a narrowing, e.g., tricuspid valve;
v = velocity of blood on either side of the narrowing; usually $v_1 \ll v_2$ so it is ignored, giving $4v_2^2$.

- Percent shortening fraction (SF) of the left ventricle.

$$SF = (LVEDD - LVESD)/LVEDD \times 100$$

LVEDD = end-diastolic dimension
LVESD = end-systolic dimension

- Ejection fraction (EF) of the left ventricle.

$$EF = (LVEDV - LVESV)/LVEDV \times 100$$

Volumes (V) are either measured by planimetry or calculated.

- Velocity of circumferential fiber shortening (Vcf): Preload is independent but changes with contractility and afterload.

$$Vcf = (SF/\text{ejection time})/(R-R \text{ interval})^{1/2}$$
Myocardial performance index

- Myocardial performance index (MPI): Independent of ventricular geometry but changes with contractility.

$$MPI = (ICT + IRT)/ET$$

Doppler interrogation of AV valve inflow and ventricular outflow give:

ICT = isovolumetric contraction time
IRT = isovolumetric relaxation time
ET = ejection time

Caution is required on several fronts when seeking these studies, because echocardiograph evaluation is easily accessed. First, these tests are expensive, frequently costing several thousand dollars for a complete study. Second, it is easy to rely on the values produced in the report, even when the clinical scenario suggests otherwise. An excellent example is the patient with a pericardial effusion. Its size and consistency can be determined by echocardiograph, and the hallmarks of a significant effusion (right atrial and right ventricular collapse with respiration) can be sought. Nevertheless, the diagnosis of tamponade is a clinical diagnosis. The timing of pericardial drainage is best made by examining the patient, not by relying on the echocardiograph report.

Caution is also required when using sedation for outpatient studies. There are inherent benefits and risks to its use (Chapter 21). Notably, in some pediatric patients, a diagnostic echocardiograph cannot be performed while they are awake and moving. Each institution must have policies and procedures for the safe use of sedatives in this setting. Practice varies: In some hospitals, inhaled agents are administered by anesthesia; in others, oral chloral hydrate is used.

Cardiac catheterization

Pediatric cardiac catheterization has a low incidence of complications and a high degree of clarity in the resultant data (Bergersen et al., 2008). It is possible to safely catheterize premature infants for both diagnostic and interventional purposes, although few centers have extensive experience with this procedure in the smallest infants. There are few indications where catheterization is essential in the diagnosis of a cardiac anatomic anomaly. One of these conditions is anomalous left coronary from the pulmonary artery. For this abnormality, diagnosis may be made by other imaging modalities; however, cardiac catheterization with direct aortic root angiography is most sensitive.

Cardiac catheterization hemodynamics

- Cardiac catheterization mean pressures (Table 22-5)
- Oxygen content:

$$(\text{Hemoglobin (gm/100 mL)} \times 1.36 \times \text{fractional saturation}) + 0.003 \times PO_2$$

- Fick cardiac index or QS (L/min-m^2) :

$$\frac{O_2 \text{ consumption (mL/min-m}^2)}{(\text{aortic content} - \text{mixed venous content}) \times 10}$$

- Pulmonary flow or QP (L/min-m^2):

$$\frac{O_2 \text{ consumption (mL/min-m}^2)}{(\text{pulmonary vein content} - \text{pulmonary artery content}) \times 10}$$

- Ratio of pulmonary to systemic blood flow (QP/QS)

$$QP/QS: (\text{Aortic sat} - \text{SVC sat})/(\text{pulmonary vein sat} - \text{pulmonary artery sat})$$

Sat = oxygen saturation by oximetry

- Pulmonary vascular resistance (PVR in indexed Wood units):

$$PVR: (\text{mean PA pressure} - \text{mean LA or wedge pressure})/QP$$

- Systemic vascular resistance (SVR in indexed Wood units):

$$SVR: (\text{mean aortic pressure} - \text{mean RA})/QS$$

TABLE 22-5

Cardiac Catheterization: Pediatric Mean Pressures				
Pressures: Mean (Standard Deviation)	**Infant to- 5 Years**	**5–10 Years**	**10–15 Years**	**15–18 Years**
Right atrial	4 (2)	3 (1)	4 (2)	3 (2)
Pulmonary wedge	8 (3)	8 (2)	8 (3)	8 (2)
Pulmonary artery	13 (5)	18 (23)	13 (3)	14 (3)
Arterial	72 (11)	83 (10)	84 (11)	87 (11)

Source: Adapted from Lock et al., 1993.

The use of sedation or general anesthesia for cardiac catheterization must be determined based on the individual needs of the patient and the proposed procedure. Children as young as 8 years of age may undergo successful catheterization, myocardial biopsy, coronary angiography, or pulmonary hypertension testing without premedication or sedation. For these patients, it is recommended that a child life specialist work with them before and during the procedure. For additional information and depth; Table 22-6 provides a list of specific recommended references.

TABLE 22-6

Recommended Cardiac Resources	
Developmental cardiology	Clark & Takao, 1990
Cardiac function	Lakatta & Maughan, 1990
Neural and hormonal control of the heart	Garfield, 1990; Levy & Pappano, 2006
Cardiorespiratory interactions	Garfield, 1990; Healy et al., 2010; Levy & Pappano, 2006
Neural and hormonal control of the vasculature	Shaddy & Wernovsky, 2005
Physical examination pertaining to pediatric cardiology	Constant, 2002

ADVANCED LIFE SUPPORT EDUCATION

Harriet S. Hawkins

PEDIATRIC ADVANCED LIFE SUPPORT (PALS)

Sponsoring organizations

American Heart Association (AHA)
American Academy of Pediatrics (AAP)

Focus of course

The PALS course is intended for HCPs who have a primary focus and responsibility to provide care for infants and children. The goal of this course is to facilitate the development of knowledge and skills necessary to efficiently and effectively manage critically ill infants and children. The focus of the course is assessment and early treatment of infants and children with respiratory distress, respiratory failure, shock, and rhythm disturbances. Skills taught include recognition and treatment of infants and children at risk for cardiopulmonary arrest; a systematic approach to pediatric assessment; effective respiratory management; defibrillation and synchronized cardioversion; intraosseous access and fluid bolus administration; and effective resuscitation team dynamics. Because good pediatric life support depends on good basic life support (BLS), infant and pediatric basic life support skills are reviewed and practiced in every PALS course (Ralston et al., 2006).

History of the course

In 1983, the AHA formed a subcommittee to develop a course in pediatric advanced life support that would address resuscitation guidelines specifically for children. At the time, the resuscitation of children was discussed minimally in the Advanced Cardiac Life Support (ACLS) course. The first edition of the *PALS Provider Manual* was published in 1988, and PALS courses began that same year (Quan & Seidel, 1997).

Evidence that supports the course

All AHA guidelines for resuscitation are the result of an evidence evaluation process. The AHA works in collaboration with the International Liaison Committee on Resuscitation (ILCOR), an international consortium of experts from resuscitation councils throughout the world. ILCOR was formed in 1992 to provide a forum for review of resuscitation science with the goal of developing evidence-based guidelines for worldwide use. The guidelines are updated every 5 years and are based on the most current resuscitation science available at the time. The evidence

evaluation process is a continual effort, with work on the next set of guidelines starting almost as soon as the current set is published.

Representatives of ILCOR and the AHA establish task forces to address various resuscitation topics including basic life support, pediatric life support, neonatal life support, advanced life support for adults, stroke, and education. Members of each task force then identify topics that they feel require evidence evaluation. Hypotheses are formulated on each topic and international experts are assigned as worksheet authors for each hypothesis. Worksheet authors search for, critically evaluate, and determine the level of evidence based on methodology, using eight levels of evidence. They summarize the evidence related to the hypothesis and suggest treatment recommendations (AHA, 2005) (Table 22-7). Treatment recommendations are classified using a system with five levels. The classification system takes into consideration the weight of the scientific evidence, the efficacy of the recommendation, educational/training challenges, cost, and implementation difficulties (Table 22-8).

The AHA requires that all editors and volunteers fully disclose any potential conflict of interest. These disclosures are mandated in the published guidelines as well as in any presentation given by speakers. In the last 10 years, all AHA committees have included experts in the field of education. Changes have been made to the course that are educational sound and that will enhance both initial learning and retention (AHA, 2005).

TABLE 22-7

Levels of Evidence	
Evidence	**Definition**
Level 1	Randomized clinical trials or meta-analyses of multiple clinical trials with substantial treatment effects
Level 2	Randomized clinical trials with smaller or less significant treatment effects
Level 3	Prospective, controlled, nonrandomized cohort studies
Level 4	Historic, nonrandomized cohort or case-control studies
Level 5	Case series; patients compiled in serial fashion, control group lacking
Level 6	Animal studies or mechanical model studies
Level 7	Extrapolations from existing data collected for other purposes, theoretical analyses
Level 8	Rational conjecture (common sense); common practices accepted before evidence-based guidelines

Source: American Heart Association, Inc.

TABLE 22-8

Classification of Recommendations for Procedures/Treatments or Diagnostic Tests/Assessments				
Class I	**Class IIa**	**Class IIb**	**Class III**	**Class Indeterminate**
Benefit >>> risk	Benefit >> risk	Benefit ≥ risk	Risk ≥ benefit	Risk/benefit unknown
Should be performed	Is reasonable to perform	May be considered	Should not be performed/ administered; not helpful and may be harmful	Cannot recommend for or against; new research starting or continuing area or research

Source: American Heart Association, Inc.

Intended participants

The PALS course is intended for HCPs who are responsible for the initiation and direction of advanced life support in pediatric patients. The goal of the course is to facilitate the development of knowledge and skills that will enable the provider to evaluate and manage seriously ill infants and children in a timely manner (Doto et al., 2006). The PALS provider course is designed for the HCP who has not previously taken a PALS course. HCPs who have a current or prior PALS card may take the PALS renewal course.

PALS course topics

The PALS course includes a combination of video-directed discussions and hands-on skills stations. Topics covered in the course include pediatric and infant cardiopulmonary resuscitation (CPR), management of respiratory emergencies, rhythm disturbances and treatment, defibrillation and cardioversion, vascular access, and management of shock. Students practice assessment and care in simulated team sessions using manikins and equipment. A discussion of team dynamics is included as part of the course. Students must pass a written examination and participate in team skills testing in respiratory, shock, and cardiac stations.

The PALS renewal course is recommended every two years and covers the same topics as the PALS provider course but in less detail. Both skill and written testing is required to receive a PALS provider card.

HeartCode PALS

An alternative method for obtaining PALS training is the HeartCode PALS. HeartCode PALS is a self-directed online learning program that delivers the PALS course information and is approved for use by new and renewal students. The program includes the pre-course self-assessment, the team dynamics lesson, the full texts of the *PALS Provider Manual,* the current guidelines, the supplementary AHA PALS videos, 12 interactive pediatric patient scenarios, and the PALS multiple-choice exam.

The student, working independently, successfully completes the cognitive portion of the program, including passing all of the scenarios and the multiple-choice exam. Debriefing of actions performed in the online scenarios provides instant feedback, including suggestions for improvement. This program is approved for continuing education credit by the American Medical Association, American Nurses Credentialing Center Commission on Accreditation, Continuing Education Coordinating Board for Emergency Medical Services, and American Association of Physician Assistants. For the convenience of the reader, please refer to Table 22-9 for an abbreviated comparison of the described courses.

After completion of the online program, a certificate is printed and taken to a PALS instructor for whom the skills portion of the PALS class is performed and tested. This part of the course takes from 1 to 1.5 hours and includes the core case testing of cardiac, respiratory, and shock cases (AHA, 2010b).

ADVANCED PEDIATRIC LIFE SUPPORT (APLS)

Sponsoring organizations

American Academy of Pediatrics
American College of Emergency Physicians (ACEP)

Focus of course

The focus of the APLS course is the identification and treatment of a variety of pediatric illnesses and injuries seen in the emergency setting, including respiratory distress, shock, chronic diseases, and acute medical illnesses. More than 90 skills are covered in the course, including endotracheal intubation, placement of a variety of vascular access lines, sedation, pain management, wound care, suturing, splinting, casting, and thoracic procedures. The revised fourth edition of APLS is described by the authors as "the body of knowledge in pediatric emergency medicine" (AAP & ACEP, 2010).

History of the course

The first edition of the APLS course was published in 1989, although the first APLS course was actually presented in 1984. The work toward APLS began in the late 1970s as health care organizations sought to develop guidelines for the care of children in the emergency setting. This effort evolved into the American Academy of Pediatrics Section on Emergency Medicine and resulted in a manual on pediatric emergency care. In 1983, two groups emerged, both with a focus on pediatric life support education. One group became the American Heart Association Subcommittee on Pediatric Resuscitation, and the other became the APLS Steering Committee of the American College of Emergency Physicians.

Evidence that supports the course

The APLS course is based on the most current science information from the AHA as well as other well-recognized professional publications. References are included at the end of each chapter in the book (Fuchs et al., 2007).

Intended participants

The APLS course is designed for the knowledge level and advanced skills of physicians who handle pediatric illness and injury in an emergency setting. It is open to nurses, paramedics, and other HCPs who care for critically ill and injured children.

APLS course topics

The APLS course can be customized according to the educational needs of the student. Course directors can adjust the schedule and use any of the didactic sessions or skill station modules in the course. The two requirements for the customized course include that the course must be a total of 14.5 hours long and that at least 2 hours must be consist of training at skill stations covering airway procedures and cardiovascular procedures.

The recommended two-day course schedule includes 14.5 hours of class time. Topics include pediatric assessment, airway and cardiovascular assessment and procedures, medical emergencies, trauma, surgical emergencies, children with special health care needs, metabolic issues, child maltreatment, toxicology, and CNS problems. The course involves a combination of skill stations, lecture, and small-group discussions. Each course may be somewhat different, as the course director may provide multiple optional lessons. An alternative to the full two-day course is a one-day course of classroom instruction along with self-study of six chapters from the APLS student manual.

Students verify completion of their self-study by answering questions online prior to attending the course. The recommended one-day schedule includes 7.5 hours of class time and includes pediatric assessment, airway and cardiovascular procedures, central nervous system issues, medical emergencies, and trauma. Regardless of the format, students have the option of receiving a course attendance card or a course completion card. To receive the course completion card, the student must take the course examination.

The ACEP has approved the course for continuing education credit. The APLS "Check Your Knowledge" online continuing education program provides one credit per module. Students planning to take a one-day course can have their online test results send directly to the APLS course director (AAP & ACEP, 2010).

ADVANCED CARDIOVASCULAR LIFE SUPPORT (ACLS)

Sponsoring organization

American Heart Association

Focus of course

The goal of the ACLS course is to improve the care of the adult victim of cardiac arrest, symptomatic cardiac arrhythmias, or stroke. The focus of this course is the identification and treatment of potentially life-threatening symptoms and pre-arrest conditions as well as the management of cardiac arrest as a member or leader of a resuscitation team. Given that good BLS care is the basis of effective ALS care, chest compression proficiency and automated external defibrillator (AED) use are demonstrated throughout the course (Field, 2006).

History of the course

Cardiopulmonary resuscitation was developed in 1960 but was first taught only to physicians. Three years later, the AHA formed the first CPR Committee and published a formal endorsement of CPR as a life-saving technique. It was not until 1974 that the first guidelines for advanced cardiovascular life support were published, however. These guidelines have since been updated in 1980, 1986, 1992, 2000, 2005, and 2010.

Evidence that supports the course

The evidence process for the ACLS course is the same process delineated previously for the PALS course (AHA, 2005).

Intended participants

The ACLS provider course is intended for HCPs who participate in the assessment and resuscitation of adult patients. The course is appropriate for both hospital and prehospital providers of care.

Acls course topics

The ACLS provider course includes the BLS primary survey and ACLS secondary survey, adult CPR practice, management of respiratory arrest, and assessment and management of tachycardic and bradycardic rhythm disturbances, acute coronary syndrome, and stroke. A review of current defibrillator technology is included in each course, and students must participate in a megacode skill station using principles of good team dynamics. Both written and skill tests are given at the end of the course. The provider course is typically 10 to 12 hours long (Field & Doto, 2006).

The ACLS renewal course is typically 6 hours long and includes the BLS primary survey and ACLS secondary survey, adult CPR practice, management of respiratory arrest, assessment and management of tachycardic and bradycardic rhythm disturbances, and the megacode skill station. Both written and skill tests are given at the end of the course (Field & Doto, 2006).

HeartCode ACLS

An alternative method for obtaining ACLS training is the HeartCode ACLS program. Like the PALS program, this self-paced interactive program incorporates all cognitive requirements for the ACLS course and is approved for use by both new and renewal students. The program includes the pre-course self-assessment, the lesson in team dynamics, and 10 interactive patient scenarios. The full texts of the *ACLS Provider Manual,* the guidelines, and the ACLS core drugs list are included. The AHA's ACLS multiple-choice examination is completed online after the student completes the learning activities.

The HeartCode ACLS program is approved for continuing education credit from the American Association of Physician Assistants, American Nurses Credentialing Center Commission on Accreditation, Accreditation Council for Pharmacy Education, and Continuing Education Coordinating Board for Emergency Medical Services.

After completion of the online program, a certificate is printed and taken to an ACLS instructor, who observes as the skills portion of the ACLS class is practiced and tested. This part of the course takes from 1 to 1.5 hours and includes the core case testing of ACLS (AHA, 2010a).

NEONATAL RESUSCITATION PROGRAM (NRP)

Sponsoring organizations

American Heart Association
American Academy of Pediatrics

Focus of course

The NRP is focused on the resuscitation of the neonate at the time of delivery, with emphasis on assistance with the transition from intrauterine to extrauterine life that is needed by some neonates (Kattwinkel, 2006).

History of the course

In 1978, the AHA Emergency Cardiac Care Committee formed a Working Group on Pediatric Resuscitation. That group determined the need for a course that specifically spoke to the unique needs of the newly born. At the same time, the specialty of neonatology was growing. In recognition of the importance of this area, in 1985 the AHA and the AAP joined to form a work group to develop such a course. The first NRP course was published in 1987, with revisions in 1990, 1994, 2000, and 2006 (Kattwinkel, 2006).

Evidence that supports the course

The evidence process for the NRP is the same process as delineated previously for the PALS course (AHA, 2005).

Intended participants

The NRP is intended for any HCP who is responsible for the care of the newly born infant. The course consists of nine lessons, and students need take only those lessons that apply to their profession and responsibility.

NRP course topics

The NRP provider course includes an overview of the principles of neonatal resuscitation, the initial steps in neonatal resuscitation, use of resuscitation devices for ventilation, chest compressions, intubation of the neonate, medications use in neonatal resuscitation, special situations that may affect resuscitation and post-resuscitation management, problems related to prematurity, and ethical issues in neonatal resuscitation. The course consists of self-study, discussion, skill practice, and skill testing. Detailed review of ventilation techniques and resuscitation equipment is included in the skill practice stations. The testing may be done either online prior to class or as a paper test during the class. Skill testing focuses on the student's ability to perform both independently and as a member of a team (Zaichkin, 2006).

The NRP renewal course is intended for students who have a current NRP card. Experienced students may not need review or discussion and may take the test online prior to coming to class. The class then consists of a megacode testing station that may be completed individually or as a small group.

EMERGENCY NURSING PEDIATRIC COURSE (ENPC)

Sponsoring organization

Emergency Nurses Association (ENA)

Focus of course

The focus of ENPC is the assessment and care of the pediatric patient in the emergency department setting. This course emphasizes the pathologies of pediatric illness, assessment of the pediatric patient (including infants and neonates), initial and ongoing management, and specific nursing interventions.

History of the course

In 1991, the ENA formed a Pediatric Committee in response to member requests. A primary charge of this committee was to assess the need for a course specifically designed for pediatric emergency nursing. The first ENPC book was published in 1993, and courses began that same year. The course was revised in 1998 and in 2004. Another revision is in process (ENA, 2004a, 2004b).

Evidence that supports the course

The ENPC course is based on current evidence-based practice in pediatric emergency nursing as well as on the guidelines from the AHA.

Intended participants

The ENPC is written by registered nurses and is intended for registered nurses. Although other disciplines may audit the course, only registered nurses may participate in the testing and receive verification in ENPC.

ENPC course topics

The ENPC provider course is typically 16 hours long and comprises a combination of lectures and hands-on skill stations. Topics include dealing with children, initial assessment, pediatric triage, respiratory distress and failure, shock, rhythm disturbances, trauma, child maltreatment, neonatal specific assessment and common illnesses, children with special health care needs, poisonings, psychiatric emergencies, crisis intervention, and stabilization for transport. Skill stations include a review of various nursing clinical interventions for children, pediatric triage, and management of the ill or injured pediatric patient. A key part of the ENPC is teaching a systematic approach to the nursing assessment of the pediatric patient. To receive verification in ENPC, the participant must pass a written examination and two skill stations, *Management of the Ill or Injured Pediatric Patient* and *Pediatric Triage* (ENA, 2004a, 2004b).

The ENPC renewal (reverification) course is 6 hours long; it includes a review of basic pediatric assessment and care, as well as highlights of specific illnesses and trauma. The student completes a pre-course assessment prior to coming to the ENPC reverification course, and this self-study prepares the individual for testing. Skill stations include pediatric triage and management of the ill or injured pediatric patient. Testing is the same as in the ENPC provider course.

PEDIATRIC EMERGENCY ASSESSMENT, RECOGNITION, AND STABILIZATION (PEARS)

Sponsoring organizations

American Academy of Pediatrics
American Heart Association

Focus of course

The PEARS course is intended to enhance the assessment and recognition skills of the HCP professional who provides acute—not resuscitative—care to children.

History of the course

The PEARS course was developed in 2007 and is based on information in the PALS course. It was developed because HCPs were taking the PALS course, even though their responsibilities did not include the actual resuscitation of pediatric patients. The AHA Subcommittee on Pediatric Resuscitation recognized the need for a course that was not as heavily focused on resuscitation. The PEARS course was developed with input from third-year medical students at the University of Arkansas College of Medicine (Ralston et al., 2007).

Evidence that supports the course

The evidence process for the PEARS course is the same process as delineated previously for the PALS course (AHA, 2005).

TABLE 22-9

Quick Reference to Courses					
	Focus of Course	**Intended Audience**	**Course Content**	**Course Format**	**Online Options**
Pediatric Advanced Life Support (PALS)	Assessment/treatment of pediatric patients with a focus on resuscitation.	Health care professionals who are responsible for the initiation and direction of advanced life support in pediatric patients.	Pediatric respiratory distress and failure, shock, rhythm disturbances.	Video/discussion, small-group skill practice.	Online course review and test.
Advanced Pediatric Life Support (APLS)	Identification and treatment of a variety of pediatric illnesses and injuries seen in the emergency setting.	Physicians who handle pediatric illness and injury in an emergency setting.	Respiratory distress, shock, chronic diseases and acute medical illnesses.	Lecture, small-group discussion, skill practice.	Online course review.
Advanced Cardiac Life Support (ACLS)	Identification and treatment of pre-arrest conditions and management of cardiac arrest in adults.	Health care professionals who participate in the assessment and resuscitation of adult patients.	Rhythm disturbances, stroke, acute coronary syndrome, resuscitation management, defibrillation.	Lecture/discussion, video, small-group skill practice.	Online course review and test.
Neonatal Resuscitation Program (NRP)	Resuscitation of the neonate at the time of delivery.	Health care professionals with responsibilities for the care of the newly born infant.	Transitional physiology, management of the neonatal airway, ventilation of the neonate, neonatal chest compressions.	Small-group didactic and skill practice.	Self-review and online test.
Emergency Nursing Pediatric Course (ENPC)	Assessment and care of the pediatric patient in the emergency department setting.	Registered nurses.	Multiple pediatric pathologies, trauma, child maltreatment, nursing assessment and care.	Lecture, small-group skill practice.	None.
Pediatric Early Assessment, Recognition, and Stabilization (PEARS)	Assessment and recognition of the pediatric patient with respiratory distress or with shock but does not focus heavily on management.	Health care professionals who care for pediatric patients but do not routinely encounter patients who need resuscitation.	Pediatric assessment with a focus on airway, breathing, circulation and disability.	Video, small-group skill practice.	None.

Intended participants

The PEARS course was developed for HCPs who care for pediatric patients but do not routinely encounter patients who need resuscitation (Doto et al., 2007).

PEARS course topics

The PEARS Provider course is 6 to 7 hours long and includes pediatric CPR and AED competency testing; an overview of pediatric assessment with a focus on airway, breathing, circulation, and disability (neurological assessment); respiratory case discussions and skills stations; and shock case discussions and skill stations. Case simulations are practiced at the end of the course, with the students working as a team and the instructor taking the role of the team leader. Students must complete a short video-based test to receive validation of their PEARS training (Doto et al., 2007).

The PEARS renewal course is approximately 4 to 5 hours long and is intended for students who have a current PEARS card. The topics are the same as in the provider course, but less time is spent on review. Case simulations are practiced and the same video-based test is taken to receive a new PEARS card.

ARRHYTHMIAS AND PACEMAKERS

Patricia R. Lawrence

Arrhythmias seen in the pediatric setting require rapid diagnosis to optimize patient outcomes. Most pediatric patients diagnosed with arrhythmias have structurally normal hearts (Hanisch, 2001), while specific arrhythmias are intrinsic to certain congenital lesions, such as intra-atrial reentrant tachycardia (IART) as commonly seen with tetralogy of Fallot (Walsh,

2007). Pediatric patients who undergo cardiothoracic surgical procedures survive longer, but can develop arrhythmias as sequelae to surgery that may require medical intervention (Park & Guntheroth, 1992). Other causes of arrhythmia generation include cellular injury from hypoxia and cardiopulmonary bypass (CPB) and direct trauma to specialized conduction tissue during intracardiac interventions (Walsh, 2007). Understanding of pediatric rhythm disturbances combined with advances in pharmacologic and interventional electrophysiologic techniques have led to improved outcomes and enhancement of the quality of life for patients with these conditions.

RHYTHMS ORIGINATING IN THE SINUS NODE

In general, the sinus node determines the heart's rate and rhythm (Table 22-10 and Figure 22-2). All rhythms that originate in the sinoatrial (SA) or sinus node have a P wave before every QRS complex, and a normal P-wave axis (Figure 22-3 and Figure 22-4).

Sinus tachycardia

In sinus tachycardia, the heart rate is higher than expected, while electrocardiograph (ECG or EKG) complexes and intervals remain normal. Common causes of this arrhythmia include pain, anxiety, excitement, fever, sepsis, anemia, hypovolemia, shock, and medications such as albuterol and steroids. Management is aimed at treating the underlying cause.

Sinus arrhythmia

Sinus arrhythmia is a normal and predictable irregularity in heart rate that occurs with respiration. The heart rate increases during inspiration and slows with expiration, while maintaining normal ECG complexes and intervals (Figure 22-5). Sinus arrhythmia can be rather pronounced

in adolescence and is usually appreciated as a sign of cardiac health (Park & Guntheroth, 1992). This variation in heart rate is a normal finding.

Sinus bradycardia

In sinus bradycardia, the sinus node functions properly and the ECG complexes are normal, but the heart rate is lower than expected for the patient's age. Causes of this arrhythmia include increased intracranial pressure, hypothermia, hypoxia, hypothyroidism, hyperkalemia, sedation, sleep, and drugs such as digoxin. Unless the degree of sinus bradycardia is contributing to hemodynamic instability, management is directed toward correcting the underlying cause.

Sinus pause

Sinus pauses occur when the sinus node fails to initiate an impulse. The pause is of short duration, and no P wave or QRS complex is recorded (Figure 22-6). Causes may include hypoxia, increased vagal tone, and digoxin toxicity. Therapeutic management of this condition is rarely indicated. However, in the case of prolonged or increased frequency of sinus pauses, perfusion and hemodynamic stability need to be more closely monitored while investigative measures are under way.

Sick sinus syndrome

Sick sinus syndrome (SSS) is predominantly seen in children with congenital heart disease who have undergone cardiac surgery involving the atria. In this subset of patients, the sinus node performs abnormally slowly, or may completely fail to function as the primary pacemaker of the heart. Surgical procedures such as the Fontan, Senning, and Mustard procedures require extensive suturing in the atrium, which may leave behind scars that affect sinus node function and result in SSS. Other causes include inflammatory diseases such

TABLE 22-10

Vital Sign Normal Values in Pediatric Patients				
Age	Mean Weight (kg)	Minimun Systolic BP	Normal Heart Rate	Normal Respiratory Rate
Premature	<2.5	40	120–170	40–60
Term	3.5	60	100–170	40–60
3 months	6	60	100–170	30–50
6 months	8	60	100–170	30–50
1 year	10	62	100–170	30–40
2 years	13	74	100–160	20–30
4 years	15	78	80–130	20
6 years	20	82	70–115	16
8 years	25	86	70–110	16
10 years	30	90	60–105	16
12 years	40	94	60–100	16

Source: Aghababian, R. (Ed.) (2006). *Essential emergency medicine.* Sudbury, MA: Jones and Bartlett.

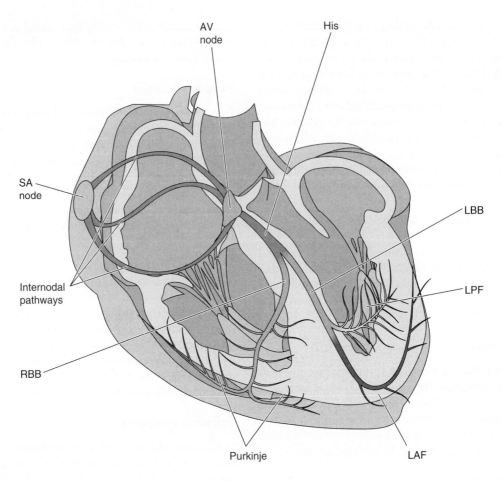

FIGURE 22-2

Conduction System.

Source: Garcia, T., & Holtz, N. (2001). 12-Lead ECG. Sudbury, MA: Jones & Bartlett.

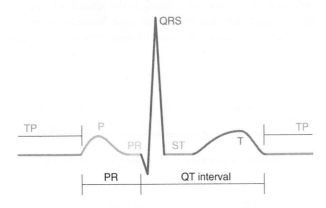

FIGURE 22-3

Basic Components of the ECG complex.

Source: Garcia, T., & Holtz, N. (2001). 12-Lead ECG. Sudbury, MA: Jones & Bartlett.

as myocarditis, pericarditis, and rheumatic heart disease; increased vagal tone and conditions that cause right atrial dilatation; and medications such as antiarrhythmic agents (Hanisch, 2001).

SSS may lead to a variety of atrial arrhythmias, and patients may or may not be symptomatic. The most worrisome of these arrhythmias is bradytachyarrhythmia, which can cause syncope or death (Park, 2008). Permanent pacemaker therapy may be indicated in bradycardic patients who are symptomatic or in patients who are affected by tachyarrhythmias. National practice guidelines that specify the indications for permanent pacemaker therapy for pediatric patients are published and updated regularly by the AHA and the American College of Cardiology (ACC) (Epstein et al., 2008).

RHYTHMS ORIGINATING IN THE ATRIUM

Rhythms that occur elsewhere in the atrium and that do not originate in the SA node are classified as "rhythms originating in the atrium." Atrial arrhythmias are characterized by unusually contoured P waves and/or an abnormal number of P waves per QRS complex; they follow a QRS complex of normal duration (Park, 2008).

Premature atrial contraction

A premature atrial contraction, or complex (PAC), is an atrial beat that occurs too early (Figure 22-7). This condition is common in healthy children, but can also be

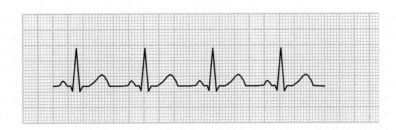

FIGURE 22-4

Normal Sinus Rhythm (NSR).

Source: Garcia, T., & Holtz, N. (2001). 12-Lead ECG. Sudbury, MA: Jones & Bartlett.

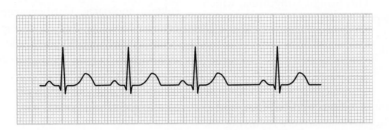

FIGURE 22-5

Sinus Arrhythmia.

Source: Garcia, T., & Holtz, N. (2001). 12-Lead ECG. Sudbury, MA: Jones & Bartlett.

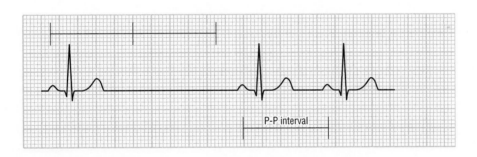

FIGURE 22-6

Sinus Pause.

Source: Garcia, T., & Holtz, N. (2001). 12-Lead ECG. Sudbury, MA: Jones & Bartlett.

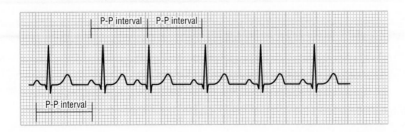

FIGURE 22-7

Premature Atrial Contraction (PAC).

Source: Garcia, T., & Holtz, N. (2001). 12-Lead ECG. Sudbury, MA: Jones & Bartlett.

associated with congenital heart disease. PACs may occur after cardiac surgery and can be associated with digitalis toxicity (Park, 2008). The premature atrial beats are usually of no clinical significance and do not require management unless digitalis toxicity is the primary cause. When PACs are consecutive, are incessant, or produce bradycardia, the HCP should consider checking serum chemistry and consider existing intracardiac lines as a possible cause.

Wandering pacemaker

A wandering pacemaker occurs when the site of electrical impulse gradually shifts between the SA node, the atrioventricular (AV) node, or within the adjacent atrial tissue between these two nodes. This benign arrhythmia, which requires no therapy, is depicted by transient changes in the size, shape, and direction of the P waves, while the QRS complex remains normal.

Atrial flutter

Atrial flutter (AF) is rare in infants and children, and is more likely to occur after cardiac surgery involving the atria (Park & Guntheroth, 1992). It has a "saw-tooth appearance" on the ECG, with an average atrial rate of 300 beats per minute (bpm) and normal QRS complexes (Figure 22-8). Because the AV node cannot respond quickly, varying degrees of AV block may occur; fortunately, they cause heart rates to be closer to 150 bpm.

Other causes of AF include structural heart disease that leads to atrial dilation and digitalis toxicity. The clinical presentation depends on the corresponding ventricular rate. Patients with a slow ventricular rate in the face of AF may be asymptomatic, whereas children with faster rates may complain of palpitations, fatigue, and exercise intolerance. Congestive heart failure (CHF) can ensue if diagnosis is delayed.

Management consists of slowing the ventricular rate, primarily with the use of medications such as amiodarone or procainamide. Occasionally, acute management such as cardioversion may be required, depending on the pediatric patient's symptoms and vital signs. Stable blood pressure and other vital signs allow for a less aggressive, pharmacologic approach. Cardioversion should be avoided in patients receiving digoxin therapy unless the arrhythmia is life threatening. Digoxin and cardioversion are associated with malignant ventricular arrhythmias (Doninger & Sharieff, 2006). In the rare instance that cardioversion is contraindicated, trasvenous or transesophageal pacing may be effective (Park, 2008).

Atrial fibrillation

Another rare arrhythmia in pediatrics is atrial fibrillation. Its presence suggests significant pathology (Park, 2008). This condition is described as a very rapid atrial rate ranging from 350 to 600 bpm (Figure 22-9), and an irregularly

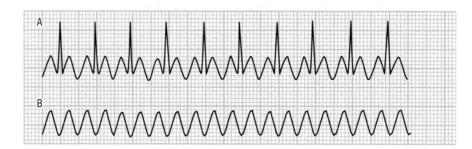

FIGURE 22-8

Atrial Flutter.

Source: Garcia, T., & Holtz, N. (2001). 12-Lead ECG. Sudbury, MA: Jones & Bartlett.

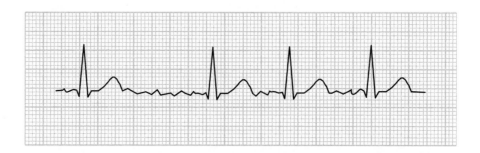

FIGURE 22-9

Atrial Fibrillation.

Source: Garcia, T., & Holtz, N. (2001). 12-Lead ECG. Sudbury, MA: Jones & Bartlett.

irregular ventricular response that is best recognized in lead V$_1$ (Doninger & Sharieff, 2006). The QRS complex is normal. Causes of atrial fibrillation are similar to those of atrial flutter.

The concerning clinical manifestations of atrial fibrillation include the high potential for thrombus formation and decreased cardiac output due to the combination of fast ventricular rates and discoordination between the atria and ventricles (Park, 2008). Because management modalities will depend on hemodynamic stability, all pediatric patients must be rapidly assessed. Hemodynamically unstable patients require immediate cardioversion, whereas those who are stable can be given digoxin. Propranolol may be added, if after 24 hours, digoxin therapy has been ineffective.

Supraventricular tachycardia

Supraventricular tachycardia (SVT), the most common rhythm disturbance in the pediatric population, is a broad category that includes any rapid rhythm that occurs above the bundle of His (Hanisch, 2001). The classifications of SVT may be confusing, owing at least in part to the detailed mechanisms demonstrated during electrophysiologic testing and ablation. For most patients, the initial management will be the same, regardless of the precise mechanism involved. The response to initial therapy often clarifies the underlying mechanism and aids in determining the most beneficial therapeutic approach.

Because a variety of mechanisms of SVT exist, the most pragmatic way of grouping these tachycardias are by atrial, nodal, and AV reentrant types. The atrial and nodal types are automatic tachycardias that exist without an additional circuit. The atrial type of SVT, in which rapid firing of a single focus in the atria is responsible for the tachycardia, is a rare mechanism of SVT (Park, 2008). An example of this type of SVT is ectopic atrial tachycardia (EAT). In the nodal type of SVT, there is rapid firing of a single focus in the AV node. An example of this type of SVT is junctional ectopic tachycardia (JET).

Reentrant SVT. The majority of pediatric cases of SVT are due to AV reentrant tachycardias. In this type of SVT, two circuits are involved. In addition to the normal conduction pathway from the SA node to the AV node and then to the bundle of His and Purkinje fibers, a second accessory pathway communicates with the AV node (Figure 22-10). This accessory pathway leads to a reentrant circuit in which conduction travels first down either of the two circuits and then up the other, with conduction through the accessory pathway occurring more rapidly. The accessory pathway may be either anatomically separate, as with Wolff-Parkinson-White (WPW) syndrome, or it can be functionally separate, as in a dual AV node pathway. The best-known type of reentrant SVT is WPW, in which an accessory pathway can be seen on surface ECG by in the form of a delta wave (Figure 22-11), but only when the patient is in a normal sinus rhythm.

Atrioventricular reciprocating tachycardia (AVRT) is a type of reentrant SVT with an accessory pathway; atrioventricular nodal reentrant tachycardia (AVNRT) is a type of reentrant SVT without an accessory pathway, but with two distinct AV node pathways. Both AVRT and AVNRT are clinically similar and respond in the same fashion to therapeutic interventions. Both types are seen on ECG as narrow-complex tachycardias that have a sudden onset and termination. Heart rates in infants can be as high as 300 bpm, becoming slower with age (up to 220 bpm in the adolescent). The main difference between these two mechanisms of reentrant SVT is the age of onset: AVRT is more common in infants and young children, whereas AVNRT is seen in older children and adolescents (Hanisch, 2001). Approximately 50% of all patients diagnosed with SVT have an idiopathic cause, while fewer cases (23%) are associated with congenital heart disease, such as Ebstein's anomaly, or L-transposition (Doninger & Sharieff, 2006).

Most pediatric patients can tolerate prolonged periods of SVT, but it is nonetheless critical to rapidly assess the pediatric patient's cardiorespiratory status. Some patients in SVT may have decreased cardiac output and go on to develop CHF. Infants generally present with a history of irritability, pallor, or diaphoresis with poor feeding. Older pediatric patients may describe palpitations, chest pain, dizziness, and shortness of breath.

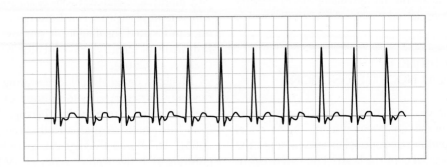

FIGURE 22-10

Supraventricular Tachycardia (SVT).

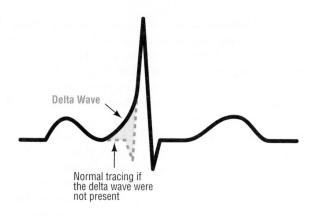

FIGURE 22-11

Delta Wave.

Source: Garcia, T., & Holtz, N. (2001). 12-Lead ECG. Sudbury, MA: Jones & Bartlett.

For unstable pediatric patients with poor perfusion, synchronized cardioversion should be administered, without delay, beginning with 0.5 to 1 joules per kilogram (J/kg) and increased to a maximum of 2 J/kg if necessary. If intravenous (IV) access has already been established, adenosine 0.1 mg/kg/dose can be rapidly administered, but cardioversion should never be delayed while awaiting IV placement in the unstable patient (Doninger & Sharieff, 2006). Adenosine, whose half-life is less than 1½ seconds, transiently blocks AV conduction, thereby terminating most all SVT in which the AV node forms part of the reentry circuit. Caution should be used when this medication is given, as adenosine can induce severe bronchospasm in the asthmatic patient (Taketomo, Hodding, & Kraus, 2010). Stable pediatric patients can be initially treated with vagal stimulatory maneuvers to terminate the SVT. A bag of ice can be placed, for up to 10 seconds, on the younger patient's forehead to induce the diving reflex, or the older patient can be asked to perform a Valsalva maneuver.

Chronic management of SVT varies with the patient's age, the presence of congenital heart disease, the frequency and types of symptoms, and the risk for sudden death (Hanisch, 2001). Pharmacologic management may include digoxin or propranolol, and in some cases amiodarone or flecainide when the SVT is refractory to first-line agents. If medical management fails, radiofrequency (RF) catheter ablation should be considered.

RHYTHMS ORIGINATING IN THE ATRIOVENTRICULAR NODE OR JUNCTION

The dysfunction of the sinus node creates a response by the distal portions of the conduction system. The AV node, which has the second-fastest pacemaker rate, assumes the role as the main pacemaker of the heart. This can occur in the setting of sinus node slowing, disease, or dysfunction. Junctional arrhythmias can also occur as a result of abnormal automaticity in the AV node leading to JET. These rhythms are characterized by (1) inverted P waves following the QRS complex or (2) absent P waves while the QRS complex remains normal.

Junctional rhythm

In junctional rhythm, the heart rate can be as low as 40 to 60 bpm (Park, 2008). This arrhythmia may be seen in pediatric patients with a structurally normal heart (Figure 22-12). Junctional rhythm can also be seen after cardiac surgical procedures that involve the atria, in any condition that increases vagal tone (such as increased intracranial pressure), and in digoxin toxicity. Junctional rhythm is considered clinically significant only if the patient becomes hemodynamically unstable. If the patient is asymptomatic and remains well perfused, no therapy is needed, except in digoxin-toxic patients. In contrast, pharmacologic therapy with atropine or some form of temporary pacing is required in patients who exhibit symptoms of poor perfusion and decreased cardiac output.

Junctional ectopic tachycardia

The most common arrhythmia that occurs acutely after cardiac surgery in the pediatric patient younger than 2 years of age is JET (also known as accelerated junctional rhythm) (Beke et al., 2005). This condition is rarely seen in patients with a structurally normal heart (Hanisch, 2001). The JET arrhythmia is an automatic tachycardia that originates within the AV node. Ventricular rates range from 150 to 300 bpm, and the QRS complex is narrow, often making it difficult to distinguish this condition from atrial tachycardia (Figure 22-13). Some clinicians and reference books may categorize JET as a type of SVT. Central to accurate diagnosis is AV dissociation on ECG; ventricular rates are faster than the atrial rate (Hanisch). It is this combination of rapid ventricular rates and dissociated atrial contraction that leads to hemodynamic compromise and high mortality if the arrhythmia is not adequately controlled (Hanisch). JET is better tolerated when junctional rates are only mildly accelerated (Keene et al., 2006). If atrial pacing wires are in place after cardiac surgery, an atrial wire tracing can be used for diagnostic purposes when the P wave is difficult to identify or is obscured by the QRS complex (Beke et al., 2005).

Management goals include restoring AV synchrony and slowing ventricular rates to improve cardiac output. With the development of effective therapies for JET, mortality from this cause has dramatically decreased (Keene et al., 2006). Atrial wire tracings can assist in not only distinguishing JET from other types of SVT, but can also be

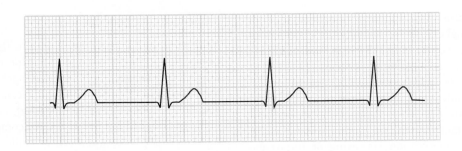

FIGURE 22-12

Junctional Rhythm.

Source: Garcia, T., & Holtz, N. (2001). 12-Lead ECG. Sudbury, MA: Jones & Bartlett.

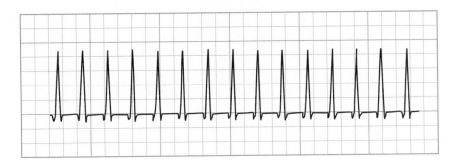

FIGURE 22-13

Junctional Ectopic Tachycardia (JET).

used to restore AV synchrony by overdrive pacing at a rate slightly higher than the intrinsic junctional rate. Inducing hypothermia to as low as 34°C can slow the junctional rate; this goal is best achieved with a cooling blanket while the patient remains intubated and chemically paralyzed (Park, 2008; Plammatter et al, 2001). Because JET is catecholamine sensitive, every effort should be made to reduce the patient's exposure to exogenous sources of catecholamines while balancing the need for inotropic therapy to support hemodynamic compromise caused by the arrhythmia itself. Pharmacologic management includes procainamide or amiodarone.

RHYTHMS ORIGINATING IN THE VENTRICLE

Ventricular arrhythmias are much less common in pediatric patients than they are in adults (Beke et al., 2005). These abnormalities are characterized by bizarre, wide QRS complexes that are long in duration, with T waves extending in the opposite direction. QRS complexes may be inconsistently related to P waves.

Premature ventricular contraction

A premature ventricular contraction, or complex (PVC), is characterized by a wide QRS complex with a distinct morphology that is not preceded by a P wave (Figure 22-14). Bigeminy occurs when PVCs are present with every other beat, alternating with a normal QRS impulse. Premature ventricular contractions that occur with every third beat, separated by two normal QRS impulses, are known as trigeminy. PVCs can also occur consecutively: A couplet consists of two PVCs occurring consecutively, while three or more PVCs occurring consecutively is considered ventricular tachycardia. Unifocal PVCs occur from a single focus within the ventricle (also known as uniform, monophasic PVCs), giving rise to a consistent QRS pattern in the same lead. Multifocal PVCs (also known as multiform, polymorphous, or pleomorphic PVCs), are assumed to originate from different foci within the ventricle, resulting in varying configurations of the QRS pattern in the same lead. (Park, 2008).

Causes of premature ventricular contractions include electrolyte imbalances, drug toxicities (amphetamines, general anesthesia), cardiac injury and tumors, cardiomyopathies (both dilated and hypertrophic), myocarditis, acidosis, and hypoxia. PVCs are more common in pediatric patients with congenital heart disease, prolonged QT syndrome, and mitral valve prolapse (Doninger & Sharieff, 2006).

In the absence of congenital heart disease, pediatric patients with isolated, unifocal PVCs require no therapy. Multifocal and frequent PVCs—particularly those precipitated by activity—can be more serious, especially in the pediatric patient with congenital heart disease. These patients are at higher risk for hemodynamic decompensation and for developing lethal rhythms, and need more careful monitoring and ongoing assessment.

Management of PVCs should be geared toward correcting the underlying cause, such as an electrolyte imbalance, hypoxia, or acidosis. Patients who are especially vulnerable to hemodynamic compromise should receive swift therapeutic intervention consisting of intravenous (IV) lidocaine at 1 mg/kg/dose, followed by a lidocaine infusion at 20–50 mcg/kg/min (Doninger & Sharieff, 2006). Pediatric patients who are refractory to lidocaine may require amiodarone, procainamide, or beta blockade.

Ventricular tachycardia

Ventricular tachycardia (VT) is a wide-complex tachycardia defined as a series of three or more PVCs with a heart rate between 120 and 200 bpm, but usually less than 250 bpm (Hanisch, 2001). VT can be nonsustained, lasting 9 seconds or less, or sustained, lasting 10 seconds or longer (Figure 22-15). The QRS complexes that make up ventricular tachycardia can be unifocal or multifocal. A distinct form of multifocal or polymorphic VT known as torsades de pointes (twisting of the points) is characterized by "undulating QRS complexes that appear to be spiraling around an axis" (Hanisch, p. 356) (Figure 22-16).

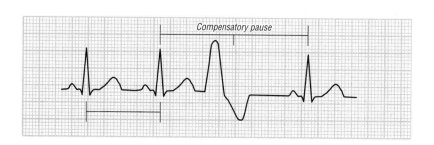

FIGURE 22-14

Premature Ventricular Contraction (PVC).

Source: Garcia, T., & Holtz, N. (2001). 12-Lead ECG. Sudbury, MA: Jones & Bartlett.

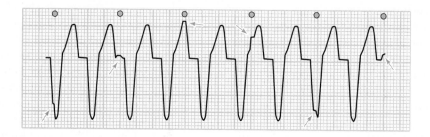

FIGURE 22-15

Ventricular Tachycardia (VT).

Source: Garcia, T., & Holtz, N. (2001). 12-Lead ECG. Sudbury, MA: Jones & Bartlett.

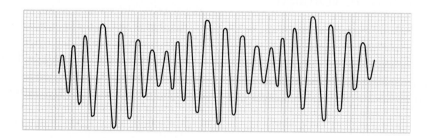

FIGURE 22-16

Torsades de Pointes.

Source: Garcia, T., & Holtz, N. (2001). 12-Lead ECG. Sudbury, MA: Jones & Bartlett.

The causes of VT are similar to those of PVC. Pediatric patients who have undergone cardiac surgery—particularly procedures involving a right ventriculotomy—are at increased risk for early and late postoperative VT. Torsades de pointes can be caused by drugs or chemicals that prolong the QT interval such as antiarrhythmics, tricyclic antidepressants, certain antibiotics (macrolides), and organophosphate insecticides (Park, 2008).

Ventricular tachycardia can lead to significant hemodynamic compromise and quickly deteriorate to ventricular fibrillation. For this reason, wide-complex tachycardias must be assumed to be ventricular tachycardia until proven otherwise, and investigative measures should not be delayed. Reversible causes of VT should be treated as quickly as possible, while assessing the stability of the patient. The acute management of VT in the hemodynamically unstable or unconscious pediatric patient must focus on prompt termination of the arrhythmia with synchronized cardioversion of 0.5 to 1 J/kg. Pulseless VT necessitates immediate defibrillation at 2 to 4 J/kg. In the rare instance of uncontrollable VT, extracorporeal membrane oxygenation (ECMO; described later in this chapter) may be required (Hanisch, 2001). Conscious, hemodynamically stable pediatric patients should receive IV lidocaine of 1 mg/kg/dose over 1 to 2 minutes, followed by an IV infusion of lidocaine at 20–50 mcg/kg/min.

Standard therapy for torsades de pointes is directed at shortening the QT interval by increasing the heart rate through the use of cardiac pacing or isoproterenol infusion. Hemodynamically unstable pediatric patients with torsades de pointes should be treated with IV magnesium.

The treatment of documented or suspected VT in pediatric patients with congenital heart disease has moved away from medication therapy and toward the use of implantable defibrillators and ablation procedures (Walsh, 2007). An implantable cardioverter–defibrillator (ICD) is indicated in patients with cardiomyopathy, long QT syndrome, and life-threatening VT, and in resuscitated patients following sudden cardiac death (Hanisch, 2001).

Ventricular fibrillation

Ventricular fibrillation (VF) is an uncommon pediatric arrhythmia that results from an erratic firing of multiple foci within the ventricles, leading to death if not immediately recognized and treated. On ECG, it is characterized by a bizarre, wavy ventricular pattern with varying sizes and configurations of the QRS complex (Figure 22-17). Causes of VF include hypoxia, hyperkalemia, digoxin or quinidine toxicity, myocardial infarction, myocarditis, or complications from cardiothoracic surgery for congenital heart disease (Park, 2008). Acute management involves immediate CPR and defibrillation following PALS guidelines.

DISTURBANCES OF ATRIOVENTRICULAR CONDUCTION

Atrioventricular conduction disorders (also known as AV block) occur when there is a disturbance between the normal sinus impulse and the ventricle's response to that impulse, whether it be by conduction delay or incomplete conduction. AV block can be either congenital or acquired. These conduction abnormalities are classified based on their severity as either first degree (the least severe), second degree, or third degree (the most severe and extreme form of AV block).

First-degree AV block

First-degree AV block is described as a prolongation of the PR interval due to an abnormal delay in conduction through the AV node. The pediatric patient remains in normal sinus rhythm with a P wave present before each QRS complex, while the QRS complex is normal in duration and appearance (Figure 22-18). There is 1:1 conduction with no dropped beats. Although first-degree AV block can occur in healthy children, it is more commonly seen in pediatric patients with rheumatic fever, cardiomyopathies, and certain types of congenital heart disease such as atrial septal defect, endocardial cushion defect, and Ebstein's anomaly.

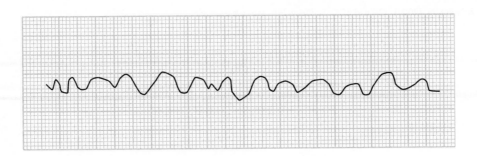

FIGURE 22-17

Ventricular Fibrillation (VF).

Source: Garcia, T., & Holtz, N. (2001). 12-Lead ECG. Sudbury, MA: Jones & Bartlett.

First-degree AV block is a sign of digoxin toxicity, which is the most common cause of this condition in pediatric patients. Patients with first-degree heart block typically are hemodynamically stable and asymptomatic. Therapeutic management, except in patients with digoxin toxicity, is not required (Park, 2008). Lyme disease should be a consideration when the PR interval is greater than 280 seconds.

Second-degree AV block

In pediatric patients with second-degree AV block, some (but not all) P waves are followed by QRS complexes, resulting in dropped beats. There are several types of second-degree AV block, the most common of which are Mobitz type I block and Mobitz type II.

Mobitz type I. Mobitz type I AV block, also known as the Wenckebach phenomenon, has a characteristic pattern in which the PR interval becomes progressively prolonged until one QRS complex is eventually dropped, resulting in a missed beat (Figure 22-19). Causes of this subtype of second-degree AV block include congenital heart disease, myocarditis, myocardial infarction, cardiomyopathies, and drug toxicity (digoxin, beta blockers, calcium-channel blockers, quinidine). In addition, this condition may occur in patients following cardiac surgery. Mobitz type I AV block can also occur in otherwise healthy children (Doninger & Sharieff, 2006). Mobitz type I block occurs

at the level of the AV node, may reflect dysfunction of the AV node, and usually does not progress to complete heart block (Park, 2008). Management of this variant AV block is directed at treating the underlying cause when applicable, as in cases of drug toxicity. Therapy is often unnecessary, as second-degree AV block does not compromise hemodynamic stability (Park).

Mobitz type II. Mobitz type II AV block has a distinct characteristic pattern in which there is either normal AV conduction with a normal PR interval or the conduction is completely blocked, giving rise to a ventricular rate that depends solely on the number of normally conducted atrial impulses (Figure 22-20). Mobitz type II AV block occurs at the level of the bundle of His, and its causes are the same as the causes of Mobitz type I AV block. Although therapy also focuses on the causes of this type of AV block, prophylactic pacemaker therapy is always a consideration in asymptomatic patients because of the higher likelihood of progression to complete heart block. In pediatric patients who are symptomatic with Mobitz type II AV block, pacemaker therapy is indicated (Hanisch, 2001).

Third-degree AV block

In third-degree AV block, also known as complete heart block, there is complete failure of conduction from the atrial impulses to the ventricles, leading to the atria and

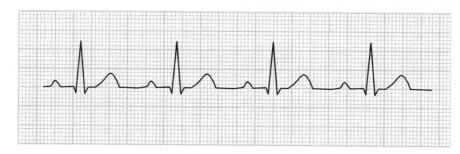

FIGURE 22-18

First-Degree Heart Block.

Source: Garcia, T., & Holtz, N. (2001). 12-Lead ECG. Sudbury, MA: Jones & Bartlett.

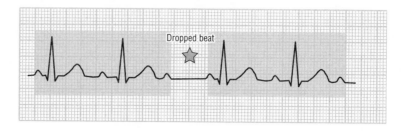

FIGURE 22-19

Mobitz I Second-Degree Heart Block (Wenckebach).

Source: Garcia, T., & Holtz, N. (2001). 12-Lead ECG. Sudbury, MA: Jones & Bartlett.

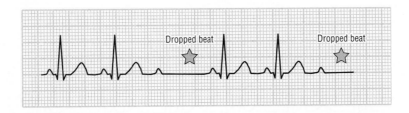

FIGURE 22-20

Mobitz II Second-Degree Heart Block.

Source: Garcia, T., & Holtz, N. (2001). 12-Lead ECG. Sudbury, MA: Jones & Bartlett.

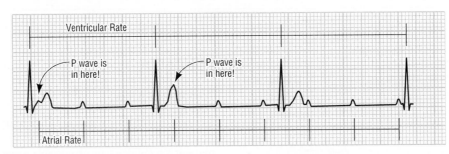

FIGURE 22-21

Third-Degree Heart Block.

Source: Garcia, T., & Holtz, N. (2001). 12-Lead ECG. Sudbury, MA: Jones & Bartlett.

ventricles beating independently from each other. On ECG, the P waves appear regular, with a normal PP interval for the pediatric patient's age. The QRS complexes are also regular, with a normal RR interval, but at a much slower rate than would be expected given the pediatric patient's age (Figure 22-21). This type of AV block may be either congenital (with or without structural heart disease) or acquired.

In the congenital type of complete heart block (CHB), causes can include maternal lupus erythematosus and certain congenital heart defects such as L-transposition (Keene et al., 2006). The QRS duration and impulse appear normal, but the ventricular rate is higher than expected, at 50 to 80 bpm (Park, 2008). Acquired cases of temporary or permanent CHB most often result as a complication from various cardiac surgical procedures. Disruption of ventricular structures, such as a repair of a ventricular septal defect (VSD) and tetralogy of Fallot, or an inflammatory disease such as rheumatic fever or Lyme disease, may also lead to CHB. In acquired CHB, the QRS duration is prolonged and the ventricular rate is slower, at 40 to 50 bpm, giving the appearance of a PVC.

Clinical concerns related to CHB stem from low cardiac output if the ventricular rate is low, with symptoms including fatigue, dizziness, syncope, and exercise intolerance. Infants may present with severe CHF. For symptomatic pediatric patients diagnosed with congenital CHB, permanent pacemaker therapy is indicated (Hanisch, 2001). Postoperative pediatric patients with surgically induced

CHB are managed by temporary AV sequential pacing, and permanent pacemaker therapy is viewed as an indication when heart block persists for more than 7 days (Walsh, 2007). National practice guidelines that specify the indications for permanent pacemaker therapy for pediatric patients are published and updated regularly by the AHA and American College of Cardiology (ACC) (Epstein et al., 2008).

LONG QT SYNDROME

Long QT syndrome (LQTS), also known as prolonged QT syndrome, is a disorder of delayed ventricular repolarization that is characterized by prolongation of the QT interval on ECG (Figure 22-22). When measured manually in lead II, a worrisome corrected QT interval (QTc) is greater than 0.46 second, with the upper limit of normal being 0.44 second (Park, 2008). T-wave formation frequently appears abnormal, with the waves being notched or biphasic. Note that the diagnosis of LQTS is not based on ECG findings alone, but rather is made in conjunction with specific signs and symptoms and a careful family history. Long QT syndrome can be either congenital or acquired.

Patients with the eventual diagnosis of LQTS may present, at any age, with seizures or syncope along with ECG findings as previously described. Other signs and symptoms include palpitations, dizziness, and even cardiac arrest, with the majority of symptoms coinciding with exercise,

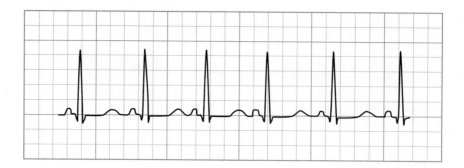

FIGURE 22-22

Long QT Syndrome.

emotion, or sudden auditory stimuli (alarm, doorbell). Understandably, these symptoms can be confused with vasovagal syncope or seizures, underscoring the importance of an ECG as part of the initial evaluation for a pediatric patient with these presenting symptoms. Family history is an essential component of the evaluation. As many as 60% of patients with this arrhythmia have a positive family history for LQTS or premature, sudden death and 5% have an associated hearing deficit (Hanisch, 2001; Park, 2008).

More than seven distinct gene defects can cause LQTS (Keene et al., 2006). One of these causes is Jervell and Lange-Nielsen syndrome, which is associated with congenital deafness and is an autosomal recessive form; by comparison, Romano-Ward syndrome is an autosomal dominant form that is not associated with deafness. All blood relatives of patients with congenital LQTS, regardless of symptoms, should have a screening ECG.

Causes of acquired LQTS can include medications such as some antibiotics, antidepressants, and antipsychotics; electrolyte disturbances such as hypokalemia, hypocalcemia, and hypomagnesemia; and medical conditions such as hypothyroidism, anorexia nervosa, and head trauma (Park, 2008).

Management is individualized, but is directed at reducing sympathetic activity of the heart with surgical or pharmacologic therapy. Pharmacologic management typically begins with beta blockade using propranolol (2–4 mg/kg/day) or atenolol (0.5 mg/kg/day) (Doniger & Shareiff, 2006). Surgical therapy consists of either the placement of a demand cardiac pacemaker, ICD implantation, or left cardiac sympathetic denervation surgery. Pacemaker therapy and ICD placement are considered for patients at high risk, who have experienced a previous cardiac arrest, or who have failed medication therapy (Hanisch, 2001). Acute management for the pediatric patient with LQTS presenting with ventricular tachycardia or torsades de pointes consists of IV magnesium (25–50 mg/kg, maximum 2 gm); the HCP must also obtain serum electrolytes and a toxicology screen.

PACEMAKER THERAPY

Temporary pacing

The use of temporary pacing is necessary in certain pediatric patients after cardiac surgery, in patients with failed permanent pacemakers awaiting replacement, in patients with temporary or reversible second- or third-degree heart block, and in patients with symptomatic bradycardia. Several types of temporary pacemaking modalities exist—namely, esophageal, epicardial, and transcutaneous.

Esophageal pacing is used mainly to diagnose and terminate SVT.

Epicardial pacing is used in pediatric patients after cardiac surgery. Temporary pacing wires are placed on the epicardial surface of the heart in the operating room prior to chest closure, and can be used for temporary pacing and for aiding in the diagnosis of atrial arrhythmias (Jowett et al., 2007). These wires must be carefully labeled and secured in a way that can allow immediate access to them in emergency situations (Figure 22-23). Atrial wires emerge from the chest in a rightward position, while ventricular wires emerge from the chest toward the left of the pediatric patient's chest. Care must be used when removing epicardial pacing wires in postoperative patients, due to the risk of bleeding and cardiac tamponade. When Jowett et al. (2007) studied the ideal time for removal of epicardial wires, they found that no patients in normal sinus rhythm for more than 24 hours after surgery required pacing prior to discharge. Their findings suggest that epicardial pacing wires may be safely removed after 24 hours in patients in normal sinus rhythm after surgery.

Transcutaneous pacing is achieved with self-adhesive anteroposterior electrode pads and a pulse generator. This technique is useful in emergency settings because it does not require central access, is noninvasive, can be done rapidly, and requires little training (Timothy & Rodeman, 2004).

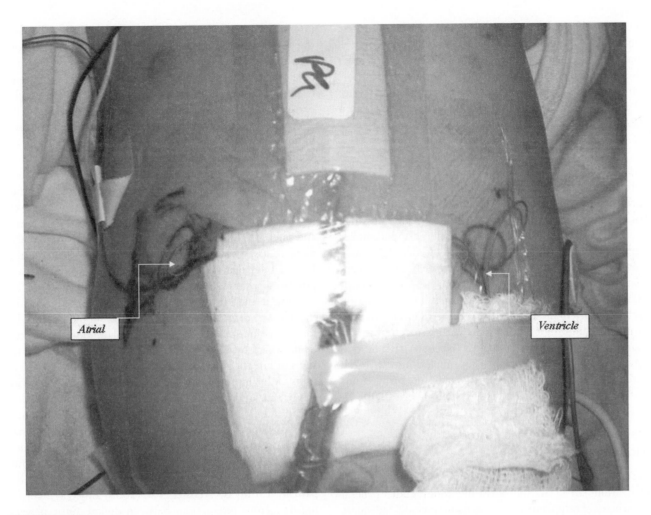

FIGURE 22-23

Location of Epicardial Pacemaker Wires.

Source: Courtesy of Patricia Lawrence.

Types of permanent pacemakers and defibrillators

A permanent pacemaker is a battery-operated device that delivers electrical stimuli to the heart through leads that can be placed either transvenously or directly onto the epicardium (Figure 22-23). Batteries last for 3 to 15 years depending on the device used. Fortunately, as device and lead sizes have become smaller and as technological capabilities have improved, there has been a trend toward less restrictive permanent pacer indications in pediatric patients (Silka & Bar-Cohen, 2006). National guidelines specify the indications for permanent pacemaker therapy for pediatric patients (Epstein et al., 2008).

Patient size, weight, growth potential, and coexisting complex congenital heart defects present the biggest challenges for pacemaker therapy in pediatric patients. Lead implantation considerations must also be considered when selecting device implantation. Leads may be epicardial or transvenous. Pediatric patients with scarring from repeated cardiac surgical interventions may have poorly suited lead attachment points for epicardial placement (Walsh, 2007). Transvenous lead wires may be outgrown in children, yet are advantageous because of the lack of lead fractures and the need for lower pacing thresholds compared to epicardial wires (Keene et al., 2006).

Types of pacemakers.   Pacemakers can be single- or dual-chamber devices, and may offer numerous programming features. A generic letter code has been devised by the North American Society of Pacing and Electrophysiology (NASPE) and British Pacing and Electrophysiology Group (BPEG) to allow for a common language in describing the types and functions of pacemakers. The letter in the first position stands for the chamber paced, the letter in the second position stands for the chamber sensed, and the third letter stands for the response of the device to an intrinsic cardiac event (Table 22-11). The choice of pacemaker mode (Table 22-12) in the pediatric patient is based on many factors, including anatomy and the system's ability to ensure AV synchrony, which is preferred when possible. More recently, cardiac pacing has been used to improve the quality of life in pediatric patients with congenital heart disease, and in heart failure patients as a bridge to heart transplantation (Villain, 2008). A multicenter review of 73 patients with CHD who underwent resynchronization therapy demonstrated a mean increase in systemic ventricular ejection of 12% (Dubin et al., 2005).

Implantable cardioverter–defibrillator. The implantable defibrillator, also known as an ICD, has been a valuable therapy option for pediatric patients with sustained ventricular arrhythmias, and those at risk for sudden cardiac death. While the ICD is larger than most pacemaker devices (because larger batteries are needed for shock energy), the reduction in hardware size of ICDs in recent years has allowed for their greater use in the pediatric population (Keene et al.). Indications for ICD implantation include aborted sudden cardiac death, spontaneous sustained VT, and high-risk patients with hypertrophic cardiomyopathy or congenital LQTS (Keene et al.). Several routes of ICD placement are used, including epicardial patch systems, pericardial ICD lead systems, transvenous systems, and subcutaneous array systems (Berul, 2008).

Operative placement and postoperative care: pacemakers and ICDs

Pacemaker generators and ICDs can be placed in the catheterization lab or in the operating room under general anesthesia. Postoperative management includes adequate pain control and mitigation of the side effects from general anesthesia. Temporary feeding intolerance may be seen in infants whose intraperitoneal pacemaker devices lie over the stomach. Toddlers and older children are often troubled by surgical site pain, because tissue stretching occurs to accommodate placement of these devices. Most patients receive prophylactic antibiotic therapy at the time of device placement for 48 hours post-device implantation (Selke et al., 2005). Duration of prophylactic antibiotics depends on surgeon preference, but should be used judiciously, given the increase in drug-resistant organisms.

The most common complication in the early postoperative period is lead malfunction and/or dislodgement; thus patients should receive telemetry monitoring while recovering from this surgery (Selke et al., 2005). A posteroanterior and lateral CXR should be obtained the day after placement to assess lead and generator positions (Selke et al.). Device interrogation and final settings should occur just prior to discharge.

Patient and family education prior to discharge should include care of the incision. The wound should be kept dry for at least one week after device implantation and should be inspected by the pediatric patient or family regularly for signs of infection (Selke et al., 2005). Education related to signs and symptoms of infection is critical to discuss with the patient and family, as this is the most common complication following device placement. Pain should improve each postoperative day, and adequate pain control may need to continue after discharge. The type of pacemaker placed and final device settings used should be communicated to the patient, family, and all HCPs caring for the patient. A study by Webster et al. (2008) aimed at identifying dangerous interactions between digital music players, pacemakers, and ICDs concluded that while there was no interference between the function of ICDs or pacemakers and digital music players, there was interference during device interrogation. Thus digital music players should not be used during interrogation, but can otherwise be safely operated by pediatric patients with pacemakers and ICDs.

Device implantation complications occur in fewer than 2% of patients. Early procedural complications may include bleeding, infection, pneumothorax, tamponade, and pocket hematoma (Selke et al., 2005). Late complications may include device pocket or lead infections, lead fracture, migration of the generator, and pocket skin erosion. When revisions are necessary, they are often related to device battery depletion or lead failure. Some patients will require device upgrades as their clinical condition changes.

TABLE 22-11

Pacemaker Codes		
First Letter: Chamber Paced	**Second Letter: Chamber Sensed**	**Third Letter: Sensed Response**
V: Ventricle	V: Ventricle	D: Dual (trigger and inhibit pacing)
A: Atrium	A: Atrium	I: Inhibit pacing
D: Dual (A and V)	D: Dual (A and V)	O: None
O: None	O: None	

TABLE 22-12

Pacemaker Modes				
AAI	**VVI**	**DDD**	**DVI**	**AOO**
Atrial demand pacing	Ventricular demand pacing	Atrial/ventricular demand pacing, senses and paces both chambers; trigger or inhibit	Atrial/ventricular pacing, senses ventricle only; pacing inhibited by ventricular rate only	Atrial asynchronous pacing

Follow-up with the primary cardiologist or electro-physiology specialist should occur within one month of device placement. The primary cardiologist should be alerted to sudden, unexpected pain, as it could be a sign of infection. The patient and family should also alert the cardiologist if the patient experiences episodes of syncope, dizziness, chest pain, or shortness of breath, as any of these symptoms can be related to lead or device malfunction (Silka & Bar-Cohen, 2006).

Long-term prognosis

In 2007, a study of the long-term outcomes after epicardial pacemaker insertion in neonates and infants concluded that modern pacemaker therapy was safe and effective with low morbidity and rare complications (Aellig et al., 2007).

CARDIAC TRANSPLANTATION

Katheryn Gambetta

The first pediatric heart transplant was performed in1967 by Dr. Adrian Kantrowitz three days after the first adult heart transplant was performed. Since then, the field of heart transplantation has made great strides in immunosuppression, management of the donor and recipient, surgical transplantation techniques, and detection and treatment of complications of heart transplantation, which have given heart transplant recipients hope, a longer survival, and an improved quality of life. Between 1982 and 2007, 8,058 heart transplants in pediatric patients (age younger than 18 years) were reported (Kirk et al., 2009). This section provides an update on conditions that lead to heart transplantation, the stages of the heart transplantation process (preoperative, operative, and postoperative), the complications of heart transplantation, and the long-term management of heart transplant recipients.

EPIDEMIOLOGY AND ETIOLOGY

Heart transplantation is performed for pediatric patients with end-stage heart failure refractory to medical therapy and for children with congenital heart disease that is not amenable for surgical palliation. Approximately 25% of all pediatric heart transplants are performed in infants younger than 1 year of age, with the remainder divided between the 1- to 10-year age group and the greater than 10-year age group (Boucek et al., 2006). For infants younger than 1 years old, the most common reason for heart transplantation is a congenital heart defect (63%), followed by cardiomyopathy (31%). However, in older children aged 1 to 10 years, the reverse becomes true, with cardiomyopathy (55%) predominating over congenital heart defects (36%)

as the reason for heart transplant. In adolescents aged 11 to 17 years, 64% were transplanted for cardiomyopathy and 24% for congenital heart disease. The retransplantation rate has remained approximately 6% for children between 1 and 10 years of age and 7% for children between 11 and 17 years of age (Kirk et al., 2009).

There are no established criteria for heart transplantation in children. Because of the relatively smaller number of pediatric patients who are potential candidates for heart transplantation and because of their diversity of diagnosis and pathology, it has been difficult to establish guidelines. In the past, consensus guidelines regarding the indications for pediatric heart transplantation have been relatively broad:

- Need for ongoing intravenous inotropic or mechanical circulatory support
- Complex congenital heart disease not amenable to conventional surgical palliation or repair or where the surgical procedure carries a higher short- and mid-term risk of mortality than transplantation
- Progressive deterioration of ventricular function or functional status despite optimal medical care with digitalis, diuretics, or angiotensin-converting enzyme (ACE) inhibitors, plus beta blockade
- Malignant arrhythmia or survival after cardiac arrest that is unresponsive to medical treatment, catheter ablation, or an automatic implantable defibrillator
- Progressive pulmonary hypertension secondary to systemic ventricular failure that may preclude cardiac transplantation later
- Growth failure secondary to severe CHF unresponsive to conventional medical treatment
- Unacceptably poor quality of life secondary to heart failure
- Progressive deterioration in functional status or the presence of certain high-risk conditions following the Fontan procedure (Hsu et al., 2007).

The AHA recently reaffirmed the earlier guidelines and added restrictive cardiomyopathy (associated with reactive pulmonary hypertension) as an indication for heart transplantation (Canter et al., 2007).

The U.S. national transplant system was established following the National Organ Transplant Act of 1984. This legislation mandated the creation of the Organ Procurement and Transplantation Network (OPTN). Under the OPTN contract, United Network of Organ Sharing (UNOS) maintains information on all individuals listed in the United States as needing organ transplants. As donated organs become available, the OPTN system matches them with the most suitable candidates. The process of organ donor identification is required in all hospitals and the management of organ donors is regulated by government-regulated local agencies called Organ Procurement Organizations (OPOs). OPOs coordinate organ procurement in designated service areas, evaluate potential donors, discuss donation with family members, arrange for the surgical removal and preservation of donated organs, and arrange for their distribution according to national organ-sharing policies. The distributions of organs is guided by a patient's medical urgency, blood type, size match with the donor, time on the waiting list, and proximity to the donor.

PRETRANSPLANT

Once a child is being considered for heart transplantation, an extensive evaluation (Table 22-13) is conducted by an interdisciplinary team consisting of transplant cardiologists, social workers, medical psychologists/psychiatrists, and other medical subspecialists. During this evaluation process, careful assessment is performed to determine whether the child meets appropriate indications for transplantation, to identify and treat potentially reversible causes of the child's end-stage heart failure, and to ascertain if any problematic issues or risks might affect the child's posttransplant outcome or even preclude candidacy for heart transplantation.

Cardiac catheterization is often performed to delineate cardiac anatomy and assess hemodynamics. Importantly, cardiac catheterization can assess pulmonary vascular resistance and reactivity of the pulmonary vascular bed. Pulmonary vascular resistance, which is usually indexed to body surface area (PVRI), is of paramount importance prior to listing a patient as a candidate for heart transplantation. A PVRI greater than 6 Wood units/m^2 or a transpulmonary gradient greater than 15 mmHg has previously been considered a contraindication for transplantation secondary to potential donor right ventricular failure upon implantation of the donor heart (Gajarski et al., 1994). Children found to have a PVRI greater than 6 Wood units/m^2 must undergo evaluation of their pulmonary vascular reactivity—an examination that can be performed with administration of 100% O_2 or administration of a pulmonary vasodilator such as nitric oxide. Elevated PVRI with a nonreactive pulmonary vascular bed is considered more important in determining suitability for orthotopic heart transplantation; a heterotopic heart transplant or heart lung transplant may be considered as an option in such situations (Khaghani et al., 1997). In addition, if elevated PVRI is found, treatment with pulmonary vasodilators or intravenous afterload reduction can be initiated.

A comprehensive history and physical examination of the patient is mandatory, with data collected including age, height, weight, and body surface area. A thorough laboratory assessment of kidney, hepatic, and pulmonary function is necessary because irreversible dysfunction can potentially preclude the child from consideration for heart transplantation. Consultation with other medical specialties such as pulmonary, nephrology, and gastrointestinal disorders may be considered as well. An extensive infectious disease

TABLE 22-13

General Components of Pretransplant Recipient Evaluation

Cardiac Assessment

- Echocardiograph
- Electrocardiograph
- Cardiac catheterization
- MRI/MRA or CT
- Exercise testing

Assessment of End-Organ Function

- Kidney function
- Liver function
- Pulmonary function testing
- Lipid profile

Infectious Disease Exposure

- Viral serologies
- Cytomegalovirus titers
- Epstein-Barr virus titers
- Herpes
- HIV-III
- Varicella
- Toxoplasmosis
- Hepatitis panel
- Purified protein derivative for exposure to tuberculosis

Immunological Status

- HLA tissue typing
- Panel reactive antibody
- Determination of isohemagglutinin titers

Hematology

- Complete blood count with differential
- Prothrombin time, partial thromboplastin with international normalized ratio
- Fibrinogen

Psychosocial

- Assessment of family dynamics, coping strategies, and support network
- Psychiatric evaluation if indicated

Financial

- Insurance and resource evaluation

Magnetic resonance imaging/angiography (MRI/MRA), computed tomography (CT), human immunodeficiency virus (HIV), human leukocyte antigen (HLA).

evaluation is necessary to exclude active infection and to determine potential latent infection with organisms such as Epstein-Barr virus (EBV) or cytomegalovirus (CMV). An accurate and documented blood type is one of the primary and critical components that determines donor recipient matching.

Evaluation of the immune system is an integral part of the pretransplantation evaluation. Each candidate should undergo human leukocyte antigen (HLA) typing. Screening panel reactive antibody (PRA) is performed on all patients before transplantation in an effort to determine the recipient's degree of sensitization. PRA screening tests for the presence of preformed HLA antibodies to a random panel of donor lymphocytes. High PRA titers (greater than 10%) are associated with an increased incidence of antibody-mediated rejection, early graft failure, and reduced survival following cardiac transplantation. Patients with a significantly elevated PRA levels undergo further HLA antibody specification testing in an effort to determine which antibodies the patient has already formed. In such situations, the need for a prospective cross-match or a virtual cross-match prior to acceptance of a donor organ can be determined. In addition, immunization status should be determined through either history or serology, and any incomplete immunizations should be updated according to the child's age.

Finally, a psychosocial evaluation is a critical component of the pretransplant assessment. The recipient, along with his or her family members and members of his or her support system, generally undergo a complete psychosocial evaluation to assess their coping abilities when confronted with the many emotional and physical stresses that transplant recipients inevitably encounter. A strong and reliable support system is vital to help the child go through this process because family members must often have to restructure their daily routines to care for the young child. It is important that both family and child maintain a positive attitude toward mandatory follow-up and medication compliance because failed adherence can lead to rejection. Any risk factors for nonadherence should be determined. Illicit drug use and medical noncompliance may be considered a contraindication to transplantation because these pretransplant behaviors have been associated with poor outcomes. Financial needs and resources of the patient and family should also be evaluated.

An important component of the pretransplant evaluation is to identify factors that may complicate the posttransplant outcome or be significant enough to preclude heart transplantation candidacy. There are no established contraindications for heart transplantation and the list of potential contraindications has changed over the past years. In children with congenital heart disease, the technical issues that arise from unusual anatomy such as abnormal situs, systemic venous abnormalities, anomalous pulmonary venous drainage without stenosis, and some pulmonary artery anomalies are no longer contraindications for transplantation. More generally, potential contraindications to heart transplantation include presence of elevated and nonreactive pulmonary vascular resistance, active uncontrolled infection, ongoing malignancy, irreversible failure of multiple organs, systemic diseases that limit life expectancy, and untreatable metabolic diseases or mitochondrial disorders.

Each candidate listed for heart transplantation is assigned a status code established by UNOS, which corresponds to how medically urgent it is that the candidate receive a heart transplant. Medical urgency is assigned to a heart transplant candidate who is younger than 18 years of age at the time of listing as follows: 1A, 1B, 2, or 7 (UNOS, 2010). Status 1A candidates are the most urgent candidates and must meet one of the following criteria:

- Requires ventilator assistance
- Requires assistance with a mechanical assist device
- Requires assistance with a balloon pump
- Is younger than six months of age with congenital or acquired heart disease exhibiting reactive pulmonary hypertension at more than 50% of the systemic level
- Requires infusion of high-dose inotropes or be on multiple inotropes

A candidate who does not meet these criteria may be listed as status 1A if he or she has a life expectancy without a heart transplant of less than 14 days, such as due to refractory arrhythmia.

The waiting time for donor hearts is unpredictable. Some children may wait for extensive periods of time, during which time the child may rapidly deteriorate or sustain significant end-organ damage. In some situations, end-organ damage can be serious enough to render such children potentially unsuitable candidates for heart transplantation. Death while waiting still occurs. Given these possibilities, management of the pediatric heart transplant candidate requires close vigilance and understanding of the problems inherent to the patient's medical condition, and knowledge of available therapeutic approaches to optimize the child's overall health prior to undergoing the rigors of heart transplantation.

Some children with heart failure may be stable enough to receive outpatient treatment prior to transplant. Medical care for heart failure should be maximized and typically includes optimization of diuretics, afterload-reducing agents (ACE inhibitors), potassium-sparing agents (spironolactone), and beta blockers (metoprolol, carvedilol). All of these agents have been used with some success in improving symptoms and cardiac function in select children. In these instances, frequent visits to the transplant center are required to optimize heart failure management and to preserve end-organ function. Children with elevated pulmonary vascular resistance may be treated with oxygen or pulmonary vasodilators. Right heart catheterization may need to be performed serially to confirm that pulmonary vascular resistance is still within an acceptable range. The nutritional status of the candidate should also be optimized to best prepare the child for transplant surgery, wound healing, and recovery. In addition, physical therapy and exercise suited to the patient's level of debilitation should be prescribed.

Atrial and ventricular arrhythmias are not uncommon in patients with heart failure. Arrhythmias should be treated appropriately, and the use of agents that may have negative inotropic effects must be balanced against the risk of lethal arrhythmias. The placement of an ICD may be considered in some children with severely reduced cardiac function. Adult guidelines recommend placement of prophylactic ICDs for patients with stage C heart failure from ischemic or nonischemic cardiomyopathy and a left ventricular ejection fraction of less than 35% (Dickstein et al., 2008). However, pediatric patients with nonischemic cardiomyopathies awaiting heart transplant are at a lower risk of sudden death.

Children with poor cardiac output and chronic heart failure are at risk for thromboembolism. The poorly contractile heart is also at risk for the development of intracardiac thrombi. Venous or right heart thrombi may embolize to the lungs and result in potentially fatal pulmonary embolus, whereas left heart thrombi may embolize to the systemic circulation and result in renal or neurologic injury. For this reason, anticoagulation with either warfarin or aspirin should be considered in children with severe ventricular dysfunction.

Children with chronic heart failure are also at risk for the development of anemia of chronic disease. Frequent blood draws and poor diet tend to exacerbate such anemia. Severe anemia is not tolerated well in children with severe ventricular dysfunction, such that children may require blood transfusions. If possible, transfusions should be given judiciously to transplant candidates' to avoid the risk of unnecessary exposure to foreign HLA antigens.

Despite aggressive medical management, some children deteriorate while awaiting transplants, to the point that they require hospitalization and intensive care management for treatment of symptoms of worsening cardiac output and hemodynamic compromise. Approximately 72% of pediatric patients are status 1A at the time of transplantation, meaning that they require at least some form of ventilator assistance, need high-dose inotropy, or have a life expectancy of less than 14 days (Duncan et al., 2007).

The Frank-Starling curve describes the relationship between preload and stroke volume. Children with chronic heart failure require meticulous and judicious management of their fluid status, as any derangements in fluid status can adversely affect cardiac output. Children with underfilled ventricles require preload to maximize cardiac output, while children with volume overload require diuretics to decrease preload: Both scenarios can occur in children with heart failure awaiting heart transplantation. The use of a central venous catheter or Swan-Ganz pulmonary catheter allows for estimation of preload. Diuretic therapy with furosemide, metolazone, or chlorothiazide may be instituted if necessary.

Contractility may be augmented by the use of intravenous inotropes. These agents, which are described in depth later in this chapter, are titrated to maximize contractility and decrease afterload, while striving to avoid excessive tachycardia.

An important adjunct to the cardiac support of children with end-stage heart failure is endotracheal intubation and mechanical ventilation—therapies that can decrease the work of breathing and oxygen consumption. In addition, positive-pressure mechanical ventilation can reduce left ventricular afterload and pulmonary edema. Adequate sedation will also decrease oxygen consumption. Mechanical ventilation may aid in the management of pulmonary hypertension by allowing the induction of hypocarbia and facilitation of nitric oxide and high inspired oxygen concentration. Finally, the decrease in respiratory workload with intubation and ventilation may reduce caloric requirements and improve the child's catabolic status. Unfortunately, prolonged intubation may also have deleterious effects. It can lead to bacterial or candidal colonization of airways because the normal host defenses for clearing airways are impaired. Moreover, mechanical ventilation contributes to atrophy of the respiratory muscles.

Children with chronic heart failure may develop end-organ dysfunction because of low cardiac output as heart failure worsens. Elevated serum levels of liver enzymes can reflect the severity of cardiac-induced hepatic venous congestion, although this condition is rarely associated with irreversible cardiac cirrhosis. Children with low cardiac output are also susceptible to compromised kidney dysfunction that is usually reversible after heart transplantation. However, a significant elevation of serum creatinine before transplant (greater than 2 mg/dL) is associated with an increased risk of postoperative kidney failure and death (Duncan et al., 2007). Severe decreases in cardiac output can also lead to intestinal ischemia and the inability to tolerate enteral feeding, especially in the newborn. Such children may require parenteral nutrition and should be routinely treated with intravenous proton pump antagonists as prophylaxis against gastritis and gastric stress ulcers.

Mechanical circulatory support should be considered when low cardiac output results in end-organ dysfunction despite maximal medical therapy. Extracorporeal membrane oxygenation (ECMO) is the most commonly used form of pediatric circulatory support in the United States and has been used successfully as a short-term bridge to transplant (Blume et al., 2006).

Previous sensitization to HLA antibodies can occur following pregnancy, blood transfusions, or prior cardiac surgery, especially those procedures necessitating the placement of homograft material. Elevated PRA titers (greater than 10%) are associated with an increased incidence of rejection and reduced survival post cardiac transplantation (Tambur et al., 2000). The most conservative approach in such cases is to only list patients with the requirement of performing a prospective cross-match prior to donor acceptance. Cross-matching involves reacting serum from the recipient with serum from the potential donor. A positive cross-match reaction suggests that the potential transplant recipient has preexisting anti-donor HLA antibodies and in certain situations will preclude use of that particular donor. Cross-matching is time consuming because the recipient serum must be transported to wherever the donor is located. This also limits the geographic radius within which the donor organ can be harvested. Newer methods are being implemented to allow transplant centers to perform "virtual" cross-matches on donors without obtaining donor serum using the recipient's known anti-HLA antibody specification.

Highly sensitized children should be considered for pretransplant interventions aimed at decreasing the antibody levels. However, there are no uniform protocols to manage patients who have high PRAs prior to transplant. Various strategies have been employed to reduce the level of preformed recipient anti-HLA antibodies, including use of intravenous immunoglobulin (IVIG) as well as agents that inhibit antibody production by B cells. Recently introduced therapies include oral methotrexate, mycophenolate mofetil, oral and intravenous cyclophosphamide, and, in some centers, monthly rituximab or use of plasmapheresis (Duncan et al., 2007). None of these modalities completely eliminates the antibodies associated with a high PRA; but these agents have been observed to lower the antibody titers.

In children who are critically ill and highly sensitized, a negative cross-match may not be achieved. In such a case, the decision must be made as to whether an organ from the first suitable ABO-compatible donor should be used regardless of the cross-match results. These highly sensitized candidates may be managed with plasma exchange intraoperatively and postoperatively in combination with a specialized post-transplantation immunosuppression regimen. Despite these measures, children with these characteristics may still be at increased risk for humoral rejection and the early development of allograft vasculopathy. Longitudinal studies are needed to determine the long-term outcomes of these children.

There is an ongoing shortage of donor organs for pediatric recipients, and this shortage is one of the main limitations to the use of heart transplantation as a modality to treat end-stage heart failure. In the United States, pediatric donors have represented a declining percentage (14%) of all organ donors in the past decade (Sweet et al., 2006). Because of this shortage, many efforts have been made to increase public awareness and to optimize donor resuscitation, management, and allocation techniques. Increasing the number of potential donors remains an important goal to ensure that all sick children in need of a new heart have that second chance. More recently, use of non-heart-beating donation as an additional source of donors for both adults and children has drawn increased attention.

Once a potential heart donor has been identified, contraindications to accepting the donor organ must be determined. These conditions include significant cardiac dysfunction or congenital heart disease, transmissible diseases, or malignancies except for primary tumors of the central nervous system (Alkhaldi et al., 2006). Cardiac anatomy and function in the donor is assessed by echocardiography and 12-lead ECG. Serum enzyme markers such as troponin I and creatine phosphokinase–MB fraction can be evaluated for evidence of myocardial injury. In addition, for male donors older than 40 years of age and female donors older than 45 years of age, coronary angiography is usually performed in the donor hospital to determine whether the donor has any preexisting coronary artery disease. Once a potential donor has been accepted, the next step is to match the donor with a suitable heart transplant candidate.

Donor blood type, size, and age; donor mechanism of death; degree of inotropic support; and ischemic time are all important considerations when assessing the suitability of a donor organ for any transplant recipient. The current standard in cardiac transplantation has been to match a recipient with a donor who has a compatible ABO blood type. In a series of pediatric patients, donor gender did not appear to predict post-transplant outcome. Although the mechanism is unclear, advanced-age donor hearts greater than 40 years appear to carry significantly higher one-year post-transplant mortality than use of younger donor hearts (Chin et al., 1999). Because of this finding, UNOS now specifies that adolescent donor hearts should be preferentially allocated to adolescent recipients (UNOS, 2010).

The size of the donor can also affect the post-transplant outcome. Recent reports suggest that donor-to-recipient weight ratios of less than 0.5 and more than 2.5 are associated with a significantly increased risk of one-year mortality in pediatric heart transplant recipients (Boucek et al., 2006). The problems encountered with a graft when the weight ratio is greater than 2.5 include a higher incidence of delayed chest closure, transient lobar collapse, and greater left ventricle mass index (Razzouk et al., 2005).

Domestic trauma and asphyxia are the most common causes of brain death in pediatric donors. Brain death is associated with many complex processes that include hemodynamic, neuroendocrine, and metabolic physiologic derangements; these conditions can detrimentally affect heart function, especially the function of the right ventricle. In a potential donor, the goal is to maintain ventricular function and prevent further myocardial ischemia. Inotropic support may be required to maintain donor cardiac function. High-dose inotropic support is not an absolute contraindication for heart donation, but it must be placed in the context of other factors such as length of donor cardiopulmonary resuscitation, age of donor, donor left ventricle ejection fraction, potential complexity of the recipient transplant operation, and presence of elevated pulmonary vascular resistance in the recipient. Hormonal resuscitation using vasopressin, thyroid hormone, steroids, and insulin is frequently employed to optimize donor cardiac function and contractility. Pediatric recipients with allografts obtained from donors with long periods of time from brain injury to declaration of brain death or from death to organ removal appear to have significantly improved freedom from rejection but no difference in overall survival (Odim et al., 2005).

After the donor heart has been procured, it is stored in a cardioplegia solution and then cooled and prepared for transport to the recipient hospital. In multicenter studies, donor ischemic times of more than 4 hours using current organ preservation techniques have been shown to be a risk factor for reduced short- and long-term survival in adult heart transplant recipients. In pediatric transplantation, however, difficulty of obtaining hearts has led many centers to consider the use of donor organs with longer ischemic times. Several studies have demonstrated that donor ischemic times exceeding 4 hours do not correlate with long-term cardiac function or primary graft failure. In contrast, a smaller study of 165 pediatric heart transplant recipients did find a relationship between donor ischemic times and primary graft failure; even so, the patients with primary graft failure did survive with aggressive management, so there was no overall effect on mortality. Nevertheless, current practices still reflect the consensus that ischemic times up to 6 hours may be tolerated depending on additional factors such as recipient pulmonary vascular resistance, the complexity of the reconstruction at implantation, and the extent of expected bleeding in complex reoperations.

Organ donors of appropriate size for infants have always been limited. In addition, infant heart transplant candidates are at greater risk for death before transplantation than older recipients. However, humoral responses are not effective in early infancy, and this phenomenon has clear advantages in heart transplantation. Newborns do not produce isohemagluttinins, and the complement system is not fully developed immediately after birth. Isohemagluttins to nonself A and/or B antigens remain absent until a child reaches approximately 4 to 6 months of age. ABO-incompatible heart transplants have been performed in infants younger than 1 year old and occasionally older children (West et al., 2001). Infants who receive an ABO-incompatible graft do not develop antibodies against the incompatible blood group from the donor, but do make antibodies normally to other incompatible blood groups. The advantage of ABO-incompatible transplantation is a reduction in waiting time and waiting list mortality by expanding the pool of eligible donors for these infants. Ten-year follow-up of the largest single-center cohort revealed no differences in survival, rejection, kidney dysfunction, allograft vasculopathy, or post-transplant lymphoproliferative disorder between ABO-compatible and ABO-incompatible transplants in newborns (Dipchand et al., 2009).

TRANSPLANT

The surgical approach to be used in cardiac transplant is determined prior to transplantation and depends on many factors, such as the size of the child, cardiac position, atrial arrangement, systemic venous anatomy, and pulmonary venous anatomy. In some children with congenital heart disease, portions of the right and left pulmonary arteries, aorta, inferior vena cava, or brachiocephalic veins may need to be harvested from the donor to help reconstruct anastomoses within the recipient. This surgery is usually planned before the transplantation.

A variety of surgical approaches are used for heart transplantation. *Orthotopic* heart transplantation typically occurs via the biatrial technique or the bicaval technique. The biatrial technique involves anastomoses of the donor and recipient aorta, pulmonary arteries, and atrial cuffs. Studies have associated the biatrial technique with higher risk of thrombus formation, arrhythmias, conduction disturbances, and residual atrioventricular valve regurgitation.

In 1991, the bicaval technique was introduced in an attempt to better preserve atrial anatomy. It involves completely excising the right atrium by leaving a 2- to 3-cm cuff around each vena cava. The left atrium is separated, leaving only a small margin of atrial cuff around the pulmonary veins. The interatrial septum is also removed. The donor left atrial cuff is sutured to the pulmonary vein stump and the donor right atrium is kept intact with separate caval anastomoses. Theoretically, the bicaval technique allows maintenance of normal-shaped atria, which may preserve atrial contractility, sinus node function, and atrioventricular valve competence (Sun et al., 2007). In addition, compared to the biatrial technique, the bicaval approach has been associated with fewer tachyarrhythmias, slightly better hemodynamics, less tricuspid regurgitation, lower incidence of pacemaker support, and better exercise tolerance (Aziz et al., 1999).

Heterotopic heart transplantation has not been used frequently in the pediatric population. This surgical technique involves closure of systemic veins of the donor heart, and connection of the donor pulmonary artery to the right atrium of the recipient. The right pulmonary veins are usually closed off connecting the donor left pulmonary veins via an incision to make a cuff, which is then connected to the recipient's left atrium on the side of the right mediastinum. The donor aorta is then connected to the recipient aorta as an end-to-side connection. Indications for which this surgical technique has been used include severe pulmonary hypertension and a significant donor–recipient mismatch where the donor/recipient ratio is less than 75% (Alkhaldi et al., 2006). In patients with irreversible pulmonary hypertension, the donor left ventricle provides the systemic flow while the native right ventricle, which is already accustomed to high pulmonary artery pressures, provides the pulmonary blood flow.

POST-TRANSPLANT

The first 72 hours after heart transplantation are often the most critical period of the transplantation course. It is during this time that the once-ischemic donor heart is reperfused, the new heart is exposed to varying yet often elevated levels of pulmonary vascular resistance, immunosuppression is initiated, and the recipient is subjected to all of the sequelae of a major open heart surgery and CPB. In addition, the transplanted heart is denervated and has an impaired heart rate response, often in the form of a transiently slow sinus or junctional rhythm.

Immediate postoperative management strategies are aimed at maintaining coronary arterial perfusion, systemic blood pressure, and adequate cardiac output. Inotropic support is often required. Most children also benefit from an elevated heart rate initially to overcome diastolic filling abnormalities. Temporary pacing is often employed for this purpose. Stenosis can develop at the sites of systemic venous anastomoses, pulmonary vein anastomoses, pulmonary arterial anastomoses, and aortic arch reconstruction anastomoses. Ideally, these sites should be evaluated in the operating room at the time of the postoperative transesophageal echocardiograph prior to leaving the operating room. Finally, two serious conditions may occur immediately after heart transplantation: primary graft failure and right heart failure with elevated pulmonary vascular resistance.

Primary graft failure

Primary graft failure is defined as severe dysfunction of the cardiac allograft without any anatomic or immunologic cause. It is characterized by the need for mechanical circulatory support or the use of multiple inotropes or vasopressors within the first 24 hours after transplantation. Primary graft failure is the most common cause of death in the first 30 days after transplant and accounts for approximately one-fourth of all cardiac deaths in the pediatric transplant age group (Boucek et al., 2006). Graft failure accounts for 10% of the mortality in recipients undergoing heart transplantation due to hypoplastic left heart syndrome, 5% of the mortality in patients undergoing transplantation for other congenital heart diseases, and 1% of deaths in transplant recipients who do not have congenital heart disease (Frazier et al., 1999).

Risk factors for primary graft failure include both donor and recipient issues. Donor issues may lead to poor donor quality as manifested by decreased left ventricular ejection fraction on the donor echocardiograph, requirement of high inotropic support, and elevated blood troponin I level. Other donor issues include prolonged ischemic time, large donor with a donor-to-recipient weight ratio greater than 2.0, small donor with a donor-to-recipient weight ratio less than 1, prolonged donor cardiopulmonary resuscitation times, anoxia as a cause of death, and advanced donor age.

Recipient risk factors include pretransplantation diagnosis of congenital heart disease, previous sternotomy, preexisting elevated pulmonary vascular resistance, pretransplantation need for ECMO, and pretransplantation need for ventilatory support. However, in contrast to the findings with use of ECMO, transplantation in children who were maintained on ventricular assist devices is not associated with a higher risk of graft failure. This difference may be due in part to the stability provided by these devices, which allow for end-organ recovery and more general rehabilitation (Blume et al., 2006; Stiller et al., 2003).

The initial management of primary graft failure incorporates the principles and treatment for children with low cardiac output, including administration of the pharmacologic agents that are commonly used to improve contractility and adjust afterload. If low cardiac output is refractory to these agents, then mechanical circulatory support must be considered. ECMO and ventricular assist devices have been employed in these situations for short durations. Retransplantation is not always practical because of the waiting time required to find a suitable donor. Avoidance of graft failure is the primary goal: Thus donor selection, organ procurement techniques, identification of risk factors, and pretransplant recipient management are crucial.

Right heart failure

Early right heart failure associated with elevated pulmonary vascular resistance is a major cause of mortality after pediatric heart transplant. The donor right ventricle may not be adapted to elevated pulmonary vascular resistances. Thus some degree of right heart failure is common in these patients, especially 3 to 5 days after transplant. Perioperative issues, including ischemia reperfusion, cardioplegia, and surgical trauma, may also impair the function of the donor right heart and lead to donor-related myocardial strain. Moreover, the donor right heart must contend with high afterload immediately during weaning from CPB as well as any preexisting elevated pulmonary vascular resistance in the recipient.

Treatment options include prolonged sedation (sometimes in combination with neuromuscular blockade), avoiding hypercapnia, avoiding hypoxia, maintaining coronary perfusion pressure (by avoiding systemic hypotension), and using pulmonary vasodilators such as inhaled nitric oxide and prostaglandins. Unfortunately, once established, right heart failure may become irreversible. Therefore, proactive prophylactic measurements started immediately after transplantation and before weaning from bypass may be more advantageous than reactive treatment. A preventive strategy consisting of pulmonary vasodilators, phosphodiesterase inhibitors, and use of mechanical assist devices such as ECMO or ventricular assist devices can allow the right heart to recover and adapt to the recipient's habitus.

IMMUNOSUPPRESSION MANAGEMENT

Without adequate immunosuppression, antigens from the allograft or donor heart will be recognized by the recipient's CD4 T cells as foreign, thereby triggering a host response that eventually leads to rejection of the organ. The goal of immunosuppression is to prevent rejection and promote tolerance to foreign antigens. The ideal immunosuppressive agent is one that inhibits alloantigen immune responses, prevents allograft rejection, and is without major adverse effects. Most pediatric programs use a triple-drug regimen in the immediate postoperative period, extending to as long as the first 6 months following transplantation, to prevent rejection. Different regimens may be employed for immunosuppression based on the reason for their use—that is, as induction therapy, maintenance therapy, or therapy for rejection.

Induction immunosuppression

Induction immunosuppression is defined as intensive prophylactic immunotherapy administered in the perioperative period that is not part of maintenance immunotherapy. Immediately after transplant, stimuli such as donor brain death, ischemia/reperfusion, and surgical trauma increase donor antigen expression, thereby augmenting the recipient's immune response. The intense induction therapy is designed to reduce rejection in the early postoperative period when graft dysfunction can be problematic and allow HCPs to delay the introduction of potentially nephrotoxic immunosuppressants. Cytolytic agents available for use as induction therapy include polyclonal antibodies, monoclonal antibodies, and anticytokine receptor antibodies (Table 22-14).

Polyclonal antithymocte antibodies are most commonly used for induction and are directed against numerous B- and T-cell surface antigens. Antithymocyte globulin is a polyclonal antibody preparation derived from the hyperimmune serum of animals inoculated with human thymus lymphocytes. Commercially available preparations include Thymoglobulin, which is prepared using rabbits, and Atgam, which is produced using horses. Administration of either agent leads to prompt lymphocytolysis and impairment of proliferative responses of T cells. Monitoring of T-cell subsets and immune function with flow cytometry may be useful to guide therapy. Polyclonal antithymocyte antibodies have been shown to reduce the incidence of acute rejection and mortality significantly in pediatric heart transplant recipients (Di Filippo et al., 2003; Parisi et al., 2003).

Muromonab (OKT3) is a murine monoclonal antibody preparation that is directed against the epsilon chain of the CD3 molecule, which is a critical component of the T-cell activation cascade. By disrupting T-cell receptors, OKT3

TABLE 22-14

Typical Induction Agents				
Medication	**Brand Name**	**Mechanism**	**Side Effects**	**Suggested Pediatric Dosing**
Polyclonal Antibody Preparations				
Antithymocyte globulin	Thymoglobulin (rabbit ATG)	Targets numerous T- and B-cell surface antigens	Anaphylaxis	1–1.5 mg/kg/day for 3–5 days
	ATGAM (equine ATG)	Same as thymoglobulin		5–25 mg/kg/day for 3–5 days
Monoclonal Antilymphocyte Preparations				
Muromonab (OKT3)	Orthoclonal OKT3	Targets CD3 receptors on T cells	Anaphylaxis, cytokine release syndrome	0.1 or 5 mg/kg/day
Monoclonal Anti-IL2R Antibodies				
Basiliximab	Simulect	Chimeric antibody that inhibits activation and clonal expansion	Hypersensitivity	Two doses at 12 mg/m^2 intravenously on postoperative days 0 and 4
Daclizumab	Zenapax	Humanized antibody that inhibits activation and clonal expansion	Hypersensitivity	Five doses at 1 mg/kg intravenously every 14 days

The use of brand name is for product identification purposes only and does not imply endorsement.

renders T cells incapable of responding to an antigen challenge. The incidence of side effects is greater with OKT3 than with polyclonal agents, so relatively few centers now use OKT3 as a means of induction. Many centers use OKT3 to treat hemodynamically significant rejection that is refractory to corticosteroids.

Using these polyclonal and monoclonal antibody preparations is not without risks, and both classes are associated with a host of adverse effects. Additionally, children may suffer from anaphylaxis due to the xenophobic origin of the polyclonal antibody preparations. Symptoms may include fever, chills, rash, diarrhea, or headache. In addition, some children may develop a "cytokine release syndrome" that occurs due to opsonization of the target cells and the subsequent immune response that results in a release of cytokines. This syndrome, which may occur following the first or second dose, is associated with symptoms including headache, nausea, fever, chills, dyspnea, and chest pain. A more serious manifestation is pulmonary edema. Cytokine release syndrome is rare with polyclonal antibody preparations, but occurs more commonly with OKT3. Finally, another side effect that has been observed with OKT3 includes aseptic meningitis. To alleviate possible reactions, patients may be pretreated with antipyretics, antihistamines, steroids, and histamine-2 receptor blockade. In addition, HCPs should be aware that intense immunosuppressive therapy places children at increased risk of infection and malignancies.

Anticytokine receptor antibodies bind the interleukin-2 (IL-2) receptor expressed on antigen-activated T cells, thereby inhibiting proliferation of T cells. Daclizumab is a humanized antibody containing murine antigen-binding sequences. Basiliximab is a chimeric antibody with murine variable regions fused to human immunoglobulin G (IgG) constant regions. These newer agents are attractive because they are specific to T cells, have a longer half-life, carry minimal risk of side effects, and are useful in preventing early rejection. Neither agent has been shown to increase the risk of infection or malignancy.

Intravenous methylprednisone is also initiated as part of induction immunosuppression. Corticosteroids are nonspecific anti-inflammatory agents that act by several mechanisms, including decreasing the release of cytokines and cell-surface molecules that are necessary for inflammation. Corticosteroids upregulate IkB protein synthesis, which binds nuclear factor-kB in the cytoplasm, thereby preventing it from translocating to the nucleus. Corticosteroids also inhibit phospholipase A_2 activity by decreasing the inflammatory response. These agents are used routinely by all transplant centers in the immediate postoperative period, with the goal of discontinuing their use within the first year following transplant (Lindenfield, 2004).

Photophoresis or extracorporeal photochemotherapy (ECP) is a new type of immunomodulatory therapy in which patients' lymphocytes are removed by leukopheresis, treated with methoxalen and ultraviolet A (UVA) light in an extracorporeal system, and then reinfused into the patient. Methoxalen's activity is limited to those cells that are exposed to the UVA. The ECP-treated lymphocytes undergo apoptosis, which also elicits an autologous suppressor response to non-irradiated T cells of similar clones (Wolf et al., 1994). Preliminary adult data indicate that when this technique is combined with the standard triple-drug immunosuppression regimen, rejection may be decreased in the first six months post-transplant and that the development of transplant coronary artery disease may be inhibited (Barr et al., 1998).

Maintenance immunosuppression

Most maintenance immune suppressive regimens include a combination of an antiproliferative agent and a calcineurin inhibitor. A significant number of patients also receive corticosteroids (Table 22-15).

Antiproliferative agents inhibit the pathways leading to purine synthesis and DNA replication, resulting in the prevention of synthesis and proliferation of both T and B lymphocytes. Historically, the most commonly used agent for this purpose was azathioprine, a nonselective inhibitor that caused the undesirable side effect of nonspecific bone marrow suppression. Mycophenolate mofetil (MMF) is a newer antiproliferative agent that is rapidly converted to mycophenolic acid, which selectively inhibits the inosine monophosphate dehydrogenase in the de novo pathway of guanine nucleotide synthesis, thereby impairing proliferation of lymphocytes without producing nonspecific bone marrow suppression. MMF also inhibits antibody production by plasma cells. Monitoring for MMF is performed by measuring mycophenolic acid levels in blood or serum (goal trough levels are in the range of 2.5–5 mcg/mL); however, this testing is not performed often, and most centers rely on leukocyte count instead (Sulemanjee et al., 2008). MMF is rapidly replacing azathioprine in many transplant protocols. Gastrointestinal side effects such as vomiting and diarrhea are common with mycophenolic acid.

Calcineurin inhibitor therapy has long been the cornerstone of transplant immunosuppression, based on the strategy of inhibiting T-cell activation. Calcineurin is a calcium-dependent phosphatase located in the T-cell cytoplasm between the T-cell receptor and the IL-2 gene. Cyclosporine binds cyclophilin in the T-cell cytoplasm, forming a complex that inhibits calcineurin. Cyclosporine can be given intravenously or orally. Higher doses of this agent are given immediately post-transplantation (trough of 250–350 ng/mL), but then doses are tapered based on the time post-transplant to achieve blood levels of 100–300 ng/mL. Cyclosporine levels should be monitored to ensure efficacy and avoid toxicity.

Tacrolimus acts at a different site along the IL-2 activation pathway of lymphocytes by binding FK-binding protein 12 in cells, thereby inhibiting calcineurin. This agent

TABLE 22-15

Typical Maintenance Immunosuppresants				
Medication	**Mechanism of Action**	**Dosing**	**Therapeutic Level**	**Adverse Effects**
Calcineurin Inhibitors				
Cyclosporine	Csa–cyclophilin complex inhibits T-cell activation	IV: 0.03–to 0.1 mg/kg/hr Oral: 2–6 mg/kg/day divided every 8 h for infants and every 12 hr for older children	Adjusted to serum levels, depends on time since transplant	Nephrotoxicity, neurologic toxicity, hypertension, hyperlipidemia, diabetes mellitus, gingival hyperplasia, hypertrichosis, hypomagnesemia
Tacrolimus	Tacrolimus FKBP-12 complex inhibits T-cell activation	0.05–0.1 mg/kg/day	Adjusted to serum levels. 10–15 mcg/mL initially, depends on time since transplant	Similar to cyclosporine, diabetes mellitus and neurologic toxicity more common
Antiproliferative Agents				
Azathioprine	Purine analogue incorporated into DNA inhibits proliferation	1–2 mg/kg/day once a day	Follow CBC	Bone marrow suppression, rare pancreatitis and hepatitis
Mycophenolate mofetil	Inhibits de novo synthesis of guanine nucleotides	20 mg/kg BID orally	> 3 mcg/mL, follow CBC	Vomiting, diarrhea
Corticosteroids				
Methylprednisolone, prednisone	Nonspecific immunosuppression	10 mg/kg IV daily with taper		Peptic ulcer, osteoporosis, glucose intolerance, hypertension, cataracts, hyperlipidemia, salt and water retention, cushingoid facies, aseptic hip necrosis
Target of Rapamycin Inhibition				
Sirolimus	Arrests cell cycle, inhibits proliferation	1–2 mg/m^2/day	Adjusted to serum levels	Bone marrow suppression, hyperlipidemia, hypertriglyceridemia, poor wound healing

Intravenous (IV), complete blood count (CBC), twice daily (BID).

is increasingly replacing cyclosporine in maintenance immunosuppression. It can be given intravenously or orally. Tacrolimus is given orally with starting doses ranging from 0.05 to 0.1 mg/kg/day initially, with trough blood levels being monitored to ensure efficacy while minimizing toxicities. Initial goal levels of tacrolimus concentration are between 10 and 15 ng/mL; however, goal levels decrease based on time since transplant and rejection history.

The side-effect profiles of cyclosporine and tacrolimus are comparable, though there are some notable differences. Cyclosporine is associated with nephrotoxicity (both acute and chronic), hypertension, hyperlipidemia, diabetes mellitus, and neurologic toxicities (seizures and tremors).

Nausea and vomiting, hypertrichosis, gingival hyperplasia, cholelithiasis, and cholestasis may occur as well. An increased incidence of osteoporosis has also been observed. Tacrolimus shares many of the same side effects, but is not associated with hypertrichosis or gingival hyperplasia. The incidence of type 1 diabetes mellitus, anemia, and neurologic toxicities is greater in patients receiving tacrolimus. Drug and food interactions are common with both agents, and their levels should be carefully monitored when the patient starts taking any other new drugs, especially antibiotics or foods such as grapefruit.

Sirolimus (rapamycin) is a macrolide antibiotic with a similar structure to tacrolimus. Like tacrolimus, it binds a member of the FK-binding protein family. However, sirolimus inhibits cytokine-induced signal transduction distal to calcineurin and inhibits several kinases critical to cell division. The sirolimus/FK-binding protein complex inhibits the target of rapamycin (TOR), a cytoplasmic kinase involved in the T-cell activation cascade. By interrupting this pathway, sirolimus holds the T cell in the G_1–S transition phase of the cell cycle, thereby preventing clonal expansion of activated T cells. In addition, sirolimus inhibits smooth muscle and endothelial cell proliferation, which are processes that have significant implications for the development of coronary allograft vasculopathy. The dosing and monitoring of sirolimus in the pediatric population is not well defined. Sirolimus is most often used in combination with tacrolimus. Notable side effects with use of sirolimus include hyperlipidemia, hypertriglyceridemia, thrombocytopenia, neutropenia, anemia, and inhibition of wound healing.

Immunosuppression for rejection

Immunosuppression given during an episode of rejection has also been referred to as rescue therapy (rejection) therapy; its purpose is to acutely reverse an episode of rejection. In such cases, treatment options generally include augmentation or intensification of current management, addition of corticosteroids, or change the immunosuppression protocol regimen. Generally, the severity and grade of rejection and the clinical status of the patient will determine the treatment given during the episode of rejection.

POST-TRANSPLANT COMPLICATIONS

The average survival is 11 years for those who receive an allograft as teenagers and 18 years for those who receive a cardiac transplant as infants (Kirk et al., 2009). The risk of death is highest in the first 6 months after transplant. By estimating survival for those who have exceeded this high-risk period and including only those who survived at least 1 year after transplant (conditional survival), researchers have shown that the average conditional survival is 15 years for teenagers and nearly 19 years for those who undergo transplantation between age 1 and 10 years (Kirk et al., 2009). The threat of acute rejection is always present, accounting for approximately 20% of all deaths through 3 years after transplant, with a gradual decline thereafter. The risk of infection is highest in the first year post transplant, but declines rapidly afterward. An increasing number of deaths from cardiac allograft vasculopathy (CAV) and graft failure occur 3 years after transplant, such that by 5 years after transplant the leading cause of death in the long term is CAV. Post-transplantation malignancy is another important cause of morbidity and mortality in pediatric heart transplant recipients. Families are counseled on these important risks and complications both prior to the heart transplant and after transplant occurs.

Rejection

Rejection of the transplanted organ is an immune response mediated through both T-cell and humoral mechanisms of the recipient targeting the donor myocytes and endothelial cells. Rejection is one of the most common causes of death in the first five years after transplantation, although its incidence is decreasing as a result of improvements in perioperative immunosuppression. The incidence of acute rejection peaks in the first month after transplant and then tapers off by three months. The early peak is delayed by induction immunosuppression, but acute rejection still occurs. By six months after transplant, 60% of patients have had at least one episode of acute cellular rejection; the majority of recipients will have at least one further episode of acute cellular rejection in the first year found on surveillance biopsy, but will usually be asymptomatic (Dodd et al., 2007). These episodes are easily treatable and do not incur significant morbidity or mortality. Nevertheless, rejection is the most important morbidity associated with pediatric heart transplantation, as rejection can not only cause acute graft injury but also promote the development of the most frequent cause of long-term graft failure: CAV.

Cellular rejection, which is mediated by T cells, usually develops within the first few weeks and is present to some degree in most patients. It is initiated by antigen-presenting cell (APC) contact with T-helper lymphocytes. This is the most common type of rejection seen post-transplant. Cellular rejection is characterized by varying degrees of lymphocytic infiltration and necrosis.

Antibody-mediated humoral or vascular rejection (AMR) is initiated by alloantibodies directed against donor HLA or endothelial cell antigens and is mediated by B cells' response rather than by T cells. It is characterized by presence of donor-specific antibodies in the recipient serum, little evidence of cellular rejection on biopsy, and left ventricular dysfunction. Biopsy may reveal endothelial swelling, endothelial macrophage infiltration, and evidence of complement fixation with capillary deposition of C3d and C4d complement fragments.

AMR can occur immediately upon transplantation, as in hyperacute (humoral) rejection. In this relatively rare form of rejection, tissue destruction occurs within minutes to hours of transplantation due to the presence of preformed antibodies within the recipient to donor antigens. Serologic detection of preformed or de novo newly formed donor anti-HLA antibodies has been closely linked to AMR and poor outcomes (Kfoury & Hammond, 2010). AMR can also present with hemodynamic compromise necessitating administration of inotropes. More than 50% of episodes of rejection with hemodynamic compromise are attributable to AMR (Webber et al., 2003). Furthermore, rejection with hemodynamic compromise is associated with a higher incidence of graft failure and mortality, with only one-half of patients being alive at one year after experiencing such an episode (Chin et al., 2004).

Late rejection refers to rejection occurring more than one year after transplant. Episodes of late rejection are more often associated with AMR and hemodynamic compromise requiring inotropic support. Mortality among patients experiencing late rejection is significantly higher than mortality among patients who have not had late rejection (Dodd et al., 2007). Risk factors for late rejection include two or more episodes of rejection in the first year, African American race, and older age at transplant (more than 1 year). Finally, late rejection has been attributed to nonadherence with medication dosing and monitoring.

Clinical manifestations of rejection may range from no symptoms at all to a wide variety of nonspecific symptoms that include tachycardia, tachypnea, abdominal pain, lethargy, irritability, fatigue, poor feeding, and fever. Additional physical findings may include new murmur, gallop rhythm, jugular venous distention, or hepatomegaly.

The gold standard for diagnosis of rejection remains the endomyocardial biopsy. Transplanted patients routinely undergo percutaneous intravascular endomyocardial biopsies with hemodynamic assessment for evaluation of allograft rejection and function.

Treatment for rejection depends on many factors, including the type of rejection (cellular or antibody mediated), the grade, the timing post-transplant, the clinical and hemodynamic status of the child, and baseline immunosuppression. For mild asymptomatic cellular rejection, treatment may not be required given the high rate of spontaneous improvement observed in such cases. Moderate cellular rejection generally will require intensification of immunosuppression, which traditionally includes a high-dose intravenous course of corticosteroids and an increase in the maintenance immunosuppression dose. Treatment for AMR includes high-dose corticosteroids and antilymphocytic therapies. Any rejection with hemodynamic compromise requires support commensurate with the child's clinical status and aggressive intensification of immunosuppression. Two studies have demonstrated resolution of heart failure and rejection using combination of corticosteroids, anthymoglobulin, plasmapheresis, and the use of OKT3 or cyclophosphamide (McComber et al., 2004; Pahl et al., 2000). However, despite improvement in the short term, long-term follow-up revealed a high prevalence of transplant coronary artery disease in these patients. Recently, rituximab has been used in a small number of patients to treat humoral rejection (Garrett et al., 2005).

Coronary artery vasculopathy

Coronary artery vasculopathy is a diffuse chronic vascular coronary arteriopathy that occurs in heart transplant recipients and affects both children and adults. It is the leading cause of mortality among pediatric recipients surviving for more than 5 years. Ischemia results from circumferential proliferation of the vascular intima, which can eventually involve the entire coronary artery, resulting in stenosis or occlusion of large and small branches of the artery.

The exact pathogenesis of CAV is multifactorial but does appear to be related to both immunological and non-immunological factors. Both a chronic allogeneic response to the donor organ and non-immunologic issues likely contribute to endothelial injury and disease progression. There appears to be a correlation between the number of acute rejection episodes and the risk of vasculopathy (Pahl et al., 2005). In addition, the presence of donor-specific HLA antibodies has been found to be associated with the development of transplant coronary artery disease (TCAD) as well as graft loss (Stasny et al., 2007). Non-immunological factors are related to both donor and recipient characteristics as well as surgery-related variables. Non-immune considerations include both donor factors—age, hypertension, and undiagnosed atherosclerosis—and recipient factors—graft ischemia/reperfusion injury, hypertension, hyperlipidemia, obesity, smoking, diabetes, and infection with cytomegalovirus (Pahl et al., 2007). In children, major potential risk factors for the development of CAV include older recipient, older donor age, *two or more* episodes of rejection in the first year post-transplant, late rejection, CMV infection, and earlier year of heart transplant (Pahl et al., 2007).

Classical signs of ischemia are rare in heart transplant recipients. Because the transplanted heart is denervated, characteristic chest pain—even in the face of significant myocardial ischemia—may not occur. Consequently, the first signs may be symptoms of advanced disease with heart failure, syncope, arrhythmias, or death.

Coronary angiography is used to diagnose CAV; however, it may underestimate the vasculopathy when compared with pathological examination or intravascular ultrasound (IVUS). In addition, angiography provides minimal information on the impact of CAV on cardiac function. Moreover, although IVUS is one of the more sensitive modalities to detect CAV, it is also one of the most invasive. In adults, IVUS has been utilized to detect CAV; compared with angiography, it appears to be more sensitive at detecting epicardial disease (Pahl et al., 2007). Intimal thickening can be seen diffusely even in patients with angiographically normal coronary arteries (Costello et al., 2003). However, the use of and experience with IVUS is limited in pediatric patients. Unfortunately, once CAV is diagnosed angiographically, the short-term mortality is high, with the development of moderate or severe TCAD portending a poor prognosis: fewer than 30% of patients avoid death or graft loss within 4 years (Pahl at al., 2005) (Figure 22-24).

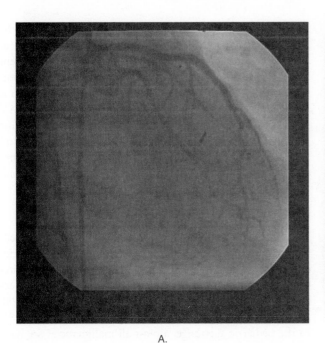

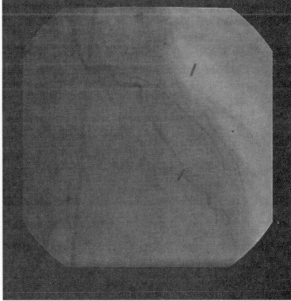

A.

B.

FIGURE 22-24

Coronary Allograft Vasculopathy. A. Coronary angiography of left main coronary artery, left anterior descending coronary artery, and left circumflex coronary artery of child ten years post transplant. There is no gross focal or diffuse narrowing of the major branches. B. Coronary angiography of left main, left anterior descending artery, and left circumflex coronary artery one year later. Note occlusion of the proximal left main coronary artery and diffuse narrowing of the left anterior descending artery and left circumflex artery.

Source: Courtesy of Kathryn Gambetta.

Treatment of established CAV is challenging and limited. Due to the diffuse nature of the intimal thickening, interventional procedures such as coronary angioplasty or coronary stents have limited utility. Nevertheless, two reports have recently described the application of coronary stenting and angioplasty in pediatric patients (Shaddy et al., 2000; Tham et al., 2005). Medical treatment for CAV has been directed toward preventive measures and manipulation of immunosuppression. Lipid-lowering agents (pravastatin, atorvastatin) have proven useful to lower the incidence of TCAD (Chin et al., 2002; Pahl et al., 2005). Sirolimus has been shown to inhibit arterial smooth muscle and endothelial proliferation, and has both antiproliferative and immunosuppressive effects. Despite these beneficial changes, many children with moderate to severe disease and evidence of graft dysfunction may require retransplantation.

Infection following heart transplantation

Infection remains an important source of morbidity and mortality after pediatric heart transplantation, and is the second most common cause of death within the first year after transplantation (Kirk et al., 2009). It can be difficult to recognize serious infections in transplant recipients because the usual symptoms of infections, such as fever, are often diminished. In addition, rejection may present with fever.

The risk of infection after transplantation changes over time, especially with any modifications in immunosuppression. Therefore, HCPs must assess a recipient's risk of infection while also considering the risk of allograft rejection, the recipient's present state of immunosuppression, and other factors that may contribute to increased susceptibility to infection. Three time-periods of different susceptibilities have been recognized: the first month after transplant, an intermediate period between one and six months after transplant, and an extended period beyond the first six months post transplant.

During the first month after transplant, all cardiac transplant recipients are at risk for nosocomial infections. The most common infections within the first month after cardiac transplantation include bacterial and candidal infections of suture sites, urinary catheters, lungs, and vascular access devices. Therefore, it is important to minimize the time foreign bodies are present to decrease the risk of infection.

Between one and six months after transplant, patients are susceptible to infection with reactivated viruses such as herpes simplex virus (HSV), Epstein-Barr virus (EBV), and most notably cytomegalovirus (CMV). In addition, opportunistic infections such as *Pneumocystis jirovecii* pneumonia (formerly known as *Pneumocystis carinii* pneumonia [PCP]) and infections due to *Nocardia* and *Aspergillus* may become clinically more important at this time. Given that the risk for serious opportunistic infections includes fungal, bacterial, viral (especially CMV), and protozoal (notably, PCP) infections, particularly in the first six months after heart transplantation when immunosuppression is greatest, many centers use prophylaxis against such infections consisting of nystatin, ganciclovir, or trimethoprim/sulfamethoxazole, respectively.

In the period after six months, post-transplant patients are susceptible to community-acquired pathogens such as respiratory viruses. Opportunistic infections are less common, but patients who are still receiving high-dose immunosuppressants are at high risk for these diseases. In addition, patients with chronic viral infections who are at risk for progressive organ dysfunction and viral-associated malignancy may develop viral-related complications.

Transplant patients are especially susceptible to common viral upper respiratory infections that do not require antibiotic therapy. Gastroenteritis with vomiting and diarrhea is another common childhood illness that is prevalent in this population; it can typically be managed with supportive therapies such as oral rehydration. An added challenge in children who are transplant recipients is the administration and absorption of immunosuppressant medications when acutely ill. Generally, these illnesses are tolerated well; however, in cases where the illness is protracted or clinically severe, the HCP must have a low threshold to treat more aggressively and search for uncommon pathogens. Every effort must be made to stabilize the pediatric patient and determine the specific diagnosis. Appropriate viral, bacterial, fungal, and protozoal samples should be obtained. In some situations, consultation with an infectious diseases specialist familiar with caring for transplant patients is required.

Cytomegalovirus infection. CMV is a major cause of mortality and morbidity for all solid-organ transplant recipients, largely because of its association with potentially serious specific disease syndromes such as fever, hepatitis, thrombocytopenia, pneumonia, myocarditis, retinitis, and gastrointestinal inflammation. It is important particularly to heart transplantation for several reasons. First, CMV is one of the most common infectious agents identified in pediatric heart transplant recipients. Second, CMV is associated with the development of acute rejection, CAV, and post-transplant lymphoproliferative disorder (PTLD) (Rubin, 2000). Transplant recipients at highest risk of CMV disease are recipients who are seronegative and receive an allograft from a seropositive donor as well as recipients who are seropositive and received antilymphocytic antibody therapy.

Due to its high morbidity, the approach to CMV has been focused on prophylaxis and more recently on pre-emptive therapy based on routine laboratory surveillance. CMV prophylaxis with oral valganciclovir or intravenous ganciclovir is now used routinely for the first 3 to 12 months after heart transplantation in all high-risk patients (Sulemanjee et al.,

2008). Some centers also use CMV prophylaxis during the first 3 months after transplantation for patients who are at low risk, meaning the patient was a seronegative recipient and received an organ from a seronegative donor. Frequent monitoring for CMV seroconversion and active infection is necessary. Methods of surveillance currently include CMV polymerase chain reaction (PCR) detection of viral genome and the PP65 antigenemia test. From these tests, CMV viral load can be assessed and can guide decisions regarding preemptive therapy when viral load exceeds a certain threshold.

Post-transplant malignancy

An increased risk of malignancy is an important and well-known complication of organ transplantation. Malignancies may either occur as a new cancer, may involve a reactivation of a previous cancer, or may result from chronic viral infections. The cumulative prevalence in transplant patients is 2% at 1 year, 5% at 5 years, and 8% at 10 years (Kirk et al., 2009). In the pediatric age range, almost all malignancies are lymphomas. *Post-transplant lymphoproliferative disorder* (PTLD) is the term used to describe all clinical syndromes associated with lymphoproliferation; manifestations can range from an infectious mononucleosis-like illness to an aggressive monoclonal lymphoma that may be fatal. The clinical presentation is variable. For example, children may present with an asymptomatic localized adenopathy or tonsillar hypertrophy, oral ulcerations, or a specific organ-related syndrome such as a pneumonitic process, diarrhea, or malabsorption. Hematologic abnormalities or neurologic or nonspecific constitutional complaints such as fever, lethargy, abdominal pain, and failure-to-thrive may also be presenting signs.

The most important risk factor for the development of PTLD is EBV serologic status. EBV is a member of the herpes virus family, which has the ability to remain latent in the host and transform and immortalize B cells. Immunosuppression prevents the normal host cytotoxic T cells from controlling this infection. Transplant recipients who were seronegative and contract EBV from their donor organ or after transplant are at increased risk for developing PTLD compared with recipients who were seropositive before transplant. In addition, studies have shown that increases in serial quantitative EBV viral load can be used to identify patients who are greater risk of developing PTLD (Allen et al., 2005). For this reason, routine screening for EBV with PCR on peripheral blood samples is performed routinely in certain transplant centers.

The development of a very high viral load should alert the clinician to evaluate the patient for signs or symptoms of disease, even in the asymptomatic child. The diagnosis of PTLD is made based on clinical suspicion, rising EBV viral load, risk factors, and tissue sample histology. Staging should consist of CT scanning of the head, neck, chest, abdomen, and pelvis; bone marrow aspiration; and lumbar puncture. Table 22-16 outlines a suggested surveillance regimen for PTLD.

TABLE 22-16

Suggested Surveillance Regimen for Post-transplant Lymphoproliferative Disorder		
	Diagnostic Labs	**Plan**
New heart transplant patient	• EBV PCR every 3 months • Annual CXR • EBV titers on donor and recipient	• If rising, repeat in 2 weeks to confirm • If still rising, CT scan of neck through pelvis (with and without contrast)
Known transplant with large tonsils	• Obtain EBV PCR and determine plan based on result	• If low, monitor every 3 months • If elevated, CT scan and biopsy
New lymphadenopathy	• EBV PCR immediately • Obtain CT scans	• Obtain CT scan • Consult oncology • Monitor closely • Consider biopsy
Suspicious symptoms	• EBV PCR, LDH, uric acid, CBC with differential	• Consider CT scan of neck through pelvis • Consult oncology

Epstein-Barr virus (EBV), polymerase chain reaction (PCR), computed tomography (CT), complete blood count (CBC), chest radiograph (CXR).

Treatment for PTLD is always performed in consultation with an oncologist with experience in treating this disease. First-line treatment generally entails the reduction of immunosuppression. During this time, the patient is monitored closely for signs of regression and for signs of rejection. Other aggressive treatments include chemotherapy, tumor debulking, radiation therapy, administration of antiviral agents, and use of monoclonal antibodies such as rituximab (Herman et al., 2002; Pescovitz, 2004).

LONG-TERM MORBIDITIES

In addition to rejection, infection, CAV, and malignancies, the adverse effects of immunosuppressant medications may result in specific long-term medical morbidities such as hypertension, kidney insufficiency, lipid abnormalities, diabetes mellitus, and neurotoxicity.

Hypertension is defined as systolic or diastolic blood pressure that is at or above the 95 percentile for age, gender, and height on three or more occasions. This condition is highly prevalent in pediatric heart transplant recipients, and its prevalence increases even more with time post-transplant. Approximately 50% of children have hypertension by one year post-transplant (Boucek et al., 2005). Hypertension is usually first diagnosed in children within days of transplantation, when co-administration of calcineurin inhibitors and steroids is commonplace; however, it can also appear over time. Calcineurin inhibitors cause hypertension by activating the renin–angiotensin system and stimulating the release of renin from the juxtaglomerular apparatus. They also cause afferent arteriolar constriction and decrease renal blood flow, which results in further renin release. Transplant patients also tend to lose the pattern of diurnal variation and nocturnal decline in blood pressure seen in normal children.

It is imperative to treat hypertension effectively because it is a known risk factor for left ventricular hypertrophy, atherosclerosis, and chronic kidney disease. Moreover, aggressive control of hypertension may have beneficial effects on preventing CAV (Singh, 2007). Salt restriction and diuretic therapy are important, but usually more intensive drug therapy is required. Medications commonly used for treating hypertension include ACE inhibitors, calcium-channel blockers, and (less commonly) beta blockers.

Kidney dysfunction can be a significant source of morbidity post-transplant. Severe kidney dysfunction, defined as a patient requiring renal dialysis or kidney transplant, or presenting with a serum creatinine level greater than 2.5 mg/dL, shows a linear increase after transplantation, occurring in as many as 11% of pediatric transplant recipients 10 years after transplant (Kirk et al., 2009). The deterioration in kidney function is likely multifactorial. For example, it may stem from antecedent pretransplant renal dysfunction from low cardiac output, chronic diuretic therapy, mechanical support, ischemia/reperfusion injury following CPB, and use of nephrotoxic medications post-transplant (Dipchand & Blume, 2010). In the long term, cumulative use of calcineurin inhibitors can produce structural changes in the kidney characterized by glomerular sclerosis, tubular atrophy, interstitial fibrosis, and afferent arteriopathy. Early kidney dysfunction can be seen within days of transplant and presents with azotemia, hypertension, and (in some cases) acute kidney failure. No difference has been observed between the use of cyclosporine or tacrolimus in terms of the decline in creatinine clearance (English et al., 2002).

Unfortunately, kidney dysfunction in pediatric transplant recipients is not uncommon and can be progressive. Monitoring for renal function with estimations of creatinine clearance, glomerular filtration rate, and screening for renal tubular acidosis should be performed on a regular basis. Strategies to improve kidney function should be directed toward reducing exposure to nephrotoxic agents, including reduction in calcineurin inhibitors, if feasible. If renal dysfunction is developing, switching to a kidney-sparing immunosuppression regimen should be considered. Recently, the combination of sirolimus with lowered doses of calcineurin inhibitors has been reported to improve renal function (Singh, 2007).

A high prevalence of lipid abnormalities has been reported among pediatric heart transplant recipients. Hyperlipidemia is present in more than one-fourth of recipients by 5 years after heart transplantation (Boucek et al., 2005). These abnormalities are related to the direct effects of immunosuppressants, such as cyclosporine, steroids, and sirolimus, along with coexisting factors of obesity and diabetes. Small-center studies have demonstrated the safety and efficacy of statin use in children after transplantation (Chin et al., 2002; Penson et al., 2001).

Other morbidities include post-transplant diabetes mellitus, which has been observed in approximately 2% of children treated with cyclosporine and 8% of children treated with tacrolimus (Paolillio et al., 2001). Neurotoxicities such as tremors, restlessness, dyesthesias of the palms and sole, seizures, and altered mental status have been observed with cyclosporine and tacrolimus immunosuppression, especially in the early postoperative period.

Osteopenia is another morbidity that can become significant if it leads to osteoporosis and pathologic fractures. Prior to transplant, many children will have had preexisting osteopenia due to chronic diuretic use, poor nutrition, lack of mobility, and inability to exercise. Post-transplant, the use of calcineurin inhibitors and steroids further increases the risk of osteopenia by altering bone metabolism. Screening for osteopenia (i.e., measurement of bone mineral density) should be performed, and prophylaxis and treatment provided as appropriate.

DISPOSITION AND DISCHARGE PLANNING

After heart transplantation, children require close follow-up and meticulous attention to detail to achieve a good long-term outcome. Therefore, good prognosis for the pediatric patient is contingent upon close communication between the family and child, the heart transplant team, and the child's primary care provider. The heart transplant team usually consists of a medical social worker, a medical psychologist or psychiatrist, a nurse practitioner, a transplant pharmacist, and a transplant cardiologist.

Prior to discharge home, the pediatric patient and his or her family require extensive counseling about the required medication regimen, potential medical complications, and the importance of adherence to medications and to the mandatory medical clinic evaluations. At least two designated caregivers should be instructed on medication administration and basic CPR. Ideally, caregivers should be identified

prior to transplantation, and education should occur both before and after transplantation. In some centers, prior to discharge from the hospital, the two designated caregivers are given the opportunity to administer medications while being supervised by the nursing staff. Many transplant centers discharge families and heart transplant recipients to a nearby care facility prior to going to their actual home so that families have an opportunity to care for their child unaided, yet still be in very close proximity to the transplant center should any concerns arise.

Initially, cardiac evaluations are performed at least weekly after discharge. The intervals between these visits are increased over time, depending on the child and the comfort of his or her caregivers. Echocardiographs are performed to assess for any changes in systolic or diastolic function, left ventricular wall thicknesses, or evidence of valvular regurgitation that can be a harbinger of rejection or CAV. ECGs are performed to assess for signs of ischemia or rhythm abnormalities. In addition, 24- or 48-hour Holter monitoring may be performed to assess for any changes in heart rhythm. In the beginning, each of these tests is performed quite frequently. Once the child has been stabilized from a cardiac perspective, echocardiographs are performed approximately every 3 to 6 months, ECGs every 3 to 6 months, and Holter monitoring yearly depending on the institution and the child.

It is important to recognize that children with transplanted hearts may not complain of the typical symptoms of chest pain, even in the face of significant myocardial ischemia, as transplanted hearts are denervated. Other symptoms that can be ominous for rejection or ischemia include fatigue, syncope, abdominal pain, arm pain, or back pain. For HCPs, it is important to maintain a high index of suspicion in transplant recipients and to perform such tests as clinically warranted.

Diagnostic studies are also performed to assess kidney function, to monitor for appropriate levels of immunosuppressants, to assess electrolyte levels, and to monitor viral loads of EBV and CMV. The frequency with which these laboratory values are obtained depends on the medical history of the child as well as the institution's policies.

Transplanted patients routinely undergo percutaneous intravascular endomyocardial biopsies with hemodynamic assessment for evaluation of allograft rejection and function. The frequency of biopsies varies between institutions. Given the high risk of rejection in the first 2 months after transplant, endomyocardial biopsy is usually performed either weekly or every other week during this time. Infants younger than 1 year are not usually biopsied until they are 6 months post-transplant unless clinical suspicion for rejection is raised. After the first 3 months, routine biopsies may be performed less frequently, depending on the rejection history of the child.

Endomyocardial biopsies are taken in the cardiac catheterization lab using a bioptome device. Usually, three to six biopsy specimens are taken each time to ensure minimization of false negative results. Although there have been many efforts to identify noninvasive methods of diagnosis of rejection including echocardiography, profiling of gene expression, and intramyocardial electrocardiography, to date no noninvasive test has been found to consistently and accurately diagnose rejection. Therefore, despite the lack of reproducibility, the risk of false negatives, and the risk for complications such as development of tricuspid regurgitation, endomyocardial biopsy remains the gold standard for diagnosing rejection.

Usually, beginning the first year after heart transplantation, coronary angiography is performed annually to assess for any evidence of CAV. Angiography remains the standard for diagnosis, but its sensitivity is low. Stress echocardiography—in the form of both exercise and dobutamine induced—has also been used to evaluate for any wall motion abnormalities that might signal the presence of CAV.

Exercise restriction is not necessary after heart transplantation once patients are recovered from surgery and the incision healed, which generally occurs 6 to 8 weeks post-transplant. Following heart transplantation, physiological responses to exercise may be impaired due to several factors—age at transplantation, deconditioning prior to transplantation, degree of reinnervation of the donor heart, chronotropic incompetence, and the presence of other comorbidities such as kidney dysfunction. However, regular aerobic exercise should still be encouraged at least 30 minutes a time for at least three to four times a week. Cardiopulmonary exercise testing is usually performed annually once the child is more than 8 years old and able to understand to understand the mechanics of performing the exercise test. The purpose is to assess the ability of the transplanted heart to increase cardiac output in response to an increased workload and to assess for evidence of ischemia with exercise, arrhythmias with exercise, changes in endurance time, or symptoms that can be a sign of allograft vasculopathy.

Numerous advances have been made in the management of children who have required heart transplantation. Although survival has improved, heart transplantation appears to be time limited, and surviving children will likely need to be considered for retransplantation. An increasing number of children have undergone retransplantation over the last several years, with most of these procedures being performed more than 5 years after the initial transplant. Retransplantation now accounts for 5% of all pediatric transplants performed (Kirk et al., 2009).

The most common indications for retransplantation include CAV, nonspecific graft failure, acute rejection, and chronic rejection. Overall survival following retransplantation approaches that of primary transplantation when retransplantation occurs more than one year after primary transplantation. However, for children who receive a second transplant within one year of the first transplant,

actuarial survival is 60% compared to 90% for those transplanted more than three years later (Boucek et al., 2007). In addition, retransplantation for early failure or acute rejection has a high mortality. Thus the assessment for retransplantation is an important and ongoing component to the management and surveillance of children who have undergone their first transplantation.

Transplantation programs work closely with primary care providers to meet pediatric patients' routine health maintenance needs. Children who have had heart transplants should resume general pediatric care with their provider on a regular basis. In addition, many children have other complex comorbidities that develop as a consequence of the immunosuppressants or their preceding heart failure and require long-term follow-up and consultation with other medical specialties. Therefore, the primary care clinician can be extremely beneficial to the child and family as the central focal point of care for the pediatric patient post-transplant.

Vaccines should be administered to recipients prior to transplantation. Most children have not finished their routine vaccination schedule prior to their heart transplant. After transplantation, immunizations are administered at routine age-appropriate time intervals using only killed vaccines. Resumption of vaccination schedules is recommended at approximately 6 months after transplantation. Family members of recipients should be immunized fully and receive injectable influenza vaccine yearly. Most centers rely on primary care physicians to administer immunizations.

Delayed growth is common in children after heart transplantation. Rate of growth in terms of height for children undergoing heart transplantation falls between the time of listing and the time of transplantation. Although catch-up growth is seen during the first year after transplant, children remain shorter on average than their peers 6 years after transplant (Ibrahim et al., 2002). Children transplanted for reasons other than congenital heart disease maintain steady linear growth after transplantation but may fail to achieve normal height. Pubertal development does appear to progress at normal expected time intervals.

The mean developmental scores for both mental and psychomotor indices in infants falls within normal limits, although they tend to be at the lower end of normal (Baum et al., 2000). Reports of children transplanted beyond infancy also reveal cognitive scores at the lower limit of normal. Many older children have been able to return to mainstream school after transplant, although their educational success has been found to vary.

Despite the potential risks that many children with heart transplants face, their prospects for good quality of life are excellent. Approximately 92% of children who survive at least 10 years have no limitations on physical activity, and only 1% require total assistance (Kirk et al., 2009). The majority of patients do not require rehospitalization for transplant-related problems. Most patients return to age-appropriate activities, including a physical education class, within the first 6 months after transplantation (Fricker, 2002).

While most children and their families do report a good quality of life post-transplant, evidence of adverse psychosocial functioning has also been reported. Most children and adolescents seem to demonstrate good psychological adjustment after transplant, yet behavioral problems, anxiety, school difficulties, depression, and poor adherence have been identified. In one study, 25% of children were reported to have emotional adjustment difficulties at some stage regardless of diagnosis (DeMaso et al., 2004). These problems included illness-related stress, symptoms of post-traumatic stress, and nonadherences, especially in the adolescent population. Oftentimes, the primary care provider is the first to identify such problems. Therefore, a coordinated effort between the child's primary care provider, the transplant team, and the family must be established to help identify children at risk.

CARDIOMYOPATHY

Stephen G. Pophal

PATHOPHYSIOLOGY

The majority of pediatric cardiomyopathies are idiopathic. They may lead to decompensated heart failure, arrhythmia, and sudden death by different mechanisms. Because each type of pediatric cardiomyopathy is associated with heart chamber enlargement, all can be described as an "enlarged heart."

Heart failure is defined as the heart's inability to maintain the body's demands. The heart has two major roles: to receive blood and to pump blood. In *dilated cardiomyopathy* (DCM), the ventricle (pump) is dysfunctional and cannot maintain adequate output for increasing demands. Over time, the ventricles become stiff and do not fill, leading to a backup of blood. This phenomenon can lead to pulmonary edema, atrial enlargement with arrhythmias, or pulmonary hypertension.

In *hypertrophic cardiomyopathy* (HCM), the ventricular function is adequate, if not hyperactive. The ventricular chambers become thick and stiff, and lack the diastolic filling properties essential to maintain cardiac output. In addition, progressive muscular outflow obstruction compromises cardiac output. Therapies that enhance the pump's systolic function, such as inotropes, worsen a stiff heart's ability to fill, further reducing cardiac output.

The physiology of *restrictive cardiomyopathy* (RCM) is similar to HCM, but occurs without the outflow obstruction. Typically RCM is associated with grossly elevated atrial pressure and size. This leads to complex atrial arrhythmias and significant pulmonary hypertension.

Arrhythmias more commonly occur secondary to the myopathy, but chronic primary arrhythmias can also lead to cardiomyopathy. This is a very important distinction, as the cardiomyopathy is reversible after control of the rhythm disturbance. In addition, each cardiomyopathy can be associated with stasis of blood, leading to thromboembolic phenomena. Stroke, pulmonary emboli, or another systemic embolic episode can be catastrophic.

EPIDEMIOLOGY AND ETIOLOGY

In contrast to adults, ischemic and hypertensive cardiomyopathies are rarely seen in pediatric patients. In large multicenter studies of cardiomyopathies, more than 50% of cases involved dilated conditions, 25% to 40% were hypertrophic in nature, and less than 4% were restrictive. Males are more susceptible to cardiomyopathy than females. The overall incidence is between 1 and 2 cases per 100,000 children (Lipshultz et al., 2003; Towbin et al., 2006; Wilkinson et al., 2008).

Certain malformation syndromes, neuromuscular disorders, and inborn errors of metabolism are highly associated with cardiomyopathy; however, genotype-positive/phenotype-negative scenarios are also common (Colan et al., 2007; Kane et al., 2007). Multiple mutant genes with hundreds of specific mutations are linked to these types of abnormalities, none of which are relevant for acute management. HCM is highly associated with Noonan's syndrome in addition to dysplastic pulmonary valve, lymphedema, and pathologic branch pulmonary stenosis. Duchene's and Becker's muscular dystrophy produce inevitable deteriorations in the cardiopulmonary system (Connuck et al., 2008). Inborn errors of metabolism with metabolic crisis can be indistinguishable from septic shock, although the treatment pathways for these conditions markedly differ.

PRESENTATION

The presentation of cardiomyopathy may vary. Rapid identification of a cardiomyopathy and, more importantly, the type of cardiomyopathy is paramount in deciding upon early treatment strategies. A detailed history might elucidate clues about poor cardiac function. Past medical history frequently contains recurrent respiratory illnesses, asthma, abdominal pain, and failure-to-thrive. Presentation complaints of dizziness, orthostatic hypotension, syncopal episode, angina, palpitations, or any symptoms of CHF should be further explored. The patient with compensated cardiomyopathy commonly has longstanding elevated pulmonary venous pressures that often lead to "cardiac wheezing." Any history of cancer should prompt a discussion of the cumulative anthracycline dose, which is directly related to the development of dilated cardiomyopathy. Active cancer is a contraindication to cardiac transplantation, should that treatment be recommended. Family history continues to be the mainstay of cardiomyopathy screening in healthy subjects. A direct relative with early, sudden death, an enlarged heart, or a pacemaker should prompt further investigation.

The consequences of ventricular dysfunction, hypertrophy, or restriction can range from mild limitations in exercise with a nondescript murmur, to classic anginal chest pain with exertion, to near sudden death from ventricular fibrillation (Nadkarni et al., 2006). Dyspnea with exertion, orthopnea, and systemic or pulmonary edema may occur in pediatric patients as well as adults, although these symptoms are frequently confused with more common childhood illnesses in young patients. A heart murmur or gallop is typically noted on careful examination. The systolic murmur is either from left ventricular outflow tract (LVOT) obstruction in HCM or from mitral insufficiency in DCM or HCM. In decompensated heart failure, pulses are thready and capillary refill is delayed. Extremities may be cool, with the degree of coolness correlating with the degree of compromised cardiac output.

DIFFERENTIAL DIAGNOSIS

Sepsis can be associated with transient cardiac dysfunction. Pericarditis or pericardial effusions with tamponade physiology can also present with shock and cardiomegaly on CXR. All left-sided obstructive congenital heart lesions can mimic the presenting signs and symptoms of cardiomyopathy. Critical aortic stenosis or coarctation of the aorta can present in a manner similar to a dilated cardiomyopathy.

PLAN OF CARE

Abnormalities on CXR are typically the first indication of a cardiac muscle disorder. Electrocardiograph lacks diagnostic accuracy, but may be helpful as an adjunct to CXR to confirm a cardiac abnormality. More importantly, ECG aids with the assessment of three important, potentially treatable causes of cardiomyopathy: (1) myocarditis; (2) anomalous origin of the left coronary artery from the pulmonary artery (ALCAPA); and (3) ectopic atrial tachycardia-induced cardiomyopathy. Myocarditis and acute rejection in heart transplantation share similar microscopic findings of lymphocytic infiltrates into the myocardium with edema, which leads to diffusely low voltage on ECG. Rarely, myocarditis may present with similar

ECG and serological findings of myocardial infarction (Lindblade et al., 2006). ALCAPA ECG findings are consistent with profound ischemia or, more commonly, infarct patterns in the left coronary distribution. Ectopic atrial tachycardia can present with unusually high heart rates (160 to 200 bpm) with abnormal or inverted P waves in leads II and a VF. All patients with suspected cardiomyopathy should be placed on 24-hour telemetry to monitor for potential life-threatening arrhythmias.

Laboratory assessments are not diagnostic of cardiomyopathy but may aid in distinguishing a primary pulmonary process from a cardiac one. B-type natriuretic peptide (BNP) is a useful serologic tool (Law et al., 2009; Maher et al., 2008) for making the initial diagnosis and for regulating therapeutic management. Standard laboratory tests for infection and for assessing end-organ function are important as well.

Echocardiographic findings are distinctly different for each of the three most common cardiomyopathies. In DCM, the left ventricle is grossly dilated and has decreased systolic function. Left ventricular (LV) size, as indexed for body surface area, is found to be considerably greater than normal (z score > 3) and systolic function (LV shortening or ejection fraction) is considerably less than normal (z score < 2) (Singh et al., 2009). In HCM, LV cavity size is normal to small, but the walls (interventricular septum, posterior wall) are thick (z score > 2). LV systolic function is normal or enhanced. In RCM, the LV appears normal in its size and function, but it lacks normal filling patterns. In contrast to the situation with DCM or HCM, the atria are grossly enlarged.

Treatment strategies vary considerably based on whether the patient has a dilated, hypertrophic, or restrictive cardiomyopathy. Performing echocardiographic assessment early and often is an important diagnostic strategy to improve survival for pediatric patients presenting to the intensive care unit with cardiomyopathy.

DCM accounts for nearly 50% of all cardiomyopathies but leads to more than 75% of all transplant referrals for cardiomyopathy (Canter et al., 2007; Singh et al., 2009; Tsirka et al., 2004). Early transplant referral (described earlier in this chapter) and mechanical support can drastically reduce mortality in these patients (Huang et al., 2008). Cardiorespiratory support should be a calculated and coordinated effort involving multiple experienced critical care team members, as cardiac arrest may be imminent (Tsirka et al., 2004). In patients with DCM, volume resuscitation can be hazardous, leading to pulmonary edema and respiratory failure. Early inotropic support and continuous telemetry is recommended. It is important to initiate early diuresis, *avoiding* significant volume shifts. Afterload reduction may be difficult at first as blood pressure can be tenuous, although administration of milrinone (a phosphodiesterase enzyme inhibitor) may improve survival.

Therapeutic management for HCM differs significantly from the approach used in DCM. Both therapies are aimed at optimizing cardiac output; however, in HCM, enhancing systolic function with inotropes can lead to worsening LVOT obstruction and impaired filling. Strategies should be directed, instead, at decreasing the heart rate and systolic function while carefully monitoring systemic output. Beta and calcium-channel blockade should be introduced early, in tandem with careful volume management.

A limited number of therapies other than transplant are available for RCM. Early respiratory failure, difficult-to-manage rhythm disturbances, and pulmonary hypertensive crisis should be anticipated. Careful volume management with central venous and possible wedge pressure monitoring can be efficacious.

Myocarditis may resolve over time, but supportive care prior to its resolution can be challenging. All patients suspected or proven to have myocarditis may be candidates for mechanical support as a bridge to recovery or heart transplantation (Lindblade et al., 2006; Vashist & Singh, 2009). Endomyocardial biopsy or MRI assessment for myocarditis should be considered depending on the level of institutional expertise with these measures. Patients with DCM and RCM who are resistant to conventional therapies may also be candidates for mechanical support.

Surgical palliations for most cardiomyopathy are limited in the acute care setting. Septal myomectomy, however, is an established and traditional therapy for symptomatic HCM patients with LVOT obstruction who are refractory to medical therapy (Rhee et al., 2008). Significant LVOT obstruction as measured by echocardiography is one of the strongest independent predictors of disease progression to severe heart failure and death. If LVOT obstruction cannot be relieved, patients with HCM or severe DCM may require automatic implantable cardioverter–defibrillator (AICD) implantation prior to discharge to minimize their risk of sudden death.

Prompt recognition is critical to survival. To ensure that patients receive the best possible care, early consultation of the following subspecialties should be initiated: critical care, pulmonology, cardiology, cardiothoracic surgery, mechanical cardiac support team, cardiac transplant team, and infectious disease specialists. Although nutritionists may not be consulted immediately, they should become involved in the patient's plan of care as soon as it is reasonably possible. Additional subspecialists may be called upon depending on the etiology of the underlying disorder. The diagnosis of cardiomyopathy in a child may be overwhelming for his or her family and any of a number of support services may prove valuable in assisting them, such as social work, spiritual support, and child life. As the patient begins his or her recovery period, the rehabilitative team should be consulted to promote return to developmental baselines.

Patient and family education may initially address the acute illness, the diagnostic studies and their findings, and health care team members who are involved in the plan of care. If the patient's acuity worsens, discussions about life support and transplant may be required.

DISPOSITION AND DISCHARGE PLANNING

In addition to implantable defibrillators, activation of a care system that is responsive to a high-risk patient population is necessary to avoid outpatient morbidity and mortality due to cardiomyopathy. The mortality rate for pediatric patients with HCM is 1% per year, whereas mortality rates for idiopathic restrictive cardiomyopathy are particularly high in the absence of heart transplantation. Prognosis for the pediatric patient is poor, with two-year actuarial survival rates of 50% (Denfield, 2002; Denfield et al., 1997; Rivenes et al., 2000). This rate decreases to 29% to 39% at –three to five years after presentation (Russo & Webber, 2005). Overall actuarial one-year survival for DCM is 90%, and five-year survival is 83%, however, actuarial freedom from "heart death" (death or transplantation) is only 70% at one year and 58% at five years (Tsirka et al., 2005).

Patients with myocarditis may make a full recovery or be left with impaired function and require chronic heart failure management. Patients who present in cardiogenic shock due to cardiomyopathies may likewise survive with chronic heart failure. Referral to a specialized pediatric heart failure management program optimizes outcomes for such children (Margossian, 2008). Those who require cardiac transplantation constitute a distinct group; their longevity and quality of life will depend on the services of an integrated transplant management program.

CARDIOGENIC SHOCK

Michael Worthen

PATHOPHYSIOLOGY

Cardiogenic shock is a shock state resulting from primary cardiac pump failure. Implicit in this definition is normal (or normalized) preload and regulation of vascular tone, to distinguish this condition from hypovolemic and vasodilatory shock.

The source of cardiogenic shock is the inability of the heart to provide enough forward flow of oxygenated blood to meet tissue demands. Despite compensatory vasoconstriction (where possible), tachycardia, hypotension, and tissue ischemia develop. Without successful intervention, cardiogenic shock rapidly becomes a vicious cycle of impaired pump function, hypotension, reduced coronary perfusion, and systemic acidosis. These factors further impair myocardial performance, worsen pump function, and, if left untreated, lead to cardiac arrest and death.

Reduced contractility decreases left ventricular (LV) ejection at any given afterload. In addition, myocardial compliance decreases under ischemic and metabolic stress (diastolic dysfunction), which leads to increased LV end-diastolic volumes and pressures. The increased wall stress raises myocardial O_2 demand; when the heart cannot meet this demand, performance deteriorates more and a second vicious cycle of distension and elevated end-diastolic pressure follows. Subendocardial ischemia and necrosis may ensue as well. High-pressure edema from pulmonary venous congestion produces hypoxemia, and numerous systemic circulatory reflexes may generate counterproductive effects. Renal fluid retention exacerbates pulmonary edema and ventricular distention. Sympathetic activation results in tachycardia, which increases O_2 demand and decreases diastolic filling. Pathologic arrhythmias may be exacerbated. Increased afterload from vasoconstriction further impairs ejection of the impaired ventricle, perpetuating the cycle of failure.

EPIDEMIOLOGY AND ETIOLOGY

The incidence of cardiogenic shock in children is unknown. Recent studies have estimated the incidence of new-onset heart failure in children at 0.87 case per 100,000 population (Webber, 2008). The one-year mortality in this group is significant, which suggests that many of these patients may have developed cardiogenic shock at some time. Fulminant viral myocarditis may present with shock. Reports of such cases associated with H1N1 influenza A (Bratincsak et al., 2010) suggests that the incidence may vary during pandemics. Large congenital cardiac surgical programs report significant numbers of patients who require mechanical cardiac support perioperatively, allowing researchers to estimate how many members of this population are at risk for cardiogenic shock (Duncan et al., 1998).

Myocardial abnormalities

Cardiac pump failure may start at the myocardial level. and congenital myocardial abnormalities may produce heart failure. Ventricular noncompaction is a genetically determined failure of endomyocardial development that results in structural disarray of ventricular muscle. Hypertrophic cardiomyopathies, which often have a genetic etiology, result in myocardial thickening and disorganization. Many cardiomyopathies, however, are idiopathic. Inborn errors of metabolism may produce myocardial failure owing to failure of cellular energy production (mitochondrial beta-oxidation abnormalities) or myocardial

infiltration due to diseases of glycogen storage (Pompe's, Andersen's) or lysosomal storage (Niemman-Pick, Gaucher's, muccupolysaccharidosis, Sandhoff's) (Guertl et al., 2000). In addition, many forms of congenital muscular dystrophies may result in myocardial failure (Duchene, Fukuyama). Both progressive systolic and diastolic dysfunction may culminate in pump failure in all these conditions.

In addition to congenital conditions, acquired myocardial injury may produce heart failure and shock. For example, myocarditis impairs heart function through myocyte inflammation and necrosis. Viral causes (adenovirus, enterovirus, H1N1) predominate as the source of these injuries, although many cases remain idiopathic. Myocarditis is a common cause of fulminant cardiogenic shock. Hypermetabolic states (thyrotoxicosis, pheochromocytoma) may produce catecholamine-mediated heart failure. Drug-induced heart failure may result from side effects of therapeutic use (anthracycline chemotherapy), accidental or deliberate overdose of prescription drugs (tricyclic antidepressants, beta blockers, digoxin) or from use of drugs of abuse (cocaine, methamphetamine). Trauma may cause cardiogenic shock via blunt mechanisms (myocardial contusion or chamber rupture) or penetrating injury (chamber perforation or tamponade).

The most common situation in which children develop acquired myocardial failure and shock is following CPB. As a result of this surgery, patients may have residual anatomic defects or arrhythmias. Repair of these intracardiac defects creates direct muscle trauma and ischemia. Cardiopulmonary bypass produces a state of systemic inflammation that worsens myocardial edema, depresses function, and impairs compensatory reflexes. Mediastinal hemorrhage may create tamponade. Both length and complexity of the repair are primary risk factors for cardiogenic failure following heart surgery for a congenital abnormality. Notably, mechanical cardiac support is an important treatment option in this population.

Coronary abnormalities

In adults, the most common cause of cardiogenic shock is acute myocardial infarction due to atheromatous coronary artery disease. Although this condition is uncommon in children, coronary artery insufficiency may occur and produce ischemic cardiogenic shock. Anomalous origin of the left coronary artery from the pulmonary artery (ALCAPA syndrome) is a congenital malformation in which the left coronary arises from the pulmonary trunk. Coronary steal and myocardial ischemia develop postnatally in patients with this abnormality. Children with Williams syndrome may develop severe occlusion of the coronary ostia associated with supravalvar aortic stenosis. Ischemic chest pain, heart failure, or sudden death may ensue. Acquired coronary artery disease due to aneurysm formation is the most feared complication of Kawasaki syndrome.

Heart transplant recipients may develop coronary artery narrowing (transplant vasculopathy) as a manifestation of chronic rejection. The incidence of this condition is more than 50% at 10 years post-transplant (Taylor et al., 2007).

Electrical abnormalities

Adequate cardiac output depends on a cardiac rhythm of adequate rate and organization, such as atrial–ventricular (A-V) synchrony. In contrast, severe bradycardia from sinus node dysfunction or intoxication may produce shock. High-degree A-V block attributed to congenital, postoperative, or drug-induced causes may result in inadequate cardiac output if the ventricular rate is too slow. The loss of atrial contraction with appropriate A-V synchrony may be quite detrimental in children with valvular disease or with impaired ventricular compliance.

Tachyarrhythmias are more commonly a cause of pump failure in pediatric patients than slow rhythms, with ventricular fibrillation being the extreme case of a nonperfusing rapid rate. Even organized cardiac rhythms may critically impair cardiac output if they are rapid enough to prevent adequate diastolic filling. Acute rhythms may originate in the ventricle, such as ventricular tachycardia (VT) and junction ectopic tachycardia (JET), or from the atrium, such as supraventricular tachycardia (SVT) and atrial ectopic tachycardia (AET). Although most commonly associated with structural heart disease, severe rhythm disturbances may be primary. The electric cardiomyopathies (long QT syndrome, Brugada syndrome) are congenital abnormalities of myocardial electrical function that predispose patients to poorly perfusing or nonperfusing rhythms, syncope, and sudden death (Veltmann et al., 2009). Sustained, chronic tachycardias may lead to ventricular dysfunction, heart failure, and shock (tachycardia-mediated cardiomyopathy) (Gopinathanniar et al., 2009).

Structural abnormalities

Both congenital and acquired lesions may produce cardiogenic shock via obstruction, regurgitation, or shunting. Critical aortic stenosis (AS), hypoplastic left heart syndrome (HLHS), and critical coarctation may present with shock after ductal closure. As noted with tamponade, some experts would not consider AS, HLHS, or critical coarctation to represent primarily cardiogenic shock, although myocardial failure may develop if these conditions go untreated. The problem with these lesions is obstruction to systemic output; hence, prompt improvement is possible if the patient is treated rapidly with prostaglandins to reopen the ductus arteriosus. Thrombosis of a mechanical valve may produce heart failure due to obstruction. Although progressive left-sided valve insufficiency may be

well tolerated, acute aortic or mitral valve insufficiency, due to either endocarditis or trauma, may produce shock in the uncompensated ventricle. Likewise, the acute presentation of a ventricular septal defect (VSD) as a result of trauma, post infarction, or patch dehiscence may critically impair forward cardiac flow.

Extra-cardiac lesions causing obstruction to flow

Cardiac tamponade is an accumulation of fluid within the pericardium that results in depression of cardiac output. Although large volumes of pericardial fluid that accumulate gradually may be tolerated, rapid accumulation of fluid can result in critical impairment of ventricular filling and shock. Causes of hydropericardium include infectious pericarditis, postpericardotomy syndrome, uremia, and extravasations from central venous catheters. Hemopericardium results from blunt or penetrating trauma and perioperative bleeding in cardiac surgery. Tension pneumothorax is another intrathoracic extra-cardiac lesion that may critically reduce cardiac output.

Acute obstruction to pulmonary blood flow may cause right-sided heart failure and produce left-sided failure and shock via ventricular interdependence. Massive pulmonary embolism secondary to deep vein thrombosis (DVT) or in thrombophilic states (protein C and S deficiency, factor V Leyden, systemic lupus erythematosus) may produce cardiogenic shock. Pulmonary hypertensive crises, if severe, can also lead to biventricular failure and shock. In newborns, primary pulmonary hypertension (PPHN), congenital diaphragmatic hernia (CDH), and severe meconium aspiration may present with cardiogenic shock. Such severe vasospasm in older children is most often seen following surgical repair of congenital cardiac lesions, typically in patients with large preexisting left-to-right shunts such as with ventricular septal defect (VSD) or complete atrioventricular canal (CAVC), although exacerbation of chronic pulmonary hypertension may also precipitate heart failure and shock.

PRESENTATION

The signs of cardiogenic shock are the same as those associated with other modes of shock—hypotension, vasoconstriction, clouded sensorium, and oliguria. Infants may present with irritability, lethargy, or poor feeding. Tachycardia will occur except in cases of sinus node failure or heart block. Signs of profound vasodilatation will typically be absent, as the primary cause of this condition is low cardiac output and compensatory reflexes will predominate. Specific signs may be present depending on the etiology of cardiac failure.

Physical examination may reveal distant heart sounds, jugular venous distention, gallop rhythms, and pulsus paradoxus in tamponade. Murmurs may suggest structural lesions such as valvular stenosis, valvular insufficiency, or VSD. Pulse palpation reveals the heart rate and may suggest the presence of coarctation or important aortic insufficiency.

DIFFERENTIAL DIAGNOSIS

Cardiogenic shock must be distinguished from hypovolemic, vasodilatory, or distributive shock, because the course of treatment depends on correctly identifying the cause of the pump failure. As a consequence, differential diagnosis and treatment must proceed in parallel.

PLAN OF CARE

Cardiogenic shock is identified by demonstration of pump failure. If the shock state is unresponsive or poorly responsive to aggressive volume loading and inotropic/vasopressor support, then evidence of the source of pump failure must be sought.

Laboratory studies should include basic screening studies to exclude severe anemia and electrolyte abnormalities as physiologic causes. Blood gas analysis will reveal any associated impairment of pulmonary gas exchange and the degree of metabolic acidosis. Serum lactate more specifically measures deficiency of tissue oxygen delivery and is easily tracked. Troponin levels, as a measure of myocyte injury, will be elevated in trauma, ischemia, and myocarditis (Sukova et al., 2007). BNP is a marker of heart failure; its levels will be elevated in many etiologies of cardiogenic shock (Mutlu et al., 2006).

Initial diagnostic studies include an ECG and CXR. The ECG allows pathologic rhythms to be identified. In particular, severe bradycardia or heart block will be obvious in cardiogenic shock. Most pediatric patients in shock are tachycardic; therefore, distinguishing causative pathologic tachycardia (SVT, AET, JET) from reflex sinus tachycardia secondary to heart failure may require specialist consultation. Important points are the presence of sinus rhythm, QRS morphology, and response to volume support. The CXR reveals heart size; significant cardiomegaly suggests that HCPs investigate the possibility of heart failure or tamponade. Pulmonary edema may also suggest the presence of heart failure. Tension pneumothorax may also be excluded. These examinations may be done rapidly and will direct care toward the necessary specialized investigations and care.

Echocardiography is the critical diagnostic study required, because it characterizes cardiac systolic dysfunction. In particular, this technique may identify pericardial fluid and tamponade physiology. Structural lesions, either congenital or acquired, are rapidly defined and their physiologic impact assessed. Most important, ventricular

function may be rapidly estimated. Short- and long-axis views of the heart allow measurement of ventricular ejection and shortening fractions and will show segmental wall motion abnormalities. Impaired ventricular relaxation, as in diastolic dysfunction, may be detected. Coronary artery lesions may be identifiable. Pulmonary hypertension may be suggested by predominant right ventricular dysfunction and estimates of RV pressure. Treatable lesions, if present, may be rapidly addressed. Identification of severely depressed myocardial function both defines the clinical state and should set in motion the necessary steps to provide options for definitive support.

Invasive measurement of cardiac performance is typically used to both diagnose and treat cardiogenic shock. For example, arterial catheterization allows precise beat-to-beat measurement of blood pressure in patients who may be hemodynamically labile and in whom noninvasive blood pressure measurements may be inaccurate. Central venous catheterization (CVC) provides direct evidence of right-sided filling pressures and permits safe infusion of inotropes and vasopressors. Flow-directed pulmonary thermodilution catheters provide the best bedside estimates of left-sided filling pressure, systemic and pulmonary vascular resistance, and cardiac output. When these measures are considered, the benefit to a given patient must be carefully weighed against the risks, especially of induced arrhythmia, and in light of the quality of other information available. In rare cases, cardiac catheterization may be indicated for diagnosis (coronary abnormalities, pulmonary hypertension, intracardiac lesions), biopsy (myocarditis, cardiomyopathy), or therapy (balloon dilatation, atrial septostomy).

Although accurate diagnosis of the many possible etiologies of cardiogenic shock is vital to successful management of this condition, immediate support is necessary: diagnosis and treatment must occur in parallel. It is worth repeating that *the earliest indication that shock in a pediatric patient is cardiogenic is the poor or absent response to standard fluid resuscitation.* Prompt recognition of cardiogenic shock is critical to survival and allows early involvement of experts in critical care, cardiology, and mechanical cardiac support. Once shock is recognized, the basics of monitoring, intravenous access, volume support, supplemental oxygen, and assisted ventilation (if needed) are provided. Further treatment is best organized according to the components of cardiac output.

Rate and rhythm

Severe bradycardia may be treated with anticholinergic agents and/or chronotropic infusions. Isoproterenol effectively accelerates heart rate, but the ensuing vasodilatation may be detrimental; thus epinephrine may at times be a better choice. If conduction block is present and ventricular response to catecholamines is inadequate, pacing may be needed—use of the transcutaneous, transesophageal, or transvenous routes may ensure that this treatment is rapidly initiated.

Tachycardia unresponsive to volume support, especially if sinus rhythm cannot be verified, must be carefully evaluated. Wide-complex tachycardia with unstable hypotension requires synchronized cardioversion. Adenosine may be safely used to diagnose and (sometimes) treat SVT. Treatment of primary tachyarrhythmias in shock patients is a treacherous enterprise, as almost all antiarrhythmic drugs have negative inotropic effects or other potential toxicities. Expert electrophysiologic consultation is critically important in arrhythmia-mediated cardiogenic shock.

Preload

Central venous access and pressure monitoring are mandatory in shock patients who do not rapidly improve with intravenous volume support. If the central venous pressure (CVP) is still low, additional volume should be given. Preload must be optimized by correlating volume administration, CVP, and response (improved measures of blood pressure and apparent cardiac output). Once an adequate CVP (in the range of at least 10–12 cm H_2O) is obtained, a Starling response (cardiac output/preload relationship) from additional volume should be sought. If administration of additional volume increases blood pressure and cardiac output, CVP may be increased until a plateau of benefit is seen. If increasing the CVP does not improve circulatory function, other therapeutic interventions are needed.

Cardiac function

To treat cardiogenic shock, the patient's metabolic state should be optimized. Appropriate ionized calcium and phosphorus levels are important for myocardial contractility. Normal sodium and potassium levels reduce the risk of arrhythmias. Correction of acidemia and treatment of hypoxemia may improve cardiac function.

Pharmacologic inotropic support is usually required in cardiogenic shock. Catecholamines are the mainstay of treatment. Dopamine is a common initial treatment but an enlightened empiricism must be used: An individual patient's response must be monitored and drugs added or changed according to his or her therapeutic response. Dobutamine, epinephrine, and norepinephrine may also be used singly or in combination. The relative changes in contractility, rate, and vasoconstriction produced by the chosen catecholamines will determine the efficacy. Tachycardia may be a detrimental consequence of catecholamine therapy, and increased arrhythmias may limit the choice or dose of a given drug. Antiarrhythmic therapy and catecholamine support may need to be combined and titrated in unison. Signs of increasing cardiac output (urine output, decreasing lactate, improved capillary refill) in addition to rising blood pressure signal therapeutic success.

Noncatecholamine therapy may be helpful in selected cases. For example, the phosphodiesterase inhibitor milrinone reduces afterload and increases inotropy, which is theoretically the ideal support combination for the failing myocardium, however, this agent may be poorly tolerated in the presence of hypotension and is difficult to titrate. Vasopressin may raise blood pressure, yet the vasoconstriction it produces may further impair cardiac function (Hollenberg, 2009). High-dose corticosteroids and triiodothyronine (T_3, the active form of thyroid hormone) may improve heart function in some scenarios (Cini et al., 2009). If pulmonary hypertension is suspected or demonstrated, therapy may include metabolic and respiratory alkalinization, hyperoxygenation, and administration of specific pulmonary vasodilators (INO, inhaled or intravenous prostacyclin) (Suesawalak et al., 2010).

Mechanical support

Recognizing the need for mechanical cardiac support is a difficult but a mandatory step in the algorithm of care for patients with cardiogenic shock. Most patients will respond to the interventions previously detailed. However, if the trajectory of the disease is not improved by conventional support, and if the underlying cause of the myocardial failure is believed to be reversible, then mechanical support should be considered if available. He pediatric patient in progressive cardiogenic shock who suffers cardiac arrest is *unlikely* to be successfully resuscitated.

Emergent mechanical cardiac support is provided with veno-arterial ECMO. Vascular access is gained surgically or percutaneously, though the sites of access will vary by patient size and institutional preference (as described later in this chapter). Extracorporeal support provides gas exchange and oxygen delivery independent of native cardiac function, allowing for organ system recovery while relieving cardiac workload. Emergent provision of ECMO in children is a technically demanding task that requires planning, training, interprofessional cooperation, and institutional commitment; however, improved patient soutcomes after emergent cardiac mechanical support justify the effort (Raymond et al., 2010).

A mandatory step in successful rescue ECMO is recognition by the HCP at the bedside that conventional support has failed to stabilize the course of the patient in cardiogenic shock. As therapy proceeds, all of the previously noted parameters of diagnosis must be integrated into the plan of care. If blood pressure, rhythm, urine output, Starling performance, acid–base status, and lactate clearance improve, then the therapy is working. If the patient in cardiogenic shock fails to improve despite escalating inotropic therapy and higher filling pressures or continues in a pathologic rhythm after antiarrhythmic treatment, then the local protocol for securing access to mechanical support should be initiated.

Given the time required at most institutions to assemble the team and equipment for ECMO, proactive decision making at the bedside is vital. It is far better to ask the ECMO team to stand down when the patient unexpectedly improves than to initiate mechanical support after prolonged delivery of CPR (Lin et al., 2008). Nevertheless, more centers are using, and reporting, acceptable outcomes using ECMO during active CPR (Huang et al., 2008; Kelly & Harrison, 2010). At institutions without ECMO capability, rapid and difficult decisions will be required to facilitate transport of patients who may require mechanical support to ECMO-capable centers. Expectant action and a high index of suspicion for treatment failure are required to save pediatric patients with refractory cardiogenic shock.

The patient who is stabilized on mechanical cardiac support may follow several paths. Some patients—typically those with acute myocarditis or arrhythmia-mediated cardiomyopathy—may recover cardiac function over time and transition off support. Surgical or interventional correction of structural lesions may then proceed. For other patients, ECMO may serve as a direct bridge to cardiac transplantation when functional recovery is not expected. However, the waiting period for a donor organ is typically longer than the period for which ECMO support can be provided without life-threatening complications. At institutions that provide patients with long-term mechanical support, these patients may be transitioned to a left ventricular assist device (LVAD) or right ventricular assist device (RVAD). Bridge to transplantation (or in some cases long-term recovery) therapies may be provided for months in patients who are awake and mobile (Imamura et al., 2009). Other patients who have no recovery, who are not candidates for transplantation, or who suffer irreversible organ injury may ultimately require withdrawal of mechanical support without hope of survival.

Prompt recognition of cardiogenic shock is critical to the patient's survival. Early consultation of the following subspecialties should be initiated: critical care, pulmonology, cardiology, cardiothoracic surgery, mechanical cardiac support team, cardiac transplant team, and infectious disease specialists. Although nutrition specialists may not be consulted immediately, they should become involved in the patient's plan of care as soon as it is reasonably possible. Additionally, other subspecialists may be called upon depending on the etiology of the underlying disorder. The diagnosis of cardiogenic shock and failure may be overwhelming for the family; thus, a number of support services may be necessary to assist them, such as social work, spiritual support, and child life. As the patient begins his or her recovery period, the rehabilitative team should be consulted to promote return to developmental baselines.

Patient and family education may initially address the acute illness, the diagnostic studies and their findings, and health care team members who are involved in the plan of care. If the patient's acuity worsens, discussion about life-support options and possible transport may be required.

DISPOSITION AND DISCHARGE PLANNING

Recoveries from cardiogenic shock are as diverse as the causes of this condition. For example, a pediatric patient with an acute hydropericardium and tamponade may recover fully shortly after treatment. Surgically treated structural lesions may likewise be completely corrected. Arrhythmia-mediated heart failure may fully resolve with drug or ablation therapy. Patients with myocarditis may either make full recovery or be left with impaired function and require chronic heart failure management. Patients who present in shock due to cardiomyopathies may likewise survive with CHF. Referral to a specialized pediatric heart failure management program optimizes outcome for such children (Margossian, 2008). Those who require cardiac transplantation represent a distinct group; their longevity and quality of life will depend on the services of an integrated transplant management program.

> **Critical Thinking**
> An index of suspicion for cardiogenic causes is critical in children who do not respond well to resuscitation.

CARDIOVASCULAR AGENTS

Jennifer L. Fuller and Justin T. Hamrick

Cardiovascular disease is multifaceted in etiology and often associated with complex underlying pathophysiology. Since Sir William Withering first described the therapeutic benefits of foxglove (digitalis) in 1785, cardiovascular agents have steadily evolved to encompass an expansive arsenal of medications with diverse mechanisms of action. Cardiovascular agents are used to ultimately optimize the four determinants of cardiac output: preload, contractility, afterload, and heart rate (Costello & Almodovar, 2007). This section reviews vasopressors and inotropes, antihypertensives, antiarrhythmics, and several other medications commonly used in pediatric acute care.

ADRENOCEPTORS

The term "adrenoceptor" is widely used to describe receptors that respond to catecholamines (Katzung, 2001). Endogenous catecholamines include dopamine, epinephrine, and norepinephrine; synthetic catecholamines are referred to as sympathomimetics. Three major classes of adrenoceptors are distinguished: α-adrenergic, β-adrenergic, and dopaminergic. The effector cell response to endogenous or exogenous catecholamines is related primarily to their interaction with these receptors (Shekerdemian & Redington, 1998). In particular, the molecular heterogeneity of the complex transmembrane glycoprotein is the foundation of receptor specificity (Latifi et al., 2000). The vasopressin receptor, although not an adrenoceptor, is included here to provide a comprehensive review. The roles of the various receptors in homeostatic control of the cardiovascular system are summarized in Table 22-17.

α-adrenoceptor

Two distinct subtypes of α-adrenoceptors exist: α_1 and α_2.

α_1 *receptor.* α_1-Adrenoceptors are found in coronary, cutaneous, uterine, intestinal, and splanchnic vascular smooth muscle (Johnson et al., 2009). They are exclusively postsynaptic. In vascular smooth muscle, their activation affects vasomotor tone. In resistance and capacitance vessels, their activation results in vasoconstriction. In intestinal beds, their activation results in vasodilation (Johnson et al.). Activation of myocardial α-adrenoceptors results in increased contractility, also known as positive inotropy.

α_2 *receptor.* α_2-Adrenoceptors can be located on either the presynaptic or postsynaptic cell membrane. Presynaptic α_2-adrenoceptors are found in sympathetic nerve terminals

TABLE 22-17

Adrenoceptors and Vasopressin Receptors				
Receptor	**Receptor Site**	**Physiologic Action**	**Clinical Significance**	**Agonist Potency**
α_1	• Vascular smooth muscle • Heart	• Arterial vasoconstriction • Increased myocardial contractility	• ↑ Afterload via ↑ SVR • ↓ Distal perfusion with risk of tissue and end-organ ischemia • ↑ Myocardial oxygen demand	NE ≥ E > D
α_2	• Vascular smooth muscle • Presynaptic sympathetic nerve terminals	• Vasoconstriction of venous capacitance vessels • Feedback inhibition of NE release	• ↑ Preload by shifting venous capacitance centrally • Vasodilation and ↑ PS tone (↓ SVR, ↓ CO, ↓ HR)	NE ≥ E
β_1	• Heart	• ↑ Inotropy • ↑ Chronotropy • ↑ AV node conduction velocity	• ↑ Myocardial oxygen demand	I > E ≥ NE ≥ D
β_2	• Vascular smooth muscle • Bronchial smooth muscle	• Vasodilation • Bronchodilation	• ↓ Preload by shifting venous capacitance distally • ↓ Afterload via ↓ SVR	I ≥ E >> D > NE
D_1	• Vascular smooth muscle (kidney, splanchnic, cerebral, coronary) • Kidney tubules	• Vasodilation • Inhibition of sodium absorption, leading to natriuresis and diuresis	• ↑ Preload and afterload as above • ↑ Kidney, cerebral, splanchnic, and coronary perfusion • ↓ Preload via ↓ CBV	D
D_2	• Presynaptic sympathetic nerve terminals • Kidney and mesenteric vasculature	• Inhibits NE release with resultant vasodilation • Vasoconstriction	• ↑ Preload and afterload • ↑ Preload and afterload • ↓ Kidney & mesenteric perfusion	D
V_1	• Vascular smooth muscle (skin, skeletal muscle)	• Arterial vasoconstriction	• ↑ Afterload via ↑ SVR • ↓ Cutaneous and skeletal muscle perfusion	V
V_2	• Vascular smooth muscle (mesenteric) • Renal tubular cells	• Arterial vasoconstriction • Enhanced free water resorption	• ↑ Afterload via ↑ SVR • ↓ Mesenteric perfusion • ↓ Preload via ↑ CBV	V

Cardiac output (CO), circulating blood volume (CBV), dopamine (D), epinephrine (E), isoproterenol (I), norepinephrine (NE), parasympathetic (PS), systemic vascular resistance (SVR), vasopressin (V).

Sources: Dager et al., 2006; Hoffman, 2001a, 2001b; Johnson et al., 2009; Latifi et al., 2000.

in the coronary and peripheral vascular smooth muscle; their activation triggers a negative feedback loop that results in inhibition of norepinephrine release into the synaptic cleft. The overall result is decreased sympathetic and increased parasympathetic tone, which culminates in local vasodilation, decreased cardiac output, decreased inotropy, and decreased heart rate (Johnson et al., 2009). Postsynaptic α_2-adrenoceptors are similar to the α_1-adrenoceptors; they are located in vascular smooth muscle and their activation results in vasoconstriction.

β-adrenoceptor

Two subtypes of β-adrenoceptors are significant to the cardiovascular system: β_1 and β_2.

β_1 receptor. β_1-Adrenoceptors are located in the myocardium, sinoatrial (SA) node, and ventricular conduction system (Johnson et al., 2009). Like the α_1-adrenoceptors, they are exclusively postsynaptic. Activation of these receptors ultimately results in an increase in both contractility and heart rate—known as positive inotropy and chronotropy, respectively.

β_2 receptor. Like α_2-adrenoceptors, β_2-adrenoceptors can be located on either the presynaptic or postsynaptic cell membrane. Presynaptic β_2-adrenoceptors are found in the myocardium, SA node, and ventricular conduction system. They counteract presynaptic α_2-adrenoceptors; that is, their activation results in an increase in norepinephrine release into the synaptic cleft (Johnson et al., 2009). This effect ultimately results in increased sympathetic and decreased parasympathetic tone, which culminates in local vasoconstriction, increased cardiac output, increased inotropy, and increased heart rate. Postsynaptic β_2-adrenoceptors are located in the myocardium and in both vascular and bronchial smooth muscle. Activation of postsynaptic myocardial β_2-adrenoceptors results in positive inotropy and chronotropy, whereas activation of postsynaptic vascular and bronchial β_2-adrenoceptors results in vasodilation and bronchodilation, respectively.

Dopaminergic adrenoceptor

Two distinct subtypes of D-adrenoceptors are relevant to the cardiovascular system: D_1 and D_2.

D_1 receptor. D_1-adrenoceptors are postsynaptic receptors that are found in renal, mesenteric, cerebral, and coronary vascular smooth muscle; sympathetic ganglia; renal tubules; and juxtaglomerular cells (Johnson et al., 2009). Activation of vascular D_1-adrenoceptors results in vasodilation, whereas activation of renal tubular D_1-adrenoceptors results in natriuresis and diuresis (Table 22-17).

D_2 receptor. D_2-adrenoceptors can be either presynaptic or postsynaptic. Like the presynaptic α_2-adrenoceptors, presynaptic D_2-adrenoceptors are located in sympathetic nerve terminals and inhibit norepinephrine release into the synaptic cleft (Johnson et al., 2009). Postsynaptic D_2-adrenoceptors are found in renal and mesenteric vasculature; their activation results in vasoconstriction of these vessels.

Vasopressin receptor

Two subtypes of vasopressin receptors are distinguished: V_1 and V_2.

V_1 receptor. The V_1 receptors are located in vascular smooth muscle of the skin and skeletal muscle (Dager et al., 2006). Their activation ultimately results in arterial vasoconstriction, shunting blood to more vital organs.

V_2 receptor. The V_2 receptors are located in vascular smooth muscle of the mesenteric circulation and in renal tubular cells (Dager et al., 2006). Activation of mesenteric vascular receptors results in arterial vasoconstriction, whereas activation of renal tubular receptors results in free water resorption and, ultimately, increased circulating blood volume (Reid, 2001).

VASOPRESSORS AND POSITIVE INOTROPES

Vasopressors are endogenous or synthetic substances that produce a vasoconstriction effect and result in increased systemic vascular resistance. Positive inotropes are endogenous or synthetic substances that result in improved cardiac contractility. In general, different combinations of these medications are used in three scenarios (Ceneviva et al., 1998):

- ↓ Cardiac output and ↑ systemic vascular resistance: inotrope ± vasodilator
- ↑ Cardiac output and ↓ systemic vascular resistance: vasopressor
- ↓ Cardiac output and ↓ systemic vascular resistance: inotrope + vasopressor

The medications are summarized in Table 22-18.

Digoxin (digitalis)

Digoxin is the most commonly used cardiac glycoside. It is prescribed in the treatment of CHF as a positive inotrope and in the treatment of cardiac dysrhythmias. Digoxin acts via inhibition of the sarcolemmal sodium–potassium ATPase, resulting in an increased concentration of myocyte intracellular calcium, which is required for myocardial

TABLE 22-18

Vasopressors and Positive Inotropes

Drug	Receptor Specificity	Physiologic Effects	Clinical Use	Dosage	Adverse Effects
Digoxin	Na$^+$/K$^+$ ATPase	• Inotrope: ++ • Vasopressor: — • Chronotrope: — • Vasodilator: — • Other: Indirect antiadrenergic effects (causes ↑ PS tone)	• CHF • Supraventricular arrhythmias	Recommended oral doses: DD (mcg/kg): • PRE: 20 • FT: 30 • C < 2 yr: 40–50 • C > 2 yr: 30–40 MD (mcg/kg): • PRE: 5 • FT: 8–10 • C < 2 yr: 10–12 • C > 2 yr: 8–10 TR: 1–2 ng/mL *NOTE: IV dose is 75% of the oral dose*	• Bradycardia • SA and AV node blockade • Atrial and ventricular arrhythmias • N/V, anorexia • Altered mental status • Hypersensitivity reaction • Caution: Hypokalemia, hypercalcemia, hypomagnesemia • C/I: AV block, hypertrophic cardiomyopathy, constrictive pericarditis
Dobutamine	β$_1$ > β$_2$ >>> α	• Inotrope: +++ • Vasopressor: +/− • Chronotrope: ++ • Vasodilator: + • Other: Lusitrope, does not significantly ↑ pulmonary vascular resistance	• CHF • Cardiogenic shock • First line if ↓ CO and ↑ SVR • Good agent to ↑ inotropy without significant ↑ HR • Good agent for patients with PHTN	• Infusion: 2–20 mcg/kg/min	• Tachycardia • Arrhythmias • Cardiac ischemia • Extravasation injury • Caution: On BBx (unmask α-effects) • C/I: Dynamic outflow obstruction
Dopamine	D$_1$ = D$_2$ >> β >> α	• Inotrope: +++ • Vasopressor: ++ • Chronotrope: + • Vasodilator: + • Other: Dose-related activity, ↑ pulmonary vascular resistance	• Hypotension • Cardiogenic shock • Distributive shock (first line) after adequate fluid resuscitation	• Infusion: 2–20 mcg/kg/min	• Tachydysrhythmias • Hypertension • Cardiac and peripheral (especially limb and cutaneous) ischemia • Extravasation injury • Caution: PHTN • C/I: Pheochromocytoma
Epinephrine	α$_1$ = α$_2$ β$_1$ = β$_2$	• Inotrope: ++++ • Vasopressor: +++ • Chronotrope: +++ • Vasodilator: +/− • Other: Bronchodilation	• Pulseless arrest, bradycardia • Hypotension • Distributive shock • DA + fluid-refractory shock • Anaphylaxis • Severe asthma	• Bolus: 0.01 mg/kg 1:10,000 IV/IO q 3–5 min (maximum 1 mg/dose) • Infusion: 0.1–1 mcg/kg/min	• Tachycardia • Hypertension • Cardiac ischemia • Arrhythmia • C/I: Acute-angle glaucoma, cardiac dysrhythmias

Drug	Receptor	Pharmacologic effects	Indications	Dose	Adverse effects/Cautions
Isoproterenol	$\beta_1 = \beta_2$	• Inotrope: ++++ • Vasopressor: — • Chronotrope: ++++ • Vasodilator: +++ • Other: Bronchodilation, pulmonary vasodilation	• Use limited by adverse effects on myocardial O_2 balance • Bradycardia • AV block • PHTN • Right ventricular myocardial dysfunction	• Infusion: 0.05–0.5 mcg/kg/min	• Tachycardia • Cardiac ischemia • Arrhythmia • Hypotension • C/I: Outflow tract obstruction, unrepaired tetralogy of Fallot, diastolic hypotension
Milrinone	PDE III	• Inotrope: + • Vasopressor: — • Chronotrope: — • Vasodilator: + • Other: Lusitrope, pulmonary vasodilation	• Myocardial dysfunction with ↑ SVR or PVR • Diastolic dysfunction • LCOS • PHTN	• Loading dose: 50–75 mcg/kg • Infusion: 0.5–0.75 mcg/kg/min	• Ventricular and supraventricular dysrhythmias • Hypotension • Cardiac ischemia • Caution: Renal failure • C/I: Severe aortic or pulmonary obstructive disease
Norepinephrine	$\alpha_1 = \alpha_2$ $\beta_1 \gg \beta_2$	• Inotrope: ++++ • Vasopressor: ++++ • Chronotrope: +++ • Vasodilator: — • Other: Compensatory vagal reflexes may overcome (+) chronotropy	• Hypotension • Distributive shock • DA + fluid-refractory shock • Hypercyanotic tet spells	• Infusion: 0.1–2 mcg/kg/min	• Hypertension • Bradycardia • Cardiac and peripheral ischemia
Phenylephrine	$\alpha_1 > \alpha_2$	• Inotrope: — • Vasopressor: ++++ • Chronotrope: — • Vasodilator: — • Other: Reflex bradycardia	• Hypercyanotic Tet spells • SVT • Refractory hypotension	• Infusion: 0.1–0.5 mcg/kg/min	• Bradycardia • Cardiac ischemia • Caution: Ischemic heart disease
Vasopressin	$V_1 = V_2$	• Inotrope: — • Vasopressor: ++++ • Chronotrope: — • Vasodilator: — • Other:	• Persistent hypotension despite adequate fluids and NE in distributive shock • Pulseless arrest • Neurogenic diabetes insipidus	• Bolus: 40 IU × 1 dose • Infusion: 0.003–0.002 IU/kg/min	• Cardiac and peripheral ischemia • Caution: SIADH

Atrioventricular (AV), beta blocker (BBx), cardiac output (CO), child (C), congestive heart failure (CHF), contraindication (C/I), digitalizing dose (DD), dopamine (DA), full-term infant (FT), international unit (IU), international unit /kilogram/minute (IU/kg/min), low cardiac output state (LCOS), maintenance dose (MD), micrograms/kilogram/minute (mcg/kg/min), milligrams (mg), nausea/vomiting (N/V), norepinephrine (NE), parasympathetic (PS), phosphodiesterase (PDE), premature infant (PRE), pulmonary artery pressure (PAP), pulmonary hypertension (PHTN), sinoatrial (SA), supraventricular tachycardia (SVT), systemic vascular resistance (SVR), therapeutic range (TR), years of age (yr).

Sources: AHA, 2006; Dellinger et al., 2008; Hoffman, 2001a, 2001b; Johnson et al., 2009; Latifi et al., 2000; Shekerdemian & Redington, 1998; Wessel & Fraisse, 2008.

contraction (Shekerdemian & Redington, 1998). The potential for digitalis toxicity requires closely monitoring patients, however, as life-threatening arrhythmias may be the first and only presenting symptom of this problem (Shekerdemian & Redington). Additional symptoms of digitalis toxicity include bradycardia, SA or atrioventricular (AV) block, atrial or nodal ectopy or tachycardia, ventricular arrhythmias, nausea or vomiting, anorexia, diarrhea, headache, blurred vision, and generalized fatigue (Latifi et al., 2000).

Dobutamine

Dobutamine is a synthetic catecholamine that is derived (modified) from the classic inodilator isoproterenol (Johnson et al., 2009). This agent's actions are primarily mediated via stimulation of β-adrenoceptors, resulting in positive inotropy and chronotropy (Wessel & Fraisse, 2008). Other beneficial effects include pulmonary vasodilation, enhanced diastolic relaxation (lusitropy), and significantly increased coronary blood flow when compared to dopamine (Shekerdemian & Redington, 1998). Dobutamine is used primarily in the treatment of depressed cardiac output associated with high systemic vascular resistance (cold shock) (Dellinger et al., 2008).

Dopamine

Dopamine is an endogenous catecholamine that acts via dose-dependent stimulation dopaminergic-, α-, and β-adrenoceptors. Historically, dopamine has been described as low-dose, medium-dose, or high-dose therapy based on receptor specificity and activation within the dose range. In pediatrics, however, there is a great deal of variability in patients' response to this agent, making this classification less relevant in this patient population. Dopamine doses ranging from 5 to 10 mcg/kg/min begin to activate β-adrenoceptors, with resultant positive inotropy and chronotropy; by comparison, dopamine doses greater than 10 mcg/kg/min begin to activate α-adrenoceptors, causing an increase in afterload and pulmonary vascular resistance (Shekerdemian & Redington, 1998). Dopamine is used as a first-line agent in the treatment of fluid-refractory hypotension, and it is a good single-agent therapy for depressed cardiac output states associated with low systemic vascular resistance (Dellinger et al., 2008).

Epinephrine

Epinephrine is an endogenous catecholamine that is synthesized and released from the adrenal medulla; it acts via stimulation of α- and β-adrenoceptors in a dose-related manner. Low-dose infusions have more β-adrenergic effects—that is, positive inotropy and chronotropy. Additionally,

decreased systemic vascular resistance may occur due to vasodilation of splanchnic and skeletal muscle vascular beds. Higher-dose infusions begin to promote α-adrenergic effects, resulting in increased systemic vascular resistance (Shekerdemian & Redington, 1998). Epinephrine is the most widely used catecholamine in the treatment of cardiac arrest, but is also used in the treatment of hypotension, anaphylaxis, and asthma (Johnson et al., 2009).

Isoproterenol

Isoproterenol is a synthetic isopropyl derivative of norepinephrine (Latifi et al., 2000). A selective, balanced β-**adre**nergic agonist, its use results in positive inotropy and chronotropy and peripheral and pulmonary vasodilation. Although its clinical use is limited secondary to its adverse effects on myocardial oxygen balance, this agent is very effective in the treatment of bradycardia and AV block (Shekerdemian & Redington, 1998).

Milrinone

Milrinone is a synthetic phosophodiesterase (PDE) inhibitor. Inhibition of PDE III in myocardial cells results in increased intracellular calcium levels and positive inotropy. In vascular smooth muscle, increased stores of intracellular calcium lead to vasodilation and decreased systemic vascular resistance. In addition, milrinone is a positive lusitropic agent; its use promotes diastolic relaxation, which in turn stimulates diastolic filling (Johnson et al., 2009). Milrinone is used in the treatment of low cardiac output states associated with high systemic vascular resistance, isolated diastolic dysfunction, and pulmonary hypertension (Shekerdemian & Redington, 1998).

Norepinephrine

Norepinephrine, which is the immediate precursor of epinephrine, is an endogenous catecholamine that is derived from dopamine. It primarily acts through activation of α-adrenoceptors, although it has some β-adrenergic activity. This dual action results in an increase in systemic vascular resistance with little to no inotropic or chronotropic effect (Shekerdemian & Redington, 1998). Norepinephrine is primarily used in the treatment of hyperdynamic cardiac output states associated with low systemic vascular resistance (warm shock) (Johnson et al., 2009).

Phenylephrine

Phenylephrine is a synthetic catecholamine that is specific to α-adrenoceptors. It increases systemic vascular resistance in a dose-dependent manner, but has little effect on cardiac output or inotropy (Johnson et al., 2009). In pediatrics, phenylephrine is most frequently used in the treatment of hypercyanotic "Tet" spells, although it has successfully been used for chemical cardioversion of SVT (Shekerdemian & Redington, 1998). The resting vagal tone in pediatric patients is higher than that in adults, so reflex bradycardia with this agent may be more profound.

Vasopressin

Vasopressin is an exogenous analogue of antidiuretic hormone that acts on vasopressin receptors. In addition to causing free water resorption at the renal level, vasopressin receptors are found in vascular smooth muscle and cardiac myocytes; activation of the receptors in these areas results in positive inotropy and vasoconstriction (Johnson et al., 2009). Vasopressin may be used in the treatment of pulseless arrest and refractory hypotension.

ANTIHYPERTENSIVES

Antihypertensive agents are classified into four broad categories based on the final common pathway of their mechanism of action: diuretics, agents that block the production or action of angiotensin II, sympathoplegic agents, and direct vasodilators (Benowitz, 2001) (Table 22-19).

Diuretics

Diuretics act by depleting total body sodium via the kidney. This effect decreases the circulating blood volume and lowers the blood pressure. This medication class includes thiazide and loop diuretics.

Agents that block the production or action of angiotensin II

Inhibition of either the production or action of angiotensin II results in decreased peripheral vascular resistance, which may also decrease effective circulating blood volume via indirect inhibition of aldosterone secretion. This medication class includes angiotensin-converting enzyme inhibitors (ACE or ACEI) and angiotensin-receptor blockers (ARBs).

Sympathoplegic agents

Sympathoplegic agents act to decrease systemic vascular resistance and cardiac output, via depressed cardiac function and increased venous pooling in capacitance vessels. This medication class includes centrally acting α-adrenoceptor antagonists, α-adrenoceptor antagonists, β-adrenoceptor antagonists, and mixed α- and β-adrenoceptor antagonists.

Direct vasodilators

Direct vasodilators act via relaxation of arterial and/or venous smooth muscle, thereby decreasing systemic vascular resistance and/or increasing venous capacitance. This medication class includes calcium-channel blockers, fenoldopam, hydralazine, nitroglycerin, and sodium nitroprusside.

ANTIARRHYTHMICS

The classification of antiarrhythmic drugs is based on the drug's effect on the two types of action potentials found in cardiac tissue: the fast-response action potential and the slow-response action potential. The fast-response action potential is predominated by sodium channels, and is found in the atrial and ventricular myocytes and in the Purkinje fibers. The slow-response action potential is predominated by slow calcium channels and is present in the SA and AV nodes (Marino et al., 2008). Although digoxin and adenosine are not included in this class, they are useful antiarrhythmics. Antiarrhythmics commonly used in pediatrics include adenosine, amiodarone, lidocaine, and procainamide (Table 22-20).

Class I: sodium-channel blockers

Class I antiarrhythmics act via blockade of the rapid sodium channel and delay the upstroke of the action potential. This results in lengthening of the QRS complex and the QT interval (Marino et al., 2008). The three subdivisions within this class—IA, IB, and IC—are based on variable degrees of sodium-channel blockade and effects on the action potential duration. Examples include procainamide (IA), lidocaine (IB), and flecainide (IC).

Class II: beta blockers

Class II antiarrhythmics result in decreased sympathetic activity via competitive β-adrenoceptor blockade. Decreased sympathetic tone slows spontaneous discharge from the SA node, decreases conduction velocity through the AV node, and decreases abnormal automaticity from ectopic sites (Marino et al., 2008). The members of this class differ in their receptor selectivity and intrinsic sympathomimetic activity (Perry & Walsh, 1998). Examples include esmolol, atenolol, and propofol.

Class III: potassium-channel blockers

Class III agents act on the blockade of potassium channels, resulting in a prolonged action potential duration and effective refractory period (Perry & Walsh, 1998). Members of this class are pharmacologically complex, with additional

TABLE 22-19

Antihypertensives

Class	Mechanism of Action	Physiologic Effects	Clinical Use	Adverse Effects	Examples and Dosage
Agents That Block the Production or Action of Angiotensin II					
ACE inhibitors	• Prevents conversion of AT-I to AT-II via inhibition of ACE • Prevents breakdown of bradykinin • Aldosterone production is usually maintained by ACTH	• Balanced vasodilation • ↓ SVR • Little to no change in CO or HR • ↑ Renal blood flow • No change in coronary or cerebral perfusion	• Hypertension • CHF • Left ventricular hypertrophy • Dilated cardiomyopathy • Postischemic systolic dysfunction • Diabetes mellitus	• Hypotension • Angioedema • Chronic cough • Renal insufficiency • Self-limited proteinuria • Fetotoxicity in the second and third trimesters • Hyperkalemia	Captopril: • 0.3–0.5 mg/kg/dose in 2–4 divided doses • Maximum dose: 6 mg/kg/day
ARBs	• Competitive blockade of AT-I receptors	• Balanced vasodilation • ↓ SVR • Little to no change in CO or HR	• Hypertension • CHF	• Hypotension • Angioedema • C/I in pregnant and breastfeeding mothers • Hyperkalemia	Losartan: • 0.7 mg/kg/day once daily • Maximum dose: 50 mg / day
Sympathoplegic Agents					
Centrally acting α agonists	• Activates central α_2-receptors in the medulla • ↓ Central SNS outflow • Indirect ↑ PS tone	• Vasodilation • ↓ SVR • ↓ CO • ↓ Plasma renin concentrations • ↓ Plasma NE and EPI concentrations	• Hypertension • CRPS • Anxiety	• Hypotension • Orthostatic hypotension • Bradycardia • AV block • Sedation • Xerostomia • Withdrawal syndrome	Clonidine: • Children ≥ 12 yr/age: • 0.2 mg/day in 2 divided doses • Maximum dose: 2.4 mg/day
α Receptor antagonists	• Blockade of peripheral α-adrenoceptors	• Balanced vasodilation • ↓ SVR • Little to no change in CO	• Hypertension • Preoperative treatment of pheo • Treatment of α-adrenergic agonist drug extravasation	• Hypotension • Orthostatic hypotension • Reflex tachycardia • Interferes with pressor effects of α-agonists	Phentolamine: • 0.05–0.1 mg/kg/dose IV q 2–4 hr • Maximum dose: 5 mg
β Receptor antagonists	• Blockade of peripheral β-adrenoceptors • Cardioselective (β_1—esmolol), versus nonspecific (β_1 and β_2—propranolol)	• Balanced vasodilation • ↓ SVR • ↓ HR • ↓ Contractility • ↓ Automaticity • ↓ Nodal conduction velocity • ↓ Renin release	• Hypertension • CHF • Angina • Post-MI • PVCs • Ventricular rate control in AFib and AFlutter • AV-reentrant tachycardia • VTach in patients with prolonged QT syndrome • Thyroid storm	• Hypotension • Bradycardia • Bronchospasm (nonspecific) • AV block • Withdrawal syndrome	Esmolol: • Loading dose: 500 mcg/kg/min over 1 min • Maintenance dose: 50–250 mcg/kg/min

Drug class	Mechanism	Indications	Adverse effects	Dosing

Combined α and β receptor antagonists	• Blockade of both peripheral α- and β-adrenoceptors
	• Relative α : β blockade:
	  • PO 1:3
	  • IV 1:7
	• Balanced vasodilation
	• ↓ SVR
	• ↓ HR or unchanged
	• Little to no change in CO
		• Hypertensive crisis	• Hypotension
			• Orthostatic hypotension
			• Bradycardia
			• Bronchospasm
			• Headache
			• Fatigue
				Labetalol:
				• PO: 1–3 mg/kg/day in 2 divided doses
				• Maximum: 10–12 mg/kg/day or 1,200 mg/day
				• IV: 0.3–1 mg/kg/dose

Direct Vasodilators				
Calcium-channel antagonists	• Blockade of L-type calcium channels in vascular SM, SA and AV nodes, and cardiac myocytes • Prevents calcium influx • Arterial vasodilation • ↓ SVR • ↓ HR • ↓ Contractility • ↓ Nodal conduction velocity • ↑ Coronary BF	• Hypertension • SVT • AFib and AFlutter • Hypertrophic cardiomyopathy	• Hypotension • Bradycardia • Question of coronary steal phenomenon • Avoid in SSS, AV block, and CHF • Use limited in pediatrics as can cause asystole or cardiac arrest in neonates and infants	Nifedipine: • 0.25–0.5 mg/kg/day in 1–2 divided doses • Maximum 3 mg/kg/day or 120 mg/day Nicardipine: • Loading dose: 5–10 mcg/kg • Maintenance: 1–3 mcg/kg/min
Fenoldopam	• Selective D_1-adrenergic agonist • Balanced vasodilation • ↑ Renal BF and UOP • Natriuresis • Diuresis	• Hypertension • Hypertensive crisis with renal impairment • Improved renal perfusion	• Hypotension • Reflex tachycardia • Cutaneous flushing • Dizziness • Headache	• Initial dose: 0.1–0.2 mcg/kg/min • Titrate up every 20–30 min to maximum dose 0.8 mcg/kg/min
Hydralazine	• Unknown • Direct smooth muscle relaxation without interacting with adrenergic or cholinergic receptors • Arterial vasodilation • ↓ SVR • Baroreflexly mediated ↑ SNS tone • ↑ Renal, coronary, splanchnic, and cerebral BF	• Hypertensive crisis • LVH • Myocardial dysfunction	• Tachycardia • Palpitations • Angina • Lupus-like syndrome • Polyneuropathy	• PO: 0.75–1 mg/kg/day in 2–4 divided doses • Maximum 7.5 mg/kg/day or 200 mg/day • IV: 0.1–0.2 mg/kg/dose (up to 20 mg) q 4–6 hr • Maximum 3.5 mg/kg/day

(Continued)

TABLE 22-19

Antihypertensives (*Continued*)

Class	Mechanism of Action	Physiologic Effects	Clinical Use	Adverse Effects	Examples and Dosage
Direct Vasodilators (*Continued*)					
Nitroglycerin	• Converted to NO in vascular endothelial cell	• Venodilation • ↑ Venous capacitance • ↓ Preload	• Hypertension • Angina • CHF • PHTN	• Hypotension • Orthostatic hypotension • Reflex tachycardia • Tachyphylaxis • Headache	• IV: 0.25–0.5 mcg/kg/min • ↑ by 0.5–1 mcg/kg/min q 3–5 min to maximum dose 10 mcg/kg/min or 200 mcg/min
Sodium nitroprusside	• Nonreceptor stimulant of guanylate cyclase • Nitric oxide donor, similar to nitroglycerin	• Balanced vasodilation • ↓ SVR • Reflex ↑ HR	• Hypertensive crisis • CHF • Postischemic systolic dysfunction • Dilated cardiomyopathy • Acute aortic dissection • PHTN • Controlled hypotension in the OR	• Tachycardia • Palpitations • Question of coronary steal • Cyanide/Thiocyanate intoxication (tachyphylaxis, ↑ mixed venous PaO₂, and metabolic acidosis)	• Weight < 40 kg: 1–8 mcg/kg/min • Weight ≥ 40 kg: 0.1–5 mcg/kg/min

Angiotensin-receptor blockers (ARBs), angiotensin (AT), angiotensin-converting enzyme (ACE), atrial fibrillation (AFib), atrial flutter (AFlutter), atrioventricular (AV), blood flow (BF), cardiac output (CO), complex regional pain syndrome (CRPS), congestive heart failure (CHF), contraindications (C/I), epinephrine (EPI), heart rate (HR), left ventricular hypertrophy (LVH), micrograms/kilogram/minute (mcg/kg/min), milligrams/kilogram/day (mg/kg/day), myocardial infarction (MI), nitric oxide (NO), norepinephrine (NE), operating room (OR), parasympathetic (PS), pheochromocytoma (pheo), premature ventricular contraction (PVC), pulmonary hypertension (PHTN), sick sinus syndrome (SSS), sinoatrial (SA), smooth muscle (SM), sympathetic nervous system (SNS), systemic vascular resistance (SVR), urine output (UOP), ventricular tachycardia (VTach).

Sources: Benowitz, 2001; Hoffman, 2001a, 2001b; Johnson et al., 2009; Lexi-Comp Online, Pediatric Lexi-Drugs Online, 2009; Shekerdemian & Redington, 1998.

TABLE 22-20

Antiarrhythmics

Drug	Mechanism of Action	Physiologic Effects	Clinical Use	Dosage	Adverse Effects
Adenosine	• Unclassified antiarrhythmic • Hyperpolarizes SA and AV nodes via ↑ K$^+$ conductance	• ↓ Conduction velocity • ↑ Effective refractory period	• Terminate SVT • Determine cause of SVT	First dose: 0.1 mg/kg IVP (maximum 6 mg) Second dose: 0.2 mg/kg IVP (maximum 12 mg)	• Bradycardia or asystole • Hypotension • AV block • Ventricular ectopy • Flushing • Bronchospasm
Amiodarone	• Class III antiarrhythmic • Primary action: K$^+$ channel blockade • Also has Na$^+$ and Ca$^+$ channel and β-receptor blocking properties	• ↑ Action potential duration • ↑ Effective refractory period • ↓ Automaticity in SA node • Prolonged PR, QRS, and QT intervals	• AFib • AFlutter • Reentry SVT • Ectopic AT • JET • VTach • VFib	5 mg/kg IV load over 20–60 min (maximum 300 mg) Repeat to maximum daily dose of 15 mg/kg (or 2.2 g) Therapeutic range: 0.5–2.5 mg/L	• Bradycardia • AV block • Torsades de pointes • Pneumonitis, pulmonary fibrosis • Corneal deposits • Peripheral neuropathy • Hypothyroidism or hyperthyroidism
Lidocaine	• Class IB antiarrhythmic • Blockade of rapid Na+ channel • Works on depressed myocardium/ischemia	• ↓ Action potential duration • ↓ Effective refractory period • ↓ Automaticity in partially depolarized (abnormal) tissue	• Ventricular ectopy • VT • VF • Arrhythmias in presence of prolonged QT • Re-entrant tachycardia	1 mg/kg IV bolus Maintenance: 20–50 mcg/kg/min Therapeutic range: 1.5–5 mcg/mL Toxic range: > 9 mcg/mL	• CNS depression • Seizures • Arrhythmia • Allergic reaction • Methemoglobinemia • Bronchospasm • Tinnitus
Procainamide	• Class IA antiarrhythmic • Blockade of rapid Na+ channel • Metabolite, NAPA, also blocks K$^+$ channels (class III activity) • Anticholinergic effects	• ↑ Action potential duration • ↑ Effective refractory period • ↓ Automaticity of fast fibers • ↑ SA and AV node conduction (anticholinergic effect) • Prolonged PR, QRS, and QT intervals	• AFib • AFlutter • SVT • VT with pulses • Lidocaine-resistant VT • JET in conjunction with hypothermia	15 mg/kg IV load over 30–60 min Therapeutic range: • Procainamide: 4–10 mcg/mL • NAPA: 15–25 mcg/mL • Combined: 10–30 mcg/mL Toxic range: Procainamide: > 10–12 mcg/mL	• Hypotension • Myocardial depression • Torsades de pointes • Ventricular arrhythmias • Lupus-like syndrome • Thrombocytopenia • Allergic reaction

Atrial fibrillation (AFib), atrial flutter (AFlutter), atrial tachycardia (AT), atrioventricular (AV), calcium (Ca$^+$), central nervous system (CNS), junctional ectopic tachycardia (JET), micrograms/kg/min (mcg/kg/min), N-acetyl-procainamide (NAPA), potassium (K$^+$), sodium (Na$^+$), supraventricular tachycardia (SVT), sinoatrial (SA), ventricular fibrillation (VF), ventricular tachycardia (VT).

Sources: AHA, 2006; Johnson et al., 2009; Lexi-Comp Online, Pediatric Lexi-Drugs Online, 2009; Marino et al., 2008; Otto, 2008; Perry & Walsh, 1998.

TABLE 22-21

Other Commonly Used Cardiovascular Agents					
Drug	**Mechanism of Action**	**Physiologic Effects**	**Clinical Use**	**Dosage**	**Adverse Effects**
Nesiritide	• Binds to guanylate cyclase receptor on vascular SM and endothelial cells • ↑ cGMP	• Vasodilation • Enhanced diastolic relaxation (lusitropy) • Natriuresis • Diuresis • Inhibits renin and aldosterone release	• Congestive heart failure	• Loading dose: 2 mcg/kg • Maintenance: 0.01–0.03 mcg/kg/min	• Hypotension • Renal dysfunction • Headache
PGE 1	• Eicosanoid • Direct action on vascular and ductus arteriosus SM	• Vasodilation • Smooth muscle relaxation	• Ductal-dependent congenital heart disease	• Initial dose: 0.05–0.1 mcg/kg/min • Then decrease to 0.01–0.05 mcg/kg/min	• Apnea • Hypotension • Seizures • Hyperpyrexia • Flushing

Prostaglandin E₁ (PGE₁), smooth muscle (SM).

Sources: Johnson et al., 2008; Lexi-Comp Online, Pediatric Lexi-Drugs Online, 2009; Shekerdemian & Redington, 1998; Wessel & Fraisse, 2008.

sodium-channel, calcium-channel, α-adrenoceptor, and β-adrenoceptor blocking properties (Otto, 2009). Examples include amiodarone and sotalol.

Class IV: calcium-channel blockers

Class IV agents act by slowing the inward movement of ions through calcium channels of nodal tissue, especially AV nodal tissue. This results in decreased conduction velocity and an increased effective refractory period in the AV node (Marino et al., 2008). Examples include verapamil and diltiazem.

OTHER COMMONLY USED CARDIOVASCULAR AGENTS

Nesiritide

Nesiritide is a recombinant human B-type natriuretic peptide that is identical to the endogenous hormone released by the ventricles in response to volume overload and increased wall tension (Johnson et al., 2009). The natriuretic hormone system is an important regulator of neurohormonal activation, vascular tone, diastolic function, and fluid balance (Wessel & Fraisse, 2008). It is primarily used as an afterload reducer in the treatment of CHF with poor perfusion (Table 22-21).

Prostaglandin E₁

Prostaglandin E₁ (PGE₁) is an eicosanoid that causes vasodilation by acting directly on vascular and ductus arteriosus smooth muscle. In pediatrics, it is used to reopen or

maintain the patency of the ductus arteriosus in the setting of cyanotic congenital heart disease (Table 22-21). It is effective up to four months of life, but is most efficacious when used in the first three days of life (Shekerdemian & Redington, 1998).

CARDITIS

Julie Kuzin

ENDOCARDITIS

Pathophysiology

Infective endocarditis (IE) refers to an infection of the endothelial surface of the heart. It can develop at any site within the heart structures, including mural endocardium, valves, septum, septal defects, foreign material, thrombus, or chordae tendineae. The development of IE begins with a key substrate of endocardial cell damage, which may result from either a congenital or acquired abnormality. Congenital heart disease, and its accompanying structural anomalies, predisposes pediatric patients to this problem. For example, turbulent blood flow from a congenital structural abnormality may course against a septum and damage the endothelium. Alternatively, after surgical alteration, sutured shunts and patches may attract fibrin and platelet deposition, which result in a thrombus formation with microbial adherence (Allen et al., 2007; Wilson et al., 2007).

Once a thrombus forms and microbes adhere to it, deposition of fibrin and platelets continue, providing a protected environment for organisms to flourish. The infected thrombus is referred to as a *vegetation*. Vegetations on the left side of the heart demonstrate higher densities of colony-forming units in comparison to lesions on the right side. Microbes in older vegetations become deeply embedded, reducing their exposure (and vulnerability) to antibiotics (Wilson et al., 2007).

IE is now thought to be a systemic process. Immune complexes and rheumatoid factors have been found in the serum of affected individuals for weeks following infection—a finding that supports the theory that IE creates a hyperimmune response. Microembolism occurs, with the resulting emboli migrating both peripherally and to larger organs. Many patients with IE develop nephritis. Sterile emboli are often noted within the kidney and are usually associated with cellular proliferation, complement, and immunoglobulin deposition (Allen et al., 2007).

Epidemiology and etiology

IE has a reported incidence rate of 0.3 per 100,000 children, with a mortality rate of 11.6% (Caviness et al., 2004). IE admissions account for approximately 1 in every 1,300 to 2,000 admissions per year, although the mortality rate has consistently decreased from 35% to 11%. This decline is attributed to the dramatic decreases (50%) in rheumatic heart disease (RHD) and increasing survival (8% to 26%) of children with congenital heart disease. Nevertheless, endocarditis remains a major complicating factor in developing countries, where RHD persists as an active disease (Day et al., 2009; Wilson et al., 2007). A recent study reported that in 1,480 cases of IE, there was no difference in gender incidence; the two peak occurrences of its onset were noted at 1–11 months and 17–20 years of age. Forty-two percent of patients with IE had preexisting heart disease. Tetralogy of Fallot was found to have the highest incidence (19.8%) and the highest mortality rate at 48% (Day et al.). The following factors are associated with the highest risk of developing IE: prosthetic valves, previous episode of endocarditis, complex cyanotic congenital heart disease, surgically placed systemic-to-pulmonary shunts, injection drug use, and indwelling central catheters. In these high-risk groups, the incidence of IE is 300 to 2,160 per 100,000 cases per year (Allen et al., 2007).

IE is caused by a relatively small group of organisms. Those considered least virulent include α-hemolytic streptococci, enterococci, and coagulase-negative staphylococci. Organisms with greater virulence include bacteria such as *Staphylococcus aureus, Streptococcus pneumoniae, and β-hemolytic streptococci,* as well as fungal sources such as *Aspergillus*. Rapid destruction of valve tissue and myocardial infiltration can occur with the more virulent organisms (Allen et al., 2007; Wilson et al., 2007). Fifty-seven percent of IE cases are caused by *S. aureus* infection, 20% by the *viridans* group of streptococci, and 14% by coagulase-negative staphylococci (Allen et al.; Day et al., 2009).

Presentation

Clinical examination findings are a reflection of toxic bacterial effects, immunologic vascular effects, or microembolism. A toxic presentation is most commonly seen in acute, rapidly progressing IE in which the patient presents with high fever and hemodynamic instability. Subacute presentations in children may include arthralgia, myalgia, headache, malaise, relapsing fever, or decreased appetite. For both acute and subacute infections, fever is the most commonly described symptom. Neonates, however, may present as either afebrile or hypothermic. Symptoms of CHF may be observed and changes in a murmur may be appreciated. Valve destruction may increase the grade of a murmur, whereas shunt murmurs obscured by vegetation may become less obvious. Dental caries may be the source of infection; thus a thorough dental examination should be completed in a patient with IE (Allen et al, 2007; Baddour et al., 2005).

Complications of IE include CHF, structural cardiac injury, abscess, and embolism. In particular, the existence of CHF predicts a poor prognosis. The degree of CHF depends on the valve involved and degree of damage. In general, tricuspid regurgitation is better tolerated than aortic regurgitation. Mild CHF may progress to a severe form of the disorder during therapy. Pericardial effusion, mycotic aneurysms, and myocarditis are rare complications of IE.

In the case of embolization, symptoms will be based on the location of the IE vegetation. Left heart vegetations produce systemic emboli, whereas right heart lesions embolize to the lungs. Systemic emboli may include lesions to the brain, kidneys, spleen, and peripheral tissue. Although embolism is difficult to predict, the risk may decrease after the first two to three weeks of antimicrobial therapy. Petechiae may be seen as a result of systemic emboli or sepsis. Abnormal neurologic symptoms may suggest an abscess or infarction, whereas renal emboli may cause hematuria, leukocyturia, and proteinuria. Renal dysfunction is more common in adults than in pediatric patients. Osler nodes, Janeway lesions, Roth spots, and splinter hemorrhages are rare findings, but their presence suggests systemic emboli versus immune complex formation. Osler nodes are small, painful, raised lesions that appear on the toe and finger pads. Janeway lesions are small, flat, nontender, erythematous lesions that are observed on the palms or soles. Roth spots are retinal hemorrhages with central whiting. Splinter hemorrhages are tiny red/brown lines running vertically under the nail (Allen et al., 2007; Baddour et al., 2005).

Differential diagnosis

Differential diagnoses should be considered based on the patient's history and presenting symptoms. Insidious IE may be difficult to identify, but should be suspected in children with congenital heart disease presenting with fever and nonspecific symptoms. The symptoms of IE are common to many childhood diseases. Arthritis or arthralgia may suggest an indolent viral infection such as EBV infection, or rheumatic fever, rheumatoid disease, Kawasaki disease, or connective tissue disorder. Patients presenting with neurologic symptoms secondary to cerebral embolism or abscess may appear similarly to those with meningitis or toxic encephalopathy. Hematuria or renal insufficiency may mimic nephritis; CHF associated with IE may be mistaken for myocarditis (Danilowicz, 1995).

Plan of care

The Duke criteria are a standardized approach to diagnosis of IE first proposed in 1994 and modified in 2000. These criteria organize patients into one of three categories: definite, possible, or rejected. The diagnosis of IE is also based on satisfaction of major and minor criteria. *Major criteria* include two positive blood cultures or histological evidence of infection and significant echocardiographic findings. *Minor criteria* include history of injection drug use, predisposition to IE, fever, vascular phenomena, immunologic phenomena, or microbiologic evidence that does not satisfy the major criteria (Baddour et al., 2005).

Evaluation of the pediatric patient with suspected IE should include three peripheral blood cultures from different locations within a 24-hour period. The recommended blood volume is 1–3 mL for infants, 5–7 mL for children, and 20–30 mL for adolescents. These volumes will enhance organism recovery. Two repeat cultures may be obtained the second day if the first cultures are negative for growth at the 24-hour reading. Cultures should be drawn prior to antibiotic administration to prevent sterilization. Although acute-phase reactants are not considered diagnostic, they may be of value in monitoring disease course. A complete blood count may reveal anemia, which is common in IE. Leukocytosis is not routinely present. Urinalysis should be evaluated for microhematuria or macrohematuria suggesting renal embolization or nephritis (Allen et al., 2007; Baddour et al., 2005).

Echocardiography may reveal the presence of CHF. A transthoracic echocardiogram is 80% sensitive in detecting IE, although false negatives are possible. Findings may include vegetation/mass, annular abscess, partial dehiscence of a prosthetic valve, or new valvular insufficiency. The discovery of these findings satisfies a major criterion in the Duke modified criteria. Patients with CHF should be considered for surgical intervention, as mortality is significantly decreased if the valve is repaired. Medical therapy for CHF may include diuretics, beta blockers, or ACE inhibitors (Allen et al., 2007; Baddour et al., 2005).

Extended-course intravenous antimicrobials are recommended, and long-term IV access should be secured. The plan for antimicrobial therapy depends on the sensitivities of the isolated microorganism and should be developed in collaboration with the infectious diseases service. Negative blood cultures are encountered in as many as 20% of patients, which presents a significant therapeutic challenge. In culture-negative IE, empiric therapy should be planned in consultation with infectious diseases experts and based on epidemiological features as well as the patient's clinical course.

Surgical referral is generally indicated for patients with persistent infection, significant embolic events, new heart block, an abscess that is large or increasing in size, vegetation, or progressive CHF (Allen et al., 2007; Baddour et al., 2005).

Consultations with the following subspecialists are encouraged to promote a comprehensive therapeutic management plan: cardiology, cardiothoracic surgery, critical care, and infectious diseases. Should various symptoms suggest alternative or systemic sequelae associated with IE, then consultations may include nephrology, neurology, gastroenterology, dermatology, and pulmonology specialists. Because patients may be hospitalized for long-term care, consultation with child life and occupational and physical therapy may be required.

Individuals with IE are at high risk for recurrence, a phenomenon that is associated with increased morbidity and mortality (Wilson et al., 2007). Infection with *Clostridium difficile* is a major risk for those receiving long-term antibiotics and can develop several weeks following discontinuation of therapy. Fever in the child with a history of IE requires immediate medical attention. Prescribing empiric antibiotics for nonspecific febrile syndromes is inappropriate, because this therapy may mask IE recurrence and lead to culture-negative endocarditis (Baddour et al., 2005). Patients and families require teaching on care both during and following therapy.

Disposition and discharge planning

Outpatient completion of therapy can be considered for many patients with IE. Outpatient parenteral antimicrobial therapy has been shown to be safe, effective, and cost saving. The stable pediatric patient without symptoms of CHF, who has received at least 2 weeks of IV antibiotic therapy, has access to medical care, has a reliable home environment and social situation, and has low risk factors for developing complications, may be considered for outpatient therapy. Arrangements for the pediatric school-age patient to continue schoolwork should also be made (Baddour et al., 2005).

Echocardiographs should be repeated as needed based on the child's status and just prior to completion of antimicrobial therapy to define a baseline for future comparison. Drug-level monitoring to avoid toxicity should be completed as recommended, and audiograms should be performed for those patients receiving aminoglycosides. The indwelling intravenous catheter should be discontinued as soon as antimicrobial therapy is complete.

Follow-up with cardiology and infectious diseases specialists may be indicated. In addition, good dental hygiene is important in preventing recurrent IE by decreasing bloodstream exposure to microbes. The AHA continues to recommend prophylactic antibiotics prior to dental procedures for individuals at highest risk of developing endocarditis, which includes individuals with a history of IE (Baddour et al., 2005).

MYOCARDITIS

Pathophysiology

Myocarditis is categorized as a type of inflammatory cardiomyopathy. It is defined as inflammation of the heart muscle in conjunction with cardiac dysfunction, which can be established by histologic, immunologic, and immunohistochemical criteria (Richardson et al., 1996). The mechanism of myocarditis varies depending on the cause, although animal studies reveal that viruses invade myocytes, release myocardial toxin, and induce immune-mediated myocardial damage (Chang & Towbin, 2006; Magnani & Dec, 2006; Schultz et al., 2009).

Three phases of viral myocarditis onset and progression are identified: first phase (days 0–3), second phase (days 4–14), and third phase (days 15–90). In the *first phase*, the virus enters, disrupts, and kills myocytes. Myocyte necrosis triggers the host's immune response, including antibody production that results in viral clearance for some patients. In susceptible individuals, however, immune activation is perpetuated and cytotoxic T lymphocytes and cross-reactive antibodies further damage the myocytes.

Patients who progress to the *second phase* experience a systematic immune assault to eliminate the virus through complex mechanisms involving natural killer cells, major histocompatibility complexes (MHC), and cytotoxic T lymphocytes. Nitric oxide, a known cardiac depressant, is produced during this phase, and is suspected to have both positive and negative effects in patients. The cumulative effect of this attack is necrosis of healthy and infected myocytes (Chang & Towbin, 2006; Wheeler & Kooy, 2003).

Over time, the diffuse cell injury progresses into the *third phase* of myocarditis, which encompasses myocardial fibrosis and ventricular dysfunction. This phase is the bridge from myocarditis to dilated cardiomyopathy (DCM). There are many proposed pathways for the development of DCM. In particular, defects in dystrophin—a key component in the myocardial cytoskeleton—have been implicated in mouse models when exposed to coxsackie B viral myocarditis. Persistence of viral RNA in the myocardium may stimulate prolonged immune activation, in addition to local inflammation, antiheart antibodies, and apoptosis, thereby stimulating further fibrosis and myocardial injury (Chang & Towbin, 2006; Magnani & Dec, 2006; Schultz et al., 2009; Wheeler & Kooy, 2003).

Cardiac function in the murine model with viral myocarditis has been described as normal to hyperdynamic ventricular function during the first phase, followed by a marked change in cardiac performance in the second phase. In phase 2, ventricular contractility, stroke volume, and cardiac output are severely depressed, which corresponds with a dilated left ventricle and an increased end-diastolic pressure. During the latter part of this phase, compliance and stroke volume improve, although only minimal improvement in contractility may occur (Chang & Towbin, 2006).

Epidemiology and etiology

The diverse presentations of myocarditis make accurate diagnosis and incidence reporting for this condition challenging. Estimates of incidence range from 1 to 10 per 100,000 children (Chang & Towbin, 2006). In 1,426 cases of DCM recorded in the Pediatric Cardiomyopathy Registry, only 34% of DCM cases had an identified cause. The majority of those with an identified etiology (222 cases, or 46%) were caused by myocarditis. Of the patients with myocarditis, 9.4% died and 14.4% required cardiac transplantation. Overall, DCM had an incidence of 0.57 per 100,000 children, with an increased incidence in males, infants, and African (Towbin et al., 2006). Myocarditis pathology has been seen in 42% of pediatric sudden cardiac deaths (SCD) and 9% of SCD in athletes (Allen et al., 2007).

Many agents and conditions have been linked to myocarditis, including infections, toxins, hypersensitivity reactions, and systemic disorders (Table 22-22) (Magnani & Dec, 2006; Shultz et al., 2009; Wheeler & Kooy, 2003). The vast majority of studies, however, have focused on viral myocarditis. Invading pathogens are suspected to interact with the host in varied ways, as suggested by the histopathologic differences associated with adenovirus myocarditis versus enterovirus myocarditis.

Of the viral causes of myocarditis, enteroviruses—specifically coxsackie viruses A and B—were reported most often. More recently, an increasing trend of non-enterovirus-associated myocarditis has been observed. In the 1990s, adenovirus activity increased, and as the year 2000 approached parvovirus B19 was the most frequently identified viral genome (Chang & Towbin, 2006; Schultz et al., 2009). Influenza A virus, herpes simplex virus, respiratory syncytial virus, human immunodeficiency virus, cytomegalovirus, and EBV have been less frequently identified in cases of acute and chronic myocarditis (Schultz et al.). Viral predominance varies by geographic location. For example, hepatitis C myocarditis remains more common in Japan, whereas parvovirus B19 is most prevalent in Germany (Magnani & Dec, 2006; Mahrhodt et al., 2006).

TABLE 22-22

Etiologies of Myocarditis

Infectious			Other	
Viral	**Bacterial**	**Spirochetal**	**Cardiotoxin**	**Systemic Disease**
Adenovirus	*Brucella*	*Borrelia*	Alcohol	Celiac disease
Arbovirus	*Chlamydia*	Leptospirosis	Anthracyclines	Churg-Strauss
Coxsackie A and B	Cholera	Lyme disease	Arsenic	Diabetes mellitus
CMV	*Clostridia*	Syphilis	Carbon monoxide	Giant cell myocarditis
Dengue virus	Corynbacterium		Catecholamines	Hypereosinophilia
Echovirus	Diphtheria	**Fungal**	Cocaine	Inflammatory bowel
Epstein-Barr	*Hemophilus influenzae*	*Actinomyces*	Heavy metals	disease
Hepatitis A and C	*Legionella*	*Aspergillus*	Interleukin-2	Kawasaki disease
Herpes simplex	*Meningococcus*	*Blastomyces*		Sarcoidosis
Herpes zoster	*Mycobacterium*	*Candida*	**Hypersensitivity**	Systemic lupus
HIV	*Mycoplasma*	*Coccidiodes*		erythematosus
Influenza A and B	*Neisseria gonorrhoeae*	*Cryptococcus*	Anticonvulsants	Takayasu's arteritis
Measles	*Pneumococcus*	*Histoplasma*	Cephalosporins	Thyrotoxicosis
Mumps	*Psittacosis*	Mucomycosis	Clozapine	Wegener's
Parvovirus B19	*Salmonella*	*Nocardial*	Diuretics	granulomatosis
Poliomyelitis	*Serratia marcescens*	Sporotrichosis	Digoxin	
Rabies	*Staphylococcus*		Dobutamine	
Rubella	*Streptococcus pyogenes*	**Protozoal**	Insect bites	
Rubeola	Tetanus	African sleeping sickness	Lithium	
RSV	*Treponema pallidum*	Amebiasis	Mesalamine	
Varicella zoster	(Chagas disease)	Leishmaniasis	Snakebites	
Variola	Tuberculosis	Malaria	Sulfonamides	
Yellow fever	Tularemia	Toxoplasmosis	Smallpox vaccine	
		Trypanosoma cruzi (Chagas	Tetanus toxoid	
Parasitic		disease)	Tricyclic	
Ascaris			antidepressants	
Echinococcosis		**Rickettsial**		
Filariasis		*Coxiella burnetti* (Q fever)		
Larva migrans		Rocky Mountain spotted fever		
Paragonimiasis		Typhus		
Schistosomiasis				
Strongyloides				
Trichinella				

Cytomegalovirus (CMV), human immunodeficiency virus (HIV), respiratory syncytial virus (RSV).

Sources: Magnani & Dec, 2006; Schultz et al., 2009; Wheeler & Kooy, 2003.

Presentation

The symptoms most commonly noted in pediatric patients with myocarditis are tachypnea, wheezing, and dyspnea to severe respiratory distress. Tachypnea, increased work of breathing, and wheezing may occur secondary to pulmonary edema associated with heart failure (Durani et al., 2009; Freedman et al., 2007; Schultz et al., 2009; Wheeler & Kooy, 2003). Pediatric patients with myocarditis may also present asymptomatic and may quickly advance to cardiac arrest (Cooper, 2009). Nontraditional cardiac symptoms may predominate in infants, including vomiting, poor feeding, fever, diaphoresis, irritability, or upper respiratory symptoms. Both younger children and adolescents may present with fever, anorexia, respiratory distress, syncope, lethargy, or abdominal or chest pain. Vomiting

and feeding intolerance may be the first sign of heart failure (Allen et al., 2007; Durani et al.; Schultz et al.).

The patient's health history, which includes his or her activity level, may indicate a decreased activity level and inability to keep up with peers, suggesting heart failure. A report of a recent viral infection can also support the diagnosis of myocarditis, whereas a family history of sudden death, premature heart failure, or the need for defibrillators/pacemakers may suggest the existence of familial cardiomyopathy (Allen et al., 2007).

The HCP may find an abnormality in the cardiac physical examination or cardiomegaly on CXR (Durani et al., 2009; Freedman et al., 2007; Wheeler & Kooy, 2003). Cardiac-specific symptoms depend on the degree of heart failure. Resting tachycardia, arrhythmias, mitral regurgitation murmur, laterally displaced point of maximal impulse, gallop, hepatomegaly, jugular venous distention, or decreased pulses or perfusion may also be present on examination. Any of these findings alone, or in combination, should stimulate further investigation (Schultz et al., 2009). Four-extremity blood pressure measurements may rule out aortic coarctation as a cause for cardiac dysfunction, and an oxygen saturation measurement can aid in ruling out congenital cyanotic heart disease (Allen et al., 2007).

Differential diagnosis

Any condition that mimics or is associated with heart failure may be considered in the differential diagnosis for myocarditis (Table 22-23). Diagnosis of myocarditis requires a comprehensive history, physical examination, diagnostic studies, and elimination of differential diagnoses.

Plan of care

Initial diagnostic studies for myocarditis include CXR, ECG, echocardiography, oxygen saturation, and four-extremity blood pressure measurements. The CXR may reveal cardiomegaly or pulmonary vascular congestion. The ECG classically demonstrates sinus tachycardia, low-voltage QRS complexes, and ST-T wave flattening. However, ECG has a low sensitivity (47%) in myocarditis (Cooper, 2009). Other, more ominous ECG findings include Q waves or left bundle branch block, as these findings may be predict the need for transplant or death. Atrial arrhythmias, varying degrees of AV block, prolonged QT interval, supraventricular or ventricular tachycardia, and atrial or ventricular ectopy may be seen (Allen et al., 2007; Chang & Towbin,

TABLE 22-23

Differential Diagnoses for Myocarditis	
Bacterial or viral sepsis	Idiopathic DCM
Endocardial fibroelastosis	X-linked DCM
Meningitis	Autosomal dominant DCM
Bronchiolitis	Barth syndrome
Pneumonia	Anomalous origin of LCA
Reye's syndrome	Hyperthyroidism
Connective tissue disorders	Pericarditis
Kawasaki disease	Cerebral arteriovenous
Acute rheumatic fever	malformation
Methemoglobinemia	Congenital syphilis*
Drug toxicity	Hypoxia*
Tachyarrhythmia	Hypoglycemia*
Infant of diabetic mother	Hypocalcemia*
Inborn errors of metabolism	Structural heart disease*

*Indicates condition specific to infants.
Left coronary artery (LCA), dilated cardiomyopathy (DCM).
Sources: Allen et al., 2007; Wheeler & Kooy, 2003.

2006). Ventricular tachycardia is rarely present in the early stages of myocarditis, but may be seen during the recovery phase (Magnani & Dec, 2006; Schultz et al., 2009).

Echocardiographic findings cannot differentiate myocarditis from other forms of cardiomyopathy. A dilated left ventricular cavity, though, is suggestive of dilated cardiomyopathy as opposed to acute onset myocarditis (Cooper, 2009). A recent study of patients with myocarditis found an overwhelming number with abnormal echocardiography (Durani et al., 2008). Echocardiography, therefore, is useful in assessing important features of the myocardium, including regional wall motion abnormalities, hypertrophy, chamber dilation, effusion, and structural abnormalities (Magnani & Dec, 2006; Schultz et al., 2009). Left ventricular dysfunction is present in most patients with myocarditis, regardless of the presence of cardiomegaly on CXR. Other key findings may include mitral regurgitation due to valve annulus dilation, pericardial effusion, and mural thrombus. Coronary artery origin must be identified in infants presenting with ventricular dysfunction so as to distinguish an anomalous origin of the left coronary artery from myocarditis.

Cardiac biomarkers such as troponin I have a reported sensitivity of 34% and specificity of 89% in myocarditis (Cooper, 2009). Other serologic markers, such as creatinine phosphokinase MB isoenzyme and C-reactive protein (CRP), are commonly elevated and are followed as part of trend monitoring of myocardial inflammation. Serum B-type natriuretic peptide (BNP) and pro-BNP have been under investigation in recent years as biomarkers for heart failure. Although these proteins have not been evaluated in myocarditis, their negative predictive values in heart failure are influenced by many variables. Given this fact, interpretation of elevated levels of BNP and pro-BNP should be conservative, and taken within context of all other clinical data (Law et al., 2009).

MRI is becoming more popular as a diagnostic tool, as this technology can provide a description of myocardial tissue and aids in visualization of small myocardial injury, thereby increasing the sensitivity for detecting myocyte injury and active myocarditis (Magnani & Dec, 2006; Schultz et al., 2009).

Although endomyocardial biopsy (EMB) has significant limitations, it remains the the diagnostic study of choice for definitive determination of myocarditis (Magnani & Dec, 2006). Advances in quantitative and qualitative PCR techniques have increased the detection of viral genomes in the myocardium. Special handling precautions must be maintained to avoid degradation and contamination of specimens which might lead to false positive results (Cooper et al., 2007). PCR detection of viral genomes in tracheal aspirate has shown a strong correlation with myocarditis diagnosis. Collectively, the American College of Cardiology Foundation, American Heart Association, and European Society of Cardiology recommend a limited role for EMB in patients with cardiomyopathy, however. Class I EMB is indicated in patients who meet the following criteria: (1) two weeks of new-onset heart failure with a normal or dilated left ventricle and hemodynamic compromise; (2) new-onset heart failure within two weeks to three months with a dilated left ventricle, ventricular arrhythmia, or high-degree atrioventricular block; and (3) failure to respond to medical therapy within three weeks. EMB is not without risks, which include vasovagal reaction, arrhythmia, conduction abnormality, perforation, and death (Cooper et al., 2007).

Therapeutic management in the acute phase depends on the patient's stability, and should be guided by current American Heart Association and American College of Cardiology guidelines. A beneficial effect from intravenous immunoglobulin (IVIG) may be found if administered in the initial phase of myocarditis. In retrospective studies evaluating the use of IVIG in pediatric patients (albeit with limited data), beneficial effects have been appreciated. Furthermore, IVIG has been associated with reduced myocellular necrosis, plasma catecholamines, and interferon-gamma in murine mouse models. Although immunosuppressive therapy for myocarditis remains controversial, patients with autoimmune disease may benefit from the therapy. Antiviral therapy with ribavirin and interferon-alpha is under investigation, and may be recommended for acute myocarditis in the future (Chang & Towbin, 2006; Magnani & Dec, 2006; Schultz et al., 2009; Wheeler & Kooy, 2003).

Supportive therapies should be considered if the patient is hemodynamically stable; ACE inhibition or angiotensin receptor blockade may provide afterload reduction and myocardial remodeling. Likewise, angiotensin and adrenergic pathway inhibition with aldosterone antagonists may be beneficial. Diuretics can decrease edema and symptoms associated with heart failure, but must be used judiciously in patients with compromised cardiac output. Beta blockade therapy is used to improve left ventricular function, heart failure symptoms, and decrease inflammation; however, use of beta blockers in pediatric patients should be closely monitored and is contraindicated with decompensated heart failure (Magnani & Dec, 2006; Schultz et al., 2009; Wheeler & Kooy, 2003). Prophylactic anticoagulation should be considered in infants and children with severe ventricular dysfunction or dilation; recommended agents include aspirin, warfarin, or intravenous heparin. Pharmacologic management of ventricular arrhythmias should be approached with intravenous lidocaine or amiodarone during the decompensated phase. Patients with hemodynamically significant atrioventricular blocks may require transvenous pacing.

Pediatric patients with decompensated heart failure may require intensive care monitoring and management with vasopressors, including phosphodiesterase inhibitors, adrenergic agonists, and/or vasodilators. Ultimately,

mechanical circulatory support may be needed as a bridge to transplantation (Magnani & Dec, 2006; Schultz et al., 2009). Given that ventricular tachycardia have been known to develop during the recovery phase of myocarditis, routine surveillance for arrhythmias is important in the long-term care plan. In patients with ventricular arrhythmias, an implanted cardiac defibrillator maybe required.

Consultations with the following subspecialists are recommended to promote development of a comprehensive therapeutic management plan: cardiology, cardiothoracic surgery, critical care, infectious diseases, and cardiac transplant program. Because patients may be hospitalized for long-term care, the addition of child life, nutrition, and occupational and physical therapy specialists to the health care team may be required.

Patient and family education relies on good communication, with the interprofessional team clearly delineating the ongoing therapeutic management strategies. These children often have activity and lifestyle limitations, deconditioning, growth failure, nutritional deficiencies, and comorbid conditions, and emotional and psychosocial strain may be appreciated among the patient and family (Miller et al., 2007; Sadof & Nazarian, 2007; Somarriba et al., 2008).

Disposition and discharge planning

Perhaps unexpectedly, children presenting with fulminant myocarditis are more likely to recover left ventricular function and have better long-term outcomes, when compared to those presenting with acute, nonfulminant myocarditis. According to research, one-third of patients with myocarditis experience complete recovery, one-third die or need transplantation, and the remaining one-third have chronic cardiac dysfunction. The future care of pediatric myocarditis depends on the development of a reliable, standardized diagnostic criteria and recognition of the pathogenesis of the myocarditis (Wheeler & Kooy, 2003).

PERICARDITIS

Pathophysiology

Pericarditis is an inflammatory process affecting the pericardium. Although the pathophysiology is dependent of the cause, this type of carditis remains a potentially life-threatening disorder. Pericarditis is complicated by supraphysiologic fluid accumulation; the resulting pericardial effusion may lead to cardiac tamponade. The pericardium contains both a parietal layer and a visceral layer. The visceral pericardium is composed of one or two cell layers of mesothelial cells and adheres closely to the epicardium. In healthy adults, the pericardial sac usually contains 15 to 30 mL of fluid (proportionally less in pediatric patients). If the effusion collects slowly, the pericardium compensates by stretching to accommodate it, and hemodynamics may be unaffected. In contrast, if the effusion collects rapidly, the pericardium is unable to stretch; in this case, the heart becomes compressed and cardiac tamponade ensues. The inability of the ventricles to adequately fill during diastole results in a decreased cardiac output (Allen et al., 2007; Maisch et al., 2004).

Epidemiology and etiology

The incidence of pericarditis is difficult to assess due to the prevalence of subclinical episodes. Rates reported by autopsy range from 1% to 6%. Some sources estimate that pericarditis accounts for 5% of patients who present with chest pain in emergency centers (Lange & Hillis, 2004). Some individuals experience chronic or recurrent forms of this condition. Chronic pericarditis persists longer than three months and is generally associated with a chronic condition (Maisch et al., 2004).

Constrictive pericarditis can be a complication of many types of pericarditis. In such patients, the pericardium becomes thickened and inflamed, leading to myocardial constriction and diastolic dysfunction. These patients present with symptoms of CHF and will require surgical pericardiectomy. Other etiologies of pericarditis include Kawasaki disease, drug reaction, kidney failure, hypothyroidism, chylopericardium, intrapericardial tumors, cancer, radiation, cardiac transplantation, congenital pericardial defects, trauma, and idiopathic causes (Allen et al., 2007; Troughton et al., 2004).

Presentation

The pediatric patient with pericarditis may present with a variety of symptoms. The patient nearing cardiac tamponade will be tachycardic with evidence of decreased cardiac output, such as poor perfusion and decreased level of consciousness. Pulsus paradoxus occurs when the systolic blood pressure decreases more than 10 mmHg with inspiration; its emergence indicates a hemodynamically significant pericardial effusion. If the effusion has developed chronically, tachycardia may not be present, regardless of effusion size (Allen et al., 2007; Maisch et al., 2004; Troughton et al., 2004).

Precordial chest pain is the most commonly reported symptom of pericarditis. Notably, movement and respirations are likely to exacerbate this pain. Fever is also a common presenting sign in acute pericarditis, and may occur secondary to infection, collagen vascular disease, or rheumatic fever. The presence of a friction rub and muffled or distant heart tones strongly suggests a pericardial effusion. However, if the effusion is particularly large, the rub may be absent or difficult to auscultate. Patients who present with bacterial pericarditis generally appear in extremis (Allen et al., 2007; Troughton et al., 2004).

Differential diagnosis

A variety of conditions should be considered in the context of pericarditis. Viral symptoms are often reported in pediatric patients. Therefore, if an etiology is not identified, viral pericarditis is presumed. Patients presenting with CHF and pericarditis should be evaluated for underlying congenital heart or rheumatic heart disease. Pericarditis is also a feature of postpericardiotomy syndrome, which can occur following cardiac surgery (Allen et al., 2007; Maisch et al., 2004; Troughton et al., 2004). Additional differential diagnoses that warrant consideration include Lyme disease, tuberculosis, hypothyroidism, nephritic syndrome, pneumonia, pneumothorax, systemic lupus erythematosus, thalassemia, and radiation pericarditis.

Plan of care

Chest radiograph may reveal a normal to enlarged cardiac silhouette. ECG findings change as pericarditis worsens: Initially the ECG reveals diffuse PR depression and ST elevation, but these segments then normalize, which is followed by widespread T-wave inversion. Pericardial effusions are easily detected by echocardiography. Right atrium and ventricle compression are seen in hemodynamically insignificant effusions. Findings associated with greater hemodynamic instability include (1) a large effusion wherein the heart appears to swing within the collection, (2) septal motion abnormalities, (3) inferior vena cava dilation, and (4) decrease in mitral inflow variation. Although no biomarkers specific to pericarditis have been identified, cardiac enzyme levels are often obtained to evaluate patients for prolonged inflammation and cardiac muscle stress (Allen et al., 2007; Troughton et al., 2004).

Hemodynamic compromise or cardiac tamponade requires emergent stabilization. Pericardiocentesis should be performed to relieve cardiac compression. In preparation for the pericardiocentesis, volume resuscitation should be administered to maximize preload and increase cardiac output (Maisch et al., 2004; Troughton et al., 2004).

Purulent pericarditis carries a mortality rate in the range of 25% to 75% and generally requires drainage or surgical intervention, as antibiotics do not adequately penetrate large abscesses. Prior to identification of the microorganism, antibiotic coverage should include agents targeting *S. aureus,* coverage for methicillin-resistant *Staphylococcus* (MRSA), and Gram-negative bacilli coverage with penicillinase-resistant penicillins or vancomycin, and a third-generation cephalosporin. Antifungal coverage may also be indicated if a fungal organism is suspected; an aminoglycoside may be added if the patient is immunocompromised or recuperating from recent cardiac surgery. Drainage should be considered in all cases of pericarditis with effusion. In purulent pericarditis, drainage is particularly important for microbe identification and antimicrobial penetration of the abscess. Constrictive pericarditis is a potential long-term complication of bacterial (Allen et al., 2007; Maisch et al., 2004).

When pericardial fluid is obtained, it should be analyzed for cell count and differential, glucose, protein, triglycerides, and gram stain and culture to isolate for bacteria, viruses, *Mycobacterium tuberculosis*, and fungi. Specific studies may be ordered for particular bacterial antigens, viral PCR panels, and inflammatory markers (Allen et al., 2007).

Inflammatory types of pericarditis—as in the case of rheumatic fever or systemic lupus erythematosus—are treated with anti-inflammatory therapies. The combination of colchicine with anti-inflammatory therapy has shown beneficial effects in recurrent pericarditis (Imazio et al., 2005). Drug-induced pericarditis usually resolves with discontinuation of the inciting agent (Allen et al., 2007).

Those presenting with pericardial effusion following cardiac surgery should be suspected of having postpericardiotomy syndrome or a chylopericardium. Chylous effusions can be a complication of cardiac surgery secondary to direct injury of the thoracic duct or elevated central venous pressure. Chylous effusions present a therapeutic challenge; treatment for this condition includes a fat-free diet, strict nothing-by-mouth (NPO) status, or surgical intervention with pleurodesis or thoracic duct ligation (Allen et al., 2007; Troughton et al., 2004). Placement of a pericardial window or pericardiectomy may be indicated in effusions that recur frequently or in the case of constrictive pericarditis (Allen et al.; Maisch et al., 2004).

Consultations with the following subspecialists are recommended to promote development of a comprehensive therapeutic management plan: cardiology, cardiothoracic surgery, critical care, and infectious diseases. If the patient is experiencing a rheumatic- or autoimmune-associated pericarditis, an immunologist and a rheumatologist may be consulted. Because patients may be hospitalized for long-term care, the addition of child life, nutrition, and occupational and physical therapy specialists to the health care team may be required.

Patient and family education relies on good communication, with the interdisciplinary team clearly delineating the ongoing therapeutic management strategies. These children often have activity and lifestyle limitations, deconditioning, growth failure, nutritional deficiencies, and comorbid conditions, and emotional and psychosocial strain may be appreciated in both the patient and family (Miller et al., 2007; Sadof & Nazarian, 2007; Somarriba et al., 2008).

Disposition and discharge planning

Follow-up depends on the etiology of the pericarditis. Pericarditis associated with inflammatory processes should be monitored for recurrence. Additionally, development of constrictive pericarditis is possible in infectious pericarditis,

connective tissue disorders, neoplastic disorders, radiation, trauma, and some metabolic and genetic syndromes. The prognosis for patients with pericarditis is generally excellent, with the exception of bacterial pericarditis; in the latter cases, patients are usually very ill and there is a significant risk of mortality (Allen et al., 2007; Maisch et al., 2004; Troughton et al., 2004).

CHYLOTHORAX

Karen Corlett

PATHOPHYSIOLOGY

Chylothorax is the accumulation of chylous lymphatic fluid in the space between the visceral and parietal pleura. Chyle is a component of lymphatic fluid; it is created in response to dietary intake of fat. Large volumes of chyle, as much as 2.5 liters per day in adults, are produced and reabsorbed via the lymphatic system (Agrawal & Sahn, 2006). Not all dietary fats require chyle for absorption. For example, medium-chain triglycerides (MCTs) diffuse, along with other dietary nutrients, from the gastrointestinal (GI) tract to the portal system and on to the liver, thereby not producing chyle.

In the GI tract, small lymphatic vessels, called lacteals, absorb chylomicrons created in response to non-MCT dietary fat intake, and transport them via the lymphatic channels to the bloodstream. The small chylous vessels converge, travel through the diaphragm near the aorta, enter into the posterior mediastinal space, course up around the aortic arch, and empty into the bloodstream via the thoracic duct at the confluence of the left subclavian and left jugular veins (Agrawal & Sahn, 2006). Chylothorax occurs when excess production of chyle overwhelms the lymphatic system's resorptive capacity, or when damage or blockage affects some portion of the lymphatic drainage system.

EPIDEMIOLOGY AND ETIOLOGY

Four main causative categories of chylothorax are noted in pediatric patients: congenital, spontaneous, oncologic, and postsurgical or trauma.

Congenital chylothoraces most often occur in hydropic fetuses. The list of reported causes is exhaustive, ranging from chromosomal abnormalities, to structural abnormalities such as vascular atresias, to congenital heart disease, to infectious etiologies (Rocha, 2007).

Spontaneous chylothorax most commonly occurs with an acquired blockage in the lymphatic or vascular systems. Blockage can be pressure related; in particular, high central venous pressure (CVP) may create a relative obstruction to thoracic duct drainage. Thrombosis of the central vessels may also obstruct outflow from the lymphatic system. Presence of tumors or other masses may directly obstruct the lymph or vascular channels.

Oncologic chylothorax is the most common form of this disorder in adults, but is less frequently observed in pediatric patients. Lymphomas are the malignancy most closely associated with chylous effusions.

Post-trauma effects, including *postsurgical* causes, are the most common etiology of chylothorax in pediatric patients. Direct trauma from chest tube placement, penetrating injuries, and blunt forces may also damage the lymphatic system. Ultimately, the majority of chylothoraces are related to surgical trauma. Any surgery in the thoracic cavity can result in damage or disruption to the lymph channels. Due to the typical course of the chylous channels, cardiac procedures, followed by thoracic surgery, carry the highest risk, even though chylothorax is an overall rare postsurgical complication. At particular risk are patients who undergo surgeries for repair or palliation of congenital heart lesions with manipulation or reconstruction around the aortic arch.

PRESENTATION

Chylothorax is most often suspected when an effusion appears on CXR or ultrasound, or the patient produces milky-appearing chest tube drainage. If the patient is not receiving enteral fat, copious, serous chest tube drainage may be a clue to disruption or blockage to normal lymphatic drainage. Large effusions may present with tachypnea, increased work of breathing, and respiratory distress or failure. Chest pain is rare with chylous effusions, as this condition does not involve an inflammatory process.

Pleural effusions in general may be bloody, serous, purulent, or chylous in nature. Direct sampling of the pleural fluid from an indwelling chest drain or via thoracentesis is necessary for examination and determination of its character. Visual examination of the color and consistency of the fluid is typically illustrative.

DIFFERENTIAL DIAGNOSIS

The first level of differential diagnosis is to determine whether the radiographic findings indicate a pleural effusion. Other possibilities include pneumonia, atelectasis, pleural thickening, and thoracic mass or abscess. A lateral decubitus film may show dependent layering of the fluid, thereby confirming pleural effusion.

Once the differential diagnosis has been narrowed to pleural effusion, the character of the effusion can be determined. The possibilities are empyema, hemothorax, and hydrothorax including transudative or exudative effusions.

PLAN OF CARE

Diagnostic evaluation confirming chyle includes a triglyceride level greater than 110 mg/dL and presence of chylomicrons (Agrawal & Sahn, 2006). Supporting evidence includes a pleural fluid white cell count greater than 1,000 microL with more than 80% lymphocytes (Rocha, 2007). With large-volume or long-term chylothoraces, immune compromise can occur secondary to lymphocyte losses.

Conservative management of chylothorax includes restriction of dietary fat and administration of MCTs to decrease chyle production. If these measures prove successful in decreasing drainage, the MCT diet is maintained for 3 to 6 weeks after resolution of chylous drainage. It is often a challenge to maintain adequate protein and caloric intake in patients owing to the limitations on dietary fat, particularly considering ongoing protein losses via the chylous leak. More aggressive management includes restricting all enteral dietary intake and providing nutrition exclusively through the parenteral route. Intravenous lipid solutions do not promote chyle production, as no enteral absorption is required with this type of feeding. Once enteral intake is allowed, an MCT-fat-only diet is maintained for an additional 3 to 6 weeks.

Octreotide, a somatostatin analogue, is an antisecretory agent that is effective in the GI tract; it has been used on an off-label basis with varied results in the treatment of neonatal and post cardiac surgery chylothoraces. Langdvoigt and Mullet (2006) reported minimal success with the use of octreotide post cardiac surgery, but postulated success may be greatest when the patient's central venous pressure is low and the triglyceride level of the pleural fluid is high. Lim et al. (2005) reported excellent success with the use of octreotide for chylothoraces occurring post cardiac surgery; however, a significantly higher dosing range was used in this study. Octreotide may be given either subcutaneously or parenterally as a continuous infusion. The dose is increased in a stepwise approach, observing for GI and other side effects. Neonates—and particularly premature neonates—may be at risk for vasoconstrictive side effects in the GI tract when this agent is used.

Diuretics may be a helpful adjunct in chylothorax, particularly on a postsurgery basis when pulmonary edema may be an additional source of fluid accumulation in the pleural space. In cases where vascular obstruction inhibits emptying of the thoracic duct into the central venous system, anticoagulation or attempts at thrombolysis may also be appropriate.

Large chylothoraces that hinder respiratory functioning require drainage. This may be accomplished by thoracentesis or chest tube placement (see Chapter 42). An indwelling chest tube allows continued surveillance of drainage volume, and its use avoids reaccumulation if the drainage tube remains patent. Dietary restriction and pharmacologic management represent therapy options if drainage persists or if chylothorax recurs.

Chemical or mechanical pleurodesis may be considered as a treatment for persistent chylous drainage. The goal is to adhese the visceral and parietal pleura together to obliterate potential space where chyle may accumulate, thereby shunting drainage into the appropriate channels. Minimizing chylous output around the time of pleurodesis keeps the pleural space dry, optimizing the chances that this approach will be successful. If chyle continues to escape the lymphatic system post pleurodesis, loculated chylous effusions may occur.

Surgical options for persistent chylothorax focus on direct repair or ligation of the thoracic duct. Identification of a specific site of leakage and repair is often difficult. Intraoperative administration of enteral fat to elucidate the chylous leak has been used with anecdotal success. More commonly, the thoracic duct is surgically ligated. Chemical or mechanical pleurodesis may be performed in conjunction with thoracic duct ligation.

Identification and management of chylothorax may create stress among pediatric patients and their caregivers, as both require vigilance and patience. Chylothorax is often associated with another event such as congenital heart surgery or oncologic diagnosis. Education regarding the reason for chylous drainage, rationale for management strategies, careful instruction regarding dietary limitations if instituted, and any plans for escalation to surgical management should be discussed with both the patient and family.

DISPOSITION AND DISCHARGE PLANNING

Resolution of chylothoraces depends on the treatment. Congenital chylothorax is most often associated with hydrops, which has a high mortality rate. Treatment of spontaneous chylothorax focuses on reestablishing normal lymph or vascular drainage channels and has varying success rates. Chylothoraces associated with oncologic presentation are typically large, requiring drainage, and the focus rapidly shifts to oncologic needs. Traumatic (including postsurgical) chylothoraces are the most common subgroup in pediatrics. Outcomes range from success with single thoracentesis to recurrence after surgical ligation and pleurodesis.

Initial radiologic follow-up should occur on a daily schedule to evaluate the size of the pleural effusion. After several days of minimal to no fluid reaccumulation, the frequency of radiologic surveillance may be decreased. As chylothorax is most often a comorbidity, its recurrence risk is only one factor in determining discharge timing. Discharge criteria include freedom from pleural effusion with the patient taking either no or only enteral diuretics. Timing of initial follow-up is influenced by the temporal relationship to the last occurrence, recent pleural effusion, and HCP determination of whether chylothorax is a resolved or potentially recurrent problem.

Prior to the patient's discharge, caregivers should be educated regarding the importance of scheduled follow-up care, such as radiological examinations. Education should also be provided about dietary restrictions, with caregivers being instructed to seek medical attention for the patient if signs of respiratory distress occur, as such signs are an indicator of effusion recurrence.

CONGENITAL HEART LESIONS

Dawn Tucker, Kristen T. Sullivan, Valarie Eichler, Laurie Beth Williams, and Joseph J. Amato

EMBRYOLOGY

Congenital heart disease (CHD) begins with in utero malformations of the heart structure and/or circulatory system. Failure of embryonic structures to develop normally results in altered circulatory flow patterns, which are otherwise required for later stages of cardiac development; thus the idiom "no flow—no grow." Normal cardiac development begins in the third week of gestation and is complete by day 45, before many women even know that they are pregnant. It starts when a straight heart tube is formed from the cardiogenic crescent of the precardiac mesoderm. The left and right halves of the crescent migrate cephalad and medial to form the tube. Normally, the tube then loops or folds to the right, forming a D-loop with normal anatomic organization, and normally related ventricles. In abnormal, or L-loop, formation, the tube folds to the left, which results in ventricular inversion, with the right ventricle (RV) lying to the left of the left ventricle (LV).

During the fourth week of gestation, loop formation is complete. The ventricles then begin to develop, as does the primitive arterial trunk; circulation commences. During the fifth week of gestation, the ventricles continue to grow and divide as the ventricular septum begins to develop. The great vessels (arteries) separate from the trunk into the pulmonary artery (PA) and the aorta; in the endocardial cushion, the initial common atrioventricular (AV) valve separates into the mitral and tricuspid valves. The atria separate into right and left portions with the closure of the ostium primum, and positioning of the pulmonary and aortic valves occurs. By the sixth to seventh week of gestation, the development of the heart structure is complete (Clark et al., 2000; Van Praagh, 1972).

ANATOMY

Cardiac situs refers to the relationship of the atria to the thoracic viscera, as well as the relationship of the ventricles to each other. *Situs solitus* means that the atria and mainstem bronchi have developed in the usual relationship to each other: The right atria is to the right of the left atria, the left atria is to the left of the right atria, and the mainstem bronchi are in the normal positions (Landing et al., 1971). In *situs inversus*, the opposite relationships occur. *Situs ambiguous* refers to the absence of lateralization of the atria and the thoracic organs. When there are two right or left atrial chambers, the condition is referred to as *atrial isomerism*. Atrial isomerism is commonly associated with a lack of lateralization of the abdominal organs; patients are usually asplenic or polysplenic (Lev et al., 1971; Liberthson et al., 1973; Partridge et al., 1975; Stanger et al., 1968; Van Mierop & Wiglesworth, 1962).

As in atrial relationships, the ventricles are in a normal relationship to each other (situs solitus) when the right ventricle is to the right of the left, and the left ventricle is to the left of the right. Ventricular situs solitus may also be referred to as D-loop. Ventricular inversion, also known as L-loop ventricles, occurs when the right ventricle is more posterior and to the left of the left ventricle (Van Praagh et al., 1979).

In atrial inversion, L-loop is the concordant or normal situs, while D-loop is the inverted situs. The definition of looping is independent of atrial situs. Given that there are two possible ventricular positions and two possible atrial positions, there are four basic hearts, each capable of providing "normal" cardiac blood flow (Van Praagh et al., 1980).

Each portion of the heart connects with adjoining structures—the atria to the ventricles, and the ventricles to the great arteries. The atrioventricular connections may be *concordant*, whereby the right atrium (RA) connects to the right ventricle, and vice versa. Alternatively, they may be *discordant*, which occurs when the right atrium attaches to the left ventricle, and the left atrium (LA) to the right ventricle. These relationships may also be *univentricular*, such that the atria connect to only one ventricle. Finally, the elements of the heart may be *ambiguous*; when an AV valve is either straddling or overriding, it is described as being committed to whichever ventricle is receiving more than 50% of its output (Stanger et al., 1968).

Much of the same nomenclature applies when describing connections from the ventricles to the great vessels. Concordant ventriculoarterial connections occur when the right ventricle connects with the pulmonary artery, and the left ventricle with the aorta. Similarly, disconcordant ventriculoarterial connections occur when the aorta arises from the right ventricle, and the pulmonary artery from the left—a condition also known as transposition of the great arteries. As in atrioventricular connections, if the pulmonary or aortic valve is overriding a ventricular septal defect (VSD), it is considered to arise from the ventricle from which greater than 50% of the valve is committed. In such a "double outlet" connection, both of the great arteries arise completely, or for the most part, from one ventricle. Just as the connection may involve only one ventricle, so it may also consist of only one great vessel or a common arterial

trunk, a phenomenon known as "single outlet" physiology (Milo et al., 1979; Van Praagh & Van Praagh, 1966).

The assignment of the correct morphology of the atria is determined not based on the status of the systemic or pulmonary venous return to the chamber, but rather by the morphology of the atrial appendage. The right atrial appendage is wide based and blunt ended, whereas the left atrial appendage is long and narrow. Clinically, it may be difficult to differentiate the atria. However, if the patient's anatomy is studied in the cardiac catheterization lab, certain aspects of the atrial septum may be visualized under angiography, particularly the structure of the right atrial septum. The limbus of the fossa ovalis, or primum septum, may be visible. The outline of the shape of the atrial appendage may also assist in delineating the morphology of the atrium. Generally, determination of the location of the left atrium is determined by exclusion after the right atrium has been identified (Brandt & Calder, 1977; Partridge et al., 1975; Soto et al., 1978; Van Mierop et al., 1970; Van Mierop & Wiglesworth, 1962).

The atrioventricular valves separate the atria from the ventricles. The morphologic right-sided valve is termed the tricuspid valve, and the morphologic left-sided valve is known as the mitral valve. The atrioventricular valve associated with each ventricle is characteristic of that ventricle; in other words, regardless of position of the morphologic ventricle, the associated valve will follow that ventricle. The tricuspid valve is a trileaflet structure, while the mitral valve is a bileaflet valve. The valve leaflets are supported by papillary muscles, which attach to the leaflets via chordae tendinae.

The three leaflets of the tricuspid valve are known as the anterior, posterior, and septal leaflets. Visualizing all three leaflets can be challenging. The anterior leaflet is the largest of the three leaflets, and the posterior the smallest. The septal leaflet is usually slightly larger than the posterior leaflet, and as its name implies, the majority of this leaflet attaches to the membranous and muscular portions of the ventricular septum. Of importance when considering the anatomical landmarks of the tricuspid valve is the proximity of the conduction system to the septal leaflet (Barry & Patten, 1968; Gross, 1931; Sherman, 1963).

While the tricuspid valve consists of three leaflets, the mitral valve is made up of just two, known as the anterior and posterior leaflets. The anterior or septal leaflet is larger than the posterior or mural leaflet, and is triangular in shape. The septal leaflet is in continuity with the aortic valve, and forms a boundary of the left ventricular outflow tract. The septal leaflet has a more scalloped appearance. The mitral valve is designed to allow for the largest orifice possible during diastole so that no obstruction hinders blood flow from the left atrium to the left ventricle. This valve opens as the anterior leaflet moves anterior and away from the posterior leaflet. During systole, the mitral valve closes as the anterior leaflet extends toward the posterior leaflet (Ranganathan et al., 1970).

The morphologic right ventricle is triangular, and consists of inlet, trabecular, and outlet portions. The inlet portion has attachments from the septal leaflet of the tricuspid valve, and it surrounds and supports the valve. Just inferior to the inlet portion is the moderator band, a trabeculation running from the septum to the free wall of the ventricle. The right ventricle is heavily trabeculated, which represents a major anatomical difference from the left ventricle. The outlet portion of the ventricular septum consists of three components. First, the infundibular septum (conal septum) separates the aortic valve from the pulmonary valve. Second, the ventriculoinfundibular fold (crista supraventricularis) separates the tricuspid valve from the pulmonary valve. Third, the anterior and posterior limbs of the trabecula septomarginalis form a "Y" shaped muscle bundle that extends apically to become continuous with the moderator band (Anderson et al., 1977; Anderson & Weinberg, 2005; Bartelings & Gittenberger-de Groot, 1989).

The morphologic left ventricle is elliptical in shape and, in contrast with the right ventricle, is finely trabeculated. It consists of two portions: the inlet or sinus portion of the ventricle, which supports the mitral valve and also includes the apex, and the outlet portion, which sits beneath the aortic valve (Brandt & Calder, 1977).

The ventricles are separated by the ventricular septum, an asymmetric structure that is positioned secondary to the presence of an infundibulum in the right ventricle. Due to higher pressures in the left ventricle, the septum maintains a concave surface on the left side of the septum, and a convex surface on the right that is accentuated during systole. The membranous portion of the septum separates the left ventricular outflow tract from both the right ventricle and, to some degree, the right atrium. Specific anatomical variations are determined by the attachment of the tricuspid valve to the septum. This portion of the septum continues upward, forming the septum between the LV outflow tract and the right atrium. Meanwhile, the lower portion of the ventricular septal wall is composed of thicker, muscular tissue (Bargeron et al., 1977).

The semilunar valves, which consist of the ventricular outflow valves, separate the ventricles from the great arteries. The pulmonary valve separates the RV from the pulmonary artery; likewise, the aortic valve separates the LV from the aorta. Both valves are trileaflet in structure. The ostia of the coronary arteries arise from the left and right cusps of the aortic valve, whereas the noncoronary cusp lacks any coronary artery structure. Of note, the noncoronary cusp of the aortic valve is in continuity with the anterior leaflet of the mitral valve and the membranous portion of the ventricular septum. The aortic sinuses, or sinuses of Valsalva, are "pockets" at the base of the aortic root that are responsible for "trapping" regurgitant blood in the aorta (Kerr & Goss, 1956; Yacoub et al., 1999; Zimmerman, 1969).

The pulmonary valve is similar in structure to the aortic valve, but it lacks coronary ostia and the arteries that arise from them. Unlike the aortic valve, the pulmonary valve is not in fibrous continuity with the tricuspid valve, nor does it have any direct relationship with the ventricular septum. The subpulmonary infundibulum separates the pulmonary valve from the ventricular septum (Gray, 1973).

The great arteries (vessels) arise from the ventricles through the pulmonary and aortic valves. The aorta gives rise to the systemic and coronary arterial circulation. The aorta may be identified by its attachment to the brachiocephalic arteries, which never arise from the pulmonary arteries. In contrast, the coronary arteries may not always arise from the base of the aorta; one of these arteries, and very rarely both, may arise from the base of the PA. The normal course of the aortic arch is toward the left, and the pulmonary valve and artery sit anterior and to the right of the aortic valve and the aorta (Ogden, 1970).

In normal cardiac anatomy, systemic venous return is directed to the morphologic right atrium. The superior vena cava receives blood from the head and upper extremities, and empties into the roof of the right atrium. The inferior vena cava empties into the inferior portion of the right atrium, and returns blood from the trunk and lower extremities of the body. The coronary veins drain into the coronary sinus, which in turn empties into the right atrium.

In similar manner, pulmonary venous return is directed to the morphologic left atrium. Four pulmonary veins drain blood from the lungs—two to the right side, and two to the left side of the left atrium. They drain in inferior and superior locations on each side (Figure 22-25). Pulmonary vascular

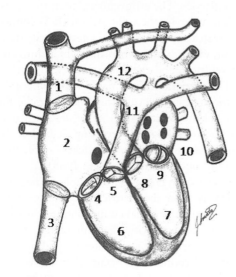

FIGURE 22-25

Normal Heart.

Note: Superior vena cava (1), right atrium (2), inferior vena cava (3), tricuspid valve (4), pulmonic valve (5), right ventricle (6), left ventricle (7), aortic valve (8), mitral valve (9), pulmonary veins (10), pulmonary artery (11), aortic arch (12).

Source: Used with permission. Courtesy of Joseph J. Amato, MD MJ. All Rights Reserved.

resistance (PVR) is high in the newborn and decreases over the first few days to months of life. Depending on the cardiac lesion, when the PVR drops, the infant's heart defect may be detected as flow patterns change.

SHUNT LESIONS

Patent ductus arteriosus

The ductus arteriosus is part of normal fetal circulation. The vessel connects the left main pulmonary artery with the descending aorta below the left subclavian artery. In utero, the ductus shunts blood from the main pulmonary artery to the descending aorta, bypassing the nonaerated lungs. Under normal circumstances, the ductus arteriosus closes functionally postnatally within 48 hours and anatomically at approximately 2 weeks of age. The increase in arterial oxygen saturation with the first breath is thought to be the initiating step in ductal closure. In addition, other factors, such as decreasing prostaglandin levels, influence the ductus to close. Prostaglandin levels decrease due to the removal of the placenta (the major source of prostaglandin in utero), and an increase in metabolism by the lungs. Premature infants are at greater risk for patent ductus due to poor metabolism of prostaglandins secondary to immature lung tissue.

Patent ductus arteriosus (PDA) is a common congenital heart problem accounting for approximately 10% of the total number of cardiac defects in newborns. PDA occurs more frequently in females, and is commonly found in infants born to mothers who were exposed to rubella in the first trimester of pregnancy. Approximately 15% of all children with PDA have an associated congenital heart defect.

Pathophysiology. Shortly after birth, pulmonary vascular resistance begins to fall, reversing the direction of shunt flow to primarily left to right across the PDA. Left-to-right shunting leads to increased pulmonary blood flow, left atrial dilation, and left ventricular volume overload. The degree of shunting is determined by the size of the communication and the relative resistances between the systemic and pulmonary circulations. A large PDA leads to considerable aortic runoff, lowering diastolic pressure; in turn, this effect may lead to organ hypoperfusion (Heidl et al., 2010).

Presentation. Clinical manifestations of PDA depend on the amount of left-to-right shunting. A small PDA produces a machinery-type murmur heard best at the left upper sternal border. A large PDA produces symptoms of CHF and/or pulmonary hypertension, wide pulse pressure with a low diastolic pressure, and bounding peripheral pulses. Because premature infants have fewer compensatory mechanisms to adjust to the stress of a large PDA, they are at higher risk for necrotizing enterocolitis (NEC), kidney failure, and

pulmonary vascular disease. In the full-term infant and child, pulmonary vascular disease, infective endocarditis, and aneurysm formation are potential problems (Shimada et al., 1994).

Plan of care. Chest radiograph findings will include increased pulmonary vascular markings and cardiomegaly from increased left atrial and left ventricular volumes. Electrocardiography will show left atrial enlargement and biventricular hypertrophy. Echocardiograph is the diagnositic study of choice; it enables the visualization of the PDA, and color Doppler outlines shunting. The presence of a large PDA results in left atrial and ventricular dilation. Echocardiograph is also a useful technology if serial evaluations are required.

The approach to treatment in patients with PDA varies considerably due to the lack of evidence-based resources that might recommend one approach as superior. In addition, the effect of PDA on the outcome of premature infants is unclear due to the lack of clinical trials in this population. Historically, medical management has included the prophylactic use of cyclooxygenase (COX) inhibitors such as indomethacin, which inhibit prostaglandin synthesis, thereby resulting in smooth muscle contraction at the ductus arteriosus (Tefft, 2010). However, a recent report suggests monitoring for spontaneous closure rather than using prophylactic indomethacin. This recommendation is made based on the side effects of COX inhibitors and the possibility of spontaneous closure even in very-low-birth-weight (VLBW) infants (Laughon et al., 2004).

PDA closure can also be accomplished with minimal risk using a variety of invasive techniques. Surgical management involves performing a left posterior thoracotomy, isolating the vessel, and either ligating or dividing the PDA. Newer surgical techniques include the use of video-assisted thoracoscopic surgery. Closure via interventional catheterization has been increasing over the past decade. Detachable coils are widely used to close small PDAs, while Amplatzer Duct Occluders are used for moderate to large PDAs (Figure 22-26).

Postoperative care and discharge planning. The postoperative course following closure of isolated PDA is usually benign. The length of hospitalization following closure is typically 1 to 2 days. Invasive hemodynamic monitoring and vasoactive infusions are usually unnecessary.

Atrial septal defect

Atrial septal defect (ASD) is an opening in the atrial septum. Isolated ASDs account for 5% to 10% of all congenital heart defects and occur more frequently in females (Hoffman & Kaplan, 2002). Four types of ASDs are distinguished, based on their location in the atrial

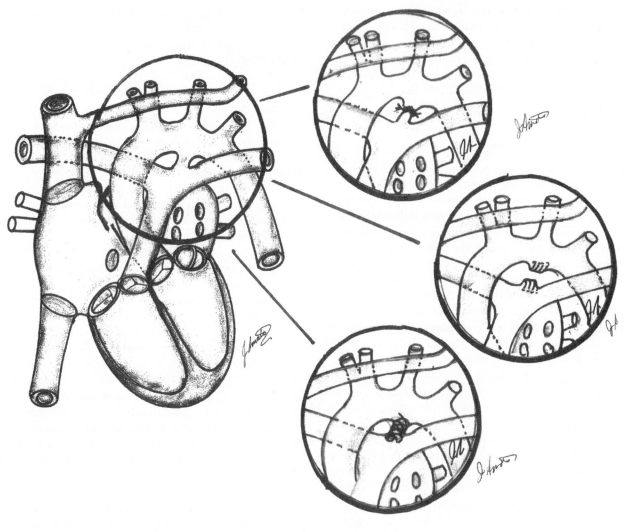

FIGURE 22-26

Patent Ductus Arteriosus Repairs: Ligation, Ligation and Division, or Coil.

Source: Used with permission. Courtesy of Joseph J. Amato, MD MJ. All Rights Reserved.

septum: ostium secundum, sinus venosus, ostium primum, and coronary sinus. An *ostium secundum* defect is located in the center of the atrium and is the most commonly occurring ASD. A *sinus venosus* ASD is located near the superior vena cava and is often associated with abnormal drainage of the right pulmonary veins. *Ostium primum* defects are often associated with abnormalities of the atrioventricular valves. *Coronary sinus* defects are a rare type of interatrial communication in which the septum between the coronary sinus and left atrium is either partially or completely unroofed; these ASDs are associated with left-sided superior vena cava.

Pathophysiology. Pathophysiologic findings with ASD include left-to-right shunting at the atrial level, leading to right atrial dilation, right ventricular volume overload, and increased pulmonary blood flow. The degree of shunting depends on the size of the defect and the relative compliances of the left and right ventricles during diastole. Prolonged ventricular and atrial dilation leads to right ventricular dysfunction and atrial arrhythmias.

Presentation. Infants and children with ASD are usually asymptomatic, though most will be noted to have a slender body build. CHF usually does not occur until the second or third decade of life. A soft systolic ejection murmur with a fixed S_2 heart sound may be present. The ECG findings may be normal; however, right axis deviation and right ventricular hypertrophy may be noted. Radiographic findings reveal an enlarged heart with a cardiothoracic ratio greater than 0.5 and increased Pulmonary vascular markings. If the defect is left unrepaired, radiographic changes consistent with pulmonary hypertension may be evident, such as an enlarged main pulmonary artery. Lung fields may be clear or oligemic.

Plan of care. ASDs are monitored via echocardiograph for spontaneous closure. Ostium secundum defects smaller than 3 mm are likely to close spontaneously. In contrast, a defect measuring 8 mm or greater in size requires intervention. Medical management is often not indicated, given that CHF typically does not develop until after the second decade of life. Instead, closure of a secundum defect may be accomplished surgically or by a catheter device. King and Millis first performed transcatheter closure in 1976 (King et al., 1976). The Amplatzer Septal Occluder has been used since 1995 and continues to be the most utilized ASD closure device (Knepp et al., 2010). Approximately 85% of secundum ASDs can be closed using the device.

Larger defects require surgical intervention. Specifically, primum, venosus, and coronary sinus defects require surgical intervention. Surgical closure of ASD entails a median sternotomy or submammary thoracotomy incision and CPB with aortic cross clamping (AoX). The defect is closed via a right atriotomy and patch closure using Dacron, pericardium, or suture for small defects. Sinus venosus defects require an additional baffling of the anomalous pulmonary veins to the left atrium.

Postoperative care and discharge planning. Postoperative care following surgical closure is usually uneventful. Extubation often occurs in the operating room or shortly after the patient's arrival to the intensive care unit. Monitoring includes arterial and central venous catheters. Vasoactive support is rarely indicated. Typically, patients remain hospitalized for 2 to 4 days. Potential postoperative complications include sinoatrial node dysfunction, heart block, postpericardiotomy syndrome, left ventricular dysfunction, and venous obstruction. Patients with isolated ASDs are expected to make a full recovery without sequelae.

Ventricular septal defect

Ventricular septal defect (VSD) is an opening in the ventricular septum. VSDs are the most common forms of congenital heart disease, accounting for approximately 21% of all cases. Multiple types of VSDs exist (Figure 22-27). The nomenclature is often dependent on institutional preferences. Most institutions classify VSDs into four categories based on their location in the ventricular septum: muscular, inlet, perimembranous, and infundibular (Roguin et al., 1995).

Pathophysiology. VSD allows for left-to-right shunting, across the septum, leading to left atrial dilation, left ventricular volume overload, and increased pulmonary blood flow.

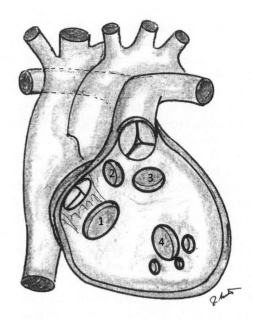

FIGURE 22-27

Ventricular Septal Defects.

Note: Inlet (1), perimembraneous (2), infundibular (3), muscular (4).

Source: Used with permission. Courtesy of Joseph J. Amato, MD MJ. All Rights Reserved.

The determinants of shunting are size of defect and pulmonary vascular resistance. In small restrictive defects, the degree of shunting is determined by the size of the defect. Shunt flow from small defects causes little to no hemodynamic effect. In large unrestrictive defects (i.e., the defect is more than 50% of the aortic diameter), equilibration of pressures between the two ventricles occurs. As a consequence, the amount of left-to-right shunting is determined by the resistances in the pulmonary and systemic systems. The hemodynamic changes, which occur over time, are a result of excess blood flow and pressure loading conditions. As pulmonary blood flow increases, left ventricular diastolic preload increases, causing CHF. VSD shunting occurs during systole, causing pressure-loading conditions on the right ventricle. The transmission of systemic pressure on the pulmonary vasculature may ultimately lead to pulmonary hypertension or pulmonary vascular obstructive disease (Hayworth, 1987).

Presentation. Clinical findings are determined by the size of defect and amount of pulmonary over-circulation. Often the presenting complaint is failure-to-thrive and/or respiratory infections, accompanied by CHF signs and symptoms. A left ventricular heave may be noted as left ventricular volumes increase. A holosystolic murmur is often accompanied by a diastolic rumble indicative of LV volume overload. Pulmonary over-circulation ultimately causes the manifestations of pulmonary hypertension.

Plan of care. Clinical evaluation for VSD includes echocardiograph, CXR, B-type natriuretic peptide (BNP) serum level, ECG, and infrequently cardiac catheterization. Increased pulmonary vascular markings and enlarged left atrium are noted on CXR. Levels of BNP, which is secreted from the chambers in the heart in response to stretched myocardium, are increased in large VSDs. Although the ECG may be normal in small VSDs, large VSDs will be evident as left ventricular hypertrophy and possibly right ventricular hypertrophy if RV pressures are elevated. Echocardiograph allows for the identification of the VSD location and is the standard for diagnosis. In addition, it quantifies jet flow across the VSD and tricuspid valve, allowing for the evaluation of pulmonary and right ventricular pressures. When significant pulmonary hypertension is a concern, a cardiac catheterization is performed to determine the feasibility of closing the VSD.

Initial therapy is directed at controlling CHF symptoms through medical management. As mentioned earlier, surgery is indicated for large defects. The timing of surgery is determined by CHF symptoms and weight gain (Kostolny et al., 2006). Children who are experiencing CHF symptoms and not gaining weight despite medical management are referred for surgery. Spontaneous closure is possible with perimembranous and muscular defects; therefore, surgical repair is avoided prior to the child reaching one year of age. Other defects, such as an infundibular or inlet defect, should be repaired within the first year of life to ensure optimal pulmonary and ventricular recovery (Moe & Guntheroth, 1987).

In recent years, successful closure by catheterization devices has been reported with muscular VSDs. This technique is evolving and not all institutions are yet utilizing catheterization for VSD closure (Knauth et al., 2004).

Surgical closure requires CPB bypass. The VSD is typically approached through the tricuspid or pulmonary valve and closed using a patch technique (Hannan et al., 2009). In the past, pulmonary artery banding was used as palliation to protect the pulmonary vasculature until definitive repair could be completed. Currently, this procedure is reserved for children who are at high risk for undergoing CPB.

Postoperative care and discharge planning. The postoperative course following surgical closure is typically uncomplicated. Care includes arterial and central venous catheter monitoring, near-infrared spectroscopy (NIRS), and occasional vasoactive support. Most patients are extubated shortly after surgery. Patients who present late for surgery with large VSDs, or who have comorbidities such as trisomy 21, may require positive-pressure ventilatory support for longer periods or inhaled nitric oxide due to pulmonary hypertension. Atrioventricular conduction disturbances can be seen postoperatively; therefore, atrial and ventricular temporary pacing wires are usually placed

during surgery. The length of hospitalization averages 3 to 6 days, and full recovery is expected without sequelae.

Atrioventricular canal

Atrioventricular canal (AVC) results from the failure of the endocardial cushion to develop normally. AVC defects account for approximately 4% to 5% of all CHD cases (Allan et al., 1994). Typically, AVC has three components: ASD, most often ostium primum; an inlet VSD; and abnormal formation of the atrioventricular valves. Several types of canal defects are possible, ranging on a continuum from complete to partial. A complete AVC includes ASD, large inlet VSD, and a single atrioventricular valve. Complete AVCs may also have ventricular asymmetry, and are known as unbalanced AVCs. A partial AVC consists of an ASD with a cleft in the anterior leaflet of the left atrioventricular valve, usually associated with valve insufficiency; there is no VSD component, and two atrioventricular valves are present. A transitional AVC has an associated ASD with partially separated atrioventricular valves and small ventricular communication (Backer et al., 2007).

Pathophysiology. Varying degrees of left-to-right shunting may be noted at the atrial and ventricular levels, depending on the type of AVC. The degree of shunting determines the pathophysiologic findings. For instance, a partial AVC resembles an ASD, whereas a complete AVC resembles a large VSD. Atrioventricular regurgitation may increase the left-to-right shunt and promote atrial and ventricular volume overload.

Presentation. Clinical manifestations depend on the type of AVC. Patients with complete AVC often have a presentation similar to that of patients with a large VSD in which CHF symptoms predominate. Tachypnea and poor weight gain are associated with moderate to severe mitral valve regurgitation. Mitral regurgitation will produce a holosystolic murmur. Patients with partial AVC have a presentation similar to that of patients with an ASD. The heart size is often enlarged and pulmonary vascularity is prominent on chest radiograph. Trisomy 21 is often associated with this lesion.

Plan of care. Diagnostic evaluation for AVC is similar to that for ASD and VSD. Echocardiograph is an invaluable tool to delineate the AV valves, ventricular and atrial septums, and presence of associated lesions. Initial management is aimed at controlling CHF symptoms and improving weight gain. The timing of surgical repair is determined by type of defect. Surgical repair for complete AVC is recommended in the first 6 months of life to avoid hemodynamic and pulmonary vascular compromise in the growing child (Kobayashi et al., 2007). Repair requires CPB. The atrial and ventricular defects are closed using a one- or two-patch technique, and the available valve tissue is fashioned into functioning mitral and tricuspid valves.

Postoperative care and discharge planning. Immediate postoperative care is aimed at lowering atrial pressures to prevent atrioventricular valvar regurgitation (Ten Harkel et al., 2009). The newly repaired AV valves may become regurgitant in the presence of volume loading. Improvement in cardiac output is achieved by reducing afterload, improving inotropy, and ensuring AV association. In addition to arterial and central venous monitoring, left atrial pressure monitoring may be useful. Near infrared spectroscopy (NIRS) monitoring aids in assessing regional and global perfusion. Positive-pressure ventilation is applied, and inhaled nitric oxide may be indicated in the immediate postoperative period. The duration of positive-pressure ventilation is determined by the patient's preoperative condition, the amount of AV valve regurgitation, and the reactivity of the pulmonary vasculature. Sinoatrial node dysfunction and heart block can occur postoperatively; therefore, atrial and ventricular temporary pacing wires are usually placed during the surgery (Jonas, 2004). The length of hospitalization is commonly 7 to 10 days, depending on the type of AVC.

Patients with AVC should receive subacute bacterial endocarditis (SBE) prophylaxis for the rest of their lives, due to the defects in the AV valves. Detailed guidelines, last updated in 2007, are available from the AHA at http://circ. ahajournals.org/cgi/content/full/116/15/1736. Long-term follow-up includes observing for development of AV regurgitation, subaortic stenosis, and dysrhythmias.

Truncus arteriosus

Truncus arteriosus (TA) is a rare congenital heart disease that accounts for only 1% to 4% of all congenital heart lesions (Swanson et al., 2009). TA represents failure of the primitive arterial trunk to septate and divide into a distinct aorta and pulmonary artery. Instead, a single arterial vessel originates from the heart, overrides the ventricular septum, and supplies the coronary, pulmonary arterial, and systemic circulations. TA is always associated with a VSD, and an interrupted aortic arch is present in approximately 13% of patients. The truncal valve is often abnormal, with the number of leaflets varying from two to six. In addition, the valve is often stenotic or regurgitant. The aortic arch may be right sided (Konstantinov et al., 2006). TA usually occurs as an isolated heart defect, but may be may be associated with other disorders—in particular, DiGeorge syndrome.

Four types of TA are distinguished, based on the relationship of the pulmonary arteries to the trunk (i.e., the size and site of origin of the pulmonary arteries). Type I has a short pulmonary trunk from which both pulmonary arteries arise. In Type II, the pulmonary arteries arise very close to one another and separate from the truncus. When the pulmonary arteries are at a distance from one another and separate from the truncus it is Type III. Type IV truncus is a form of pulmonary atresia with a ventricular septal defect (Cabalka et al., 2008).

Pathophysiology. Pathophysiologic findings are similar to single-ventricle physiology. In TA, complete admixture of the systemic and pulmonary venous return occurs. Pulmonary and systemic blood flow is determined by the presence of pulmonary stenosis and pulmonary vascular resistance. In the absence of PA stenosis, as pulmonary vascular resistance falls, pulmonary over-circulation ensues. When pulmonary arteries are exposed to increased flow and systemic pressure, early pulmonary vascular obstructive disease may result. The volume and pressure overload can be further increased by truncal valve stenosis or regurgitation. Coronary ischemia may develop secondary to low diastolic pressure caused by pulmonary circulation run-off. Pulmonary over-circulation occurs at the expense of systemic blood flow; therefore, systemic oxygen transport is decreased (Fuglestad et al., 1988).

Presentation. Signs of CHF are present shortly after the normal fall of pulmonary vascular resistance (PVR). The degree and severity of symptoms are determined by the amount of pulmonary over-circulation. Bounding peripheral pulses are evident, and the patient may be cyanotic if pulmonary stenosis is present. Once pulmonary vascular obstructive disease has developed, the clinical findings are consistent with increased PVR. The second heart sound may be single, with a harsh systolic murmur. Chest radiograph reveals cardiomegaly with pulmonary edema and increased pulmonary vascular markings. Left atrial enlargement and biventricular hypertrophy may be present on ECG. If this defect goes undiagnosed in utero, the patient often presents in shock due to an elevated pulmonary to systolic ratio of blood flow (Qp:Qs), which causes low systemic cardiac output.

Plan of care. Confirmation of TA is made by echocardiograph. Cardiac catheterization is indicated only if the anatomy cannot be delineated by echocardiograph or if pulmonary vascular obstructive disease is suspected. Once the diagnosis is confirmed, therapeutic management is directed toward reversing shock states, managing CHF symptoms, and correcting cyanosis if present. Cyanosis, which is usually due to pulmonary stenosis, is treated with the administration of prostaglandin E_1, which relaxes smooth muscle in the ductus arteriosus, thereby maintaining its patency (Brizard et al., 1997). Surgery is indicated once the patient is stabilized and any shock states are reversed. Palliation by pulmonary artery banding is no longer used due to the incidence of hypoplasia and obstruction of vessels. Definitive repair requires CPB and includes VSD closure via right ventriculotomy and placement of a valved homograft from the right ventricle to the detached pulmonary arteries. Correction of other anomalies such as interrupted aortic arch or coarctation is completed as part of the same procedure (Adachi et al., 2009) (Figure 22-28).

Postoperative care and discharge planning. Postoperative care requires monitoring of arterial, central venous, and left atrial pressures, and NIRS. Vasoactive support, positive-pressure ventilation, and inhaled nitric oxide are commonly required.

Patients with dysfunctional truncal valves are often difficult to manage. Afterload reduction may be useful in treating truncal valve regurgitation. Severe regurgitation or stenosis is not well tolerated, so patients who experience these conditions may require a return to the operating room for a valvuloplasty.

Low cardiac output is relatively common following TA repair. Due to the right ventriculotomy, patients often experience right bundle branch block. Temporary complete heart block can occur, requiring atrioventricular pacing. In addition, right ventricular dysfunction can occur and is exacerbated when pulmonary hypertension is present.

Monitoring for postoperative bleeding is important given the high risk of bleeding, because suture lines are exposed to systemic pressure. Systemic arterial oxygen saturations should be normal.

Many factors contribute to the length of hospitalization including shock states, truncal regurgitation and stenosis, and incidence of necrotizing enterocolitis (NEC). Patients with TA are at risk for NEC due to pulmonary over-circulation causing preoperative distributive shock, leaving the bowel with inadequate perfusion (Thomas et al., 2001). The length of hospitalization averages 10 to 14 days.

Patients with TA will require lifelong follow-up. Replacement of the right ventricular to pulmonary homograft will be required at least once in the patient's lifetime. Interventional catheterization procedures are being developed to enable replacement of RV to PA homografts in the catheterization lab instead of the operating room. Many patients will develop pulmonary artery stenosis or aortic stenosis (if a coarctation was present in the initial surgery), which may be palliated by interventional cardiac catheterization (Tlaskal et al., 2010).

Total anomalous pulmonary venous return

Anomalous pulmonary venous return is the drainage of the pulmonary veins into a systemic venous structure or right atrium instead of the left atrium. The anomalous drainage can be partial or complete (total) and classified as supracardiac, infracardiac, intracardiac, or mixed cardiac types. In addition, the veins can be obstructed or unobstructed.

Total anomalous pulmonary venous return (TAPVR) is the focus of this section. The most common TAPVR is supracardiac (Figure 22-29), in which the common pulmonary vein drains into the superior vena cava (SVC) via the left vertical and innominate veins. The second most common type is intracardiac, in which the common pulmonary vein drains into the coronary sinus. In infracardiac TAPVR, the common pulmonary vein drains into the portal vein, ductus venosus, hepatic vein, or inferior vena cava. Finally, mixed drainage is a combination of two or more TAPVR types (Herlong et al., 2000).

Pathophysiology. The pathophysiology for TAPVR may be classified into unobstructed and obstructed types. Unobstructed TAPVR produces left-to-right shunting with increased pulmonary blood flow, causing right atrial and ventricular dilation similar to that observed with a large ASD. TAPVR with obstruction creates pulmonary venous hypertension with resultant pulmonary edema. In addition, pulmonary arteriolar vasoconstriction and pulmonary hypertension develop with right heart failure (Wang et al., 2004).

Presentation. Clinical manifestations of TAPVR differ, depending on whether there is obstruction to the pulmonary venous return and whether there is total versus partial anomalous venous return. Without obstruction, patients

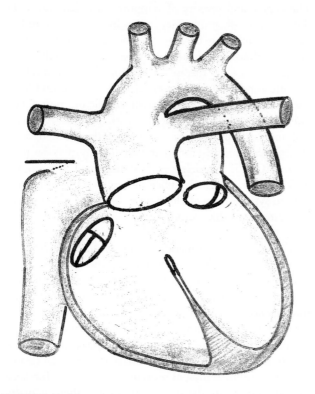

FIGURE 22-28

Truncus Arteriosus Type II.

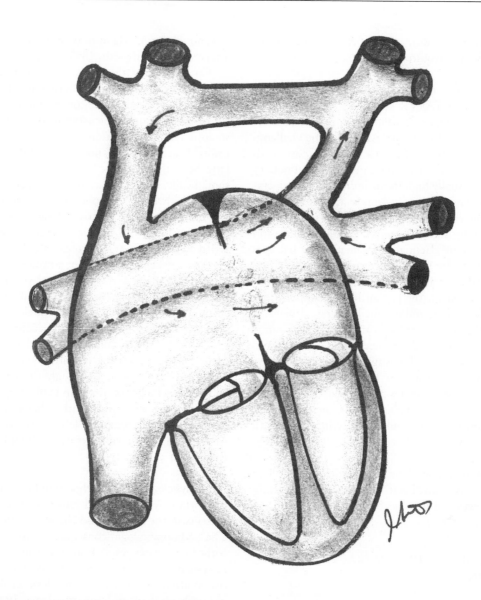

FIGURE 22-29

Total Anomalous Pulmonary Venous Return: Supracardiac.

Source: Used with permission. Courtesy of Joseph J. Amato, MD MJ. All Rights Reserved.

may present with CHF, inadequate growth, and frequent pulmonary infections. They may also exhibit mild cyanosis. Chest radiograph will reveal marked cardiomegaly involving the right atrium RA and RV, and increased pulmonary vascular markings. The "snowman" sign may be seen with supracardiac TAPVR after a child reaches 4 months of age, due to widening of the mediastinum by dilated vessels; this development gives the illusion of the snowman's head and the body from the enlarged RA.

Patients with pulmonary venous obstruction present with marked cyanosis and respiratory distress in the neonatal period. Chest radiograph demonstrates normal heart size with linear opacities of fluid collection or pulmonary edema (Kerley B lines). Echocardiograph will reveal a large RV with compressed LV. An interatrial communication

is present. If interatrial communication is small, the left atrium and left ventricle may be small (Wang et al., 2004).

Plan of care.   A thorough echocardiograph is needed to delineate the anatomy and evaluate for pulmonary vein obstruction. Patients with TAPRV and pulmonary venous obstruction require emergent care directed at providing ventilatory support and surgical intervention. Nitric oxide increases pulmonary blood flow to the lungs; thus it is contraindicated in patients with obstructed pulmonary veins. In the event that atrial communication is restrictive, an atrial septostomy is indicated.

Patients with unobstructed TAPVR receive therapies to decrease CHF symptoms, and surgical repair is completed by the time the child reaches 2 to 3 years of age.

The surgical repair procedure used depends on the type of TAPVR, but all types require CPB.

Postoperative care and discharge planning.   Postoperative care of patients with TAPVR and unobstructed veins is usually benign. In contrast, postoperative care of patients undergoing repair of obstructed TAPVR can be challenging. These patients often experience severe acidosis with profound pulmonary edema prior to surgery. Pulmonary artery pressure is usually high in the immediate postoperative period, requiring ventilatory support and often inhaled nitric oxide to increase pulmonary blood flow to the lungs. Invasive monitoring such as arterial, central venous, and left atrial catheters are essential for evaluating cardiac output. NIRS is helpful for monitoring cerebral and renal perfusion. Because the left atrium and ventricle sizes are often small and noncompliant, the patient has less opportunity to increase stroke volume and is more heart rate dependent in response to the need to increase cardiac output. Volume administration should be administered cautiously to avoid excessive and rapid left atrial pressure elevation. Vasoactive infusions are often required for hemodynamic management. Pulmonary vascular resistance usually decreases gradually following repair. Persistence in increased PVR may indicate reobstruction of pulmonary veins. The length of hospitalization for patients with obstructed TAPVR is usually 2 to 3 weeks.

Patients require follow-up by their cardiologists at least every 6 months. Visits are directed at evaluating for pulmonary vein obstruction at the anastomosis site.

LEFT VENTRICULAR OUTFLOW TRACT OBSTRUCTION

Coarctation of the aorta

Coarctation of the aorta (coarc, COA) is a term used to describe a range of clinical pathologies occurring anywhere along the aortic arch. This diagnosis may be applied to the finding of a discrete narrowing in the aorta, usually in close proximity to the ductus arteriosus, or a generalized hypoplasia of the arch.

The most common presentation of the lesion, a discrete coarctation, is caused by a narrowing or shelf along the posterolateral aorta opposite the ductus arteriosus. The pathogenesis of discrete coarctation of the aorta has been hypothesized to be related to an abnormal extension of ductal tissue into the aorta. The location of the coarctation is described in relation to the ductus arteriosus—that is, preductal, postductal, or juxtaductal. The presentation of coarctation of the aorta in the neonatal period is much more commonly associated with hypoplasia of the arch, usually at the isthmus or along the transverse arch. Nevertheless, coarctation of the aorta may be found as far distally as the abdominal aorta, where it is often associated with renal artery stenosis (Edwards, 1953; Isner et al., 1987).

Coarctation of the aorta occurs between two to five times more commonly in males than in females (Campbell, 1961). It may occur alone, or in combination with other cardiac defects such as bicuspid aortic valve, VSD, or mitral stenosis. Aortic coarctation accounts for 5% to 10% of congenital heart defects (Tanous et al., 2009). Although it has long been thought that most cases of coarctation occur sporadically, recent data suggest a genetic influence, as this anomaly has been reported in identical twins, siblings, and other first-degree relatives. Coarctation of the aorta is often associated with Turner syndrome (Cripe et al., 2004; Loffredo et al., 2004; McBride et al., 2005).

Two concepts have been advanced as the cause of coarctation of the aorta: the ductus tissue theory and the hemodynamic theory. As noted, the ductus tissue theory accounts for those discrete lesions in close proximity of the ductus arteriosus, but it does not account for those lesions that occur at any distance from the ductus. The hemodynamic theory proposes that coarctation develops as a result of altered flow patterns through the embryonic arterial trunk. This theory is useful in explaining the presence of coarctation in association with other intracardiac defects that diminish the volume of left ventricular outflow (Ho & Anderson, 1979; Hornberger et al., 1994; Kim et al., 2009; Rudolph et al., 1972).

Pathophysiology.   The pathophysiology of coarctation of the aorta may be classified into two types: The first type presents in the neonate and the second in the older child. The pathophysiologic consequences of coarctation of the aorta in neonates result from the acute-onset obstruction to systemic blood flow. Neonates do not tolerate an acute rise in afterload; therefore, this elevation leads to LV failure with resultant pulmonary edema. In the older child, chronic LV pressure overload arises in conjunction with the development of concentric hypertrophy. Systemic hypertension occurs and thoracic aortic collaterals develop.

Presentation.   The presentation of the lesion will vary greatly, ranging from heart failure and shock in the neonate to an asymptomatic murmur or hypertension in an older child or adolescent. In a newborn with a significantly obstructed lesion, once the ductus arteriosus closes, the infant may present in shock and acidosis. Multisystem organ failure, particularly kidney failure and NEC, may occur. Whereas a neonate may present with critical symptomology, an older child or adolescent may be completely asymptomatic, except for a murmur or systolic hypertension.

The findings during physical examination will likewise vary greatly, depending on the severity of the lesion. In any patient, the hallmark finding consists of discrepancies in the blood pressure and quality of the pulses between the four extremities. The systolic blood pressure will be elevated proximal to the obstruction, and the quality of the pulses will be weaker distal to the obstruction. It is not wise to assume the discrepancy will exist solely between the upper and lower extremities, however; depending on the location of the lesion, the discrepancy may also be noted between the upper extremities. Consequently, blood pressures in children should be performed on the right extremity. If there are any pulse discrepancies, or if pressure is high, then blood pressures should be taken on all four extremities.

In a symptomatic neonate, the signs and symptoms of CHF will be present, including tachycardia, tachypnea, and hepatomegaly. The quality and location of the murmur will vary based on the severity and location of the coarctation, along with any other associated cardiac lesions. The usual murmur arising from the coarctation itself is a grade 2 to 3/6 systolic ejection murmur best heard at the left upper sternal border, at the base, or radiating to the left interscapular area. If cardiac output is significantly diminished, there may be little to no murmur appreciated; instead, a gallop rhythm may be a more prominent finding.

Plan of care. Electrocardiographic and radiographic findings will be nonspecific, particularly in the neonate. The ECG changes in an older child may have features of left ventricular hypertrophy—in particular, deep S waves in the right chest leads. The CXR in the neonate with CHF is also nonspecific; cardiomegaly may be present, as well as increased pulmonary vascular markings. However, in an older child or adolescent, the "3" sign may be present on an anterioposterior film. The abnormal contour of the aortic arch results in a "3" sign at the localized site of the indentation of the aorta. Rib notching may also be present in older children; the inferior surfaces of the posterior ribs become eroded from dilated arterial collateral vessels that may have developed following long-standing obstruction.

Definitive diagnosis may be made with the use of a number of different imaging modalities. Echocardiograph with Doppler studies provides the information needed to diagnose the majority of patients, including data related to the hemodynamic severity of the lesion. For patients requiring additional study, MRI provides clear, high-quality images of the aorta. MRI images in the sagittal and parasagittal views will define the location and the severity of the coarctation. Three-dimensional enhancement of contrast-enhanced CT images has also been found to be of diagnostic value with regard to defining the anatomy of the aortic arch (Di Sessa et al., 2009; Secchi et al., 2009).

For those infants who present in a shock-like state, the initial vital therapy includes an infusion of prostaglandin E$_1$ to restore patency to the ductus arteriosus. In addition, the patient may benefit from inotropic support as well as other efforts to improve perfusion to the areas distal to the coarctation. As soon as hemodynamic stability has been established, the infant should be taken to the operating room for definitive repair.

The treatment plan for an older, asymptomatic child allows for a more elective timing of repair or intervention. If the child's condition will allow, timing of the intervention after the age of 2 to 3 years is preferable. The risk of coarctation recurrence is increased in children who have undergone intervention prior to the age of 2. By the age of 3 years, the aortic diameter has attained approximately 55% of its final adult size (Moss et al., 1959). However, repair should be undertaken prior to the adolescent years to decrease the risk of chronic residual hypertension.

Although surgical intervention is most likely indicated in the neonate or young infant with coarctation, older children and adolescents may have the opportunity to undergo intervention in the cardiac catheterization laboratory. Balloon angioplasty was long thought to be useful only in addressing recoarctation following surgical repair. More recently, in patients with discrete narrowing, balloon angioplasty has been used in treating native coarctation with mixed results. Although this technique may immediately reduce the gradient across the coarctation, it is associated with a high incidence of recoarctation. Aortic wall injury, such as dissection and aneurysm formation, has also been reported. This procedure has not been found to be a successful therapy in neonates with CHF or shock-like states, or in those with generalized arch hypoplasia (Liang et al., 2009).

The opportunity for stent placement has long been limited by the size of the stents themselves, but current research and practice have found stents to be tolerated in smaller children. In particular, the advancement in technology from bare metal stents to covered stents has made their use more attractive. Many centers consider the stent to be a superior option over balloon angioplasty (Qureshi, 2009). There may be less aneurysm formation with stent placement than occurs with balloon angioplasty, as the stent itself reduces elastic recoil and thus the amount of balloon stretch required. Residual gradients have been documented to be less in stent placement than in balloon angioplasty (Hornung et al., 2002; Mohan et al., 2009).

For those children requiring surgical intervention, several techniques may be used and depend on the characteristics of the coarctation. In isolated lesions, the aorta is almost universally approached from a left-sided thoracotomy and repaired without the use of CPB. The surgical approach of choice in most centers for patients with a discrete lesion is a resection with end-to-end anastomosis. The benefits of this technique include resection of ductal tissue, sparing of the subclavian artery, and avoidance of prosthetic materials. The disadvantage of the procedure is that it results in a circumferential suture line, which historically led to an increase in the incidence of recoarctation (Horvath et al., 2008). To meet this challenge, improved surgical techniques and suture material have been developed.

Prosthetic patch angioplasty is no longer a common procedure. It is associated with increased incidence of late aneurysm formation. Nevertheless, the technique is still described in the literature, and may be encountered from time to time, particularly in long-segment coarctation or hypoplasia. In this procedure, a longitudinal incision is made on the aorta at the site of the coarctation, extending to the left subclavian artery if necessary. The area is then enlarged with either a Dacron or Gore-Tex graft. Compared with end-to-end anastomosis, this technique offers the advantage of avoiding a circumferential suture line (Kaushal et al., 2009).

Left subclavian flap aortoplasty requires sacrificing the left subclavian artery in the repair of the coarctation. The artery is ligated and divided, and a longitudinal incision is made from the proximal portion of the subclavian artery through the aorta distal to the coarctation. Used as an autologous patch, the proximal stump of the artery is turned down to cover the area of the coarctation. The benefits of this approach include the avoidance of a circumferential suture line and use of prosthetic material. Use of living tissue as a patch offers benefit of growth potential. This repair is useful in long-segment coarctation as well as arch hypoplasia. The obvious disadvantage is the sacrifice of the left subclavian artery, which carries the risk of altered blood flow to the left upper extremity (Hager et al., 2008). After undergoing this procedure, patients should not have blood pressures taken in their left arm.

Postoperative care and discharge planning.   The long-term prognosis for children having had repair of coarctation of the aorta is excellent. Initial postoperative care centers on control of blood pressure and rebound hypertension. Systemic hypertension in the early postoperative period is common. Paradoxic hypertension may arise due to imbalances in sympathetic discharge, baroreceptor activity, and renin–angiotensin system disarrangement. Continuous infusions of nitroprusside or beta blockers such as esmolol are often required in the immediate postoperative period. The patient often needs to be transitioned to oral therapy with an ACE inhibitor (such as captopril or enalapril) or a beta blocker (such as propranolol or atenolol) prior to discharge home (Tabbutt et al., 2001).

Monitoring includes arterial and central venous catheters. Oral feedings should be initiated slowly to protect the patient's intestinal tract from ischemic injury caused by postcoarctectomy syndrome. This syndrome, which is not well understood, may occur within the first days after surgery and is suspected to be related to pressure changes in the mesenteric arteries. Patients may experience abdominal pain, distention, and vomiting—symptoms that may cause postcoarctectomy syndrome to be confused with an acute abdomen.

In those patients who have undergone a left subclavian flap repair, it is important to remember that blood pressures should not be obtained from the left arm, as they will not be accurate. Other potential postoperative complications include phrenic nerve damage, spinal cord ischemia, and chylothorax due to proximity to the thoracic duct. Recurrent laryngeal nerve damage should be suspected in patients who experience prolonged voice hoarseness (Yuan & Raanani, 2008) (Figure 22-30).

Pediatric patients who have undergone repair will require a lifetime of follow-up with a cardiologist. Long-term complications can include recoarctation, hypertension, aortic aneurysm or dissection, and diminished left arm growth in those who have undergone left subclavian flap repair (Burch et al., 2009; Swan et al., 2008).

The rate of recoarctation of the aorta is reported to be in the range of 15% to 30% (Hager et al., 2009). The rate is lower in children whose defect was not repaired in infancy. In some centers, the incidence of recoarctation has been reported to be lower in those who underwent repair via an end-to-end anastamosis.

Chronic hypertension may occur either at rest or with exercise following repair of these defects (Hager et al., 2008). Patients who have undergone coarctation repair are at increased risk for atherosclerosis. In long-term follow-up, those who undergo repair via end-to-end anastomosis experience a reduced incidence of late hypertension (Bassareo et al., 2008).

The incidence of postoperative aortic aneurysm is highest among those who have undergone repair via patch aortoplasty. Delayed complication rates associated with patch angioplasty have been reported to be as high as 50% (Piciucchi et al., 2008). The length of hospitalization varies depending on the patient's age at the time of surgery.

Interrupted aortic arch

Interrupted aortic arch is defined as a complete lack of luminal continuity between the ascending and descending aorta. It is classified as Type A, B, or C depending on the position of the interruption. In Type A, the interruption is distal to the left subclavian artery; in Type B, the interruption is between the carotid and subclavian arteries; and in Type C, the interruption occurs between the carotid arteries.

In utero, there are initially six aortic arches, and they either regress or transform into permanent structures. The first, second, and fifth arches completely regress. The sixth arch becomes the pulmonary arteries and the ductus arteriosus. The third arch forms the connection between the carotid arteries, and the fourth arch forms the connection between the left carotid and subclavian arteries. Any disruption in this development process will lead to anomalies of the aortic arch, with interruption occurring where embryogenesis was disrupted. Type A interruptions tend to occur in combination with an aortopulmonary connection and an intact ventricular septum; Type B defects in general have normally related great vessels and a large malalignment ventricular septal defect with some degree of aortic obstruction (Braunlin et al., 1982; Moerman et al., 1987).

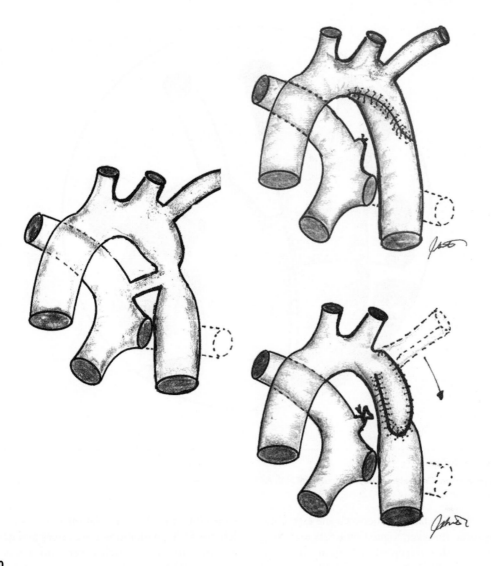

FIGURE 22-30

Coarctation of Aorta and Repairs.

Note: Clockwise from lower left, coarctation, extended end-to-end (Amato) procedure, subclavian turn down.

Source: Used with permission. Courtesy of Joseph J. Amato, MD MJ. All Rights Reserved.

Type B is by far the most common type of interruption, while Type C is relatively rare. Type B interrupted aortic arch is found in 43% of children with DiGeorge syndrome, or microdeletion of chromosome 22q11.2; conversely, 68% of children with interrupted arch have DiGeorge syndrome (Ziolkowska et al., 2008) (Figure 22-31).

Interrupted aortic arch is a ductal-dependent lesion that requires an infusion of prostaglandin E_1 to maintain the patency of the ductus arteriosus. Infants with interrupted arch will present with cardiovascular collapse upon ductal closure. Fluid resuscitation, along with vasoactive support and possible intubation with ventilatory support, may be required in those infants who are not diagnosed prenatally. Physical examination may reveal differential pulses depending on the site of interruption (Mishra, 2009).

Pathophysiology. Similar to coarctation of the aorta, acute onset of obstruction to systemic blood flow results in left ventricle failure with pulmonary edema.

Plan of care. Diagnosis of interrupted aortic arch is made by echocardiograph, although both CT and MRI may be useful in further delineating anatomy and planning for surgical repair. Echocardiograph findings may reveal a discrepancy in size between the pulmonary artery and the ascending aorta. Imaging of the arch may help determine the branching pattern of the brachiocephalic arteries and the patency of the arch. CT is a fast, noninvasive imaging modality whose findings may add value to the echocardiograph, which may be limited due to adequate windows. MRI 3-D reconstruction can also demonstrate the branching

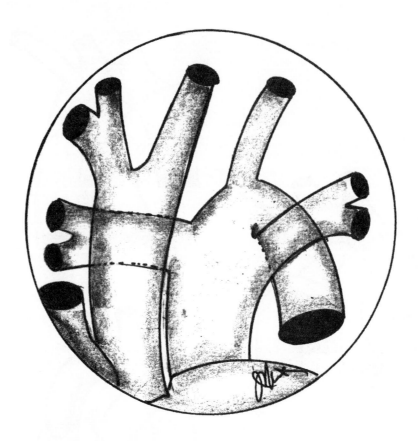

FIGURE 22-31

Interrupted Aortic Arch Type B.

Source: Used with permission. Courtesy of Joseph J. Amato, MD MJ. All Rights Reserved.

pattern and the point of separation between the ascending and descending aorta; however, a question exists regarding its ability to distinguish interrupted arch from arch hypoplasia (Dillman et al., 2008; Yang et al., 2008).

Medical management is appropriate for initial stabilization and maintenance of hemodynamic stability once the diagnosis has been made. However, interrupted aortic arch must be approached with a sense of urgency when patients are referred for surgical repair. Surgical repair is directed at addressing both the arch anomaly and any other associated defects. The arch can almost always be reconstructed with dissection of the ends of the two arch components and reanastamosis in an end-to-end fashion. Arch augmentation with homograft may be necessary to achieve adequate arch size (Joynt et al., 2009).

The degree of left ventricular outflow obstruction associated with VSD will dictate the surgical approach that is best suited for the patient. The VSD associated with interrupted arch is malaligned, with a degree of posterior deviation of the infundibular septum. Subaortic diameters greater than 5 mm are usually compatible with patch closure of the VSD and aortic arch repair. In contrast, if the subaortic diameter is less than 3 mm, the heart will be unable to generate adequate cardiac output to sustain cardiovascular function. In this type of defect, conversion to a Norwood type circulation is necessary. The VSD is left open, the main pulmonary artery and descending aorta are anastamosed to each other, and a modified Blalock-Taussig (BT) shunt is placed to assure pulmonary blood flow (Kobayashi et al., 2009). The Norwood procedure is described in more detail later in this section.

Postoperative care and discharge planning. Postoperative morbidity and mortality have both been found to be significantly elevated for children with DiGeorge syndrome (22q11.2 deletion) (Carotti et al., 2008). Patients with this deletion may also have neurodevelopmental disabilities, depressed immunological function (hypoplastic or absent thymus), or hypocalcemia secondary to poorly functioning parathyroid glands (Kyburz et al., 2008). Regardless of any genetic comorbidities, the surgical repair for interrupted arch can potentially be an intricate procedure with its own risks. Hospital stays for patients undergoing such surgery can be prolonged.

Aortic stenosis

Aortic stenosis (AS) may occur above, below, or at the level of the valve. Valvar aortic stenosis is more common in males than in females (4:1). Subvalvar AS is also more common in males than in females (2:1) (Campbell, 1968; Frank et al., 1973). Approximately 20% of patients will have other associated congenital heart defects, such as PDA, coarctation of the aorta, pulmonary stenosis, or VSD. While 10% of patients are diagnosed with this defect in infancy. AS may present at any time during childhood (Braunwald et al., 1963). Familial clustering that is consistent with an autosomal dominant inheritance has been observed; thus first-degree relatives of an affected patient should undergo screening echocardiograph (Lewin et al., 2004). The appearance of an isolated membrane is uncommon in infancy: The earlier the age of presentation, the more likely that the child will require repeated interventions to relieve the obstruction, particularly in children with a tunnel-like lesions (Kerr & Goss, 1956; Pyle et al., 1976).

Pathophysiology. In AS, the valve is thickened and rigid, with varying degrees of commissure separation. A bicuspid aortic valve is the most common finding, although the valve may be unicuspid or tricuspid. Bicuspid aortic valves are associated with a defect in collagen metabolism, which affects both the valve and the wall of the aorta (Friedman et al., 2008). Although congenital bicuspid valves may be stenotic, they are rarely responsible for serious outflow tract obstruction in childhood. Instead, the bicuspid nature of the valve leads to increased turbulence, which over time traumatizes the valve leaflets, leading to fibrosis and rigidity, and eventually calcification (Sabet et al., 1999). Prolonged obstruction of the left ventricular outflow tract may lead to hypertrophy of the ventricular wall and dilation of the ascending aorta (Wessels et al., 2005). The severity of the obstruction is determined by the pressure gradient between the left ventricle and the aorta during systole. Unless significant ventricular dysfunction exists, end-diastolic pressure in the left ventricle should be normal.

Subvalvar AS may present along a spectrum of anomalies, all of which lead to obstruction of the left ventricular outflow tract. The most common form is a discrete obstruction, usually consisting of a fibrous ring or a membrane encircling the outflow tract, or leading to a narrowing in the outflow tract. The obstruction may also occur as a result of "tunnel" narrowing of the left ventricular outflow tract. The tunnel may form secondary to hypoplasia of the tract, or from hypertrophy of the ventricular muscle. It may exist as an isolated lesion, or it may be found with other lesions—most commonly aortic valvar disease, complex left-sided lesions, or a VSD (Newfeld et al., 1976).

Supravalvar aortic stenosis occurs above the level of the aortic valve, and presents as either a discrete obstruction or a diffuse hypoplasia. Discrete obstructions occur just proximal to the aortic valve. Most common is the "hourglass" type, which is caused by a thickening of the aortic media, leading to constriction of the aorta at the superior border of the sinus of Valsalva. In addition, discrete narrowing may be due to a membranous covering with a small opening,

over the aortic valve. Diffuse hypoplasia of the ascending arch may also exist. Peripheral pulmonary artery stenosis is also found in those patients with Williams syndrome (McDonald et al., 1969; O'Connor et al., 1985; Stamm et al., 2001). There is a strong association between supravalvar aortic stenosis and Williams syndrome, and approximately half of all patients with supravalvar AS will suffer from this genetic defect (Williams et al., 1961).

Presentation. Symptoms may range from mild to severe for neonates with aortic stenosis. Mild, in utero AS may result in a small amount of left ventricular hypertrophy and little else. Moderate AS may lead to left ventricular hypertrophy, but normal LV size and dimensions. In contrast, in the infant with severe AS, the size of the LV cavity may be decreased, as are the mitral and aortic valves, much as in hypoplastic left heart syndrome (HLHS). At birth, the workload of the left ventricle increases slightly. In an infant with mild AS, this increase is well tolerated. In an infant with moderate AS, some increased left heart failure may be evident. However, a child born with severe AS will not be able to produce the cardiac output necessary to support circulation, and will depend on a patent ductus arteriosus to meet that need.

Valvar AS presents with a wide range of manifestations depending on the severity of the obstruction, and the age of the child. An infant with severe stenosis will present with CHF. The patient may be irritable with poor feeding; there may be hypotension and tachycardia with poor perfusion. Physical examination may reveal a systolic murmur, which is usually loudest at the left upper sternal border. If cardiac function is significantly reduced, however, a murmur may or may not be appreciated. Crackles, tachypnea, and respiratory distress with retractions may also be present.

Older children with aortic valve stenosis are asymptomatic, and the disease is often not diagnosed until they are evaluated for a murmur. When they are symptomatic, they usually present with exercise intolerance, chest pain, or syncope. The symptomology reflects the degree of obstruction. For example, the degree of obstruction may be moderately severe in the child who presents with dyspnea on exertion and exercise intolerance, or severe in the child who presents with syncope due to inadequate cerebral blood flow during exercise (Dodge-Khatami et al., 2008). Physical examination may reveal a lift or thrill on the chest. A systolic ejection "click" may be heard on auscultation; it is indicative of mild to moderate stenosis, as the valve is mobile and not calcified. Absence of this "click" may suggest severe stenosis in a valve that has already calcified and is no longer mobile.

Clinical presentation of subvalvar AS is similar to that of valvar stenosis. As the degree of obstruction increases, the child may begin to experience increasing fatigability, dyspnea on exertion, and decrease in exercise tolerance. Children with a mild form of obstruction may be asymptomatic, and the lesion may be diagnosed on their referral to a cardiologist for assessment of a systolic murmur. The cardiac examination in supravalvar AS is similar except for the absence of an ejection click. The presence of the "Coanda effect" is specific to supravalvar AS: The systolic blood pressure in the right arm is higher than that in the left arm. Flow selectively streams to the right innominate artery as it adheres to the aortic wall (French & Guntheroth, 1970). A thrill in the suprasternal notch is found in severe forms of supravalvar AS. Peripheral pulmonary stenosis may produce a continuous murmur heard best in the lung fields, which is accentuated by inspiration.

Differential diagnosis includes other obstructive lesions to left ventricular outflow. HCPs should evaluate the sick neonate for progression of the disease beyond just the valve and HLHS. Endocardial fibroelastosis should be considered in infants presenting with severe aortic stenosis, and left subclavian stenosis should be considered in those with elevated right arm pressures.

Plan of care. Two-dimensional echocardiograph is the diagnostic tool of choice in neonates. In severe AS, the aortic valve is immobile, the ascending aorta will be dilated, and the left ventricle is hypertrophied. Varying degrees of endocardial fibroelastosis are commonly observed with poor ventricular function. Doppler assessment of gradients across the valve is not reliable if the function is poor. Chest radiograph will show evidence of increased pulmonary congestion as well as cardiomegaly. Cardiac catheterization is not routinely used as a diagnostic tool.

Left ventricular hypertrophy is found on the ECG of approximately 85% of children with AS. Nevertheless, the absence of hypertrophy does not preclude a diagnosis of AS. The most telling finding on ECG is that of left ventricular "strain"—that is, hypertrophy combined with ST-segment depression and T-wave inversion in the left precordial leads (Shem-Tov et al., 1982). Prolonged QT dispersion has been found on 12-lead ECG and 24-hour Holter monitoring in children, along with an increased pressure gradient and increased left ventricular mass (Beekman et al., 1992; Piorecka-Makula & Werner, 2009).

As in neonates, echocardiography remains the diagnostic tool of choice for all types of AS in older children. The severity of the stenosis at the level of the valve may be determined by imaging the orifice of the valve as well as by calculating the degree of calcification of the valve and assessing the function of the ventricle. To best image the valve, a transesophageal echocardiograph may be considered. Doppler measurements are useful in determining the pressure gradient from the left ventricle to the aorta. Pressure gradients must be determined by flow velocity across the valve, and can be influenced by turbulence, ventricular function, and valvar regurgitation (Beekman et al., 1992). A discrete subvalvar ridge or narrowed outflow tract will be obvious, which helps to differentiate subvalvar from valvar

obstruction (Wilcox et al., 1980). In centers where MRI is available, this modality is useful in determining ventricular size and volume as well as quantifying the severity of the AS (Caruthers et al., 2003). Cardiac catheterization is not commonly used as a primary diagnostic tool.

Initial medical management for a neonate who presents in a low cardiac output state consists of cardiovascular resuscitation (inotropic and ventilatory support, prostaglandin E_1 infusion) until the anatomy can be further delineated. If the left-sided structures appear large enough to support a biventricular repair, the infant is taken to the cardiac catheterization laboratory for intervention via balloon valvuloplasty. The introduction of smaller devices such as sheaths and introducers has improved the availability of interventional procedures to even small infants (Vogt et al., 1983); however, approximately 40% of infants at one center required re-intervention in the cardiac catheterization lab, and 13% of the infants did not survive (Han et al., 2007). Fetal balloon angioplasty has shown promise in promoting the growth of left-sided structures and improved ventricular function, although its use is limited to a few centers (McLean et al., 2006). Infants with small left-sided structures and AS are rarely candidates for biventricular repair. For these patients, surgery similar to the Norwood procedure is performed.

In older children, mild to moderate AS without symptoms may be monitored and observed. Patients with moderate AS should be restricted from severe exertion and limit their exercise to low-intensity sports activities. Some data indicate that children with mild valvar AS will remain stable and not require intervention (Ardura et al., 2006). This lesion has an excellent prognosis when diagnosed beyond the neonatal period, and mortality is nearly absent in this age group (Ten Harkel et al., 2009). However, even asymptomatic children require follow-up with a cardiologist on at least an annual or biannual basis. Dilation of the ascending aorta in children with bicuspid aortic valves is well documented, even if the child is asymptomatic and the valve functions appropriately .

In general, children with a diagnosis of subaortic membrane may be monitored as long as they remain asymptomatic and the gradient remains low. Three-fourths of patients diagnosed with subaortic membrane will experience an increase in the degree of obstruction to the point that surgical intervention becomes necessary. To avoid further damage to the left ventricle, most centers will refer the child for surgical intervention when the gradient across the outflow tract reaches 30 mmHg or more.

Children with severe valvar AS should be considered for either intervention in the cardiac catheterization lab or referral for surgery. In most cases, valvuloplasty is an acceptable primary choice of treatment unless additional factors are present, such as severe aortic regurgitation or other significant cardiac lesions. Certain risks are associated with this procedure, however—such as progression of aortic regurgitation as well as aortic valve prolapse.

The latter complication is likely due to the tearing of the valve cusp or detachment of the valve from the valve ring. The efficacy of valvuloplasty is patient specific, but some data indicate that this surgery is effective in postponing or preventing surgical intervention for as long as 10 years in 60% to 70% of patients (Fratz et al., 2008).

Should nonsurgical interventions fail, or if the child is not a candidate for such an intervention, several surgical options are available. Aortic valvotomy, also known as commissurotomy, is relatively safe and effective in relieving symptoms. However, care must be taken when dissecting the leaflets so as not to open the commissures all the way to the valve annulus, which would result in severe aortic regurgitation. Despite the apparent success of surgical valvotomy, the valve leaflets remain deformed, and the chance of restenosis due to calcification exists.

If the native aortic valve is not salvageable and a biventricular repair is possible the Ross procedure should be performed. In the Ross procedure, the native aortic valve is discarded, and a pulmonary autograft is used to replace the diseased aortic valve. The right ventricular outflow tract is then reconstructed with a right ventricle to pulmonary artery conduit (Figure 22-32). The benefits of this procedure include the avoidance of a prosthetic valve and anticoagulation. The pulmonary autograft should continue to grow as the child grows. Obstructive processes of the right ventricle to pulmonary artery homograft are one of the few long-term sequelae. The strongest predictive factor is small homograft size at the time of surgery. Short- and long-term morbidity and mortality are quite low with the Ross procedure (Brown et al., 2006; Pasquali et al., 2007; Piccardo et al., 2009).

In cases of discrete subaortic membrane, resection of the membrane is the operative procedure of choice. Although the success rate with this surgery is high, and the morbidity and mortality quite low, the recurrence rate of the membrane is relatively high. As many as 20% patients will ultimately require reoperation, often related to incomplete removal of the membrane at the time of surgery. If tunnel obstruction is severe, the patient may require myomectomy, or enlargement of the outflow tract with a Konno procedure. As rates for recurrence of outflow tract obstruction are elevated for both discrete membranes as well as tunnel obstructions, follow-up with a cardiologist is of utmost importance. The rates of reoperation are highest in those patients with tunnel-type obstructions, those with residual gradients at the time of surgery, and those requiring surgery at a younger age (Ruzmetov et al., 2006).

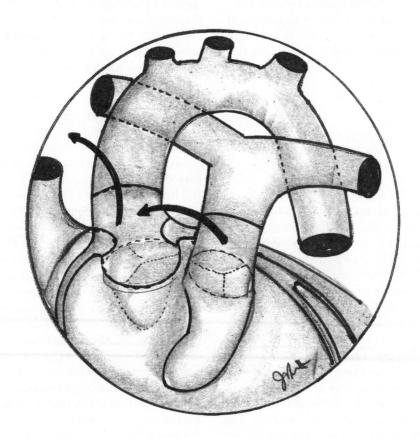

FIGURE 22-32

Ross Procedure.

Source: Used with permission. Courtesy of Joseph J. Amato, MD MJ. All Rights Reserved.

Many cardiologists consider a gradient of 40 mmHg across a supravalvar obstruction as indication that surgical intervention is necessary. Children with lower gradients may, in fact, experience regression of the obstruction without intervention—particularly those with Williams syndrome. Should surgical intervention be necessary, the surgical approach will be tailored to the individual anatomical defect of the child. In those patients with the typical hourglass deformity, a longitudinal incision is made in the ascending aorta in the shape of an inverted "Y," and a patch is placed over the area. In those patients with a more diffuse narrowing, the patch augmentation may be extended into the transverse arch. Postsurgical outcome following repair of supravalvar AS is good, and reoperation is rarely necessary (Hickey et al., 2008; Scott et al., 2009).

Postoperative care and discharge planning. Postoperative care includes arterial, central venous, and left atrial pressure monitoring. The postoperative course varies, depending on the type of AS and surgical repair. As suggested by the data collected in relation to this disease, continued, specialized follow-up is imperative for all patients with a diagnosis of aortic stenosis, whether or not they have undergone any sort of intervention. As previously noted, diagnosis beyond the neonatal period is associated with a better prognosis for relief of symptoms and slower progression of stenosis. Many children with mild aortic stenosis will live a full lifetime, without valvular intervention. Close follow-up is indicated for anyone with the diagnosis of bicuspid aortic valve and/or aortic stenosis.

RIGHT VENTRICULAR OUTFLOW TRACT OBSTRUCTION

Pulmonary stenosis

As in aortic stenosis, the obstruction may occur above, below, or at the level of the valve. Valvar pulmonary stenosis (PS) is by far a more common finding than subvalvar or supravalvar PS. When associated with an intact ventricular septum, it occurs in 25% to 30% of all patients with congenital heart disease, whether as an isolated finding or in combination with associated defects.

Pathophysiology. The main physiologic effect of pulmonary stenosis is a rise in right ventricular pressure proportional to the severity of obstruction. Patients with mild stenosis may have little to no increase in muscle mass or hyperplasia of the right ventricle. Patients with atretic valves may have severe hyperplasia of the right ventricle. The pathologic presentation of the stenotic pulmonary valve varies from a well-formed valve with three leaflets and varying degrees of fusion of the commissures, to a completely imperforate valve without outflow. The valve may also be dysplastic, with thickened cusps, disorganized tissue, and a hypoplastic valvar annulus (Edwards et al., 1948).

Subvalvar pulmonary stenosis may occur as a result of either anomalous muscle bundles (also known as a double-chambered right ventricle) or narrowing of the infundibulum that extends directly below the level of the pulmonary valve. The cause of anomalous muscle bundles is unknown, but it has been postulated to result from a localized area of growth of trabeculations in the myocardium early in fetal development. Infundibular stenosis results from fibromuscular thickening of the infundibular wall.

Isolated supravalvar PS is extremely rare. Supravalvar PS may occur in children who have undergone arterial switch procedure for transposition of the great vessels (arteries).

Presentation. The clinical presentation varies according to the degree of obstruction. Neonates with severe PS will be critically ill and appear cyanotic secondary to right-to-left shunting at the atrial level (Freed et al., 1973). They will require an infusion of prostaglandin E_1 (PGE_1) to keep the ductus arteriosus patent and assure adequate pulmonary blood flow. Children with mild to moderate stenosis are usually asymptomatic, and the diagnosis of PS is made at the time of referral for a murmur. If diagnosis is not made at an early age, symptoms may appear with an increase in the gradient across the outflow tract. Exercise intolerance and fatigue may be the initial symptoms, progressing to chest pain and syncope with strenuous exercise as the right ventricle is unable to meet the demands of increased output.

Pulmonary stenosis is associated with a variety of syndromes. Dysplastic valves are found in most patients with Noonan syndrome (Noonan, 1968). Supravalvar stenosis is associated with both Williams and Alagille syndromes. A familial incidence of pulmonary valve disease has been reported. An increased incidence of either isolated pulmonary valve disease or tetralogy of Fallot exists in siblings of children who suffer from pulmonary stenosis.

The differential diagnosis includes other defects associated with decreased outflow from the right ventricle. Symptoms in neonates with severe PS may mimic Ebstein's anomaly. Other defects to consider are tetralogy of Fallot and pulmonary atresia with intact ventricular septum.

Physical examination is unique in patients with PS. The first heart sound is normal in quality, and is followed by an ejection click heard best at the left upper sternal border, radiating to the entire precordium, neck, and back. The second heart sound is usually split, and the degree of splitting is proportional to the degree of stenosis. A soft murmur is indicative of poor cardiac output, such as occurs in a neonate with critical PS. A thrill may be palpable in patients with severe stenosis, felt best at the second to third intercostals space. On auscultation of children with infundibular stenosis, the ejection click will not be heard, but otherwise their examination findings are similar to those associated with valvar stenosis.

One-half of all patients with mild PS will have a normal ECG. In those with moderate to severe PS, right axis deviation is common, and an RV conduction delay may be noted. The ECG in neonates with severe stenosis and RV hypoplasia may be indicative of left axis deviation and LV dominance.

On CXR, heart size and pulmonary markings will be normal in a child with mild to moderate stenosis. However, a prominent main pulmonary artery is usually present. Neonates with severe stenosis usually present with cardiomegaly and reduced pulmonary vascular markings.

Plan of care. Echocardiograph is an effective study for evaluating the pulmonary valve. In PS, the leaflets will be prominent in appearance secondary to the thickening of the tissue. While the leaflets of a dysplastic valve will appear immobile, those of a stenotic valve will be dome shaped, due to reduced systolic motion and inward curving of the tips of the leaflets. Echocardiograph is the diagnostic tool of choice for confirming the diagnosis of subvalvar PS. Anomalous muscle bundles may be visualized easily with Doppler interrogation, and the degree of obstruction from infundibular stenosis may then be calculated.

Cardiac catheterization is a useful study for obtaining hemodynamic measurements and for performing nonsurgical interventions to address the stenosis; however, it is not a necessary tool in making a definitive diagnosis. Pressures of importance include the pressure in the right ventricle as compared to the systemic arterial pressure, and the pressure gradient across the pulmonary valve. Cardiac catheterization may be useful in demonstrating a pressure gradient between the inflow portion and the apex of the ventricle in a double-chambered right ventricle.

In patients with isolated pulmonary valve stenosis, percutaneous balloon valvuloplasty has excellent outcomes. This procedure is relatively simple: A catheter with a balloon attachment is threaded through the right heart, with the tip of the catheter positioned in the pulmonary arteries. The balloon itself is positioned at the valve and inflated until the "waist" is no longer seen. Long-term follow-up data, even in neonates, reveal that this approach has good efficacy. As many as three-fourths of children remain free from surgical intervention 10 years following valvuloplasty (Werynski et al., 2009).

In children for whom valvuloplasty is not effective or is not an option, surgical valvotomy may be indicated. In those with stenosis not responsive to valvuloplasty, surgical valvotomy, with or without commissurotomy, may be an option. The valve is approached through the pulmonary artery in a retrograde fashion, avoiding a ventriculotomy to the right ventricle. Although valvotomy may be an option for those patients with a dysplastic valve, the valve may need to be partially or completely resected. The patch inserted increases the size of the annulus, avoiding "free" pulmonary insufficiency when possible. Long-term follow-up following simple surgical valvotomy is excellent, with 96% of children remaining free from further surgical intervention at 10 years (Hayes et al., 1993) (Figure 22-33).

Subvalvar pulmonary stenosis is only amenable to surgical intervention, and referral is recommended when the right ventricular pressure is 60% of the systemic pressure. The right ventricle can be approached through the tricuspid

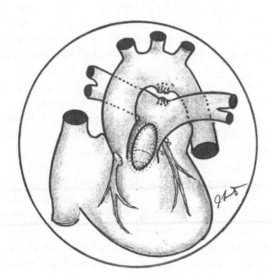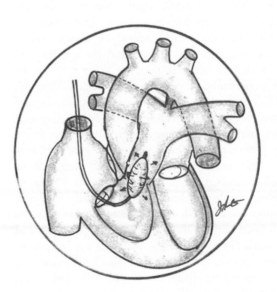

FIGURE 22-33

Pulmonary Stenosis and Repairs: Valvulotomy/Patch, Balloon.

Source: Used with permission. Courtesy of Joseph J. Amato, MD MJ. All Rights Reserved.

valve, again avoiding ventriculotomy whether or not the child requires resection of muscle bundles or has discrete infundibular stenosis (Hachiro et al., 2001; Kveselis et al., 1984).

Postoperative care and discharge planning. Long-term follow-up will depend on the child's individual anatomy; however, all children with pulmonary stenosis will require follow-up over the course of their entire lifetime. If a neonate has required placement of an aortopulmonary shunt to provide for adequate pulmonary blood flow, further intervention will be necessary. Monitoring of right ventricular size and hemodynamics, including pulmonary insufficiency, will be required. If any significant degree of ventricular hypertrophy was present prior to the relief of the obstruction, the ventricle may be hyperdynamic in the immediate post-intervention period. This hyperdynamic phenomenon may lead to a secondary form of obstruction as the hypertrophied outflow tract obstructs outflow during systole. This condition may be well controlled with a beta blocker such as propranolol.

Some patients will ultimately require replacement of the pulmonary valve. Significant advances have been made in the field of pulmonary valve replacement in recent years. Percutaneous replacement in the cardiac catheterization lab has become one such option, particularly in those patients who have had right ventricular outflow tract reconstruction (Kumar et al., 2009; Lurz et al., 2009; Oosterhof et al., 2009; Papadopoulos et al., 2009).

Tetralogy of fallot

The four characteristic findings in tetralogy of Fallot (Tet, TOF) are: outlet-type VSD, right ventricular outflow tract obstruction, overriding aorta, and right ventricular hypertrophy. However, the individual characteristics of the defect are extremely diverse, and the spectrum of associated variants is wide. Tetralogy of Fallot is by far the most common cyanotic congenital heart defect. Although its prevalence varies from study to study, the percentage of patients with congenital heart disease who have a diagnosis of TOF has been reported to be as high as 9%. The defect is equally prevalent in all races and ethnic groups. There is a very slight male predominance in affected infants. The familial recurrence rate is in the 2% to 3% range if one sibling is affected, but rises dramatically if two or more siblings are affected. Environmental factors known to be associated with TOF include maternal diabetes and phenylketouria (PKU), as well as maternal use of retinoic acids. Many genetic syndromes have also been associated with TOF, including trisomies (13, 18, 21), DiGeorge, velocardiofacial, and Alagille (Rausch et al., 2009).

Pathophysiology. The single most important characteristic of TOF is the degree of pulmonary stenosis, which is commonly infundibular. The degree of cyanosis is related to the degree of right ventricle outflow tract (RVOT) obstruction. The RVOT obstruction is caused by deviation of the infundibular septum, which in turn gives rise to the malaligned perimembranous VSD. In addition to the infundibular stenosis, the pulmonary valve is often small and stenotic, and supravalvar stenosis may be present. The pulmonary arteries may be diffusely hypoplastic or obstructed.

The VSD is usually large and nonrestrictive, and additional defects of the septum may be present. The malalignment of the VSD contributes to the aortic override. In a normal heart, the right aortic sinus may overlay the ventricular septum to some extent. By comparison, in the presence of a VSD, the overriding nature of the aorta is accentuated and contributes to the impression of an aorta that is committed to receive outflow from both ventricles.

Right ventricular hypertrophy (RVH) is a proportional measurement in relation to the left ventricle. A large, unrestrictive VSD should result in two ventricles with essentially equal pressures. Thus the degree of pulmonary blood flow should be determined by the amount of pulmonary stenosis and the systemic vascular resistance. Pulmonary artery pressures should remain low so that the pulmonary arteries are protected from excessive blood flow from the various levels of obstruction. The pulmonary vascular resistance should also remain low. The balance in pulmonary and systemic blood flow will be determined by the difference between the unimpeded but relatively high systemic pressure and the obstructed but relatively low pulmonary blood flow.

Many children will experience hypercyanotic events, or "Tet" spells, while waiting for surgical correction. These hypercyanotic events, which are characterized by profound periods of decreased arterial saturation, result from a sudden increase in right-to-left shunting through the VSD, due to a change in the ratio of systemic to pulmonary circulation. Given that surgical intervention is now possible at younger and younger ages, the occurrence and frequency of these spells may dictate the timing of intervention.

A number of anatomical defects are associated with TOF. A right-sided aortic arch occurs in approximately one of every four children with TOF. Coronary artery anomalies may be present, such as origination of the left anterior descending artery from the right coronary artery with a path that courses across the infundibulum of the right ventricle, or a single origin of the coronary arteries. Associated intracardiac defects include ASDs in more than three-fourths of children with TOF, as well as a left superior vena cava that may or may not drain into the left atrium in the setting of an unroofed coronary sinus. Children with trisomy 21 may have a coexisting AV canal. In addition, a small percentage of children will present with absence of the pulmonary valve.

Presentation. The presentation of a child with TOF will vary greatly depending on the degree of obstruction to pulmonary blood flow. In a child with a net left-to-right shunt path, there is no cyanosis. The extent of cyanosis depends on the degree of pulmonary obstruction. The precordium is active, due to an accentuated right ventricular impulse. Perfusion should be normal, with equal and full pulses throughout. The characteristic murmur of TOF is systolic, heard best at the left upper sternal border. It is usually harsh in quality, and the intensity and duration will vary inversely with the degree of pulmonary obstruction; the flow through the VSD is silent. This concept is best demonstrated during a hypercyanotic spell when little to no murmur is audible.

Characteristic findings on ECG include the persistence of RVH beyond the age of 3 months, at which time this finding is no longer normal. The axis may be deviated slightly to the right. No conduction defects or arrhythmias should be apparent in the preoperative patient. Postoperatively, a right bundle branch block is common. The CXR is often diagnostic: The cardiac silhouette resembles a "boot-shaped" heart (due to right ventricular enlargement), and the pulmonary vasculature is diminished. Polycythemia may be present in those patients with chronic cyanosis.

Definitive diagnosis is made by two-dimensional echocardiograph. The long-axis parasternal view yields an excellent view of the VSD and the overriding aorta, while the short-axis view allows for visualization of the infundibulum and proximal pulmonary arteries. The anatomy of the coronary arteries must also be visualized, paying special attention to any vessels coursing across the right ventricular outflow tract.

Cardiac catheterization is rarely indicated in TOF; its use is limited to obtaining hemodynamic data and angiography. This technique may also be useful to delineate pulmonary artery anatomy should there be a concern for stenosis or hypoplasia. MRI and MRA may also be useful in quantifying ventricular volumes, defining the anatomy of the RVOT and the pulmonary arteries, and imaging for the possible presence of major aortopulmonary collaterals (MAPCAs).

Differential diagnosis includes other malaligned VSDs, truncus arteriosus, and TOF with pulmonary atresia. If the override of the aorta is greater than 50%, the possibility of a double-outlet right ventricle should be considered.

Plan of care. Although children with TOF may be medically managed until the time at which intervention is necessary, surgical repair is the only definitive treatment for the defect. The goal of surgical intervention is to provide as much relief from RVOT obstruction as possible, and to close the VSD. Complete surgical repair has become an option for those below the age of six months with very low mortality rates. Neonates with ductal dependant blood flow will require a PGE_1 infusion until their anatomy is defined, at which time they may undergo a primary repair, or receive palliation with an aortopulmonary shunt. However, very few neonates with TOF have ductal dependant blood flow, unless the pulmonary valve is atretic. Although neonatal repair is an option, many centers prefer to wait to do complete primary repair at or about six months of age.

Many children will remain asymptomatic until the time of surgery, and will require no care other than careful monitoring. Beta blockade therapy may be initiated to treat hyperdynamic muscle (Park, 2008).

Should a child present with a hypercyanotic spell, the goal of therapy is to decrease impedance to pulmonary blood flow and increase systemic vascular resistance. First-line measures include oxygen, morphine, and sedation. If the spell persists, vasopressors—in particular, phenylephrine—will act to selectively increase the systemic vascular resistance, redirecting blood flow as the ratio between pulmonary and systemic pressures change. Unfortunately, some children will not respond to medical intervention during a hypercyanotic spell, and will need to go to the operating room emergently to provide for either palliation or repair. Some children self-treat their spells by squatting to increase systemic vascular resistance. This same technique can also be used for infants by bringing their knees to their chest.

As previously noted, primary repair of TOF consists of closing the VSD and relieving the obstruction from the right ventricular outflow tract (Figure 22-34). These goals may be achieved without the need for a ventriculotomy. The right ventricle can be accessed through the right atria

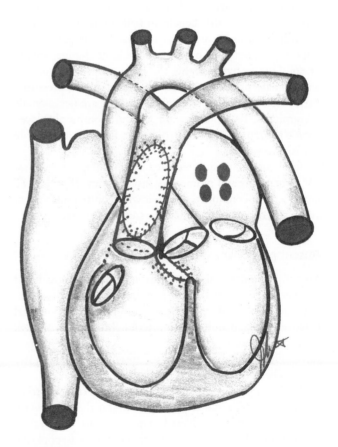

FIGURE 22-34

Tetralogy of Fallot Repair.

Source: Used with permission. Courtesy of Joseph J. Amato, MD MJ. All Rights Reserved.

and tricuspid valve; alternatively, it may be approached through the pulmonary valve. The VSD is closed with a patch, usually consisting of Dacron material. The obstruction at the infundibulum is resected, and the outflow tract is augmented. If the anatomy allows, RVOT reconstruction is attained with the use of a transannular patch across the pulmonary valve. In some patients, to sufficiently reconstruct the RVOT, a homograft or conduit, preferably with a valve, may be needed.

Postoperative care and discharge planning. Postoperative care following TOF repair varies. Arterial, central venous, and left atrial pressure monitoring are implemented, and NIRS monitoring is useful to evaluate cerebrall and renal perfusion.

Following repair of TOF, patients invariably demonstrate some degree of RV diastolic dysfunction while biventricular systolic function is generally normal. Approximately 30% to 40% of these patients develop diastolic heart failure. For them, the RV is often characterized as being "restrictive" or unfillable. This status is the result of several factors, including the adverse effects of CPB on the myocardium, the use of cardioplegia, and RV hypertrophy. Low cardiac output (CO) results from inadequate ventricular filling and not systolic dysfunction, so inotropic and vasodilatory agents are of little benefit in remedying this problem. RV filling pressures are often increased. It is particularly important to note that pressure and volume changes are not linear. Due to hypertrophy, the RV is noncompliant and an adequate preload may require higher filling pressures. Atrioventricular conduction abnormalities are occasionally encountered. Temporary pacing wires are commonly placed during the repair. The length of hospitalization ranges from one to two weeks.

Lifelong follow-up is required by cardiology to monitor RV dimensions and pulmonary insufficiency. If an RVOT homograft or conduit was used, it will require replacement as the size becomes inadequate or stenosis occurs.

Absent pulmonary valve

Absent pulmonary valve syndrome is a relatively rare defect and variant form of TOF. It is most often found in combination with a VSD, pulmonary outflow obstruction, and massively dilated pulmonary arteries. Most often, it will be referred to as tetralogy of Fallot with absent pulmonary valve. The isolated occurrence of absent pulmonary valve has also been described, but is extremely rare.

In absent pulmonary valve syndrome, the right ventricle is extremely large and hypertrophied, and the pulmonary arteries are markedly dilated, sometimes to aneurysmal proportions. The pulmonary valve annulus is hypoplastic and restrictive, with a ring of gelatinous, nodular tissue present—most likely the primitive pulmonary valve. The VSD is large and nonrestricted, just as in TOF. The aortic arch is oftentimes deviated rightward, and is usually dilated.

The central pulmonary arteries are dilated, mainly due to poststenotic dilatation from the pulmonary valve annulus. This massive dilation unfortunately leads to compression of the mainstem bronchi. Distal pulmonary arterial branching is not normal, and "tufts" of smaller vessels compress the smaller bronchioles. This abnormality in the distal airways may explain why some children continue to do poorly even after the proximal pulmonary arteries have been palliated.

As with TOF, absent pulmonary valve syndrome is associated with DiGeorge and velocardiofacial syndromes. However, the incidence of these comorbidities is extremely low.

Infants born with TOF with absent pulmonary valve syndrome will be symptomatic at birth. They present with extreme respiratory distress due to the compression of the bronchi. This distress may be relieved when the neonate is placed in the prone position. Infants are cyanotic, tachypneic, using their accessory muscles, and retracting. Inspiratory and expiratory wheezing may be heard. Auscultation of the heart will yield a systolic and diastolic murmur, heard best at the left upper sternal border, and transmitted throughout the precordium. The systolic murmur is due to the pulmonary stenosis, while the diastolic murmur occurs as a result of the pulmonary insufficiency.

RVH will be noted on ECG. Chest radiograph will reveal an enlarged heart, with massively dilated pulmonary arteries. In the presence of a right-sided aortic arch, the heart will be displaced into the left chest. Echocardiograph is sufficient to make an accurate diagnosis. Intracardiac findings will be similar to TOF. To visualize the pulmonary arteries, the parasternal short-axis view and suprasternal notch view may be used. Diagnosis may also be made prenatally by fetal echocardiograph. Cardiac catheterization is helpful to obtain additional hemodynamic data, but is not necessary to make the diagnosis.

The long-term outcome for the majority of children with absent pulmonary valve syndrome is poor: One-third will die in infancy. Surgical intervention is the only treatment. Initially, most children will require intubation and mechanical ventilation. Those children who are fortunate enough to have only mild airway obstruction may gradually improve, or may be able to wait until they are slightly older and larger to undergo surgical intervention. Surgical intervention is directed at not only repairing the VSD and pulmonary outflow tract, but also alleviating the pulmonary artery dilation and resulting airway compression. Several strategies have been proposed to address this specific issue. Translocation of the pulmonary artery and its placement anterior to the aorta has been identified as one method of relieving airway compression. In addition, reduction arterioplasty of the pulmonary arteries has found to be of use in decreasing compression on the airways.

Single ventricle

The term *single ventricle* (SV) is used to describe a physiologic state that is associated with congenital heart lesions in which children have one or two ventricles. Either one ventricle is "dominant" due to hypoplasia of the other or the AV valve alignment precludes successful partitioning of the heart into two functioning ventricles. In addition, SV is often associated with atresia of an AV or semilunar valve (Wernovsky & Bove, 1998). This section focuses on anatomy that involves one dominant ventricle.

The essential substrate for SV is the physiology of complete mixing of the systemic and pulmonary venous return. Congenital defects that are categorized in this class include tricuspid atresia, pulmonary atresia with intact ventricular septum and hypoplastic right ventricle, double-inlet LV, and hypoplastic left heart syndrome.

Pathophysiology. Single ventricle physiology involves the complete mixing of the systemic and pulmonary venous return. The SV acts as a common mixing chamber where the aortic and pulmonary artery saturations are the same. The ventricular output is the sum of the pulmonary blood flow (Qp) and the systemic blood flow (Qs); the determinants of Qp:Qs are the relative resistances in each system.

Patients with SV may be categorized into two classes: those with obstruction to pulmonary blood flow (pulmonary atresia, tetralogy of Fallot with pulmonary atresia) and those with obstruction to systemic blood flow (hypoplastic left heart, aortic atresia). Obstruction to blood flow on either side can result from vascular resistance or anatomical obstruction. After birth, there is a normal decrease in pulmonary vascular resistance (PVR). If no anatomical obstructions exist to pulmonary blood flow (PBF), the result is preferential flow to the pulmonary system leading to pulmonary over-circulation. As PVR continues to decrease, pulmonary over-circulation worsens and leads to systemic hypoperfusion. The heart must increase both stroke volume and heart rate to maintain systemic perfusion. This results in ventricular overload. Over time, as pulmonary over-circulation persists or Qp:Qs ratio approaches 2:1, systemic flow becomes inadequate and systemic oxygen delivery is compromised (Wernovsky & Bove, 1998).

Hypoplastic left heart syndrome (HLHS) is one of the most common congenital heart defects that result in SV physiology (Figure 22-35). HLHS comprises a range of

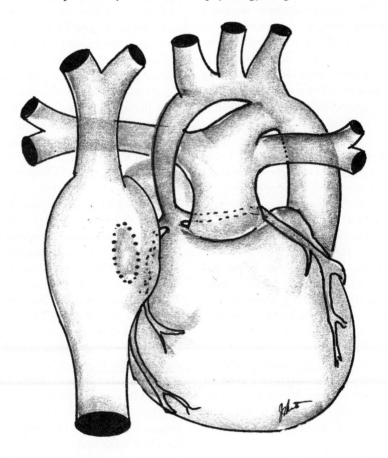

FIGURE 22-35

Hypoplastic Left Heart Syndrome.

Source: Used with permission. Courtesy of Joseph J. Amato, MD MJ. All Rights Reserved.

congenital cardiac abnormalities characterized by hypoplasia or absence of the left ventricle and significant hypoplasia of the ascending aorta. Mixing of the pulmonary and systemic circulations occurs in the right atrium. The systemic circulation depends on the right ventricle, which in turn depends on a patent ductus arteriosus (Ohye et al., 2003).

HLHS accounts for 7% to 9% of all neonatal congenital heart disease. This lesion is fatal unless unless surgical intervention is perfomed. HLHS accounts for 25% of cardiac deaths that occur within the first week of life (Ohye et al., 2003).

Presentation.   Clinical manifestations of SV are dependent on whether there is inadequate or excessive PBF. Patients with inadequate PBF present with hypoxemia. These patients may have severe pulmonary valvar or subvalvar stenosis, restrictive ductus arteriosus in ductal-dependent lesions, or elevated PVR. It is important to recognize that patients with hypoxia may not have accompanying poor blood pressure or metabolic acidosis due to adequate, albeit hypoxic systemic tissue perfusion. The Qp:Qs ratio in these patients may be 0.5:1, meaning they are hypoxic but have adequate blood flow to the systemic circulation. Patients presenting with excessive PBF initially will show symptoms related to CHF. Their arterial oxygen saturations will be greater than 85% (Tabbutt et al., 2008), but this high arterial oxygen saturations may be misunderstood in SV physiology. Pulmonary over-circulation leads to higher saturations due to the progressive increase in PBF. Excessive flow occurs at the expense of the systemic circulation, which ultimately leads to shock and death (Hoffman et al., 2004).

Plan of care.   When an infant is born with HLHS, the family has essentially three options: (1) staged reconstruction, (2) cardiac transplantation, and (3) supportive therapy only (which usually leads to rapid demise). Surgical techniques for staged reconstruction and cardiac transplantation have improved over time, leading to better outcomes when these options are chosen (Ohye et al., 2003).

The goal for all SV patients is separation of the pulmonary and systemic systems, thereby creating near-normal arterial oxygen saturations. Most centers accomplish this via three-stage procedures, with some variability in the initial procedure depending on the degree of aortic outflow obstruction and amount of PBF.

The first stage of palliation is the Norwood procedure. Recently, the classic Norwood procedure has been revised, so that it is now referred to as the *modified Norwood procedure.* This procedure is usually done within the first week of life. The essential components of surgical intervention are as follows:

- Unobstructed pulmonary venous return across the atrial septum (atrial septectomy)
- Unobstructed systemic blood flow from the right ventricle to the aorta (anastomosis of the pulmonary artery to the aorta with augmentation of the aortic arch)

- Sufficient pulmonary blood flow with minimal volume overload (aortopulmonary shunt)

Staged reconstruction for HLHS is based on the idea that effective circulation is possible in the absence of a pulmonary ventricle. Due to the high pulmonary vascular resistance that is present in the newborn period, an atrial shunt is necessary. When this happens, the right ventricle needs to account for the increased blood volume of both the pulmonary and systemic circulations; thus RV function must be preserved (Bove et al., 2004). The aortopulmonary shunt may be constructed via a right pulmonary artery to right subclavian nonvalved tube graft made of Gore-Tex®, termed a modified Blalock-Taussig (MBT) shunt. An alternative procedure is an RV to PA nonvalved Gore-Tex® graft known as the Sano shunt. The advantage to the Sano shunt is that it avoids the diastolic run-off and coronary steal that can occur with the MBT shunt. Survival is reportedly higher with the Sano shunt (Ohye & Pediatric Heart Network Investigators, 2010). The disadvantage of this technique is that it requires a ventriculotomy, which may lead to ventricular dysfunction or arrhythmias (Figure 22-36).

Stage II of the HLHS surgery involves either the bidirectional Glenn anastomosis (bidirectional cavopulmonary shunt) (Figure 22-37) or the hemi-Fontan procedure. This stage of reconstruction is usually performed when the infant is between 4 and 10 months of age (most often at 6 months of age). The procedure is performed on CPB. First, the aortopulmonary shunt is ligated and divided, and then the superior vena cava is transected and anastomosed in an end-to-side fashion to the superior aspect of the right pulmonary artery. The atrial septal defect is inspected and enlarged if necessary. The tricuspid valve is also examined and repaired if needed (Bove et al., 2004). When this stage of the surgery is completed, it provides adequate pulmonary blood flow and decreases the volume overload that the right ventricle experiences until the child is ready for the third and final stage, the Fontan completion (Ohye et al., 2003).

The hemi-Fontan procedure focuses on the same physiology as the Glenn procedure, but also includes an anastomosis of the pulmonary arteries to the atriocaval junction. The major advantage of the hemi-Fontan approach is that it shortens the time on CPB and dissection for the Fontan completion (Bove et al., 2004). There are various approaches in which the hemi-Fontan procedure can be performed, but each includes a connection between the atrium and the pulmonary artery that is occluded by a temporary intra-atrial patch (Ohye et al., 2003).

Stage III of reconstruction or palliation is called the Fontan completion. This stage is usually performed when the child is between 18 and 36 months of age. There have been many modifications to this procedure through the years. Fontan completion is achieved by redirecting inferior vena cava blood flow to the pulmonary arteries with an extracardiac conduit (Figure 22-38). This technique decreases the possibility of obstruction of the pulmonary venous

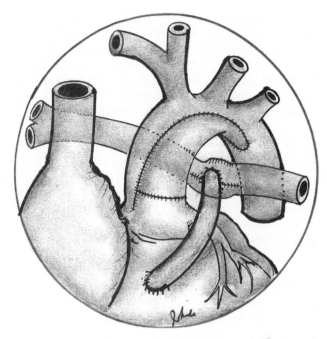

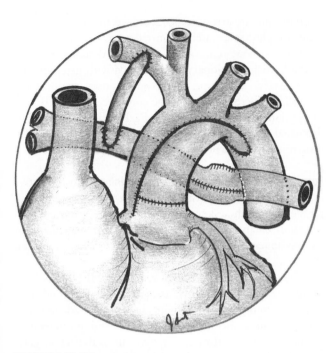

FIGURE 22-36

Stage I: Norwood Procedure.

Note: Left (modified Blalock-Taussig shunt), right (Sano shunt).

Source: Used with permission. Courtesy of Joseph J. Amato, MD MJ. All Rights Reserved.

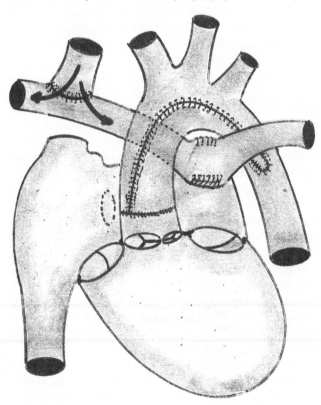

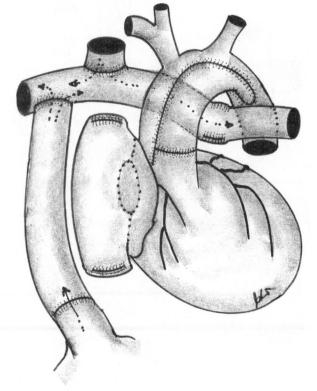

FIGURE 22-37

Bidirectional Glenn Anastomosis.

Source: Used with permission. Courtesy of Joseph J. Amato, MD MJ. All Rights Reserved.

FIGURE 22-38

Extracardiac Fontan Completion.

Source: Used with permission. Courtesy of Joseph J. Amato, MD MJ. All Rights Reserved.

return. A significant advance in this surgical approach was the creation of a fenestration (or a small hole) within the conduit. This hole functions as a "pop-off valve" if the pressure get too high within the Fontan completion, shunting blood from right to left into the right atrium. The Fontan procedure can be completed on CPB without needing to arrest the heart. The risk for atrial dysrhythmias may be reduced due to the resulting lower RA pressure and the lack of extensive atrial suturing and anastamosis that are near the sinoatrial (SA) node (Bove et al., 2004).

An alternative strategy to the stage I Norwood procedure is the less complex hybrid approach. This set of procedures combines surgical techniques (banding of the branch pulmonary arteries) and interventional cardiology techniques (stenting of the patent ductus arteriosus and ballooning of the atrial septectomy) (Figure 22-39). The advantage of the hybrid approach is that it enables the family to defer surgery and CPB until the infant is older (Galantowicz et al., 2008).

When the hybrid approach is used for stage I of palliation, stage II reconstruction becomes a combination procedure. Pizarro et al. (2008) described this stage as "amalgamation of the proximal ascending aorta with the

main pulmonary artery, removal or resection of the ductus/ stent complex, aortic arch reconstruction, atrial septectomy (with or without removal or atrial septal stent), removal of the branch pulmonary artery bands with arterioplasty, if necessary, and superior cavopulmonary connection" (p. 1385). There continue to be controversy and differing of opinions over this procedure. Each patient's anatomy is discussed on an individual basis to determine which procedure offers the best prospect for an optimal outcome.

Postoperative care and discharge planning. Postoperative management is tailored to the preoperative anatomy and physiology, with a key goal being maintaining oxygen transport balance. In-depth postoperative management for SV physiology is beyond the scope of this section. Hospital stays may be protracted.

The effectiveness of staged repair for HLHS has been limited by the high mortality associated with this condition. Although multiple advancements have been made in surgical techniques, medical management, and postoperative monitoring in an effort to improve survival after surgery, mortality between stage I and II remains in the range of 10% to 15% (Ghanayem et al., 2004). This mortality typically results from parallel circulation, volume overload of the single ventricle, cyanosis, and residual or new lesions (restrictive atrial septal defect, pulmonary artery distortion, tricuspid valve insufficiency, aortic arch obstruction). Other reasons for interstage death include acquired childhood illnesses (viral illnesses, gastroenteritis, respiratory infections) and comorbidities.

For all these reasons, transitioning infants home after stage I palliation and home monitoring is critical to their survival to the second stage of palliation. Home management takes the effort of an inter interprofessional team. Most centers have adapted a home monitoring program for children with SV defects. Ensuring adequate nutritional intake and weight gain can be difficult. Patients often experience feeding intolerance and dysphagia. Family members are trained to use monitoring devices (scales and pulse oximeters) while they are in the hospital. They should meet regularly with nutritionists and should be made aware that patients may require gastrostomy tube placement. Caregivers may be asked to weigh the infant and report to an HCP daily between the first and second stage of palliation or reconstruction, as well as to bring the child to the clinic weekly for evaluation. Close monitoring provides early detection of warning signs related to potentially fatal outcomes (Ghanayem et al., 2004).

Patients with SV lesions experience multiple hospitalizations throughout their lifetime, and the family is often subjected to significant financial burden. Consequently, families should be provided with thorough information about disease trajectory for infants with HLHS; moreover, they should be directed to support groups and discharge planning or social work for additional assistance.

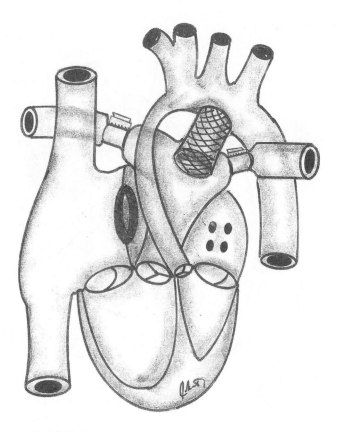

FIGURE 22-39

Hybrid Norwood Procedure.

Source: Used with permission. Courtesy of Joseph J. Amato, MD MJ. All Rights Reserved.

Pulmonary atresia with intact ventricular septum

By definition, pulmonary atresia with intact ventricular septum (PA/IVS) occurs in a left-sided heart with a normal atrial relationship, normal atrioventricular concordance, and normal ventriculoarterial concordance. Pulmonary blood flow is ductal dependent. The pulmonary valve is imperforate, and the right ventricle will vary widely in size. This type of congenital heart defect is included here because it is often considered a variant of single ventricle pathology. Connections may or may not exist between the right ventricle and the coronary arteries; coronary artery anatomy plays a major role in treatment options for these children (Selamet et al., 2004).

With PA/IVS, the heart may be mildly or massively enlarged (large right atrium). The presence of an ASD is essential, due to the obligatory right-to-left shunt at the atrial level. The pulmonary valve itself may be well formed with fusion of the commissures, or it may be primitive and poorly formed, particular in those patients with a small right ventricle. The tricuspid valve is rarely normal; it may be stenotic, regurgitant, or displaced and Ebstenoid (Ebstein's anomaly is described later in this section). The more underdeveloped the right ventricle, the more stenotic the tricuspid valve will be. The right ventricle may be well formed with the inlet, apex, and outlet components visible; poorly developed right ventricles may exhibit only an inlet portion.

The left atrium is usually normal, with normal return of the pulmonary veins. The left ventricular outflow tract may become obstructed in the setting of a hypertensive right ventricle when the septal wall protrudes into the left ventricle. The pulmonary arteries themselves are usually confluent, and a main PA trunk is usually present.

In children with a small tricuspid valve or a hypoplastic right ventricle, one must assume that ventriculocoronary artery connections exist. Coronary arteries are normally supplied via retrograde blood flow from the ascending aorta, with aortic diastolic pressure being responsible for perfusing the coronary arteries. The presence of connections between the right ventricle and the coronary arteries will lead to changes in the anatomy of the coronary arteries, and diastolic run-off from the aorta may not be sufficient to provide adequate perfusion to them. Therefore, the coronary arteries are also dependent upon retrograde blood flow from the right ventricular communication to be adequately perfused. The hypertensive nature of the right ventricle prior to unloading is responsible for this driving force. A reduction in pressure in the right ventricle of a heart that depends on right ventricle perfusion to maintain flow to the coronary arteries will result in ischemia to the myocardium, with infarction and death (Wessels et al., 2005).

Patients commonly present for diagnosis at the time of closure of the ductus arteriosus. If there is not adequate intra-atrial communication, cardiac output will be diminished, resulting in significant acidosis. Auscultation reveals a soft pansystolic murmur at the left lower sternal border, consistent with tricuspid regurgitation. Chest radiograph findings will vary widely, as this defect is extremely heterogeneous. The cardiac silhouette may be only slightly enlarged; alternatively, the heart may fill the entire chest cavity. Left-sided dominance is noted on ECG.

Although the diagnosis of PA/IVS can be made by echocardiograph alone, angiography is needed to evaluate for right ventricular dependent coronary circulation. This is particularly true in infants with a hypoplastic right ventricle, in whom the incidence of ventriculocoronary artery connections is high. A systematic approach to evaluating the anatomy via echocardiograph should begin with assessing the atrial septum to evaluate the interatrial communication, and to assure that it is not restrictive. Next, the tricuspid valve is evaluated, and the size, morphology, and the presence of regurgitation are identified. Right ventricular size is then assessed—it usually corresponds to the size of the tricuspid valve annulus. Antegrade pulmonary blood flow may be confused with flow through the ductus arteriosus.

Cardiac catheterization is indicated in the presence of either a small tricuspid valve or a hypoplastic right ventricle, although the two are usually coexistent. Angiography with a right ventriculogram will definitively reveal the presence or absence of any connections between the right ventricle and the coronary arteries. In addition, it will provide further information about the function of the tricuspid valve and the extent to which the right ventricle is apex forming. An aortogram will delineate the sidedness of the arch, and retrograde injections in the aorta will aid in elucidating the coronary arteries' anatomy.

Immediate medical management consists of initiation of PGE_1 infusion to assure ductal patency. Resuscitation and reversal of cardiogenic shock may also be necessary. Achieving these goals may require intubation and mechanical ventilation.

The surgical approaches used to treat PA/IVS vary greatly, as there is a wide spectrum of right heart morphology with this lesion. The primary concern—and, therefore, one of the deciding factors in proceeding with surgery—is the coronary artery anatomy. In addition, the size of the right ventricle and the patient's candidacy for a one- versus two-ventricle repair are important factors. Recent advances in the cardiac catheterization lab have evolved to include catheter intervention for pulmonary atresia. Radiofrequency perforation of the valve, particularly in those patients in whom two-ventricle repair appears feasible, has been practiced since the 1990s. Certain centers are also intervening prenatally in fetuses diagnosed with PA/IVS, albeit with mixed results (Figure 22-40).

Once the decision has been made that the child is a suitable candidate for surgical intervention, the appropriate approach must be selected. As previously noted , information must be obtained regarding the presence of a communication between the right ventricle and the coronary

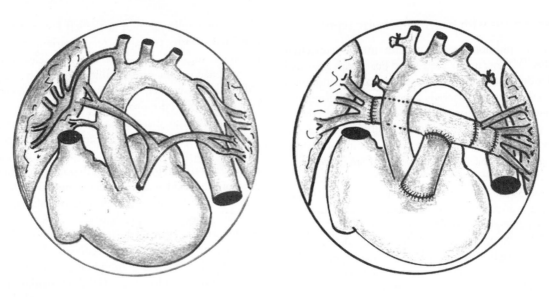

FIGURE 22-40

Pulmonary Atresia and Repair.

Source: Used with permission. Courtesy of Joseph J. Amato, MD MJ. All Rights Reserved.

arteries. Some centers electively ligate the communication while the child is off CPB, and allow the myocardium to recover and the coronary circulation to remodel prior to continuing with decompression of the right ventricle. Many centers use the size of the tricuspid valve as a guide in determining whether to attempt a two-ventricle repair: The larger the valve, the higher the likelihood of a successful two-ventricle repair. However, recent studies have shown that the tricuspid valve will continue to grow once continuity between the right ventricle and the pulmonary artery is achieved. Initial surgical treatment in those patients who are believed to be good candidates for two-ventricle repair is a decompressive intervention, either alone or in combination with a systemic to pulmonary artery shunt. Decompressive measures may include a valvotomy, with the possibility of a transannular patch.

CONOTRUNCAL LESIONS

Transposition of the great arteries (vessels)

Transposition of the great arteries (d-TGA or d-TGV) is characterized by the aorta arising from the anatomic right ventricle and the pulmonary artery arising from the anatomic left ventricle. Forty percent of patients with d-TGA will have an associated VSD. Fewer patients will have a coexisting coarctation of the aorta or obstruction to the left ventricular outflow tract. Approximately one-third will have some sort of anomaly of the coronary arteries. Without intervention, d-TGA is invariably a lethal defect. The incidence of d-TGA is 5% to 7% of all congenital anomalies, and there is a very strong male predominance,

approaching a male-to-female ratio of 2:1. In addition, infants of diabetic mothers are at higher risk for developing the defect.

Pathophysiology. The pathology of the d-tga lesion is characterized by two separate and parallel circulations. This phenomenon leads to an essential recirculation of the output of each ventricle and severe hypoxia, unless some mixing occurs at either the atrial or ventricular level. The principal factors that determine arterial oxygen saturations in d-TGA include the size and number of communications between the pulmonary and systemic circuits. Infants with intact ventricular and atrial septums will require pge₁ infusions to maintain ductal flow. In addition, balloon septostomy should be performed as soon as possible to maintain mixing and cardiac output.

Plan of care. Surgical repair is completed in the first few days to week of life. Prior to operating, a full evaluation of the right and left ventricular outflow tracts should be undertaken. This may be achieved by echocardiograph. Also of importance is the evaluation of the coronary artery anatomy. If the coronaries cannot be visualized by echocardiograph, a cardiac catheterization may be necessary to further delineate the anatomy. Surgical repair is the arterial switch operation. This is performed on CPB. The great vessels are transected, and the coronary arteries are translocated from the native aortic root to the neoaorta. The pulmonary arteries are then moved anterior to the aorta (Lecompte maneuver), and reconstruction of the outflow tracts completed. The right atrium is opened, and the atrial and ventricular septa are examined for any possible defects (Figure 22-41).

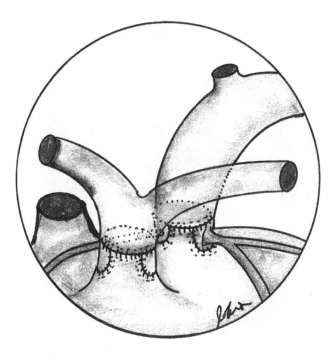

FIGURE 22-41

d-Transposition of the Great Arteries Repair.

Source: Used with permission. Courtesy of Joseph J. Amato, MD MJ. All Rights Reserved.

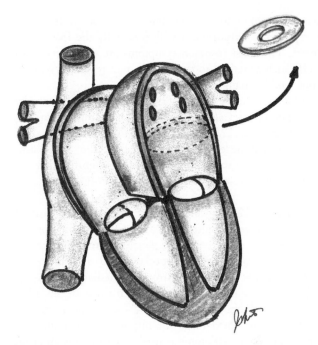

FIGURE 22-42

Cor Triatriatum Sinister Repair.

Source: Used with permission. Courtesy of Joseph J. Amato, MD MJ. All Rights Reserved.

Postoperative care and discharge planning. Postoperative monitoring includes arterial, central venous, and (often) left atrial pressures. Left atrial pressure monitoring may provide details about left ventricular failure, as evidenced by poor compliance and dysfunction. In addition, careful monitoring for postoperative arrhythmias is important due to the manipulation of the coronary arteries. Transposed coronary arteries may become occluded or kink, which can lead to myocardial ischemia or infarction. Monitor ST segments closely on ECG. For most children with d-TGA, long-term outcomes are very good.

Cor triatriatum sinister

Cor triatriatum sinister is a rare congenital cardiac lesion that is surgically correctable. It accounts for 0.1% of all congenital cardiac malformations. This anomaly results from an obstruction between the common pulmonary vein and the left atrium, most commonly in the form of a fibromuscular membrane. This membrane divides the atrium into two chambers. The proximal portion of the chamber receives the pulmonary veins, whereas the distal chamber contains the left atrial appendage and the mitral valve (Brown & Hanish, 2003). The membrane that divides the atrium can vary in size and shape.

Approximately 30% to 50% of children are found to have cor triatriatum as an isolated defect. In 12% to 50% of patients, this lesion occurs concomitantly with a ventricular septal defect, tetralogy of Fallot, double-outlet right ventricle, or atrioventricular septal defect (Figure 22-42).

Pathophysiology. The pathophysiology and symptoms associated with cor triatriatum sinister are closely connected. The flow through the pulmonary veins into the left atrium and mitral valve are abnormal due to the presence of the membranous barrier. As a consequence, cor triatriatum symptoms mimic those of severe mitral stenosis and causes of CHF. The degree of symptoms is directly correlated with the presence and size of the atrial septal defect or the number of fenestrations within the membrane. Severe pulmonary hypertension occurs if the opening within the membrane restricts forward blood flow. Conversely, if the atrial septal defect is large, or if the communication between the atria is large, then there will be minimal impediment to blood flow. Pulmonary hypertension will not be seen due to left-to-right shunting of blood across the atria. Because cor triatriatum is comorbid with other congenital heart defects, it is often initially overlooked (Brown & Hanish, 2003).

Presentation. The communication between the two atrial chambers will determine the onset and severity of symptoms in cor triatriatum. If the membrane between the atria is less than 3 mm in size, the child will present with symptoms within the first year of life. When larger communications are present, symptoms may not occur and this defect may go unnoticed. As many of 75% of children with unrepaired cor triatriatum will eventually die from their defect. The most common symptoms are those seen with CHF, such as failure-to-thrive, recurrent respiratory infections, and tachypnea.

ECG will show evidence of right ventricular hypertrophy and right axis deviation. A CXR will show right ventricular enlargement. Echocardiograph is the diagnostic tool of choice. When the left atrial appendage is in the same chamber as the mitral valve ring, this findings signifies that cor triatriatum is present (Brown & Hanish, 2003).

Plan of care. Management of cor triatriatum consists of surgical intervention, although balloon catheter dilation has been used successfully in some patients. Cardiopulmonary bypass is used with systemic hypothermia to surgically repair this defect. The approach is through a median sternotomy, although a left atriotomy is used when there are no other associated defects. The obstructing membrane is excised carefully as to not damage the mitral valve or injure the atrial wall. Right atriotomy is used when there is an atrial septal defect through which to approach the left atrium.

Postoperative care and discharge planning. Postoperative care depends on the specific repair. Results from surgical repair are very good. Long-term survival rates are excellent with early diagnosis.

Ebstein's anomaly of the tricuspid valve

Ebstein's anomaly of the tricuspid valve was first described in 1866. This rare cardiac anomaly accounts for less than 1% of all congenital heart disease. Children with this defect have a limited life expectancy; when Ebstein's anomaly is diagnosed in infancy, prognosis is poor (Dearani & Danielson, 2003).

Pathophysiology. Multiple presentations are possible with Ebstein's anomaly. One variant is characterized by downward displacement of the posterior and septal leaflets of the tricuspid valve. This phenomenon occurs in combination with a "sail-like" anterior leaflet in less severe cases. Part of the tricuspid valve is abnormally thin. In another presentation, the tricuspid leaflets are adhered to the underlying myocardium, with malformation of the right ventricle. The severity of the tricuspid valve, right atrium, and right ventricle abnormality is variable (Dearani & Danielson, 2003) (Figure 22-43).

Presentation. Hemodynamic alterations that occur in Ebstein's anomaly vary greatly. Symptoms are associated with the severity of the tricuspid regurgitation, the presence (or absence) of an atrial septal defect, and the presence of any other cardiac anomalies.

Neonatal presentation of Ebstein's anomaly presents with unique challenges. The infant may suffer from severe

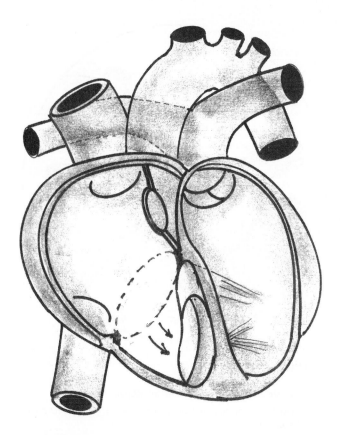

FIGURE 22-43

Ebstein's Anomaly.

Source: Used with permission. Courtesy of Joseph J. Amato, MD MJ. All Rights Reserved.

heart failure due to high pulmonary resistance and low cardiac output. A right-to-left atrial shunt due to the foramen ovale and severe tricuspid regurgitation will cause the infant to be severely cyanotic. As the pulmonary vascular resistance decreases over time, the degree of cyanosis and symptoms will decrease. In older patients, symptoms usually consist of fatigability, dyspnea with exercise, and cyanosis. Older patients may also experience palpitations caused by premature ventricular beats. If the regurgitation is severe, peripheral edema may be present (Dearani & Danielson, 2003).

Echocardiograph allows for accurate evaluation of the tricuspid leaflets and the sizes of the right atrium and ventricle. ECG findings are usually abnormal but not diagnostic (Dearani & Danielson, 2003).

Plan of care. There is no one approach to surgical reconstruction in Ebstein's anomaly; instead, each surgery is customized to the individual anatomy. Prosthetic valve replacement is the most widely employed surgical procedure, although the results obtained with this approach vary. Mechanical valves are used less often due to the possibility of valve malfunction and complications with thrombus formation. Valve replacement is less desirable in young children, due to the need to replace the valve as the child grows (Dearani & Danielson, 2003).

Postoperative care and discharge planning.   The postoperative course for an infant who undergoes surgical repair of Ebstein's anomaly varies depending on the type of repair. Invasive monitoring of arterial, central venous, and left atrial pressures is common. Postoperative arrhythmias are not uncommon due to the placement of sutures near the atrioventricular conduction pathways.

Vascular ring/pulmonary artery sling

Vascular ring is a term used to describe an anomaly of the aortic arch that causes compression of the esophagus, trachea, or both structures. Vascular rings are classified as complete vascular rings, partial vascular rings, or complete tracheal rings. Most children with vascular ring present in the first few months of life and undergo surgical repair.

A *pulmonary artery sling* is a very rare vascular anomaly in which the left pulmonary artery originates from the right pulmonary artery and encircles the right mainstem

bronchus and distal trachea. The most common vascular ring involves a dominant right arch with a left ductus arteriosus (Backer & Mavroudis, 2003b).

In double aortic arch, two aortic arches are present. The posterior, right aortic arch develops into the right common carotid artery and the right subclavian artery. The anterior, left aortic arch becomes the left carotid artery and the left subclavian artery. With a double aortic arch, the esophagus and trachea are encircled and compressed by the two arches.

A pulmonary sling develops when the developing left lung gets its arterial blood supply from the right sixth arch through capillaries caudad (rather than cephalad) to the developing tracheobronchial tree. In this case, the left pulmonary artery comes from the right pulmonary artery instead of coming from the main pulmonary artery. With a sling, the left pulmonary artery comes around the right main bronchus and goes between the trachea and the esophagus (Figure 22-44).

Presentation.   Symptoms usually occur within the first weeks of life, but can be noted to develop over time. These symptoms may include respiratory distress, stridor,

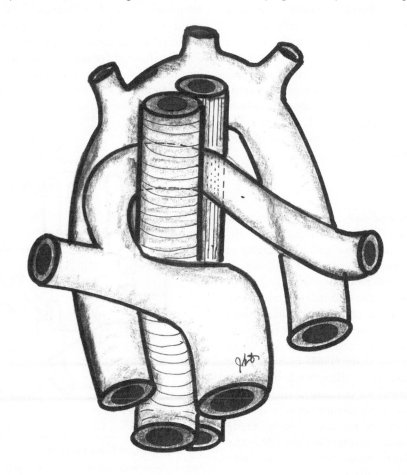

FIGURE 22-44

Pulmonary Artery Sling.

Source: Used with permission. Courtesy of Joseph J. Amato, MD MJ. All Rights Reserved.

classic "seal bark" cough, apnea, dysphagia, wheezing, and recurrent respiratory infections. Other children will present with feeding difficulties, slow feeding, or hyperextending their head to lessen the obstruction and help with their breathing).

Diagnosis of a vascular ring often starts with a CXR to evaluate for arch positioning and tracheal narrowing. Several other diagnostic studies may be useful, including barium esophagram, bronchoscopy, and CT with contrast. Esophagraph may reveal esophageal compression; bronchoscopy may illuminate trachea compression. Nevertheless, CT with contrast provides the greatest detail of the aortic arch and great vessels (Backer & Mavroudis, 2003b).

Plan of care. Surgical intervention is indicated in children who are symptomatic, as delayed intervention can lead to further tracheobronchial damage. Most vascular rings and slings are surgically repaired through a left thoracotomy incision. Cardiopulmonary bypass is usually not required for this anomaly (Backer & Mavroudis, 2003b).

Postoperative care and discharge planning. Children who undergo vascular ring/sling repair usually have an uneventful intensive care course. Care usually includes high humidity to loosen excess secretions, oxygen therapy, oxygen saturation monitoring, and nasopharyngeal suctioning to keep the airway clear. Early postoperative extubation is the goal in all children except those in whom tracheal reconstruction was performed. Complete relief from all symptoms usually occurs within months of surgery (Backer & Mavroudis, 2003b).

Shunts and banding

The word "palliative" in medicine and surgery refers to relief or reduction of the symptoms of a disease or disorder without effecting a cure. Most palliative surgery is performed in neonates who are too small for full surgical repairs. The primary palliative procedures that are done in such patients are aortopulmonary shunts and pulmonary artery banding. A few of the aortopulmonary shunts used historically are the Blalock-Taussig shunt (1944; right subclavian artery to right PA), Potts shunt (1946; left PA to descending aorta), Waterston shunt (1962; main or right PA to ascending aorta), and Cooley shunt (1966; ascending aorta to right PA). Successful use of many of these shunts relied on matching the size of the opening between the vessels to the needs of the child. The modified Blalock-Taussig shunt (graft from right subclavian artery to right PA) spares the subclavian artery and is the most commonly used shunt today (Backer & Mavroudis, 2003a).

Pulmonary artery banding is an option in infants with large left-to-right shunts (single ventricle) or excessive pulmonary blood flow until more permanent repair or reconstruction can be performed. This technique may be used in the following circumstances: (1) muscular VSDs, (2) multiple VSDs with coarctation of the aorta, and (3) single ventricle with increased pulmonary blood flow (in preparation for Fontan completion). As with shunts, matching the size of the band restriction to the child's anatomy can be difficult. Pulmonary artery narrowing may follow band removal. Pulmonary artery banding can be done through either a left thoracotomy incision or a median sternotomy, based on surgeon preference.

Cardiopulmonary bypass

Cardiopulmonary bypass (CPB) provides tissue perfusion and oxygenation by bypassing the patient's own heart and lungs and using a mechanical pump and oxygenator (Figure 22-45). To reroute blood, cannulas are placed in the right atrium and/or superior/inferior vena cava and the ascending aorta. Arterial blood is returned to the patient from the oxygenator via the arterial cannula, and venous blood is drained from the patient to the bypass system via the venous cannulas.

Most open-heart surgeries require the heart to be completely stopped or "arrested." To achieve safe cardiac arrest, a "cross-clamp" is placed across the aorta between the aortic valve and the site of insertion of the aortic cannula distal to the origin of the coronary arteries. A small cannula is placed in the aortic root proximal to the aortic cross-clamp and is used to inject a cold, high-potassium solution called cardioplegia into the aortic root. The cardioplegia

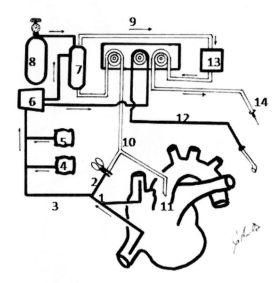

FIGURE 22-45

Cardiopulmonary Bypass Circuit.

Note: Superior vena cava cannula (1), bridge (2), venous line (3), fluids (4), heparin (5), monitor/heater (6), oxygenator (7), oxygen (8), roller pump (9), arterial line (10), aortic cannula (11), suction (12), cardioplegia reservoir (13), cardioplegia cannula (14).

Source: Used with permission. Courtesy of Joseph J. Amato, MD MJ. All Rights Reserved.

then enters into the coronary arteries, where it is distributed to the heart muscle. The hypothermia decreases cardiac metabolism, and the potassium terminates electrical and muscular activity. Following repair, the heart is reperfused by removing the aortic cross-clamp. The removal of the cross-clamp allows blood from the bypass machine to perfuse the coronary arteries, thereby restarting of the electrical and muscular activity of the heart.

A heat exchanger is also incorporated into this system to allow the perfusionist to adjust the blood and body temperatures. Most surgical procedures are carried out using moderate hypothermia (26–34°C [78.8–93.2°F]). Some procedures, however, require the cessation of all blood flow, including that from the bypass machine. This technique is called deep hypothermic circulatory arrest (DHCA). Some surgeons will choose DHCA for defects such as interrupted aortic arch or TAPVR. DHCA requires cooling at extremely low temperatures (less than 15°C [59°F]). In addition to cooling and potassium, heparin is used to provide anticoagulation in the circuit (Castaneda et al., 1994).

CPB has allowed for significant advancement in cardiac surgical techniques for children with congenital heart disease. Despite its utility, certain adverse effects occur with the use of CPB, aortic cross-clamping, and DHCA. Many studies have demonstrated inflammatory mediator release with the use of CPB. Exposure of blood elements to the non-endothelialized circuit and oxygenator leads to activation of pro-inflammatory plasma proteins. Amplification of the inflammatory cascade results from ischemia–reperfusion injury following restoration of oxygen delivery to the myocardium and lung. Inflammatory mediators increase microvascular permeability, alter vasomotor function, and stimulate neutrophils to release proteolytic enzymes and reactive oxygen species, all of which may lead to multiple organ dysfunction.

Low cardiac output is common after CPB and cardiac surgery. Ischemia experienced during CPB leads to increased intracellular calcium concentrations in the heart and vasculature (Kozik & Tweddell, 2006). Calcium extrusion pumps, which remove calcium from the cells, are more ATP dependent than the calcium channels that bring calcium into the cell. The result is a noncompliant, poorly functioning heart and high systemic vascular resistance. Milrinone has been shown to reduce the incidence of low cardiac output syndrome after CPB.

Coagulopathy may be seen post CPB secondary to heparin administration, hepatic dysfunction from hypoperfusion, or platelet dysfunction. Platelets are consumed during CPB and partially degranulate, reducing their function; hypothermia has the same effect (Wypij et al., 2003).

Mediastinitis and delayed sternal closure

Mediastinitis is a postoperative complication associated with cardiothoracic surgery. In these procedures, undesirable outcomes may include purulent drainage within the mediastinal space, positive wound cultures from the mediastinal space, or instability of the sternum in conjunction with positive blood cultures (Straumanis, 2008). Despite the use of prophylactic antibiotics, mediastinitis occurs in approximately 1% of all patients after cardiothoracic surgery (Allpress et al., 2004).

Current thought is that the surgical wound is seeded with the patient's own flora. These bacteria spread throughout the wound, causing a localized infection. Gram-positive pathogens such as *Staphylococcus aureus* and coagulase-negative *Staphylococcus* are responsible for approximately two-thirds of postsurgical infections, while the remaining one-third of infections are caused by Gram negative organisms such as *Pseudomonas aeruginosa*. Fungal and multimicrobial infections are rare in postoperative mediastinitis but the incidence of *Candida* is increasing (Straumanis, 2008; Van Schooneveld & Rupp, 2009).

Mediastinitis has been directly correlated with the following factors:

- Delayed sternal closure
- Underlying comorbidities
- Prolonged stay in an intensive care unit
- Postoperative use of inotropes
- Long CPB time
- Need for a repeat surgical procedure more than 24 hours after the original surgery
- Low cardiac output for more than 24 hours
- Prolonged mechanical ventilation
- Postoperative bleeding
- Transfusion of blood products
- Age younger than 1 month (Allpress et al., 2004; Costello et al., 2010, Mehta et al., 2000; Rosanova et al., 2009)

In an attempt to augment myocardial support following extensive or complex pediatric cardiac procedures, the sternal wall may be left open. This technique is referred to as *delayed sternal closure* (DSC). While it does improve both pulmonary and cardiac function postoperatively, this approach increases the patient's risk for prolonged mechanical ventilation, longer stay in the intensive care unit, and infection, particularly mediastinitis (Johnson et al., 2010). The sternum is usually left open until adequate hemostasis has been achieved and there is reduced edema around the myocardium. A negative fluid balance is desirable, but not entirely necessary prior to closure. Generally, the time frame for closure is as early as 2 to 3 days to as long as 2 weeks after the initial surgery (Riphagen et al., 2005).

Presentation. Children with mediastinal infections often have fever, tachycardia, crepitus, or localized cellulitis with purulent drainage and chest pain. Sternal dehiscence or instability may sometimes be the only sign of infection. Leukocytosis with a left shift is observed in the white blood cell count; radiographically, widening of the mediastinum may be apparent. Pleural effusion and pneumoperitoneum are late complications of mediastinal infection (Van Schooneveld & Rupp, 2009).

Plan of care. In addition to supportive measures and prompt surgical debridement if indicated, administration of antimicrobial therapy is imperative in mediastinitis. Empiric coverage with broad-spectrum antibiotics or antifungals is essential. Once the infectious organism is identified and the susceptibility pattern elucidated, antimicrobial coverage may be narrowed. The duration of therapy is variable and based on pathogen virulence and patient response to treatment (Van Schooneveld & Rupp, 2009).

Negative-pressure wound therapy (NPWT) has shown remarkable promise in the therapeutic management of mediastinitis. NPWT is used either for primary closure or as a bridge to debridement and flap closure . As compared to traditional treatment, NPWT leads to shorter hospitalizations, fewer wound dressing changes, reduced need for soft-tissue flaps, and earlier sternal wiring. C-reactive protein levels also return to normal more quickly in patients using NPWT than in those receiving traditional therapy (Van Schooneveld & Rupp, 2009). The combination of continuous irrigation and NPWT has proven an effective treatment to decrease morbidity and mortality in postoperative pediatric cardiac patients. The continuous irrigation flushes out the wound and debrides it of purulent and necrotic tissue, while the NPWT maintains the surgical wound by removing the fluid, increasing perfusion locally, and enhancing the growth of granulation tissue (Ugaki et al., 2010).

Disposition and discharge planning. Postoperative mediastinitis mortality is approximately 5% If the child survives the initial surgical phase, his or her chance of survival is equal to that of a patient who has a noncomplicated cardiac surgical repair (Van Schooneveld & Rupp, 2009). Because postoperative mediastinal infections are considered preventable, the Center for Medicaid and Medicare Services no longer reimburses hospitals for costs related to treatment of postoperative infections. A more comprehensive review of risk factors prior to surgery, immaculate handwashing and surgical site preparation, empiric use of antibiotics, and early sternal closure are measures that can decrease the risk of postoperative mediastinitis.

CONGESTIVE HEART FAILURE

Dana M. Connolly and Valarie Eichler

PATHOPHYSIOLOGY

Traditionally, the "C" in the acronym "CHF" has stood for the pulmonary "congestive" element of heart failure symptoms. This is a symptom-limited acronym. The "C" more

accurately stands for "chronic" or "compensated" because of the marked variation in disease etiology.

Heart failure in pediatric patients is well summarized by Hsu and Pearson (2009a, 2009b) as a progressive clinical and pathophysiological syndrome caused by cardiovascular and noncardiovascular abnormalities that results in characteristic signs and symptoms such as edema, respiratory distress, growth failure, and exercise intolerance. It is accompanied by circulatory, neurohormonal, and molecular derangements. Conceptually, heart failure syndrome is cyclical, with underlying pathways and compensatory mechanisms that result in a compensated state with associated deleterious effects (Figure 22-46).

The CHF cycle is initiated by myocardial disease or injury that causes changes in loading conditions and cardiac output. A number of physiologic scenarios can cause these changes. For example, systolic dysfunction results in decreased cardiac output and increased venous pressures. Commonly seen in pediatric patients is a left-to-right shunt, which results in decreased pulmonary vascular resistance and increased cardiac output. Diastolic heart failure results from decreased ventricular compliance and can occur either alone or in combination with systolic heart failure. Diastolic stiffness, distensibility, or dysfunction may lead to abnormal ventricular filling. Causes of primary diastolic dysfunction include an anatomic obstruction that prevents ventricular filling (pulmonary venous obstruction), a primary reduction in ventricular compliance (cardiomyopathy, transplant rejection), external constraints (pericardial effusion), and poor hemodynamics after the Fontan surgical procedure (elevated pulmonary vascular resistance).

The CHF cycle maintains cardiac output and perfusion pressure to vital organs to prevent acute heart failure or cardiogenic shock by activating the sympathetic nervous system and renin–angiotensin system to increase myocardial contractility, selective peripheral vasoconstriction, sodium and fluid retention, and blood pressure maintenance. The CHF cycle is progressive, with deterioration of both the myocardium and the patient occurring over time. This deterioration is a result of energy starvation, cytotoxic mechanisms leading to necrosis, or acceleration of apoptosis (programmed cell death). Disease progression leads to decompensation, acute heart failure, cardiogenic shock, and multiple organ dysfunction. The period of time during which the chronic or compensated heart failure cycle is in motion, either forward or in reverse, represents a dynamic continuum of signs and symptoms and responses to treatment.

EPIDEMIOLOGY AND ETIOLOGY

Heart failure caused by congenital heart disease and cardiomyopathy affects approximately 12,000 to 35,000 children in the United States each year (Hsu & Pearson, 2009a,

PROGRESSION ➡ ⬅ REGRESSION

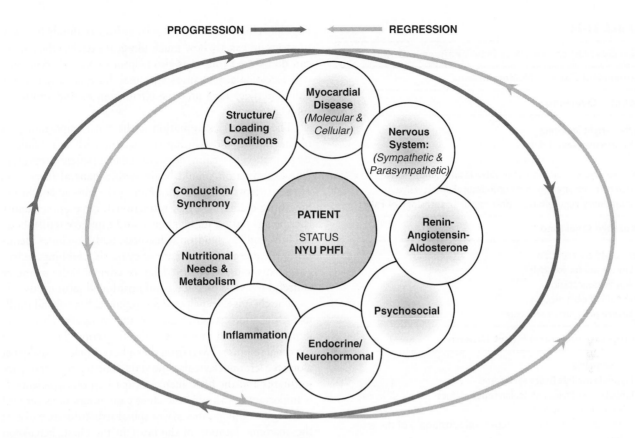

FIGURE 22-46

Pathways Comprising Clinical Status within the CHF Cycle. The figure illustrates the complex interplay of pathophysiologic and compensatory mechanisms and modifiers (M & M's) shown in the blue circles that comprise CHF. In the center is the patient, who manifests the signs and symptoms. The outer circle shows the bidirectional nature of the cycle, driven by the M & M's. It is in this outer circle where heart failure severity can be measured at any given point in time.

2009b). Patients with either congenital or acquired heart disease often develop heart failure at various stages of their illness.

The etiology of heart failure in pediatric patients today is most often either structural congenital heart lesions or cardiomyopathy. Patients with congenital heart lesions may have volume overload malformations, pressure overload malformations, or complex combinations of both. Cellular features of ventricular myocytes from hypoplastic left and right heart syndrome patients include disorganized, focally small cells with scant myoplasm; abundant and loose connective tissue; and scattered, dilated, thin-walled blood vessels. Surgically palliated patients with a single ventricle defect have abnormal loading conditions; they can be considered to be in heart failure simply by definition, although these patients usually feel and appear asymptomatic at rest and during nonexertional daily activities.

In the structurally normal heart, primary cardiomyopathies and other primary conditions that give rise to cardiomyopathies can occur due to inflammation from infections, genetic factors, toxins, or chemotherapy. In developing nations, many cases of CHF are related to anemia, often secondary to malaria and malnutrition. Hypocalcemia and

vitamin D deficiency may also cause heart failure in infants. CHF in the fetus, or hydrops, may represent underlying anemia (e.g., Rh sensitization, fetal–maternal transfusion), arrhythmias, or myocardial dysfunction. Structural heart disease is rarely a cause of congestive heart failure in the fetus, although it does occur. Atrioventricular valve regurgitation in the fetus is often associated with poor fetal outcomes.

Postnatally, clinical presentation will vary case by case, according to the etiology, the severity of the CHF, and the patient's age (Table 22-24).

PRESENTATION

The characteristic history of the pediatric patient with CHF includes growth failure, respiratory distress, and feeding or exercise intolerance. However, a comprehensive history should start with the family. Inquire about sudden death, miscarriages, congenital malformations, or congenital deafness. The prenatal, perinatal, and postnatal histories are often informative. Siblings' health histories also may provide clues into the origins of the disease. The presence

TABLE 22-24

Cardiovascular Causes of Heart Failure in Children

Congenital Cardiac Malformations

Volume Overload

Left-to-right shunting
- Ventricular septal defect
- Patent ductus arteriosus

Atrioventricular or semilunar valve insufficiency
- Aortic regurgitation in bicommissural aortic valve
- Pulmonary regurgitation after repair of tetralogy of Fallot

Pressure Overload

Left-sided obstruction
- Severe aortic stenosis
- Aortic coarctation

Right-sided obstruction
- Severe pulmonary stenosis

Complex Congenital Heart Disease

Single ventricle
- Hypoplastic left heart syndrome
- Unbalanced atrioventricular septal defect

Systemic right ventricle
- One-transposition ("corrected transposition") of the great arteries

Structurally Normal Heart

Primary Cardiomyopathy

Dilated
Hypertrophic
Restrictive

Secondary Cardiomyopathy

Malnutrition
Arrhythmogenic
Ischemic-anomalous origin of left coronary artery
Toxic
Infiltrative
Infectious
Anemia
Anthracyclines in childhood cancer survivors

Source: Modified from Hsu, D., & Pearson, G. (2009). Heart failure in children: Part I: History, etiology, and pathophysiology. *Circulation: Heart Failure, 2,* 63–70.

or absence of maternal systemic lupus erythematosus, gestational diabetes, substance abuse, infections, medications, or other complications must be ascertained.

For infants, a detailed feeding history is typically the most illuminating in describing CHF symptoms. What is the patient eating? How much? How often? Over what period of time? A history of severe colic can suggest anginal pain, from anomalous origin of the left coronary artery.

For older children, a detailed activity history should be taken to ascertain exactly how much physical exertion the patient can do before tiring. It is also helpful to ask questions that will elucidate any changes that may have occurred in the child's activity level and the circumstances and timing of such changes.

The physical examination is the most important part of diagnosing and treating the patient with heart failure. Examination of a calm, quiet, or sedated patient is optimal. The examination should begin with a general inspection of the patient. This includes noting the airway condition, breathing quality (flaring, retractions), circulation quality (peripheral pulses, jugular veins, and capillary refill), body habitus, and any syndromic features. It also includes identifying the presence or absence of cyanosis, clubbing, pulsus paradoxus, radial–femoral delay, or edema. Pulse oximetry is useful to assess preductal and postductal saturations.

The chest is then palpated for impulses, heaves, and thrills using the more sensitive area of the metacarpophalangeal joints of the hand rather than the fingertips. The point of maximal impulse (PMI) from the right ventricle is usually felt along the left midclavicular line at the fourth intercostal space in infants and the fifth intercostal space in older patients. It is important to examine the chest configuration, as surgical scarring or cardiopulmonary or spinal structures may distort the anatomic location of the heart in the chest. Percussion helps define the size of the heart or diaphragmatic excursion to assess the phrenic nerve. While examining the abdomen, it is easy to palpate the location of the liver's edge and note any hepatomegaly, splenomegaly, distention, or acites.

Accurate auscultation can be done only with a stethoscope placed directly on the patient's skin, not through the shirt or patient gown. First, listen for hepatic and cranial bruits. Auscultate the lungs, and then the heart. Maneuvers to change the systemic venous return or cardiac output during the physical examination can be diagnostically useful. For example, the Valsalva maneuver increases intrathoracic pressure and decreases systemic venous return and blood pressure, which can bring out the click of a mitral valve prolapse, or accentuate the murmurs of mitral valve regurgitation or obstructive hypertrophic cardiomyopathy.

The first manifestation of CHF is usually tachycardia, unless it is masked by sinus node dysfunction, heart block, mechanical pacing, or beta blockade. CHF is characterized by fluid retention with subsequent respiratory symptoms (tachypnea, retractions, nasal flaring or grunting, abnormal breath sounds) resulting from pulmonary edema, activity intolerance, and failure-to-thrive. Patients with right heart dysfunction or single ventricle physiology may present with hepatosplenomegaly, jugular venous distention, edema, ascites, and pleural effusions. Other signs of low cardiac output include fatigue or low energy, pallor, diaphoresis, syncope, and poorly perfused extremities (cool, mottled, slow capillary refill, weak pulses). Signs of pulmonary venous congestion in an infant generally include tachypnea, respiratory distress (retractions), grunting, and difficulty with feeding. Often, infants with CHF have diaphoresis during feedings, which is possibly related to a catecholamine surge that occurs when they are challenged with eating while in respiratory distress.

Clinical findings may include hypotension, cool extremities with poor peripheral perfusion, a thready pulse, and decreased urine output—all of which are signs of cardiogenic shock. Evidence of kidney and liver dysfunction may be present, as well as a diminished level of consciousness. Right-sided venous congestion is characterized by hepatosplenomegaly and, less frequently, by edema or ascites. Jugular venous distention is not a reliable indicator of systemic venous congestion in infants, as the jugular veins are difficult to observe due to the distance from the right atrium to the angle of the jaw (no more than 8 to 10 cm), even when the patient is in a sitting position. Uncompensated CHF in an infant is primarily manifested as a failure-to-thrive. In severe cases, failure-to-thrive may be followed by signs of kidney and hepatic failure.

In older children, left-sided venous congestion causes tachypnea, respiratory distress, and wheezing (cardiac asthma). Right-sided congestion may result in hepatosplenomegaly, jugular venous distention, edema, ascites, and pleural effusions.

Pediatric heart failure index

One of the greatest challenges to investigation of pediatric CHF therapies has been the selection of an accurate primary endpoint that reflects degree of CHF, even in the absence of significant symptomatology. The New York University Pediatric Heart Failure Index (PHFI) was developed to reflect a quantifiable determination of disease severity by measuring the location of each patient within the bidirectional cycle at any given point in time, such that higher PHFI scores reflect disease progression. The PHFI has been used to assess CHF severity in children of all ages (Table 22-25). This index comprises a weighted, linear cumulative score based on physiologic indicators and need for medical treatment. It requires only a cardiopulmonary exam, with or without an echocardiograph and CXR. Patients with diastolic dysfunction, such as those with restrictive cardiomyopathy, are also assessed using the PHFI, even in the absence of symptoms; in such patients, the "ventricular dysfunction or gallop" can be used to score systolic or diastolic dysfunction (Connolly et al., 2001).

DIFFERENTIAL DIAGNOSIS

Infants younger than 2 months are the most likely group to present with CHF related to structural heart disease. The systemic or pulmonary circulation may depend on the patency of the ductus arteriosus, especially in patients

TABLE 22-25

The NYU Pediatric Heart Failure Index	
Signs and Symptoms	
+2	Abnormal ventricular function by echocardiograph OR gallop
+2	Dependent edema OR pleural effusion OR ascites
+2	Failure-to-thrive OR cachexia
+1	Marked cardiomegaly by radiograph OR by physical examination
+1	Reported physical activity intolerance OR prolonged feeding time
+2	Poor perfusion by physical examination
+1	Pulmonary edema by radiograph OR by auscultation
+2	Resting sinus tachycardia
+2	Retractions
+1	Hepatomegaly:
+2	< 4 cm below costal margin > 4 cm below costal margin
+1	Observed tachypnea OR dyspnea:
+2	Mild to moderate Moderate to severe
Medications	
+1	Digoxin
+1	Diuretics:
+2	Low to moderate dose High dose OR more than one diuretic
+1	ACE inhibitors OR non-ACE-inhibitor vasodilators OR angiotensin receptor blockers
+1	Beta blockers
+2	Anticoagulants not related to prosthetic valve
+2	Antiarrhythmics OR ICD
Physiology	
+2	Single ventricle

New York University (NYU), angiotensin-converting enzyme (ACE), implantable cardioverter–defibrillator (ICD).

presenting with CHF in the first few days of life. In these patients, prompt cardiac evaluation is mandatory. Myocardial disease due to primary myopathic abnormalities or inborn errors of metabolism must be investigated. Respiratory illnesses, anemia, and known or suspected infection must be considered and managed appropriately.

In older children, CHF may be caused by left-sided obstructive disease (aortic stenosis or coarctation), myocardial dysfunction (myocarditis or cardiomyopathy), hypertension, kidney failure, or, more rarely, arrhythmias or myocardial ischemia. Illicit drugs such as inhaled cocaine and other stimulants are becoming more common precipitating causes of CHF in adolescents; therefore, an increased suspicion of drug use is warranted in unexplained CHF. Although CHF in adolescents can be related to structural heart disease (including complications after surgical palliation or repair), it is usually associated with chronic arrhythmia or acquired heart disease, such as cardiomyopathy.

PLAN OF CARE

A CHF diagnosis is a culmination of findings that include the history, physical examination, and the PHFI. By the end of the history and cardiopulmonary exam, it is possible to produce a PHFI score. Documenting this simple quantification of disease severity can also be helpful in guiding clinical care within the CHF cycle. The diagnostic evaluation includes laboratory findings, such as noninvasive imaging and biomarker profiling (Table 22-26).

Evaluation and management of the pediatric patient with heart failure is best accomplished in an intensive care setting. In many cases, patients will require cardiopulmonary resuscitation, pericardiocentesis, and continuous infusion of intravenous inotropes or PGE_1 to maintain patency of a ductus arteriosus. Mechanical ventilatory support or mechanical circulatory support may be required. Once the patient is stabilized, a thorough diagnostic evaluation may begin.

Therapeutic decisions are based on the underlying cause of CHF and the patient's age. Treatment goals include meeting metabolic needs, correcting underlying causes, preventing unnecessary health care utilization, and improving and prolonging the patient's life. Modification of the underlying pathways and compensatory mechanisms through targeted interventions can slow and even reverse the CHF cycle.

The majority of the medication guidelines set forth by the International Society for Heart and Lung Transplantation (Rosenthal et al., 2004) are based on expert consensus. Even today, few medications used in the treatment of pediatric CHF have demonstrated evidence-based efficacy or received regulatory approval for use in children. However, the mainstay of contemporary CHF treatment has to date included diuretics, digoxin, angiotensin-converting enzyme (CE inhibitors, beta blockers, and inotropic and mechanical support [Table 22-27]).

Diuretics increase sodium and water loss. Digoxin increases calcium levels in heart muscle by inhibiting ATPase, which should theoretically increase the heart's contraction. It also slows heart rate, allowing for a more optimal balance of oxygen supply and demand, and inhibits the sympathetic nervous system and release of renin.

ACE inhibitors reduce the activation of the renin–angiotensin–aldosterone (RAA) system, a perpetuator of

TABLE 22-26

Diagnostic Evaluation

Vital Signs

Respiratory rate and quality
Heart rate, pulses, and quality
Blood pressures
Oximetry and hyperoxia test

Electrophysiology

Electrocardiograph rhythm strip
Holter monitor
Electrophysiology studies

Imaging

Chest radiography
Echocardiograph/wall stress (EF with biplane)
Magnetic resonance imaging/angiography (MRI/A)
Computed tomography (CT)
Fluorodeoxyglucose positron emission tomography
Cardiac catheterization with root injection and endomyocardial biopsy

Labs Studies

Arterial blood gas (pH, anion gap)
Complete blood count with differential
Sedimentation rate
Comprehensive metabolic panel
Thyroid function tests
Liver function tests
BNP/N-terminal pro-BNP
Cardiac enzymes (CK-MB, troponin I)
Lactate dehydrogenase
Amino acids
Free fatty acids
C-reactive protein
Blood for cell lines
Serum carnitine, acylcarnitine profiles
Serum selenium, thiamine, and zinc
Ammonia, lactate and pyruvate levels
Insulin level
Urinalysis
Urine carnitine, amino acids, acyglycines, organic acid profiles
Blood or urine toxicology screen
Chlamydia pneumoniae
Helicobacter pylori
EBV, CMV, toxoplasmosis, herpes titers
Coxsackie A, B1–B6, influenza A and B, mumps, polio 1–3, adenovirus, H_1N_1
Nose and throat for enterovirus (coxsackie, echo, polio viruses), PCR for viral genome

Other

Maximal oxygen consumption
Exercise test
6-minute walk test
Skeletal bone radiographs
Skeletal muscle biopsy
Skin fibroblast culture for enzyme assays

Epstein-Barr virus (EBV), cytomegalovirus (CMV), polymerase chain reaction (PCR).

TABLE 22-27

Therapeutic Agents in Congestive Heart Failure

Agent	Pediatric Dose	Comment
Digoxin	Preterm infants: 5–10 mcg/kg/day PO divided BID IV is 75% of oral dose: < 10 yr: 10 mcg/kg/day PO divided BID or 75% of this dose IV > 10 yr: 5 mcg/kg/d PO daily or 75% of this dose IV	Load: Preterm infant: 10 mcg/kg PO Term infant: 10–20 mcg/kg PO
Preload Reduction		
Furosemide	1–2 mg/kg PO or IV	Every 4–12 hr
Torasemide	Not established (one small study in pediatrics suggested beneficial results; Senzaki et al., 2008)	10–40 mg once daily to BID
Bumetanide	0.01–0.05 mg/kg/dose IV or PO daily or every other day	Maximum 0.1 mg/kg/day
Chlorothiazide	20–40 mg/kg/day PO divided into BID 1–4 mg/kg/dose IV q 6–12 hr	
Ethacrynic acid	0.5–1 mg/kg IV q 12–24 hr	
Hydrochlorothiazide	2 mg/kg/day PO divided BID	May increase to QID
Mannitol	0.5–1 gm/kg IV After urine flow is established, lower doses (0.25–0.5 gm/kg) are recommended, q 6 hr as needed	Use with caution in newborns due to hyperosmolarity
Metolazone	0.2–0.4 mg/kg/dose PO once daily	Used with loop diuretic, may increase to BID
Spironolactone	1–3.5 mg/kg/day PO	Caution in combination with ACE inhibitors (may produce hyperkalemia)
Inotropes		
Dopamine	5–28 mcg/kg/min IV	Gradually titrate upward to desired effect
Dobutamine	5–28 mcg/kg/min IV	Gradually titrate upward to desired effect
Agents to Increase Systemic Vascular Resistance		
Phenylephrine	0.5–5 mcg/kg/min IV	
Epinephrine	0.01–1 mcg/kg/min IV	Not to exceed 0.1–0.3 mcg/kg/min
Isoproterenol	0.05–1 mcg/kg/min IV	Not to exceed 0.1–0.3 mcg/kg/min
Norepinephrine	0.05–1 mcg/kg/min IV	Not to exceed 0.1–0.3 mcg/kg/min
Amrinone	5–10 mcg/kg/min IV	Load: 1–3 mg/kg IV over 30 minutes, may cause hypotension
Milrinone	0.5–1 mcg/kg/min IV	Load: 0.1 mg/kg IV over 15–30 min Typically used without loading dose, especially in unstable patients due to hypotension
Vasodilators and Antihypertensives		
Captopril	0.3–1.5 mg/kg/day PO divided q 8 hr	Maximum neonatal dose 3 mg/kg/24 hr
Enalapril	0.1–0.5 mg/kg/day PO once daily or divided into BID	Adults: 2.5–5 mg/day PO daily or BID, not to exceed 40 mg/day
Enalaprilat	0.01–0.05 mg/kg/dose IV	Q 8–24 hr
Hydralazine	0.1–0.5 mg/kg/dose IV; 0.25–0.75 mg/kg/dose PO	For chronic therapy, q 6–8 hr PO or q 4–6 hr IV
Losartan	0.3–1.4 mg/kg	Adults: 25–100 mg/day PO Daily or divided BID
Nifedipine	0.1–0.5mg/kg PO q 8 hr	May depress cardiac contractility in neonates
Nitroprusside	0.5–10 mcg/kg/min IV	May need to monitor cyanide level
Nitroglycerin	0.1–0.5 mcg/kg/min IV	Vasodilator

(Continued)

TABLE 22-27

Therapeutic Agents in Congestive Heart Failure *(Continued)*		
Vasodilators and Antihypertensives *(Continued)*		
Nesiritide	0.01–0.03 mcg/kg/min IV	Initiate with 0.01 mcg/kg/min May cause dose-related hypotension
Nitric oxide	1–40 ppm via inhalation	
Phentolamine	0.05–0.1 mg/kg/dose IV; 2.5–15 mcg/kg/min	Treatment of extravasation (due to dopamine, dobutamine, norepinephrine, or phenylephrine); dilute 5–10 mg in 10 mL normal saline and infiltrate area subcutaneously. Do not exceed 0.1–0.2 mg/kg or 5 mg total.
Prostaglandin E	Initial dose 0.05 mcg/kg/min; 0.01–0.15 mcg/kg/min IV	Tapering to lowest effective dose is recommended because it can cause apnea and hypotension
Beta Blockers		
Atenolol	0.5–4 mg/kg/day PO	Adults: 50–100 mg PO BID
Carvedilol	Limited data suggest a therapeutic dosage range of 0.2–0.4 mg/kg/dose PO BID; initiate with lower dose and gradually increase dose q 2–3 wk to therapeutic range	Adults: 12.5–25 mg PO BID Initiate with 3.125 mg PO BID
Propranolol	0.5–1 mg/kg/day PO	
Esmolol	25–250 mcg/kg/min Can increase in 50–100 mg/kg/min in increments up to 1,000 mcg/kg/min	Load: 500 mcg/kg IV over 2–4 min

Congestive heart failure (CHF), twice daily (BID), by mouth (PO), intravenous (IV), four times daily (QID), angiotensin-converting enzyme (ACE).

the CHF cycle. Studies of ACE inhibitors in pediatric CHF patients are well summarized by Momma (2006):

> ACE inhibitors lower aortic pressure and systemic vascular resistance, do not affect pulmonary vascular resistance significantly, and lower left atrial and right atrial pressures . . . In infants with a large ventricular septal defect and pulmonary hypertension, ACE inhibitors decrease left-to-right shunt in those infants with elevated systemic vascular resistance. ACE inhibitors induce a small increase in left ventricular ejection fraction, left ventricular fractional shortening, and systemic blood flow in children with left ventricular dysfunction, mitral regurgitation, and aortic regurgitation. These beneficial effects usually persist long-term without the development of tolerance. Therapeutic trials of ACE inhibitors have been reported in children with heart failure and divergent hemodynamics, including myocardial dysfunction, left-to-right-shunt . . ., aortic or mitral regurgitation, and Fontan circulation. Hypotension and renal failure usually occur within 5 days after starting ACE inhibition or increasing the dose and, in most cases, recovery is seen after reduction or cessation of the drug. (p. 55)

Angiotensin receptor blockers reduce some of the effects of the RAA system, such as vasoconstriction, sodium and water retention, inhibition of nitric oxide release, and myocardial fibrosis. Aldosterone antagonists act similarly to the angiotensin receptor blockers and reduce myocardial apoptosis. Although they also have an antiarrhythmic effect, these agents predispose patients to hyperkalemia.

Beta blockers counter the activation of the sympathetic nervous system and also slow heart rate, prevent arrhythmias, reduce myocardial apoptosis and fibrosis, and reduce afterload. Developmental differences in patients need to be taken into account when beta blocker therapy is contemplated. The heart begins to beat as early as the fourth week of gestation and is fully formed between 6 and 7 weeks' gestation. The myocardium continues to develop until approximately 6 months after birth. Beta receptors are tonically stimulated in the fetal/newborn heart, and this stimulation is necessary for cardiomyocyte proliferation. Beta blockade would, therefore, reduce the number of cardiomyocytes in the young heart.

The concept of intervening medically at the level of inflammatory pathways, by inhibiting the systemic inflammatory response, has only recently been examined. Modified ultrahemofiltration during CPB has proven beneficial. Pharmacologic agents under study for this indication include steroids, nonsteroidal anti-inflammatory drugs (NSAIDs), and interferon.

It would seem logical to treat reduced cardiac contractility with strategies that would increase cardiac contractility, but doing so accelerates CHF cycle progression. More favorable longer-term outcomes have been achieved by administering drugs that transiently reduce contractility while maintaining adequate perfusion pressure and that block longer-term deleterious effects of neurohormonal stimulation. Inotropes, for example, stimulate cardiac contractility and/or produce peripheral vasoconstriction to maintain tissue perfusion. Inotropes, calcium-channel blockers, and antiarrhythmics may all increase morbidity and mortality in this population, however, and should be used with caution. Myofilament Ca sensitizers have shown promise in adult patients, but some evidence indicates that signal transduction and calcium homeostasis affects contractility differently in the immature myocardium; thus this approach requires formal study in children before it is recommended. There are currently no data as to whether antiarrhythmic, anticoagulant, or antiplatelet agents have any effect on morbidity and mortality in either children or adults with heart failure. (Refer to Table 22-27 for a list of therapeutic agents used to treat CHF.)

The institution of mechanical cardiac support should be considered primarily as a bridge to transplant in patients with acute decompensation. Mechanical support may be considered in patients who have experienced cardiac arrest, hypoxia with pulmonary hypertension, or severe ventricular dysfunction with low cardiac output after surgery, including those who fail to wean off CPB or have myocarditis (Rosenthal et al., 2004).

Medical therapies will not be successful if basic human needs are not first met. Therefore, the most important treatment for pediatric heart failure is nutrition in the form of maximized caloric density and necessary nutrients. Other basic needs include physical closeness to family members, exercise as tolerated, consistency of daily activities, exposure to sunlight, music, meticulous dental hygiene, and psychosocial expression from play.

In CHF, myocardial cells die from energy starvation. Pediatric CHF patients have increased metabolic demands, requiring a minimum of require 120 to 160 kcal/kg/day to thrive. The quality of those calories is as important as the quantity. Attention should be given to the nutritional status of the breastfeeding mother, as well as the contents of formulas and supplementations given to infants in CHF. Likewise, attention must be paid to the contents of enteral formulas for tube-fed infants and children and parenteral formulas for critically ill children. The practice guidelines set forth by the International Society for Heart and Lung Transplantation (Rosenthal et al., 2004) provide pharmaceutical management strategies, but do not include specific essential nutrient requirements for pediatric patients with heart failure.

The scientific community is now beginning to recognize the importance of micronutrients and to study bioavailability and supplemental formulations. A vast body of literature exists that provides specific information about the scientific basis and clinical trials of nutritional supplements. The best and safest way for any person to ingest bioactive nutrients is through a varied, healthy diet.

A healthy diet consists of fruits, vegetables, whole grains, fish, beans, eggs, nuts, lean meat, and poultry. Foods to be avoided are high in fat, cholesterol, salt, and sugar. Intake of fried foods and hydrogenated oils results in ignition of the systemic inflammatory response as measured by rise in C-reactive protein (CRP). By contrast, fiber intake can counteract the inflammatory response and lower CRP levels. For example, cocoa may help activate nitric oxide to improve endothelial function and can be easily added to milk. Omega-3 fatty acids have anti-inflammatory attributes and are available now in fruit-flavored gummies for children.

Vitamins C, E, and B-complex are important for fetal development, cardiac function, and cell repair and have recently been shown to improve heart failure. Necessary minerals include zinc, chromium, magnesium, calcium, and selenium. Many nutrients traditionally used for their beneficial effects on the cardiovascular system have recently been scientifically validated. One example is nattokinase, a natural potent fibrin inhibitor. Similarly, serrepeptase digests thrombi and possibly arterial plaque; it has been used in Asia and Europe for more than 25 years. Glutamine reduces infectious complications. Eicosapentaenoic acid has significant anti-inflammatory effects. Ethylene diaminetetracetic acid, alpha lipoic acid, quercetin, policosanol, phytosterols, lecithin, bilberry, ginkgo biloba, garlic, curcumin, and the amino acids L-argine, L-taurine, and L-carnitine bring in long-chain fatty acids across the mitochondrial membrane, where they produce biological energy in the form of adenosine triphosphate (ATP). D-Ribose, a sugarlike molecule, is a powerful substrate for L-carnitine and coenzyme Q10 (CoQ10).

CoQ10 is a micronutrient that provides nourishment for the cellular mitochondria. Levels of this nutrient begin to decrease after age 20 years, and supplementation in adult patients with CHF has produced impressive results. Cardiac metabolism is directly associated with this mitochondrial respiratory chain, and as many as 25% of all cardiomyopathies are associated with mitochondrial disease. In a small study presented at the Third World Congress on Pediatric Cardiology and Cardiac Surgery, researchers reported treating three children with dilated cardiomyopathy with CoQ10. These patients, who were 4 to 12 months of age with New York Heart Association (NYHA; Connolly et al., 2001) class III heart disease, were given CoQ10 mixed with soya oil, 10 mg/day, twice daily, and were followed for a mean of 6 months. The CoQ10 was delivered as an adjunct to their standard therapy, which consisted of an ACE inhibitor, diuretics, and digoxin. After receiving CoQ10, the severity of the patients' heart disease classification decreased from NYHA class III to NYHA class I. They also experienced a significant change in fractional shortening (a measure of ventricular function) and a significant increase in left ventricular ejection fraction. Chest radiograph revealed a decrease in cardiothoracic ratio. ECG also revealed a regression of left ventricular hypertrophy and a complete disappearance of left ventricular strain. Other antioxidants are still in evaluation, awaiting well-designed clinical trials to elucidate their value in this indication.

Regardless of the etiology of CHF, the clinical presentation of the infant or child can range from an early stage of mild tachycardia to fully decompensated failure and hemodynamic instability. The child should be admitted to the intensive care unit and stabilized. Once the patient is stable, the cardiology service should be consulted to assist with management. The diagnostic evaluation should include a baseline CXR, echocardiograph, ECG, and labs including viral and bacterial studies. Depending on the findings, a cardiac catheterization or endomyocardial biopsy may be scheduled (Breinholt et al., 2008). Based on the limited availability of pediatric donor organs, consultation with the cardiac transplant service should be considered early in the course of the disease. Care is interdisciplinary and coordinated between the critical care and cardiology services, with support from nutrition, pharmacy, and child life specialists as needed.

There are many opportunities throughout the intensive care and inpatient stay to educate the patient and family about the etiology for the CHF, the expected trajectory of illness, and the goals of care. Exercise limitations, fluid and dietary restrictions, medication administration, illness prevention, and the child's ability to return to school are all questions that families have in regard to their children at discharge. A list of basic signs and symptoms of CHF should be given to the caregivers as well as a detailed list of medications and the rationale for their use.

DISPOSITION AND DISCHARGE PLANNING

The discharge planner or social worker provides expertise to arrange home care for those patients who need durable medical equipment (DME) or home health services after discharge. Care needs vary widely based on the reversability of the CHF and its underlying cause.

Prognosis also varies depending on the etiology of CHF. In infants presenting with acute myocarditis, the mortality rate can exceed 75%. By comparison, in the older infant and child, the mortality rate is in the range of 10% to 25%. However, those children who do not have resolution of cardiac dysfunction will often be left with chronic dilated cardiomyopathy (DCM) and may require heart transplantation. In the child with DCM, there can be complete resolution of the dysfunction, progression of ventricular dysfunction requiring heart transplantation, or death (Jefferies, 2008). In children who present with CHF secondary to structural abnormalities, such as anomalous left coronary artery from the pulmonary artery (ALCAPA) or aortic arch obstruction, there may be full resolution of the CHF after surgical correction. Children who have nonsurgical causes of CHF may initially do well with medical management

but become resistant over time to therapy and relapse. Some require ICDs to prevent sudden cardiac death.

Close monitoring by cardiology services and primary care providers, and attention to details of nutrition and medication administration by the patient and family, will lessen the number of CHF relapses.

EXTRACORPOREAL LIFE SUPPORT

Steven A. McDonald

Initially described as extracorporeal membrane oxygenation (ECMO), the new term *extracorporeal life support* (ECLS) better reflects the expanded group of available devices used to support the heart and lungs.

EXTRACORPOREAL MEMBRANE OXYGENATION

ECMO is a short-term use resuscitative tool to enhance cardiac or pulmonary function when the underlying condition is reversible. ECMO was first developed to sustain the pulmonary system in the immediate postoperative period following cardiopulmonary bypass. It was not until 1971 that this technology was described as a life-saving therapy for patients outside of the postoperative setting (Van Meurs, 1999). Since then, ECMO has gone through a series of improvements and is now used for patients of all ages and conditions. As of 2008, some 36,466 patients worldwide had been supported with ECMO, with an overall survival rate of 64% (Mayock, 2009).

ECMO technology is highly invasive and requires dedicated professionals who have specialized training—one person to manage the circuit and another person to manage the patient. For medium- and long-term needs, a second device, the ventricular assist device (VAD), was developed.

Indications

Pediatric patients who experience critical primary or secondary cardiac failure, respiratory failure, septic shock, submersion injury, or severe hypothermia may be candidates for ECMO (Guenther et al., 2009). ECMO has also been applied to support pediatric patients in a low cardiac output state following heart surgery, idiopathic cardiomyopathy, cardiac failure secondary to viral illness, or chemotherapy (Farouk et al., 2009; Freilich et al., 2009; Suzuki et al., 2009). This strategy also allows for reduction in adverse effects by minimizing therapeutic ventilator and cardiovascular agent support. It can be considered for use as a therapeutic bridge to cardiac transplant (Imamura et al., 2009).

Congenital diaphragmatic hernia in the newborn is the second most common cause of respiratory failure treated by ECMO (Haricharan et al., 2009). However, as high-frequency oscillatory ventilation and therapeutic strategies to manage persistent fetal circulation have gained widespread acceptance, the number of patients requiring ECMO has steadily declined (Pawlik et al., 2009). Contraindications in the neonatal population have been better established through collection of evidence associated with poor outcomes (Table 22-28).

Description and management

Two types of ECMO exist: veno-arterial (VA) and veno-venous (VV). *Veno-arterial* ECMO is more common and provides heart and lungs support; consequently, it is used primarily for patients with cardiopulmonary failure. In contrast, *veno-venous* ECMO supports oxygenation and ventilation and is based on the premise that the patient has sufficient cardiac output. Although there is no direct cardiac support with VV ECMO, cardiac function may improve as a result of the better oxygenation, left-sided filling pressures, and pulmonary flow. Occasionally, patients require transition from VV ECMO to VA ECMO if subsequent cardiac failure ensues.

VV ECMO circuits can use either a single two-phase cannula with both an inlet and an outlet or two separate venous cannulation sites. The advantage of using two sites is that very limited recirculation occurs; the disadvantage is the risk to reduced distal extremity venous blood flow (Haley et al., 2009). Recirculation occurs when oxygenated blood flowing from the ECLS circuit to the patient is returned in the direction of the pump through the inflow lumen of the cannula. VV ECMO provides a higher level of oxygenated blood to the pulmonary circulation, thereby relaxing the smooth muscle, and is optimal if increased pulmonary vascular resistance is contributing to the pulmonary hypertension.

VA ECMO differs from VV support in that it provides both cardiac and pulmonary support (Figure 22-47). VA ECMO supports the patient with no recirculation; it maximizes efficiency and provides the patient with a higher partial pressure of oxygen in the arterial blood (PaO_2).

TABLE 22-28

Relative Contraindications of Extracorporeal ECLS

- Neonatal ECLS
  - Birth weight < 2,000 grams
  - Gestational age < 34 weeks
  - Significant bleeding or coagulopathy
  - Major intracranial hemorrhage (> grade 1)
  - Ventilator days > 10–14 days
  - Lethal malformations or irreversible condition
- Pediatric ECLS
  - Irreversible condition

Extracorporeal life support (ECLS).

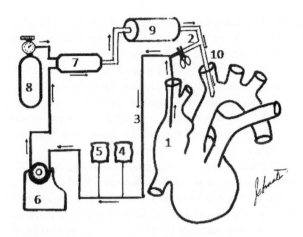

FIGURE 22-47

Extracorporeal Membrane Oxygenation Circuit.

Note: Superior vena cava cannula (1), bridge (2), venous line (3), fluids (4), heparin (5), roller pump (6), oxygenator (7), oxygenator (8), membrane (9), aortic cannula (10).

Source: Used with permission. Courtesy of Joseph J. Amato, MD MJ. All Rights Reserved.

Higher efficiency allows the VA ECMO pump to spin at lower speeds, thereby minimizing red blood cell damage. In the patient with elevated pulmonary artery pressures, VA ECMO directly decreases the volume of blood entering the pulmonary circulation, whereas VV ECMO provides a higher level of oxygenated blood to the pulmonary circulation.

The primary disadvantage of VA ECMO is the requirement to access a major artery to return blood from the ECMO circuit to the patient. This technique increases the risk of embolism of air, thrombus or other foreign material (Haines et al., 2009). The majority of patients are supported with VA ECMO despite these risks because of the clear benefit they receive from its cardiac and pulmonary support. It is often difficult to determine if or when a patient who presents in pulmonary failure will progress to cardiopulmonary failure, so many patient are placed directly onto VA ECMO.

Cannulation is based on the specific need for the therapy and the age and size of the patient. Patients who require ECMO for cardiac support after cardiac surgery are often cannulated centrally, with the venous cannula placed in the right atrium and the arterial return placed near the ascending aorta. Occasionally, a left atrial cannula is added to assist in decompression of the left side of the heart. Essential aspects of the cannula positioning affect monitoring requirements and ECMO circuit venous saturations. Although there may be institutional variation in the ECMO equipment deployed, the premise and application of its use are consistent.

Neonates tend to require only respiratory support; thus they are most often placed on VV ECMO. This support is accomplished through a single cannula placed percutaneously in the internal jugular and positioned to limit recirculation. If the patient also requires cardiac support, he or she is instead placed on VA ECMO. This support is accomplished by placing the cannulae through the internal jugular vein and the internal carotid artery. Although access can be obtained without a sternal incision, the services of a trained surgeon are required to cannulate the vessels.

Oxygenators vary in both construction and design. The common feature in all models, however, is blood flow on one side of a semipermeable membrane and a gas on the other side. The blood and gas flow in opposite directions to optimize the interface. Ventilation is controlled by the speed at which the gas travels through the oxygenator; and oxygen delivery is determined by the percentage of oxygen present in the gas phase. The efficiency of the oxygenator can be determined by measuring premembrane and post-membrane blood gases, specifically the decrease in the carbon dioxide and the increase in oxygen concentrations (Zwischenberger et al., 2000). The efficiency of gas exchange will decrease with older oxygenators.

Exposure of blood to artificial surfaces activates clotting cascades and requires intervention to prevent thrombus formation; this factor affects oxygenator effectiveness. Management of the patient on ECMO requires balancing stable anticoagulation with prevention of acute hemorrhage. The ECMO circuit components are often heparin bonded to decrease the likelihood of thrombus formation. Unfractionated heparin, which is easily titrated, is the standard medication used for this purpose. A disadvantage is that it requires frequent blood sampling to monitor effectiveness.

Normal cardiac function is pulsatile. The nonpulsatile, continuous flow from ECMO results in decreased pulse pressure due to the significant portion of the patient's cardiac output that goes through the circuit rather than through the heart. A disadvantage of this type of flow is that it can result in lower end-organ perfusion and higher risk for systemic inflammatory response syndrome (Ji & Undar, 2006). Mean arterial blood pressure, rather than systolic pressure, is monitored to guide therapy. Preload and afterload remain essential concepts for management of patient hemodynamics even while the patient is on ECMO, because the same principles apply to the ECMO pump as to the heart. Decreased preload will decrease the amount of blood the ECMO pump can deliver, whereas increased afterload will decrease cardiac output of the pump due to the increased resistance to flow (Zwischenberger et al., 2000).

Emergencies associated with ECMOS

Invasive cardiopulmonary support increases risk for significant morbidity and mortality; thus, the HCP must be ready to identify and respond to emergencies (Table 22-29).

Weaning

Weaning the patient off ECMO requires decreasing the amount of support provided by the ECMO circuit while monitoring the patient's response. In this step-by-step process, the patient's response provides information about the probability of success (Table 22-30). The ECMO perfusionist or technician adjusts the circuit flow or pulse over time. Serial monitoring of the patient's hemodynamics and oxygenation is required throughout the weaning effort.

VENTRICULAR ASSIST DEVICES

Indications

The development of VADs has allowed for moderate- to long-term therapeutic cardiac support. The VAD supports univentricular or biventricular heart function through the use of either one or two pumps, respectively. If two pumps are used to provide biventricular support, they are placed in series. Pulsatile pumps can be set to eject simultaneously or synchronized to provide the patient with maximal support.

Contraindications for VADs are similar to those for ECMO (Table 22-28), although this issue has not been examined as vigorously for VADs owing to the limited experience with these devices. Individual devices also vary in design, size, and function, so each will have its own set of limitations and device-specific contraindications. For instance, implantable VADs require the patient to be significantly larger than VADs that incorporate an external pump design.

Description and management

Univentricular assist device consist of either a *left ventricular assist device* (LVAD) or a *right ventricular assist device* (RVAD) (Figure 22-48). Placement of a LVAD requires adequate right heart function and normal pulmonary vascular resistance to ensure left ventricular filling or preload. Likewise, placement of a RVAD requires adequate left ventricular function and adequate systemic venous return.

The original pumps used nonpulsatile, continuous flow via roller pump or centrifugal technology, and were adapted from traditional CPB or ECMO circuits. More recently, axial flow or impeller pumps have been developed to provide pulsatile flow (more similar to the heart's natural flow) and reduce the problems associated with continuous flow.

Pulsatile pumps provide a flow that resembles the physiologic flow within a solid housing. The components of this housing, which is divided into a blood cavity and an air chamber, are separated by a flexible membrane. These VADs are attached to a driver, which supplies air pressure

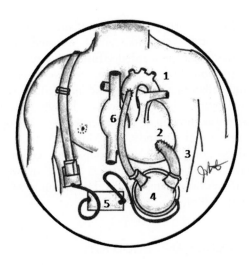

FIGURE 22-48

Left Ventricular Assist Device.

Note: Aorta (1), left ventricle (2), in-flow hose (3), prosthetic left ventricle (4), system control (5), out-flow hose (6).

Source: Used with permission. Courtesy of Joseph J. Amato, MD MJ. All Rights Reserved.

essential for pump flow. Air forces the membrane to move; pumping a bolus of blood at the same time that forward flow is ensured by valves built into the device. Pulsatile VADs have a set rate that is independent of the patient's intrinsic heart rate, which creates varying degrees of synchrony between the VAD and the patient's intrinsic cardiac output. Either the two pumps may work in concert to augment systolic pressure, or the VAD may eject blood into the aorta as the heart is simultaneously attempting to eject blood. The latter approach creates asynchrony and is important to consider when weaning from the device, or during normal monitoring of pulse oximetry and peripheral pulses.

Many VADs can be implanted in a corporeal manner, so that only the electrical or pneumatic drive line exits the patient and attaches to the mechanical driver. Most infants and small children, however, require paracorporeal VADs. With these devices, the inflow and outflow cannulae exit through the patient's soft tissue and dermis. This approach creates unique and challenging skin care issues and is associated with an increased risk of bleeding and infection.

For patients on VADs who require longer-term anticoagulation, low-molecular-weight heparin or warfarin, as well as platelet inhibition, are used to prevent thrombus formation. Aspirin and dipyridamol may be used as platelet inhibition agents, and their effectiveness is monitored with a thromboelastogram test. Expect each institution and device to have specific guidelines and monitoring recommendations for thrombus prevention.

Ventricular devices assist cardiac function and improve oxygen delivery to tissues; therefore, patients require frequent monitoring of end-organ perfusion and oxygen delivery (regional tissue) for early recognition of suboptimal therapy. Diagnostic markers used for monitoring global ischemia include venous blood saturation, lactic acid level, and evaluation of metabolic acidosis.

To compensate for compromised regional tissue perfusion, the VAD flow rate can be increased. This acceleration results in increased blood flow through the cannula and decreased ventricular afterload. However, an increased flow rate may also lead to greater red blood cell damage and increased free hemoglobin in the plasma. Medications such as milrinone or sodium nitroprusside, which decrease afterload, may improve tissue perfusion and have the desired effect or can be used in combination with increased pump flow (Zwischenberger et al., 2000).

Emergencies associated with VAD

Invasive cardiopulmonary support increases risk for significant morbidity and mortality; thus, the HCP must be ready to identify and respond to emergencies (Table 22-29).

Weaning

Weaning of the patient off a VAD shares many of the same principles as weaning of the patient off ECLS (Table 22-30).

TABLE 22-29

Emergencies Scenarios on Extracorporeal Life Support or with a Ventricular Assist Device
• Emergencies include:
• Bleeding
• Hypotension
• Air in the circuit
• Embolism
• Device failure
• Chest compressions are generally contraindicated because of the cannula
• Volume restoration is important to ensure adequate pump filling
• Especially important with single ventricle VADs
• Blood products should be constantly available at the bedside
• Dysrhythmias will affect all patients except those on total ventricular-assisted ECLS
• Medication to increase native heart function may be needed for device failure
• Emergency ventilator settings should be readily available at the bedside for device failure
• Emergency drills ensure effective staff response

Extracorporeal life support (ECLS), ventricular assist device (VAD).

TABLE 22-30

Weaning of Extracorporeal Life Support

- Ensure adequate cardiac recovery:
  - Pulse pressure represents the patient's own cardiac function
  - Pulsatile pumps require other testing: heart catheterization or echocardiography
- Pulmonary recovery for patient on VA ECLS:
  - ECLS gas flow rates and FiO_2 can be weaned
  - A traditional ventilator a used to support the patient
  - Blood gas analysis is used to monitor adequacy of support
- Preparing for a trial off support:
  - Ensure ready access to emergency medications and intravascular volume
  - Start inotropic medications early to ensure adequate delivery
  - Institute emergency ventilator settings prior to trial off support
  - Continuously monitor the patient during the weaning process
- Decrease the flow rate if on continuous flow:
  - Full support = 100–150 mL/kg/min
  - Minimal flow = 50 mL/min
- Lower flow rates will require more aggressive anticoagulation
- Decrease the rate of VAD support if on pulsatile flow
- Serial blood gas analysis to monitor end-organ perfusion and oxygen delivery
- Success is the patient being supported with conventional therapies off ECLS

Extracorporeal life support (ECLS), ventricular assist device (VAD).

Due to the long-term support provided with VADs, the weaning process may occur at much less frequent intervals and take much longer to accomplish. Device-specific factors dictate the weaning process to be used. Whereas continuous-flow pumps are weaned through a decrease in the flow rate, pulsatile pumps have the rate of pulsation deceased to ensure that the pump continues to empty completely.

POSTPERICARDIOTOMY SYNDROME

Karen Corlett

Postpericardiotomy syndrome (PPS) occurs after tissue injury to the myocardium, most commonly after cardiopulmonary bypass. It has also been reported after thoracic trauma, myocardial infarction (Dressler's syndrome), pacemaker placement, and repair of pectus excavatum (Berberich et al., 2004; Cabalka et al., 1995; Cheung et al., 2003; Muensterer et al., 2003; Zeltser et al., 2004).

At first PPS was attributed to an inflammatory response associated with fever, leukocytosis, elevated inflammatory markers, and pericardial effusion due to postoperative reactivation of rheumatic fever; however, pretreatment with anti-inflammatory drugs did not reduce the incidence (Maisch et al., 1979; Mott et al., 2001). Later, this syndrome was thought to be associated with the opening of the pericardial sac and CPB. More recently, antiheart antibodies, complement activation, and cell-mediated immunity have been postulated as having an important role in the development of PPS (Hoffmann et al., 2002; Meri et al., 1985).

EPIDEMIOLOGY AND ETIOLOGY

The frequency rate of PPS in adults and older pediatric patients is similar. Nevertheless, its incidence varies significantly with the patient's age, gender, and type of inciting event, and has been reported to be as low as 2% and as high as 50%. The variation in reported rates of occurrence may be influenced by the lack of a standard set of diagnostic criteria or postoperative monitoring with echocardiography (Mott et al., 2001; Zeltser et al., 2004). PPS occurs less frequently in infants, and more frequently in females and patients following closure of atrial or ventricular septal defects. What triggers the cascade of events remains unclear. Viral exposure—to organisms such as coxsackie B, adenovirus, and cytomegalovirus, for example—has been found in approximately two-thirds of patients with PPS; in prospective studies, however, a viral etiology for this condition was not confirmed (Cabalka et al., 1995; Descheerder et al., 1984; Engle et al., 1980; Maisch et al., 1979; Webber et al., 2001).

PRESENTATION

Presentation of PPS most commonly occurs within 1 to 2 weeks after surgery or the inciting event—typically, after the patient is discharged home. The most common symptom is fever. Other early symptoms include irritability, decreased appetite, and anterior pleuritic chest pain. Young children often cannot isolate the chest pain in the same way as older children or young adults, resulting instead in a report of listlessness by the caregiver.

The symptoms of PPS are associated with the accumulation of pericardial fluid. As the volume of the fluid in the pericardial sac increases, the initial symptoms may progress to fatigue at rest and mild respiratory distress or shortness of breath. On physical examination, an audible pericardial friction rub may be noted with smaller fluid accumulations. Heart sounds become more distant and friction rubs may become inaudible as the volume of pericardial fluid increases.

Pericardial tamponade occurs when the pericardial effusion is of a size whereby venous return is impeded and contractility impaired. Physical examination findings associated with tamponade include significantly muffled heart sounds, jugular vein distention, and hypotension—a pattern collectively referred to as Beck's triad. Other findings of decreased venous return and poor cardiac output include respiratory failure, tachycardia, narrowed pulse pressure, and poor peripheral perfusion.

DIFFERENTIAL DIAGNOSIS

The following disorders and diseases have similar presenting findings to PPS: endocarditis, myocarditis, pericarditis, and congestive heart failure.

PLAN OF CARE

Most patients with presumed PPS have had a cardiac surgical instrumentation of some kind; consequently, the immediate evaluation must include diagnostic studies focusing on cardiac function and infection. Obtain a complete blood count (CBC) with differential, blood cultures, and wound cultures if drainage is present. Cardiac enzymes such as troponin 1, creatine phosphokinase MB (CKMB), brain natriuretic peptide (BNP), and lactate levels provide insight into myocardial injury and systemic perfusion. Associated findings for PPS include leukocytosis and elevated inflammatory markers such as erythrocyte sedimentation rate (ESR) and C-reactive protein (CRP).

Chest radiographs (anterior-posterior, lateral) may reveal enlargement in the size of the cardiac silhouette indicative of a pericardial effusion. This finding may be best appreciated when comparisons to previous radiographs can be made. CXRs are also helpful to evaluate for other causes of fever and respiratory distress, such as pleural effusions, atelectasis, or pneumonia. Electrocardiograph tracings may reveal diffuse ST-segment elevation early in the course of PPS, or flattened T waves and decreased QRS amplitude as the pericardial effusion enlarges and causes further compression of the ventricles (Tanel, 2005). Echocardiograph is diagnostic and will define the size of the effusion and its impingement on cardiac function.

The therapeutic management of PPS is empirical and initially based on use of anti-inflammatory medications and rest. Postoperative prophylaxis with acetylsalicylic acid (ASA) or methylprednisolone administered prior to or following CPB has not been proven effective in reducing the incidence of PPS (Gill et al., 2009; Mott et al., 2001).

Once PPS is diagnosed, a 5- to 7-day course of NSAIDs such as ibuprofen or ketorolac is well tolerated in pediatric patients; however, therapy may be required for several weeks. Systemic steroids may also be administered as first-line therapy, but are often reserved for recurrent or recalcitrant pericardial effusions due to their adverse side effects (Muensterer et al., 2003). Methotrexate has been used successfully for chronic PPS (Zucker et al., 2003). Colchicine, which is typically used for joint inflammation, has shown promise in treating PPS in studies of patients who are older than 18 years of age (Finkelstein et al., 2002; Imazio et al., 2007). Diuretics are a useful adjunct therapy for larger effusions.

Patients presenting with effusions not controlled by medication, with significantly compromised cardiac output, or with cardiac tamponade require drainage of the pericardial effusion via echocardiograph-guided pericardiocentesis. Isotonic intravenous fluids should be immediately available at the time of the procedure: Upon relief of the restrictive pericardial effusion, circulating volume will likely be insufficient. A pericardial catheter may be left in place to allow for ongoing drainage of fluid from the pericardial space, although it is removed once drainage volume is minimal. A fluid sample can be examined for infectious etiology, however, most such samples are sterile. For recurrent pericardial effusions, surgical creation of a pericardial window, allowing for drainage of fluid without restriction to the pericardial space, may be performed (Zeltser et al., 2004).

Consultation with the following subspecialties will enhance the care of a patient with PPS: cardiology, cardiothoracic surgery, critical care, pulmonology, surgery services, and infectious disease. Given that patients may require additional hospital care, social and spiritual support, child life, nutrition, and the rehabilitative team may be consulted as needed.

Caregiver education should include review of recurrent PPS or pericardial effusion symptomology such as chest pain, fever (less likely), decreased endurance, fatigue, respiratory distress, and cardiac collapse. Also, specific direction as to when to seek emergency care should be given. Caregivers should also be informed about the importance of continuing therapy for the prescribed time period and instructed to watch for signs of gastrointestinal irritation or bleeding and kidney problems. Inform families that many of the medications used for PPS may mask a fever. Patients on a steroid taper require a written schedule and review of potential side effects of transient immunosuppression, hyperglycemia, hunger, hypertension, and compromised wound healing.

DISPOSITION AND DISCHARGE PLANNING

Most cases of PPS resolve completely after treatment or drainage, with defervescence, relief of chest pain, and resolution of pericardial effusion. Because recurrence is possible, patients should return to the pediatric cardiologist for follow-up after discharge to evaluate resolution of effusion by echocardiograph.

PULMONARY HYPERTENSION

Deborah Walter

PATHOPHYSIOLOGY

Pulmonary hypertension (PH) is defined as a mean pulmonary artery pressure greater than 25 mmHg at rest. To qualify as the subcategory of pulmonary arterial hypertension (PAH), the pulmonary arterial wedge pressure must be 15 mmHg or less (Badesch et al., 2007).

Pulmonary vascular reactivity is maintained by a complex interaction or synthesis and/or by the activation or inactivation of vasoactive hormones. Balance among these substances influences vascular tone and reactivity in the normal and pathologic state. An important factor in the regulation of pulmonary vascular tone is the balance of nitric oxide (NO, a vasodilator), prostacyclin (a vasodilator), and endothelin (a vasoconstrictor). Over time, impaired production of these vasoactive mediators can adversely affect vascular tone and promote vascular remodeling. Predominant vascular changes include vasoconstriction, smooth muscle and endothelial cell proliferation, and thrombosis.

PH is caused by vasoconstriction of the pulmonary vascular bed as well as proliferation of endothelial and smooth muscle cells. Development of medial hypertrophy of the arterioles can lead to muscularization, resulting in decreased size of the vessel lumen and eventually leading to the loss of small pulmonary arterioles. Histopathologic studies will reveal medial hypertrophy, intimal proliferation and fibrosis, and thrombotic lesions, which can be unevenly distributed throughout the pulmonary vasculature (Pietra et al., 1989).

Vasoconstriction reduces alveolar oxygen tension, resulting in alveolar hypoxia that eventually leads to reduced nitric oxide production and increased endothelin production. Pulmonary vascular resistance (PVR) is significantly increased when acidosis is present, as acidosis and hypoxia work synergistically. An increase in pulmonary blood flow or PVR can, therefore, result in PH. The normally thin-walled right ventricle is unable to sustain a rapid increase in pulmonary artery pressure (PAP) of more than 40 to 50 mmHg, thereby resulting in right heart failure. However, if PAP increases gradually, the RV hypertrophies and may tolerate higher pressures, at times approaching systemic to suprasystemic pressures.

EPIDEMIOLOGY AND ETIOLOGY

The incidence of PH in children and adults is largely unknown. The estimated incidence of idiopathic pulmonary arterial hypertension (IPAH) ranges from 1 to 2 new cases per 1 million people in the general population (Ivy et al., 2009; Rosenzweig et al., 2004). Pediatric patients with PH commonly present with nonspecific symptoms and subtle physical examination findings; as a consequence, the disease may go undiagnosed or be misdiagnosed as another condition. Technological advances have aided in making earlier diagnoses and definitive determinations of severity. In addition, new therapeutic options have improved quality of life, exercise capacity, hemodynamics, and survival among persons with PH.

The classification of PH has undergone a number of changes since first proposed and endorsed by the World Health Organization (WHO) in 1973. Since that time, meetings in France in 1998 (Evian Classification), Venice in 2003, and Dana Point, California, in 2008 have further modified the classification to better reflect current research and knowledge as to the etiology of PH (Beghetti, 2006; Simonneau et al., 2009) (Table 22-31).

Category 1 of the PH classification system has histopathological similarities to PAH associated with congenital heart disease lesions. This group of patients is grossly identical to those patients with IPA; therefore, the pathobiological mechanisms are thought to be similar (Beghetti, 2006). Patients with increased pulmonary blood flow or pressure are at risk to develop increased pulmonary vascular resistance. In patients with CHD, determining the degree and reversibility of pulmonary vascular disease (PVD) related to systemic-to-pulmonary shunts is important, as it allows for prediction of best outcome after surgical repair. Four variables affect the likelihood of reversal of PVD after cardiac repair: (1) type of cardiac lesion, (2) age of the patient at time of repair, (3) PVR at time of repair, and (4) interaction of genetic and environmental factors unique to the patient (Kulik et al., 2009).

PRESENTATION

The most successful approach in identifying and developing a therapeutic PH management plan is to determine and treat the underlying cause (Depta & Krasuski, 2009). Obtaining a thorough history to evaluate for known causes of PH and performing a comprehensive physical examination (Table 22-32) will direct the HCP as to necessary diagnostic studies and treatment strategies (Rosenzweig et al., 2009).

TABLE 22-31

Clinical Classifications of Pulmonary Hypertension, 2008

1. Pulmonary arterial hypertension (PAH)
   1.1 Idiopathic PAH
   1.2 Heritable
       1.2.1 BMPR2
       1.2.2 ALK-1 endoglin (with or without hereditary hemorrhagic hemangiomatosis)
       1.2.3 Unknown
   1.3 Drug and toxin induced
   1.4 Associated with
       1.4.1 Connective tissue diseaseHuman immunodeficiency virus (HIV) infection
       1.4.2 Portal hypertension
       1.4.3 Congenital heart disease
       1.4.4 Schistomasomiasis
       1.4.5 Chronic hemolytic anemia
   1.5 Persistent pulmonary hypertension of the newborn.
   1.6 Pulmonary veno-occlusive disease (PVOD) and/or pulmonary capillary hemangiomatosis (PCH)

2. Pulmonary hypertension due to left heart disease
   2.1 Systolic dysfunction
   2.2 Diastolic dysfunction
   2.3 Valvular disease

3. Pulmonary hypertension due to lung disease and/or hypoxia
   3.1 Chronic obstructive pulmonary disease
   3.2 Interstitial lung disease
   3.3 Other pulmonary diseases with mixed restrictive and obstructive pattern
   3.4 Sleep disordered breathing
   3.5 Alveolar hypoventilation disorders
   3.6 Chronic exposure to high altitude
   3.7 Developmental abnormalities

4. Chronic thromboembolic pulmonary hypertension (CTEPH)

5. Pulmonary hypertension with unclear multifactorial mechanisms
   5.1 Hematologic disorders: myeloproliferative disorders, splenectomy
   5.2 Systemic disorders: sarcoidosis, pulmonary Langerhans cell histiocytosis, lymphangioleiomyomatosis, neurofibromatosis, vasculitis
   5.3 Metabolic disorders: glycogen storage disease, Gaucher disease, thyroid disorders
   5.4 Others: tumoral obstruction, fibrosing mediastinitis, chronic kidney failure on dialysis

Pulmonary arterial hypertension (PAH), bone morphogenetic protein receptor type II (BMPR2), activin receptor-like kinase I (ALK-I).

Source: Adapted from Simonneau et al., 2009.

TABLE 22-32

Pulmonary Hypertension History and Physical Examination

History

Family history of pulmonary hypertension
Drug use (diet pills, contraceptives, methamphetamines)
Prior cardiac and other surgeries
Complete review of systems
Residence at high altitude

Signs and Symptoms

Infants: Poor feeding, tachypnea, cyanotic spells, failure-to-thrive, irritability, syncope
Children: dyspnea, chest pain, shortness-of-breath, decreased exercise tolerance, syncope, seizures

Physical Examination

Right ventricular lift
Loud second heart sound
Tricuspid regurgitation murmur
Pulmonary insufficiency murmur
Jugular venous distention
Signs of right heart failure:
• Hepatosplenomegaly
• Gallop rhythm
• Peripheral edema
Cyanosis

Source: Adapted from Rosenzweig et al., 2009.

DIFFERENTIAL DIAGNOSIS

The differential diagnosis for PH may vary depending on the presenting acuity and known comorbidities. Refer to Table 22-31 for a list of recognized diagnoses.

PLAN OF CARE

Cardiac catheterization is the considered the study of choice for diagnosis of PH, as it can define the following structural and functional components of the cardiopulmonary system:

• Anatomy: measuring pressures and oxygen saturations throughout the heart
• Pulmonary arteries and pulmonary veins: calculating shunts and pulmonary vascular resistance

A comprehensive list of laboratory and diagnostic imaging studies appears in Table 22-33 (Mullen, 2010; Rosenzweig et al., 2009).

Determining the vasoreactivity of the pulmonary vascular bed facilitates decision making based on the consensus

TABLE 22-33

Pulmonary Hypertension Diagnostic Studies and Evaluation

Chest radiograph (cardiomegaly and enlarged pulmonary arteries)

Electrocardiograph (right ventricular hypertrophy and/or ST-T changes)

Echocardiograph (right ventricular hypertrophy, exclude congenital heart disease, quantify right ventricular systolic pressure)

Cardiac Catheterization with acute vasodilator testing (evaluate pulmonary artery pressure and resistance and degree of pulmonary vasoreactivity)

Liver evaluation:
- Liver function tests
- Abdominal ultrasound (portopulmonary hypertension)
- Hepatitis profile

Complete blood count

Urinalysis

Hypercoagulable evaluation:
- DIC screen
- Factor V Leiden
- Antithrombin III
- Prothrombin mutation 22010
- Protein C and protein S
- Anticardiolipin IgG or IgM
- Russell viper venom test

Collagen vascular disease evaluation (autoimmune disease):
- Antinuclear antibody with profile (DNA, Smith, RNP, SSA, SSB, centromere, SCL-70)
- Rheumatoid factor
- Erythrocyte sedimentation rate (ESR)
- Complement

Evaluation of pulmonary disease:
- Pulmonary function tests with DLCO or bronchodilators (to exclude obstructive/restrictive disease)
- Sleep study and pulse oximetry (degree of hypoxemia or diminished ventilatory drive)
- CT or MRI scan of chest (evaluation of thromboembolic or interstitial lung disease)
- Ventilation/perfusion scan
- Lung biopsy

Six-minute walk test or cycle ergometry

HIV test

Thyroid function tests

Toxicology screen (cocaine, methamphetamine)

Computed tomography (CT), disseminated intravascular coagulation (DIC), diffusing capacity for carbon monoxide (DLCO), deoxyribonucleic acid (DNA), human immunodeficiency virus (HIV), immunoglobulin G (IgG), immunoglobulin M (IgM), magnetic resonance imaging (MRI), ribonucleoprotein (RNP), scleroderma-70 (SCL-70), Sjogren's syndrome A (SSA); Sjogren's syndrome B (SSB).
Sources: Adapted from Mullen, 2010; Rosenzweig et al., 2009.

definition. A favorable response is now defined as a reduction in the pulmonary artery pressure mean (PAPm) of 10 mmHg or more or a PAPm of 40 mmHg or less with an unchanged or increased cardiac output (Badesch et al., 2007).

Antipyretics

For patients presenting with a fever greater than 101°F (38°C), antipyretics such as acetaminophen should be administered to minimize the consequences of increased metabolic demands. Nonsteroidal anti-inflammatory drugs should be administered only after discussion with a PH specialist.

Anticoagulation

Anticoagulation should be considered in children with PH, but especially when this state is associated with low cardiac output, as this combination may lead to sluggish flow through pulmonary arteries and increase the risk of thrombus formation. Administration of warfarin in adults with PH has been reported to improve survival (Rich et al., 1992). The use of anticoagulation has not been studied widely in pediatric patients, yet is usually recommended in this population. Anticoagulation dosing should aim to achieve an International Normalized Ratio (INR) in the range of 1.5 to 2.0. In patients with known hypercoagulability, the INR may need to be maintained at a higher level. Coordination with the hematology service is recommended.

Oxygen

The use of low-flow supplemental oxygen in patients with PH and pulmonary disease alleviates alveolar hypoxemia and attenuates pulmonary pressures. However, because patients with Eisenmenger's syndrome or IPAH do not seem to exhibit resting alveolar hypoxia, they do not derive the same hemodynamic benefits from this therapy. Some patients will demonstrate oxygen desaturation with activity and may benefit from supplemental oxygen therapy. Patients with significant right heart failure and resting hypoxemia should be treated with continuous oxygen. In addition, some patients demonstrate modest oxygen desaturation at night (without evidence of obstruction or apnea), which appears to be the result of mild hypoventilation; these patients would benefit from wearing an oxygen mask when sleeping (Rosenzweig et al., 2004). Patients with Eisenmenger's syndrome also appear to benefit from delivery of oxygen at night, as this therapy has been associated with slower progression of polycythemia (Bowyer et al., 1986).

Diuretics and cardiac glycosides

The use of digitalis for the treatment of isolated right heart failure associated with PH has been controversial, although patients may benefit from its judicious use (Rich et al., 1998). Decreasing intravascular volume and hepatic congestion in patients with right heart failure may be achieved through the use of diuretics. However, the HCP is cautioned that in patients with severe PH, the right ventricle is highly preload dependent and excessive diuresis may result in decreased cardiac output. Close monitoring of electrolytes is warranted, as potassium, magnesium, or phosphorus imbalance may contribute to arrhythmias.

Calcium-channel blockade

Calcium-channel blockers (CCBs) inhibit calcium influx through the slow channel into cardiac and smooth muscle cells. The use of these agents in patients with PH is based on their ability to cause pulmonary vasodilation. This response is tested during the cardiac catheterization and is considered a part of the initial diagnostic evaluation. Patients who do not demonstrate an acute response to vasodilator testing in the cardiac catheterization lab are not candidates for this therapy. Sitbon and colleagues (2005) reported that only 13% of patients were true responders to CCB therapy; of those patients, approximately 7% had a sustained response after one year. Thus patients treated with CCBs require close follow-up to assess for worsening clinical condition.

Targeted management for pulmonary hypertension

Various strategies exist for targeted management of pulmonary hypertension. These therapies may be offered in limited settings and under the guidance of PH specialists. Figure 22-49 describes an algorithm for use of the following management strategies.

Prostaglandins

Continuous intravenous epoprostenol was approved for use in patients with IPAH in 1995. When administered on a long-term basis, it has been shown to improve survival and quality of life, with the 5-year survival rate in children who receive this therapy exceeding 80% (Rashid & Ivy, 2005). Epoprostenol is administered by an infusion pump 24 hours a day through a central venous catheter. It is chemically unstable at neutral pH and room temperature, and has a half-life of 6 minutes or less when mixed daily. This medication must be kept cold, with ice packs placed around the cassette. Interruption of the infusion may result in a pulmonary hypertensive crisis; if delivery of this agent is interrupted, reinitiating the infusion as soon as possible is recommended. The mean dose in pediatric patients is approximately 50–80 ng/kg/min; however, there is significant patient variability in optimal dosing (Rosenzweig et al., 2004). Dosage will also vary based on whether the patient is on single-agent versus combination therapy (Preston, 2008).

Treprostinil (Remodulin) is a prostacyclin analogue that was initially approved for subcutaneous infusion, and is now approved for intravenous infusion. It is similar in action to epoprostenol, yet has important differences. Specifically, treprostinil has a longer half-life, estimated at 4 hours. It is also stable at room temperature for 48 hours. Dosage comparison to epoprostenol is estimated to be approximately 1.5–2 ng/kg/min treprostinil versus 1 ng/kg/min epoprostenol.

The decision to use an intravenous prostacyclin is based on the severity of PH and the quality of life issues associated with administration of this therapy. It is considered the therapy of choice for patients in right heart failure or those who clinically worsen when receiving alternative, less invasive therapies. Only one specialty pharmacy (Accredo Therapeutics) is approved to provide the IV prostacyclins, supplies, and home care. Instructions as to completing the referral paperwork are available at www.accredo.com.

Prostaglandins may also be administered via inhalation. Iloprost was the first formulation approved for inhalation. It utilizes a specialized administration system, the I-neb Adaptive Aerosol Delivery (ADD) system, to precisely and reproducibly deliver the correct dose. Dosing begins at 2.5 mcg initially, and if tolerated, is increased to 5 mcg, with inhalations performed 6 to 9 times per day. Iloprost is also provided by a specialty pharmacy (Actelion); referral paperwork is available at www.phpathways.com.

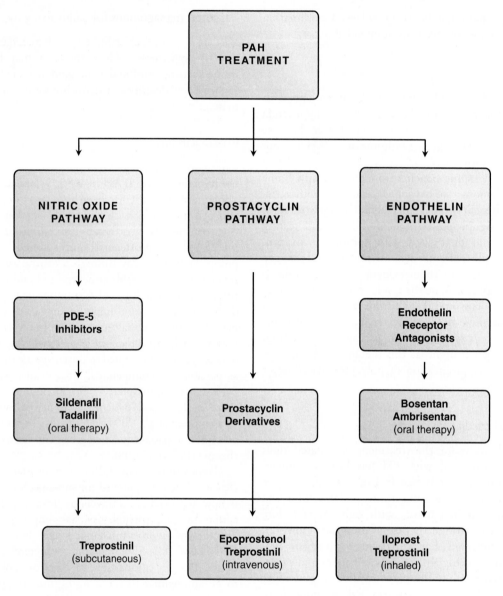

FIGURE 22-49

Targeted Management of PAH.

Note: Phosphodiesterase type 5 (PDE-5), Pulmonary Arterial Hypertension (PAH)

Sources: Adapted from Preston, 2008; Depta & Krasuski, 2009.

Treprostinil (Tyvaso) is also available in an inhaled form. Dosing is based on the number of breaths per session. It is recommended that the patient begin with three breaths (6 mcg per breath), taken four times per day. Dosing can be increased as tolerated by increasing to six breaths per session. Inhaled treprostinil is supplied by a specialty pharmacy; referral forms are available at www. tyvaso.com.

Endothelin antagonists

The first oral medication specifically approved for the treatment of PH was bosentan (Tracleer), which received U.S.

Food and Drug Administration (FDA) approval in 2001. Bosentan, an endothelin A and B receptor blocker, acts on the vascular endothelium and smooth muscle. Endothelin receptor stimulation is associated with vasoconstriction and proliferation. In clinical trials, bosentan increased cardiac output and decreased PAP, PVR, and mean right atrial pressure. It also decreased the rate of clinical worsening, and improved exercise capacity and PH symptoms (Adatia, 2005; Barst et al., 2003).

The FDA requires monthly monitoring of liver function and pregnancy testing while the patient is taking bosentan. Specific guidelines determine dosing (Table 22-34).

TABLE 22-34

Bosentan Dosing	
< 10 kg	15.6 mg daily × 4 weeks then increase to 15.6 mg BID
10–20 kg	31.25 mg daily × 4 weeks, then increase to 31.25 mg BID
20–40 kg	31.25 mg BID × 4 weeks, then increase to 62.5 mg BID
> 40 kg	62.5 mg BID × 4 weeks, then increase to 125 mg BID

Twice-daily dosing (BID).

Sources: Adapted from Adatia, 2005; Barst et al., 2003.

If elevations in the previously noted serum components occur, recommendations are as follows:

- AST/ALT more than 3 times but less than 5 times upper limits of normal: Confirm the elevation and then reduce the dose or interrupt treatment. Monitor transaminase levels every 2 weeks. When levels return to normal, reintroduce the medication at the initial dose and recheck transaminase levels within 3 days.
- AST/ALT more than 5 times but 8 times or less the upper limits of normal: Confirm the elevation and stop treatment. Monitor transaminase levels at least every 2 weeks. Consider restarting treatment if levels return to pretreatment values.
- AST/ALT more than 8 times upper limits of normal: Stop treatment.

Ambrisentan is an endothelin A receptor antagonist that was approved by the FDA in June 2007. Dosing begins at 5 mg daily and may be increased to 10 mg daily if the initial dose is well tolerated. It is currently approved for patients who weigh more than 40 kg, and also requires monitoring liver function.

Phosphodiesterase type 5 inhibitor

Two phosphodiesterase type 5 (PDE5) inhibitor medications have been approved for treatment of PH: sildenafil (Revatio) and tadalafil (Adcirca). PDE5 is found in the pulmonary vascular smooth muscle and breaks down cyclic guanosine monophosphate (cGMP). Nitric oxide activates the enzyme guanylate cyclase, which increases levels of cGMP. Inhibition of PDE5 increases cGMP levels, thereby promoting smooth muscle relaxation. Sildenafil is available in 20 mg tablets and may be compounded into a suspension of 2.5 mg/mL. Dosing begins at 0.5 mg/kg/dose and can be increased to 4 mg/kg/day. Tadalafil dosing is 20 to 40 mg once a day; this agent is approved for use in patients who weigh more than 40 kg.

Inhaled nitric oxide

Nitric oxide is a low-molecular-weight, lipophilic molecule that has a rapid onset of action and a very short intravascular half-life (within seconds). Inhaled NO (iNO) increases cGMP, which leads to smooth muscle relaxation, and is recognized as an effective acute pulmonary vasodilator. As an inhaled gas, it has a quick mechanism of action but produces minimal systemic effects. This therapy has proven to be valuable in treating postoperative pulmonary vascular crisis, which is represented by an acute rise in PVR (Kulik et al., 2009). Inhaled NO may be administered in postoperative patients with a known history of PH or patients who have the potential for pulmonary vasoreactivity after cardiac surgery. In patients with PH refractory to conventional management, iNO has had a dramatic effect on decreasing PAP acutely. It is dosed in parts per million (ppm) and usually is administered at 20 ppm, with titration to 80 ppm. Measurement of methemoglobin levels is required with monitoring for toxicity.

The patient presenting with or being readmitted for PH will require a comprehensive interprofessional team to facilitate swift evaluation and therapeutic management. Consultation with a PH specialist, cardiologist, cardiothoracic surgeon, pulmonologist, and critical care team is advised to promote best outcomes. In addition, the underlying etiology may predicate involvement by hematology, rheumatology, immunology, and infectious diseases specialists. Given that PH may involve lengthy hospitalization, additional team members may become involved in the care of the patient, such as nutrition, rehabilitation, child life, social work, and spiritual support members.

In the acute care setting, patient and family education involves information about diagnostic studies and their results, inclusion of consultants to facilitate a comprehensive plan, and medication choices based on effect and lifestyle. As the therapeutic plan evolves, medication administration, care of long-term venous access, and recognition of poor response or illness are discussed.

DISPOSITION AND DISCHARGE PLANNING

Pulmonary artery pressure is an important determinant of morbidity and mortality. In a 1965 series of 35 patients with idiopathic ("primary") pulmonary hypertension, 22 died within 1 year of symptom onset, with the remaining patients dying within 7 years of diagnosis. In 1995, the prognosis for this disorder remained dismal, with a median survival of 4.12 years in a smaller study of 18 children (Rashid & Ivy, 2005). In data from the Primary Pulmonary Hypertension National Institute of Health Registry, a similarly dismal prognosis for children as compared to adults was noted, with a median survival for all 198 patients of 2.8 years and 10 months in children (D'Alonzo et al., 1991).

The Pulmonary Hypertension Association (PHA; www.phassociation.org) was initially founded as a support group in 1985 by 4 patients with PH. Since its launch, it has grown to more than 10,000 members, including PH patients, caregivers, family members, and medical professionals. With its programs and services expanding to serve the needs of the growing population of patients, families, and PH-focused medical professionals, PHA has also become an international hub for the PH community. This organization provides online resources for therapies, access to HCPs, educational events, and patient resource books. Every 2 years, it sponsors an international conference that hosts patients, families, and HCPs.

Patients started on intravenous prostacyclins receive intensive education before hospital discharge. This education focuses on mixing the medication, operation of the home infusion pump, central venous catheter care, medication administration, dosing and side effects, and emergency management should the medication be interrupted for any reason. Access to the specialty pharmacy providing the medication and supplies is available to patients and families 24 hours a day, 7 days a week. Patients should be cared for by PH specialists or HCPs who are knowledgeable in the management of the therapies for PH. All PH patients require close and frequent follow-up.

Pulmonary hypertension patients have a more reactive pulmonary vascular bed; thus any respiratory infection has the potential to cause ventilation/perfusion mismatch, resulting in alveolar hypoxia and precipitating a catastrophic event. Annual influenza and pneumococcal immunizations are recommended, providing there are no existing contraindications to these measures.

RHEUMATIC FEVER

Julie Kuzin

PATHOPHYSIOLOGY

The pathogenesis of rheumatic fever (RF) is not clearly defined, despite extensive study of the disease. The association of group A beta-hemolytic *Streptococcus* (GAS) pharyngitis preceding RF is well established (Veasy & Hill, 1997; World Health Organization [WHO], 2004). Fortunately, all individuals who experience GAS pharyngitis do not develop RF. The genetic disposition of the host, environmental factors, and the virulence or rheumatogenicity of the GAS strain all contribute to determining the development of RF. While several streptococcal serogroups can cause pharyngitis (including B, C, F, and G), group A is uniquely associated with progression to RF (Stollerman, 2001; WHO).

RF and the subsequent development of rheumatic heart disease (RHD) are nonsuppurative complications of GAS pharyngitis. RF and RHD are widely believed to be autoimmune-mediated diseases triggered by untreated GAS pharyngitis (Gerber et al., 2009). A landmark event in discovering the pathogenesis of RF occurred in the 1930s, when Lancefield identified subgroups of streptococci and M protein variability in the cell wall. Since that time, the focus of RF research has centered on the M protein and the many other self-defense mechanisms of the GAS species (Fischetti, 1989; Lancefield, 1941).

The composition of the M molecule has been revealed through researchers' successful efforts to define the M6 (emm-6) protein (Figure 22-50). When viewed with electron microscopy, M proteins are fine, asymmetrical projections on the cell wall. The M protein is formed from two polypeptide chains composing an alpha-helical coiled-coil structure with fimbriae attachments of amino acid

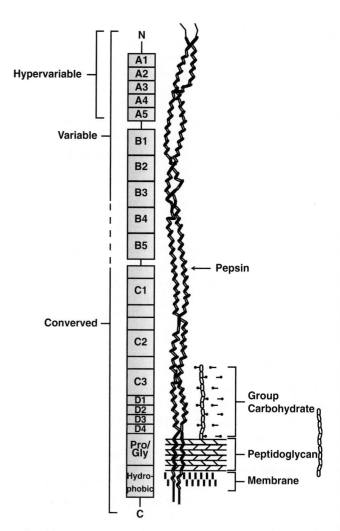

FIGURE 22-50

M6 Protein.

Source: Used with permission: Fischetti, V. (Ed).(2006). *Gram Positive Pathogens.* Washington D.C.: ASM Press.

sequences (Fischetti et al., 1988). The M protein has both distal and proximal portions. The proximal portion (C terminal) is highly conserved, in contrast to the distal portion (N terminal), which is highly variable. This highly variable region allows for the Lancefield classification (Fischetti, 1989; Veasy & Hill, 1997).

M protein has emerged as one of the key indicators of virulence in the streptococcal species. It has several features that lend resilience to the GAS organism, including avoidance of phagocytosis, antigenic variation, adherence, encapsulation, thermal stability, colonization, and internalization. The GAS strains that exhibit encapsulation are covered in hyaluronic acid; they are described as having opacity factor, which refers to the mucoid appearance of the organism when grown in media. Some researchers refer to the particularly virulent M types as "rheumatogenic," as they have been associated with RF outbreaks in the United States (Fischetti, 1989; Veasy & Hill, 1997). Aside from the M protein and intracellular virulence properties, the GAS organism possesses an arsenal of extracellular weapons, including toxins streptolysin O and S, pyrogenic exotoxins, streptokinase, and superantigen activation (Bessen & Hollingshead, 2006; WHO, 2004).

To explore the M protein's resistance to phagocytosis, Fischetti (1989) demonstrated that GAS with few M proteins were readily removed by human neutrophils when exposed to blood, whereas those with sufficient M protein flourished. This finding suggests that less virulent GAS are eliminated by the body's defenses, while the more virulent may thrive unabated (Stollerman, 2001).

M proteins are able to express antigenic variation by changing their size and resequencing their genes, resulting in a variety of M proteins. These features allow the M protein to readily alter its immunodeterminants and delay host recognition (Fischetti, 1989, 2006).

Five chromosomal constellations are known to be based on the *emm* subfamily (*emm* refers to the genetic code for M protein): A, B, C, D, and E. Each group has a tissue tropism. Groups A, B, and C are prone to pharyngitis, group D is prone to impetigo, and group E is found in both regions (Bessen & Hollingshead, 2006). Group A streptococci have been categorized into class I or class II organisms based on the presence of opacity factor, tissue tropism, and response to antibodies against the C repeat region on the M protein (Cunningham, 2000).

Finally, the complex condition of molecular mimicry is an important factor to consider in RF and RHD. Molecular mimicry is the term used to describe the close resemblance of some features of the GAS organism to the molecular design of certain mammalian proteins. This concept may explain epitope formation and the subsequent cross-reaction between mammalian and microbe proteins (Cunningham; Fischetti, 1989). Researchers have suggested varying sites of antigen reactivity might exist, including the streptococcal membrane or cell wall, M antigen, and M-associated protein (Cunningham). This evidence lends support to the theory that RHD and RF are autoimmune-mediated processes.

The pathway from what is understood at the molecular level of GAS infection to the development of the clinical manifestations of RHD remains theoretical. The development of RF is suggested to be similar to other autoimmune processes. First, the host experiences exposure to an antigen. In the case of GAS pharyngitis, the susceptible host is likely to be repeatedly exposed to GAS pharyngitis. At some point along the disease course, the host's immune defense tolerance fails. The immune system loses its ability to distinguish between invading antigens and similarly appearing proteins belonging to the host. Following this break in immune defense, there is a latency period—usually 1 to 5 weeks in RF—in which the immune system initiates a systematic assault (Cunningham, 2000; Stollerman, 2001; Veasy & Hill, 1997).

Further evidence in support of an autoimmune mechanism for RF and RHD includes identification of human autoantibodies that are cross-reactive with streptococcal antigens, antiheart antibodies, and complement deposition in rheumatic hearts (Adderson et al., 1998; Cavelti, 1945; Kaplan & Frengley, 1969; Zabriski et al., 1970). Additionally, Adderson et al. (1998) found that M protein antibodies had direct, cytotoxic effects on myocytes. The presence of immune complexes in the synovial, basal ganglia, skin, and other tissues may account for the nondestructive system effects of RF (Stollerman, 2001).

EPIDEMIOLOGY AND ETIOLOGY

The factors that predispose certain individuals to develop RF remain elusive. Genetics, demographics, environment, and GAS pharyngitis are all recognized as contributing disease factors (Cunningham, 2000). WHO (2004) reported that only 0.3% to 3% of people with GAS pharyngitis progress to developing RF. A significant body of evidence suggests that the progression to RF is ultimately genetically mediated (WHO, 2004). In addition, research supports the idea that specific HLA antigens are associated with many autoimmune disorders. Several international studies have investigated the relationship between HLA antigens and RF, during which a wide variety of HLA antigen types have been identified; some have been shown to have a greater association with RF than others (Haffejee, 1992).

The host environment is known to be a factor in the development of RF and RHD. GAS pharyngitis most often affects children aged 5 to 15 years. It is predominant in temperate climates, whereas *Streptococcus* serogroups C and G prevail in tropical climates. RF has also shown a seasonal preference among people living in temperate climates, with peak disease rates occurring in early fall, late winter, and early spring. Living conditions associated with low socioeconomic status have also been associated with increased incidence of RF (WHO, 2004).

While RF and RHD have been rare in the United States since the 1950s, rates of respiratory tract infections caused by GAS have not declined. RF and RHD continue to be significant health problems in developing countries. WHO (2004) estimates rates of RF to be less than 1 case per 100,000 population in developed countries. Table 22-35 summarizes estimated death rates secondary to RF (WHO, 2004).

A notable resurgence of RF in the United States occurred in the 1980s, particularly in Utah and the Rocky Mountains. Taubert and colleagues (1994) reported a 56% increase in RF in certain areas of the United States during the 1985–1986 period, followed by a gradual decrease in incidence from 1986 to 1990. Shortly after the 1985 increase, there was an outbreak of severe streptococcal disease, manifested as toxic shock syndrome and necrotizing fasciitis. Because rheumatogenic strains (M1, M3, M18) were found among contacts of affected individuals, organism virulence was suspected as the culprit in these RF outbreaks (Kaplan, 1993). The population affected by this outbreak consisted of middle-class, Caucasian families, suggesting that the risk factor of low socioeconomic status and crowded living conditions was changing (Gerber et al., 2009; Taubert et al., 1994). Appropriate treatment of GAS pharyngitis serves as secondary prophylaxis for RF, and hygienic practices have contributed to the near disappearance of RF in the United States (Gerber et al.; Veasy & Hill, 1997).

PRESENTATION

Symptoms of GAS pharyngitis are similar to those of pharyngitis caused by other pathogens, and no particular symptom is sensitive for GAS infection. Symptoms suggestive of GAS pharyngitis include sudden-onset sore throat; painful swallowing; fever (usually 101–104°F [38.3–40°C]); scarlatina rash; headache; nausea; vomiting; abdominal pain; tonsillopharyngeal erythema and exudate; soft palate petechiae; beefy, swollen, or red uvula; and tender or enlarged anterior lymph nodes. When children younger than 3 years of age have GAS pharyngitis, the symptoms may be less specific, such as purulent nasal discharge and excoriated nares. Because it is unusual for a child within this age group to contract GAS pharyngitis, a high rate of occurrence in the community or a case in a close contact should be evaluated (Gerber et al., 2009).

Evidence of a GAS pharyngitis infection within 45 days prior to the development of rheumatic symptoms is important in satisfying criteria for RF. In many cases, pharyngitis may go unreported or unidentified in young children, making the diagnosis of RF challenging. If RF is suspected, rapid antigen detection, throat culture, or streptococcal antibody tests can be performed to provide evidence of recent GAS infection (Gerber et al., 2009).

While the RF criteria are well known, diagnosis can be difficult because symptoms are nonspecific and do not present concurrently. The Jones criteria were developed as a guide to accurately identify acute and recurrent RF. These criteria were initially introduced in 1944, and have been revised by the WHO and AHA several times, most recently in 2004 (Table 22-36). The Jones criteria divide symptoms of RF into major and minor categories (WHO, 2004) (Table 22-37).

Just as GAS pharyngitis is rare in children younger than 3 years of age, so is RF. Tani and colleagues.(2003) reported that RF in this age group commonly presents with moderate to severe carditis, erythema marginatum, or arthritis, and affected children are unlikely to have chorea. Those who present with carditis commonly go on to develop RHD (Tani et al., 2003).

Regarding the Jones criteria, subcutaneous nodules are considered major symptoms due to their association with RF carditis, which is oftentimes severe when nodules are present. The nodules are round, firm, freely mobile, and painless, and range in size from 0.5 to 2 cm. They are often found over bony prominences, the scalp, or extensor tendons (WHO, 2004).

Rheumatic carditis is unique among the features of RF, as it leads to permanent damage and can cause significant morbidity and mortality. Resting tachycardia and a murmur of valvulitis may be the first signs of carditis. A systolic murmur of mitral regurgitation or diastolic murmur of aortic regurgitation may be auscultated. Significant carditis will also result in increased precordial activity and tachypnea, in addition to varying symptoms of congestive heart failure. Presenting symptoms in pediatric patients with carditis vary, ranging from asymptomatic to florid heart failure with the majority of children developing carditis within the first 2 weeks (Allen et al., 2007).

TABLE 22-35

Estimated Incidence of Death Secondary to Rheumatic Heart Disease, 2000	
WHO Region	**Deaths per 100,000 Population**
Africa	4.5
The Americas	1.8
Eastern Mediterranean	4.4
Europe	4.3
South-east Asia	7.6
Western Pacific	6.8
World	5.5

Source: World Health Organization (WHO). (2004). Rheumatic fever and rheumatic heart disease. Retrieved from www.who.int/ cardiovascular_diseases/resources/trs923/en/

TABLE 22-36

Revised Jones Criteria	
Diagnostic Categories	**Criteria**
Primary RF episode	Two major OR one major and two minor manifestations AND evidence of preceding GAS infection‡
Recurrent attack of RF (in patient without RHD)*	Two major OR one major and two minor manifestations AND evidence of preceding GAS infection‡
Recurrent episode of RF in a patient with RHD	Two minor manifestations AND evidence of a preceding GAS infection‡
Rheumatic chorea. Insidious-onset rheumatic carditis	Other major manifestations or evidence of GAS infection not required
Chronic valve lesions of RHD (patients presenting for first time with mitral stenosis or mixed mitral valve and/or aortic valve disease)†	Other criteria NOT required to be diagnosed with RHD

* Infective endocarditis should be excluded.
† Congenital heart disease should be excluded.
‡ Elevated or rising streptococcal antibody, positive throat culture, positive rapid antigen test for GAS, or scarlet fever.
Group A beta-hemolytic *Streptococcus* (GAS), rheumatic fever (RF), rheumatic heart disease (RHD).
Source: World Health Organization (WHO). (2004). Rheumatic fever and rheumatic heart disease. Retrieved from www.who.int/cardiovascular_diseases/resources/trs923/en/

TABLE 22-37

Jones Major/Minor Criteria		
Major	**Minor**	**Special Consideration**
Carditis	Prolonged PR interval	Evidence of streptococcal infection within last 45 days*
Arthritis	Arthralgia	Pre-existing rheumatic fever, rheumatic heart disease
Subcutaneous nodules	Fever	
Chorea	Abdominal pain	
Erythema marginatum	Anemia	
	Epistaxis	
	Pulmonary findings	
	Leukocytosis, elevated erythrocyte sedimentation rate (ESR), elevated C-reactive protein (CRP)	

*Elevated or rising streptococcal antibody, positive throat culture, positive rapid antigen test for Group A *Streptococcus* (GAS), or scarlet fever.
Source: World Health Organization (WHO). (2004). Rheumatic fever and rheumatic heart disease. Retrieved from www.who.int/cardiovascular_diseases/resources/trs923/en/

Rheumatic carditis causes interstitial and perivascular inflammation, without myocyte necrosis, as in myocarditis. Auscultation of a friction rub may raise the suspicion of a pericardial effusion, suggesting the presence of associated pericarditis. The effusion of RF reveals lymphocytic and mononuclear infiltration. Pericarditis is rare in RF; however, when present, it is always associated with valvular disease. While myocarditis and pericarditis may be present in RF, they do not meet the criteria for RF diagnosis in the absence of valvular changes. Endocarditis is responsible for the pathologic valvular changes noted in RF. Vegetations develop along the mitral and aortic valve, with underlying histiocyte and lymphocyte infiltration. The mitral valve is most commonly affected in RF. Over time, the mitral valve leaflets thicken and fibrose and the annulus dilates, leading to poor leaflet coaptation and mitral regurgitation. Mitral stenosis is a result of chronic RF disease. Mitral valve chordae elongate, fuse, and may rupture. The aortic valve affected by RF becomes regurgitant, likely as a result of valve prolapse. Only 20% to 25% of patients will have an affected aortic valve, and this finding is most often noted in association with mitral valve disease (Allen et al., 2007).

Mild mitral regurgitation is generally well tolerated. Children who experience moderate or severe regurgitation will present with symptoms of pulmonary edema and left heart failure. Overtime, pulmonary hypertension may develop secondary to pulmonary venous congestion and cause right heart failure. Pulmonary hypertension is suspected when a loud S_2 heart sound is auscultated (Allen et al., 2007).

Noncardiac major manifestations of RF occur in varying constellations. Arthritis is the most common major manifestation, seen in as many as 75% of patients presenting with the first episode of RF, and always affecting the large joints. The degree of pain associated with RF arthritis ranges from mild to severe. Rheumatic arthritis is generally migratory, beginning in one joint and then moving to other large joints as the originally affected joint inflammation resolves. Less often, the arthritis may occur in more than one joint concurrently. The entire episode of arthritis usually resolves within 1 month (WHO, 2004).

Sydenham's chorea, which almost exclusively affects females, is rare after patients reach 20 years of age. Features of chorea include emotional lability, uncoordinated movements, and muscular weakness. The onset of this condition may be subtle, consisting of irritability or lack of focus to schoolwork. These subtle findings are then followed by physical incoordination, which may be unilateral and affect all muscle groups. Chorea may present 1 to 7 months following GAS infection. Resolution of chorea ranges from 1 week to 2 years, with 75% of patients recovering in 6 months (WHO, 2004).

Erythema marginatum occurs in fewer than 15% of patients. The rash initially presents as bright pink macules on the trunk or proximal extremities (never on the face). The lesion then spreads outward in a circular fashion. The nonpainful, nonpruritic lesions can come and go within hours. Erythema marginatum tends to present with subcutaneous nodules, and is also associated with carditis (WHO, 2004).

Regarding the minor criteria, fever is present during the onset of most rheumatic attacks, with the patient's temperature usually being in the range of 101–104°F [38.3–40°C]. Abdominal pain and epistaxis are reported to occur in approximately 5% of patients. Many patients with RF experience minor-criteria symptoms in the days preceding the development of major symptoms (WHO, 2004).

DIFFERENTIAL DIAGNOSIS

The diagnosis of RF requires satisfying certain criteria over time; therefore differential diagnoses for individual symptoms as well as systemic diseases must be considered. Arthritis and fever may be suggestive of an infection, such as septic arthritis, endocarditis, Lyme disease, or other problems such as gout, inflammatory bowel disease, mucocutaneous disorders, collagen vascular disease, or cancer (WHO, 2004).

Post-streptococcal reactive arthritis should not be confused with the arthritis that occurs in RF. Post-streptococcal reactive arthritis occurs approximately 1 week following streptococcal infection, is minimally affected by anti-inflammatory agents, and is not associated with any other symptoms of RF (WHO, 2004).

Sydenham's chorea is specific to RF and can occur as long as 6 months after GAS infection. Chorea without symptoms of RF is associated with collagen vascular disease (e.g., systemic lupus erythematosus), cerebrovascular accident, hyperthyroidism, hypoparathyroidism, Lyme disease, atypical seizures, Wilson's disease, or a familial chorea. Chorea has also been associated with oral contraceptive use, pregnancy, or drug intoxication (WHO, 2004).

Subcutaneous nodules may be present in RF, specifically in patients who develop severe carditis. The nodules may also be found in systemic lupus erythematosus or rheumatoid arthritis. Erythema marginatum is not commonly reported in RF; if it occurs, other diseases should be considered in the differential diagnosis, such as glomerulonephritis, sepsis, drug reaction, juvenile rheumatoid arthritis, or Lyme disease (WHO, 2004).

PLAN OF CARE

Untreated GAS pharyngitis is the precursor to developing RF in at-risk individuals. When GAS pharyngitis is suspected, a rapid antigen detection test may be performed. False positive results are rare in rapid antigen testing. If a negative result is obtained in a patient suspected of having GAS pharyngitis, a throat culture in blood agar should be obtained, as culture remains the study of choice for diagnosis. Some evidence suggests that starting penicillin as late as 9 days after the onset of pharyngitis does not increase the incidence of RF; therefore withholding antibiotics while awaiting throat culture results is both safe and appropriate.

Endomyocardial biopsy is not indicated for diagnosis of RF; however biopsy sample may yield Aschoff bodies, which are pathognomic for RF. An echocardiograph is useful and should be employed to assess valvular abnormalities when available. Echocardiograph findings specific to RF include progressive mitral valve thickening, chordae tendonae lengthening, aortic valve insufficiency, mitral valve insufficiency, and stenosis or cardiac chamber enlargement (Allen et al., 2007; Williamson et al., 2000). Electrocardiograph may reveal low-voltage QRS complexes, ST-T wave changes, and PR interval prolongation. Heart block may occur, but is rare. Cardiomegaly may be seen on CXR in the case of a pericardial effusion associated with pericarditis or with congestive heart failure. CHF is present in severe cases of carditis and is a result of valvular incompetence leading to ventricular dysfunction (Allen et al., 2007; WHO, 2004).

The Jones criteria for diagnosis of RF are outlined in Table 22-36. Whether the concern is for a primary or recurrent attack of RF, these criteria require evidence of prior GAS infection. Evidence of such GAS infection can be established by the following methods:

- Anti-streptolysin O titers begin to rise within 1 week and peak at 3 to 6 weeks following GAS infection, whereas anti-deoxyribonuclease B titers rise in 1 to 2 weeks and peak 6 to 8 weeks after the GAS infection. Both titers may remain elevated for months.
- A rapid antigen test or throat culture may be obtained; however, a positive result may reflect colonization and not true infection (Gerber et al., 2009).
- A CXR, ECG, and echocardiograph should be performed to evaluate for cardiac involvement. Blood cultures may help to evaluate for infective endocarditis.

Treatment of GAS pharyngitis consists of a single intramuscular dose of benzathine benzylpenicillin, or an oral course of penicillin VK or amoxicillin. If penicillin allergy exists, then a first-generation cephalosporin, clindamycin, or a macrolide may be effective (Gerber et al., 2009; WHO, 2004).

The patient who is diagnosed with RF should be given antibiotics to treat GAS infection regardless of the throat culture results. Long-term prophylactic antibiotics are needed to prevent recurrent exposure to streptococcal antigens. Anti-inflammatory therapy with high-dose acetylsalicylic acid (i.e., ASA/aspirin) should be prescribed for 2 weeks, with the dose then reduced over a minimum of 3 to 6 more weeks. Salicylate levels should be monitored, with goal levels of 20–30 mg/dL. Corticosteroid therapy is recommended for patients who develop severe carditis or who otherwise fail to improve on aspirin therapy. There is little evidence to support a particular length of anti-inflammatory therapy; instead, therapy should be tailored based on the patient's clinical response and trend of acute-phase reactants (Gerber et al., 2009; WHO, 2004). Special precautions with at least 4 weeks of bed rest should be implemented if carditis is present (Gerber et al.; WHO).

If the patient has progressed to CHF, first-line therapy includes bed rest and steroids. Depending on the degree of CHF, therapies such as diuretics, ACE inhibitors, and digoxin may be considered (Gerber et al., 2009; WHO, 2004).

Management of chronic RHD depends on the severity of the disease. Mitral valve disease is unaffected by medical therapy, although symptoms of pulmonary edema may be alleviated by diuretic therapy. Atrial fibrillation (AF), thromboembolism, and pulmonary hypertension are potential complications of mitral valve disease. Patients with AF or a history of embolus should be anticoagulated with warfarin to a goal INR in the range of 2 to 3. Accordingly, mitral regurgitation puts patients at risk for AF due to left atrial dilation, but they are less likely to experience thromboembolism (Gerber et al., 2009; WHO, 2004). Surgical intervention may be indicated for patients with severe valvular incompetence or heart failure refractory to medical therapy (Allen et al., 2007).

The development of chest pain, syncope, or heart failure attributable to aortic stenosis generally necessitates referral for valve replacement. Patients with moderate or severe aortic stenosis should be restricted from strenuous activity, secondary to the risk of sudden death. By comparison, aortic regurgitation is generally well tolerated. These patients tend to develop hypertension, which increases pressure and volume loading of the left ventricle. Timely referral for surgical intervention is important when aortic valve disease is present. Referral prior to deterioration of left ventricular function is recommended, as the onset of dysfunction is a predictor of postoperative survival (Gerber et al., 2009; WHO, 2004).

Infective endocarditis prophylaxis is indicated only for those individuals with RF who have a prosthetic valve, who have undergone a valve repair with prosthetic material, or who have previously had bacterial endocarditis (Wilson et al., 2007).

RF requires early consultation of the following subspecialties: cardiology, infectious diseases, and critical care. Although nutritionists may not be consulted immediately, they should become involved in the patient's plan of care as

soon as it is reasonably possible. Additional subspecialists may be called upon depending on the etiology of the underlying disorder. As the diagnosis of RF may be overwhelming for the family, a number of support services may be necessary to assist them, such as social work, spiritual support, and child life specialists. As the patient begins his or her recovery, the rehabilitative medicine team should be consulted to promote the child's return to developmental baselines.

Patient and family education may initially address the acute illness, the diagnostic studies and their findings, and health care team members who are involved in the plan of care. If the patient's acuity worsens, discussion about life support options and possible transport may be required.

DISPOSITION AND DISCHARGE PLANNING

Most of the conditions associated with RF will resolve over time. Carditis, however, is unique in that it does not improve, and in many patients is progressive. Individuals affected by rheumatic carditis need to maintain appropriate follow-up with a cardiologist for care and appropriately timed surgical referral if necessary (Gerber et al., 2009; WHO, 2004).

Primary RF prevention is targeted at appropriate treatment of GAS pharyngitis. Vaccine prophylaxis against GAS does not exist (Cunningham, 2000; WHO, 2004). Once RF is present, secondary prevention in the form of long-term, prophylactic antibiotics is required to avoid recurrent episodes of GAS pharyngitis. Recurrences of GAS infection in individuals with RF may not cause symptoms of pharyngitis; however, reinfection will trigger an episode of rheumatic fever and is associated with worsening carditis (Gerber et al., 2009).

Critical Thinking
Infective endocarditis prophylaxis is indicated only for those individuals with RF who have a prosthetic valve, who have undergone a valve repair with prosthetic material, or who have previously had bacterial endocarditis.

SYNCOPE

Mary E. McCulley

PATHOPHYSIOLOGY

Syncope is marked by a temporary loss of consciousness and postural tone as a result of what is usually a brief, transient decrease in cerebral blood flow due to systemic hypotension (Strickberger et al., 2006; Willis, 2000). The most common cause of syncope in pediatric cases is known as *neurocardiogenic*, or *vasovagal*, syncope (Strieper, 2005); it may also be referred to as neuroregulated or vasodepressor syncope. The pathophysiology in this type of syncope is not completely defined, but is thought to be due to a reflex-mediated response to relative hypovolemia (Strieper).

In neurocardiogenic syncope, peripheral venous pooling in the lower extremities leads to decreased ventricular filling and stroke volume. Mechanoreceptors (C-fiber afferent nerves) in the inferoposterior wall of the left ventricle detect this drop in volume, which is then transmitted to the carotid baroreceptors, triggering autonomic signals that increase cardiac rate and contractility (Sapin, 2004). Simultaneously, conflicting signals are sent to the medulla from these mechanoreceptors that trigger parasympathetic activity, leading to bradycardia; sympathetic withdrawal, which results in vasodilation, hypotension, and bradycardia; and serotonin increase, which results in peripheral vasodilatation and hypotension. This hypotension leads to cerebral hypoperfusion, resulting in loss of consciousness and postural tone. Once the affected patient is supine, venous return is quickly restored and circulating blood volume increases in the heart and lungs, followed by the return of normal blood pressure and heart rate (Strieper, 2005).

EPIDEMIOLOGY AND ETIOLOGY

In the pediatric population, syncope is most often seen in children who are older than 10 years of age. Approximately 15% of children have at least one syncopal event before the end of adolescence (Massin et al., 2004; Willis, 2000). Approximately 0.1% of emergency department visits made by children are due to syncope. The incidence of syncope is higher in females than males, and peaks between 15 and 19 years of age. Seventy-five percent of children who "faint" have vasovagal syncope, with the remaining 25% of episodes in part due to seizures, migraines, or cardiac disease (Strickberger et al., 2006).

Most syncopal episodes in children are of a benign nature; in some patients, however, they may be a symptom of a serious cardiovascular disease or other illnesses (McBride, 2007). Prolonged standing, dehydration, and limited fluid intake are just a few factors that may precipitate syncope (McBride). Emotional or physical stress-related events (such as pain or fear) might also trigger a sympathetic response, as these events lead to tachycardia and increased cardiac contractility (Strieper, 2005).

Cardiac syncope is typically a result of an outflow obstruction in the heart (such as aortic or pulmonic stenosis) or arrhythmias, which lead to reduced perfusion to the brain. Noncardiac syncope may be due to neurological entities, such as epilepsy, migraines, or metabolic disorders such as hypoglycemia. These entities have a similar pathway of hyperperfusion to the cerebral circulation (Willis, 2000).

PRESENTATION

A thorough and complete history and physical examination is more valuable than diagnostic studies g in determining the cause of syncope (Strickberger et al., 2006). A primary area of focus is the family history, with attention to "red flags" such as syncope, early or sudden deaths, arrhythmias, heart disease, or exercise-related syncope (Goble et al., 2008). A genogram may be a helpful tool in elucidating an accurate family history.

Most patients will present with an episodic loss of consciousness. These individuals may experience nausea, flushing, perspiration, visual disturbances, or lightheadedness prior to the loss of consciousness (presyncope). Sometimes the patient is noted to demonstrate brief tonic–clonic motions and eye-rolling.

Additional historical should include the following:

- Situation and any triggering factors—dehydration, nutritional status
- Onset—any presyncopal symptoms, activity prior to the event
- Frequency
- Duration
- Loss of consciousness
- Postsyncopal state—weak, dizzy, nausea, headache
- Palpitations

The cardiovascular and neurological systems are the most important systems of the physical examination in the patient with syncope. Ilicit blood pressures in each extremity and while in supine and upright positions to determine possible structural abnormalities and orthostatic changes. Any loss of consciousness for longer than 5 minutes, frothing at the mouth, head turning, tongue biting, or defecation, should raise concern for seizure activity and requires a neurological evaluation (Sapin, 2004).

DIFFERENTIAL DIAGNOSIS

In addition to neurocardiogenic (normal faint) syncope, differential diagnoses should include cardiac, neurologic, and other noncardiac causes. Table 22-38 outlines conditions other than neurocardiogenic that require consideration (McBride, 2007; Strieper, 2005; Willis, 2000).

PLAN OF CARE

Most patients with syncope present in an outpatient setting. Although laboratory studies are not necessary unless the history and physical examination suggest a concerning issue (McBride, 2007), an ECG should be obtained on every patient, to completely evaluate for arrhythmia or cardiac

TABLE 22-38

Differential Diagnoses for Non-neurocardiogenic Syncope		
Cardiac Causes of Syncope		**Other Causes**
Arrhythmias	**Hemodynamic**	

• Supraventricular tachycardia
• Wolff-Parkinson-White syndrome
• Ventricular tachycardia
• Ventricular fibrillation
• Atrial fibrillation
• Atrial tachycardia with rapid ventricular response
• Heart block
• Long QT syndrome
• Brugada syndrome
	• Hypertrophic obstructive cardiomyopathy
	• Dilated cardiomyopathy
	• Aortic or pulmonic stenosis
	• Pulmonary hypertension
	• Congenital coronary abnormalities (anomalous coronary artery)
	• Myocarditis
	• Previous congenital heart repair
	• Right ventricular outflow tract obstructionPericardial tamponade
	• Mitral valve prolapsed
	• Anemia
		• Neurologic
		  • Migraines
		  • Seizures
		  • Dysautonomia
		• Metabolic
		  • Hypoglycemia
		  • Hypoadrenalism
		  • Hypothyroidism
		• Medications
		  • Drugs or intoxicant ingestion
		• Psychogenic
		  • Conversion syndrome
		  • Breath-holding spells

issues, such as long QT syndrome, Wolff-Parkinson-White syndrome, or ventricular hypertrophy (Sapin, 2004). ECG findings of any concern should be evaluated by a pediatric cardiologist (Goble et al., 2008; Strieper, 2005). Hospitalization and a more extensive evaluation are required for those patients whose presentation suggests a life-threatening cardiac or neurological condition (Goble et al.).

Holter monitoring should be obtained if the patient experienced a cluster of occurrences, experienced a sudden loss of consciousness, palpitations, is taking medications associated with arrhythmias, has known heart disease, or has a history of abnormal ECG findings (Sapin, 2004).

Tilt-table testing may be used to evaluate patients who have a normal heart, those who experience infrequent syncope, if symptoms indicate vasovagal response but no defined precipitating event exists, or if the history is unclear (Sapin, 2004). This technique may also be used when Holter monitoring has been nondiagnostic. However, routine pediatric tilt-table testing has not been shown to have a high diagnostic yield, and it is no longer recognized as the study of choice for diagnosis. This approach may be useful to evaluate for a psychiatric cause, such as "conversion syndrome," in which the patient appears unconscious but blood pressure and heart rate remain within normal limits (Strieper, 2005).

A video electroencephalograph (EEG) may be indicated if seizures are suspected. To evaluate for metabolic disorders, blood sugar, fasting blood sugar, or abbreviated glucose tolerance testing may be required (McBride, 2007).

Decisions to admit the patient from the outpatient to the inpatient setting for further monitoring or evaluation (Strieper, 2005) may be related to the indications identified in Table 22-39.

Life-threatening arrhythmia management may include antiarrhythmic medications, ablation procedures via

TABLE 22-39

Admission for Syncope to the Inpatient Setting
• Chest pain
• Palpitations
• Any history or signs of congestive heart failure or valvular disease
• Focal neurological deficit
• Any injury present
• Sudden loss of consciousness without presyncope symptoms
• Moderate to severe orthostasis
• Electrocardiograph showing tachycardia, ischemia, arrhythmia, bundle branch block, or prolonged QT (cardiology confirmed)
• Sudden syncope that frequently occurs with exercise

cardiac catheterization, or pacing. Long QT syndrome may respond to beta blocker therapy. In some patients, a pacemaker or ICD may be required if bradycardia occurs concurrently with severe long QT syndrome. For structural heart problems, surgery may be required to correct causes of outflow obstruction, such as occurs with pulmonic and aortic stenosis (Strickberger et al., 2006).

Both seizures and migraines management may also require pharmacologic therapy. Psychiatric intervention may be required if causes are found to be due to hysteria, with appropriate patient and family intervention. Breath-holding spells are more common in young children, and patients who exhibit this behavior may benefit from caregiver counseling and a trial of anticholinergic agents (Strieper, 2005).

Uncomplicated neurocardiogenic (vasovagal) syncope may be prevented with simple techniques such as lying down if prodromal symptoms occur, wearing elastic hose to prevent venous pooling, and avoiding any stimuli that may cause syncope. The mainstay of management is adequate hydration by adequate fluid intake (60–90 oz [1.8–2.7 L] per day for adolescents), adequate salt intake, and avoidance of diuretics such as caffeine (Strieper, 2005).

Referral to a pediatric neurologist or cardiologist should be made if the diagnosis of neurocardiogenic syncope cannot be made with certainty. A cardiology referral is also necessary if the syncope is associated with exercise or is recurrent, or if the family history includes recurrent syncope or sudden death (Strieper, 2005). Additional consultations may involve metabolic, psychiatry, behavioral medicine, genetics, child life, or social work specialists if the diagnosis supports a psychiatric or behavioral component.

Patient and family education should address the diagnostic studies, their results, consultation services, and the therapeutic management plan. Both patients and families should be provided with information regarding syncope, potential evaluation of other family members if a cardiac etiology is identified, and social support. Education should also include a list and description of triggering factors, need for increased fluid intake, and teaching the patient to make positional adjustments when symptoms occur (Goble et al., 2008).

DISPOSITION AND DISCHARGE PLANNING

Syncope often recurs, but once the cause is determined, treatment is usually very effective. Follow-up should be arranged with the patient's primary care provider for neurocardiogenic responses, and with the appropriate specialist for all other conditions. The main tenet of follow-up management for neurocardiogenic syncope is reassurance that the condition is not serious.

Critical Thinking

- If loss of consciousness lasts for more than 1 minute, the etiology of the syncopal episode is likely to be more serious, such as a life-threatening arrhythmia.
- If the loss of consciousness lasts for more than 10 minutes with spontaneous recovery, it may indicate a psychological etiology, such as factitious fainting.

REFERENCES

1. Adachi, I., Seale, A., Uemura, H., McCarthy, K. P., Kimberley, P., & Ho, S. Y. (2009). Morphologic spectrum of truncal valvar origin relative to the ventricular septum: Correlation with the size of ventricular septal defect. *Journal of Thoracic Cardiovascular Surgery, 138*, 1283–1289.

2. Adatia, I. (2005). Improving the outcome of childhood pulmonary arterial hypertension: The effect of bosentan in the setting of a dedicated pulmonary hypertension clinic. *Journal of the American College of Cardiology, 46*(4), 705–706.

3. Adderson, E., Shikhman, A., Ward, K., & Cunningham, M. (1998). Molecular analysis of polyreactive monoclonal antibodies from rheumatic carditis: Human anti-*N*-acetyl-glucosamine/antimyosin antibody V region genes. *Journal of Immunology, 161*, 2020–2031.

4. Aellig, N. C., Balmer, C., Dodge-Khatami, A., Rahn, M., Pretre, R., & Bauersfeld, U. (2007). Long-term follow-up after pacemaker implantation in neonates and infants. *Society of Thoracic Surgeons, 83*(4), 1420–1424.

5. Agrawal, V., & Sahn, S. A. (2006). Lipid pleural effusions. *American Journal of the Medical Sciences, 335*, 16–20.

6. Alkhaldi, A., Chin, C., & Bernstein, D. (2006). Pediatric cardiac transplantation. *Seminars in Pediatric Surgery, 15*, 188–198.

7. Allan, L., Sharland, G., & Milburn, A. (1994). Prospective diagnosis of 1006 consecutive cases of congenital heart disease in the fetus. *Journal of the American College of Cardiology, 23*, 1452–1458.

8. Allen, H., Driscoll, D., Shaddy, R., & Feltes, T. (Eds.). (2007). *Moss and Adams' heart disease in infants, children, and adolescents including the fetus and young adult* (7th ed.). Philadelphia: Lippincott, Williams & Wilkins.

9. Allen, U., Farkas, G., Hébert, D., Weitzman, S., Stephens, D., Petric, M., et al. (2005). Risk factors for post-transplant lymphoproliferative disorder in pediatric patients: A case-control study. *Pediatric Transplantation, 9*, 450–455.

10. Allpress, A. L., Rosenthal, G. L., Goodrich, K. M., Lupinetti, F. M., & Zerr, D. M. (2004). Risk factors for surgical site infections after pediatric cardiovascular surgery. *Pediatric Infectious Diseases Journal, 2*, 231–234.

11. American Academy of Pediatrics & American College of Emergency Physicians. (2010). APLS online. Retrieved from http://www.aplsonline.com/index.cfm

12. American Heart Association (AHA). (2005). Guidelines for cardiopulmonary resuscitation and emergency cardiovascular care. *Circulation, 112*(suppl), 24.

13. American Heart Association (AHA). (2006). 2005 American Heart Association (AHA) guidelines for cardiopulmonary resuscitation (CPR) and emergency cardiovascular care (ECC) of pediatric neonatal patients: pediatric advanced life support. *Pediatrics, 117*(5), e1005–e1028.

14. American Heart Association (AHA). (2010a). HeartCode ACLS. Retrieved from http://www.americanheart.org/presenter.jhtml?identifier=3070655

15. American Heart Association (AHA). (2010b). HeartCode PALS. Retrieved from http://americanheart.org/presenter.jhtml?identifier=3069224

16. Anderson, R., Becker, A., & Van Mierop, L. (1977). What should we call the "crista"? *British Heart Journal, 39*, 856.

17. Anderson, R., & Weinberg, P. (2005). The clinical anatomy of tetralogy of Fallot. *Cardiolgy Young, 15*(suppl 1), 38–47.

18. Ardura, J., Gonzalez, C., & Andres, J. (2006). Does mild valvular aortic stenosis progress during childhood? *Journal of Heart Valve Disease, 15*(1), 1–4.

19. Aziz, T., Burgess, M., Khafagy, R., Wynn Han, A., Campbell, C., Rahman, A. et al. (1999). Bicaval and standard techniques in orthotopic heart transplantation: Medium term experience in cardiac performance and survival. *Journal of Thoracic and Cardiovascular Surgery, 118*, 115–122.

20. Backer, C., & Mavroudis, C. (2003a). Palliative operation. In C. Mavroudis & C. Backer (Eds.). *Pediatric cardiac surgery* (3rd ed., pp. 160–170). Philadelphia: Mosby.

21. Backer, C., & Mavroudis, C. (2003b). Vascular rings and pulmonary artery sling. In C. Mavroudis & C. Backer (Eds.). *Pediatric cardiac surgery* (3rd ed., pp. 234–249). Phildalphia: Mosby.

22. Backer, C., Stewart, R., & Mavroudis, C. (2007). Overview: History, anatomy, timing, and results of complete atrioventricular canal. *Seminars in Thoracic and Cardiovascular Surgery and Pediatric Cardiac Surgery Annuals*, 3–10.

23. Baddour, L., Wilson, W., Bayer, A., Fowler, V., & Bolger, A., Levison, M., et al. (2005). Infective endocarditis diagnosis, antimicrobial therapy, and management of complications: A statement for healthcare professionals from the Committee on Rheumatic Fever, Endocarditis, and Kawasaki Disease, Council on Cardiovascular Disease in the Young, and the Councils on Clinical Cardiology, Stroke, and Cardiovascular Surgery and Anesthesia, American Heart Association. *Circulation, 111*, e394–e433.

24. Badesch, D., Abman, S., Simonneau, G., Rubin, L., & McLaughlin, V. (2007). Medical therapy for pulmonary arterial hypertension: Updated ACCP evidence-based clinical practice guidelines. *Chest, 131*, 1917–1928.

25. Bargeron, L., Elliott, L., Soto, B., Bream, P., & Curry, G. (1977). Axial cineangiography in congenital heart disease. I. Concept, technical and anatomic considerations. *Circulation, 56*, 1075.

26. Barr, M., Meiser, B., Eisen, H., Roberts, R., Livi, U., Dall'Amico, R., et al. (1998). Photopheresis for the prevention of rejection in cardiac transplantation. *New England Journal of Medicine, 339*, 1744–1751.

27. Barry, A., & Patten, B. (1968). The structure of the adult heart. In S. Gould & S. Gould (Eds.). *Pathology of the heart and blood vessels* (5th ed., p. 91). Springfield, IL: Charles C. Thomas.

28. Barst, R., Ivy, D., Dingemanse, J., Widlitz, A., Schmitt, K., Doran, A., et al. (2003). Pharmokinetics, safety and efficacy of bosentan in pediatric patients with pulmonary arterial hypertension. *Clinical Pharmacology & Therapeutics, 73*(4), 372–382.

29. Bartelings, M., & Gittenberger-de Groot, A. (1989). The outflow tract of the heart: Embryologic and morphologic correlations. *International Journal of Cardiology, 22*, 289.

30. Bassareo, P., Marras, A., Manai, M., & Mercuro, G. (2008). The influence of different surgical aproaches on arterial rigidity in children after aortic coarctation repair. *Pediatric Cardiology, 30*(4), 414–418.

31. Baum, M., Freier, C., Freeman, K., Chinnock, R. (2000). Developmental outcomes and cognitive functioning in infant and child heart transplant recipients. *Progress in Pediatric Cardiology, 11*, 159–163.

32. Beekman, R., Rocchini, A., & Gillon, J. (1992). Hemodynamic determinants of the peak systolic left ventricular–aortic pressure gradient in children with valvar aortic stenosis. *American Journal of Cardiology, 69*, 813–815.

33. Beghetti, M. (2006). A classification system and treatment guidelines for PAH associated with congenital heart disease. *Advances in Pulmonary Hypertension, 5*(2), 31–35.

34. Beke, D. M., Braudis, N. J., & Lincoln, P. (2005). Management of the pediatric postoperative cardiac surgery patient. *Critical Care Nursing Clinics of North America, 17*(4), 405–416.

35. Benowitz, N. L. (2001). Antihypertensive agents. In B. G. Katzung (Ed.). *Lange: Basic and clinical pharmacology* (8th ed., pp. 155–180). New York: McGraw-Hill.

36. Berberich, T., Haecker, F., Kehrer, B., Erb, T., Gunthard, J., Hammer, J., et al. (2004). Postpericardiotomy syndrome after minimally invasive repair of pectus excavatum. *Journal of Pediatric Surgery, 39*, e1–e3.

37. Bergersen, L., Foerster, S., Marshall, A. C., & Meadows, J. (2008). *Congenital heart disease: The catheterization manual*. London: Springer.

38. Berul, C. I. (2008). Defibrillator indications and implantation in young children. *Heart Rhythm, 5*(12), 1755–1757.

39. Bessen, D., & Hollingshead, S. (2006). Molecular epidemiology, ecology, and evolution of group A streptococci. In V. Fischetti, R. Novick, J. Ferretti, D. Portnoy, & J. Rood (Eds.). *Gram positive pathogens book* (2nd ed., pp.143–148). Washington, DC: American Society for Microbiology Press.

40. Blume, E., Naftel, D., Bastardi, H., Duncan, B., Kirklin, J., Webber, S., for the Pediatric Heart Transplant Study Investigators. (2006). Outcome of children bridged to transplantation with ventricular assist devices: A multi-institutional study. *Circulation, 113*, 2313–2319.

41. Boucek, M., Aurora, P., Edwards, L., Taylor, D., Trulock, E., Christie, J., et al. (2007). Registry of the International Society for Heart and Lung Transplantation: Tenth official pediatric heart transplantation report—2007. *Journal of Heart and Lung Transplantation, 26*, 796–807.

42. Boucek, M., Edwards, L., Keck, B., Trulock, E., Taylor, D., & Hertz, M. (2005). Registry of the International Society for Heart and Lung Transplantation: Eighth official pediatric report—2005. *Journal of Heart and Lung Transplantation, 24*(8), 968–982.

43. Boucek, M., Waltz, D., Edwards, L., Taylor, D., Keck, B., Trulock, E., et al. (2006). Registry of the International Society for Heart and Lung Transplantation: Ninth official pediatric report—2006. *Journal of Heart and Lung Transplantation, 25*(8), 893–903.

44. Bove, E., Ohye, R., & Devaney, E. (2004). Hypoplastic left heart syndrome: Conventional surgical management. *Pediatric Cardiac Surgery Annual of the Seminars in Thoracic and Cardiovascular Surgery, 7*, 3–10.

45. Bowyer, J., Busst, C., Denison, D., & Shinbourne, E. (1986). Effect of long-term oxygen treatment at home in children with pulmonary vascular disease. *British Heart Journal, 55*, 385–390.

46. Brandt, P., & Calder, A. (1977). Cardiac connections: The segmental approach to radiologic diagnosis in congenital heart disease. *Current Problems Diagnostic Radiology, 7*, 1.

47. Bratincsak, A., El-Said, H., Bradley, J., Shayan, K., Grossfeld, P., & Cannavino, C. (2010). Fulminant myocarditis associated with pandemic H1N1 influenza A virus in children. *Journal of the American College of Cardiologists, 55*, 928–929.

48. Braunlin, E., Peoples, W., & Freedom, R. (1982). Interruption of the aortic arch with aorticopulmonary septal defect: An anatomic review. *Pediatric Cardiology, 3*, 329–335.

49. Braunwald, E., Goldblatt, A., & Aygen, M. (1963). Congenital aotic stenosis. I. Clinical and hemodynamic findings in 100 patients. II. Surgical and the results of operation. *Circulation, 27*, 426–462.

50. Breinholt, J., Nelson, D., & Towbin, J. (2008). Heart failure in infants and children: Myocarditis. In D. Nichols (Ed.). *Rogers' textbook of pediatric intensive care* (4th ed., pp. 1082–1092). Philadelphia: Lippincott.

51. Brizard, C., Cochrane, A., & Austin, C. (1997). Management strategy and long term outcome for truncus arteriosus. *European Journal Cardiothoracic Surgery, 11*, 687–695.

52. Brown, J., & Hanish, S. (2003). Cor triatriatum sinister, atresia of the common pulmonary vein, pulmonary vein stenosis and cor triatriantum dexter. In C. Mavroudis & C. Backer (Eds.). *Pediatric cardiac surgery* (3rd ed., pp. 625–633). Phildelphia: Mosby.

53. Brown, J., Ruzmetov, M., Vijay, P., Rodefeld, M., & Turrentine, M. (2006). The Ross-Konno procedure in children: Outcomes, autograft and allograft function, and reoperations. *Annual Thoracic Surgery, 82*(4), 1307.

54. Burch, P., Crowley, C., Holubkov, R., Null, D., Lambert, L., Kouretas, P., et al. (2009). Coarctation repair in neonates and young infants: Is small size or ow weight stil a risk factor? *Journal of Thoracic Cardiovascular Surgery, 138*(3), 547–552.

55. Cabalka, A. K., Edwards, W. D., & Dearani, J. A. (2008). Truncus arteriosus. In H. Allen, D. Driscoll, R. Shaddy, & T. Feltes (Eds.). *Moss and Adams' heart disease in infants, children, and adolescents* (7th ed., pp. 911–987). Philadelphia: Lippincott, Williams & Wilkins.

56. Cabalka, A., Rosenblatt, H., Towbin, J., Price, J., Windsor, N., Martin, A., et al. (1995). Postpericardiotoy syndrome in pediatric heart transplant recipients. *Texas Heart Institute Journal, 22*, 170–175.

57. Campbell, M. (1961). The aetiology of coarctation of the aorta. *Lancet, 1*, 463–468.

58. Campbell, M. (1968). The natural history of congenital aortic stenosis. *British Heart Journal, 30*, 514–526.

59. Canter, C., Shaddy, R., Bernstein, D., Hsu, D., Chrisant, M., Kirklin, J., et al. (2007). Indications for heart transplantation in pediatric heart disease. *Circulation, 115*(5), 658–676.

60. Carotti, A., Digilio, M., Piacentini, G., Saffirio, C., Di Donato, R., & Marino, B. (2008). Cardiac defects and results of cardiac surgery in 22q11.2 deletion syndrome. *Developmental Disability Research Review, 14*(1), 35–42.

61. Caruthers, S., Lin, S., & Brown, P. (2003). Practical value of cardiac magnetic resonance imaging for clinical quantification of aortic valve stenosis: Comparison with echocardiogramy. *Circulation, 108,* 2236–2243.

62. Castaneda, A., Jonas, R., Mayer, J., & Hanley, F. (1994). Cardiopulmonary bypass, hypothermia, and circulatory arrest. In A. Castaneda, R. Jonas, J. Mayer, & F. Hanley (Eds.). *Cardiac surgery of the neonate and infant* (pp. 23–39). St. Louis: W. B. Saunders.

63. Cavelti, P. (1945). Autoantibodies in rheumatic fever. *Proceedings of the Society of Experimental Biology and Medicine, 60,* 379–381.

64. Caviness, A., Cantor, S., Allen, C., & Ward, M. (2004). A cost-effectiveness analysis of bacterial endocarditis prophylaxis for febrile children who have cardiac lesions and undergo urinary catheterization in the emergency in the emergency department. *Pediatrics, 113,* 1291–1296.

65. Ceneviva, G., Paschall, J. A., Maffei, F., & Carcillo, J. A. (1998). Hemodynamic support in fluid-refractory pediatric septic shock. *Pediatrics, 102*(2), e19.

66. Chang, A., & Towbin, J. (Eds.). (2006). *Heart failure in children and young adults.* Philadelphia: W. B. Saunders.

67. Cheung, E., Ho, S., Tang, A., Chau, A., Chiu, C., & Cheung, Y. (2003). Pericardial effusion after open heart surgery for congenital heart disease. *Heart, 89,* 780–783.

68. Chin, C., Gamberg, P., Miller, J., Luikart, H., & Bernstein, D. (2002). Efficacy and safety of atorvastatin after pediatric heart transplantation. *Journal of Heart and Lung Transplantation, 21,* 1213–1217.

69. Chin, C., Miller, J., Robbins, R., Reitz, B., & Bernstein, D. (1999). The use of advanced age donor hearts adversely affects survival in pediatric heart transplantation. *Pediatric Transplantation, 3*(4), 309–314.

70. Chin, C., Naftel, D., Singh, T., Blume, E., Luikart, H., Bernstein, D., et al. (2004). The Pediatric Heart Transplant Study Group. Risk factors for recurrent rejection after pediatric heart transplantation: A multicenter experience. *Journal of Heart and Lung Transplantation, 23,* 178–185.

71. Cini, G., Carpi, A., Mechanick, J., Cini, L., Camici, M., Galetta, F., et al. (2009). Thyroid hormone and the cardiovascular system: Pathophysiology and interventions. *Biomedical Pharmacotherapy, 63*(10), 742–753.

72. Clark, E., Nakazawa, M., & Takao, A. (2000). *Etiology and morphogenesis of congenital heart disease: Twenty years of progess in genetics and developmental biology.* (E. N. Clark, Ed.). Armonk, NY: Futura.

73. Clark, E., & Takao, A. (1990). *Developmental cardiology: Morphogenesis and function.* Mount Kisco, NY: Futura.

74. Colan, S., Lipshultz, S., Lowe, A., Sleeper, L., Messere, J., Cox, G., et al. (2007). Epidemiology and cause-specific outcome of hypertrophic cardiomyopathy in children: Findings from the Pediatric Cardiomyopathy Registry. *Circulation, 115*(6), 773–781.

75. Connolly, D., Rutkowski, M., Auslender, M., & Artman, M. (2001). The New York University pediatric heart failure index: A new method of quantifying chronic heart failure severity in children. *Journal of Pediatrics, 138,* 644–648.

76. Connuck, D., Sleeper, L., Colan, S., Cox, G., Towbin, J., Lowe, A., et al. (2008). Characteristics and outcomes of cardiomyopathy in children with Duchenne or Becker muscular dystrophy: A comparative study from the pediatric cardiomyopathy registry. *American Heart Journal, 155*(6), 998–1005.

77. Constant, J. (2002). *Essentials of bedside cardiology (contemporary cardiology).* Totowa, NJ: Humana Press.

78. Cooper, L. (2009). Myocarditis. *New England Journal of Medicine. 360,* 1526–1538.

79. Cooper, L., Baughman, K., Feldman, A., Frustaci, A., Jessup, M., Kuhl, U., et al. (2007). The role of endomyocardial biospys in the management of cardiovascular disease: A scientific statement from the American Heart Association, the American College of Cardiology, and the European Society of Cardiology endorsed by the Heart Failure Society of America and the Heart Failure Association of the European Society of Cardiology. *Journal of the American College of Cardiology, 50*(19), 1914–1931.

80. Costello, J. M., & Almodovar, M. C. (2007). Emergency care for infants and children with acute cardiac disease. *Clinical Pediatric Emergency Medicine, 8*(3), 145–155.

81. Costello, J. M., Grahm, D. A., Morrow, D. F., Morrow, J., Potter-Bynoe, G., Sandora, T. J., et al. (2010). Risk factors for surgical site infection after cardiac surgery in children. *Annals of Thoracic Surgery, 89,* 1833–1842.

82. Costello, J., Wax, D., Binns, J., Backer, C., Mavroudis, C., & Pahl, E. (2003). A comparison of intravascular ultrasound with coronary angiography for evaluation of transplant coronary artery disease in pediatric heart transplant recipients. *Journal of Heart and Lung Transplantation, 22,* 44–49.

83. Cripe, L., Andelfinger, G., & Martin, L. (2004). Bicuspid aortic valve is heritable. *Journal of Amican College of Cardiology, 44,* 138–143.

84. Cunningham, M. (2000). Pathogenesis of group A streptococcal infections. *Clinical Microbiology Reviews, 13*(3), 470–511.

85. Dager, W. E., Sanoski, C. A., Wiggins, B. S., & Tisdale, J. E. (2006). Pharmacotherapy considerations in advanced cardiac life support. *Pharmacotherapy, 26*(12), 1703–1729.

86. D'Alonzo, G., Barst, R., Ayres, S., Bergofsky, E., Detre, K., Fishman, A., et al. (1991). Survival in patients with primary pulmonary hypertension: Results from national prospective registry. *Annals of Internal Medicine, 115,* 343–349.

87. Danilowicz, D. (1995). Infective endocarditis. *Pediatrics in Review, 16,* 148–154.

88. Davignon, A. (1980). ECG standards for children. *Pediatric Cardiology, 1,* 133–152.

89. Day, M., Gauvreau, K., Shulman, S., & Newburger, J. (2009). Characteristics of children hospitalized with infective endocarditis. *Circulation, 119,* 865–870.

90. Dearani, J., & Danielson, G. (2003). Ebstein's anolmaly of the tricuspid valve. In C. Mavroudis & C. Backer (Eds.). *Pediatric cardiac surgery* (3rd ed., pp. 524–536). Philadelphia: Mosby.

91. Dellinger, R. P., Levy, M., Carlet, J., Bion, J., Parker, M., Jaeschke, R., et al. (2008). Surviving Sepsis Campaign: International guidelines for management of severe sepsis and septic shock: 2008. *Intensive Care Medicine, 34*(1), 17–60.

92. DeMaso, D., Kelley, L., Bastardi, H., O'Brien, P., & Blume, E. (2004). The longitudinal impact of psychological functioning, medical severity, and family functioning in pediatric heart transplantation. *Journal of Heart and Lung Transplantation, 23*(4), 473–480.

93. Denfield, S. (2002). Sudden death in children with restrictive cardiomyopathy. *Cardiac Electrophysiology Review, 6*(1 & 2), 1385–2264.

94. Denfield, S., Rosenthal, G., Gajarski, R., Bricker, J., Schowengerdt, K., Price, J., et al. (1997). Restrictive cardiomyopathies in childhood: Etiologies and natural history. *Texas Heart Institute Journal, 24*(1), 38–44.

95. Depta, J., & Krasuski, R. (2009). Evidence-based medical management of pulmonary hypertension 2008: Review of updated 2007 ACCP guidelines. *Advances in Pulmonary Hypertension, 7*(1), 222–227.

96. Descheerder, I., Renterghem, L., Sabbe, L., Robbrecht, D., Clement, D., Derom, F., et al. (1984). Association of anti-heart antibodies and circulating immune complexes in the post-pericardiotomy syndrome. *Clinical & Experimental Immunology, 57,* 423–428.

97. Dickstein, K., Cohen-Solal, A., Filippatos, G., McMurray, J., Ponikowski, P., Poole-Wilson, P., et al. (2008). ESC guidelines for the diagnosis and treatment of acute and chronic heart failure 2008. *European Journal of Heart Failure, 8,* 933–989.

98. Di Filippo, S., Boissonnat, P., Sassolas, F., Robin, J., Ninet, J., Champsaur, G., et al. (2003). Rabbit antithymocyte globulin as induction therapy in pediatric heart transplantation. *Transplantation, 75*(3), 354–358.

99. Dillman, J., Yarram, S., D'Amico, A., & Hernandez, R. (2008). Interrupted aortic arch: Spectrum of MRI findings. *American Journal of Roentgenology, 190*(6), 1467–1474.

100. Dipchand, A., Pollock BarZiv, S. M., Manlhiot, C., West, L. J., VanderVliet, M., McCrindle, B. W. (2009). Equivalent outcomes for pediatric heart transplant recipients: ABO blood group incompatible versus ABO compatible *American Journal of Transplantation, 10*(2), 389–397.

101. Dipchand, A., & Blume, E. (2010). Transplantation of the heart, and heart and lungs. In R. Anderson, E. Baker, et al. (Eds.). *Paediatric cardiology* (3rd ed., pp. 269–289). Philadelphia: Churchill Livingstone, Elsevier.

102. Di Sessa, T., Di Sessa, P., Gregory, B., & Vranicar, M. (2009). The use of 3D contrast-enhanced CT reconstructions to project images of vascular rings and coarctation of the aorta. *Echocardiograpy, 26*(1), 76–81.

103. Dodd, D., Cabo, J., & Dipchand, A. (2007). Acute rejection: Natural history, risk factors, surveillance, and treatment. In C. Canter & J. Kirklin (Eds.). *ISHLT monograph series: Pediatric heart transplantation* (2nd ed., pp 139–156). Philadelphia: Elsevier.

104. Dodge-Khatami, A., Schmid, M., Rousson, V., Fasnacht, M., Doell, C., Bauersfeld, U., et al. (2008). Risk factors for reoperation after relief of congenital subaortic stenosis. *European Journal of Cardiothoracic Surgery, 33*(5), 885–889.

105. Doniger, S. J., & Sharieff, G. Q. (2006). Pediatric dysrhythmias. *Pediatric Clinics of North America, 53*(1), 85–105.

106. Doto, F., Zaritsky, A., Schexnayder, S., Kleinman, M., & Hazinski, M. (Eds.). (2007). *Pediatric emergency assessment, recognition, and stabilization instructor manual.* Dallas: American Heart Association.

107. Doto, F., Zaritsky, A., Terry, M., Schexnayder, S., Kleinman, M., & Hazinski, M. (Eds.). (2006). *Pediatric advanced life support instructor manual.* Dallas: American Heart Association.

108. Dubin, A. M., Janousek, J., Rhee, E., Strieper, M. J., Cecchin, F., Law, I. H., et al. (2005). Resynchronization therapy in pediatric and congenital heart disease patients: An international multicenter study. *Journal of the American College of Cardiology, 46*(12), 2277–2283.

109. Duncan, B., Burch, M., Kirklin, J., & Price, J. (2007). Management of patients awaiting transplantation: Medical, immunologic, and mechanical support. In C. Canter & J. Kirklin (Eds.). *ISHLT monograph series: Pediatric heart transplantation* (2nd ed., pp. 33–54). Philadelphia: Elsevier.

110. Duncan, B., Ibrahim, A., Hraska, V., del Nido, P., Laussen, P., Wessel, D., et al. (1998). Use of rapid-deployment extracorporeal membrane oxygenation for the resuscitation of pediatric patients with heart disease after cardiac arrest. *Journal of Thoracic and Cardiovascular Surgery, 116*, 305–309.

111. Durani, Y., Egan, M., Baffa, J., Selbst, S., & Nager, A. (2009). Pediatric myocarditis: Presenting clinical characteristics. *American Journal of Emergency Medicine, 27*, 942–947.

112. Edwards, J. (1953). Congenital malformations of the heart and great vessels. In S. Gould & S. Gould (Eds.). *Pathology of the heart.* Springfield, IL: Charles C. Thomas.

113. Edwards, J., Christensen, N., & Clagett, O. (1948). Pathologic considerations in coarctation of the aorta. *Mayo Clinic Proceedings, 23*, 324–332.

114. Emergency Nurses Association. (2004a). *Emergency nursing pediatric course* (3rd ed.). Des Plaines, IL: Author.

115. Emergency Nurses Association. (2004b). *Emergency nursing pediatric course* (3rd ed.): *Instructor supplement.* Des Plaines, IL: Author.

116. Engle, M., Zabriskie, J., Senterfit, L., Gay, W., O'Loughlin, J., & Ehlers, K. (1980). Viral illness and the postpericardiotoy syndrome: A prospective study in children. *Circulation, 62*, 1151–1158.

117. English, R., Pophal, S., Bacanu, S., Fricker, J., Boyle, G., Ellis, D., et al. (2002). Long-term comparison of tacrolimus and cyclosporine-induced nephrotoxicity in pediatric heart transplant recipients. *American Journal of Transplantation, 2*(8), 769–771.

118. Epstein, A. E., DiMarco, J. P., Ellenbogen, K. A., Estes, N. A. 3rd, Freedman, R. A., Gettes, L. S., et al. (2008). ACC/AHA/HRS 2008 guidelines for device-based therapy of cardiac rhythm abnormalities: A report of the American College of Cardiology/American Heart Association Task Force on Practice Guidelines (Writing Committee to Revise the ACC/AHA/NASPE 2002 Guideline Update for Implantation of Cardiac Pacemakers and Antiarrhythmia Devices) developed in collaboration with the American Association for Thoracic Surgery and Society of Thoracic Surgeons. *Journal of the American College of Cardiology, 5*(6), e1–e62.

119. Farouk, A., Zahka, K., Siwik, E., Golden, A., Karimi, M., Uddin, M., et al. (2009). Anomalous origin of the left coronary artery from the right pulmonary artery. *Journal of Cardiac Surgery, 24*, 49–54.

120. Field, J. (Ed.). (2006). *Advanced cardiovascular life support provider manual.* Dallas: American Heart Association.

121. Field, J., & Doto, F. (Eds.). (2006). *Advanced cardiovascular life support: Instructor manual.* Dallas: American Heart Association.

122. Finkelstein, Y., Shemesh, J., Mahlab, K., Abramov, D., Bar-El, Y., Sagie, A. (2002). Colchicine for the prevention of postpericardiotomy syndrome. *Herz, 27*(8), 791–4.

123. Fischetti, V. (1989). Streptococcal M protein: Molecular design and biological behavior. *Clinical Microbiology Reviews, 2*(3), 285–314.

124. Fischetti, V., Jones, K., Hollinghead, S., & Scott, J. (1988). Structure, function and genetics of streptococcal M protein. *Review of Infectious Disease, 10*(suppl 2): S356–S359.

125. Frank, S., Johnson, A., & Ross, J. (1973). Natural history of valvular aaortic stenosis. *British Heart Journal, 35,* 41–46.

126. Fratz, S., Gildein, H., Balling, G., Sebening, W., Genz, T., Eicken, A., et al. (2008). Aortic valvuloplasty in pediatric patients substantially postpones the need for aortic valve surgery: A single-center experience of 188 patients after up to 17.5 years of follow-up. *Circulation, 117*(9), 1201–1206.

127. Frazier, E., Naftel, D., Canter, C., et al. (1999). Death after cardiac transplantation in children: Who dies, when and why. *Journal of Heart and Lung Transplantation, 18*, 69–70.

128. Freed, M., Rosenthal, A., & Bernhard, W. (1973). Critical pulmonary stenosis with diminutive right ventricle in neonates. *Circulation, 48*, 875–882.

129. Freedman, S., Haldyn, J., Floh, A., Kirsh, J., Taylor, G., & Thull-Freedman, J. (2007). Pediatric myocarditis: Emergency department clinical findings and diagnostic evaluation. *Pediatrics, 120*, 1278–1285.

130. Freilich, M., Stub, D., Esmore, D., Negri, J., Salamonsen, R., Bergin, P., et al. (2009). Recovery from anthracycline cardiomyophathy after long-term support with a continuous flow left ventricular assist device. *Journal of Heart and Lung Transplantation, 28,* 101–103.

131. French, J., & Guntheroth, W. (1970). An explanation of asymmetric upper extremity blood pressures in supravalvar aortic stenosis: The Coanda effect. *Circulation, 52*, 31–36.

132. Fricker, F. (2002). Should physical activity and/or competitive sports be curtailed in pediatric heart transplant recipients? *Pediatric Transplantation, 6*(4), 267–269.

133. Friedman, T., Mani, A., & Elefteriades, J. (2008). Bicuspid aortic valve: Clinical approach and scientific review of a common clinical entity. *Expert Review of Cardiovascular Therapy, 6*(2), 235–248.

134. Fuchs, S., Gausche-Hill, M., & Yamamoto, L. (Eds.). (2007). *APLS: The pediatric emergency medicine resource* (rev. 4th ed.). Sudbury, MA: Jones and Bartlett.

135. Fuglestad, S., Puga, F., & Danielson, G. (1988). Surgical pathology of the truncal valve: A study of 12 cases. *American Journal of Cardiovascular Pathology, 2*, 39–47.

136. Gajarski, R. J., Towbin, J. A., Bricker, J. T., Radovancevic, B., Frazier, O. H., & Price, J. K. (1994). Intermediate follow up of pediatric heart transplant recipients with elevated pulmonary vascular resistance index. *Journal of the American College of Cardiology, 23*(7), 1682–1687.

137. Galantowicz, M., Cheatham, J., Phillips, A., Cua, C., Hoffman, T., Hill, S., & Rodeman, R. (2008). Hybrid approach for hypoplastic left heart syndrome: Intermediate results after the learning curve. *Society of Thoracic Surgeon, 85,* 2063–2071.

138. Garfield, O. (1990). *Current concepts in cardiovascular physiology.* San Diego: Academic Press.

139. Garrett, H., Duvall-Seaman, D., Helsley, B., & Groshart, K. (2005). Treatment of vascular rejection with rituximab in cardiac transplantation. *Journal of Heart and Lung Transplantation, 24*(9), 1337–1342.

140. Gerber, M., Baltimore, R., Eaton, C., Gewitz, M., Rowley, A., Shulman, S., et al. (2009). Prevention of rheumatic fever and diagnosis and treatment of acute streptococcal pharyngitis: A scientific statement from the American Heart Association Rheumatic Fever, Endocarditis, and Kawasaki Disease Committee of the Council on Cardiovascular Disease in the Young, the Interdisciplinary Council on Functional Genomics and Translational Biology, and the Interdisciplinary Council on Quality of Care and Outcomes Research: ndorsed by the American Academy of Pediatrics. *Circulation, 119*, 1541–1551.

141. Ghanayem, N., Cava, J., Jaquiss, R., & Tweddell, J. (2004). Home monitoring of infants after stage one palliation for hypoplastic left heart syndrome. *Pediatric Cardiac Surgery Annual of the Seminars in Thoracic and Cardiovascular Surgery, 7,* 32–38.

142. Gill, P., Forbes, K., & Coe, J. (2009). The effect of short-term prophylactic acetylsalicylic acid on the incidence of postpericardiotomy syndrome after surgical closure of atrial septal defects. *Pediatric Cardiology, 30*(8), 1061–1067.

143. Goble, M., Benitez, C., Baumgardner, M., & Fenske, K. (2008). ED management of pediatric syncope: Searching for a rationale. *American Journal of Emergency Medicine, 26*(1), 66–70.

144. Gopinathanniar, R., Sullivan, R., & Olshansky, B. (2009). Tachycardia-mediated cardiomyopathy: Recognition and management. *Current Heart Failure Reports, 6,* 257–645.

145. Gray, H. (1973). *Anatomy of the human body.* (C. Goss, Ed.). Philadelphia: Lea & Febiger.

146. Gross, L. (1931). Topographic anatomy of the histology of the valves of the human heart. *American Journal of Pathology, 7,* 445.

147. Guenther, U., Varelmann, D., Putensen, C., & Wrigge, H. (2009). Extended therapeutic hypothermia for several days during extracorporeal membrane-oxygenation after drowning and cardiac arrest: Two cases of survival with no neurological sequelae. *Resuscitation, 80,* 379–381.

148. Guertl, B., Noehammer, C., & Hoefler, G. (2000). Metabolic cardiomyopathies. *International Journal of Experimental Pathology, 81*(6), 349–372.

149. Hachiro, Y., Takagi, N., & Koyanagi, T. (2001). Repair of double-chambered right ventricle: Surgical results and long-term follow-up. *Annual of Thoracic Surgery, 72,* 1520–1522.

150. Haffejee, I. (1992). Rheumatic fever and rheumatic heart disease: The current status of its immunology, diagnostic criteria, and prophylaxis. *Quality Journal of Medicine, 2*(84) 641–658.

151. Hager, A., Kanz, S., Kaemmerer, H., & Hess, J. (2008). Exercise capacity and exercise hypertension after surgical repair of isolated aortic coarctation. *American Journal of Cardiology, 101*(12), 1777–1780.

152. Haines, N., Rycus, P., Zwischenberger, J., Bartlett, R., & Undar, A. (2009). Extracorporeal life support registry report 2008: Neonatal and pediatric cardiac cases. *ASAIO Journal, 55,* 111–116.

153. Haley, M., Fisher, J., Ruiz-Elizalde, A., Stolar, C., Morrissey, N., & Middlesworth, W. (2009). Percutaneous distal perfusion of the lower extremity after femoral cannulation for venoarterial extracorporeal membrane oxygenation in a small child. *Journal of Pediatric Surgery, 44,* 437–440.

154. Han, R., Gurofsky, R., Lee, K., Dipchand, A., Williams, W., Smallhorn, J., et al. (2007). Outcome and growth potential of left heart structures after neonatal intervention for aortic valve stenosis. *Journal of the American College of Cardiology, 50*(25), 2406–2414.

155. Hanisch, D. (2001). Pediatric arrhythmias. *Journal of Pediatric Nursing,* 16(5), 351–361.

156. Hannan, R., Zabinsky, J., Stanfill, R., Ventura, R., Rossi, A., Nykanen, D., et al. (2009). Midterm results for collaborative treatment of pulmonary atresia with intact ventricular septum. *Annals of Thoracic Surgery, 87* (4), 1227–1233.

157. Haricharan, R., Barnhart, D., Cheng, H., & Delzell, E. (2009). Identifying neonates at a very high risk for mortality among children with congenital diaphragmatic hernia managed with extracorporeal membrane oxygenation. *Journal of Pediatric Surgery, 44,* 87–93.

158. Hayes, C., Gersony, W., & Driscoll, D. (1993). Second natural history study of congenital heart defects: Results of treatment of patients with pulmonary valvar stenosis. *Circulation, 87*(suppl), 128–137.

159. Hayworth, S. (1987). Pulmonary vascular disease in ventricular septal defects: Structure and functional correlation in lung biopsies from 85 patients with outcome of intracardiac repair. *Journal of Pathology, 152,* 157–168.

160. Healy. F., Hanna, B., & Zinman, R. (2010). Clinical practice: The impact of lung disease on the heart and cardiac disease on the lungs. *European Journal of Pediatrics, 169*(1), 1–6.

161. Heidl, S., Schwepcke, A., Weber, F., & Genzel, O. (2010). Microcirculation in preterm infants: Profound effects of patent ductus arteriosus. *Journal of Pediatrics, 156*(2), 191–196.

162. Herlong, J., Jaggers, J., & Ungerleider, R. (2000). Congenital heart surgery nomenclature and database project: Pulmonary venous anomalies. *Annals of Thoracic Surgery, 69*(4), 56–69.

163. Herman, J., Vandenberghe, P., van den Heuvel, I., Van Cleemput, J., Winnepenninckx, V., & Van Damme-Lombaerts, R. (2002). Successful treatment with rituximab of lymphoproliferative disorder in a child after cardiac transplantation. *Journal of Heart and Lung Transplantation, 21*(12), 1304–1309.

164. Hickey, E., Jung, G., Williams, W., Manlhiot, C., Van Arsdell, G., Caldarone, C., et al. (2008). Congenital supravalvar aortic stenosis: Defining surgical and nonsurgical outcomes. *Annals of Thoracic Surgery, 86*(6), 1919–1927.

165. Ho, S., & Anderson, R. (1979). Coarctation, tubular hypoplasia and the ductus arteriosus. *British Heart Journal, 41,* 268–270.

166. Hoffman, B. B. (2001a). Adrenoceptor-activating and other sympathomimetic drugs. In B. G. Katzung (Ed.). *Lange: Basic and clinical pharmacology* (8th ed., pp. 120–137). New York: McGraw-Hill.

167. Hoffman, B. B. (2001b). Adrenoceptor antagonist drugs. In B. G. Katzung (Ed.). *Lange: Basic and clinical pharmacology* (8th ed., pp. 138–154). New York: McGraw-Hill.

168. Hoffman, G., Tweddell, J., & Ghanayem, N. (2004). Alteration of the critical arteriovenous oxygen saturation relationship by sustained after load reduction after Norwood procedure. *Journal of Thoracic and Cardiovascular Surgery, 127,* 738–745.

169. Hoffman, J., & Kaplan, S. (2002). The incidence of congenital heart disease. *Journal of the American College of Cardiology, 39,* 1890.

170. Hoffman, M., Fried, M., Jabareen, F., Vardinon, N., Turner, D., Burke, M., et al. (2002). Anti-heart antibodies in postpericardiotomy syndrome: Cause or epiphenomenon? A prospective, longitudinal pilot study. *Autoimmunity, 35*(4), 241–245.

171. Hollenberg, S. (2009). Inotrope and vasopressor therapy of septic shock. *Critical Care Clinics, 25*(4), 781–802.

172. Hornberger, L., Sahn, D., & Kleinman, C. (1994). Antenatal diagnosis of coarctation of the aorta: A multicenter experience. *Journal of the American College of Cardiology, 23,* 417–423.

173. Hornung, T., Benson, L., & McLaughlin, P. (2002). Interventions for aortic coarctation. *Cardiology in Review, 10*(3), 139–148.

174. Horvath, R., Towgood, A., & Sandhu, S. (2008). Role of transcatheter therapy in the treatment of coarctation of the aorta. *Journal of Invasive Cardiology, 20*(12), 660–663.

175. Hsu, D., & Pearson, G. (2009a). Heart failure in children, part I: History, etiology, and pathophysiology. *Circulation, 2,* 63–70.

176. Hsu, D., & Pearson, G. (2009b). Heart failure in children, part II; Diagnosis, treatment, and future directions. *Circulation, 2,* 490–498.

177. Huang, S-C., Wu, E-T., Chen, Y-S., Chang, C-I., Chiu, I-S., Wang, S-S., et al. (2008). Extracorporeal membrane oxygenation

rescue for cardiopulmonary resuscitation in pediatric patients. *Critical Care Medicine, 36*(5), 1607–1613.

178. Ibrahim, J., Cantera, C., Chinnock, R., Kirklin, J., Naftel, D., Basile, S., et al. (2002). Linear and somatic growth following pediatric heart transplantation. *Journal of Heart and Lung Transplantation, 21*(1), 63.

179. Imamura, M., Dossey, A., Prodhan, P., Schmitz, M., Frazier, E., Dyamenahalli, U., et al. (2009). Bridge to cardiac transplant in children: Berlin heart versus extracorporeal membrane oxygenation. *Annals of Thoracic Surgery, 87,* 1894–1901.

180. Imazio, M., Bobbio, M., Cecchi, E., Demarie, D., Demichelis, B., Pomari, F., et al. (2005). Colchicine in addition to conventional therapy for acute pericarditis. *Circulation, 112*(13), 2012–1016.

181. Imazio, M., Cecchi, E., Demichelis, B., Chinaglia, A., Coda, L., Ghisio, A., et al. (2007). Rationale and design of the COPPS trial: Arandomized, placebo-controlled, multicentre study on the use of colchicines for the primary prevention of postpericardiotomy syndrome. *Journal of Cardiovascular Medicine, 8*(12), 1044–1048.

182. Isner, J., Donaldson, R., & Fulton, D. (1987). Cystic medial necrosis in coarctation of the aorta: A potential factor contributing to adverse consequences observed after percutaneous balloon angioplasty of coarctation sites. *Circulation, 75,* 689–695.

183. Ivy, D., Feinstein, J., Humpl, T., & Rosenzweig, E. (2009). Non-congenital heart disease associated pediatric pulmonary arterial hypertension. *Progress in Pediatric Cardiology, 27,* 13–23.

184. Jefferies, J. L., Denfield, S. W., & Dreyer, W. J. (2008). Heart failure in infants and children: Cardiomyopathy. In Nichols (ed.) Rogers' textbook of pediatric intensive care. (4th ed., pp. 1075–1081). Philadelphia: Lippincott .

185. Ji, B., & Undar, A. (2006). An evaluation of the benefits of pulsatile versus nonpulsatile perfusion during cardiopulmonary bypass procedures in pediatric and adult cardiac patients. *ASAIO Journal, 52*(4), 357–361.

186. Johnson, J. N., Jaggers, J., Shuang, L., O'Brien, S. M., Li, J. S., Jacobs, J. P., et al. (2010). Center variation and outcomes associated with delayed sternal closure after stage 1 palliation for hypoplastic left heart syndrome. *Journal of Thoracic and Cardiovascular Surgery, 139,* 1205–1210.

187. Johnson, J. O., Grecu, L., & Lawson, N. W. (2009). Autonomic nervous system. In P. G. Barash, B. F. Cullen, R. K. Stoelting, M. K. Cahalan, & M. C. Stock (Eds.). *Clinical anesthesia* (6th ed., pp. 326–368). Philadelphia: Lippincott, Williams & Wilkins.

188. Jonas, R. (2004). *Complete atrioventricular canal in comprehensive surgical management of congenital heart disease.* London: Arnold Publishers of Oxford University Press.

189. Jowett, V., Hayes, N., Sridharan, S., Rees, P., & Macrae, D. (2007). Timing of removal of pacing wires following paediatric cardiac surgery. *Cardiology in the Young, 17*(5), 512–516.

190. Joynt, C., Robertson, C., Cheung, P., Nettel-Aguirre, A., Joffe, A., Sauve, R., et al. (2009). Two-year neurodevelopmental outcomes of infants undergoing neonatal cardiac surgery for interrupted aortic arch: A descriptive analysis. *Journal of Thoracic and Cardiovascular Surgery, 138*(4), 924–932.

191. Kane, J., Rossi, J., Tsao, S., & Burton, B. (2007). Metabolic cardiomyopathy and mitochondrial disorders in the pediatric intensive care unit. *Journal of Pediatrics, 151*(5), 538–541.

192. Kaplan, E. (1993). Global assessment of rheumatic fever and rheumatic heart disease at the close of the century. *Circulation, 88*(4; part 1), 1964–1972.

193. Kaplan, M., & Frengley, J. (1969). Autoimmunity to the heart in cardiac disease: Current concepts of the relation of autoimmunity to rheumatic fever, postcardiotomy and post infarction syndromes and cardiomyopathies. *American Journal of Cardiology, 24,* 459–473.

194. Kattwinkel, J. (Ed.). (2006). *Textbook of neonatal resuscitation* (5th ed.). Elk Grove Village, IL: American Academy of Pediatrics & American Heart Association.

195. Katzung, B. G. (2001). Introduction to autonomic physiology. In B. G. Katzung (Ed.). *Lange: Basic and clinical pharmacology* (8th ed., pp. 75–91). New York: McGraw-Hill.

196. Katzung, B. G., & Parmley, W. W. (2001). Cardiac glycosides and other drugs used in congestive heart failure. In B. G. Katzung (Ed.). *Lange: Basic and clinical pharmacology* (8th ed., pp. 200–218). New York: McGraw-Hill.

197. Kaushal, S., Backer, C., Patel, J., Patel, S., Walker, B., Weigel, T., et al. (2009). Coarctation of the aorta: Midterm outcomes of resection with extended end-to-end anastomosis. *Annals of Thoracic Surgery, 88*(6), 1932–1938.

198. Keene, J. F., Lock, J. E., & Fyler, D. C. (2006). *Nadas' pediatric cardiology* (2nd ed.). Philadelphia: Saunders Elsevier.

199. Kelly, R., & Harrison, R. (2010, February 10). Outcome predictors of pediatric extracorporeal cardiopulmonary resuscitation. *Pediatric Cardiology.* [Epub ahead of print.]

200. Kerr, A. Jr., & Goss, C. (1956). Retention of embryonic relationship of aortic and pulmonary valve cusps and a suggested nomenclature. *Anatomical Record, 125,* 777.

201. Kfoury, A., & Hammond, M. (2010). Controversies in defining cardiac antibody-mediated rejection: Need for updated criteria. *Journal of Heart and Lung Transplantation, 29*(4), 389–394.

202. Khaghani, A., Santini, F., Dyke, C., Onuzu, O., Radley-Smith, R., & Yacoub, M. (1997). Heterotopic cardiac transplantation in infants and children. *Journal of Thoracic and Cardiovascular Surgery, 113*(6), 1042–1048.

203. Kim, J., Kim, E., Kim, W., Shim, G., Kim, H., Park, J., et al. (2009, June 8). Abnormally extended ductal tissue into the aorta is indicated by similar histopathology and shared apoptosis in patients with coarctation. *International Journal of Cardiology.* [Epub.]

204. King, T., Thompson, S., & Steiner, C. (1976). Secundum atrial septal defect: Nonoperative closure during cardiac catheterization. *Journal of the American Medical Association, 6,* 2506–2509.

205. Kirk, R., Edwards, L., Aurora, P., Taylor, D., Christie, J., Dobbels, F., et al. (2009). Registry of the International Society for Heart and Lung Transplantation: Eleventh official pediatric heart transplantation report—2009. *Journal of Heart and Lung Transplant, 28*(10), 993–1006.

206. Knauth, A., Lock, J., & Perry, S. (2004). Transcatheter device closure of congenital and postoperative residual ventricular septal defects. *Circulation, 110,* 501–507.

207. Knepp, M., Rocchini, A., Lloyd, T., & Aiyagari, R. (2010). Long term follow up of secundum atrial septal defect closure with the amplatzer septal occluder. *Congeniatal Heart Disease, 5*(1), 32–37.

208. Kobayashi, M., Ando, M., Wada, N., & Takahashi, Y. (2009). Outcomes following surgical repair of aortic arch obstructions with associated cardiac anomalies. *Euopean Journal of Cardiothoracic Surgery, 35*(4), 565–568.

209. Kobayashi, M., Takahashi, Y., & Ando, M. (2007). Ideal timing of surgical repair of isolated complete atrioventricular septal defect. *Interactive Cardiovascular and Thoracic Surgery, 6*(1), 24–26.

210. Konstantinov, I., Karamlou, T., Blackstone, E., Mosca, R., Lofland, G., & Caldaronn, C. (2006). Truncus arteriosus associated with interrupted aortic arch in 50 neonates: A Congenital Heart Surgeons Society study. *Annals of Thoracic Surgery, 81*(1), 214–222.

211. Kostolny, M., Schreiber, C., von Arnim, V., Vogt, M., Wottke, M., & Lange, R. (2006). Timing of repair in ventricular septal defect with aortic insufficiency. *Thoracic and Cardiovascular Surgery, 54* (8), 512–515.

212. Kozik, D., & Tweddell, J. (2006). Characterizing the inflammatory response to cardiopulmonary bypass in children. *Annals of Thoracic Surgery, 81*(6), 47–54.

213. Kulik, T., Mullen, M., & Adatia, I. (2009). Pulmonary arterial hypertension associated with congenital heart disease. *Progress in Pediatric Cardiology, 27,* 25–33.

214. Kumar, A., Kavinsky, C., Amin, Z., & Hijazi, Z. (2009). Percutaneous pulmonic valve implantation. *Current Treatment Options in Cardiovascular Medicine, 11*(6), 483–491.

215. Kveselis, D., Rosenthal, A., & Ferguson, P. (1984). Long-term prognosis after repair of double-chamber right ventricle with ventricular seeptal defect. *American Journal of Cardiology, 54,* 1292–1295.

216. Kyburz, A., Bauersfeld, U., Schnizel A., Riegel, M., Hug, M., Tomaske, M., et al. (2008). The fate of children with microdeletion 22q11.2 syndrome and congenital heart defect: Clinical course and cardiac outcome. *Pediatric Cardiology, 29*(1), 76–83.

217. Lai, W., Mertens, L., Cohen, M., & Geva, T. (2009). *Echocardiography in pediatric and congenital heart disease: From fetus to adult.* Hoboken, NJ: Wiley-Blackwell.

218. Lakatta, E., & Maughan, W. (1990). Cardiovascular function. In O. Garfield (Ed.). *Current concepts in cardiovascular physiology* (pp. 351–466). San Diego: Academic Press.

219. Lancefield, R. (1941). Specific relationship of cell composition to biological activity of hemolytic streptococci. *Harvey Lectures, 36,* 251–260.

220. Landing, B., Lawrence, T., Payne, V., & Wells, T. (1971). Bronchial anatomy in syndromes with abnormal visceral situs, abnormal spleen, and congenital heart disease. *American Journal of Cardiology, 128,* 456.

221. Landvoigt, M., & Mullett, C. (2006). Octreitide efficacy in the treatment of chylothoraces following cardiac surgery in infants and children. *Pediatric Critical Care Medicine, 7,* 245–248.

222. Lange, R., & Hillis, D. (2004). Acute pericarditis. *New England Journal of Medicine, 351,* 2195–2202.

223. Latifi, S., Lidsky, K., & Blumer, J. L. (2000). Pharmacology of inotropic agents in infants and children. *Progress in Pediatric Cardiology, 12*(1), 57–79.

224. Laughon, M., Simmons, M., & Bose, C. (2004). Patency of the ductus arteriosus in the premature infant: Is it pathologic? Should it be treated? *Current Opinion in Pedatrics, 16*(2).

225. Law, Y., Hoyer, A., Reller, M., & Silberbach, M. (2009). Accuracy of plasma B-type natriuretic peptide to diagnose significant cardiovascular disease in children: The Better Not Pout Children! study. *Journal of the American College of Cardiology, 54*(15), 1467–1475.

226. Lev, M., Liberthson, R., Golden, J., Eckner, F., & Arcilla, R. (1971). The pathologic anatomy of mesocardia. *American Journal of Cardiology, 28,* 428.

227. Levy, M., & Pappano, A. (2006). *Cardiovascular physiology: Mosby physiology monograph series* (9th ed.). St. Louis: C. V. Mosby.

228. Lewin, M., McBride, K., & Pignatelli, R. (2004). Echocardiogramic evaluation of asymptomatic parental and sibling cardiovascular anomalies associated with congenital left ventricular outflow tract lesions. *Pediatrics, 114,* 691–696.

229. Lexi-Comp Online, Pediatric Lexi-Drugs Online. (2009). Hudson, OH: Lexicomp-Inc. Retrieved from http://www.crlonline.com

230. Liang, C., Su, W., Chung, H., Hwang, M., Huang, C., Lin, Y., et al. (2009). Balloon angioplasty for native coarctation of the aorta in neonates and infants with congestive heart failure. *Pediatric Neonatology, 50*(4), 152–157.

231. Liberthson, R., Hastreiter, A., Sinha, S., Bharati, S., Novak, G., & Lev, M. (1973). Levocardia with visceral heterotaxy-isolated levocardia: Pathologic anatomy and its clinical implications. *American Heart Journal, 85,* 40.

232. Lim, K., Kim, S., June, H., Kang, I., Lee, H., Jun, T., et al. (2005). Somatostatin for postoperative chylothorax after surgery for children with congenital heart disease. *Journal of Korean Medical Science, 20,* 947–951.

233. Lin, F., Ko, W., Huang, S., Wu, E., Chen, Y., Chang, C., et al. (2008). Extracorporeal membrane oxygenation rescue for cardiopulmonary resuscitation in pediatric patients. *Critical Care Medicine, 36*(5), 1607–1613.

234. Lindblade, C., Kirkpatrick, E., & Ebenroth, E. (2006). Eosinophilic myocarditis presenting with pediatric myocardial infarction. *Pediatric Cardiology, 27*(1), 162–165.

235. Lindenfeld, J., Miller, G., Shakar, S., Zolty, R., Lowes, B., Wolfel, E., et al. (2004). Drug therapy in the heart transplant recipient: Part I: Cardiac rejection and immunosuppressive drugs. *Circulation,* (110), 3734–3740.

236. Lipshultz, S., Sleeper, L., Towbin, J., Lowe, A., Orav, E., Cox, G., et al. (2003). The incidence of pediatric cardiomyopathy in two regions of the United States. *New England Journal of Medicine, 348*(17), 1647–1655.

237. Lock, J., Keane, J., & Fellows, A. (1993). Diagnostics and interventional catheterizations in congenital heart disease. Boston: Martinus Nijhoff Publishing.

238. Loffredo, C., Chokkalingam, A., & Sill, A. (2004). Prevalence of congenital cardiovascular malformations among relatives of infants with hypoplastic left heart, coarctation of the aorta, and d-transposition of the great arteries. *American Journal of Medical Genetics Part A, 124,* 225–230.

239. Lurz, P., Bonhoeffer, P., & Taylor, A. (2009). Percutaneous pulmonary valve implantation: An update. *Expert Review in Cardiovascular Therapy, 7*(7), 823–833.

240. Magnani, J., & Dec, W. (2006). Myocarditis: Current trends in diagnosis and treatment. *Circulation. 113,* 876–890.

241. Maher, K., Reed, H., Cuadrado, A., Simsic, J., Mahle, W., Deguzman, M., et al. (2008). B-type natriuretic peptide in the emergency diagnosis of critical heart disease in children. *Pediatrics, 121*(6), 1484–1488.

242. Mahrholdt, H., Wagner, A., Deluigi, C., Kispert, E., Hager, S., Meinhardt, G., et al. (2006). Presentation, patterns of myocardial damage, and clinical course of viral myocarditis. *Circulation, 114,* 1581–1590.

243. Maisch, B., Berg, P., & Kochsiek, K. (1979). Clinical significance of immunopathological findings in patients with postpericardiotomy syndrome. *Clinical & Experimental Immunology, 38,* 189–193.

244. Maisch, B., Seferovic, P., Ristic, A., Erbel, R., Reienmuller, R., Adler, Y., et al. (2004). Guidelines on the diagnosis and management of pericardial diseases: Executive summary. *European Heart Journal, 25,* 587–610.

245. Margossian, R. (2008). Contemporary management of pediatric heart failure. *Expert Review of Cardiovascular Therapy, 6*(2), 187–197.

246. Marino, B. S., Kaltman, J. R., & Tanel, R. E. (2008). Cardiac conduction, dysrhythmias, and pacing. In D .G. Nichols (Ed.). *Rogers' textbook of pediatric intensive care* (4th ed., pp. 1126–1148). Philadelphia: Lippincott, Williams & Wilkins.

247. Massin, M., Bourguignont, A., Coremans, C., Comte, L., Lepage, P., & Gerard, P. (2004). Syncope in pediatric patients presenting to an emergency department. *Journal of Pediatrics, 145*(2), 223–228.

248. Mayock, D. (2009). ECMO statistics. Retrieved from http://depts.washington.edu/nicuweb/NICU-WEB/ecmo2.stm#elso_statistics

249. McBride, K., Pignatelli, R., & Lewin, M. (2005). Inheritance analysis of congenital left ventricular outflow tract obstruction malformations: Segregation, multiplex relative risk, and heritability. *American Journal of Medical Genetics Part A, 134,* 180–186.

250. McBride, S. (2007). Syncope. In L. Zaoutis & V. Chang (Eds.). *Comprehensive pediatric hospital medicine* (pp. 223–226). Philadelphia: Mosby.

251. McComber, D., Ibrahim, J., Lublin, D., Saffitz, J., Ong-Simon, J., Mendeloff, E., et al. (2004). Nonischemic left ventricular dysfunction after pediatric cardiac transplantation: Treatment with plasmapheresis and OKT3. *Journal of Heart and Lung Transplantation, 23*(5), 552–557.

252. McDonald, A., Gerlis, L., & Somerville, J. (1969). Familial arteriopathy with associated pulmonary and systemic arterial stenosis. *British Heart Journal, 31,* 375–385.

253. McLean, K., Lorts, A., & Pearl, J. (2006). Current treatments for congenital aortic stenosis. *Current Opinion in Cardiology, 21*(3), 200–204.

254. Mehta, P. A., Cunningham, C. K., Colella, C. B., Alferis, G., & Weiner, L. B. (2000). Risk factors for sternal wound and other infections in pediatric cardiac surgery patients. *Pediatric Infectious Disease Journal, 19*(10), 1000–1004.

255. Meri, S., Verkkala, K., Miettinen, A., Valtonen, V., & Linder, E. (1985). Complement levels and C3 breakdown products in open-heart surgery: Association of C3 conversion with the postpericardiotomy syndrome. *Clinical & Experimental Immunology, 60,* 597–604.

256. Miller, T., Neri, D., Extein, J., Somarriba, G., & Strickman-Stein, N. (2007). Nutrition in pediatric cardiomyopathy. *Progress in Pediatric Cardiology, 24*(1), 59–71.

257. Milo, S., Ho, S., Macartney, F., Wilkinson, J., Becker, A., Wenink, K., et al. (1979). Straddling and over-riding atrio-ventricular valves: Morphology and classification. *American Journal of Cardiology, 44,* 1122.

258. Mishra, P. (2009). Management strategies for interrupted aortic arch with associated anomalies. *European Journal of Cardiothoracic Surgery, 35*(4), 569–576.

259. Moe, D., & Guntheroth, W. (1987). Spontaneous closure of uncomplicated vetricular septal defect. *American Journal of Cardiology, 60,* 674–678.

260. Moerman, P., Dumouln, M., & Lauweryns, J. (1987). Interrupted right aortic arch in DiGeorge syndrome. *British Heart Journal, 58,* 274–278.

261. Mohan, U., Danon, S., Levi, D., Connolly, D., & Moore, J. (2009). Stent implantation for coarctation of the aorta in children < 30 kg. *JACC Cardiovascular Intervention, 2*(9), 877–883.

262. Momma, K. (2006). ACE inhibitors in pediatric patients with heart failure. *Pediatric Drugs, 8*(1), 55–69.

263. Moss, A., Adams, F., & O'Loughlin, B. (1959). The growth of the normal aorta and the anastomotic site in infants following sugical resection of coarctation of the aorta. *Circulation, 19,* 338–349.

264. Mott, A., Frase, C., Kusnoor, A., Giesecke, N., Reul, G., Drescher, K., et al. (2001). The effect of short-term prophylactic methylprednisolone on the incidence and severity of postpericardiotomy syndrome in children undergoing cardiac surgery with cardiopulmonary bypass. *Journal of the American College of Cardiology, 17,* 1700–1706.

265. Muensterer, O., Schenk, D., Praun, M., Boehm, R., & Till, H. (2003). Postpericardiotomy syndrome after minimally invasive pectus excavatum repair unresponsive to nonsteroidal anti-inflammatory treatment. *European Journal of Pediatric Surgery, 13*(3), 206–208.

266. Mullen, M. (2010). Diagnostic strategies for acute presentation of pulmonary hypertension in children: Particular focus on use of echocardiography, cardiac catheterization, magnetic resonance imaging, chest computed tomography, and lung biopsy. *Pediatric Critical Care Medicine, 11,* S23–S26.

267. Mutlu, B., Bayrak, F., Kahvecl, G., Degerterkin, M., Eroglu, E., & Basaran, Y. (2006). Usefulness of N-terminal pro-B-type naturetic peptide to predict clinical course in patients with hypertrophic cardiomyopathy. *American Journal of Cardiology, 98*(11), 1504–1506.

268. Nadkarni, V., Larkin, G., Peberdy, M., Carey, S., Kaye, W., Mancini, M., et al. (2006). First documented rhythm and clinical outcome from in-hospital cardiac arrest among children and adults. *Journal of the American Medical Association, 295*(1), 50–57.

269. Newfeld, E., Muster, A., & Paul, M. (1976). Discrete subvalvar aortic stenosis in childhood: Study of 51 patients. *American Journal of Cardiology, 38,* 53–61.

270. Noonan, J. (1968). Hypertension with Turner phenotype: A new syndrome with associated congenital heart disease. *American Journal of Diseases of Children, 116,* 373–380.

271. O'Connor, W., Davis, J., & Geissler, R. (1985). Supravalvar aortic stenosis: Clinical and oathological observation in six patients. *Archives of Pathology and Laboratory Medicine, 109,* 179–185.

272. Odim, J., Laks, H., Banerji, A., Mukherjee, K., Vincent, C., Murphy, C., et al. (2005). Does duration of brain injury affect outcome after pediatric orthotopic heart transplantation? *Journal of Thoracic and Cardiovascular Surgery, 130*(1), 187–193.

273. Ogden, J. (1970). Congenital anomalies of the coronary arteries. *American Journal of Cardiology, 25,* 474.

274. Ohye, R., Mosca, R., Bove, E., Backer, C., & Mavroudis, C. (2003). Hypoplastic left heart syndrome. In C. Mavroudis & C. Backer (Eds.). *Pediatric cardiac surgery* (3rd ed., pp. 560–575). Philadelphia: Mosby.

275. Ohye, R., & Pediatric Heart Network Investigators. (2010). Comparison of shunt types in the Norwood procedure for single-ventricle lesions. *New England Journal of Medicine, 362*(21), 1980–1992.

276. Oosterhof, T., Hazekamp, M., & Mulder, B. (2009). Opportunities in pulmonary valve replacement. *Expert Review of Cardiovascular Therapy, 7*(9), 1117–1122.

277. Otto, C. W. (2009). Cardiopulmonary resuscitation. In P. G. Barash, B. F. Cullen, R. K. Stoelting, M. K. Cahalan, & M. C. Stock (Eds.). *Clinical anesthesia* (6th ed., pp. 1532–1558). Philadelphia: Lippincott, Williams & Wilkins.

278. Pahl, E., Caforio, A., & Kuhn, M. (2007). Allograft vasculopathy: Detection, risk factors, natural history, and treatment. In C. Canter & J. Kirklin (Eds.). *ISHLT monograph series* (2nd ed., pp. 173–185). Philadelphia: Elsevier.

279. Pahl, E., Crawford, S., Cohn, R., Rodgers, S., Wax, D., Backer, C., et al. (2000). Reversal of severe late left ventricular failure after pediatric heart transplantation and possible role of plasmapheresis. *American Journal of Cardiology, 85*(6), 735–739.

280. Pahl, E., Naftel, D., Kuhn, M., Shaddy, R., Morrow, W., Canter, C., et al. (2005). The impact and outcome of transplant coronary artery disease in a pediatric population: A 9 year multi-institutional study. *Journal of Heart and Lung Transplantation, 24*(6), 645–651.

281. Paolillo, J., Boyle, G., Law, Y., Miller, S., Lawrence, K., Wagner, K., et al. (2001) Post-transplant diabetes mellitus in pediatric thoracic organ recipients receiving tacrolimus based immunosuppression. *Transplantation, 71*(2), 252–256.

282. Papadopoulos, N., Esmaeili, A., Zierer, A., Bakhtiary, F., Ozaslan, F., & Moritz, A. (2009). Secondary repair of incompetent pulmonary valves. *Annals of Thoracic Surgery, 87*(6), 1879–1884.

283. Parisi, F., Danesi, H., Squitieri, C., Di Chiara, L., Rava, L., & Di Donato, R. (2003). Thymoglobuline use in pediatric heart transplantation. *Journal of Heart and Lung Transplantation, 22*(5), 591–593.

284. Park, M. K. (2008). *Pediatric cardiology for practitioners.* Philadelphia: Mosby.

285. Park, M. K., & Guntheroth, W. G. (1992). *How to read pediatric ECGs.* St. Louis: Mosby Year Book.

286. Partridge, J., Scott, O., Deverall, P., & Macartney, F. (1975). Visualization and measurement of the main bronchi by tomography as an objective indicator of thoracic situs in congenital heart disease. *Circulation, 51,* 188.

287. Pasquali, S., Shera, D., Wernovsky, G., Cohen, M., Tabbutt, S., Nicholson, S., et al. (2007). Midterm outcomes and predictors of reintervention after the Ross procedure in infants, children, and young adults. *Journal of Thoracic and Cardiovascular Surgery, 133*(4), 893–899.

288. Pawlik, T., Marcos Porta, N., Steinhorn, R., Ogata, E., & deRegnier, R. (2009). Medical and financial impact of a neonatal extracorporeal membrane oxygenation referral center in the nitric oxide era. *Pediatrics, 123,* e17–e24.

289. Penson, M., Fricker, F., Thompson, J., Harker, K., Williams, B., Kahler, D., et al. (2001). Safety and efficacy of pravastatin therapy for the prevention of hyperlipidemia in pediatric and adolescent cardiac transplant recipients. *Journal of Heart and Lung Transplantation, 20*(6), 611–618.

290. Perry, J. C., & Walsh, E. P. (1998). Diagnosis and management of cardiac arrhythmias. In A. C. Chang, F. L. Hanley, G. Wernovsky, & D. L. Wessel (Eds.). *Pediatric cardiac intensive care* (pp. 461–481). Baltimore: Lippincott, Williams & Wilkins.

291. Pescovitz, M. (2004). The use of rituximab, anti-CD20 monoclonal antibody, in pediatric transplantation. *Pediatric Transplantation, 8,* 9–21.

292. Pfammatter, J., Paul, T., Viemer, G., & Kallfelz, H. (1995). Successful management of junctional tachycardia by hypothermia after cardiac operation in infants. *Annals of Thoracic Surgery, 60,* 556–560.

293. Piccardo, A., Ghez, O., Gariboldi, V., Riberi, A., Collart, F., Kreitmann, B., et al. (2009). Ross and Ross-Konno procedures in infants, children, and adolescents: A 13 year experience. *Journal of Heart Valve Disease, 18*(1), 76–82.

294. Piciucchi, S., Goodman, L., Earing, M., Nicolosi, A., Almassi, H., Tisol, W., et al. (2008). Aortic aneurysms: Delayed complications of coarctation of the aorta repair using Dacron patch aortoplasty. *Journal of Thoracic Imaging, 23*(4), 278–283.

295. Pietra, G., Edwards, W., Kay, J., Rich, S., Kernis, J., Schloo, B., et al. (1989). Histopathology of primary pulmonary hypertension: A qualitative and quantitative study of pulmonary blood vessels from 58 patients in the National Heart, Lung, and Blood Institute, Primary Pulmonary Hypertension Registry. *Circulation, 80,* 1198–1206.

296. Piorecka-Makula, A., & Werner, B. (2009). Prolonged QT dispersion in children with congenital valvular aortic stenosis. *Medical Science Monitor, 15*(10), CR534–CR538.

297. Pizarro, C., Murdison, K. A., Derby, C. D., & Radtke, W. (2008). Stage II reconstruction after hybrid palliation for high-risk patients with single ventricle. *Society of Thoracic Surgeons, 85,* 1382–1388.

298. Preston, I. (2008). Combination therapies in pulmonary arterial hypertension. *Advances in Pulmonary Hypertension, 7*(1), 235–242.

299. Pyle, R., Patterson, D., & Chacko, S. (1976). The genetics and pathology of discrete subaortic stenosis in the Newfoundland dog. *American Heart Journal, 92,* 324–334.

300. Quan, L., & Seidel, J. (Eds.). (1997). *Pediatric advanced life support: Instructor's manual.* Dallas: American Heart Association.

301. Qureshi, S. (2009). Use of covered stents to treat coarctation of the aorta. *Korean Circulation Journal, 39,* 261–263.

302. Ralston, M., Hazinski, M., Schexnayder, S., Zaritsky, A., & Kleinman, M. (Eds.). (2007). *Pediatric emergency assessment, recognition, and stabilization provider manual.* Dallas: American Heart Association.

303. Ralston, M., Hazinski, M. F., Zaritsky, A., Schexnayder, S., & Kleinman, M. (Eds.). (2006). *Pediatric advanced life support provider manual.* Dallas: American Heart Association.

304. Ranganathan, N., Lam, J., Wigle, E., & Silver, M. (1970). Morphology of the human mitral valve. II. The valve leaflets. *Circulation, 41,* 459.

305. Rashid, A., & Ivy, D. (2005). Severe paediatric pulmonary hypertension: New management strategies. *Archives of Diseases in Childhood, 90,* 92–98.

306. Rausch, R., Hofbeck, M., Zweier, C., Koch, A., Zink, S., Hoyer, J., et al. (2009). Comprehensive genotype–phenotype analysis in 230 patients with tetralogy of Fallot. *Journal of Medical Genetics.* [Epub.]

307. Raymond, T., Cunnyngham, C., Thompson, M., Thomas, J., Dalton, H., & Nadkami, V. (2009, . Outcomes among neonates, infants and children after extracorporeal cardiopulmonary resuscitation for refractory in-hospital cardiac arrest: A report from the National Registry of Cardiopulmonary Resuscitation. *Pediatric Critical Care Medicine. 11*(3), 362–371.

308. Razzouk, A., Johnston, J., Larsen, R., Chinnock, R., Fitts, J., & Bailey, L. (2005). The effect of oversizing cardiac allografts on survival in pediatric patients with congenital heart disease. *Journal of Heart and Lung Transplantation, 24*(2), 195–199.

309. Reid, I. A. (2001). Vasoactive peptides. In B. G. Katzung (Ed.). *Lange: Basic and clinical pharmacology* (8th ed., pp. 292–310). New York: McGraw-Hill.

310. Rhee, E., Nigro, J., & Pophal, S. (2008). Therapeutic options in hypertrophic cardiomyopathy: A pediatric perspective. *Current Treatment Options in Cardiovascular Medicine, 10,* 433–441.

311. Rich, S., Kaufmann, E., & Levy, P. (1992). The effect of high doses of calcium-channel blockers on survival in primary pulmonary hypertension. *New England Journal of Medicine, 327,* 76–81.

312. Rich, S., Seidlitz, M., Dodin, E., Osimani, D., Judd, D., Genthner, D., et al. (1998). The short-term effects of digoxin in patients with right

313. Richardson, P., Rapporteur, M., Bristow, M., Maish, B., Mautner, B., O'Connell, J., et al. (1996). Report of the 1995 World Health Organization/International Society and Federation of Cardiology Task Force on the definition and classification of cardiomyopathies. *Circulation, 93*(5), 841–842.

314. Riphagen, S., McDougall, M., Tibby, S. M., Alphonso, N., Anderson, D., Austin, C., et al. (2005). "Early" delayed sternal closure following pediatric cardiac surgery. *Annals of Thoracic Surgery, 80,* 678–685.

315. Rivenes, S., Kearney, D., O'Brian Smith, E., Towbin, J., & Denfield, S. (2000). Sudden death and cardiovascular collapse in children with restrictive cardiomyopathy. *Circulation, 102*(8), 876–882.

316. Rocha, G. (2007). Pleural effusions in the neonate. *Current Opinion in Pulmonary Medicine, 13,* 305–311.

317. Roguin, N., Du, Z., & Barak, M. (1995). High prevelence of muscular ventricular septal defects in neonates. *Journal of American College of Cardiology, 26,* 1545–1548.

318. Rosanova, M. R., Allaria, A., Santillan, A., Hernandez, C., Snadry, L., Ceminara, R., et al. (2009). Risk factors for infection after cardiovascular surgery in children in Argentina. *Brazilian Journal of Infectious Diseases, 13*(6), 414–416.

319. Rosenthal, D., Chrisant, M., Edens, E., Mahony, L., Canter, C., Colan, S., et al. (2004). International Society for Heart and Lung Transplantation: Practice guidelines for management of heart failure in children. *Journal of Heart Transplantation, 23,* 1313–1333.

320. Rosenzweig, E., Feinstein, J., Humpl, T., & Ivy, D. (2009). Pulmonary hypertension in children: Diagnostic workup and challenges. *Progress in Pediatric Cardiology, 27,* 7–11.

321. Rosenzweig, E., Widlitz, A., & Barst, R. (2004). Pulmonary arterial hypertension in children. *Pediatric Pulmonology, 38,* 2–22.

322. Rubin, R. (2000). Prevention and treatment of cytomegalovirus disease in heart transplant patients. *Journal of Heart and Lung Transplantation, 19,* 731–735.

323. Rudolph, A., Heymann, M., & Spitznas, U. (1972). Hemodynamic considerations in the development of narrowing of the aorta. *American Journal of Cardiology, 30,* 514–525.

324. Russo, L., & Webber, S. (2005). Idiopathic restrictive cardiomyopathy in children. *Heart, 91*(9), 1199–1202.

325. Ruzmetov, M., Vijay, P., Rodefeld, M., Turrentine, M., & Brown, J. (2006). Long-term results of surgical repair in patients with congenital subaortic stenosis. *Interactive Cardiovascular and Thoracic Surgery, 5*(3), 227–233.

326. Sabet, H., Edwards, W., & Tazelaar, H. (1999). Congenitally bicuspid aortic valves; A surgical pathology study of 542 cases (1991 through 1996) and a literature review of 2,715 additioal cases. *Mayo Clinic Proceedings, 74,* 14–26.

327. Sadof, M., & Nazarian, B. (2007). Caring for children who have special health-care needs: A practical guide for the primary care practitioner. *Pediatrics in Review, 28*(7), e36–e42.

328. Sapin, S. (2004). Autonomic syncope in pediatrics: A practice-oriented approach to classification, pathophysiology, diagnosis, and management. *Clinical Pediatrics, 43*(1), 17–23.

329. Schultz, J., Hilliard, A., Cooper, L., & Rihal, C. (2009). Diagnosis and treatment of viral myocarditis. *Mayo Clinic Proceedings, 84*(11), 1001–1009.

330. Scott, D., Campbell, D., Clarke, D., Goldberg, S., Karlin, D., & Mitchell, M. (2009). Twenty-years surgical experience with congeniatal supravalvular aortic stenosis. *Annals of Thoracic Surgery, 87,* 1501–1508.

331. Secchi, F., Iozzelli, A., Papini, G., Aliprandi, A., Di Leo, G., & Sardanelli, F. (2009). MR imaging of aortic coarctation. *Radiological Medicine, 114*(4), 524–537.

ventricular dysfunction from pulmonary hypertension. Chest, 114, 787–792.

332. Selamet, S., Hsu, D., & Thaker, H. (2004). Complete atresia of coronary ostia in pulmonary atresia and intact ventricular septum. *Pediatric Cardiology, 25,* 67–69.

333. Selke, F. W., del Nido, P. J., & Swanson, S. J. (2005). *Sabiston & Spencer: Surgery of the chest* (7th ed., Vol. 2). Philadelphia: Elsevier Saunders.

334. Senzaki, H., Kamiyama, M., Masutani, S., Ishido, H., Taketazu, M., Kobayashi, T., et al. (2008). Efficacy and safety of torasemide in children with heart failure. *Archives of Diseases of Childhood, 93,* 768–771.

335. Shaddy, R., Revenaugh, J., Orsmond, G., & Tani, L. (2000). Coronary interventional procedures in pediatric heart transplant recipients with cardiac allograft vasculopathy. *American Journal of Cardiology, 85*(11), 1370–1372.

336. Shaddy, R., & Wernovsky, G. (2005). *Pediatric heart failure (fundamental and clinical cardiology).* Boca Raton, FL: Taylor & Francis Group.

337. Shekerdemian, L. S., & Redington, A. (1998). Cardiovascular pharmacology. In A. C. Chang, F. L. Hanley, G. Wernovsky, & D. L. Wessel (Eds.). *Pediatric cardiac intensive care* (pp. 45–65). Baltimore: Lippincott, Williams & Wilkins.

338. Shem-Tov, A., Schneeweiss, A., & Motro, M. (1982). Clinical presentation and natural history of mild discrete subaortic stenosis. Follow-up of 1–17 years. *Circulation, 66,* 509–512.

339. Sherman, F. (1963). Ventricular septal defect. In F. Sherman & F. Sherman (Eds.). *An atlas of congenital heart disease* (p. 170). Philadelphia: Lea & Febiger.

340. Shimada, S., Kasai, T., & Konishi, M. (1994). Effects of patent ductus arteriosus on left ventricular output and organ blood flows in premature infants with respiratory distress syndrome treated with surfactant. *Journal of Pediatrics, 125,* 270–277.

341. Silka, M. J., & Bar-Cohen, Y. (2006). Pacemakers and implantable cardioverter–defibrillators in pediatric patients. *Heart Rhythm, 3*(11), 1360–1366.

342. Simonneau, G., Robbins, I., Beghetti, M., Channick, R., Delcroix, M., Denton, C., et al. (2009). Updated clinical classification of pulmonary hypertension. *Journal of the American College of Cardiology, 54,* S43–S54.

343. Singh, T. (2007). Long-term medical morbidities: Hypertension, lipids, renal dysfunction, arrhythmias. In C. Canter & J. Kirklin (Eds.). *ISHLT monograph series: Pediatric heart transplantation* (2nd ed., pp. 215–225). Philadelphia: Elsevier.

344. Singh, T., Sleeper, L., Lipshultz, S., Cinar, A., Canter, C., Webber, S., et al. (2009). Association of left ventricular dilation at listing for heart transplant with postlisting and early posttransplant mortality in children with dilated cardiomyopathy. *Circulation: Heart Failure, 2*(6), 591–598.

345. Sitbon, O., Humbert, M., Jais, X., Ioos, V., Hamid, A., Provencher, S., et al. (2005). Long term response to calcium channel blockers in idiopathic pulmonary arterial hypertension. *Circulation, 111,* 3105–3111.

346. Somarriba, G., Extein, J., & Miller, T. (2008). Exercise rehabilitation in pediatric cardiomyopathy. *Progress in Pediatric Cardiology, 25*(1), 91–102.

347. Soto, B., Pacifico, A., Souza, A. Jr., Bargeron, L. Jr., Ermocilla, R., & Tonkin, I. (1978). Identification of thoracic isomerism from the plain chest roentgenogram. *American Journal of Roentgenology, 131,* 995.

348. Stamm, C., Friehs, I., & Ho, S. (2001). Congenital supravalvar aortic stenosis: A simple lesion? *European Journal of Cardiothoracic Surgery, 19,* 195–202.

349. Stanger, P., Benassi, R., Korns, M., Jue, K., & Edwards, J. (1968). Diagrammatic portrayal of variations in cardiac structure, reference to transposition, dextrocardia and the concept of four normal hearts. *Circulation, 37,* IV1.

350. Starr, J. (2009, Nov 29). Tetralogy of Fallot: yesterday and today. World J Surg, Epub.

351. Stasny, P., Lavingia, B., Fixler, D., Yancy, C., & Ring, W. (2007). Antibodies against donor human leukocyte antigens and the outcome of cardiac allografts in adults and children. *Transplantation, 84*(6), 738–745.

352. Stiller, B., Hetzer, R., Weng, Y., Hummel, M., Hennig, E., Nagdyman, N., et al. (2003). Heart transplantation in children after mechanical circulatory support with pulsatile pneumatic assist device. *Journal of Heart and Lung Transplantation, 22*(11), 1201–1208.

353. Stollerman, G. (2001). Rheumatic fever in the 21st century. *Clinical Infectious Diseases, 33,* 806–814.

354. Straumanis, J. P. (2008). Nosocomial infections in the pediatric intensive care unit. In D. G. Nichols (Ed.). *Rogers' textbook of pediatric intensive care* (4th ed., p. 1417). Philadelphia: Lippincott Williams & Wilkins, Wolters Kluwer.

355. Strickberger, S., Benson, D., Biaggioni, I., Callans, D., Cohen, M., Ellenbogen, K., et al. (2006). AHA/ACCF scientific statement on the evaluation of syncope. *Journal of the American College of Cardiology, 47*(2), 473–484.

356. Strieper, M. (2005). Distinguishing benign syncope from life-threatening cardiac causes of syncope. *Seminars in Pediatric Neurology, 12*(1), 32–38.

357. Suesawalak, M., Cleary, J., & Chang, A. (2010). Advances in diagnosis and treatment of pulmonary arterial hypertension in neonates and children with congenital heart disease. *World Journal of Pediatrics, 6*(1), 13–31.

358. Sukova, J., Ostadal, P., & Widimsky, P. (2007). Profile of patients with acute heart failure and elevated troponin 1 levels. *Experimental and Clinical Cardiology, 12*(3), 153–156.

359. Sulemanjee, N., Merla, R., Lick, S., Aunon, S., Taylor, M., Manson, M., et al. (2008). The first year post heart transplantation: Use of immunosuppressive drugs and early complications. *Journal of Cardiovascular Pharmacology and Therapeutics, 13,* 13–31.

360. Sun, J., Niu, J., Banbury, M., Zhou, L., Taylor D., Starling, R., et al. (2007). Influence of different implantation techniques on long-term survival after orthotopic heart transplantation: An echocardiographic study. *Journal of Heart and Lung Transplantation, 26*(12), 1243–1247.

361. Suzuki, Y., Yamauchi, S., Daitoku, K., Fukui, K., & Fukuda, I. (2009). Extracorporeal membrane oxygenation circulatory support after congenital cardiac surgery. *ASAIO Journal, 55,* 53–57.

362. Swan, L., Kraidly, M., Muhll, I., Collins, P., & Gatzoulis, M. (2008, December). Surveillance of cardiovascular risk in the normotensive patient with repaired aortic coarctation. *International Journal of Cardiology.* [Epub.]

363. Swanson, T., Selamet, E., Tworetzky, W., Pigula, F., & McElhinney, D. (2009). Truncus arteriosus: Diagnostic accuracy, outcomes, and impact of prenatal diagnosis. *Pediatric Cardiology, 30*(3), 256–261.

364. Sweet, S., Wong, H., Webber, S., Horslen, S., Guidinger, M., Fine, R., et al. (2006). Pediatric transplantation in the U.S., 1995–2004. *American Journal of Transplantation, 6*(Pt 2), 1132–1152.

365. Tabbutt, S., Nicolson, S., Adamson, P., Zhang, X., Hoffman, M., Wells, W., et al. (2008). The safety, efficacy, and pharmacokinetics of esmolol for blood pressure control immediately after repair of coarctation of the aorta in infants and children: A multicenter, double-blind, randomized trial. *Journal of Thoracic and Cardiovascular Surgery, 136*(2), 321–328.

366. Tabbutt, S., Ramamoorthy, C., & Montenegro, L. (2001). Impact of inspired gas mixtures on preoperative infants with hypoplastic left heart syndrome during controlled ventilation. *Circulation, 104,* 1159–1164.

367. Taketomo, C., Hodding, J., & Krause, D. (2010). Pediatric Dosage Handbook. (17th ed.). Hudson, OH: LexiComp.

368. Tambur, A., Bray, R., Takemoto, S., Mancini, M., Costanzo, M., Kobashigawa, J., et al. (2000). Flow cytometric detection of HLA specific antibodies as a predictor of heart allograft rejection. *Transplantation, 70*(7), 1055–1059.

369. Tanel, R. (2005). ECG's in the ED. *Pediatric Emergency Care, 21,* 281–282.

370. Tani, L., Veasy, L., Minich, L., & Shaddy, R. (2003). Rheumatic fever in children younger than 5 years: is the presentation different? *Pediatrics, 112*(5), 1065–1068.

371. Tanous, D., Benson, L., & Horlick, E. (2009, August 6). Coarctation of the aorta: Evaluation and management. *Current Opinion in Cardiology.* [Epub.]

372. Taubert, K., Rowley, A., & Shulman, S. (1994). A seven-year United States nationwide hospital survey of Kawasaki disease. *Pediatric Infectious Disease Journal, 13*(8), 675–762.

373. Taylor, D., Edwards, L., Boucek, M., Trulock, E., Aurora, P., Christie, J., et al. (2007). Registry of the International Society for Heart and Lung Transplantation: Twenty-fourth official adult heart transplant report—2007. *Journal of Heart and Lung Transplantation, 26*(8), 769–781.

374. Tefft, R. (2010). The impact of an early ibuprofen treatment protocol on the incidence of surgical ligation of the ductus arteriosus. *American Journal of Perinatology, 27*(1), 83–90.

375. Ten Harkel, A., Berkhout, M., Hop, W., Witsenburg, M., & Wa, H. (2009). Congenital valvular aortic stenosis: Limited progression during childhood. *Archives of Diseases of Children, 94*(7), 531–535.

376. Tham, E., Yeung, A., Cheng, C., Bernstein, D., Chin, C., & Feinstein, J. (2005). Experience of percutaneous coronary intervention in the management of coronary allograft vasculopathy. *Journal of Heart and Lung Transplantation, 24*(6), 769–763.

377. Thomas, L., McElhinney, D., Reddy, M., Petrossian, E., Silverman, N., & Hanley, F. (2001). Neonatal repair of truncus arteriosus: Continuing improvement in outcomes. *Annals of Thoracic Surgery, 72*, 391–395.

378. Timothy, P. R., & Rodeman, B. J. (2004). Temporary pacemakers in critically ill patients: assessment and management strategies. *AACN Clinical Issues: Advanced Practice in Acute and Critical Care, 15*(3), 305–325.

379. Tlaskal, T., Chaloupecky, V., Hucin, B., Gebauer, R., Krupickova, S., Reich, O., et al. (2010). Long term results after correction of persistent truncus arteriosus in 83 patients. *European Journal of Cardiothoracic Surgery.* [Epub.]

380. Towbin, J., Lowe, A., Colan, S., Sleeper, L., Orav, E., Clunie, S., et al. (2006). Incidence, causes, and outcomes of dilated cardiomyopathy in children, *Journal of the American Medical Association, 296*(15), 1867–1876.

381. Troughton, R., Asher, C., & Klein, A. (2004). Pericarditis. *Lancet, 363,* 717–727.

382. Tsirka, A., Trinkaus, K., Chen, S., Lipshultz, S., Towbin, J., Colan, S., et al. (2004). Improved outcomes of pediatric dilated cardiomyopathy with utilization of heart transplantation. *Journal of the American College of Cardiologists, 44*(2), 391–397.

383. Ugaki, S., Kasahara, S., Arai, S., Takagaki, M., & Sano, S. (2010, April 30). Combination of continuous irrigation and vacuum-assisted closure is effective for mediastinitis after cardiac surgery in small children. *Interactive Cardiovascular and Thoracic Surgery, icvts 235903.* Retrieved from www.icvts.org

384. United Network of Organ Sharing. (2010). Policies: Organ distribution: Allocation of thoracic organs and pediatric candidate status (Policy 3.7). Retrieved from http://www.unos.org/PoliciesandBylaws2/policies/pdfs/policy_9.pdf

385. Van Meurs, K. (1999). *ECMO specialist training manual.* Ann Arbor, MI: Extracorporeal Life Support Organization.

386. Van Mierop, L., Eisen, S., & Schiebler, G. (1970). The radiographic appearance of the tracheobronchial tree as an indicator of visceral situs. *American Journal of Cardiology, 26*, 432.

387. Van Mierop, L., & Wiglesworth, F. (1962). Isomerism of the cardiac atria in the asplenia syndrome. *Lab Investigations, 11*, 1303.

388. Van Praagh, R. (1972). The segmental approach to diagnosis in congenital heart disease. (D. Bergsma, Ed.). *Birth Defects: Original Article Series, 8,* 4–23.

389. Van Praagh, S., LaCorte, M., & Fellows, K. (1980). Superoinferior ventricles, anatomic and angiocardiographic findings in 10 postmortem cases. In R. Van Praagh, A. Takao, R. Van Praagh, & A. Takao (Eds.). *Etiology and morphologenesis of congenital heart disease* (pp. 317–378). Mt. Kisco, NY: Futura.

390. Van Praagh, R., Plett, J., & Van Praagh, S. (1979). Single ventricle: Pathology, embryology, terminology, and classification. *Herz, 4,* 113.

391. Van Praagh, R., & Van Praagh, S. (1966). Isolated ventricular inversion: A consideration of the morphogenesis, definition, and diagnosis of non-transposed and transposed great arteries. *American Journal of Cardiology, 13,* 510.

392. Van Praagh, R., Van Praagh, S., Vlad, P., & Keith, J. (1964). Anatomic types of congenital dextrocardia: Diagnostic and embryologic implications. *American Journal Cardiology, 13,* 510.

393. Van Schooneveld, T., & Rupp, M. (2009). Mediastinitis. In G. L. Mandell, J. E. Bennett, & R. Dolin (Eds.). *Mandell: Mandell, Douglas, and Bennett's principles and practice of infectious diseases* (7th ed., pp. 1173–1182). Philadelphia: Churchill Livingstone, Elsevier.

394. Vashist, S., & Singh, G. (2009). Acute myocarditis in children: Current concepts and management. *Current Treatment Options in Cardiovascular Medicine, 11,* 383–391.

395. Veasy, G., & Hill, H. (1997). Immunologic and clinical correlations in rheumatic fever and rheumatic heart disease. *Pediatric Infectious Disease Journal, 16*(4), 400–407.

396. Veltmann, C., Schimpf, R., Borggefe, M., & Wolpert, C. (2009). Risk stratification in electrical cardiomyopathies. *Herz, 34*(7), 518–527.

397. Villain, E. (2008). Indications for pacing in patients with congenital heart disease. *Pacing and Clinical Electrophysiology, 31*(suppl 1), S17–S20.

398. Vogt, J., Rupprath, G., & De Vivie, R. (1983). Discrete subaortic stenosis: The value of cross-sectional sector echocardiogramy in evaluating different types of obstruction. *Pediatric Cardiology, 66,* 253–258.

399. Walsh, E. P. (2007). Interventional electrophysiology in patients with congenital heart disease. *Circulation, 115*(25), 3224–3234.

400. Wang, P., Hwang, B., Lu, J., Lee, P., Tiu, C., Weng, Z., et al. (2004). Significance of pulmonary venous obstruction in total anomalous pulmonary venous return. *Journal of Chinese Medical Association, 67*(7), 331–335.

401. Webber, S. (2008). New-onset heart failure in children in the absence of structural congenital heart disease. *Circulation, 117,* 11–12.

402. Webber, S., Naftel, D., Parker, J., Mulla, N., Balfour, I., Kirklin, J., et al. (2003). Late rejection episodes more than one year after pediatric heart transplantation: Risk factors and outcomes. *Journal of Heart and Lung Transplantation, 22*(8), 869–875.

403. Webber, S., Wilson, N., Junker, A., Byrne, S., Perry, A., Thomas, E., et al. (2001). Postpericardiotomy syndrome: No evidence for a viral etiology. *Cardiology in the Young, 11*(1), 67–74.

404. Webster, G., Jordao, L., Martuscello, M., Mahajan, T., Alexander, M. E., Cecchin, F., et al. (2008). Digital music players cause interference with interrogation telemetry for pacemakers and implantable cardioverter–defibrillators without affecting device function. *Heart Rhythm, 5*(4), 545–550.

405. Wernovsky, G., & Bove, E. L. (1998). Single ventricle lesions. In A. Chang, F. Hanley, & G. Wernovsky (Eds.). *Pediatric cardiac intensive care* (pp. 271–287). Baltimore: Williams & Wilkins.

406. Werynski, P., Rudinski, A., Krol-Jawien, W., & Kuzma, J. (2009). Percutaneous balloon valvuloplasty for the treatment of pulmonary valve stenosis in children: A single centre experience. *Kardiologia Polska, 67*(4), 369–375.

407. Wessel, D. L., & Fraisse, A. (2008). Postoperative care of the pediatric cardiac surgical patient: General considerations. In D. G. Nichols (Ed.). *Rogers' textbook of pediatric intensive care* (4th ed., pp. 1159–1180). Philadelphia: Lippincott, Williams & Wilkins.

408. Wessels, M., Berger, R., & Frohn-Mulder, I. (2005). Autosomal dominant inheritance of left ventricular outflow tract obstruction. *American Journal of Medical Genetics Part A, 134*, 171–179.

409. West, L., Pollock-Barziv, S., Dipchand, A., Lee, K., Cardella, C., Benson, L., et al. (2001). Incompatible heart transplantation in infants. *New England Journal of Medicine, 344*(11), 793–800.

410. Wheeler, D. S., & Kooy, N. (2003). A formidable challenge the diagnosis and treatment of viral myocarditis in children. *Critical Care Clinics, 19*(3), 365–391.

411. Wilcox, W., Plauth, W., & Williams, W. (1980). Discrete subaortic stenosis: Two-dimensional echocardiogramic features with angiographic and surgical correlation. *Mayo Clinic Proceedings, 55*, 425–433.

412. Wilkinson, J., Sleeper, L., Alvarez, J., Bublik, N., Lipshultz, S., & Pediatric Cardiomyopathy Study Group. (2008). The pediatric cardiomyopathy registry: 1995–2007. *Progress in Pediatric Cardiology, 25*(1), 31–36.

413. Williams, J., Barratt-Boyes, B., & Lowe, J. (1961). Supravalvar aortic stenosis. *Cirulation, 24*, 1311–1318.

414. Williamson, L., Bowness, P., Mowat., A., & Ostman-Smith, I. (1999). Lesson of the week Difficulties in diagnosing acute rheumatic fever-arthritis may be short lived and carditis silent. *British Medical Journal, 320*(7231), 362–365.

415. Willis J. (2000, June). Syncope. *Pediatrics in Review, 21*(6), 201–203.

416. Wilson, W., Tauber, K., Gewitz, M., Lockhart, P., Baddour, L., Levison, M., et al. (2007). Prevention of infective endocarditis: Guidelines from the American Heart Association: A guideline from the American Heart Association Rheumatic Fever, Endocarditis, and Kawasaki Disease Committee, Council on Cardiovascular Disease in the Young, and the Council on Clinical Cardiology, Council on Cardiovascular Surgery and Anesthesia, and the Quality of Care and Outcomes Research Interdisciplinary Working Group. *Circulation, 116*(15), 1736.

417. World Health Organization (WHO). (2004). Rheumatic fever and rheumatic heart disease. Retrieved from http://www.who.int/cardiovascular_diseases/resources/trs923/en/

418. Wypij, D., Newburger, J., & Rappaport, L. (2003). The effect of duration of deep hypothermic circulatory arrest in infant heart surgery on late neurodevelopment: The Boston Circulatory Arrest Trial. *Journal of Thoracic Cardiovascular Surgery, 126*(5), 1397–1403.

419. Yacoub, M., Kilner, P., Birks, E., & Misfeld, M. (1999). The aortic outflow and root: A tale of dynamism and crosstalk. *Annuals of Thoracic Surgery, 68*, S37.

420. Yang, D., Goo, H., Seo, D., Yun, T., Park, J., Park, I., et al. (2008). Multislice CT angiography of interrupted aortic arch. *Pediatric Radiology, 38*(1), 89–100.

421. Yuan, S., & Raanani, E. (2008). Late complications of coarctation of the aorta. *Cardiology Journal, 15*(6), 491–492.

422. Zabriskie, J., Hsu, K., & Seegal, B. (1970). Heart-reactive antibody associated with rheumatic fever: Characterization and diagnostic significance. *Clinical & Experimental Immunology, 7*, 147–159.

423. Zaichkin, J. (Ed.). (2006). *Neonatal resuscitation instructor manual.* Elk Grove Village, IL: American Academy of Pediatrics & American Heart Association.

424. Zeltser, I., Rhodes, L., Tanel, R., Vetter, V., Gaynor, J., Spray, T., et al. (2004). Postpericardiotomy syndrome after permanent pacemaker implantation in children and young adults. *Annals of Thoracic Surgery, 78*(5), 1684–1687.

425. Zimmerman, J. (1969). The functional and surgical anatomy of the aortic valve. *Israel Journal of Medical Sciences, 5*, 862.

426. Ziolkowska, L., Kawalec, W., Turska-Kmiec, A., Krajewska-Walasek, M., Brzezinska- Rajszys, G., Daszkowska, J., et al. (2008). Chromosome 22q11.2 microdeletion in children with conotruncal heart defects: Frequency, associated cardiovascular anomalies, and outcome following cardiac surgery. *European Journal of Pediatrics, 167*(10), 1135–1140.

427. Zucker, N., Levitas, A., & Zalzstein. E. (2003). Methotrexate in recurrent postpericardiotomy syndrome. *Cardiol Young, 13*(2), 206–208.

428. Zwischenberger, J., Steinhorn, R., & Bartlett, R. (2000). *ECMO: Extracorporeal cardiopulmonary support in critical care* (2nd ed.). Ann Arbor, MI: Extracorporeal Life Support Organization.

Dermatologic Disorders

PHYSIOLOGY AND DIAGNOSTICS

Julie Edwards

The skin is the largest organ or body system, accounting for 20% of total body weight. It functions as a barrier and first line of bodily defense against microorganisms, ultraviolet radiation, and physical forces. In addition, the skin plays a vital role in the maintenance of body fluid balance. The physiology of the skin in the pediatric patient is not markedly different than that in the adult; however, manifestations of skin alterations may present differently (Heer & Huether, 2010a). The skin of infants—especially premature infants—may be significantly different than that of older children and adults. This is largely related to the poorly developed epidermis and slower keratin production in this population (Agren, et al., 2006).

PHYSIOLOGY OF THE SKIN

The skin is divided into two major section: the epidermis and the dermis. Subcutaneous tissue lies below the skin. The epidermis has two substantial layers—the stratum corneum and the cellular stratum. The stratum corneum maintains hydration, restricts water loss, and protects the body against harmful environmental influences. The cellular stratum is the layer of the epidermis where keratin cells, which serve as the building blocks of the skin, hair, and nails, are synthesized. The epidermis is avascular and receives nutrients from the dermis below. The epidermis ranges in thickness from 0.33 mm to 1.5 mm in adults. However, there are no specific references to the thickness of the epidermis in infants and children (Heer & Huether, 2010b; Seidel et al., 2003).

The dermis measures between 1 and 4 mm in thickness. It is made up of connective tissues (collagen, elastin, and reticulum fibers), which are arranged in a "haphazard" manner. This characteristic allows the skin to be elastic and mobile, smoothly moving with the body as it changes position. The dermis is extremely vascular, supporting the epidermis and separating it from the subcutaneous tissue below. The sensations of pain and touch are mediated via this layer of the skin, as it is innervated by nerve fibers, both sensory and autonomic (Heer & Huether, 2010b; Seidel et al., 2003).

Located within the dermis are the appendages or accessory portions of the main structure—namely, the sweat glands, sebaceous glands, hair, and nails (Seidel et al., 2003). Eccrine sweat glands allow for regulation of body temperature through secretion of water. Most are located on the axillae, palms, and feet. The apocrine sweat glands are located mostly in the axillae and genital areas. Their function is unclear but is often thought to be related to scent production (Heer & Huether, 2010b). Sebaceous glands are also located within the dermis; their major function is secretion of sebum, a substance important in protecting the skin and hair from dryness (Seidel et al., 2003).

Hair follicles are paired with the sebaceous glands within the matrix portion of the dermis. Hair growth, color, pattern, and distribution all vary with age (Heer & Huether, 2010b).

When epidermal cells become hard plates of keratin, nails are formed. A highly vascular bed located beneath each nail provides the nail bed with a "pink" color (Seidel et al., 2003) (Figure 23-1).

DEVELOPMENTAL DIFFERENCES

The skin of premature infants is both anatomically and physiologically immature (Korner et al., 2009). It is estimated that an extremely premature infant (less than 26 weeks' gestation) is composed of 80% to 90% water (Modi, 2004). Transepidermal water loss (TEWL) is a term used to describe the propensity of the skin of the premature infant to lose fluid based on the large surface area to weight ratio inherent in this population. The skin of the extremely premature infant can be described as very "porous" and without keratin. Keratin cell synthesis takes place within the stratum corneum of the skin, which develops at approximately 34 weeks' gestation (Modi). Absence of keratin production is associated with a high risk for dehydration, as the skin is the primary resource of fluid hydration and heat loss mitigation following birth (Agren, et al., 2006). Thus the extremely preterm infant is at high risk for skin breakdown, excoriation, infection, and water loss.

As pediatric patients become more mature, their skin becomes increasingly similar to that of their adult counterparts. Fluhr et al. (2000) examined the physiological differences in the skin of small children (ages 1 to 6 years) as compared to their parents. Results indicated that in general the children's skin had significantly lower hygroscopicity (water-holding capacity), was paler in color, and had increased cutaneous microperfusion. No differences were noted in stratum corneum hydration, pH value, or skin color on the blue–yellow axis. Likewise, there were no differences in atopy. The conclusion was that very little difference exists in the barrier function of the skin of the young child as compared to the parent counterpart on the most basic physiological level.

DIAGNOSTIC EVALUATION

Diagnostic evaluation of skin trauma, diseases, and abnormalities in infants and pediatric patients is most commonly accomplished through history and physical examination

(Heer & Huether, 2010a). Patterns of skin abnormalities are best assessed by a systematic examination of the entire body (Berkowitz, 2008). The reader is encouraged to review any of a number of excellent pediatric physical examination texts for further information on this process.

Skin seroreaction testing may be used for diagnostic screening, such as the Mantoux tuberculin skin test for tuberculosis or allergy testing. In this type of testing, reagents are injected intradermally or by prick/puncture. The extent of inflammatory response and induration to the site of injection are then measured based on a predetermined length of time. Intradermal testing has been shown to have a higher sensitivity than prick/puncture testing (Leung, 2007). Skin tests for delayed hypersensitivity are used diagnostically to assess previous infection or to evaluate cellular immune function by testing anergy. Anergy, a defect in cell-mediated immunity, is characterized by a depressed response or lack of response to skin testing with injected antigens. Anergy has been associated with congenital and acquired immunodeficiencies, viral infections, febrile illness, and malnutrition.

The placement of an intradermal puncture involves the following steps:

1. Inject the reagent in the flexor surface of the forearm.
2. Describe the wheal after injection, and repeat the injection if no wheal is demonstrated.
3. Space multiple puncture tests 5 cm apart.
4. Evaluate ("read") the skin for induration at 24, 48, and 72 hours. An immediate response is considered to be one that occurs less than 24 hours after the injection; reactions that occur beyond this point are classified as delayed hypersensitivity responses.

A false positive may occur because of sensitivity to the solution, cross-sensitivity between antigens, or improper testing procedures. Side effects of such testing may include pain, blisters, erythema, and necrosis. Emergency equipment for allergic reactions should be available (Taketomo et al., 2010).

Skin biopsy is rarely indicated in the pediatric patient. When used, "punch" biopsy is the most common technique. In a punch biopsy, all layers of the skin are removed in a specimen approximately 3–4 mm in diameter after a topical anesthetic has been applied (Darmstadt & Sidbury, 2004).

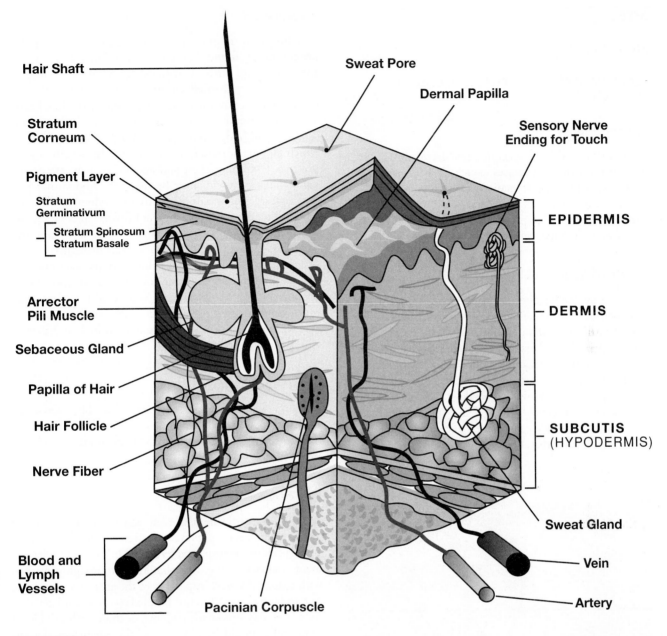

Hair Shaft

Sweat Pore

Dermal Papilla

Sensory Nerve Ending for Touch

Stratum Corneum

Pigment Layer

Stratum Germinativum

Stratum Spinosum
Stratum Basale

EPIDERMIS

Arrector Pili Muscle

Sebaceous Gland

DERMIS

Papilla of Hair

Hair Follicle

SUBCUTIS (HYPODERMIS)

Nerve Fiber

Sweat Gland

Blood and Lymph Vessels

Vein

Pacinian Corpuscle

Artery

FIGURE 23-1

Anatomy of the Skin.

Source: Courtesy of the U.S. National Institutes of Health; National Cancer Institute.

BITES

Milton Meadows

BLACK WIDOW SPIDER BITES (*LATRODECTUS MACTANS*)

Pathophysiology

Black widow spider venom contains ∝-latrotoxin, an excitatory neurotoxin that causes increased neurotransmitter release from presynaptic neurons (Shannon et al., 2007). The clinical picture of *Latrodectus* envenomation results from this excess stimulation at the neuromuscular junction, sympathetic, and parasympathetic synapses.

Epidemiology and etiology

Black widow spider bites are the leading cause of death by spider bites in the United States (Fleisher et al., 2006). These spiders are found throughout the continental United States and southern Canada. The female black widow spider is larger than the male, and is black with a bright red mark on the abdomen that is shaped like an hourglass or two red spots (Figure 23-2). Only the female is able to envenomate humans (Shannon et al., 2007). These spiders usually may be found in out-of-the-way places, and are not aggressive unless provoked or threatened.

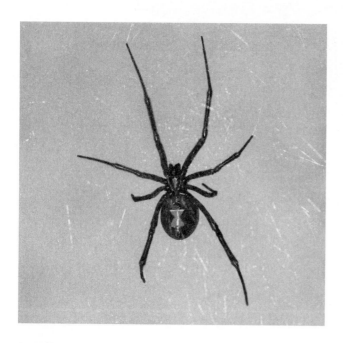

FIGURE 23-2

Black Widow.

Source: © Brian Chase/ShutterStock, Inc.

Presentation

Any history of recent exposure to locations where spiders are commonly found should raise suspicion of a bite. Often the bite is not directly witnessed, and patients may or may not notice a small pinprick sensation when the bite occurs. Dull, cramp-like pain at the site of the bite begins 15 to 60 minutes after envenomation, and may spread to the entire body (Marx et al., 2009). The "tap test," in which tapping at the suspected bite site elicits pain, may be positive. Cramping chest and abdominal pain are prominent, but all muscles may be involved. Abdominal pain and rigidity might mimic a surgical abdomen, although rebound tenderness is not present (Townsend et al., 2008). Associated symptoms may include nausea and vomiting, dizziness, ptosis, headache, dyspnea, dysarthria, facial swelling, and conjunctivitis. More serious reactions may include significant hypertension, increased intracranial pressure, or respiratory failure (Marx et al.). Patients with mild to moderate symptoms generally begin to resolve in 8 to 12 hours, with complete resolution in 1 to 2 days in adults (Townsend et al.).

Differential diagnosis

The presentation of a spider bite may resemble a new-onset infection such as community-acquired methicillin-resistant *Staphylococcus aureus* (CA-MRSA), or another spider or insect bite.

Plan of care

Initial therapeutic management consists of local wound care and tetanus prophylaxis. First responders should apply a cold pack to the suspected bite site. On emergency department evaluation, the area should be thoroughly washed with soap and water. Inspection of the area may reveal one or two fang marks. Tetanus prophylaxis is administered as indicated. Asymptomatic patients, or those with mild local symptoms, should be observed in the emergency department (ED) for 6 hours and may be discharged home if stable (Marx et al., 2009). Patients with progressive symptoms or patients with risk factors should be admitted for further observation or therapy. Patients at increased risk for developing a severe reaction include pregnant patients, small children, and patients with underlying cardiac disease or hypertension (Marx et al.).

Initial emergency department evaluation includes a complete blood count (CBC), metabolic panel, coagulation studies, electrocardiograph (ECG), and urinalysis. Intravenous (IV) access should be obtained and maintenance IV fluids administered.

Latrodectus antivenin treatment should be started as soon as possible in children weighing less than 40 kg, pregnant women, and patients with severe symptoms.

Because the antivenin is derived from horse serum, the package insert recommends skin testing before administration to evaluate for hypersensitivity reactions (Fleisher et al., 2006). The usual dose is one 2.5 mL vial in 50 mL normal saline administered over 15 minutes. Although a single vial is usually sufficient, a second vial may be needed in severely affected patients (King & Henretig, 2008). Serum sickness may develop after antivenin administration.

Symptomatic treatment may also be required in patients with moderate to severe reactions. Hypertension should be aggressively controlled with nitroprusside. Muscle cramping may be treated with benzodiazepines, morphine, or dantrolene (Marx et al., 2009). Calcium gluconate was traditionally given for muscle cramps, but recent data indicate that this measure is ineffective (Fleisher et al., 2006).

In patients with severe symptoms requiring aggressive blood pressure control and those with impending respiratory failure, early consultation with a critical care specialist is indicated. Consultation with a toxicologist may also be helpful.

Education regarding locations where black widow spiders are found may be helpful in preventing future bites. For patients discharged from the emergency department, instructions should include what symptoms to watch for and when to return if symptoms progress.

Disposition and discharge planning

Although black widow spider bites have a 4% to 5% mortality rate overall, this rate may approach 50% in young children (Fleisher et al., 2006). Mild pain or neurologic symptoms may persist for a few weeks after the bite. No special discharge planning or follow-up is required for these patients, but patients should seek medical attention for any worsening symptoms.

BROWN RECLUSE SPIDERS (LOXOSCELES RECLUSA)

Pathophysiology

Brown recluse spider venom is a complex mixture of many compounds, the most significant of which is sphingomyelinase D. Sphingomyelinase D is a phospholipase enzyme that damages the cell membranes of erythrocytes, endothelial cells, and platelets. Cell membrane damage leads to hemolysis, platelet aggregation, and coagulation, with resultant local tissue damage and occasional systemic toxicity (Shannon et al., 2007). Local injury is exacerbated by vasoconstriction, which is caused by a substance in the venom that is similar to norepinephrine.

Epidemiology and etiology

Brown recluse spiders are commonly found in the southern and midwestern United States but may be found in other regions of North and South America as well. They are brown in color, can be from 1 to 2 cm in length, and have a small violin-shaped dark area on the upper cephalothorax (Figure 23-3). These spiders are not aggressive by nature and will attack only if provoked. Brown recluse spiders are usually found outdoors under rocks or woodpiles, but may also be found indoors inside closets or other dark areas.

There are no reliable data on the number of brown recluse bites, as there is no requirement for reporting these bites to monitoring agencies. Additionally, brown recluse spider bites can mimic other disease processes and so may not be properly identified. Some effort has been made by the American Association of Poison Control Centers to quantify the number of bites. From 1983 to 2002, this organization recorded 30,816 envenomations with 6 deaths (Marx et al., 2009).

Presentation

A history of the events leading up to the bite, time elapsed since the bite, and history of any allergic reactions to bites or stings should be obtained in addition to a standard history and physical examination.

Local symptoms begin with pain in the area of the bite, usually within 3 to 4 hours of the envenomation. A white ring of tissue ischemia secondary to vasoconstriction may develop, followed by a pustule or blister. This pustule and ring of erythema gives a bull's-eye appearance to the lesion. Over the next few days this pustule may darken, become necrotic, and expand up to 10–15 cm in diameter. The pustule then drains, leaving a dark, necrotic, ulcerated

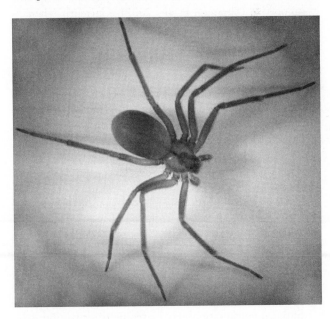

FIGURE 23-3

Brown Recluse.

Source: Courtesy of Kenneth Cramer, Monmouth College.

crater (Fleisher et al., 2006). Necrosis is often worse in areas with increased subcutaneous fat, such as the buttock, thigh, or abdomen (Marx et al., 2009).

Systemic symptoms may develop in patients without severe local signs, usually appearing 24 to 48 hours after the bite. These symptoms can include hemolysis, thrombocytopenia, shock, jaundice, kidney failure, bleeding, or pulmonary edema. Most deaths from brown recluse bites are due to severe intravascular hemolysis or respiratory failure (Fleisher et al., 2006).

Differential diagnosis

Brown recluse spider bites should be differentiated from other causes of skin lesions, including faruncle, viral or fungal infections, foreign body reactions, chemical burns, and pyoderma gangrenosum.

Plan of care

There is no definitive laboratory test for brown recluse spider envenomation. If the spider cannot be located and brought with the patient and the patient's history is atypical, diagnosis can be quite challenging.

Any patient showing signs of systemic toxicity should have a CBC, metabolic panel, coagulation studies, and urinalysis (Fleisher et al., 2006). Urine output should be monitored closely to evaluate for kidney failure secondary to hemolysis. Intravenous (IV) access should be obtained and the patient should be admitted for further observation and management. Treatment of systemic symptoms is supportive (Shannon et al., 2007). Currently, there is no antivenin for brown recluse spider bites available in the United States.

For local reactions, the area should be washed with soap and water. The wounded extremity should be splinted and elevated, with a cold compress placed on the site of the bite (Townsend et al., 2008). Tetanus prophylaxis should be given as indicated. Dapsone (diamino-diphenyl sulfone) given to adult patients within 48 hours of the bite may reduce the amount of necrosis, but its use is not recommended in children. As necrosis develops, conservative surgical debridement may be beneficial. Large areas of necrosis may require skin grafting, which is best undertaken once the area of necrosis is fully demarcated and stable (Townsend et al., 2008). Excision of the wound does not decrease the total amount of necrosis and is generally not indicated.

Patients with suspected brown recluse spider bite, but no symptoms, can be discharged after 6 hours of observation in an emergency department.

Surgical consultation may be required for wound debridement. Consultation with a toxicologist may help guide therapy. For patients with systemic symptoms, critical care consultation may be indicated.

Families should be educated about signs and symptoms of systemic toxicity in a patient who is being discharged from the emergency department, and told to return if any of these conditions develop. For open wounds, local wound care instruction is indicated.

Disposition and discharge planning

Outcomes from brown recluse spider bites are generally good if no necrosis develops at the bite site. With necrosis, some degree of scarring can be expected. Patients with systemic manifestations will likely do well if their symptoms are mild, but severe systemic symptoms can be life-threatening.

Follow-up should be arranged with the patient's primary care provider to follow progress of the wound and direct therapy or provide any education as needed. Surgical follow-up is indicated in patients with necrosis requiring debridement.

MAMMALIAN BITES

Pathophysiology

The pathophysiology of mammal bites varies with the species of animal and the location of the bite. Victims of bites are at risk for blunt or penetrating injuries, and certain anatomic locations are more prone to complications than others (Townsend et al., 2008).

Dog bites tend to comprise larger lacerations and abrasions with more associated crush injury than bites from other species. Crush injury occurs secondary to the immense pressures that dogs may generate with their jaws (Marx et al., 2009). These wounds are generally very accessible to good wound hygiene, and consequently are associated with fewer infections than other bite types. In infants and younger children, dog bites may involve deep structures and bone, though this is rare in older children.

Cats have sharp teeth that cause puncture wounds in bitten areas. These wounds are less accessible to cleaning and wound hygiene, and have higher rates of infection as a result (Fleisher et al., 2006).

Human bites in young children are mostly abrasions that have a low infection rate (Fleisher et al., 2006). A notable exception is the "fight bite" or closed fist injury (CFI), which is most often seen in older children and adolescents. These lacerations of the metacarpophalangeal joints classically result from a closed fist striking the teeth of an opponent (Marx et al., 2009). Injury with the fist clenched may include tears of the extensor tendon and bacterial contamination of the wound from human oral flora. This contamination may then be pulled back into the fascial layers of the hand once the fist is relaxed. The lacerations often penetrate into the joint space, and the risk of infection for this type of wound is high (Marx et al., 2009).

Bites in anatomic locations with a high risk of infection include any bite on the hands or feet and bites involving deep structures (Townsend et al., 2008). Bites from cats and delayed presentation are also considered factors increasing the risk for infection. Bites from dogs in anatomic locations other than the hands and feet, bites to the face and head not involving deeper structures, and abrasions resulting from human bites are considered to pose a lower risk for infection (Marx et al., 2009).

The most common infectious agents in dog and cat bites are *Staphylococcus aureus*, *Streptococcus*, *Pasteurella multocida*, and *Capnocytophaga canimorsus*, which is more rarely found but has been the cause of numerous cases of septic shock in bite victims (Marx et al., 2009). In human bites, mixed flora may be present, including *Streptococcus viridans*, *S. aureus*, *Bacteroides*, *Peptostreptococcus*, and *Eikenella corrodens* (Marx et al.).

Epidemiology and etiology

Most mammal bites, with the exception of human bites, occur in children. Approximately 80% to 90% of all bites presenting for care involve dog bites (Fleisher et al., 2006). Of those incidents, the owner is known in most cases, and in as many as 30% of cases the dog is owned by the family of the victim (Fleisher et al.). Males are bitten more often than females. In children younger than age 5, the majority of bites occur to the head and neck regions; overall, however, one-third of bites are to the lower extremity, one-third are to the upper extremity, and one-third are to the face or multiple areas (Fleisher et al.).

Presentation

The health care professional (HCP) should elucidate in the history which type of animal was involved, whether it was captive or wild, and whether the attack was provoked or unprovoked. Pertinent patient history includes any increased risk factors for sepsis or poor wound healing such as chronic corticosteroid use, as well as tetanus status (Marx et al., 2009).

On physical examination, bites may range from minor scratches to deep lacerations of multiple sites. A thorough neurovascular exam should be performed of the affected extremity, followed by local anesthesia and exploration to look for any retained foreign body or deep structure involvement. Plain radiographs of the extremity may be needed to further assess for foreign body or bony involvement (Marx et al., 2009). In infants with dog bites of the face and head, a CT scan is indicated to evaluate for depressed skull fractures that may place the patient at increased risk for intracranial infection (Marx et al.). For closed fist injuries, the hand should be examined throughout the full range of motion of the fingers to evaluate for deep structure involvement (Townsend et al., 2008).

Differential diagnosis

Mammal bites should be distinguished from all other causes of trauma, which is done primarily based on mechanism of injury. Any suspicion for nonaccidental trauma should be thoroughly investigated.

Plan of care

Diagnostic studies are rarely indicated in patients who receive a bite unless symptoms of infection exist. In those cases, appropriate cultures from the wound and blood may be warranted, along with a CBC and differential.

First aid for bite wounds includes application of ice to the wound, elevation, and direct pressure to stop any bleeding. All wounds should be cleaned well with soap and water and copiously irrigated with normal saline. Good wound hygiene is the most important step in reducing the risk of infection with all types of bites (Fleisher et al., 2006). Wounds with signs of infection should be drained, have cultures sent, and be treated with antibiotics. Any devitalized tissue should be debrided during wound exploration. The wound may then be evaluated for suturing.

Suturing of bite wounds should be carefully considered in the context of the wound's anatomic location and the risk of wound infection. Generally, only wounds with a low infection risk or those in cosmetically or functionally sensitive areas should be sutured. Wounds of the head, neck, arm, or leg may be sutured at presentation if the patient is seen within 6 to 12 hours of the bite (Marx et al., 2009). If 12 to 24 hours has elapsed since the bite occurred, a reasonable approach may be to cover the wound with a moist dressing and reevaluate it for suturing in 3 to 5 days if no signs of infection are present. Wounds of the face may be sutured up to 24 hours after the injury (Townsend et al., 2008).

Suturing is not indicated for wounds with a high risk of infection. These injuries include wounds of the hands and feet, as well as wounds from cat or human bites. They should have a bulky dressing applied, be elevated, and be reevaluated in 1 to 2 days.

Antibiotic prophylaxis should be provided for wounds with a high infection risk. A 3- to 5-day course of amoxicillin–clavulanic acid at 30–50 mg/kg/day is sufficient first-line prophylaxis for high-risk bites (Fleisher et al., 2006). In penicillin-allergic patients, combination therapy with clindamycin and trimethoprim–sulfamethoxazole may be used. The first dose of antibiotics should be administered at the time of wound evaluation. Tetanus immunization should be administered as indicated.

All patients with bite wounds should be evaluated for risk of rabies exposure. The clinician should inquire about the apparent health of the biting animal, whether the attack was provoked or unprovoked, and the animal's rabies immunization status (if available). No rabies prophylaxis is needed if the bite is from a domestic animal that appeared healthy and remains in good health over the next 10 to 14 days. Bat exposure warrants prophylaxis even if there was no apparent bite (Fleisher et al., 2006).

Rabies prophylaxis consists of a combination of rabies immune globulin and human diploid cell rabies vaccine (HDCV). Rabies immune globulin is given at a dose of 20 IU/kg, with one half of the dose infiltrated around the wound and the other one half injected intramuscularly (IM) at a site remote from the injury. HDCV (1 mL IM) is given at presentation, then again 3, 7, 14, and 28 days after the bite (Townsend et al., 2008).

Plastic surgery consultation for extensive facial wounds will improve cosmetic outcomes. Orthopedic surgery should be consulted for patients with bony involvement. Consultation with a neurosurgeon is indicated in cases of skull fracture from dog bites.

Families should be educated to look for signs of local infection of the wound as well as systemic infections.

Disposition and discharge planning

Patients with serious facial or scalp bites, skull fracture, systemic infectious symptoms, or severe bites that threaten life or limb should be admitted for monitoring and treatment. Most patients may be discharged home with follow-up wound evaluation in 2 to 4 days.

SNAKEBITES

Pathophysiology

The mechanisms by which snake venom causes injury in the victim vary among species. Two major families— subfamily Crotalinae (the pit vipers) and family Elapidae (the coral snakes)—account for most snakebites in the United States. These families vary in their identification, venom delivery mechanisms, toxicity of their venom, and treatment of envenomation.

The venom of the pit vipers contains approximately 90% protein by dry weight (Shannon et al., 2007). The two broad classes of venom include larger-molecular-weight enzymatic components, such as hyaluronidase, and lower-molecular-weight polypeptides. The larger enzymatic components, which function as digestive enzymes, are mainly responsible for the local effects of snakebite, yet they may have systemic consequences as well. The smaller polypeptide components of Crotaline venom cause systemic effects on organ systems that may occur distant from the bite site.

Protein components of Crotaline venom include hyaluronidase and other digestive enzymes, as well as glycoproteins that affect the coagulation system. The digestive proteins cause local tissue destruction, edema, and damage to the vascular basement membrane at the site of envenomation. Red blood cell extravasation into the tissues results from the basement membrane damage, and platelet exposure to damaged blood vessels causes local platelet aggregation and thrombocytopenia (Shannon et al., 2007). Glycoproteins contained in Crotaline venom act on the victim's coagulation system to produce a disseminated intravascular coagulation (DIC)–like syndrome. This syndrome differs from true DIC in that these glycoproteins produce fibrin monomers without consuming the victim's own thrombin or activating factor XIII. Although laboratory tests may reveal abnormalities of the coagulation system, clinical bleeding is rare (Shannon et al.).

The widespread effects of polypeptide venom components are mainly the result of damage to vascular endothelial cells, which allows leakage of intravascular fluid into the tissues. This leakage depletes intravascular volume and can lead to shock and circulatory collapse. In addition, damage to pulmonary capillaries results in pulmonary edema with subsequent hypoxia and respiratory failure. Polypeptide components of Mojave rattlesnake venom also have neurotoxic effects (Fleisher et al., 2006).

The venom of the coral snake exerts its effect through neurotoxins and phospholipase A_2. Direct neurotoxins bind the postsynaptic membrane of the neuromuscular junction, causing a flaccid paralysis that can be long-lasting. Phospholipase A_2 causes myonecrosis (Shannon et al., 2007).

Epidemiology and etiology

Reports of the total number of snakebites and deaths vary in the United States, with most sources reporting between 7,000 and 8,000 bites and 5 to 15 deaths per year. Approximately 25% of all snakebites occur in the pediatric population (Fleisher et al., 2006). Most occur in the warmer months of the year from April to October, and males are bitten more often than females.

Members of the Crotalinae family include rattlesnakes (*Crotalus* sp.) (Figure 23-4), copperheads (*Agkistrodon contortrix*) (Figure 23-5), and cottonmouths (*Agkistrodon piscivorus*) (Figure 23-6), which collectively account for more than 95% of all snakebites in the United States (Marx et al., 2009). These snakes have variations in markings that can make their identification a challenge, especially in the absence of the classic "rattle" of a rattlesnake. The most reliable identifying mark is the presence of a heat-sensing pit located between the nostril and eye, from which the pit viper gets its name. Other markings that signal a venomous snake include an elliptical pupil, presence of fangs, and a triangular head, although these distinctions are not as reliable as the presence of a pit for identification of venomous species (Marx et al., 2009). Nonvenomous snakes tend to have round pupils, multiple small teeth instead of fangs, and a more oval-shaped head.

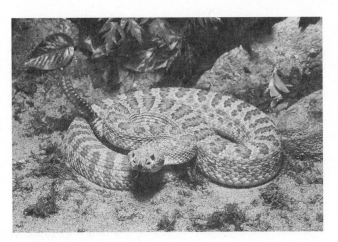

FIGURE 23-4

Rattlesnake.

Source: © Photos.com

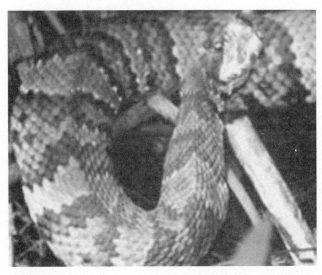

FIGURE 23-6

Cottonmouth Snake.

Source: Courtesy of U.S. Fish and Wildlife Service.

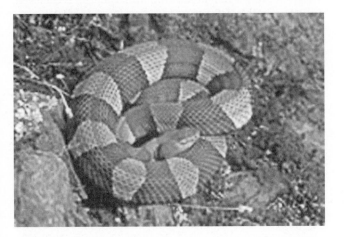

FIGURE 23-5

Copperhead Snake.

Source: Courtesy of U.S. Fish and Wildlife Service.

Coral snakes account for 1% to 4% of reported bites in the United States, and can be identified by a black snout and the presence of red, yellow, and black bands alternating along the body of the snake. Positive identification can be made if the band of red is bordered on either side by yellow, which is the origin of the expression "red on yellow, kill a fellow; red on black, venom lack." Of note, this mnemonic is valid only for coral snakes in the United States (Marx et al., 2009). If the red band is bordered by black on either side, the snake is the king snake, a nonvenomous mimic.

Presentation

History of snakebite is relatively simple to obtain in verbal children and adolescents, but may not be forthcoming in toddlers and the developmentally delayed. A high index of suspicion is required and a thorough search for fang marks

should be undertaken in these patients. A history of allergic reactions should be sought.

With Crotaline snakebites, the first symptom is immediate burning pain at the bite site. This is followed within 5 to 10 minutes by edema and erythema that increases over the next 8 to 10 hours and may progressively extend proximally from the bite. Within hours of the bite, ecchymoses or blebs may form on the affected extremity. Some blebs may be hemorrhagic. There is often lymphadenopathy or lymphangitis (Townsend et al., 2008). Necrosis of the extremity occurs if no treatment is given. Compartment syndrome, though rare, is most often seen with intracompartmental injection of venom. Local edema may cause airway compromise if the bite is located on the patient's face or neck.

Systemic signs of Crotaline envenomation initially may include perioral paresthesias or metallic taste occurring within minutes of a severe bite (Townsend et al., 2008). Weakness, nausea, vomiting, diaphoresis, dizziness, syncope, and tachycardia are also seen. Severe envenomations result in pulmonary edema with respiratory failure, hypotension, shock, and cardiovascular collapse (Fleisher et al., 2006). Kidney failure may occur as a consequence of other physiologic derangements. Venom is antigenic, and victims may develop life-threatening anaphylactic reactions.

Coral snakebites are initially minimally painful at the site, with little observed swelling. Teeth marks may be noted on physical examination, but no large fang punctures are found. Systemic symptoms predominate and may develop hours after a bite. Malaise and nausea are followed by muscle fasciculations, ptosis, diplopia, difficulty swallowing or talking, and respiratory failure from muscle paralysis (Marx et al., 2009).

Differential diagnosis

Snakebite must be differentiated from other causes of puncture wounds—notably, thorn wounds or rodent bites. Additionally, wound infection, cellulitis, sepsis, deep vein thrombosis (DVT), and DIC from other causes should be considered.

Plan of care

The diagnosis of snakebite is made clinically. Laboratory studies are undertaken to evaluate the systemic effects of the venom, the severity of the envenomation, and the patient's response to treatment. For Crotaline envenomation, initial studies should include a CBC, type and cross, urinalysis, coagulation profile, electrolytes with BUN and creatinine, fibrinogen, and fibrin split products. These studies should be repeated every 4 to 6 hours to monitor systemic effects and response to treatment. No laboratory studies are needed for coral snake envenomation, although many HCPs will obtain a set of baseline electrolytes, and a CBC with differential for those patients undergoing treatment.

The cornerstone of treatment for Crotaline bites is rapid antivenin therapy, which is based on the severity of the bite (Shannon et al., 2007). Mild bites will show local signs adjacent to the bite without proximal progression of edema. Patients may have perioral paresthesias, and laboratory study results are within normal limits (Marx et al., 2009). Moderate bites have edema extending proximally from the bite, as well as more severe systemic signs including nausea, vomiting, diarrhea, dizziness, weakness, and diaphoresis. In these patients, prothrombin time (PT) and partial thromboplastin time (PTT) will be increased, platelets will be decreased, and hemoglobin may be increased secondary to hemoconcentration from hypovolemia (Shannon et al.). Severe bites include all the preceding signs and symptoms of edema and erythema affecting the entire extremity. Patients have signs of impending respiratory failure, shock, bleeding, and altered mental status. Laboratory study findings will be significantly abnormal with elevated PT and PTT, decreased fibrinogen and platelets, and increased hemoglobin (Shannon et al.).

Initial assessment and therapeutic management of patients should focus on support for the airway, breathing, and circulation (ABCs). Early intubation is indicated for any patient with impending respiratory failure and is especially important for those with head or neck bites, as rapidly progressive local edema may make later establishment of a secure airway impossible (Shannon et al., 2007). Hypotension is treated with rapid administration of IV fluids and rarely requires vasopressor therapy. Any signs of allergic reaction should be treated aggressively.

Antivenin therapy is given based on the severity of the bite, not the weight of the patient. This relationship is based on a specific dose of antivenin neutralizing a specific amount of venom. Wyeth-Ayerst's Crotalidae Polyvalent Antivenin (ACP), an equine-derived antivenin that has been available for decades, is no longer in production and has been supplanted by Crotalidae Polyvalent Immune Fab (CroFab), a sheep-derived product that is less immunogenic. CroFab consists of the antigen-binding fragments of sheep antibodies to four species of North American crotalids. It carries some risk of hypersensitivity reactions, and risk of its use in patients with a history of allergy to sheep products, latex, papain or papaya, and dust mites must be carefully weighed.

Dosage of CroFab antivenin is based on the severity of the bite as previously described. For mild bites, 4 to 6 vials are given every 1 to 2 hours until initial control is achieved. Initial control is defined as the normalization of laboratory values and a halt of the progression of edema. For moderate bites, 8 to 12 vials may be given, with an additional 6 vials given every 1 to 2 hours until initial control is achieved. Severe bites require 12 to 18 vials initially, with 6 to 12 vials given every 1 to 2 hours to achieve initial control (Marx et al., 2009). For patients in all severity categories, an additional 2 vials every 6 hours for 3 doses are given after initial control is achieved. These subsequent doses are recommended because the antibody fragments are cleared more rapidly than the venom's duration of action. If allergic reactions to the antivenin are noted, they may be treated according to standard protocols (see Chapter 29). The antivenin infusion may be restarted at a slower rate once allergic reactions are controlled (King & Henretig, 2008). In severely bitten patients with allergic reaction to antivenin, an epinephrine infusion may be required to mitigate reactions in the setting of a need for antivenin administration.

Once systemic manifestations are controlled, attention turns to local wound care at the bite site. Most first-aid treatments for snakebite—such as suction, tourniquets, incision of fang marks, and constriction bands—are unproven or even harmful. If a constricting band is found around an effected extremity, it may be loosened once antivenin therapy is started (Fleisher et al., 2006). If a tourniquet is present and the limb appears ischemic, the tourniquet should be released immediately. The HCP should be prepared to deal with systemic signs of venom upon release of constricting bands or tourniquets. Any band left in place should be loose enough to admit a finger between the band and the patient's skin, and should be checked frequently, as progressive limb edema may cause the band to obstruct deep venous or arterial flow. If a constricting band is placed in this setting, it should be released once antivenin therapy is started.

Complete exposure of the affected extremity is essential for management. Multiple bites have been known to occur in children, and in the nonverbal patient a thorough search for multiple bites is essential. The extremity should be immobilized in a comfortable position at or slightly below heart level, and should be marked and measured at multiple locations to follow progression of edema (King & Henretig, 2008; Townsend et al., 2008). Serial measurements should be undertaken at least once hourly until no more edema progression is observed. The leading border of edema should be marked and timed with each measurement. Distal pulses should be checked hourly by palpation or Doppler imaging; if none are found, compartment pressures should be measured with consideration of fasciotomy in patients with pressures higher than 30 mmHg (Townsend et al.). Tetanus prophylaxis is given as indicated.

The wound should be washed with soap and water and examined for any remaining teeth or fangs. If any tissue necrosis develops, debridement may be indicated, although it is difficult to tell the extent of tissue destruction early in the disease course. Any bullae that form should be left intact unless they are on the digits and interfere with distal perfusion. If the patient's cardiopulmonary status is stable, pain control can be provided with narcotic agents. The occasional patient will require skin grafting for large areas of tissue breakdown.

Any patient with suspected coral snake bite should get antivenin, which is administered according to the instructions on the package insert. It is important to note that once symptoms of envenomation start, they may not be reversible with antivenin therapy (Marx et al., 2009). The HCP should be prepared to fully support the patient's breathing if needed.

Early involvement of a toxicologist for any but mild bites is beneficial to guide therapy, especially in the patient with a severe bite who has an allergic reaction to the antivenin. Surgical consultation is indicated for debridement, skin grafting, or fasciotomy if necessary. Critical care consult is needed for any patient with shock or respiratory failure, and for patients with moderate or severe envenomations who are admitted to the intensive care unit.

Disposition and discharge planning

All patients who are receiving antivenin therapy should be monitored in an intensive care setting for adverse reactions or deterioration in status. Patients who have no signs or symptoms of envenomation after 12 hours' observation may be discharged home with instructions to return if they experience any increased pain, redness, swelling, bloody nose, hematuria, diaphoresis, bruising, respiratory distress, or dizziness. Families should be informed that coagulopathy may recur in some patients, and that repeat antivenin therapy in otherwise clinically well patients is controversial.

Patients should follow up with their primary care provider in 2 to 5 days after discharge to evaluate the continued healing of the wounds. Early physical therapy is indicated for patients at risk for functional sequelae. Patients may also need follow-up with a plastic surgeon for skin grafting.

ERYTHEMA MULTIFORME

Ruth Abelt

PATHOPHYSIOLOGY

Erythema multiforme (EM), Stevens-Johnson syndrome (SJS), and toxic epidermal necrolysis (TEN) are all conditions that are attributed to a severe immune response. The exact mechanism of injury and pathophysiology is unknown; however, inflammatory cytokines such as tumor necrosis factor alpha and interleukin-6 have been found in the fluid and dermal tissue samples of patients with SJS and TEN (Murata et al., 2008). Cytotoxic T lymphocytes and natural killer cells also infiltrate skin lesions in patients diagnosed with SJS and TEN (Chung et al., 2008). These cytotoxic, immune complex–mediated reactions result in vascular injury and epithelial cell death. In one comparison of exudative fluid taken from bullous lesions of SJS and TEN patients versus burn patients, researchers found that the fluid from patients with SJS/TEN contained granulysin and cytotoxic lymphocytes, whereas the fluid from those patients with burns did not (Chung et al.). These inflammatory factors may contribute to the overwhelming keratinocyte apoptosis that is observed in SJS and TEN.

Patients with TEN have keratinocytes that produce a lytic fas ligand, which binds to a fas receptor on the cell surface, resulting in keratinocyte apoptosis (Viard et al., 1998). The production of this lytic ligand appears to be upregulated in patients with TEN. Murata and colleagues found an increase in soluble serum fas ligand levels in patients with SJS and TEN as compared to patients with the milder form of EM and healthy control subjects. SJS and TEN patients had the highest serum fas ligand levels before evidence of bulla and mucosal lesions appeared; these levels then decreased rapidly after the onset of symptoms (Murata et al., 2008).

EPIDEMIOLOGY AND ETIOLOGY

EM, SJS, and TEN are often described as a disease process continuum, representing a spectrum of severity. EM has been referred to as erythema multiforme minor, owing to its relative lack of severity. Mortality is low with this disease, and visceral organ involvement with EM is extremely rare. SJS, often referred to as erythema multiforme major, is a rare disease affecting only 1.2 to 6 persons per million per year and has a mortality as high as 15% (French, 2006). Mortality is related to subsequent infections or organ failure (Hurwitz, 1993). TEN is described as the most severe form of the immune-mediated disease. Its incidence is approximately 1.2 persons per million per year, with a mortality rate of 25% to 75% (Hurwitz). TEN is most commonly seen in adult patients, and affects women almost 2 times more often than men. Controversy persists in whether SJS and TEN are completely separate diseases or just more severe forms of EM (Auquier-Dunant et al., 2002).

Many etiologies have been linked to EM, SJS, and TEN. Viral and bacterial infections, sunlight, and certain medications are common triggers that are responsible for the vast majority of diagnosed patients. Herpes simplex virus (HSV) is a common cause of EM minor in children, accounting for more than one-half of presenting cases in children. In recurrent cases of HSV-related EM, the virus can be isolated in target lesions. HSV is not commonly a causative factor in the more severe forms, SJS and TEN (Morelli, 2007).

Bacterial infections such as *Mycoplasma pneumoniae* have been shown to cause SJS and TEN in children and young adults. In a review of the literature, Schalock et al. (2006) found *M. pneumoniae* to be a cause of EM minor and SJS in as many as 5% of pediatric and adult patients. However, one study suggested *M. pneumoniae* infection was responsible for almost two-thirds of the occurrences of SJS in children (Schalock et al., 2006). Children who are immunodeficient are at a higher risk of developing SJS and TEN.

Medications are another trigger for development of SJS and TEN in pediatric patients. The agents most commonly associated with these disorders are antibiotics (specifically sulfonamides) and antiepileptics (lamotrigine, phenobarbital, carbamazepine), although analgesic medications and anti-inflammatory agents have also been reported to trigger SJS in children (Levi et al., 2009). The use of sulfamethoxazole–trimethoprim for outpatient treatment of soft-tissue infections involving MRSA could potentially pose an increased risk for the development SJS or TEN in the pediatric population. Medications used weeks prior to presentation of symptoms may be responsible for an outbreak; recurrent exposure to the offending medication may cause symptoms to appear within 2 days (Levi et al.).

PRESENTATION

EM is characterized by an acute onset of target lesions on the extremities, palms, and soles, with little or no mucosal involvement. If mucosal involvement is present, the vermilion border of the lips is the most common place

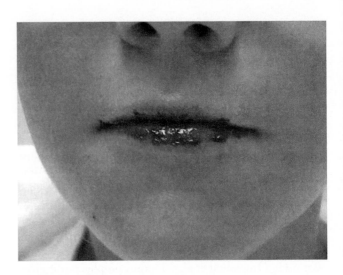

FIGURE 23-7

Erythema Multiforme.

Source: Courtesy of Alanna Bree MD.

lesions may occur (Figure 23-7). The face, trunk, and legs are typically spared or have sparse lesions. Lesions are symmetrical, fixed, round, erythematous, macular, and bullous in nature. There may be areas of central pallor, purpura, or necrosis. A burning sensation may be described prior to skin outbreak. Target or iris lesions typically evolve over approximately 1 week and self-resolve within approximately 4 weeks (Hurwitz, 1990).

SJS cutaneous lesions are often preceded by a prodrome of flu-like symptoms, fever, malaise, cough, rhinorrhea, and myalgias. Edema, erythema, and pain often precede ulceration development and subsequent hemorrhage of the oral mucosal. Lesions cover 10% or less of the body surface area (BSA), leading to large areas of denuded skin and predisposing patients to infection, electrolyte disturbances, and fluid imbalance (Figure 23-8 and Figure 23-9). Over a 1-week period, crops of target lesions appear on the face and trunk, then spread and rapidly develop into vesicles, bullae, and epidermal detachment (Morelli, 2007). A positive Nikolsky sign (dermal exfoliation with mild friction) may be seen in 93% to 100% of patients who have two or more mucosal surfaces involved (Letko et al., 2005). Ocular, buccal, urogenital, pulmonary, and gastrointestinal involvement are frequently seen and can lead to long-term sequelae. Visceral organ involvement may induce multisystem organ failure, including, but not limited to, respiratory failure, renal failure, and cardiac dysfunction. Sloughing of the buccal, gastrointestinal, and respiratory tract mucosa increases the risk of complications and mortality (Morelli). The cutaneous eruptions may take several months to completely heal (Morelli).

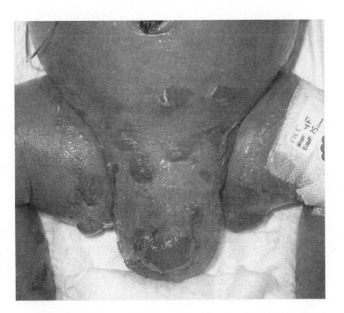

FIGURE 23-8

Stevens Johnson Syndrome (SJS).

Source: Courtesy of Ruth Abelt.

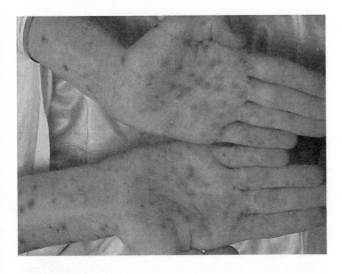

FIGURE 23-9

Stevens Johnson Syndrome (SJS).

Source: Courtesy of Ruth Abelt.

TEN involves epidermal detachment of more than 30% of the BSA. Patients who have involvement of 10% to 30% of BSA are diagnosed as having SJS and TEN overlap (Bastuji-Garin et al., 1993). TEN is often preceded by fevers exceeding 39°C (102.2°F), extreme skin tenderness and burning, and influenza-like symptoms; within approximately 24 hours, skin eruptions begin to appear. Unlike in EM and SJS, no target lesions are present; however, there are widespread purpuric macules, which quickly evolve into flaccid fluid-filled bullae. These lesions progress to confluent masses, which lead to large areas of full-thickness epidermal necrosis. The epidermis is lost in large sheets, with a loss of 100% occurring in some patients (Hurwitz, 1990). Severe ocular lesions, purulent conjunctivitis, buccal erosions, and visceral organ involvement are present in almost 100% of patients (French, 2006).

A study of 159 patients with SJS or TEN found that 74% of patients suffered mild to severe ocular involvement and that 15 months after hospital discharge 63% of patients had long-term complications ranging from chronic dry eye to blindness (Gueudry et al., 2009). More than 25% of patients develop fulminant respiratory failure secondary to sloughing of the tracheal and bronchial tree (French, 2006). Patients are also at severe risk of overwhelming bacterial infections, sepsis, dehydration, and multisystem organ failure.

DIFFERENTIAL DIAGNOSIS

Several other diseases have symptomatology similar to EM, SJS, and TEN. The mucosal involvement and the desquamation of the hands and feet in children with Kawasaki's disease can appear similar to the signs and symptoms of SJS. Drug eruptions with urticaria produce erythematous lesions similar to those seen in EM, but the former lesions are not fixed and symmetrical. Graft-versus-host disease, toxic shock syndrome, staphylococcal scalded skin syndrome, and phototoxic eruptions also bear similarities to EM, SJS, and TEN.

PLAN OF CARE

Diagnostic studies for patients with EM minor include obtaining bacterial and viral cultures from skin lesions to identify treatable causes. If HSV is suspected, then hospitalization is required to provide therapeutic management of the infection. It is paramount to have the patient discontinue medications that may have contributed to an outbreak.

Hospitalization and monitoring in an intensive care unit are indicated for patients with SJS and TEN. A robust diagnostic work-up would include an arterial blood gases, CBC with differential, erythrocyte sedimentation rate (ESR), C-reactive protein (CRP), liver function studies, amylase, lipase, tracheal aspirate, and viral/bacterial wound cultures (Morelli, 2007). *M. pneumoniae* serology should be sent for analysis, and a chest radiograph (CXR) should be obtained. Initially, peripheral and central serum blood cultures should be obtained to evaluate for systemic infection, with subsequent cultures drawn if infection is suspected. Electrolyte imbalances and renal dysfunction are common in SJS and TEN; thus monitoring of a complete metabolic chemistry panel should be performed frequently.

A skin biopsy should be obtained to rule out other diseases. Histological findings in SJS show a full-thickness necrosis of the epidermis and detachment from the dermis, with T-lymphocyte infiltration in the surrounding vasculature (Letko et al., 2005). TEN histology is similar to that found in SJS, and ductal necrosis in the sweat ducts may also be observed (Ringheanu & Laude, 2000). Fluid from lanced bullae should be sent for HSV direct fluorescent antibody (DFA) and viral cultures; if HSV is a contributing factor, evidence of the virus may be present as early as 1 day after the outbreak of skin lesions (American Academy of Pediatrics, 2009).

Therapeutic management is mostly supportive. If the causative agent is medication, then the drug should be stopped and listed as an allergy for the patient. Some practitioners have found the use of intravenous immunoglobulin (IVIG) effective in halting the progression of the disease in SJS and TEN and leading to a more rapid recovery (Metry et al., 2003). A case series of 10 patients with TEN IVIG blocked the fas-mediated cell death of the keratinocytes (Viard et al., 1998). Plasmapheresis and corticosteroids have also been used to treat patients with SJS and TEN, although they are neither widely used nor a broadly accepted management strategy (French, 2006). Use of routine antimicrobial therapies is not recommended; however, a course of antibiotics and/or antivirals should be initiated if a bacterial or viral infection is identified (Morelli, 2007).

Patients with severe mucositis, severe disease, or pulmonary complications should be intubated to maintain a patent airway. Sloughing of the tracheal and bronchial tree can lead to occluded endotracheal tubes; frequent suctioning is required to prevent complications. Patients' oxygenation and ventilation should be monitored closely. Escalation of therapy from a conventional ventilator to high-frequency ventilation may be required.

Hypovolemic dehydration and shock may present secondary to an increase in insensible fluid losses from skin lesion weepage. Meticulous fluid and electrolyte management is required in such circumstances. Fluids can be managed by administering crystalloids based on the patient's percentage of BSA involvement. Replacement fluids are typically administered at a rate of 4 mL/kg/day in addition to maintenance intravenous fluids. Replacement fluids should be administered incrementally over 24 hours, then titrated according to urine output (Jarjosa, 2009). Placement of a urinary drainage catheter facilitates accurate measurements of urine output. Because most patients with SJS and TEN will be unable to take oral feeds secondary to extreme buccal lesions, total parenteral nutrition should be initiated early to aid in proper nutrition for healing and recovery.

Wound care is paramount in identifying and preventing secondary infections. Reverse isolation should be instituted. Exposed skin will be extremely painful, so strict attention to pain control prior to wound care and throughout hospitalization is essential. Wounds should be cleansed with isotonic saline and covered with biologic dressings to help diminish ongoing fluid loss. Oral care may require rinsing with normal saline or oral rinses suggested by the infectious diseases team. If possible, patients with severe disease should be transferred to and managed by a burn unit team.

Consultation by the interprofessional HCP team would include the following specialists:

- Infectious diseases and immunology, to address the likely inciting agent and best therapeutic management approach
- Nutritionist, to ensure the patient is receiving adequate protein and calories
- Wound care team and plastic surgery, if wounds are extensive and involve joints
- Specialized kinetic or "air" beds, to prevent further damage to skin and tissues
- Physical, occupational, and speech therapy and rehabilitation medicine (early in the hospital course), to begin rehabilitation as soon as possible to keep muscles and joints mobile, and to promote speech articulation
- Ophthalmology, if there is evidence of ocular involvement and for recommendations to treat and prevent long-term ocular injury
- Pain team, to ensure appropriate and best-practice pain control is provided
- Child life and behavioral medicine, to support the patient's developmental and psychological health while hospitalized
- Social services and spiritual team to ensure patient and family support

Additionally, consultation with the renal, pulmonary, otolaryngology, and general surgery services may be required if systemic dysfunction occur.

Initially the patient, family, and caregivers will require ongoing communication with the intensive care and interprofessional teams regarding the diagnostic studies and therapies that may be required. Discussion should also focus on addressing all physical changes that the patient may be experiencing during the hospitalization. Educating patients and families on wound care, signs of infection, oral care, and long-term complications allows for discussion and sharing of accurate information. If an allergen is identified as having activated the disease process, then education regarding the allergy is essential.

DISPOSITION AND DISCHARGE PLANNING

SJS has a mortality rate as high as 15% (French, 2006), while TEN has a mortality rate of 25% to 75% (Hurwitz, 1993).

Patients who survive often have long-term chronic conditions that must be addressed on an outpatient basis. Skin lesions may take several months to heal, but patients may be medically ready for discharge prior to entire skin healing. Patients may need outpatient therapy if they developed excessive skin loss and subsequent scarring, leading to body image disturbances. HCPs should monitor these patients for depression and other psychosocial sequelae associated with long-term illness. Outpatient physical and occupational therapies should continue if there are still limitations to range of motion or physical disabilities. Patients should be closely followed by an ophthalmologist to evaluate for long-term effects of ocular lesions and vision screens.

STINGS

Milton Meadows

BEES AND WASPS (HYMENOPTERA)

Pathophysiology

The pathophysiology of bee and wasp stings is a direct result of the chemical components of their venom and, to a lesser degree, the anatomic location of the sting. Insect venom contains a variety of active components, the most toxic of which are bradykinin, acetylcholine, histamine, and dopamine (Marx et al., 2009). Bee and wasp venom also contains a variety of antigens that can cause immunoglobulin E–mediated hypersensitivity reactions that range from mild local inflammation to life-threatening anaphylaxis (Shannon et al., 2007).

Epidemiology and etiology

The total number of insect stings is difficult to estimate because most go unreported. The overwhelming majority of patients who are stung by a bee or wasp require no or minimal medical interventions. Despite this fact, bee and wasp stings account for approximately 50% of all deaths from bites and stings; and therefore, prompt recognition and therapeutic management of serious reactions is essential (Fleisher et al., 2006).

The stinging apparatus is located on the caudal end of the insect. In bees, the stinger is barbed and can remain in the skin after the sting is delivered. In wasps, the stinger does not have a barb and does not remain within the dermis; thus the same wasp may sting the patient multiple times (Marx et al., 2009).

Presentation

Historical information of a bee or wasp sting varies, depending on whether it was a witnessed or unwitnessed sting. If witnessed, often the time of the sting and the patient's reaction are recounted in more detail. In unwitnessed stings, caregivers may be able to report only that the patient was outdoors or in locations where insects are likely to nest.

The most common presenting symptom is pain at the location of the sting with associated redness, swelling, or itching. The stinger may be found embedded in the skin at the site. The severity of systemic symptoms varies and can be classified by grouping reactions (Fleisher et al., 2006):

- Group I: only a local response at the site of the sting. This local reaction can be quite impressive, covering a large area and lasting from 2 to 5 days (Figure 23-10).
- Group II: Group I symptoms *and* mild systemic symptoms of generalized pruritis and urticaria.
- Group III: Group I and II symptoms *and* wheezing, angioedema, shortness of breath, cough, nausea, vomiting, or abdominal pain.
- Group IV: life-threatening, with Group I–III symptoms *and* laryngoedema, hypotension, shock, respiratory arrest, or coma.

Most serious reactions are seen within 30 minutes of the sting, but the local effects may last for several days and delayed hypersensitivity reactions may occur up to 10 days after a sting (Marx et al., 2009).

Differential diagnosis

Bee and wasp stings may be confused with bites from arachnids (e.g., spiders) and other insects such as flies. The HCP should also evaluate for other possible causes of allergic reactions (Shannon et al., 2007).

Plan of care

There are no diagnostic studies that can confirm a sting by bee or wasp. Embedded stingers should be removed as

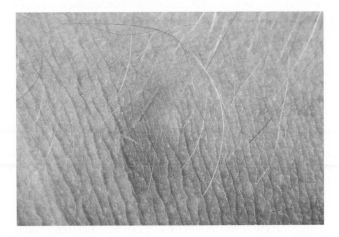

FIGURE 23-10

Bee Sting: 24 Hours Old.

Source: © Stéphane Bidouze/ShutterStock, Inc.

soon as possible by scraping the dermis with a scalpel edge. The blade should be placed as close to parallel with the dermal layer so that the stinger may be lifted and further envenomation may be avoided (Marx et al., 2009).

Additional therapeutic management focuses on aborting or mitigating the anaphylactic response elicited by antigens in the venom. Local reactions (Group I) can be treated with cool compresses to the site as needed to reduce pain and swelling (Townsend et al., 2008). Mild systemic reactions (Group II) are treated with diphenhydramine at a dose of 4 mg/kg/day (divided into four doses) for several days (Fleisher et al., 2006).

More severe reactions (Group III) may require intramuscular epinephrine. Intramuscular epinephrine is more rapidly absorbed than subcutaneous injection and is the preferred route. A dose of epinephrine 1:1,000 concentration at 0.01 mL/kg (up to 0.3 mL) should be injected intramuscularly, followed by oral or IV diphenhydramine. An H_2 receptor antagonist such as ranitidine 4–5 mg/kg/day (divided twice daily) by mouth may reduce the severity of symptoms (Fleisher et al., 2006). These patients should be observed as inpatients for 24 hours. Wheezing can be treated with inhaled β-agonists or IV aminophylline 6 mg/kg over 20 minutes followed by 0.7–1 mg/kg/hr infusion if needed.

Life-threatening reactions (Group IV) may require endotracheal intubation and mechanical ventilation, IV fluid boluses of 20–60 mL/kg, and epinephrine continuous infusion (Townsend et al., 2008). In these patients, hydrocortisone 2 mg/kg/dose IV may be given every 6 hours for 2 to 4 days. Patients with Group IV reactions should be admitted to the intensive care unit and stabilized accordingly. Consultation with an allergist is indicated in any patient who experiences a systemic reaction to a bee or wasp sting. In patients with life-threatening reactions, early involvement of a pediatric critical care specialist is crucial; otolaryngology services should be consulted if the airway is considered difficult to stabilize.

Families should be instructed to avoid behaviors and situations that place the child at risk for future bee or wasp stings. They should also be instructed on the use of all medications (including use of an EpiPen) and adverse effects. They should keep the sting site clean and dry, and watch for any signs of infection or continued irritation.

Disposition and discharge planning

Patients with local or mild systemic reactions can be observed in the ED for response to therapy. Patients with only local pain, redness, or itching can be discharged home from the ED after one hour of observation and supportive care. A patient with mild systemic symptoms may be discharged home if no further systemic signs are appreciated

within one hour of the last dose of medication (Shannon et al., 2007). These patients should continue to take diphenhydramine for 2 to 3 days after the sting.

Patients with more severe reactions should be admitted to an appropriate inpatient unit depending on their acuity. Patients with severe systemic reactions that are responsive to antihistamines, intramuscular epinephrine, and H_2 blockers in the ED should be admitted to the hospital and observed for 24 hours. Those requiring continuous infusions of epinephrine or aminophylline, or with severe life-threatening reactions, should be admitted to the intensive care unit.

Any patient with systemic reactions to bee or wasp stings should be prescribed an EpiPen (if the patient weight is more than 30 kg) or an EpiPen Junior (for patients weighing less than 30 kg) (Fleisher et al., 2006). Instructions on the identification of allergic reactions should be provided. Patients who are discharged from the ED should be instructed to return immediately if they develop any shortness of breath, wheezing, or hives.

Referral to an allergist is essential for all patients who experience systemic reactions. Allergists can conduct skin testing and initiate desensitization therapy if indicated, which is highly effective at preventing future anaphylactic reactions.

JELLYFISH STINGS

Pathophysiology

All major U.S. species of the animals commonly known as "jellyfish" deliver venom through specialized structures called nematocysts. Nematocysts are located on the tentacles and number in the hundreds of thousands per tentacle in some species (Marx et al., 2009). Contact with potential prey or predators causes the nematocysts to fire, driving barbed toxin-carrying spines into the victim. Nematocysts on tentacles separated from the animal remain capable of firing, and may fire even after the animal dies (Marx et al.).

The venom of jellyfish is poorly characterized. It contains toxic proteins that lead to paralysis and other central nervous system (CNS) effects. Pain and urticaria result from inflammatory mediators in the venom (Shannon et al., 2007). Allergic reactions may be mild and localized or (rarely) systemic and life threatening.

Epidemiology and etiology

Deaths from jellyfish stings are exceedingly rare. The only reported deaths in the United States have been associated with stings of the Portuguese man-of-war. It is important to note that species differ in other parts of the world and that knowledge of the local population is important. Three major species account for the majority of stings brought to medical attention in the United States: the Portuguese man-of-war, the purple jellyfish, and the lion's mane.

The Portuguese man-of-war (*Physalia physalis*) is not a true jellyfish, but rather a floating hydrozoan colony. It is composed of a floating body with long underwater tentacles that may reach up to 75 feet in length (Figure 23-11). These tentacles may extend behind the main body such that some victims may be stung without ever seeing the jellyfish (Shannon et al., 2007).

The common purple jellyfish (*Pelagia noctiluca*) is minimally toxic. Its stings usually cause only local skin irritation or pain (Fleisher et al., 2006).

The lion's mane (*Cyanea capillata*) is found on the Atlantic and Pacific coasts. This jellyfish has golden-yellow tentacles that surround its body that are similar to the mane of a lion. This animal's toxic venom causes immediate burning on initial contact, and prolonged exposure to the venom may result in muscle cramps or respiratory failure (Fleisher et al., 2006).

Presentation

Jellyfish stings cause immediate pain in the victim. The site of the sting will demonstrate local irritation, redness, and pain or burning that may extend up the extremity (Townsend et al., 2008). A row of urticarial lesions or adherent tentacles may be noted. Signs of more severe systemic envenomation may include headache, nausea or vomiting, fever, abdominal rigidity, arthralgias, respiratory distress, hemolysis, kidney failure, coma, or hypotension (Marx et al., 2009). The severity of symptoms depends on the size of the area stung in proportion to the size of the victim, the power of the venom, and the victim's sensitivity to the venom.

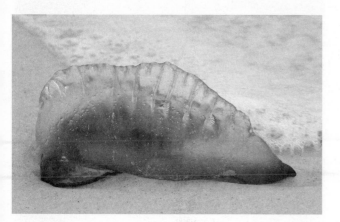

FIGURE 23-11

Jellyfish: Portuguese Man-O-War.

Source: © SaraJo/ShutterStock, Inc.

Differential diagnosis

Jellyfish stings should be differentiated from other sting-related causes. A row of urticarial lesions with or without an attached tentacle confirms the diagnosis. Differentiating between the various types of jellyfish stings is not necessary in the United States (Shannon et al., 2007).

Plan of care

There are no definitive diagnostic studies for jellyfish stings. Patients with signs of severe envenomation should have a CBC, electrolytes, BUN, creatinine, and urinalysis. Therapies should focus initially on management of systemic manifestations, with careful attention being paid to the patient's cardiopulmonary status. Local treatment is all that will be required for most victims.

Any patient with systemic symptoms should be admitted for observation and treatment if required. Management of local irritation for jellyfish stings begins with removal of any adherent tentacles. This should be done with a double-gloved hand or instrument to prevent discharging nematocysts from injuring the HCP (King & Henretig, 2008). After tentacle removal, any remaining nematocysts can be inactivated by soaking or washing the extremity with 3% acetic acid for 30 minutes.

Another treatment technique involves application of baking soda slurry to the site for 30 minutes, then shaving the area or scraping with a dull instrument (King & Henretig, 2008). The area should not be rinsed with fresh water, as this may cause firing of nematocysts. Use of sea water or normal saline is recommended.

Local painful reactions may be treated with narcotics such as morphine or fentanyl. Tetanus prophylaxis should be administered if indicated. Many patients will benefit from systemic antihistamine therapy and topical steroid creams until irritation resolves (Fleisher et al., 2006). Prophylactic antibiotics have not proven to be beneficial and are not recommended in the treatment of these patients.

More severe or exotic stings may require consultation with a toxicologist or critical care specialist. Extensive skin involvement may require consultation by dermatology and/or plastic surgery.

The family should be educated to watch the patient for systemic signs or symptoms of severe envenomation. They should be informed that urticaria and irritation at the site may occur from 1 to 4 weeks after the sting (Shannon et al., 2007).

Disposition and discharge planning

Patients may be discharged after 4 hours observation for systemic symptoms (Shannon et al., 2007). Referral to their primary care provider for follow-up is recommended anytime the patient has been admitted. Follow-up with any subspecialists involved in the patient's care while hospitalized is also recommended.

WOUNDS AND WOUND CARE

Julie Edwards

PATHOPHYSIOLOGY

An *abscess* is an area of nonfunctioning tissue that is contained or "walled off," most often resulting from a persistent bacterial infection. The abscess is characterized by leukocyte accumulation and formation of purulent exudate or pus. Specifics of the disease processes of an abscess are related to the anatomical location and associated etiology (Rote & Huether, 2010).

Lacerations are an insult to skin integrity usually attributed to trauma. This insult might be described as a "tear" or "rip" where the tissue is divided in a jagged manner, often with irregular edges (Figure 23-12). Laceration depths vary, and small vessels and nerves may be present within the separated tissue. Abrasions and contusions may accompany lacerations. An *avulsion* (Figure 23-13) is a complicated laceration in which the tissue is pulled away from the body, creating a flap-like appearance (McCance & Grey, 2010). Foreign bodies may be present within lacerated or avulsed tissue and may prove difficult to visualize (Levine et al., 2008). Abdominal or thoracic trauma may result in deep lacerations to major organs.

Puncture wounds are created by objects without sharp edges, such as that of a knife (Figure 23-14). A typical example is a foot injury caused by stepping on a nail. Puncture wounds are prone to deep wound infection and can appear to be relatively minor. *Bites* are usually classified as a subtype of puncture wound, although they may have multiple characteristics (such as avulsion or crush injury). *Envenomations* are puncture wounds caused by snakes, spiders, and other venomous animals. Venom poses an increased danger to the pediatric patient as compared to the adult due to the smaller volume of distribution (Holve, 2004).

Pressure ulcers are localized areas of tissue compromised by pressure or compression of a bony prominence against the tissue. The National Pressure Ulcer Advisory Panel (NPUAP, 2010) describes pressure ulcers as "an area of localized injury to the skin caused by pressure or pressure in tandem with shear or friction" (p. 4).

EPIDEMIOLOGY AND ETIOLOGY

Immunosuppressed patients are at the highest risk for developing an abscess (McCance & Grey, 2010). In the pediatric patient, many abscess types are possible: brain, dental, epidural, gingival, hepatic, lateral pharyngeal, pelvic, perianal, peritoneal, peritonsillar, pilonidal, psoas, pulmonary, renal, and retropharyngeal (Behrman et al., 2004). Internal abscesses usually arise following surgical intervention, infection, or consolidation. Etiological agents and epidemiology for the most common abscesses in pediatric patients are outlined in Table 23-1.

Approximately 8.2% of all ED visits are due to lacerations, and one-third of these injuries involve children. Some 3.7% of patients present with multiple lacerations.

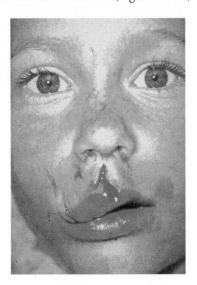

FIGURE 23-12

Laceration.

Source: Courtesy of the National EMSC Resource Alliance.

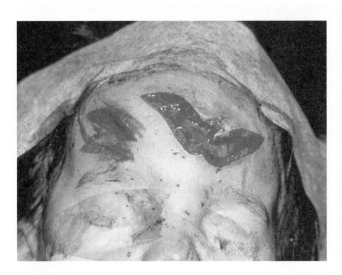

FIGURE 23-13

Avulsion.

Source: Courtesy of the National EMSC Resource Alliance.

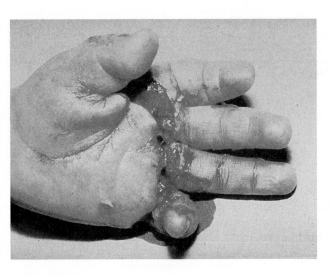

FIGURE 23-14

Puncture/amputaton.

Source: Courtesy of the National EMSC Resource Alliance.

Most lacerations are to the extremities. The leading causes of lacerations are cutting and piercing tools (28.6%), falls (19.3%), motor vehicle collisions (6.3%), and unknown (15.5%) (Singer et al., 2006). Lacerations account for 1 in every 4 childhood injuries and are most significant in the 4- to 7-year-old age group, with males being more likely to experience such an injury than females (Singer et al.). The most common soft tissue foreign bodies consist of metal, glass, or ceramic (Levine et al., 2008). Animal bites account for 0.7% to 1% of all emergency room visits in the United States each year (Ginsburg, 2004).

Pressure ulcers occur at the rate of 27% in pediatric intensive care units (PICUs) and at a rate of 23% in neonatal intensive care units (NICUs). Risk factors for the pediatric patient include terminal illness, sedation, hypotension, sepsis, spinal cord injury, impaired mobility/chemical paralysis, previous cardiopulmonary bypass surgery or vasopressor therapy, young age, prolonged length of ICU stay, and use of traction devices. Specifically, the pediatric patient who has a PICU stay of more than 8 days or mechanical ventilation

TABLE 23-1

Common Abscesses in the Pediatric Patient

Location	Etiology	Pathogen	Diagnostic Study	Presentation
Brain	Embolization due to congenital heart disease; viral or bacterial disease of the CNS	*Staphylococcus aureus*, *Streptococcus*, anaerobic organisms, Gram-negative aerobic bacilli	Peripheral WBC: may be normal or elevated Blood culture: positive in 10% of patients CSF examination: shows variable results Glucose: slightly lowered EEG: corresponding focal slowing CT and MRI: most reliable for demonstrating abscess formation	Nonspecific symptoms initially, followed by vomiting, severe headache, seizures, papilledema, hemiparesis, and coma
Hepatic	Infancy: sepsis, umbilical vein infection, and vessel cannulation After infancy: immunosuppressed patients or patients status post-abdominal disease or surgery Cat scratch disease or fungal infection	*Staphylococcus aureus*, *Escherichia coli*, *Salmonella*, anaerobic organisms	ALT/AST: slight elevation WBC and ESR: elevated Needle biopsy guided by CT or ultrasound for culture of abscess	Nonspecific symptoms initially, followed by potential right upper quadrant pain, enlarged and tender liver
Retropharyngeal and lateral pharyngeal	Children younger than 3–4 years of age: most common	Polymicrobial, Group A *Streptococcus*, oropharyngeal anaerobic bacteria, *Staphylococcus aureus* common	Soft-tissue neck radiographs CT, I & D for positive identification of organism	Nonspecific, including fever, malaise, and decreased oral intake; neck stiffness, torticollis, and refusal to move neck; complaints of sore throat and neck pain, muffled voice, stridor and respiratory distress possible

(Continued)

TABLE 23-1

Common Abscesses in the Pediatric Patient *(Continued)*				
Location	**Etiology**	**Pathogen**	**Diagnostic Study**	**Presentation**
Peritonsillar	Adolescents: most common with an acute history or pharyngitis Bacteria invasion via capsule of the tonsil is the precise etiology	Group A *Streptococcus* and mixed oropharyngeal anaerobes	CT, I & D for positive identification of organism	Recent history of pharyngitis; nonspecific symptoms, including lethargy and fever, sore throat, dysphasia, and trismus
Pulmonary	Related to lung infections: pneumonia, cystic fibrosis, gastroesophageal reflux disorder, esophageal fistulas, immunosuppression, seizures, aspiration	*Streptococcus* species, *Staphylococcus aureus*, *Escherichia coli*, *Klebsiella pneumoniae*, *Pseudomonas aeruginosa*, and anaerobic bacteriodes	Chest radiography, CT of the chest, bronchoscopic aspiration of identified area	Cough, fever, tachypnea, dyspnea, chest pain, vomiting, sputum production, hemoptysis, and weight loss
Skin and soft tissue	Community exposure to pathogen Break in skin integrity a risk factor but not always present	*Staphylococcus aureus*, methicillin-resistant *Staphylococcus aureus* (MRSA), community-acquired MRSA (CA-MRSA)	Wound culture and antibiotic susceptibility Bedside ultrasonography, I & D	Acute onset (within one week), fluctuance, erythema, induration, tenderness with or without purulent drainage

Alanine aminotransferase (ALT), aspartate aminotransferase (AST), central nervous system (CNS), cerebrospinal fluid (CSF), computed tomography (CT), electroencephalograph (EEG), erythrocyte sedimentation rate (ESR), incision and drainage (I & D), magnetic resonance imaging (MRI), white blood cell count (WBC).

of more than 7 days is at increased risk for pressure ulcers (Baharestani & Ratliff, 2007; Curley et al., 2003a).

In addition, urticaria, obesity, edema, trauma, surgical incisions, insensate areas, poor nutrition, incontinence, severe illness, and impaired cognition have been associated with the development of pressure ulcers (Pallija et al., 1999). Devices such as pulse oximetry probes, nasal cannulas, bi-level positive airway pressure (BiPAP) masks, endotracheal tubes, tracheotomy tubes, catheters, splints, and gastrostomy tubes are all frequently the cause of compromised skin integrity. An estimated 50% of ulcerations in the pediatric patient occur secondary to use of equipment and medical devices (Baharestani & Ratliff, 2007).

PRESENTATION

In general, a cutaneous abscess is diagnosed when there is erythema, tenderness, pain, warmth, induration, fluctuance, and/or drainage (Koehler & Nakayama, 2009). Symptoms of an internal abscess may initially be nonspecific, such as fever, general malaise, and fatigue. As the infectious process progresses, symptoms become more specific to the area of the abscess. Internal abscesses are often considered as a diagnosis when the patient has a pertinent history, fever, elevated white blood cell count (WBC), pain, and symptoms associated with the physiology of the site (Rote & Huether, 2010).

All lacerations, avulsions, and puncture wounds should be measured and explored for the presence of foreign material. Physical examination is sufficient for identification of these items in 78% of patients (Levine et al., 2008).

Many tools and scales for assessment of pediatric skin breakdown and pressure ulcers have been published; however, only the Braden Q (Curley et al., 2003b), Glamorgan Scale, and Neonatal Risk Assessment Scale (NSRAS) have been tested for statistical sensitivity and specificity. Both the Braden Q and NSRAS scales are based on the Braden Scale (developed for the adult population), but are modified to consider the developmental and physiological differences in pediatric patients. The NSRAS has a specificity of 81% and sensitivity of 83%. The Glamorgan Scale is based on literature review and meta-analysis. Its sensitivity rate is the highest of the three tools—98.4%. It is widely recommended that a thorough skin assessment be conducted using one of these tools upon admission, and at least daily, for all neonates and children with wounds (Baharestani & Ratliff, 2007).

For the purpose of diagnosis, documentation, and therapeutic management, staging of pressure ulcer wounds is recommended. The NPUAP (2007) recommends the following criteria be used for staging of pressure ulcers:

- *Stage I:* Intact skin with nonblanchable redness of a localized area; usually over a bony prominence. Darkly pigmented skin may have visible blanching; its color may differ from that of the surrounding area (Figure 23-15).

- *Stage II:* Partial-thickness loss of dermis presenting as a shallow, open ulcer with a red–pink wound bed, without slough. It may also present as intact or open/ruptured serum-filled bleb. This stage should be used to describe skin tears, tape burns, perineal dermatitis, maceration, or excoriation. Bruising indicates deep tissue injury (Figure 23-16).
- *Stage III:* Full-thickness tissue loss extending through dermis to involve subcutaneous tissue. Slough may

be present, but does not obscure the depth of tissue loss. Undermining and tunneling may be noted. The depth of this type of pressure ulcer differs with the anatomical location. The bridge of the nose, ear, occiput, and malleolus do not have subcutaneous tissue; consequently, the depth of a Stage III wound in these areas may be shallow (Figure 23-17).
- *Stage IV:* Deep tissue destruction extending through subcutaneous tissue to fascia; may involve muscle layers, joints, and/or bone. Undermining and tunneling are often present. The depth of the damage depends on the anatomical location (Figure 23-18).

STAGE 1

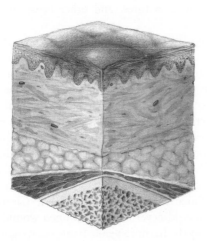

FIGURE 23-15

Stage 1 Pressure Ulcer.

Source: Courtesy of the National Pressure Ulcer Advisory Panel.

STAGE 2

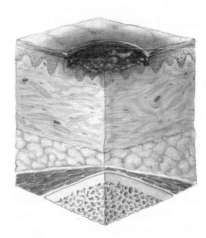

FIGURE 23-16

Stage 2 Pressure Ulcer.

Source: Courtesy of the National Pressure Ulcer Advisory Panel.

STAGE 3

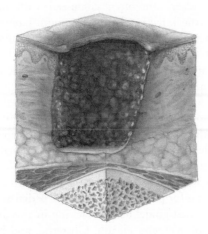

FIGURE 23-17

Stage 3 Pressure Ulcer.

Source: Courtesy of the National Pressure Ulcer Advisory Panel.

STAGE 4

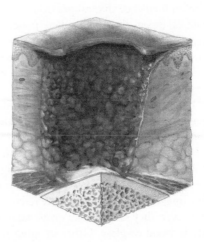

FIGURE 23-18

Stage 4 Pressure Ulcer.

Source: Courtesy of the National Pressure Ulcer Advisory Panel.

Initial wound evaluation should include size (length × width × depth), stage, tissue type in the wound bed, wound edges, margins (undermining, tracts, tunneling), periwound skin (should be intact), exudate (color, content, amount, odor), wound pain, infection (signs of acute or chronic infection), wound age, and frequency of evaluation (Conley, 2009).

PLAN OF CARE

For abscesses, the diagnostic testing depends on the wound's size and location. Most smaller cutaneous lesions are not cultured. However, if resistant organisms are suspected based on community prevalence, then culture for susceptibilities may be valuable. White blood cell count and blood culture are nonspecific, but nevertheless useful for characterizing large cutaneous and suspected internal lesions. Ultrasound (US), computed tomography (CT), and magnetic resonance imaging (MRI) are useful diagnostic studies for internal lesions, and US and CT may provide direction for needle aspiration of the abscess for purposes of culture and drainage. Cerebrospinal fluid (CSF) culture should be obtained in neonates and patients with severe illness, as should hepatic function studies such as alanine aminotransferase (ALT) and aspartate aminotransferase (AST) (Behrman et al., 2004). Table 23-1 provides details on diagnostic studies and findings specific to common abscesses in the pediatric patient.

Therapeutic management for an abscess includes administration of antibiotics based on the presumed or identified causative organism, basic wound care if the site is cutaneous, and monitoring for progression of infection. Incision and drainage of cutaneous lesions will often hasten their resolution, although there are few evidence-based studies to prove this relationship (Levine et al., 2008; Koehler & Nakayama, 2009). Surgical drainage of internal abscesses is usually required.

Infection develops in many lacerations and puncture wounds, with an incidence that ranges from 1.1% to 12%; this outcome is especially likely when patients present days, weeks, or months after the initial injury. Resistant organisms are common (Valente et al., 2003). It is estimated that almost one-third of foreign bodies are missed in the initial examination of wounds containing such contaminants. This diagnostic error has been identified as a high medical liability risk for both hospitals and HCPs. A missed foreign body potentially may result in infection, structural damage, loss of function, or chronic pain. A high index of suspicion for the presence of a foreign body is required for many wounds based on mechanism of injury. Radiographic images (standard x-rays) are reliable for some materials; however, they are of lesser or no value when the foreign body is wood or glass. Other imaging techniques may be more valuable with certain types of foreign bodies.

Consultation with radiology may be necessary for selection of the most appropriate study. CT examination is recommended for all suspected foreign-body injuries of the scalp. Approximately 10% of wounds with foreign bodies require consultation with surgical services (Levine et al., 2008; Singer et al., 2006).

Regardless of the foreign body risk, all wounds should be thoroughly cleansed. Chapter 51 provides anesthetic, wound irrigation, and closure recommendations for wound management. Without vigorous detail to cleansing, no dressing, medication, or surgical treatment will be effective. Cleansing with antibacterial agents, hydrogen peroxide, or iodine is contraindicated, as these processes are both ineffective and may do potential damage to healthy tissue (Small, 2000). No single dressing can be recommended for lacerations, punctures, and other types of traumatic wounds.

Cleansing is also a vital step in the therapeutic management of pressure ulcers. It is recommended that normal saline solution be used for cleansing and debridement in the pediatric patient. Sterile water is the preferred solution for cleansing and debridement in the neonate. A 20 mL syringe with a polytetrafluoroethylene catheter is suggested for flushing the wound and surrounding tissue. This method of cleansing and debridement enhances the removal of bacteria and decreases infection rates. Solutions should be warmed to body temperature when used in neonates (Baharestani & Ratliff, 2007). Cleansers and antiseptics should never be used on open wounds or pressure ulcers, as the harm to viable tissue outweighs the benefit from this therapy (Baharestani & Ratliff; Maklebust & Sieggreen, 2001).

Wound debridement is usually necessary. This step includes mechanical elimination of the eschar if it is overlying the calcaneal region without obvious indication of infection. Irrigation is the preferred method of debridement. Topical enzymes are not routinely used in young children (Baharestani & Ratliff, 2007).

Pressure ulcers are often colonized with numerous organisms; true infection is not common. Consequently, wound cultures are indicated only when infection is suspected and susceptibility testing is desired. The following ointments have been suggested for use in the pediatric patient: mupirocin (nasal treatment), polymyxin B, and Bacitracin. Silver sulfadiazine is contraindicated in neonates and should be used with caution in older children due to its potential toxicity. Evaluation by a wound specialist is recommended for wounds requiring antimicrobial therapy (Baharestani & Ratliff, 2007).

Caution should be used when determining which dressing to use for pressure ulcers in the pediatric patient, as evidence-based guidelines are lacking in this area. The Association of Women's Health, Obstetric, and Neonatal Nurses (AWHONN) has recommended that only three dressing types be used in neonates: hydrogels, hydrocolloids, and film dressings. Dressing choices for pediatric patients are based on the following principles:

- Cleansing
- Debridement
- Eradication or infection
- Absorption of excess exudates
- Obliteration of dead space
- Maintenance of a moist environment
- Protection from trauma and bacterial invasion
- Insulation
- Protection against percutaneous toxicity
- Pain management (Baharestani & Ratcliff, 2007, p. 218)

Refer to Table 23-2 for details regarding dressing options for the pediatric patient.

Exudate management, a variably moist wound environment, and excess bacterial burden are significant barriers to wound healing in both pediatric and adult populations.

Negative-pressure wound therapy (NPWT)—a technique initially used predominantly for adult venous stasis ulcers—is now considered a viable modality to facilitate healing and closure in the pediatric population. Using controlled suction, NPWT gently evacuates wound drainage, providing an evenly moist environment for optimal wound granulation. This approach is frequently used as an adjunct therapy to prepare a wound for surgical closure with either skin graft or tissue flap.

Vacuum Assisted Closure (VAC) is a trade name for NPWT, introduced in 1995, by KCI (Kinetic Concepts Inc., San Antonio, Texas). With the exception of a supplemental interface layer used in some wounds, dressings, supplies, and the suction unit are provided by KCI with the initiation of therapy. A polyurethane foam sponge is hand-cut to fit the exact dimensions of the wound, including any undermined or tunneled areas. Two types of foam that encourage granulation at different rates are available, depending on the needs of the individual wound. A clear occlusive dressing is placed over

TABLE 23-2

Dressing Guidelines for the Pediatric Patient				
Dressing Type	**Trade Name**	**Description**	**Indications for Use**	**Practice Notes**
Hydrocolloids	Comfeel, Cutinova, Hydro, Curaderm, Duoderm, Intrasite, Restore, Replicare, Tegasorb, Hydrocol, Ultec	Hydrophilic colloid bound to foam; impermeable to bacteria; minimal to moderate absorption	Stage I–IV pressure ulcers; preventive dressing for high-risk areas; secondary dressing under taping	Facilitates autolytic debridement; not to be used in wounds with significant drainage; difficult removal; use caution with delicate skin
Sheet and amorphous hydrogels	Biolex, Curafil, Curasol, Carrsyn Gel, Hypergel, Lamin IntraSite, Restore, Hydrogel, Tegagel, Vigalon	Water based and nonadherent; maintain a moist environment	Stage II–IV pressure ulcers; dermabrasion; painful wounds; donor sites; necrotic wounds	Nonadherent; no risk for skin irritation with removal; may require secondary dressing for reinforcement
Transparent films	Bioclusive, Flexifilm, Opsite, Tegaderm-Poly-skin	Polyurethane with porous adhesive layer; allows escape of moisture and exchange of oxygen	Donor sites; partial-thickness wounds; Stage I–II pressure ulcers; secondary dressing; burns	Allows for easy wound inspection; impermeable to external fluids; nonabsorbtive; may adhere to wounds
Polyurethane foams	Alleyvn, CarraSmart, Curafoam, Cutinova Foam, Flexzan, Hydrosorb, Lyofoam, Polyderm, Border, Teille	Hydrophilic polyurethane coated foam; nonadherent; absorptive	Stage II–IV pressure ulcers; surgical wounds; infected and non-infected wounds; tunneled and cavity wounds	Nonadherent; trauma-free removal; absorptive; not recommended for nondraining wounds
Gauze	Manufactured by many companies	Woven; nonwoven; impregnated	Draining wounds; debridement, packing, tunnel management; pressure ulcers	Readily available in many sizes; most effective as a packing agent; not recommended for moist wound treatment

Source: Adapted from Baharestani & Ratliff, 2007; Maklebust & Sieggreen, 2000.

the foam, and a specially designed suction catheter disk is placed over the sponge and secured with additional occlusive dressing for an airtight seal. The computerized pump unit, which contains a drainage receptacle, is connected to the suction tubing and provides either continuous or intermittent suction.

The benefits of NPWT occur on many levels. The even distribution of negative pressure applied to the wound provides physical stretch that draws the wound edges together as the foam contracts. On the cellular level, the stretch reduces edema, promotes perfusion, and facilitates cell migration and proliferation. NPWT evacuates excess wound fluid, thereby preventing maceration and decreasing the bacterial count. In addition, quantity and quality of wound drainage are more easily monitored with this technique, which can be critical in managing fluid loss and replacement in the neonatal population (Baharestani & Ratliff, 2007). The sponge and occlusive dressing help decrease evaporative fluid loss in less exudative wounds, providing a more evenly moist wound bed and protected wound edges. In wounds with close proximity to stool or stoma drainage, the occlusive dressing can provide extra protection from contamination. Dressing changes are typically performed every 48 hours, which increases patient comfort and decreases caregiver time.

Contraindications to NPWT include presence of necrotic wound tissue; untreated osteomyelitis; malignancy involving the wound site; coagulopathy; nonenteric and unexplored fistulas; exposed blood vessels, organs, or nerves; and anastomotic sites (Rogers, 2007).

The standard pressure setting for adult NPWT therapy is 125 mmHg, but lower pressures are often used for pediatric patients. The settings are modified based on a combination of patient age, pain response, nutritional status, coagulation status, underlying structure, and type and quality of tissue of the wound bed. Suction pressures of 50–75 mmHg are common in infants, 75–100 mmHg in children, and 125 mmHg in adolescents.

NPWT offers a safe, cost-effective alternative to traditional complex wound care in children. Its total costs have been found to be comparable to those of modern wound dressing, but its many nonfinancial advantages make NPWT the more desirable treatment in many pediatric wounds.

Painful dressing changes and anxiety of both the child and the parent factor into overall healing. Consequently, management of pain and anxiety for the pediatric patient undergoing wound therapy is essential.

Eliminating the source of pressure, however, is the cornerstone of any pressure ulcer treatment plan. Simple strategies such as rotating the site of any contacting equipment (such as an oxygen saturation probe) and turning patients routinely reduce the incidence of pressure ulcer. Adequate nutrition will optimize skin integrity and promote healing. Many supportive surfaces have proven effective in adult trials for reducing the frequency of pressure ulcers; however, caution should be used in extrapolating these recommendations to children due to developmental differences. AWHONN recommends the use of water, air, and gel mattresses and gel pads placed at points of pressure (behind the ears, behind the occiput, at the joints), although some clinical success has been achieved using visoelastic foam (VEF) or gel mattresses with neonates (Baharestani & Ratcliff, 2007).

Consultation with wound care specialists and/or plastic surgery may be indicated for poorly healing wounds or ulcerations that place the patient at risk for bacteremia. Patients who are immunocompromised may require extensive evaluation and surgical wound care. The use of NPWT may be implemented by these specialists.

Wound care patient and family education depends on the type of wound (i.e., abscess, laceration, avulsion, puncture wounds, or pressure ulcer), if antimicrobials have been prescribed, and the type of dressing and need for dressing changes. Written instructions are helpful, especially when patients have complicated wounds that may require weeks or months of therapy. Families should be informed of signs and symptoms of infection and educated about the circumstances in which they should return for follow-up.

DISPOSITION AND DISCHARGE PLANNING

Many wounds are significant enough to warrant home health care. In such circumstances, working with discharge planning staff is warranted. Follow-up with consultative services such as plastic surgery, pediatric surgery, or wound management should be determined before discharge. For wounds presenting to the emergency setting, a follow-up evaluation within 48 hours with the primary care provider is recommended.

REFERENCES

1. Agren, J., Sjors, G., & Sedin, G. (2006). Ambient humidity influences the rate of skin barrier maturation in extremely preterm infants. *Journal of Pediatrics, 148*(5), 613–617.

2. American Academy of Pediatrics. (2009). Summaries of infectious diseases: Herpes simplex virus. In L., Pickering, C., Baker, D., Kimberlin, & S., Long (Eds.). *Red book: 2009 Report of the Committee on Infectious Diseases* (28th ed., pp. 363–73). Elk Grove Village, IL: Author.

3. Auquier-Dunant, A., Mockenhaupt, M., Naldi, L., Correia, O., Schroder, W., & Roujeau, J. (2002). Correlations between clinical patterns and causes of erythema multiforme majus, Stevens-Johnson syndrome, and toxic epidermal necrolysis. *Archives of Dermatology, 138*(8), 1019–1024.

4. Baharestani, M., & Ratliff, C. (2007). Pressure ulcers in neonates and children: An NPUAP white paper. *Advances in Skin and Wound Care, 20*(4), 208–220.

5. Bastuji-Garin, S., Rzany, B., Stern, R., Naldi, L., & Roujeau, J. (1993). Clinical classification of cases of toxic epidermal necrolysis, Stevens-Johnson syndrome, and erythema multiforme. *Archives of Dermatology, 129*(1), 92–96.

6. Behrman, R., Kliegman, R., & Jenson, H. (Eds.). (2004). *Nelson's textbook of pediatrics* (17th ed.). Philadelphia: Saunders.

7. Berkowitz, C. (2008). *Pediatrics: A primary care approach* (3rd ed.). Elk Grove Village, IL: American Academy of Pediatrics.

8. Chung, W., Hung, S., Yang, J., Su, S., Huang, S., Wei, C., et al. (2008). Granulysin is a key mediator for disseminated keratinocyte death in Stevens-Johnson syndrome and toxic epidermal necrolysis. *Nature Medicine, 14*(12), 1343–1350.

9. Conley, M. (2009). Pressure ulcer evaluation: Best practice for clinicians. *Long Term Living Magazine, 58*(10), 12.

10. Curley, M., Quigley, S., & Lin, M. (2003a). Pressure ulcers in pediatric intensive care: Incidence and associated factors. *Pediatric Critical Care Medicine, 4*(3), 284–290.

11. Curley, M., Razmus, I., Roberts, K., & Wypij, D. (2003b). Predicting pressure ulcer risk in pediatric patients: The Braden Q Scale. *Nursing Research, 52*(1), 22–31.

12. Darmstadt, G., & Sidbury, R. (2004). Evaluation of the patient. In R., Behrman, R., Kliegman, & H., Jenson (Eds.). *Nelson's textbook of pediatrics* (17th ed., pp. 2154–2155). Philadelphia: Saunders.

13. Fleisher, G., Ludwig, S., & Henretig, F. (2006). *Textbook of pediatric emergency medicine* (5th ed.). Philadelphia: Lippincott Williams & Wilkins.

14. Fluhr, J., Pfisterer, S., & Gloor, M. (2000). Direct comparison of skin physiology in children and adults with bioengineering methods. *Pediatric Dermatology, 17*(6), 436–439.

15. French, L. (2006). Toxic epidermal necrolysis and Stevens Johnson syndrome: Our current understanding. *Allergology International, 55*, 9–16.

16. Ginsburg, C. (2004). Animal and human bites. In R., Behrman, R., Kliegman, & H., Jenson (Eds.). *Nelson's textbook of pediatrics* (17th ed., pp. 2385–2387). Philadelphia: Saunders.

17. Gueudry, J., Roujeau, J., Binaghi, M., Soudrane, G., & Muraine, M. (2009). Risk factors for the development of ocular complications of Stevens-Johnson syndrome and toxic epidermal necrolysis. *Archives of Dermatology, 145*(2), 157–162.

18. Heer, N., & Huether, S. (2010a). Alterations of the integument in children. In K., McCance, S., Huether, V., Brashers, & N., Rote (Eds.). *Pathophysiology: The biological basis for disease in children and adults* (pp. 1680–1696). Maryland Heights, MO: Mosby.

19. Heer, N., & Huether, S. (2010b). Structure, function, and disorders of the integument. In K., McCance, S., Huether, V., Brashers, & N., Rote (Eds.). *Pathophysiology: The biological basis for disease in children and adults* (pp. 1644–1679). Maryland, MO: Mosby.

20. Holve, S. (2004). Envenomations. In R., Behrman, R., Kliegman, & H., Jenson (Eds.). *Nelson's textbook of pediatrics* (17th ed., pp. 2387–2392). Philadelphia: Saunders.

21. Hurwitz, S. (1990). Erythema multiforme: A review of its characteristics, diagnostic criteria, and management. *Pediatrics in Review, 11*(7), 217–222.

22. Hurwitz, S. (1993). *Clinical pediatric dermatology: A textbook of skin disorders of childhood and adolescence.* Philadelphia: Saunders.

23. Jarjosa, J. (2009). Trauma, burns and common critical care emergencies. In J., Custer & R., Rau (Eds.). *Johns Hopkins: The Harriet Lane handbook* (18th ed., pp. 109–114). Philadelphia: Mosby.

24. King, C., & Henretig, F. (2008). *Textbook of pediatric emergency procedures* (2nd ed.). Philadelphia: Lippincott Williams & Wilkins.

25. Koehler, M., & Nakayama, D. (2009). Treatment of cutaneous abscesses without postoperative dressing changes. *AORN Journal, 90*(4), 569–574.

26. Korner, A., Dinten-Schmid, B., Stoffel, L., Hirter, K., & Kappeli, S. (2009). Skin care and skin protection in preterm babies. *PFLEGE, 22*(4), 266–276.

27. Letko, E., Papaliodis, D., Papaliodis, G., Daoud, Y., Ahmed, A., & Foster, S. (2005). Stevens-Johnson syndrome and toxic epidermal necrolysis: A review of the literature. *Annals of Allergy, Asthma, and Immunology, 94*(4), 419–436.

28. Leung, D. (2007). Allergy and the immunologic basis of atopic disease. In R., Behrman, R., Kliegman, & H., Jenson (Eds.). *Nelson's textbook of pediatrics* (17th ed., pp. 958–972). Philadelphia: Saunders.

29. Levi, N., Bastuji-Garin, S., Mockenhaupt, M., Roujeau, J., Flahault, A., Kelly, J., et al. (2009). Medications as risk factors of Stevens-Johnson syndrome and toxic epidermal necrolysis in children: A pooled analysis. *Pediatrics, 123*(2), e297–e304.

30. Levine, M., Gorman, S., Young, C., & Courtney, M. (2008). Clinical characteristics and management of wound foreign bodies in the ED. *American Journal of Emergency Medicine, 26*, 918–922.

31. Maklebust, J., & Sieggreen, M. (2001). *Pressure ulcers: Guidelines for prevention and management* (3rd ed.). Springhouse, PA: Springhouse.

32. Marx, J., Hockberger, R., & Walls, R. (2009). *Marx: Rosen's emergency medicine* (7th ed.) St. Louis: Mosby.

33. McCance, K., & Grey, T. (2010). Altered cellular and tissue biology. In K. McCance, S. Huether, V. Brashers, & N. Rote (Eds.). *Pathophysiology: The biological basis for disease in adults and children* (6th ed., pp. 46–93). St. Louis: Mosby.

34. Metry, D., Jung, P., & Levy, M. (2003). Use of intravenous immunoglobulin in children with Stevens-Johnson syndrome and toxic epidermal necrolysis: Seven cases and review of the literature. *Pediatrics, 112*(6), 1430–1436.

35. Modi, N. (2004). Management of fluid balance in the very immature neonate. *Archives of Diseases in Childhood Fetal Neonatal Edition, 89*, 108–111.

36. Morelli, J. (2007). Vesiculobullous disorders. In R., Kliegman, R., Behrman, H., Jenson, & B., Stanton (Eds.). *Nelson textbook of pediatrics* (18th ed., pp. 2685–2688). Philadelphia: Saunders.

37. Murata, J., Riichiro, A., & Shimizu, H. (2008). Increase soluble Fas ligand levels in patients with Stevens-Johnson syndrome and toxic epidermal necrolysis preceding skin detachment. *Journal of Allergy and Clinical Immunology, 122*(5), 992–1000.

38. National Pressure Ulcer Advisory Panel (NPUAP). (2010). Retrieved from https://www.npuap.org

39. Pallija, G., Mondozzi, M., & Webb, A. (1999). Skin care of the pediatric patient. *Journal of Pediatric Nursing, 14*(2), 80–87.

40. Ringheanu, M., & Laude, T. (2000). Toxic epidermal necrolysis in children: An update. *Clinical Pediatrics, 39*(12), 687–694.

41. Rogers, V. (2007). Wound management in neonates, children, and adolescents. In N. Browne, L. Flanigan, C. McComiskey, & P. Piper (Eds.). *Nursing care of the pediatric surgical patient.* (pp. 477–494). Sudbury, MA: Jones and Bartlett.

42. Rote, N., & Huether, S. (2010). Innate immunity: Inflammation. In K., McCance, S., Huether, V., Brashers, & N., Rote (Eds.). *Pathophysiology: The biological basis for disease in adults and children* (6th ed., pp. 183–215). St. Louis: Mosby.

43. Schalock, P., Dinulos, J., Pace, N., Schwarzenberger, K., & Wenger, J. (2006). Erythema multiforme due to *Mycoplasma pneumoniae* infection in two children. *Pediatric Dermatology, 23*(6), 546–555.

44. Seidel, H., Ball, J., Dains, J., & Benedict, G. W. (2003). *Mosby's guide to physical examination* (5th ed.). St. Louis: Mosby.

45. Shannon, M., Borron, S., & Burns, M. (2007). *Shannon: Haddad and Winchester's clinical management of poisoning and drug overdose* (4th ed.). Philadelphia: Saunders Elsevier.

46. Singer, A., Thode, H., & Hollander, J. (2006). National trends in ED lacerations between 1992 and 2002. *American Journal of Emergency Medicine, 24*, 183–188.

47. Small, V. (2000). Management of cuts, abrasions, and lacerations. *Nursing Standard, 15*(5), 41–44.

48. Taketomo, C., Hodding, J., & Kraus, D. (2010). *Pediatric dosage handbook* (16th ed.). Hudson, OH: Lexi-Comp.

49. Townsend, C., Beauchamp, R., Evers, B., & Mattox, K. (2008). *Sabiston textbook of surgery* (18th ed.). Philadelphia: Saunders Elsevier.

50. Valente, J., Forti, R., Freundlich, L., Zandieh, S., & Crain, E. (2003). Wound irrigation in children: Saline solution or tap water? *Annals of Emergency Medicine, 41*(5), 609–616.

51. Viard, I., Wehrli, P., Bullani, R., Schneider, P., Holler, N., Salomon, D., et al. (1998). Inhibition of toxic epidermal necrolysis by blockade of CD95 with human intravenous immunoglobulin. *Science 282*, 490–492. Retrieved from www.sciencemag.org

Endocrine Disorders

PHYSIOLOGY AND DIAGNOSTICS

Marianne Buzby

PHYSIOLOGY

The endocrine system regulates growth; pubertal development and reproduction; homeostasis of the organism; and production, storage, and utilization of energy. This is primarily accomplished through the secretion of hormones—chemical signals secreted into the bloodstream that act on tissues throughout the body. Hormonal action occurs primarily from chemical signals secreted by glands into the circulatory system, which are directed toward target cells in organs or tissues at a distance. Paracrine action occurs when chemical signals act on the cells adjacent to the hormone-secreting cells. Autocrine action occurs when the hormone acts on the same cells that secrete it.

The major glands in the endocrine system are the pituitary, thyroid, parathyroids, adrenals, and pineal. The hypothalamus, pancreas, and gonads (ovaries, testes) are organs that contain specialized tissue that secretes hormones; they are also part of the endocrine system. Protein hormones—such as growth hormone, parathyroid hormone, prolactin, insulin, and glucagon—are produced in specialized secretory cells. Steroid hormones, which are derivatives of cholesterol, include glucocorticoids, androgens, and estrogens.

Hormones are synthesized in response to biochemical signals generated from other organ systems. Some, such as insulin, are fully active when they enter the circulatory system; others, such as thyroxine, require activation prior to exerting their intended effect.

Hormone synthesis is generally regulated by a negative feedback loop. One endocrine gland releases a hormone (trophic hormone), which acts on another endocrine gland (target gland) to release a peripheral hormone. The peripheral hormone then provides feedback to the gland secreting the trophic hormone as well as acting on other body tissue. When the first endocrine gland senses a low level of the target gland hormone, it increases production of the trophic hormone. This feedback system allows hormone synthesis to occur as required. It is modulated by the central nervous system (CNS; neuroendocrine pathways) and other hormones as well as enzymes involved in the metabolic pathway of the target glandular cells.

The interaction of the pituitary gland with the thyroid, adrenals, and gonads is regulated by the peripheral endocrine organ hormones' (thyroid hormones, androgens, glucocorticoids) feedback on the hypothalamus–pituitary system. Serum cation (calcium) levels influence parathyroid hormone (PTH) secretion. Metabolites, other hormones, serum osmolarity, and extracellular volume also affect the secretion of specific hormones. In addition, nerve cells and the immune system may regulate hormone secretion.

Patterns of hormone release may change with age. Examples of hormonal rhythmicity include the prolactin secretion stimulated by an infant nursing and menses.

Disorders of the endocrine system are primarily categorized as hyposecretion, hypersecretion, altered tissue response to hormones, and tumors of endocrine glands. Hyposecretion—or hormone underproduction—can occur for a variety of reasons, including surgical removal of the gland, infectious destruction of the gland, and autoimmune disorders. Hypersecretion—or hormone overproduction—may occur because of genetic abnormalities that result in abnormal regulation of hormone synthesis or release. More commonly, however, this outcome reflects an increase in the number of hormone-producing cells. Altered tissue response to hormones may occur due to production of abnormal hormones, defects in hormone receptors, abnormalities of hormone transport or metabolism, and hormone abnormalities. Tumors of endocrine glands are more likely to result in hypersecretion of hormones. Other tumors may be pathologic due to their location, and produce very little hormone.

The hypothalamus

The hypothalamus is a collection of specialized cells embedded at the base of the brain stem. It has both neurologic and hormonal functions, making it a neuroendocrine organ. The hypothalamus regulates hormone secretion from the pituitary gland by secretion of specific stimulating and inhibiting hormones. This mechanism is referred to as the hypothalamic–pituitary axis. The hypothalamic hormones, which are also referred to as factors, include growth hormone–releasing hormone (GHRH), somatotropin release–inhibiting factor (SRIF) or somatostatin, prolactin-inhibiting factor (PIF), thyroid-releasing factor (TRF), corticotropin-releasing factor (CRF), and gonadotropin-releasing hormone (GnRH).

The pituitary gland

The pituitary gland responds to hypothalamic hormones by releasing trophic hormones that affect target glands. These target glands produce hormones that feed back to the hypothalamus and the pituitary gland to regulate the trophic hormone production. As a result, the pituitary gland is referred to as the "master gland." It consists of two lobes, anterior and posterior.

Anterior pituitary gland. The anterior pituitary gland (adenohypophysis) secretes growth hormone (GH), prolactin (PRL), thyroid-stimulating hormone (TSH), adrenocorticotropic hormone (ACTH), luteinizing hormone (LH), and follicle-stimulating hormone (FSH).

Human growth hormone (GH) secretion is stimulated by GHRH and inhibited by SRIF from the hypothalamus.

The balance between these hormone levels produces the pulsatile secretion pattern of GH. Growth hormone is secreted from the anterior pituitary, and it targets bones and muscles to promote linear growth, bone density, and soft-tissue growth. In addition, GH stimulates protein, fat, and carbohydrate metabolism. Much of this action is accomplished via insulin-like growth factor 1 (IGF-1), whose levels in the circulation primarily represent secretion by the liver. However, IGF-1 is synthesized by essentially all tissues, including at the physeal growth plates responsible for linear growth, thereby acting on a panacrine system. Various physiologic and pathophysiologic factors influence the secretion pattern of GH. For example, sleep, physical stress, trauma, acute illness, and hypoglycemia enhance the secretion of GH, whereas hyperglycemia, hypothyroidism, and glucocorticoids inhibit the release of GH.

Prolactin is secreted by the anterior pituitary gland. This hormone is unique in that its secretion is tonically inhibited by the hypothalamus, via dopamine (prolactin inhibitory factor). During pregnancy, prolactin stimulates the development of the secretory system in the mammary glands. Lactation does not occur at this point due to high levels of estrogen and progesterone. After delivery, when these hormone levels decrease and in response to suckling, prolactin stimulates the production of human milk.

Thyrotropin-releasing hormone (TRH) is produced by the hypothalamus and stimulates the release of TSH, also a protein, from the anterior pituitary. The thyroid gland is the target for TSH. TSH stimulates the release of thyroxine (T_4) and tri-iodothyronine (T_3) from the thyroid gland. TSH also promotes growth of the thyroid gland and is actively involved in the uptake and clearance of iodine. Collectively, the thyroid hormones influence growth and development, brain development, and protein, fat, and carbohydrate metabolism. These hormones are essential for normal secretion of GH.

Secretion of ACTH from the anterior pituitary gland is regulated primarily by CRF released from the hypothalamus. ACTH targets the adrenal glands to stimulate the synthesis of corticosteroids, which are important in the body's response to stress. The primary hormones produced in the adrenal cortex are cortisol (glucocorticoid), aldosterone (mineralocorticoid), and androgens. This pathway is controlled by the negative feedback loop to maintain homeostasis.

Cortisol stimulates gluconeogensis, maintains blood pressure, and affects mood. As a result of the diurnal secretion pattern of CRF, the levels of ACTH and cortisol vary during the course of the day. Stress, fasting, and hypoglycemia stimulate CRF and ACTH release, increasing cortisol levels. A similar response occurs to other hormones, including arginine vasopressin, oxytocin, angiotensin II, and cholecystokinin.

Aldosterone production is regulated by the renin–angiotensin system. This hormone targets the distal renal tubules and is involved in the regulation of sodium, blood pressure, and renal blood flow. In response to hypotension or hyponatremia, renin acts on angiotensinogen to form angiotensin I, which is subsequently converted to angiotensin II by an enzyme in the lung. Angiotensin II stimulates aldosterone production and secretion, which promotes sodium and chloride reabsorption and potassium loss.

Adrenal androgens—that is, testosterone and its precursors, especially dehydroepiandrosterone (DHEA)—influence growth and pubertal development. Specifically, they govern the development of secondary sex characteristics, including pubic and axillary hair.

The adrenal medulla (the inner portion of the adrenal gland) produces catecholamines in response to stress, such as exercise, hypoglycemia, trauma, and the "flight or fight" response. This production is mediated by preganglionic fibers of the sympathetic nervous system originating at the T5–T11 levels and is enhanced by high cortisol levels. Dopamine is the precursor to epinephrine and norepinephrine. Norepinephrine targets adrenergic receptors, increasing the heart rate, increasing blood pressure, and mobilizing fatty acids from storage. Epinepherine targets the heart, liver, lungs, brain, kidneys, and arteries, increasing blood flow to skeletal muscle and stimulating glycogenesis.

Luteinizing hormone and follicle-stimulating hormone are the gonadotropic hormones released from the anterior pituitary in response to GnRH from the hypothalamus. In the ovary, LH promotes maturation of ovarian follicles, ovulation of the mature ovum, formation of the corpus luteum, and secretion of progesterone. FSH stimulates follicular development in the ovary. In the testes, LH stimulates the Leydig cells to produce testosterone and FSH stimulates gametogenesis.

Posterior pituitary gland. The posterior pituitary gland (neurohypophysis) contains neural tissue that connects it directly to the hypothalamus. Antidiuretic hormone (ADH; also known as arginine vasopressin [AVP]) and oxytocin precursors are produced in the hypothalamus and stored in the posterior pituitary. An increase in plasma osmolarity triggers the release of AVP, which in turn targets the renal tubules, promoting water retention. As osmolarity normalizes, less AVP is secreted. Stretch receptors in the right atrium and the carotid baroreceptors also regulate the release of AVP, stimulating arterial muscle contraction. AVP secretion changes from moment to moment throughout the day in response to signals from the carotid baroreceptors. AVP is also involved in the stimulation of ACTH secretion.

Oxytocin production is also controlled by the posterior pituitary gland. This hormone stimulates uterine smooth muscle contractions during childbirth and is also associated with sexual orgasm. In addition, oxytocin stimulates smooth muscle contractions of the mammary glands in response to suckling resulting in the milk letdown reflex.

The parathyroid gland

Parathyroid hormone is produced by the parathyroid gland and is essential to calcium metabolism. PTH is secreted in response to low serum ionized calcium and high phosphorus concentrations. It targets the gastrointestinal tract, the distal renal tubules, and bone. This hormone mobilizes calcium from the bones, promotes intestinal calcium absorption, and increases calcium reabsorption by the kidneys. PTH also increases magnesium reabsorption by the kidneys; magnesium is a cofactor regulating PTH secretion. 1,25- Dihydroxyvitamin D is another essential component of calcium metabolism: It assists PTH in reabsorption of bone, thereby increasing the body's calcium and phosphorus stores. Calcitonin, which is secreted by the medulla parafollicular "C" cells of the thyroid gland, opposes PTH, acting to lower calcium levels. A complicated feedback loop controls the interaction of these components.

The pancreas

The islets of Langerhans are a small cluster of endocrine tissue located in the pancreas. The alpha cells in the islets produce glucagon, a protein hormone whose secretion is triggered by hypoglycemia. This hormone targets liver cells and promotes glycolysis. If glycolysis does not bring the blood sugar back into a normal range quickly enough, glucagon stimulates gluconeogensis. Glucagon also promotes relaxation of the smooth muscle in the gastrointestinal tract.

As the blood sugar rises, the beta cells in the islets of Langerhans secrete insulin. Insulin binds to receptors on the target cells, thereby facilitating the movement of glucose into the cells. In addition, insulin inhibits fat and protein metabolism and promotes fat synthesis so as to maintain appropriate blood sugar levels. Insulin also stimulates the conversion of glucose to glycogen.

A third set of cells secrete somatostatin (SRIF), which targets the alpha and beta cells in the pancreas; this hormone is also secreted in the hypothalamus and the intestine. Somatostatin inhibits the secretion of glucagon and insulin, as well as the secretion of growth hormone and thyrotropin in the pituitary. In the gastrointestinal tract, it inhibits the secretion of a broad range of gut peptides.

The pineal gland and the thymus

The pineal gland secretes melatonin, a hormone which contributes to control of the sleep–wake cycle. The thymus produces hormones that are important in the development of the immune responses.

DIAGNOSTICS

Assessment of endocrine function must take into consideration the feedback regulation and rhythmicity of hormone production. Diagnostic studies include basal circulating hormone levels, hormone-binding proteins, and hormone levels based on stimulation or suppression testing (Table 24-1). Stimulation tests evaluate hypofunction disorders; suppression tests evaluate hyperfunction disorders. Peripheral hormone receptor function must also be considered when ordering diagnostic studies to evaluate endocrine function. Radiographic studies may be useful as well (Table 24-2).

Growth charts

Height, weight, and head circumference are best plotted on appropriate growth charts. Plotting as close to the accurate age as possible allows for better comparisons with serial measurements. Growth charts have been established based on different methodological categories such as distance (stature plotted against age), velocity (annual increments), cross-sectional (entire age range of a large sample size), and longitudinal (small sample over several years). Standards provided in growth charts and growth velocity can be compared to standard mean rates of weight gain and linear growth. Centers for Disease Control and Prevention (CDC) growth charts are available for patients from birth to 20 years of age (CDC, 2000). Additionally, specialized growth charts are available for patients with conditions such as very low birth weight (less than 1,500 gm; intended for use for 120 days' uncorrected age or until the child reaches 2,000 gm), Down syndrome, Turner syndrome, Cornelia de Lange syndrome, and achondroplasia. According to the CDC (2000), special health care needs growth charts were developed with small samples and, therefore, may have limitations. For this reason, it is recommended that patients be plotted on both specialized growth charts and CDC growth charts for comparison.

Height velocity (linear growth rate). Growth dysfunction calculations may be used to determine growth delay; however, the evaluation must be considered within the context of normal standards. Although there is considerable variation in height velocity in children of different ages, there is some level of predictability between the age of 2 and the onset of puberty. Properly used calculations may inform abnormal growth. Growth velocity is determined by a minimum of two height (H) determinations taken at least 3 months apart in time (T), expressed as centimeters per year. From 2 years of age until puberty, linear growth of approximately 4 to 5 cm per year is considered normal. The following equation applies:

$$\frac{H2 - H1}{T2 - T1}$$

annualized to 12 months = linear growth velocity

Parental height. Height stature of the child and parent may also determine growth dysfunction. The first 2 years of life do not closely relate to parental height, yet by age 2 years

TABLE 24-1

Diagnostic Studies for Endocrinology			
Adrenal Function	**Glucocorticoid Excess**	**Adrenal Insufficiency**	**Congenital Adrenal Hyperplasia**
	24-hour urinary free cortisol	8 A.M. plasma cortisol and ACTH concentration	High-dose ACTH stimulation test
	Midnight salivary or plasma cortisol	Low-dose ACTH stimulation test	17-hydroxyprogesterone
	Overnight low-dose dexamethasone suppression test	High-dose stimulation test	*cyp21* analysis
		Metyrapone test	
		Serum renin level	
		Aldosterone level	
Calcium and Bone Homeostasis	**Calcium Homeostasis**	**Vitamin D Status**	**Markers of Bone Turnover**
	Total calcium	25-OH	Osteocalcin
	Ionized calcium	$1,25\text{-}(OH)_2 D$	Bone-specific alkaline phosphatase
	Parathyroid hormone		N-telopeptides
	PTH-related protein		
	Urine calcium: creatinine ratio		
Glucose Metabolism	**Diabetes Risk/Diagnosis**	**Hypoglycemia**	**Other**
	Type 1 diabetes autoantibodies	Prolonged supervised fast	Hemoglobin A_{1c}
	HLA type	Glucagon stimulation test	Serum glucose
	Oral glucose tolerance test (OGTT)	Hypoglycemic clamp	Metabolic screen for DKA
	Insulin antibodies	C-peptide and fasting serum glucose	
Growth Hormone	**Sufficiency**	**Excess**	
	Growth hormone assays	Insulin-like growth factor 1 (IGF-1)	
	Growth hormone provocative testing	OGTT	
	IGF-1	TRH stimulation test	
	IGF-binding protein 3 (IGFBP-3)		
	IGF generation test		
	IGF-binding protein 2 (IGFBP-2)		
	Growth hormone-binding protein		
	Acid-labile subunit		
	12- or 24-hour growth hormone sampling		
	Growth hormone stimulation tests: arginine; L-dopa/propranolog; glucagon		

(Continued)

TABLE 24-1

Diagnostic Studies for Endocrinology *(Continued)*			
Pubertal Disorders and Sexual Differentiation	**Gonadal Function**	**Gonadotropin Secretion**	
	Testosterone, total and free	Luteinizing hormone (LH, lutropin)	Karyotype
	Estradiol	Follicle-stimulating hormone (FSH)	
	Sex hormone-binding globulin (SHBG)	GnRH stimulation test	
	hCG stimulation test		
	Progesterone withdrawal		
Thyroid Status	**Thyroid Hormone Concentrations and TSH**	**Autoimmune Thyroid Disease**	**Central TSH Secretion**
	Thyroid-stimulating hormone (TSH)	Thyroid-stimulating immunoglobulin (TSI)	TSH diurnal testing
	Total triiodothyronine (T_3)	Thyroid receptor antibody (TRAb)	TRH stimulation test
	Free thyroxine (T_4)	Antithyroglobulin (ATG)	
		Thyroid peroxidase antibodies (TPO)	
Water Homeostasis			
	Serum and urine osmolality		
	Urine specific gravity		
	Water-deprivation test		
	Vasopressin challenge		
	Serum vasopressin levels		

Adrenocorticotropic hormone (ACTH), diabetic ketoacidosis (DKA), human leukocyte antigen (HLA), thyrotropin-releasing hormone (TRH).

Source: Adapted from Miller & McAtee, 2009.

TABLE 24-2

Radiographic Studies for Endocrinology	
Bone Age	**Short Stature**
Ultrasound	Thyroid nodules; adrenal insufficiency; ambiguous genitalia; Turner syndrome; primary amenorrhea; ovarian neoplasm; testicular tumors; cryptorchidism
Magnetic resonance imaging	Hypopituitarism; pituitary tumors; large thyroid mass; ambiguous genitalia; cryptorchidism
CT scan	Hypopituitarism; pituitary tumors; large thyroid mass; parathyroid adenoma; adrenal tumors; pancreatic tumors; ovarian neoplasm
Scintigraphy	Congenital or acquired hypothyroidism; hyperthyroidism; thyroid nodule; parathyroid adenoma; hyperparathyroidism; adrenal tumors
Plain film	Osteoporosis; osteomalacia
DEXA scan	Osteoporosis; osteomalacia

Computed tomography (CT), dual energy x-ray absorptiometry (DEXA).

Source: Adapted from Sane & Sane, 2009.

correlation between their heights are relatively predictable based on calculation. Different measurements apply based on gender as follows:

Midparental height calculation: target height

For males: [paternal height + maternal height]/2 + 5 cm
For females: [paternal height + maternal height]/2 − 5 cm

Skeletal maturation. Growth potential may be measured by the ossification of the epiphyses; therefore, radiographs of the left hand and wrist may be sought to determine chronological age. Bone age interpretation is best performed by a pediatric radiologist, and findings may indicate remaining bone growth. Height and growth predictions become less accurate if marked deviations are found between chronological and bone age.

Sexual maturity rating: tanner staging

Sexual maturity rating (SMR) describes the sequence of pubertal milestone attainment. The stages of development for males and females are predictable, as one stage follows another. However various racial–ethnic groups develop their sexual maturation differently than others based on body mass index, minimal increases in circulating hormones (estrogen) independent of gonadotropin stimulation, or hormone-like stimulation. Table 24-3, Table 24-4, Figure 24-1, and Figure 24-2 illustrate general SMR criteria.

ADRENAL DISORDERS

Valarie Eichler

PATHOPHYSIOLOGY

The adrenal gland consists of two main sections: the outer cortex and the inner medulla. The cortex is further subdivided into three zones: glomerulosa, fasciculate, and reticularis. Within these zones, three important classes of hormones are produced. The glomerulosa secretes aldosterone, a mineralocorticoid that is responsible for regulation of sodium and water balance; the fasciculata secretes cortisol, a glucocorticoid that regulates the level of carbohydrate; and the reticularis secretes progesterone, oestrogen, and androgens, which are sex hormones that interact in the development of sexual characteristics. Glucocorticoids are responsible for regulating the body's response to stress primarily by increasing gluconeogenesis, increasing cardiac output, and suppressing immune function (Donohoue, 2006a, 2006b; Hassoun & Oberfield, 2008). Mineralocorticoids control intravascular volume and maintain hemodynamic stability by regulating sodium and water balance. The chromaffin cells located within the inner medulla secrete small, nonsteroid hormones called catecholamines. These catecholamines—epinephrine and norepinephrine—are accountable for the "fight or flight" response that occurs when the body perceives a threat.

The secretion of cortisol and aldosterone are controlled by two very different mechanisms. When the body senses that the level of cortisol is low or stressed, a message is sent to the hypothalamus to release corticotrophin-releasing hormone (CRH). CRH then travels to the anterior pituitary to release adrenocorticotrophic hormone (ACTH). ACTH, in turn, travels to the adrenal cortex via the bloodstream, releasing cortisol. This mechanism is known as activation of the hypothalamus–pituitary–adrenal (HPA) axis (Figure 24-3). When cortisol is no longer needed, it travels to the hypothalamus and anterior pituitary, inhibiting further release.

The secretion of aldosterone is controlled primarily by the renin–angiotensin system and circulating serum potassium levels. In response to low circulating volume, renin is released from the kidney. This hormone is then converted into angiotensinogen in the liver, forming angiotensin I. Angiotensin-converting enzyme (ACE) in the lungs converts angiotensin I into angiotensin II. Angiotensin II travels via the bloodstream to the adrenal cortex, which releases aldosterone; the increased aldosterone level causes the kidney to reabsorb sodium and water, thereby increasing circulating blood volume.

EPIDEMIOLOGY AND ETIOLOGY

The anatomy of the adrenal gland was first described by Bartholomeo Eustachius in 1563. In 1805, Cuvier defined the medulla and cortex of the adrenal gland. In 1849 Thomas Addison described the central physiological role of the adrenal gland, and in 1856 Charles Brown-Séquard demonstrated the vital role of the adrenal glands by performing adrenalectomies on animals. He described the adrenals as "organs essential for life" (Brown-Séquard, 1856).

Adrenal insufficiency (AI) has received increased attention in the past decade in the pediatric population. AI secondary to congenital adrenal hyperplasia (CAH) occurs in approximately 1 in 16,000 infants. A Canadian study of seven tertiary care pediatric intensive care units reported the prevalence of AI to be more than 30% (Menon et al., 2010). In another study, researchers found a 56% incidence of neonatal AI based on random cortisol levels of less than 15 mcg/dL (Fernandez et al., 2008); however, the incidence of AI is likely underestimated by this study, as the definition for normal adrenal response in critical illness is not clearly defined.

Adrenal dysfunction can be categorized into one of four groups: (1) primary adrenal insufficiency, (2) secondary adrenal insufficiency, (3) tertiary adrenal insufficiency, or (4) relative adrenal insufficiency. The clinical presentation varies depending on which hormone is affected.

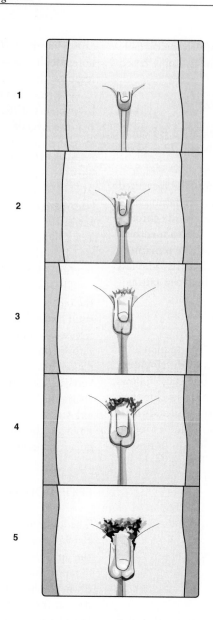

FIGURE 24-1

Sexual Maturity Rating (Tanner Staging): Male.

Source: Courtesy of M. Komoniczak.

TABLE 24-3

Sexual Maturity Rating (Tanner Staging): Male				
Stage	**Age/Development**	**Pubic Hair**	**Penis**	**Testes**
1	Early adolescence	None	Preadolescent	Prepubescent
2	(10.5–14 years)	Scanty	Slight increase in size	Enlarging
3	Middle adolescence	Darker with curls	Longer	Larger
4	(12.5–15 years)	Coarse and curly	Larger	Scrotum darkens
5	Late adolescence (14–16 years)	Adult	Adult	Adult

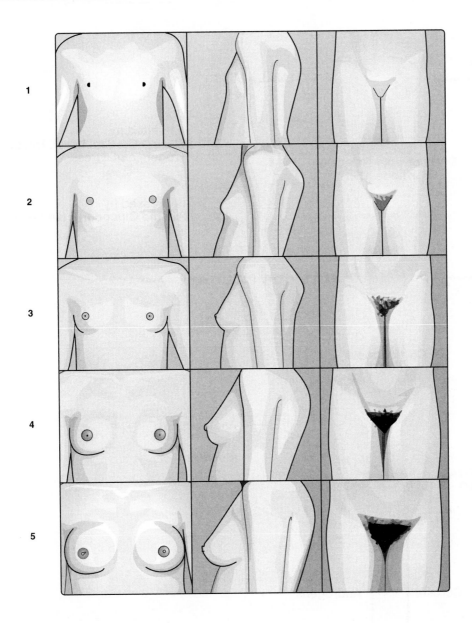

FIGURE 24-2

Sexual Maturity Rating (Tanner Staging): Female.

Source: Courtesy of M. Komoniczak.

TABLE 24-4

Sexual Maturity Rating (Tanner Staging): Female			
Stage	**Age/Development**	**Pubic Hair**	**Breasts**
I	Early adolescence	Preadolescent	Prepubescent
2	(10–13 years)	Sparse, straight	Small mound
3	Middle adolescence (12–14 years)	Dark curls	Larger with no overt contour separation
4		Coarse and curly	Secondary mound of areola
5	Late adolescence (14–17 years)	Adult Triangle-shape appearance	Adult Nipple projects, areola becomes a part of the breast

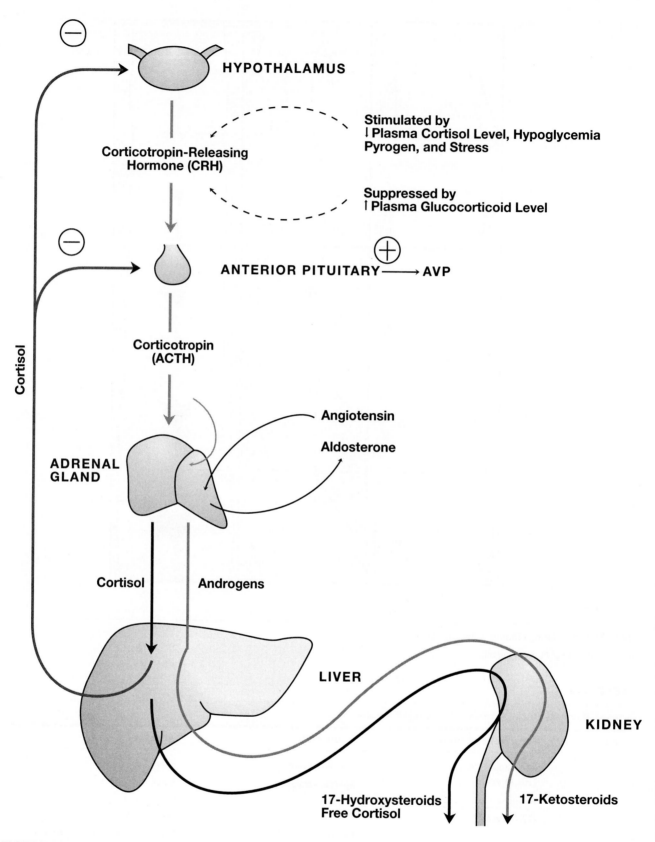

FIGURE 24-3

Adrenal Function.

Source: Courtesy of Kenneth L. Campbell, PhD, University of Massachusetts, Boston.

Primary adrenal insufficiency

Primary AI can be the result of a destroyed or inactive adrenal gland or hormone production failure. Destruction or deactivation can be related to an autoimmune process such as Addison's disease, adrenal hemorrhage as seen in Waterhouse-Friderichsen syndrome (Figure 24-4), severe sepsis, metastatic infiltration, surgical removal, or granulomatous lesions such as tuberculosis.

Although the precise mechanisms leading to adrenal hemorrhage are unclear in nontraumatic cases, available evidence implicates ACTH, adrenal vein spasm and thrombosis, and the normally limited venous drainage of the adrenal in the pathogenesis of this condition. The adrenal gland has a rich arterial supply, in contrast to its limited venous drainage, which is critically dependent on a single vein. Furthermore, in stressful situations, ACTH secretion increases, which stimulates adrenal arterial blood flow that may exceed the limited venous drainage capacity of the organ and lead to hemorrhage. In addition, adrenal vein spasm induced by high catecholamine levels secreted in stressful situations, and by adrenal vein thrombosis induced by coagulopathies, may lead to venous stasis and hemorrhage. Adrenal vein thrombosis has been found in several patients with adrenal hemorrhage, and it may occur in association with sepsis, heparin-induced thrombocytopenia, primary antiphospholipid antibody syndrome, or disseminated intravascular coagulation (DIC).

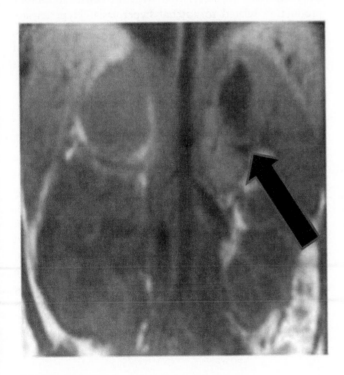

FIGURE 24-4

Left Adrenal Hemorrhage.

Source: Courtesy of Valarie Eichler.

Regardless of the precise mechanisms involved, extensive, bilateral adrenal hemorrhage commonly leads to acute adrenal insufficiency and adrenal crisis, unless it is recognized and treated promptly. The most common infection associated with AI is meningococcemia.

Primary AI as the result of hormone production failure is associated with CAH. Less often, it may be attributed to congenital adrenal hyperplasia known to be linked to Duchenne's muscular dystrophy. In infancy, CAH is the most common cause of primary AI (Hassoun & Oberfield, 2008).

Secondary adrenal insufficiency

Secondary AI is associated with a deficiency of ACTH. Hypopituitarism secondary to primary pituitary disease, congenital pituitary lesions, and developmental anomalies such as anencephaly, holoprosencephaly, and craniopharyngiomas are all causes of ACTH deficiency. Craniopharyngiomas are the most common etiology of ACTH deficiency in childhood (Hassoun & Oberfield, 2008).

Tertiary adrenal insufficiency

Tertiary AI can be defined as a hypothalamic decrease in corticotrophin-releasing hormone (CRH) secretion or production. This decrease is seen most often with the suppression of the HPA axis from prolonged use of glucocorticoids. Other drugs that have been implicated in its etiology include spironolactone, etomidate, and ketoconazole (den Brinker et al., 2005; Hassoun & Oberfield, 2008; Vinclair et al., 2008). Tertiary AI is usually the result of either a rapid steroid taper or an abrupt steroid withdrawal.

Patients at risk for tertiary AI are those using glucocorticoids for management of diseases such as asthma, immunosuppression in organ transplant, leukemia, neurosurgical conditions (preoperatively and postoperatively), nephrotic syndrome and other kidney diseases, and collagen vascular diseases such as lupus and rheumatoid arthritis. The HPA axis may not return to normal until more than one month after therapy is stopped (Felner et al., 2000). In the event such patients undergo additional stressors such as a surgical procedure or severe infections, they are assumed to be adrenal deficient for one year after cessation of therapy unless a normal ACTH stimulation test documented. Conversely, even in the face of a normal response, stress-dose glucocorticoids should be considered if a patient becomes hemodynamically unstable while undergoing a surgical procedure (Petersen et al., 2003).

Relative adrenal insufficiency

Relative AI is experienced to some degree by every critically ill patient; thus it is difficult to diagnose this condition secondary to the many changes normally occurring as a response of the HPA axis during illness (Arafah, 2006). The term "relative" is used when high absolute cortisol levels are present, but they are "relatively" insufficient to overcome the degree of physiologic stress on the patient. Critically ill children with sepsis and catecholamine-resistant shock commonly show absolute and relative AI; however, AI is absent in children with fluid-responsive shock (den Brinker et al., 2005; Pizarro et al., 2005).

Neonatal adrenal insufficiency

Children of any age may have an inadequate response related to preexisting HPA disease, exhaustion of adrenocortical reserve, or suppression of cortisol and ACTH production by inflammatory mediators during critical illness. The critically ill neonate, however, has an immature HPA axis that may further limit the infant's ability to increase cortisol production in response to stress (Langer et al., 2006).

Adrenal crisis

Adrenal crisis is defined as a rapid, overwhelming, and potentially fatal adrenocortical insufficiency. It may occur secondary to a state of chronic adrenal hypofunction, acute damage to a previously normal adrenal gland, congenital deficiency, or abrupt withdrawal of chronic steroid administration.

Congenital adrenal hyperplasia

Genetic newborn screening routinely tests for the presence of CAH. This condition usually presents in the first few weeks of life. The most common form is 21-hydroxylase deficiency, which accounts for approximately 95% of all cases. Males typically present in a salt-wasting crisis or shock at 1 to 2 weeks of age. The missing enzyme, 21-HD, reduces the production of cortisol and aldosterone by the adrenal glands, resulting in AI. The pituitary perceives that not enough cortisol is coming through, so more cholesterol is delivered. As there is still reduced production of cortisol and aldosterone, all of the surplus cholesterol is converted into androgen. This excessive androgen production, in turn, leads to ambiguous genitalia, making CAH easier to recognize in female infants (Hassoun & Oberfield, 2008; White et al., 1997).

ADRENAL HYPERFUNCTION

Cushing syndrome is commonly observed in patients who have received large doses of glucocorticoids for AI, kidney, or rheumatologic disease. In the small child, the adrenal gland is usually the origin of Cushing syndrome; in the adolescent population, an ACTH-secreting pituitary tumor is the more likely cause. Clinical appearance includes cushingoid features such as moon face, centripetal obesity, hirsutism, acne, thin extremities, and fragile

capillaries. The treatment for adrenal-related tumors is frequently surgical removal of the adrenal gland, while pituitary-related conditions are treated with transsphenoidal pituitary resection. Long-term remission is determined by postoperative serum or urine cortisol concentrations. Patients who have adrenocortical tumors frequently have metastasis, primarily to the lung and the liver; thus primary tumor removal may not improve their prognosis (Hassoun & Oberfield, 2008).

Virilizing tumors

In childhood, virilizing tumors are the most common tumor of the adrenal gland. Virilization is the most common presentation, including precocious development of pubic and axillary hair, penile enlargement without testicular growth in males, and clitoral enlargement in females. Other symptoms may include acne, muscular growth, and accelerated growth rate. Surgical removal of the tumor is the treatment of choice. In patients in whom excessive cortisol was found on presentation, AI may develop postoperatively and must be treated to prevent adrenal crisis (Hassoun & Oberfield, 2008).

Hyperaldosteronism

Hyperaldosteronism is rare in the pediatric patient but has been described in association with increased aldosterone production related to adrenal hyperplasia. Hypertension may be seen secondary to the increased aldosterone level, causing an increased reabsorption of sodium, chloride, and water in the renal collecting tubules. Hyperaldosteronism is initially treated with low-dose glucocorticoids, followed by administration of a diuretic such as spironolactone.

PRESENTATION

Generally patients with AI present with hypotension, tachycardia, fatigue, abdominal pain, vomiting, salt craving, muscle pain, weakness, anorexia, weight loss, and, in chronic AI (Addison's disease), hyperpigmentation. Specifically, if there is a cortisol deficiency, the child may present with hypotension, hypoglycemia, weakness, anorexia, nausea, and vomiting. This deficit is responsible for the lack of responsiveness to volume and catecholamine infusions during the preshock and shock states. Patients with aldosterone depletion may demonstrate hypotension, hyperkalemia, and hyponatremia (Carcillo & Fields, 2002; White et al., 1997).

DIFFERENTIAL DIAGNOSIS

A list of differential diagnoses is provided in Table 24-5.

TABLE 24-5

Differential Diagnoses for Adrenal Insufficiency

Adrenal hypoplasia

Birth trauma

Hyponatremia

Hypokalemia

Failure-to-thrive

Adrenal hemorrhage

ACTH receptor defect

Hypopituitarism

Chronic fatigue syndrome

Ambiguous genitalia

PLAN OF CARE

Electrolyte disturbances such as hyponatremia, hyperkalemia, hypocalcemia, and hypercalcemia are frequently seen in aldosterone deficiency, while anemia, acidosis, lymphocytosis, and eosinophilia are seen with cortisol deficiency. Hyponatremia is the result of too much sodium excretion by the kidney. Normally cortisol exhibits anti-inflammatory effects by suppressing the immune system and decreasing the number of circulating eosinophilia (EOS); however, with the lack of cortisol in AI, the immune system allows for increased production of EOS (Beishuizen et al., 1999).

Immediate goals of treatment are glucocorticoid replacement, correction of electrolyte and metabolic abnormalities, volume repletion, and correction of the precipitating events when possible. Diagnostic studies include ACTH stimulation testing, cortisol levels, and imaging to evaluate for adrenal or pituitary hemorrhage or tumor (Figure 24-5 and Figure 24-6). The ACTH stimulation test prompts the adrenal cortex to secrete adrenal steroids and a small amount of aldosterone. The testing ACTH doses used are as follows: neonates, 15 mcg/kg; infants younger than 2 years of age, 125 mcg; and children older than 2 years of age, 250 mcg. Cortisol levels are sent at baseline, 30 minutes, and 60 minutes after the administration of the ACTH. If the cortisol response is less than 9 mcg/dL after stimulation, the patient is considered to have adrenal insufficiency and glucocorticoids should be administered. If the cortisol response is more than 9 mcg/dL, then no steroids are required (Carcillo & Fields, 2002).

Hydrocortisone is the glucocorticoid of choice in the treatment of AI. Initial intravenous dosing in the infant and child consists of 1–2 mg/kg, followed by 25–50 mg/day divided every 6–8 hours; adult-sized patients receive 100 mg initially, followed by 150–250 mg/day

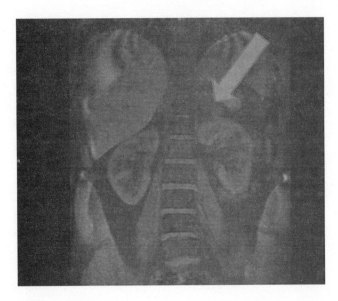

FIGURE 24-5

Left Adrenal Mass.

Source: Courtesy of Valarie Eichler.

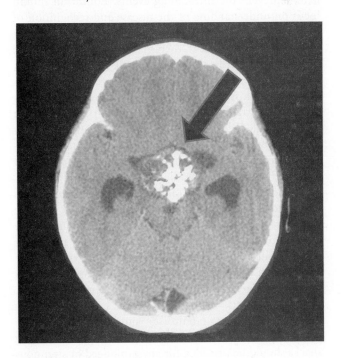

FIGURE 24-6

Craniopharyngioma.

Source: Courtesy of Valarie Eichler.

divided every 6–8 hours. Alternative dosing for shock is 50 mg/kg followed by the same dose as a 24-hour continuous infusion. Wean hydrocortisone by 20% to 30% per day until physiologic doses are reached and then continue further weaning over several weeks. This slow wean will allow the adrenal cortex to recover without redevelopment of AI. Normal daily cortisol production is in the range of 12–15 mg/m^2/day. Stress dosing is approximately 5 times the daily production; physiologic replacement is 10 mg/m^2/day. Once the patient is stable and is tolerating enteral nutrition, and the hydrocortisone dose is less than 100 mg/day, fludrocortisone may be added to the treatment regimen.

Initially, patients with AI are monitored in the intensive care unit. After initial treatment of AI has been started, the endocrinology service should be consulted to assist with long-term patient management. Once they are hemodynamically stable, patients may be transferred from intensive care to the inpatient unit.

Patient and family education is specific to the type of adrenal disorder. It should include the signs and symptoms of insufficiency and identify the circumstances in which stress-dosing of steroids will be needed.

DISPOSITION AND DISCHARGE PLANNING

Discharge teaching for patients and families is crucial, as it may prevent life-threatening events. Education should focus on understanding of the disease and recognition of symptoms. The patient and family should appreciate that if adequate replacement therapy is not provided, there is a potential for death. Prior to being discharged home, patients or their caregivers should receive instruction on how to administer supplemental glucocorticoid in times of illness or traumatic stress, and how to administer an injectable glucocorticoid if the patient is vomiting or unable to take oral stress doses. Patients and their caregivers should be advised to immediately seek medical help if the patient becomes ill, and to ensure medical alert accessories are worn when possible. Written instructions and a letter indicating the patient's disease and rescue therapy may be recommended for families who are uncomfortable with administering injectable medications, as this letter may be utilized by rescue personnel. Additionally, written instructions should be provided to the patient and family if any adjustments in glucocorticoid therapy are required. In some patients, hypoglycemia may be monitored by home blood glucose monitoring and administer glucose gel as needed. For the active patient, sugar-containing snacks should be provided for any prolonged or strenuous exercise.

Follow-up with the endocrinologist initially occurs within 1 to 2 weeks, then takes place periodically, and at least yearly so that medications may be adjusted as the patient grows. Patients who require long-term exogenous glucocorticoid therapy should be weaned to doses that are less than physiologic or given every other day to help avoid the risk of adrenal insufficiency (Shulman et al., 2007).

Patients with untreated AI have a poor prognosis, with death being the most common outcome unless replacement

> ### Critical Thinking
> - Consider AI in patients with shock refractory to volume and/or vasoactive drugs.
> - Patients who undergo additional stressors such as a surgical procedure or severe infections are assumed to be adrenal deficient for one year after cessation of therapy unless a normal ACTH stimulation test is documented. Conversely, in the face of a normal response, stress-dose glucocorticoids should still be considered if a patient becomes hemodynamically unstable while undergoing a surgical procedure.

steroid therapy is initiated. With appropriate therapeutic management and follow-up, most patients live an average life span.

DIABETES INSIPIDUS, SYNDROME OF INAPPROPRIATE ANTIDIURETIC HORMONE, AND CEREBRAL SALT WASTING

Shari Simone

DIABETES INSIPIDUS

Pathophysiology

Diabetes insipidus (DI) is a disorder characterized by excretion of large volumes of dilute urine (polyuria) as a result of antidiuretic hormone (ADH) deficiency. The ADH deficiency is most often caused by insufficient production or failure of the pituitary gland to secrete ADH (central DI), but it may also be caused by resistance of the renal collecting ducts to normal circulating levels of ADH (nephrogenic DI). Central and nephrogenic DI result in lack of water reabsorption despite increased plasma osmolarity and contraction of blood volume.

In healthy pediatric patients, volume and osmolarity of body fluids are normally regulated with extraordinary precision. Serum osmolarity is maintained within a range of 275 to 290 mosm/kg by normal pituitary response and ADH regulation (Lin et al., 2005). ADH is a polypeptide that is synthesized in the supraoptic and paraventricular nuclei of the hypothalamus as a preprohormone precursor, and stored and released from the posterior pituitary after it is packaged into granules and secreted along with carrier proteins called neurophysins (Figure 24-7). When a patient experiences dehydration, osmolar receptors surrounding the supraoptic and paraventricular nuclei sense an increase in serum osmolarity, which stimulates the release of ADH from the posterior pituitary gland. Circulating ADH then binds to V$_2$ receptors, which are functionally coupled to acquaporin channels in the apical membrane of the renal collecting ducts, resulting in an increased permeability and reabsorption of free water

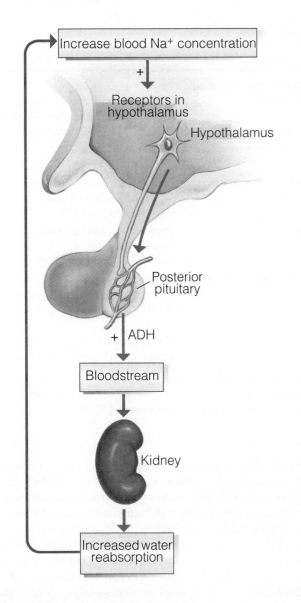

FIGURE 24-7

The Role of ADH in Regulating Fluids.

Source: Chiras, D. (2008). *Human biology* (6th ed.). Sudbury, MA: Jones and Bartlett Publishers.

(Majzoub & Srivatsa, 2006). With normal ADH secretion and renal function, urine osmolarity ranges between 100 and 1200 mosm/kg based on the body's need to excrete or retain free water (Arvanitis & Pasquale, 2005).

Epidemiology and etiology

The cause of central DI may be genetic, congenital, or acquired. The genetic association is typically x-linked recessive. Wolfram syndrome—a rare inherited autosomal recessive condition affecting 1 in 770,000 children—is characterized by central DI, diabetes mellitus, optic atrophy, and deafness (Ganie & Bhat, 2009). Central DI in

this disorder is caused by loss of ADH-secreting neurons in the supraoptic nucleus and impaired processing within the hypothalamus (Majzoub & Srivatsa, 2006).

Congenital causes of DI are often associated with midline craniofacial defects such as holoprosencephaly and septo-optic dysplasia (Bajpai et al., 2008). A recent prospective study examining the developmental outcomes of 73 children with optic nerve hypoplasia found a high prevalence of hypopituitarism, cerebral abnormalities, and developmental delay in these children (Srinivas et al., 2010). Central DI is often acquired secondary to damage to the pituitary or posterior hypothalamus from neurosurgery, trauma, tumors, meningitis, or encephalitis (Maghnie, 2003). Central DI may be either a temporary condition (lasting a few days) or a permanent disorder (Arvanitis & Pasquale, 2005). Central DI affects fewer than 1% of those individuals with traumatic brain injury (Majzoub & Srivatsa, 2006), but it is important to recognize that it may occur abruptly in those patients.

Nephrogenic DI may be either congenital or acquired as a result of renal disease (polycystic disease, pyelonephritis), metabolic conditions (hypokalemia, hypercalcemia), or medication (amphotericin B, lithium). Congenital nephrogenic DI is a rare hereditary disease that is associated with a number of genetic mutations of the vasopressin V_2 receptor in the kidney causing resistance of the renal tubules to vasopressin (Maghnie, 2003). Nephrogenic DI that is medication induced or that results from a metabolic condition may be reversed if the medication is stopped or the metabolic condition corrected.

Presentation

The hallmark findings of DI include polyuria, polydipsia, and inappropriately low urine osmolarity with a urine specific gravity of less than 1.005 and increased serum sodium and osmolarity (Table 24-6). In addition, signs and symptoms of volume depletion may be seen if water loss is greater than fluid intake. Pediatric patients with a known history of DI who present with an acute illness may rapidly develop severe symptoms of dehydration, including hypotension, seizures, and coma.

Polyuria is defined as a urine output of more than 3 L per day in adults and more than 2 L/m² in children or a 24-hour urine volume relatively more than necessary for the patient's circulating blood volume or serum sodium level (Arvanitis & Pasquale, 2005). The degree of polyuria will depend on the degree of ADH suppression, and may vary from mild to severe (more than 15 L per day) (Majzoub & Srivatsa, 2006). Polydipsia is defined as a patient consuming free water intake that is greater than necessary for maintaining a normal serum sodium concentration or arterial blood volume (Arvanitis & Pasquale).

TABLE 24-6

Presentation of Diabetes Insipidus	
Symptoms	**Key Physical Examination Findings**
Lethargy, seizures, coma	Midline craniofacial defects (suggests presence of pituitary or hypothalamus defects, central DI) Developmental delay Growth retardation

Polyuria
 Infants: soaking diapers
 Older children: nocturnal enuresis
	Dilute urine
	 Urine output:
	    > 4 mL/kg/hr
	    150 mL/kg/day
	    4–10 L/day

Polydipsia	Signs of dehydration: tacky mucous membranes, tachycardia, delayed capillary refill, cool extremities, hypotension
Headache, visual changes	Decreased pupillary reaction, visual disturbances such as nystagmus, extraocular movement defects

Diabetes insipidus (DI).

TABLE 24-7

Diagnosis of Diabetes Insipidus	
Clinical signs and symptoms	Polyuria and polydipsia Altered mental status/irritability Signs and symptoms of dehydration Failure-to-thrive Constipation
Serum laboratory studies	Sodium > 150 mEq/L Osmolarity ≥ 295 mOsm/kg
Urinary laboratory studies	Sodium < 30 mEq/L Osmolarity < 200 mOsm/L Specific gravity < 1.005
Head CT/MRI	Presence of intracranial mass, abnormal findings of hypothalamic–pituitary stalk
Water deprivation test	Diagnosis of central DI: concentrated urine and decreased urine output following ADH administration
	Nephrogenic DI: Excessive, dilute urine despite hypernatremia and hyperosmolarity

Computed tomography (CT), magnetic resonance imaging (MRI), diabetes insipidus (DI), antidiuretic hormone (ADH).

Differential diagnosis

The primary causes of polyuria and polydipsia are diabetes mellitus and central (versus nephrogenic) DI. Other potential causes include urinary tract infection, relief of renal obstruction, and psychogenic polydipsia (characterized by excessive water intake).

Once hyperglycemia has been excluded as the origin of the symptoms, the health care professional (HCP) should begin attempting to distinguish the likelihood of central versus nephrogenic DI (Table 24-7). The patient's history is often suggestive of either one or the other type of DI; therefore, inquiry should focus on determining the age of initiation and the rate of onset of polyuria, which may reflect the probability of a primary versus a secondary cause. The majority of infants with congenital nephrogenic DI present with severe polyuria in the first week of life, whereas children with familial central DI most often present after the first year of life. Identifying a family history of polyuria is also helpful, as familial forms of both central and nephrogenic DI are known to exist.

Plan of care

Management goals are to restore hemodynamics, replace water deficits, correct electrolyte abnormalities, and decrease urinary output to within a normal range. The HCP must

quickly identify presenting signs and symptoms of moderate to severe dehydration and immediately begin initial stabilization measures focusing on airway management, intravenous (IV) access, and fluid resuscitation. Although IV normal saline (NS) boluses of 20 mL/kg are recommended to restore adequate blood pressure, typically smaller amounts of such an isotonic solution are required because the intravascular volume loss associated with hypernatremic dehydration is only a small percentage of the total body water loss (Lin et al., 2005).

Diagnostic study begins with laboratory analysis, which includes a chemistry panel, serum osmolarity, urinalysis, and urine electrolytes and osmolarity. The diagnosis of DI is supported by findings of hypernatremia and hyperosmolarity, without hyperglycemia, indicating inappropriate water loss. Diagnostic imaging includes magnetic resonance imaging (MRI) of the brain to identify potential causes of central DI such as tumors or abnormalities of the pituitary–hypothalamus stalk. MRI of the brain is the preferred imaging study instead of a computed tomography (CT), because the former images provide greater detail and are more sensitive in detecting lesions within the posterior fossa (Maghnie, 2003).

Diagnostic evaluation to differentiate nephrogenic from central DI includes a water deprivation test and administration of exogenous ADH (desmopressin or DDAVP). However, if nephrogenic DI is strongly suspected in an infant with polyuria, the water deprivation test should not be performed. The water deprivation test is performed in infants and children only in an acute care setting under close medical supervision. The purpose of this test is to restrict fluids until as much as 5% of body weight has been lost and determine the urinary response when the plasma osmolarity exceeds 295 mOsm/kg. The patient's vital signs, serum sodium and osmolarity, and urine osmolarity, specific gravity, and output, along with the child's weight, are monitored hourly to prevent significant dehydration. If the urinary response continues to be abnormal (i.e., no increase in urine osmolarity or decrease in urine output) despite plasma osmolarity of more than 295 mOsm/kg or serum sodium of more than 150 mEq/L, desmopressin is administered and urinary output and urinary osmolarity are monitored to determine the response to ADH. A failure of urine osmolarity to increase by more than 100 mOsm/kg over baseline is considered diagnostic for nephrogenic DI, whereas a decreased urine output and an increased urinary concentration support the diagnosis of central DI.

A comprehensive DI therapeutic plan may require consultation with subspecialty services such as nephrology, endocrinology, neurology, neurosurgery, critical care, and genetics. Fluid and electrolyte management for patients presenting with moderate to severe hypernatremic dehydration requires accurate calculation of the free water deficit to determine the appropriate rehydration fluids. An outline of the steps undertaken to determine the solution and rate of administration to correct deficits, to provide maintenance fluid and electrolytes, and to compensate for ongoing water losses is provided in Chapter 25.

In the pediatric patient presenting with seizures secondary to severe hypernatremia and hypertonicity, aggressive therapy is needed to prevent CNS injury. Management strategies include protecting the airway, administration of NS bolus (20 mL/kg) to restore blood volume, and anticonvulsant therapy (e.g., midazolam or lorazepam) to treat the seizure. Diagnostic evaluation should include CT of the brain to evaluate for CNS injuries associated with rapid cerebral parenchymal dehydration from hypernatremia such as subcortical and subarachnoid hemorrhages, subdural hematomas, and venous sinus thrombosis (Lin et al., 2005).

The challenge in the management of children with hypernatremia is determining the appropriate rate of sodium and water correction to prevent neurological complications. Hypernatremia that has developed acutely over a few hours from rapid sodium loading may be corrected quickly. In contrast, imbalances in children presenting with chronic hypernatremia of more than 48 hours' duration should be corrected slowly to prevent shifting of water into brain cells as a result of a rapid decrease in plasma osmolarity, which can cause cerebral edema and potentially lead to seizures, permanent brain injury, and death (Lin et al., 2005). The goal is to gradually decrease sodium levels by 1–2 mEq/L every 2 to 4 hours (10 mEq/L/24 hr). Frequent monitoring of neurological signs, fluid balance, and serum and urine electrolytes and osmolarity are necessary to prevent complications.

The primary plan for central DI is ADH hormone replacement to control polyuria. The ADH preparation will depend on acuity of illness, other medical conditions, and ability to tolerate oral intake. Dosages vary based on the preparation (Table 24-8). Intravenous vasopressin is used for the management of central DI in critical care or perioperative settings due to its short plasma half-life and easy titration. Desmopressin (DDAVP) is used in all other settings, as it is available in multiple forms, including oral and nasal, and is highly effective and well tolerated (Kim et al., 2004). The ideal dosage is determined by allowing the child to drink fluids freely, then administering a low dose of DDAVP and monitoring the observed decrease in urine output. When polyuria begins to reoccur, the next dose is given. Subsequent doses are increased as needed to establish a twice-daily schedule. The major concerns with administration of DDAVP are the risks of hyponatremia and water intoxication as a result of administering too large or too frequent a dose. Symptoms are related to the degree of hyponatremia and the speed with which it has developed. Urine output, serum sodium, osmolarity, and neurologic signs should be monitored closely while establishing a stable DDAVP dose.

Nephrogenic DI may be very difficult to manage, especially if it is congenital in origin. If DI is medication induced or related to a metabolic disorder, withdrawal

TABLE 24-8

Vasopressin Replacement for Central Diabetes Insipidus				
Medication	**Route**	**Dosage**	**Onset of Action/Peak Effect**	**Duration of Effect**
Vasopressin	Intravenous infusion	0.5–10 mU/kg/hr	10–15 min/30 min to 1 hr	2–3 hr
Desmopressin (DDAVP)	Oral	0.1–0.8 mg/day	1 hr/2–7 hr	6–8 hr
	Nasal	5–30 mcg/day	1 hr/1.5 hr	5–24 hr
	Intravenous	(divided into 2–3 doses/day)	40–55 min	3.5 hr

of the medication or correction of the metabolic disturbance often reverses renal sensitivity to ADH (Majzoub & Srivatsa 2006). Patients who are able to tolerate oral intake should receive liberal fluids to alleviate their thirst and prevent dehydration. Pediatric patients who are unable to tolerate oral intake require IV delivery of hypotonic fluids at rapid rates to maintain fluid balance. Sodium restriction combined with a thiazide diuretic has been reported to reduce urine output by 40% in infants (Majzoub & Srivatsa). The addition of indomethacin, a prostaglandin inhibitor, has been shown to decrease urine output (Cheetam & Baylis, 2002). Successful management of nephrogenic DI requires collaboration with the nephrology service to achieve effective dosing regimens.

Consultation with specialists depends on the cause of DI. Management of the pediatric patient with central DI requires collaboration with an endocrinologist. If the central DI is due to an intracranial tumor, additional services, including oncology, neurosurgery, and neurology specialists, are needed. In addition, families may require support from social services and case management to effectively transition to the home environment.

Patient and family education may begin as soon as the diagnosis is made. Determining the caregivers' cognitive and emotional readiness is imperative for successful outcomes. The HCP is instrumental in facilitating interprofessional team management, identifying educational needs, and evaluating outcomes.

Disposition and discharge planning

Readiness for discharge will differ for patients who are newly diagnosed with DI versus those who have a history of the condition. Care of the pediatric patient with DI at home, regardless of the cause, may be extremely challenging for families. Discharge preparation should include comprehensive caregiver education and a documented plan of care related to medications, dietary restrictions, signs and symptoms of recurrence or poor medication tolerance, home monitoring, and follow-up. The need for ongoing, meticulous monitoring may prove overwhelming to the caregivers. Consultation with case management and social work should be initiated early to identify and ensure provision of necessary resources upon discharge.

General criteria for discharge include the following:

- Resolution or stabilization of intercurrent illness
- Adequate oral intake
- Stable doses of all medications (based on sodium, osmolarity, and urine output)
- Patient/family education completed (including demonstration of medication administration, rationale for and side effects of medications, understanding of dietary restrictions, recognition of signs and symptoms, and need for regular follow-up)

- Initial follow-up appointments scheduled with specialists—endocrinologist (for central DI) or nephrologist (for nephrogenic DI)—to monitor and adjust medications

Caregivers should also be instructed to replace water in pediatric patients who cannot express thirst or access fluids without assistance and to seek medical attention promptly and for any illness that causes decreased fluid intake or increased losses (stool, emesis, diaphoresis) to prevent life-threatening water and electrolyte imbalances. In addition, caregivers should be instructed to limit heat exposure and to moderate activities that might result in increased insensible water loss so as to prevent dehydration.

SYNDROME OF INAPPROPRIATE ANTIDIURETIC HORMONE

Pathophysiology

Syndrome of inappropriate antidiuretic hormone (SIADH) is a disorder characterized by hyponatremia and decreased urine output as a result of excessive release of ADH from the posterior pituitary. Despite normal osmolarity and euvolemia, ADH continues to be secreted and is not suppressed by further decreases in osmolarity (e.g., levels less than 280 mOsm/kg). The excess ADH secretion results in excessive water reabsorption in the renal tubules, leading to a dilutional hyponatremia and weight gain without signs of edema. Postulated mechanisms for the inappropriate ADH secretion include alteration in the hypothalamus–pituitary axis as a result of CNS disorders, including stimulation by tumor cells, medications, or afferent pain receptors following surgery (Arvantis & Pasquale, 2005).

Epidemiology and etiology

SIADH is one of the most common causes of hyponatremia in pediatric patients (Moritz & Ayus, 2002). The wide array of causes of SIADH in pediatric patients may be organized into four broad categories: CNS disorders (e.g., infections, traumatic brain injury, tumors), pulmonary disorders, surgery, and medications (Table 24-9). The most common etiology of SIADH is a brain tumor; chemotherapeutic agents such as vincristine, cyclophosphamide, and cisplatin have also been shown to precipitate SIADH (Arvantis & Pasquale, 2005). In addition, the incidence of SIADH in pediatric patients with bacterial meningitis is reported to be as high as 88% (Rauf & Roberts, 1999).

Positive-pressure ventilation is an underappreciated contributor to SIADH because it may decrease venous return, thereby reducing cardiac volume and atrial stretch. The reduced volume stimulates baroreceptors and causes enhanced ADH and atrial natriuretic peptide (ANP) secretion, ultimately resulting in fluid retention (Haviv et al., 2005).

TABLE 24-9

Causes of Syndrome of Inappropriate Antidiuretic Hormone	
Category	**Cause**
Central nervous system disease	Infections: meningitis, encephalitis Hydrocephalus Traumatic brain injury Tumors Conditions altering hypothalamus function
Pulmonary disease	Pneumonia Empyema Bronchiolitis Acute respiratory failure Positive-pressure ventilation
Surgery	Neurosurgical procedures Spinal surgery
Medications	Vincristine Cyclophosphamide Carbamazepine Serotonin reuptake inhibitors

TABLE 24-10

Diagnosis of Syndrome of Inappropriate Antidiuretic Hormone	
Clinical signs and symptoms	Hypervolemia, normal blood pressure, skin turgor, no edema Urine output ≤ 1 mL/kg/hr Nausea and vomiting Irritability, lethargy, altered mental status Seizures, coma
Laboratory studies	Serum sodium < 135 mEq/L Serum osmolarity < 280 mOsm/L BUN usually < 10 mg/dL Urine specific gravity > 1.020 Urine sodium > 25 mEq/L Urine osmolarity > 200 mOsm/L
Diagnostic studies	Head CT scan or MRI is indicated if cerebral edema or CNS disease is suspected

Computed tomography (CT), magnetic resonance imaging (MRI), central nervous system (CNS).

Presentation

The hallmark findings of SIADH include hyponatremia, decreased serum osmolarity, decreased urine output, and increased urinary osmolarity and concentration (Table 24-10). A detailed history of the fluid balance, weight changes, and medications such as diuretics should be elicited. Signs and symptoms of hypervolemia may be present without edema. Patients who experience a rapid decrease in serum sodium to less than 125 mEq/L may exhibit signs and symptoms of cerebral edema, including headache, nausea, vomiting, lethargy, pupillary changes, apnea, and seizures.

Differential diagnosis

The primary differential diagnosis of SIADH is cerebral salt wasting (CSW). The accurate differentiation between the two is crucial, as the treatments for the conditions are very different. CSW is caused by renal salt loss that is partially mediated by ANP, leading to serum hyponatremia and hypo-osmolality. Unlike in SIADH, therapeutic management of CSW includes fluid and sodium replacement. Other conditions causing hyponatremia and volume overload must be also considered, such as water intoxication, adrenal insufficiency, hypothyroidism, congestive heart failure, and liver and kidney disease.

Plan of care

Laboratory studies to establish the diagnosis of SIADH include serum sodium, glucose, blood urea nitrogen (BUN), plasma osmolarity, urine osmolarity, and urine sodium (Table 24-10). Establishing the combination of hyponatremia and hypo-osmolarity is the first step. Solutes such as glucose, protein, and lipids may cause a "pseudo" or "artificial" hyponatremia in which the serum sodium is low but the measured serum osmolarity is normal or high as a result of these substances contributing to increased plasma volume. For example, this condition may be observed in the pediatric patient with diabetic ketoacidosis. In this situation, the hyperglycemia associated with insulin deficiency causes hyperosmolarity and a pseudohyponatremia due to the expanded plasma volume. Direct and calculated measurement of serum osmolarity should be evaluated as well as potential etiologies causing a pseudohyponatremia (Table 24-11). Serum osmolarity may be calculated by the formula presented in Table 24-12.

Once plasma hypo-osmolarity has been confirmed, urine electrolytes and osmolarity are evaluated. A urinary sodium level greater than 25 mEq/L is consistent with SIADH, but other etiologies must also be considered, including renal tubular dysfunction and diuretic use. Another important distinction in SIADH is that the urine osmolarity is increased inappropriately compared with the serum osmolarity. Typically the urine osmolarity is greater than 100 mOsm/L.

Euvolemia or hypervolemia is another important characteristic in pediatric patients with SIADH and eliminates other potential causes of hyponatremia. A normal BUN is consistent with SIADH; in contrast, in CSW, BUN is typically elevated due to volume depletion. Diagnostic studies confirming normal kidney, thyroid, and adrenal

TABLE 24-11

Serum Sodium Correction for Pseudohyponatremia

Hyperlipidemia: Na^+ decreased by $0.002 \times$ (lipid mg/dL)

Hyperproteinemia: Na^+ decreased by $0.25 \times$ (protein gm/dL) -8

Hyperglycemia: Na^+ decreased by 1.6 mEq/L for each 100 mg/dL rise in glucose

TABLE 24-12

Calculation for Serum Osmolarity

Calculated serum osmolarity =
2 (serum sodium) + (glucose mg/dL ÷ 18) + (BUN mg/dL ÷ 2.8)

TABLE 24-13

Treatment of Syndrome of Inappropriate Antidiuretic Hormone

1. Manage underlying cause
2. Fluid restriction: < 75% of daily maintenance fluid requirement
3. Treat acute hyponatremia with 3 % hypertonic saline (513 mEq of Na^+/L)
   - Correct serum Na^+ to 125 mEq/L quickly
   - Na^+ deficit = (body weight in kg) $\times 0.6$ (% in ECF) $\times$ (desired serum sodium level [125] − actual serum Na^+ level) = mEq

Example: 10-kg infant with serum Na^+ 118 mEq/L

10 kg $\times 0.6 \times$ (125 − 118) = 42 mEq

42 mEq $\times$ 0.513 mEq/mL (3% saline) = 21.5 mL

Extracellular fluid (ECF).

function include serum creatinine, thyroid function tests (e.g., thyroid-stimulating hormone, free T_4), and a morning cortisol level. In addition, a head CT scan or MRI is indicated if CNS disease is suspected or if the presentation includes a seizure.

The management of SIADH begins with correction of the hyponatremia (Table 24-13). If the patient presents with seizures and hyponatremia, the serum sodium must be acutely raised to 125 mEq/L to stop seizure activity. Further management requires definitive diagnosis of the etiology of the SIADH. Treatment is based on the serum sodium level and the extent of the symptoms exhibited by the patient. The duration of SIADH is typically brief and resolves with treatment of the underlying disorder or discontinuation of the offending medication. The primary therapy in the asymptomatic patient is fluid and salt restriction; however, this approach results in a slow correction of sodium and volume overload and may be impractical for infants. Intravenous fluids should contain normal saline; in particular, hypotonic fluids must be avoided. The rate of sodium correction will depend on the patient's presentation. *In general, hyponatremia is corrected slowly, at a rate of 0.5–1 mEq/hr to avoid rapid intracellular fluid shifts that might cause cerebral edema. The patient also should receive no more than 8–10 mmol of sodium and the sodium level should rise no more than 10 mEq per 24-hour period to avoid central pontine myelinolysis.* If more rapid sodium correction is needed, administration of a loop diuretic (e.g., furosemide) facilitates urine output. However, the pediatric patient presenting with seizures or depressed mental status requires rapid correction to quell seizure activity and to achieve a serum sodium level of more than 125 mEq/L, which is best achieved with the use of hypertonic saline (Table 24-13).

Consultation with specialists may be required to determine the etiology of the hyponatremia, and consultation with a pediatric intensivist is recommended for patients presenting with acute or postoperative hyponatremia. Patients with SIADH due to an intracranial tumor or CNS disease require interprofessional management involving HCPs from services such as oncology, neurosurgery, and neurology. Other consultations may include a pediatric endocrinologist or nephrologist if the cause of SIADH is not CNS disease. In addition, families may require support from social services and case management for the underlying disease process to ensure a smooth transition of the patient to the home environment.

Patient and family education may begin as soon as the diagnosis is made. SIADH is primarily a self-limiting condition; therefore, education includes information on this condition's probable cause, treatment, and expected response. The HCP is instrumental in facilitating interprofessional team management, identifying educational needs, and evaluating outcomes.

Disposition and discharge planning

Disposition depends on the pathological nature and management of the underlying cause of the SIADH, including the severity of symptoms, laboratory evaluation, therapeutic interventions required, and the response to treatment. Pediatric patients with SIADH occurring following surgery, in conjunction with CNS infections, stemming from a medication-related cause, or supported by mechanical ventilation generally experience rapid recovery. In contrast, patients with SIADH secondary to intracranial hemorrhage or brain tumor may have recurrence. Also, complications associated with severe hyponatremia may significantly prolong hospitalization and affect disposition and discharge planning needs. Follow-up with specialists is determined by the underlying etiology of SIADH. In general, SIADH resolves with treatment and does not require further outpatient management but post-discharge recurrence is possible, especially in pediatric oncology patients requiring chemotherapy.

CEREBRAL SALT WASTING

Pathophysiology

Cerebral salt wasting is defined as the renal loss of sodium during intracranial disease leading to hyponatremia and volume depletion. The exact mechanism underlying renal salt wasting in this syndrome remains unclear. In the original report of CSW in 1950, Peters and colleagues theorized that renal salt wasting occurred when adrenocorticotropic hormone secretion was disrupted, leading to decreased adrenal mineral corticoid secretion (aldosterone) or an alteration in direct neuronal control over the kidneys. Since then, case reports and small case series have produced conflicting results regarding the etiology of CSW. Research supports the role of circulating brain and atrial natriuretic factors; however, the presence of other factors or direct neural effects on the kidneys are likely to be necessary for the development of CSW (Harrigan, 2001; Singh et al., 2002). Atrial natriuretic peptide is a hormone with natriuretic and aldosterone-inhibiting characteristics that is released from the atria in response to activation of the stretch receptors. Natriuretic peptides are also present in the brain (BNP), albeit in lower concentrations than in the heart; this difference suggests that cerebral secretion of this hormone is not responsible for CSW (Donati-Genet et al., 2001). In addition, although activation of the atrial stretch receptors is the principal mechanism for release of ANP, a growing body of evidence suggests that the cerebral nervous system also affects atrial secretion and may be the source of hormonal dysfunction (Donati-Genet et al.; Kappy & Ganong, 1996).

Epidemiology and etiology

Cerebral salt wasting occurs primarily in the setting of acute CNS disease. In pediatric patients, conditions leading to CSW may include traumatic brain injury (TBI), brain tumor, intracranial surgery, meningitis, and encephalitis. Although the prevalence of CSW in children is unknown, Jimenez and colleagues (2006) reported the prevalence in postoperative neurosurgical pediatric patients to be 11.3 per 1,000 cases. Almost 79% of patients manifested CSW during the first 48 hours postoperatively, with the mean duration of the CSW episode lasting 6.3 ± 5.4 days. The most common admitting diagnosis was brain tumor followed by hydrocephalus.

Hyponatremia is defined as a serum sodium level less than 135 mEq/L. It is well recognized as one of the most common electrolyte disturbances in hospitalized patients, occurring in approximately 3% of all pediatric patients (Moritz & Ayus, 2002). In addition, hyponatremia commonly occurs in pediatric patients with CNS injuries such as meningitis, intracranial hemorrhage, or tumors, and is an important cause of morbidity in hospitalized patients (Harrigan, 2001; Rivkees, 2008).

Presentation

The severity of presenting symptoms reflects the magnitude and rate of decrease in serum sodium concentration. Symptoms range from headache, agitation, and lethargy, to depressed mental status, seizures, and coma. Research reveals that the emergence of hyponatremia with CSW occurs earlier in pediatric patients as compared to adults (Harrigan, 2001). Reports in adults suggest that CSW syndrome is a delayed phenomenon occurring in the second week following the initial CNS insult. However, three reports in pediatric patients indicated that they were diagnosed CSW within the first week (2 to 6 days) following CNS injury (Berkenbosch et al., 2002; Donati-Genet et al., 2001; Kappy & Ganong, 1996). Therefore, it is important that the HCP considers CSW as a possibility in all neurologically injured patients with early-onset hyponatremia.

Differential diagnosis

Although various pathophysiologic mechanisms cause hyponatremia, the most important differential diagnoses include SIADH and acute adrenocortical insufficiency. Often the clinical picture and the laboratory data may be initially misleading, as the diagnostic criteria for CSW correspond to the diagnostic criteria for SIADH. These diagnostic criteria include serum sodium less than 135 mEq/L; serum osmolarity less than 280 mosm/L; high urine sodium, greater than 60–80 mmol/L; urinary osmolarity greater than serum osmolarity; and normal thyroid, adrenal, and kidney function. To date, the literature describing CSW consists of adult or small case series with limited pediatric representation (Berkenbosch et al., 2002; Bussman et al., 2001; Donati-Genet et al., 2001).

As with SIADH, differential diagnoses for CSW include other etiologies of hyponatremia, such as SIADH, congestive heart failure, kidney or liver disease, hypothyroidism, adrenal insufficiency, water intoxication, and pseudohyponatremia. It is also imperative that the HCP consider physiologic causes for natriuresis, such as inborn errors of metabolism (e.g., congenital adrenal hyperplasia, Fanconi and Bartter syndromes), renal tubular dysfunction, and diuretic administration.

It is essential to differentiate CSW from SIADH because the treatments for the two conditions are different (Table 24-14). The pediatric patient with CSW exhibits signs and symptoms of dehydration due to salt wasting, whereas the patient with SIADH has signs of fluid overload due to water retention.

TABLE 24-14

Diagnosis Summary for Diabetes Insipidus, Syndrome of Inappropriate Antidiuretic Hormone, and Cerebral Salt Wasting			
Parameter	DI	SIADH	CSW
Serum Na$^+$	> 150 mEq/L	< 135 mEq/L	< 135 mEq/L
Serum osmolarity	> 295 mOsm/kg	< 280 mOsm/kg	< 280 mOsm/kg
Urine Na$^+$	< 30 mEq/L	> 30 mEq/L	> 80 mEq/L
Urine osmolarity	< 200 mOsm/kg	> 200 mOsm/kg	> 200 mOsm/kg
Urine specific gravity	< 1.005	> 1.020	> 1.010
Urine output	≥ 4 mL/kg/hr	≤ 1 mL/kg/hr	2–3 mL/kg/hr

Plan of care

Diagnostic studies are similar to those obtained in patients suspected of having SIADH (Table 24-15). Measurements of serum ADH and ANP are not helpful in distinguishing between CSW and SIADH (Harrigan, 2001). Although plasma ANP levels have been reported to be high in patients with CSW, this has not been a consistent finding (Berkenbosch et al., 2002; Jimenez et al., 2006; Rivkees, 2008). In addition, although serum ADH is usually high in SIADH and low in CSW, many factors may promote ADH secretion, including stress, pain, and increased intracranial pressure.

Management is aimed at identifying the underlying cause of CSW and instituting prompt and appropriate treatment to prevent complications associated with hyponatremia and volume depletion. Close monitoring of the patient's sodium and fluid balance to prevent hemodynamic and neurologic complications may dictate the admission to a higher level of care.

Treatment begins with volume and sodium replacement. As with all causes of hyponatremia, serum sodium should be replaced slowly, at a rate of 0.5–1 mEq/hr and limited to an increase of the sodium level to no more than 10 mEq/day. Following urine sodium measurements, in addition to serum sodium, may help determine the patient's sodium replacement needs. For example, a urine sodium of 75 mEq/L is equivalent to a concentration of 0.45 NS. The route of replacement is based on the patient's acuity and ability to tolerate oral intake. Evidence of significant volume depletion dehydration of 10% or more or hypotension should prompt administration of a fluid bolus of 20 mL/kg normal saline. The response to saline infusion also helps the HCP distinguish between CSW and SIADH. In CSW, sodium administration corrects volume depletion and hyponatremia; in SIADH, it is of no benefit. Next, replacement fluid is initiated intravenously with NS (dextrose may be also needed, especially in infants to prevent hypoglycemia) and administered over 24 hours. The fluid rate is calculated based on maintenance requirements and fluid deficit. If the pediatric patient is able to tolerate oral intake, sodium replacement may be determined based on urinary sodium losses plus maintenance sodium needs and replaced in divided doses. Meticulous monitoring of fluid intake and output and clinical parameters as well as serum and urinary sodium is essential to guide management.

Consultation with neurosurgery, oncology, and neurology services is customary because the precipitating cause of CSW is CNS disease. Other subspecialists may be required to determine the etiology of hyponatremia; in particular, consultation with a pediatric intensivist is necessary for pediatric patients presenting with acute presentation of hyponatremia. In addition, families frequently require support from social services and case management because discharge planning for these patients is often complex.

Patient and family education may begin as soon as the diagnosis is identified. CSW, like SIADH, is primarily a self-limiting condition; therefore, education includes information about its probable cause, treatment, and expected response. The HCP is instrumental in facilitating interprofessional team management, identifying educational needs, and evaluating outcomes.

Disposition and discharge planning

Disposition depends on both success of the treatment of CSW and management of the complications associated with the underlying intracranial pathology. Severe neurological injury, such as may be seen with severe traumatic brain injury, will significantly prolong hospitalization and affect disposition and discharge planning needs. CSW usually occurs early in the hospital course and does not prolong hospitalization. Pediatric patients typically respond to replacement therapy and infrequently require oral sodium replacement at discharge (Jimenez et al., 2006). Patients with pituitary dysfunction as sequelae of their disease

TABLE 24-15

Diagnosis of Cerebral Salt Wasting Syndrome	
Clinical signs and symptoms	Signs and symptoms of dehydration
	Nausea and vomiting
	Lethargy, weakness
	Seizures and/or coma
Laboratory studies	Serum Na$^+$ < 135 mEq/L
	Serum osmolarity < 280 mOsm/L
	Elevated BUN > 15 mg/dL
	Urine Na$^+$ > 80 mEq/L
	Urine osmolarity > 200 mOsm/L
	Urine specific gravity ≥ 1.020
	Urine output > 1 mL/kg/hr
Diagnostic studies	Head CT scan or MRI to determine CNS pathology
	Lumbar puncture is suspect meningitis or encephalitis

Computed tomography (CT), magnetic resonance imaging (MRI), central nervous system (CNS), blood urea nitrogen (BUN).

process may require electrolyte and hormone replacement therapy.

Correction of hyponatremia in patients with CNS disease may be also associated with significant morbidity secondary to the development of cerebral edema or central pontine myelinosis. Those patients who present with seizure or coma are more likely to have poor neurological outcomes, including paralysis and death (Arieff et al., 1992; Donati-Genet et al., 2001).

> **Critical Thinking**
>
> Sodium correction: reduction or increase in serum sodium by a rate *no faster than* 0.5–1 mEq/hr or 10 mEq in 24 hours.

DIABETIC KETOACIDOSIS

Rosemary Briars

PATHOPHYSIOLOGY

Insulin deficiency is the main stimulus in diabetic ketoacidosis (DKA). For glucose to enter the cell, insulin must be present and bind with the specific cellular receptor site. Insulin deficiency creates a starvation state that triggers a cascade of metabolic responses as the body attempts to liberate stored glucose in an effort to feed the cells (Figure 24-8). Levels of counter-regulatory hormones (glucagon, catecholamines, cortisol, growth hormone) increase, as do lypolysis, proteolysis, and glycogenolysis, resulting in hyperglycemia and cellular insulin resistance.

Low serum insulin levels and/or insulin resistance lead to decreased glucose uptake in the periphery (glucose utilization) and increased hepatic and renal glucose production (gluconeogensis), resulting in hyperglycemia. Hyperglycemia leads to osmotic diuresis, electrolyte loss, dehydration, decreased glomerular filtration, and hyperosmolarity. Lipolysis liberalizes free fatty acids, which are then converted to glucose by the liver. Free fatty acid oxidation generates acetoacetic and beta-hydroxybutyric acids—that is, it creates ketones (ketogenesis). Ketone body formation coupled with lactic acidosis from decreased tissue perfusion results in metabolic acidosis (Wolfsdorf et al., 2006).

With decreased peripheral glucose uptake and the compensatory liver/kidney gluconeogenesis and glycogenolysis, hyperglycemia begets hyperglycemia in a self-perpetuating cycle of metabolic decline. This cycle cannot be broken until insulin is replaced, allowing glucose to enter the cells and thus ending the starvation state. DKA is deadly without rapid recognition, careful insulin replacement, and fluid and electrolyte therapy.

Their immature cerebral and autoregulatory mechanisms predispose pediatric patients to more severe DKA presentations and complications such as cerebral edema (Wolfsdorf et al., 2006). It was once thought that cerebral edema was directly related to the administration of bicarbonate and/or the phenomenon of over-hydration creating osmotic cellular shifts. However, this theory has been confounded by the evidence that cerebral edema may occur prior to any treatment at all and the lack of a significant change in the overall incidence of cerebral edema despite guidelines restricting the use of bicarbonate and limiting volumes for fluid resuscitation.

Glaser and associates (2004) examined cerebral water distribution and perfusion measurements both during DKA and after treatment, using diffusion- and perfusion-weighted MRI. Their findings included a significant elevation in cerebral perfusion during DKA treatment, suggesting an expansion in the extracellular space as opposed to the intracellular space. The researchers concluded that a vasogenic process may represent the predominant mechanism of edema formation, rather than osmotic cellular swelling (Glaser et al., 2004). While recent data have provided helpful evidence in favor of various theories for the pathogenesis of cerebral edema, these data remain the topic of current review.

EPIDEMIOLOGY AND ETIOLOGY

Undiagnosed diabetes is the leading cause of DKA in children. In children with an established diagnosis of diabetes, insulin dose omission is the most common cause of DKA. The stress of an intercurrent illness can increase

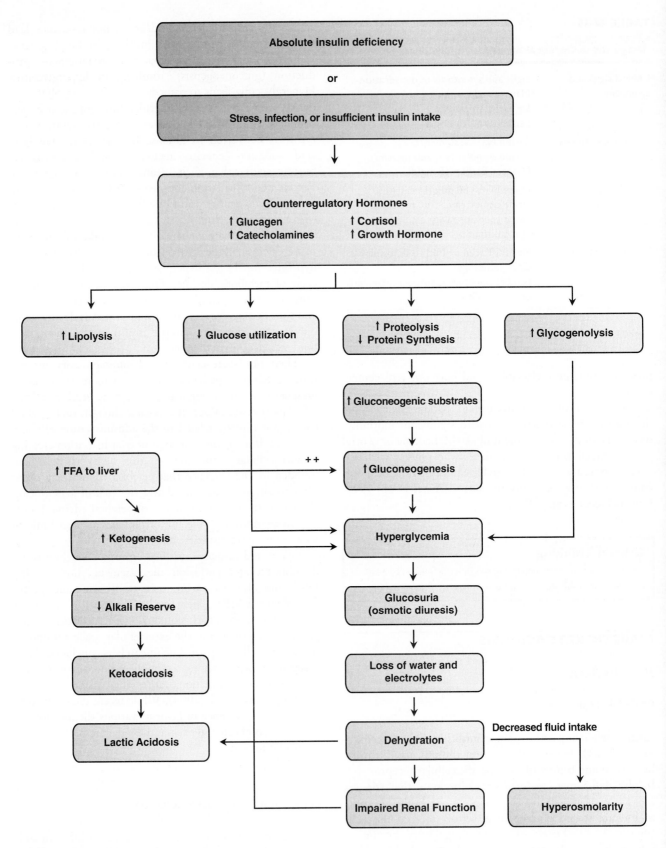

FIGURE 24-8

Pathophysiology of DKA, FFA, and Free Fatty Acid.

Source: Reprinted with permission. Copyright 2006. American Diabetes Association. From Wolfsdorf, J., Glaser, N., & Sperling, M. (2006). American Diabetes Association consensus statement diabetic ketoacidosis in infants, children and adolescents. *Diabetes Care, 29*(5), 1150–1159.

insulin requirements due to counter-regulatory hormone excess, which in turn promotes gluconeogenesis and insulin resistance, ultimately resulting in DKA. DKA can also occur with incorrect administration of insulin leading to under-dosing. Children on insulin pump therapy can develop DKA rapidly if an unplanned or unnoticed interruption of the insulin infusion or problem at the insertion site occurs.

By definition, diabetes is a group of metabolic diseases characterized by hyperglycemia resulting from defects in insulin secretion, action, or both. The abnormalities in carbohydrate, fat, and protein metabolism that are found in diabetes are due to deficient action of insulin on target tissues (Craig et al., 2009). Diabetes is divided into types. The variations most common in children include *type 1*, *type 2*, *atypical*, and *monogenic* (rare genetic mutation causing beta-cell dysfunction). In patients who are newly diagnosed type 1 diabetes, insulin deficiency is the initial event in progressive pancreatic beta-cell failure. With type 2 diabetes, insulin resistance creates hyperglycemia that, over time, can lead to insulin deficiency. Unlike their adult counterparts, it is not uncommon for children with type 2 diabetes to present with DKA, despite having only a relative insulin deficiency. As the number of children with type 2 diabetes increases, it has become increasingly important to differentiate the diabetes type so as to provide accurate therapeutic and educational interventions.

Type 1 diabetes

While the exact cause of type 1 diabetes is unknown, the current theory is that children with immune-mediated type 1 diabetes are born with a genetic susceptibility that is activated in response to an environmental trigger. This environmental trigger initiates the development of diabetes-associated autoantibodies that eventually destroy the pancreatic beta cells located in the islets of Langerhans. This immune-mediated pancreatic beta-cell destruction eventually leads to absolute insulin deficiency.

Susceptibility to immune-mediated type 1 diabetes is determined by multiple genes with strong human leukocyte antigen (HLA) associations. There is linkage to specific combinations of alleles at the DRB, DQA, and DQB loci. These HLA-DR/DQ alleles can be either predisposing or protective. The environmental triggers that initiate the process of beta-cell destruction are not completely understood. Enterovirus infection has been associated in some populations. The T-cell–mediated beta-cell destruction occurs at a variable rate, and presenting symptoms become apparent when only 10% of the beta cells remain functional. Serum markers of the immune process include anti-islet cells, glutamic acid decarboxylase (GAD65), tyrosine phosphatases IA-2 and IA-2β, and insulin autoantibodies; such markers are present in 85% to 90% of children with type 1 diabetes at the time of diagnosis (Craig et al., 2009). Autoimmune type 1 diabetes is associated with other autoimmune conditions, such as thyroid disorders, celiac disease, adrenal disease, vitiligo, or pernicious anemia.

At diagnosis, a child with immune-mediated type 1 diabetes usually has a rapid onset of symptoms with ketosis due to the insulin deficiency. Such children test positive for diabetes-associated autoantibodies, and are usually lean with no physical signs of insulin resistance. Approximately 90% of children with type 1 diabetes have immune-mediated type 1 disease. There may or may not be a family history of type 1 diabetes, as there is not a recognizable pattern of inheritance. Only 2% to 4% of these children have a parent with diabetes. When the clinical features are typical of type 1 diabetes, as described, but the antibodies are negative, the diabetes is classified as type 1B or idiopathic (Craig et al., 2009).

Type 2 diabetes

Type 2 diabetes is becoming more common in children. Children with this variant tend to be overweight or obese (85%) but may present at normal weight. Most will have hyperglycemia and glycosuria without ketonuria, yet as many as 33% have ketonuria at diagnosis and 5% to 25% of patients who are subsequently classified as having type 2 diabetes have ketoacidosis at presentation (American Diabetes Association [ADA], 2000). They have no evidence of autoimmunity, but will have normal to elevated fasting insulin and C-peptide levels. A high insulin level is suggestive of insulin resistance. The presence of C-peptide indicates endogenous insulin production. Disorders associated with insulin resistance and obesity such as polycystic ovarian syndrome (PCOS), lipid disorders, and hypertension also occur in children with type 2 diabetes. Finally, a family history of type 2 diabetes is almost always present in at least one parent (45–80%) or in a first- or second-degree relative (74–100%) (ADA, 2000).

PRESENTATION

Presentation of DKA requires a detailed history, review of systems, and physical examination to confirm the diagnosis, identify the cause, and provide insight into the duration of the prodrome. Complaints of vomiting and increased urine output may trigger early recognition during triage; otherwise, inquiry should include the onset and duration of nausea and vomiting plus the classic triad of symptoms—polyuria, polydipsia, and polyphagia—as well as the amount of weight lost. Polyuria may present as enuresis, nocturia, overflowing diapers, or bedwetting in a previously toilet-trained child. The younger the child, the more difficult it is to assess the classic symptoms; and polyuria may go unnoticed in the infant or toddler who is not yet toilet trained. Caregivers may describe the urine as sweet-smelling or sticky. Complaints may also include nonspecific weakness, blurred vision, abdominal pain, lethargy, malaise, and signs of mental status change. History of infections, illness exposures, or other chronic conditions should be explored. Patients may present with an exacerbation of their chronic illness or a coexisting acute illness.

A patient presenting with type 2 diabetes may not exhibit symptoms of overt polyuria and polydipsia, and may have inconspicuous weight loss; however, onset of these markers may vary from slow and insidious to severe DKA. Additionally, a common and abnormal physical finding is acanthosis nigricans, described as a velvety hyperpigmented lesion noted in intertriginous regions such as the axillae, the groin, and at the nape of the neck. This painless skin lesion may also be found in those persons at risk of developing type 2 diabetes.

If the patient has a known history of diabetes, the history should include an assessment of the current regimen, current insulin dose, timing of last self-administered dose, meal plan, adherence to the plan, degree of adult support, supervision of the home care, and any previous episodes of DKA. Make sure the insulin dose is appropriate for the child's age and stage of development.

Check all home equipment, insulin pens, pumps, and meters for malfunction. Ask to see the home blood glucose meter. Most home meters have an easily accessible memory and downloading capability to find evidence of self-care and assess the degree of control prior to admission. Insulin pumps also store historical data on what has been done in terms of insulin self-administration, an alarm history to indicate pump malfunction, and a record of infusion settings. Caregivers should know how to access historical information from the meter and/or pump. Almost all meters and pumps have a 24-hour toll-free customer support number placed on the back of the device that caregivers can call for assistance with accessing data stored in the memory, retrieving data, or reprogramming settings. Identify interruptions or delays in insulin delivery listed in the pump's historical information. Insulin omission is not uncommon in patients with a long duration of diabetes or lack of adult supervision due to "burnout." Find out how long the child has been on the pump. Patients new to the pump might not be well versed on troubleshooting problems with hyperglycemia or inadvertent disconnection of the infusion set. Remove the pump before starting therapy for DKA.

The physical examination should focus on the cardiopulmonary and neurological systems. Evaluate the work of breathing and measure pulse oximetry on room air. Kussmaul respirations or deep and labored breathing with fruity-smelling breath are late symptoms of DKA. Assess perfusion, cardiovascular function, and hemodynamics.

Signs of dehydration include tachycardia, weak pulses, pale cool skin, enophthalmos, dry mucous membranes, poor skin turgor, and hypotension. The greater the number of symptoms present, the greater the severity of dehydration. Clinical determination of dehydration severity

may be challenging due to the patient's hyperosmolar state and osmotic diuresis. The following criteria, which are based on a combination of physical signs, are most useful in assessing dehydration and acidosis in young children:

- 5%: prolonged capillary refill time $\geq$ 1.5–2 seconds, abnormal skin turgor, hyperpnea
- > 10%: weak or impalpable peripheral pulses, hypotension, oliguria (Wolfsdorf et al., 2009, p. 120)

Evaluation of the patient's mental status and Glasgow Coma Scale (GCS) score requires vigilance, as evidence of a decline may be subtle. Signs of irritability, behavior change, vomiting, and lethargy are indications of possible cerebral edema and require immediate attention.

Examine the ear, nose, throat, and dermis for a focal infection. For the child with a known history of diabetes, assessment of injection sites for signs of hypertrophy may indicate overuse or impaired insulin absorption, which may lead to erratic insulin action. Alternatively, evidence of blood glucose monitoring on the fingertips or on alternate sites may provide information about the cause of DKA.

DIFFERENTIAL DIAGNOSIS

Several conditions may cause similar abnormalities at presentation in the pediatric population (Table 24-16). Stress hyperglycemia in pediatric patients can be associated with an acute illness, injury, trauma, febrile seizures, or elevated

TABLE 24-16

Differential Diagnoses for Diabetic Ketoacidosis
Metabolic acidosis
Hypokalemia
Dehydration
Flu, viral illness, sepsis
Salicylate toxicity
Acute respiratory distress syndrome
Respiratory acidosis
Asthma
Pneumonia
Acute abdomen
Pancreatitis
Pyloric stenosis
Constipation
Stress hyperglycemia
High-dose steroids
Hyperosmolar hyperglycemia nonketotic coma

TABLE 24-17

Criteria for Hyperglycemic Hyperosmolar State

- Plasma glucose > 600 mg/dL
- Arterial pH > 7.30
- Serum bicarbonate > 15 mmol/L
- Small ketonuria, absent to mild ketonemia
- Effective serum osmolality > 320 mOsm/kg
- Stupor or coma

body temperature (Craig et al., 2009). Hyperglycemia under this type of stress may be transitory and should not be considered diagnostic for diabetes.

Hyperosmolar hyperglycemic state (HHS) may be differentiated from DKA when the serum glucose and osmolality are very high in the absence of severe ketoacidosis (Table 24-17). Patients with HHS have severe dehydration and altered mental status. This condition may also occur in type 2 diabetes. It is important to distinguish this state from type 2 diabetes, as its treatment requires different fluids, insulin dose, electrolyte content, and fluid volumes to correct the severe dehydration, hyperglycemia, and electrolyte disturbance.

PLAN OF CARE

The diagnostic evaluation begins with laboratory studies that include electrolytes, BUN, creatinine, calcium, magnesium, phosphate, pH analysis (arterial or venous blood gas), serum ketones, urinalysis, osmolality, and hemoglobin A_{1c}. A high percentage of hemoglobin A_{1c} in a child previously diagnosed with diabetes indicates poor compliance with insulin therapy. Autoimmune markers such as GAD65, IA-2, IA-2β, and insulin antibodies may be evaluated for evidence of associated autoimmune conditions such as antithyroglobulin and antithyroperoxidase antibodies, celiac disease, and adrenal antibodies.

The primary diagnostic evidence of DKA consists of hyperglycemia greater than 200 mg/dL with ketoacidosis, ketones in the serum (ketonemia) and urine (ketonuria), plus pH less than 7.3 or bicarbonate less than 15 mmol/L. Wolfsdorf et al. (2009) categorize the severity of DKA by the degree of acidosis:

- Mild: venous pH < 7.3 or bicarbonate < 15 mmol/L
- Moderate: pH < 7.2 and bicarbonate < 10 mmol/L
- Severe: pH < 7.1 and bicarbonate < 5 mmol/L

A complete blood count (CBC) with differential is required; however, leukocytosis is not a reliable indicator of infection, as elevation of the stress hormones epinephrine and cortisol in DKA may mimic an infection (Cooke &

Plotnick, 2008). Therefore, antibiotics should be started in a patient with an identified infection or in a febrile patient after cultures are obtained. If cough, fever, or respiratory distress is present, a chest radiograph (CXR) should be performed. A baseline electrocardiograph (ECG) will assess any electrophysiologic changes.

Pediatric DKA therapy typically begins in an emergency department or ambulance. Due to the complexities of DKA and its life-threatening nature, the pediatric patient with DKA should be transferred to a facility that is affiliated with a pediatric diabetes specialty program. A pediatric intensive care unit (PICU) should be considered for patients with moderate to severe presentation or any mental status changes. Vital signs and neurological checks should be performed every 1 to 2 hours for at least the first 24 hours or until the patient is stable.

In patients with severe DKA and an altered level of consciousness, mechanical airway support and a nasogastric tube may be needed to decrease the risk of aspiration. Supplemental oxygen should be given for any respiratory distress, increased work of breathing, severe circulatory impairment, or shock. Establishing multiple peripheral IV catheters will facilitate fluid infusion and frequent blood sampling. An arterial pressure infusion may be required to provide accurate pH and prevent IV infiltration from frequent blood sampling. A cardiac monitor should be used to assess T waves for alterations due to hyperkalemia or hypokalemia. Catheterize the bladder if the child is unconscious or unable to void on demand. Strict measurement of intake and output and nothing by mouth (NPO) status is required until the severity of DKA is known. All urine should be checked for ketones.

The patient's response to each phase of treatment needs to be carefully monitored for dynamic metabolic changes. During the first hour of treatment, the goal is volume expansion to treat dehydration and diagnostic study to confirm DKA. In the second hour, the aim is correction of acidosis, reversal of ketosis, restoration of electrolyte balance, and slow, gradual correction of hyperglycemia, in addition to continued rehydration. Throughout the course of management, the overall goal is to avoid complications of therapy and to identify and treat any precipitating event.

The therapeutic management plan includes serial laboratory studies, individualized intravenous fluid and electrolyte therapy, insulin, dextrose, and ongoing monitoring. A DKA flow sheet is most helpful for tracking all of the important details of DKA management, including hour-by-hour clinical and laboratory findings. Serum glucose should be checked hourly until the patient demonstrates neurologic and hemodynamic stability, normal pH, and serial normoglycemia. After the initial diagnostic studies, basic metabolic panel, pH, and serum ketones are assessed at least every 3 to 6 hours depending on the severity of the patient's condition and until acidosis has cleared. The baseline calcium, phosphate, and magnesium should be rechecked in 12 hours.

TABLE 24-18

Calculations of Anion Gap, Corrected Sodium, and Effective Osmolality

$$\text{Anion gap} = [Na^+ + K^+] - [Cl^- + HCO_3] \textbf{ or } [Na^+] - [Cl^- + HCO_3^-]$$

Normal AG range is 8–16 mEq/L.

This calculation helps to quantify unmeasured anions (i.e., ketones and lactate) in ketoacidosis. The anion gap will vary in response to the changes in serum concentrations of anions and cations that contribute to acid–base balance. Normally, there are more unmeasured anions so the anion gap is usually positive.

$$\text{Corrected sodium} = [Na^+] + [1.6 \times (\text{plasma glucose mg/dL} - 100)]/100$$

This calculation adjusts the sodium according to the glucose value so as to more accurately evaluate sodium concentration. With hyperglycemia, water is pulled into the extracellular space, which tends to cause a dilutional hyponatremia. As hyperglycemia is corrected, the corrected sodium should rise accordingly.

$$\text{Effective osmolality} = 2\ [\ \text{measured } Na^+\ (mEq/L)] + [\text{glucose (mg/dL)}/18]$$

The effective osmolality measures deviation in serum water content. With diabetic ketoacidosis, the patient develops an extracellular fluid deficit that is clinically hard to measure. Calculation of the effective osmolality is useful during therapy to monitor this fluid volume.

Fluid replacement

All patients with DKA require supplemental fluids. Fluid and electrolyte replacement is administered very carefully to ensure restoration of circulating volume, replacement of sodium and the extracellular and intracellular fluid deficit of water, restoration of glomerular filtration with enhanced clearance of serum glucose and ketones, and avoidance of over-hydration (Wolfsdorf et al., 2009). Due to the hemodynamic derangements noted in DKA, special calculations are used throughout the process of correction to ensure precise biochemical monitoring and interpretation of the patient's clinical status (Table 24-18).

For moderate to severe DKA with poor perfusion, the fluid therapy starts with a 10–20 mL/kg bolus of 0.9% saline given over 1 to 2 hours. If poor tissue perfusion and hypotension persist, the fluid bolus may be repeated. In pediatric DKA treatment, it is important to avoid overaggressive fluid administration and instead opt for frequent reevaluations, and repeat boluses as necessary.

After the initial fluid bolus, repeat the blood gas, finger-stick blood glucose, and basic metabolic panel, as these results may change significantly with volume expansion. Following the initial fluid resuscitation, the remaining calculated deficits are replaced evenly over 36 to 48 hours using an isotonic fluid such as 0.9% normal saline with 30–40 mEq potassium per liter. Hold the supplementation of potassium until evidence of adequate kidney function appears and the serum potassium level is less than 6 mEq/L. The volume of fluids used for volume expansion should be subtracted from the total 24 hours' fluid calculation and the remainder administered over the first 24 hours. Urinary losses should not be replaced. Using traditional calculations for fluid volumes of maintenance plus dehydration replacement will yield excessive volumes for older children with severe dehydration. The total fluid rate should not exceed 1.5 to 2 times the typical daily maintenance fluid requirement based on age and weight or body surface area.

Introduction of oral fluids should occur when substantial clinical improvement is noted. When oral fluids are tolerated, the IV rate may be reduced. As the serum ketones have cleared, pH is normal, the serum bicarbonate is greater than 18 mmol/L, there is a normal anion gap, and oral intake is tolerated, transition from IV fluids and insulin to oral feeding and subcutaneous insulin may occur. If IV hydration continues during this transition, remove any dextrose from the base fluid; otherwise, the patient will experience persistent hyperglycemia.

Insulin

Insulin is usually started at 1 to 2 hours after initiation of fluid and electrolyte therapy. The continuous intravenous insulin infusion is delivered at 0.1 unit/kg/hr. *A loading dose or bolus of insulin is not recommended, as the goal of insulin therapy is to gradually replace effective circulating insulin, normalize blood glucose, and correct the ketoacidosis.* Hypoglycemia needs to be avoided because it will complicate the clinical picture with its concomitant hormonal counter-regulation. Mix the insulin infusion with 50 units of regular insulin added to 50 mL of normal saline to create an infusion in which there is 1 unit/1 mL. Insulin adheres to intravenous tubing; therefore, *flush the solution completely through the tubing with 20 mL to saturate binding sites and prevent further insulin adherence during therapy.* Omitting this step will lead to a much lower concentration of insulin given than desired and no improvement in the patient's biochemical state.

Continue to follow hourly serum glucose, pH, ketonemia, and serum electrolytes. Do *not* allow the glucose to fall faster than 100 mg/dL/hr. Glucose may be added to the maintenance IV fluids to maintain the blood glucose within the range of 200–250 mg/dL. Adjust the amount of glucose in the maintenance fluids (rather than decrease the insulin) to control the level and rate of fall of the blood glucose. The insulin infusion needs to remain continuous to treat the acidosis. Decrease the insulin infusion rate to 0.05 unit/kg/hr, or less, only if the patient shows significant sensitivity to insulin, as occurs in some very young children or patients with HHS, as long as the metabolic acidosis continues to resolve. The insulin infusion should be continued until the pH is greater than 7.3, the bicarbonate level is greater than 18 mmol/L, the serum ketones have cleared, or there is closure of the anion gap (Wolfsdorf et al., 2006).

Glucose

When the serum glucose is less than 250 mg/dL, 5% dextrose should be added to the maintenance fluid. Maintain serum glucose in the range of 200–250 mg/dL; if necessary, add higher concentrations of glucose. Switch to 10% dextrose when the serum glucose is less than 200 mg/dL.

Glucose supplementation provides a substrate for the insulin and prevents hypoglycemia as normal glucose metabolism is restored. If the patient is clinically improving and is no longer nauseated, supplemental oral intake may also be given to maintain the blood glucose in the target range. Remove the glucose from the IV fluid when it is time to stop the insulin infusion and the patient is ready to eat. This process of glucose titration is easier to accomplish if a multiple-bag IV system is used at the bedside, as it reduces the interruption in glucose administration when switching from one glucose concentration to another. Electrolyte supplements should be equal in each bag.

Electrolytes

Sodium.   Restoring electrolyte balance in DKA is a delicate process. Serum sodium deficits must be replaced by using 0.9% normal saline or Ringer's lactate as fluid deficit replacement for the first 4 to 6 hours of treatment. This treatment is followed with 0.45% normal saline with additional electrolytes. Hyperglycemia depresses serum sodium concentration because of movement of water into the extracellular fluid, causing a dilutional hyponatremia. It is important to calculate the corrected sodium concentration using the formula shown in Table 24-18 and to monitor changes in this level throughout therapy. The corrected sodium concentration is a much more accurate measure of dehydration in DKA because it takes into account the effect of hyperglycemia. As the hyperglycemia improves with treatment, the measured and corrected serum sodium should rise. Failure of the sodium level to rise or a decrease in serum sodium with DKA treatment is a worrisome sign and has been associated with cerebral edema, the most common cause of death in pediatric DKA (Wolfsdorf et al., 2009).

Potassium.   DKA is associated with total body depletion of potassium, regardless of the initial serum level. The largest loss of potassium comes from the intracellular space. As water leaves the cells due to increased serum osmolality, cellular potassium becomes increasingly more concentrated. This increased concentration drives up the potassium gradient, drawing potassium out of the cell. Potassium is also lost from the body with vomiting and renal excretion through elimination of ketones in the urine. Renal impairment in advanced DKA may also contribute to hyperkalemia through decreased elimination. Thus the potassium level can be high, low, or normal depending on these multiple factors.

Correction of acidosis and supplemental insulin both cause an intracellular shift of potassium back into the cells, resulting in a fall in serum concentration. Insulin administration should not start until severe hypokalemia is corrected. This shift may occur abruptly, after several hours of treatment, causing a precipitous fall in serum potassium and leading to fatal cardiac arrhythmias. The ECG will show flattening of the T wave, widening of the QT interval, and the appearance of U waves with hypokalemia (Wolfsdorf et al., 2006). As long as the patient is voiding, potassium replacement is started right after the initial volume expansion, or sooner, if the patient is hypokalemic; this treatment continues throughout IV therapy. The replacement potassium concentration should be 40 mEq/L and may be divided and given as 20 mEq/L of potassium chloride plus 20 mEq/L of potassium phosphate.

Phosphorus and calcium.   Depletion of intracellular phosphate also occurs in DKA due to acidosis, osmotic diuresis, and an intracellular shift caused by insulin given during treatment. Replacing phosphate with 20 mEq/L of potassium phosphate plus 20 mEq/L of potassium chloride minimizes the amount of chloride given, which in turn decreases the hyperchloremic metabolic acidosis that occurs in most patients. Hyperchloremic acidosis can complicate the interpretation of biochemical measurements made during the process of DKA therapy. Monitor the calcium and phosphorus levels every 12 hours, as phosphate replacement may cause hypocalcemia and tetany.

Bicarbonate.   In the majority of patients, DKA is reversible with fluid and insulin administration. Insulin addresses the source of acidosis by halting ketoacid production. It also stimulates the body's own production of bicarbonate from the metabolism of ketones.

Clinical trials have not been able to demonstrate any benefit of bicarbonate administration during the treatment for DKA. The risks of bicarbonate administration are well documented and include CNS acidosis, hypokalemia, and an association with cerebral edema. Therefore, the use of bicarbonate to correct acidosis is rarely necessary, except under the most extreme circumstances. These cases may include patients who experience shock, hypoxia, kidney failure, sepsis, cardiac insufficiency, severe academia, and life-threatening hyperkalemia. Give bicarbonate *only* if absolutely necessary (Cooke & Plotnick, 2008).

Cerebral edema recognition and therapy

Cerebral edema is the most serious complication of pediatric DKA and the most frequent diabetes-related cause of death in this population. Survivors are often left with serious neurological deficits. Symptomatic cerebral edema occurs in approximately 1% of patients with DKA, although asymptomatic cerebral swelling is believed to occur more frequently (Glaser et al., 2004). Typically, cerebral edema occurs 4 to 12 hours after the initiation of therapy, but it may occur earlier or later, and has been reported even before treatment is initiated. Risk factors for cerebral edema include younger age, new-onset diabetes, and a longer duration of symptoms. Risk factors at diagnosis and during treatment include a high BUN, severe acidosis, and hypocapnia. Patients may experience a gradual deterioration in level of consciousness or, more commonly, a gradual general improvement followed by sudden neurological deterioration (Table 24-19).

Cerebral edema requires rapid recognition and treatment. Reduce the rate of fluid administration by one-third and elevate the head of the bed. Hyperosmolar therapy with mannitol, 0.5–1 gm/kg IV over 20 minutes, should be immediately given. The mannitol therapy may be repeated if there is no response in 30 minutes to 2 hours. Hypertonic saline (3%), 5–10 mL/kg over 30 minutes, may be given as an alternative to mannitol, or as a second line of therapy if the patient did not respond to the initial dose of mannitol.

TABLE 24-19

Signs and Symptoms of Cerebral Edema

Headache

Bradycardia

Increasing blood pressure

Decreased oxygen saturation

Change in neurological status:

- Restlessness
- Irritability
- Increased drowsiness
- Incontinence
- Cranial nerve palsies
- Abnormal papillary responses
- Posturing

Intubation and mechanical ventilation may be necessary with progression of symptoms. A CT scan should be obtained after treatment has been initiated to evaluate for other causes of neurologic deterioration that may require additional therapy (Wolfsdorf et al., 2009).

Transitioning to subcutaneous insulin

The best time to convert to subcutaneous insulin is just before a meal. Because IV insulin lasts only a few minutes, give the rapid-acting subcutaneous insulin 10 to 15 minutes before discontinuing the insulin infusion so as to avoid rebound hyperglycemia.

Most newly diagnosed pediatric patients are started on a multiple daily injection regimen with basal and bolus insulin. Basal insulin is given once a day and has a 24-hour action profile with no peak. This insulin meets the body's basal needs for insulin, including hepatic glucose output, and provides blood glucose control throughout the night and between meals. At meal time, the blood glucose is checked and a dose of bolus insulin is calculated based on the pre-meal glucose and the carbohydrate content of the meal.

The amount of the total daily starting dose will vary based on the patient's stage of development and depending on whether he or she is in the recovery phase of DKA. After DKA treatment, a prepubertal child will need approximately 0.8 unit/kg/day of insulin. One-half of this dose is given as the once-a-day basal dose; the other one-half is used for pre-meal bolus dosing. The patient is given guidelines on how to dose the pre-meal bolus insulin. For example, the patient may need 1 unit for every 15 gm of carbohydrate in the meal plus one additional unit to correct hyperglycemia, for every 50 mg/dL over 150 mg/dL. The blood glucose should be checked prior to consuming a meal and two hours after the meal ends to evaluate the efficacy of the insulin-to-carbohydrate ratio and the correction factor. Bedtime glucose is compared to the fasting measurement to evaluate the basal dose.

Mild DKA: outpatient management

In some cases, DKA is very mild and the patient may be treated in the outpatient setting. These mild, early-onset cases are typically characterized by hyperglycemia with mild ketonemia or ketonuria and no evidence of serum acidosis. Patients can be started on subcutaneous insulin and oral hydration to clear the ketones.

Once the target blood glucose is identified, the patient is sent home with instructions to check the blood glucose before meals and at 2 A.M. and to notify the diabetes specialist on call of the evening blood glucose result. Patients are scheduled to return the next morning. Day 2 starts with a blood glucose check, an insulin dose, and breakfast in a supervised setting. After lunch, the patient and family may meet with the social worker for a family assessment and referrals to any needed resources. A plan is then outlined for return to maintenance management.

Patient and family education

Most caregivers are devastated at the time of the initial diagnosis of diabetes. Support systems aim to focus the family's and patient's energy on learning how to care for themselves and their child. Diabetes education should be ongoing throughout the hospitalization. Make families aware that they will need to know how to manage diabetes at home prior to the patient's discharge. The importance of insulin replacement should be highlighted by explaining that the often dramatic improvement in the child's condition was almost exclusively due to insulin. The action of insulin should be described, as well as the importance of eating after taking an insulin injection. Teach the patient and caregivers how to identify carbohydrate food servings on their child's meal tray. Caregivers need to make arrangements to stay with their child in the hospital to learn about appropriate diabetes care. Explaining these expectations will help prepare families to participate in the diabetes education process.

Four main skills need to be mastered before discharge:

- How to draw up and give insulin
- How to check the blood glucose and urine for ketones
- What to do if the blood glucose is too high or too low, or if the patient becomes ill
- What, when, and how to eat and keep a log

Caregivers should be taught to perform finger-stick sampling and measure blood glucose on the bedside meter, as they will need to master this skill prior to the patient's discharge, even if they may go home with a different meter. The procedures for finger-stick sampling are very similar for the various meters. Education with written instructions about maintaining the patient's blood glucose with the target range (80–180 mg/dL in most cases) and the signs and symptoms of hyperglycemia should begin while the child is receiving inpatient care. Glucose results need to tracked and analyzed by the caregivers so that they eventually can determine when a change in the dose is needed. Families with a member who is newly diagnosed with diabetes need to be in daily phone contact with the diabetes specialty team to get advice on insulin dose adjustments.

In patients with an established diagnosis of diabetes, the DKA admission creates an opportunity to evaluate their self-care skills and have the caregiver and child demonstrate their self-injection technique. In a child with known diabetes, the most common cause of DKA is omitted insulin injections. Emotional stress may be a clue to insulin omission (Silverstein

et al., 2005). Intercurrent illness may result in DKA, especially if sick-day management is not followed. Many patients will inadvertently stop insulin administration if they are too ill to eat. This behavior indicates a need for further education. Insulin should not be withheld, especially when the child is ill. Assess the events that occurred prior to the patient's admission. Ask about roles, including who is responsible for giving shots and how that was decided. Given the shortened lengths of stay in hospitals today, all teaching opportunities need to be optimized. Communicate all findings to the diabetes team who will continue to manage the patient after discharge.

DISPOSITION AND DISCHARGE PLANNING

Discharge criteria for the patient with new-onset diabetes are met when the DKA has resolved, education is complete, the child has appropriate adult supervision of care in the home and at school, the caregivers have been trained and have demonstrated competency with diabetes skills and knowledge, the family knows who to call and when to seek medical intervention, and the family has all required equipment and supplies. Eight basic supplies are needed for home care:

- Basal and bolus insulin
- Syringes
- Blood glucose meter with test strips and lancets
- Urine ketone testing strips
- Glucagon emergency kit

Follow-up care includes an appointment 2 weeks after discharge, with daily phone contact until the scheduled appointment with the endocrinology service.

As the patient is learning to master the basic concepts of diabetes self-care and develop a basic understanding of his or her blood glucose pattern, insulin pump therapy may be an option. Insulin pump therapy requires a highly motivated patient who has a good understanding of hypoglycemia and hyperglycemia management. The pump requires constant programming for meal doses and maintenance, including regular site changes. Blood glucose must be tested frequently and acted upon to utilize the pump to its fullest potential. Patients who follow safe pumping self-care guidelines may obtain excellent blood glucose control that is not possible with traditional insulin injection therapy.

The patient with recurrent DKA cannot be discharged until the cause of DKA is identified and resolved to prevent rehospitalization. Social services should be consulted to assess the family. Caregivers are ultimately responsible for providing appropriate diabetic care. Home care contracts that outline caregiver tasks of providing diabetes care support and supervision can help clarify these roles and responsibilities. A complete educational assessment and plan should be in place to manage the diabetes care at home.

If the patient has recurrent DKA, and after all supportive attempts have been provided, a report to child protective services should be made if evidence of caregiver medical neglect is present. This report should be initiated while the child is in the intensive care unit to underscore the severity and risk associated with insulin omission. The diabetes team can follow up on the report, as they will likely have an established relationship with the family. DKA is potentially a life-threatening situation that in most cases is completely preventable. Some families are unable to cope with the burden of managing a chronic illness in addition to other socioeconomic or emotional stressors that take priority. Diabetes self-management requires a great deal of self-discipline to perform all of the required care. Many barriers may impede a person's ability to perform the repetitive diabetes self-care skills 24 hours a day, 7 days a week. The child protective services team and community workers may be able to provide families with referrals and resources to relieve some of their social stressors so that more attention can be given to the diabetes home care.

Unlike type 1 diabetes, type 2 diabetes can be prevented in people at risk through lifestyle modification, including maintenance of normal body weight and regular exercise. In a recent study, Perreault et al. (2009) demonstrated that establishing healthy habits early in life before age-related changes in insulin secretion occur is most likely the best strategy for type 2 diabetes prevention in the pediatric population.

THYROID AND PARATHYROID DISORDERS

Rani Ganesan, Yasir Kazmi, and Richard Levy

The thyroid gland is located in the anterior aspect of the neck, just below and lateral to the thyroid cartilage. The primary role of the thyroid gland is to secrete thyroid hormones, including tri-iodothyronine (T_3) and thyroxine (T_4). These hormones are vital in regulating linear growth and development; carbohydrate, protein, and fat metabolism; and stimulation of protein synthesis.

The synthesis and release of T_3 and T_4 are regulated through feedback mechanisms. The beginning of the feedback loop starts at the hypothalamus, where thyrotropin-releasing hormone (TRH) is produced and secreted. The release of TRH stimulates the anterior pituitary to release thyroid-stimulating hormones (TSH). TSH then stimulates receptors located on the thyroid, which results in an increase uptake of iodine. This chain of reactions leads to the production and release of thyroid hormones. When high levels of thyroid hormones are present, the feedback loop is reversed: The high levels of T_3 and T_4 decrease the production of TRH, which leads to the slowed release of TSH and ultimately decreased synthesis and release of thyroid hormones. T_3 and T_4 are produced in the thyroid gland by the iodination of tyrosine. Iodine is primarily transported to the thyroid gland, where it is stored for thyroid hormone production. Iodination of tyrosine, by the enzyme known as thyroid peroxidase, forms both mono-iodotryosine (T_1) and di-iodotryosine (T_2). The combination of two T_2 molecules forms T_4, and the coupling of T_1 and T_2 forms T_3. T_3 and T_4 are stored in the thyroid as thyroglobulin, a thyroprotein found in material within the lumen of the thyroid follicle called colloid. When the thyroid is signaled by TSH, proteases and peptidases act upon the colloid collection to release T_4 and T_3 into the body's circulation.

Although there is approximately 50 times more T_4 available in the circulation, T_3 is the active thyroid hormone that acts upon target cells; it is three to four times more potent than T_4. The deiodination of T_4 at peripherally located target cells results in the formation of T_3. However, only the free (nonbound) thyroid hormone is able to enter cells and induce a cellular response. Approximately 99% of the circulating T_3 and T_4 are bound to carrier proteins (Chang et al., 2008). T_3 and T_4 are primarily bound to thyroxine-binding globulin (TBG)—50% and 70%, respectively. The remaining T_3 and T_4 are bound to transthyretin (prealbumin) and albumin. Only 0.03% of T_4 and 0.3% of T_3 are available in an unbound form. These unbound molecules are the active hormones. T_3 is able to freely enter cells and directly acts on the cellular nucleus, resulting in gene transcription modification. The amount of free hormone depends on the production of carrier proteins, which should be considered when analyzing hormone serum levels because these levels can change in various disease processes.

HYPERTHYROIDISM: THYROTOXICOSIS AND THYROID STORM

Pathophysiology

In normal physiologic states, thyroid hormone is responsible for maintaining the basal metabolic rates/demands at the cellular levels. When an excess of the T_3 and T_4 hormones is present in serum, the patient is deemed to be in a hyperthyroid state. The illness and severity spectrum of hyperthyroid diseases vary from mildly symptomatic to life threatening, as in a thyroid storm of thyrotoxicosis. The elevated levels of hormone act systemically by increasing cellular metabolism of fats and proteins (Nayak & Burman, 2006). Although the increased metabolism of these substrates consumes more energy, the thermal energy produced is markedly greater and is physiologically more significant. This thermal energy increases basal metabolic rates at the cellular level. While thyroid hormone works directly at the cellular level, elevated hormone levels also potentiate β-adrenergic receptors, thereby exaggerating sympathetic nervous system activity. This generalized hypermetabolic state of hyperthyroidism affects all of the body's organ systems.

Epidemiology and etiology

Incidence of hyperthyroidism varies among different pediatric age groups. The incidence in children 0 to 11 years of age is reported at 0.44 case per 1,000 population, whereas the group including 12- to 17-year-olds was reported to have an incidence of 0.59 case per 1,000 population (Emiliano et al., 2010).

Hyperthyroidism results from an increase in the synthesis, release, and/or intake of thyroid hormone. Furthermore, the etiology of hyperthyroidism can be classified as primary, secondary, or exogenous. *Primary* hyperthyroidism is characterized by increased synthesis and/or secretion of thyroid hormone related to the thyroid gland itself. *Secondary* hyperthyroidism refers to the increased production and secretion of hormone due to increased stimulation of the thyroid gland by the hypothalamus or pituitary. *Exogenous* causes refer to hyperthyroidism attributable to increased intake of supplemental hormone in patients with chronic hypothyroid states or medications that may alter the hypothalamus–pituitary–thyroid axis. The most common cause of hyperthyroidism in the pediatric population is primary thyroid disease of autoimmune etiology.

Graves' disease.
Graves' disease is the most common cause of thyrotoxicosis in children, with an incidence of 1 case per 5,000 population. This condition commonly emerges in early adolescence. Like most other autoimmune diseases, it is more prevalent in females, with a 5:1 female-to-male ratio; a positive family history of autoimmune thyroid disease is often present.

Graves' disease results from the production of thyroid-stimulating immunoglobulin (TSI) produced by B lymphocytes. TSI stimulates the production of thyroid hormone as it competes with TSH to bind at TSH receptor sites on the thyroid gland. Studies have demonstrated the placental transmission of TSI and the presence of thyrotoxicosis in 2% to 3% of neonates born to mothers with Graves' disease (Moshang, 2005), with neonatal morbidity rates as high as 20% (Strange et al., 2009), despite the transient nature of this condition.

The treatment of Graves' disease includes symptomatic management, antithyroid medications, radioactive iodine, and surgery. Radioactive iodine and surgery typically result in hypothyroidism and require chronic thyroid hormone supplementation.

Hashimoto's thyroiditis.
Another autoimmune insult to the thyroid gland that can cause hyperthyroid activity is chronic autoimmune (Hashimoto's) thyroiditis, which typically presents as a painless goiter. With Hashimoto's thyroiditis, the autoimmune destruction of the thyroid gland causes an initial surge of thyroid hormone, which may result in a severe hyperthyroid state. After this initial phase, the thyroid levels decline, often resulting in a chronic state of hypothyroidism.

Subacute thyroiditis.
Subacute thyroiditis is an uncommon, self-limiting inflammatory process of the thyroid gland, which may present with a painful goiter and fever secondary to viral infection or granulomatous disease. This inflammation of the thyroid gland has three physiologic phases: an initial period of hyperthyroidism, followed by hypothyroidism, with subsequent return to normal serum thyroid hormone levels and function. As autoimmunity is thought to be unlikely, the possibility of cell-mediated immunity against thyroid cell antigens must be considered. The exact etiology and pathophysiology of subacute thyroiditis remain unclear.

Mass lesions, exogenous hyperthyroidism, and other causes of hyperthyroidism.
Unlike their adult counterparts, children rarely present with thyroid nodules as a cause for hyperthyroidism; although rare, single nodules, or toxic adenomas, may be observed in children. Multinodule goiters are unusual (Chang et al., 2008) and are typically associated with neck irradiation. Although uncommon, some pituitary adenomas may secrete TSH, thereby directly increasing the synthesis and release of thyroid hormone. Theoretically, administration of iodine-containing dyes or medications might increase thyroid hormone levels by providing abundant iodine substrate, but this outcome is unlikely. Intentional or unintentional intake of thyroid replacement can produce a presentation similar to that noted with thyrotoxicosis. Many recent studies have demonstrated a relationship between amiodarone intake and hyperthyroidism.

Autosomal dominant hyperthyroidism is caused by genetic mutations occurring at TSH receptors, which is also known as central thyroid hormone resistance (reset "thyrostat"). As the negative feedback mechanism fails, it leads to a presentation similar to that noted in children with neonatal Graves' disease, except on a permanent basis. If peripheral tissues are also resistant, the patient may appear euthyroid despite the elevated levels of thyroid hormone and TSH.

Other special cases include McCune-Albright syndrome, a rare disease associated with hyperthyroidism and linked with a mutation of GNAS1 gene in 38% of cases (Dumitrescu & Collins, 2008). Molar pregnancies produce high levels of TSH and put those expectant mothers at risk for thyrotoxicosis. Teratomas of the ovary are also known to secrete T_4 from ectopic thyroid tissue.

Presentation

Children with thyrotoxicosis generally present in two age groups: the newborn period and early adolescence. The most common cause of congenital hyperthyroidism is placental transmission of TSH receptor antibodies from mothers suffering from Graves' disease to their unborn fetuses. In the first few days of life, newborns with this condition demonstrate nonspecific findings including irritability, wide-eye stares, and tachycardia. Other symptoms include irritability, poor feeding and weight gain, diarrhea, insomnia, goiter, hepatosplenomegaly, jaundice, and craniosynostosis. This presentation may last for weeks as levels of TSI persist in the infant's circulation. However, thyroid-binding inhibitory immunoglobulins (TBII) may also cross over to the fetus and block TSH receptors, causing transient hypothyroidism in the newborn.

It is important to elicit a family history of autoimmune disease, history of any recent viral infections, and a detailed medication history. Children with hyperthyroidism may have a history of developmental delays, behavior changes, declining academic performance, poor weight gain, increased appetite, frequent stools, vomiting, and fatigue. The physical examination of these children may include neurologic, cardiovascular, gastrointestinal, and ophthalmologic findings. Neurologically, patients may have an altered mental status, tremors, brisk deep tendon reflexes, delirium, psychosis, seizures, and eventual coma. Flow murmurs, various forms of supraventricular tachycardia, heart block, mitral valve prolapse, and an overactive precordium may be appreciated during cardiovascular evaluation. If left untreated, congestive heart failure and, in its most severe form, cardiac arrest may occur. Hepatic dysfunction is a commonly associated with jaundice. The presence of a goiter on neck exam is often considered a nonspecific finding. Compared to adults with hyperthyroidism, children have notably milder findings of exophthalmos on physical examination.

The overall history and physical examination findings of a child in a hyperthyroid state are consistent with a state of hypermetabolism.

Differential diagnosis

Because a patient with hyperthyroidism may initially present with a toxic appearance, such as high fever and signs of high cardiac output failure, the presentations may be similar to that of patients with septic shock or malignant hyperthermia. Hyperthyroidism can also imitate toxic ingestions of adrenergic agonists and anticholinergics, most commonly pesticides. Various neuropsychiatric etiologies should be considered when a patient presents with altered mental status, encephalopathy, and behavior changes. In addition to hyperthyroidism, gastrointestinal hyperactivity may be caused by severe gastroenteritis, liver dysfunction, and metabolic and electrolyte disturbances. Thyrotoxicosis is associated with many cardiovascular findings that can be confused with inherent arrhythmias (atrial flutter, atrial fibrillation, ventricular tachycardia), anatomic defects producing flow murmurs (mitral valve prolapse, valvular heart disease), and progressive congestive heart failure.

Plan of care

Thyroid function tests—usually TSH and free T_4 thyroxine levels—are obtained to assess the status of the patient's hypothalamic–pituitary–thyroid axis. TSH levels provide information about the function of the feedback mechanism of thyroid hormone to the pituitary. If the TSH level by itself is normal, it usually indicates normal thyroid function. TSH levels are very sensitive to free T_4 levels, so they are commonly used alone as a screening test for both hyperthyroidism and hypothyroidism. Low TSH levels are seen with hyperthyroidism, secondary hypothyroidism, L-thyroxine administration, critical illnesses, starvation, severe depression, and use of other drugs such as dopamine, serotonin agonists, glucocorticoids, opiates, and α-adrenergic antagonists.

The free T_4 level is measured to estimate the amount of biologically active thyroid hormone in circulation and is a reflection of thyroid gland function. The total T_4 (bound and unbound) level is difficult to interpret given its dependence on the amount of circulating carrier proteins. This amount varies from patient to patient.

Other thyroid laboratory tests useful in selective circumstances include total or free T_3, TBG, thyroid antibodies (thyroglobulin, thyroid peroxidase), and anti-TSH receptor antibodies (TSI, TBII).

Newborn screening results are often misinterpreted due to physiological changes occurring over the initial 3 to 5 days of life. It is also important to understand that premature infants have immature hypothalamus–pituitary–thyroid axes, which results in varying levels of TSH and free T_4. Preterm infants born before 30 weeks' gestation generally have low free T_4 levels, with normal to low TSH levels. This transient hypothyroidism typically corrects itself as the hormone axis matures between 4 and 8 weeks of age and as the thyroid hormone axis matures. Term and near-term infants demonstrate a TSH surge at birth that lasts approximately 2 to 3 days after birth, leading to increased levels of free T_4 and T_3. After 3 to 5 days of life, the TSH level usually falls into the normal range.

Newborn screening tests may measure only free T_4, only TSH, or both. The combination of the two screens reduces the false positive rates that would be seen if each individual test were used exclusively. Generally, TSH levels are normal after 72 hours of life.

Radiological testing may be performed to further delineate the cause of hypothyroidism or hyperthyroidism after initial evaluation with thyroid function tests. Sonography is used to evaluate soft-tissue structures of the thyroid. Scintigraphy is a nuclear medicine scan that uses radioactive tracers, consisting of technetium-99m (Tc-99m), which are coupled to various isotopes of iodine. Unlike sonography, scintigraphy is used to evaluate the thyroid gland's actual function, as it measures the gland's ability to take up iodine and produce thyroid hormone.

In Graves' disease, sonography reveals a diffuse, heterogeneous enlargement of the thyroid gland that appears hypoechoic (Chang et al., 2008). In contrast, the thyroid gland suffering from Hashimoto's thyroiditis will have a coarse echotexture. An actual abscess may be identified using sonography in patients with subacute thyroiditis.

Finally, when goiters or distinct nodules are present, ultrasound can aid with fine-needle aspiration (FNA) to sample single nodules and nodular hyperplasia (multiple nodules) for pathological analysis. When used in conjunction with scintigraphy, FNA can help delineate hormone-producing (hot) nodules from nodules that do not produce hormone (cold).

Initial diagnosis and management of thyroid storm should take place in hospital units with high monitoring capabilities, typically emergency departments and intensive care units. Basic and advanced life support algorithms are to be followed in regard to airway, breathing, and circulatory management (ABCs). Oxygen supplementation, venous access, and appropriate fluid resuscitation are critical components of care in these patients. Simultaneously, a patient's core temperature should be reduced with cooling blankets, ice packs, and administration of antipyretics. Salicylates should be avoided, as they can displace protein-bound thyroid hormone in circulation (Nayak & Burman, 2006).

First-line treatment in thyroid storm is methimazole or propylthiuracil (PTU) to block thyroid hormone synthesis. PTU has a rapid onset of action and works to block thyroid hormone synthesis and to decrease peripheral conversion of T_4 to T_3 (Strange et al., 2009). However, administration of PTU places the patient at high risk for severe liver injury and acute liver failure. Methimazole can block thyroid hormone synthesis but does not decrease conversion of T_4 to T_3 (Strange et al). Relative to PTU, this agent provides the advantage of less frequent dosing because of its longer half-life. However, its use should be avoided in pregnancy as it linked to a number of birth defects.

To block the release of thyroid hormone already synthesized in the thyroid, iodine compounds should be administered at least 1 hour after initiation of PTU or methimazole therapy. Examples include sodium iodide and Lugol's solution, which consists of 5% iodine (Strange et al., 2009). When given in large doses in a short period, iodine supplementation blocks the release of prestored hormone and decreases iodine transport. This inhibition of thyroid hormone synthesis usually persists for 48 hours as the thyroid adapts to higher levels of serum iodine (Nayak & Burman,

2006). If these agents are unavailable, a viable substitute is a radio contrast dye containing iodine, but it should be used with caution in patients with kidney disease.

Due to the aggressive nature of thyroid storm and the stress it places on the cardiovascular system, prompt administration of antiadrenergics, such as intermittent propranolol or continuous intravenous esmolol, is critical in these patients. Cardiac arrhythmias and congestive heart failure should be treated accordingly.

Finally, corticosteroids such as dexamethasone or hydrocortisone can be administered to decrease peripheral conversion of T_4 to T_3 (Strange et al., 2009).

In rare cases that are refractory to the treatment described previously, plasamapheresis has been used to physically remove thyroid hormone from circulation.

Disposition and discharge planning

Patients should be admitted to pediatric intensive care units for management of thyroid storm and its associated complications of congestive heart failure, severe liver injury, arrhythmias, and electrolyte management. Consultation with a pediatric endocrinologist should be obtained to tailor treatment needs for patients based on the underlying etiology. Finally, after stabilization and resolution, patients are discharged home, often with propranolol prescribed as deemed necessary.

HYPOTHYROIDISM

Hypothyroidism is defined as the presence of low levels of circulating thyroid hormone. Diagnosing hypothyroidism in a newborn can be difficult because of associated nonspecific clinical findings. The presenting signs of congenital hypothyroidism can be subtle and sometimes infants appear asymptomatic. For this reason, many states have adopted various types of thyroid screening tests to detect hypothyroidism early.

For newborns, the cause of hypothyroidism is usually primary—due to a dysfunctional thyroid gland or to the actual absence of the gland itself. Due to the varying degrees of serum thyroid hormone levels, the disease spectrum ranges from mild to severe. Normal thyroid hormone function in the fetus and during the early newborn period is necessary for optimal CNS development (Knobel, 2007). Congenital hypothyroidism (CH) may be considered a critical newborn condition due to its potentially irreversible and deleterious impact on the infant's neurodevelopment. Early identification via newborn screening has virtually eliminated mental retardation caused by hypothyroidism (Rovelt & Ehrlich, 2000). However, delayed treatment of hypothyroidism in the newborn leads to poor neurological outcomes with decreased cognitive functioning.

Pathophysiology

As mentioned in the section on hyperthyroidism, thyroid hormone availability is extremely important for neurodevelopment; linear growth; and carbohydrate, protein, and fat metabolism. Both β-adrenergic and sympathetic nervous system activity are slowed by low levels of circulating thyroid hormones, resulting in slower substrate metabolism. In contrast to hyperthyroidism, patients who are hypothyroid are in a hypometabolic state.

Epidemiology and etiology

The actual incidence of all cases of hypothyroidism in the pediatric population in the United States is unclear. Congenital hypothyroidism occurs in approximately 1 in every 4,000 live births, with a female-to-male ratio of 2:1 (Park & Chatterjee, 2005). The majority of cases are identified through government-mandated newborn screening tests. Hashimoto's thyroiditis is the most common cause of hypothyroidism in the United States after individuals reach 6 years of age, with a reported incidence of 13 cases per 1,000 population.

Similar to hyperthyroidism, there are many causes of hypothyroidism that should be considered when the suspicion for this condition is high.

Congenital hypothyroidism. Congenital hypothyroidism is the most common cause of hypothyroidism in the pediatric population, accounting for 85% of all cases (Park & Chatterjee, 2005); 98% of cases occur sporadically and 2% are familial (Chang et al., 2008). Down syndrome patients often have hypothyroidism due to thyroid dysgenesis (Polk & Fisher, 1998). There are three recognized forms of CH:

- *Aplastic thyroid* refers to the complete lack of structural thyroid tissue.
- *Hypoplastic thyroid dysgenesis* refers to a normally located thyroid gland with poor uptake and function.
- Abnormal location of functioning thyroid tissue is called *ectopic thyroid dysgenesis*. Ninety percent of the time, the glands are located at the base of the tongue and serve as the only source of functional thyroid tissue in 75% of patients (Chang et al., 2008).

CH patients also may have an inability to produce and secrete functional thyroid hormone. This inborn error of thyroxine synthesis, which is known as thyroid dyshormonogenesis, accounts for 10% of CH cases. Thyroid peroxidase (TPO) deficiency is the most common cause of thyroid dyshormonogenesis. In addition to structural and functional thyroid gland abnormalities, inadequate production or secretion of TRH or TSH by the hypothalamus and pituitary gland, respectively, may result in congenital hypothyroidism. In this case, both free T_4 and TSH levels are low.

Acquired hypothyroidism. Acquired hypothyroidism occurs later in childhood and is typically autoimmune in origin. This disorder has an increased prevalence in adolescent females. The child typically has a period of normal thyroid function but then suffers an insult to the thyroid gland, which eventually leads to thyroid dysfunction. Chronic lymphocytic thyroiditis (Hashimoto's) is the most common cause of acquired hypothyroidism.

Exogenous and other causes of hypothyroidism. Iodine is the primary substrate for thyroid hormone synthesis. Poor intake, such as is often seen in underdeveloped countries, can be associated with hypothyroid states.

Some medications and exogenous hormone supplements may lead to low levels of circulating thyroid hormone by directly affecting the thyroid gland. Medications that have been associated with decreased thyroid hormone production include lithium, iodide, and amiodarone. Dopamine, octreotide, and glucocorticoids have been associated with decreased TSH secretion by the pituitary gland.

Because thyroid function is largely regulated by the hypothalamus and pituitary, any disruption of the hypothalamus–pituitary–thyroid axis, such as might occur with trauma, surgery, radiation therapy, or other intracranial process, can lead to a decrease in hormone production by the gland. Along with the normal production and adequate secretion of thyroid hormone from the gland, normal peripheral utilization of thyroid hormone is essential to maintain cellular homeostasis. Although rare, peripheral target cells can become resistant to thyroid hormone and lead to a hypothyroid state in the presence of normal TSH and thyroid hormone levels.

Transient hypothyroidism in the newborn is another significant cause of concern. This condition occurs in as many as 3% to 5% of neonates, such that a state of hypothyroidism persists for a variable period of time (Knobel, 2007). A state of transient hypothyroidism is more prevalent in preterm infants due to hypothalamic immaturity or in critically ill pediatric patients. As the preterm infant approaches term gestation, thyroid hormone production typically reaches normal levels when the child is 4 to 8 weeks of age. Transient hypothyroidism may also arise when transmitted maternal TBII in Grave's disease blocks neonatal TSH receptors. Antithyroid drugs, such as PTU (used during pregnancy by affected mothers), can also result in transient hypothyroidism of the newborn.

Presentation

The presence of CH is often detected by newborn screening tests. Congenital hypothyroidism can lead to severe mental retardation if it goes untreated. Some of the hallmark physical examination findings associated with CH include a protuberant and large tongue, widened posterior fontanel, dry skin, large for gestational age status, hypotonia, bradycardia, and cool extremities. A rapid reduction in growth rate within the first week of life can be seen (Polk & Fisher, 1998). Behavioral abnormalities include difficulty feeding, difficulty with salivary secretion clearance, and the presence of a hoarse cry.

A high index of suspicion for acquired hypothyroidism is generally elicited through history of symptoms. Symptoms typically include weight gain, cold intolerance, constipation, lethargy, dry skin, and delayed puberty. In addition to symptoms elicited in history, poor growth velocity, presence of a goiter, enlarged or small thyroid gland, decreased pulse strength, bradycardia, and delayed bone age on radiograph objectively support the diagnosis of acquired hypothyroidism. Diffusely enlarged glands are usually due to lymphocytic invasion, which more commonly presents with autoimmune thyroiditis. Palpation of the gland is generally painless, and it is noted to have a rough consistency. Diffusely enlarged thyroids are typically present in patients who are hypothyroid due to iodine deficiency.

Although extremely rare in the pediatric population, myxedema coma results from a longstanding hypothyroid state and is considered a medical emergency. Implementation of newborn screening has led to decline in the incidence of this potential neurologic catastrophe (Dang & Kearney, 2006).

Differential diagnosis

Due to the nonspecific signs and symptoms associated with hypothyroidism, it is important to investigate other abnormalities commonly observed in children. Diseases associated with poor weight gain and feeding difficulties, such as congenital cardiac and pulmonary etiologies, should be investigated. The symptoms of malabsorption and nutritional deficiencies mimic those of hypothyroidism. Although chronic constipation may be evident in an individual with undiagnosed hypothyroidism, behavioral constipation remains the most common cause of constipation in the pediatric population. As linear growth delay is a common symptom of hypothyroidism, caregivers and pediatricians should have a higher level of suspicion for constitutional growth delay and growth hormone deficiencies.

Plan of care

Thyroid function tests, usually measuring TSH and free T_4 levels, are obtained to assess the hypothalamic–pituitary–thyroid axis. TSH tests measure the efficiency of the feedback mechanism between thyroid hormone and the pituitary gland. If serum TSH is normal, this finding usually represents normal thyroid function. TSH levels are very sensitive to free T_4 levels; thus they are commonly used alone as a screening test for both hyperthyroidism and hypothyroidism.

Other thyroid laboratory tests useful in selective circumstances include total or free T_3, TBG, thyroid antibodies (thyroglobulin, thyroid peroxidase), and anti-TSH receptor antibodies (TSI, TBII).

Newborn screening results are often misinterpreted due to physiological changes occurring over the initial 3 to 5 days of life. It is also important to understand that premature infants have immature hypothalamus–pituitary–thyroid axes, which results in varying levels of TSH and free T_4. Preterm infants born before 30 weeks' gestation generally have low free T_4 levels, with normal to low TSH levels. This transient hypothyroidism typically corrects itself as the hormone axis matures between 4 to 8 weeks of age and as the thyroid hormone axis matures. Term and near-term infants demonstrate a TSH surge at birth that lasts approximately 2 to 3 days after birth, leading to increased levels of free T_4 and T_3. After 3 to 5 days of life, the TSH is usually within the normal range.

Newborn screening tests measure only free T_4, only TSH, or both. The combination of the two screens reduces the false positive rates that might otherwise be seen if each individual test were used exclusively. Since TSH levels are normal after 72 hours of life, an elevated TSH level after this time, with a low or normal free T_4 level, is consistent with congenital hypothyroidism and should be dealt with promptly. Marginal TSH elevations may represent transient hypothyroidism and require further follow-up and evaluation.

Radiologic testing. Radiological testing is not commonly used for screening purposes, but rather is employed to further delineate the cause of hypothyroidism or hyperthyroidism after initial evaluation with thyroid function tests. Sonography is generally used to evaluate soft-tissue structures of the thyroid. Scintigraphy is a nuclear medicine scan that uses a radioactive tracer, technetium-99m (Tc-99m), which is coupled to various isotopes of iodine. Unlike sonography, scintigraphy is used to evaluate the thyroid gland's actual function as it measures the gland's ability to take up iodine and to produce thyroid hormone.

Profound neurological impairment is one of the most severe morbidities associated with hypothyroidism; thus immediate hormone supplementation, in the cases of high clinical suspicion or at the time of diagnosis, is critical. Exogenous T_4, in the form of levothyroxine, is supplemented because it is peripherally converted to active T_3. During the initial treatment of congenital hypothyroidism, the goal is to reach normal T_4 concentrations by 2 weeks of life and normal TSH levels at one month of age (Knobel, 2007). For newborns and critically ill pediatric patients with transient hypothyroidism, there is no consensus on the most appropriate treatment strategy. However, if T_4 levels remain low at 6 weeks of life in preterm infants, initiation of treatment is recommended (Rose et al., 2006). In all cases of CH, treatment delayed beyond 6 weeks of life leads to risk of delayed cognitive development.

Disposition and discharge planning

Children with hypothyroidism need follow-up care with a pediatric endocrinologist. In the early phases of treatment, the intensity of follow-up depends on the frequency of medication adjustments, symptoms, and the age of the patient. Because long-term neurologic prognosis largely depends on the timing of treatment in CH, it is critical to follow the patient's neurodevelopment and linear growth during the first year of treatment (Park & Chatterjee, 2005). Communication with the primary care provider is encouraged to reinforce the need for overall care for the child.

PARATHYROID GLAND FUNCTION

The four parathyroid glands are located posterior to the thyroid gland and lie in close proximity to the thymus. Their primary responsibilities are to tightly regulate the amount of calcium present in serum and in bone, and to some degree, the body's stores of phosphate. Derailments in parathyroid function lead to hypocalcemic or hypercalcemic states, which may be life-threatening.

Similar to what occurs with thyroid hormone, production and secretion of parathyroid hormone are regulated through feedback mechanisms. When serum calcium levels drop, the calcium-sensitive receptors of the parathyroid gland initiate the release of parathyroid hormone (PTH) into circulation.

PTH released into circulation works to regulate serum calcium levels at primarily three different organ systems: musculoskeletal, kidney, and gastrointestinal. This hormone indirectly stimulates osteoclast-induced bone resorption. Over time, this destruction of bone results in an increase in serum calcium and, to a lesser degree, serum phosphate. PTH also stimulates calcium absorption and phosphate excretion at the distal tubules of the kidney. In the setting of chronic kidney failure, the patient's ability to retain calcium and eliminate phosphate is significantly impaired, resulting in an increased level of circulating parathyroid hormone. PTH also upregulates the enzyme involved in the activation of vitamin D. In its active form, vitamin D controls absorption of intestinal calcium through its relationship with calbindin.

When caring for critically ill patients, consideration of the parathyroid gland's role in electrolyte disturbances is important.

Hyperparathyroidism

Elevation of serum intact PTH levels is referred to as hyperparathyroidism. The incidence of primary hyperparathyroidism in the pediatric population is unclear, but its diagnosis should raise suspicion for parathyroid adenomas and multiple endocrine neoplasia (MEN) I and II syndromes. Both of these conditions are rare in children. Secondary hyperparathyroidism typically occurs in patients with chronic kidney failure who have lower calcium and higher phosphate levels.

As there are no current treatments to block the effects of elevated PTH in primary hyperparathyroidism, symptomatic treatment of hypercalcemia is important. Patients with mildly elevated serum calcium levels are often asymptomatic. Nonspecific symptoms include constipation, bone pain, depression, altered mental status, anorexia, vomiting, kidney stones, and arrhythmias. Severe hypercalcemia can lead to life-threatening arrhythmias, cardiac arrest, and coma. Treatment is directed at managing the elevated serum calcium levels. Hydration, diuretics (for their calcium-losing properties), phosphate binders in patients with kidney failure, and rarely dialysis may be used as therapies.

Hypoparathyroidism

When serum PTH levels are low, patients are considered to be in a hypoparathyroid state. Although uncommon in children, primary hypoparathyroidism in the pediatric population has been associated with aplastic development of the parathyroid. These disorders are typically abnormalities that occur during embryonologic development of midline structures, including the thymus and parathyroids. Velocardiofacial defects, including DiGeorge syndrome, are the most common of these syndromes. Hypoparathyroidism can also occur with any throat or neck trauma, surgery involving the neck/throat, and thyroid surgeries. The hypocalcemia that results from hypoparathyroidism can lead to tetany, seizures, and life-threatening cardiac arrhythmias if left untreated. Timely calcium and vitamin D supplementation are required to manage this condition.

REFERENCES

1. American Diabetes Association (ADA). (2000). Consensus statement: Type 2 diabetes in children and adolescents. *Diabetes Care, 23,* 381–389.
2. Arafah, M. (2006). Review: Hypothalamic–pituitary–adrenal function during critical illness limitations of current assessment methods. *Journal of Clinical Endocrinology and Metabolism, 91,* 3725–3745.

3. Arieff, A., Ayus, J., & Fraser, C. (1992). Hyponatremia and death or permanent brain damage in healthy children. *British Medical Journal, 304*(6836), 1218–1222.

4. Arvanitis, M., & Pasquale, J. (2005). External causes of metabolic disorders. *Emergency Medicine Clinics of North America, 23*(3), 827–841.

5. Bajpai, A., Kabra, M., & Menon, P. (2008). Central diabetes insipidus: Clinical profile and factors indicating organic etiology in children. *Indian Pediatrics, 45*(6), 463–468.

6. Beishuizen, A., Vermes, I., Hylkema, B., & Haanen, C. (1999). Relative eosinophilia and functional adrenal insufficiency in critically ill patients. *Lancet, 353*, 1675–1676.

7. Berkenbosch, J., Lentz, C., Jimenez, D., & Tobias, J. (2002). Cerebral salt wasting syndrome following brain injury in three pediatric patients: Suggestions for rapid diagnosis and therapy. *Pediatric Neurosurgery, 36*(2), 75–79.

8. Brown-Séquard, C. (1856). Recherchés experimentales sur la physiologic et la pathologie des capsules surrenales. *Archives Générales de Médecine*, ser 5(8), 385–401.

9. Bussmann, C., Bast, T., & Rating, D. (2001). Hyponatremia in children with acute CNS disease: SIADH or cerebral salt wasting? *Nervous System, 17*(9), 58–62.

10. Carcillo, J., & Fields, A. (2002). Clinical practice parameters for hemodynamic support of pediatric and neonatal patients in septic shock. *Critical Care Medicine, 30*(60), 1365–1378.

11. Centers for Disease Control and Prevention (CDC). (2000). Growth charts. Retrieved from http://www.cdc.gov/growthcharts/charts.htm

12. Chang, Y., Hong, H., & Choit, D. (2008). Sonography of the pediatric thyroid: A pictorial essay. *Journal of Clinical Ultrasound, 37*(3), 149–157.

13. Cheethan, T., & Baylis, PH. (2002). Diabetes insipidus: pathophysiology, diagnosis & management. *Pediatric Drugs, 4*(12), 785–796.

14. Cooke, D., & Plotnick, L. (2008). Management of diabetic ketoacidosis in children and adolescents. *Pediatric Review, 29*, 431–436.

15. Craig, M., Hattersley, A., & Donaghue, K. (2009). ISPAD clinical practice consensus guidelines 2009: Compendium definition, epidemiology and classification of diabetes in children and adolescents. *Pediatric Diabetes, 10* (suppl 12), 3–12.

16. Dang, C., & Kearney, T. (2006). Diabetic and endocrine emergencies. *Postgraduate Medical Journal, 83*, 79–86.

17. den Brinker, B., Joosten, K., Liem, O., de Jong, F., Hop, W., Hazelzet, J., et al. (2005). Adrenal insufficiency in meningococcal sepsis: Bioavailable cortisol levels and impact of interleukin-6 levels and intubation with etomidate on adrenal function and mortality. *Journal of Clinical Endocrinology and Metabolism, 90*, 5110–5117.

18. Donati-Genet, P., Dubuis, J., Giradin, E., & Rimensberger, P. (2001). Acute symptomatic hyponatremia and cerebral salt wasting after head injury: An important clinical entity. *Journal of Pediatric Surgery, 36*(7), 1094–1097.

19. Donohoue, P. (2006a). Adrenal cortex. In McMillan, J. (Ed.), *Oski's principles and practice* (4th ed., pp. 2133–2143). Philadelphia: Lippincott.

20. Donohoue, P. (2006b). Adrenal medulla. In McMillan J. (Ed.), *Oski's principles and practice* (4th ed., pp. 2143–2145). Philadelphia: Lippincott.

21. Dumitrescu, C., & Collins, M. (2008). McCune-Albright syndrome. *Orphanet Journal of Rare Diseases, 3*, 1–12.

22. Emiliano, A., Governale, L., Parks, M., & Cooper, D. (2010, March 24). Shifts in propylthiouracil and methimazole prescribing practices: Antithyroid drug use in the United States from 1991 to 2008. *Journal of Clinical Endocrinology and Metabolism, 95*(5), 2227–2233.

23. Felner, E., Thompson, M., Ratliff, A., White, P., & Dickson, B. (2000). Time course of recovery of adrenal function in children treated for leukemia. *Journal of Pediatrics, 137*, 21–24.

24. Fernandez, E., Montman, R., & Watterberg, K. (2008). ACTH and cortisol response to critical illness in term and late preterm newborns. *Journal of Perinatology, 28*(12), 797–802.

25. Ganie, M. A., & Bhat, D. (2009). Current developments in Wolfram syndrome. *Journal of Pediatric Endocrinology & Metabolism, 22*(1), 3–10.

26. Glaser, N., Wootton-Gorges, S., Marcin, J., Buonocore, M., DiCarlo, J., Neely, K., et al. (2004). Mechanism of cerebral edema in children with diabetic ketoacidosis. *Journal of Pediatrics, 145*, 164–171.

27. Harrigan, M. R. (2001). Cerebral salt wasting syndrome. *Critical Care Clinics, 17*(1), 125–138.

28. Hassoun, A., & Oberfield, S. (2008). Adrenal dysfunction. In Nichols D. (Ed.), *Rogers' textbook of pediatric intensive care* (4th ed., pp. 1584–1597). Philadelphia: Lippincott.

29. Haviv, M., Haver, E., Lichtstein, D., Hurvitz, H., & Klar, A. (2005). Atrial natriuretic peptide in children with pneumonia. *Pediatric Pulmonology, 40*(4), 306–309.

30. Jimenez, R., Casado-Flores, J., Nieto, M., & Garcia-Teresa, M. A. (2006). Cerebral salt wasting syndrome in children with acute central nervous system injury. *Pediatric Neurology, 35*(4), 261–263.

31. Kappy, M. S., & Ganong, C. A. (1996). Cerebral salt wasting in children: The role of atrial natriuretic hormone. *Advances in Pediatrics, 43*, 271–308.

32. Kim, R. J., Malattia, C., Allen, M., Moshang, T., & Maghnie, M. (2004). Vasopressin and desmopressin in central diabetes insipidus: Adverse effects and clinical considerations. *Pediatric Endocrinology Reviews, 2*(1), 115–123.

33. Knobel, R. (2007). Thyroid hormone levels in term and preterm neonates. *Neonatal Network, 26*(4), 253–259.

34. Langer, M., Modi, B., & Agus, M. (2006). Adrenal insufficiency in the critically ill neonate and child. *Current Opinion in Pediatrics, 18*(4), 448–453.

35. Lin, M., Liu, S., & Lim, I. (2005). Disorders of water imbalance. *Emergency Medicine Clinics of North America, 23*(3), 749–770.

36. Maghnie, M. (2003). Diabetes Insipidus. *Hormone Research, 59*(suppl 1), 42–54.

37. Majzoub, J., & Srivatsa, A. (2006). Diabetes insipidus: Clinical and basic aspects. *Pediatric Endocrinology Reviews, 4*(suppl 1), 60–65.

38. Menon, K., Ward, R., Lawson, M., Gabourg, J., Hutchison, J., Hebert, P., et al. (2010). A prospective multi-center study of adrenal function in critically ill children. *American Journal of Respiratory and Critical Care Medicine 182*, 246–251.

39. Miller, B., & McAtee, I. (2009). Endocrine testing. In K., Sarafoglou, G., Hoffmann, & K. Roth (Eds.). *Pediatric endocrinology and inborn errors of metabolism*. New York: McGraw-Hill.

40. Moritz, M., & Ayus, J. (2002). Disorders of water metabolism in children. *Pediatrics in Review, 23*(11), 371–380.

41. Moshang, T. (2005). *Pediatric endocrinology: The requisites in pediatrics*. St. Louis: Elsevier Mosby.

42. Nayak, B., & Burman, K. (2006). Thyrotoxicosis and thyroid storm. *Endocrinology and Metabolism Clinics of North America, 35*, 663–686.

43. Park, S., & Chatterjee, V. (2005). Genetics of congenital hypothyroidism. *Journal of Medical Genetics, 42*, 379–389.

44. Perreault, L., Kahn, S., Christophi, C., Knowler, W., & Hamman, R. (2009). Regression from pre-diabetes to normal glucose regulation in the diabetes prevention program. *Diabetes Care, 32*(9), 1583–1588.

45. Peterson, K., Muller, J., Rasmussen, M., & Schmiegelow, K. (2003). Impaired adrenal function after glucocorticoid therapy in children

with acute lymphoblastic leukemia. *Medical and Pediatric Oncology, 41,* 110–114.

46. Pizarro, C., Troster, E., Damiani, D., & Carcillo, J. (2005). Absolute and relative adrenal insufficiency in children with septic shock. *Critical Care Medicine, 33,* 855–859.

47. Polk, D., & Fisher, D. (1998). Disorders of the thyroid gland. In H. Taeusch & R. Ballard (Eds.). *Avery's diseases of the newborn* (7th ed., pp. 1224–1233). Philadelphia: Saunders.

48. Rauf, S., & Roberts, N. (1999). Supportive management in bacterial meningitis. *Infectious Disease Clinics of North America, 13*(3), 647–659.

49. Rivkees, S. (2008). Differentiating appropriate antidiuretic hormone secretion, inappropriate antidiuretic hormone secretion and cerebral salt wasting: The common, uncommon, and misnamed. *Current Opinion in Pediatrics, 20*(4), 448–452.

50. Rose, S., Kaplowitz, P., Kaye, C., Sudararajan, S., & Varma, S. (2006). Update of newborn screening and therapy for congenital hypothyroidism. *Pediatrics, 117*(6), 2290–303.

51. Rovelt, F., & Ehrlich, R. (2000). Psychoeducational outcome in children with early-treated congenital hypothyroidism. *Pediatrics, 105,* 515–522.

52. Sane, K., & Sane, S. (2009). Radiographic imaging. In K., Sarafoglou, G., Hoffmann, & K. Roth (Eds.). *Pediatric endocrinology and inborn errors of metabolism.* New York: McGraw-Hill.

53. Shulman, D., Palmert, M., & Kemp, S. (2007). Adrenal insufficiency: Still a cause of morbidity and death in childhood, *Pediatrics, 119*(2), e484–e494.

54. Silverstein, J., Klingensmith, G., Copeland, K., Plotnick, L., Kaufman, F., Laffel, L., et al. (2005). Care of children and adolescents with type 1 diabetes. *Diabetes Care, 28*(1), 186–212.

55. Singh, S., Bohn, D., Carlotti, A., Cusimano, M., Rutka, J., & Halperin, M. (2002). Cerebral salt wasting: Truths, fallacies, theories, and challenges. *Critical Care Medicine, 30*(11), 2575–2579.

56. Srinivas, R., Brown, S. D., Chang, Y. F., Garcia-Fillion, P., & Adelson, D. (2010). Endocrine function in children acutely following severe traumatic brain injury. *Childs Nervous System, 26*(5), 647–653.

57. Strange, G., Ahrens, W., Schafermeyer, R., & Wiebe, R. (2009). *Pediatric emergency medicine* (3rd ed.). New York: McGraw Hill.

58. Vinclair, M., Broux, C., Faure, P., Brun, J., Genty, C., Jacquot, C., et al. (2008). Duration of adrenal inhibition following a single dose of etomidate in critically ill patients. *Intensive Care Medicine, 34*(4), 714–719.

59. White, P., Gonzalez, J., & Marks, J. (1997). Acute adrenocortical insufficiency. In D. Levin & F. Morriss (Eds.). *Essentials of pediatric intensive care* (2nd ed., pp. 571–576). New York: Churchill.

60. Wolfsdorf, J., Craig, M., Daneman, D., Dunger, D., Edge, J., Lee, W., et al. (2009). ISPAD clinical practice consensus guidelines 2009: Compendium definition, epidemiology and classification of diabetes in children and adolescents. *Pediatric Diabetes, 10*(suppl 12), 118–133.

61. Wolfsdorf, J., Glaser, N., & Sperling, M. (2006). American Diabetes Association consensus statement: Diabetic ketoacidosis in infants, children and adolescents. *Diabetes Care, 29*(5), 1150–1159.

Fluid, Electrolytes, and Nutrition

PHYSIOLOGY AND DIAGNOSTICS

Sammé Fuchs

Nutrition is a crucial component of the clinical management of hospitalized pediatric patients. Suboptimal nutritional intake can result in malnutrition as well as poor recovery and outcomes. Malnutrition is defined as a deficiency or excess of energy substrate, protein, and micronutrients that results in measurable adverse outcomes on tissue, anthropometrics, and physical function. Malnutrition can be acute, chronic, or a combination of the two. Preexisting or chronic malnutrition may occur in patients due to underlying chronic illness, poor food choices, or neglect. As many as 44% of pediatric patients with various types of congenital heart disease are chronically malnourished. Although few studies have been published in the literature, it has been reported that the prevalence of acute malnutrition in hospitalized pediatric patients with assorted diagnoses ranges from 6.1% to 40.9% (Joosten & Hulst, 2008).

Events that can lead to acute malnutrition include decreased appetite due to pain, nausea, or pharmacotherapeutics, resulting in subsequent suboptimal oral intake. Nothing by mouth (NPO) status for procedures or surgery, malabsorption, increased energy expenditure, and failure to adequately monitor nutrition status may also contribute to acute malnutrition.

Ongoing nutritional screening should be implemented to identify children at risk of malnutrition during hospitalization (Gibbons & Fuchs, 2009). The Joint Commission (TJC) mandates that all hospitalized patients receive initial nutrition screening within 24 hours of admission (TJC, 2009).

EBB AND FLOW PHASES OF METABOLISM

Hospitalized pediatric patients experience mild to significant alterations in metabolism. In severe injury, such as burns or major trauma, physiologic events proceed through two phases: the ebb and the flow.

The initial, or ebb, phase lasts 3 to 5 days post injury. It is characterized by shock, loss of plasma volume, poor tissue perfusion, and a decrease in blood pressure, plasma insulin, oxygen consumption, cardiac output, and body temperature. Decreased oxygen consumption results in hypometabolism and decreased basal energy expenditure. Basal energy expenditure is the minimum amount of energy required to maintain basic body function such as breathing, temperature regulation, circulation, and peristalsis.

Following the ebb phase, the body enters the state known as the flow phase. This phase is characterized by prolonged hypermetabolism, primarily as a result of the release of catecholamines, glucocorticoids, and glucagon (Gottschlich & Mayes, 2005). This counter-regulatory hormone cascade is proportional to the magnitude and nature of the injury and has significant nutritional implications.

CATECHOLAMINES

The release of catecholamines results in the reduction of insulin secretion and peripheral insulin action. It also stimulates the production of both glucagon and adrenocorticotrophic hormone (ACTH). The release of ACTH causes increased production of corticosteroids, which inhibits insulin activity. In contrast, the increased glucagon levels mobilize amino acids from skeletal muscle for gluconeogenesis. Cortisol facilitates the mobilization of amino acid from skeletal muscle, stimulates glucagon production, and mediates lipolysis and release of free fatty acids. In addition, release of epinephrine causes increased levels of free fatty acids and glucose and suppresses insulin. This counter-regulatory hormonal cascade results in glycogen storage depletion, hyperglycemia, lipid intolerance, and protein catabolism (Kinney, 1995).

GLUCOSE

Glycogen reserves—the stored form of glucose—become depleted quickly during acute illness and injury. Glucose is the primary source of fuel for the brain and is useful in the repair of injured tissues. It also provides fuel for erythrocytes and the renal medulla. Rapid glycogen depletion results in gluconeogenesis. The provision of dietary glucose in metabolically stressed pediatric patients does not attenuate gluconeogenesis, so protein catabolism tends to persist in these individuals. Hence, the practice of providing increased intake of carbohydrates in an attempt to spare protein has been abandoned (Mehta et al., 2009b).

HYPERGLYCEMIA

Hyperglycemia occurs frequently in acutely and chronically stressed hospitalized pediatric patients. It occurs through multiple mechanisms, including the counter-regulatory hormone-mediated upregulation of gluconeogenesis and glycogenolysis, as well as downregulation of glucose transporters resulting in decreased utilization of glucose by tissues such as skeletal muscle and liver. Historically, a hyperglycemic state was thought to be beneficial, providing energy substrate to vital organs, such as the brain and myocardium. Hyperglycemia had also been thought to compensate for volume loss by promoting the shift of cellular fluid into the intravascular compartment (Faustino & Apkon, 2005).

More recently, these beliefs have been challenged by the results of studies examining morbidity and mortality outcomes. Despite a paucity of research in the area of hyperglycemia in hospitalized pediatric patients, some studies have demonstrated that hyperglycemia is associated with poor outcomes, and suggested that maintaining glycemic control may improve morbidity and mortality rates in certain pediatric populations (Preissig & Rigby, 2009). Additional studies in the pediatric population are needed to elucidate the effects that tight glycemic control may have on morbidity and mortality rates.

ACUTE-PHASE PROTEINS

Hepatic protein synthesis changes during periods of inflammation. Notably, production of positive acute-phase proteins such as C-reactive protein (CRP) increases and production of negative acute-phase proteins such as albumin and prealbumin decreases (Gabay & Kushner, 1999). Alterations in protein metabolism can predict mortality in postoperative pediatric patients, intensive care outcomes, and response to nutrition support during inflammation with acute illness and injury. Specifically, an inverse relationship exists between preoperative serum albumin and hospital length of stay, infection, and mortality in surgical pediatric patients. Growth is stunted during periods of inflammation (Skillman & Wischmeyer, 2009).

LIPIDS

Lipid turnover increases in surgery, trauma, and critical illness, suggesting that the primary energy source in metabolically stressed pediatric patients is fatty acids (Coss-Bu et al., 2001). The limited fat reserves of infants and children, paired with the increased demand for fatty acids, can result in essential fatty acid deficiency (EFAD) if insufficient amounts of fat are administered as part of the diet. Indeed, EFAD can develop within days in neonates receiving parenteral nutrition without intravenous fat emulsion. Linoleic and alpha-linolenic fatty acids are considered essential, as the body does not synthesize them.

The clinical presentation of essential fatty acid deficiency consists of alopecia, scaly dermatitis, hepatomegaly, thrombocytopenia, fatty liver, anemia, and increased susceptibility to infection. A triene:tetratriene ratio of greater than 0.4 is the biochemical marker used to diagnose EFAD. To prevent EFAD, provision of 1% to 2% of daily energy needs from linoleic acid and 0.5% of daily energy needs from linolenic acid is recommended (Canada et al., 2009).

ENERGY EXPENDITURE

Energy expenditure varies widely in acute injury and illness due to wide ranges of metabolic alterations, though there is a marked tendency toward hypermetabolism in the early phase. Pediatric patients with extreme thermal injury become significantly hypermetabolic. Conversely, critically ill patients who are sedated, pharmacologically paralyzed, and ventilated may have significantly reduced energy expenditure due to decreased activity and stunting of growth during inflammation (Mehta et al., 2009b).

ENERGY REQUIREMENTS

Estimating energy requirements accurately in hospitalized pediatric patients is essential to provide adequate nutrition. The use of predictive equations to estimate energy needs is unreliable (Mehta et al., 2009a). Indirect calorimetry is a method used to more accurately predict energy expenditure; it measures oxygen consumed (V_{O_2}) and carbon dioxide produced (V_{CO_2}). The results of the measurement of these gases are then used to calculate resting energy via the Weir equation (Table 25-1). Indirect calorimetry also measures the respiratory quotient (V_{CO_2}/V_{O_2}).

ADVANTAGES AND LIMITATIONS OF INDIRECT CALORIMETRY

Indirect calorimetry measurements provide useful information about substrate metabolism and help prevent overfeeding or underfeeding. Some of these measurements are performed using a continuous metabolic monitor, but measurements as short as 15 minutes can elucidate 24-hour energy expenditures. Indirect calorimetry should not be used during hemodialysis or continuous renal replacement therapy, when the fraction of inspired oxygen (FiO_2) is greater than 60%, or if endotracheal tubes have significant air leaks, as results will be inaccurate in these scenarios (Skillman & Wischmeyer, 2009). Cost and need for technical support are limiting factors that may rule out the routine use of indirect calorimeters in the hospital setting. Therefore, it is recommended that indirect calorimetry be performed on patients who are at highest risk of metabolic

TABLE 25-1

The Weir Equation
REE = $[V_{O_2} (3.941) + V_{CO_2} (1.11)] \times 1440$ min/day

Source: American Association for Respiratory Care, 2004.

alterations (Table 25-2) (Mehta et al., 2009a). If indirect calorimetry results are not available, predictive equations may be used to estimate energy needs. Nevertheless, very close monitoring of anthropometric, biochemical, clinical, and dietary data is essential to prevent overfeeding or underfeeding (Table 25-3).

OVERFEEDING AND UNDERFEEDING

Both overfeeding and underfeeding can have deleterious effects on hospitalized pediatric patients. Overfeeding places additional stress on organ systems and can increase the risk of morbidity and mortality. Carbohydrate intake in significant excess of what the patient expends promotes hyperglycemia, lipogenesis, and increased CO_2 production, and can prolong the requirement for mechanical ventilation and increase the hospital length of stay. When nutrition goals are based on predictive equations in critically ill, mechanically ventilated patients, overfeeding of parenteral or enteral solutions can easily occur.

TABLE 25-2

Suggested Criteria for Selecting Patients for Indirect Calorimetry in the Pediatric Intensive Care Unit

- Underweight (BMI < 5th percentile for age), at risk of overweight (BMI > 85th percentile for age), or overweight (BMI > 95th percentile for age)
- Greater than 10% weight gain or loss during medical–surgical intensive care unit stay
- Failure to consistently meet prescribed caloric goals
- Failure to wean or escalation in ventilatory support
- Need for muscle relaxants for fewer than 7 days
- Neurologic trauma (traumatic, hypoxic, ischemic) with evidence of dysautonomia
- Oncologic diagnoses (including stem cell or bone marrow transplantation)
- Need for mechanical ventilatory support for more than 7 days
- Suspicion of severe hypermetabolism (status epilepticus, hyperthermia, systemic inflammatory response syndrome, dysautonomic storms) or hypometabolism (hypothermia, hypothyroidism, phenobarbital or midazolam coma)
- Intensive care unit length of stay of more than 4 weeks

Body mass index (BMI).
Source: Mehta, M., Bechard, L., Leavitt, K., & Duggan, C. (2009). Cumulative energy imbalance in the pediatric intensive care unit: Role of targeted indirect calorimetry. *Journal of Parenteral and Enteral Nutrition, 33*(3), 336–344. Reprinted with permission from Sage Publishing.

Underfeeding is common in the hospital setting and is multifactorial in origin. In enterally fed pediatric patients, inappropriate nutrition prescription, intermittent tube feed holds, NPO status for procedures, fluid restriction, and inappropriate delivery of nutrition may all contribute to underfeeding macronutrients and micronutrients. Underfeeding can result in weight loss or poor weight gain, protein-energy malnutrition, and increased infections. Nutritional interventions such as the use of indirect calorimetry, calculation of actual nutritional intake, use of concentrated enteral formulas when fluids are restricted, prokinetic agents, and acceptance of higher gastric residual volumes could potentially improve nutritional intake (Skillman & Wischmeyer, 2009).

REFEEDING SYNDROME

Refeeding syndrome occurs when previously malnourished patients are aggressively fed; this condition results in metabolic disturbances. Pediatric patients who present with recent weight loss, prolonged poor nutritional intake, or malnutrition are at risk of refeeding syndrome. Oral, enteral, or parenteral nutrition should be initiated and advanced slowly in patients deemed at risk for this problem. Any electrolyte abnormalities should be corrected prior to initiating a nutritional regimen. Serum electrolytes, phosphorus, magnesium, calcium, glucose, fluid status, and cardiopulmonary function should be monitored closely during nutrition advancement. As an integral part of the interprofessional team, the registered dietitian plays an important role in the prevention and management of refeeding syndrome (Dunn et al., 2003).

NUTRITION PARAMETERS

Nutrition monitoring is essential to evaluate patients for overfeeding or underfeeding. Anthropometric, biochemical, clinical, and dietary data may be used to determine nutritional adequacy. In particular, serial weights should be obtained daily or weekly as the patient's condition permits. Weights should be interpreted with regard to fluid status.

Biochemical markers such as albumin and prealbumin may be used to assess nutritional status. Prealbumin is more reliable to assess acute nutritional changes, as it has a half-life of only 24 to 48 hours. Baseline and weekly prealbumin levels should be checked to trend the patient's nutritional status and assess response to nutritional support. Prealbumin may be elevated in patients on steroids or hemodialysis. Albumin is a less reliable means by which

TABLE 25-3

Estimated Energy and Protein Requirements for Infants, Children, and Adolescents

	Age	Protein (gm/kg/day)	DRI (calories/kg/day)	REE (calories/kg/day): WHO Equation	REE (calories/kg/day): Schofield Equation
Infants	0–3 months	1.52	102	**Males 0–3 years:** 60.7W − 54	**Males 0–3 years:** 0.17W + 15.17H − 617.6
	4–6 months	1.52	82		
	7–12 months	1.2	80	**Females 0–3 years:** 61W − 51	**Females 0–3 years:** 16.25W + 10.232H − 413.5
	13–35 months	1.05	82		
Children	3 years	1.05	85	**Males 3–10 years:** 22.7W + 495	**Males 3–10 years:** 19.6W + 1.303H + 414.9
	4 years	0.95	70		
	5–6 years	0.95	65	**Females 3–10 years:** 22.5W + 499	**Females 3–10 years:** 16.97W + 1.618H + 371.2
	7–8 years	0.95	60		
Boys	9–13 years	0.95	47		
	14–18 years	0.85	38	**Males 10–18 years:** 17.5W + 651	**Males 10–18 years:** 16.25W + 1.372H + 515.5
	>18 years	0.8	36		
Girls	9–13 years	0.95	40	**Females 10–18 years:** 12.2W + 746	**Females 10–18 years:** 8.365W + 4.65H + 200
	14–18 years	0.85	32		
	>18 years	0.8	34		

Activity Factors
Paralyzed 1.0 Confined to bed 1.2
Ambulatory 1.3

Stress Factors
Surgery 1.2–1.3 Sepsis 1.4–1.5
Trauma 1.1–1.8 Catch-up growth 1.5–3
Fever 12% per degree > 37° C

Resting energy expenditure (REE), World Health Organization (WHO), Dietary Reference Intake (DRI), weight (W; in kg), height (H; in cm).

Sources: Bunting, D., D'Souza, S., Nguyen, J., Phillips, S., Rich, S., & Trout, S. (2008). *Texas Children's Hospital pediatric nutrition reference guide* (8th ed., p. 18); Schofield, W. N. (1985). Predicting basal metabolic rate: New standards and review of previous work. *Human Nutrition: Clinical Nutrition, 39c*(1s), 5–41; World Health Organization. (1985). Energy and protein requirements. *World Health Organization Technical Support Series 724.* Geneva, Switzerland: Author.

to assess acute nutritional changes, as it has a longer half-life (14 to 20 days) and is affected by dehydration, sepsis, trauma, liver disease, and albumin infusions.

Hair, eyes, skin, mouth, and extremities should be examined regularly for changes that may reveal macronutrient or micronutrient deficiencies. Daily oral, enteral, and parenteral intake should be reviewed and compared with estimated needs to assess adequacy of nutritional intake (Golts et al., 2007).

Critical Thinking
A counter-regulatory hormonal cascade occurs in response to illness or injury and results in glycogen storage depletion, hyperglycemia, lipid intolerance, and protein catabolism.

ASSESSMENT OF NUTRITION

Dana Palermo and Karen LeRoy

Nutrition assessment is an important facet of the care of acutely ill pediatric patients. Maintaining adequate nutrient intake from birth through adolescence is vital for growth and development, but is especially important during acute illness and injury. The goal of a nutrition assessment is to identify those patients who are at risk for poor nutrition and to elucidate their nutrient requirements and deficiencies (Canada et al., 2009; Kleinman, 2009). Depending on the degree and duration of illness or injury, nutrition risk may be either temporary or long term. A patient's nutrition risk can change during the course of treatment and should continue to be reassessed throughout his or her hospital course as appropriate.

A nutrition assessment traditionally includes the evaluation of anthropometric, biochemical, clinical, and dietary data (Leonberg, 2008). When conducting a nutrition assessment, both preadmission and current nutrition status should be evaluated. Nutrition-related concerns commonly transpire in the acute care setting when patients have prolonged NPO status, feeding intolerances, inadequate supplementation, and nutrient inadequacies secondary to medical treatments (Corkins, 2010; Kleinman, 2009). The most common nutrition-related risks are malnutrition or the potential to develop malnutrition and nutrient deficiencies and excesses.

ANTHROPOMETRICS

Anthropometric measurements are the most important parameter when conducting a nutrition assessment in a pediatric patient. Weight, height or length, and head circumference are the most commonly assessed anthropometric measures (Corkins, 2010; Leonberg, 2008). These measurements should be taken using the appropriate equipment, and compared to standards for age, to allow for an accurate assessment of growth. If a measurement is taken a single time, the patient can be compared to other children of the same age group. If he or she is measured over time, growth velocity can be assessed. Other anthropometric measurements, such as midarm circumference, fat-fold measurements, hydrodensitometry, air-displacement plethysmography, and total body water, can be used to assess body fat percentages (Kleinman, 2009).

The most frequently used growth standards are those provided by the Centers for Disease Control and Prevention (CDC) and the World Health Organization (WHO) (Leonberg, 2008). As part of patient assessment, standards provided in the form of growth charts or growth velocity can be compared to standard mean rates of weight

gain and linear growth. CDC-developed growth charts are available for patients from birth to 20 years of age (CDC, 2009a). They are based on data from the National Health and Nutrition Examination Survey (NHANES), and include infants who are both formula fed and breast-fed. WHO-developed growth standards are available for children between the ages of 0 and 60 months and are based on healthy breastfed infants from various socioeconomic statuses (WHO, 2010). Additionally, specialized growth charts have been developed for multiple conditions, including very-low-birth-weight infants (i.e., those weighing less than 1,500 gm; intended for use for 120 days' uncorrected age or until the child reaches a weight of 2,000 gm), Down syndrome, Turner syndrome, Cornelia de Lange syndrome, and achondroplasia. According to the CDC (2009a), special health care needs growth charts were developed with small samples and may have limitations. Therefore, it is recommended that patients be plotted on both specialized growth charts and CDC growth charts for comparison.

Weight should be taken on a calibrated, level scale (Leonberg, 2008). When a pediatric patient younger than 18 months of age is weighed, the measurement should be taken while the child is either naked or in a clean, dry diaper. Patients older than 18 months of age should be weighed wearing minimal clothing. After the patient's weight is determined, it should be plotted on the appropriate growth chart to allow for comparison of that patient to others of the same age. If serial weights are available, average daily or monthly weight gain can be calculated.

Table 25-4 and Table 25-5 illustrate mean rates of weight gain for boys and girls from birth to 20 years of age. If their weight trends are greater or less than the average, they may be at nutrition risk. It is important to note that a pediatric patient cannot be classified as underweight or overweight from weight measurements alone.

TABLE 25-4

Mean Rates of Daily Weight Gain Based on 50% CDC Growth Charts for Infants 0–36 Months		
Age (months)	Males (gm/day)	Females (gm/day)
0–3	28	24
3–6	21	19
6–9	15	14
9–12	11	11
12–18	8	8
18–36	5	5

Centers for Disease Control and Prevention (CDC).

Source: Adapted from Leonberg, 2008.

TABLE 25-5

Mean Rates of Monthly Weight Gain Based on 50% CDC Growth Charts for Youths 3–20 Years		
Age (years)	Males (gm/month)	Females (gm/month)
3–4	150	150
4–5	175	183
5–6	192	192
6–7	200	208
7–8	217	242
8–9	242	275
9–10	283	325
10–11	325	367
11–12	383	367
12–13	425	350
13–14	458	292
14–15	433	225
15–16	392	150
16–17	300	108
17–18	217	83
18–19	167	100
19–20	125	75

Centers for Disease Control and Prevention (CDC).

Source: Adapted from Leonberg, 2008.

TABLE 25-6

Mean Rates of Monthly Stature Gain Based on 50% CDC Growth Charts for Infants 0–36 Months		
Age (months)	Males (cm/month)	Females (cm/month)
0–3	3.6	3.3
3–6	2.0	2.0
6–9	1.6	1.5
9–12	1.3	1.3
12–18	1.1	1.1
18–24	0.9	0.9
24–36	0.8	0.8

Centers for Disease Control and Prevention (CDC).

Source: Adapted from Leonberg, 2008.

TABLE 25-7

Mean Rates of Yearly Stature Gain Based on 50% CDC Growth Charts for Children 3–16 Years		
Age (years)	Males (cm/year)	Females (cm/year)
3–4	7	6
4–5	6	7
5–6	7	7
6–7	6	7
7–8	6	6
8–9	6	5
9–10	5	5
10–11	5	6
11–12	6	8
12–13	7	6
13–14	7	3
14–15	6	1
15	4	1
16	2	1

Centers for Disease Control and Prevention (CDC).

Source: Adapted from Leonberg, 2008.

Length should be measured using a length board or stadiometer (Corkins, 2010). Pediatric patients younger than the age of 24 to 36 months should be measured recumbently. To ensure accuracy, two health care professionals (HCPs) should measure recumbent length, as this technique allows for the patient's head and feet to be held as straight as possible on the length board. Patients who are older than 24 to 36 months should be measured without shoes and with their heels, buttocks, shoulders, and head touching the vertical measurement device surface. For older pediatric patients who cannot stand, arm span, sitting height, and upper-arm or lower-leg length can be used to estimate stature. After taking an accurate measurement, the value should be plotted on the appropriate growth chart. Stunting or a low percentage length for age (less than 5%) may reflect long-term nutritional or caloric insufficiency (Leonberg, 2008). Conversely, over-nutrition may accelerate linear growth.

Table 25-6 and Table 25-7 outline mean rates of stature gain for boys and girls from birth to 20 years of age. These tables can be used to assess growth velocity in pediatric patients over time.

To determine if a pediatric patient is underweight, of normal weight, overweight, or obese, weight-for-length and body mass index (BMI) should be used. Weight-for-length growth charts are for patients younger than 36 months of age. If a child plots as less than 5% or more than 95% for age, it may indicate under- or over-nutrition (Leonberg, 2008). BMI should be used for patients who are older than 2 years of age. This value can be calculated as follows:

$$BMI = [weight(kg)/height^2(cm^2)] \times 10,000 \text{ or}$$
$$BMI = [weight(lb)/height^2(in^2)] \times 703$$

Four weight classifications are distinguished based on percentage BMI for age:

- Underweight: < 5%
- Healthy weight: 5–84.9%
- Overweight: 85–94.9%
- Obese: > 95% or BMI > 30 kg/m², whichever is lower (Barlow, 2007; CDC, 2009c)

BMI percentiles can be used at a single point in time, but are also used to assess growth over time. Pediatric patients should be monitored for early adiposity rebound, which is seen naturally around 5 to 6 years of age, as well as for sudden changes in BMI to prevent malnutrition and obesity (Barlow, 2007; Leonberg, 2008). If a patient is at risk of becoming or is underweight, overweight, or obese, he or she will likely benefit from continued nutrition monitoring. These patients should be referred to a dietician in an outpatient setting or to appropriate nutrition classes upon the time of discharge.

If a pediatric patient is underweight according to weight-for-length or BMI classification, it may be beneficial to determine his or her degree of wasting. To assess the degree of wasting, the percentage ideal body weight (IBW) should be calculated using the following equation (Corkins, 2010):

$$[\text{Measured weight}/50\% \text{ weight for age}] \times 100$$

The Waterlow criteria classify patients into four groups based on IBW: ≥ 90% IBW, normal; 80–90% IBW, mild wasting; 70–80% IBW, moderate wasting; and < 70% IBW, severe wasting (Waterlow, 1972). Those patients who are severely wasted (less than 70% IBW) or have had a 10% or more weight loss in 2 to 3 months are at the greatest risk for refeeding syndrome (Corkins, 2010). When risk of refeeding syndrome exists, any oral, enteral, or parenteral nutrition should be advanced to meet the nutritional goal slowly to prevent changes in the patient's blood glucose, electrolytes, and vital signs. Percentage IBW can also be used as a short-term monitoring tool to evaluate response to nutrition interventions because it changes more quickly than BMI (Leonberg, 2008).

Head circumference, also known as frontal occipital circumference (FOC), can be used to monitor brain growth until a child reaches 36 months of age (Leonberg, 2008). To make this measurement, a flexible tape measure should surround the point of the head with the largest circumference. It should lie above the eyebrows and ears. Impaired brain growth is a symptom of chronic malnutrition, and head circumference will be the final anthropometric measure to be affected by inadequate nutrient intake. FOC can also be affected by genetic disposition, microcephaly (less than 5% of the normal size for age), macrocephaly (more than 95% of the normal size for age), and other disorders affecting brain or skull size.

BIOCHEMICAL ANALYSIS

Biochemical analyses can be used to assess malnutrition, nutrient deficiencies and excesses, and response to nutrition interventions. Commonly evaluated nutrition-related laboratory values include serum proteins, electrolytes, lipids, blood glucose, vitamins, and minerals (Kleinman, 2009). The fecal fat test, breath hydrogen test, sweat chloride test, plasma amino acids, and nitrogen balance studies are other medical tests that can be important parts of a nutrition assessment (Leonburg, 2008). If nutrition-related biochemical testing is suggested after clinical and dietary data are collected, careful selection should be used to ensure that the benefits of these tests outweigh their cost and invasiveness.

Albumin, transferrin, and prealbumin (transthyretin) are all indicators of visceral protein status. Although these markers can be affected by inadequate calorie and protein intake, they are also affected by infection, altered fluid status, kidney and liver disease, pregnancy, and inflammation (Canada et al., 2009). Prealbumin is commonly used to monitor protein status, because it has a relatively short half-life (2 to 3 days) compared to albumin (Corkins, 2010; Kleinman, 2009). Albumin has a longer half-life (21 days) and is also affected by fluid status, which can falsely elevate or decrease plasma concentrations. During acute states of inflammation, the liver reprioritizes protein synthesis by increasing production of positive acute-phase proteins, such as CRP, and decreasing synthesis of negative acute-phase proteins, such as albumin and prealbumin. Therefore, prealbumin and CRP should be monitored concomitantly (Gabay & Kushner, 1999).

Iron deficiency is commonly observed in pediatric patients. To determine if the patient is truly anemic, hemoglobin, hematocrit, and mean corpuscular volume (MCV) are evaluated (Corkins, 2010). Iron-deficiency anemia should be differentiated from other causes of anemia, including vitamin B_{12} (folate) deficiency and anemia from chronic disease. If iron deficiency is suspected, iron studies can be ordered, including transferrin saturation, serum ferritin, and total iron binding capacity, for confirmation.

PHYSICAL EXAMINATION

Clinical assessments consist of a physical examination focused on nutrition-related findings. Physical examination of the patient's hair, eyes, skin, tongue, fingernails, and general physical appearance can provide information on body composition, edema, hydration status, nutrient deficiencies, and toxicities (Canada et al., 2009). Table 25-8 outlines possible signs and symptoms of nutrition-related concerns. Physical findings can be further evaluated later with biochemical tests (Leonburg, 2008).

TABLE 25-8

Nutrition-Focused Physical Examination

Location	Examination Findings	Potential Nutritional/Metabolic Relevance
Skin	Delayed wound healing	Insufficient calories, protein, vitamin C, or zinc
	Dermatitis	Essential fatty acid, zinc, niacin, riboflavin, or tryptophan deficiency
	Pallor	Iron, folate, vitamin B_{12}, or vitamin C deficiency
	Petechiae	Vitamin C or K deficiency
	Poor turgor	Inadequate fluids
Hair	Dull, dry, thin, sparse	Insufficient calories, protein, iron, or zinc or essential fatty acid deficiency
Nails	Thin, spoon shaped	Iron deficiency
	Mottled, pale, poor blanching	Vitamin A or C deficiency
Face	Moon face	Protein-calorie deficiency
	Bilateral temporal wasting	Protein-calorie deficiency
Neck	Thyroid gland enlarged	Iodine deficiency
Eyes	Cracks in brows, lids	Riboflavin or niacin deficiency
	Night blindness	Vitamin A deficiency
	Bitot's spots	Vitamin A deficiency
Mouth	Cracked lips	Riboflavin, niacin, or pyridoxine deficiency
	Spongy, bleeding gums	Vitamin C deficiency
	Magenta color tongue	Riboflavin deficiency
	Red, slick, loss of papillae tongue	Folate, niacin, iron, riboflavin, or vitamin B_{12} deficiency
	Excessive caries	Excessive simple carbohydrate intake, insufficient flouride
Abdomen	Round, distended	Gas, edema, ascites, obesity
Urine	Dark concentrated	Sign of dehydration
	Light diluted	Sign of overhydration

Sources: Canada et al., 2009; Leonberg, 2008.

DIET HISTORY

Evaluation of food and diet history is an important part of a nutrition assessment. Looking at patterns of typical and recent intake can provide insight into potential insufficient or excessive intakes of macronutrients and micronutrients. Pediatric diet histories can be complicated by the use of multiple caregivers, possibly limited development and education, and variations in independence.

Several methods may be used to obtain a diet history, including diet interview, 24-hour recall, 3-day food record, and calorie count (Leonburg, 2008). All of these methods have both advantages and disadvantages, and should be used in combination with anthropometric, biochemical, and clinical information when assessing the patient's nutritional status. Diet histories should include type and quantities of foods and beverages/formula consumed, preparation methods of food and formulas, feeding methods (by mouth or by feeding tube), frequency and length of meals, food availability, food allergies, use of nutritional supplements, and typical activity level.

After collecting appropriate anthropometric, biochemical, clinical, and dietary data, the patient's nutritional needs may be assessed and a nutrition care plan can be developed. When developing a nutrition care plan, current illness and injury, past medical history, medications, and drug–nutrient interactions should also be considered. Care plan development can be challenging in pediatric patients because energy and nutrient requirements for growth vary based on age and can change depending on the patient's acute state. For example, a patient under moderate stress with wound healing issues will require more calories, protein, and micronutrients compared to a healthy patient of the same age (Corkins, 2010). Additionally, due to various inherited and genetic syndromes and complex pediatric diseases, nutrient and growth needs can differ from one patient to the next. When nutrition concerns are apparent, a dietician should be consulted to provide evidence-based nutrition recommendations to the interprofessional team.

DEHYDRATION AND FLUID MANAGEMENT

Karen LeRoy

PATHOPHYSIOLOGY

Seventy percent of the lean body mass (LBM) in infants and the malnourished patient is water. For these patients, LBM and weight are the same. The water is distributed as follows:

- 25% extracellular (ECF)
  - 19% interstitial (skin and cellular)
  - 6% plasma, protein, and lipids
- 45% intracellular (ICF)

As children grow, these proportions change, and LBM is reduced to approximately 60% water as 10% of body weight moves to fat. By the time a child reaches 5 years of age, LBM approximates that of an adult, with 20% of the water being extracellular and 50% intracellular.

Infants are more vulnerable to dehydration from fluid losses or decreased oral intake because they have a higher water/LBM ratio, greater ECF volume, and greater excretion of fluid per day than older pediatric patients or adults. In the first days of illness, the volume losses are primarily from the extracellular compartment (80%) rather than from the intracellular compartment (20%). However, after approximately 3 days, the proportion changes to approximately 60% extracellular losses and 40% intracellular losses (Finberg, 2002; Reid & Losek, 2009).

Daily maintenance fluid requirements for healthy children include fluid for physiologic needs, daily excretions (urine, stool), and insensible losses, closely approximating expended caloric requirements at 100 mL/kcal/day. Insensible losses account for approximately 45 mL/100 kcal expended and, under normal conditions, can be further divided into 15 mL/100 kcal from respiratory losses and 30 mL/100 kcal from skin evaporation. Urine (50 mL/kcal/day) and stool (5 mL/kcal/day) account for the remaining daily losses, for a total loss of 100 mL/100 kcal (Finberg, 2002; Friedman & Ray, 2008). Fever is common in ill children and increases insensible water loss by 12% for every 1°C over 38°C (100.4°F). Insensible losses that may increase daily fluid requirements include respiratory distress, overheating, or sweating. Other concerns that may require recalculation of daily fluid requirements include diabetes insipidus, oliguric kidney failure, and increased gastric fluid or stool losses (Friedman & Ray).

A formula for determining the volume of fluid required by healthy children for daily maintenance therapy, based on kilocalories expended per day, was first published by Holliday and Segar in 1957. An adaptation of this calculation is the most frequently used formula today (Table 25-9). Other commonly used formulas are 1,600 mL/m² and a further adaptation of the Holliday-Segar calculation that converts volume per day to volume per hour (Table 25-9).

There has been significant controversy regarding the ideal maintenance fluid to use with these formulas. By extension, such management affects the treatment of dehydration. The concern is that hypotonic intravenous fluid ($D_5.2$ NS, $D_5.45$ NS), which is commonly used in the United States for maintenance and replacement fluid, may lead to hyponatremia; if this condition is severe, hyponatremic encephalopathy may arise in ill or injured children. Those patients with increased levels of antidiuretic hormone (ADH) seem to be at the greatest risk of developing this complication. Circumstances that may lead to elevated levels of ADH can be divided into osmotic and non-osmotic causes. Osmotic causes include hypovolemia and the administration of hypotonic fluids. Non-osmotic causes include pain, nausea, vomiting, stress, CNS and pulmonary infections, medications (e.g., diuretics), and anesthetics, with the immediate postoperative period being a time of particularly high risk (Friedman & Ray, 2008; Holliday et al., 2007; Moritz & Ayus, 2003).

A moderate or severe dehydration leads to hypovolemic shock, as a result of a decrease in circulating intravascular volume and a decrease in venous return

TABLE 25-9

Holliday and Segar Maintenance Fluid Calculation		
Patient Weight	**Fluid Dose**	**Infusion Rate**
3–10 kg	100 mL/kg/day	4 mL/kg/hr
10–20 kg	1,000 mL + 50 mL for each additional kg over 10 kg	40 mL/hr + another 2 mL/hr for each additional kg over 10 kg
20–70 kg	1,500 mL + 20 mL for each additional kg over 20 kg	60 mL/hr + 1 mL/hr for each additional kg over 20 kg
Volume should be decreased for kidney insufficiency and increased for abnormal insensible losses.		

Source: Holliday et al., 2007.

with inadequate delivery of oxygen to the tissues. Catecholamines are released in response to the decrease in venous return—a phenomenon that leads to tachycardia, peripheral vasoconstriction, and increased myocardial contractility. Uncorrected profound hypovolemia progresses to hypotension and myocardial failure due to reduced cardiac output and impaired coronary perfusion. As perfusion worsens, anaerobic metabolism generates lactic acidosis. If this combination of acidosis and myocardial failure continues unabated, or uncorrected, it can progress to multisystem collapse. Contributing to this collapse may be leukocyte- and platelet-adhesion-releasing humoral and cellular mediators. The increased levels of these mediators further impair blood flow to the splanchnia (Kreimeier, 2000).

EPIDEMIOLOGY AND ETIOLOGY

More than 1.5 million outpatient visits, 200,000 hospitalizations, and 300 deaths occur each year in the United States as a consequence of gastroenteritis and dehydration (Centers for Disease Control and Prevention [CDC], 2003). Dehydration is listed as one of the top three preventable hospitalizations in children younger than age 5 years and accounts for more than 333 hospitalizations per 100,000 population younger than 18 years of age (Agency for Healthcare Research and Quality, 2004). The

severity of dehydration is classified into three categories based on the percentage of plasma volume lost (Table 25-10).

Dehydration can be attributed to either an infectious or non-infectious etiology. Infectious causes of dehydration include both viral and bacterial pathogens. The most common causes of dehydration are vomiting and diarrhea due to viral gastroenteritis.

Non-infectious causes of dehydration include antibiotic therapy, urinary tract and respiratory infections, malnutrition, overfeeding, allergies to proteins, and chronic nonspecific diarrhea (toddler's diarrhea) related to low-residue, low-fat, or high-carbohydrate diets. Other causes of dehydration include osmotic diuresis (e.g., diabetic ketoacidosis), capillary leak (sepsis, burn injury), hemorrhage, increased insensible loss (e.g., sweating), and inadequate fluid intake. Antibiotic-related diarrhea can be due to a decrease in carbohydrate transport and lactase levels or elimination of normal gut flora and overgrowth of *Clostridium difficile*. Malnourished patients also have altered gastrointestinal motility and changes in intestinal flora. Young infants have comparatively less pancreatic amylase, which contributes to the occurrence of diarrhea in these patients after their ingestion of starchy foods. Consumption of high-fructose fruit juices and sorbitol may cause osmotic diarrhea. Spices and high-fiber foods, as well as histamine-containing or histamine-releasing foods, such as citrus fruits, tomatoes, certain cheeses, and fish, may also cause diarrhea in young children. Dietary protein allergies may cause diarrhea,

TABLE 25-10

Symptoms Associated with Dehydration			
Symptom	**Minimal or no dehydration** (<3% loss of body weight)	**Mild to moderate dehydration** (3%–9% loss of body weight)	**Severe dehydration** (>9% loss of body weight)
Mental status	Well; alert	Normal, fatigued or restless, irritable	Apathetic, lethargic, unconscious
Thirst	Drinks normally; might refuse liquids	Thirsty; eager to drink	Drinks poorly; unable to drink
Heart rate	Normal	Normal to increased	Tachycardia, with bradycardia in most severe cases
Quality of pulses	Normal	Normal to increased	Weak, thready, or impalpable
Breathing	Normal	Normal; fast	Deep
Eyes	Normal	Slightly sunken	Deeply sunken
Tears	Present	Decreased	Absent
Mouth and tongue	Moist	Dry	Parched
Skin fold	Instant recoil	Recoil in <2 seconds	Recoil in >2 seconds
Capillary refill	Normal	Prolonged	Prolonged; minimal
Extremities	Warm	Cool	Cold; mottled; cyanotic
Urine output	Normal to decreased	Decreased	Minimal

Sources: Courtesy of Centers for Disease Control and Prevention. (2003). Managing acute gastroenteritis among children oral rehydration, maintenance, and nutritional therapy. *MMWR, 52*(16).

particularly in children younger than 12 months of age. These allergies usually resolve over time. Older infants and toddlers may have chronic nonspecific diarrhea as a result of diet, abnormalities in bile acid absorption, or atypical motor function.

PRESENTATION

Important information gathered from the patient's history can assist in the initial assessment of the dehydrated pediatric patient:

- Etiology of the fluid loss (e.g., vomiting, diarrhea, sweating, respiratory distress)
- Concurrent chronic illness
- Exposures to heat or sunlight
- Fever
- Intake and volume of fluids taken
- Level of activity
- Medications that may contribute to the dehydration (e.g., diuretics)
- Number of days ill
- Number of wet diapers or frequency of urinary output
- Possibility of ingestion errors (metabolic or toxic)
- Recent surgery
- Type of fluids and diet

The physical signs of dehydration directly reflect fluid losses and the body's compensatory mechanisms for these losses. Poor skin turgor is a sign of loss of interstitial fluid, while tachycardia and delayed capillary refill indicate the body's compensation for maintaining perfusion (Table 25-11). The percentage of body weight loss approximates the percentage of the child's lost fluid volume (Finberg, 2002).

Other physical findings in dehydration include mottled skin, sunken fontanel in infants, sunken eyes, and increased respiratory and heart rate. The skin may feel soft, with subcutaneous doughiness being noted. Most patients with moderate dehydration and all patients with severe dehydration will present with signs of compromised circulation, categorized as hypovolemic shock with signs of end-organ dysfunction (e.g., decrease or absent urine output, altered level of consciousness).

DIFFERENTIAL DIAGNOSIS

Dehydration is differentiated based on the serum sodium level and is identified as isonatremic, hypernatremic, or hyponatremic.

Isonatremic dehydration (serum sodium 130–150 mEq/L) is the most common form and is often related to gastroenteritis, where losses of water and salt in the stool are typically balanced. If the pediatric patient also has vomiting, however, a decrease in water consumption may occur; thus the balance shifts, and more water is lost than salt, resulting in volume contraction and hypernatremic dehydration (Finberg, 2002).

In *hypernatremic dehydration* (serum sodium >150 mEq/L), rapid reduction in brain volume, due to the loss of brain water, creates shearing forces on the falx cerebri and venous sinuses. These forces can cause subarachnoid hemorrhage or subdural hematomas; infants appear to be most at risk of this complication. Other symptoms include neuromuscular excitability, hyperreflexia, confusion, seizure, or coma.

The opposite occurs in *hyponatremic dehydration* (serum sodium < 130 mEq/L). Hyponatremic dehydration results from a loss of fluid, especially salt, in the stool or sweat. Severe hyponatremia may present with seizures, noncardiogenic pulmonary edema, respiratory arrest, or cerebral herniation (Moritz & Ayus, 2003). Generally the patient presenting with mild hyponatremic dehydration looks like a patient with serious isonatremic dehydration, until the sodium level drops below 125 mEq/dL, at which time seizures may occur. The hypernatremic dehydrated patient has better preserved circulatory status, but more evident neurological findings.

PLAN OF CARE

Diagnostic studies are not as useful for quantifying volume loss through weight changes or capillary refill for mild dehydration, although they can be useful to establish a baseline for therapy (CDC, 2003; Emond, 2009; Finberg, 2002). Blood urea nitrogen (BUN) may increase with the severity of dehydration (kidney compromise) and is a more sensitive marker than creatinine concentration. The bicarbonate level may reflect the extent of metabolic acidosis but has a poor specificity and sensitivity to the degree of dehydration. Blood pH has also not proved predictive of the degree of dehydration.

Measurement of sodium is important, however, as the sodium level determines the type of dehydration

TABLE 25-11

Capillary Refill Time and Plasma Volume Loss	
Capillary Refill Time	**Loss of Plasma Volume (mL/kg)**
< 2 seconds	Normal
2–2.9 seconds	50–90 mL/kg
3–3.5 seconds	90–110 mL/kg
3.5–3.9 seconds	110–120 mL/kg
≥ 4 seconds	150 mL/kg

Source: Finberg, 2002.

(isonatremic, hypernatremic, or hyponatremic). An elevated serum anion gap (AG) suggests a metabolic acidosis and may be calculated using the following formula:

$$AG = [Na^+ + K^+] - [Cl^- + HCO_3^-] \text{ or } [Na^+] - [Cl^- + HCO_3^-]$$

The normal AG range is 8–16 mEq/L. Prolonged illness and longer hospital stays have been associated with high anion gaps (Shaoul et al., 2004). Daily weights, accurate intake and output measurements, blood pressure measurements, observing for signs of edema, and monitoring of serum sodium levels are recommended for those patients requiring hospitalization (Moritz & Ayus, 2003, p. 230).

Mild to moderate dehydration, especially from gastroenteritis, is generally managed with oral rehydration therapy (ORT; see Chapter 26). More than 90% of dehydrated patients can be rehydrated orally (CDC, 2003). Contraindications to oral rehydration include severe dehydration or shock, severe vomiting or ileus, and lack of caregiver supervision in the administration of ORT (CDC). Moderately dehydrated children should be monitored for ongoing losses that should be added to the rehydration volume. Rapid rehydration restores plasma volume, corrects acidosis, and improves perfusion to tissues. The moderately dehydrated child should be reassessed every hour at home, in the primary care office, in the observation unit, or in the emergency department. Rarely will hospitalization be required. Feeding can be started as soon as initial hydration is complete (Diggins, 2006). Oral rehydration therapy is equally as effective as and less costly than intravenous rehydration therapy (Bellemare et al., 2004).

In contrast, severe dehydration is a medical emergency. Management is divided into two phases: initial resuscitation and repletion or replacement therapy. The initial management consists of a 20 mL/kg IV fluid bolus, which is repeated until restoration of plasma volume and normal perfusion occurs (e.g., improved level of consciousness [LOC], improved pulse quality, decreased capillary refill time). Achieving this goal may require up to 60 mL/kg in the first hour, with therapy typically being initiated before diagnostic studies are available. An isotonic fluid such as normal saline (NS) or lactated Ringer's (LR) must be used; do not use hypotonic fluids or fluids containing glucose. If the history is suggestive of hyperchloremic dehydration, then LR is preferable to NS (CDC, 2003). If the severe dehydration occurs secondary to thermal injury, an additional loss of plasma proteins is expected (see Chapter 38). In hemorrhagic shock, LR is commonly used as the temporizing solution to sustain stroke volume and, therefore, cardiac output, in anticipation of either control of hemorrhage or administration of blood transfusion (Holliday, Friedman, & Wassner, 1999).

The evidence for use of isotonic solutions without glucose (NS, LR) for initial volume resuscitation and replenishment of the extracellular compartment is strong and not the focus of the controversy. However, which IV solution to administer during the repletion or replacement therapy phase remains subject to debate. Because many pediatric patients receiving IV fluids will have alterations in ADH excretion, especially from non-osmotic causes, the current thinking is that only isotonic fluid should be administered to prevent potentially poor outcomes associated with hyponatremia, while recognizing that no one solution will meet every child's needs. Two examples of isotonic solutions that can be used for maintenance therapy are D_5 NS and D_5 LR. There are caveats to this strategy, such as in the setting of hypernatremia, hyperchloremia, risk for fluid overload, or kidney problems, and consultation with critical care, nephrology, or pulmonology specialists to devise individualized therapeutic plans may be required (Friedman & Ray, 2008; Holliday et al., 2007; Moritz & Ayus, 2003).

Unless the patient's glucose stores are depleted, 5% glucose IV solution concentrations are usually enough to prevent ketosis when nutrition interruption is limited to a few days (Holliday et al., 2007). When adequate kidney function has been confirmed, 20 mEq/L of potassium may be added to the solution. Physiologic dosing of bicarbonate, lactate, or acetate in the isotonic IV fluid for the acidotic patient may be considered, whereas only chloride should be administered to the patient with alkalotic dehydration (e.g., pyloric stenosis) (Finberg, 2002).

After initial management of severe dehydration, replacement therapy specific to the type of dehydration (isonatremic, hypernatremic, or hyponatremic) should be initiated.

Isonatremic dehydration

In patients with isonatremic dehydration, fluid therapy is based on repletion, maintenance, and treatment of ongoing losses as needed. It is usually designed to be completed over 24 hours and to replace ECF and ICF in proportions related to the severity of dehydration. Templates for calculation are readily available. Replacement therapy is based on the patient's fluid, sodium, and potassium deficits. When fluid boluses have been administered as part of initial management, this fluid volume should be subtracted from that calculated for the 24-hour period (Table 25-12). Ongoing losses should be measured at least every 4 to 6 hours and replaced with a solution similar to the drainage (Table 25-13) over the next 4 to 6 hours.

Hypernatremic dehydration

The goal of therapy for patients with hypernatremic dehydration is to improve perfusion based on the degree of dehydration and to safely lower the serum sodium to approximately 155 mEq/L, as lowering the serum sodium level too rapidly can lead to cerebral edema and a poor outcome. Serum sodium levels should be decreased no faster than 10 mEq/L in 24 hours. This rate usually

TABLE 25-12

Sample Calculations for Isonatremic Dehydration

A 10-kg infant (pre-illness weight) has diarrhea for 4 days. His mucous membranes are dry, eyes are sunken, pulse rate is elevated, and urine output is reportedly less than usual. His current weight is 9 kg and serum sodium is 136 mEq/L.

When fluid boluses have been administered as part of initial management, this fluid volume should be subtracted from that calculated for the 24-hour period as noted in this example.

The infant is 10% dehydrated by weight and physical examination and has *isonatremic* dehydration.

Fluid Deficit

10% dehydration (0.1) × pre-illness wt in kg (10) × 1,000 mL/kg = 1,000 mL or 1 L
Illness < 3 days: 80% from ECF and 20% ICF
Illness ≥ 3 days: 60% from ECF and 40% from ICF
For this child, 60% is from ECF and 40% is from ICF.

Na$^+$ Deficit

Normal Na$^+$ in ECF 145 and normal K$^+$ in ICF 150
1 L (fluid deficit) × 0.6 (% from ECF) × 145 (normal ECF sodium) = 90 mEq Na$^+$

K$^+$ Deficit

1 L (fluid deficit) × 0.4 (% from ICF) × 150 (normal ICF potassium) = 60 mEq K$^+$

Maintenance Fluid Requirement

10 kg × 100 mL/kg/day = 1,000 mL or 1 L

Maintenance Na$^+$ Requirement

1L maintenance fluid/day × 3 mEq/100 mL = 30 mEq Na$^+$/day

Maintenance K$^+$ Requirement

1L maintenance fluid/day × 2 mEq/100 mL = 20 mEq K$^+$/day

Fluid Management Plan

Correct fluid losses over 24 hr

Our patient received 20 mL/kg NS (200 mL, 31 mEq Na$^+$) IV as part of initial management. This needs to be subtracted from the total fluid volume for the day.

First 8 hr: give $^1/_3$ maintenance (333 mL) + ½ replacement (500 mL) = 833 mL – 67 mL ($^1/_3$ IV bolus) = 766 mL or 32 mL/hr

Do the same for the Na$^+$ and K$^+$ maintenance and replacement.

First 8 hr: Na$^+$ give $^1/_3$ maintenance (10 mEq) + ½ replacement (45 mEq) – 10 mEq ($^1/_3$ IV bolus) = 45 mEq

K$^+$ give $^1/_3$ maintenance (7 mEq) + ½ replacement (30 mEq) = 37 mEq

Na$^+$ 45/0.766 L = 59 mEq/L

K$^+$ 37/0.766 L = 48 mEq/L

The premade solution that comes closest to this mixture is D$_5$ .45 NS with 40 mEq KCl/L or Potassium acetate at 32 mL/hr × 8 hr.
(Refer to Table 25-13.)

Next 16 hr: give $^2/_3$ maintenance (666 mL) + ½ replacement (500 mL) = 1,166 mL – 133 ($^2/_3$ IV bolus) =1,033 mL or 43 mL/hr

Next 16 hr: Na$^+$ give $^2/_3$ maintenance (20 mEq) + ½ replacement (45 mEq) – 21 mEq ($^2/_3$ IV bolus) = 44 mEq

K$^+$ give $^2/_3$ maintenance (14 mEq) + ½ replacement (30 mEq) = 44 mEq

Na$^+$ 44/1.033 L = 43 mEq/L

K$^+$ 44/1.033 L = 43 mEq/L

The pre-made solution that comes closest to this mixture is D$_5$ .2 NS with 40 mEq KCl/L or Potassium acetate at 43 mL/hr × 16 hr.

After the completion of the maintenance + replacement fluids for 24 hr, consider maintenance fluid at D$_5$ .2 NS with or without 20 mEq KCl/L or Potassium acetate at 40 mL/hr unless there have been ongoing losses.

See the text for discussion regarding isotonic saline.

Potassium can be added as desired after adequate urine output has been established.

Ongoing losses should be measured at least every 4–6 hours and replaced with a solution similar to the drainage (review Table 25-14) over the next 4–6 hours.

Source: These calculations were completed using commonly available values modified from the original work of Holliday and Segar, 1957.

TABLE 25-13

Electrolyte Composition of Body Fluids				
Body Fluid	**Na^+ (mEq/L)**	**K^+ (mEq/L)**	**Cl^- (mEq/L)**	**HCO_3^- (mEq/L)**
Saliva	30–80	20	70	30
Gastric	20–80	5–20	100–150	0
Pancreatic	120–140	5–15	90–120	40–100
Bile	120–140	5–15	80–120	40
Small bowel	100–140	5–15	90–130	25–50
Ileostomy	45–135	3–15	20–115	NA
Diarrhea	10–90	10–80	10–110	NA
Sweat: normal	10–30	3–10	10–35	0
Sweat: cystic fibrosis	50–130			
Burns (with additional protein loss)	140	5	110	0

Sources: *The Merck Manual*, www.merck.com; Grogan, 2006; *The Harriet Lane Handbook*, 2009.

requires that fluid replacement be extended over 48 hours for hypernatremic dehydration. When fluid boluses have been administered as part of initial management, this fluid volume should be subtracted from that calculated for the 24-hour period (Table 25-14). Ongoing losses should be measured at least every 4 to 6 hours and replaced with a solution similar to the drainage (refer to Table 25-13) over the next 4 to 6 hours.

Hyponatremic dehydration

Hyponatremic dehydration, with no neurological symptoms, is managed in the same way as isonatremic dehydration. Mild neurologic symptoms (headache, nausea/vomiting, generalized weakness) may not be obvious with serum sodium greater than 125 mEq/L (Lauriat & Berl, 1997). The goal of therapy is to improve perfusion based on the degree of dehydration and to safely raise the serum sodium to at least 125 mEq/L, as raising the serum sodium level too quickly can lead to osmotic demyelination syndrome (previously called central pontine myelinolysis). When fluid boluses have been administered as part of the initial management plan, this fluid volume should be subtracted from that calculated for the 24-hour period (refer to Table 25-15). Ongoing losses should be measured at least every 4 to 6 hours and replaced with a solution similar to the drainage (refer to Table 25-13) over the next 4 to 6 hours.

After initial resuscitation, the dehydrated patient may require further evaluation and consultation by the critical care team, gastroenterology, infectious diseases, and metabolic specialists depending on the presentation and etiology of the dehydration. Patients admitted to the hospital

may require social services, child life, and nutrition support until they are ready for discharge.

If ORT is used in the outpatient setting, caregivers will need education on how to appropriately administer oral fluid replacement (see Chapter 26). The following information will help families decide when to seek help from their primary care provider and when it is necessary to return for a second visit:

- Patient who is younger than 6 months of age or weighs less than 8 kg
- History of prematurity, chronic medical condition, or concomitant illness
- Fever of 38°C (100.4°F) or higher in infants younger than 3 months of age or 39°C (102.2°F) or higher in children 3 to 36 months of age
- Blood in the stool
- Large amounts of output, including frequent and large amounts of diarrhea
- Continual vomiting
- Signs of dehydration such as sunken eyes, decreased tears, dry oral mucosa, or decreased urine output
- Irritability, listlessness, disinterest in drinking, or lethargy
- Inability of the caregiver to provide oral rehydration or poor response to oral rehydration (CDC, 2003)

DISPOSITION AND DISCHARGE PLANNING

Patients with mild to moderate dehydration may be discharged home once they have successfully completed oral rehydration over a 3- to 4-hour period if the caregivers are able to continue with the home fluid plan. Patients who

TABLE 25-14

Sample Calculations for Hypernatremic Dehydration

A 10-kg infant (pre-illness weight) has had diarrhea for 4 days. His mucous membranes are dry, eyes are sunken, skin recoil is more than 2 seconds, pulse rate is elevated, and urine output is reportedly less than usual. His current weight is 9 kg and serum sodium is 162 mEq/L.

The infant is 10% dehydrated by weight and physical examination and has *hypernatremic* dehydration.

Free Water Deficit

4 mL/kg × 10 (pre-illness wt in kg) × 162 – 145 (actual Na⁺ – normal Na⁺ in ECF) = 680 mL

Total Fluid Deficit

10 (pre-illness wt in kg) – 9 (actual wt in kg) × 1,000 mL/kg = 1,000 mL

Solute Deficit

1,000 mL (total fluid deficit) – 680 mL (free water deficit) = 320 mL or 0.32 L
Illness < 3 days: 80% from ECF and 20% ICF
Illness ≥ 3 days: 60% from ECF and 40% from ICF
For this child 60% is from ECF and 40% is from ICF.

Solute Na⁺ Deficit

Normal Na⁺ in ECF 145 and normal K⁺ in ICF 150
0.32 L (solute deficit) × 0.6 (% from ECF) × 145 (normal ECF sodium) = 28 mEq Na⁺

Solute K⁺ Deficit

0.32 L (solute deficit) × 0.4 (% from ICF) × 150 (normal ICF potassium) = 19 mEq K⁺

Maintenance Fluid Requirement

10 kg × 100 mL/kg/day = 1,000 mL or 1 L

Maintenance Na⁺ Requirement

1L maintenance fluid/day × 3 mEq/100 mL = 30 mEq Na⁺/day

Maintenance K⁺ Requirement

1L maintenance fluid/day × 2 mEq/100 mL = 20 mEq K⁺/day

Fluid Management Plan

Correct fluid losses over 48 hr

First 24 hr: give maintenance (1,000 mL) + ½ free water deficit (340 mL) + solute deficit (320 mL)+ Na⁺ deficit
(28 mEq) + Na⁺ maintenance (30 mEq) + K⁺ deficit (19 mEq) + K⁺ maintenance (20 mEq) = 1,660 mL + 58 mEq Na⁺ + 39 mEq K⁺

Na⁺ 58/1.66 = 35 mEq/L

K⁺ 39/1.66 = 24 mEq/L

The pre-made solution that comes closest to this mixture is D₅ .2 NS with 20 mEq KCl/L or potassium acetate at
69 mL/hr × 24 hr.

Next 24 hr: give maintenance (1,000 mL) + ½ free water deficit (340 mL) + Na⁺ maintenance (30 mEq) + K⁺ maintenance
(20 mEq) = 1,340 mL + 30 mEq Na⁺ + 20 mEq K⁺

Na⁺ 30/1.34 = 22 mEq/L

K⁺ 20/1.34 = 15 mEq/L

The pre-made solution that comes closest to this mixture is D₅ .2 NS with 20 mEq KCl/L or potassium acetate at
56 mL/hr × 24 hr.

Do not reduce serum sodium levels by more than 10 mEq/L in 24 hr; count the fluid bolus in the total volume given.

After the completion of the maintenance + replacement fluids for 48 hr, consider maintenance fluid at D₅ .2 NS with
or without 20 mEq KCl/L or potassium acetate at 40 mL/hr unless there have been ongoing losses. See the text for discussion
regarding isotonic saline.

Potassium can be added as desired after adequate urine output has been established.

Ongoing losses should be measured at least every 4–6 hours and replaced with a solution similar to the drainage (review
Table 25-13) over the next 4–6 hours.

Note: These calculations were completed using commonly available values modified from the original work of Holliday and Segar, 1957.

TABLE 25-15

Sample Calculations for Hyponatremic Dehydration

A 10-kg infant (pre-illness weight) has had diarrhea and vomiting for 4 days. His mucous membranes are dry, eyes sunken, pulse rate elevated, and urine output is reportedly less than usual. His current weight is 9 kg and serum sodium is 123 mEq/L.

When fluid boluses have been administered as part of initial management, this fluid volume should be subtracted from that calculated for the 24-hour period as noted in this example.

The infant is 10% dehydrated by weight and physical examination and has *isonatremic* dehydration.

Fluid Deficit

10% dehydration (0.1) × pre-illness wt in kg (10) × 1,000 mL/kg = 1,000 mL or 1 L
Illness < 3 days: 80% from ECF and 20% from ICF
Illness ≥ 3 days: 60% from ECF and 40% from ICF
For this child, 60% is from ECF and 40% is from ICF,

Na$^+$ Deficit

Normal Na$^+$ in ECF 145 and normal K$^+$ in ICF 150
1 L (fluid deficit) × 0.6 (% from ECF) × 145 (normal ECF sodium) = 90 mEq Na$^+$

Additional Na$^+$ Deficit

135 (low normal Na$^+$) − 123 (actual Na$^+$) = 12 mEq × 0.6 (% from ECF) × 10 (pre-illness wt in kg) = 72 mEq Na$^+$

K$^+$ Deficit

1 L (fluid deficit) × 0.4 (% from ICF) × 150 (normal ICF potassium) = 60 mEq K$^+$

Maintenance Fluid Requirement

10 kg × 100 mL/kg/day = 1,000 mL or 1 L

Maintenance Na$^+$ Requirement

1L maintenance fluid/day × 3 mEq/100 mL = 30 mEq Na$^+$/day

Maintenance K$^+$ Requirement

1L maintenance fluid/day × 2 mEq/100 mL = 20 mEq K$^+$/day

Fluid Management Plan

Replace over 24 hr

Your patient received 20 mL/kg NS (200 mL, 31 mEq Na$^+$) IV as part of initial management. This needs to be subtracted from the total fluid volume for the day.

First 8 hr: give 1/3 maintenance (333 mL) + ½ replacement (500 mL) = 833 mL − 67 mL (1/3 IV bolus) = 766 mL or 32 mL/hr

Do the same for the Na$^+$ and K$^+$ maintenance and replacement.

First 8 hr: Na$^+$ give 1/3 maintenance (10 mEq) + ½ replacement (81 mEq) − 10 mEq (1/3 IV bolus) = 81 mEq

K$^+$ give 1/3 maintenance (7 mEq) + ½ replacement (30 mEq) = 37 mEq

Na$^+$ 81/0.766 L = 105 mEq/L

K$^+$ 37/0.766 L = 48 mEq/L

The pre-made solution that comes closest to this mixture is D$_5$ .45 NS with 40 mEq KCl/L or Potassium acetate at 32 mL/hr × 8 hr (see Table 25-13).

Next 16 hr: give 2/3 maintenance (666 mL) + ½ replacement (500 mL) = 1,166 mL − 133 (2/3 IV bolus) = 1,033 mL or 43 mL/hr

Next 16 hr: Na$^+$ give 2/3 maintenance (20 mEq) + ½ replacement (81 mEq) − 14 mEq (2/3 IV bolus) = 87 mEq

K$^+$ give 2/3 maintenance (14 mEq) + ½ replacement (30 mEq) = 44 mEq

Na$^+$ 87/1.033 L = 84 mEq/L and K$^+$ 44/1.033 L = 43 mEq/L

The pre-made solution that comes closest to this mixture is D$_5$ .45 NS with 40 mEq KCl/L or Potassium acetate at 43 mL/hr × 16 hr.

After the completion of the maintenance + replacement for 24 hr, fluids consider maintenance fluid at D$_5$ .2 NS with or without 20 mEq KCl/L or Potassium acetate at 40 mL/hr unless there have been ongoing losses. See the text for discussion regarding isotonic saline.

Potassium can be added as desired after adequate urine output has been established.

Ongoing losses should be measured at least every 4–6 hours and replaced with a solution similar to the drainage (refer to Table 25-13) over the next 4–6 hours.

Source: These calculations were completed using commonly available values modified from the original work of Holliday and Segar, 1957.

receive IV volume replacement must successfully complete an oral hydration challenge prior to discharge home.

Any child evaluated for dehydration in an emergency department or urgent care center should have follow-up the next day to evaluate whether the ORT has been successful. Diagnostic studies are usually not required unless the etiology of the dehydration is unknown or the patient's physical examination findings are unimproved (Finberg, 2002).

The children most at risk for poor prognosis are those who present with severe hyponatremic or hypernatremic dehydration. The greatest risk in both populations is too rapid a correction of the serum sodium, ultimately resulting in cerebral edema, seizures, and death from CNS injury. Children with mild to moderate isonatremic or hyponatremic dehydration who tolerate ORT should not have any sequelae.

EATING DISORDERS

Daniel Goodman, John D. Mead, Gary R. Strokosch

PATHOPHYSIOLOGY

The two most common eating disorders are anorexia nervosa (AN) and bulimia nervosa (BN) (Table 25-16 and Table 25-17). Although many people think of bulimia nervosa in terms of its binge–purge cycle, its most important feature is restriction of calories. Much of the breakthrough and frank binge eating that occurs within this disorder is likely a result of hunger, secondary to restriction of caloric intake. Thus AN and BN disorders have this characteristic in common. When calorie restriction alone or purging by any of several various means results in significant weight loss, the

psychological and emotional sequelae can be devastating. It is common in emaciated patients to see examples of idiosyncratic thought, most commonly food preoccupation.

As early as the mid-1940s, when Ancel Keys first conducted his research on the effects of dietary deprivation (Keys et al., 1950), the behaviors associated with starvation were noted. His group of conscientious objectors looked very similar to the starving, eating-disordered patients one might encounter today. These individuals spent time talking about food, looking at pictures of food in magazines, exchanging recipes, chewing gum and ice, and smoking. Additionally, modern-day families of anorexics often report that these individuals engage in preparation and service of food, without ever eating themselves. The engagement is a result of preoccupation with food.

Clinically, HCPs who treat eating disorders have found that food obsession does not lead to increased eating. In fact, it appears that increased weight loss is accompanied by an increased drive to push one's weight down further. This cycle renders these individuals incapable of recovering from these disorders without intervention.

Weight loss also interferes with a person's ability to modulate emotions. Starving patients are often anxious, depressed, agitated, or distractible. They can also be confused and combative at times.

Thus the main thrust of treatment must be restoration of weight. In essence, a better way of understanding anorexia nervosa is to think of it as a *weight disorder* rather than an *eating disorder*. Weight gain is the key to recovery.

TABLE 25-16

Anorexia Nervosa

- Refusal to maintain a body weight over a minimal normal weight for age and height:
  - Weight loss leading to maintenance of body weight less than 85% of that expected
  - Failure to make expected weight gain during period of growth, leading to body weight less than 85% of that expected
- Intense fear of gaining weight or becoming fat, even though underweight
- Disturbance in the way in which one's body weight, size, or shape is experienced; undue influence of body weight or shape on self-evaluation; or denial of the seriousness of the current low body weight
- In postmenarchal females, absence of at least three consecutive menstrual cycles when otherwise expected to occur (primary or secondary amenorrhea)

Source: American Psychiatric Association, 2000.

TABLE 25-17

Bulimia Nervosa

- Recurrent episodes of binge eating. An episode of binge eating is characterized by both:
  - Eating, in a discrete period of time (within any 2-hour period), an amount of food that is definitely larger than most people would eat during a similar period of time and under similar circumstances
  - A sense of lack of control over eating during the episode (a feeling that one cannot stop eating or control what or how much one is eating)
- Recurrent inappropriate compensatory behavior in an attempt to prevent weight gain, such as self-induced vomiting; misuse of laxatives, diuretics, enemas, or other medications; fasting; or excessive exercise
- The binge eating and inappropriate compensatory behaviors that both occur, on average, at least twice a week for 3 months
- Self-evaluation that is unduly influenced by body shape and weight
- A disturbance that does not occur exclusively during episodes of anorexia nervosa

Source: American Psychiatric Association, 2000.

PRESENTATION

While severely emaciated individuals may present to the emergency department, it is best to stabilize them medically and schedule an outpatient evaluation to more thoroughly assess the situation. More commonly, evaluations are scheduled after an initial phone call is made to a professional or program by an eating-disordered individual or a concerned family member. Evaluations should include the identified patient as well as family members, especially parents or caregivers. Due to the secretive nature of eating disorders, it is helpful to conduct separate interviews; the HCP should meet with the patient individually to obtain a history and complete a physical examination, while the psychologist meets with family and other interested parties. This separation allows all parties more freedom to share information at the outset.

A follow-up appointment should be scheduled, during which the pertinent findings are shared in a sensitive and respectful manner. Additionally, a therapeutic plan may be discussed at the second meeting. Critical to the patient's overall success are an effective programmatic approach and commitment from, and involvement of, many individuals. It also helps to establish the expectation that the family and loved ones will be a part of the interprofessional therapeutic team, thereby allowing for more communication during treatment.

In general, the information gathered from the identified patient and from those accompanying him or her should include a developmental history, family history, the patient's medical history, and the history of the present illness. This history may be collected somewhat differently from the patient than from the family, but it can be very helpful to have multiple informants when trying to understand the individual's current situation.

A few patterns are worth noting in the history taking. It is common for the identified patient to underestimate the duration or the severity of the current symptoms. As a consequence, the input of the other informants may prove very useful. In addition, any findings on the physical examination that are inconsistent with the history warrant further consideration. Examiners should inquire about any history of anxiety, especially with respect to examples of trouble with separation from parents. It is common for individuals with eating disorders to fail at camps and sleepovers. Extracurricular activities should be discussed as well. Questions should focus on the nature of the individual's involvement, his or her ability to handle increased responsibility, and any recent changes. Finally, peer relationships should be discussed. Often, these are misrepresented or exaggerated by the patient. In truth, such relationships are often lacking in individuals with eating disorders.

Eating-disordered individuals and their families will typically report periods of emotional lability alternating with times of flat affect. In particular, increases in sadness, depression, irritability, and anxiety are observed. Likewise, these individuals experience obsessional thinking, increased perfectionism, feelings of guilt, and ritualistic or compulsive behaviors, especially with respect to food. Social withdrawal, loss of sexual libido, and overall dysphoria are common and likely related to the state of semistarvation. Again, the relationship between weight loss and overall mood cannot be overstated. The need for nutritional rehabilitation in eating disorders is paramount.

As previously noted, many of the physical findings with eating-disordered patients result from their state of starvation. These findings may include the following signs and symptoms:

- Decreased weight and cachectic appearance
- Decreased body temperature
- Bradycardia and hypotension (with significant postural changes)
- Acrocyanosis
- Edema
- Dry skin with discoloration or dirty-looking areas
- Cold extremities
- Loss of scalp hair
- Increased lanugo
- Diminished deep tendon reflexes

Most of these physical examination findings can be explained by the weight loss. Families appreciate hearing that these findings represent the body's attempt to compensate for decreased energy intake and that they are reversible with proper therapy.

With bulimic patients, given their tendency toward more normal weight, vital signs may be normal. However, tachycardia and hypotension reflect volume depletion. Other signs of dehydration may be noted, along with enlarged parotid glands or tonsils, and possible erosion of tooth enamel. Occasionally, signs of self-induced vomiting, ranging from superficial ulceration to calluses or scarring on the dorsum of the fingers (Russell sign), may be observed. Additionally, a decreased or absent gag reflex may be further evidence of vomiting. Swelling of the hands and feet may also be noted if serum albumin levels are low.

Other physical complaints frequently noted by eating-disordered patients include fatigue, muscle weakness, cramps, abdominal pain, constipation, headaches, chest pain, heart palpitations, easy bruising, and sore throat. These patients may also report sleep disturbances, problems with concentration, increased physical activity, and dizziness with or without fainting.

DIFFERENTIAL DIAGNOSIS

The majority of individuals who are evaluated by eating disorder specialists display the typical features of anorexia nervosa or bulimia nervosa and are actually suffering from one of these two disorders. However, one must consider other conditions, particularly in those patients who are genuinely concerned about their low weight and general health. These conditions would include such disease processes as malignancy, inflammatory bowel disease, malabsorption syndrome (celiac disease), diabetes mellitus, hyperthyroidism, hypopituitarism, or other chronic disease. In addition, mood disorders such as anxiety or depression, and obsessive–compulsive disorder should be considered.

PLAN OF CARE

While there are no definitive diagnostic tests available for anorexia nervosa, several laboratory findings may be of interest, most of which are related to malnutrition and conservation of energy. They include increased BUN, aspartate aminotransferase (AST), alanine aminotransferase (ALT), cholesterol, and serum carotene levels, as well as decreased serum magnesium, phosphate, calcium, zinc, and copper concentrations. Thyroid function tests may reveal low thyroxine and low T_3 levels. Additionally, estradiol levels are often low to the point of being immeasurable if the weight loss is not more recent. Patients with bulimia nervosa tend to exhibit elevated serum amylase secondary to parotid gland overstimulation.

While these data may help support a diagnosis of an eating disorder, the interprofessional team typically makes its judgments and subsequent recommendations based on the history. The plan for treatment should be described to the family, with particular emphasis on family members' roles in the recovery of the identified patient. Due to the very nature of eating disorders, most patients present to the HCP against their will to at least some degree. Thus the commitment to a treatment program of those persons accompanying the individual is much more useful than the promise of compliance from the patient in the throes of these disorders.

As part of this therapeutic alliance, a decision regarding the most appropriate treatment setting is made. Three situations would necessitate inpatient hospitalization on an acute care unit. The first is a significantly low body weight (e.g., BMI below the 5th percentile). The second condition is a significant weight loss without an alarmingly low BMI. These patients may not appear especially emaciated, but will likely be suffering some of the same physical symptoms as a function of the amount of weight lost. Finally, it may be necessary to admit the individual to the inpatient unit based on the degree of struggle at home or a family's inability to manage the symptoms of the eating disorder. In certain cases, this decision is built into a management plan that starts with an attempt at outpatient treatment with an agreement at the outset of treatment to move to the inpatient level of care if the patient fails to make progress in at a lower level of care.

At present, the most commonly used inpatient settings for the treatment of eating disorders are psychiatric hospitals or psychiatric units of medical centers. This makes intuitive sense, given that these disorders are psychiatric in nature. It would not be atypical for a patient to be admitted to a psychiatric unit once he or she has been stabilized medically, or to be admitted directly to the psychiatric unit with medical consultation for management of any medical problems. Problems can arise, however, when patients present with, or develop, more significant medical problems in these settings. Consequently, based on this factor and on the emergence of some innovative management strategies being used in a handful of eating disorders programs, the acute care unit is an extremely useful setting for the initial phase of a comprehensive approach to treatment. This type of program goes well beyond the monitoring and medical stabilization traditionally used simply as a step toward transfer to the psychiatric unit. Instead, it begins with the understanding that the patient is to be admitted to a medical unit under a psychiatric diagnosis (most often anorexia nervosa or bulimia nervosa) specifically for treatment of the eating disorder. Additionally, it is understood that the inpatient portion of the program functions as one of several steps. In fact, it is often the briefest of these steps.

Along with medical stabilization, which is typically achieved relatively quickly, actual treatment of the eating disorder is undertaken. It comprises an integrated management model under the co-direction of a physician and a psychologist. It also involves participation from any number of other professionals—most notably the nursing staff on the unit. The approach is behavioral in nature, and food is the key to rehabilitation. As part of this phase of treatment, the family or other loved ones are quite heavily involved, becoming an essential part of the treatment team. Specifically, they participate in training to prepare for the next phase of treatment, which begins as soon as the patient is discharged home. The same strategies and techniques employed on the inpatient unit are taught and used at home. Symptom management remains the focus of treatment, with weight gain constituting the central issue in recovery.

DISPOSITION AND DISCHARGE PLANNING

It is widely reported that anorexia nervosa has the highest mortality rate of any mental disorder (usually agreed to be 10%). Patients with a younger age of onset, as well as those receiving earlier intervention, have better outcomes, and those with BN often do better than those with AN. Experienced treatment programs are effective at restoring weight, but relapse remains all too common. For some patients, this outcome may be attributed to a changing cast of HCPs involved in the different phases of care. When continuity of care is achieved, outcomes improve and prognosis becomes less dependent on the severity of symptoms or the willingness of the patient to improve. The ability of a coordinated, interprofessional program to help manage symptoms across inpatient and outpatient settings is the critical factor and may actually be a better predictor of long-term success.

ELECTROLYTE IMBALANCES

CALCIUM

Randall Ruppel

Pathophysiology

Calcium is involved in many important functions of the body, including neuronal activity, muscular contraction, myocardial conduction, and blood coagulation. Moreover, it is involved in many intracellular processes, and has an obvious role in bone formation. The concentration of calcium in the plasma, therefore, is tightly regulated, primarily by the actions of parathyroid hormone (PTH). Approximately 1 to 2 kg of calcium is present within the average adult body, 98% of which is found within the skeleton (Holick et al., 1998). The plasma concentration of calcium ranges from 9 to 10 mg/dL (2.4 mmol/L).

Plasma calcium exists in three forms: (1) combined with plasma proteins—specifically albumin; (2) diffusible, nonionic complexes, such as calcium citrate or calcium phosphate; and (3) unbound ion. As a significant amount of plasma calcium is bound to proteins, the measurement of total calcium is affected by albumin levels. The ionized form is not bound to albumin and direct measurement of ionized calcium is not affected by albumin levels; therefore, it may be a more accurate assessment of plasma calcium concentration. The ionized form of calcium is of primary importance for most functions in the body, with its normal concentration ranging from 1.1 to 1.3 mmol/L. Alternatively, the following formula may be used to determine the corrected total calcium concentration (Avent, 2007):

$$\text{Corrected Ca}_{total} = \text{Measured Ca}_{total} + 0.8 \times (4 - \text{Albumin level})$$

Regulation of calcium concentration is a complex interaction between the gastrointestinal (GI), renal, and skeletal systems. Primarily regulation is controlled by parathyroid hormone (PTH). Increasing concentration of PTH causes increasing concentration of serum calcium. It does so by promoting calcium absorption from the bone and decreasing renal excretion of calcium. PTH also triggers the process by which vitamin D is converted into its active form, thereby increasing intestinal absorption of calcium. This is a much slower means of increasing plasma calcium concentration than the former two mechanisms, however.

Hypocalcemia

Etiology. A number of conditions may cause hypocalcemia. In the acute care setting, the underlying reason is often secondary to other aspects of care. One of the more common causes in pediatric patients is binding of ionized calcium to the citrate of banked blood—a condition seen frequently during or after cardiac bypass, with massive transfusion after trauma, or during plasmapharesis. Although transient, this binding may produce dramatic effects on an irritable myocardium and may require acute replacement.

Renal replacement therapy may lead to hypocalcemia, either by an imbalance between clearance and replacement of calcium or by binding to the citrate sometimes used for anticoagulation. Again, this condition may lead to acute, symptomatic hypocalcemia, sometimes referred to as "citrate lock." Citrate lock occurs when the amount of citrate used exceeds the metabolic potential of the liver, resulting in increasing total calcium levels but concomitant decreasing ionized calcium levels.

Tumor lysis syndrome is a potentially acute complication of cancer chemotherapy, most commonly associated with treatment for leukemia, lymphoma, and bulky solid tumors (Colen, 2008). The massive lysis of tumor cells creates electrolyte disturbances, especially an acute rise in phosphorus levels. Sudden hyperphosphatemia may cause calcium to precipitate out of the plasma, leading to symptomatic hypocalcemia.

Other acute illnesses are also associated with hypocalcemia. Pancreatitis may cause breakdown of intra-abdominal fat via released lipase, which then binds to calcium. Rhabdomyolysis causes both an acute rise in phosphorus levels, with subsequent calcium binding, and movement of calcium into damaged muscle cells. Sepsis is associated with hypocalcemia (particularly meningococcemia) by means that are unclear.

The neonate is at risk for hypocalcemia. Transient physiologic hypoparathyroidism occurs during the first 3 days of life and may lead to neonatal seizures. Multiple factors contribute to this electrolyte imbalance, including a reduced intake of calcium, a temporary parathyroid suppression by a high fetal calcium level, and tissues that are refractory to PTH. Prematurity and low birth weight increase the neonate's risk of developing symptomatic hypocalcemia.

Hypocalcemia of a more chronic nature may result from a number of disorders. Several illnesses are associated with hypoparathyroidism, which lead to subsequent low PTH levels and consequent hypocalcemia. DiGeorge syndrome, also known as velocardiofacial syndrome, may be detected perioperatively. It results from partial deletion of chromosome 22 and may be associated with cardiac malformations, facial anomalies, and aplasia of the parathyroid glands and thymus. Hypocalcemia from hypoparathyroidism in the perioperative period is sometimes the first symptom of this diagnosis.

Pseudohypoparathyroidism is a condition characterized by normal PTH levels but an end-organ resistance to PTH effects. Vitamin D deficiency is defined by both an inadequate intake of vitamin D and an insufficient amount of ultraviolet light exposure. Certain medications may create a calcium imbalance, particularly furosemide, phenytoin, and radiocontrast agents. Hypomagnesemia may lead to hypocalcemia; it is reviewed later within this section. Kidney failure is often associated with low calcium levels, owing to both inappropriate utilization of calcium by the kidneys and poor hydroxylation of vitamin D into its active form.

Presentation. Low plasma calcium concentration leads to instability of cellular membrane potentials and results in increased firing of action potentials. The clinical manifestations of hypocalcemia, therefore, reflect the irritability of the neuromuscular complex. Also, the cardiac action potential is acutely affected, with a lengthening of phase 2 of the action potential and lengthening of the QT interval (Ariyan & Sosa, 2004).

Symptoms of hypocalcemia are largely related to the neuromuscular irritability that develops. Early symptoms include numbness and tingling, muscle cramps, and mild mental status changes such as irritability or confusion. Later, as symptoms become more severe, Chvostek's and Trousseau's signs may be elicited. Chvostek's sign is a contraction of the upper lip or side of the face that occurs when the facial nerve is tapped near the earlobe, just below the zygomatic bone. Trousseau's sign is a carpal spasm (adducted thumb, flexed wrist with fingers extended and together) that occurs when a blood pressure cuff is inflated on the arm. The QT interval is prolonged on an electrocardiograph (ECG) tracing with severe hypocalcemia, and hypotension and bradycardia may develop. Other severe signs include laryngospasm, seizures, and tetany.

Plan of care. Laboratory evaluation of hypocalcemia that is of unclear etiology should include measurement of total and ionized calcium, phosphorus (elevated in hypoparathyroidism, decreased in vitamin D deficiency), magnesium, alkaline phosphatase (high in vitamin D deficiency, normal or low in hypoparathyroidism), PTH, BUN, and creatinine levels. If vitamin D deficiency is suspected, levels of 25-hydroxyvitamin D and 1,25-hydroxyvitamin D should be evaluated. Ankle and wrist radiographs may show bone density in rickets, and a chest radiograph (CXR) may demonstrate the absence of a thymus (suspected DiGeorge syndrome).

Treatment of symptomatic hypocalcemia requires IV replacement. Calcium chloride (10 mg/kg) provides more calcium (13.6 mEq/gm) than calcium gluconate (100 mg/kg, 4.6 mEq/gm), yet carries a much higher risk of tissue necrosis with extravasation; thus this medication should be given only via a central venous catheter when possible (Taketomo et al., 2010). Careful monitoring is important during calcium infusion, as sudden, high concentrations of calcium may inhibit the sinus node and lead to bradycardia or arrest.

For chronic treatment, calcium carbonate or calcium citrate may be given as oral supplements. Patients with vitamin D deficiency may require vitamin D supplementation. The patients who do not convert vitamin D appropriately (e.g., because of kidney failure or hypoparathyroidism) require supplementation with 1,25-hydroxyvitamin D (Greenbaum, 2004).

Certain illnesses necessitate care when considering calcium replacement. In patients with pancreatitis and rhabdomyolysis, resolution of the process results in release of calcium, and hypercalcemia may subsequently result (Greenbaum, 2004). Of note, the American Heart Association (AHA, 2005) does not recommend the routine use of calcium during resuscitation.

Hypercalcemia

Etiology. Compared to hypocalcemia, hypercalcemia is a relatively uncommon finding. In the inpatient setting, the cause is most likely to be malignancy; this imbalance occurs in as many as 1.3% of childhood cancers (Kerdudo et al., 2005), although it is far less common than in adults (Shepard & Smith, 2007). Elevated calcium may occur as a result of bony destruction by cancer cells or secretion of humoral factors. Neoplastic cells may secrete parathyroid hormone-related protein (PTHrP), which has many of the biological effects of PTH (Inukai et al., 2007). Tumor cells may also secrete humoral factors, such as interleukin-6 (IL-6) or tumor necrosis factor (TNF), that result in an elevated calcium level. With bone marrow involvement, these factors may directly affect osteoclastic activity (Trahan et al., 2008).

Hypercalcemia may occur from immobility, injuries such as leg fractures, spinal cord damage, or critical illness. Bone resorption leads to an elevated calcium level and bone density loss. PTH and 1,25-hydroxyvitamin D levels are decreased in this case (in response to the elevated calcium level), and nephrocalcinosis may result from calcium deposition in the kidney.

Infants who have a history of perinatal asphyxia may develop subcutaneous fat necrosis, which in rare cases may contribute to hypercalcemia. These lesions are typically firm, erythematous plaques or nodules located on the cheeks, buttocks, thighs, and/or arms. Either prostaglandin E or macrophage production of 1,25-hydroxyvitamin D are hypothesized to cause the elevated calcium level.

Children with Williams syndrome (chromosome 7 microdeletion) who experience associated cardiac or renovascular problems may develop hypercalcemia in infancy. The cause of this calcium abnormality is unknown.

Patients with sarcoidosis frequently have hypercalcemia. The granulomatous tissue that occurs as a result of the disease produces 1,25-hydroxyvitamin D independent of the normal feedback loop, which ultimately results in an elevated calcium level. Other granulomatous diseases may have the same effect, such as tuberculosis or histoplasmosis, albeit not as commonly as in sarcoidosis.

Excessive intake of both vitamin A and vitamin D intake leads to increased osteoclastic activity, and excess vitamin D intake causes increased intestinal absorption of calcium, leading to hypercalcemia. The excessive intake has to occur over an extended period for this effect to appear.

Familial hypocalciuric hypercalcemia is an inherited disorder in which the calcium sensors in the parathyroid gland are dysfunctional. It is similar to neonatal hyperparathyroidism but is less severe, as the individual has at least some functioning sensors. The PTH level is normal in the face of hypercalcemia, or slightly elevated with normocalcemia. The abnormal calcium sensors are also found in the kidneys, where they increase calcium resorption due to the body's (erroneous) perception of calcium deficiency.

Abnormalities of hyperparathyroidism can be associated with calcium derangements and may be of primary or secondary etiology. Primary hyperparathyroidism may be the result of a parathyroid adenoma or hyperplasia and is rare in pediatric patients. It may be associated with multiple endocrine neoplasia (MEN) syndromes. Secondary hyperparathyroidism occurs in response to a hypocalcemic state, such as arises with chronic kidney failure. Vitamin D metabolism is impaired in the setting of chronic kidney failure, which results in hypocalcemia and a compensatory elevated PTH level. The excess secretion of PTH may persist after correction of the kidney failure, as in kidney transplants, leading to hypercalcemia. Intestinal malabsorption of calcium may create a similar scenario, as may vitamin D–deficient rickets. Neonatal hyperparathyroidism may be severe in infants who have an absence of calcium sensors in the parathyroid gland. This imbalance may also occur in children born to mothers with hypoparathyroidism.

Presentation. Symptoms of hypercalcemia may be vague and difficult to separate from the symptoms of the underlying disease. Mild to moderate hypercalcemia is usually asymptomatic. The gastrointestinal effects as a result of smooth muscle relaxation include constipation and anorexia. Neurologic symptoms include lethargy, headache, depression, anxiety, hypotonia, and coma. Renal tubular dysfunction may occur with resulting polyuria and dehydration. Nephrolithiasis and nephrocalcinosis are also risks of hypercalcemia.

Physical examination usually shows only signs of the underlying disorder. It is rare to see calcium deposits on the cornea under slit-lamp exam. The ECG shows a shortened QT interval or possibly first-degree heart block.

Plan of care. Many causes of hypercalcemia may be determined based on the patient's history. When the etiology of hypercalcemia is unknown, PTH, 25-hydroxyvitamin D, phosphorus, and urinary calcium levels will help determine its cause. BUN and creatinine measurements are important to assess kidney function. When a malignancy is suspected, the PTHrP level may be measured in addition to completing diagnostic studies for cancer. Williams syndrome may be diagnosed by fluorescent in situ hybridization (FISH).

Ensuring hydration with normal saline is the first step in treating hypercalcemia. Polyuria may occur from elevated calcium levels and lead to dehydration. Because increased sodium excretion in the urine improves calcium excretion, the combination of normal saline and loop diuretics aids in increasing calcium clearance. Health care professionals should *not* prescribe or administer thiazide diuretics to patients with hypercalcemia, as these agents decrease renal calcium excretion.

Glucocorticoids may be useful to treat hypercalcemia. Steroids reduce both the level and the effects of vitamin D and, therefore, are particularly helpful when excess amounts of vitamin D are the main cause of the elevated calcium. Steroids are also particularly useful in malignancies such as sarcoidosis, as they treat the underlying disease, Although care must be taken that use of these medications does not impede the diagnosis of the underlying malignancy.

Calcitonin may be administered when rapid correction of the calcium is required, or if hydration and diuresis prove ineffective in rectifying the imbalance. Calcitonin inhibits bone resorption and is safe, but of limited effectiveness, as resistance to therapy often develops. Bisphosphonates, therefore, have become the mainstay of therapy when rapid treatment of severe hypercalcemia is required (Mittal, 2007). Pamidronate (0.5–2 mg/kg as an infusion) is effective in pediatric patients if administered within 3 to 4 days of the development of hypercalcemia. Bisphosphonates also act by reducing bone resorption. Phosphate and magnesium levels may be affected by this therapy, however, so they should be monitored along with calcium levels.

CHLORIDE

Randall Ruppel

Pathophysiology

Chloride is the most abundant anion in the extracellular fluid. Its level is regulated by the kidneys and the intestine. Chloride generally passively follows sodium reabsorption in the kidney, so it is indirectly affected by aldosterone. It also passively follows sodium absorption in the gastrointestinal system, although this anion may be actively absorbed when bicarbonate is excreted in the intestine. Note that chloride is actively secreted in the stomach in the form of hydrochloric acid.

Chloride is important for maintaining electrical neutrality in the body. As the primary extracellular anion, it is responsible for balancing cations—primarily sodium—in the bloodstream. It therefore generally follows sodium levels: When sodium is elevated, chloride is usually elevated; concomitantly, when sodium is low, chloride is usually low. Chloride has an inverse relationship with bicarbonate. Altered bicarbonate levels with subsequent acid–base abnormalities compel the chloride level to adjust independent of the sodium level so as to maintain the electrical balance. Therefore, chloride is closely related to the acid–base balance in the body.

Hypochloremia

Etiology. Hypochloremia is associated with metabolic alkalosis. Because chloride and bicarbonate have an inverse relationship, the chloride level drops and the bicarbonate level increases to maintain electrical neutrality. An excess of bicarbonate results from hypochloremia, with the subsequent development of metabolic alkalosis.

Emesis or nasogastric suctioning is a common cause of hypochloremia, owing to the loss of hydrochloric acid through the gastric fluid. Initially, a metabolic alkalosis develops as a result of hydrogen ion loss. Later, volume depletion maintains the metabolic alkalosis through a number of factors. First, the decreased glomerular filtration rate results in less bicarbonate filtration and less bicarbonate excretion. Second, volume depletion results in a reflexive increase in sodium reabsorption in an effort to reclaim volume. In hypochloremia, the sodium reabsorption is accompanied primarily by bicarbonate reabsorption. Third, aldosterone secretion increases in response to volume depletion, causing bicarbonate reabsorption.

A common cause of hypochloremia in hospitalized pediatric patients is diuretic use. This complication is accompanied by a contraction alkalosis in which the fluid loss from diuretics causes primarily chloride (not bicarbonate) excretion. The remaining total bicarbonate load is contained in less total fluid, with a consequent higher concentration of bicarbonate that results in alkalosis.

Both respiratory and cardiac failure may lead to hypochloremia. Patients with chronic hypercarbia, whether from chronic lung disease or hypoventilation while on a ventilator, may develop a compensatory metabolic alkalosis and an associated hypochloremia. Permissive hypercapnia in the management of acute lung injury may also be associated with these findings. The fluid retention and excess fluid buildup that occurs in congestive heart failure may lead to hyponatremia and hypochloremia.

Unusual causes of hypochloremia include chloride-losing diarrhea, or congenital chloridorrhea—an autosomal recessive illness that results in excessive chloride loss in the stool. Cystic fibrosis may cause hypochloremia through excessive sodium and chloride loss in sweat. Bartter's syndrome is a defect of the renin–angiotensin system that results in tubular dysfunction and loss of chloride in the urine.

Ulimia with excessive vomiting and surreptitious diuretic use may present with hypochloremia, metabolic alkalosis, and hypokalemia. A patient with bulimia will have a low urine chloride level as a result of his or her volume-depleted state. Diuretic use produces a high urinary chloride level after the medication is administered, but a low level in between doses.

Presentation. Signs and symptoms of hypochloremia are usually those of metabolic alkalosis and the underlying disorder (Powers, 1999). In states with associated volume depletion, signs and symptoms may include thirst, lethargy, tachycardia, tachypnea, or delayed capillary refill. Alkalosis enables increased binding of calcium to albumin, so signs and symptoms of hypocalcemia may be present. Arrhythmias are a possible complication of alkalosis and hypokalemia; note that anti-arrhythmic medications are less effective in alkalotic states. Respiratory effort may be slow and shallow with a metabolic alkalosis, in a natural attempt to compensate and normalize the pH. Severe hypochloremia may present with seizures.

Plan of care. Diagnosis of the etiology of hypochloremia is usually apparent from the history. A diagnostic work-up is more likely to be aimed at determining the cause of metabolic alkalosis than the cause of hypochloremia. Chloride is rarely measured in isolation; sodium, potassium, calcium, and bicarbonate levels should also be evaluated when a chloride imbalance exists. An arterial blood gas measurement may be indicated, especially if hypercarbia is suspected. Urine chloride is a useful test for volume depletion in the face of metabolic alkalosis (Greenbaum, 2004). Given that bicarbonate is excreted in the urine during metabolic alkalosis, and sodium is excreted along with it, the urine sodium level may be high despite the patient being in a volume-depleted state when concomitant alkalosis is present. A low urine chloride level, therefore, is a better indicator of volume depletion in this circumstance.

Treating the underlying problem is the first step in correcting hypochloremia. This therapy usually involves volume repletion, except in patients with congestive heart failure. Nasogastric suctioning or diuretic use may need to be reduced or stopped. Alternatively, a proton-pump inhibitor may reduce the acid loss if nasogastric suction is still required. Refeeding nasogastric secretions into a jejunal tube may help avoid excessive hydrogen and potassium losses. With diuretic use, the addition of a potassium-sparing diuretic may help mitigate the resulting alkalosis. Also, acetazolamide may help correct metabolic alkalosis by decreasing reabsorption of bicarbonate through its action as a carbonic anhydrase inhibitor, although it may not have an effect on chloride levels.

Replacement of chloride may be accomplished by administration of a number of solutions. Sodium chloride and potassium chloride are both options, depending on which of the cations requires replacement. Sodium chloride must be used with caution in patients with congestive heart failure, as the sodium load may increase the total body fluid level. Ammonium chloride is another option. Ammonium is acidifying: It releases hydrogen ions. For this reason, it is not recommended in patients with liver or kidney failure, as it is poorly metabolized and excreted.

In the rare case of severe hypochloremia associated with seizures, arrhythmias, or respiratory depression, arginine hydrochloride or hydrochloric acid may be infused for rapid correction of the imbalance. Administration of these acids is dangerous, however, and this treatment should be reserved for emergent situations in a setting with resuscitation equipment and monitoring capabilities.

Hyperchloremia

Etiology. Hyperchloremia may be associated with a metabolic acidosis. The most common cause of this chloride imbalance is diarrhea resulting in excessive bicarbonate loss. This condition produces a non-anion gap or hyperchloremic acidosis. Distal renal tubular acidosis (RTA), along with a number of other electrolyte abnormalities, is associated with a hyperchloremic acidosis, arising from the body's inability to acidify the urine.

Urinary diversion into the colon—which, in pediatric patients, is usually for congenital malformations—may cause a non-anion gap acidosis. The chloride in the urine is absorbed in the colon and exchanged for bicarbonate, resulting in hyperchloremic acidosis. Urinary diversions are more commonly performed into the ileum for this reason, although acidosis may still develop.

Excessive treatment with chloride-containing substances may result in hyperchloremia. In the case of ammonium chloride, acidosis may be exacerbated by the presence of excessive amounts of ammonium.

When recovering from respiratory alkalosis, there may be a lag time before pH normalizes. Specifically, the compensatory metabolic acidosis that develops in response to the respiratory alkalosis may persist for a few days after resolution of the alkalosis, resulting in a lingering metabolic acidosis.

Presentation. Hyperchloremia does not produce specific symptoms in itself; rather, most of the symptoms may be attributed to the accompanying acidosis. Hypernatremia and hyperkalemia are common findings in this state. Hyperkalemia occurs secondary to hydrogen ion shifts into the cells to compensate for the altered pH, with potassium subsequently moving out of the cells.

Acidosis impairs cardiac contractility and cardiac response to inotropes, although this effect probably requires a severe acidosis (Handy & Soni, 2008). Respiratory compensation for a metabolic acidosis may lead to Kussmaul breathing. Brain metabolism is affected by acidosis and may result in lethargy, headache, confusion, or coma if severe.

Plan of care. Treatment of hyperchloremia is directed at correcting the underlying cause and the accompanying acidosis. The use of IV bicarbonate is generally recommended only for patients with severe acidosis.

MAGNESIUM

Randall Ruppel

Pathophysiology. Approximately 50% of the body's magnesium stores are found in bone. Most of the remainder is found in intracellular spaces or in soft tissue. Only 1% of the total magnesium is extracellular fluid; thus serum magnesium levels are poor indicators of total body magnesium stores.

Magnesium is involved in a multitude of important processes, including ATP generation, DNA transcription, and protein synthesis. It is a cofactor in ion transport channels and is important for membrane stabilization. Magnesium deficiency may be an important component of hypokalemia, as magnesium is an important cofactor in the regulation of potassium excretion, and hypokalemia is often refractory to treatment in the face of hypomagnesemia (Huang & Kuo, 2007).

Approximately 40% of dietary magnesium is absorbed in the upper small intestine. The amount absorbed varies depending on the serum magnesium level. Excretion and regulation occur primarily through the kidneys. Unlike sodium and calcium, which are reabsorbed in the proximal tubules, magnesium is mainly reabsorbed in the thick ascending limbs. Magnesium movement in the thick ascending limbs is passive, depending on the electrical gradient formed by sodium and potassium (Yucha & Dungan, 2004).

No single hormone plays a principal role in magnesium regulation. Factors that affect sodium excretion may also affect magnesium excretion; therefore, diuretics may increase magnesium excretion. Magnesium excretion is also affected by the calcium level, with reduced reabsorption occurring in the setting of hypercalcemia. This relationship likely reflects signaling by a calcium–magnesium sensor in the glomeruli. Alterations in pH, PTH, calcitonin, and vasopressin levels may all affect magnesium regulation. The most important regulator of magnesium excretion is the magnesium concentration itself.

Hypomagnesemia

Etiology. Either GI or renal losses primarily cause hypomagnesemia. Diarrhea, for example, may cause significant magnesium losses. Steatorrhea is particularly troublesome due to the formation of magnesium–lipid complexes. A number of illnesses, therefore, may lead to magnesium deficiency, including inflammatory bowel disease, cystic fibrosis, celiac disease, or intestinal failure (short gut syndrome). A rare condition called primary intestinal hypomagnesemia is a genetic disorder that leads to malabsorption of magnesium in the intestine.

A common cause of hypomagnesemia in hospitalized patients is medications. Amphotericin and cisplatin both cause magnesium wasting in the kidney. Diuretics, as previously described, may induce increased urinary magnesium excretion; potassium-sparing diuretics seem to decrease this effect. Osmotic diuretics also cause magnesium loss. Treatment with calcium is thought to stimulate the calcium–magnesium sensor, which results in increased magnesium excretion.

Treatment of diabetic ketoacidosis may lead to hypomagnesemia. Total body stores of magnesium may become depleted during DKA as a result of the osmotic diuresis that takes place during this imbalance. Treatment with insulin stimulates increased uptake of magnesium by the cells, resulting in low serum magnesium levels.

Excessive uptake of magnesium into bone is possible in "hungry bone syndrome," which usually occurs after parathyroidectomy. This effect occurs in conjunction with the hypocalcemia and hypophosphatemia that result from the same condition. Refeeding syndrome may have a similar effect, with increased uptake occurring in the face of total body depletion. Pancreatitis may trap magnesium in the process of saponifying necrotic fat tissue.

A number of rare genetic renal disorders may cause hypomagnesemia. Bartter syndrome and Gitelman syndrome are the most common of these conditions, and both are associated with defects of tubular transport. Gitelman syndrome, in particular, is usually associated with a low serum magnesium concentration. Other illnesses characterized by hypomagnesemia include hypercalciuria and nephrocalcinosis, autosomal dominant hypoparathyroidism, dominant hypomagnesemia, and mitochondrial hypomagnesemia (Weglicki et al., 2005).

IV fluids may cause hypomagnesemia by two different mechanisms. First, volume expansion may result in less sodium reabsorption, which in turn leads to decreased magnesium reabsorption. Second, extended therapy with magnesium-deficient fluids may result in insufficient magnesium intake.

Newborns may develop a transient or idiopathic hypomagnesemia. Hypomagnesemia is commonly seen in newborns of diabetic mothers, and may be associated with any maternal condition that results in magnesium depletion.

Presentation. Most of the symptoms associated with hypomagnesemia are attributable to the concomitant hypo-calcemia and hypokalemia; therefore, neuromuscular excitability may present as seizures, paresthesias, ataxia, tetany, muscle weakness, and delirium. The most important consequence of magnesium depletion is arrhythmia. Specifically, a low magnesium level may predispose pediatric patients with heart disease or those undergoing cardiopulmonary bypass to serious arrhythmias, including torsades de pointes. Hyperglycemia may be seen when magnesium levels are low secondary to insulin resistance.

Plan of care. Diagnosis of hypomagnesemia requires an index of suspicion, as it may not be included in standard electrolyte panels. Generally, the cause of low serum magnesium will be apparent based on the patient's history. If it is unclear where the magnesium losses are occurring, a fractional excretion (FE) of magnesium may be measured using the following formula:

$$FE_{Mg} = (U_{Mg} \times P_{Cr})/(0.7 \times P_{Mg} \times U_{Cr})$$

where U equals urine magnesium or creatinine and P equals plasma magnesium or creatinine. This number should be low when serum magnesium is low, usually less than 2%. A higher number implies renal losses, whereas a low (appropriate) number probably implies GI losses.

Severe hypomagnesemia should be treated with parenteral magnesium replacement. Magnesium sulfate is most commonly used for this purpose, although magnesium chloride is available. Both forms may be given intravenously or intramuscularly. Given that kidney excretion of magnesium is regulated primarily by the serum magnesium concentration, a rapid increase in the serum magnesium level may cause an increase in the amount excreted, making the replacement less effective. Therefore, a slow infusion rate will be more effective at raising the serum magnesium level. Emergent bolus dosing of magnesium is recommended in symptomatic hypomagnesemia associated with seizure or arrhythmia and should be performed only in a setting with available resuscitation equipment and monitoring capabilities.

Oral magnesium replacement is available in several forms. Magnesium gluconate, magnesium oxide, and magnesium sulfate are preparations used for such treatment. Doses must be divided to avoid diarrhea.

Magnesium has some therapeutic uses outside of hypomagnesemia. For example, it is indicated as a primary drug for the treatment of torsades de pointes or other polymorphic ventricular tachycardias characterized by a prolonged QT interval. Magnesium may also be used to treat ventricular arrhythmias that are unresponsive to other antiarrhythmics. Magnesium is a common therapy for preeclampsia, as it acts as a calcium antagonist. In addition, its relaxation effects on bronchial smooth muscle make this medication a suggested therapy in the management of status asthmaticus.

Hypermagnesemia

Etiology. Hypermagnesemia is almost invariably due to excessive intake of magnesium. Because intestinal absorption of this anion is largely unregulated, use of magnesium-containing laxatives or antacids may cause an elevated serum magnesium level. When the patient is receiving total parenteral nutrition, hypermagnesemia may be related to either an inappropriate concentration or impaired kidney function. Newborns are at risk for hypermagnesemia if maternal magnesium therapy was used for preeclampsia. Neonates are at particular risk for this imbalance due to their naturally reduced glomerular filtration rate.

Chronic kidney failure, tumor lysis syndrome, milk alkali syndrome, and lithium ingestion may all be associated with a mild elevation in magnesium level. Diabetic ketoacidosis may initially present with mild hypermagnesemia before insulin therapy is initiated despite a total body depletion of magnesium.

Presentation. Hypermagnesemia may impair the functioning of the neuromuscular junction, leading to hypotonia, decreased reflexes, weakness, and even paralysis. Other neurologic effects include lethargy and CNS depression. Magnesium also affects vascular tone and may lead to hypotension and flushing when elevated. Prolonged PR, QRS, and QT intervals may be seen with hypermagnesemia, which may progress to heart block in severe cases. Abdominal cramping, nausea, and vomiting are other possible side effects.

Plan of care. In severe cases of hypermagnesemia, basic stabilization is the first consideration. Inotropes may be needed for hypotension, and ventilatory assistance for severe muscle weakness. Calcium chloride or calcium gluconate may be of temporary benefit with magnesium-induced heart block. For rapid removal of excess magnesium, dialysis is most effective, although it is reserved for life-threatening hypermagnesemia. Exchange transfusion may also be used, especially in neonates who may not be dialyzed. Loop diuretics may increase magnesium excretion, as may fluid expansion.

Mild or asymptomatic hypermagnesemia should resolve spontaneously, as long as kidney function is normal, with the cessation of the magnesium intake.

PHOSPHORUS

Randall Ruppel

Pathophysiology

Phosphate is the most abundant intracellular anion. It shifts easily between intracellular and extracellular compartments and plays important roles in membrane structure, energy storage, and transport. It is involved in some way in most metabolic processes and is an important part of glycolysis as well as a key component of ATP, 2,3-DPG, and CPK. Most of the phosphorus obtained from the diet is absorbed passively in the jejunum, although some active transport of this anion is vitamin D dependent. The kidney primarily controls phosphate excretion, where phosphorus is filtered and reabsorbed. Phosphaturia increases under the influence of an increased PTH level by reduction of tubular reabsorption.

Unlike calcium, approximately 12% of phosphorus is bound to proteins (Holick et al., 1998). Inorganic phosphate is present in several forms, including HPO_4^{2-}, $NaHPO_4^-$, and $H_2PO_4^-$, and, therefore, is usually expressed in terms of the elemental phosphate concentration. Phosphorus levels vary according to a circadian rhythm, reaching a low point between about 9 A.M. and 12 P.M., and then peaking in the afternoon and again around midnight. The concentration of phosphorus also varies with age—more so than any other electrolyte.

Hypophosphatemia

Etiology. One percent of the total body phosphorus store is extracellular, therefore the serum phosphate level may not reflect total body depletion of this anion. A classic example of hypophosphatemis is diabetic ketoacidosis (DKA). Intracellular stores are sometimes depleted with DKA due to the extracellular shift of phosphorus from acidosis and insulin deficiency, leading to an increase in urinary losses. As insulin is administered, more phosphorus is drawn into the cells for the beginning of glycolysis, which may lead to a subsequent drop in the serum phosphate level. Similarly, the refeeding syndrome after protein starvation may lead to hypophosphatemia. When a malnourished patient receives carbohydrates, the insulin level rises, which in turn induces a shift of phosphorus into the cell. The demand for phosphorus increases as anabolic metabolism increases and may lead to low serum phosphorus levels. Such an effect typically occurs within three days of starting nutrition (Marinella, 2003). This degree of malnutrition may be observed in illnesses such as severe anorexia nervosa, cystic fibrosis, Crohn's disease, or neglect.

Respiratory alkalosis, or recovery from respiratory acidosis, causes an intracellular shift of phosphorus. The acute drop in carbon dioxide stimulates glycolysis, which again increases the need for intracellular phosphate and may lead to low serum phosphorus. Hyperventilation and the subsequent induced respiratory alkalosis are associated with pain, panic attacks, sepsis, salicylate poisoning, and mechanical ventilation. Intracellular pH is less affected by metabolic alkalosis (because carbon dioxide moves more freely in and out of the cells compared to bicarbonate), so this imbalance will not typically lead to acute hypophosphatemia.

Rapidly growing tumors may consume a significant amount of phosphorus and lead to deficiency. Notably, hypophosphatemia may occur after bone marrow transplant as the new bone marrow begins to grow, or due to a tumor-induced osteomalacia that causes kidney phosphorus wasting as a result of factors secreted by the tumor.

Chronic use of aluminum-containing antacids may cause phosphorus depletion. Antacids bind phosphate and increase excretion in the stool. In addition, medication used for the purpose of binding phosphate, as in chronic kidney failure, may occasionally lead to iatrogenic hypophosphatemia. Pediatric patients may also develop rickets as a response to chronic phosphorus depletion.

Extensive burns are often accompanied by severe hypophosphatemia. This finding may be associated with increased incidence of sepsis in burn patients (Subramanian & Khardori, 2000) and may worsen in hyperventilation states.

Hyperparathyroidism causes kidney phosphate wasting, as PTH inhibits tubular reabsorption. Although many of the symptoms of hyperparathyroidism are attributable to hypocalcemia, some of the symptoms—including weakness and fatigue—may also result from hypophosphatemia. Following parathyroidectomy, both hypocalcemia and hypophosphatemia may occur due to "hungry bone syndrome," in which massive deposition of calcium and phosphorus into the bone results from removal of the stimulus for bone dissolution.

Two forms of rickets, x-linked hypophosphatemic rickets and autosomal dominant hypophosphatemic rickets, are associated with kidney phosphate wasting, inappropriately low or normal 1,25-hydroxyvitamin D levels, and hypophosphatemia. The x-linked form may occur in both males and females. In addition to these genetic conditions, the tubular defect associated with Fanconi syndrome leads to urinary losses of a number of substances, including phosphorus, and may cause rickets. Similar urinary losses may be seen after kidney transplant.

Vitamin D deficiency causes impaired calcium absorption with subsequent hyperparathyroidism. The combination of increased kidney wasting of phosphorus from elevated PTH, along with decreased absorption of phosphorus from the gut with low vitamin D, may also lead to rickets. Although dietary causes of hypophosphatemia are unusual, premature infants have an increased need for phosphorus for purposes of rapid bone growth and may have a relative deficiency if fed regular formula or human breastmilk without supplementation.

Presentation. The most severe effects of hypophosphatemia were described with refeeding syndrome during World War II (Marinella, 2003). When severely malnourished patients were fed carbohydrates too quickly, the resulting hypophosphatemia led to edema and cardiac failure, likely due to ATP depletion in the myocytes. Presenting symptoms include muscle weakness (including diaphragmatic weakness) and rhabdomyolysis, likely due to CPK dysfunction. This weakness may be profound enough to

lead to respiratory failure. Dysfunction of 2,3-DPG may be attributed to both neurologic effects (hypoxia, delirium, coma) and hematologic effects (hemolytic anemia, impaired granulocyte activity, thrombocytopenia).

Phosphorus has numerous important roles in the body, and it affects every major system. Several studies have shown an association between hypophosphatemia and mortality in hospitalized patients (Brunelli & Goldfarb, 1999). Although evidence is lacking, hypophosphatemia has been implicated in prolonged need for mechanical ventilation, cardiac dysfunction, and decreased tissue oxygen delivery.

Chronic hypophosphatemia may lead to rickets. Early signs of rickets include craniotabes (a ping-pong ball effect noted when pressing on the occiput), rachitic rosary (enlargement of the costochondral junctions), and thickening of the wrists and ankles. As the disease progresses, the individual may develop malformation of the skull, bowing of arms and legs, delayed eruption of teeth with enamel defects, long bone fractures, and abnormalities of the spine and pelvis. Radiologic exams may be confirmatory.

Plan of care. Intravenous phosphorus supplements are available, with both sodium and potassium being used as the balancing ion; the appropriate supplement is often chosen based on the patient's potassium level. IV supplementation is recommended for severe hypophosphatemia, as large oral supplements may cause diarrhea and have unreliable absorption. Rapid infusion of phosphate may cause kidney failure, hypocalcemic tetany, hyperphosphatemia, and ECG changes; given these risks, infusions should be administered over 4 to 6 hours (Brunelli & Goldfarb, 1999).

Oral supplements are effective for milder or chronic hypophosphatemia. Doses are divided to avoid diarrhea and GI distress. Nutritional causes of phosphate may usually be corrected simply with dietary changes. Rickets, depending on the form, may require vitamin D supplementation.

Hyperphosphatemia

Etiology. The main cause of hyperphosphatemia is kidney failure. Phosphorus is readily absorbed from the GI tract, and the kidney regulates excretion. Failure of the kidney to maintain phosphorus excretion may lead to hyperphosphatemia. Increased PTH secretion may decrease renal phosphorus reabsorption and compensate for mild to moderate kidney failure. As kidney function continues to decline, however, the compensatory mechanisms eventually become overwhelmed. Conversely, the decreased secretion of PTH in hypoparathyroidism leads to increased phosphorus retention and hyperphosphatemia. An inherited disorder of phosphorus excretion, known as tumoral calcinosis, causes calcifications around large joints (Weisinger & Bellorin-Font, 1998).

Disorders that cause cellular disruption may induce hyperphosphatemia by releasing large amounts of intracellular phosphorus into the extracellular space. An important example is tumor lysis syndrome, which is most commonly associated with treatment of leukemia, lymphoma, or bulky solid tumors (Colen, 2008). When tumor cells are rapidly destroyed, intracellular products such as phosphorus, potassium, and uric acid are released and temporarily overwhelm the ability of the body to excrete them. Other illnesses that cause hyperphosphatemia by a similar mechanism include rhabdomyolysis, which is associated with muscle cell destruction and elevated CPK, and massive hemolysis, which leads to red cell destruction and elevated bilirubin and lactate dehydrogenase (LDH) level.

Kidneys with normal function may generally manage increased intake of phosphorus. Neonates have a limited kidney function; therefore, consumption of a high phosphorus load, like that present in cow's milk, may lead to hyperphosphatemia. In addition, some laxatives and enemas have high phosphorus content and may be absorbed if the child has intestinal dysmotility. Treatment of hypophosphatemia and vitamin D intoxication may also lead to hyperphosphatemia.

Phosphorus utilization is reduced in diabetic ketoacidosis, such that a shift of phosphorus to the extracellular compartment may occur. Patients in DKA may present with hyperphosphatemia. The elevation in extracellular phosphorus may also be associated with increased phosphorus excretion. Total body stores of phosphorus may actually be low despite the high serum concentration, and treatment may subsequently cause hypophosphatemia. Disorders causing lactic acidosis may have a similar effect.

Presentation. An abrupt rise in serum phosphorus concentration may cause precipitation of calcium and produce symptoms of hypocalcemia, including tetany. Chronic elevation of phosphorus may lead to calcium precipitation or, more likely, result in calcium deposition in soft tissues. Serum calcium (albumin corrected) times serum phosphate ($Ca \times PO_4$) greater than 72 mg^2/dL^2 is actually associated with increased mortality in adults (Ganesh et al., 2001).

Phosphorus has an important role in the development of renal osteodystrophy. First, the concomitant decrease in the calcium level, along with the elevated phosphorus level, causes increased production of PTH and secondary hyperparathyroidism, with subsequent osteoclastic activity to help raise the serum calcium level. In addition, increased phosphorus concentration in the kidney inhibits vitamin D production; this effect, in conjunction with downregulation of vitamin D receptors in kidney failure, leads to decreased osteoblastic activity. This combination of events results in abnormal bone formation (Schucker & Ward, 2005).

Plan of care. Mild hyperphosphatemia, especially when the patient has normal kidney function, may not require treatment. The combination of phosphate restriction in the diet, which may be achieved by reducing protein intake,

and IV fluids may help reduce a mild elevation in the individual's phosphorus level.

With kidney disease, ongoing problems with phosphate overload warrant management with phosphate binders that reduce GI phosphorus absorption. Although aluminum-containing salts are excellent phosphate binders, the chronic absorption of aluminum may lead to toxicity. Specifically, aluminum deposited into bone may lead to osteomalacia. Systemic aluminum may cause anemia and encephalopathy (Schucker & Ward, 2005).

Calcium salts are the usual agent of choice for treating hyperphosphatemia. Calcium carbonate and calcium acetate are commonly administered for this purpose. Clinical trials comparing the two have not shown a definitive advantage of one medication over the other (Schucker & Ward, 2005). However, calcium carbonate is most effective in an acid environment, so it will be less effective if acid-reducing medications such as proton-pump inhibitors are a part of the pediatric patient's treatment regimen.

Sevelamer hydrochloride is a phosphate binder that does not contain a metal. Clinical trials have failed to show a distinct advantage of this medicine over calcium-containing salts, although it is clearly preferable in the face of hypercalcemia. Lanthanum carbonate is a metal-containing substance that has excellent phosphate-binding properties and minimal gastrointestinal absorption.

Dialysis has limited effectiveness in removing phosphorus. Thus, in patients suffering from kidney failure; phosphorus absorption from the more efficient GI tract is required.

POTASSIUM

Randall Ruppel

Pathophysiology

Potassium, the most abundant cation in the body (Rastegar & Soleimani, 2001), is primarily found within the intracellular space. However, this ion is a major determinant of the cellular resting membrane potential, affecting the level of potassium in the extracellular concentration, so it is modulated under strict control. The primary route for potassium excretion is through the kidneys, which serves as the main route for overall regulation of total body serum stores. The balance between intracellular and extracellular potassium concentration is regulated by several key hormones. Insulin and β-adrenergic catecholamines cause an intracellular shift of potassium, whereas α-adrenergic catecholamines cause an extracellular shift. Aldosterone plays an important role in kidney regulation of potassium, but has only a mild effect on this ion's transcellular distribution. Parathyroid hormone also has a mild effect on this electrolyte, causing a decrease in intracellular potassium, whereas mineralocorticoids cause a mild increase in this level.

Acid–base balance and osmolarity have an important effect on potassium homeostasis. A sudden increase in serum osmolarity causes water to shift out of the cells, producing a concurrent shift of potassium out of the cells by solvent drag. Acid–base variations affect serum potassium differently depending on the underlying cause of the irregularity. A metabolic acidosis from an organic acid, such as is seen with diabetic ketoacidosis, usually leads to little change in the total concentration of potassium. Conversely, nonorganic acidosis (as in kidney failure) produces a dramatic increase in serum potassium level (Rastegar & Soleimani, 2001). In general, acidosis may cause a rise in serum potassium and alkalosis may cause a decrease in extracellular potassium level.

Hypokalemia

Etiology. Hypokalemia is usually a result of abnormal potassium loss, and is most frequently drug induced. The class of drugs that most commonly causes hypokalemia by potassium wasting is the diuretics (Gennari, 1998). Diuretics allow more sodium to be delivered to the collecting tubules, where reabsorption creates a favorable gradient for potassium excretion. Penicillin may also cause potassium loss by increasing sodium delivery to the distal nephrons. Laxatives and enemas may waste potassium in the stool, leading to low potassium stores. Other drugs may cause hypokalemia by promoting a shift into the intracellular compartment if they have β-sympathetic activity. Agents that have this effect include bronchodilators, decongestants, dopamine, and dobutamine. Theophylline and caffeine increase Na^+/K^+ ATPase activity, so their use may result in hypokalemia, especially if they are taken in large doses. Several drugs cause magnesium depletion, including amphotericin B, cisplatin, and aminoglycosides; this depletion subsequently leads to hypokalemia.

Another common cause of excessive potassium loss in pediatric patients is diarrheal illnesses. Although only 10% of total potassium excretion normally occurs in the stool, in diarrheal states these losses may become significant. The addition of vomiting, or nasogastric suctioning, results in chloride depletion and metabolic alkalosis, which may further exacerbate hypokalemia by increasing renal potassium excretion.

Some diseases may lead to metabolic alkalosis and hypokalemia. The most dramatic of these disorders is hyperaldosteronism, in which increased sodium reabsorption in the distal tubules creates an environment favorable for potassium excretion. Liddle's syndrome may have a similar effect on sodium reabsorption despite the presence of a low aldosterone level; as a consequence, it may lead to alkalosis and hypokalemia. Other diseases that have similar effects include Bartter's syndrome and Gitelman's syndrome, both of which are due to an intrinsic kidney defect and are associated with hypotension and volume depletion. Type I renal tubular acidosis is also associated with hypokalemia.

Presentation. Hypokalemia is generally asymptomatic. It has several adverse consequences, however, that may affect different systems. The main cardiovascular effect of note is hypokalemia-induced ventricular arrhythmias in patients with underlying heart disease. Patients with ischemic heart disease, heart failure, or left ventricular hypertrophy are at highest risk for developing arrhythmias (Schulman & Narins, 1990). In addition, the risk of digoxin toxicity is heightened in the face of a low serum potassium level. Experimental evidence suggests that potassium depletion may contribute to diastolic dysfunction (Srivastava & Young, 1995). Finally, hypokalemia may contribute to hypertension (Weiner & Wingo, 1997). Due to the numerous detrimental effects of this imbalance, it has been suggested that in adult cardiovascular patients potassium levels be maintained above 4.5 mmol/L (Macdonald & Struthers, 2004).

In addition to its cardiovascular effects, potassium depletion may affect other systems. Potassium is very important for the resting membrane potential, and a low serum potassium level may impair depolarization and muscle contraction. In addition, severe hypokalemia may reduce the blood flow to muscle, leading to muscle necrosis. Subsequently, muscle weakness, cramping, and fatigue may develop. Hypokalemic periodic paralysis is a rare disorder associated with recurrent episodes of weakness or paralysis. Other effects of hypokalemia include impaired insulin release, polyuria, kidney cystic disease, and worsening hepatic encephalopathy (Weiner & Wingo, 1997).

Plan of care. Hypokalemia is corrected by potassium replacement. Supplemental potassium replacement is the most common cause of hyperkalemia in hospitalized patients (Rimmer et al., 1987); thus care must be exercised in administering this treatment. In emergent situations (cardiovascular patients at risk for arrhythmia), IV supplementation with potassium chloride at 0.5–1 mEq/kg may be given, up to a maximum dose of 20 mEq. Cardiac monitoring is required during IV replacement, and the supplement should be given through a central vein when possible. Institutional policy should be followed for all administration of IV potassium.

For nonemergent therapy, oral supplementation may be used. Three formulations of oral potassium exist: potassium chloride, potassium phosphate, and potassium bicarbonate. The majority of the time, potassium chloride is the formulation of choice. The latter two formulations are typically used only for patients who require phosphate supplementation or correction of acidosis, respectively.

Hyperkalemia

Etiology. The first consideration when a high serum potassium level is noted is to determine if it might be a spurious result due to hemolysis of the sample, muscle activity during the blood draw, thrombocytosis, or leukocytosis.

Repeating the blood draw is warranted if any of these confounding factors is suspected while preparing to treat the patient.

The most common cause of hyperkalemia in hospitalized patients is supplementation or use of potassium-sparing diuretics (Rimmer et al., 1987). As the kidneys generally excrete large amounts of potassium, hyperkalemia is usually associated with impaired renal excretion. However, it is possible to overload normal kidney excretion capacity, especially with IV supplementation.

An acute rise in potassium may occur from acidosis, especially in the face of renal failure or decreased renal perfusion. An abrupt shift from intracellular stores may occur that may temporarily overwhelm the ability of the kidneys to manage the potassium level. This imbalance may also occur with an acute rise in osmolarity, especially when combined with insulin deficiency, such as is seen with diabetic ketoacidosis.

Hyperkalemia of a more chronic nature most commonly results from impairment of kidney excretion. Decreased aldosterone production occurs in Addison's disease and in congenital adrenal hyperplasia, resulting in decreased potassium excretion. In addition, treatment with angiotensin-converting enzyme (ACE) inhibitors, angiotensin II receptor blockers, or nonsteroidal anti-inflammatory drugs (NSAIDs) may reduce aldosterone production. Aldosterone resistance is seen in pseudohypoaldosteronism, as well as with therapeutic administration of potassium-sparing diuretics, trimethoprim, or pentamidine. Kidney failure may lead to both decreased aldosterone production and sensitivity. This hyporeninemic hypoaldosteronism, especially when it is accompanied by decreased glomerular filtration rate, may lead to hyperkalemia in patients with even mild to moderate kidney failure.

Presentation.   Hyperkalemia may be a life-threatening emergency. Its most serious complication is arrhythmia. The first ECG change that may be seen with a high serum potassium level is a peaked T wave; with continued elevation of serum potassium, the PR and QRS intervals subsequently become prolonged, leading to a loss of the PR interval, and merging of the QRS and T waves to produce a sine wave pattern. This arrhythmia is the precursor to ventricular fibrillation or asystole.

Because the resting membrane potential depends on the transcellular concentration of potassium, muscle weakness may be seen with hyperkalemia. Hyperkalemic periodic paralysis is a rare disorder associated with recurrent muscle weakness or paralysis.

Plan of care.   Hyperkalemia with ECG changes is an emergency and should be treated immediately. Membrane stabilization occurs with use of calcium chloride (10 mg/kg) or calcium gluconate (100 mg/kg). Calcium should be

effective within minutes and lasts 30 to 60 minutes; however, the dose may be repeated in 5 to 10 minutes if no change is seen with the initial therapy (Taketomo et al., 2010). A combination of insulin and glucose will help shift the potassium intracellularly until a more definitive form of therapy may be used. Insulin will cause a potassium shift within 15 to 30 minutes, an effect that should last a few hours. Bicarbonate is useful in the acidotic patient and has the same effect. β-Agonists may be given in IV or aerosolized form, will have an onset of action within 30 minutes, and usually produce an effect that lasts 2 hours, depending on the form administered. In addition to these therapies, all exogenous potassium and any confounding medications must be stopped.

More definitive therapy focuses on potassium removal. Diuretics may help increase potassium excretion when kidney function is normal. Cation exchange resin, given enterally or rectally, helps remove potassium by exchanging it for sodium in the gastrointestinal tract. Each gram of sodium polystyrene sulfonate binds 1 mmol of potassium in exchange for 2 to 3 mmol of sodium. The most effective therapy for potassium removal is hemodialysis. This treatment is usually reserved for hyperkalemia that either is unresponsive to conventional therapy or occurs secondary to kidney failure.

After the acute management of hyperkalemia is ensured, the underlying cause must be treated, whether it is by medication change, hormone replacement, or kidney failure management.

SODIUM

Maureen A. Madden

Pathophysiology

Sodium (Na^+), the primary extracellular cation, is the principal osmotically active solute responsible for the maintenance of intravascular and interstitial volumes. It is associated with functioning of skeletal muscle, nerve and myocardium action potentials, and maintenance of acid–base balance. The normal serum sodium concentration range is approximately 135 to 145 mEq/L.

A complex balance of intake and excretion regulates sodium stores in the body. The regulatory mechanism for sodium intake is poorly developed, although it may respond to large changes in sodium levels. Alterations in sodium and fluid balance often occur in tandem and affect serum osmolality. Absorption of sodium occurs throughout the GI tract, maximally in the jejunum and minimally in the stomach, with absorption facilitated by way of a sodium- and potassium-activated adenosine triphosphate (ATP) transport mechanism that is affected by aldosterone or desoxycorticosterone acetate (DCA). Excretion of sodium occurs through urine, sweat, and stool, with the kidney being the principal organ regulating sodium output.

The renal regulation of sodium excretion depends on a balance between glomerular and tubular functions, in concert with the actions of osmoreceptors in the hypothalamus that control secretion of antidiuretic hormone (ADH, vasopressin). This fine balance of water maintains the narrow range for normal serum sodium concentration, despite great variation in water intake. The kidney filters sodium, 99% of which is reabsorbed along the length of the renal tubule and only 1% of which is excreted in the urine. Normally changes in glomerular filtration rate (GFR) do not affect sodium homeostasis. When an alteration in GFR occurs, changes in the filtered load of sodium are compensated for by changes in tubular reabsorption of sodium. Approximately two-thirds of the filtered sodium is reabsorbed by the proximal convoluted tubules. With ECF volume contraction, the fraction of absorbed sodium increases; in contrast, with volume expansion, sodium absorption decreases. The percentages of filtered sodium and water reabsorbed in the proximal tubules are proportional; therefore, fluid passing through the proximal convoluted tubules maintains a sodium level comparable to the serum level in the blood.

A significant amount of sodium reabsorption occurs in the loop of Henle; this process is essential for determining water balance and the concentration of urine. Water reabsorption occurs in the descending limb of the loop of Henle, while the ascending limb is responsible for sodium reabsorption. When the sodium load is increased in the loop, either through changes in GRF or sodium reabsorption in the proximal tubules, most of the excess load is reabsorbed within the loop.

In many disease states, the body loses its ability to regulate sodium normally. Such abnormalities result in changes in volume rather than changes in sodium concentration. When a higher level of sodium occurs, the body compensates by retaining an equal amount of water; the result is edema, with sodium concentration remaining in or near the normal range. Excessive losses of sodium may cause hyponatremia but are often accompanied by comparable water losses, resulting in volume contraction with minimal changes in sodium concentration.

Alterations in sodium concentration most often are related to an abnormality in the body's handling of water. A defect in the urinary diluting capacity, in conjunction with excess water intake, results in hyponatremia. A defect in urinary concentration, when accompanied by inadequate water intake, results in hypernatremia.

Hyponatremia

Etiology. Hyponatremia defined as a serum sodium level less than 135 mEq/L, indicating that there is relatively less sodium than water in the ECF space. This imbalance often occurs as a complication of disease or therapy. The pediatric patient may develop hyponatremia from increased free water intake, excess water retention, increased sodium loss, or a combination of these factors. Hyponatremia may occur in relation to hypervolemia, euvolemia, or hypovolemia.

Hypervolemic hyponatremia is associated with congestive heart failure, acute or chronic renal failure, nephrotic syndrome, water intoxication (e.g., ingestion of powdered formula diluted with an excessive amount of water, ingestion of excessive amounts of water), and cirrhosis. Hypovolemic hyponatremia can occur with either renal losses (e.g., osmotic diuresis, renal tubular acidosis) or extrarenal losses (e.g., diarrhea, vomiting, burns, pancreatitis). Hyponatremia may also be seen in conjunction with normovolemic states. Potential causes include syndrome of inappropriate antidiuretic hormone (SIADH), adrenal insufficiency, CNS disease (e.g., cerebral salt wasting syndrome, meningitis, intracranial tumors), pulmonary disease (e.g., cystic fibrosis), and excessive use of diuretics.

Presentation. In the pediatric patient, signs and symptoms of hyponatremia may include irritability, poor feeding, nausea, vomiting, lethargy, seizures, and coma.

A laboratory value of hyponatremia can be misleading, secondary to the existence of "pseudo" hyponatremic states that are associated with hyperlipidemia, hyperproteinemia, or hyperglycemia. When an elevated level of a lipid or protein is present in the circulating blood, the substance displaces fluid from serum, which in turn decreases the relative volume of water and electrolytes. As a result, the reported sodium concentration will be low, because the concentration of sodium is reduced, although the total body sodium may actually be normal.

Serum osmolality is determined by the combined effects of solutes in the serum, especially sodium, glucose, and BUN. Establishing hyponatremia with hypoosmolarity is necessary to evaluate and guide management of hyponatremia.

The volume of water shift and the severity of clinical symptoms associated with hyponatremia are related to the acuity and the rate of the drop in serum sodium and osmolality. Pediatric patients who develop hyponatremia over several days or weeks may be asymptomatic until the serum sodium level reaches a very low point (Ralston et al., 2006). Acute hyponatremia that develops over hours or days (e.g., over a period less than 48 hours) is more likely to produce cerebral edema and produce significant alterations in neurologic status. Seizures and coma are associated with lower serum sodium concentrations.

Plan of care. If the pediatric patient is at risk for hyponatremia, the HCP should closely monitor the serum sodium concentration to detect and promptly treat hyponatremia and prevent progression. Urgent treatment of hyponatremia should be instituted in all patients who exhibit neurological changes. If the patient presents with seizures and hyponatremia, the serum sodium must be acutely raised to 125 mEq/L to stop seizure activity. A hypertonic saline chloride solution (e.g., 3% NaCl [513 mmol/L] contains 0.5 mEq/L Na$^+$) should be administered if available. It is necessary to calculate the amount of sodium required to correct to a desired mEq/L; the following equation may be used for this purpose:

$$\text{Total mEq Na}^+ \text{to raise sodium to target level}$$
$$= 0.6 \times (\text{wt in kg}) \times (\text{target Na}^+ - \text{measured Na}^+)$$

To raise the serum sodium level, the calculated amount of hypertonic saline should be administered over 15 to 20 minutes to gain rapid control of the seizures. A 1.2 mL/kg aliquot of 3% NaCl will raise the serum sodium level by 1 mEq/L and increase serum osmolality sufficiently to slow the intracellular water shift. If hypertonic saline is unavailable, a 20 mL/kg bolus of 0.9% NaCl (normal saline) may be given to raise the serum sodium.

Once the acute correction is completed or if the pediatric patient is no longer experiencing neurological changes, correction of hyponatremia should proceed more slowly, at a rate of approximately 10 mEq/L per day (0.5–1 mEq/L every hour). Management of hyponatremia includes restoration of appropriate intravascular volume, replacement of sodium deficit, and identification and treatment of the underlying cause. Symptomatic hypovolemia is treated with boluses of normal saline or lactated Ringer's solution. Management of hyponatremia with hypervolemia may include fluid restriction and administration of loop diuretics.

If the serum sodium and osmolality are raised too rapidly, the resulting water shift from the intracellular to the extracellular (including intravascular) compartments can produce neurologic complications, including intracranial bleeding. Additional important assessments include strict monitoring of intake and output, urine specific gravity, serum electrolytes, serum osmolality, and daily weights.

Hypernatremia

Etiology. Hypernatremia is defined as serum sodium greater than 145 mEq/L. This imbalance may result from derangements of sodium or water balance either alone or in combination. Hypernatremia occurs when excessive sodium intake or loss of too much free water results in an increase in ECF sodium in relation to the amount of water in this space.

One of the body's major defenses against hypernatremia is thirst. The groups at greatest risk for hypernatremia, therefore, are infants, small children, and patients with significant developmental delay, decreased level of consciousness,

or critical illness, as they may not be able to signal thirst during episodes of fluid loss. Pediatric patients who develop hypernatremia may have received concentrated formula, been breastfed without supplementation, been treated with salt supplements, or received sodium bicarbonate. Water loss can be due to diarrhea, diabetes insipidus (central and nephrogenic), renal tubular disorders, and post obstructive diuresis.

Hypernatremia may be associated with hypovolemia, hypervolemia, or euvolemia. For this reason, it is important to assess the patient's fluid volume status when investigating the cause of the hypernatremia.

Presentation. Signs and symptoms of hypernatremia include irritability, high-pitched cry, lethargy, seizures, fever, renal failure, and rhabdomyolysis. In infants, these symptoms mimic those associated with infections and sepsis. A focused history, in addition to physical examination, is important in elucidating the diagnosis.

Hypernatremia typically increases serum osmolality. This rise in osmolality stimulates the posterior pituitary to release ADH, causing the renal water reabsorption until the osmolality returns to normal. The increased osmolality also leads to a shift in water from the intracellular to the extracellular compartment, including the vascular space. Such water movement from the cells can cause cellular dehydration and CNS dysfunction). Permanent CNS dysfunction can result when the serum sodium concentration is extremely high (e.g., greater than 165–170 mEq/L) (Hellerstein, 1993).

Pediatric patients who are unable to produce or respond to ADH (e.g., those with diabetes insipidus) are at risk for significant hypernatremia. These patients must be closely monitored to detect and treat hypernatremia before it becomes severe.

Plan of care. It is essential that hypernatremia is treated slowly and carefully. When the sodium concentration increases, serum osmolality increases concomitantly. In response, fluid moves from inside the cells to the serum in an attempt to balance the osmolality. In addition, the cells use amino acids or small protein peptides, further increasing the internal serum osmolality. Administration of free water would mean that water goes from the area of low osmolality (i.e., serum) to the area of higher osmolality (i.e., inside the cells), causing the cells to swell. In the brain, this effect can result in cerebral edema.

If the patient with hypernatremia demonstrates signs of inadequate tissue perfusion (i.e., shock), administer isotonic crystalloid by bolus (20 mL/kg) until perfusion is adequate. Avoid a rapid fall in serum sodium and osmolality, such as is associated with excessive bolus fluid administration, as it may contribute to the development of cerebral edema and other neurologic complications.

Once shock is corrected, estimate the fluid deficit and plan to replace the deficit over a period of 48 to 72 hours, while providing for maintenance fluid requirements and replacement of any ongoing additional fluid losses (e.g., through persistent diarrhea). The type of IV fluids administered will vary depending on the rate at which the serum sodium is falling. Generally, the serum sodium should decrease at a rate no faster than 0.5 to 1.0 mEq/L/hr throughout the course of treatment. Management of the hypervolemic hypernatremic patient includes the administration of loop diuretics and decreased sodium.

ENTERAL NUTRITION

GENERAL PRINCIPLES

Sammé Fuchs

Enteral nutrition in this section refers to the provision of manufactured nutrition products or human breastmilk into a functioning gastrointestinal (GI) tract via an enteral access device (A.S.P.E.N., 2009). The benefits and nutrient composition of human breastmilk are reviewed in detail later in this section.

Benefits of enteral nutrition

When an alternate feeding route is required, enteral nutrition is the preferred route of nutrition (over parenteral nutrition), as it is more physiologic, provides fuel to enterocytes, helps to maintain the protective barrier function of the gut, is associated with fewer infectious complications, and is more cost-effective (Mehta, 2009). Enteral nutrition provides key nutrients that are essential for growth and may mitigate inflammation by decreasing the release of cytokines, specifically IL-6 (Sanderson & Croft, 2005). Although the preferential use of enteral nutrition has not been substantiated by randomized control trials, it has been consistently promoted by consensus-based guidelines in the pediatric population (Mehta).

Indications and contraindications of enteral feeding

Pediatric patients requiring an alternate feeding route due to the refusal or inability to ingest, digest, or absorb adequate amounts of nutrients orally are potential candidates for enteral feeding (A.S.P.E.N., 2009). In the acute care setting, common indications for enteral feeding include mechanical ventilation, medication- or treatment-induced anorexia, hypermetabolism, or impaired swallowing ability. In the neonatal intensive care unit, the most common indication for enteral feeding is prematurity (i.e., neonates born at less than 32 to 34 weeks' gestational age with impaired inability to suck/swallow). Some hospitalized pediatric patients have preexisting gastrostomy tubes due to conditions such as failure-to-thrive or neurologic impairment that prevent adequate oral nutritional intake (A.S.P.E.N., 2002).

Contraindications to enteral nutrition may include inability to gain enteral access, bowel obstruction, postoperative ileus, active upper GI bleed, or intractable vomiting or diarrhea. In the critical care setting, the provision of enteral nutrition is often delayed in patients who require vasopressor support, have evidence of ischemic bowel, or require intubation (Mehta, 2009). Parenteral nutrition may be considered if establishment of enteral nutrition must be delayed for more than 5 days. Patients with preexisting malnutrition or low-birth-weight neonates may need parenteral nutrition earlier than 5 days (A.S.P.E.N., 2002).

Early enteral feeding

Hospitalized pediatric patients with conditions that warrant the use of enteral nutrition should be fed within 24 to 48 hours whenever possible. In the critical care setting, early enteral nutrition has been found to be safe and well tolerated in most pediatric patients with a functional GI tract, even in those who require vasopressor support (Skillman & Wischmeyer, 2009). Early enteral nutrition reduces the time needed to achieve goals related to calorie and protein intake. Some studies suggest that early enteral nutrition is associated with improved clinical outcomes, shorter hospital length of stay, decreased infection rates, and improved immune function (Petrillo-Albarano et al., 2006). Enteral feeding protocols optimize early enteral nutritional intake and improve tolerance of enteral feedings (Petrillo-Albarano et al.)

Enteral access

Selection of the proper enteral access device is essential to the success of enteral nutrition. When selecting this device, the patient's medical condition or disease state, GI anatomy, and gastric and intestinal function should all be considered. The HCP must decide whether to place the enteral access device into the stomach or the small bowel. Gastric feeding is indicated in patients with absence of delayed gastric emptying, obstruction, or fistula. When medically feasible, gastric feeding is preferred, as it allows for physiologic digestion. Transpyloric (also referred to as postpyloric) feeds are indicated in patients with gastric outlet obstruction, gastroparesis, pancreatitis, or documented aspiration. Transpyloric feeds may also be indicated in patients who do not tolerate gastric feeds well. A dual-lumen gastrojejunal tube is indicated in patients who need gastric decompression simultaneously with transpyloric feeds (A.S.P.E.N., 2009).

Nasogastric and orogastric feeding tubes are often placed blindly at the bedside. Placement of nasojejunal tubes is often accomplished using interventional radiology with fluoroscopy or endoscopy. Transpyloric tubes can be successfully placed at the bedside (Joffe et al., 2000) (see Chapter 47). Proper placement of the enteral access device is required prior to administering enteral nutrition or medication. Several bedside tests are used to confirm correct tube placement, though they vary in their accuracy. The method of choice used to confirm proper placement of a blindly placed enteral access device is a radiograph (A.S.P.E.N., 2009). It is not feasible to obtain several radiographs throughout the day and feeding tubes may migrate after initial of enteral feeds, so bedside methods may be used to confirm tube placement. Some useful bedside methods include checking for any changes in the external length of the tube since the time of radiographic confirmation, measuring the pH of the feeding tube aspirates, observing for negative pressure when withdrawing fluid from the feeding tube, and observing for any unforeseen changes in residual volumes (Methany et al., 2005).

Delivery

The specific method used to administer enteral nutrition depends on the clinical condition of the patient and the location of the feeding tube. Continuous-infusion feeds and intermittent-bolus feeds are the two methods most commonly used to deliver enteral nutrition; they are sometimes used in combination to optimize nutritional intake. Patients with transpyloric feeding tubes should be fed continuously. Patients with gastric feeding tubes may be fed by either method. In terms of tolerance, there is no evidence that continuous gastric feeds are superior to intermittent bolus gastric feeds (Mehta, 2009).

Decisions related to initiating and advancing enteral feeds in pediatric patients depend on clinical judgment and institutional practices. In general, isotonic formulas may be initiated at 1–2 mL/kg/hr for smaller children and 1 mL/kg/hr for larger children weighing 35 to 40 kg. Preterm, critically ill, or malnourished patients at risk of refeeding syndrome may initially need a lower volume of 0.5–1 mL/kg/hr. Feedings are advanced to meet nutritional goals based on tolerance, increasing by 0.5–1 mL/kg/hr every 6 to 24 hours. Bolus feeds may be initiated with a volume of 2.5–5 mL/kg given five to eight times per day, with a gradual increase occurring to condense feeds closer to five feedings per day; alternatively, they may be initiated with 25% of the goal volume divided equally into desired number of feedings per day and increased by 25% per day as tolerated until the goal volume is achieved (Table 25-18) (A.S.P.E.N., 2009). Patients receiving bolus feeds who cannot tolerate the goal volume during the day may be given supplemental continuous nocturnal feeds.

TABLE 25-18

Initiation and Advancement of Enteral Feeds		
	Initiation	**Advancement**
Continuous Feeds		
Smaller children (< 35 kg)	1–2 mL/kg/hr	0.5–1 mL/kg/hr every 6–24 hr
Larger children (> 35–40 kg)	1 mL/kg/hr	0.5–1 mL/kg/hr every 6–24 hr
Critically ill, preterm, or malnourished (at risk of refeeding syndrome) pediatric patients	0.5–1 mL/kg/hr	0.5–1 mL/kg/hr every 6–24 hr
Bolus Feeds		
Children	2.5–5 mL/kg, 5–8 feeds per day **or** 25% of goal volume divided equally into desired number of feeds as tolerated	Gradual increase in volume to condense number of feeds closer to 5 per day. Use supplemental continuous night feeds if unable to achieve goal with day bolus feeds.

Source: Enteral Nutrition Practice Recommendations Task Force, 2009.

Formula selection

Proper selection of nutrition products is important to optimize tolerance to enteral feeds. Age, underlying medical condition, and GI function should be considered when selecting an enteral formula. Human breastmilk is recommended as the preferred source of nutrition in infants whenever possible.

When human breastmilk is not available, several commercial infant formulas are available (Table 25-19). Infant formulas have higher concentrations of selected nutrients than breastmilk due to lower bioavailability. Standard formulas for infants less than 1 year of age include intact proteins and require intact GI function for their digestion. Specialized infant formulas are available for patients with specific diseases or malabsorption of or intolerance to carbohydrate, protein, or fat. Infant formulas are generally intended to provide 20 calories per 30 mL consumed. Infants who are fluid restricted or who require more calories or protein may need a concentrated formula. Infant formula may be concentrated with caution to a maximum of 30 calories per 30 mL by adding less water to concentrated liquid or powdered formula and/or by using modular additives (Sapford, 2000).

TABLE 25-19

Selected Term Infant Formulas (20 calories/30 mL)					
Trade Name	**Calories/mL**	**Grams pro/mL**	**Manufacturer**	**Features**	**Indications**
Milk Based					
Enfamil A.R. Lipil	0.67	0.017	Mead Johnson	Milk based, added rice starch	Frequent spit-up
Enfamil Gentlease	0.67	0.015	Mead Johnson	Hydrolyzed protein, reduced lactose	Fussiness, gas
Enfamil Lactofree Lipil	0.67	0.014	Mead Johnson	Lactose free	Lactose sensitivity
Enfamil Premium with Triple Health Guard	0.67		Mead Johnson	Milk based, contains prebiotics, nucleotides, DHA/ARA	Healthy term infant
Good Start Supreme	0.67	0.015	Nestlé	100% whey protein, hydrolyzed protein	Healthy term infant, fussiness, gas
Similac Advance Early Shield	0.67	0.014	Abbott Nutrition	Milk based	Healthy term infant
Similac Organic	0.67	0.014	Abbott Nutrition	Organic, milk based	Healthy term infant
Similac Sensitive	0.67	0.014	Abbott Nutrition	Milk based, lactose free	Fussiness, gas, lactose sensitivity
Similac Sensitive R.S.	0.67	0.014	Abbott Nutrition	Milk based, lactose free, added rice starch	GERD, fussiness, gas, lactose sensitivity
Soy Based					
Enfamil Prosobee	0.67	0.017	Mead Johnson	Soy based	Fussiness, gas, sensitivity to milk-based formula, vegetarian
Good Start Supreme Soy DHA and ARA	0.67	0.017	Nestlé Nutrition	Soy based	Fussiness, gas, sensitivity to milk-based formula, vegetarian
Similac Isomil Advance	0.67	0.017	Abbott Nutrition	Soy based	Fussiness, gas, galactosemia, vegetarian
Semi-elemental					
Similac Alimentum	0.67	0.021	Abbott Nutrition	Hydrolyzed casein, lactose free, 33% of fat as medium-chain triglycerides	Milk protein allergy
Nutramigen Lipil	0.67	0.019	Mead Johnson	Hypoallergenic, lactose free, sucrose free	Milk protein allergy/ sensitivity
Pregestimil Lipil	0.67		Mead Johnson	Hypoallergenic, lactose free, sucrose free, 55% of fat from medium-chain triglyceride oil	Intact protein sensitivity, fat malabsorption, galactosemia
Elemental					
EleCare	0.67	0.021	Abbott Nutrition	Hypoallergenic, 100% free amino acids, 33% of fat as medium-chain triglycerides	Short bowel syndrome, eosinophilic GI disorders, GI tract impairment, severe food allergies, protein maldigestion, malabsorption

(Continued)

TABLE 25-19

Selected Term Infant Formulas (20 calories/30 mL) *(Continued)*					
Trade Name	**Calories/mL**	**Grams pro/mL**	**Manufacturer**	**Features**	**Indications**
Neocate Infant	0.67	0.021	Nutricia	Hypoallergenic, 100% free amino acids	Short bowel syndrome, eosinophilic GI disorders, GI tract impairment, severe food allergies, protein maldigestion, malabsorption
Disease Specific					
Enfaport (20 calorie/ounce)	0.67	0.023	Mead Johnson	84% of fat as medium-chain triglyceride oil	Chylothorax, long-chain 3-hydroxyacyl-CoA-dehydrogenase deficiency
Portagen	0.67		Mead Johnson	87% of fat from medium-chain triglycerides, *not* nutritionally complete	Chylothorax, fat malabsorption, intestinal lymphatic obstruction
Similac 60/40	0.67	0.015	Abbott Nutrition	Mineral levels close to mineral content of breastmilk	Impaired renal function, requirement for lowered mineral intake

Gastroesophageal reflux disease (GERD).

Sources: Abbott Nutrition. (2009). *Pediatric nutrition product guide.* Columbus, OH: Author, pp. 2–161; Nutricia. (2008). *2008 product reference guide.* Gaithersburg, MD: Author, pp. 4–186; www.abbottnutrition.com; www.mjn.com; www.nestlenutrition.com/us.

Many standard and specialized formulas are available for the school-age, adolescent, and adult patient populations (Table 25-20). Modular additives may be needed to meet specific nutrient needs. Semi-elemental formulas may be indicated in patients with impaired absorption, diarrhea, or food allergy. Elemental formulas are indicated in patients with malabsorption, intestinal failure (short gut syndrome), or severe food allergy. Disease-specific formulas have modified nutrient profiles and are used under special circumstances such as kidney failure, chylothorax, or metabolic disorders.

Immunonutrition

Immunonutrition refers to the potential to modulate immune system activity by way of delivering specific nutrients. Immune-modulating enteral formulas are commercially available. Nutrients commonly found in these immune-modulating formulas include arginine, glutamine, aminopeptides, omega-3 fatty acids, and antioxidants.

The role of immune-modulating enteral nutrition formulas has not been well studied in the pediatric patient population. Based on the data available, immune-modulating enteral nutrition is not yet recommended in the pediatric patient population (Mehta et al., 2009).

Hang time for enteral formula

Enteral nutrition formulas can become contaminated at any point in the delivery process. To guide against this possibility, the manufacturer's guidelines should be followed in the storage, preparation, and administration of all enteral formulas.

Formulas used in a closed system offer a hang time of 24 to 48 hours. By comparison, human breastmilk and formula reconstituted from powder or liquid concentrate in an open system offer a hang time of only 4 hours. Table 25-21 summarizes appropriate hang times of various types of formulas.

TABLE 25-20

Selected Pediatric Formulas					
Trade Name	**Calories/mL**	**Grams pro/mL**	**Manufacturer**	**Features**	**Indications**
Standard					
Boost Kid Essentials 1.5	1.5	0.045	Nestlé Nutrition	Concentrated, lactose free, low residue, gluten free, kosher	Children ages 1–10 years, fluid restriction
Nutren Junior	1	0.03	Nestlé Nutrition	Lactose free, low residue, gluten free, kosher	Children ages 1–10 years
Nutren Junior Fiber	1	0.03	Nestlé Nutrition	Fiber containing, lactose free, low residue, gluten free, kosher	Children ages 1–10 years, when fiber-containing formula needed
Pediasure Enteral	1	0.03	Abbott Nutrition	Lactose free, gluten free, kosher	Children ages 1–13 years
Pediasure Enteral with Fiber	1	0.03	Abbott Nutrition	Fiber containing, lactose free, gluten free	Children ages 1–13 years, when fiber-containing formula needed
Semi-elemental					
Peptamen Junior	1	0.03	Nestlé Nutrition	Hydrolyzed whey protein, 100% whey based, 60% of fat as medium-chain triglycerides	Children ages 1–10 years, malabsorption, chronic diarrhea, pancreatitis, delayed gastric emptying
Peptamen Junior Fiber	1	0.03	Nestlé Nutrition	Hydrolyzed whey protein, 100% whey based, 60% of fat as medium-chain triglycerides, fiber containing	Children ages 1–10 years, malabsorption, chronic diarrhea, pancreatitis, delayed gastric emptying
Peptamen Junior 1.5	1.5	0.045	Nestlé Nutrition	Concentrated, hydrolyzed whey protein, 100% whey based, 60% of fat as medium-chain triglycerides	Children ages 1–10 years, fluid restriction, malabsorption, chronic diarrhea, pancreatitis, delayed gastric emptying
Vital jr.	1	0.03	Abbott Nutrition	Whey protein hydrolysate, 50% of fat as medium-chain triglycerides	Children ages 1–13 years, malabsorption, maldigestion
Elemental					
EleCare (30 calories per 30 mL)	1		Abbott Nutrition	Hypoallergenic, 100% free amino acids, 33% of fat as medium-chain triglycerides	Intestinal failure (short gut syndrome [SGS]), eosinophilic GI disorders, GI tract impairment, severe food allergies, protein maldigestion, malabsorption

(Continued)

TABLE 25-20

Selected Pediatric Formulas (*Continued*)

Trade Name	Calories/mL	Grams pro/mL	Manufacturer	Features	Indications
Neocate Junior	1	0.033	Nutricia	100% non-allergenic free amino acids, additional vitamins and minerals for malabsorption	Children ages 1–10 years, malabsorption, soy and milk allergy, intestinal failure (SGS), eosinophilic esophagitis
Vivonex Pediatric	0.8	0.024	Nestlé Nutrition	100% free amino acids, 68% of fat as medium-chain triglycerides	Severe intestinal failure (SGS), Crohn's disease, intestinal failure, malabsorption
Disease Specific					
Novasource Renal	2	0.074	Nestlé Nutrition	High calorie, reduced electrolyte content,	Acute renal failure, chronic renal failure, electrolyte restriction, fluid restrictions
Nepro with Carb Steady	1.8	0.081	Abbott Nutrition	High calorie, reduced electrolyte content	Dialysis
Suplena	1.8	0.045	Abbott Nutrition	High calorie, reduced electrolyte content, low protein	Impaired kidney function

Selected Enteral Formulas for Older Children (More Than 10 Years Old) and Adults

Trade Name	Calories/mL	Grams pro/mL	Manufacturer	Features	Indications
Standard					
Nutren 1.0	1	0.04	Nestlé Nutrition	Nutritionally balanced	Normal calorie and protein requirements
Nutren 1.0 Fiber	1	0.04	Nestlé Nutrition	Nutritionally balanced, fiber containing	Normal calorie and protein requirements
Nutren 1.5	1.5	0.06	Nestlé Nutrition	High calorie, 50% of fat as medium-chain triglycerides	Increased calorie needs, fluid restriction
Nutren 2.0	2	0.08	Nestlé Nutrition	High calorie, 75% of fat as medium-chain triglycerides	Increased calorie needs, fluid restriction
Osmolite 1 Cal	1.06	0.044	Abbott Nutrition	Nutritionally balanced, low residue	Normal calorie and protein requirements
Osmolite 1.5 Cal	1.5	0.063	Abbott Nutrition	High calorie, low residue	Increased calorie needs, fluid restriction
Jevity 1.2 Cal	1.2	0.056	Abbott Nutrition	Concentrated calories, fiber containing	Increased calorie and protein needs, fluid restriction
Promote	1	0.063	Abbott Nutrition	Very high protein	Low calorie needs, burns, trauma, pressure ulcers
Replete	1	0.063	Nestlé Nutrition	High protein	Low calorie needs, burns, trauma, pressure ulcers
TwoCal HN	2	0.084	Abbott Nutrition	High calorie, contains prebiotics	High calorie needs, fluid restriction

(Continued)

TABLE 25-20

Selected Enteral Formulas for Older Children (More Than 10 Years Old) and Adults *(Continued)*					
Trade Name	**Calories/mL**	**Grams pro/mL**	**Manufacturer**	**Features**	**Indications**
Semi-elemental					
Crucial	1.5	0.094	Nestlé Nutrition	Very high peptide-based protein, arginine, omega-3 fatty acids, antioxidants	Burns and wounds, stage 3 and 4 pressure ulcers, critical illness with GI dysfunction
Peptamen	1	0.04	Nestlé Nutrition	Hydrolyzed whey protein, 100% whey based, 70% of fat as medium-chain triglycerides	Malabsorption, pancreatitis, intestinal failure (SGS), chronic diarrhea, Crohn's disease
Peptamen AF	1.2	0.076	Nestlé Nutrition	Hydrolyzed whey protein, high protein, prebiotic fiber, omega-3 fatty acids	Intestinal failure (SGS), inflammatory conditions, sepsis, ARDS
Peptamen 1.5	1.5	0.068	Nestlé Nutrition	High calorie, hydrolyzed whey protein, 100% whey based, 70% of fat as medium-chain triglycerides	Malabsorption, pancreatitis, intestinal failure (SGS), chronic diarrhea, Crohn's disease, fluid restriction
Pivot 1.5	1.5	0.094	Abbott Nutrition	High calorie, high protein, arginine, omega-3 fatty acids, glutamine	Metabolic stress, severe wounds
Elemental					
Tolerex	1	0.021	Nestlé Nutrition	100% free amino acid, 1.3% fat	Severe protein and fat malabsorption
Vivonex T.E.N	1	0.038	Nestlé Nutrition	100% free amino acid, 3% of calories from fat	Intestinal failure (SGS), chylothorax, severe protein and fat malabsorption
Disease Specific					
Nepro with Carb Steady	1.8	0.081	Abbott Nutrition	High calorie, reduced electrolyte content	Dialysis
Novasource Renal	2	0.074	Nestlé Nutrition	High calorie, reduced electrolyte content,	Acute renal failure, chronic renal failure, electrolyte restriction, fluid restrictions
Nutrihep	1.5	0.4	Nestlé Nutrition	High branched-chain amino acids, low protein	Hepatic disease
Oxepa	1.5	0.063	Abbott Nutrition	Marine oils, borage oil	Acute respiratory distress syndrome, systemic inflammatory response syndrome, acute lung injury

(Continued)

TABLE 25-20

Selected Enteral Formulas for Older Children (More Than 10 Years Old) and Adults *(Continued)*					
Trade Name	**Calories/mL**	**Grams pro/mL**	**Manufacturer**	**Features**	**Indications**
Suplena	1.8	0.045	Abbott Nutrition	High calorie, reduced electrolyte content, low protein	Impaired kidney function

Sources: Abbott Nutrition. (2009). *Pediatric nutrition product guide.* Columbus, OH: Author, pp. 2–161; Nutricia. (2008). *2008 product reference guide.* Gaithersburg, MD: Author, pp. 4–186; www.abbottnutrition.com; www.mjn.com; www.nestlenutrition.com/us.

TABLE 25-21

Hang Time for Enteral Nutrition	
Type of Enteral Nutrition	**Hang Time**
Human breastmilk Reconstituted formula from a liquid concentrate Reconstituted formula from a powder Sterile formula in an open system (neonates) Formulas with modular additives	4 hours
Sterile formula in an open system	8 hours
Sterile formula in a closed system	24–48 hours

Source: Adapted from Enteral Nutrition Practice Recommendations Task Force, 2009.

The use of sterile, liquid enteral formulas is preferred to reconstituted formulas whenever possible (A.S.P.E.N., 2009). In the hospital setting, powdered and liquid concentrate formulas should always be reconstituted with sterile water (A.S.P.E.N.).

Nutrition monitoring

Patients receiving enteral nutrition must be monitored regularly to evaluate the nutritional adequacy of feeds and tolerance. Tube feeds are often intermittently held so that tests, procedures, intubation, and extubation can be performed. Continuous nasojejunal feeds do not need to be held during extubation (Lyons et al., 2002).

Actual intake of the enteral nutrition regimen should be reviewed routinely, and the tube feed rate or concentration should be adjusted accordingly. Serial weights and heights should be obtained to monitor nutritional adequacy. Weights should be interpreted with regard to the patient's fluid status. Trends of biochemical markers such as prealbumin and nitrogen balance studies may also be used to evaluate nutritional adequacy and the patient's response to nutrition support. These biochemical markers should be interpreted with regard to actual nutritional intake, medications, and underlying medical conditions. Steroid use and hemodialysis, for example, may cause elevated prealbumin levels. Thus biochemical markers should be used in combination with anthropometrics to assess the patient's nutritional status (Golts et al., 2007). Single nitrogen balance studies may not be reliable in patients with burns or multiple open wounds, as they do not account for nitrogen loss from the wounds.

Gastrointestinal assessment should be done routinely to assess for tolerance of enteral feeds. Tolerance is based on absence of emesis, diarrhea, constipation, and increased abdominal distention. Many clinicians monitor gastric residual volume with the presumption that it correlates with aspiration risk and predicts feeding tolerance and gastric emptying. However, studies have demonstrated that gastric residual volume is not reliable as a marker for feeding tolerance, aspiration risk, and gastric emptying, and its use may result in unnecessary interruptions of enteral feeds (Mehta, 2009).

Complications of enteral feeds

Mechanical, GI, and metabolic complications can occur with enteral feeds. For example, malpositioned or migrated feeding tubes may perforate the pharynx, esophagus, or intestine. Inadvertent tracheobronchial placement of the feeding tube can cause pneumothorax (Mehta, 2009). GI intolerance to feeds—evidenced by vomiting, diarrhea, and abdominal distention—can lead to frequent interruption of feeds. Metabolic complications may include hyperglycemia, fluid overload, dehydration, and electrolyte imbalances. Collectively, these complications of enteral feeds may lead to suboptimal nutritional intake. Table 25-22 summarizes strategies to manage complications associated with enteral feeds.

TABLE 25-22

Management and Prevention of Enteral Feeding Complications	
Complication	**Management/Prevention**
Mechanical	
Malpositioning of tube Obstructed tube	• Reposition or replace the tube. Confirm tube placement radiographically • Use sterile water or saline to flush the tube after medication administration, before and after aspirating residuals, after bolus feeds, and every 4–8 hours during continuous feeds.
Gastrointestinal	
Diarrhea (more than 4 loose stools in 24 hours)	• Check stool cultures. • Discontinue any medications that contain sorbitol. • Evaluate for malabsorption. • Review the osmolarity of the formula. • Consider a fiber-containing, isotonic, semi-elemental, and/or lactose-free formula. • Consider decreasing the concentration or rate of enteral formula. • Discontinue laxatives and stool softeners. • Consider parenteral nutrition and bowel rest for intractable diarrhea.
Constipation (no stool after 48 hours of enteral nutrition initiation)	• Ensure that the patient is receiving adequate fluid. • Consider a fiber-containing formula. • Consider starting a bowel program (prune juice, glycerin suppository, senna, polyethylene glycol).
Vomiting	• Hold feeds for 1 hour, then restart them at the same rate. If vomiting continues, hold feeds for 4 hours, then restart them at a slower rate. • Review the osmolarity of the enteral formula. Change to an isotonic formula if feasible. • Consider transpyloric tube placement.
Abdominal distention	• Evaluate for constipation. • Evaluate for acute abdomen.
Aspiration pneumonia	• Ensure that the head of the bed is elevated 30° unless contraindicated. • Evaluate for risk of aspiration (gastroesophageal reflux, delayed gastric emptying, severe bronchospasm, depressed gag/cough, history of aspiration). • Consider transpyloric feeds.
Metabolic	
Hyperglycemia	• Review actual enteral nutrition intake to ensure the patient is not being overfed. • Consider underlying causes such as surgery, infection, or trauma.
Dehydration	• Routinely monitor hydration status. • Increase free water as appropriate.
Fluid overload	• Consider a concentrated formula.
Electrolyte imbalance	• Consider diluting or concentrating formula as appropriate. • Evaluate the adequacy of the electrolytes in the formula.

Sources: Mehta, 2009; Nevin-Folino & Miller, 2005.

Transitional feeds

Weaning from enteral nutrition may be initiated when it is medically feasible to begin oral feeds. In some instances, the patient may need a swallow evaluation prior to advancing to oral feeds. Transitioning back to full oral feeds requires cooperation from the patient and support of the caregiver and interprofessional team (Nevin-Folino & Miller, 2005). Enteral nutrition should not be completely weaned until the patient achieves satisfactory nutrition status and demonstrates the ability to consume adequate nutrients consistently (Nevin-Folino & Miller). High-calorie snacks and oral supplements may be needed to help the patient achieve adequate nutritional intake.

Some patients may need to continue enteral feeds upon discharge. If a prolonged need for enteral nutrition support is anticipated, the placement of a percutaneous endoscopic gastrostomy tube should be considered. Collaboration with the dietitian and the discharge planner is important to ensure that the caregiver receives appropriate education on proper administration of home enteral feeds. Good candidates for home enteral feeds will meet the criteria outlined in Table 25-23.

HUMAN BREASTMILK AS A THERAPY

Marguerite Degenhardt and Nancy A. Rodriguez

Health outcomes

Numerous studies have linked human milk feedings with enhanced short- and long-term health outcomes, including a lower incidence of infection, enhanced feeding tolerance, enhanced visual acuity, and higher scores on tests that measure neurocognitive function (Arifeen et al., 2001; Furman et al., 2003; Lucas et al., 1992; Lucas et al., 1998; Meinzen-Derr et al., 2009; Ronnestad et al., 2005; Singhal et al., 2007; Uraizee & Gross, 1989). Human milk feedings appear to be especially beneficial for preterm infants, protecting them from costly sources of prematurity-associated morbidities including necrotizing enterocolitis (NEC) and retinopathy of prematurity (Hylander et al., 2001; Lucas & Cole, 1990; Mcguire & Anthony, 2003; Schanler, 2001; Schanler et al., 2005; Sisk et al., 2007). Based on these benefits, exclusive human milk feeding is recommended for all infants during the first year of life, particularly for premature and ill infants (American Academy of Pediatrics [AAP], 2005).

TABLE 25-23

Criteria for Home Enteral Feeds

- The patient has demonstrated tolerance to feeds prior to discharge.
- The home is safe and has running water, electricity, refrigeration, and adequate storage space.
- The caregiver is competent and willing to administer the feeding.
- A funding source is available for the enteral formula and associated equipment; supplies and equipment are available.
- The patient has a primary care provider who assumes responsibility for following the patient after discharge.
- The caregiver has been provided with appropriate education and discharge instructions.
- A nutrition care plan is implemented by the dietitian.
- A home health agency is available to provide service to the patient. If an agency is not available, a hospital dietitian, pharmacist, or pediatric nurse who follows home care patients takes responsibility for the patient.
- Ongoing follow-up care is arranged.

Protective factors in human milk

Recent studies have associated the *degree* of prematurity with the composition of mother's milk and found an inverse relationship between the duration of pregnancy and the concentration of protective factors in the milk (Araujo et al., 2005; Dvorak et al., 2003; Koenig et al., 2005; Ronayne de Ferrer et al., 2000). Thus, the milk that is expressed by women who deliver the smallest, extremely premature infants contains the highest level of protection. These differences are most dramatic in the early milk, or colostrum, that is expressed during the first days after delivery.

The protective properties of human milk are attributed to a multitude of biological factors, including nutritional, enzymatic, epigenetic, antioxidant, antimicrobial, anti-inflammatory, and immunomodulatory components that work synergistically and have overlapping functions. Some of these factors have multiple functions. For example, lipids provide substrate for energy but also promote retinal and brain development. Once metabolized, the products of lipid digestion promote the development of "normal" GI microflora, which help protect the infant from GI infections including NEC (Rodriguez et al., 2005).

The ongoing identification of new human milk factors, which includes a better understanding of their biological functions, is a rapidly expanding area of lactation research. The in vivo effects of many immunologically derived human milk factors remain unclear as yet. However, current evidence suggests that protection is afforded through several distinct mechanisms, including barrier protection, receptor-site binding, bacterial cell lysis, anti-inflammatory effects, immunomodulatory functions, and the creation of a GI environment that inhibits the proliferation of pathogenic species while encouraging the growth of beneficial (commensal) bacteria (Rodriguez et al., 2005). Many of these protective factors are more highly concentrated in colostrum, as a result of mammary gland immaturity and the open para-cellular pathways between the mammary epithelium (the milk-producing cells) that allow the easy movement of protective substances into the milk (Patel et al., 2007). Recent evidence suggests that the use of exclusive human milk feedings during critical exposure periods post birth may have the greatest impact on health outcomes for premature infants (Meier et al., in press).

Colostrum is the milk that is produced when the tight junctions between the mammary epithelial cells are open, permitting the paracellular transport of many immunologically derived factors from the mother's circulation into the milk (Neville, 2001). This process results in higher concentrations of protective immune agents in colostrum as compared to milk that is expressed later in lactation. Colostrum expressed by women who deliver extremely premature infants is especially concentrated and, therefore, might potentially serve as an "immune therapy" for high-risk, immunocompromised, extremely premature infants in the first days of life. The junctions of the paracellular pathway close gradually during the first days post delivery and eventually fuse, which corresponds to the beginning of lactogenesis II—often referred to as the "milk coming in" period (Neville, 2001). While immune agents continue to be produced and secreted in breastmilk, they are present in lower concentration in the milk, largely in part to dilution.

Hindmilk feedings

The composition of human milk remains highly dynamic well past the colostral phase. The lipid concentration is the most highly variable milk component; it changes considerably throughout the day, between the two breasts, and over the course of the milk expression session. For example, the milk that is removed from the breast during the first minutes of expressing is referred to as *foremilk*. Similar to skim milk, foremilk is low in fat and calories. The fat content and caloric density gradually change during the expressing session to a high-fat, calorie-dense *hindmilk*, which is removed during the last few minutes of pumping. The change from foremilk to hindmilk is a gradual one, similar to warm water gradually becoming hot when a faucet is turned on. Mothers often report noting a change in the color and consistency of the milk (appearing creamier) during the pumping session.

The lipid and caloric content of the milk can be accurately measured with a validated procedure known as the creamatocrit technique (Meier et al., 2006). The creamatocrit value can be utilized as an important clinical tool in diagnosing and managing slow weight gain (Meier & Engstrom, 2007; Meier et al., 2002). The ability to control and adjust the caloric content of the milk enables the HCP to optimize weight gain strategies for the infant. For example, the mother may be taught how to fractionate her milk during the milk expression procedures so as to reach a target caloric density, which will facilitate rapid weight gain for the infant during critical periods.

- The mother can separate the foremilk from the hindmilk during the pumping session by interrupting pumping and changing the milk collection containers when the color of the milk changes. The containers should be labeled as foremilk or hindmilk.
- The foremilk can be immediately frozen and saved for another time, when rapid short-term weight gain is not a priority.
- The hindmilk can be fed to the infant.

Hindmilk feedings are particularly beneficial for infants who require rapid growth or those who cannot tolerate large volumes at feedings. Infants with respiratory or cardiac disease are typically intolerant to large fluid volumes, which necessitates fluid restriction. Infants with gastroesophageal reflux, which is often exacerbated with large feeding volumes, may also benefit from this type of feeding. Hindmilk feedings enable the HCP to offer the highest-caloric-density feeding in the smallest volume. Such feedings can be especially beneficial for fluid-restricted infants being treated in a general pediatric unit or a PICU, such as those with chronic lung disease or cardiac conditions.

In contrast, infants with chylothorax may need to be fed fat-free milk. This can be accomplished by centrifuging the entire milk specimen and then, using sterile technique, removing the cream (fat) layer on the top of the milk (Chan & Lechtenberg, 2007).

Supporting lactation and breastfeeding in the hospital setting

In the case of a prolonged mother–infant separation during hospitalization, mothers should be instructed to use an efficient and effective breast pump, at regular intervals throughout the day, so as to establish and maintain breastmilk volume (Meier et al., 2008). Mothers should be instructed to pump at least eight times in a 24-hour period. The appropriate type of breast pump in this situation is a hospital-grade electric pump with a double setup collection kit. A battery-operated device cannot adequately stimulate the initiation of lactogenesis II (the onset of copious milk secretion) or adequately maintain a mother's milk supply. A double setup enables mother to pump both breasts simultaneously, which expedites the milk removal process while stimulating more prolactin release and more milk production. Equally important are optimal suction pressure from the breast pump and appropriately sized and fitted breast shields.

Oftentimes, PICU staff may be hesitant to encourage breastfeeding. This hesitation may reflect concern about the ability to adequately measure the amount of volume consumed at the breast. The use of test weights can easily address these concerns. When the infant feeds at the breast, pre- and post-feeding test weights taken with a digital scale can assist in determining appropriate milk transfer (Hurst, Meier, & Engstrom, 1999). Milk intake is calculated as follows: 1 gram of weight increase = 1 milliliter of milk intake. For the majority of infants who are PICU patients, lactation will have already been established prior to admission. These infants include chronic NICU infants, newborn surgical or cardiac infants, those with acute illness or trauma, or those admitted for elective surgery. The use of test weights in this population can be a critical component of a feeding plan that incorporates evidence-based practices and protects breastfeeding.

In the case of an infant who has a poor suck as a result of suboptimal intraoral suction pressure, a nipple shield can facilitate milk transfer during breastfeeding. A nipple shield is a thin silicone device that fits over the areola and nipple. During breastfeeding, a vacuum is created within the nipple that makes it easier for the breastfeeding infant to transfer milk without working so hard. A nipple shield may be a helpful tool with infants having a weak suck, diminished muscle tone, or decreased endurance (Meier, Furman, & Degenhardt, 2007), conditions commonly found in the critically ill population and late preterm infants.

Storage and delivery of human milk

Correct storage and delivery of expressed human milk is essential to maintain its antibacterial and nutritional qualities. Milk should be stored in sterile, food-grade, plastic containers with tightly fitting lids. Plastic storage bags or disposable bottle liners are not recommended, as they can easily leak or spill. Containers may hold 2 to 4 ounces (60 to 120 mL) depending on the volume the infant will likely consume in a single feeding, thereby avoiding waste. At least 1 inch of space should be left between the top of the milk and the top of the container to allow for milk expansion as it freezes. Colostrum should be collected in smaller containers, often as small as 11 mL.

Human milk should be refrigerated immediately after it is expressed and can be stored for 48 hours in the refrigerator at temperatures less than 4°C (less than 39°F). Milk that will not be consumed within 48 hours should be stored in a freezer at –20°C (–4°F) for up to 6 months. Milk that has been frozen should be thawed in its container in warm water. Because human milk is not homogenized, the calorically dense lipid (or cream) portion can separate, so it is important to ensure that lipid does not remain in the storage cap or other areas of the container (Meier & Engstrom, 2007). Once thawed, milk should be consumed immediately or may be refrigerated for as long as 24 hours.

The method of delivery of stored human milk depends on the needs of the infant. Studies have shown that human milk lipid adheres to plastic surfaces such as gavage infusion tubing, thereby decreasing the caloric content actually delivered to the child (Brennan-Behm et al., 1994; Greer et al., 1984). Evidence-based procedures to minimize separation of components of human milk and to ensure optimal caloric density include the following steps:

* Administer gravity gavage feedings that flow over several minutes.
* Use minibore tubing for gavage feedings administered via syringe pumps.
* Position the infusion pump vertically so that the lipid rises to the top.
* Infuse air at the end of the feeding to clear the adhered lipid in the tubing.

For infants with gastric tubes, the priority should be to administer fresh milk feedings. It is recommended that the setup be changed every 4 hours (A.S.P.E.N., 2009).

Counseling mothers

In the inpatient general pediatric and PICU settings, the HCP is often the primary source of information regarding breastfeeding. Mothers will seek out these clinical experts to obtain up-to-date information and professional guidance. Research has demonstrated that mothers want and require professional lactation advice to help them make informed decisions regarding feeding preference for their infant (Miracle et al., 2004). Mothers who receive information from a HCP are more likely to decide to express milk for their infant (Lu et al., 2001; Miracle et al.). Likewise, mothers who have already initiated lactation prior to their infant's PICU hospitalization may be more likely to sustain lactation and ultimately breastfeed successfully if they receive adequate information, guidance, and professional support.

When an infant is admitted to the PICU, there is no reason to abruptly wean the child off lactation once it has been established. Therefore, the priority must be to protect lactation and to promote breastfeeding opportunities for the infant–mother dyad. The HCP should be knowledgeable and well prepared to instruct, counsel, and support mothers who are lactating during this critical period. The involvement of lactation consultants may also support the HCP in promoting optimal breastfeeding throughout the patient's hospitalization.

FAILURE-TO-THRIVE

Cheryl Mele

PATHOPHYSIOLOGY

Failure-to-thrive (FTT) is not a disease, but rather a symptom that may result from many medical, psychosocial, and environmental conditions that lead to poor growth in a young child (Careaga & Kerner, 2000). It is the result of the interaction between the environment and the pediatric patient's health, development, and behavior (Gahagan, 2006).

EPIDEMIOLOGY AND ETIOLOGY

Failure-to-thrive is a common problem in pediatrics and usually presents in the first two years of life; however, it may also occur at any time during childhood (Stephens et al., 2008). The single most common causative factor for FTT worldwide is poor nutrition. In the United States, poor growth is more common in lower-socioeconomic communities due to the prevalence of risk factors such as the lack of adequate nutrition knowledge, financial hardship, and social problems including substance abuse and child maltreatment (Block et al., 2005). Nevertheless, FTT exists in all socioeconomic groups. In the United States, it accounts for 1% to 5% of all pediatric hospitalizations and 10% of visits to primary care practices (Careaga & Kerner, 2000). Fifteen to 30 percent of the patients seen with acute issues in inner-city emergency departments (ED) have symptoms of growth deficits (Careaga & Kerner). FTT may be associated with lower developmental scores, neurological and behavioral disorders, and an increased prevalence of infection (Black et al., 2007). FTT should be considered a medical emergency if the pediatric patient weight and length are less than < 70% of the predicted values (Block et al.).

In general, most infants and children with symptomatic growth failure are influenced by multiple factors, such that both medical and psychosocial issues affect their growth and development. These factors include physiological factors, caregiver–infant temperament, economic considerations, and social networks (Gahagan, 2006).

Definition

There is no consensus in the literature regarding the definition of failure-to-thrive; however, basic definitions of this disorder include the following points:

- Failing to grow at a rate consistent with expected standards for infants and toddlers younger than 3 years of age (Gahagan, 2006)
- A prolonged cessation of appropriate weight gain and linear growth in comparison to recognized standards after having achieved a stable pattern

The most commonly recognized standards are the growth charts developed by the U.S. National Center for Health Statistics and the Centers for Disease Control and Prevention (CDC, 2000). FTT should be considered as a possible diagnosis if the pediatric patient's growth measurements fall below the 3rd to 5th percentile or if they are two or more standard deviations below the baseline on the growth chart (Block et al., 2005).

Common terminology

The dividing of FTT into two subgroups—organic and non-organic—is no longer recognized as diagnostic (Stephens et al., 2008). For patients older than 3 years of age, the term FTT is less commonly used. Instead, the terms *growth failure* and *delayed sexual maturation* are more frequently applied (Careaga & Kerner, 2000).

DIFFERENTIAL DIAGNOSIS

Four principal pathological mechanisms leading to FFT should be considered in the differential diagnosis and clinical evaluation: (1) loss of calories through malabsorption, (2) increased caloric metabolism, (3) inadequate caloric intake, and (4) defective utilization of digestive nutrients (Table 25-24) (Bergman & Graham, 2005; Krugman & Dubowitz, 2003; Stephens et al., 2008).

PRESENTATION

History is one of the most important investigative techniques in the evaluation of FTT. The initial evaluation

TABLE 25-24

Differential Diagnosis for Failure-to-Thrive	
Inadequate Caloric Intake	**Loss of Calories Through Malabsorption**

• Incorrect preparation of formula or feeding technique
• Mechanical feeding disorders
  • Oromotor disorders
  • Congenital esophageal–facial anomalies
  • Severe gastroesophageal reflux, oral aversions
  • Central nervous system disorders
• Poverty
• Neglect
• Dysfunctional caregiver–child relationship
	• Celiac disease
	• Cystic fibrosis
	• Inflammatory bowel disorder
	• Intestinal failure
	  • Short gut syndrome
	• Biliary atresia
	• Cow's milk protein disorder
	• Parasitic or bacterial infections of the gastrointestinal tract

Increased Metabolism or Excessive Utilization of Calories	**Defective Utilization of Digestive Nutrients**

• Chronic illness
• Kidney and liver failure
• Congestive heart failure due to cardiomyopathy or congenital heart lesion
• Chronic infection
  • HIV
  • Immune deficiency disorders
  • Frequent urinary tract infections
• Perinatal infections
  • Cytomegalovirus
  • TORCH
• Tuberculosis
• Bronchopulmonary dysplasia
• Hyperthyroidism
	• Chromosomal or genetic abnormalities
	  • Trisomy-21, -18, and -13
	• Metabolic disorders
	  • Amino acid, storage abnormalities
	• Pituitary disorders
	• Growth hormone deficiency
	• Inborn error of metabolism
	• Adrenal insufficiency

Human immunodeficiency virus (HIV); toxoplasmosis, rubella, cytomegalovirus, herpes simplex, human immunodeficiency virus (TORCH).

Source: Modified from Bergman & Graham, 2005; Krugman & Dubowitz, 2003; Stephens et al., 2008.

should include the pediatric patient's dietary intake, feeding behaviors, current and past medical history, and psychosocial history (Table 25-25). The HCP must avoid judgmental questioning, as this bias may deter further evaluation.

Investigate methods of feeding, food and formula preparation, volumes of formula, and cultural food practices. Family history of short stature, constitutional delay, and potential hereditary disorders should be sought. Calorie counts, obtained with the aid of a dietary consultant, may need to be completed.

Elicit information on current and past medical illnesses with attention to delays in achievement of developmental milestones, which could indicate a neurological problem. Recurrent febrile illness without an identified source could indicate a urological or kidney problem with undiagnosed urinary tract infections. Bowel habits, especially incidences of diarrhea, may reveal malabsorption disorders such as lactose intolerance, food allergies, cystic fibrosis, or celiac disease. A history of sleep apnea and snoring could alert the HCP to tonsillar and adenoid hypertrophy, both of which have been associated with FTT (Schwartz, 2000).

TABLE 25-25

Failure-to-Thrive History	
History	**Implication**
Dietary History	
• Amount of food/formula • Quality of food/type • Preparation of formula	• Inadequate caloric intake • Inadequate nutrient quality of food • Improper preparation of formula
Feeding History and Behaviors	
• How long does it take the infant to take a bottle? • How is the infant latching on if breastfeeding? • Actions during feeding (tongue thrust, weak, unsustained suck) • Aversion behaviors (arching, emesis, spitting, coughing with feeds) • How is the child fed? • Mealtime behaviors • Feeding battles	• Oromotor dysfunction • Food aversion • Gastroesophageal reflux • Fatigue related to underlying medical condition • Inappropriate feeding techniques for the developmental stage • Distracting mealtime environment • Behavioral problems
Past and Current Medical History	
• Birth history (perinatal infections, medical disorders, prematurity) • Current or chronic illness (frequent otitis media, pharyngitis, gastroenteritis) • Chronic medical conditions (congenital heart lesion, cystic fibrosis, asthma, anemia) • Gastrointestinal symptoms (stool pattern, emesis, gastroesophageal reflux) • Past hospitalizations or injuries	• Underlying problems with malabsorption such as cystic fibrosis, celiac disease, gastroenteritis, or milk protein allergy • Decreased appetite related to frequent infections, esophagitis, or congestive heart failure • Fatigue related to respiratory distress or anemia • Child maltreatment or neglect
Family and Psychosocial History	
• Medical conditions or failure-to-thrive in siblings • Genetic short stature • Who are the caregivers? • Does the patient live at home? • Does the family feel safe? • Economic situation • Patient's temperament • History of maternal psychological disorders, depression, drug or alcohol abuse	• Predisposition for genetic or medical disorders • Sense of maternal–child attachment and behaviors • Child maltreatment or neglect

Source: Krugman & Dubowitz, 2003.

The perinatal history may be important to elicit as well. Small for gestational age (SGA) infants are more likely to have a history of problems such as infections, drug exposure, maternal disease/infection, and placental insufficiency. The infant with symmetric SGA (i.e., height, weight, and head circumference are all equally affected) may have been exposed in utero to infections such as rubella, cytomegalovirus, syphilis, toxoplasmosis, or malaria. These children rarely exhibit catch-up growth and may experience developmental delays, especially if the exposure occurred in the early stages of pregnancy. By comparison, infants with asymmetrical SGA (i.e., only weight affected) may have good potential for growth catch-up if adequate support is provided. Maternal conditions such as diabetes, hypertension, and kidney disease may also affect placental sufficiency and predispose an infant to low birth weight and height, often sparing head growth. Premature infants should have their measurements and development evaluated using their "corrected age." Corrected age is calculated by subtracting the number of weeks of prematurity from the infant's chronological age. Thus a neonate born at 31 weeks' gestation would have 9 weeks' prematurity. If the infant presents at age 3 months (12 weeks), the corrected age would be 3 weeks. There is no consensus as to when the HCP should stop using the corrected age, but many continue to adjust the child's age until the patient is 2 years old.

Psychosocial issues are critical to evaluate when assessing the pediatric patient's history. Recent data estimate that 20% of all children in the United States live below the poverty line (Schwartz, 2000). Hence, the history should include questions pertaining to the availability of food and homelessness. Other psychosocial concerns to be addressed during evaluation include domestic violence, parental employment, substance abuse, and if there is a nurturing environment in the home. Maternal drug abuse with tobacco, cocaine, alcohol, and heroin has been associated with both lower birth weight and a non-nurturing environment (Stephens et al., 2008). Infants born to mothers younger than 18 years of age have been reported to have poorer growth and are twice as likely to show signs of neglect than children born to older mothers, who may provide a more emotionally stable and cognitively stimulating home (Block et al., 2005; Schwartz). In middle- to upper-class families, an over-focus on careers or activities away from home can be detrimental to adequate nutrition (Block et al.).

More than 80% of children diagnosed with FTT do not have an organic disorder; rather, nutritional and psychosocial issues are the most common causes in these patients (Stephens et al., 2008). Observing the interaction between caregiver and pediatric patient is good way to evaluate psychosocial influences on growth (Bergman & Graham, 2005), as psychological, behavioral, and caregiver–child interaction factors are intertwined in infant feeding behaviors (Skuse, 1993). Many FTT-diagnosed infants have a history of feeding difficulties and, in combination with mismanagement of the feeding process, may have insufficient caloric intake (Wells, 2002). Thus a caregiver–child feeding observation session should note the infant cues, temperament, and caregiver's responses.

A complete physical examination starts with inspection. Evaluating the child for dysmorphic features, such as micrognanthia, major or minor anomalies (cleft lip or palate), and neurocutaneous markings, may reveal a genetic disorder or child maltreatment (Gahagan, 2006). The HCP should also look for any signs of underlying disease that has impaired growth, such as muscle wasting, congestive heart failure, or respiratory disease. Such signs include abdominal distention, flat buttocks, barrel chest, and organomegaly (Krugman & Dubowitz, 2003). Additionally, evaluation should include assessment of acute dehydration such as dry mucous membranes, sunken eyes, and poor skin turgor. A complete screen for developmental delays may indicate impaired eating abilities (Shah, 2002).

Anthropometric measurements are plotted on the standard growth charts, which include height, weight, and head circumference until the child reaches 2 years of age. A single isolated measurement should not be a basis for a diagnosis of slowing or failing growth; rather, the best measurements are those obtained over time. Length is measured until the pediatric patient is 2 years of age; after that age, height measurements via stadiometer (a wall-mounted measuring device) are used. This series of measurements allows the HCP to evaluate if a patient has fallen off his or her anticipated growth curve suddenly or if growth has been consistently suboptimal (Careaga & Kerner, 2000).

Weight for stature is a better index of fat stores than weight alone; it is measured for those younger than 2 years of age. For patients older than 2 years, the body mass index (BMI) is calculated using the same growth charts. A BMI less than 5% requires further investigation (Shah, 2002). Table 25-26 lists red flags in anthropometric measurements and several associated conditions.

FTT must also be differentiated from normal or expected growth variants. These include a pediatric patient with genetically small parents, infants with constitutional delay, premature infants, and "catch-down growth" (Bergman & Graham, 2005).

- Infants born to small genetic parents may grow along or below the lower percentile on the growth chart. An endocrine evaluation of short stature should be considered if height is more than three standard deviations below the mean or less than the 3rd percentile (Careaga & Kerner, 2000).
- Patients with constitutional delay will often experience a lag in linear growth, rather than weight, in comparison to children of the same age. There is also often a positive family history for the same trend. Constitutional delay is measured by bone age assessment; however, it

TABLE 25-26

Red Flags in Anthropometric Measurement and Associated Conditions			
Weight	**Height**	**Head Circumference**	**Associated Conditions**
Decreased	Decreased/normal	Normal	Inadequate caloric intake, increased metabolic demands or disorders, cerebral palsy, systemic illness, psychosocial issues
Decreased	Decreased	Normal	Constitutional delay, endocrine disorders, genetic dwarfism, structural bone disorders
Decreased	Decreased	Decreased	Hereditary, genetic disorders; perinatal insults or infections (e.g., TORCH, CMV); CNS disorders; metabolic abnormalities

TORCH comprises the following set of perinatal infections: toxoplasmosis, rubella, cytomegalovirus (CMV), herpes simplex, and human immunodeficiency virus.

Sources: Careaga & Kerner, 2000; Shah, 2002.

is reliable only in children older than 12 months of age (Bergman & Graham, 2005).

- Premature infants, as previously noted, are measured based on their corrected age until they reach 2 years of age. In very-low-birth-weight infants (less than 1,200 gm), this time period may be extended until 3 years of age.
- Infants with "catch-down growth" are infants born large for gestational age (LGA). These infants are often offspring of diabetic mothers. They will eventually experience catch-down growth and rejoin the expected curve (Bergman & Graham, 2005).

PLAN OF CARE

Early diagnosis and prompt medical intervention is critical for the FTT-diagnosed child. Few affected children have serious organic disease, yet all require comprehensive growth failure evaluation and a successful plan for therapeutic management (Gagahan, 2006). Thus a practical approach is to order diagnostic studies based on the history or physical examination and differential diagnostic findings (Table 25-27). For example, frequent respiratory infections, FTT, and steatorrhea should prompt the HCP to order a sweat test and stool analysis to evaluate the patient for cystic fibrosis. In young infants, the HCP should review the newborn screening tests to evaluate for an inborn error of metabolism or hypothyroidism (Gahagan). For infants 6 to 18 months of age, diagnostic studies include a blood lead level, tuberculosis screening, complete blood count, and/or urinalysis (Gahagan; Krugman & Dubowitz, 2003). Patients with identified risk factors should have screening for human immunodeficiency virus (HIV) (Schwartz, 2000). Suspected malabsorption disorders can be further investigated with stool analysis for fat, reducing substance, and celiac antibody testing (Bergman & Graham, 2005). Evaluation of endocrine function should include a thorough

TABLE 25-27

Diagnostic Studies for Failure-to-Thrive
Blood Test

- Complete metabolic panel with serum Ca^+ and phosphate
- Complete blood count and erythrocyte sedimentation rate (ESR)
- Iron studies
- Immunoglobulins
- Celiac screen
- Thyroid function panel

Stool Test

- Stool culture and microscopy
- Fat analysis

Urine

- Urinalysis
- Culture and sensitivity

Additional Studies Based on History and Physical Examination Findings

- Blood and urine for organic and amino acids
- Chromosome analysis
- Allergy testing: radioallergosorbent (RAST), skin prick test
- Sweat test
- Gastroscopy

Sources: Bergman & Graham, 2005; Stephens et al., 2008.

screening of thyroid function, with growth hormone deficiency studies being reserved for those patients with persistent hypoglycemia or microphallus (Schwartz, 2000). If a pediatric patient has dysmorphic features and identified organ disruption, chromosomal testing and brain imaging may be indicated.

The goals of therapeutic management are sixfold: (1) treat the underlying cause; (2) provide adequate calories, protein, and other nutrients; (3) provide nutritional counseling for the family; (4) monitor growth over time; (5) provide education regarding feeding and nurturing techniques; and (6) evaluate and provide economic assistance if required (Shah, 2002).

Most patients with FTT can be treated with nutritional interventions and behavior modification in an outpatient setting (Krugman & Dubowitz, 2003). Completion of three-day food diaries identifying deficient calories, limiting fruit juices, or adding taste-pleasing fats to toddler foods are common practices employed with these patients (Krugman & Dubowitz). Children with FTT need at least 150% of their recommended daily caloric intake, based on their expected weight (not their actual weight), for catch-up growth (Krugman & Dubowitz). The patient's diet is usually fortified for increased caloric density by using concentrated formula or adding glucose polymers or microlipids (Shah, 2002).

Catch–up growth requirement (kcal/kg/day)
= [Calories required for weight age (kcal/kg/day)
× Ideal weight for age (kg)] ÷ Actual weight (kg)

Vitamin and mineral replacement may also be needed. This type of supplementation is often best guided by an experienced dietitian, nutritionist, or subspecialist such as an endocrinologist. Appetite-enhancing medications, such as cyproheptadine, have been suggested to increase calories, but results when using these agents have varied (Schwartz, 2000).

Enteral tube feedings should be considered for those patients who have oromotor dysfunction or when oral feeding is insufficient due to problems such as respiratory distress or chronic fatigue. Replacing calories or refeeding with high-caloric diets too quickly (in the first few days of therapy) in the significantly undernourished pediatric patient should be done with caution.

Therapeutic management of FTT also includes behavioral manipulation. Both inefficient feeding in normal infants and subtle abnormal neurodevelopment have negative effects on growth (Ramsay et al., 2002). Feeding behavior begins with coordination of the suck and swallow reflexes; thus intervention for a breastfed infant may require instruction for assistance with latching-on behaviors (Gahagan, 2006). Formula-fed infants may require nighttime awakening to eat if they sleep long intervals between feedings. Caregivers of infants with a cleft lip or palate will require special training for feeding. Other families might misinterpret infant feeding behavioral cues or have problems with maternal–child attachment and discontinue feeding when the infant is actually still hungry.

For toddlers, their developmental stage is one of independence and increasing ability. At this age, the child wants to pursue self-feeding behaviors. Caregivers who want complete control over their toddler's feeding may experience food battles. They should be encouraged to instead make mealtimes pleasant. Families should be advised to

avoid force-feeding their child, as children will often go hungry rather than submit (Gahagan, 2006). Caregivers should instead consider foods that the child likes and encourage variety while still covering the four basic food groups. Toddlers should obtain 50% of their calories from nonmilk foods. Table 25-28 lists interventions to address feeding behaviors in infants and toddlers.

To manage the physiological and psychosocial elements of FTT, an interprofessional team that includes members from specialties such as gastroenterology, speech therapy, nutrition, occupational therapy, psychology, developmental therapy, and social work or discharge planning may be necessary to ensure successful treatment (Shah, 2002). HCPs should tailor any social service supports based on the family's unique needs. The negative impacts of poverty are evident in many indicators of a pediatric patient's growth

TABLE 25-28

Interventions for Infant and Toddler Feeding Behaviors

Breastfeeding

Newborn
- Engage specialist with assisting mothers with breast latch-on techniques
- Proper feeding techniques
  - Breastfeed infants frequently throughout the day (feed every 2–3 hours)
  - Breastfeed on each breast at least every 5–10 minutes
- Help increase mother's milk supply with breast pump, increasing fluids, and consider medications such as metoclopramide

Toddler
- Assess for caloric intake with other types of food, especially those high in iron
- Choose breastfeeding wean or increase food supply

Formula Feeding

- Verify proper formula preparation
- Verify caloric minimum intake of 110 kcal/kg/day

Toddler Feeding

- Ensure three meals a day and nutritious snacks in a social environment
- Ensure milk intake (whole milk until 2 years of age)
- Ensure milk intake of 16–32 oz/day (480–960 mL/day)
- Limited or no fruit juice (8 oz/day [240 mL/day])
- Do not force-feed and avoid food battles

Consultants

- Speech therapist referral for oromotor dysfunction, food aversion, and craniofacial abnormalities
- Referral for dietitian or nutritionist may be necessary to work with caregivers and clinicians

Source: Gahagan, 2006.

and development. The use of public assistance programs that support mother, infant, and child nutrition may be necessary (Block et al., 2007).

Education in nutrition, child development, and behavioral management is essential for the family. Caregivers should be empowered and involved in all aspects of the treatment program. Addressing nonmedical problems, including mental health disorders or depression, is also important to identify and resolve. The HCP must document interventions attempted, specific instructions to caregivers, and evidence of understanding of the therapeutic management plan.

DISPOSITION AND DISCHARGE PLANNING

Outpatient team approaches have shown to be beneficial and to decrease the frequency of hospitalization of FTT-diagnosed children (Schwartz, 2000). However, hospitalization may be required if initial management is unsuccessful, if FTT is severe, or if the child is at social risk (Berwick et al, 1982). In addition, the hospital can provide a controlled environment to assess for refeeding syndrome, caloric intake, feeding techniques, ineffective feeding behaviors, and caregiver–child interaction.

The pediatric patient with FTT should be followed by the primary care provider (PCP) at least monthly until catch-up growth is demonstrated (Krugman & Dubowitz, 2003). It is important to note that the catch-up height will lag behind the weight; hence nutritional assessment and interventions should continue until height for age is reached (Shah, 2002). Any family's nonadherence to the treatment plan is a red flag for abuse or neglect or unmet social needs. Early home intervention with strong social services support may mitigate many of the negative effects of FTT (Black et al., 2007)

Pediatric patients who return to normal growth parameters require ongoing monitoring for growth and cognitive development (Bergman & Graham, 2005). Children with FTT are at risk for adverse outcomes such as short stature, behavior problems, poor school performance, and developmental delay (Krugman & Dubowitz, 2005). It is difficult to differentiate between the effects of FTT and the impacts of poor nutrition or the problematic environment that the child encounters such as poverty, family stress, poor parental skills, or genetics (Rudolf & Logan, 2005).

PARENTERAL NUTRITION

Natalie B. Ratz

The goals of parenteral nutrition (PN) in the pediatric population are to meet nutrient needs that cannot be met by enteral intake alone, to avoid nutrient toxicity and deficiency, and to optimize the patient's nutritional status. The selection of appropriate candidates for PN is a complex process that should evaluate the patient's medical history, current clinical status, GI tract function, and nutritional status. Parenteral nutrition prescriptions may be individualized, standardized institutional, or purchased premixed solutions. The PN solution should be tailored to account for the unique needs of each patient. Determination of individual nutrient requirements may vary based on factors such as weight, age, organ dysfunction, disease state, metabolic condition, body composition, and current medication usage.

INDICATIONS

Indications for parenteral nutrition include patients who have a nonfunctional or inaccessible GI tract, who cannot meet their nutritional requirements by enteral intake alone, or who have extraintestinal disorders for which PN has been proven useful (Table 25-29) (AAP, 2009; Cox & Melbardis, 2005). PN may also be indicated in well-nourished pediatric patients who are unable to be fed for 5 to 7 days or as short a period as 1 to 2 days in neonates (August et al., 2002). The malnourished pediatric patient may require PN earlier. Protocols, policies, or decision trees may be useful in selecting appropriate candidates for PN (Figure 25-1).

VASCULAR ACCESS

Peripheral venous catheter administration

A peripheral venous catheter (PVC) is considered a temporary access line. Its use is usually limited to 10 to 14 days due to the potential for venous irritation by the PN solution (Canada et al., 2009). The maximum osmolarity tolerated by a peripheral vein is generally considered to be 900 mOsm/L, although some institutions may limit peripheral PN (PPN) to 700–800 mOsm/L (Table 25-30). It is difficult to meet the nutritional needs of a pediatric patient via this approach, as dextrose concentration is limited in peripheral PN to less than 12.5% (Cox & Melbardis, 2005). A large volume of fluid is also often required to meet nutritional requirements, which prove problematic for those patients with fluid restrictions. Examples of PVCs include peripheral canulas, midline catheters, and midclavicular catheters with the distal tip outside the central superior or inferior vena cava.

Central venous catheter administration

A central venous catheter (CVC) is a line with the catheter distal tip placed in the right atrium or the distal vena cava (Canada et al., 2009). The most commonly used veins include the subclavian, jugular, femoral, cephalic,

TABLE 25-29

Indications for Parenteral Nutrition	
Nonfunctional or Inaccessible GI Tract	**Extraintestinal Disorders**
• Intestinal failure (short gut syndrome) • Severe malabsorption • Obstruction or ileus • Intractable vomiting or diarrhea • Necrotizing enterocolitis • Congenital anomalies of the GI tract • Bowel ischemia	• Malignancies • Body surface burns • Cardiac failure • Kidney failure • Chylothorax

and basilic veins. Examples of CVCs include umbilical venous catheters (newborns), tunneled catheters (Broviac, Hickman, and Groshong), nontunneled central catheters, implanted ports, and peripherally inserted central venous catheters (PICCs). The distal tip location of the CVC

should be confirmed by chest radiograph prior to administering PN. For the pediatric patient with significant linear growth, positioning of the catheter tip should be reverified every 6 to 12 months (Reed & Phillips, 1996). Central PN is the preferred mode of PN delivery, as solutions are generally hypertonic and require a high blood flow to rapidly dilute the solution.

MACRONUTRIENTS

Protein

Protein in PN takes the form of crystalline amino acids and supplies 4 kcal/gm when oxidized for energy. Neonatal amino acid solutions are generally used for infants until they reach one year of age, after which adult amino acid products are routinely used. Based on the composition of human breastmilk, the neonatal solutions contain taurine, tyrosine, histidine, aspartic acid, and glutamic acid.

Neonatal solutions do not contain cysteine—cysteine is unstable in PN over prolonged periods of time. Cysteine

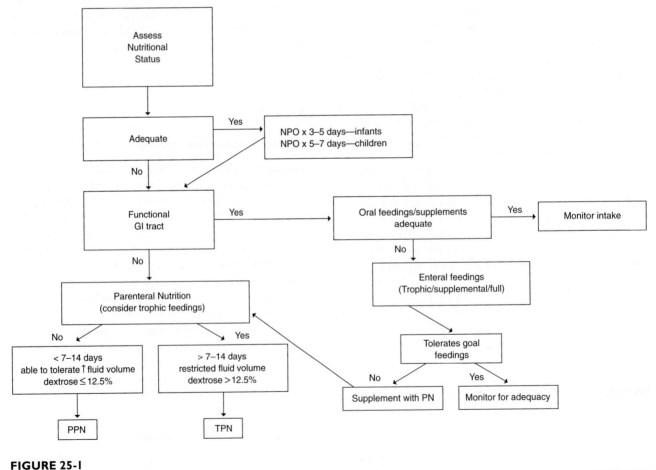

FIGURE 25-1

Pediatric Nutrition Support Algorithm.

Source: Samour, P. & King, K. (2005). *Handbook of Pediatric Nutrition.* Sudbury, MA: Jones and Bartlett Publishers.

TABLE 25-30

Calculating the Osmolarity of Parenteral Nutrition Solutions				
1. Total grams of amino acids **per liter** of solution		_____ grams × 10 =	_____ mOsm	
2. Total grams of dextrose **per liter** of solution		_____ grams × 5 =	_____ mOsm	
3. Total mEq of sodium and potassium **per liter** of solution		_____ mEq × 2 =	_____ mOsm	
4. Total mEq of calcium **per liter** of solution		_____ mEq × 1.4 =	_____ mOsm	
5. Total mEq of magnesium **per liter** of solution		_____ mEq × 1 =	_____ mOsm	
		Total osmolarity =	_____ mOsm	

For peripheral vein tolerance, total osmolarity per liter is limited to 700–900 mOsm.

is a conditionally essential amino acid; thus the addition of L-cysteine hydrochloride is recommended just prior to administration. Cysteine also decreases the pH of the solution, allowing for better calcium–phosphorus solubility (Mirtallo, 2001).

Although glutamine is also considered a conditionally essential amino acid, it is not currently available in crystalline amino acid products.

Protein is generally well tolerated in pediatric patients. Protein initiation in PN may consist of 2 gm/kg/day, advancing by 1 gm/kg/day to a maximum of 3 gm/kg/day in a term infant, 2.5 gm/kg/day in an older infant or child, and 2 gm/kg/day in the adolescent (AAP, 2009). Table 25-31 outlines the recommended protein ranges for pediatric patients. When kidney or liver dysfunction is evident, protein may need to be limited to the lower end of the recommended range.

Carbohydrates

Carbohydrate is provided as dextrose monohydrate, provides energy of 3.4 kcal/gm, and is the primary source of calories in PN solutions. Dextrose is usually limited to 12.5% for delivery through a PVC (final concentration), but can be much higher in a CVC. Gradual increases of 2.5% to 5% dextrose are generally well tolerated in pediatric patients. To avoid complications associated with excessive carbohydrate administration, the usual glucose infusion rate (GIR) upper limits with dextrose are 12–14 mg/kg/min for infants, 8–10 mg/kg/min for children 1–10 years of age, and 5–6 mg/kg/min for adolescents 11–18 years of age (Baker & Baker, 2007). Table 25-31 includes recommended carbohydrate ranges for pediatric patients. The equation for calculating GIR is as follows:

$$GIR = \% \text{ dextrose(gm/100 mL)} \times \text{volume (mL/kg/day)} \div 1.44$$

$$(1.44 = 1440 \text{ min/day} \div 1{,}000 \text{ mg/gm glucose})$$

Example: infant receiving 15% dextrose at 120 mL/kg/day

$$GIR = (0.15 \times 120) \div 1.44 = 12.5 \text{ mg/kg/min}$$

Complications of excessive carbohydrate infusion include phlebitis, refeeding syndrome, hepatosteatosis, cholestasis, CO_2 retention, hypoglycemia, and hyperglycemia (Lee & Werlin, 1997). It is not recommended to add the insulin to the PN to treat hyperglycemia. A separate infusion of insulin at a continuous rate of 0.01–0.1 unit/kg/hr has been shown to be effective and safe in the neonate; however, the AAP (2009) suggests further study of the effects of insulin is needed before routinely recommending its use. To reduce the possibility of hypoglycemia, a 1- to 2-hour taper should be used when PN is discontinued. An infusion of 5% to 10% dextrose for at least 1 hour after PN is discontinued may also be helpful (Canada et al., 2009).

Lipids

Intravenous fat emulsions (IVFEs) provide essential fatty acids, linoleic acid, and linolenic acid; these iso-osmolar substances serve as a concentrated source of energy. While IVFEs are available in both 10% and 20% solutions, 20% IVFEs are most commonly used for pediatric patients. The 10% solutions supply 1.2 kcal/mL, while the 20% solutions supply 2 kcal/mL and contains fewer surface active agents (egg phophatides) per gram of fat. This results in more normal concentrations of lipoproteins, especially low-density lipoproteins (Mirtallo et al., 2004). Neonatal patients on PN should receive IFVE within 3 days of birth, starting at 0.5 to 1 gm/kg/day. The IFVE should then be advanced by 0.5 to 1 gm/kg/day, up to the goal of 3 gm/kg/day (Canada et al., 2009). Maximum lipid infusions for older pediatric patients are 2.5 gm/kg/day for patients 1 to 10 years of age, and up to 1.8 gm/kg/day for patients 11 to 18 years of age (Cox & Melbardis, 2005) (see Table 25-31).

IVFE provides a substantial number of calories to the pediatric patient. It also prevents essential fatty acid deficiency (EFAD). Symptoms of EFAD may not appear until after 3 weeks of a fat-free diet or fat-free PN in children and adults. Infants, however, may experience a deficiency within 1 week of going without essential fatty acids (Baker & Baker, 2007).

TABLE 25-31

Recommendations for Daily Parenteral Administration of Macronutrients, Electrolytes, and Minerals

	Dose Unit	Premature Infants	Term Infants	1–3 Years	4–6 Years	7–10 Years	11–18 Years	Maximum Dose
Basal Energy[1]	kcal/kg	46–55	55	40–55	38–40	25–38	23–25	
Total Energy[2]	kcal/kg	85–105	90–108	75–90	65–80	55–70	30–55	
Dextrose[3]	mg/kg/min	5–15	5–15	5–12	5–11	6–10	4–7	see text
Carbohydrate	g/kg	8–21	8–21	8–18	8–16	8–14	6–10	see text
Protein[4]	g/kg	2.5–4	2.5–3.5	1.5–2.5	1.5–2.5	1.5–2.5	0.8–2	4
Fat[5]	g/kg	0.6–3	0.6–3	0.6–2.5	0.5–2.5	0.5–2.5	0.4–1.8	4
Sodium	mEq/kg	2–4	2–4	2–4	2–4	2–4	60–150 mEq/d	150 mEq/d
Potassium	mEq/kg	2–4	2–4	2–4	2–4	2–4	70–180 mEq/d	180 mEq/d
Chloride	mEq/kg	2–4	2–4	2–4	2–4	2–4	60–150 mEq/d	150 mEq/d
Calcium[6]	mEq/kg	2.5–3	1–2	0.5–1	0.5–1	0.5–1	10–40 mEq/d	see text
Phosphorus[7]	mmol/kg	1–1.5	1–1.5	0.5–1.3	0.5–1.3	0.5–1.3	9–30 mEq/d	see text
Magnesium[8]	mEq/kg	0.5–1	0.25–1	0.25–0.5	0.25–0.5	0.25–0.5	8–24 mEq/d	see text
Zinc[9]	mcg/kg	325–400	100–250	100	100	50	2–5 mg/d	5000 mcg/d
Copper[9]	mcg/kg	20	20	20	20	5–20	200–300 mcg/d	300 mcg/d
Chromium[9]	mcg/kg	0.14–0.2	0.14–0.2	0.14–0.2	0.14–0.2	0.14–0.2	5–15 mcg/d	15 mcg/d
Manganese[9]	mcg/kg	1	1	1	1	1	40–50 mcg/d	50 mcg/d
Selenium[9]	mcg/kg	2	2	2	2	1–2 mcg/d	40–60 mcg/d	60 mcg/d
Molybdenum[9]	mcg/kg	0.25	0.25	0.25	0.25	0.25	5 mcg/d	5 mcg/d
Iron[10]	mg/kg	see text	0.1/see text	see text	see text	see text	see text	see text

Source: Data from Teitelbaum et al., 1998; American Society for Parenteral and Enteral Nutrition, 1993; Kerner et al., 1983; Heimler at al., 1993; Tilden et al., 1989; Lowery et al., 1973; Heird et al., 1991; Greene et al., 1990; Kleinman, 1998; Khaldi et al., 1984; Sunehag et al., 2002; Prelak et al., 2001.

Serum triglyceride levels should be monitored 4 hours after initiating IVFE and 4 hours after an increase in dose. Weekly monitoring may be sufficient once the pediatric patient is stable (AAP, 2009). The American Society for Parenteral and Enteral Nutrition (A.S.P.E.N.) recommends that IVFE be suspended if the neonate's serum triglyceride levels exceed 200 mg/dL, with the infusion then being restarted at a rate of 0.5 to 1 gm/kg/day (August et al., 2002). In the neonate with a serum bilirubin greater than 8 to 10 mg/dL (with a serum albumin of 2.5 to 3 gm/dL), a low dose of IVFE to prevent EFAD may be indicated (Barnes et al., 1981). In the older pediatric patient, acceptable triglyceride levels are up to 400 mg/dL (Baker & Baker, 2007). Increased triglyceride levels may decrease immune response (especially in septic patients), alter pulmonary hemodynamics, and increase the risk of pancreatitis (Canada et al., 2009; Seidner et al., 1989).

IVFE may be infused as a separate infusion, as part of a total nutrient admixture (TNA), or as a 3-in-1 solution. The TNA approach allows for easy administration; lower costs; less manipulation of the delivery system and, therefore, decreased contamination; lower loss of vitamin A; and continuous infusion of all nutrients (AAP, 2009). The AAP does not recommend the use of TNA for neonates and infants (Barnes et al., 1981), but this feeding strategy may be used in older pediatric patients, especially for home PN. Delivery of TNA requires the use of a 1.2-micron filter, whereas an amino acid and dextrose PN solution can be infused through a 0.2-mm filter. TNA may mask calcium–phosphate precipitation when high levels of calcium and phosphorus are added to PN, as the precipitate can pass through the 1.2-micron filter. Lipids infused as part of TNA therapy have a decreased microbial growth potential (Sacks & Driscoll, 2002). When IVFEs are infused separately, it is recommended to limit hang times to 12 hours when possible (Barnes et al.; CDC, 2002; Pearson, 1996).

In the United States, soybean oil is the predominate parenteral lipid source and is rich in omega-6 polyunsaturated fatty acids (PUFA). Long-term infusion of parenteral soybean oil may be a major contributing factor to PN-associated liver disease (PNALD). PNALD is a prevalent and severe complication characterized by increased bilirubin concentrations and liver function tests (deMeijer et al., 2009). Use of fish oil–based IVFE—specifically Omegavan (Fresenius Kabi AG, bad Homburg VDH, Germany), which is rich in omega-3 PUFAs—may offer protection and reversal of PNALD (deMeijer et al.; Gura et al., 2006; Gura et al., 2008). Other formulations of IFVE offer some promise in patients receiving long-term PN, including an emulsion containing olive oil and soybean oil (Gobel et al., 2003).

MICRONUTRIENTS

Electrolytes

Electrolytes in PN may be ordered individually or in preset combinations. Preset combinations of electrolytes may be hospital prepared or provided by manufacturers. Sodium and potassium are available as chloride, acetate, or phosphate compounds. Calcium gluconate is the preferred calcium salt, as it allows for better compatibility with phosphorus. Magnesium is added as magnesium sulfate. Chloride and acetate are adjusted to help maintain acid–base balance.

Table 25-31 includes normal recommendations for electrolytes in the pediatric population. Patients who are experiencing GI and kidney losses may require higher levels of electrolytes. Conversely, electrolyte restriction may be needed in patients with conditions such as congestive heart failure, traumatic brain injury, and kidney insufficiency (Cox & Melbardis, 2005).

Vitamins

Vitamins may be added to PN as a multivitamin preparation or as single vitamins, although not all vitamins are available as a single parenteral dose. Pediatric solutions are designed for children up to 11 years of age and 40 kg in weight (Canada et al., 2009). Table 25-32 lists the recommended amounts for pediatric patients. The AAP has recommended a minimum of 400 IU/day of vitamin D for all children; thus the pediatric patient older than 11 years of age may require an additional source of vitamin D. Currently, a separate parenteral vitamin D preparation is not available in the United States, so enteral supplementation would be necessary.

Minerals and trace elements

Zinc, copper, chromium, manganese, and selenium are trace elements that are commonly added to PN. These minerals are available as a multimineral preparation or as single minerals. Table 25-33 shows the dosage for trace mineral levels for pediatric patients.

For patients with kidney or hepatic dysfunction, trace element dosages may need to be adjusted from the standards shown in Table 25-33 (Mirtallo et al., 2004). Copper and manganese may be removed from PN in patients with direct bilirubin greater than 2 mg/dL. Selenium and chromium should be removed for patients with a clinical concern for kidney failure (Green et al., 1988). Patients on long term PN therapy (more than 1 month) should have their serum trace mineral levels checked. Although iron dextran is compatible with dextrose–amino acid PN, it is not compatible with IFVE (Kumpf, 2003).

TABLE 25-32

Recommendations for Pediatric Parenteral Daily Vitamin Dosage

	A IU	D IU	E mg	K mcg	C mg	B1 mg	B2 mg	B3 mg	B6 mg	B12 mcg	FA mcg	PA mg	Biotin mcg
Recommended amount/kg/day Preterm infant (# 2.5 kg)	1700	160	2.8	80	25	0.35	0.15	6.8	0.18	0.3	56	2	6
MVI Pediatric** doses													
30% dose/day (0.5–1 kg)	700–1400	120–240	2.1–4.2	60–120	24–48	0.4–0.7	0.3–0.6	5–10	0.3–0.6	0.3–0.6	42–84	1.5–3	6–12
65% dose/day (1–2.5 kg)	600–1500	100–260	1.8–4.5	50–130	21–52	0.3–0.8	0.4–0.9	4–11	0.3–0.6	0.3–0.6	36–90	1.5–3	5–13
40% dose/kg/day (#2.5 kg)*	920	160	2.8	80	32	0.48	0.56	6.8	0.4	0.4	56	2	8
Recommended amount/day Preterm infant (2.5 kg)	700–1500	40–160	2–4	6–10	35–50	0.3–0.8	0.4–0.9	5–12	0.3–0.7	0.3–0.7	40–90	2–5	6–13
Term infant/child (age 1–11 yrs)	2300	400	5–7	200	80	1.2	1.4	17	1	1	140	5	20
MVI Pediatric,** 1 dose/day	2300	400	7	200	80	1.2	1.4	17	1	1	140	5	20
Recommended amount/day Adolescents (11–18 yrs)	3300	200	10	150–700	100	3	3.6	40	4	5	400	15	60
MVI-12,** 1 dose/day	3300	200	10	150	100	3	3.6	40	4	5	400	15	60

Note: A 5 retinol, D 5 cholecalciferol, E 5 alpha-tocopherol, K 5 phytonadione, B1 5 thiamin, B2 5 riboflavin, B3 5 niacin, B6 5 pyridoxine, B12 5 cyanocobalamin, FA 5 folic acid, PA 5 pantothenic acid.

*Maximum dose not to exceed 1 full dose per day

**Pediatric MVI (Pediatric parenteral multivitamin) and MVI-12 Injection or Unit Vial, Astra USA, Inc., Westboro, MA.

Source: Data from Teitelbaum DH, Coran AG. Perioperative nutritional support in pediatrics. Nutrition. 1998;14:130; Greene HL, Hambidge KM, Schanler R, et al. Guidelines for the use of vitamins, trace elements, calcium, magnesium, and phosphorus in infants and children receiving total parenteral nutrition: Report of the Subcommittee on Pediatric Parenteral Nutrient Requirements from the Committee on Clinical Practice Issues of The American Society for Clinical Nutrition. Am J Clin Nutr. 1988; 48:1324. (Revised in 1990.); Adamkin DH. Total parenteral nutrition. Neonatal Intensive Care. 1997; Sept/Oct:24; Pereira GR. Nutritional care of the extremely premature infant. Clin Perinatol. 1995;22:61; Moore MC, Greene HL, Phillips B, et al. Evaluation of a pediatric multiple vitamin preparation for total parenteral nutrition in infants and children. I. Blood levels of water soluble vitamins. Pediatr. 1986;77:530, and; 163. Greene HL, Moore MEC, Phillips B, et al. Evaluation of a pediatric multivitamin preparation for total parenteral nutrition. II. Blood levels of vitamins A, D, and E. Pediatr. 1986;77:539.

TABLE 25-33

Dose Concentrations and Recommendations for Combined Trace Mineral Products

Product category	Dose mL	Zinc mcg	Copper mcg	Chromium mcg	Manganese mcg	Selenium[1] mcg
Neonatal[2]	1	500	100	0.85	25	—
	0.2/kg	300/kg[3]	20/kg	0.17/kg	5/kg[4]	—
Pediatric	1	500 or 1000	100	0.85 or 1	25	0 or 15
	0.1/kg	50 or 100/kg	10/kg	~0.1/kg	2.5/kg	0 or 1.5/kg
	0.2/kg	100 or 200/kg	20/kg	~0.2/kg	5/kg[4]	0 or 2/kg
	25[5]	2000	200	2	50	30
	55[5]	2500 or 5000	500	4.25 or 5	125	0
Adult[6,7] (standard)	1	1000	400	4	100	0 or 20
	0.05/kg	50/kg	20/kg	0.2/kg	5/kg[4]	0 or 1/kg
Adult[6] (concentrate)	1	5000	1000	10	500	0 or 60
	0.01/kg	50/kg	10/kg	0.1/kg	5/kg[4]	0 or 0.6/kg

[1]Neonatal and select pediatric and adult products do not contain selenium or molybdenum. These may be added separately when total parenteral nutrition is required longer than 4 weeks.

[2]Neonatal products are generally recommended for preterm infants until term age. Maximum dose is 3 mL/day.

[3]Additional zinc is needed to meet recommendations for preterm neonates.

[4]Manganese dose may be excessive in cholestatic jaundice.

[5]Maximum dose of pediatric product with selenium is limited by the amount of selenium. Maximum dose of pediatric product with out selenium is limited by copper content.

[6]Adult products are generally used for adolescents, or children over 10 years of age.

[7]Iodine is included in one standard and one concentrated adult product in concentrations of 25 and 75 mcg/mL respectively; molybdenum is included in one standard adult product in a concentration of 25 mcg/mL.

Source: Data from Product literature and Intravenous nutritional therapy. Trace metals. Drug Facts ad Comparisons. St. Louis, Missouri: Wolters Kluwer Heath Inc. 2003; p. 125.

Aluminum is a trace mineral that is a contaminant of PN; it may be neurotoxic to premature infants and children with kidney failure (Bishop et al., 1997). Currently, parenteral products used to make PN contain excessive amounts of aluminum and do not meet the U.S. Food and Drug Administration's standard of less than 5 mcg/kg/day of aluminum exposure (Poole et al., 2008). The Safe Practices for Parenteral Nutrition published by A.S.P.E.N. states that HCPs should minimize pediatric patients' aluminum exposure when possible (Mirtallo et al., 2004).

MEDICATIONS

Ranitidine, famotidine, regular insulin, and unfractionated heparin are medications that are often added to PN despite the lack of clinical data regarding their compatability with the solution (Canada et al., 2009). Carnitine is available as a parenteral additive for pediatric patients with a carnitine deficiency and those who are susceptible to a deficiency (Borum, 1993). Dosages of 10 to 20 mg/kg/day may be used in the pediatric patient on PN more than 2 weeks (Slicker & Vermilyea, 2009).

CALORIE REQUIREMENTS

Energy requirements for parenterally fed patients are 10% to 15% less than those for enterally fed patients, because calories are not required for the digestion and absorption of nutrients with the former approach. Although predictive equations may be used to estimate energy requirements, it is important to understand that these equations are derived from resting energy expenditure (REE) values for healthy children and adults (Skillman & Wischmeyer, 2008). Basal energy needs and estimated total energy needs are provided in Table 25-31. Given that estimating energy requirements requires subjective interpretation, it is recommended to use indirect calorimetry for measurement of energy needs of the critically ill pediatric patient (Skillman & Wischmeyer). Indirect calorimetry measurements may not be as useful in the chronically PN-fed patient, as they may not account for growth. In other words, pediatric patients on chronic PN will need to be monitored to ensure that they are achieving adequate growth.

Overfeeding and underfeeding are problematic in patients fed with PN. Overfeeding (excessive energy intake) in the pediatric patient can lead to increased carbon dioxide production, increased lipogenesis, decreased lipid oxidation, hyperglycemia, and prolonged duration of mechanical ventilation and hospital stay (Skillman & Wischmeyer, 2008; Slicker & Vermilyea, 2009). Underfeeding of the pediatric patient may occur due to inadequate prescription/delivery, restriction of fluids, increased severity of illness, vasoactive medications, or procedural interruptions (Skillman & Wischmeyer).

ORDERING PARENTERAL NUTRITION

PN orders may be electronic or written, and should always be standardized for both adult and pediatric patients (Mirtallo et al., 2004). According to the Task Force for the Revision of Safe Practices for Parenteral Nutrition, the following items are mandatory for the PN order form: clarity of form, contact number for the person writing the order, contact number for assistance with PN ordering, time by which orders need to be received, location of the venous access device, patient height, patient weight/dosing weight, diagnosis, PN indication, hang time guidelines, institutional policy for infusion rates, and information regarding potential incompatibilities (Mirtallo et al.). The following information is strongly recommended for inclusion on PN order forms: nutrient dosing guidelines based on weight and age, recommended nutrient ranges, guidelines to assist in nutrient and volume calculations, monitoring guidelines, guidelines for stopping or interrupting PN infusion, specific content of multivitamin and trace element preparations, specific amino acid and IFVE brands available, and insulin guidelines (Canada et al., 2009). Ordering by percent concentration of amino acids and dextrose is discouraged, but still often used in clinical practice (Mirtallo et al.).

PN orders should be written in their entirety on a daily basis, (Mirtallo et al., 2004). Table 25-34 includes calculations for dextrose, protein, lipids and calorie count. Table 25-35 contains a suggested monitoring protocol for parenteral nutrition. Cycling PN may be appropriate in some pediatric patients to help prevent or delay liver dysfunction,

TABLE 25-34

Calculating Dextrose, Protein, and Calorie Count

Dextrose Calculations

$$\frac{_____ \text{ gm}}{100 \text{ mL}} \times _____ \text{ mL/day} = _____ \text{ gm/day}$$

$$\frac{_____ \text{ gm/day}}{\text{wt} \times 1.44} = _____ \text{ mg/kg/min}$$

Protein Calculations

$$\frac{_____ \text{ gm}}{100 \text{ mL}} \times \text{ mL/day} = _____ \text{ gm/day}$$

$$\frac{_____ \text{ gm/day}}{\text{wt}} = _____ \text{ gm/kg/day}$$

Calorie Count

Dextrose:	_____ gm/day	× 3.4 kcal/gm	=	_____	kcal/day
Fat:	_____ mL/day	× 2 kcal/mL	=	_____	kcal/day
Protein:	_____ gm/day	× 4 kcal/gm	=	_____	kcal/day

Total kcal/day = _____ kcal/day

Total kcal/kg/day = _____ kcal/kg/day

TABLE 25-35

Suggested Monitoring Protocol for Parenteral Nutrition		
Parameter	**Initial**	**When Stable**
Weight	Daily	Daily
Length, head circumference	Weekly	Weekly
BMP, with magnesium and phosphorus	Daily	2–3 times per week
CMP, ionized calcium	Weekly	Weekly
Triglyceride levels	2–3 days after starting	2 times per week
Glucose (bedside or laboratory)	1–2 hours after initiating PN or changing glucose concentration; if cycled, mid-infusion and 1 hour after stopping PN	As needed
Trace elements	One month after initiating PN	Monthly

BMP (basic metabolic panel), CMP (comprehensive metabolic panel), PN (parenteral nutrition).

although there is little evidence to support this assumption. A stable patient on PN for 2 weeks or more may be a good candidate for cycled PN (Slicker & Vermilyea, 2009).

COMPLICATIONS OF PARENTERAL NUTRITION

Complications of PN can be metabolic, mechanical, and infectious in nature. Hypoglycemia, hyperglycemia, hypertriglyceridemia, EFAD, and PNALD have been reviewed earlier in this section. In addition to the use of fish oil IVFE to prevent and manage PNALD, it is suggested to avoid overfeeding, initiate PN with a balanced macronutrient mixture (50% to 60% carbohydrate, 10% to 20% protein, 20% to 30% lipid), cycle PN when possible, and start and provide the maximum amount of enteral nutrition that will be tolerated (Slicker & Vermilyea, 2009). Other potential metabolic complications of PN include metabolic acidosis and alkalosis, hypokalemia and hyperkalemia, volume overload, hypocalcemia and hypercalcemia, hypophosphatemia and hyperphosphatemia, hypomagnesemia and hypermagnesemia, anemia, and cholestatic jaundice. Careful monitoring of electrolytes, fluids, and medications can help prevent these complications.

Refeeding syndrome may occur in the pediatric patient who is malnourished, has experienced starvation (either intentional or non-intentional), or has experienced recent weight loss. Hypophosphatemia is the classic sign of this syndrome, but patients may develop other electrolyte disorders as well as neurologic, pulmonary, cardiac, neuromuscular, and hematologic complications (Kraft et al., 2005). Symptoms include generalized fatigue, lethargy, muscle weakness, edema, cardiac arrhythmia, and hemolysis (Canada et al., 2009). Pediatric patients should be screened for refeeding syndrome risk prior to the initiation of nutrition support, and PN (especially dextrose) should be advanced cautiously.

Metabolic bone disease may be associated with prolonged use of PN as well as with endocrine disease, GI disease, malignancy, use of medications such as steroids, genetic disease, and immobilization (Canada et al., 2009). Metabolic bone disease includes osteoporosis, osteopenia, and osteomalacia. Appropriate monitoring and provision of calcium, phosphorus, protein, vitamin D, and magnesium levels are indicated in patients receiving PN to guard against development of these problems. Aluminum toxicity and copper deficiency may also be risk factors for development of metabolic bone disease. Routine skeletal radiographs are recommended in pediatric patients on long-term PN (Canada et al.).

Mechanical complications may be related to the actual placement of the venous access device, problems with the device, or occlusions. Complications related to the central line include malposition of the central line, hemorrhage, pneumothorax, brachial plexus injury, air embolism, catheter emboli, and thrombophlebitis. Pediatric patients experience central line occlusions more readily than adults (Othersen et al., 2007). Catheter occlusions may be intraluminal due to blood clotting or drug/lipid precipitation, a fibrin sleeve at the catheter tip, vessel thrombosis, or mechanical occlusions (Canada et al., 2009). Calcium–phosphorus precipitation remains a concern in the neonatal population. Factors that affect calcium–phosphorus solubility include the concentration of amino acids and dextrose in the PN solution, the composition of the amino acid solution, the type of calcium salt used, the pH of the solution, the temperature of the solution, and the order in which additives are mixed into the solution (Canada et al.). Calcium–phosphorus solubility curves have been developed to help pharmacies compound appropriate PN solutions for neonatal populations. Medications that may cause catheter occlusions include phenytoin, diazepam, and etoposide (Othersen et al.).

Catheter-related infections may consist of a localized catheter colonization, exit site infection, tunnel infection, pocket infection, infusate-related bloodstream infection, or CVC-related bloodstream infection (Othersen et al., 2007). Organisms commonly associated with catheter-related bloodstream infections (CRBSIs) include *Staphylococcus epidermidis, Staphylococcus aureus, Enterococcus faecalis, Enteroccus faecium, Enterobacter* spp., *Escherichia coli, Klebsiella pneumniae, Pseudomonas aeruginosa,* and *Candida* (Canada et al., 2009; Othersen et al.). The Institute for Healthcare Improvement has developed a "care bundle" to help combat CRBSIs; this central line bundle consists of hand hygiene, maximal barrier precautions, chlororhexidine skin antisepsis, optimal catheter site selection, and daily review of line necessity (Canada et al.).

Parenteral nutrition can be a life-saving modality for pediatric patients who have a nonfunctioning GI tract or cannot meet their enteral nutritional needs. Careful attention to detail is required to safely deliver PN to these vulnerable patients. Nutrition support teams can be instrumental in initiating and monitoring PN to ensure adequacy of nutrition support and safety of PN.

REFERENCES

1. Agency for Healthcare Research and Quality. (2004). *Preventable hospitalizations: A window into primary and preventive care, 2000.* HCUP Fact Book No. 5. AHRQ Publication No. 04-0056.

2. American Academy of Pediatrics (AAP). (2005). Policy statement: Breastfeeding and the use of human milk. *Pediatrics, 115*(2), 496–506.

3. American Academy of Pediatrics (AAP). (2009). Parenteral nutrition. In *Pediatric nutrition handbook* (6th ed., pp. 519–540). Elk Grove, IL: Author.

4. American Association for Respiratory Care. (2004). Metabolic measurement using indirect calorimetry during mechanical ventilation-2004 revision & update. *Respir Care, 49*(9),1073–1079.

5. American Heart Association. (2005). 2005 American Heart Association guidelines for cardiopulmonary resuscitation and emergency cardiovascular care. *Circulation, 112*(suppl 1), IV-1–203.

6. American Psychiatric Association. (2000). *Diagnostic and statistical manual of mental disorders* (4th ed., text revision). Washington, DC: Author.

7. Araujo, E., Goncalves, A., Cornetta, M., Cunha, H., Cardoso, M., Morais, S., et al. (2005). Evaluation of the secretory immunologlobulin A levels in the colostrum and milk of mothers of term and preterm infants. *Brazilian Journal of Infectious Diseases, 9*(5), 357–362.

8. Arifeen, S., Black, R., Antelman, G., Baqui, A., Caufield, L., & Becker, S. (2001). Exclusive breastfeeding reduces acute respiratory infection and diarrhea deaths among infants in Dhaka slums. *Pediatrics, 108*(4), e67. doi:10.1542/peds.108.4.e67

9. Ariyan, C., & Sosa, J. (2004). Assessment and management of patients with abnormal calcium. *Critical Care Medicine, 32,* S146–S154.

10. A.S.P.E.N. Board of Directors and the Clinical Guidelines Task Force. (2002). Guidelines for the use of parenteral and enteral nutrition in adult and pediatric patients. *Journal of Parenteral and Enteral Nutrition, 26*(suppl), 1SA–138SA.

11. A.S.P.E.N. Board of Directors and the Enteral Nutrition Practice Recommendations Task Force. (2009). Enteral nutrition practice recommendations. *Journal of Parenteral and Enteral Nutrition, 20*(10), 1–46.

12. August, D., Teitelbaum, D., Albina, J., Bothe, A., Guenter, P., Heitkemper, M., et al. (2002). Guidelines for the use of parenteral and enteral nutrition in adult and pediatric patients. *Journal of Parenteral and Enteral Nutrition,26*(1), 25SA–110SA.

13. Avent, Y. (2007). Managing calcium imbalance in acute care. *Nurse Practitioner, 32,* 7–10.

14. Baker, S., & Baker, R. (2007). Macronutrients. In S. Baker, R. Baker, & A. Davis, *Pediatric nutrition support* (pp. 299–312). Sudbury, MA: Jones and Bartlett.

15. Barlow, S. (2007). Expert committee recommendation regarding the prevention, assessment, and treatment of child and adolescent overweight and obesity: Summary report. *Pediatrics, 120,* 164–192.

16. Barnes, L., Dallman, P., Anderson, H., Collip, P., Nichols, B., Walker, W., et al. (1981). Use of IV fat in pediatric patients. *Pediatrics, 68,* 738–743.

17. Bellemare, W., Hartlin, L., Weibe, N., Russell, K., Craig, W., McConnell, D., et al. (2004). Oral rehydration versus intravenous therapy for treating dehydration due to gastroenteritis in children: A meta-analysis of randomized controlled trials. *BMC Medicine, 4*(2), 1–8.

18. Bergman, P., & Graham, J. (2005). An approach to failure-to-thrive. *Australian Family Physicians, 34*(9), 725–729.

19. Berwick, D., Levy, J., & Kleinerman, R. (1982). Failure-to-thrive: Diagnostic yield of hospitalization. *Archives of Disease in Childhood, 57,* 347–351.

20. Bishop, N., Morley, R., Chir, B., Day, J., & Lucas, A. (1997). Aluminum neurotoxicity in preterm infants receiving intravenous-feeding solutions. *New England Journal of Medicine, 336,* 1557–1561.

21. Black, M., Dubowitz, A., Krishnakumar, A., & Starr, R. (2007). Early intervention and recovery among children with failure-to-thrive: Follow-up at age 8. *Pediatrics, 120,* 59–69.

22. Block, R., Krebs, N., Committee on Child Abuse and Neglect, & Committee on Nutrition. (2005). Failure-to-thrive as manifestation of child neglect, *Pediatrics, 116,* 1234–1237.

23. Borum, P. (1993). Is L-carnitine stable in parenteral nutrition solutions prepared for preterm neonates? *Neonatal Intensive Care, 6,* 30–32.

24. Brennan-Behm, M., Carlson, G., Meier, P., & Engstrom, J. (1994). Caloric loss from expressed mother's milk during continuous gavage infusion. *Neonatal Network, 13*(2), 27–32.

25. Brunelli, S., & Goldfarb, S. (1999). Hypophosphatemia: Clinical consequences and management. *Journal of the American Society of Nephrology, 18,* 1999–2003.

26. Canada T., Crill C., & Guenter P. (2009). *A.S.P.E.N. parenteral nutrition handbook.* Silver Springs, MD: American Society of Parenteral and Enteral Nutrition.

27. Caraeaga, M., & Kerner, J. (2000). A gastroenterologist's approach to failure-to-thrive. *Pediatric Annals, 29*(9), 558–562.

28. Centers for Disease Control and Prevention (CDC). (2000). Clinical growth charts. Retrieved from http://www.cdc.gov/growthcharts/clinical_charts.htm

29. Centers for Disease Control and Prevention (CDC). (2002). Guidelines for the prevention of intravascular catheter-related infection. *Morbidity and Mortality Weekly Report, 51*(RR-10), 1–37.

30. Centers for Disease Prevention and Control (CDC). (2003). Managing acute gastroenteritis among children oral rehydration, maintenance, and nutritional therapy. *Morbidity and Mortality Weekly Report, 52*(16), 1–20.

31. Centers for Disease Control and Prevention (CDC). (2009a). CDC growth charts: United States. Retrieved from http://www.cdc.gov/growthcharts/background.htm

32. Centers for Disease Control and Prevention (CDC). (2009b). Frequently asked questions about 2000 CDC growth charts. Retrieved from http://www.cdc.gov/growthcharts/growthchart_faq.htm

33. Centers for Disease Control and Prevention (CDC). (2009c). Using the BMI-for-age growth charts. Retrieved from http://www.cdc.gov/nccdphp/dnpa/growthcharts/training/modules/module1/text/page10a.htm

34. Chan, G., & Lechtenberg, E. (2007). The use of fat-free human milk in infants with chylous pleural effusion. *Journal of Perinatology, 27,* 434–436.

35. Colen, F. (2008). Oncologic emergencies: Superior vena cava syndrome, tumor lysis syndrome and spinal cord compression. *Journal of Emergency Nursing, 34,* 535–537.

36. Corkins, M. (2010). *The A.S.P.E.N. pediatric nutrition support core curriculum.* Silver Springs, MD: American Society of Enteral and Parenteral Nutrition.

37. Coss-Bu, J., Klish, W., Walding, G., Stein, F., Smith, E., & Jefferson, L. (2001). Energy metabolism, nitrogen balance, and substrate utilization in critically ill children. *American Journal of Clinical Nutrition, 74*(5), 664–669.

38. Cox, J., & Melbardis, I. (2005). Parenteral nutrition. In P. Q. Samour & K. King (Eds.), *Handbook of pediatric nutrition* (3rd ed., pp. 525–557). Sudbury, MA: Jones and Bartlett.

39. deMeijer, V., Gura, K., Le, H., Meisel, J., & Puder, M. (2009). Fish oil–based lipid emulsions prevent and reverse parenteral nutrition–associated liver disease: The Boston experience. *Journal of Parenteral and Enteral Nutrition, 33*(5), 541–547.

40. Diggins, K. (2006). Treatment of mild to moderate dehydration in children with oral rehydration therapy. *Journal of the American Academy of Nurse Practitioners, 20,* 402–406.

41. Dunn, R., Stettler, N., & Mascarenhas, M. (2003). Refeeding syndrome in hospitalized pediatric patients. *Nutrition in Clinical Practice, 18,* 327–332.

42. Dvorak, B., Fituch, C., Williams, C., Hurst, N., & Schanler R. (2003). Increased epidermal growth factor levels in human milk of mothers with extremely premature infants. *Pediatric Research, 54,* 15–19.

43. Emond, S. (2009). Dehydration in infants and young children. *Annals of Emergency Medicine, 53*(3), 395–397.

44. Faustino, E., & Apkron, M. (2005). Persistent hyperglycemia in critically ill children. *Journal of Pediatrics, 146*(1), 30–34.

45. Finberg, L. (2002). Dehydration in infancy and childhood. *Pediatrics in Review, 23*(8), 277–282.

46. Friedman, A., & Ray, P. (2008). Maintenance fluid therapy: What it is and what it is not. *Pediatric Nephrology, 23,* 677–680.

47. Furman, L., Taylor, G., Minich, N., & Hack, M. (2003). The effect of maternal milk on neonatal morbidity of very-low-birth-weight infants. *Archives of Pediatrics & Adolescent Medicine, 157*(1), 66–71.

48. Gabay, C., & Kushner, I. (1999). Acute-phase proteins and other systemic responses to inflammation. *New England Journal of Medicine, 340,* 448–453.

49. Gahagan, S. (2006). Failure-to-thrive: a consequence of undernutrition. *Pediatrics in Review, 27*(1), 1–11.

50. Ganesh, S., Stack, A., Levin, N., Hulbert-Shearon, T., & Port, F. (2001). Association of elevated serum PO4, Ca × PO$_4$ product, and parathyroid hormone with cardiac mortality risk in chronic hemodialysis patients. *Journal of the American Society of Nephrology, 12,* 2131–2138.

51. Gennari, F. (1998). Hypokalemia. *New England Journal of Medicine, 339,* 451–458.

52. Gibbons, T., & Fuchs, G. (2009). Malnutrition: A hidden problem in hospitalized children. *Clinical Pediatrics, 48*(4), 356–361.

53. Gobel, Y., Koletzko, B., Bohles, H., Engelsberger, I., Forget, D., Brun, A., et al. (2003). Parenteral fat emulsions based on olive and soybean oils: A randomized clinical trial in preterm infants. *Journal of Pediatric Gastroenterology and Nutrition, 37,* 161–167.

54. Golts, E., Choi, J., Wilson, W., Fuchs, S., & Angle, A. (2007). Nutritional and metabolic evaluation and monitoring. In W. Wilson, C. Grande, & D Hoyt (Eds.), *Trauma critical care* (pp. 569–582). New York: Informa Healthcare USA.

55. Gottschlich, M., & Mayes, T. (2005). Nutrition for the burned pediatric patient. In P. Samour & K. King (Eds.), *Handbook of pediatric nutrition* (3rd ed., pp. 483–498). Sudbury, MA: Jones and Bartlett.

56. Green, H., Hambidge, K., Schanler, R., & Tsang, R. (1988). Guidelines for the use of vitamins, trace elements, calcium, magnesium, and phosphorus in infants and children receiving total parenteral nutrition: report of the Subcommittee on Pediatric Parenteral Nutrition Requirements from the Committee on Clinical Practice Issues of the American Society for Clinical Nutrition. *American Journal of Clinical Nutrition, 48,* 1324–1342.

57. Greenbaum, L. (2004). Electrolyte and acid–base disorders. In R. Behrman, R. Kliegman, & H. Jenson (Eds.), *Nelson textbook of pediatrics* (pp. 191–242). Philadelphia: Saunders.

58. Greer, F., McCormick, A., & Loker, J. (1984). Changes in fat concentration of human milk during delivery by intermittent bolus and continuous mechanical pump infusion. *Journal of Pediatrics, 105*(5), 745–746.

59. Gura, K., Duggan, C., Collier, S., Jennings, R., Folkman, J., Bistrian, B., et al. (2006). Reversal of parenteral nutrition–associated liver disease in two infants with short bowel syndrome using parenteral fish oil: Implications for future management. *Pediatrics, 118,* e197–e201.

60. Gura, K., Lee, S., Valim, C., Zhou, J., Kim, S., Modi, B., et al. (2008). Safety and efficacy of a fish-oil based fat emulsion in the treatment of parenteral nutrition associated liver disease. *Pediatrics, 121,* e678–e686.

61. Handy, J., & Soni, N. (2008). Physiological effects of hyperchloraemia and acidosis. *British Journal of Anaesthesia, 101,* 141–150.

62. Hellerstein, S. (1993). Fluids and electrolytes: Clinical aspects. *Pediatrics in Review, 14*(3), 103–115.

63. Holick, M., Krane, S., & Potts, J. (1998). Calcium, phosphorus, and bone metabolism: Calcium regulating hormones. In A. Fanci, E. Braunwald, K. Isslebacher, J. Wilson, J. Martin, D. Kasper, S. Hauser, & D. Longo (Eds.), *Harrison's principles of internal medicine* (pp. 2214–2223). New York: McGraw-Hill.

64. Holliday, M., & Segar, W. (1957). The maintenance need for water in parenteral fluid therapy. *Pediatrics, 19*(5), 823–832.

65. Holliday, M., Friedman, A., & Wassner, S. (1999). Extracellular fluid restoration in dehydration: A critique of rapid versus slow. *Pediatric Nephrology, 13,* 292–297.

66. Holliday, M., Ray, P., & Friedman, A. (2007). Fluid therapy for children: Facts, fashions and questions. *Archives of Disease in Childhood, 92,* 546–550.

67. Huang, C., & Kuo, E. (2007). Mechanism of hypokalemia in magnesium deficiency. *Journal of the American Society of Nephrology, 18,* 2649–2652.

68. Hurst, N., Meier, P., & Engstrom, J. (1999). Mothers performing in-home measurement of milk intake during breastfeeding for their preterm infants: Effects on breastfeeding outcomes at 1, 2, and 4 weeks post-NICU discharge. *Pediatric Research, 45,* 287A.

69. Hylander, M., Strobino, D., Pezzullo, J., & Dhanireddy, R. (2001). Association of human milk feedings with a reduction in retinopathy of prematurity among very low birth weight infants. *Journal of Perinatology, 21*(6), 356–362.

70. Inukai, T., Hirose, K., Inaba, T., Kurosawa, H., Hama, A., Inada, H., et al. (2007). Hypercalcemia in childhood acute lymphoblastic leukemia: Frequent implication of parathyroid hormone–related peptide and E2A-HLF from translocation 17;19. *Leukemia, 21,* 288–296.

71. Joffe, A., Grant, M., Wong, B., & Gresiuk, C. (2000). Validation of a blind transpyloric feeding tube placement technique in pediatric intensive care: Rapid, simple, and highly successful. *Pediatric Critical Care Medicine, 1*(2), 151–155.

72. Joint Commission International. (2009). *2009 comprehensive accreditation manual for hospitals.* Chicago, IL: The Joint Commission.

73. Joosten, K., & Hulst, J. (2008). Prevalence of malnutrition in pediatric hospitalized patients. *Current Opinion in Pediatrics, 20,* 590–596.

74. Kerdudo, C., Aerts, I., Fattet, S., Cherret, L., Pacquement, H., Doz, F., et al. (2005). Hypercalcemia and childhood cancer: A 7-year experience. *Journal of Pediatric Hematology Oncology, 27,* 23–27.

75. Keys, A., Brozek, J., Henschel, A., Mickelsen, O., & Taylor, H. (1950). *The biology of human starvation,* (2 volumes). Minneapolis: University of Minnesota Press.

76. Kinney, K. (1995). The metabolic responses of the critically ill patient. *Critical Care Medicine, 11,* 569–586.

77. Kleinman, R. (2009). *Pediatric nutrition handbook*. Elk Grove Village, IL: American Academy of Pediatrics.

78. Koenig, A., de Albuquerque, E., Diniz, E., Barbosa, S., & Vaz, F. (2005). Immunologic factors in human milk: The effects of gestational age and pasteurization. *Journal of Human Lactation, 21*(4), 439–443.

79. Kraft, M., Btaiche, I., & Sacks, G. (2005). Review of the refeeding syndrome. *Nutrition in Clinical Practice, 20*, 625–633.

80. Kreimeier, U. (2000). Pathophysiology of fluid balance. *Critical Care, 4*(suppl 2), S3–S7.

81. Krugman, S., & Dubowitz, H. (2003). Failure-to-thrive. *American Family Physicians, 68*(5), 879–884.

82. Kumpf, V. (2003). Update on parenteral iron therapy. *Nutrition in Clinical Practice, 18*, 318–326.

83. Lauriat, S. & Berl, T. (1997). The hyponatremic patient: Practical focus on therapy. *Journal of the American Society of Nephrology, 8*, 1599–1607.

84. Lee, P., & Werlin, S. (1997). Carbohydrates. In R. Baker, S. Baker, & D. Davis (Eds.), *Pediatric nutrition* (pp. 97–107). New York: Chapman & Hall.

85. Leonberg, B. (2008). *ADA pocket guide to pediatric nutrition assessment*. Chicago: American Dietetic Association.

86. Lu, M., Lange, L., Slusser, W., Hamilton, J., & Halfon, N. (2001). Provider encouragement of breastfeeding: Evidence from a national survey. *Obstetrics and Gynecology, 97*(2), 290–294.

87. Lucas, A., & Cole, T. (1990). Breast milk and neonatal necrotizing enterocolitis. *Lancet, 336*(8730), 1519–1523.

88. Lucas, A., Morley, R., & Cole, T. (1998). Randomized trial of early diet in preterm babies and later intelligence quotient. *British Medical Journal, 317*(7171), 1481–1487.

89. Lucas, A., Morley, R., Cole, T., Lister, G., & Leeson-Payne, C. (1992). Breastmilk and subsequent intelligence quotient in children born preterm. *Lancet, 339*(8788), 261–265.

90. Lyons, K., Brilli, R., Wieman, R., & Jacobs, B. (2002). Continuation of transpyloric feeding during weaning of mechanical ventilation and tracheal extubation in children: A randomized controlled trial. *Parenteral and Enteral Nutrition, 26*(3), 209–213.

91. Macdonald, J., & Struthers, A. (2004). What is the optimal serum potassium level in cardiovascular patients? *Journal of the American College of Cardiology, 43*, 155–161.

92. Marinella, M. (2003). The refeeding syndrome and hypophosphatemia. *Nutrition Reviews, 61*, 320–323.

93. Mcguire, W., & Anthony, M. (2003). Donor human milk versus formula for preventing necrotizing enterocolitis in preterm infants: Systematic review. *Archives of Disease in Childhood: Fetal and Neonatal Edition, 88*, F11–F14.

94. Mehta, M., Bechard, L., Leavitt, K., & Duggan, C. (2009a). Cumulative energy imbalance in the pediatric intensive care unit: Role of targeted indirect calorimetry. *Journal of Parenteral and Enteral Nutrition, 33*(3), 336–344.

95. Mehta, M., Compher, C., & A.S.P.E.N. Board of Directors. (2009b). A.S.P.E.N. clinical guidelines: Nutrition support of the critically ill child. *Journal of Parenteral and Enteral Nutrition, 33*(3), 260–276.

96. Mehta, N. (2009). Approach to enteral feeding in the PICU. *Nutrition in Clinical Practice, 24*(3), 377–387.

97. Meier, P., & Engstrom, J. (2007). Evidence-based practices to promote exclusive feeding of human milk in very low birth weight infants. *NeoReviews, 8*(11), e467–e477. doi:10.1542/neo.8-11-e467

98. Meier, P., Engstrom, J., Hurst, N., Ackerman, B., Allen, M., Motykowski, J., et al. (2008). A comparison of the efficiency, efficacy, comfort and convenience of two hospital-grade electric breast pumps for mothers of very low birthweight infants. *Breastfeeding Medicine, 3*(3), 141–149.

99. Meier, P., Engstrom, J., Murtaugh, M., Vasan, U., Meier, W., & Schanler, R. (2002). Mothers' milk feedings in the neonatal intensive care unit: Accuracy of the creamatocrit technique. *Journal of Perinatology, 22*(8), 646–649.

100. Meier, P., Engstrom, J., Patel, A., Jegier, B., & Bruns, N. (In press). Improving the use of human milk during and after the NICU stay. *Seminars in Perinatology*.

101. Meier, P., Engstrom, J., Zuleger, J., Motykowski, J., Vasan, U., Meier, W., et al. (2006). Accuracy of a user-friendly centrifuge for measuring creamatocrits on mothers' milk in the clinical setting. *Breastfeeding Medicine, 1*(2), 79–87.

102. Meier, P., Furman, L., & Degenhardt, M. (2007). Increased lactation risk for late preterm infants and mothers: Evidence and management strategies to protect breastfeeding. *Journal of Midwifery & Women's Health, 52*(6), 549–587.

103. Meinzen-Derr, J., Poindexter, B., Wrage, L., Morrow, A., Stoll, B., & Donovan, E. (2009). Role of human milk in extremely low birth weight infants' risk of necrotizing enterocolitis or death. *Journal of Perinatology, 29*(1), 57–62.

104. Methany, N., Schnelker, R., McGinnis, J., Zimmerman, G., Duke, C., Merritt, B., et al. (2005). Indicators of tubesite during feedings. *Journal of Neuroscience Nursing, 37*(6), 320–325.

105. Miracle, D., Meier, P., & Bennett, P. (2004). Mothers' decision to change from formula to mothers' milk feeding for very low birth weight infants. *Journal of Obstetric, Gynecologic, and Neonatal Nursing, 33*(6), 692–703.

106. Mirtallo, J. (2001). Parenteral formulas. In J. Rombeau & R. Rolandelli (Eds.), *Parenteral nutrition* (3rd ed., pp. 118–139). Philadelphia: W. B. Saunders.

107. Mirtallo, J., Canada, T., Johnson, D., Kumpf, V., Peterson, C., Sacks, G., et al. (2004). Safe practices for parenteral nutrition. *Journal of Parenteral and Enteral Nutrition, 28*, S39–S70.

108. Mittal, M. (2007). Severe hypercalcemia as a harbinger of acute lymphoblastic leukemia. *Pediatric Emergency Care, 23*, 397–400.

109. Moritz, M., & Ayus, J. (2003). Prevention of hospital-acquired hypnatremia: A case for using isotonic saline. *Pediatrics, 111*(2), 227–230.

110. Neville, M. (2001). Anatomy and physiology of lactation. In R. J. Schanler (Ed.), Breastfeeding 2001: The evidence. *Pediatric Clinics of North America, 48*, 13–34.

111. Nevin-Folino, N., & Miller, M. (2005). Enteral nutrition. In P. Samour & K. King (Eds.), *Pediatric nutrition* (3rd ed., pp. 499–524). Sudbury, MA: Jones and Bartlett.

112. Othersen, H., Glenn, J., Chessman, K., & Tagge, E. (2007). Central venous catheters in parenteral nutrition. In S. Baker, R. Baker, & A. Davis (Eds.), *Pediatric nutrition support* (pp. 331–346). Sudbury, MA: Jones and Bartlett.

113. Patel, A., Meier, P., & Engstrom, J. (2007). The evidence for use of human milk in very low birthweight preterm infants. *NeoReviews, 8*(11), e459–e466. doi:10.1542/neo.8-11-e459

114. Pearson, M. L. (1996). The Hospital Infections Control Practices Advisory Committee: Guidelines for prevention of intravascular-device–related infections. *Infection Control and Hospital Epidemiology, 17*, 438–479.

115. Petrillo-Albarano, T., Pettignano, R., Asfaw, M., & Easley, K. (2006). Use of a feeding protocol to improve nutritional support through early, aggressive, enteral nutrition in the pediatric intensive care unit. *Pediatric Critical Care Medicine, 7*(4), 340–344.

116. Poole, R., Hintz, S., Machenzie, N., & Kerner, J. (2008). Aluminum exposure from pediatric parenteral nutrition: Meeting the New FDA regulation. *Journal of Parenteral and Enteral Nutrition. 32*, 242–246.

117. Powers, F. (1999). The role of chloride in acid–base balance. *Journal of Intravenous Nursing, 22*, 286–291.

118. Preissig, C., & Rigby, M. (2009). Pediatric critical illness: Hyperglycemia: Risk factors associated with development and severity of hyperglycemia in critically ill children. *Journal of Pediatrics, 155*(5), 734–739.

119. Ralston, M., Hazinski, M., Zaritsky, A., Schexnayder, S., & Kleinman M. (2006). *PALS provider manual*. Dallas, TX: American Heart Association.

120. Ramsay, M., Gisel, E., McCusker, J., Bellavance, F., & Platt, R. (2002) Infant sucking ability, non-organic failure-to-thrive, maternal characteristics, and feeding practices: A prospective cohort study. *Developmental Medicine and Child Neurology, 4*(6), 405–414.

121. Rastegar, A., & Soleimani, M. (2001). Hypokalemia and hyperkalemia. *Postgraduate Medical Journal, 77*, 759–764.

122. Reed, T., & Phillips, S. (1996). Management of central venous catheter occlusions. *Journal of Intravenous Nursing, 19*, 289–294.

123. Reid, S., & Losek, J. (2009). Rehydration: Role for early use of intravenous dextrose. *Pediatric Emergency Care, 25*(1), 49–51.

124. Rimmer, J., Horn, J., & Gennari, F. (1987). Hyperkalemia as a complication of drug therapy. *Archives of Internal Medicine, 147*, 861–869.

125. Rodríguez, N., Miracle, D., & Meier, P. (2005). Sharing the science on human milk feedings with mothers of very low birth weight infants. *Journal of Obstetric, Gynecologic, and Neonatal Nursing, 34*(1), 109–119.

126. Ronayne de Ferrer, P., Baroni, A., Sambucetti, M., Lopez, N., & Cernadas, J. (2000). Lactoferrin levels in term and preterm milk. *Journal of the American College of Nutrition, 19*(3), 370–373.

127. Ronnestad, A., Abrahamsen, T., Medbo, S., Reigstad, H., Lossius, K., Kaaresen, P., et al. (2005). Late-onset septicemia in a Norwegian national cohort of extremely premature infants receiving early full human milk feeding. *Pediatrics, 115*(3), e269–e276.

128. Rudolf, M., & Logan, S. (2005). What is the longterm outcome for children who fail to thrive? *Archives of Disease in Childhood, 90*, 925–931.

129. Sacks, G., & Driscoll, D. (2002). Does lipid hang time make a difference? *Nutrition in Clinical Practice, 17*, 284–290.

130. Sanderson, I., & Croft, N. (2005). The anti-inflammatory effects of enteral nutrition. *Journal of Parenteral and Enteral Nutrition, 29*(4 suppl), S134–S140.

131. Sapford, A. (2000). Human milk and enteral nutrition products. In S. Groh-Wargo & M. Thompson (Eds.), *Nutritional care for the high risk newborn* (3rd ed., pp. 286–287). Chicago: Precept Press.

132. Schanler, R. (2001). The use of human milk for premature infants. *Pediatric Clinics of North America, 48*(1), 207–219.

133. Schanler, R., Lau, C., Hurst, N., & Smith, E. (2005). Randomized trial of donor human milk versus preterm formula as substitutes for mother's milk in the feeding of extremely premature infants. *Pediatrics, 11*(2), 400–406.

134. Schucker, J., & Ward, K. (2005). Hyperphosphatemia and phosphate binders. *American Journal of the Health System Pharmacology, 62*, 2355–2361.

135. Schulman, M., & Narins, R. G. (1990). Hypokalemia and cardiovascular disease. *American Journal of Cardiology, 65*, 4E–9E.

136. Schwartz, D. (2000). Failure to thrive: An old nemesis in the new millennium. *Pediatrics in. Review, 21*, 257–264.

137. Seidner, D., Mascioli, E., Istfan, N., Porter, K., Selleck, K., Blackburn, G., et al. (1989). Effects of long-chain triglyceride emulsions on reticuloendothelial system function in humans. *Journal of Parenteral and Enteral Nutrition, 13*, 614–619.

138. Shah, M. (2002). Failure-to-thrive in children. *Journal of Clinical Gastroenterology, 35*(5), 371–374.

139. Shaoul, R., Okev, N., Tamir, A., Lanir, A., & Jaffe, M. (2004). Value of laboratory studies in assessment of dehydration in children. *Annals of Clinical Biochemistry, 41*(3), 192–196.

140. Shepard, M., & Smith, J. (2007). Hypercalcemia. *American Journal of Medical Sciences, 334*, 381–385.

141. Singhal, A., Morley, R., Cole, T., Kennedy, K., Sonksen, P., Isaacs, E., et al. (2007). Infant nutrition and stereoacuity at age 4–6 y. *American Journal of Clinical Nutrition, 85*(1), 152–159.

142. Sisk, P., Lovelady, C., Dillard, R., Gruber, K., & O'Shea, T. (2007). Early human milk feeding is associated with a lower risk of necrotizing enterocolitis in very low birth weight infants. *Journal of Perinatology, 27*(7), 428–433.

143. Skillman, H., & Wischmeyer, P. (2009). Nutrition in critically ill infants and children. *Journal of Parenteral and Enteral Nutrition, 32*(5), 520–534.

144. Skuse, D. (1993). Identification and management of problem eaters. *Archives of Disease in Childhood, 69*, 604–608.

145. Slicker, J., & Vermilyea, S. (2009). Pediatric parenteral nutrition: Putting the microscope on macronutrients and micronutrients. *Journal of Parenteral and Enteral Nutrition, 10*, 481–486.

146. Srivastava, T., & Young, D. (1995). Impairment of cardiac function by moderate potassium depletion. *Journal of Cardiac Failure, 1*, 195–200.

147. Stephens, M., Gentry, B., & Michener, M. (2008). What is the clinical workup for failure-to-thrive. *Journal of Family Practice, 57*(4), 264–266.

148. Subramanian, R., & Khardori, R. (2000). Severe hypophosphatemia: Pathophysiologic implications, clinical presentation and treatment. *Medicine, 79*, 1–8.

149. Taketomo, C., Hodding, J., & Kraus, D. (2010). *Pediatric dosage handbook.* Hudson, OH: Lexi-Comp.

150. Trahan, A., Cheetham, T., & Bailey, S. (2008). Hypercalcemia in acute lymphoblastic leukemia: An overview. *Journal of Pediatric Hematology and Oncology, 31*, 424–427.

151. Uraizee, F., & Gross, S. (1989). Improved feeding tolerance and reduced incidence of sepsis in sick very low birth weight (VLBW) infants fed maternal milk (abstract). *Pediatric Research, 25*, 298A.

152. Waterlow, J. (1972). Classification and definition of protein energy malnutrition. *British Medicine Journal, 3*, 566–569.

153. Weglicki, W., Quamme, G., Tucker, K., Haigney, M., & Resnick, L. (2005). Potassium, magnesium, and electrolyte imbalance and complications in disease management. *Clinical and Experimental Hypertension, 1*, 95–112.

154. Weiner, I., & Wingo, C. (1997). Hypokalemia: Consequences, causes, correction. *Journal of the American Society of Nephrology, 8*, 1179–1188.

155. Weisinger, J., & Bellorin-Font, E. (1998). Magnesium and phosphorus. *Lancet, 352*, 391–396.

156. Wells, J. (2002). Growth and failure-to-thrive. *Pediatric Nursing, 14*(3), 37–42.

157. World Health Organization (WHO). (2010). The WHO child growth standards. Retrieved May 10, 2010, from http://www.who.int/childgrowth/standards/en/

158. Yucha, C., & Dungan, J. (2004). Renal handling of phosphorus and magnesium. *Nephrology Nursing Journal, 31*, 33–37.

Gastrointestinal Disorders

PHYSIOLOGY AND DIAGNOSTICS

James Pierce

The gastrointestinal (GI) tract begins at the mouth and continues to the anus (Figure 26-1). From the level of the lips to the larynx, there is considerable overlap between anatomic structure, neurologic function (such as speech and swallowing), and aerodigestive physiology. Once a food bolus passes beyond the upper esophageal sphincter, the physiology of the GI tract is recognized by its four components of action: motility, secretion, digestion, and absorption.

PHYSIOLOGY

The supraglottic digestive tract has its embryologic origin in the development of the face. Thus the lips, teeth, tongue, and pharynx are all derived from the branchial arches. As such, they receive their motor and sensory innervation by cranial nerves, receive their arterial supply from branches of the common and external carotid arteries, provide venous drainage to the internal jugular veins, and have skeletal muscle tissue under somatic control for movement. Chewing and swallowing require complex neural control. The oral cavity and pharynx are responsible for two types of actions: mixing and propulsion. Mixing consists of chewing food, allowing it to mix with oral secretions and liquid ingestions; propulsion is the act of initiating a swallowing reflex whereby the

food bolus is handed from somatic control (chewing) over to autonomic control (the enteric nervous system responsible for the remainder of the GI tract).

Once the food bolus is swallowed, it begins its trek through the GI tract. Swallowing pushes the bolus through the upper esophageal sphincter into the foregut—the first anatomical division of the GI system. The foregut consists of the esophagus and its parts—the upper esophageal sphincter, esophageal body, intra-abdominal esophagus, and lower esophageal sphincter; the stomach and its parts—the fundus, body, antrum, and pylorus; and the first part of the small intestine, commonly known as the duodenum.

The transition from the early small intestine (arterial supply by the celiac artery) to the majority of the small intestine (arterial supply by the superior mesenteric artery) defines the entry into the midgut. All structures that receive blood from this artery are considered part of the midgut. Thus the midgut consists of the distal duodenum, jejunum, ileum, cecum, appendix, ascending colon, and first portion of the transverse colon.

The final portion of the GI tract, the hindgut, includes all structures that receive blood from the inferior mesenteric artery or pelvic arteries. They include the remaining transverse colon, descending and sigmoid colon, intra-abdominal rectum, extra-peritoneal rectum, and anus.

One last group of important anatomic structures is the gut appendages derived from the foregut. They include the liver, gallbladder, biliary tree, and pancreas. Derived from ventral and dorsal buds off the future duodenum, these

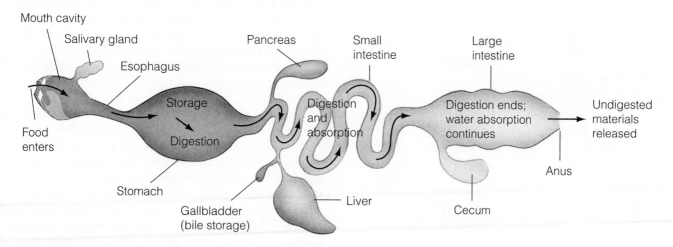

FIGURE 26-1

The Digestive System.

Source: Chiras, D. (2008). *Human Biology*, 6th edition. Sudbury, MA: Jones and Bartlett Publishing.

hepatobiliary and pancreatic structures play an important role in GI physiology.

Despite the fact that there are distinct anatomic boundaries for each gastrointestinal region (foregut, midgut, hindgut) and each organ (stomach, small intestine, colon), the physiologic "unit" of function is different. The fundamental physiologic unit of the gut is the motor–valve–reservoir system (Figure 26-2).

Each physiologic unit of the gut begins with a motor. The motor is responsible for two types of jobs—mixing and propulsion. At the end of the motor region, there is either an anatomic (such as the pylorus) or physiologic (such as the "ileal brake") barrier to the forward movement of luminal contents. The valve generally remains closed while the motor is mixing, opens when the motor is pushing contents forward, and then closes again as the reservoir fills. The reservoir for each unit is a region of gut that is capable of relaxing and accommodating inbound luminal contents. It is capable of feedback control, thereby ensuring that the proximal motor–valve system does not move food forward before completing the process, and is often responsible for initiating subsequent distal motor–valve functions as well. The upper esophageal sphincter is the valve that opens during swallowing and subsequently closes, preventing reflux aspiration of esophageal food or liquid contents. Finally, the upper esophageal body is the reservoir that serves to initiate the enteric reflexes responsible for esophageal peristalsis.

Most primary diseases of the gut start at one physiologic component (motor, valve, or reservoir), although some diseases may have secondary complications in the other components. History and physical examination can often delineate which component is the primary problem. Diseases are diagnosed by the company they keep—for example, primary aspiration due to oropharyngeal motor dysfunction secondary to neurologic disease is often associated with other neuromotor symptoms, such as poor phonation and articulation, drooling, and poor control of liquids. In contrast, aspiration due to gastroesophageal reflux is more likely to have esophageal symptoms such as heartburn.

Motility

Foregut. The first foregut physiologic unit includes the esophageal body (motor), lower esophageal sphincter (valve), and upper stomach (reservoir). The esophagus is unique—it is the only region of the gut designed strictly for transport and not for mixing. Thus the esophageal lining is a more protective stratified squamous epithelium and the only source of esophageal secretions is from swallowing.

Esophageal motor function, as expected, does not include any mixing. Instead, following a "swallow" trigger, the esophagus motor function consists of primary, secondary, and tertiary peristalsis waves designed to push solid and liquid food through the thorax, through the gastroesophageal junction, and into the stomach. The valve is the lower esophageal sphincter and consists of three parts: the length of intra-abdominal esophagus, the length and tone of the sphincter muscle, and the proper apposition of the diaphragm hiatus. Together these components allow opening only during antegrade movement of food from esophagus to stomach; they close to prevent retrograde regurgitation or reflux of material. Finally, the proximal stomach acts as a reservoir to receive and store intermittent boluses of food. At the same time the lower esophageal sphincter relaxes, the fundus of the stomach relaxes. The tone of the fundus determines gastric pressure, one of the contributing parasympathetic sensations involved in both central nervous system awareness (i.e., fullness) and distal gastric function (control of secretion and motility).

The next physiologic unit is also part of the foregut; it consists of the antrum as the motor, the pylorus as the valve, and the duodenal bulb as the reservoir. The gastric pacemaker is located between the proximal and distal stomach. The proximal reservoir, or upper stomach, and the autonomic nervous system are integrated to provide a consistent phasic gastric electrical output. The motor of this physiologic unit converts these electrical signals into mechanical gastric waves. For the motor unit to perform mixing, the pylorus remains closed. Then, the peristaltic wave causes gastric contents to collide against the closed pylorus, leading to mixing in the antrum. When appropriate, gastric contents move forward into the duodenum due to pylorus relaxation, thereby allowing antegrade ejection of luminal contents into the duodenal bulb. Thus the tone

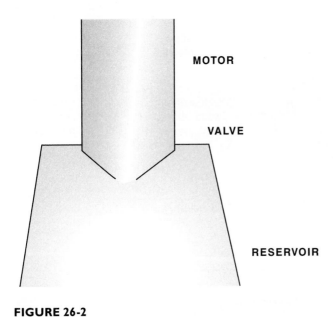

FIGURE 26-2

Motor Valve Reservoir Unit.

of the pyloric valve determines the degree of mixing and ensures only properly digested contents may move forward. The duodenal bulb—the reservoir of this unit—is responsible for sampling the luminal contents for pH, osmolarity, and lipophilicity, and for providing feedback to the motor and valve components that further ensures only properly prepared chime may move into the duodenum.

Midgut. The next two units are defined based on a physiologic valve rather than a mechanical valve. The duodenum, jejunum, and ileum all have differing abilities to digest and absorb. Therefore, luminal contents need to spend the "right amount of time" in each section of intestine. Two physiologic feedback loops facilitate this process, both of which are referred to as a brake. In the first physiologic unit, the motor is the duodenum (or proximal small intestine), the valve is the jejunal brake, and the reservoir is the jejunum. In the second physiologic unit, the motor is the jejunum (or mid small intestine), the valve is the ileal brake, and reservoir is the ileum.

In both cases, the small bowel, acting as a motor, performs two types of movements: segmentation and peristalsis. Segmentation is an intermittent squeezing pattern designed to optimize mixing. Peristalsis is a progressive squeezing pattern designed to propel chyme forward. Without a mechanical valve, the luminal contents will intermittently arrive in and be sampled by the more distal bowel. If the chyme is poorly digested or insufficient content has been absorbed, the distal bowel secretes high levels of enteric hormones. Once the luminal contents have been processed appropriately, the distal bowel hormone secretion drops, "releasing the brake." Then, the motor segment (more proximally) switches from segmentation to peristalsis. Although the exact mechanisms for the jejunal and ileal brakes are not entirely clear, current evidence suggests the hormones neurotensin and peptide YY are likely involved.

The small bowel as a whole also acts as a motor component in the next physiologic unit. The distal small bowel is the motor, the valve is the ileocecal valve, and the reservoir is the cecum. Again, the distal bowel can act in two fashions—segmentation (or mixing) and peristalsis (or propulsion). Unlike the more hormonal brakes, the conversion from segmentation to peristalsis is associated with a change in the activity of the enteric nervous system. After prolonged fasting, intestine begins to demonstrate the presence of the migrating myoelectric complex and its electromechanical result—peristaltic waves from more proximal bowel to ileocecal valve. This process helps to sweep the last luminal products and any refluxed colonic material into the cecum. The ileocecal valve, though not necessarily competent, acts to limit the degree of bacterial load reflux into the small bowel. The cecum receives the watery waste and begins facilitating the colonic role of water and salt absorption. The ileum, appendix, and cecum have a very important role in maintaining the appropriate colonic bacterial balance and facilitating proper immune development and function. However, the current understanding of the exact mechanism is unknown.

Hindgut. The last two physiologic units are located in the hindgut. The first consists of the majority of the colon as the motor, the sigmoid colon as the valve, and the upper rectum (or rectal ampulla) as the reservoir. The second consists of the rectum and pelvic floor as the motor, the anal sphincter complex as the valve, and the expelled fecal content as the reservoir. The colon also performs mixing and propulsion functions.

Interestingly, colonic antegrade movement is a large, powerful, peristaltic wave referred to as a mass movement. Once luminal contents are sufficiently thickened (i.e., water has been effectively absorbed), the mass movement pushes the stool through the sigmoid valve into the rectum. Acute distention of the reservoir—the proximal rectum—transmits a signal to the spinal cord and brain to initiate the transition from autonomic to somatic control of evacuation of stool. When a child chooses to defer defecation, after 30 to 45 seconds the rectum will relax and the rectal luminal pressure will fall. This removes the sensation of needing to pass a stool. After several deferrals, however, the rectum cannot relax and defecation must occur. Thus it is the reservoir function of the rectum that allows conscious continence. On the reverse side, during defecation the rectum and pelvic floor act as a motor unit pushing solid stool forward. The anal sphincters are the valves that are required to relax.

Secretion

Secretion begins before food consumption. Although various gut appendages will increase secretion in response to eating, basal GI secretions are of a significant volume and hypovolemia can rapidly ensue with any gastrointestinal loss. These secretions assist in all aspects of GI function: motility, digestion, and absorption, as well as excretion of waste products. Proximal secretion ensures that chyme is a liquid that is easy to segment or peristalse. More distal secretions, such as colorectal mucus, help lubricate the more solid particles to prevent injury during mass movements and defecation. Secretion of protons, bicarbonate, and enzymes assists in the digestion of food particles. Finally, secretion of certain molecules assists in the specialized absorbance of important substances, such as bile assisting in the uptake of lipophilic vitamins and intrinsic factor ensuring absorbance of vitamin B_{12}.

Gastrointestinal secretion begins with saliva production, often in response to the sight, smell, or taste of food. In addition, saliva can be produced and swallowed in response to wash gastric secretions from the esophagus or biliary secretions from the stomach. While the range of salivary production is quite large, most estimates suggest that it averages 1.5 to 2 liters per day for an adult. The esophagus lacks secretory glands; therefore, it minimally contributes to gastrointestinal secretion.

The best-studied and -understood secretion in the GI tract occurs in the stomach. The gastric mucosa consists of gastric glands and a protective mucous layer. The glands contain a number of different cell types, whose distribution varies in different regions of the stomach. The most well-understood cell is the parietal cell; other key players include the chief cells, mucous (or goblet) cells, basal cells (the progenitors), and the various hormone-secreting cells (such as G cells, which secrete gastrin).

A basal amount of mucus and acid secretion occurs, which can significantly increase in response to the three phases of gastric secretion. The first (cephalic) phase consists of gastric acid secretion in response to cerebral and oropharyngeal stimuli such as seeing, chewing, and swallowing food. The primary mediator of acid secretion is parasympathetic stimulation of the parietal cells and G cells, with a secondary mediator being G-cell-released gastrin stimulation of parietal cell mass. The second (gastric) phase consists of gastric acid secretion in response to gastric distention. Distention is sensed by afferent parasympathetic nerves; thus the primary mediators of acid secretion are local and vagal parasympathetic reflexes onto the parietal cells. The third (intestinal) phase consists of hormonal response to products of protein digestion in the duodenum. The primary mediator of acid secretion is duodenal gastrin secretion via duodenal G cells, though a number of enterogastrones play a part.

In all three phases, a combination of parasympathetic and hormonal control instructs the parietal cells to increase acid secretion. The parietal cells respond to three main stimuli: acetylcholine (from parasympathetic innervation), gastrin, and histamine. Histamine response is particularly important in maintenance of the mucous barrier, but is less important in ingestion-mediated gastric secretion.

The parietal cells are responsible for secretion of acid (protons) and intrinsic factor. The mechanism of acid secretion is the presence of proton pumps ($H^+ATPase$) on the intracellular vesicles and luminal membrane. Without stimulation, the majority of these pumps are located in the intracellular compartment. With the addition of histamine, acetylcholine, or gastrin, however, these vesicles fuse with the luminal membrane and massively increase the luminal concentration of proton pumps, leading to significant proton secretion. The chief cells are responsible for secretion of pepsinogen; in an acidic pH environment, pepsinogen self-cleaves to its active form, known as pepsin. The mucous cells secrete mucus and bicarbonate, with the bicarbonate remaining trapped under a bed of mucus,

thereby ensuring that mucosal pH remains in the 6–7 range while luminal contents are exposed to pH of 1–2.

The duodenum receives a variety of secretions, such as the chyme mixed with gastric secretions, which enters through the pylorus; in addition, Brunner's glands secrete directly into the lumen, and the pancreatic and biliary secretions enter through the ampulla of Vater. Secretions are responsible for adjusting the luminal pH, decreasing the osmolarity and thereby improving the viscosity, enhancing the lipid solubility, and continuing digestion. In addition, the duodenum is very hormonally active, secreting a number of peptide hormones for feedback control on the stomach and feedforward control on the hepatobiliary secretion. The most important hormonal secretions are gastrin, gastric inhibitory peptide (GIP), cholecystokinin, and secretin. High levels of amino acids in the duodenum lead to gastrin secretion, enhancing acid hydrolysis of protein in the stomach. High levels of fats and other lipophilic substances in the duodenum lead to cholecystokinin and GIP secretion. GIP slows gastric emptying, whereas cholecystokinin enhances biliopancreatic secretion via direct (secretogoge) and indirect (gallbladder contraction) mechanisms. Low pH leads to secretin secretion and subsequent bicarbonate release from the pancreas. In this way, the duodenal hormones enhance the influx of appropriate fluids for mixing in the duodenum.

The hepatobiliary and pancreatic systems are gut appendages that drain into the second portion of the duodenum. They develop as embryologic diverticula on the dorsal and ventral aspects of the foregut, and as a result of foregut twisting, merge to drain on the left side of the duodenum. The dorsal appendage becomes the body and tail of the pancreas, and the ventral appendage becomes the head and uncinate process of the pancreas, the bile ducts, gallbladder, and liver.

Two main paths bring these secretions to the duodenum. In one pathway, the liver drains through branched bile ducts into a common hepatic duct. In the second pathway, depending on the hormonal state, bile can either drain into the gallbladder for storage or drain from the gallbladder and liver through the common bile duct. The pancreatic ductal system consists of a main duct, comprising the ventral and dorsal main ducts, and a minor duct, comprising a small portion of the dorsal duct that carries pancreatic secretions. The common bile duct and main pancreatic duct drain through a single common channel named the ampulla of Vater into the second portion of the duodenum. The accessory pancreatic duct often drains through an accessory channel in a secondary location.

The bile that is secreted consists of three main components: bile salts, cholesterol, and lecithin. In addition, significant amounts of sodium, chloride, water, and lipophilic waste are present in bile as it is initially secreted from the liver. When bile is stored in the gallbladder, salt and water are reabsorbed, resulting in concentrated lipophilic viscous bile. The absorption of water is necessary because the liver can secrete 500 to 1,000 mL of bile per day in an adult and the gallbladder is incapable of holding such large volumes. Bile and the lipophilic substances in chyme mix in the duodenum and throughout the small intestine. A large portion of these substances will be reabsorbed in the distal ileum, with waste products and some bile salts being excreted in stool.

The pancreas can secrete bicarbonate and water in response to duodenal acidity or proenzymes in response to digestive needs. Pancreatic secretions comprise two major components: the acinar secretions, which contain large numbers of proenzymes for digestion, and the ductal secretions, which consist of large amounts of electrolytes (especially bicarbonate) and water. These secretions are governed by different hormonal control mechanisms: Acinar secretion responds to both neural (acetylcholine) and hormonal (gastrin and cholecystokinin) stimuli, whereas ductal secretion responds predominantly to secretin.

Although they are often thought of as digestive and absorptive organs, both the small bowel and the colon secrete a variety of substances. For example, the small bowel secretes antibodies (IgA) and other immunohormones and effectors for maintenance of body defenses. In addition, it secretes a number of hormones for feedforward and feedback regulation of motility. The small and large bowels also allow transcellular and paracellular movement of water, cations, and anions. This movement facilitates isotonicity of luminal contents, transcellular electroneutrality, and, most importantly, the absorption in the colon of large amounts of sodium and water. Finally, the colon, rectum, and anus secrete mucus that acts as a lubricant, allowing for the passage of solid stool without mucosal injury.

Digestion

Digestion refers to the breaking down of food into absorbable components. It begins in the mouth with mastication, during which time individual bites of food are mixed with saliva and converted into a mushy, but solid, food bolus for transport to the stomach. While some enzymatic digestion occurs as a result of salivary amylase, for the most part oropharyngeal digestion occurs on a gross level.

The stomach is responsible for ongoing gross digestion, during which food continues to mix with gastric secretions en route to becoming chyme—the thick, nearly isotonic liquid that represents the completion of gross digestion. In the stomach, microscopic digestion begins to play an increasing role in the breakdown of food into usable nutrients. On a microscopic level, two main mechanisms contribute to digestion: nonenzymatic and enzymatic. Acid-based hydrolysis leads to digestion of many biologic compounds,

and gastric-secreted pepsin enzymatically facilitates the digestion of proteins into oligopeptides.

The majority of microscopic digestion occurs in two locations in the small bowel: in the lumen and on the epithelial surface. When the pancreatic and hepatobiliary secretions mix with the chyme, the resulting basic pH and improved lipid solvability lead to denaturing of proteins and effective mixing of fats on a microscopic level. As trypsinogen becomes activated by the enteropeptidase to trypsin, it becomes capable of activating all of the enzymes secreted by the pancreas. The relatively uniform mix of chyme and enzymes allows for effective microscopic digestion to oligosaccharides, oligopeptides, and fatty acids. Digestion of oligos is predominantly performed by membrane-bound enzymes on the luminal surface of the mucosal epithelium. The effective digestive surface, like the absorptive surface, has a tremendous area due to presence of intestinal villi and cellular microvilli. Digestion occurs tightly coupled to absorption, as oligos are broken down to monosaccharides, amino acids, and dipeptides and tripeptides.

Some digestion does occur at the level of the colon and rectum, although in most cases this process is pathologic. Any complex biologic compound that arrives in the colon will be processed by the symbiotic colonic bacteria. Often, as these compounds are digested, the resulting increase in luminal osmoles draws water into the lumen and leads to a subsequent osmotic diarrhea.

Absorption

The gut epithelium is responsible for the absorption of every salvageable component in chyme. Several mechanisms for absorption exist at the epithelial level, and there are two routes by which absorbed compounds reach general circulation. The epithelium supports both paracellular diffusion and transcellular transport, and membrane transport incorporates both facilitated and active transport. Once absorbed through the epithelium, these nutritive components are either transported through the portal venous circulation to the liver or returned via lacteals (specialized villi lymphatics) through the abdominal lymphatic system to the thoracic duct, which drains into the systemic circulation at the junction of the left internal jugular and left subclavian veins. Paracellular diffusion of water and electrolytes follows both pathways; most other substances follow one or the other. The colon is the largest site of water and electrolyte absorption.

As carbohydrates are broken down to monosaccharides, the now-smaller compounds are transported into the epithelial cells via several different channels—most commonly, SGLT-1 and GLUT-5 for glucose/galactose and fructose, respectively. Subsequent basal transport occurs through GLUT-2 channels. In a similar fashion, proteins are not transported into epithelial cells until they have been broken down to single amino acids or dipeptides and tripeptides. At the intracellular level, these short peptides are degraded to individual amino acids by cellular peptidases. Ultimately, only individual amino acids are transported across the basal membrane, with all amino acids and monosaccharides subsequently entering the portal circulation for processing by the liver.

Fats and other lipophilic substances are processed differently. Although well-mixed micelles of lipids are present in the lumen of the gut, components cross individually into the epithelial cells, where they are packaged into chylomicrons and subsequently delivered to the epithelial lacteals. The distal ileum is the site of significantly increased absorption of the bile acids and smaller lipophilic substances such as vitamins. These compounds, due to their higher hydrophilicity and better dissolution, are transported through the portal vein to the liver, thereby completing the enterohepatic circulation.

ABDOMINAL PAIN AND TENDERNESS

Two major pathophysiologies contribute to abdominal pain: splanchnic and somatic. Splanchnic, or visceral pathophysiology refers to nociception via the autonomic nervous system. Somatic pathophysiology refers to nociception via the somatic nervous system. Each pain pathway possesses different characteristics of sensation, transmission, and central processing of pain—and, therefore, can be identified by a thorough history and physical examination. Thus a good clinical examination can help guide the healthcare professional (HCP) in the selection of appropriate diagnostic tests or timely consultation.

Acute splanchnic abdominal pain originates in the post-ganglionic parasympathetic neurons that innervate the dense, irregular connective tissues that make up the capsules of the solid organs and the myenteric and submucosal plexuses that innervate the GI tract. Splanchnic pain occurs in three main locations: substernal/epigastric, which includes the foregut, foregut appendages (liver, pancreas), and lower thoracic organs (heart, fibrous pericardium); periumbilical, which generally includes the small bowel, appendix, and proximal colon as well as the retroperitoneal kidney and ureters; and suprapubic, radiating to the pelvis, which contains the distal colon, rectum, and genitourinary organs.

Splanchnic nociception is unable to sense cutting or burning; instead, this type of pain is caused by tension. For example, solid organ swelling, such as occurs in hepatitis, stretches the capsule and causes pain. Distention of a hollow organ, such as a full bladder or rectum, causes pain by direct wall tension. The worst visceral pain, however, occurs during obstruction. First, at the level of the obstruction, the entity becomes distended, which causes pain. Second, in

an attempt to relieve the obstruction the organ increases secretion and peristalsis, leading to proximal organ distention and increased wall tension with each peristaltic wave. Finally, increased pressure causes mucosal ischemia, the last cause of splanchnic pain.

Somatic pain is derived from dermis, soft tissues, and, most importantly, the peritoneum. Standard somatic nociceptors in dermatomal distribution innervate the peritoneum as well as overlying abdominal wall. These nociceptors sense sharp pain, deep pressure, and temperature, and their signals are carried predominantly via the spinothalamic tract to the brain. As most somatic nerves embryologically were transferred to their final location by the migrating dermatomyotomes, frequently skin and soft tissue innervations do not match skeletal muscle and peritoneum innervations. This leads to a process known as radiation, the best example of which is the phrenic nerve (roots C3, C4, and C5), which informs the brain about pain in the diaphragm as well as pain in the shoulder's dermis (C3, C4, and C5 dermatomes).

Although radiation can give clues about the pain's origin during the patient history taking, simply understanding peritoneal structural locations allows a more comprehensive examination. The peritoneum is a three-dimensional structure. The top consists of the diaphragm, central tendon, and hiatuses. The bottom consists of the organs of the pelvis that have a peritoneal lining: the anterior pelvis (bladder, and in women the uterus, a portion of vagina, and adenexal structures), and the posterior structures (the pelvic floor at the base of the rectouterine/rectovesicular pouch and the rectum). The lateral structures consist of the iliacus muscle, and neurovascular plexus; thus splanchnic pain is generally midline in nature, and is typically caused by obstruction (partial or complete) in a tube. In contrast, somatic pain is generally focal, and is caused by inflammation of the peritoneum, fascial container of an organ (such as Glisson's capsule), or abdominal wall components.

NAUSEA, VOMITING, AND ABDOMINAL DISTENTION

Nausea is an unpleasant sensation often—but not always—associated with a sensation of needing to vomit. In the hindbrain, there is a nausea center that receives several sensory inputs and is ultimately responsible for informing the cortex that it is nauseated. This nausea center may be stimulated directly by toxins, such as chemotherapies or ingested poisons, as well as by neural input. Several neurotransmitter systems have been identified as being involved in this process and their roles in nausea characterized; this line of research has led to the development of effective antinausea and antiemetic medications. The most important neurotransmitter is serotonin, which through its receptor acts as a final common pathway for a number of different causes of nausea. Other important efferent neurotransmitters include dopamine and norepinephrine, which integrate GI motility and obstruction with cortical sensation and ensure avoidance of food and initiation of vomiting in the setting of decreased motility and partial or complete obstruction. In most cases, several mechanisms act synergistically to cause significant nausea. For example, consumption of excessive alcohol can cause pyloric spasm (partial obstruction of the stomach), gastric mucosal irritation, and toxin stimulation of the nausea center. Similarly, acute appendicitis treated with surgery can cause decreased motility by proximity to the infection, immunologic stimulation of the nausea center, and anesthetic mediated nausea.

An essential principle of nausea management is distinguishing a mechanical origin from a central etiology. Acute distention, particularly of the stomach and proximal small intestine, causes nausea. If a true obstruction (mechanical or functional) exists, the failure to pass secretions forward will, therefore, lead to nausea. Relief of obstruction or drainage of proximal secretions can reduce (and often eliminate) nausea. Thus a history of nausea should motivate the HCP to look for obstruction and ensure prompt diagnosis and therapy. Once any mechanical nausea has been addressed, then central nausea can be treated effectively with medications. Inappropriate use of antiemetics will likely be unsuccessful, however, and may lead to delay in diagnosis of the true etiology.

Vomiting is often—but not always—associated with nausea. Most importantly, the character of the vomitus should be discussed and, if possible, inspected. Vomit with large amounts of foam is almost always due to significant saliva production. By comparison, foam, burping, and regurgitation of undigested food without gastric juice are pathognomonic for esophageal outlet obstruction. Vomit often contains a combination of food, saliva, and swallowed pulmonary secretions, and its character may provide a clue about the cause of toxin-mediated nausea and vomiting.

Most important in the pediatric patient, however, is distinguishing bilious from nonbilious vomiting. Bile salts, in a chemical sense, are weak acids. When they enter the stomach, gastric acidity protonates the bile salts, causing them to become insoluble and precipitate. This reaction leads to the characteristic streaks of thick bile that occur with dry heaves. In contrast, when a small bowel or large bowel mechanical obstruction is present, the reflux of bile may exceed the gastric acid contents. Vomitus will be of larger volume and contain significant amounts of bile. This gives the vomitus a characteristic green fluorescence (as opposed to the dull, matte appearance of precipitated bile or gastric juice) known by the descriptor "bilious." The same color may be seen in a patient with a nasogastric tube who is receiving significant acid suppression therapy (such as a proton-pump inhibitor) for the same reason. Bilious vomiting should never be accepted as a normal type of nausea and vomiting; it should

always be evaluated. Because the description of bilious emesis may mean different things to different HCPs and family members, visualizing vomitus remains highly useful.

OBSTRUCTION

Mechanical obstructions refer to a partial or complete obstruction resulting from an anatomic cause, such as intraluminal (swallowed coin, intussusception) or extraluminal (hernia, adhesion) blockage. An obstruction is considered partial if any gas, liquid, or solid can pass; otherwise, it is called complete. An important physiologic effect noted with partial obstruction is enhanced secretion and motility proximal to the level of obstruction, which occurs as the body attempts to push the offending obstruction open and overcome the blockage. Thus a partial obstruction at the level of an ostomy or distal bowel may actually present with both diarrhea-like increased output and proximal distention, nausea, and vomiting. An ileus is a functional disorder of decreased motility due to some nonmechanical cause. Most commonly, an ileus occurs following an infection or widespread inflammation and is often a symptom of the severity of the underlying process rather than a reflection of the state of the bowel itself.

DIAGNOSTICS

Laboratory studies

The most useful ancillary testing for GI disorders is a complete blood count (CBC) with differential, closely followed by a urinalysis (UA) and urine pregnancy test. In the setting of dehydration from vomiting or diarrhea, or suspicion of kidney disease, electrolytes with kidney function tests are appropriate. Liver function studies that include measurement of amylase and lipase levels are useful for diagnosing foregut and biliary tract disease. On very rare occasions, coagulation studies may prove helpful (e.g., in the setting of purpura or petechiae).

The amount and character of stool can provide insight into the function of the small and large intestines. Diarrhea of intestinal origin, often due to viral infection, bacterial toxin exposure, and allergy, tends to be of significantly larger volume, watery appearance, and low pH (less than 5.5). Diarrhea of colonic origin, often due to invasive bacterial infection or parasites, tends to be of smaller volume but higher frequency, mucoid or bloody appearance, and high pH (greater than 5.5).

A large number of stool studies are available, most of which are more valuable for the insight they provide into the physiology of diarrhea rather than for the therapeutic management of an individual patient. The most useful studies are stool osmolarity, fecal leukocytes, fecal occult blood, and ova and parasites (O&P). Diarrhea should be isotonic to serum: Alterations in stool osmolarity alert the HCP to improper sampling (scooping from toilet water) or factitious diarrhea (diluting with water). While small bowel infection does not generally lead to elevations in either serum or fecal white blood cells, fecal leukocytes are elevated in acute colitis, particularly of bacterial origin. Gross blood almost always indicates colitis, and fecal occult blood tends to indicate colitis or a bacterial toxin affecting small bowel. Finally, although an O&P test is not often positive, it can be extremely helpful when the patient has a history of consumption of contaminated water, as this test has very high specificity. Other stool studies include various stool cultures (different media for isolation of different bacteria), examinations for specific toxins (e.g., *Shigella, Clostridium difficile*), and viral studies (particularly for norovirus and rotovirus). In many cases, these tests do not help in the initial management of patients but are useful in identifying endemic and epidemic trends in illness.

Plane radiographs

The most common and still extremely useful study in the setting of GI disease is the plane radiograph. With this type of imaging, a single exposure of a flat radiograph plate is performed, resulting in a two-dimensional (plane) image. Although it is possible to do a single radiograph, in almost all situations a second view is appropriate. Selecting the best radiographic views depends on the diagnostic question.

There are several plane radiograph views. The most common view is supine, or an image of a patient lying supine on a gurney. Another common view is upright, or an image of a patient standing against the radiograph plate. Synonyms for the standard anteroposterior view include "A-P" (anteroposterior), "KUB" (kidney, ureters, bladder), and even "flat plate" (a description of the radiograph plate). It is important, however, to indicate for the radiograph technician whether the patient is positioned upright or supine. Additional views include left lateral decubitus (or left side down) and cross-table views.

In all cases, the radiographs demonstrate differences in density, predominantly between bone, organ (or water density), and air. Subtle differences can often be appreciated between fat and organ, such as the kidney or psoas shadows. The most useful, highest-sensitivity, and highest-specificity examination is for radio-opaque foreign bodies, such as a coin or surgical sponge, or for bony changes, such as a spine fracture. Most commonly, however, plane radiographs are utilized to evaluate for constipation and gas (Figure 26-3). While solid stool has a characteristic appearance from the gas bubbles inside the stool, absence of the classic appearance does not imply an empty colon. Similarly, the quantity of gas in the small and large bowel that can be considered

normal varies widely. Thus the utility of the plane radiograph is really a function of the clinical question. Nevertheless, all radiographs should be evaluated for the presence and location of lines and foreign bodies.

Suspected perforation requires multiple views and proper technique to enhance the sensitivity of the imaging modality. If possible, an upright chest radiograph after two minutes of standing has the maximum sensitivity for free gas suggestive of perforation. A left lateral decubitus view also has better sensitivity than other radiographic views, as that position causes free gas to rise around the liver, enhancing the radiologist's ability to distinguish it from surrounding bowel gas (Figure 26-4). While somewhat

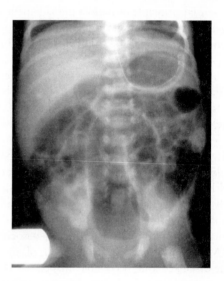

FIGURE 26-3

Anteroposterior Radiograph: Dilated Bowel Loops and Abdominal Distention.

Source: Courtesy of Sam Alaish, M.D., 2005, Baltimore, Maryland.

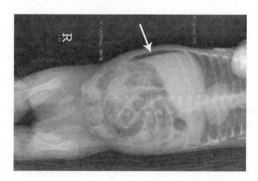

FIGURE 26-4

Left Lateral Decubitus Radiograph: Dilated Bowel Loops with Free Air.

Source: Courtesy of Sam Alaish, M.D., 2005, Baltimore, Maryland.

inferior, cross-table lateral views can sometimes show free gas along the anterior abdominal wall, and standard supine views may show the falciform ligament or bowel outline, suggesting the presence of free gas.

Findings in obstruction depend on the level and duration of obstruction and the presence of a partial versus complete obstruction. Proximal obstructions are the most difficult to confirm on a plane radiograph, as a single episode of burping or vomiting can decompress the stomach and esophagus. Plane radiographs are more useful for assessing small bowel and large bowel obstruction. In particular, the presence of differential air–fluid levels is pathognomonic. Every loop of bowel will contain some gas and some chyme: When viewed perpendicular to the vertical (gravitational) plane, liquid goes down and gas goes up, causing a horizontal line. In obstructed bowel, because liquid and gas do not pass forward and backward easily, multiple lines are likely to be present, giving the appearance of several air–fluid levels. Especially if distended bowel with the classic presence of plicae is noted in the supine view, obstruction can be confirmed.

Other useful radiographic findings in the pediatric and neonatal populations include pneumatosis intestinalis and portal venous gas, both of which suggest mucosal necrosis due to enterocolitis.

Fluoroscopy

For the most part, GI fluoroscopy has been replaced by ultrasound and CT. This preference is largely attributable to the greater amount of radiation utilized in fluoroscopy than in CT scans. Also, CT scans and ultrasound are superior in assessing for many diagnoses. Nevertheless, several types of GI fluoroscopy are still regularly performed, which are considered therapeutic as well as diagnostic.

Fluoroscopy is a continuous radiograph emission and acquisition technique that can produce live imaging, still images, and a recorded movie. In GI fluoroscopy, a contrast agent is administered under fluoroscopic guidance and a combination of still images and recorded movie is obtained. Three types of contrast agents are used: air, iodine based, and barium based. These agents may also be combined, as with air and barium. Each agent has both advantages and disadvantages. Barium is viscous and quite sticky, for example, and standard barium solutions give the optimal sensitivity and specificity for GI fluoroscopic studies. Its disadvantage is that barium, in the setting of a perforation, will coat any body cavity and be impossible to completely remove, thereby creating a difficult surgical environment and residual radiograph findings. The advantage of iodine-based agents, particularly the isotonic iodinated agents, derives from their excellent combination of good sensitivity and specificity for study findings with the ability to easily evacuate or excrete iodinated agents. Iodine is associated

with a low incidence yet still significant risk of allergy, and the hypertonic iodinated agents can induce significant fluid shifts with resulting hemodynamic changes. Air is the safest, easiest contrast agent, but has the lowest sensitivity and specificity. The contrast medium/agent should be selected to optimize results while minimizing complications.

Upper GI fluoroscopy images the process from swallowing to the small bowel. The most proximal study is the modified barium swallow study (MBSS), which typically uses thin and thick barium contrast agents, as well as barium-impregnated hamburger, to evaluate swallowing (from mouth to upper esophagus), looking for aspiration and coordination. This type of imaging is not the same thing as a "swallow" (also known as an "upper GI"), which is a study that follows the movement of a contrast agent from the esophagus, through the stomach, to the first portion of the small bowel. These studies, which may also be referred to by the anatomic location (e.g., esophagogram, gastrogram, esophagogastroduodenography), provide static and dynamic pictures that can investigate questions related to anatomy, perforation, obstruction, and, to a moderate extent, function.

The last two components of upper GI fluoroscopy are small bowel follow-through (SBFT) and enteroclysis. SBFT requires additional time in the radiology suite or delayed plane films to ensure progression (peristalsis) of the contrast to the colon. Enteroclysis is a highly specialized study in which both air and barium are injected into the small bowel; this study is rarely indicated but provides excellent images of small bowel mucosa.

Lower GI fluoroscopy consists of enemata and defecograms. A barium enema is the single most useful GI fluoroscopic study, as it provides anatomic evaluation of the colon and rectum. It is also frequently therapeutic—for example, evacuating inspissated or thickened stool and reducing ileocecal intussusception. Other contrast agents have equivalent efficacy in reducing intussusception; air, in particular, has become popular in this regard. Defecograms involve fluoroscopic evaluation during defecation of thick barium.

An important part of ordering a diagnostic GI study is ensuring good communication with the radiologist. This allows the radiologist to select the optimal agent and study method and, therefore, maximize the yield.

Computed tomography scan

Computed tomography (CT) is a radiograph-based imaging study that relies on computer processing of multiple, nearly simultaneous radiographs to create a density map of the patient. This data set can then be displayed with several different color mappings, providing two-dimensional and projection-style pictures of the patient. Classic CT scans were produced by sequential imaging of a cross-sectional "slice" of the patient inside the scanner, and the resulting images represented transverse sections of the imaged part. Modern CT scanning involves spiral acquisition on multiple-detector arrays with significantly improved computational algorithms, allowing for faster imaging with higher resolution, particularly on sagittal and coronal views.

CT scan can be performed with or without contrast. Contrast agents include intravenous iodinated compounds and enterically administered (either orally or rectally) iodinated compounds. Movement, barium, metal, and excess tissue can all cause significant artifacts on CT scan, however, and decrease the quality of imaging. Timing of the scan relative to administration of contrast can also enhance or diminish the quality of the study. The choice of timing and contrast types should be made by the radiologist and HCP based on the clinical issue in question.

The addition of intravenous contrast enhances CT in several ways. First, if timed appropriately, the scan can occur when the contrast is intra-arterial, returning through the portal vein, or returning through the systemic veins. This allows separate identification of vascular structures and nonvascular fluid-filled tubes. It also allows for determination of primary blood supply in the liver. Second, in regions of inflammation, the enhanced blood flow will bring higher amounts of IV contrast to these areas, which permits identification of regional inflammation. Third, clearance of the iodinated contrast via the kidneys allows for delayed images in which urine-filled structures can be distinguished from surrounding fluid-filled tubes or pockets.

Use of oral and rectal contrast, like intravenous contrast, facilitates identification of the bowel (filled with radio-dense luminal contents) relative to surrounding fluid-filled structures. The greatest challenge with oral contrast is getting the child to drink adequate amounts of contrast and waiting for the contrast to progress to the small bowel. Rectal contrast, by comparison, involves a rectally placed balloon and subsequent pressure-augmented insufflation, typically using a high column of fluid.

Ultrasound

Ultrasound is the most readily available nonradiation means of imaging. Unfortunately, despite its ease of access, low cost, and absence of radiograph production, ultrasonography is extremely operator dependent for quality of image acquisition and requires significant expertise to achieve high sensitivity and specificity of image interpretation. Fortunately, high demand for ultrasonography by HCPs in the emergency department and inpatient setting, as well as by caregivers, has driven most children's hospitals and pediatric radiologists to provide timely imaging and review to reduce the rate of unnecessary CT scanning.

In all cases, ultrasonography is performed by utilizing high-frequency sound waves emitted by a probe that travel through tissue. Depending on the tissue type, these sound waves are then reflected, scattered, and modified by that tissue. Returning sound waves are collected by a transducer and processed into a displayed image. Several different mathematical algorithms may be used for this processing; thus several different ultrasound modalities are available. All of these modes can be performed to acquire static images or provide "real-time" or cine movies.

A-mode, or amplitude-modulated ultrasonography produces a graph of time versus intensity of the echo, much like echophonography for displaying "heart sounds" on a graph. A-mode is not particularly useful for abdominal evaluation.

B-mode, or brightness-modulated ultrasonography, is the most useful imaging mode for the abdomen. It produces a two-dimensional gray-scale image of the tissue. Depending on the transducer type, energy emitted, and tissue characteristics, B-mode can provide an excellent view of all abdominal wall and most intra-abdominal findings. Challenges to effective B-mode imaging include very echo-dense barriers, such as the ribs, and echo-impermeable air, as is found in the bowels. In these settings, operator technique becomes extremely important in achieving appropriate imaging.

M-mode, or motion mode ultrasound, provides a time-versus-brightness graph; in other words, it produces an image of motion along a single axis. M-mode is most useful in echocardiography to look at the movement of cardiac muscle or valves, but does not have much use in the abdominal cavity.

Finally, Doppler ultrasound refers to the application of the Doppler frequency shift to identify velocities of movement within tissue. Addition of Doppler imaging to B-mode imaging can provide a useful color map of vascular flow, or Doppler-versus-time display can be used to demonstrate vascular waveforms. The greatest benefit of using Doppler ultrasound in the abdominal cavity is its ability to distinguish blood vessels from ducts. For example, if two small lumens are seen in the liver, the one with a Doppler signal is the hepatic artery and the one without such a signal is a hepatic duct.

Ultrasonography of the abdomen can image a number of different locations. In the supracolic abdomen, ultrasound is extremely useful in evaluating the liver, biliary tree, and head of the pancreas. The spleen is also well imaged by the ultrasound technique, but is less likely to have significant pathology outside of trauma. The retroperitoneum, especially the kidneys and adrenals, is also effectively imaged by ultrasound. Pelvic ultrasound can often be performed transabdominally when a child has a full bladder. There is a growing use of ultrasound to look for bowel pathology. Specifically, pathology of the bowel often creates a situation where the bowel cannot be compressed—such as an obstructed, pus-filled appendix; a hypertrophic pylorus; or a bowel distended by the presence of an intussuception.

Thus increasingly radiologists are attempting ultrasound evaluation of all abdominal processes even when a subsequent radiograph-based study will be performed. As a result, the best use of ultrasonography requires direct communication between radiology and the clinician to select the optimal mode of imaging for a given clinical question.

Magnetic resonance imaging

Abdominal magnetic resonance imaging (MRI) is not generally utilized during the initial evaluation of patients, as CT scan is more accessible, is faster, and can often be done without anesthesia. Magnetic resonance imaging studies are performed when the CT scan or ultrasound results are inconclusive. This imaging modality is most often used to stage malignancies, determine the characteristics of liver lesions, identify blunt abdominal trauma, and assess determinant adrenal, kidney, and liver masses.

APPENDICITIS

Cindy L. Kerr

PATHOPHYSIOLOGY

Appendicitis is a progressive inflammatory process that begins within the lumen of the appendix. Blockage of the appendix lumen by lymphoid hyperplasia, foreign body, stool, fecalith (calcified fecal matter), or tumor are the most common mitigating factors. When such a blockage occurs, mucosal secretions arising from the lymphoid follicles of the appendix lining are retained. As the volume of secretions increases, pressures within the lumen of the tubular appendix mount, causing swelling of the appendix. Venous congestion impedes blood flow down the length of this tubular shaped appendage. Hypoxia and bacteria proliferation in the retained secretions compromise integrity of the mucosal barrier. With the breakdown of the protective mucosal barrier, the underlying muscular layers of the appendix become open to bacterial destruction. If this process continues to progress, perforation results, with stool and bacteria being released into the peritoneal cavity. Progressive inflammation within the appendix accounts for the various pathological reports found when the appendix is removed: acute appendicitis, suppurative appendicitis, gangrenous appendicitis, and perforated appendicitis.

EPIDEMIOLOGY AND ETIOLOGY

Appendicitis is the most common surgical emergency; 4 out of every 1,000 pediatric patients in the United States will undergo an appendectomy, resulting in 70,000 appendectomies each year. Approximately 5% to 25% of these patients are ultimately found to have a normal appendix (Smink et al., 2004).

Incidence of appendicitis increases with age and is most common in the second decade of life (Bundy et al., 2007). In children younger than 2 years of age, the appendix has a larger opening and is funnel shaped. As a child grows, the appendix takes on a tubular shape, which is more susceptible to blockage. Nonverbal children who cannot contribute information regarding location and intensity of pain present a diagnostic challenge; this can delay diagnosis and makes perforation of the appendix more common in the younger patient. Goldin et al. (2007) reported that 15% to 36% of pediatric patients have a perforated appendix at the time of surgery. In 2007, Morrow and Newman reported that rates of perforation of the appendix were as high as 82% for children younger than 5 years of age and up to 100% in those 1 year of age.

PRESENTATION

In patients with appendicitis, the most common chief complaint is abdominal pain. Typically, the pain begins as vague diffuse epigastric or periumbilical pain and is associated with gastrointestinal symptoms such as nausea, vomiting, and anorexia. As inflammation increases over a period of hours to days, pain progresses in severity and changes in location. Pain assessments in suspected appendicitis include McBurney's point and Rovsing's, psoas, and obturator signs (Table 26-1). Pain arises from irritation of structures surrounding the inflamed appendix and varies depending on the location of the appendix. The most common appendix locations are intraperitoneal (either anterior to the cecum or retrocecal), extraperitoneal, or within the pelvis. Each location elicits different clinical findings (O'Neill et al., 2003a).

- Anterior to the cecum: direct contact with the parietal peritoneum:
  - Focal right lower quadrant pain
  - Rovsing's sign positive
  - McBurney's point tenderness
- Behind the cecum (retrocecal):
  - Flank and back pain
  - Iliospoas sign positive
  - Testicular pain
- Pelvis:
  - Obturator sign positive
  - Urinary frequency and dysuria
  - Rectal exam elicits heightened pain

Completion of a thorough abdominal examination may be challenging in the younger patient, and becomes even more difficult with each repetitive examination that

TABLE 26-1

Physical Examination Findings	
Physical Examination Test	**Finding**
McBurney	Located one-third of the distance from the anterior superior iliac spine to the umbilicus
Rovsing	Pain in the right lower quadrant when pressure is applied to the left abdomen
Psoas	Right lower abdominal pain with extension of the right hip
Obturator	Pain with internal rotation of the right hip

Source: Adapted from Kwok et al., 2004.

induces pain. Using distraction, caregiver support, and starting with less sensitive areas may allow for an accurate examination. Observing patient movement, willingness or refusal to walk, guarding, and facial expressions during the abdominal examination can give valuable insight into the degree of pain that is present.

The most significant symptoms are fever, abdominal pain that migrates to the right lower quadrant, and presence of vomiting or diarrhea (Bundy et al., 2007). Constipation, lethargy, and dysuria are less helpful in confirming the diagnosis.

Clinical scoring systems for the evaluation of appendicitis also rely on key physical findings. Kharbanda et al. (2005) developed a decision rule to identify children at low risk for appendicitis when the chief complaint is abdominal pain. The goal of this tool is to identify patients who can safely be observed or discharged while avoiding unnecessary imaging or surgical procedures. The six-part score includes nausea, right lower quadrant pain, migration of pain, difficulty walking, rebound tenderness/pain with percussion, and absolute neutrophil count of greater than 6.75×10^3 mcg/L.

DIFFERENTIAL DIAGNOSIS

Abdominal pain—the most common presenting symptom of appendicitis—has a wide spectrum of etiologies that can vary with age, making accurate diagnosis of its cause challenging. Diagnostic accuracy is lowest among females, very young children, developmentally delayed children, and patients hospitalized for other conditions (O'Neill et al., 2003a).

Gastroenteritis and constipation are two of the more common diagnoses that should be considered in the differential diagnosis for appendicitis. The differential list is typically categorized by systems:

- Gastrointestinal: gastroenteritis, constipation, Meckel's diverticulitis, inflammatory bowel disease, cholecystitis, pancreatitis, gastroenteritis, mesenteric adenitis, intestinal obstruction, typhlitis, pancreatitis, and abdominal trauma (Morrow & Newman, 2007)
- Gynecologic: ovarian cysts, follicle rupture, ovarian torsion, ectopic pregnancy, salpingitis, and tubo-ovarian abscess (O'Neill et al., 2003a)
- Urinary tract: cystitis, hydronephrosis, pyelonephritis, and nephrocalcinosis (O'Neill et al., 2003a)
- Other: pneumonia, diabetic ketoacidosis, Henoch-Schönlein purpura, and sickle cell disease

PLAN OF CARE

Confirming the presence of appendicitis requires an accurate history, clinical examination, radiographic imaging, and laboratory study. Making the correct diagnosis in

a timely manner can help reduce the risk of perforation and its sequelae. Bickell et al. (2006) found that in adult patients the risk of rupture was minimal (2% or less) in the first 36 hours of symptom onset; however, there was 5% risk of rupture in each ensuing 12-hr period.

Laboratory findings consistent with appendicitis include an elevated leukocyte count (more than 10,000/mm³) and an absolute neutrophil count higher than 6.75×10^3 mcg/L. Results below these levels have been found to substantially decrease the likelihood of appendicitis (Bundy et al., 2007). C-reactive protein may be elevated in appendicitis, but it has not been found to be more accurate than leukocyte count in making the diagnosis (Morrow & Newman, 2007).

Imaging has become a routine part of the appendicitis diagnostic evaluation. The imaging technique of choice for appendicitis is abdominal computed tomography (Figure 26-5). Multiple studies have confirmed the sensitivity and specificity of CT scanning to be as high as 97% and 94%, respectively (Friday, 2006). Initially CT studies were performed using intravenous, oral, and rectal contrast. The need for rectal contrast has been debated; its use may delay timely completion of the study and provide minimal diagnostic help. Studies completed without contrast avoid completion delays but are not as accurate as contrast-enhanced CT scans, which increases the risk for misdiagnosis. CT imaging is not without risk, however, due to increased organ radiosensitivity and longer lifetime risk for radiation-induced cancer (Siegel, 2008).

Abdominal ultrasound studies are often used as the first-line imaging modality for this indication and have several advantages—namely, low cost, less invasive nature, ready availability in most centers, and no radiation risk. The sensitivity and specificity of ultrasound are much lower than the same measures for CT, however; the former's sensitivity ranges from 50% to 100%, and its specificity ranges from 88% to 99% (Chang et al., 2007). Operator skill, location of

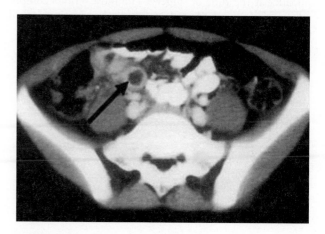

FIGURE 26-5

Abdominal CT Demonstrating Appendicitis.

Source: Courtesy of Cindy L. Kerr.

the appendix, inability of the patient to cooperate, overlying bowel gas pattern, and obesity may obscure visualization. The ultrasound criteria for appendicitis are presence of a noncompressible tubular structure that is 6 mm or larger in diameter, a complex mass in the right lower quadrant, or a fecalith (Morrow & Newman, 2007) (Figure 26-6).

The best therapeutic intervention for acute appendicitis is an appendectomy. Historically, the diagnosis of appendicitis meant an emergent operation with the goal of completing the appendectomy within hours of diagnosis. Recent practice has shown that the complication rate is not substantially affected by a 6- to 24-hr waiting period before operation during which fluid therapy and intravenous antibiotics are administered. This trend helps avoid surgery during the middle of the night and allows adequate time for stabilization prior to entering the surgical suite (Yardeni et al., 2004).

Intravenous antibiotic therapy is considered the first-line therapy for appendicitis, and its timely administration is critical to arrest progression of any infection. Choice of antibiotics should provide broad-spectrum coverage of Gram-positive, Gram-negative, and anaerobic bacteria. Single daily dosing, beta lactam and metronidazole antibiotic therapy is being used with increasing frequency in lieu of multidose aminoglycoside-based combination therapy (ampicillin, gentamicin, and metronidazole) (St. Peter et al., 2008).

Dehydration and electrolyte imbalance due to anorexia, vomiting, and diarrhea should be addressed early in the treatment course. A basic metabolic panel will determine the amount and type of fluid replacement required. A pregnancy test is best completed prior to CT or surgical intervention. Placement of a nasogastric tube for recurrent vomiting and bowel decompression may be necessary. Pain control with intravenous narcotics such as morphine should be instituted.

Postoperative care depends on the condition of the appendix at the time of surgery. The most serious complications are reported when the appendix has perforated and include postoperative intestinal obstruction, intra-abdominal abscess, sepsis, pneumonia, and prolonged ileus. Placement of a percutaneous intravenous central venous catheter (PICC) is beneficial for administration of IV antibiotics and parenteral nutrition. Postoperative CT imaging and additional laboratory studies may be required when fever and abdominal pain persist. Percutaneous drainage catheters placed by interventional radiologists are often utilized when intra-abdominal abscesses do not respond to therapy.

When the initial diagnosis is perforated appendicitis, nonoperative therapy with IV antibiotic therapy may be employed. If the patient improves in 24 to 48 hours with antibiotics alone, the surgeon plans for a 2-week course of IV antibiotics followed by an interval appendectomy in 6 to 8 weeks. Some surgeons may even opt not to operate after the course of IV antibiotics is completed if the patient remains symptom free.

A surgical consultation early in the diagnosis can help ensure a timely diagnosis without undue testing and imaging. Evaluation by a surgeon should be done before administration of IV antibiotics or pain medication, as both types of agents can significantly change the clinical examination findings. In anticipation of surgery and general anesthesia, a consult with the anesthesia service should be initiated to ensure that all significant health issues are addressed. An infectious diseases specialist may be consulted if the infectious organism is refractory to antibiotics.

After the diagnosis of acute appendicitis is made, caregivers often expect immediate surgical intervention and may become anxious when surgery is delayed. Educating the caregiver about the role of intravenous antibiotics as treatment for appendicitis can reduce or alleviate stress. With cases involving perforation of the appendix, carefully explaining complications and informing caregivers that prolonged hospitalization may be expected often helps families make appropriate plans. Caregivers should be assured that removal of the appendix will not interfere with the body's gastrointestinal tract ability to function normally, and that no diet modifications are required after such surgery.

DISPOSITION AND DISCHARGE PLANNING

Although appendicitis is one of the most common causes of abdominal pain, mortality from this disease is rare. This statistic is attributed to availability of broad-spectrum IV antibiotics. The most common postoperative complications are wound infection (3%), pelvic abscesses (less than 5%), and postoperative bowel obstruction due to adhesions (3–5%) (O'Neill et al., 2003a).

Follow-up with the surgeon for assessment of the incision sites and recovery status should be expected. Patients who undergo interval appendectomy may require several follow-up visits—just prior to the end of the IV

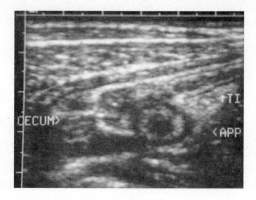

FIGURE 26-6

Abdominal Ultrasound Demonstrating Appendicitis.

Source: Courtesy of Cindy L. Kerr.

antibiotic regimen, prior to surgery, and again after the appendectomy. Caregivers of patients with a perforated appendix should be instructed to follow up with the surgeon if patient develops fever, abdominal pain, vomiting, or infection of the incision sites.

Postoperative discharge instructions should include signs and symptoms of possible complications, such as fever, increased abdominal pain or pain not controlled with oral analgesics, decreased oral intake, vomiting, or signs of infection at the surgical incision sites. A follow-up appointment with the surgeon 2 to 3 weeks after discharge should be arranged. Caregivers should be told that if future episodes of abdominal pain occur and medical attention is required, they should inform HCPs that the patient's appendix has been removed.

Prognosis depends on the condition of the appendix at the time of surgery. Patients with nonperforated appendix following laparoscopic surgery are often discharged home in 24 to 48 hours following surgery without further antibiotic coverage. When the surgical findings reveal a perforated appendix, the recovery period can be extensive and can include serious complications that may require home IV antibiotic therapy, intra-abdominal drain placement, or even a return to the operating room.

ABDOMINAL MASS

James Pierce and Karen Rodriguez

EPIDEMIOLOGY AND ETIOLOGY

Two-thirds of all abdominal masses are due to organomegaly, while one-third represent congenital abnormalities, developmental abnormalities, or neoplasms. One-third of GI congenital anomalies are found within the first month of life, and 90% have been identified by the time the child reaches 2 years of age. The one exception is congenital abnormalities of the uterus, cervix, vagina, and hymen, which may remain unidentified until onset of puberty.

Approximately one-third of the 1 to 2 cancers per 10,000 children younger than age 16 years are intra-abdominal in origin. Neuroblastoma is one of the most common extracranial solid tumors of childhood, second only to astrocytoma in the posterior fossa. The next most common solid tumor in pediatric patients is Wilms' tumor, the most common kidney tumor of childhood. Other relatively common solid tumors include germ cell tumors, rhabdomyosarcoma, and hepatoblastoma.

PRESENTATION

An abdominal mass may be detected due to contour deformity of the abdominal wall or a defined palpable fullness in the abdominal cavity. Not surprisingly, masses are often identified by caregivers during bathing or changing. An organized approach and a careful history of illness will identify risk factors for trauma, infectious diseases, and malignancies. Components of the trauma history should include maltreatment as a potential cause of an abdominal mass.

Review of systems may give insight into acute or chronic presentations. During the physical examination, the HCP should measure the child's weight, height, and head circumference (if appropriate). Chronic progressive illnesses, weight loss, loss of appetite, fever, and night sweats act as red flags for tumors, infections, and inflammatory diseases. The history should include questions regarding emesis and its character; soiling patterns; and the color, consistency, and presence of blood in the stool which all may prove valuable in determining whether an obstruction exists. Additionally, urinary excretion of bile salts may lead to cola-colored urine, and obstruction of the biliary system may present with acholic stools. Kidney and urinary tract disease may present with change in the character of urine (hematuria, dark urine, sediment, foam) as well as urinary tract irritative or obstructive symptoms. Thus frequency, urgency, dysuria, reduced urine output, weak stream, and dribbling may aid in identifying renal pathology. A gynecologic history in females should include menstruation and sexual activity. Moreover, the HCP should ask about bleeding and bruising patterns.

The physical examination should be approached systematically. The patient should be observed for jaundice, icteric sclera and oral frenulum, and pruritus. Jaundice may indicate liver disease. Pale skin may indicate anemia, flushed rosy skin may be present in sepsis, and classic exanthems may be present with viral infections. If the general appearance is of an ill-appearing child, particularly with cachexia or failure-to-thrive, chronic infections or malignant disease may be the cause. A careful examination of all lymph node basins for both lymphadenopathy and lymphadenitis is necessary.

Abdominal examination should narrow the differential diagnosis. Consider the location of the abdominal mass. Masses in the right upper quadrant most often involve the liver, gallbladder, and biliary tree—albeit to a lesser extent—bowel or retroperitoneal organs (kidney and adrenal) may present as isolated right upper quadrant masses. Epigastric masses can include both epigastric hernias and diastasis recti. Stomach masses may include bezoar or volvulus, hepatomegaly, and pancreas pathology such as pseudocyst. Left upper quadrant masses most often involve the stomach, spleen, adrenal gland, and kidney. Right lower quadrant masses include ovarian and fallopian processes and ileocecal disease, such as intestinal or colonic phlegmon, appendicitis, abscess, or inflammatory bowel disease. Suprapubic masses are most commonly genitourinary, such as full bladder, bladder distention from obstruction, and uterine pathology such as pregnancy, hydrometropcolpos, and hematocolpos.

Abdominal wall masses may be superficial to the muscular layers or, alternatively, their movement may be coupled with the contraction of the abdominal musculature. Abdominal wall hernias can often be "popped out" by restraining the very small child—who will almost always cry—or by asking the older child to elevate both legs at the same time. Characteristics such as mobility or immobility will suggest the degree of attachment or invasion to the retroperitoneum. Immobile masses are either invasive tumors or masses that arise from the retroperitoneal organs. Tenderness generally suggests a recent change; events such as hemorrhage that lead to acute increase in the volume of the mass place tension on the capsule and, therefore, nociception. Firmness, hardness, and irregularity suggest either tumor or desmoplasia (scar). Smoothness, by contrast, suggests an encapsulated mass. Tympany indicates gas, such as in a hollow viscus. Dullness can represent either fluid or solid mass.

DIFFERENTIAL DIAGNOSIS

A hernia—whether umbilical, inguinal, or ventral in location—is likely to be diagnosed on physical examination. Occasionally, soft-tissue masses from closure of omphalocele or gastroschisis are present; a careful history should indicate these causes. Trauma can lead to hematoma formation. This disorder is usually easy to diagnose except for rectus hematomas, which are hidden from view by the rectus sheath. A number of soft-tissue tumors such as fibromas and lipomas may also be diagnosed on physical examination alone.

Intra-abdominally, the omentum and mesentery may occasionally harbor masses—most often mesenteric cysts and lymphadenopathy. Occasionally, however, a fixed abdominal mass is related to mesenteric fibromatosis or retroperitoneal sarcoma. The diagnosis of these disorders is often made through CT or MRI imaging rather than ultrasound, given that bowel gas often obscures retroperitoneal ultrasonography.

In infants, crying may be associated with significant ingestion of air. This phenomenon leads to acute gastric distention and may cause vagal symptoms or respiratory embarrassment. Fortunately, the tympanic left upper quadrant and response to nasogastric drainage make gastric distension relatively easy to diagnose and treat. Less common are ingested foreign bodies, particularly hair and roughage that result in bezoars; congenital duplications; gastric tumors; and gastric torsion, which presents with acute gastric distention with the inability to pass a nasogastric tube.

Constipation, an exceedingly common disorder, may present with abdominal discomfort and a palpable mass. In addition, infectious and inflammatory diseases of the bowel will often produce a mass. This category includes abscesses (inflammatory masses) associated with perforated

appendicitis, Meckel's diverticulum, phlegmons from Crohn's disease, and palpable lead pipe colon from ulcerative colitis. Younger patients may experience symptoms of intussusception, duplications, mesenteric cysts, bowel atresias, or meconium pseudocysts. Malrotation with volvulus can occasionally present with abdominal mass. Finally, bowel tumors such as carcinoid, lymphoma, and occasionally adenocarcinoma may present with a mass.

Although in infants the kidney is occasionally palpable, in most cases a palpable kidney represents either obstructive or parenchymal kidney disease. Multiple cysts may be caused by polycystic kidney disease or multicystic dysplastic kidney disease. If a large, fluid-filled structure is present at the hilum, it may represent a dilated renal pelvis with or without associated hydroureter. Bilateral findings may suggest bladder outflow obstruction, such as posterior urethral valves or neurogenic bladder. Diffuse unilateral renal swelling may occur from renal vein thrombosis. Finally, Wilms' tumor can present as a unilateral mass.

Closely associated with the kidney is the adrenal (suprarenal) gland. Small adrenal hemorrhages can occur as the result of birth or external trauma, but are rarely large enough to produce a palpable finding. Adrenal masses are most commonly neoplastic in origin, with neuroblastoma being the most common pediatric adrenal tumor. Other endocrine tumors, such as pheochromocytoma, may occasionally be found, although these endocrine cancers rarely are of sufficient size to produce a palpable mass.

In females, gynecologic masses are extremely common. Small ovarian cysts are a physiologic requirement for menstruation. In addition to these simple or follicular cysts, a number of more heterogeneous ovarian masses can occur. They include both benign ovarian masses such as dermoid cysts and mature teratomas, as well as immature teratomas and germ cell tumors. Furthermore, torsion can occasionally produce a very edematous and swollen ovary that may occasionally present as a mass. The most common fallopian and uterine masses are those associated with pregnancy (ectopic or intrauterine). Nevertheless, obstruction of the fallopian tube at the isthmus, uterus at the cervix, or vagina at the hymen can also lead to accumulation of serum or menses and a large palpable pelvic mass, including hydrosalpynx, hematocolpos, and hydrometrocolpos.

An enlarged spleen should immediately suggest hematologic disease or malignancy, until proven otherwise. Splenomegaly is often associated with the hereditary hemolytic anemias, such as spherocytosis or elliptocytosis. It is also frequently present in new-onset hematologic malignancy such as leukemias and lymphomas. A variety of inflammatory conditions, such as acute viral infection with Epstein-Barr virus or cytomegalovirus, and rheumatologic diseases such as systemic lupus erythematosus, and Langerhans cell histiocytosis can also lead to an enlarged spleen. In addition, storage diseases such as Niemann-Pick and Gaucher's disease can be associated with splenomegaly.

A number of intrinsic liver diseases lead to hepatomegaly. The various acute viral hepatidities as well as autoimmune hepatitis can cause significant hepatic edema and enlarged, tender liver. Most metabolic disorders, such as the glycogen storage diseases or Wilson disease, can present with an enlarged, painless liver. Congenital hepatic fibrosis may also produce painless hepatomegaly. In addition, the liver can be enlarged due to the presence of simple or biliary cysts. Simple cysts may present as a single cyst diagnosed on ultrasound or as multiple or polycystic liver disease. Biliary cysts—or choledochal cysts—can be present anywhere along the biliary tree; when they are found exclusively and diffusely intrahepatically, the disorder is known as Caroli's disease. Solid hepatic masses include those of vascular origin, such as hemangioma and other lymphovascular malformations, as well as parenchymal origin, such as focal nodular hyperplasia, adenoma, or neoplasia. The most common tumors are hepatoblastoma in younger patients, hepatocellular carcinoma in older pediatric patients, and lymphoma, which can produce diffuse neoplastic infiltration of the liver. Finally, acute liver congestion and hepatomegaly are associated with vascular congestion, such as in heart failure or Budd-Chiari syndrome.

Congenital dilations of the biliary tract are classified as choledochal cysts. Acquired dilation of the biliary tree can occur secondary to obstruction, including gallbladder hydrops from chronic cystic duct obstruction, and biliary ductal dilation due to obstruction from gallstone disease or biliary strictures. Biliary obstruction can also occur from pancreatic head masses such as pseudocysts and pancreatoblastomas. Pancreatic and biliary tract malignancies are rare in children.

PLAN OF CARE

Complete blood count (CBC) with differential will indicate the presence of infection, inflammation, and anemia. A chemistry panel will identify kidney disease through blood urea nitrogen (BUN) and creatinine levels, pancreatic disease with amylase and lipase levels, and various classes of liver disease through the hepatic function panel. In addition, hypoalbuminemia, while nonspecific, is extremely sensitive for detecting significant illness. Finally, uric acid and lactate dehydrogenase (LDH) levels are particularly useful in identifying solid tumors.

Imaging is extremely valuable in making the diagnosis of an abdominal mass. A two-view radiograph of the abdomen may identify intestinal obstruction, fecal impaction, and calcifications associated with tumor. While the specificity of these findings is high, they are not particularly common; thus radiographs are often nonspecific. Ultrasound can identify the origin of the mass and differentiate between solid and cystic masses. While ultrasound may not lead to a definitive diagnosis, it can guide the selection of further imaging and laboratory evaluation.

CT scan with intravenous contrast can be particularly useful in evaluating solid abdominal masses. In addition to elucidating the characteristics of the mass, CT imaging demonstrates vascular anatomy, identifies the presence of associated lymph nodes, and helps stage many cancers. Intravenous and oral contrast agents are also particularly useful in evaluating a cystic mass to see if there is continuity with the bowel or bladder. Masses of the primary bowel or bladder are often not well characterized by CT scan; fluoroscopic studies such as upper GI series, barium enema, and voiding cystourethrogram are much more useful when the history, physical examination, and ultrasound suggest a primary bowel or bladder origin. One caveat should be noted: Barium contrast administered to the bowel will produce significant artifact and prevent immediate subsequent CT scan. Hepatobiliary and pancreatic masses can add an extra level of complexity to the imaging process, because neither ultrasound nor CT scan is effective at visualizing the biliary and pancreatic ductal system. Traditionally, the hepatobiliaryimino-diacetic acid (HIDA) scan was the first choice for identifying biliary and gallbladder pathology; however, magnetic resonance cholangiopancreatography (MRCP) is increasingly being used for diagnosing hepatobiliary and pancreatic disease.

Benign masses

The majority of benign masses are neither medical nor surgical emergencies. Emergent evaluation is appropriate for bowel obstruction, appendicitis or colitis with pending perforation, biliary tract obstruction with cholangitis and sepsis, and potential ovarian torsion or ectopic pregnancy. Standard resuscitation guidelines apply, which include prompt IV access, nasogastric drainage (mandatory for obstruction or perforations), administration of antibiotics, and support for septic shock. Finally, in all patients, prompt surgical consultation should be obtained, as many of benign masses that present in extremis require urgent surgery or radiologic intervention.

For patients who present without these warning signs, initial basic laboratory tests and radiologic imaging are warranted. Once the differential diagnosis is made, referral and follow-up can be made with a pediatric surgeon to ensure timely evaluation and intervention.

Malignant abdominal tumors

Malignant abdominal tumors warrant urgent admission for evaluation. In general, transfer to a setting where both oncologic and surgical consultations are available is warranted. Again, emergent evaluation needs to occur if any of the signs or symptoms of obstruction or perforation exist. Therapeutic management for tumor lysis syndrome, acute hemorrhage, coagulopathy, or endocrine abnormalities may be required. Provided no signs of imminent danger are present, hydration and complete laboratory and radiologic evaluation can be performed under the guidance of the oncologists and surgeons. Many of these tumors require additional imaging and diagnostic study for staging purposes. Therefore, care should be taken to involve specialists such as surgeons or oncologists as well as to follow institutional protocols so as to help children avoid repeated exposure to CT scans, iodinated contrast, and laboratory studies. Thus one of the most efficient and useful ways to start the evaluation is with a plane radiograph or an abdominal ultrasound.

DISPOSITION AND DISCHARGE PLANNING

In most cases, the pediatric patient with an abdominal mass should be admitted to the hospital for prompt evaluation and treatment. In the unusual event that the child is first discharged from an outpatient setting, the single most important aspect of patient and family education is ensuring appropriate follow-up. Providing contact information for the surgeon or oncologist receiving the patient, instructing the family to return immediately if the follow-up appointment does not occur, and providing telephone follow-up to ensure that the appointment was made are all essential to timely diagnosis.

ABDOMINAL PAIN

James Pierce and Karen Rodriguez

Abdominal pain is associated with two major pathophysiologies: splanchnic and somatic. Splanchnic, or visceral, pathophysiology refers to nociception via the autonomic nervous system. Somatic pathophysiology refers to nociception via the somatic nervous system. Each pathway has different characteristics related to sensation, transmission, and central processing of pain, which can be identified by a careful history and physical examination. Thus a good physical examination can help guide the HCP in the selection of appropriate diagnostic studies or timely consultation.

GASTROINTESTINAL PAIN

Many GI disorders produce pain. In most cases, this pain consists of a splanchnic, crampy, intermittent pain. A differential diagnosis usually follows the careful pain history. Substernal or upper abdominal pain usually derives from foregut structures (esophagus to duodenum); periumbilical pain generally occurs from midgut structures (small bowel and right colon); and low pelvic pain is indicative of a source in hindgut structures (left colon and rectum). Pain significantly off midline should suggest somatic origin and cause the HCP to question (but not exclude) the GI system as the source. In the gastrointestinal differential, it is important to

recognize that the more severe the gut distention, the worse the splanchnic pain. Furthermore, the rate of peristalsis, which varies from region to region of the gut, determines the frequency of waves of pain.

Ingestion

Ingestion often can be identified on presentation alone. A careful history will indicate supraglottic, subglottic, or GI ingestion, and often identify the type of consultant to which referral is appropriate. Physical examination and addition of plane radiographic films will identify obstruction or perforation, which requires prompt surgical consultation. Airway symptoms also indicate a need for urgent otolaryngologist consultation.

Food intolerance

One of the most common causes of GI abdominal pain is food intolerance. Most food intolerance is non-immunologic in origin; a very infrequent cause of pain is true food allergy. Generally speaking, early appearance of pain following eating is more likely to be pathologic, such as gastroesophageal reflux, gastritis, or peptic ulcer disease. Most food intolerance occurs as food traverses the small bowel and colon. Thus pain is generally crampy and occurs in waves every 5 minutes when originating from the small bowel, or every 15 minutes when originating from the colon. In many cases, pain is associated with gut distention. Small bowel pain is often associated with nausea; colonic pain is often associated with significant diarrhea and passage of flatus.

A number of pathologic mechanisms for food intolerance exist. Most common is the incomplete digestion of food particles in the small bowel, such as in lactose intolerance. When these particles arrive in the cecum, colonic bacteria complete the digestion process and produce large numbers of osmotically active particles, drawing water into the cecum and causing acute colonic distention with subsequent diarrhea. In patients with lactose intolerance, it is the absence of epithelial enzymes (such as lactase) that lead to incomplete digestion. In other patients (e.g., with consumption of beans or meat), it is an inadequate amount of enzymes relative to the foods eaten.

Other causes of food intolerance may be pharmacologic, metabolic, toxin mediated, immunologic, or psychological. All food contains some small molecules that are capable of pharmacologic action. Different individuals may have greater or lesser sensitivity to these effects due to variations in metabolism; in the extreme form, such sensitivity may result from an inborn or acquired disorder of metabolism, which allows a small molecule to circulate and cause symptoms. Examples include the inborn error of phenylketonuria as well as the acquired inability to process tyramine resulting from use of many antidepressants. More frequently noted than complete disorders of metabolism are sensitivities to various preservatives, colors, or taste enhancers, such as monosodium glutamate or salicylates. Toxin-mediated sensitivity is related to naturally present toxins or food contamination. Immunologic sensitivity, or true food allergy, is the result of IgE-mediated response to consumed allergens. Finally, much like blushing can occur following an emotion (a physiologic effect), some patients may experience significant GI symptoms when they consume certain foods.

Effective management of food intolerance requires completion of several steps. First, the more dangerous causes of abdominal pain should be excluded. Given that most food intolerance is not initially obvious, the next step is effective caregiver and patient education. Families will often benefit from keeping a food diary and obtaining regular primary care follow-up to identify and track food intolerances. It is unusual when simple dietary modification does not work to relieve symptoms; indeed, such failure is a warning sign that gastroenterology or allergy and immunology consultation should be sought.

Gastroenteritis

Acute gastroenteritis (AGE) is another very common cause of abdominal pain. The term "gastroenteritis," like "enteritis" and "colitis," is a nonspecific description of "inflammation of the gut." Nevertheless, AGE has come to represent a spectrum of illness related to transient viral infection of the GI tract. Although the manifestations vary from virus to virus, most forms of AGE have several common symptoms. Infection of the foregut (especially the stomach) leads to significant nausea, nonbilious vomiting, and dry heaves. Infection of the midgut (small bowel) leads to increased secretions and concomitant bowel distention, manifested as crampy abdominal pain. Infection of the hindgut (particularly the distal colon and rectum) also leads to increased secretions, bowel distention, and irritation of rectal muscle. Together, these effects produce crampy abdominal pain with urgency of defecation followed by loose diarrhea and gas. Finally, viral infection is often associated with release of interleukin-1 (IL-1) and interleukin-6 (IL-6); these cytokines cause fever and chills.

The classic history of AGE describes exposure to an ill contact (often shortly after starting school), followed by a progression from nausea and vomiting, to crampy abdominal pain, and finally to diarrhea. The differential diagnosis of viral AGE includes almost all of the causes described in this section. Most importantly, however, are partial bowel obstructions and the bacterial and parasite infections, whose treatment requires antibiotics and occasionally surgery. Evaluation consists of a careful history and physical examination, which often can distinguish between obvious AGE and illness that requires further evaluation.

Use of white blood count (WBC) and C-reactive protein (CRP) can help distinguish AGE (usually normal results) from bacterial infections (usually elevated results). Use of abdominal radiographs—particularly two-view images—can help distinguish AGE (ileus pattern with distal gas) from bowel obstruction (multiple differential air fluid levels, occasionally fixed loops). In some circumstances, additional studies (most often CT scan and ultrasound) can be utilized to help in a diagnostic dilemma. Most importantly, passage of time and repeat examination are the most reliable tests, as AGE is usually self-limited, whereas illnesses such as small bowel obstruction, infectious colitis, and appendicitis continue to progress.

Appendicitis

The best example of a classic pain history occurs in appendicitis. Acute appendicitis initially presents with splanchnic pain due to appendiceal obstruction. This crampy periumbilical pain seems to migrate to the right lower quadrant as the disease becomes transmural. Worsening ileus or partial obstruction leads to constipation, nausea, vomiting, and loss of appetite. Tenderness and fever indicate ischemia of the appendix and focal peritonitis, and perforation often brings worsening peritonitis with improved crampy pain. Perforation may be associated with conversion of constipation to diarrhea as rectal irritation from pelvic pus stimulates rectal secretion. Given that appendicitis is a surgical diagnosis, history, physical examination, CBC, and urinalysis are all that are necessary to prompt surgical consultation.

Mesenteric adenitis

Mesenteric adenitis is an important cause of abdominal pain that should be distinguished from appendicitis. Similar to appendicitis, it begins with splanchnic, crampy pain that is periumbilical in origin. Unlike in appendicitis, complete obstruction of the appendix or small bowel does not occur; for this reason, there is no progression to tenderness. Additional probing into the patient's history usually elicits report of a recent viral infection or exposure to viral infections, so the progression and addition of symptoms such as loss of appetite, nausea, vomiting, and fever may be noticeably lacking. Laboratory evaluation may even demonstrate a normal WBC.

No therapy is necessary for mesenteric adenitis, as the reactive lymph nodes and Peyer's patches will resolve. Rather, the most important goal is the exclusion of appendicitis as a diagnosis. Imaging may be necessary for patients with a several-day history with no associated symptoms and normal WBC. In the event that imaging is considered, it is reasonable to initiate surgical consultation. Of particular importance is discharge counseling: Because a certain number of these patients will have an early form of appendicitis, it is always necessary to counsel the family to return to be evaluated in the setting of progression of symptoms or worsening pain.

Bowel obstruction

Small bowel obstruction (SBO) requires prompt surgical evaluation, as a number of its common causes require intervention. Several key questions will help distinguish between different types of obstruction and assist in management.

- First question: a careful surgical and infection history of the abdomen.
- Second question: the color of the vomitus.
- Third question: the presence of gas, liquid, or solid passing per ano.

Asking the first question helps identify the first type of bowel obstruction: SBO in the child who has never had a surgery or severe infection of the abdominal cavity. This condition can be further delineated by addressing the second question: Presence of bile or feculent material in the vomit is a red flag that always indicates further thought and evaluation are necessary. The other types of bowel obstruction can be distinguished when the first question identifies that the patient has a history of abdominal surgery. The second and third questions help distinguish between complete obstruction (bilious or feculent vomiting, no gas or stool per ano) and partial obstruction (decreased stool and almost no gas).

Full evaluation of suspected bowel obstruction starts with history and physical examination, as noted previously. Radiologic imaging is often the most useful first diagnostic study, with the two- or three-view abdominal series being standard practice. In most patients, the pain of bowel obstruction relates to the bowel distention. Tenderness often results from bowel ischemia and peritoneal inflammation.

The child (not neonate) without prior surgery may have obstruction from several common causes. High on the list is inguinal hernia; history and physical examination usually quickly locate the bulge in the groin. Also high on the list, especially in younger children, is perforated appendicitis (where the inflammatory right lower quadrant mass is causing a distal small bowel obstruction). In the toddler and preschool child, the most common cause of painful bowel obstruction is intussusception. Finally, bilious vomiting should always raise suspicion for malrotation with volvulus; although not as common as hernia or appendicitis, the ramifications of missed volvulus are life-threatening.

Children who have undergone prior surgery may have the previously described disorders, although most commonly they will have adhesive (postoperative) bowel obstruction. The pathogenesis of adhesive bowel obstruction begins with the laying down of scar tissue in the peritoneum (adhesions). If partial blockage of the small bowel occurs due to adhesions, the resulting distention and kinking of the bowel often worsen the partial obstruction and stretch the smooth muscle in the bowel, weakening peristalsis. In addition to adhesive bowel obstruction, resection

of retroperitoneal tumors (neuroblastoma, Wilms' tumor) may lead to ileoileal intussusception through an unclear mechanism.

The most important aspect of therapy relates to whether the bowel obstruction is partial or complete. The more partial a bowel obstruction is, the greater likelihood that it will respond to nonoperative management. The more complete a bowel obstruction is, the greater likelihood that surgical intervention will be required. With complete obstruction, proximal distention and overgrowth can cause mucosal and bowel ischemia, leading to bowel necrosis and perforation. Particularly in younger children, resuscitation of severe bowel obstruction may even lead to abdominal compartment syndrome.

Intussusception

Intussusception is most common in infants and toddlers. Classically, it is characterized by a pain history without tenderness on exam. Children are brought in by parents with a history of episodes of severe pain, inconsolability, and often pulling legs up to the chest. Caregivers report that pain recurs every 15 to 30 minutes; between pain episodes, the child behaves in a completely normal fashion. Physical examination generally demonstrates a well-developed, well-nourished child who appears nontoxic, although careful inspection will find evidence of dehydration and often a right upper quadrant mass. History or physical examination finding of bloody "currant jelly" stools (associated with ischemia and mucosal sloughing of the intussusceptions) should significantly raise the suspicion for this disorder.

Intussusception occurs when a proximal piece of bowel (traditionally the ileocecal valve) telescopes inside the distal bowel. All bowel peristalses, and occasionally the bowel itself, will push forward both food and proximal squeezed bowel. Fortunately, the mesentery acts as a lasso; without something to peristalse, it keeps these tiny, asymptomatic intussusceptions from progressing. Increasing use of CT has demonstrated evidence that small ileoileal intussusceptions are quite common and self-limited. If a focal abnormality is present in the bowel, it can act as a "lead point." The abnormality predisposes the patient to intussusception, and with every peristalsis the "lead point" is pushed farther, thereby forming significant lengths of telescoping bowel. In this situation, the blood supply becomes compressed, and the intussuscepted bowel becomes ischemic. Each round of peristalsis brings the pain wave described earlier, and the mucosal ischemia and sloughing lead to the classic currant jelly stools. Because infants and toddlers have larger immunologic tissues (lymph nodes, mucosal-associated lymphoid tissue/Peyer's patches, appendix), the distal ileal tissue acts as the lead point in this process, which often progresses after reactive hypertrophy that occurs with a recent viral infection. Even upper respiratory illness can be associated with gastrointestinal hypertrophy, as phlegm is coughed to the oropharynx and swallowed, and GI lymph tissue can continue to react and generate antibodies to viral particles.

Constipation

Constipation is an extremely common condition and a final common pathway for many abdominal illnesses. The HCP needs to separate urgent constipation requiring intervention from chronic constipation that can be carefully evaluated in the clinic setting. A careful stooling history will alert the HCP to urgent constipation based on the presence of an abrupt change. Physical examination must look for mechanical obstruction, such as hernia or adhesive bowel obstruction, and the anus must be inspected. Three-view radiographs of the abdomen can assist in the identification of mechanical obstruction. Evidence of enterocolitis in the setting of constipation without perforation suggests a need for irrigations, fluid resuscitation, and antibiotics. Most importantly, significant right-side constipation should be seen as a marker for infectious process, such as pneumonia, right pyelonephritis, or appendicitis. Once these acute illnesses (obstruction, perforation, enterocolitis, infection) have been deemed unlikely, enemas and outpatient broad evaluation is appropriate. Discharge from an acute care setting requires that family be well informed regarding their follow-up appointments and contact information, as these patients often return several times when they neglect follow-up.

Inflammatory bowel disease

Among the more chronic GI problems that can present with acute abdominal pain are the inflammatory bowel diseases (IBD). These illnesses represent a spectrum of GI disease with associated nongastrointestinal symptoms that are immunologic in nature. The two classic IBD patterns are Crohn's disease and ulcerative colitis.

Crohn's disease is a pangastrointestinal inflammatory disease characterized by patchy, noncontiguous regions of inflammation separated by healthy bowel. Pathology reveals transmural inflammation and significant noncaseating granulomas. The most common presenting symptom in Crohn's disease is abdominal pain. The pain of Crohn's disease can be described as either crampy, epigastric or periumbilical, and intermittent. This pattern is most likely related to the distribution of the disease, where distal ileal and ileocolonic areas make up the bulk of affected bowel.

A careful history and physical examination will often identify symptoms suggestive of Crohn's disease. Specifically, GI history may identify multiple sites of illness, ranging from oropharyngeal involvement to perianal disease. Extraintestinal history may identify associated symptoms common in autoimmune disease, such as polyarticular arthritis and ocular, hepatobiliary,

and integumetary findings. Physical examination may also identify intestinal and extraintestinal findings that patients had not previously noticed.

Crohn's disease can present as stricturing or fistulizing disease. In the setting of a stricture, patients may present with partial or complete bowel obstruction. Similarly, fistulizing disease may present with free perforation or abscess formation, both of which require prompt evaluation and surgical consultation.

Evaluation for stable patients with Crohn's disease usually begins with laboratory and radiologic evaluation to exclude more common acute causes of abdominal pain. After exclusion of these causes, ongoing evaluation often utilizes fluoroscopic studies of the bowel (upper GI series with small bowel follow-through or barium enema) or upper and lower endoscopy with biopsy.

Ulcerative colitis (UC) is an inflammatory disease of the bowel that extends in contiguous fashion from the rectosigmoid region proximally and can be associated with abdominal pain. Pathology reveals superficial global inflammation with mucosal sloughing. Unlike with Crohn's disease, the most common presenting symptom is lower GI bleeding, but pain is also often present. Pain is classically a splanchnic colorectal pain, described as crampy, suprapubic or pelvic, and midline, and often associated with tenesmus. As with Crohn's disease, a careful GI history often demonstrates the associated symptoms of bleeding and anemia.

Evaluation of UC usually begins with laboratory and radiologic evaluation to exclude more common acute causes of colitis, particularly infectious colitis. After exclusion of these causes, ongoing evaluation requires lower endoscopy and biopsy. On occasion, autoimmune colitidies cannot be definitively identified as UC and the diagnosis is, therefore, called "indeterminate colitis." Herein lies one of the long-term challenges of IBD management: A subset of patients with indeterminate colitis managed as having UC may go on to be identified as having Crohn's disease.

Other chronic causes of abdominal pain include irritable bowel syndrome (IBS) and a variety of functional bowel disorders. This poorly understood collection of illnesses is associated with significant, intermittent pain and functional symptoms of constipation, diarrhea, or alternating constipation and diarrhea. History and physical examination are often nonspecific, and management consists of early evaluation to exclude more acute causes of abdominal pain, followed by referral to a gastroenterological specialist.

HEPATOBILIARY PAIN

Classically, hepatobiliary pain was considered to be related to the acute hepatitidies, acute pancreatitis, and infectious diseases of the hepatobiliary system. However, now it can also be attributed to cholelithiasis due to its increasing prevalence in the pediatric population.

The histories for patients with hepatobiliary pain are typically quite similar despite different pathophysiologies. Liver-mediated pain results from liver edema and resulting tension in the hepatic capsule (Glisson's capsule). It is often constant, sharp, located in the right upper quadrant, and worsened by coughing or breathing. Pain from the biliary tree and gallbladder results from a partial or complete obstruction, with subsequent colonization or infection of the biliary tree. When the obstruction is intermittent or partial, as often occurs if small gallstones travel down the ducts to the duodenum, the pain is crampy, intermittent, and transient, and usually follows consumption of fatty foods. When the obstruction is complete, the intermittent pain changes to constant and gains a sharp characteristic. If infection is present, fevers and significant jaundice (Charcot's triad) are present. Finally, pancreatic pain is often sharp, constant, and epigastric, radiating to the left side as well as to the back, and exacerbated by food intake.

A careful history can elicit the subtle differences between pain generated by the various regions of the hepatobiliary system. Physical examination coupled with laboratory investigation of liver function tests, pancreatic studies, and blood count will typically identify the correct region (liver, biliary tree, or pancreas) as the source and guide further radiologic evaluation (most commonly ultrasound).

Hepatitis

Hepatitis characteristically is associated with significant elevations in AST and ALT, with lesser derangements of bilirubin metabolism being noted. Acute hepatitis can be associated with multiple types of toxic ingestions, particularly mushrooms, acetaminophen, and tricyclic antidepressants. Initially history should focus on potential ingestions and infectious exposures. Subsequently, acute hepatitis evaluation focuses on identifying the cause, predominantly via laboratory evaluation. Screening for viral hepatidities includes hepatitis A, B, and C, as well as less common causes such as hepatitis D (associated with B) and E, Epstein-Barr virus, and cytomegalovirus. In the event that a primary exposure or infection cannot be found, additional investigation should investigate autoimmune hepatitis and chronic causes of hepatitis.

Biliary tract disorders

Biliary tract and gallbladder disorders generally present with elevations in total and direct (conjugated) bilirubin, alkaline phosphatase, and gamma-glutamyl transferase. To a lesser extent, ALT will be elevated, although not near the levels associated with hepatitis. Patients often complain of jaundice, icteric sclera, and itching (associated with deposition of bile salts in the skin). Physical examination to diagnose this disorder may be coupled with a careful abdominal ultrasound, as it is the optimal imaging study to the evaluate intrahepatic and extrahepatic biliary tree, gallbladder, and liver parenchyma. Historically, major causes of pediatric abdominal pain associated with jaundice included congenital abnormalities of the biliary tract, particularly choledocal cysts that had become secondarily infected.

Pancreatitis

Acute pancreatitis is the final common pathway to several congenital and acute illnesses. It comprises a self-sustaining process in which an initial injury leads to loss of pancreatic ducal integrity, release of exocrine secretions, and autolysis pancreatic parenchyma destruction. Its history begins with the onset and worsening of sharp epigastric pain, radiating to the left and back. Often, history combined with focal laboratory analysis will identify the cause of this disorder. Careful questioning regarding trauma, ingestions, exposures, recent viral infections, gallstones, familial pancreatitis, and elevated triglycerides is necessary. Physical examination demonstrates epigastric and left upper quadrant tenderness and is important for what it is *not*—namely, tenderness that does not require urgent surgery. Laboratory studies include amylase and lipase, total bilirubin, alcohol level (particularly in adolescents), triglyceride level, ionized calcium, and CBC. Ultrasound is often performed to exclude gallstones as a cause of pancreatitis. Although trauma, gallstones, viral etiologies, toxin-mediated etiologies, and hereditary pancreatitis remain the leading causes, in many patients the cause of the pancreatitis cannot be identified.

Trauma

Child maltreatment (i.e., inflicted trauma or nonaccidental trauma) may present with abdominal pain that may be nonspecific and disconcordant with history. If this cause is suspected, it is important to expand the assessment to a full physical examination—focusing on the neurologic examination to evaluate for traumatic brain injury and skin to evaluate for nonaccidental injury patterns. Urgent surgical consult should be obtained for signs of perforation, obstruction, or trauma.

Accidental trauma also can present with abdominal pain. Patients and families may initially report only a history of abdominal pain upon presentation to the health care system. It may take further interview to elicit the history of trauma; however, once a patient has been identified as having a traumatic injury, clinical focus should shift toward the therapeutic management of the pediatric trauma patient.

PATIENT AND FAMILY TEACHING AND FOLLOW-UP

Effective patient and family education coupled with arranged follow-up can ensure satisfaction and appropriate use of resources. Most abdominal pain situations do not require admission or acute intervention. However, many times children are unable to describe the pain, the nature of the pain changes, or concurrent symptoms become more definitive. In such circumstances, it is necessary for families to have a very clear idea of the natural course of illness and to know when to return for reevaluation. Indeed, the extra time taken to counsel families can prevent a second emergency department evaluation or delayed diagnosis. During the teaching of the natural course of disease, it is important to emphasize all the warning signs that should prompt return for care. As basic as it sounds, "Return for worsening pain" is a very appropriate statement.

In many cases, there are various options for home care of the patients previously described. Therefore, it is also appropriate to explain different solutions for caregivers—from the differences between ibuprofen and acetaminophen, to options for oral rehydration therapy or perianal care. When caregivers have a good understanding of therapies available to them, they are less likely to have inappropriate return for further evaluation and are more likely to be satisfied with the care provided to their child.

Finally, teaching should ensure that the caregivers understand the follow-up plan for their child, including ways to contact HCPs. That means providing the full name, address, and office number for new outpatient referrals as well as ensuring follow-up with the primary pediatric care provider (PCP). Indeed, a short, dictated letter to the PCP can facilitate continuity of care and ensure that the family can retrieve all referral information as needed.

CHOLECYSTITIS

Laurette Mouat

PATHOPHYSIOLOGY

Cholecystitis is characterized by inflammation and distension of the gallbladder. It is generally classified as either calculous or acalculous, based on the presence or absence of visualized gallstones, respectively. Both the calculus and acalculous types of cholecystitis are affected by hypofunction or stasis in the gallbladder.

Gallstones are categorized into cholesterol or pigmented (black or brown) types. Cholesterol stones consist of more than 50% cholesterol by weight, whereas pigmented stones contain a mixture of calcium salts and other anions (Heubi, 2007; Ostrow, 1984). Cholesterol stones, which are the most common type in adolescent and adult disease, occur when cholesterol concentrations exceed their maximum equilibrium solubility in the presence of stasis, resulting in nucleation of cholesterol crystals (Heubi). Mucin glycoproteins serve as the framework for growth of pigmented stones, in combination with supersaturation of bile and stasis. Additionally, brown stone formation requires the presence of bacteria (Heubi).

In both cholesterol and pigmented gallstone subtypes, biliary sludge formation and inflammation may lead to obstruction and edema, which in turn create more inflammation and stasis. More specifically, bile stasis and bacterial overgrowth lead to a release of lysolecithins, exacerbating inflammation. Edema can also cause ischemia of the local tissue, which furthers the release of pro-inflammatory agents. Bacterial contamination can occur as tissue damage increases; indeed, culture-positive findings are noted in most patients, most commonly *Escherichia coli* (Tabata & Nakayama, 1981). The mechanism of pain is thought to be related to the obstruction process, which results in increasing pressure in the gallbladder as it pushes against the blockage (Heubi, 2007).

EPIDEMIOLOGY AND ETIOLOGY

Acalculous cholecystitis is most often seen in pediatric patients who are critically ill or who have systemic disease. Its occurrence, however, is poorly recognized due to diagnostic complexity—these patients may have multiple underlying conditions (Imamoglu et al., 2002; Tsakayannis et al., 1996). A lack of enteral feeding, parenteral nutrition (PN), use of narcotics, previous surgical procedures, burns, multiple transfusions, trauma, ischemia, and sepsis have all been identified as risk factors for, or as being associated with, development of acalculous cholecystitis (Heubi, 2007). This disorder can present as an abdominal emergency and requires prompt recognition and treatment.

Pigmented stones are the most common in young children, accounting for 72% of pediatric cholelithiasis occurrences, especially in children younger than 5 years of age (Friesen & Roberts, 1989). The incidence of cholesterol stones gradually increases with age, with a strong predominance in females (Kaechele et al., 2006). Although the significant prevalence of gallstones in hemolytic conditions is a well-known phenomenon that increases with age (14% for individuals younger than age 10 years, increasing to 50% by early adulthood), the overall prevalence of gallstone disease in children is quite low; a rate of 0.13% was noted in one Italian series (Bond et al., 1987; Palasciano et al., 1989). However, speculation suggests that the increasing incidence of adolescent obesity may lead to a rise in rates of cholesterol stone–mediated cholecystitis, thereby making this a more common condition in the pediatric population than previously appreciated: The prevalence of gallstone disease in obese adolescents has been estimated at 2.0% (Kaechele et al.).

The most common hematologic conditions associated with development of gallstones (usually pigmented) are: hereditary spherocytosis, sickle-cell anemia, and thalassemia major (Holcomb & Holcomb, 1990). Other conditions associated with formation of stones include distal ileal resection, parenteral nutrition (PN), a fasting state, prematurity, bronchopulmonary dysplasia, prolonged immobilization, cystic fibrosis, hepatobiliary disease, adolescent pregnancy, use of oral contraceptives, and obesity (Holcomb & Holcomb; Rescorla, 1997). Drugs whose use is commonly associated with gallbladder disease include furosemide, octreotide, ceftriaxone, cyclosporin, and tacrolimus. Prematurity, small bowel disease, and sepsis are conditions that may exacerbate drug-induced stone formation (Gilger, 2006).

PRESENTATION

Gallstone disease should be considered within the differential diagnosis for any child with vague, colicky upper quadrant pain, but especially for those patients with associated risk factors (Holcomb & Holcomb, 1990). History taking for acalculous cholecystitis will most often reveal a context of sepsis or critical illness, whereas gallstone-induced disease would be suspected in patients with a history of hemolytic disease or complaints of right upper quadrant (RUQ) postprandial pain, nausea, and biliary colic. Physical examination may be significant for RUQ pain on palpation, jaundice, positive Murphy sign (pain or inspiratory arrest during inspiration when a hand is placed over the gallbladder), vomiting, fever, and on occasion a palpable mass in the right upper quadrant. Jaundice is the most common symptom in children less than 1 year of age (Friesen & Roberts, 1989). Fever greater than 40.8°C (105.4°F) and worsening pain may indicate complications such as perforation, abscess, or empyema (Gilger, 2006).

DIFFERENTIAL DIAGNOSIS

Acalculous cholecystitis in particular may be difficult to recognize in the pediatric patient with multiple systemic complications. Nevertheless, it should be considered in every critically ill patient with risk factors, physical examination findings, or suggestive diagnostic studies. Diagnoses that share overlapping signs or symptoms with cholecystitis/cholelithiasis should be consider as differential diagnoses (Table 26-2).

Biliary dyskinesia is an increasingly recognized but clinically discrete condition that can cause significant recurrent RUQ pain in the older child and adolescent (typically female) and that is characterized by abnormal contractility of the gallbladder. This condition should also be considered in a work-up of a pediatric patient with chronic symptoms mimicking cholecystitis (Haricharan et al., 2008a).

TABLE 26-2

Cholecystitis Differential Diagnosis

- Appendicitis
- Intussusception
- Infectious hepatitis
- Choledochal cyst
- Peritonitis
- Biliary atresia
- Cholangitis
- Peptic ulcer disease
- Renal colic
- Renal stones
- Gastritis
- Pneumonia
- Hepatic abscess
- Abdominal tumor
- Pyelonephritis
- Irritable bowel syndrome
- Pancreatitis
- Small bowel obstruction

PLAN OF CARE

Diagnostic studies for a pediatric patient in whom cholecystitis is suspected would include a CBC, liver function tests (LFTs), total and direct bilirubin, gamma-glutamyl transpeptidase (GGT), amylase, and lipase. Lab findings expected with cholecystitis are as follows:

- Elevated white blood count with predominance of polymorphonuclear leukocytes and bandemia
- Elevated bilirubin, alkaline phosphatase, and GGT, suggesting the possibility of stones present in the biliary tree (Gilger, 2006)
- A mild increase in the aminotransaminases, including aspartate aminotransferase (AST) and alanine aminotransferase (ALT)

Of note, concomitant elevations in amylase and lipase (pancreatitis) occurs in as many as 8% of patients.

Imaging should start with a plain abdominal film for an initial screening of abdominal pain. Cholesterol stones are radiolucent, whereas pigmented stones are usually radiopaque. An abdominal ultrasound is the diagnostic study of choice for evaluating both cholecystitis and cholelithiasis (Rescorla, 1997). Findings on ultrasound often include a discrete echo density with acoustic shadowing, gallbladder dilation, thickened gallbladder wall, and presence of sludge (Gilger, 2006). The nuclear medicine hepatobiliary imino-diacetic acid (HIDA) scan may helpful for assessing acute acalculous cholecystitis by demonstrating good hepatic uptake but nonfilling of the gallbladder. However, false-positive findings may be found in patients who are in a fasting state or in patients with hepatocellular disease. In pediatric patients with hemolytic disease, annual screening with ultrasound should be considered, as these individuals have a higher incidence of cholelithiasis (Bond et al., 1987; Holcomb & Holcomb, 1990).

Therapeutic management focuses on stabilizing and preparing the patient for laparoscopic cholecystectomy (LC), the accepted treatment for symptomatic pediatric patients. This procedure is associated with very low complication rates and rapid recovery time when performed by experienced pediatric surgeons. Dissolution of stones has been attempted with ursodeoxycholic acid (Actigall) with only limited success. Asymptomatic cholelithiasis, especially in young children, may also be considered for LC if the presence of stones has been documented for several months, although spontaneous resolution has frequently been reported in infants (Rescorla, 1997). An intraoperative cholangiogram or magnetic resonance cholangiopancreatography should be performed before cholecystectomy of common bile duct (CBD) stones are suspected. In these patients, endoscopic retrograde cholangiopancreatography (ERCP) is usually performed to dislodge CBD stones before surgery.

Emergency laparotomy for cholecystectomy or cholecystostomy may be necessary for those patients with acute acalculous cholecystitis. By comparison, surgery may be avoided if the following therapies are implemented: close monitoring of symptoms, serial ultrasounds, gastric decompression, intravenous fluids, and broad-spectrum antibiotics such as meropenum or ampicillin/gentamicin/clindamycin (Imamoglu et al., 2002; Millar, 2008).

Measures to prevent cholecystitis in high-risk populations should be ordered whenever possible. These strategies include the delivery of trophic enteral stimulation for patients who are on PN, and controlled weight loss for obese adolescents (rapid weight loss can *induce* stone formation). Therapeutic management to prevent complications in patients with hemolytic diseases deserves special considerations: Ample hydration (150% maintenance rate) and preoperative transfusions are desirable in most cases, and some specialists favor elective cholecystectomy in certain hemolytic populations (Millar, 2008).

Consultation with the following subspecialists may be necessary in the management of a patient with possible or identified cholecystitis:

- Gastroenterology
- General surgery
- Hematology
- Infectious disease
- Intensive care medicine
- Nutrition

Patient and family education should focus on awareness of signs and symptoms for the at-risk population. Patients with hemolytic disorders, in particular, should discuss yearly screening with their HCP. Weight loss counseling should be offered to obese adolescents.

DISPOSITION AND DISCHARGE PLANNING

As recovery is typically rapid and uncomplicated following LC, discharge can occur soon after surgery as long as the pediatric patient is tolerating a sustainable diet. Surgical follow-up usually occurs within 2 weeks of any operative intervention. Pediatric patients with asymptomatic gallstones should have serial ultrasounds determined by gastroenterology or hematology to assess for resolution.

CHOLESTASIS

Laurette Mouat

PATHOPHYSIOLOGY

Cholestasis is defined as a significant decrease in bile flow combined with the accumulation of substances within the hepatocytes and bile ducts. These substances are those normally excreted in bile (i.e., cholesterol, bile acids, bile salts). The conjugated bilirubin will usually make up more than 20% of the total bilirubin value on chemical analysis. Cholestasis can rapidly lead to fibrosis and eventual cirrhosis of the liver. Numerous congenital and acquired conditions can cause cholestasis.

Biliary atresia (BA) is the most common cause of obstructive jaundice in the newborn, and the leading indication for pediatric liver transplantation worldwide (Balistreri et al., 2007). BA is thought to be an inflammatory process leading to complete obstruction of bile flow due to progressive destruction and possible obliteration of part of, or the entire, extrahepatic biliary tree. In this condition, the gallbladder is absent or atretic. BA is generally thought to be acquired in late gestation or after birth, as the most common presentation is characterized by destruction of fully formed structures. An "embryonic" or "fetal" subtype, however, occurs in 10% to 35% of patients (Balistreri et al.).

Choledochal cysts are another obstructive phenomenon that can cause cholestasis. Although the pathogenesis of the obstruction is not fully understood, an abnormally long common pathway between the pancreatic and common bile ducts has been found in two-thirds of patients. This unusual pathway causes a reflux of pancreatic enzymes that can damage the biliary mucosa. An alternative theory suggests that the cysts arise from a distal common bile duct obstruction (Metcalfe et al., 2003; Millar, 2008).

Alagille syndrome, in contrast with biliary atresia, is characterized by bile duct paucity, rather than proliferation. It is associated with cardiac, ocular, facial, renal, and skeletal anomalies and leads to cholestasis secondary to bile duct damage. Other cholestatic conditions associated with bile duct paucity include α_1-antitrypsin (A1AT) deficiency (an inherited metabolic disorder), prematurity, and trisomy 21. Other types of disorders leading to cholestasis include the following:

- Cholestatic genetic syndromes such as progressive familial intrahepatic cholestasis (PFIC syndrome)
- Infectious processes such as TORCH infections (toxoplasmosis, other infections, rubella, cytomegalovirus, herpes simplex virus), HIV, and viral hepatitis
- Other metabolic disorders such as tyrosinemia, galactosemia, and glycogen storage diseases
- Bile acid synthetic defects
- Cystic fibrosis
- Endocrinopathies
- Toxins, especially parenteral nutrition
- Cardiovascular disease (Ng, 2006)

EPIDEMIOLOGY AND ETIOLOGY

In BA, the etiology remains unknown; current theories of its origin focus on viral insult versus genetic mutation, impaired immunologic response, and probable interaction among all three of these factors (Petersen, 2006). Incidence ranges between 1 in 8,000 and 1 in 18,000, with higher rates being noted among Asian populations and nonwhites in general, and a slightly higher female predominance (Basset & Murray, 2008; The et al., 2007). The literature provides conflicting evidence regarding theories supporting a seasonal variation in BA incidence (Millar, 2008; The et al., 2007).

The incidence of choledochal cysts is 1 in 15,000, but as high as 1 in 1,000 births in Japan, with a 4:1 female-to-male ratio. This entity is the causative factor in 2% of infants with obstructive jaundice (Balistreri et al., 2007). Impaired bile flow from obstruction and ductal dilatation can lead to cholestasis and other hepatic and pancreatic complications (Miele-Vergani & Hadzic, 2006).

Alagille syndrome is caused by a mutation in the *Jagged* 1 gene and has variable penetrance in family members, ranging from mild to severe (Quiros-Tejeira et al., 1999). The estimated incidence of this condition is 1 per 100,000 population. A1AT deficiency is an autosomal codominant condition that occurs in 1 per 1,600 to 2,000 live births, making it the most common genetic cause of liver disease in pediatric patients. Generally, only the PiZZ phenotype is associated with liver disease; of persons with this subtype, only 8% to 10% progress to significant cholestasis and liver damage (Perlmutter, 2007).

Parenteral nutrition–induced cholestasis is especially problematic in the premature infant requiring PN support. Onset of cholestasis can occur as early as 2 to 3 weeks after initiation of this feeding approach, and typically progresses the longer the pediatric patient requires PN. The etiology is likely multifactorial, but new research is focused on the detrimental effect of lipid products containing a predominance of omega-6 fatty acids (Gura et al., 2008).

PRESENTATION

The presentation of cholestatic patients is primarily characterized by conjugated hyperbilirubinemia and jaundice. In BA, jaundice is present at birth or soon thereafter, and persists beyond 14 days of life. The patient will initially have acholic (nonpigmented) stools and hepatomegaly, with progression to poor growth, splenomegaly, ascites, and coagulopathy (Chardot, 2006).

In patients with choledochal cysts, the "classic triad" of intermittent abdominal pain, jaundice, and right epigastric mass is actually present only 20% of the time (Balistreri et al., 2007). Most patients will present with jaundice alone, or the condition may be identified incidentally during work-up for nonspecific symptoms. The patient may also present with symptoms of pancreatitis or biliary peritonitis from perforation of the cyst (Balistreri et al.).

Alagille syndrome will present with mild to severe cholestasis, often accompanied by significant pruritus secondary to very high bile salt serum elevations. Cholesterol levels may exceed 1,000 to 2,000 mg/dL (Kamath et al., 2007). Initially synthetic function is preserved, but the patient may progress to demonstrate signs of coagulopathy, vitamin malabsorption, elevated ammonia levels, and hypoalbuminemia. Growth failure is common, and most patients also have obvious symptoms and complications from the associated system anomalies mentioned previously (Rovner et al., 2002).

A1AT deficiency can present with conjugated hyperbilirubinemia, intrauterine growth retardation, and severe cholestasis, including acholic stools. Coagulopathy and hepatomegaly are frequently seen. Adults with A1AT deficiency may develop emphysema (Perlmutter, 2007).

DIFFERENTIAL DIAGNOSIS

Cholestatic conditions can initially present similarly; therefore, a thorough and careful exploration is required to elucidate the diagnosis (Ng, 2006). Neonatal hepatitis, Alagille syndrome, BA, and A1AT deficiency can all mimic one another in the early phase of the evaluation, with the latter two often distinguishable only through liver biopsy. Metabolic disorders such as galactosemia, endocrine disorders, and sepsis may present with cholestasis but need to be considered expeditiously so that timely intervention may be implemented. BA is also an extremely time-sensitive diagnosis, with a very poor outcome if diagnosis is delayed (Petersen, 2006). Also within the differential of cholestatic conditions are those associated with systemic diseases such as ischemia, chromosomal syndromes (Down syndrome), and autoimmune conditions (Ng, 2006).

PLAN OF CARE

Diagnostic studies for the jaundiced pediatric patient should always include a fractionated serum bilirubin analysis, aminotransaminases (AST and ALT), alkaline phosphatase, and gamma-glutamyl transpeptidase. Synthetic function markers, including coagulation studies, albumin, ammonia, and glucose levels, should be obtained if any significant presentation of jaundice exists (Ng, 2006). Ultrasound is the preferred initial imaging study. Any infant with persistent jaundice beyond 14 days should be referred urgently to a center with pediatric gastroenterology and pediatric surgery.

The following additional diagnostic studies are relevant to suspicion of specific diagnoses:

- *BA:* Ultrasound will show an irregular or absent gallbladder. If the infant is less than 60 days of age, percutaneous liver biopsy should be obtained; if the patient's age is close to or beyond 60 days, however, consideration should be given to performing an intraoperative cholangiogram in preparation for immediate Kasai (hepatoportoenterostomy) procedure, which is a palliative Roux-en-Y to reestablish bile flow. This procedure can dramatically mitigate rapid onset of fibrosis and cirrhosis if performed in a timely manner. Infants well beyond 60 days of age at time of diagnosis may already have cirrhosis, so consideration might be given to proceeding straight to transplantation, although this is an area of controversy (Balistreri et al., 2007; Petersen, 2006).
- *Choledochal cyst:* An ultrasound should be obtained initially, but often magnetic resonance cholangiopancreatography and/or endoscopic retrograde cholangiopancreatography will be required for definitive evaluation and intervention. Treatment consists of surgical removal of the cyst with a Roux-en-Y loop for biliary drainage.
- *Alagille syndrome:* Evaluation for associated anomalies, such as slit-lamp eye examination for posterior embryotoxon, imaging for renal and skeletal abnormalities, cardiac work-up, and growth parameters, should be undertaken. Liver biopsy is helpful to confirm the diagnosis and differentiate this disease from other conditions (Mieli-Vergani & Hadzic, 2006).

- *A1AT deficiency:* Serum A1AT levels can be falsely elevated, as this is an acute-phase reactant. These levels can also be falsely low if there are excessive losses in the stool. Given these possible outcomes, phenotyping is a more specific assay. Liver biopsy tissue can be stained to determine the presence of this condition (A-Kader & Ghishan, 2006).

The therapeutic plan for all pediatric patients with cholestatic conditions focuses on three areas: performing any palliative or curative interventions in a timely manner, management of synthetic dysfunction, and attention to nutritional supplementation. Roux-en-Y procedures and transplant work-up need to be initiated promptly. Supportive management of synthetic dysfunction involves delivery of coagulation products for active bleeding, albumin infusions to relieve ascites, and continuous dextrose infusion for patients with end-stage liver failure. Elevated medium-chain triglyceride (MCT) content formulas are preferred for the infant and young child, and continuous nasogastric infusion may be necessary, as optimal nutrition is of utmost importance, especially for the pediatric patient awaiting transplant (Balistreri et al., 2007; Petersen, 2006). Dense caloric concentrations (120 kcal/kg or more) are often required for a slow-growing infant. Supplementation of fat-soluble vitamins (A, D, E, K) using a water-soluble formulation is standard for any persistently cholestatic pediatric patient (Petersen). Trophic enteral stimulation and reduction of lipid infusion are helpful for PN-induced cholestasis. Finally, ursodeoxycholic acid is beneficial as a choleretic agent, and may also have a cytoprotective effect.

Consultation with gastroenterology, general surgery, nutrition, and supportive interprofessional services should be instituted early into the diagnostic and therapeutic plan.

Patient and family education is necessarily specific to the cholestatic condition, but should include an extensive discussion about long-term prognosis and potential need for transplantation. Adherence to close follow-up should be emphasized. Teaching should also be provided for recognition of symptoms such as bleeding, ascites, and hypoglycemic state for patients with synthetic dysfunction. An understanding of the importance of good nutrition and careful monitoring of growth parameters should be communicated clearly.

DISPOSITION AND DISCHARGE PLANNING

The decision to allow a pediatric patient with cholestasis to be managed as an outpatient depends on the severity of the synthetic dysfunction, the patient's nutritional deficiency, and the reliability of the social context of the family in situations requiring a time-sensitive evaluation. Follow-up of the jaundiced infant should include frequent monitoring of the fractionated serum bilirubin analysis and liver function tests as well as measurement of synthetic function. Referral for transplant evaluation should be initiated if the patient's condition may lead to cirrhosis or intractable synthetic dysfunction.

CONSTIPATION

Cheryl Mele

PATHOPHYSIOLOGY

The pelvic muscles that wrap around the urethra, rectum, and anus can be voluntarily controlled to hold either urine or stool. Bowel-holding results in functional constipation or megacolon by causing muscles in the pelvis to become stronger and hypertrophy (Nicholson & Preston, 2007). As the stool-holding continues, the rectum enlarges and stretches, and the urge to defecate gradually disappears (Borowitz et al.,2005). Stool left in the rectum becomes harder due to fluid reabsorption, making it more difficult for the child to evacuate. The child often experiences abdominal pain, anal tears, and urinary dysfunction, which in turn further encourages stool retention behaviors.

Constipation can result in loss of rectal sensitivity and urge to defecate, which may lead to fecal soiling (encopresis) (Baker et al., 2006). In addition, a dilated lower colon may cause obstruction to the bladder, which can result in enuresis, urinary tract infections, and ureteral obstruction (Abi-Hanna & Lake, 1998). The expanded lower colon, which contains a large amount of stool, loses tone and may allow internal prolapse, intussusception, stasis syndrome, and ischemic ulcer of the rectal wall to develop (Abi-Hanna & Lake).

EPIDEMIOLOGY AND ETIOLOGY

Constipation is a common complaint, accounting for 3% to 10% of all pediatric primary care office visits and 25% of all pediatric gastroenterology referrals (Borowitz et al., 2005; Limbos, 2005). Normal defecatory patterns can be very diverse in the pediatric population, ranging from several bowel movements per day to one movement every few days. Constipation is often defined as difficulty passing stool, pain on defecation, decrease in frequency of stool, or passage of hard stools that is present for 2 or more weeks. The range of age at presentation is 4 to 12 years (Montgomery & Fernando, 2008).

Constipation often results in encopresis, which caregivers may misidentify as diarrhea. The social stigma associated with the malodorous smell of encopresis can be debilitating to children and may often result in "teasing" in schools. Children also may hide soiled clothing from caregivers.

Complications of constipation are listed in Table 26-3.

PRESENTATION

A thorough history and physical examination are an essential part of the evaluation of a child with constipation. The history questions pertain to potential organic and nonorganic causes based on the age of the child: presence of meconium stool after birth; any toilet training concerns; frequency and nature of the stool; any encopresis; any blood in the stool; and any urinary problems such as frequency, dribbling, nonfebrile urinary tract infections, and enuresis (Nicholson & Preston, 2007). Is the child immobile or disabled? Which treatments have the family already tried? Have they used any over-the-counter medications or complimentary therapies? In addition, inquiry should be made into the dietary history, exercise patterns, developmental milestones, and free-water intake per day. The last point is especially important to those patients on gastric tube feedings, who may be receiving only liquid nutrition.

A psychosocial history is also part of the evaluation. Questions should focus on the household environment, the child's relationship with different caregivers, family issues, and stressors. Child maltreatment may also present as constipation. If the child is in school, inquire as to his or her interactions with peers, whether the child uses the restrooms at school, and whether these facilities are readily accessible.

The physical examination must include a rectal examination. Visualization and palpation includes stool in the rectal vault, skin tags, rectal tone or "wink," rectal tears, prolapse, and hemorrhoids (Dilliway, 2001). Anal position may provide pertinent information about an anatomical or inflammatory condition (Nicholson & Preston, 2007). Neurological examination should focus on lower-extremity strength, tone, sensation, and cremestric reflex to evaluate for a spinal tumor or a symptomatic tethered cord. The presence of spinal dimpling with hair tufts, abnormal spinal alignment,

TABLE 26-3

Complications of Constipation
Abdominal pain
Rectal fissures
Encopresis
Urinary dysfunction
• Obstruction
• Enuresis
• Urinary tract infection
Rectal prolapse, intussusception, rectal ulceration
Stasis syndrome
• Bacterial overgrowth, fermentation, and maldigestion
• Steatorrhea
• Protein loss enteritis
Social stigma, exclusion, bullying

and irregular pigment of the lower spine should be noted. Abdominal distention requires palpation of all quadrants and for bladder distention and firm masses within the suprapubic region (Rosen et al., 2004). Severe impaction and abdominal distention may impede diaphragmatic excursion, resulting in respiratory insufficiency and distress.

DIFFERENTIAL DIAGNOSIS

Beyond the neonatal period, the majority of cases of constipation are more often derived from nonorganic causes than from organic disorders. The etiology of constipation depends on presentation of symptoms, patient age, history, and physical examination.

The causes of constipation are categorized as nonorganic and organic (Table 26-4). Nonorganic causes of constipation—also referred to as functional constipation—have no evidence of pathologic condition. Functional constipation frequently occurs in infancy due to dietary changes such as early introduction to rice cereal, excessive intake of cow's milk, or transitioning from breastfeeding to formula. The toddler and preschool period often results in the child demonstrating stool-holding behaviors for a number of reasons. Stool-holding behaviors include squatting, crossing ankles, stiffening of the body, holding on to a caregiver or furniture, flushing, sweating, and crying. Stool-holding behaviors may result from fear, anxiety, and avoidance of painful defecation during toilet training (Borowitz et al., 2005). Behavioral factors that may contribute to dysfunctional elimination include involvement in play, privacy issues, public phobias, and parenting issues (Nicholson & Preston, 2007). Psychological conditions can lead to constipation as well (Table 26-4).

Organic causes of constipation and encopresis account for only 5% of pediatric cases. Constipation can result from a large variety of pathological disorders. The differential diagnosis is often narrowed depending on the patient's age and symptoms. The most common pathological disorder is Hirschsprung's disease, which is characterized by a lack of ganglion cells in the colon and is often diagnosed in the newborn period. Delayed passage of meconium stool in the first 72 hours of life, along with abdominal distention, and bilious vomiting, should raise the HCP's suspicion for Hirschsprung's disease. Older children may present with ribbon-like stools, abdominal distention, or failure-to-thrive. Coexisting endocrine and metabolic conditions that may result in constipation include hypothyroidism, hypokalemia, hypercalcemia, cystic fibrosis, lead poisoning, celiac disease, diabetes mellitus, and infant botulism (Borowitz et al., 2005; Coughlin, 2003). Neuroanatomic defects of the spine and anus can also be associated with constipation and encopresis, such as spina occulta, spina bifida, tethered cord, displaced rectum, and imperforate anus with fistula (Coughlin).

TABLE 26-4

Differential Diagnosis of Constipation

Behavioral

- Functional fecal retention/withholding behaviors due to past painful experience
- Bathroom phobias
- Too involved with play and lack of time

Dietary

- Change of formula or breastmilk
- Lack of fiber
- Introduction of solids

Neurological

- Hirschsprung's disease
- Hypotonia syndromes, central nervous system disorders
- Neuronal dysplasia
- Infant botulism

Coexisting Medical Conditions/Illness

- Hypothyroidism
- Diabetes
- Cystic fibrosis
- Dehydration and electrolyte imbalance
- High fever
- Prolonged bed rest

Medicinal

- Over-the-counter medications
- Respiratory medication (pseudoephedrine)
- Antacids (aluminum based)
- Tricyclic antidepressants
- Anticonvulsants
- Narcotics, codeine
- Iron
- Lead poisoning

Obstructional

- Small left colon
- Pelvic tumor
- Rectal or sigmoid stricture (post surgery, post necrotizing enterocolitis)
- Congenital or acquired anal ring stenosis
- Imperforate anus
- Anterior displacement of the anus

Psychosocial Disorders

- Attention-deficit disorder
- Sexual abuse
- Over-demanding toilet training
- Depression
- Oppositional defiant disorder

PLAN OF CARE

For the majority of patients with constipation, diagnostic study is not required. Diagnostic testing is warranted to evaluate for organic causes of constipation when there is a history of neuroanatomic abnormalities, occult blood, absent anal wink, absent cremasteric reflex, abnormal lower-extremity tone, or failure-to-thrive (Baker et al., 2006). Laboratory studies may be useful if a metabolic derangement, such as hypothyroidism, is suspected (Abi-Hanna & Lake, 1998). Abdominal radiographs may be helpful in evaluating the amount of stool in the colon and the success of disimpaction interventions. Such imaging may also be useful for children in whom physical examination is difficult due to obesity or disability. Neurological disorders should be suspected when there is a sacral dimple with a tuft of hair, especially with persistent elimination dysfunction. Magnetic resonance imaging is the most definitive test for tethered cord (Rosen et al., 2004). Barium enema and rectal biopsy are performed when there is suspicion of a megacolon or Hirschsprung's disease.

The following diagnostic studies may also be performed based on the presentation:

- Stool guaiac
- Urinalysis and urine culture
- Immunoglobulin A (IgA) level for celiac disease
- Serum electrolytes
- Serum lead level

Therapeutic management begins with removal of impacted stool; maintenance therapy then focuses on prevention. Caution should be used in medication selection for patients with hepatic or renal failure due to the potential for drug toxicities.

Phase I: disimpaction

Disimpaction can be performed via the oral route or by enema. The oral route is more tolerable in children and less invasive, but it requires significant caregiver commitment. The rectal route provides for faster results, but it can be traumatic to the patient. The options should be discussed with the family; caregivers typically choose the oral route.

Several oral medications options exist for disimpaction (Table 26-5). An osmotic, oral electrolyte solution such as polyethylene glycol 3350 (PEG 3350) is often recommended (Baker et al., 2006).

Disimpaction via the rectal route utilizes enemas such as mineral oil, normal saline, or hypertonic phosphate solutions. Stimulants are often added to promote evacuation. Hospitalization may be required for severe impactions so that serial enemas can be administered and electrolytes monitored.

Disimpaction usually requires 3 to 5 days and is best accomplished at home, resulting in a school absence. After disimpaction, the child should start maintenance therapy and follow up with the HCP in 1 to 2 weeks. Relapse is common (Baker et al., 2006).

Phase II: maintenance

Maintenance therapy incorporates a combination of diet, medication, and behavioral modification. The goals of the maintenance phase are to establish normal bowel patterns, restore normal rectal tone, prevent painful bowel movements, and prevent another impaction episode. The success of management for chronic constipation depends on the understanding and cooperation of both the child (dependent on age) and caregivers.

Dietary changes include increasing consumption of fiber and fluids and decreasing consumption of dairy products. However, in a rectal vault that has lost its tone, dietary intake of fiber has no value and should be increased only when rectal tone has been restored (Abi-Hanna & Lake, 1998).

With simple constipation, a laxative should be instituted to enable the child to pass one or two stools a day (Table 26-5). Glycerin suppositories or juices that contain sorbitol can safely relieve constipation in infants. Other options that are safe for infants and young children have an osmotic effect; they include barley malt extracts and lactulose. Enemas should be avoided in infants due to their potential to produce rectal perforation or electrolyte imbalances. Effective options for older children (older than 4 years of age) include lubricant therapy such as mineral oil or osmotic laxative (magnesium hydroxide, lactulose, sorbitol, or PEG 3350) (Montgomery & Fernando, 2008).

Behavioral modification is a valuable adjunct to therapy, but requires caregiver commitment and patience for success. Families are counseled on normal evacuation patterns. One goal is for the child to toilet in a relaxed and nonforceful atmosphere. Another is to establish a daily toilet routine. This is preferably planned for 20 minutes after meals and before bedtime. Tips to reduce the discomfort with toileting are to rest the feet on a stool and ask the child to roar like a lion or blow bubbles through a straw. Reward systems should be encouraged, such as sticker charts and calendars to record successes.

Phase III: weaning

Tapering of laxatives is usually started after a normal bowel routine has been established. Follow-up is frequent and scheduled at 1-, 2-, 3-, and 6-month intervals to titrate medications and evaluate the success of strategies (Montgomery & Fernando, 2008). Tapering medications too quickly may cause a rebound effect; as a consequence, therapy is often required for as long as 1 year (Thompson, 2001). The family should be educated about the long-term nature of the problem and the need for consistence of routines and dietary behaviors.

TABLE 26-5

Medications for the Treatment of Constipation and Encopresis		
Type of Medication	**Selected Medications**	**Recommended Dosage**
Osmotic	Lactulose Sorbitol	1–3 mL/kg/day (once per day or twice per day dosing); maximum 60 mL
	Polyethylene glycol powder (PEG) (Miralax, Glycolax)	2–5 years of age: 5 mL in 60 mL of juice every day
		6–12 years of age: 10 mL in 120 mL of juice every day
		> 12 years of age: 15 mL in 180 mL of juice every day
	Magnesium hydroxide* (MOM)	1–3 mL/kg/day (once per day or twice per day); maximum 60 mL
	Magnesium citrate*	< 6 years of age: 1–3 mL/kg/day
		6–12 years of age: 100–150 mL/day
		> 12 years of age: 150–300 mL/day
Lubricant	Mineral oil	> 4 years of age: not recommended
		Disimpaction: 15–30 mL/year; maximum 240 mL
		Maintenance: 1–3 mL/kg/day
Stimulant	Sennodies (Senna; Senekot)	2–6 years: 2.5–7.5 mL/day
		6–12 years: 5–15 mL/day
	Bisacodyl (Dulcolax)	> 2 years: ½–1 (10 mg) suppository
	Glycerin suppository	Infant < 6 months of age: a sliver of pediatric suppository
		6–12 months of age: ½ pediatric suppository
		1–6 years of age: 1 pediatric or ½ adult suppository
		6–12 years of age: 1 adult suppository
Osmotic enema	Fleet*	2–11 years of age: 6 mL/kg/day pediatric enema
		> 11 years of age: adult enema or 135 mL
Juices	Apple, pear, or prune	1–4 months of age: 15 mL once per day
		> 4 months of age: 15 mL twice per day with high-fiber diet (peas, apricots, peaches, plums)

* Avoid in renal failure.
Sources: Baker et al., 2006; Schmitt, 2007.

Consultation with a pediatric gastroenterologist is indicated when therapy fails, as unidentified underlying organic disease may be playing a role (Baker et al., 2006). Psychological referral may need to be considered in complex stool-holding behaviors or when behavior modification fails.

DISPOSITION AND DISCHARGE PLANNING

Maintenance therapy should be followed for at least 4 to 6 months, especially if the constipation is related to toilet training or stool-holding behaviors (Thompson, 2001). Medication weaning may take an additional 6 months to complete. Relapse is common, so rigorous follow-up is important.

ESOPHAGEAL ATRESIA/FISTULA AND DUODENAL ATRESIA

Cindy L. Kerr

ESOPHAGEAL ATRESIA AND TRACHEOESOPHAGEAL FISTULA

Pathophysiology

Esophageal atresia (EA) refers to a congenitally interrupted esophagus, whereas a tracheoesophageal fistula (TEF) is a communicating fistula with the trachea. The foregut is develops into both the esophagus and the trachea. Pathogenesis theories for EA and TEF range from apoptosis and recanalization issues to aberrant biochemical and genetic signals (Beasley, 2005). These disturbances are thought to occur early in fetal development, within the first four weeks of gestation. Esophageal motility is adversely affected by these changes and tracheal cartilage is more pliable, leading to tracheomalacia (Spitz, 2005).

A range of anatomic variations and types of communication between the trachea and esophagus exist. Several classification systems are used to describe the variations, with one of the more common classifications identifying five variations (Table 26-6).

Epidemiology and etiology

The incidence of EA is 1 in 3,000 live births. Familial cases are extremely rare, but in twins EA is two to three times more common (Spitz, 2005). In 50% to 75% of patients with EA, at least one other malformation is seen (Harmon & Coran, 2006). The acronym VACTERL summarizes the most common malformations (Table 26-7).

Presentation

Prenatal clinical signs of EA include polyhydramnios and an ultrasound demonstrating a small or absent stomach bubble. After birth, signs of EA are seen within hours; excessive salivation that does not clear with suctioning and choking are the most common presentation. If allowed to feed, patients appear to have difficulty swallowing; they may vomit, cough, or become cyanotic and develop respiratory distress. When the defect includes a distal fistula—which occurs in 85% of patients with EA—the stomach will become distended as air passes through the fistula, resulting in abdominal distention. Placement of an oral feeding tube becomes difficult to advance beyond 10 to 11 cm in such patients (Spitz, 2005). Due to EA's high rate of association with other defects, the physical examination may reveal findings consistent with VACTERL anomalies.

Differential diagnosis

Difficulty with oral feeding can be a sign of a neurologic disorder. Coughing, which often occurs after feeding, may be a result of congenital infections such as cytomegalovirus and rubella pneumonia (Finder, 2007). Upper GI structural obstructions such as esophageal or pyloric stenosis, duodenal atresia, and annular pancreas should be considered as well. Hirschsprung's disease can also present as a mechanical bowel obstruction accompanied by vomiting and feeding intolerance similar to that seen in EA.

Plan of care

The feeding tube placed during the physical examination serves as an important marker during imaging studies. When a small amount of air is injected into the feeding tube, the pouch will expand and the air will serve as contrast to confirm the presence of an upper pouch. The end of the oral gastric tube is typically observed at the T2 to T3 level. When air is seen in the stomach and bowel, the presence of a distal fistula is confirmed; nevertheless, a gasless abdomen does not rule out the presence of a fistula. In some patients, blockage from a mucus plug or atretic segments may prevent the passage of air (Gedicke et al., 2007).

Imaging utilizing contrast in the upper pouch places the patient at risk for aspirating the hyperosmolar contrast into the lungs and should be avoided if possible. Tracheobronchoscopy is often used preoperatively to define the anatomy for surgical repair and to verify anomalous communication between the structures (Gopal & Woodward, 2007). Important preoperative considerations include the following:

- Clearing excessive fluids from the upper esophageal pouch with a sump catheter set to low intermittent suction
  - Goal: prevent aspiration, pneumonia, and abdominal distention when a fistula is present
- Upright or head-up prone positioning
  - Goal: control pouch overflow
- Intravenous fluids
  - Goal: maintain hydration, electrolyte balance, and adequate glucose levels

TABLE 26-6

Types of Esophageal Atresia	
Esophageal atresia and distal tracheoesophageal fistula	85%
Esophageal atresia alone (no fistula)	6%
Esophageal atresia with proximal distal fistula	2%
Esophageal atresia with double fistula	1%
"H" fistula	6%

Source: Spitz, 2005.

TABLE 26-7

VACTERL-Associated Malformations	
Vertebral	Hypoplastic vertebrae
Anorectal	Anal atresia, imperforate anus
Cardiac	Arterial septal defect, ventricular septal defect, patent ductus arteriosus, tetralogy of Fallot
Tracheoesophageal fistula	
Esophageal atresia	
Renal	Obstructive uropathy
Limb	Radial hypoplasia

- Prophylactic broad-spectrum antibiotics
  - Goal: treatment for possible aspiration pneumonia
- Avoid endotracheal intubation
  - Goal: avoid abdominal distention, especially if a distal fistula is present (Harmon & Coran, 2006)

The surgical procedure undertaken to correct EA depends on the type of defect. When a long-gap EA is found, the surgical approach is to create a cervical esophagostomy or "spit fistula." This approach allows drainage of the upper pouch; a gastrostomy tube is placed to allow enteral feedings. In these patients, surgical repair will be delayed until the patient has had time to grow, thereby making surgical repair easier (Harmon & Coran, 2006). Reanastamosis procedures are completed through a thoracotomy incision or thoracoscopically; laterality will depend on the location of the aortic arch.

Postoperatively, the patient will be intubated with a chest tube and nasogastric catheter. Extubation often occurs within days after surgery, and any reintubation should be completed with the assistance of the surgeon to avoid disruption of the surgical site. The chest tube is often kept in place until after feedings are started to evaluate for an anastomotic leak. The nasogastric catheter placed during surgery is strategically placed, with the tip either beyond the anastomosis or just above it. Maintaining the correct depth is essential to avoid disruption of the esophageal repair. Oral secretions are expected to continue until swelling of the anastomosis decreases.

Approximately 1 week after surgery, a contrast study of the esophagus is obtained to evaluate for an esophageal leak. If no leak is observed, oral feedings are slowly started and the chest tube is removed. Discharge should be planned to occur once oral feedings have successfully been established.

If the EA is identified prior to delivery, delivery at or transfer to a tertiary care center is recommended. Surgical consultation should be initiated as soon as there is suspicion for EA. Cardiology consultation and echocardiography are required preoperatively due to the high incidence of congenital heart lesions in patients with EA and to verify the side of the aortic arch. A right-sided arch is not uncommon; if present, it will determine the surgical approach to the EA repair (Allen et al., 2006). Consultation with anesthesia will also help ensure that the patient's airway status is stable prior to entering the operative suite.

Caregiver education initially focuses on the specific structural defects and on the plan for surgical repair. EA and TEF caregiver teaching sheets developed by the American Pediatric Surgical Nurses Association are available online at www.apsna.org. Long-term education should focus on the most common complications:

- Esophageal stricture
- Gastroesophageal reflux disease
- Dysphasia
- Tracheomalacia (Harmon & Coran, 2006)

Caregivers will need to be educated about the importance of long-term follow-up, as some complications may persist into adulthood. Input from multiple specialists—for example, surgery, pulmonology, gastroenterology, and nutrition—may be required depending on the type of complications encountered. Severity of symptoms such as gastroesophageal reflux is expected to improve as the patient grows and develops.

Disposition and discharge planning

Survival rates for all types of EA are in the range of 85% to 95%. Patients at the highest risk for poor outcomes include those who have severe pulmonary dysfunction requiring mechanical ventilation, severe associated anomalies (especially cardiac disease), birth weight less than 1,500 grams, and long-gap atresia (Harmon & Coran, 2006). Outcomes are also dependent on the presence of associated anomalies.

Close follow-up communication between the pediatrician and the surgeon is required. Common complications to anticipate include esophageal stricture, esophageal dysmotility, tracheomalacia, and gastroesophageal reflux, all of which can contribute to failure-to-thrive.

Esophageal stricture is reported to occur in as many as 80% of patients with EA (Harmon & Coran, 2006). Symptoms, which may be either acute or progressive, include dysphasia, gagging, drooling, and food refusal. Treatment usually entails serial esophageal dilations performed in the operating room. Esophageal dysmotility often requires a delay in diet advancement and avoiding difficult-to-swallow foods such as white bread and meats that are not ground or chopped. Food must be thoroughly cut, then chewed, before swallowing. Caregivers are advised to offer small amounts of food at a time so that the child will avoid swallowing a large food bolus that may become lodged in the esophagus.

Dysphasia often persists into adulthood; its prevalence in adult EA patients has been reported to be as high as 53% to 92%. Gastroesophageal reflux disease is a significant long-term problem for EA patients, which is seen in 35% to 58% of children and 46% of adult patients. Although most patients with this disorder will respond to pharmacologic intervention, 44% will require antireflux surgery to correct their condition. The major concern is that chronic reflux might develop into Barrett esophagus (Kovesi & Rubin, 2004).

Tracheomalacia is found more commonly in patients with TEF. It can be a source of significant long-term issues, including chronic cough, stridor, decreased lung capacity, and recurrent pneumonia.

DUODENAL ATRESIA

Pathophysiology

Duodenal atresia (DA) occurs in the first four weeks of gestation, when the duodenum is formed through the merger of the foregut and the midgut. Disruption or failure of recanalization of this segment is thought to be the etiology of DA (Poki et al., 2005). Such disruption results in intrinsic anomalies such as atresia, stenosis, and formation of mucosal webs. Intrinsic obstructions are commonly associated with other congenital anomalies (Table 26-8). Extrinsic obstructions can also occur, including malrotation, preduodenal portal vein, cysts, or pseudocysts of the pancreas and biliary tree (Applebaum et al., 2006).

Epidemiology and etiology

The incidence of DA is 1 per 10,000 live births. Intrinsic congenital duodenal obstruction accounts for the majority of cases and is also more likely to be accompanied by concurrent significant congenital anomalies. Neither intrinsic nor extrinsic causes are regarded as familial conditions (Mustafawi & Hassan, 2008).

Presentation

Polyhydramnios may be the first indication that a problem in the duodenum exists. Prenatal ultrasonography findings include a dilated amniotic-filled stomach and duodenum, often called the "double bubble" sign (Coliste et al., 2008). The double bubble sign becomes visible when the stomach and proximal duodenum are distended on either side of the narrow pylorus (Figure 26-7). These findings are not typically seen until the seventh or eighth month of pregnancy (O'Neill et al., 2003b).

A history of prematurity and low birth weight is common among patients with DA. In the neonatal period, frequent vomiting that starts within hours after birth is a diagnostic indicator that some form of intestinal obstruction exists. In 85% of patients with DA, emesis will appear bilious because the obstruction is located distal to the entry of the bile duct into the duodenum (O'Neill et al., 2003b). Physical examination may reveal epigastric fullness from stomach dilation, but overall the abdomen will appear flat and nondistended or scaphoid. Placement of a nasogastric tube will produce aspirate volumes larger than 20 mL. This volume exceeds the expected volume of 5 mL found in neonates without obstruction (Millar et al., 2005).

TABLE 26-8

Anomalies Associated with Duodenal Atresia	
Cardiac	Atrial septal defect, ventricular septal defect, patent ductus arteriosus
Anorectal	Vestibular anus, imperforate, cloaca
Intestinal	Malrotation, Meckel's diverticulum, small intestine atresia, annular pancreas, tracheoesophageal fistula
Genitourinary	Ectopic kidney, incomplete duplex system
Chromosomal	Trisomy 21
Hepatic	Anterior portal vein

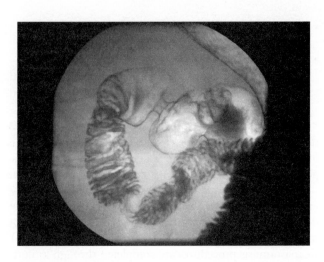

FIGURE 26-7

Duodenal Atresia: Double Bubble Sign.

Source: © Medical Body Scans/Photo Researchers, Inc.

Physical findings may also suggest trisomy 21 (Down syndrome), as approximately 30% of these patients will have DA (Mustafawi & Hassan, 2008).

Differential diagnosis

Bilious emesis in a neonate is considered a surgical emergency until proven otherwise, with the most concerning diagnosis being malrotation with volvulus. Other possible diagnoses are summarized here:

- Esophageal stenosis
- Pyloric stenosis
- Annular pancreas
- Preduodenal portal vein
- Duodenal duplication cyst
- Hirschsprung's disease (O'Neill et al., 2003b)

Plan of care

Presence of an air-filled stomach proximal to an air-filled first portion of the duodenum on an abdominal radiograph confirms the diagnosis of duodenal atresia. Absence of gas in the remaining small and large bowel is more conclusive to the presence of this abnormality. Contrast-enhanced studies are not required for diagnosis when the double bubble sign is observed.

Once the diagnosis of DA has been made, the goal is to prepare the patient for surgical repair. Adequate fluid replacement, monitoring of glucose level, and correction of electrolyte imbalance due to frequent vomiting are all needed. The nasogastric tube should be set to provide low intermittent suction to prevent recurrent vomiting and help decompress the dilated stomach and duodenum. Special attention should be given to ruling out other anomalies associated with DA, specifically cardiac anomalies.

Duodenal atresia and stenosis require surgical intervention to create intestinal continuity. Duodeno-duodenostomy, in which a diamond-shaped incision is used to join the proximal bowel to the distal bowel, is the most common surgical approach and is used in more than 80% of DA repairs (Applebaum et al., 2006). This procedure is routinely completed through an incision in the left abdominal wall or laparoscopically through three abdominal port sites.

Postoperatively, the nasogastric tube will remain in place, thereby enhancing gastric decompression. It is important that the nasogastric tube not be advanced inadvertently, as this maneuver may disrupt the surgical site. Parenteral nutrition may be required, given that initiation of feedings should not start until bowel function is demonstrated. This is accomplished by the passing of stool, decreased volume of nasogastric tube output, and clear nasogastric drainage. These signs are reassuring that bowel peristalsis has resumed, propelling gastric contents and bile forward. Oral feedings are usually started as small, 5-mL bolus feedings. The volume is slowly advanced over a period of days, with HCPs watching closely for vomiting and abdominal distention. This advancement continues until the patient's caloric needs are met. Some patients cannot tolerate larger volumes; in such circumstances, increasing the caloric concentration of the formula can help satisfy their metabolic needs using limited volumes.

Prenatal ultrasound consistent with duodenal atresia should prompt fetal medicine and pediatric surgical consultation. An in utero transfer to a tertiary center where neonatal and surgical care is available should be considered (Piper et al., 2008).

Reassure the caregiver that in the vast majority of patients, the bowel will function as intended, allowing for normal growth and development without nutritional supplements or dietary adjustments. After repair and discharge, however, these patients are at risk for development of bowel adhesions, which may potentially cause bowel obstruction. Caregivers should be instructed to seek medical care if bilious emesis is seen at any time throughout the patient's life and to alert HCPs to the patient's surgical history.

Disposition and discharge planning

Postoperative feeding intolerance is the most common complication following DA surgery. It is anticipated that normal feeding patterns will be achieved within 2 to 3 weeks post repair. Gastrointestinal motility issues can arise from stomach and duodenal dilation and surgical manipulation. Prokinetic medications may be useful in alleviating this problem (Applebaum et al., 2006). Frequent weight checks are needed during hospitalization and after discharge to ensure adequate growth is being achieved. Once full feedings are achieved and weight gain is adequate, follow-up can be planned to occur yearly. All care should be coordinated with the primary care provider.

The survival rate for patients with duodenal obstruction is 95%. Risk factors are mainly attributed to the associated anomalies, rather than to the presence of the atresia itself. Long-term complications include narrowing at the surgical site, dysfunctional peristalsis, and gastroesophageal reflux disease (Applebaum et al., 2006).

FOREIGN BODY INGESTION

Minnette Markus-Rodden

PATHOPHYSIOLOGY

The most common site of esophageal foreign body impaction is at the thoracic inlet. Radiographically, the thoracic inlet is located between the clavicles. It is also the point at which the muscle of the esophagus changes from skeletal muscle to smooth muscle (Louie & Bradin, 2009). A normal physiologic narrowing of the esophagus at the cricopharyngeus muscle contributes to the risk of foreign body impaction. The next most common sites of impaction are the gastroesophageal junction and then the aortic arch (Delghani & Ludemann, 2008). Pediatric patients with underlying esophageal disorders such as repaired tracheoesophageal fistulas are at higher risk to have esophageal foreign body impactions.

Foreign bodies that have passed safely into the stomach or lower GI tract typically pass without complication. The exceptions to this rule occur when the objects are more than 5 cm in size or very sharp (Schunk, 2006).

EPIDEMIOLOGY AND ETIOLOGY

Ingestion of foreign bodies is a common occurrence. More than 125,000 foreign body ingestions are reported each year in the United States in individuals younger than 19 years of age. Pediatric patients aged 9 to 30 months are at increased risk of foreign body ingestion due to several factors: their immature neuromuscular swallowing mechanisms, their mobility to gain access to small objects, their lack of molar teeth, and their oral orientation (Hill & Voight, 2000). The male-to-female ratio of foreign body ingestion in young children is 1:1.

Coins are the most common nonfood ingested foreign bodies, and pennies represent 45% of all coins ingested (Chen et al., 2006). In addition to coins, the most common foreign body ingestions, in order of frequency, are fibrous foods (meats, string vegetables), small toys, and batteries. Alkaline disk batteries pose an additional threat of leakage of caustic material or emissions of electrical currents, which may cause further tissue damage (Nowicki, 2000). Many toys now include small magnets, and reports of ingestions with significant morbidity are increasing despite the attempt to heighten public awareness of the danger posed by this problem.

PRESENTATION

Pediatric patients with foreign body ingestions typically present to a HCP after a witnessed ingestion, an ingestion suspected by the child or caregiver, or signs and symptoms of foreign body ingestion. Symptoms depend on the type and size of item ingested as well as the location of the foreign body.

Most ingested foreign bodies will pass without incident. Pediatric patients with foreign body ingestions may have no symptoms and caregivers may present the child for medical care only after signs and symptoms develop as a result of complications. Symptoms of foreign body ingestion vary, but may present differently depending on the location involved (Table 26-9). The most common areas for impaction, perforation, or obstruction are found at anatomic regions of narrowing, such as the cricopharyngeus muscle and the ileocecal valve (Ginsberg, 1995). It is also possible for foreign body ingestions impacted within the esophagus to distend the esophagus so that they cause airway compression (Figure 26-8). These patients may present with symptoms of airway obstruction, prompting emergency intervention and removal (Nowicki, 2000).

DIFFERENTIAL DIAGNOSIS

The differential diagnosis of pediatric patients with foreign body ingestion will vary based on the location of the object, the physical properties of the object, and the local tissue reaction to the object (Schunk, 2006). Symptoms of foreign body ingestion such as drooling, dysphagia, anorexia, abdominal pain, abdominal distention, and fever are similar to many common childhood illnesses. Therefore the differential diagnoses of pediatric patients without a witnessed or communicated foreign body ingestion are similar to typical childhood infectious illnesses such as gastroenteritis, pharyngitis, or gastroesophageal reflux (Schunk). Foreign

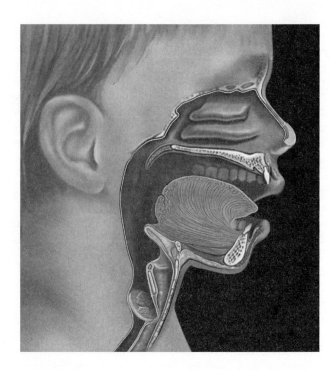

FIGURE 26-8

Airway Compression from an Esophageal Foreign Body.

body ingestions that have distended the esophagus to cause airway compromise will lead to a differential diagnosis that includes foreign body aspiration, asthma, pneumonia, or epiglottitis. In addition, patients with repeated foreign body ingestions should be evaluated for anatomic anomalies, psychiatric disorders such as bulimia and toothbrush ingestion, or air bezoars with trichillomania.

PLAN OF CARE

Diagnostic studies in a pediatric patient with a history of possible foreign body ingestion may include posterior–anterior and lateral chest radiographs (CXRs), "wide" chest radiographs including the oropharynx, soft-tissue lateral neck radiographs, and abdominal radiographs. Handheld metal detectors have also been used to identify the presence of metallic foreign bodies (Delghani & Ludemann, 2008).

Chest radiographs can be used to diagnose the location of the foreign body if the object is radiopaque. Radiographic findings typically reveal esophageal foreign bodies lying in the transverse plane, whereas tracheal foreign bodies are typically oriented vertically. The presence of mediastinal or peritoneal free air is indicative of perforation.

The appropriate therapeutic plan for the ingested foreign body depends on the location of the object, the physical properties of the object, and the symptoms the

TABLE 26-9

Symptoms of Foreign Body Ingestion	
Esophageal Foreign Body	**Stomach/Lower GI Tract Foreign Body**
Dysphagia	Abdominal pain
Drooling	Abdominal distention
Pain	Emesis, hematemesis
Emesis, hematemesis	Melena, hematochezia
Anorexia/weight loss	Unexplained fever
Stridor, cough, respiratory distress	Weight loss
Sore throat, chest pain	
Unexplained fever	

pediatric patient is exhibiting. Most objects located at the gastroesophageal junction will pass spontaneously. A stepwise treatment plan should be established. In the case of a known or suspected ingestion, CXR and/or abdominal radiograph should be obtained. Foreign bodies impacted within the esophagus or causing symptoms should be removed, using any of the several methods recommended for removal of esophageal foreign bodies (Table 26-10). Foreign bodies within the stomach or within the distal GI tract may be managed by observation only. Exceptions to this management are when the object poses a threat, such as with magnets and sharp or long objects. In these circumstances, surgical removal may be necessary.

Consultation with general surgery, otolaryngology, gastroenterology, and radiology services may inform the therapeutic plan. Patients at risk for airway obstruction or toxic/corrosive ingestion may require intensive care.

Even the most fastidious caregiver can miss foreign body ingestions in young children. Education should be provided to the caregiver regarding prevention of foreign body ingestion in the context of the patient's age and risk factors. This information should include anticipatory guidance regarding food types, careful supervision during meals, keeping dangerous objects out of reach, and attention to toy safety and labeling. Not all ingested objects occur in young children, however: Adolescents and adults can also accidently ingest items such as pen caps and safety pins. Persons of all ages should be taught ingestion prevention measures. Caregivers should also be offered training in first aid and choking rescue procedures.

DISPOSITION AND DISCHARGE PLANNING

The discharge criteria for retained foreign body ingestions remain controversial. In general, the discharge criteria are dictated by the object ingested and the resulting injury, the patient's condition, and the bodily threat posed by the object. Consideration of removal of esophageal foreign bodies should be made if the patient is exhibiting symptoms or if the object does not pass into the gastroesophageal junction after 16 to 24 hours. Serial radiographs and abdominal examinations every 5 to 7 days can follow retained foreign objects through to the stomach or lower GI tract if questions about safe passage arise (Schunk, 2006).

Pediatric patients who have undergone endoscopic removal of esophageal foreign bodies with no operative complications and with minimal postoperative risk factors are typically discharged home within 24 hours. Complications and the previous health state of the patient with foreign body ingestion, such as a history of tracheoesophageal fistula, may require further medical management.

TABLE 26-10

Recommendations for Removal of Esophageal Foreign Bodies

Rigid or Flexible Endoscopy

Rigid endoscopy is performed under general anesthesia and should be used to retrieve objects that pose a threat, such as sharp objects, and for objects lodged at the level of the hypopharynx or cricopharyngeus muscle (Ginsberg, 1995).

Balloon-Tipped Catheters

This method is typically performed using fluoroscopy. The pediatric patient is placed in Trendelenberg position; the catheter is inserted and passed beyond the foreign body. The balloon is then inflated and the catheter is withdrawn, bringing the foreign body with it. This method has been criticized for its associated lack of airway control, episodes of vomiting, esophageal perforation, and inadequate visualization of the esophagus (Schunk, 2006; Waltzman, 2006).

Esophageal Bougienage

This method is performed by using a semi-rigid esophageal Bougie dilator and slowly advancing the object distally. It has been successful in cases of single coin ingestions, but complications have occurred when it was used to remove multiple ingested objects.

Medications

Historically, many medications, such as glucagon, have been used in an attempt to enhance passage of the foreign body from the esophagus. More recent studies show little or no advantage of administering these medications to aid in the passage of esophageal foreign bodies.

> **Critical Thinking**
>
> Neither a negative history nor the absence of symptoms excludes the possibility of foreign body ingestion. Any patient exhibiting symptoms of foreign body ingestion or having ingested a foreign body that is longer than 5 cm, has sharp edges, or contains corrosive material should receive prompt evaluation.

HEPATITIS

Randolph M. McConnie

PATHOPHYSIOLOGY

The liver is irrigated by the portal vein and the hepatic arteries, and drained by the hepatic veins. Bile is drained via the biliary system. The liver also has a lymphatic drainage system. Hepatic function regulates the metabolism of glucose, lipids, nitrogen, and drugs and is involved in the synthesis of proteins such as albumin and coagulation factors. The liver forms bile and bile acids, both of which are important in assisting in gastrointestinal digestion.

Hepatitis implies an inflamed liver, rather than elevated aminotransferase levels. Older terminology differentiates between acute (less than 6 months' duration) and chronic (more than 6 months' duration) hepatitis. Chronic hepatitis can present with acute symptoms; thus this terminology may at times be misleading.

EPIDEMIOLOGY AND ETIOLOGY

The liver can be damaged by many different means—toxins, viral and bacterial infections, hemodynamic instability, passive congestion, storage diseases (copper, iron, fat, glycogen), or autoimmune injury (Table 26-11). With viral forms of hepatitis, incubation periods can vary from 2 to 20 weeks. Toxin exposure can injure the liver either acutely or after prolonged exposure.

TABLE 26-11

Drugs and Toxins Causing Hepatocellular Injury

Acute Injury

Acarbose
Acetaminophen
Allopurinol
Amoxicillin/clavulanate
Bromfenac
Buproprion
Ciprofloxacin
Diclofenac
Fluoxetine
Isoniazid
Itraconazole
Ketoconazole
Lisinopril
Losertan
Nefazodone
Nevirapine
Nitrofurantoin
Paroxetene
Pyrazinamide
Rifampin
Risperidone
Ritonavir
Sertraline
Statins
Tetracycline
Trazodone
Trimethoprim–sulfamethoxazole
Troglitazone
Trovafloxacin
Valproic acid

TABLE 26-11

Drugs and Toxins Causing Hepatocellular Injury (Continued)

Cholestatic Injury

Anabolic steroids
Azathioprine
Chlorpromazine
Clopidogrel
Cytarabine
Erythromycin
Estrogen
Flucloxacillin
Fosinopril
Irbesartan
Minocycline
Nitrofurantoin
Phenothiazines
Sulindac
Terbinafine
Tricyclics
Trimethoprim–sulfamethoxazole

Mixed Injury

Amitryptilline
Azathiprine
Captopril
Carbamazepin
Clindamycin
Cyproheptadine
Enalapril
Flutamide
Ibuprofen
Nitrofurantoin
Phenobarbital
Phenytoin
Sulfonamides
Traxodone
Trimethoprim–sulfamethoxazole
Verapamil

Steatohepatitis

Amatoxins (from poisonous mushrooms)
Amiodarone
Carbon tetrachloride
Chlorinated hydrocarbons
Chloroform
Cynaobacterium toxins
Nucleoside reverse transcriptase inhibitors
Tamoxifen
Tetracycline
Trichloroethylene
Valproic acid
White phosphorus

(Continued)

TABLE 26-11

Drugs and Toxins Causing Hepatocellular Injury (Continued)

Granulomatous Hepatitis

Amoxicillin/clavulanate
Diltiazem
Pyrazinamide
Quinine
Sulfa drugs

Sinusoidal Obstruction

Busulfan
Cyclophosphamide

Fibrosis

Methotrexate

Hepatic Adenoma

Oral contraceptives

Autoimmune Hepatitis

Minocycline
Nitrofurantoin

Herbs Causing Hepatotoxicity

Atractylis gummifera from the Mediterranean region
Black cohosh (*Actaea racemosa/Cimicifuga racemosa*) from the United States and Canada
Camphor
Cascara sagrada
Chaparral (*Larrea tridentate*) from the Southwest United States and Mexico
Chinese herbal medicines
    Chaso and onshido from China
    Dai-saiko-to and sho-saiko-to from China and Japan (Kampo medicine)
    Jin bu huan (*Lycopodium serratum*) from China and found worldwide
    Ma huang (*Ephedra sinica*) from Mongolia
    Shou-wa-pian (*Polygonum multiforme*) from China
Cloves (oil)
Comfrey/pyrrolizidine alkaloids (*Heliotropium, Senecio, Crotalaria*) in bush tea from Jamaica
Germander (*Teucrium chamaedrys*) in Europe and the Middle East
Greater celandine (*Chelidonium majus*) from Europe
Impila (*Callilipis laureola*) from South Africa
Isabgol
Kava (*Piper methysticum*) from the South Sea Islands
Margosa oil
Mistletoe (*Viscum album*)
Paeonia spp,
Pennyroyal (a mint oil)
Sassafras

TABLE 26-11

Drugs and Toxins Causing Hepatocellular Injury (Continued)

Herbs Causing Hepatotoxicity

Skullcap (*Scutellaria*) from North America
Usnic acid
Valerian (*Valeriana officinalis*) from Europe and parts of Asia

Sources: Adapted from Chang & Shiano, 2007; Polson, 2010; Seef, 2007.

PRESENTATION

Hepatitis may present in a silent, asymptomatic way, often recognized only when elevation in the aminotransferase levels is found incidentally on laboratory study for another purpose. Alternatively, it may present with acute onset of jaundice, fever, joint pains, right upper quadrant pain, generalized weakness, malaise, altered mental status, nausea, vomiting, kidney failure, elevated central nervous system pressure, or cardiovascular collapse. The presence of dark urine (bilirubin excretion) may coincide with the onset of jaundice. In terms of patient history, exposure to sick individuals, chemicals, drugs, herbs, and travel should be explored as pertinent to this disorder.

Physical examination findings can range from none to jaundice, palmar erythema, spider angiomata, asterixis, joint inflammation, a distended abdomen from hepatosplenomegaly or ascites, peripheral edema, ecchymosis skin, petechiae, altered mental status, poorly reactive pupils (a sign of cerebral edema), and tenderness to palpation of or percussion over the liver.

DIFFERENTIAL DIAGNOSIS

Once the liver is established as the source of the elevated enzymes, the cause of the hepatitis needs to be determined. The differential diagnoses for hepatitis are extensive (Table 26-12).

PLAN OF CARE

Diagnostic study findings include elevated aminotransferases (ALT/AST), direct bilirubin, and elevated alkaline phosphatase, though not all patients with an elevated ALT and AST have hepatitis. Patients with muscular injury such as muscular dystrophy and rhabdomyolysis may present with elevated enzymes, normal alkaline phosphatase, and normal GGT. These transaminases are also produced by muscle; thus, in the absence of cholestasis (elevated bilirubin and alkaline phosphatase or GGT), the HCP should question the possibility of the increased ALT and AST levels

TABLE 26-12

Differential Diagnoses for Hepatitis

Viral

Hepatitis A
Hepatitis B
Hepatitis D
Hepatitis E
Hepatitis G
Cytomegalovirus
Epstein-Barr virus
Enterovirus
Echovirus
Coxsackievirus
Rubella
Varicella
Human immunodeficiency virus

Autoimmune (Nonviral)

Type 1 (positive ANA, anti-SMA)
Type 2 (positive anti-LKM1)
Serum sickness/drug reaction (immune complex illness)

Vascular/Ischemic Injury

Budd-Chiari syndrome
Passive congestion of the liver
Ischemic injury due to shock

Toxins

Heavy metals
Antiepileptic drugs
Other drugs
Alcohol
Chemicals (teas, chemical toxins)

Bacterial

Metabolic/Genetic

Wilson disease
Hemochromatosis
Cystic fibrosis
α_1-Antitrypsin deficiency
Progressive familial intrahepatic cholestasis
Mitochondrial disorders
Alagille syndrome
Fatty liver

Anatomic

Primary sclerosing cholangitis
Obstructive cholangitis
Secondary sclerosing cholangitis (related to surgery)
Neoplasm

Antinuclear antibody (ANA), anti-smooth muscle antibody (anti-SMA), anti-liver/kidney microsoma-1 (anti-LKM1).

originating as a result of muscle injury by checking the creatine phosphokinase (CPK) level. A very rapid rise in aminotransferase levels may present with a vascular or

TABLE 26-13

Diagnostic Studies for Hepatitis

Complete blood count (CBC) with differential
Reticulocyte count
Blood smear examination
Albumin, total protein
Prothrombin time (PT)/partial thrombin time (PTT)
Alanine aminotransferase (ALT), aspartate aminotransferase (AST)
Alkaline phosphatase
Gamma-glutamyl transpeptidase (GGT)
Electrolytes
Blood urea nitrogen (BUN), creatinine
Viral serologies: HbsAg, anti-HbsAg, anti-HB core, hepatitis C, anti-HAV, HIV (human immunodeficiency virus), EBV (Epstein-Barr virus), CMV (cytomegalovirus), hepatitis D (if positive for HbsAg)
Ceruloplasmin level
Iron, total iron-binding capacity, ferritin
Antinuclear antibody (ANA), antimicrosomal antibody (AMA), anti-LKM1 (anti-liver, kidney, microsomal 1 antibody), SMA (smooth muscle antibody)
Toxicology screen (acetaminophen level)
Abdominal ultrasound with Doppler of the hepatic vessels
Evaluation of stool color and stool hemoccult
Liver biopsy

hemodynamic insult (as in shock or acute obstruction to hepatic drainage), an acute viral infection, or exposure to a toxin. A rapid drop in aminotransferase levels may indicate recovery or worsening hepatic failure if it is accompanied by a worsening prothrombin time (PT) or a rising bilirubin level and collapsing liver size.

Whenever hepatitis is suspected, liver functions should be assessed and monitored (Table 26-13). Sick individuals with vomiting, hemodynamic instability, altered mental status, or failing hepatic function require inpatient care and close monitoring.

Assessment of factors that are produced in the liver (Table 26-14)—such as, bilirubin, PT, albumin, and ammonia—may help to determine the status of hepatic function. Glucose, which is also produced in the liver, is important in gluconeogenesis; a low sugar value may suggest hepatic failure or a glycogen storage disease. A normal factor VIII level (not produced in the liver) in light of low concentrations of liver-produced factors argues in favor of liver dysfunction. A low factor VIII level (in the absence of hemophilia) with low liver-produced factors argues for disseminated intravascular coagulation (DIC), rather than liver failure. An elevated PT may indicate poor hepatic function or malabsorption of vitamin K. The HCP can distinguish vitamin K malabsorption from hepatic insufficiency by giving the patient vitamin K subcutaneously to see whether the PT returns to a normal range or

TABLE 26-14

Clotting Factors Produced in the Liver
Fibrinogen
Prothrombin (Vitamin K dependent)
Factor V
Factor VII (Vitamin K dependent)
Factor IX (Vitamin K dependent)
Factor X (Vitamin K dependent)

by checking levels of vitamin K–dependent factors. A low factor VII level (vitamin K dependent) with a normal factor V level (not vitamin K dependent) would argue for vitamin K deficiency, rather than liver dysfunction. Low factor V and VII levels suggest the presence of liver dysfunction or DIC. However, a normal factor VIII level would negate the possibility of DIC, while a low factor VIII level would support a diagnosis of DIC or hemophilia.

Declining platelet levels may indicate DIC or onset of portal hypertension with spleen sequestration of platelets. A high total protein-to-albumin ratio suggests an autoimmune process as the etiology.

An abdominal ultrasound with Doppler studies of the hepatic vessels may be useful to determine the patency of the hepatic vessels and the velocity and direction of portal vein flow, thereby evaluating vascular etiologies of hepatic injury. Liver echogenicity can suggest an etiology of the inflammation, as in the case of fatty infiltration. A liver biopsy is sometimes necessary to ascertain the exact etiology of the hepatitis.

The goal of the therapy should be to keep the patient hemodynamically stable, with a normal glucose level and stable or normal hepatic function. The patient who has hemodynamic stability, normal clotting studies, no vomiting, and a normal mental status can be assessed and monitored on an outpatient basis. In contrast, the patient who is hemodynamically unstable or demonstrates mental status changes needs to be hospitalized and monitored closely for signs of acute hepatic failure and cerebral edema.

Therapeutic management for hepatitis is initially supportive. Patients who show signs of hepatic insufficiency or failure may need aggressive supportive intervention. By comparison, patients with vomiting and dehydration may need only bowel rest and hydration. In patients presenting with an abnormal PT, admission to the hospital for close monitoring may be indicated, because such patients may progress to fulminant hepatic failure. For those patients suspected of having autoimmune hepatitis, steroids may be beneficial. In patients with hepatitis B, hepatitis C, and HIV, antiviral treatment options may need to be considered.

Consultation with gastroenterology or hepatology specialists is recommended for those patients requiring hospital admission. Subspecialty referral may be needed based on the underlying cause, including consultation with toxicology, pulmonology, and infectious diseases specialists.

Patient and family education should be provided regarding disease progression and ways to prevent further transmission of the disease for those patients with infectious etiologies. Patients with acute hepatitis A can shed virus and be infectious via the fecal–oral route. Patients with hepatitis B or C need to be on needle precautions, practice safe sex with their non-immune sexual partners, and avoid the sharing of objects such as razors and toothbrushes. All patients should be encouraged to immunize themselves against viruses (e.g., hepatitis A, hepatitis B) that may produce liver disease.

DISPOSITION AND DISCHARGE PLANNING

If the patient's hepatitis resulted from an overdose of medication, appropriate psychiatric support needs to be provided. The patient's hepatic function should be tracked after discharge, and depending on the etiology of the hepatitis, compliance with medications such as steroids for autoimmune hepatitis should be monitored. If the patient remains cholestatic, fat-soluble vitamins should be supplemented. For patients with portal hypertension, evaluation for esophageal or gastric varices should be performed and prophylaxis with propranolol considered. If the patient has developed hepatic encephalopathy, treatment with antibiotics or lactulose may be warranted.

Autoimmune hepatitis, hepatitis B, and hepatitis C may lead to chronic hepatitis and predispose patients to liver cancer if they develop cirrhosis. Given this possibility, such patients need to be monitored for an extended period of time. If the patient survives acute hepatitis A and does not develop aplastic anemia during recovery, hepatitis A should cause no long-lasting injury to the liver.

GASTROENTERITIS

Jill Marks

PATHOPHYSIOLOGY

Gastroenteritis is generally acquired via the fecal–oral route, and can be transmitted through person-to-person contact, contaminated food or water, or fomites. The pathophysiology of infectious gastroenteritis differs depending on the causative agent.

Bacterial enteropathogens may cause an inflammatory or non-inflammatory response in the intestinal mucosa by adherence, invasion, cytotoxic production, or enterotoxin production. Bacteria produce toxins that bind directly to enterocyte receptors, stimulating secondary messengers and resulting in increased fluid secretion, loss of water, stool, and electrolytes, and/or decreased absorption (Bhutta, 2007; Centers for Disease Control and Prevention [CDC], 2003).

Viral enteropathogens promote lysis of mucosal enterocytes, which interferes with the function of micovilli brush border and results in electrolyte and carbohydrate malabsorption (Barnes & Townley, 1973). In viral gastroenteritis, the direct inoculation of mature enterocytes on the villi of the small intestine leads to cell death, sloughing, and shortening of villi, resulting in diminished absorptive function. Mature enterocytes are replaced with immature secretor cells. The decreased absorption and increased secretion results in osmotic diarrhea (Bhutta, 2007). Certain viruses, especially rotavirus, can alter water and electrolyte transport by opening calcium channels, resulting in cellular gain of calcium and loss of sodium and water; this process may ultimately lead to cell death. Furthermore, inhibition of sodium chloride (NaCl)–coupled transport and cell loss of chloride result in increased secretion and loss of water to the intestinal lumen. Stimulation of the enteric nervous system also produces increased secretion of electrolytes and intestinal water loss (Wilhelmi et al., 2003).

Parasitic organisms invade gastrointestinal mucosal epithelial cells and cause villus atrophy. This phenomenon may lead to fluid loss via enterotoxin-induced secretions and eventual malabsorption (Bitterman & Zich, 2006).

EPIDEMIOLOGY AND ETIOLOGY

Gastroenteritis is a common illness in children worldwide, with an estimated 1.5 billion episodes and 1.2 to 2.5 million deaths occurring in children younger than the age of 5 years. Morbidity and mortality vary widely based on geographic location and industrialization. In the United States, acute gastroenteritis and dehydration are responsible for more than 1.5 million outpatient visits, 200,000 hospitalizations, and 300 deaths per year, resulting in approximately $1 billion per year in economic costs to society (CDC, 2003). While the hospitalization rate for gastroenteritis decreased between the years 1994 and 2000, the hospitalization rate for dehydration did not (Agency for Healthcare Research and Quality [AHRQ], 2004).

The most common organisms associated with gastroenteritis are viruses including rotavirus, adenovirus, astrovirus, calcivirus, coronavirus, sapovirus, and parvovirus. Subtypes exist for each class of virus, and epidemiology differs depending on location and season (Wilhelmi et al., 2003).

Bacterial causes of gastroenteritis include *Staphylococcus, Escherichia coli, Campylobacter, Salmonella, Shigella, Yersinia, Vibrio parahaemolyticus, Aeromonas, Bacillus cereus, Clostridium perfringens,* and *Clostridium difficile* (Bitterman & Zich, 2006). Bacterial infections may cause GI symptoms in the same manner as viral infections.

Protozoa and parasites such as *Cryptosporidium, Isospora,* and *Cycospora* may cause infection resulting in fluid loss and malabsorption. *Giardia* and *Enteromonas hominis* parasites directly infect the small bowel, leading to malabsorption (Bitterman & Zich, 2006).

PRESENTATION

The most common symptoms of gastroenteritis include fever, vomiting, and diarrhea, although these three symptoms need not occur simultaneously to make a diagnosis. Other systemic symptoms may be present, such as myalgias, headache, fatigue, rashes, and upper respiratory symptoms; these symptoms are usually related to the underlying infection.

Because diarrhea may be defined differently by caregivers and HCPs, the HCP should ask the caregiver to be very specific in his or her description of the child's symptoms. Definitions of diarrhea may include (1) a normal bowel movement that has an increased frequency and larger water content or (2) a stool output of more than three 3 episodes per day. Diarrhea can be classified as acute (lasting 14 days or less), persistent (more than 14 days), or chronic (more than 30 days) (Guerrant et al., 2001). Determining the classification of diarrhea will narrow the differential diagnosis.

If vomiting is present, its quantity, timing, color (in particular, noting any bloody or bright green color), consistency, and relation to food intake should be established. The time of the most recent episode of vomiting should be noted. If the patient describes diarrhea, quantify the number of episodes, color, consistency, and presence of blood. Inquire about the usual bowel habits, including the date of the patient's last "normal" bowel movement, any history of straining with stool, hard stools, prior episodes of diarrhea, and any previous blood in the stool. If the patient is febrile, note the duration of fever as well as the use, dose, timing, and patient's response to antipyretics.

Abdominal pain is a common symptom of gastroenteritis, but may also be a symptom of many other pediatric disorders; thus a thorough history of the pain may help narrow the differential diagnosis. A pain history should elicit the onset, duration, quality, and location of pain as well as any aggravating or alleviating factors. Any recent trauma or exposure to toxins or exposure to other sick individuals should be noted. A travel history is important and should be further investigated, especially if the travel occurred outside the United States or to an area in the United States with a known outbreak of GI illness.

Inquire about any underlying medical conditions, allergies, or food intolerance the patient has. The patient's medications, especially antidiarrheals, including any herbal and over-the-counter (OTC) medications, should be noted. Recent antibiotic use should prompt concern for *C. difficile* infection.

TABLE 26-15

Symptoms Associated with Dehydration

Symptom	Minimal or no dehydration (<3% loss of body weight)	Mild to moderate dyhdration (3%–9% loss of body weight)	Severe dehydration (>9% loss of body weight)
Mental status	Well; alert	Normal, fatigued or restless, irritable	Apathetic, lethargic, unconscious
Thirst	Drinks normally; might refuse liquids	Thirsty; eager to drink	Drinks poorly, unable to drink
Hearth rate	Normal	Normal to increased	Tachycardia, with bradycardia in most severe cases
Quality of pulses	Normal	Normal to decreased	Weak, thready, or impalpable
Breathing	Normal	Normal; fast	Deep
Eyes	Normal	Slightly sunken	Deeply sunken
Tears	Present	Decreased	Absent
Mouth and tongue	Moist	Dry	Parched
Skin fold	Instant recoil	Recoil in <2 seconds	Recoil in >2 seconds
Capillary refill	Normal	Prolonged	Prolonged; minimal
Extremities	Warm	Cool	Cold; mottled; cyanotic
Urine output	Normal to decreased	Decreased	Minimal

Source: Courtesy of Centers for Disease Control and Prevention. (2003). Managing acute gastroenteritis among children oral rehydration, maintenance, and nutritional therapy. MMWR, 52(16).

Given that the symptoms of gastroenteritis may mimic those associated with other conditions and may be somewhat vague, a full review of systems and pertinent family history should be completed. Particular attention should be paid to any gynecological or genitourinary symptoms the patient reports, as similar symptoms are often noted. Any positive findings on the review of systems that are not consistent with gastroenteritis should prompt the HCP to consider other diagnoses when determining the therapeutic management for the patient.

In the pediatric patient, a comprehensive physical examination should include ongoing mental status assessment. Physical examination findings of mild to moderate dehydration are also common with gastroenteritis and directly related to the degree of fluid loss and the body's compensatory mechanisms to manage the losses (Table 26-15). Skin turgor and tissue perfusion should be assessed, and will help classify degree of dehydration. Sunken eyes and pupillary reaction may identify possible CNS illness and aid in classification of dehydration.

Any concern for variation or abnormality should prompt a more complete neurological examination. Periorbital edema associated with bloody diarrhea may be indicative of hemolytic uremic syndrome. Ear infections may cause fever, vomiting, and diarrhea; thus it is important that the HCP visualize the tympanic membranes. Examination of the mouth and oropharynx should be performed, as dry mucous membranes may be a sign of dehydration. Any oral lesions should be noted, as they may be a sign of inflammatory bowel disease or certain viral illnesses. Erythema in the oropharynx or malodorous breath may be evidence of sinusitis or pharyngitis, both of which can present with fever, abdominal pain, and vomiting.

Particular attention should be paid to the abdominal examination. External inspection may reveal signs of trauma or injury, although lack of external evidence does not exclude the possibility of internal injury. Any abdominal distention or visible masses should be noted. Auscultation should reveal bowel sounds in four quadrants, although in gastroenteritis these sounds may be either hypoactive or hyperactive. Palpation of the abdomen should be done last, and each quadrant should be palpated individually in an attempt to localize the pain if reported. Examine the patient for any peritoneal signs, including rebound tenderness, hepatomegaly, splenomegaly, and abdominal masses. Any tenderness to the right lower quadrant should raise concern for appendicitis, while right upper quadrant pain may indicate a liver or gallbladder etiology. Pain to the left upper quadrant may be associated with the pancreas or spleen, pain at the costovertebral angle may indicate kidney infection, and flank pain may be related to pyelonephritis. Localized pain is a red flag that the patient may have pathology other than gastroenteritis.

Evaluation in the primary care provider's office, urgent care, or emergency department is recommended in the following circumstances:

- Infants who are younger than 6 months of age or who weigh less than 8 kg
- Chronic illness, prematurity, or concurrent illness
- Fever of 38°C (104.4°F) or higher in infants or 39°C (102.2°F) or less in children 3 to 36 months of age

- Bloody stool
- High stool output or persistent vomiting
- Report of symptoms consistent with dehydration
- Changes in mental status
- Lack of response to oral rehydration (CDC, 2003)

DIFFERENTIAL DIAGNOSIS

Infectious gastroenteritis, as previously noted, generally causes vomiting, diarrhea, and fever. While deviation from this classic triad does not exclude a diagnosis of gastroenteritis, it should prompt the HCP to carefully consider other possibilities in the differential diagnosis, especially for those patients with underlying chronic illnesses or developmental delays that may complicate the physical exam findings. Additional causes to consider (not previously described) include chronic nonspecific diarrhea (toddler's diarrhea), food allergy, lactose intolerance, intussusception, ileus, pseudomembranous colitis, and bowel obstruction. Radiation colitis, cystic fibrosis (CF), hemolytic uremic syndrome (HUS), malabsorption, and various medication side effects may also present with symptoms of diarrhea.

PLAN OF CARE

If the patient is diagnosed with infectious gastroenteritis and presents with minimal or moderate dehydration, diagnostic studies are rarely indicated. Stool cultures for bacterial and parasitic infections or stools for leukocyte count are usually indicated only for patients with bloody diarrheal stools. Such studies are not necessary in those individuals with watery diarrhea unless illness persists, the patient does not respond to rehydration efforts, or the patient experiences worsening illness. For those patients in whom the diagnosis is less clear, diagnostic studies will be based on the results of the history and clinical examination (CDC, 2003). Review the discussion of dehydration and fluid management in Chapter 25 for a detailed description of the diagnostic studies and therapeutic management for severe dehydration.

For most patients with acute gastroenteritis, care can be managed at home, especially those children with minimal or no dehydration. The CDC published guidelines in 2003 for the treatment of acute gastroenteritis, which were subsequently endorsed by the American Academy of Pediatrics (AAP) in 2004. These guidelines suggest oral rehydration as the primary treatment for mild to moderate dehydration. Contraindications to oral rehydration include severe dehydration/shock, severe vomiting or ileus, or lack of caregiver supervision in the administration of oral rehydration therapy (ORT).

ORT is divided into two phases—rehydration and maintenance. In the rehydration phase, pediatric patients should receive water and electrolytes in the form of an oral rehydration solution (ORS) administered over 3 to 4 hours to quickly replace what has been lost. The maintenance phase follows, including reinstitution of nutrition. Gut rest is not recommended. Breastfed infants should continue nursing even during the rehydration phase. Additional fluid should be provided for ongoing losses during both phases of ORT (AAP, 2004; CDC, 2003). The World Health Organization (WHO) developed a standard ORS that can be used with ORT and has a sodium concentration of 75 mEq/L, a glucose concentration of 75 mmol/L, and a total osmolarity of 245 mOsm/L. In the United States and other developed countries, similar solutions are commercially available (Table 26-16).

The CDC guidelines for ORT can be divided into those for patients with minimal or no dehydration, mild to moderate dehydration, and severe dehydration. For patients with minimal or no dehydration, the goal is to provide fluids and nutrition while preventing dehydration:

- Use ORS for maintenance fluids. Provide an additional 60 to 120 mL of replacement fluid for each episode of vomiting or diarrhea in a patient weighing less than 10 kg, or 120 to 240 mL in a patient weighing more than 10 kg.
- Offer an age-appropriate diet.
- Home management is feasible.

For patients with mild to moderate dehydration, the goal is to first replace fluid deficits and then maintain hydration and nutrition throughout the illness:

- Give 50 to 100 mL/kg ORS for replacement of fluid deficits over 2 to 4 hours.
- Give an additional 60 to 120 mL of replacement fluid for each episode of vomiting or diarrhea in a patient weighing less than 10 kg, or 120 to 240 mL in a patient weighing more than 10 kg during both the replacement and maintenance phases.
- Start with small ORS volumes (5–10 mL), offer them every 5 to 10 minutes, and slowly increase the volume as tolerated.
- If the patients refuses to take ORS by mouth, ORS via nasogastric tube is recommended and proven safe and effective in patients who are vomiting.
- Once losses have been replaced and vomiting has subsided, an age-appropriate diet should begin immediately, as ORS does not contain sufficient calories or nutrition when used alone. Continue ORS as maintenance fluid.
- Observation until signs of dehydration are resolved is needed, after which home management is feasible if the caregivers are able to demonstrate efficient delivery of ORT; they can return to the hospital if the patient's condition warrants more complex care.

TABLE 26-16

Oral Rehydrating Solutions

Solution	Carbohydrate (gm/L)	Sodium (mmol/L)	Potassium (mmol/L)	Chloride (mmol/L)	Base* (mmol/L)	Osmolarity (mOsm/L)
ORS						
World Health Organization (WHO) (2002)	13.5	75	20	65	30	245
WHO (1975)	20	90	20	80	30	311
European Society of Paediatric Gastroenterology, Hepatology, and Nutrition	16	60	20	60	30	240
Enfalyte®	30	50	25	45	34	200
Pedialyte®§	25	45	20	35	30	250
Rehydralyte®¶	25	75	20	65	30	305
CeraLyte®**	40	50–90	20	NA‡	30	220
Commonly Used beverage (not appropriate for diarrhea treatment)						
Apple juice§§	120	0.4	44	45	N/A	730
Coca Cola¶¶ Classic	112	1.6	N/A	N/A	13.4	650

* Actual or potential bicarbonate (e.g., lactate, citrate, or acetate).

‡ Mead-Johnson Laboratories, Princeton, New Jersey. Additional information is available at http://www.meadjohnson.com/products/cons-infant/enfalyte.html

§ Ross Laboratories (Abbott Laboratories), Columbus, Ohio. Data regarding Flavored and Freezer Pop Pedialyte are identical. Additional information is available at http://www.pedialyte.com

¶ Ross Laboratories (Abbott Laboratories), Columbus, Ohio. Additional information is available at http://rpdcon40.ross.com/pn/PediatricProducts.NSF/web_Ross.com_XML_PediatricNutrition/96A5745B1183947385256A80007546E5?OpenDocument

** Cera Products, LLC, Jessup, Maryland. Additional information is available at http://www.ceralyte.com/index.htm

‡ Not applicable.

§§ Meeting U.S. Department of Agriculture minimum requirements.

¶¶ Coca-Cola Corporation, Atlanta, Georgia. Figures do not include electrolytes that might be present in local water used for bottling. Base = phosphate.

Source: Courtesy of Centers for Disease Control and Prevention. (2003). Managing acute gastroenteritis among children oral rehydration, maintenance, and nutritional therapy. *MMWR, 52*(16).

In patients with severe dehydration, the initial fluid replacement is administered intravenously. Once the patient is stabilized and alert, ORS may be administered by mouth or nasogastric tube.

Antidiarrheal medications are not recommended for pediatric patients, as no studies that prove their effectiveness have been published and their side-effect profile (drowsiness, opiate-induced ileus) may limit their safety in children. Antibiotics are usually not indicated because most gastroenteritis is of viral origin. Disease-specific recommendations for bacterial gastroenteritis are outlined in the AAP's (2009a) *Red Book.*

Limited evidence exists regarding the use of antiemetics to reduce vomiting associated with gastroenteritis. However, a single dose of ondansetron or metoclopramide will reduce the amount of vomiting and ameliorate the need for intravenous rehydration in many children. In one study, while a slight increase in diarrhea was associated with the use of the medications, it did not appear to lead to an adverse outcome (Alhashimi et al., 2009). HCPs should be aware of the potential for side effects when administering any antiemetic and consider the risk versus the benefit of using such drugs. Antinausea medications such as ondansetron may be used for a short duration to provide relief from vomiting and allow for oral rehydration. Patients should not be prescribed home doses, however, as re-evaluation of the patient is indicated if vomiting persists (Alhashimi et al.).

Evidence is emerging regarding the efficacy of the use of zinc supplements and probiotics for patients with acute gastroenteritis. While more studies are needed to firmly establish their benefits, these treatments show encouraging potential to help decrease diarrhea and improve outcomes for pediatric patients with diarrhea (CDC, 2003; Thomas et al., 2010).

Skin care therapy may be required for perianal excoriation. Various topical OTC agents exist to aid with healing, drying, and providing a barrier while the diarrheal illness persists. Secondary skin infections should be treated with appropriate topical medications. In cases of extreme skin breakdown, exposing the skin, air drying, oxygen directed therapy to the buttocks, or a wound care consultant may be necessary.

Consultation with any of a number of specialists, such as emergency medicine, gastroenterology, pediatric surgery, critical care, neurosurgery, nephrology, and oncology, may be considered as circumstances warrant.

Caregivers should be given instructions that clearly outline how to perform ORT at home, when to seek further evaluation and care, and when to see the PCP for a follow-up visit. Signs and symptoms of dehydration and other concerns should be well understood. Caregivers must be educated regarding infection control, especially given that the vast majority of gastroenteritis is viral in origin and spread easily in households and day care facilities. Proper hand washing technique should be reviewed, along with the need to refrain from sharing beverages, glasses, utensils, towels, and toothbrushes.

In children with positive stool cultures, recommendations for return to school or day care depend on which organism has been cultured from the stool and which state-specific public health guidelines apply. For instance, pediatric patients with *Salmonella* serotype *Typhi*; *Shiga* toxin-producing *E. coli* (STEC), including *E. coli* O157:H7; or *Shigella* infection may need to demonstrate several negative stool cultures before return to school or day care is permitted. In general, afebrile patients with viral gastroenteritis or other types of bacterial gastroenteritis may return to school or day care when they have fewer than three episodes of loose stools each day. Additional disease-specific return to school or day care guidelines are outlined in the AAP's (2009a) *Red Book*.

DISPOSITION AND DISCHARGE PLANNING

For most routine cases of gastroenteritis, whether viral or bacterial, disease will be self-limited and no medications are indicated. Most patients will not require overnight hospital stay. Once the child has received adequate fluid resuscitation and demonstrated the ability to maintain hydration by drinking and retaining oral fluids, he or she may be discharged home. Caregivers should be educated on the importance of continuing rehydration strategies and age-appropriate diet at home. Adherence to published guidelines for ORT by caregivers is poor (50%); therefore, reinforcement teaching may be required (Tieder et al., 2009). Caregivers should be encouraged not to use juices, sugar-based drinks, or soda for rehydration due to their osmotic properties. Instead, ORS should be used for rehydration whenever possible.

Gastroenteritis may lead to a minor secondary lactose deficiency and malabsorption. Studies suggest that infants should continue taking standard (undiluted) formulas and/or human breastmilk while receiving rehydration. Temporarily changing to lactose-free or soy formula is not recommended (CDC, 2003; Heyman, 2006).

Preventive education and vaccination may help avoid many cases of gastroenteritis in pediatric patients. Each year in the United States, *rotavirus* alone is responsible for nearly 600,000 visits to HCPs, upward of 70,000 hospitalizations, and 20 to 70 deaths. The cost of care for such infections exceeds $1 billion. HCPs should follow the guidelines on routine immunizations that are published and updated each year by the CDC's Advisory Committee on Immunization Practices (CDC, 2009) and the AAP (2009b).

GASTROESOPHAGEAL REFLUX DISEASE

Sherri L. Adams and Sanjay Mahant

PATHOPHYSIOLOGY

Gastroesophageal reflux (GER) is the passage of gastric contents into the esophagus, whereas gastroesophageal reflux disease (GERD) is diagnosed when the reflux is associated with symptoms or complications (Vandenplas et al., 2009). GER is commonly associated with transient relaxation of the lower esophageal sphincter (LES), which allows the passage of gastric material back up into the esophagus. Gastric secretions and their acidity are traumatic to the gastric mucosa. Several factors potentiate GER, resulting in GERD. They include delayed gastric emptying, impaired esophageal peristalsis resulting in ineffective clearing of refluxed gastric contents from the esophagus, and lower esophageal dysfunction that may be transient or persistent. When GERD causes erosion of the esophageal wall, it is termed erosive reflux disease (ERD). When there is no erosion, it is termed nonerosive reflux disease (NERD) (Sherman et al., 2009). While histological changes of eosinophilia, elongation of papillae, basal hyperplasia, and dilated intercellular spaces are often associated with GERD, these changes are not always diagnostic.

EPIDEMIOLOGY AND ETIOLOGY

GER, or regurgitation, occurs in as many as 70% of all healthy infants, prompting the idiom "happy spitters." Ninety-five percent of all cases resolve without treatment by the time the infant is 12 to 14 months of age. Infants who spit up, but continue to feed and gain weight, are not considered to have GERD (Sherman et al., 2009).

GERD is the most common pediatric esophageal disorder. While the condition is reported worldwide, there are few data to suggest any gender or ethnic prevalence. Notably, diagnosis rates are 8% in infants and children, and 3% to 5% in adolescents. Several disorders are thought to predispose a child to chronic GERD, including neurological impairment, cystic fibrosis, hiatal hernia, congenital esophageal abnormalities, obesity, and a positive family medical history of severe GERD.

PRESENTATION

The patient with GERD may present with vomiting, food refusal or feeding aversion, unexplained crying, sleeping disturbances, abdominal pain, choking, coughing, or gagging (Sherman et al., 2009). School-age children and adolescents are generally able to provide a description of their symptoms, which may include heartburn, regurgitation, sore throat, cough, epigastric pain, or reporting that their mouth tastes like vomit. The typical reflux syndrome seen in older children and adolescents presents as epigastric pain or heartburn. Many patients with special health care needs have gastrostomy tubes (GT) for nutritional delivery. On occasion, the placement of these tubes exacerbates reflux; consequently, the HCP should elicit whether symptoms worsened after GT insertion.

Some patients may experience extra-esophageal symptoms of reflux such as dental erosion or dystonic head posturing (Sandifer's syndrome). Other illnesses that may be associated with GERD include reactive airway disease, recurrent pneumonia, chronic cough, otitis media, chronic hoarseness, and sinusitis (Sherman et al., 2009). Apparent life-threatening events (ALTEs) are often associated with GERD; however, there is little evidence to support anything but a causal relationship (Vandenplas et al., 2009).

In most patients with GERD, the physical examination is unremarkable. Severe dental erosion secondary to acid reflux or odors from the child's mouth may be noted. Nonspecific finding related to the upper or lower respiratory tract may be identified, but are not diagnostic for GERD. Growth is the most important examination finding, as poor weight gain or weight loss may be an indication of GERD.

DIFFERENTIAL DIAGNOSIS

The differential diagnoses for GERD are vast and include many of the same components of the differential diagnoses for vomiting or failure-to-thrive (Rudolph et al., 2001). Other conditions should be considered as indicated from the history and physical examination findings (Table 26-17).

PLAN OF CARE

A caregiver history is essential in determining the diagnosis. Although there is currently no one good diagnostic

TABLE 26-17

Differential Diagnosis for Gastroesophageal Disease by Systems	
Neurologic	Increased intracranial pressure
	• Hydrocephalus
	• Meningitis
	• Intracranial mass
	Seizures
Gastrointestinal	Malrotation
	Pyloric stenosis
	Cow's milk allergy/eosinophilic esophagitis
	Peptic ulcer disease
	Hepatitis
	Pancreatitis
	Malabsorption (e.g., celiac disease)
	Inflammatory bowel disease
Genitourinary	Urinary tract infection
	Urinary tract obstruction
Functional/psychiatric	Rumination
	Anorexia
	Bulimia
Genitourinary	Urinary tract infection
	Urinary tract obstruction
Others	Cyclic vomiting syndrome

study for GERD, response to empiric medical treatment may be considered diagnostic. The use of pH monitoring is common, even though its sensitivity and specificity for GERD are not well established. Combined multiple-lumen impedance (MII) is considered more effective at detecting both acid and non-acid episodes of reflux in adults; however, its effectiveness in children has not yet been determined. Endoscopy and biopsy, once thought to be the gold standard for diagnosing reflux, are reliable only if changes to the epithelial mucosa have occurred. A biopsy excludes other diagnoses such as eosinophilic or infectious esophagus, and complications of reflux esophagitis (strictures and Barrett esophagus) (Vandenplas et al., 2009). Table 26-18 compares the various diagnostic studies and their utility.

Diet and position changes are often effective in relieving GERD-related symptoms in the infant population. Prone positioning is helpful; however, due to the risk of sudden infant death syndrome (SIDS), it is not recommended when the infant is asleep. A trial of hydrolyzed protein formula (in an already formula-fed infant) may be considered for 2 to 4 weeks (Vandenplas et al., 2009). Symptom reduction has not been shown with either thickening of feeds or diet restriction of specific foods (Rudolph et al., 2001). In older children and adolescents, prone or left-sided sleeping with the head of the bed elevated may be helpful (Vandenplas et al.).

TABLE 26-18

Diagnostic Studies for Gastroesophageal Reflux Disease

Diagnostic Study	Description	Diagnostic Utility
Barium contrast radiography	Radiographic films of the upper gastrointestinal tract using barium contrast	Evaluating anatomic abnormalities of the upper gastrointestinal tract Not sensitive or specific for GERD
24-hour esophageal pH monitoring	Probe passed through the nose into the esophagus to measure lower esophageal acidity over time	Good measure of esophageal acid exposure but will not establish relationship with symptoms or disease Helpful in monitoring efficacy of antisecretory medications
Combined multiple intraluminal impedance (MII) and pH monitoring	MII and pH probe passed through the nose into the esophagus to measure pH exposure of lower esophagus	Measures esophageal acid and non-acid exposure Utility is still uncertain, but is superior to pH monitoring alone
Esophageal manometry		Measures esophageal peristalsis, upper and lower esophageal sphincter pressuresDoes not diagnose GERD Useful to diagnose achalasia or other motor disorders of the esophagus
Endoscopy and biopsy	Visualization and biopsies of the esophagus with an endoscope	Not sensitive in diagnosis of GERD Useful to rule out other disorders (eosinophilic esophagitis) or complications of esophagitis
Radionuclide scintigraphy	Radioactive isotope is added to age-appropriate meal and esophagogastric area	Not diagnostic for GERD Used to measure gastric emptying May have a role in detecting pulmonary aspiration
Empiric trial of acid suppression	Empiric trial of a proton pump inhibitor for up to 4 weeks	Useful in an older child or adolescent with typical symptoms of GERD

TABLE 26-19

Differential Diagnoses for Gastrointestinal Bleeding

Infant		Young Child		Older Child and Adolescent	
Site		**Site**		**Site**	
Upper	Hemorrhagic gastritis/gastritis Stress ulcer Vascular malformation Reflux esophagitis	Upper	Hemorrhagic gastritis/gastritis Stress ulcer Gastric/duodenal ulcer Esophageal varices Mallory-Weiss tear Epistaxis Reflux esophagitis Foreign body Toxic ingestion	Upper	Hemorrhagic gastritis/gastritis Mallory-Weiss tear Stress ulcer Gastric/duodenal ulcer Esophageal varices Epistaxis Reflux esophagitis
Lower	Infectious colitis Midgut volvulus Anal fissures Necrotizing enterocolitis Intussusception Milk protein allergy Hirschsprung's disease Lymphonodular hyperplasia	Lower	Infectious colitis Midgut volvulus Anal fissures Hemorrhoid Ulcer Polyps Hemolytic-uremic syndrome Juvenile polyp Pseudomembranous colitis Inflammatory bowel disease Henoch-Schönlein purpura Meckel's diverticulum Ischemic colitis Intussusception Angiodysplasia Graft-versus-host disease	Lower	Infectious colitis Anal fissures Hemorrhoid Ulcer Polyps Juvenile polyp Inflammatory bowel disease Henoch-Schönlein purpura Meckel's diverticulum Hemolytic-uremic syndrome Bacterial enteritis Angiodysplasia Graft-versus-host disease

Acid-suppressing medications are the mainstay of therapy. These agents are recommended over antacids, which do not decrease acid production. Potential risks of acid suppression therapy include pulmonary and gastrointestinal infections.

Histamine-2 receptor antagonists (H_2RA) inhibit histamine-2 receptors on the gastric parietal cells, thereby decreasing acid secretion. These medications have a rapid onset of action; however, tachyphylaxis may occur. Commonly used medications in this category are ranitidine and cimetidine, both of which can be purchased as over-the-counter (OTC) products. Their use in children and adolescents should be under the guidance of a HCP.

Proton-pump inhibitors (PPI) are the most effective medications for acid suppression. They block the final common pathway of acid section on the parietal cells, the enzyme sodium–potassium ATPase. Unlike with H_2RAs, tachyphylaxis does not occur with administration of PPIs. Commonly used medications in this category are omeprazole, lansoprazole, and esomeprazole.

Prokinetic therapies (e.g., metoclopramide) are not routinely recommended for the treatment of pediatric GERD due to their lack of effectiveness and potential side effects. Buffering agents, such as sucralfate, may be of value for intermittent use but are not recommended for long-term therapy. They should be used with caution in infants (Vandenplas et al., 2009).

If medical management has failed or if pulmonary aspiration of refluxed contents is a problem, surgical management is considered. The most common surgical intervention is the Nissen fundoplication. In this procedure, the fundus of the stomach is wrapped around the lower esophagus to improve LES function. The evidence of fundoplication effectiveness is unclear, and complication rates are higher in neurologically impaired children.

Children who fail first-line treatment with a PPI should be referred to a gastroenterologist for further evaluation. Children with a predisposing condition for GERD, such as neurologic impairment, should be considered for early referral to a gastroenterologist, as they may not respond to conventional therapy.

It is important to educate the family regarding the natural history of GER and to explain that in healthy infants it most often resolves without treatment. In parents of infants who are "happy spitters," education regarding how much, and how often, to feed a child is important. Overfeeding can also result in spillage.

DISPOSITION AND DISCHARGE PLANNING

In most children who are previously healthy, GERD will respond to treatment with medical management. Parents should be educated on warning signs such as inadequate weight gain, vomiting blood, and feeding refusal that require reevaluation by a HCP. In most healthy patients, treatment resolves symptoms and disease. Nevertheless, in children with predisposing conditions for GERD, such as neurologic impairment, this disorder may be a lifelong condition. Parents should be educated as to the complications and natural history of the disease.

GASTROINTESTINAL BLEEDING

Randolph McConnie

PATHOPHYSIOLOGY

The ligament of Treitz is the divide between the upper and lower sections of the nonobstructed GI tract. Bleeding sources proximal to the ligament usually present as hematemesis or bloody drainage from a gastric tube, although some of the blood passes on to the lower GI tract. Bleeding sources distal to the ligament of Treitz commonly present with melena (stool that is liquid tarry in consistency, black in color, and offensive odor), maroon-colored stool, bright red bloody stool, red blood-streaked stool, or a stool that is normal in color and consistency yet guaiac positive. The color of the blood in the stool depends on the location of the intestinal segment involved.

EPIDEMIOLOGY AND ETIOLOGY

Blood in the GI track is never normal. GI bleeding is uncommon in pediatric patients. Even patients with profound coagulopathy rarely experience GI bleeding. The vast majority of patients with upper GI bleeding have lesions of the GI mucosa or esophageal varices secondary to liver disease. Infectious colitis is the most common cause of colonic bleeding worldwide. In countries with good water supplies, colon polyps, allergic colitis, anal fissures, ulcerative colitis, and Crohn's disease account for the majority of lower GI bleeding arising from the colon. Few patients with either upper or lower pathology require transfusion or operative therapy.

PRESENTATION

The history should focus on the patient's symptoms, diet, medications, recent travel, ill contacts, and social and family history. An infant who is fed cow's milk or soy-based formula may have allergic colitis. Recent antibiotic therapy may lead to *Clostridium difficile* toxin-induced colitis. A history of dry heaves, followed by hematemesis or melena, suggests a Mallory-Weiss tear. Recent illness may lead one to suspect hemolytic uremic syndrome (HUS). Ingestion of nonsteroidal anti-inflammatory drugs (NSAIDs) can lead to gastritis, duodenitis, or ileal and right colonic lesions.

A family history of inflammatory bowel disease (IBD), intestinal cancers at an early age, or liver disease should be noted. Liver disease may be related to an inherited α_1-antitrypsin deficiency, and hepatitis B may be transmitted vertically at birth.

The complaint of heartburn in the older child or adolescent, or an apparent life-threatening event in an infant, suggests an upper GI source such as esophagitis, gastritis, or ulcer. Urgency to defecate and tenismus suggests colitis. Delayed passage of meconium, or constipation in infancy, can be symptoms of cystic fibrosis or Hirschsprung's disease. Instrumentation of the umbilical vein at birth can result in cavernous transformation of the portal vein and portal hypertension and esophageal varices. The presence of spider angiomata, palmar erythema, fetor hepaticus, or splenomegaly suggests chronic liver disease and portal hypertension. In patients with hematemesis or melena who receive nothing-by-mouth (NPO), are on nasogastric (NG) suction, and are receiving antibiotics, consider coagulopathy from low vitamin K levels and/or NG tube-induced gastritis.

A comprehensive physical examination will provide information regarding the patient's hemodynamic stability associated with blood loss. Assess for oxygen saturation, tachycardia, postural changes in pulse and blood pressure, and hypotension. Skin, conjunctivae, or nail beds may be pale. Skin manifestations of other diseases may also provide useful information to help determine the etiology of the GI bleeding. A rectal examination is performed to assess for hemorrhoids, rectal tears, or other perianal disease. Finding melena or bright red blood in the digital exam suggests the source of the blood. Finding a palpable movable rectal mass might identify polyps as another etiology. The patient's smell might lead one to suspect chronic liver disease (fetor hepaticus) or acute alcohol-induced gastritis.

DIFFERENTIAL DIAGNOSIS

The differential diagnoses for GI bleeding are vast. In the newborn, blood may be seen in vomitus or stool and may not be that of the patient, but rather come from the mother. Various ingestants, such as commercial dyes (numbers 2 and 3), blueberries, beets, and bismuth, may present with a red-tinted or -colored stool, which can be confused with blood. Table 26-19 summarizes some of the diagnoses to consider for GI bleeding. The following distinctions help determine the source of the bleeding:

- Age at presentation
- Upper or lower intestinal tract
- Hemorrhage or slow rate of bleeding
- Bright red blood or dark blood
- Underlying medical conditions

PLAN OF CARE

If the patient shows signs of hemodynamic instability, IV access is obtained and fluid volume administered. Initial IV fluids that support hemorrhagic hypovolemia include normal saline, lactated Ringer's solution, or packed red blood cells (PRBCs). The patient should be kept NPO and admitted to a monitored bed or the intensive care unit. An urgent upper endoscopy should be considered in the patient presenting with significant upper-GI bleeding. A colonoscopy should be considered in the patient with bright red lower-GI bleeding. These studies should be performed only after the patient has been stabilized and coagulopathies corrected.

In a stable patient with guaiac-positive stools, the source of the blood may be from either the upper or lower GI track. Thus a non-urgent upper endoscopy and colonoscopy should be considered. An endoscopy assesses for duodenal or gastric ulcer and provides the ability to cauterize visible bleeding vessels and test for *Helicobacter pylori* infection. Bleeding esophageal varices or esophageal varices that have recently bled should be sclerosed or banded to decrease the risk of rebleeding.

Administration of an agent that decreases central venous pressure, such as octreotide, is thought to be useful in the management of bleeding esophageal varices before endoscopic intervention. In the case of variceal bleeding that is not controlled by endoscopic or tamponade intervention, emergency transjugular intrahepatic portosystemic shunting (TIPS) or surgical shunting to decrease portal hypertension may be warranted.

In patients with significant gastrointestinal bleeding in whom an upper endoscopy and colonoscopy have failed to show the source of bleeding, a nuclear medicine tagged red blood cell (RBC) bleeding study may help define the source of the blood loss, assuming the loss of blood is brisk enough to detect it with the scan. If the patient is actively bleeding, an angiogram with selective vessel embolization may be required. A single- or double-balloon enteroscopy may help identify a radiographically silent lesion or one beyond the reach of the conventional upper or lower endoscope.

The method for determining the source of the bleeding depends on the urgency of the patient's condition and its suspected origin (i.e., upper versus lower). For stable patients with mild bleeding, diagnostic study is elective. It may involve passing a NG tube for a gastric lavage to evaluate the upper GI tract. A negative lavage does not always negate an upper GI bleeding, as bleeding may have stopped or a pylorospasm may be preventing blood from reaching the duodenum from refluxing back into the stomach. Nasogastric lavage is not routinely performed for a stable patient with formed, brown guaiac-positive stools. Lavage with cold fluids does not improve outcome. The use of a NG tube for continuous suction is controversial, as the very placement or presence of suction may exacerbate bleeding.

Polyps are usually removed with snare electrocautery at the time of colonoscopy. Ulcerative colitis and Crohn's disease are treated medically or with surgery. GI bleeding from Henoch-Schönlein purpura and HUS usually resolves with resolution of the disorders.

DISPOSITION AND DISCHARGE PLANNING

Further education and follow-up depends on the source of bleeding and the nature of the illness. Patients should be informed if there is a low or high risk for rebleeding, which symptoms are associated with recurrence, and when to seek emergency care. For patients with upper GI bleeds, consumption of the normal diet may resume within 24 hours. If the patient remains stable, then discharge on a proton-pump inhibitor for gastritis or beta blocker (e.g., propranolol) for esophageal varices may be considered. Close outpatient follow-up with the GI service is warranted.

Discharge of patients with lower GI bleeding depends on the etiology of the bleeding, underlying chronic illness, and response to therapy. Patients require close follow-up with the GI service and other subspecialists as needed.

GASTROINTESTINAL TRANSPLANTATION

Barbara V. Wise

Liver transplantation (LT) has been an accepted treatment for end-stage liver disease in children since 1983. In 2008, 613 children from 0 to 17 years of age underwent LT (United Network for Organ Sharing [UNOS], 2009). Until the mid-1990s, survival rates for children were limited by the lack of available size-matched donors. To alleviate the problem of high mortality rates in infants, reduced-size liver transplantation—using the right lobe, left lobe, or left lateral segment from a cadaveric donor—was recommended for this population. Initially this procedure was used in critically ill children who required immediate transplantation, and improved survival rates were demonstrated. Today multiple procedures for LT exist, including living-related donor transplants, split-liver grafts, and whole-liver grafts.

Intestinal transplantation (IT) was initially performed in the late 1980s as a curative therapy for intestinal failure. Referral criteria for IT include life-threatening complications of parenteral nutrition such as dehydration, multiple episodes of sepsis and impending liver failure, high risk of death due to gastrointestinal disease, and intestinal failure with high morbidity (American Gastroenterological Association [AGA], 2003). In 2008, 93 children from 0 to 17 years of age underwent an isolated intestinal transplant,

TABLE 26-20

Pediatric End-Stage Liver Disease Scoring
Age (months, years)
Albumin (gm/dL)
Total bilirubin (mg/dL)
International Normalized Ratio (INR)
Growth failure (z score, length/height)

6 children underwent a liver-intestine transplant, and 94 children underwent a multivisceral transplant (UNOS, 2009). The majority of patients listed for IT are children younger than 5 years of age (63%) who are diagnosed with short gut syndrome (Berg et al., 2009). The median wait time for IT is 257 days.

INDICATIONS FOR TRANSPLANT

The pediatric end-stage liver disease (PELD) score was developed simultaneously with the adult model (MELD) to create an effective system for donor liver allocation and reflect 3-month mortality rates accurately (Table 26-20). Clinical situations for listing criteria that deviate from standard PELD scores include children with chronic liver disease with recurrent gastrointestinal bleeding, acute liver failure, urea-cycle disorders, and hepatic tumors.

Pediatric donors maintain priority for allocation to pediatric patients, and regional boards maintain discretion to upgrade patients to status 1 if the PELD score does not reflect the urgency of transplantation (McDiarmid et al., 2004). In 2005, the PELD allocation policy criteria were modified to limit the additional points to children younger than 12 years of age rather than the more inclusive age of younger than 18 years (Berg et al., 2009). Long wait periods and high mortality rates led to a recent change in MELD/PELD allocation criteria giving pediatric combined intestinal and liver candidates (younger than 18 years of age) an additional 23 points. Liver transplant recipients are listed as status 1A or 1B if admitted to the intensive care unit (ICU) with fulminant liver failure, hepatic artery thrombosis, primary graft dysfunction, or acute decompensated Wilson's disease. Status 1B candidates have "chronic" liver failure, hepatoblastoma, or a metabolic disease and are recertified every 90 days. Other potential recipients are assigned a PELD score that determines the frequency of recertification. Intestinal organ allocation is determined by degree of urgency. Status 1 candidates have liver function abnormalities and/or no vascular access through the subclavian, jugular, or femoral veins for intravenous feeding. Status 2 candidates do not meet criteria for status 1 (UNOS, 2009).

Timing and referral for liver transplantation in children with end-stage liver disease (ESLD) vary. Signs and symptoms associated with ESLD include portal hypertension associated with ascites, digital clubbing, pallor, caput medusa (prominent abdominal wall vessels), anorexia, nausea and vomiting, fever, fatigue, weight loss, jaundice, bleeding, pruritus, rickets, fractures, cutaneous xanthoma, bacterial peritonitis, hypersplenism, hepatic encephalopathy, and variceal bleeding (Leonis & Balistreri, 2008a).

The clinical signs and symptoms of IT failure vary widely depending on the pediatric patient's overall health. When liver disease accompanies intestinal failure, jaundice and ecchymosis are present. Additional skin findings may include pruritus, thinning hair, decreased skin turgor, edema, stomas, feeding tube sites, and surgical scars. Spider angioma, ascites, hepatosplenomegaly, and distended abdominal veins are commonly found in the presence of liver failure. Most children referred for IT are rated at less than the 25th percentile on the growth charts for height and weight. The serum albumin is less than 3 mg/dL. Oral aversion is a common finding related to prolonged periods of no, or limited, oral intake. Adolescents present with decreased muscle mass and weight loss (Kosmach-Park & De Angelis, 2008).

Certain medical problems are frequent complications of liver and intestinal failure. Failure to gain weight in children with ESLD is multifactorial in origin, being related to increased energy expenditure, malabsorption of macronutrients and micronutrients, and decreased caloric intake. Malnutrition hinders infant brain growth and overall development, and it may also be a factor in delayed puberty and amenorrhea found in adolescent females. The problem of poor weight gain in infants is further impeded by generalized malaise, early satiety, delayed gastric emptying, gastroesophageal reflux secondary to ascites, and increased incidence of emesis. Increasing caloric intake to 120% to 150% of the estimated daily requirements and providing caloric-density formulas with medium-chain triglycerides are two strategies to maximize fat absorption. Feedings administered as nighttime feedings either via nasogastric or nasojejunal tubes are used in infants with frequent emesis or ascites.

Cholestasis associated with malabsorption deprives the patient of essential fat-soluble vitamins (A, D, E, K) and may induce diarrhea, necessitating supplementation with fat-soluble vitamins. Although some infants develop an aversion to oral feeds, this problem is best addressed after transplantation with the assistance of speech/occupational therapists (Leonis & Balistreri, 2008a). Derusso et al. (2007) reported that growth failure is an important risk factor for pre- and post-transplant death and graft failure.

Gastric erosions, ulcers, varices, portal hypertension, and infection in this population may all cause GI bleeding. Children with portal hypertension have functional asplenia, which increases their risk of developing infection,

especially from encapsulated organisms such as *Streptococcus pneumoniae* and *Neisseria meningitidis* (Cochran & Losek, 2007). Vitamin K may be administered to prevent coagulopathy in chronic liver failure that is associated with decreased synthesis of clotting factors.

Infants are at high risk for developing ascites that leads to gastrointestinal and pulmonary compromise. Contributing factors to this finding are hypoalbuminemia, excessive fluid administration, and infection. Tense ascites results in gastric outlet obstruction that further limits adequate nutritional intake (Leonis & Balistreria, 2008a; Squires, 2008). Initial management of ascites involves administration of diuretics and a modestly salt-restricted diet (Debray et al., 2006). Initially a potassium-sparing diuretic such as spironalactone is prescribed. Care should be taken to avoid hyponatremia or other electrolyte abnormalities and fluid shifts. When the ascites does not respond to diuretic therapy, a therapeutic abdominal paracentesis may be performed; however, it is likely to produce only a short-term benefit. In addition, this procedure carries an increased risk of hypotension and infection (Leonis & Balistreri, 2008a). Portal hypertension occurs secondary to decreased blood flow to the liver and increased flow from collateral circulation from the stomach and spleen.

Impaired kidney function or hepatorenal syndrome (HRS) is a complication of ascites that is associated with chronic liver failure and occasionally acute liver failure (ALF). Early identification of children with impaired kidney function by screening with a urinalysis, glomerular filtrate rate, and monitoring for hypertension may prevent complications. HRS is considered a "functional" reversible form of kidney failure characterized by impaired renal function (elevated creatinine—double the baseline—and BUN) with arterial vasodilatation and renal vasoconstriction. Precipitating factors for HRS may include an episode of spontaneous bacterial peritonitis or a therapeutic paracentesis. Vasoconstrictors (ornipressin and terlipressin), somatostatin analogues, and alpha-adrenergic analogues with concomitant administration of volume expansion (albumin) are used in the medical management of HRS. Children with progressive kidney failure may require renal replacement therapy with continuous veno-venous hemofiltration or dialysis (Squires, 2008). Transplantation is the only effective treatment for HRS, but worse outcomes are reported in patients undergoing transplantation in kidney failure (Kiser et al., 2009; Møller et al., 2008; Turban et al., 2007).

Hepatic encephalopathy (HE) is less common in ESLD compared with ALF. Additionally, HE associated with ESLD can be managed with a protein-restricted diet (2–3 gm/kg/day), but care should be taken that such a diet does not further impair growth or cause other nutritional deficits in children with chronic liver failure.

Table 26-21 lists potential causes of liver and intestinal failure.

TABLE 26-21

Diagnoses Leading to End-Stage Disease

Liver Diseases	Intestinal Diseases
Biliary atresia	**Neonates**
Hemochromatosis	Gastroschesis
Parenteral nutrition–induced cholestasis	Necrotizing enterocolitis
α_1-Antitrypsin deficiency	Atresia
Wilson's disease	Midgut volvulus
Alagille syndrome	Total aganglionosis, a rare form of Hirschsprung's disease
Tyrosinemia	
Viral hepatitis	**Older Children**
Primary sclerosing cholangitis	Dysmotility syndrome
Glycogen storage disease	Microvillus inclusion disease
Urea-cycle disorders	Abdominal trauma
Hepatoblastoma/hepatocellular cancer	Crohn's disease
Hepatotoxic drugs	
Veno-occlusive liver disease	
Bile acid synthetic defects	
Primary sclerosing cholangitis	
Idiopathic neonatal hepatitis	

TABLE 26-22

Transplant Evaluation

Laboratory Data

CBC with differential	HLA typing
Chemistry panel (electrolytes, liver function studies)	Blood type
Viral studies: CMV, EBV, VZV, syphilis, toxoplasmosis	HIV
Hepatitis A, B, C	Coagulation studies
Ammonia level	

Radiographic Studies

Chest radiograph	Echocardiograph
Duplex ultrasound of liver/abdomen	Upper gastrointestinal study
Electrocardiograph	Liver biopsy

Consults

Hepatology	Psychiatry/social work
Surgery	Occupational/physical therapy
AnesthesiaNutrition	Child life

Educational information is provided for the family and patient depending on the age of the recipient to describe the process of listing, waiting for an organ, potential complications, surgery, hospitalization, and the organ allocation system.

Complete blood count (CBC), human leukocyte antigen (HLA), cytomegalovirus (CMV), Epstein-Barr virus (EBV), varicella zoster virus (VZV), human immunodeficiency virus (HIV).

TRANSPLANTATION

The pediatric hepatologist and transplant surgeon evaluates children referred for LT with ESLD or ALF. A series of laboratory tests and radiographic studies is obtained prior to listing a patient for liver transplantation. Consultations with a transplant social worker or psychologist are necessary to identify family or financial problems that may interfere with transplant outcomes. Immunization records should be requested. Potential recipients are listed by blood type, weight, and PELD score on the UNOS list.

Absolute contraindications for IT include profound neurological disability, life-threatening irreversible disease unrelated to the gastrointestinal tract, HIV infection, and unresectable malignancy. Similar to what happens with LT recipients, an interprofessional team performs a pretransplant evaluation. Additional studies performed as part of this assessment include quantitative immunoglobulin levels; an upper gastrointestinal series to identify bowel anatomy, estimate bowel length, and evaluate gastric transport; and an abdominal ultrasound to identify patency of the hepatic vasculature, biliary system, and the presence of varices or hepatosplenomegaly. A liver biopsy is performed to assess the extent of liver failure. An echocardiograph and electrocardiograph are obtained to evaluate cardiomyopathy or other contraindications to surgery. Many children referred for IT have a history of prematurity; therefore a careful assessment for chronic respiratory problems is essential. Pretransplant care focuses on managing acute problems such as infection, monitoring for fluid electrolyte abnormalities, determining organ deterioration or dysfunction, and administering parenteral nutrition and early enteral feeding to promote adequate growth and development. Table 26-22 lists specific tests and consults to obtain when evaluating recipients for liver and intestinal transplantation.

Once a donor liver is available, the child is brought to the hospital and preoperative laboratory tests are obtained. The liver transplant procedure takes approximately 8 to 12 hours. Procurement of the donor liver occurs according to the standard procedure for whole-liver transplantation and is prepared at the back table simultaneously with hepatectomy of the native liver by a second surgical team. In a reduced-liver transplant, the liver is reduced through a formal lobectomy (right or left) or trisegmentectomy for left lateral segment implants, with ligation of the main vessels and ducts. The biliary and vascular structures along the cut edge are ligated, and the remaining vascular structures are flushed with preservation solution.

The child receiving the transplant is brought to the operating room, where he or she undergoes intubation and placement of one or two large-bore catheters in the upper extremities. Intubation is performed with a cuffed tube to allow for adjustments in pulmonary compliance during the procedure. A bilateral subcostal incision is made to visualize major structures, known as the "Mercedes incision." The vena cava, portal vein, and hepatic artery are cross-clamped prior to hepatectomy. Hemodynamic instability is a risk during this anhepatic phase secondary to the decreased intravascular volume, ongoing fluid and blood losses, and decreased venous return to the heart.

The graft is implanted in the usual orthotopic position. Vascular anastamoses are performed in the following manner: suprahepatic inferior vena cava, infrahepatic inferior vena cava, portal vein, and hepatic artery. The liver graft is flushed prior to reperfusion but after the portal vein anastamosis to prevent air emboli. During reperfusion, fluid shifts can result in intestinal edema, third spacing, and renal compromise. Children generally tolerate the caval clamping and reperfusion well, however, because of collateral circulation.

The last step is bile duct reconstruction using an end-to-side Roux-en-Y limb (hepaticocholedochojejunostomy) of the jejunum or duct-to-duct (choledochcholedochostomy) anastomosis. Two or three Jackson-Pratt drains are inserted. Duct-to-duct biliary reconstruction is often performed in children with an adequate biliary tree (i.e., recipients diagnosed with metabolic disorders or fulminant hepatic failure).

Other surgical options include the split-liver transplant and living-related liver transplantation. Split-liver grafts differ from reduced-size grafts in their approach to separating the vascular and biliary structures, which seeks to produce two viable grafts for separate recipients. The goal with this procedure had been to address donor shortages by providing a two-for-one application. However, a higher incidence of postoperative complications such as biliary leaks and bleeding has made this procedure a less viable option. In contrast, studies comparing outcomes in living-related donor transplants with reduced-size or whole-liver transplants indicate improved outcomes with living-related liver transplantation. The arterial reconstruction necessary in a living-donor liver transplant creates a surgical challenge because of the many normal variants found in the hepatic arterial system.

Several different types of grafts are possible for IT:

- Isolated intestinal
- Composite liver–intestine–liver
- Intestine with or without the colon, the duodenum, a potion of the pancreas, and biliary tree
- Noncomposite liver–intestine–pancreas
- Multivisceral (stomach, liver, pancreas, and intestine)
- Modified multivisceral (native spleen and pancreas are preserved)

The composite liver–intestine–pancreas transplant was developed to avoid back-table work and prevent injury to the hepatic hilar structure when removing the pancreas from the graft. The Noncomposite liver–intestine procedure was developed to accommodate size discrepancies between the donor and the recipient (Kato et al., 2006; Reyes et al., 2002; Selvaggi & Tzakis, 2009). Another controversial option is the combined living-related intestinal or liver and intestinal transplant performed simultaneously if liver function is adequate (Gangemi et al., 2009).

The intestinal graft is flushed with University of Wisconsin solution or histidine–tryptophan–ketoglutarate solution at procurement. Operative times range from 6 to 18 hours, depending on the type of transplant, the patient's history of previous surgeries, and the child's current health status.

With IT, a midline incision is made with unilateral or bilateral transverse extension for exposure and based on the type of transplant. The diseased intestine is removed from the ligament of Treitz to the ileocecal valve. The healthy intestine is preserved when appropriate, because it provides protection from parenteral nutrition–associated injury in the post-transplant period. In cadaveric IT, the donor graft usually includes the entire jejunum and ileum. Vascular anastomoses connect the donor iliac arterial vessel to the infrarenal aorta using an interpositional graft, while venous drainage is performed by connecting the portal system to the inferior vena cava. The intestinal graft is implanted into the orthotopic position. A terminal eneterostomy (Bishop-Koop) is created at the end of the intestinal graft that allows access for future intestinal biopsies to monitor rejection (Pascher et al., 2008).

The abdomen is closed with staples or sutures that remain in place for 2 to 3 weeks. In children with a small abdominal cavity or fistulas, primary closure may not be possible (Selvaggi & Tzakis, 2009). Instead, a prosthetic graft using a Silastic sheet or grafted fascia may be necessary temporarily, followed by serial reduction until the abdomen can be permanently closed.

A feeding tube is inserted at the end of the IT procedure because oral intake is inconsistent in the immediate postoperative period. A nasogastric tube is placed for abdominal decompression and two to four Jackson-Pratt drains are inserted for drainage of residual fluid from the abdomen (Kosmach-Park & De Angelis, 2008).

POST-TRANSPLANTATION

Postoperatively, the recipient is taken to the pediatric intensive care unit (PICU) while still intubated. Some recipients have impaired respiratory function prior to transplantation that influences the duration of mechanical ventilation. Most isolated IT recipients can be extubated within 24 to 48 hours of surgery. In contrast, the patient with a multivisceral graft may require a longer period of mechanical ventilation secondary to graft-size mismatch or diaphragmatic dysfunction.

Liver and intestinal transplant recipients are at risk for hypothermia because of exposure of the abdominal viscera during the surgical procedure. Hypothermia can predispose the patient to arrhythmias, clotting abnormalities, impaired kidney function, and delayed wound healing.

Hemorrhage is an early sign of technical problems following LT or IT. Its presenting signs are pallor, tachycardia, hypotension, and increased output from the Jackson-Pratt drains. Other causes may include preexisting coagulopathy or bleeding at the anastamoses. Low-molecular-weight dextran and subcutaneous heparin are administered in the immediate postoperative period when coagulation factors are normalizing to prevent thromboses. Frequent monitoring of output from the Jackson-Pratt drains, increasing abdominal girth, and oozing from the suture line are all indications of bleeding. Fresh frozen plasma is used to correct coagulopathies; the usual goal is to maintain a slightly prolonged prothrombin time (PT) or an International Normalized Ratio (INR) between 2 and 3, with a platelet count of 40,000 cells/microliter, to prevent bleeding (Hauser et al., 2008). Thrombocytopenia may occur if more than 2 blood volumes are transfused during the procedure, necessitating a platelet transfusion. If the bleeding is unresponsive to other therapies, cryoprecipitate should be given for low fibrinogen levels or factor VII for persistent nonsurgical bleeding. A duplex ultrasound of the liver is obtained in the first 24 hours to assess for vessel patency. Regardless of the source of the hemorrhage, emergent surgical reexploration is necessary.

Impaired kidney function is found in children with a history of cirrhosis, delayed liver function, and previous exposure to nephrotoxic drugs. Often low-dose dopamine is administered at 0.03–0.1 mcg/kg/min to maintain adequate perfusion. Other supportive therapies include renal replacement with continuous veno-venous hemofiltration (CVVH) to prevent rapid shifts of fluid. Electrolytes are monitored frequently per the center's routine to identify and manage potential problems with hypokalemia, hyperkalemia, acidosis, hypocalcemia, hypomagnesemia, and hyperglycemia. Either hypertension or hypotension may occur in the postoperative period related to altered kidney function and volume losses. The child with hypotension presents with decreased capillary refill, a weak pulse, and low systolic blood pressures (Hauser et al., 2008).

Fluids are administered at 80% of maintenance and electrolytes are monitored every 6 hours. Decreased urine output of less than 1 mL/kg/hr may indicate early graft dysfunction or nephrotoxicity related to calcineurin inhibitors (CNIs). Hypotension secondary to hypovolemia results from fluid shifts out of the intravascular space and high peritoneal fluid losses. Administration of albumin is necessary to manage protein losses from the peritoneal fluid

(Hauser et al., 2008). By day 3 to 5, the IT recipient's fluids and electrolytes should be stable and allow for resumption of parenteral nutrition. A nasogastric tube remains in place for several days to decompress the stomach, but is removed when the child's diet is advanced. Once the ileus has resolved, enteral feedings can be initiated via the jejunal route secondary to the delayed gastric emptying found postoperatively.

Neurological assessments are performed every 2 hours in the immediate postoperative using a modified Glasgow Coma Scale depending on the age of the child. Seizures are rare except in the most ill children. Neurotoxic side effects are common with tacrolimus administration, presenting with tremor, confusion, or headache if the trough level is elevated.

Liver function guides the use of sedatives and analgesics in the immediate postoperative period. Intravenous continuous narcotics are administered. The child should be assessed for excessive sedation, respiratory depression, hypotension, and constipation. An alternative approach entails placement of an epidural catheter. Oral narcotics can be administered once the child is tolerating oral feeds.

Cardiovascular monitoring following IT focuses on maintaining adequate perfusion of the graft with bedside Doppler monitoring of the stoma, ensuring adequate capillary refill, keeping oxygen saturations greater than 95%; maintaining hematocrit between 27% and 30%; ensuring hypertension control (due to CNIs); observings for hypervolemia or hyperperistalsis; and monitoring the QT interval to avoid torsades de pointes. Tachycardia may be a sign of dehydration that requires administration of additional fluids. In contrast, bradycardia may indicate hyperkalemia or be a side effect of narcotics or calcium-channel blockers (Hauser et al., 2008).

IMMUNOSUPPRESSIVE THERAPY

The goal of immunosuppressant therapy is to avoid over immunosuppressing the child. A challenge in pediatrics is considering the lifetime risk of immunosuppression in regard to its impact on future malignancies, growth and development, and fertility. The risk of acute rejection is greatest during the first 1 to 2 months after transplantation.

The approach is slightly different for liver and intestinal transplant recipients; however, most recipients receive a combination of drugs. Initially patients receive triple therapy with a CNI (tacrolimus 0.1–0.3 mg/kg/day BID or cyclosporine 5–10 mg/kg/day BID), corticosteroids (1 mg/kg/day tapered), and cell toxins that inhibit purine biosynthesis (mycophenalate mofetil 15 mg/kg BID or azathioprine 2 mg/kg) (Tredger et al., 2006). Since 2005, fewer than 5% of liver recipients have been treated with cyclosporine. Initially cyclosporine levels are maintained between 200 and 300 ng/mL and tacrolimus levels range from 5 to 15 ng/mL (McGuire et al., 2009). In the immediate IT postoperative period, tacrolimus levels are maintained in the range of 15 to 18 ng/dL.

CNIs have a similar side-effect profile that includes nephrotoxicity, neurotoxicity (tremors, headaches, seizures), diabetes mellitus (DM), hypertension, and lipid abnormalities. Campbell et al. (2006) reported a 32% rate of kidney dysfunction (GFR < 80 mL/min/1.7 3m^2) in children receiving cyclosporine post liver transplant at a mean of 7.6 years of age. DM occurs in 13.4% of gastrointestinal transplant recipients receiving CNIs. The primary risk factors for developing DM are obesity, African American or Hispanic ethnicity, family history, hepatitis C infection, and multiple transplant procedures (Greenspan et al., 2004).

In stable patients 6 months post-transplant, tacrolimus levels are commonly in the range of 5 to 7 ng/mL and cyclosporine levels are in the range of 100 to 200 ng/mL. CNIs are administered twice daily, but a modified release form of tacrolimus will be available soon, simplifying administration to a once-daily regimen. The antimetabolites are frequently discontinued within a year of transplantation. Mycophenalate mofetil is not recommended in IT because of the gastrointestinal side effects. Table 26-23 describes the side effects, drug interactions, and mechanisms of action of various classes of immunosuppressant agents.

Other maintenance options include rapamycin (0.02–0.35 mg/kg) and afinitor (0.8 mg/m^2), both of which are mammalian target of rapamycin (mTOR) inhibitors that inhibit T-cell proliferation during the cell cycle. Rapamycin is usually not administered in the immediate postoperative period secondary to concerns with delayed wound healing. This agent has also been used effectively as a rescue agent in abdominal transplant recipients. Rapamycin has a long half-life, approximately 21.5 hours, that affects its absorption and trough levels.

Induction immunosuppression is commonly used in IT, typically consisting of an anti IL-2 receptor antibody, antilymphocyte globulin, or alemtuzumab. Alemtuzumab is not recommended in children younger than 4 years of age because its use is associated with cytopenias, increased infection rates, acute respiratory distress syndrome, and delayed growth and development of bones. New immunosuppressant management strategies include the use of induction therapy with antithymocyte globulin (1.5 mg/kg) for 1 to 2 weeks post-transplant (dose is dependent on age at transplant), daclizumab (1 mg/kg times 5 doses every other week), and basiliximab (12 mg/m^2 on days 0 and 4) to provide IL-2 suppression (Pascher et al., 2008; Pirenne & Kawai, 2009; Tredger et al., 2006).

Liver transplant recipients are good candidates for steroid withdrawal. Nevertheless, the timing when initiating steroid wean is controversial, with some centers starting at 3 months post-transplant and other centers waiting until 1 year post-transplant. Providers must carefully identify patients at low immunological risk who are suitable candidates for steroid and CNI withdrawal or avoidance. During immunosuppressant weaning, children must be carefully monitored because acute rejection can occur at any time (Bucuvalas & Alonso, 2008).

The goal in developing new immunosuppressant agents is to prevent the long-term toxicities associated with currently used drug regimens. New agents in Phase II and III clinical trials with adult renal recipients include targeted small-molecule agents and biologic agents (belatacept-CTLA-4) that are being developed as maintenance therapy in hopes of avoiding the toxicity associated with use of daily oral agents (Sarwal, 2008; Vincenti & Kirk, 2008).

POST-TRANSPLANT COMPLICATIONS

Infection is a common complication following LT and IT, and accounts for high levels of post-transplant morbidity and mortality, occurring in 52% of patients (Kotton, 2008). Potential sites of infection include central venous catheters, the abdominal cavity, the bloodstream, the urinary tract, and the lungs, which account for 56% of deaths related to infection. Several factors influence the incidence and timing of infection, including the immunosuppressant regimen (dose, duration, timing), drug-related neutropenia, the presence of invasive objects (catheters) that impact on cutaneous barriers, metabolic abnormalities such as malnutrition, low albumin levels, viral exposures pre- and post-transplant, donor organ type, anhepatic time, and race (African Americans have lower risk of infectious complications) (Tredger et al., 2006). In the first 30 days post-transplant, infection is typically related to organisms not eradicated pretransplant, those acquired from the donor, or infections found in a general surgical population (e.g., pneumonia, bacterial or fungal surgical wounds, vascular access). Prevention of infection following IT involves administration of prophylactic antibiotic and antifungal agents.

The herpes group of viruses (HHV-6 and HHV-7, parvovirus, adenovirus, roseoloviruses) are a frequent cause of major infections from 1 to 6 months post-transplant. Signs and symptoms of infections with these pathogens should be investigated particularly if the child has pyrexia, rash, or bone marrow suppression.

Cytomegalovirus (CMV) is the most commonly occurring viral infection in the early post-transplant period, particularly in the recipient-negative/donor-positive group; nevertheless, all transplant recipients are potentially at risk of CMV infection (Shepherd et al., 2008). There is an association between CMV infection and rejection. Surveillance for this disease, with or without prophylactic therapy, may be undertaken, depending on institutional protocols. CMV disease presents as fever, hepatitis, enteritis, pneumonia, or a

TABLE 26-23

Immunosuppressant Medications Used in Gastrointestinal Transplantation				
Name	**Mechanism of Action**	**Indication**	**Common Side Effects**	**Medication Interactions**
Calcineurin inhibitors • Cyclosporine • Sandimmune • Neoral • Tacrolimus	Suppress activation of T cells	Primary or maintenance immunosuppression	Hypertension Hyperlipidemia Hirsutism Tremor Gingival hyperplasia Hyperkalemia Hypomagnesemia Nephrotoxicity Headache Diarrhea Insomnia	Elevate blood levels: • Fluconazole • Nifedipine • Erythromycin • Omeprazole • Grapefruit juice Lower blood levels: • Naficillin • Octreotide • Caspofungin • Phenobarbital • St. John's wort
Antiproliferative/ antimetabolites • Azathioprine • Mycophenalate mofetil • Myfortic	Block purine synthesis to B- and T-cell proliferation	Used in conjunction with maintenance immunosuppression to prevent graft rejection	BM depression Nausea Vomiting Pancreatitis Gastrointestinal BM depression Pharyngitis	Elevate blood levels: • Allopurinal • Aminosalicylates • Warfarin Lower blood levels: • Antacids with magnesium • Ganciclovir
mTOR inhibitors • Rapamycin • Everolimus	Inhibit cell-cycle activity from G_1 to S phase Inhibit IL-2 T-lymphocyte proliferation	Maintenance therapy or minimize side-effect profile of CNIs	Hypercholesterolemia Hyperlipidemia Acne Rash Nephrotoxicity Delayed wound healing HUS	Phenytoin Rifampin Dexamethasone Azithromycin Ketaconazole Grapefruit juice Fatty foods impair absorption; administer with or without food consistently
Corticosteroids • Methylprednisolone	Inhibit secretion of IL-1 and IL-2 Inhibit cytotoxic T-cell formation	Induction agent Maintenance Treat acute rejection Used in combination with CNIs	Cumulative SE Glucose intolerance Acne Mood changes Hypertension Osteoporosis Cataracts/glaucoma Fluid retention Weight gain GI distress Inhibits bone growth in children Suppress HPA axis Increased risk for infection	BCP Erythromycin Phenobarbital Warfarin NSAIDs
Polyclonal antilymphocyte globulins • Atgam • Thymoglobulin	Not completely understood Depletes T cells from circulation	Prevention or treatment of acute rejection	Fever Chills Headache Leukopenia Rash Pruritus Anaphylaxis Thrombocytopenia	Influenza nasal vaccine Live virus vaccines

Bone marrow (BM), bovine cornea protein, calcineurin inhibitor (CNI), gastrointestinal (GI), hemolytic uremic syndrome (HUS), nonsteroidal anti-inflammatory drugs (NSAIDs), steroid effect (SE).

viral syndrome with neutropenia and thrombocytopenia. In the liver transplant recipient, CMV may contribute to vanishing bile duct syndrome, accelerate the development of chronic rejection, and increase the patient's risk of contracting other serious infections such as *Pneumocystis* pneumonia or aspergillosis. Primary CMV infection occurs secondary to direct exposure to pathogen-carrying bodily fluids such as saliva, tears, urine, stool, or breastmilk. The highest rate of active transmission is in children aged 13 to 24 months (Campbell & Herold, 2004; Kotton, 2008).

Treatment of CMV is divided into universal prophylaxis versus preemptive therapy. Universal prophylaxis involves the administration of antiviral agents with or without an immunological agent to all transplant recipients regardless of CMV risk. The use of universal CMV prophylaxis delays the onset of symptoms for several months following solid-organ transplant. There is no consensus among experts regarding the best route of administration of antiviral agents (oral versus intravenous) or the use of immunoglobulin prophylaxis. In contrast, pre-emptive therapy involves administering effective treatment to high-risk recipients for a short course of therapy. Preemptive therapy requires the ability to detect changes in the viral load with tests that demonstrate sufficient sensitivity and specificity to differentiate latent from active replicating virus. Polymerase chain reaction (PCR) tests are sensitive predictors of CMV disease in solid-organ transplant recipients. Prophylactic therapy has traditionally consisted of intravenous ganciclovir; however, concerns about its cost and the safety of long-term administration have led to implementation of other management strategies. Valganciclovir can be used interchangeably with ganciclovir and is administered orally with minimal resistance. The bioavailability of valganciclovir in children is lower than in adults, however, so patients may require pharmacokinetic monitoring to assure adequate therapy (Kotton, 2008). Another option, foscarnet, is comparable to intravenous ganciclovir, but is associated with significant side effects (Campbell & Herold, 2004).

Epstein-Barr virus (EBV) is another common viral infection that can lead to post-transplant lymphoproliferative disease (PTLD). Risk factors for PTLD include lifelong immunosuppression, young age at time of transplantation (increasing the risk in liver and intestinal transplant recipients), and recipient seronegative status. The World Health Organization classifies PTLD into four classifications: early lesions (presenting less than 1 year post-transplant), polymorphic PTLD, monomorphic PTLD, and other types (Harris et al., 1997). The incidence of PTLD is highest in IT recipients—19%—but occurs in only 3% of liver recipients (Everly et al., 2007). When PTLD presents with polycolonal features, the virus is more likely to respond to a dose reduction in immunosuppression. Children who present with monoclonal features such as a diffuse large B-cell lymphoma (Burkitt's lymphoma) have no response to reduction in immunosuppression. Common sites affected

by this disease include the tonsil, adenoids, cervical nodes, lung, and abdomen.

The clinical presentation of PTLD is highly variable. Early symptoms consist of fever, malaise, sore throat, abdominal pain or palpable mass, diarrhea with protein or blood loss in the stool, graft dysfunction, or headache. Serial monitoring of quantitative EBV PCR titers every 2 to 4 weeks in the first 3 months post-transplant and every 1 to 3 months in patients who are more than 3 months post-transplant throughout the first year is recommended. Patients with more than 4,000 copies/mcg DNA or EBV biopsy-proven infection should undergo weaning of immunosuppression, radiological monitoring with computed tomography, and ongoing assessment of their EBV viral load (Lee et al., 2005a). Preemptive treatment with antiviral agents—specifically, ganciclovir and acyclovir—has not demonstrated a clear reduction in the incidence of PTLD.

Localized disease is managed with reduction or withdrawal of immunosuppression combined with surgical excision and/or localized radiation. Children with extensive PTLD may undergo a 50% reduction in CNIs and discontinuation of other immunosuppressant agents. Adjuvant therapy with rituximab and other chemotherapy agents (CHOP: cyclophosphamide, doxorubicin, vincristine, prednisone) may be necessary to achieve remission; it is effective in 69% of patients with B-cell tumors (Bucuvalas et al., 2008; Everly et al., 2007). Antiviral agents administered for treatment of PTLD have shown evidence of efficacy in small retrospective reviews, but this practice is controversial and is not recommended as solo therapy.

Post-transplant solid-organ recipients are also at risk for common childhood illnesses. Fever should be completely evaluated, with both a history and physical examination being undertaken. A septic evaluation is required if no source of the fever is immediately identified, including complete blood count, blood and urine cultures, and metabolic panel. Acetaminophen is recommended in the treatment of temperature elevation because NSAIDs may impair compromised hepatic/kidney function. The "common cold" and gastroenteritis occur frequently in the fall and winter months. If pneumonia is suspected, a chest radiograph should be obtained. The symptoms of a cough, cold, and gastrointestinal illness are likely to "hang on" for a longer period in IT and LT recipients than the same symptoms in well siblings. Parents should avoid the use of OTC cough and cold medications in children who have received liver or intestinal transplant. Supportive care to prevent dehydration and keep secretions thin is important. If the child is unable to orally hydrate, intravenous fluids should be provided to prevent abnormally elevated calcineurin levels in the face of dehydration.

Influenza is an acute illness characterized by coryza, cough, fever, pharyngitis, headache, myalgia, and malaise. Transplant recipients are likely to experience more short- and long-term complications related to influenza than the general population; in addition, the immunologic response often results in acute allograft rejection. Prevention is enhanced by encouraging immunization of all household contacts and HCPs on transplant units. In one study, Madan et al. (2008) reported similar antibody seroconversion rates in transplant recipients compared to their healthy siblings following administration of the influenza vaccine. Antiviral medications in addition to vaccines may be required to prevent or treat influenza. Infected transplant patients require isolation or should be cohorted to prevent the transmission of virus.

Hepatic artery thrombosis (HAT) is the most common post-transplant surgical complication, occurring in 8.3% of pediatric liver recipients (Bekker et al., 2009; McGuire et al., 2009) and representing the major cause of graft loss. Factors affecting the likelihood of HAT include the small vasculature found in infants and small children, the CMV status of the donor and the recipient, retransplantation versus primary transplantation, and prolonged operative times. HAT may present with elevated transaminase and bilirubin levels, a change in mental status, biliary leak, or sepsis. Diagnosis of HAT in the first 1 to 6 days postoperatively is possible with a duplex ultrasound; however, if collateral vessels have developed, angiography may be necessary. HAT is managed with observation, thrombectomy to restore blood flow, or retransplantation.

Similarly, thrombosis of the intestinal graft is a rare complication, presenting with a dusky stoma or deteriorating function. Prevention and treatment is institution specific, but may include administration of low-molecular-weight heparin, aspirin, or enoxaprin. Abdominal ultrasounds are obtained in the immediate postoperative period to assess for thrombus formation that requires surgical intervention.

Another potential vascular complication is portal vein (PV) thrombosis. This problem presents with variceal bleeding or a slowly enlarging liver or spleen and decreasing platelet counts. Recipients of living-related liver transplantation are at higher risk for developing a PV thrombosis because of the shorter vessel pedicles compared to patients who receive whole-liver grafts from cadaveric donors or cryopreserved vein grafts. Usually no intervention is required and children resolve the ascites as the spleen size decreases. Occasionally an interventional venoplasty is performed to correct the obstruction (Ueda et al., 2005).

Biliary leaks are a leading cause of morbidity and mortality in liver recipients, occurring in 14% to 38% of living-related liver transplants (Kling et al., 2004). A postoperative change in the color of fluid in the Jackson-Pratt drain, fever, elevated liver function tests, and cholangitis indicate a leak. Abdominal pain may or may not be present because the transplanted liver has been innervated. Bacterial contamination is possible if the leak occurs at the Roux-en-Y anastamosis. The risk of HAT increases significantly when a biliary leak is noted in the immediate postoperative period. Diagnosis is made by ultrasound or percutaneous transhepatic cholangiogram. Nonoperative management of biliary leaks is possible with percutaneous cholangiographic intervention (Kling et al., 2004). Similarly, bile leaks associated with the T tube are managed with percutaneous drainage, stent placement, or surgical revision of the biliary connection and broad-spectrum antibiotics (McGuire et al., 2009).

NUTRITION AFTER INTESTINAL TRANSPLANTATION

The long-term goal of IT is to provide nutrition that contributes to gut trophicity. Prior to initiating enteral feedings, an upper gastrointestinal study is obtained to evaluate for an intestinal leak. Abdominal distention, fever, and peritonitis are signs of a gastrointestinal leak.

Several weeks after IT, a combination of parenteral and enteral feedings are offered through the gastric or jejunal route, using a low-osmolar formula (isotonic amino acid or peptide-based formula) that contains medium-chain triglycerides. The volume is advanced first, followed by the formula concentration—starting with a one-fourth strength formula and advancing to full strength as tolerated. Once lymphatic drainage is reestablished, the formula should include standard long-chain triglycerides.

Chylous ascites and fat malabsorption may impair both short- and long-term outcomes. Supplementation with fat-soluble vitamins and zinc is required in children with fat malabsorption and high ostomy output. Prokinetic and motility agents are administered in children with abdominal cramping and rapid transit time. Small oral feeding with water should be offered when jejunal feedings are initiated and advanced as tolerated (Hauser et al., 2008; Kosmach-Park & De Angelis, 2008).

Oral aversion is a very real problem in children who receive parenteral nutrition for extended periods. Referral to an occupational or speech therapist can assist the child in obtaining oral motor skills. There is a potential risk of developing food allergies with alternative feeding methods, so avoidance of eggs and milk is recommended. Improved linear growth and weight gain are observed following IT, but most patients do not attain full "catch-up" growth owing to early stunting (Colomb & Goulet, 2009; Encinas et al., 2006).

REJECTION

Risk factors affecting the likelihood of transplant rejection include the recipient's age (older age is associated with increased risk), gender, primary diagnosis, donor organ type, and primary immunosuppression and early use of monoclonal or polyclonal antibodies (Shepherd et al., 2008). Early signs of rejection in liver transplant recipients are low-grade fever, increased liver enzymes and bilirubin levels, pain over the graft, irritability, and ascites. Diagnosis is confirmed with a percutaneous liver biopsy. This procedure is usually performed under conscious sedation with local anesthesia. Prior to performing a liver biopsy, the HCP should type and cross-match the child for one unit of blood and obtain a prothrombin and partial thromboplastin time. A hemoglobin level should be obtained 4 to 6 hours after the procedure, and the child should remain flat in bed for 4 to 6 hours.

The incidence of acute rejection in IT is higher than with transplantation of other solid organs because of the high degree of lymphoid tissue found in the graft. The incidence of severe rejection is reduced in multivisceral grafts compared with intestine-only grafts. Two variables that predict graft survival are progression to severe rejection and prolonged rejection lasting more than 21 days. Repeated episodes of acute rejection lead to chronic rejection with a slow loss of intestinal function over a prolonged period of time (Pascher et al., 2008).

The hallmark of IT rejection is increased stomal output, which is frequently accompanied by fever, diarrhea, and bloody discharge. Other markers of early rejection include new-onset feeding intolerance, emesis, and cramping change in the color and consistency of ileostomy drainage. In the early postoperative period, prior to initiating feeds, output is approximately 20 mL/kg/day in children and 300 mL/day in adolescents. Ostomy output greater than 50 mL/kg/day indicates acute rejection. In the case of multivisceral or composite transplantation, appropriate serum markers of liver or kidney function may aid in the diagnosis of rejection (Hauser et al., 2008). Surveillance endoscopies and biopsies are performed through the ileostomy to monitor for rejection. Immediate biopsy for new symptoms of rejection may also be obtained by this route. New, less invasive strategies (e.g., zoom video endoscopy) are under evaluation for monitoring of early rejection (Hauser et al.; Kato et al., 2006; Pascher et al., 2008). IT biopsies indicate the presence of increased apoptotic bodies, blunted villa, and ulceration in patients who experience rejection.

Acute rejection is treated with a bolus of steroids (intravenous solumedrol or oral methylprednisolone). Rapidly progressive or severe acute rejection in the intestinal transplant recipient may require treatment with OKT3 or antithymocyte globulin. Late acute rejection is histologically different from early acute rejection. Liver biopsies demonstrate centrilobular necrosis in these circumstances, and patients' response to treatment is not as rapid as in patients with early acute rejection.

Chronic rejection is another important cause of graft loss. In such patients, the liver biopsy demonstrates bile duct loss with fibrosis and cirrhosis. The cause is unknown, but is most likely multifactorial, including multiple episodes of acute rejection, CMV infection, or inconsistent immunosuppressant levels. Similarly, chronic rejection in

IT occurs over a long period of time and may result from inadequate treatment of acute rejection. The biopsy demonstrates villous blunting, focal ulcerations, and limited cellular infiltrates. Initial treatment involves changing immunosuppressant agents. If this measure fails, the child should be relisted for transplantation. Late intestinal graft rejection presents with progressive weight loss, chronic diarrhea, intermittent fever, and blood in the stoma effluent. Rejection that is not responsive to available treatment may require enterectomy and/or retransplantation.

GRAFT-VERSUS-HOST DISEASE

Three factors contribute to the development of graft-versus-host disease (GvHD) following IT:

- Presence of immunologically active cells in the graft
- Host tissues lacking in the donor
- Recipient with an immunologic response

The incidence of GvHD in both IT and multivisceral transplantation is approximately 7% to 8%. Affected children present with skin rashes, ulceration of the oral mucosa, diarrhea, lymphadenopathy, or native liver malfunction. Management is similar to the approaches used for rejection—namely, administration of corticosteroids and optimization of CNIs (Pascher et al., 2008). Increased mortality is reported in children with acute and chronic GvHD (Kato et al., 2006).

OUTCOMES OF LIVER AND INTESTINAL TRANSPLANTATION

In one study, between 1996 and 2001, LT patient and graft survival rates in 2,291 children were found to be 89.8% and 84.8%, respectively (Ng et al., 2008) with no significant differences being noted based on graft type. However, a recent larger review indicated increased morbidity in children who received reduced or split grafts. In this study, 55 patients (12%) required retransplantation, most commonly for HAT, biliary complications, chronic rejection, and primary graft dysfunction. Survival rates for children undergoing retransplant at 1 and 5 years are 60% and 50%, respectively. Variables that predict improved outcomes for this group are older age at retransplantation, ethnicity (African American recipients experience greater morbidity than Caucasians recipients), and not currently requiring life-support and type of graft (Davis et al., 2009). Variables that predict late mortality (1 year after transplantation) are malignancy (hepatoblastoma or PTLD), ALF, history of HAT, more than 5 hospitalizations in the first year posttransplant, and weight deficit at transplant (Bucuvalas & Alonso, 2008).

In 2007, the 1-year IT graft survival was 70% and the patient survival rate was 78% (Berg et al., 2009). It is likely that administration of newer immunosuppressant agents will contribute to improved results and shift the focus from short-term to long-term outcomes. Five years after IT, 73% of patients were reported to have linear growth below that of the normal population. This factor is related to long-term steroid use and poor nutrition prior to transplantation. In one study (Barshes et al., 2006), the height z score was correlated with both longer duration of hospitalization during the transplant and increased costs.

Another long-term complication of gastrointestinal transplantation is the development of chronic kidney failure related to the use of CNIs, perioperative complications, primary liver diseases with potential renal involvement, and arterial hypertension (Ng et al., 2008). Approximately 28% of pediatric LT recipients have a GFR of 90 mL/min/ 1.73 m² 1 year after transplantation. The risk of kidney failure increases over time, with an estimated incidence of 25% in recipients 10 years after LT (Harambat et al., 2008). Few studies of the reversibility of kidney failure after LT have been performed, however. Signs and symptoms of chronic kidney failure are anemia, osteodystrophy, and electrolyte abnormalities. Monitoring for hypertension and obtaining a urinalysis are early screening tools for kidney failure on a post-transplant basis. Early referral to nephrology is recommended when proteinuria and hypertension are present (Bucuvalas & Alonso, 2008; McGuire et al., 2009). Exposure to parenteral nutrition, nephrotoxic medications, dehydration, and sepsis are risk factors for kidney insufficiency in IT recipients prior to transplantation. Similar to LT recipients, a GFR less than 70 mL/min/1.73 m² at 1 year post IT is associated with long-term kidney insufficiency and poor outcome. CNI-sparing regimens that substitute rapamycin for tacrolimus may positively affect patients' chances of developing renal dysfunction (Campbell et al., 2006; Watson et al., 2008).

DISPOSITION AND DISCHARGE PLANNING

Discharge planning includes providing education about side effects of immunosuppressant medications, reviewing signs and symptoms of rejection and infection, and monitoring for wound infections and ostomy output. As adolescents near adulthood, specific programs focusing on the transition to an adult or primary care specialist should be initiated. Key program goals center on discussing risk-taking behaviors regarding sexual behavior and drug and alcohol use, counseling patients about birth control, identifying a source of health insurance, developing disease management skills, and counseling patients in relation to their career and education plans. Table 26-24 provides information on discharge planning and follow-up for recipients of gastrointestinal transplants.

TABLE 26-24

Discharge Planning and Long-Term Management of Patients with Gastrointestinal Transplants
Monitor for graft function
Update/resume immunization schedule
Twice-yearly dental visits
Once-yearly ophthalmology examination
Return to school
Neuropsychological testing/school evaluation
Monitor for growth and development
Screen for kidney dysfunction
• Monitor blood pressure and treat hypertension aggressively
• Urinalysis
Obtain a lipid profile
Nutrition counseling for weight management
Monitor for adherence with immunosuppression regimen
Recommend participation in rehabilitation to improve strength and endurance
Recommend sunblock use

Adolescents

Transition to adult health care team
Career/school counseling
Avoid smoking
Counseling about birth control

In the past, live virus vaccines were contraindicated after transplantation; however, more recent studies have shown that these vaccines may be safely administered in a select group of patients receiving low-dose immunosuppression. In one study, more than 80% of such patients achieved both humoral and cellular immunity (Weinberg et al., 2006). Children do not require revaccination, but should resume the previous schedule recommended by the American Academy of Pediatrics. Recipients should avoid oral polio, measles/mumps/rubella (MMR), varicella, oral typhoid, intranasal influenza, yellow fever, and bacillus Calmette-Guérin (BCG) vaccines. Children younger than 2 years of age should be considered for pavilizumab. The AAP recommends two doses of pneumococcal conjugate vaccine (PCV7), followed by a single dose of 23V (pneumococcal) vaccine.

Care should be taken when prescribing antibiotics to LT and IT recipients. Avoid the use of macrolide antibiotics whenever possible, as these medications interact with CNIs and produce elevated levels of tacrolimus and cyclosporine (Tredger et al., 2006). Nonsteroidal medications and agents metabolized through the cytochrome P450 pathway should also be avoided in children receiving CNIs or mTOR immunosuppressant agents. Indiscriminate use of antibiotics in the transplant recipient increases the risk of developing a fungal infection. In addition, families should be instructed to avoid the use of herbal supplements and OTC medications because of the possibility that they might interact with immunosuppressant medications.

In a study of post-transplant quality of life in adolescents, Taylor et al. (2009) found that adolescents' self-reported health-related quality of life (HRQL) was 10 points lower than the values reported by adolescents without transplants, irrespective of acute or chronic presentation of liver failure. Variables associated with a lower HRQL include older age at transplantation, frequency of symptoms (weight gain, difficulty with sleep, painful joints, headaches), and distress related to immunosuppressive medications. The most important variable that leads to a low HRQL is development of a second chronic illness after transplantation. Teens are also at risk for suicidal thoughts, concerns about fertility, financial security, and the inability to obtain health insurance.

Many children have significant problems following a liver or intestinal transplant, such as poor academic performance, low self-esteem, depression, and anxiety. In one study, 18% of transplant-recipient children reported repeating a grade or being held back in school at least 1 year (Ng et al., 2008). Adëback et al. (2003) studied cognitive and emotional outcome after liver transplantation. They found that one-half of the children evaluated had IQ scores less than 85, indicating learning difficulties that required additional academic resources. Gilmour et al. (2009) reported similar findings—specifically, a 27% delay and 27% borderline delay in children undergoing LT prior to 6 years of age. Children had the lowest test scores in mathematics and numeric operations. When compared to age-matched peers, the most significant differences were found in higher function skills such as abstract thinking, logical analyses, and memory (Bucuvalas et al., 2008).

Transplantation dramatically improves a young person's quality of life, but often changes an acute or life-threatening illness into a chronic disease. Adherence to a mutually agreed plan of therapy can be very difficult. Nonadherence with immunosuppressive therapy is common problem in this population, with estimated rates ranging from 5% to 71% (Bucuvalas et al., 2008; Dew et al., 2009). Standard measures to monitor blood levels of CNIs that have a narrow therapeutic range results are a poor proxy for monitoring adherence to immunosuppression. In addition, the inconsistent pharmacokinetics of immunosuppressant agents found in children compounds the problems associated with dosing, monitoring, and follow-up care in this population (Dew et al.; Venkat et al., 2008).

Shemesh (2004) reported preliminary data on a clinical adherence monitoring program consisting of five different types of monitoring. Subjective ratings of adherence by the patient, caregiver, physician, and nurse were compared, along with medication blood levels. The findings indicated that HCPs were accurate in identifying the most severe cases of nonadherence, but missed patients who continued to do well medically. Psychosocial predictors of nonadherence included the existence of post-traumatic stress symptoms, described as anxiety, nightmares, or intrusive thoughts.

Failure to attend clinic appointments and complete tests may be another indicator of nonadherence and should be evaluated.

Treatment involves consultation with a mental health professional or social worker, along with ongoing education. Health care professionals need to be vigilant in assessing children for risk factors for nonadherence and making timely referrals. Defining a reliable measure of adherence will allow for the development of targeted interventions (Stuber et al., 2008; Venkat et al., 2008). Currently few data are available on nonadherence in IT recipients.

INDIRECT HYPERBILIRUBINEMIA IN THE NEONATE

Terri L. Russell

PATHOPHYSIOLOGY

During fetal life, the placenta and maternal circulation efficiently clear bilirubin from amniotic fluid, even in the presence of significant fetal hemolysis resulting from maternal–fetal hemorrhage or blood-type incompatibility. A number of factors that promote fetal-to-maternal transfer of indirect bilirubin severely limit the newborn's ability to maintain low levels of unconjugated, or indirect, bilirubin after birth.

Bilirubin is formed primarily from the degradation of hemoglobin from erythrocytes, which occurs normally as aged cells are removed from circulation. The degradation of erythrocytes produced earlier in gestation increases bilirubin production in late gestation by as much as 150%. As a result, the newborn produces more than twice as much bilirubin as in an adult, up to 8 to 10 mg/kg/day (Blackburn, 2007).

Heme is released from hemoglobin and converted to biliverdin heme oxygenase in the reticuloendothelial system (Figure 26-9). This step in bilirubin metabolism produces free iron, which is stored for hemoglobin synthesis, and carbon monoxide (CO), which is excreted by the lungs. Biliverdin is reduced to unconjugated bilirubin by biliverdin reductase and rapidly bound to albumin.

Other elements of bilirubin production, conjugation, and excretion impede the neonate's ability to effectively handle a bilirubin load. The placenta transports bilirubin only in its fat-soluble form for removal by the maternal liver; thus enzyme systems (or lack thereof) favor maintaining bilirubin in an unconjugated state after birth and impede clearance. In the liver, UDP-glucuronyl transferase conjugates indirect bilirubin to water-soluble forms (monoglucuronides and diglucuronides) to facilitate excretion in urine and stool. This enzyme activity is low in the newborn—less than 1% of adult activity when an infant

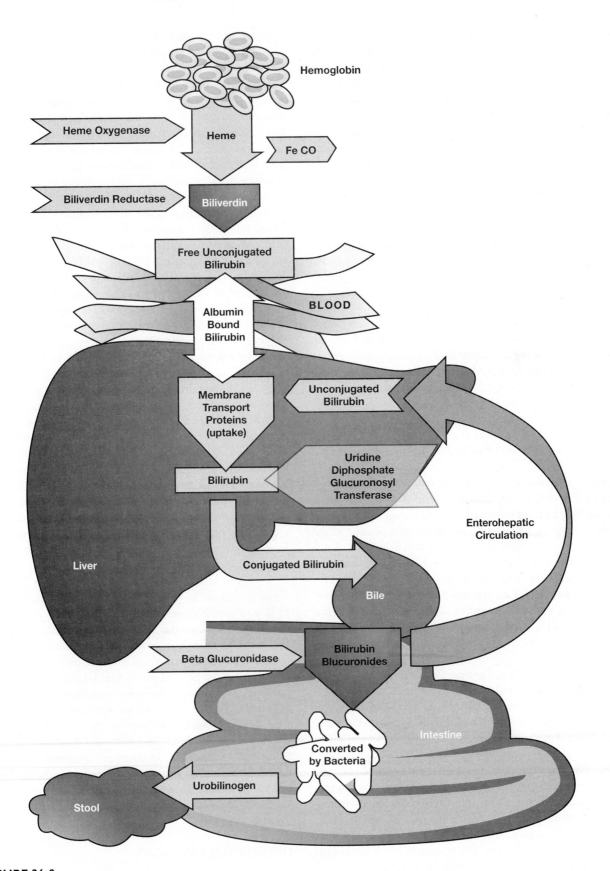

FIGURE 26-9

Neonatal Bilirubin Metabolism.

Source: Courtesy of Mary Puchalski.

is born at term (Blackburn, 2007). β-Glucuronidase, an enteric mucosal enzyme in the intestines, hydrolyzes the conjugated monoglucuronides and diglucuronides of bilirubin back to the unconjugated form, which is then reabsorbed across the intestinal mucosa and returned to the liver via portal circulation. This process—known as the enterohepatic shunt—is responsible for the increased recirculation of bilirubin. High β-glucuronidase concentrations promote placental transfer of unconjugated bilirubin into maternal circulation and remain elevated after birth.

Meconium, which is present in the newborn intestine, may contain as much as 200 mg of bilirubin. Decreased intestinal motility is common in the newborn, delaying passage of meconium and promoting deconjugation of bilirubin by β-glucuronidase, which in turn results in increased indirect bilirubin levels.

Direct or conjugated hyperbilirubinemia is uncommon in the neonate during the time when indirect hyperbilirubinemia is likely to occur. Cholestasis resulting from altered hepatic function leads to decreased excretion of bilirubin into the bile and the development of direct hyperbilirubinemia. When an increase in the direct bilirubin accompanies severe indirect hyperbilirubinemia, evaluation for infection should be included in the investigation.

EPIDEMIOLOGY AND ETIOLOGY

Routine evaluation for hyperbilirubinemia occurs in all neonatal settings and takes the form of both universal screening and early follow-up after discharge. Despite this widely accepted practice, some infants may present to the emergency department or an outpatient setting with significant jaundice. For others, evaluation for hyperbilirubinemia may be forgotten while the neonate is being treated for a life-threatening illness in a non-neonatal pediatric setting, such as the pediatric intensive care or pediatric surgical heart unit. The development of bilirubin encephalopathy in these infants has been called "critical illness kernicterus" (Shapiro, 2008).

Nearly all newborns develop total bilirubin levels well above the norm for older children and adults, reaching a mean peak of 5–6 mg/dL within the first 2 to 5 days of life (Wong et al., 2006). Some infants—especially Asian and Asian American infants—develop levels in the range of 10–14 mg/dL in the first 3 to 5 days after birth, before gradually declining. For most newborns, this physiologic jaundice is nothing more than a transient rise that resolves spontaneously and without intervention. However, unrecognized progressive hyperbilirubinemia, in which levels exceed 20–25 mg/dL, may occur in a small percentage of infants. This may lead to the development of hazardous indirect bilirubin levels and result in kernicterus, an irreversible encephalopathy that leaves the infant neurologically devastated. To prevent this most dreaded complication, identification of risk factors for the development of severe

hyperbilirubinemia, combined with close surveillance of bilirubin levels, are fundamental practices in the care of any newborn.

Non-immune and immune factors may superimpose on the already limited ability of the neonate to handle a bilirubin load and lead to abnormally high serum bilirubin levels. Hemolysis is common in bacterial and viral infections and results in increased breakdown of red blood cells and increased bilirubin production. Extravascular blood resulting from ecchymoses, cephalohematoma, and polycythemia may all increase bilirubin availability.

G6PD deficiency is the most common inherited red blood cell (RBC) enzyme defect and results in hemolysis after exposure to oxidative stress from a chemical trigger or infection (Gallagher, 2000). G6PD deficiency occurs in nearly 13% of African American males and a smaller percentage of African American females (Maisels, 2009). Hyperbilirubinemia requiring phototherapy is more likely to develop in G6PD-deficient infants than in their G6PD-sufficient counterparts. Oxidative stress can lead to acute, severe hemolysis and produce a rapid rise in bilirubin levels. G6PD deficiency was identified as the cause in 21% of severe hyperbilirubinemia cases reported to the U.S. Kernicterus Registry (Maisels).

ABO incompatibility is an isoimmune reaction occurring when antibodies (anti-A, anti-B) from a mother with type O blood react against the A or B antigens on her infant's RBCs, resulting in hemolysis and an increased bilirubin production. Although this condition does not guarantee the development of hyperbilirubinemia, ongoing systematic assessment of the newborn for jaundice is required to prevent dangerously high bilirubin levels from occurring when ABO incompatibility, G6PD deficiency, or other risk factors are present.

Bilirubin unbound to albumin, called free bilirubin, easily crosses the blood–brain barrier, is deposited in brain cells, and results in permanent brain damage. Areas of the brain vulnerable to the toxic effects of bilirubin include the basal ganglia, the structure controlling movement, brain stem auditory pathways, and oculomotor nuclei. The level of bilirubin beyond which brain damage occurs is not absolute; underlying conditions associated with hypoproteinemia, hypoxia, and acidosis may lower the threshold. *Kernicterus* is the classic term to describe this neuropathology, which includes choreathetoid cerebral palsy, sensorineural hearing loss, impairment of upward gaze, and dental dysplasia (Shapiro, 2008). Intellect is thought to be normal in individuals with this condition, but severe physical handicaps impede education and rehabilitation.

DIFFERENTIAL DIAGNOSIS

Jaundice is classified into two categories: physiologic and pathologic. By definition, in physiologic jaundice, the bilirubin level does not exceed 12 mg/dL (Wong et al., 2006).

When higher levels are present, the etiology of indirect hyperbilirubinemia becomes the differential diagnosis. One or more conditions previously described in this section may add to the normal immaturity of neonatal conjugating ability, and appropriate treatment may depend on the identification of a pathologic process.

PRESENTATION

Frequent assessment and evaluation of an infant with any of a number of conditions known to exacerbate the already limited ability of the neonate to metabolize bilirubin are necessary to detect bilirubin levels requiring treatment. For example, feeding promotes stooling and elimination of bilirubin-rich meconium. Nothing-by-mouth (NPO) status promotes β-glucuronidase activity, deconjugation of bilirubin in the intestine, and an exaggerated enterohepatic circulation of bilirubin. Therefore, a newborn who remains NPO is at higher risk for increased bilirubin levels and warrants more frequent evaluation.

Jaundice is frequently assessed in the newborn by blanching the skin to reveal the underlying color. Physiologic jaundice usually appears on the second or third day of life. Jaundice appearing within the first 24 hours is more likely to have a pathologic origin, so that immediate evaluation is warranted. Following a cephalocaudal pattern, jaundice first appears in the face and progresses caudally to the chest, abdomen, and extremities. Increased involvement of body surfaces correlates with higher bilirubin levels.

Although jaundice is an important clinical sign, visual assessment alone is not a reliable indicator of bilirubin levels and may underestimate the actual level. The presence of extensive jaundice on plantar and palmer surfaces and the mucous membranes, including the tongue and gums, is associated with dangerously high bilirubin levels. An infant presenting with such findings, particularly when combined with signs of encephalopathy, requires immediate treatment with intensive phototherapy while awaiting laboratory confirmation of the bilirubin level.

PLAN OF CARE

When an infant presents with jaundice, a number of clinical tests may be performed to diagnose the underlying etiology (Table 26-25). First, is the bilirubin level, which determines therapeutic management. In 2004, the American Academy of Pediatrics published a clinical practice guideline for the management of hyperbilirubinemia in the newborn of 35 weeks' or more gestation; this document has since been updated (Maisels et al., 2009). All HCPs providing care to newborns should be familiar with these guidelines. When an infant presents to the acute care setting with an extremely high bilirubin measurement that is either nearing or at the level for exchange transfusion, consultation with a neonatal HCP should be sought.

TABLE 26-25

Diagnostic Studies
Total and direct serum bilirubin
Blood type and Rh of infant and mother
Direct Coombs test
Complete blood count and reticulocyte count
Peripheral smear for red blood cell morphology
G6PD screen
Urinalysis and urine culture
Check newborn thyroid and galactosemia screen
Evaluate for signs or symptoms of hypothyroidism
Sepsis evaluation if indicated by history and physical examination

Important components of the practice guideline include graphs identifying age-in-hours–specific total serum bilirubin levels indicating the need for phototherapy treatment (Figure 26-10) or an exchange transfusion (Figure 26-11). A high degree of vigilance on the part of HCPs is required to prevent extreme hyperbilirubinemia from unknowingly occurring.

Phototherapy has been used for more than 30 years in treating indirect hyperbilirubinemia and is a commonly employed therapy in hospital settings. The total serum bilirubin level at which phototherapy is indicated varies based on the child's gestational age and the presence of risk factors. Phototherapy may be provided by banked units, tungsten–halogen lamps, or fiber-optic systems where light from a high-intensity lamp is delivered to a fiber-optic blanket. Light predominantly in the blue–green spectrum (400–520 nm) treats neonatal jaundice by using visible light to stimulate photoisomerization of bilirubin (Stowkowski, 2006). The photoproducts produced are water soluble and can be excreted in urine and bile (stool), thereby effectively lowering the circulating bilirubin concentration (Figure 26-12). Photoisomerization begins as soon as phototherapy is instituted. Because photoproducts are water soluble, they are not neurotoxic. Consequently, phototherapy may confer some amount of neuroprotection, even in situations when serum bilirubin levels have reached or exceeded exchange transfusion levels.

Increased irradiance is provided by moving the light source closer to the infant. A naked near-term or term infant receiving phototherapy will maintain a normal temperature in a bassinet and does not need to be placed in an incubator, as that practice will increase the distance from the light. Fluorescent tubes can be safely brought within 10 cm of an infant in a bassinet. Halogen-spot phototherapy lamps, however, may increase the risk of burning, and should not be positioned closer than specified in the manufacturer's recommendations.

Maximum skin exposure increases effectiveness of phototherapy; for this reason, the infant should be naked while receiving phototherapy, with only a minimal diaper area covered. The surface area treated may be increased by placing one or more fiber-optic pads under the infant and

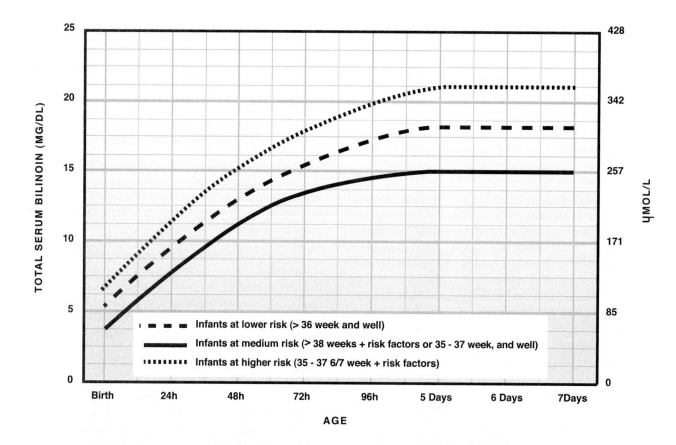

- Use total bilirubin. Do not subtract direct reacting or conjugated bilirubin.
- Risk factors = isoimmune hemolytic disease, G6PDf deficiency, asphyxia, significant lethargy, temperature instability, sepsis, acidosis, or albumin > 3.0g/dL (if measured).
- For well infants 35 - 37 6/7 week can adjust TSB levels for intervention around the medium risk line. It is an option to intervene at lower TSB levels for infants closer to 35 weeks and at higher TSB levels for those closer to 37 6/7 weeks.
- It is an option to provide conventional phototherapy in hospital or at home at TSB levels 2 - 3 mg/dL (35 - 50 mmol/L) below those shown but home phototherapy should not be used in any infant with risk factors.

FIGURE 26-10

Guidelines for Phototherapy in Hospitalized Infants of 35 or More Weeks' Gestation.

Source: Reproduced with permission. From American Academy of Pediatrics, Subcommittee on hyperbilirubinemia. (2004). Clinical practice guideline: management of hyperbilirubinemia in the newborn infant ≥ 35 or more weeks of gestation. Pediatrics, 114, 297–316. Copyright © 2004 American Academy of Pediatrics.

multiple phototherapy lamps above the infant. Lining the sides of the bassinet with aluminum foil adds to surface area exposure.

Dehydration related to inadequate breastfeeding may be related to the development of high serum bilirubin levels; thus assessment of hydration should include evaluation of skin turgor, mucous membranes, urine output, and current weight compared to birth weight. Unless dehydration is present, parenteral fluids are generally not indicated; however, enteral feedings with an elemental formula in a nonencephalopathic infant may help promote excretion of bilirubin in the stools.

Infants with isoimmune hemolytic disease, and a rising serum bilirubin despite intensive phototherapy, should receive intravenous immunoglobulin (IVIG). IVIG reduces hemolysis by blocking maternal antibody destruction of neonatal red blood cells. Less hemolysis results in a decreased bilirubin load.

The bilirubin level at which treatment is discontinued depends on the age at which phototherapy was initiated and the cause of hyperbilirubinemia. Generally, once a steady decline in bilirubin levels is observed and values are well below the exchange level, phototherapy may be discontinued. A repeat bilirubin within 24 hours

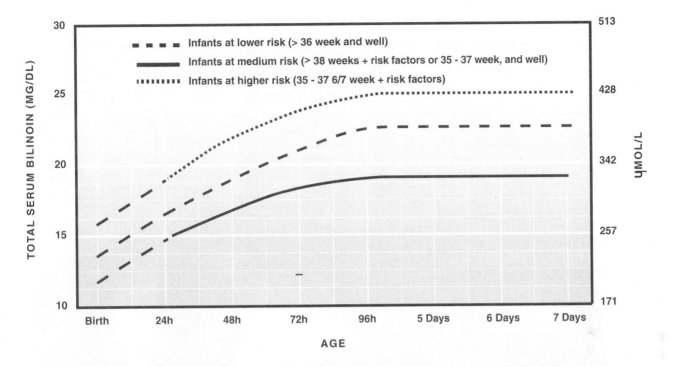

- The dashed lines for the first 24 hours indicate uncertainty due to a wide range of clinical circumstances and a range of responses to phototherapy.
- Immediate exchange transfusion is recommended if infant shows signs of acute bilirubin encephalopathy (hypertonia, arching, retrocollis, opisthotonos, fever, high pitched cry) or if TSB is > 5 mg/dL (85 uml/L) above these lines.
- Risk factors - isoimmune hemolytic disease, G6PDF deficiency, asphyxia, significant lethargy, temperature instability, sepsis, acidosis.
- Measure serum albumin and calculate B/A ratio (See legend)
- Use total bilirubin. Do not subtract direct reacting or conjugated bilirubin.
- If infant is well and 35 - 36 6/7 week (median risk) can individualize TSB levels for exchange based on actual gestational age.

FIGURE 26-11

Guidelines for Exchange Transfusion in Infants of 35 or More Weeks' Gestation.

Source: Reproduced with permission. From American Academy of Pediatrics, Subcommittee on hyperbilirubinemia. (2004). Clinical practice guideline: management of hyperbilirubinemia in the newborn infant ≥ 35 or more weeks of gestation. Pediatrics, 114, 297–316. Copyright © 2004 American Academy of Pediatrics.

should be considered, but discharge does not need to be postponed for continued observation or follow-up bilirubin measurement.

Exchange transfusion is indicated when serum bilirubin levels rise to the indicated levels despite phototherapy, or when levels are sustained at or above exchange levels after a period of intensive phototherapy. A neonate's circulating blood volume is approximately 80–85 mL/kg. During an exchange transfusion, a double-volume exchange consisting of two times the infant's blood volume (160–170mL/kg)ismade,usingaliquotsofwholebloodnotexceeding 10 mL/kg. Approximately 85% of the circulating blood volume is replaced during an exchange transfusion, which reduces the bilirubin level by as much as 50% (Wong et al.,

2006). An exchange transfusion also aids in the elimination of circulating maternal antibodies when hyperbilirubinemia occurs secondary to an isoimmune cause.

This procedure may be accomplished using a number of vessel configurations—an umbilical vein, a combination of umbilical artery to draw blood and umbilical vein to replace blood, or a peripheral arterial line (drawing) and umbilical vein (replacing). An umbilical cord stump may be successfully catheterized for more than a week after an infant leaves the hospital. Umbilical exchange transfusion trays contain special umbilical catheters with an open end that permit easier withdraw of blood when only umbilical venous access is utilized. Intensive phototherapy should continue throughout the exchange. Clear plastic whole-body

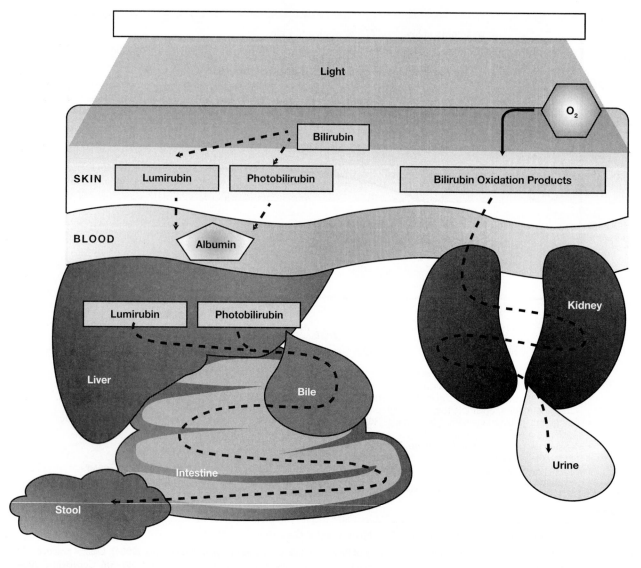

FIGURE 26-12

Mechanism of Phototherapy.

Source: Courtesy of Mary Puchalski.

drapes may be available to provide the necessary aseptic field while permitting light penetration.

More recently, the term *bilirubin-induced neurologic disorders* (BIND) has been used to describe the spectrum of encephalopathy, from mild to severe, associated with excess bilirubin levels. The BIND score is a simple method for tracking clinical progression from subtle symptoms to severe toxicity (Table 26-26). When an infant presents in an outpatient setting or emergency department with evidence of severe jaundice, neurologic evaluation should be performed. Signs of encephalopathy in an infant should be considered a neurologic emergency, and the initiation of intensive phototherapy should not be delayed while laboratory investigation is performed (Shapiro, 2008). When such an infant requires transfer from one hospital to another for a higher level of care, intensive phototherapy should be continued during transport.

Family education in the immediate newborn period focuses on teaching parents warning signs of hyperbilirubinemia such as jaundice, poor feeding, or lethargy. Mothers are taught how to breastfeed effectively, and early follow-up is emphasized. When an infant is admitted for treatment of severe hyperbilirubinemia, thorough explanations of the infant's condition and plan of care should be provided. Depending on the infant's condition, explanations

TABLE 26-26

Bilirubin-Induced Neurologic Disorders (BIND) Score					
	0	1	2	3	Score
Mental status	Normal	Sleepy, poor feeding	Lethargic, irritable	Semicoma, coma, seizures	
Muscle tone	Normal	Neck stiffness, mild hypertonia or hypotonia	Arching neck and/or trunk	Opisthotonos	
Cry	Normal	High-pitched	Shrill	Inconsolable	
				Total	

Scores:
0–3 = subtle encephalopathy.
4–6 = progressive encephalopathy.
7–9 = advanced toxicity.

Source: Shapiro, 2008.

as to neurologic evaluations are necessary so that caregivers understand the potential lifelong consequences of bilirubin encephalopathy and the need for long-term neurodevelopmental follow-up.

DISPOSITION AND DISCHARGE PLANNING

Once stable with a decreasing bilirubin, the infant with severe hyperbilirubinemia should undergo MRI evaluation to assess the child for findings consistent with kernicterus. However, a normal MRI does not exclude the diagnosis, and long-term follow-up is still needed. Auditory brain stem response (ABR) can detect damage to the cochlea, auditory nerve, and the brain stem auditory pathways. Hearing evaluation by acoustic emissions (OAE) should not be used for the infant with potential bilirubin toxicity. OAE detects peripheral auditory problems of the inner ear and may be normal in an infant with auditory nerve deafness.

For the infant with suspected bilirubin encephalopathy, an interprofessional approach to discharge planning includes serial neurologic evaluations during the first several months of life, and treatment with physical, occupational, and speech therapy. Infants with hyperbilirubinemia are at high risk for failure-to-thrive secondary to feeding difficulties; therefore, ongoing nutritional evaluation is warranted.

Every neonatal contact in any setting should include an evaluation for possible hyperbilirubinemia. Health care professionals should be familiar with current guidelines,

know how to institute prompt treatment, and be ready to contact neonatal providers for assistance when an infant presents with severe hyperbilirubinemia.

INFLAMMATORY BOWEL DISEASE

Elizabeth L. Yu

PATHOPHYSIOLOGY

Increasing evidence supports the hypothesis that inflammatory bowel disease (IBD) results from a genetic predisposition of the gastrointestinal tract to interact abnormally with an environmental stimulus. This abnormal interaction, in turn, leads to excess immune activation and the chronic intestinal inflammation that is the hallmark of IBD. Abnormal GI immunoregulatory function is an important contributor to pathophysiology in IBD. Immunologically active cells in the GI tract are stimulated continuously by dietary and microbial antigens and, therefore, are in a constant state of physiologic inflammation. These immunologically active cells work in conjunction with epithelial cells to form a barrier to toxic external stimuli. In IBD, the constant physiologic inflammation becomes pathologic in nature, causing tissue damage.

On a cellular level, mucosal inflammation in IBD is manifested as increased mononuclear cell infiltration of the lamina propria. In addition, polymorphonuclear leukocytes (PMNs) may infiltrate crypts and cause distortion of crypt architecture, creating similarities to infectious colitis.

Definitions

Inflammatory bowel disease is an umbrella term used to describe the two distinct disorders associated with inflammation of the GI tract: Crohn's disease (CD) and ulcerative colitis (UC). Differentiation between CD and UC is based on the location and characteristics of the inflammation.

Crohn's disease manifests as inflammation that may involve any part of the GI tract—from mouth to anus. The terminal ileum is the most likely affected area of bowel in Crohn's disease, with 30% of patients having disease limited to the terminal ileum, 60% having disease limited to the terminal ileum and colon, and only 10% to 20% having disease limited to the colon. Microscopic characteristics include transmural extension of fibrosis, histiocytic proliferation of bowel mucosa, and granuloma formation. Inflammation in CD is generally transmural and patchy with "skip lesions," but can become more generalized later in the disease course. The transmural nature (extending from mucosa, to submucosa, to muscularis, and finally to serosa) of inflammation may result in fistula formation. Aphthous lesions, superficial ulcers overlying lymphoid follicles, may be found anywhere; oral lesions are common early manifestations of CD. Noncaseating granulomas are considered pathognomic for this disease.

Ulcerative colitis consists of generalized, confluent inflammation confined to the mucosa. Microscopic features include distortion of crypt architecture, decreased crypt density, diffuse transmucosal lamina propria cell increase, and severe mucin depletion. A variable extent of colon is involved, with classification of UC based on the area of involvement (Table 26-27).

EPIDEMIOLOGY AND ETIOLOGY

IBD has no gender specificity; males and females are equally affected by the disease. Peak incidence is bimodal, with a first peak between the ages of 15 and 30 years and the second peak between the ages of 50 and 80 years. Twenty-five percent of patients with CD and 20% of patients with UC present before the age of 20. The incidence of CD generally exceeds that of UC. Incidence rates of CD and UC in North America are approximately 3.1 to 14.6 cases per 100,000 person-years and approximately 2.2 to 14.3 cases per 100,000 person-years, respectively. The prevalence is also similar, with 26 to 201 cases per 100,000 people for CD and 37 to 246 cases per 100,000 people for UC. In the United States and Europe, the incidence of IBD decreases in a north-to-south direction. Incidence rates of IBD are relatively lower in Asia, Japan, and South America. Also reported is a higher incidence of IBD in people with Jewish ancestry. Lower rates are found in Africa Americans and Hispanics compared to Caucasians. To date, the incidence of IBD has been increasing in parallel with overall population trends, although the rate of increase in ulcerative colitis incidence greater than the rate of increase in Crohn's disease incidence.

TABLE 26-27

Ulcerative Colitis Classification			
	Ulcerative Proctitis	Left-Sided Colitis	Pancolitis
Involvement	≤ 15 cm of rectum	Rectal, sigmoid, descending colon	Involvement past the splenic flexure
Prevalence in patients with ulcerative colitis	10%	30%	40–50%

The etiology of IBD is still not fully elucidated, although both genetic and environmental factors are suspected to contribute to development of IBD. First-degree relatives of patients with IBD (more so with CD than with UC) are 3 to 20 times more likely to develop the disease. Nevertheless, the majority of patients (more than 85%) do not have any family history of IBD. If family history is present, genetic anticipation can be expected, with earlier age of diagnosis in subsequent generations of patients.

Several genes have been shown to contribute to the IBD phenotype. Mutations of *IBD1*, which encodes the NOD-2 protein, increase susceptibility to ileal Crohn's disease. Other genes involved are ATG I6L-1 (CD) and several major histocompatibility complex (MHC) loci: HLA-DR2 increases susceptibility to UC, whereas HLA-A2, HLA-DR1, and HLA-DQw5 confer increased risk of extraintestinal manifestations of CD. While these specific genes may confer increased susceptibility to IBD, the actual disease presentation depends on the presence of appropriate environmental factors in combination with the presence of specific genes.

Additionally, certain antibodies may be markers of disease. For example, peripheral antineutrophil cytoplasmic antibodies (pANCA), which are believed to be markers of genetically controlled immunoregulatory disturbance, are present in approximately 70% of patients with UC and approximately 6% of patients with CD. Anti-*Saccharomyces cerevisiae* antibodies (ASCA) are present in 50% to 60% of patients with CD and correlate with the presence of small bowel involvement as well as fibrostenosing and perforating disease.

Similar to genetic factors, environmental factors are more likely to contribute to disease in predisposed individuals. Smoking/nicotine has a mixed relationship with IBD, having a positive correlation with CD and a negative correlation with UC. Other environmental influences associated with increased risk of development of IBD include oral contraceptives, infectious colitis, and infectious agents. Infectious agents are thought to lower the threshold for development of IBD in susceptible individuals and may be the inciting factor.

Diseases associated with a higher frequency of IBD include Turner syndrome, Hermansky-Pudlak syndrome, glycogen storage disease type IB, and inborn errors of leukocyte adhesion.

PRESENTATION

Intestinal symptoms of IBD include abdominal pain (95%), diarrhea (77%), hematochezia (50%), and perirectal inflammation with fistulization (25%). Other symptoms include fevers (38%), failure-to-thrive (30%), and weight loss (80%). Abdominal pain is a common presenting symptom in CD and is generally more severe than that found in UC. Localization may depend on intestinal involvement. Pain localized to the right lower quadrant may be found in those patients who have ileal or ileocecal disease, whereas epigastric pain may signify gastroduodenal involvement, and periumbilical pain may indicate colonic or generalized small bowel disease. Ulcerative colitis may present with bloody diarrhea as well tenesmus and urgency if proctitis is involved. Aphthous lesions are often a presenting sign in CD. Other clinical symptoms that may increase clinical suspicion for Crohn's disease include perianal skin tags, fistulae, or abscesses, growth failure, weight loss, and pubertal delay.

Aside from intestinal manifestations, extraintestinal manifestations occur in approximately 25% to 35% of patients with IBD and are more often associated with colonic disease; therefore, these findings may be the first indication of IBD. Joints, skin, the hepatobiliary tract, and ocular involvement are the systems most commonly affected.

Arthralgias and arthritis are the most common extraintestinal manifestation, with arthralgias being noted more often than arthritis. Arthralgias and arthritis are divided into two types based on location and symmetry. Type I involves large peripheral joints such as the hips, knees, and ankles. Usually asymmetric in nature, this variant is termed "colitic arthritis." The associated joint swelling directly parallels inflammatory activity in the intestines. This type of arthritis improves with treatment of intestinal inflammation. Type II arthritis typically presents as symmetrical inflammation of small joints that is unrelated to disease activity. Axial arthritis in the form of ankylosing spondylitis and sacroiliitis is rare in children and is not correlated with IBD activity.

Erythema nodosum (EN)—acute, nodular, painful, erythematous lesions usually 1 to 3 cm in diameter—may sometimes be found on the extensor aspects of the lower extremities (i.e., shins) in IBD-affected individuals. EN occurs in approximately 8% to 15% of all patients with IBD and reflects disease activity; that is, it emerges only when intestinal disease is active. EN is more common among patients with CD. Pyoderma gangrenosum—a severe ulcerating rash—is another dermatological manifestation of IBD; it occurs in 1% to 3% of patients, is more common in patients with UC, and unlike EN, is not associated with disease activity.

The hepatobiliary tract may also be affected in patients with IBD. Approximately 3% of patients with UC develop primary sclerosing cholangitis (PSC). Although PSC is more common in patients with UC, patients with CD and colonic involvement may also develop this extraintestinal manifestation. Persistent elevation of gamma-glutamyl transpeptidase (GGT) combined with fatigue, pruritus, and intermittent jaundice in the setting of IBD should raise HCP suspicion and prompt further investigation. Development of PSC is unrelated to disease activity. Autoimmune hepatitis, nonspecific mild elevations of liver function tests (LFTs) and increased risk for cholelithiasis are other hepatic manifestations of IBD.

Nephrolithiasis, especially oxalate stone formation, is yet another extraintestinal manifestation of IBD. Increased risk of nephrolithiasis formation exists in diseased bowel. The oxalate stones form secondary to malabsorption of fat and bile salts in patients with ileal inflammation that impedes normal absorption. Calcium binds to oxalates; because the resulting calcium oxalate is poorly absorbed, oxalate is fecally excreted. With malabsorption, increased fatty acids become available. Calcium preferentially binds to fatty acids. Thus oxalate binds to sodium, forming sodium oxalate; this compound is then absorbed in the colon. Subsequent ureteric obstruction and hydronephrosis may result from the increased incidence of oxalate kidney stones.

Ocular manifestations of IBD include episcleritis, with bilateral burning, itching, and uveitis. Ocular manifestations are less common in pediatric patients with IBD in comparison to adult patients.

Finally, growth failure occurs in approximately 10% of patients with UC and 20% to 30% of patients with CD. Growth failure is multifactorial in nature: It is associated with undernutrition, the effects of proinflammatory cytokines from diseased bowel on bone metabolism, and subsequent treatment with corticosteroids. Osteopenia may also occur secondary to vitamin D deficiency, which in turn occurs secondary to malabsorption.

DIFFERENTIAL DIAGNOSIS

Other possibilities that should be included in the differential diagnosis for inflammatory bowel disease are infection (e.g., *Amebiasis, Salmonella, Yersinia*), hemolytic uremic syndrome (HUS), Henoch-Schönlein purpura (HSP), ischemic colitis, irritable bowel syndrome, and Behçet syndrome.

PLAN OF CARE

Diagnosis of inflammatory bowel disease may be subdivided into five major steps. First, the HCP completes a detailed clinical and family history, a comprehensive physical examination, and initial screening studies to exclude diagnoses. These studies include the following tests:

- Complete blood count (CBC) with manual differential. Pertinent positives may include anemia secondary to decreased iron as a result of chronic intestinal losses and thrombocytosis secondary to the inflammatory state in IBD. Additionally, thrombopoiesis is stimulated by IL-6. The white blood count (WBC) may or may not be elevated depending on the chronicity of inflammation.
- Erythrocyte sedimentation rate (ESR), which is elevated in 80% of patients with CD and approximately 40% of patients with UC.
- C-reactive protein (CRP) to evaluate for the presence of active bowel inflammation.
- Albumin, which is usually low due to enteric protein loss and poor nutritional status.
- Serum aminotransferases and GGT to evaluate for possible hepatic involvement.

Second, to exclude other possible diagnoses, stool studies to evaluate for infectious causes should be sent to the lab. Infectious pathogens such as *Clostridium difficile, Salmonella, Shigella, Campylobacter, E. coli* O157:H7, *Yersinia,* and *Aeromonas* may be ruled out with stool samples. Fecal WBCs are usually a result of inflammation. Placement of a tuberculin skin test is also useful in evaluation of possible tuberculosis in patients with isolated terminal ileum infection. Normal laboratory findings do not exclude the diagnosis of IBD.

Third, endoscopic visualization of the intestinal tract is performed to establish and differentiate the diagnosis. With endoscopy, biopsy and histology are also paramount to diagnose IBD and differentiate between CD and UC. Grossly, endoscopic features indicative of CD are ulceration and stenosis of the ileocecal valve, cobblestoning or linear ulcerations in the terminal ileum, and stricture and fistulae formation. Discontinuous colitis with intervening areas of normal mucosa, small ulcerations (aphthous lesions) in the small or large bowel, and relative rectal sparing are additional endoscopic features of CD. Gastritis may be present in either patients with either UC or CD at the time of diagnosis. Endoscopically, UC may present as a diffuse, continuous process starting at the rectum and extending proximally. The colonic mucosa usually appears friable and erythematous, and it may contain small erosions and ulcerations. Pseudopolyps and periappendiceal inflammation may be found in patients with more chronic UC. Additionally, "backwash ileitis" or ileal erythema may be a feature associated with a diagnosis of UC. Histologically, noncaseating granulomas on biopsy are pathognomonic for CD.

Fourth, because CD and UC may have large bowel involvement, imaging modalities may help to further differentiate and localize the region of disease. An upper GI with small bowel follow-through (SBFT) barium study may help identify small bowel involvement and demonstrate mucosal irregularity, cobblestoning, narrowing, or presence of fistulae (often found in CD). Pill or video-capsule endoscopy allows for visualization and severity of small bowel disease that may not be evident by upper GI with SBFT. Additionally, CT and MRI may detect small bowel disease in areas that are inaccessible to endoscopy. These modalities may also identify intra-abdominal complications of CD such as fistulae. Such imaging techniques help in localization of disease, which is important for optimal therapeutic management.

Additional modalities used in differentiating between CD and UC include antibody testing for anti-saccharomyces cerevesiae antibody (ASCA) and peripheral antineutrophil cytoplasmic antibodies (pANCA). The ASCA test is positive in 40% to 80% of patients with CD and may identify patients with disease in the terminal ileum and cecum. ASCA is unusual in UC patients. pANCA, by comparison, is positive in 60% to 80% of patients with UC, but only 10% to 27% of patients with CD. Patients with pANCA positivity often exhibit colonic disease. Other measured antibodies are anti-ompC antibody, which is an outer membrane porin derived from *E. coli* and a potential serological marker of IBD and anti-CBir1 ab, an antibody to bacterial flagellin CBIR1. Anti-CBir1 is associated with small bowel disease and fibrostenosing disease. Antibody testing is a supplement to standard diagnostic evaluation and must be interpreted in combination with endoscopic evaluation. A caveat with antibody testing is the possibility of false-positive results. Patients with low levels of symptoms and less likelihood of disease are more likely to have false-positive results.

Fifth and last, the HCP seeks to identify extraintestinal manifestations, such as those described in the "Presentation" section. If these symptoms exist, then diagnostic studies and further investigation are necessary to choose the most effective treatment for the patient.

The primary goal of therapy is to reduce bowel inflammation, eliminate symptoms, and promote healing and prevention of worsening of disease or further complications. Other goals are to promote normal growth and development, optimize the patient's nutritional status, and minimize the potential psychological impact of new diagnosis of chronic disease on both the patient and family. Both pharmacological and nutritional routes of therapy are available. The initial therapy selected depends on the severity of disease at presentation.

Nutrition

Therapy may be divided into three broad phases: induction, remission, and maintenance. Nutritional therapy may be an option for induction therapy; it consists of ingestion of an elemental or polymeric formula as the sole source of nutrition for 6 to 8 weeks. Nutritional therapy may be used as either induction therapy or adjunctive therapy in CD, and has been shown to produce remission in as many as 80% of patients. It is only adjunctive therapy in UC, however. Consumption of an elemental diet is advantageous in that it allows avoidance of steroids and subsequent adverse effects (e.g., stunting of growth). The difficulty with elemental diet is adherence: Ingesting only formula for as long as 8 weeks is often difficult to achieve. Furthermore, maintenance of remission following discontinuation of enteral therapy is difficult.

Medication therapy

Pharmacological therapy can be divided into six categories: (1) aminosalicylates, (2) corticosteroids, (3) immunomodulators, (4) biologic agents, (5) antibiotics, and (6) probiotics.

Aminosalicylates and the 5-aminosalicylates (e.g., mesalamine, sulfasalazine) are effective in reducing inflammation in both induction and maintenance of remission in mild to moderate UC. They may also be useful in mild Crohn's colitis or mild distal small bowel disease. Aminosalicylates are site-specific and locally active medications; they work by scavenging oxygen metabolites and inhibiting 5-lipoxygenase, which in turn decreases production of leukotriene-B4 and IL-1 as well as activation of PPARgamma. Both oral and rectal forms are available. Sulfasalazine, mesalamine, olsalazine, and balsalazide—the oral forms—are active in the distal small bowel and colon. Mesalamine enemas and suppositories are useful in treatment of proctosigmoiditis and may help in alleviation of associated symptoms such as tenesmus, urgency, and rectal bleeding. Adverse effects of the aminosalicylates include pancreatitis, allergic reactions to the sulfa component (occurring in approximately 10% of patients), and rare pulmonary or kidney toxicity.

Corticosteroids (i.e., prednisone, methyprednisolone) are used as first-line therapy for induction of remission after initial diagnosis in moderate or severe disease or for induction or remission in IBD flares. Both oral and IV forms are available. Unfortunately, multiple systemic adverse effects may develop with the use of these agents, including osteoporosis, glucose intolerance, Cushing syndrome, hypertension, mood disturbances, adrenal insufficiency, and pancreatitis.

6-MP and azathioprine are examples of immunomodulators. Because these agents have a slow onset of action (approximately 3 months), they are used in maintenance instead of induction of remission. They are effective in the long-term maintenance and prevention of relapse of active disease in both CD and UC. Additionally, immunomodulators are steroid sparing. Their mechanism of action relies on incorporation of 6-thioguanine nucleotide metabolites of 6-MP into leukocyte DNA or induction of lymphocyte apoptosis via inhibition of the *rac-1* gene. Azathioprine is converted, in vivo, to 6-MP.

Prior to starting 6-MP or azathioprine, it is important to assess the patient's thiopurine S-methyltransferase (TPMT) genetics for dose determination purposes. TPMT is an enzyme that metabolizes thiopurine drugs. Patients with homozygous or heterozygous genotypes and, therefore, reduced enzymatic activity levels are at risk for developing leucopenia and should be given a reduced amount of drug. Monitoring is also required after initiation of treatment with immunomodulators to prevent adverse effects and to adjust dosing as necessary. 6-MMP and 6-TGN metabolites are measured approximately 8 weeks after initiation of therapy, as increased 6-MMP metabolite levels are associated with hepatotoxicity and increased 6-TGN levels are associated with leucopenia. Alternatively, to evaluate for hepatotoxicity and leucopenia, regular testing of CBC and liver enzymes may be performed. Other possible adverse effects of immunomodulators include allergic hypersensitivity reactions and pancreatitis.

Methotrexate is another drug in the immunomodulator category. Considered a second-line therapy in IBD, it is used in steroid-dependent patients with CD who are intolerant or unresponsive to 6-MP. This agent, which is useful in severe small or large bowel disease and fistulizing disease, has a faster onset of action than the other immunomodulators, so it may be used in either induction or maintenance therapy. As it is also steroid-sparing, methotrexate is useful in cases of growth failure. The disadvantage to utilization of methotrexate is its adverse effects, which include bone marrow suppression, nausea, possibility of hepatotoxicity, and ulcerative stomatitis.

Inhibitors of IL-2 (a pro-inflammatory cytokine), cyclosporine, and tacrolimus are used in severe or fulminant UC or fistulizing CD. These drugs are usually reserved for severely ill, corticosteroid-resistant patients. Given the severity of their adverse effects (kidney/neurologic toxicities) and multiple drug–drug interactions, cyclosporine and tacrolimus are not used as maintenance therapy. Instead, they are administered to control severe inflammation while waiting for thel the onset of action for other immunomodulators (i.e., methotrexate, 6-MP).

Infliximab and adalimumab are biologic agents that are useful in the treatment of IBD refractory to other therapies. These monoclonal antibodies bind to the pro-inflammatory cytokine TNF-alpha present in both CD and UC, resulting in mucosal healing and reduction of symptoms that may last as long as 2 months. Infliximab and adalimumab are both intravenous medications that must be infused routinely—initially more frequently, but eventually every 2 months. Infliximab is a mouse chimeric IgG monoclonal antibody, whereas adalimumab is a human chimeric monoclonal antibody. They are used for both induction and maintenance of remission in IBD patients with severe disease; these agents may also be used in steroid-refractory patients suffering from disease flares and are usually initiated after lack of response to a 10- to 12-day course of IV steroids. These biologic agents are also effective in control of extraintestinal manifestations of IBD—that is, fistulizing CD, metastatic CD, arthritis, and pyoderma gangrenosum.

As with other medications, infliximab and adalimumab produce adverse side effects. Sporadic and inconsistent use increases the risk of antibody development to infliximab, which in turn may increase the patient's risk for developing an infusion reaction and decrease the response to treatment. Other potential adverse effects include lupus-like syndrome, cardiac failure, and hepatosplenic T-cell lymphoma (rare) in patients using infliximab in combination with immunomodulators (i.e., 6-MP, azathioprine). Evaluation for latent tuberculosis should be performed prior to initiation of treatment with infliximab or adalimumab given these monoclonal antibodies' propensity for reactivation of latent TB.

Finally, antibiotics such as metronidazole or ciprofoloxacin may be useful in patients with CD and perirectal fistulas or abscess pouchitis. Probiotics (e.g., lactobacillus, *Saccharomyces*) have also been used as adjunctive therapy to ensure optimal bowel health as well as for treatment of recurrent pouchitis.

Surgery

If the previously described dietary and pharmacological therapies do not adequately control intestinal inflammation, surgical measures are a last option. In addition to refractory disease, uncontrolled GI bleeding and bowel perforation or obstruction are indications for bowel resection as therapy for IBD. In UC, colectomy is curative and the patient is left with an ileal pouch and anal anastomosis. In CD, however, despite segmental bowel resection, disease often recurs at the same site. The most commonly resected sites in CD are the terminal ileum with adjacent inflamed colon.

Involvement of an interprofessional team for patients with suspected inflammatory bowel disease is optimal. Consultation with a pediatric gastroenterologist during the patient's initial presentation will facilitate the steps to diagnosis and treatment. When diagnosis is confirmed, involvement of nutritionists, social workers, and child life specialists for patient and family support is ideal.

Multiple resources are available for patient and family education. With the pediatric gastroenterologist, disease etiopathology, course, and prognosis may be discussed in detail. The nutritionist will provide education to the patient and family as well. Additionally, websites such as the Crohn's and Colitis Foundation of America (www.ccfa.org) are very useful in terms of providing both practical disease education and support from other patients and families with IBD.

DISPOSITION AND DISCHARGE PLANNING

IBD is a chronic disease that is marked by periods of both remission and exacerbation. Most children with UC are in remission by 3 months after initiation of initial therapy. Approximately 50% of these children will remain in remission over the next year. The eventual outcome is reflects the severity of disease, with colectomy being required in one-fourth of patients with severe disease compared to fewer than 10% of patients with mild disease. Most patients with CD have relapses after initial diagnosis and treatment, with only 1% of patients remaining in remission.

Prognosis depends on the severity of presentation as well as the area of bowel affected. Patients with ileocolitis do not respond as well to medical therapy and have a greater need for eventual surgical measures compared to patients with isolated small bowel disease. A long-term risk for IBD is intestinal adenocarcinoma. The most important risk factors to take into consideration are the duration of colitis (greater risk with more than 10 years' duration) and the extent of the colitis. Patients with pancolitis are at greater risk than those with left-sided colitis. Patients with left-sided colitis are at greater risk, in turn, than those patients with isolated proctitis. Annual screening via colonoscopies is important for patients with colonic disease for more than 10 years to look for any evidence of dysplasia. If dysplasia is found, colectomy is suggested. Patients should follow up regularly with their pediatric gastroenterologist.

INTESTINAL FAILURE (SHORT GUT SYNDROME)

Pamela Ruppel and Keli Hansen

PATHOPHYSIOLOGY

Intestinal failure (IF) is the most current term used for the condition of malabsorption and metabolic complications from intestinal resection or malfunction. Former terms for the same condition included short gut syndrome and short bowel syndrome. In IF, pathophysiologic changes occur after resection of the bowel; their extent depends on the amount of absorptive surface area that remains and the presence or absence of the ileocecal valve and colon.

A full-term neonate has approximately 240 cm of small bowel and 40 cm of colon. In the last trimester of pregnancy, the length of the jejunum, ileum, and colon doubles. A preterm infant, therefore, does not have the same length of absorptive surface area as a term neonate (Bradshaw, 2009).

The duodenum and jejunum are the chief sites for absorption of fat, carbohydrates, minerals (including vitamin D and iron), and protein. The jejunum is the site of the most nutritional absorption because of the greater length of its villi and its increased surface area. It also has the greatest number of digestive enzymes, which are required for the breakdown and absorption of enteral nutrition. The ileum has shorter villi and less absorptive capability, yet is the only area of the bowel that absorbs vitamin B_{12} and bile salts through receptor-mediated transport. The ileum is the primary location of fat-soluble vitamin absorption and gastrointestinal hormone production affecting the motility of the entire digestive tract (Abad-Sinden & Sutphen, 2003).

The presence of the ileocecal valve and the colon are important to the nutritional management of a neonate with IF. The transit time through the digestive tract is greatly increased without the presence of either, which can dramatically affect fluid and electrolyte losses. The ileocecal valve regulates the flow of *chyme*, or food content of the small intestine, into the colon and plays a key role in regulating transit and absorptive time (Abad-Sinden & Sutphen, 2003).

The ability to survive on a completely enteral diet in the neonate with IF depends on the length of remaining bowel and the presence or absence of the ileocecal valve. A neonate is able to have a good clinical outcome and be fed entirely with enteral feedings with as little as 15 cm of jejunum and ileum as long as the ileocecal valve is present, but must have 40 cm if the valve is missing. The condition of the remaining bowel and its absorptive capability are also important in determining the outcome (Abad-Sinden & Sutphen, 2003).

In an adult, the normal length of the small intestine is approximately 600 to 100 cm; 100 cm is considered to be the minimum length of healthy bowel needed to survive on a completely enteral diet without a colon (Scolapio, 2003). Patients with less than 100 to 150 cm of small bowel and no colon often need parenteral nutrition (PN) to meet fluid and nutritional requirements. With 50 cm of small bowel and even part of their colon, most patients can survive without PN. The colon can convert complex carbohydrates

to short-chain fatty acids and stimulate sodium and water absorption to provide additional calories. Patients with colons, therefore, require a diet rich in complex carbohydrates (60% of total intake). Patients without colons do not usually benefit from a special diet but often require antimotility agents to slow transit through the remaining bowel and to manage absorption of fluids and electrolytes (Scolapio).

EPIDEMIOLOGY AND ETIOLOGY

Intestinal failure is characterized by dysfunction of all or part of the digestive tract. Malabsorptive diarrhea, which is characteristic of this syndrome, causes fluid, electrolyte, and weight loss. In addition to the impact that the bowel length has on clinical outcome in IF, the function of the small bowel is essential to understanding this disorder. A number of conditions, both surgical and medical, cause IF. For example, several medical conditions mimic bowel resection in that they diminish the absorptive ability of the small bowel or lead to deterioration of the villi and mucosal surface area. Such medical conditions include allergic enteropathy, Crohn's disease of the small bowel, and celiac disease (Scolapio, 2003).

In addition, formation of eosinophils in the digestive tract from allergen exposure can reduce the surface area of nutritional absorption in the digestive tract, leading to intestinal failure. Crohn's disease, with its associated disrupted villi from inflammation and destruction of the mucosa, may alter the patient's ability to obtain adequate nutrition. Celiac disease or other types of gluten enteropathy cause smoothing of the villi in the small intestine, reducing its absorptive ability. All of these conditions can lead to the weight loss, diarrhea, malnutrition, osteoporosis, acute liver failure, and anemia commonly seen with IF (Scolapio, 2003).

A vast number of congenital conditions may also lead to intestinal failure, including gastroschesis, omphalocele, congenital atresias, cloacal extrophy, congenital short bowel syndrome, and intrauterine growth retardation resulting in poor bowel growth. Moreover, the presence of an umbilical arterial catheter, which is associated with the potential for thrombosis and decreased perfusion to the small intestine, has been implicated as a causative factor for ischemia leading to IF (Abad-Sinden & Sutphen, 2003). Neonates with congenital heart disease affecting bowel perfusion also can have issues with ischemia, and segmental bowel resection is sometimes needed if malperfusion time is lengthy and the bowel does not regain function after the perfusion to the bowel is restored.

Necrotizing enterocolitis (NEC) is the most common condition seen in the neonate leading to surgical resection in IF. The NEC process involves inflammation and necrosis of the bowel wall. It affects approximately 12% of all preterm neonates weighing less than 1,200 grams. This disease is most common in preterm infants between 3 and 10 days of age but can be seen even in term infants who are several months old (Bradshaw, 2009).

NEC most commonly involves the right upper quadrant of the abdomen and usually affects the duodenum, jejunum, and cecum. It is precipitated by an ischemic event and in approximately one-third of infants require surgery and bowel resection. As many as 25% of these infants have long-term sequelae related to the loss of bowel function (Bradshaw, 2009).

Malrotation of the small and large intestines and volvulus can lead to ischemic bowel, necessitating the resection of portions of the digestive tract as well. Although this condition can occur in the neonate, it most commonly occurs in the infant and young child.

Following resection of the small bowel, adaptation occurs over 1 to 2 years. Adaptation includes lengthening of the villi and crypts in the small bowel and occurs to a greater extent in the ileum than in the jejunum. Adaptation in the remaining bowel is important to nutrition, although PN is often required on a short-term basis as the process of absorptive and digestive capabilities are evolving (Bradshaw, 2009).

PRESENTATION

Patients with IF may present with malabsorption, diarrhea, dehydration, electrolyte abnormalities, seizures, failure-to-thrive, and vomiting. Malabsorption is attributed to the condition of the intestinal mucosa, the ability to absorb nutrients, and the length of the intestine and its overall function. Diarrhea can be related to acquired enteropathies such as gluten intolerance or food sensitivities, bacterial overgrowth, or rapid transit due to surgical resection. Patients are vulnerable to diarrhea-related skin breakdown due to their impaired nutritional status. Ongoing fluid losses due to diarrhea can lead to dehydration, electrolyte imbalances, and seizures if the electrolyte imbalance is severe enough.

DIFFERENTIAL DIAGNOSIS

Intestinal failure is typically due to surgical resection of the intestine for the conditions previously noted. If a patient does not have IF as a result of a surgical resection, the medical differential diagnosis can include congenital short bowel syndrome, congenital enteropathies such as microvillus inclusion disease and "tufting" enteropathy, acquired enteropathies such as autoimmune or Crohn's disease, and motility disorders (particularly chronic intestinal pseudo-obstruction). The challenge for patients with acquired short bowel lies not in making the diagnosis itself, but rather in determining how well the remaining bowel

is functioning, what degree of IF is present, and how to manage the medical complications.

PLAN OF CARE

Frequent diagnostic studies will be required to monitor for nutrient absorption, unmet metabolic needs, and infection. Serum electrolyte levels, CBC, and liver and kidney function should be checked regularly. Calcium, albumin, prealbumin, magnesium, and phosphorus levels are also important and should be assessed at least weekly in the initial period, and then periodically once the treatment regimen is stable. Adequate magnesium and phosphorus levels are important to maintain gut motility and transit time.

Iron studies, including reticulocyte count, total iron binding capacity (TIBC), and ferritin levels are important to monitor, as are vitamin B_{12} and folate levels. Periodic supplementation with intranasal or subcutaneous vitamin B_{12} is commonly required after ileum resection. Fat-soluble vitamins (vitamins A, D, E, and K) are typically administered on a daily basis, with periodic adjustment for weight changes and to normalize serum levels. Prothrombin time is used to determine the need for vitamin K supplementation. Additionally, laboratory studies such as carnitine levels (important for muscular function), vitamin D, copper, zinc, and selenium levels should be periodically assessed. Triglyceride levels are important, especially in the patient receiving PN with intralipids and to determine the need for supplementation with intralipid therapy. An acute elevation in triglyceride level is often an early indicator of infection and inflammation in the digestive tract.

Intestinal failure and surgical intervention carry the risk of inflammation at the sites of surgical anastomoses, strictures, and adhesions causing dysmotility. Blood loss can be significant in those patients with IF across anastomoses, at gastrostomy sites, at enteral tube sites, and with gastric ulcers. Bacterial overgrowth and protein-losing enteropathy can exacerbate blood loss. Inadequate bowel length for absorption of iron, folic acid, vitamin B_{12} and copper may prevent the resolution of secondary anemia associated with IF (Abad-Sinden & Sutphen, 2003).

In addition to the direct effects of IF, patients with this disorder are at an increased risk of bacterial translocation from the intestine into the bloodstream. Translocation most often occurs with cholestasis, pharmacologic acid suppression, dysmotility, and absence of an ileocecal valve due to backwash of colonic bacteria into the small intestine. Patients who have had one or more line infections are at an increased risk of cholestasis and hyperbilirubinemia (Abad-Sinden & Sutphen, 2003).

Some patients who have a remaining colon are at increased risk of hyperoxaluria and calcium oxalate urinary stone formation and should be placed on a low-oxalate, low-fat diet. In the former case, foods such as spinach, chocolate, tea, cola, and rhubarb should be avoided. Lactic acidosis and elevated anion gap are associated with fermentation of malabsorbed carbohydrates and can be caused by bacterial overgrowth. Antibiotics and carbohydrate-restricted diets are needed in patients with bacterial overgrowth (Scolapio, 2003).

Doppler flow studies and abdominal ultrasounds are often useful if hepatic- or kidney-specific laboratory values are abnormal to assess portal venous, liver, and kidney function and size. Ultrasound may be used in identification of ascites, central venous catheter tip fungal masses, and biliary tract stones and function. A hepatobiliary imino-diacetic acid (HIDA) scan is sometimes needed to identify dyskinesia of the biliary tract. CT scanning for identification of a source of infection such as an abscess may also be employed. CT volumetric scanning and angiography are useful when bowel-altering surgery is being considered.

Endoscopy with biopsy helps to identify peptic disease, celiac disease, lactose intolerance, allergic enteropathy, hypertensive gastropathy, and esophageal varices, which are frequently observed in conjunction with small bowel disease and associated liver disease. Adaptation of the small bowel can be monitored by biopsy and pathologist's tissue evaluation of the small intestinal mucosa. Colonoscopy is helpful in monitoring colonic mucosa for function and disease. Kidney, ureter, and bladder (KUB) radiograph and small bowel barium studies can be useful to identify areas of obstruction or ileus, malrotation, size, and transit time. When bowel obstruction is a concern, barium or air enemas may be employed to identify the function and size of the sigmoid colon and rectum.

Liver biopsy is rarely indicated unless liver dysfunction is present and hyperbilirubinemia persists after PN discontinuation (Sudan et al., 2005). Liver biopsy for identification of IF-related liver disease, cirrhosis, and fibrosis may be indicated if the patient's serum bilirubin levels remain abnormally high even after the patient has transitioned off PN. It is also recommended in those patients who are being considered for transplantation to evaluate the presence and degree of portal hypertension (Sudan et al.). Motility evaluation of the stomach and small bowel with barium studies or nuclear medicine scans may be indicated to assess transit time. Many patients require antidiarrheal medications on a regular basis to slow transit time and allow nutrients and fluids to be absorbed in the small intestine and colon; thus transit studies can be helpful to monitor baseline transit time and response to medications.

Therapeutic management of the patient with IF must be tailored to the individual, based on the amount and type of bowel remaining and the presence or absence of an ileocecal valve. PN is often required for a short time period (see Chapter 25), with a combination of enteral and PN being used while transitioning the patient to complete enteral feedings.

Medications to treat patients with IF include antibiotics such as metronidazole, sulfamethoxazole–trimethoprim, ciprofloxacin, and nitazoxanide. These agents are often used to reduce bacterial overgrowth and malabsorption as well as to reduce the incidence of lactic acidosis; lactic acidosis can lead to ataxia, dysarthria, and confusion (Abad-Sinden & Sutphen, 2003). Phenobarbital and ursodiol are used as choleretic agents. Many gastroenterologists are proponents of probiotic use to control the problem of bacterial overgrowth and diarrhea, and studies have shown favorable outcomes with this regimen (Sudan, 2009). Proton-pump inhibitors are used to treat gastrointestinal reflux disease, which is common in this population. They have a secondary effect of slowing intestinal transit time. Loperamide, an antidiarrheal medication, helps to slow motility and reduce fluid and electrolyte losses. Cholestyramine is used for bile salt binding and to treat diarrhea. Octreotide is frequently prescribed to reduce secretory diarrhea. Vitamin B_{12} levels and other vitamin levels are often affected by use of these agents and must be checked on a regular basis (Abad-Sinden & Sutphen).

Cholestasis is a common side effect of PN usage and intestinal failure; and liver disease associated with intestinal failure is usually cholestatic in origin. It may be the result of decreased enteral intake with resultant decreased stimulation and emptying of the gallbladder. Central venous catheter (CVC) infections and thrombosis are common complications of long-term therapy. Patients also often experience the need for multiple replacements of their CVCs to maintain function (Abad-Sinden & Sutphen, 2003).

The diarrhea associated with IF will resolve over time with adaptation of the remaining bowel. Constipation may then become a problem, especially in patients with cerebral palsy or those who do not receive bolus feedings that stimulate the gastrocolic reflex. Inadequate fluid intake can be a contributing problem to constipation (Abad-Sinden & Sutphen, 2003).

In the early 1990s, intestinal transplantation was introduced and is now considered by many pediatric intestinal surgeons to be the standard of care for patients with IF who are failing PN (Sudan et al., 2005). Surgical procedures other than transplantation include tapering and lengthening the remaining bowel through the Bianchi lengthening procedure, serial transverse enteroplasty (STEP) procedure, and recruitment of bypassed or unused intestine (Sudan et al.).

Surgical approaches to controlling the rapid transit of nutrients from the stomach to the colon have been described. To meet the goal of improving mucosal contact time and nutrient absorption, surgeons focus on reversal of short segments of jejunum or ileum (i.e., antiperistaltic), which are usually placed just proximal to the small bowel–colonic junction. An alternative procedure involves inserting a small segment of colon approximately halfway through the remaining length of small bowel (Sudan et al., 2005).

Management of intestinal failure takes the work of an interprofessional team, whose members include specialists from areas such as nutrition, pharmacy, gastroenterology, surgery, critical care, child life, and social work. Family education should address current and ongoing management plans. Long-term care goals, home care, and equipment training are also required prior to successful transition to home.

DISPOSITION AND DISCHARGE PLANNING

Efforts should be focused on promoting intestinal adaptation in pediatric patients with intestinal failure. This process can take up to 2 years, or even longer in rare cases. An interprofessional strategy should be used to minimize the complications associated with long-term PN whenever possible and to facilitate early discharge to home PN. Transitioning to a combination of PN and enteral feedings, with the aim of eventually providing nutrition with entirely enteral feedings, is the ultimate goal. Intestinal transplant is reserved for patients who develop complications related to PN and who have been given sufficient time for the remaining bowel to adapt and develop absorptive mucosa (Sudan, 2009).

In the hospital setting, ongoing monitoring includes accurate measurement of intake and output and daily weights. Stool should be tested for reducing substances, as their presence indicates malabsorption of carbohydrate. At home, caregivers are encouraged to keep track of intake and output, and patients should be weighed frequently on the same scale to assess weight changes. Height velocity should also be assessed both in and out of the hospital on a regular basis. Adjustments in PN and enteral feedings should be made with nutritionist support to assure adequate caloric and fluid intake. If the patient with IF is unable to take enough by mouth to provide adequate caloric intake, feeding tubes are recommended. Feeding tubes are usually placed prior to discharge but may be placed later if the patient fails to thrive at home.

INTESTINAL OBSTRUCTIONS

Sarah Martin and Kelly Finkbeiner

HIRSCHSPRUNG'S DISEASE

Pathophysiology

Hirschsprung's disease (HD) is the absence of ganglion cells of the enteric nerve plexus of the intestines. The aganglionosis, which begins at the anus and continues proximally, results in absent peristalsis in the affected bowel and causes a functional intestinal obstruction. Ganglion cells are normally located throughout the intestines from the mouth to the rectum. Along with the lack of peristalsis, HD is characterized by loss of the rectosphincter reflexes, so the internal sphincter does not relax to allow stool to be evacuated.

Epidemiology and etiology

HD occurs in 1 per 5,000 live births and affects males four times more often than females (Dasgupta & Langer, 2007). In 75% to 80% of patients, the aganglionosis is limited to the rectosigmoid colon. As many of 30% of cases involve a familial occurrence; in these circumstances, the diseased segment is usually more extensive than in nonhereditary cases (Kapur, 2009).

The exact reason for this aganglionosis is unknown. Eighty percent of HD cases involve an autosomal dominant genetic mutation with incomplete penetrance. To date, research for "Hirschsprung's gene" mutations has identified 11 different genes. The rearranged-during-transfection (RET) proto-oncogene has been identified most commonly in nonsyndromic patients (Kapur, 2009). The RET proto-oncogene functions in the development of the myenteric nervous system, which in turn aids in the development of ganglion cells (Teitelbaum & Coran, 2006). Ongoing research continues in an attempt to further delineate the specific genetic mutation to help in the diagnosis and treatment of HD.

Presentation

HD can present at any age. Approximately 50% to 90% of pediatric patients are diagnosed with HD in the neonatal period (Dasgupta & Langer, 2007). The classic presentation consists of failure to pass meconium in the first 8 hours of life. Other presenting symptoms frequently noted during the neonatal and infant period are bilious emesis, abdominal distention, failure-to-thrive (FTT), and sepsis. On physical examination, patients may have visible bowel loops with peristalsis. A rectal examination may reveal a spastic rectum with no stool in the rectal vault, and the rectal exam itself may cause the patient to have explosive diarrhea.

Infants and older children may present differently and can be more difficult to manage, as many of the obstructive symptoms may have been present since birth. The diagnosis of HD after the age of 2 years is very rare (Teitelbaum & Coran, 2006). Children who are diagnosed at an older age commonly have a shorter segment of intestine affected by HD. They typically present with a long and tenuous history of constipation, malnutrition, FTT, and chronic abdominal distention. Many times infants will present to HCPs around the time that solid foods are introduced into their diet.

Differential diagnosis

Hirschsprung's disease should be in the differential diagnosis for any patient who presents with obstructive symptoms. Table 26-28 lists differential diagnoses for HD.

TABLE 26-28

Differential Diagnoses for Hirschsprung's Disease

Meconium ileus
Malrotation with volvulus
Jejunoileal atresia
Colonic atresia
Intestinal duplication
Small left colon syndrome
Low imperforate anus
Necrotizing enterocolitis
Constipation
Sepsis
Hypothyroidism
Functional bowel obstruction

Plan of care

The diagnosis of HD is made based on clinical findings and radiologic studies, and is confirmed by pathology from a rectal biopsy. The first study done on a patient with obstructive symptoms is a plain abdominal radiograph. In HD, this imaging usually reveals large dilated loops of intestines that may have air–fluid levels (Figure 26-13).

After an abdominal radiograph, the next diagnostic imaging test is a barium enema (BE), which is helpful in making the diagnosis in 75% of affected children. A BE is done by inserting a small catheter into the rectum, instilling contrast into the colon, and taking several radiographs. In HD, the BE will reveal dilation of the area of normal ganglionic colon. This area is followed by a funnel-shaped

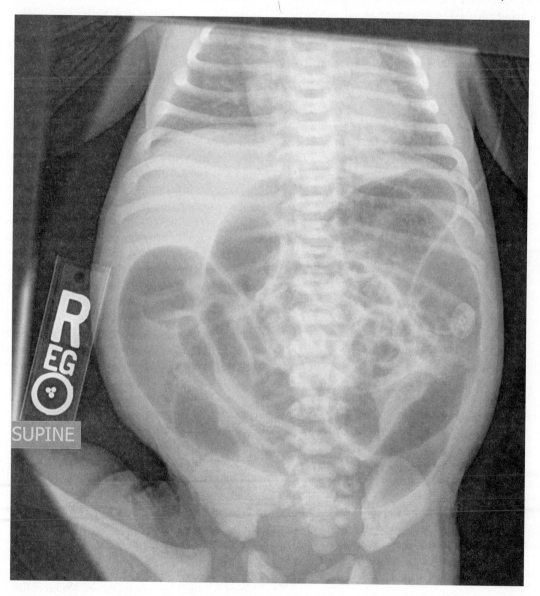

FIGURE 26-13

Plain Film of the Abdomen in a Child with Hirschsprung's Disease. The abdominal radiograph reveals dilated loops of intestine and air-fluid levels.

Source: Courtesy of Sarah Martin and Kelly Finkbeiner.

area, which is the transition zone. The transition zone is an area of the colon that has some ganglion cells, but not an adequate amount. It is followed by an area of dilation that narrows into the aganglionic bowel, which will not be dilated (Figure 26-14). The BE may not be helpful in neonates because they will not have had enough time to develop noticeable dilation of the colon. A BE test should not be done if there are concerns for perforation or enterocolitis (Teitelbaum & Coran, 2006).

Anorectal manometry may be helpful in diagnosing HD. This noninvasive test assesses for the absence of the relaxation reflex after distending the rectum; however, it carries a false-positive rate as high as 62% (Klar, 2007). Anorectal manometry also measures resting anal sphincter pressure and in older children, it can assess for the sensation of being full. This technique is frequently used in developing bowel continence in children with HD (Teitelbaum & Coran, 2006).

The study of choice for definitive diagnosis of HD is a rectal biopsy, which has a sensitivity of 93% in diagnosing this disease (Lorijn et al., 2005). A suction rectal biopsy is performed at the bedside on neonates and infants. During this procedure, the submucosal layer of the rectum is excised. The most common problem encountered with a suction rectal biopsy is inadequate sample or a sample taken too close to the sphincter. Specifically, the sample must be obtained 2 cm above the anus. A full-thickness rectal biopsy is perfomed if an inadequate sample is obtained or in an older child. This type of biopsy takes all of the musculature layers of the colon and must be sutured closed.

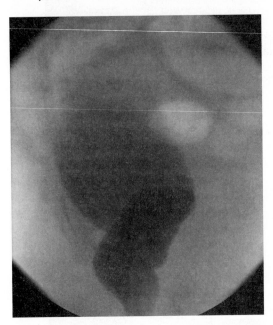

FIGURE 26-14

Barium Enema Suggestive of Hirschsprung's Disease. The barium enema shows an area of dilation that narrows in to the aganglionic bowel, which will not be dilated.

Source: Courtesy of Sarah Martin and Kelly Finkbeiner.

Unfortunately, this procedure requires general anesthesia and poses the greatest risks (i.e., bleeding, infection, and scar tissue formation) to patients, but it also provides the most accurate results (Teitelbaum & Coran, 2006).

The goal of any treatment is that the child be allowed to grow and thrive. Many times the initial treatment is to resuscitate the child with intravenous fluids, ensure bowel decompression via a nasal gastric tube, rectal irrigations, and provide antibiotics if enterocolitis or sepsis is a concern. Caregivers may be taught how to perform rectal irrigations. If the child is able to tolerate a diet without abdominal distention, the surgeon may wait for adequate weight gain and bowel decompression prior to undertaking surgical intervention.

Over the years, the surgical correction for HD has evolved from a three-stage procedure involving a colostomy at the time of diagnosis to a single-stage surgery performed on neonates. Regardless of whether the surgery is done laparoscopically, transanally, or by laparotomy, three surgical options are available: the Swenson pull-through, the Soave endorectal pull-through, and the Duhamel procedure.

The Swenson pull-through, the first definitive surgical therapy for HD, was initially reported in 1948. This procedure removes the aganglionic segment of bowel, with an end-to-end anastamosis then being done at the rectum. Careful dissection of the bowel is required to prevent injury to the pelvic nerves responsible for rectal, bladder, and sexual function. Of the three procedures for HD repair, the Swenson procedure resects the largest amount of aganglionic bowel. This procedure has been proven safe and effective laparoscopically on neonates weighting as little as 3.4 kg (Nasr & Langer, 2007).

The Soave endorectal pull-through is performed by dissecting the mucosal layer of the aganglionic segments and then pulling the ganglionic segment through the muscular cuff of the aganglionic segment. The ganglionic segment is then anastomosed to the rectum. This procedure is thought to preserve the integrity of the internal sphincter and decrease the risk of damage to the pelvic nerves (Klar, 2007; Teitelbaum & Coran, 2006).

The Duhamel procedure, which is also known as a retrorectal pull-through, limits the dissection of the aganglionic segment of colon to the retrorectal space. The surgeon brings the ganglionic bowel down and makes a side-to-end anastomosis with the aganglionic bowel. A significant portion of the aganglionic colon is left in place to form a neorectum. This procedure is technically the easiest to perform and may reduce the risk of anastomotic leak, stricture, and damage to the pelvic nerves (Teitelbaum & Coran, 2006). It is often used in patients who have had a failed Swenson pull-through. The disadvantage is that patients may have complications associated with the retained aganglionic segment, such as constipation, enterocolitis, and stool incontinence.

The surgical procedure chosen depends on the surgeon's training and experience with each procedure. Given the increased comfort of most surgeons in performing minimally invasive surgery, most procedures today are being done laparoscopically, transanally, or using a combination of the two. The transanal approach is performed by dissecting the aganglionic segment from the rectum; it leaves the patient without any abdominal incision, which decreases complications of a laparotomy. Using a minimally invasive approach has been proven to decrease hospital length of stay, decrease cost, lessen pain, and shorten time to eating in patients with shorter aganglionic segments (Zhang et al., 2005). The transanal pull-through approach is contraindicated in infants with dilated colon, enterocolitis, or long-segment HD (Sauer et al., 2005).

The complications associated with surgical repair may be divided into two categories: those occurring in the early postoperative period and long-term complications. The initial postoperative complications include anastomotic leak, bleeding, bowel obstruction, wound infection, abscess, sphincter spasm or stricture, and perianal excoriation. An anastomotic leak can occur whenever a surgeon is anastomosing two segments of bowel together. Patients with an anastomotic leak may develop fever, irritability, or abdominal distention. Bowel obstruction is reported in 8% to 13% of patients. Wound infection may occur in as many as 15% of cases—a rate similar to that for most other abdominal surgeries (Teitelbaum & Coran, 2006). An abscess may occur if poor hemostasis causes a hematoma that becomes infected. Stricture of the sphincter may occur when retracting the sphincter muscle during surgery; a sign of stricture is delayed passage of stool postoperatively. This defect may be fixed by gently dilating the anus with a lubricated Hegar dilator. Perianal excoriation will usually occur once a patient has started stooling. One study showed patients had a 30% increase in stool output after pull-through procedures (Pratap et al., 2007). Over time, however, the patient's stooling pattern returns to normal. It is very important that each patient has his or her vital signs, nasogastric output, urine output, abdominal girth, and pain control monitored closely in the initial postoperative period. If complications are missed during this time, it can have devastating effects on patient outcomes.

Common long-term complications of HD surgery include anal stenosis or stricture, incontinence, constipation, and enterocolitis. Complications such as retained aganglionic segment, impotence, and urinary dysfunction are rare. Stenosis or strictures occur in as many as 20% of patients and usually respond to rectal dilations. Although the overall incidence of incontinence is low, this complication has the biggest impact on the patient's quality of life. Incontinence typically occurs due to poor sphincter tone after surgery. Sometimes the rectal nerves may be damaged during surgery, so that patients do not feel the need to stool. Constipation is a common problem after a pull-through procedure. It is important for families of a patient who experiences either constipation or incontinence to continue to work with the surgeon to establish an effective bowel regimen.

HD-associated enterocolitis is linked to the highest rates of morbidity and mortality. Rates of enterocolitis are reported to range from 12% to 37% (Haricharan et al., 2008b; Singh et al., 2007). Enterocolitis is defined as inflammation of the lining of the colon or small intestines; as it progresses, it erodes into the lining of the intestines, which then becomes infected. Patients with this complication will usually have fever, abdominal distention, and classically explosive diarrhea. Prompt medical treatment is imperative, consisting of bowel decompression with a nasogastric tube, rectal irrigations, and broad-spectrum intravenous antibiotics followed by oral metronidazole. Preventing enterocolitis is difficult, however, and ongoing research is attempting to identify methods to decrease enterocolitis. In their study, Singh et al. (2007) reported an enterocolitis rate of 12%, which is lower than the rates obtained in other studies; this difference may be related to caregivers performing rectal dilations at 2 weeks post surgery. Caregivers must be educated regarding the signs of enterocolitis and the need for prompt medical care.

HD can be a complex illness requiring an interprofessional team approach to its management. If the patient is diagnosed with HD, it is important to get a dietician involved early—ensuring that the patient has appropriate weight gain can be difficult for families to achieve without support. It may be appropriate to have a social worker involved to help the family cope with the diagnosis and provide them with appropriate resources. To manage the complex stooling issues that patients with HD have, consultation with gastroenterology may be of help.

Caregivers of patients with HD require significant education and support. Rectal irrigations will be required at least daily until the surgical repair is performed. Caregivers must know the signs of enterocolitis and know what to do if they suspect their child has it.

Prognosis and discharge planning

The most common and concerning complications of HD are enterocolitis, constipation, and incontinence. Enterocolitis is the leading cause of HD-related mortality. The important thing is to prevent enterocolitis after the surgical repair or, at a minimum, to diagnose and treat the enterocolitis early. The majority of patients with HD are able to establish normal bowel function and achieve bowel continence, although functional delay is not uncommon.

HD requires long-term management and follow-up. Many pediatric surgeons are developing clinics that emphasize an interprofessional approach to care, with team members including gastroenterologists, nurse practitioners, dieticians, social workers, and a psychologist. Most pediatric patients with HD experience fewer disease-associated complications by adolescence. Some patients have psychological problems associated with all of the stooling issues. Consequently, patients may be prescribed polyethylene glycol 3350, antegrade continence enema, or loperamide to improve stool regularity. It is important for families to be informed that HD is not cured with the surgical intervention and, that patients will require close monitoring of bowel function, nutritional status, and overall health for their lifetime.

The surgical correction for HD has a very low morbidity and mortality. The prognosis of HD is highly dependent on the amount of colon affected. At one extreme of the disease spectrum, a pediatric patient with a short segment will usually have a good outcome with very few interventions required. At the other end of the spectrum, patients with total-colon HD may require multiple procedures; in rare cases, an intestinal transplant may be needed. The vast majority of patients fall between these two extremes, however, and have a good prognosis.

ILEUS

Pathophysiology

An ileus is a *functional* obstruction, which occurs when the peristalsis of the GI tract is impaired. It is characterized by failure of the normal flow of chyme through the intestinal lumen from intestinal immotility in the absence of an obstructing lesion. When an ileus occurs, the portion of the bowel proximal to the obstruction becomes distended, as fluid and air accumulate due to the bowel's inability to reabsorb fluid and from both oral ingestion and bacterial overgrowth gas production.

The pathophysiologic basis of an ileus is unknown, but is thought to be related to an interaction between inhibitory neural impulses, inflammatory mediators, and endogenous and exogenous opioids (Person & Wexner, 2006). Sympathetic stimulation inhibits GI motility in contrast to parasympathetic stimulation, which stimulates bowel motility by inducing the release of acetylcholine. Following surgery, there is greater sympathetic stimulation from pain and tissue trauma than parasympathetic stimulation, resulting in decreased GI motility (Mattei & Rombeau, 2006).

Although the specific mechanism underlying ileus is not known, the inflammatory response appears to be related to the migration of leukocytes into the gut mucosa from tissue trauma. This process leads to the release of prostaglandins, nitric oxide, and cytokines (e.g., tumor necrosis factor-α, interleukin-1b, interleukin-6, monocytes chemotactic protein-1) that act directly upon the enteric nervous system. Nitric oxide acts locally on the myenteric plexus and is a potent inhibitor of GI motility. Inflammatory mediators most likely play a prominent role, and with known tissue trauma postoperative ileus (POI) tends to be prolonged (lasting more than 5 days).

Both exogenous and endogenous opioids decrease GI activity, due to their direct effect on the μ_2-opioid receptors.

The effect on the receptors leads to decreased GI motility, including a decrease in the propulsive peristaltic waves. The effect of endogenous opioids is thought to be minimal as compared to exogenous opioids; however, these medications remain the mainstay of treatment for pain in the postoperative period.

Epidemiology and etiology

Ileus following abdominal surgery is universal. The extent of POI is thought to be related to the amount of tissue manipulation and handling of the patient's bowel. Specifically, POI tends to be more sustained following laparotomy as compared to minimally invasive procedures. The presence of peritonitis in patients with a perforated appendix or traumatic bowel injury contributes to a prolonged ileus. Causes of ileus are listed in Table 26-29 and Table 26-30.

Presentation

Symptoms of ileus vary depending on the affected bowel segment and the length of the intestinal tract proximal to the obstruction. Abdominal distention, absent or hypoactive bowel sounds due to lack of peristalsis, and constant pain that worsens with increased bowel distention are commonly reported. Unfortunately, the postoperative patient may have pain associated with the ileus coupled with the expected postoperative pain.

TABLE 26-29

Causes of Functional Bowel Obstruction
Abdominal surgery
Peritonitis
Sepsis
Trauma
Head injury
Medications (e.g., opioids, anesthetic agents)
Metabolic imbalances (hypokalemia, hyponatremia, hypomagnesemia, acidosis)

TABLE 26-30

Causes of Mechanical Bowel Obstruction
Postoperative adhesions
Intussusception
Distal intestinal obstruction syndrome
Malrotation with volvulus
Tumors
Congenital abnormalities:
• Duodenal atresia
• Duodenal web
• Annular pancreas
• Jejunoileal atresia

Vomiting is typically a late sign of ileus and is preceded by distention and accumulation of GI fluids. The higher the obstruction, the more rapid and frequent the emesis episodes may be. If the distal intestine is involved, there is more space to accommodate fluid and air; however, the distention may be more apparent because a greater bowel length is involved. Vomiting proximal to the sphincter of Oddi will more likely be nonbilious. Bilious emesis represents an obstruction occurring beyond the sphincter of Oddi. Emesis will be green in color.

The more distal the location of the operative intervention, the longer it should be anticipated that the patient will exhibit signs of POI. Symptoms that may be present with resolution of POI include the passage of flatus and stool. Perhaps the best indicator of resumption of bowel function is the ability to tolerate an oral diet. As compared to adults, children tend to recover from ileus more quickly.

Differential diagnosis

Simple obstruction (mechanical blockage) of the lumen by a lesion, hematoma, bezoar, volvulus, or intussusception may be considered based on patient history. Consideration should be given to a mechanical bowel obstruction from adhesions or other surgical complication in patients with a sustained POI.

Plan of care

An abdominal radiograph is usually the first diagnostic study. With an ileus, the bowel becomes distended. As air and fluid accumulate, air–fluid levels become visible, as would also be seen with a mechanical obstruction. Serial radiographs may be of use in identifying the buildup. If the patient is experiencing significant gastric fluid losses, electrolyte levels are warranted.

There are no useful studies and a paucity of data related to caring for POI in children; thus clinical experience guides care (Mattei & Rombeau, 2006). The usual treatment for an ileus is bowel rest, decompression with a nasogastric tube to low intermittent suction or gravity, and replacement of fluid and electrolytes. Generally, it is appropriate to replace the fluid lost from nasogastric decompression with intravenous fluids (e.g., 0.45 normal saline with 20 mEq KCl/L). If it is anticipated that a patient will require bowel rest for more than 3 days, consideration should be given to initiating parenteral nutrition.

Nasogastric tubes are placed more often in younger children as compared to older children and adults. Particularly in premature and young infants, abdominal distention may interfere with diaphragmatic excursion, hampering adequate ventilation. Mechanical ventilation should be provided as needed in these children.

Pain control may affect the duration of POI by minimizing sympathetic stimulation. To reduce the effects of opioids on gastric motility, other classes of analgesics should be considered to provide pain relief. In adults, bupivicaine thoracic epidurals have proven useful to shorten the duration of POI; this approach minimizes sympathetic stimulation. NSAIDs may be of use in younger patients to treat both pain and inflammation; however, consideration should be given to the possible side effect of GI bleeding.

Routine postoperative care practices such as early ambulation and enteral feeding may aid in the resolution POI. Motility agents (metocloprimide, neostigmine), however, have been studied in adults and a proven benefit has not been reported. Their side-effect profile is also a source of concern (Zeinali et al., 2009). In contrast, μ-opioid receptor antagonists such as alvimopan and methylnaltrexone have shown early promise in their ability to shorten the duration of POI and reduce hospital stays for adult patients (Maron & Fry, 2008). Low-dose oral naloxone may also minimize the GI effects of opioids, although its dosing presents a concern regarding the impedance of the desired analgesic effect as this medication also acts on central μ-opioid receptors. Even chewing (sugar-free) gum has been studied. Researchers have speculated that the act of chewing may stimulate digestion-producing hormones associated with bowel motility; it might also act as a sham feeding that stimulates the motility of the duodenum, stomach, and rectum or that stimulates the secretion of saliva and pancreatic juices (Tandeter, 2009).

For most patients, postoperative ileus will resolve with time. Educating the patient and family of what to expect in the postoperative period may allay anxiety, which can further contribute to development of an ileus. If it can be anticipated that a nasogastric tube will be placed intraoperatively, this information should be shared with the patient and family prior to surgery.

Disposition and discharge planning

The prognosis for POI depends on its cause. The usual pattern of resolution is for the small bowel function to return within 12 to 24 hours, for the stomach within 24 to 48 hours, and for the colon within 3 to 5 days (Livingston & Passaro, 1990).

Usual postoperative follow-up is 1 to 2 weeks after discharge. For medical causes of a functional obstruction, follow-up would depend on the underlying diagnosis.

INTUSSUSCEPTION

Pathophysiology

Intussusception is the invagination or telescoping of the intestines. The telescoping proximal portion of bowel (intussusceptum) invaginates into the adjacent distal bowel (intussuscepiens). The mesentery of the intussusceptum becomes compressed, and the swelling of the bowel wall leads to obstruction. Venous engorgement and ischemia of the intestinal mucosa cause bleeding, followed by an outpouring of mucus, which may result in "currant jelly" stool.

Epidemiology and etiology

Intussusception most commonly occurs in the ileocecal region; it is the most common cause of bowel obstruction in children (Fagerman & Faber, 2007). Intussusception occurs in 1 of 2,000 infants and children, with a slightly increased incidence being noted in white males. Although intussusceptions occur throughout the age spectrum, 75% of these cases occur before the age of 2 years and 40% of cases emerge by 9 months of age (Ein & Daneman, 2006).

Three categories of intussusception are distinguished: idiopathic, lead point, and postsurgical. *Idiopathic* intussusceptions are seen more commonly in infants and children (Ein & Daneman, 2006). Their exact cause is unknown, but may correlate with viral gastroenteritis or an upper respiratory infection. According to one theory, a viral infection leads to hypertrophy of Peyer's patches (a type of lymph nodes found in the intestines), which acts as a lead point causing the intussusception.

Lead point intussusception has an identifiable cause in the intestinal mucosa. The incidence of a lead point causing intussusception in children 5 to 14 years of age is 60% (Ein & Daneman, 2006). An inverted Meckel's diverticulum, polyps, duplication cyst, and hemangiomas are the most common causes (Bailey et al., 2007). Pediatric patients with cystic fibrosis are at increased risk of intussusception due to the changes that occur in the intestines from mucus and thick inspissated stool, which acts as a lead point (Fagerman & Faber, 2007).

Postsurgical intussusception, the least common type, is seen in patients after abdominal and thoracic operations. It is thought to result from anesthesia's effect on the intestines and bowel manipulation during surgery (Fagerman & Faber, 2007). Surgical intussusception can be difficult to diagnose, as the underlying surgical process may mask an invagination.

Presentation

Intussusception can present with a wide range of symptoms. It frequently presents in a healthy, well-nourished infant or child. The classic signs and symptoms include crampy abdominal pain, emesis, bloody stool, and a mass in the right lower quadrant. Eighty-five percent of children will present with severe colicky abdominal pain, which forces the child to retract his or her legs into the abdomen and usually lasts for a few minutes (Ein & Damen, 2006). All four of the classic signs and symptoms are seen in fewer than 25% of patients. Notably, the child may become lethargic and irritable as the bowel's blood flow becomes compromised.

Prompt diagnosis will help decrease the need for surgical intervention. According to Kaiser et al. (2007), 61% of patients require operative intervention due to delay in diagnosis. If a patient has classic signs and symptoms of intussusception, it is important to obtain immediate appropriate diagnostic imaging so that HCPs can initiate the prompt management necessary to decrease mortality and morbidity.

Differential diagnosis

The following diagnoses should be considered when intussusception is suspected: gastroenteritis, malrotation with midgut volvulus, appendicitis, Meckel's diverticulum, and incarcerated hernia.

Plan of care

In approximately 50% of patients, the diagnosis of intussusception is made based on clinical findings. Further investigation with an abdominal radiograph, ultrasound, and contrast/air enema is needed for the remaining 50% (Byrne et al., 2005). Abdominal radiographs are useful because they are rapid and noninvasive, but lack the sensitivity needed to diagnose an intussusception. A right upper quadrant soft-tissue density with the absence of colonic gas may indicate an intussusception (Figure 26-15), which should be followed by a contrast/air enema.

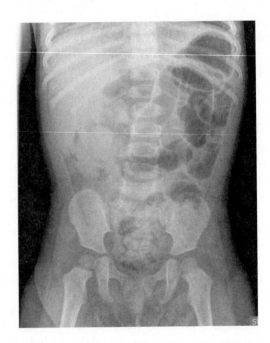

FIGURE 26-15

Plain Film of the Abdomen in a Child with Intussusception. A right upper quadrant soft-tissue density with the absence of colonic gas.

Source: Courtesy of Sarah Martin and Kelly Finkbeiner.

An ultrasound or enema may be both diagnostic and therapeutic (Byrne et al., 2005). Ultrasound has been proven to be effective in diagnosing intussusception; and it has 98% sensitivity and 98% specificity for this condition (Hryhorczuk & Strouse, 2009). On ultrasound, an intussusception has a characteristic appearance of a 3- to 5-cm mass called a "doughnut" or "target sign" (Figure 26-16). In some instances, ultrasound may be helpful in diagnosing other pathology if the patient does not have an intussusception.

If the HCP strongly suspects that a patient has intussusception, he or she may opt for a contrast enema. An enema is 100% accurate in diagnosing intussusception and has a 70% success rate for reduction of the mass. The success rate, however, declines as the duration of symptoms increases (Kaiser et al., 2007). If the intussusceptum is not fully reduced on the first attempt, a second or third attempt may be performed. After the third unsuccessful attempt, it is likely that the intussusception will need to be surgically reduced (Chua et al., 2006).

The contrast enema is performed by instilling air or contrast medium into the rectum via a rectal tube. The pressure from the air/contrast pushes the intussusceptum proximally, which reduces the obstruction. Fluoroscopy is used to assess whether the air or contrast has fully refluxed into the small intestine. During fluoroscopy, a filling defect or lead point may be appreciated and will require further investigation.

Patients may be dehydrated when they present for care, such that they require fluid resuscitation with ongoing evaluation. Once a patient is diagnosed with intussusception,

and prior to having an air/contrast study or surgical reduction, the surgeon may recommend broad-spectrum antibiotics to prevent systemic bacteremia associated with bacterial translocation and/or perforation.

The therapeutic management choice for intussusception is nonsurgical reduction by air or contrast enema. If this treatment fails, or if the patient becomes unstable or perforation is noted, surgical intervention is required. Ultimately, surgical re-reduction is required in approximately 20% of all patients with intussusception (Jen & Shew, 2009). A pathologic lead point is seen in 14% of all patients with intussusception, most of whom require surgical intervention (Kaiser et al., 2007). Two surgical techniques are currently used in this population: laparoscopic and open reduction of the intussusception. Both methods have proven to be safe and effective in treating intussusception.

Historically the most common surgical procedure was an open laparatomy during which the surgeon made a transverse right lower quadrant incision. The intussusception was brought out of the abdominal cavity, and was reduced by slowly and steadily milking the intussusceptum proximally (like a tube of toothpaste). If the surgeon was unable to completely reduce the intussusception or if necrosis was present, a small bowel resection was performed with an end-to-end anastomosis. Often an incidental appendectomy was performed. The surgeon also inspected the intestines for a lead point and resected any such points identified.

The use of laparoscopy is proving to be a safe and effective alternative way to treat an unreducible intussusception. Laparoscopy allows for better visualization of the intestine with less manipulation than with the open laparotomy technique. It is performed by placing three laparoscopic ports in the abdomen: a 5-mm port in the umbilicus (for the camera) and two 3- to 5-mm ports in the left upper and lower abdomen. When reducing the intussusception laparoscopically, it is safe to use traction on the proximal bowel and pull the intussusceptum out from the distal bowel. The intestines are inspected to assure complete reduction and to assess for necrosis, serosal tear, or lead point. When less manipulation occurs, patients have a quicker return of bowel function. A retrospective analysis of laparoscopic reduction of intussusception revealed that this technique was associated with decreased postoperative pain, length of hospitalization, and overall hospital cost (Bailey et al., 2007).

Care of patients after reduction of the intussusception will vary depending on the type of reduction (i.e., radiologic versus surgical). With radiologic reduction, patients will remain NPO for a short time post procedure, followed by introduction of clear liquids with diet progression as tolerated. Twenty-four-hr observation after reduction is recommended to closely monitor the patient for signs of perforation. If recurrence is suspected, an abdominal ultrasound should be performed. If present, an additional contrast enema could be performed to attempt re-reduction.

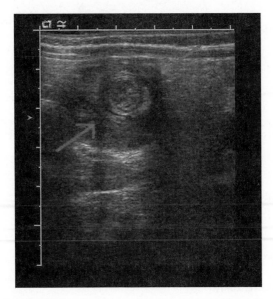

FIGURE 26-16

Ultrasound of an Intussusception. Characteristic appearance of a target sign.

Source: Courtesy of Sarah Martin and Kelly Finkbeiner.

The care of a patient after surgical reduction is more complicated than that after radiologic reduction. Following surgery, patients remain NPO until the return of bowel function, and receive intravenous fluids and antibiotics. It is important to monitor hydration status by monitoring heart rate and urine output, which should be at least 1 mL/kg/hr. Patients will also require pain management.

When a patient presents to an emergency department and is suspected of having an intussusception, a surgical consult should be obtained. It is very important that a surgeon see the patient prior to performing the air/contrast enema procedure due to the risk of perforation. If the enema is unsuccessful in reducing the intussusception, the patient will require an emergent surgical procedure. The longer the symptoms are present, the more frequent the need for operative intervention and bowel resection.

Caregivers need to be educated regarding recurrence, including what to do if it is suspected. They should be instructed on the classic signs of intussusception and told that if these symptoms emerge, they must seek medical treatment for the child promptly. There are no known methods to reduce the risk of recurrence.

Disposition and discharge planning

The most common complication associated with an intussusception is recurrence, which occurs in 10% to 20% of patients (Grosfeld, 2005). Recurrence is more common with nonsurgical reduction and typically takes place within the first 24 hours after a reduction, with most recurrence occurring within 6 months of the initial diagnosis (Kaiser et al., 2007).

Patients who require a surgical reduction of the intussusception will have a longer recovery period. These individuals may require opioid-containing pain medications at discharge for a short period. Because the surgical incision is closed with dissolving sutures, most patient can bathe 24 to 48 hours after surgery. They will require a postoperative visit with the pediatric surgeon. If the intussusception is reduced nonsurgically, follow-up with the pediatrician in a week is advised.

Intussusception is a self-limiting illness with a good prognosis and very few negative outcomes following nonsurgical or surgical reduction. Most morbidity and mortality related to the intussusception are a consequence of delayed diagnosis and treatment, due to the associated intestinal ischemia. In rare situations, this ischemia can lead to intestinal failure (short gut syndrome) and necessitate small bowel transplant.

Intussusceptions cannot be prevented, and many times they have no specific cause. It is possible that by preventing viral illnesses such as rotavirus, some cases of intussusception might be prevented. The most important consideration when dealing with a patient with possible intussusception is prompt diagnosis and reduction of the intussusceptum.

MALROTATION/VOLVULUS

Pathophysiology

Malrotation is an abnormal rotation and fixation of the bowel during embryologic development. The classic form of malrotation is a result of an abnormal rotation of the duodenojejunal and cecocolic loop and a high, medially positioned cecum (Lampl et al., 2009). The distal duodenum, jejunum, ileum, cecum, appendix, ascending colon, and proximal part of the transverse colon develop from the midgut (Kenner & Lott, 2003). Midgut development begins as a short, straight continuous tube suspended from the superior mesenteric artery (SMA). As early as the fifth gestational week, a series of rotations involving the forming bowel and SMA occurs outside of the abdomen. This rotation places the duodenum behind the SMA, the ligament of Treitz (duodenojejunal junction) to the left of the spine, and the right colon (with the cecum) to the right of the abdomen. Normally there is a 270-degree rotation; once rotation is completed, fixation occurs (Figure 26-17). This fixation is necessary to prevent the bowel from

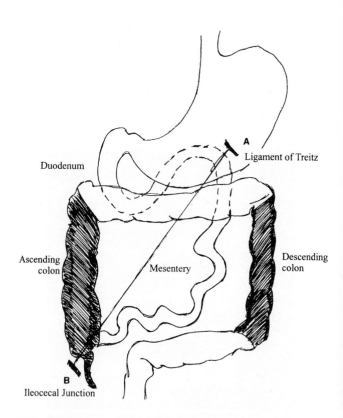

FIGURE 26-17

Normal Fixation of the Mesentery.

Source: Diana-Zerpa, J. & Shapiro-Stolar, T. (2007). Malrotation and volvulus. In N. Browne, L. Flanigan, C. McComiskey, & P. Pieper (Eds.). *Nursing Care of the Pediatric Surgical Patient.* 2nd edition. Sudbury, MA: Jones and Bartlett Publishers.

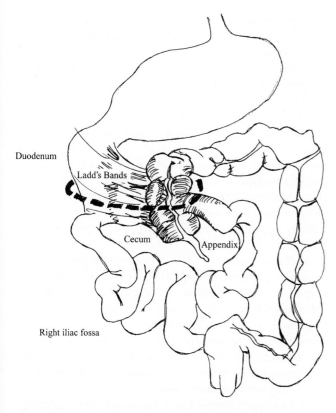

FIGURE 26-18

Ladd's Bands with Duodenal Obstruction.

Source: Diana-Zerpa, J. & Shapiro-Stolar, T. (2007). Malrotation and volvulus. In N. Browne, L. Flanigan, C. McComiskey, & P. Pieper (Eds.). *Nursing Care of the Pediatric Surgical Patient.* 2nd edition. Sudbury, MA: Jones and Bartlett Publishers.

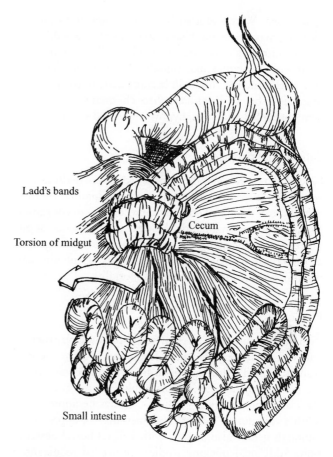

FIGURE 26-19

Midgut Volvulus.

Source: Diana-Zerpa, J. & Shapiro-Stolar, T. (2007). Malrotation and volvulus. In N. Browne, L. Flanigan, C. McComiskey, & P. Pieper (Eds.). *Nursing Care of the Pediatric Surgical Patient.* 2nd edition. Sudbury, MA: Jones and Bartlett Publishers.

twisting on itself, thereby creating a midgut volvulus. With malrotation, there are aberrant attempts at fixation and the intestine attaches with abnormal tissue known as a Ladd's band (Figure 26-18).

Volvulus occurs when malrotation is present and the midgut twists in a clockwise direction around the SMA, leading to occlusion of the SMA. It is thought to occur in part from the abnormal attachment with the Ladd's bands, when the twist occurs and blood flow to the intestines is reduced (Figure 26-19). If the obstruction is not addressed quickly, bowel necrosis rapidly ensues.

Epidemiology and etiology

The incidence of malrotation is not known, as the majority of people with this disorder are asymptomatic. Autopsy studies indicate that the disorder may occur in as many as 1% of the population (Kapfer & Rappold, 2004). An increased incidence of malrotation is observed in children with the following syndromes: heterotaxy; trisomies 13, 18, and 21; Marfan's disease, and prune belly. Diaphragmatic hernia, duodenal web, and abdominal wall defects

(gastroschisis, omphalocele) are some of the most common anatomic abnormalities associated with malrotation.

Volvulus is most often diagnosed in infancy. In infants diagnosed with volvulus, approximately one-third are less than 1 week old, and more than one-half are less than 1 month old (American Pediatric Surgical Association, 2009). However, malrotation and volvulus may both present in adulthood, leading to delays in their diagnosis.

Presentation

When a pediatric patient presents with a malrotation, there are three possibilities: no symptoms, complaints of intermittent symptoms, or an acute presentation. Commonly manifested symptoms include vomiting, abdominal pain, and failure-to-thrive. The classic presentation is that of a neonate discharged home who later develops bilious emesis. Initially the emesis will be clear; however, as the bowel becomes obstructed, the emesis will take on a bilious appearance. With eventual bowel ischemia, intraluminal bleeding may occur and bloody stool may be passed.

In contrast, a child with a volvulus will have emesis. A child with a volvulus may initially appear nontoxic; however, with time the child will become toxic in the presence of ischemic bowel. Eventually these children will develop a firm, distended abdomen, hypovolemia, and shock.

Differential diagnosis

Several diagnoses may be considered when malrotation/volvulus is suspected, including sepsis, abdominal trauma, some type of duodenal obstruction secondary to congenital bands, or an internal hernia. However, the presence of bilious emesis in the neonate or infant mandates investigation, as the failure to make a timely diagnosis of volvulus can result in significant morbidity and mortality.

Plan of care

Two-view abdominal films may suggest a bowel obstruction with the presence of air–fluid levels and is often the first study obtained. Although plain films for duodenal atresia are nondiagnostic, the "double bubble" sign—considered the classic presentation—may not always be appreciated. With a volvulus, a "gasless" abdomen may be appreciated, although it may also be seen with a distal bowel obstruction. Additional imaging studies are needed to diagnose malrotation, whereas the diagnosis of volvulus may be revealed through imaging.

The upper GI study is considered the study of choice for diagnosis of malrotation. In most situations, the radiologist is able to determine the normal position of the small bowel with the ligament of Treitz (duodenojejunal junction). The normal position is to the left of the left-sided pedicle of the vertebral bodies, at the level of the duodenal bulbs on frontal, posterior, and lateral views (Applegate et al.). Nevertheless, approximately 15% of upper GI studies are equivocal, leading to both false-positive and false-negative interpretations. For these pediatric patients, a barium enema may be performed to evaluate the relationship of the cecum, as the cecum has been shown to be abnormally positioned 80% of the time in malrotation (Applegate et al.).

Depending on the presentation of a child suspected of having a volvulus, no imaging may be able to expedite the needed surgical intervention. Again, radiologic findings may not be confirmatory, although an ultrasound may reveal an abnormal SMA and superior mesenteric vein orientation. A CT scan of the abdomen may reveal a "swirl sign" that radiologists consider diagnostic.

If time permits before surgery, a chemistry panel should be obtained and electrolyte abnormalities addressed. It is common for patients with malrotation and volvulus to have a metabolic acidosis. Given that intraluminal bleeding may

occur preoperatively, a complete blood count and type and screen should be obtained and—blood transfusion may be indicated in some cases.

Surgical intervention is required to correct volvulus. Whether it is necessary to surgically repair all malrotations remains controversial. Sometimes malrotations have been incidentally diagnosed while patients were in the process of having abdominal imaging studies done for unrelated symptoms. Many surgeons will advocate for correction of the defect with a Ladd procedure, as there is no way to predict which children will go on to develop a life-threatening volvulus. Other surgeons choose to avoid surgical repair of an asymptomatic malrotation. When the diagnosis of a volvulus is suspected, urgent operative intervention is always indicated.

Pediatric patients with asymptomatic malrotation undergoing an elective surgical repair may be treated with outpatient surgery. Pediatric patients who present with a volvulus will generally require fluid resuscitation, need correction of electrolyte abnormalities, and should have blood products readied for surgery. The priority is operative intervention; therefore, the patient should be promptly transferred to the operating room, with resuscitative efforts continuing in the operative suite.

A Ladd procedure is the surgical approach performed for both malrotation and volvulus. This procedure can be performed via laparoscopy or laparotomy. Some surgeons perform the procedure using an open laparotomy technique, which is associated with the development of fewer postoperative adhesions and, therefore, minimizes the risk of subsequent occurrence of a volvulus. A recent retrospective analysis concluded that the laparoscopic Ladd procedure should be the initial approach in malrotation in the absence of volvulus, with a low threshold for conversion to an open approach if concern for volvulus arises (Fraser et al., 2009).

The standard Ladd procedure includes the following components:

- Detorsion of the bowel by a counterclockwise rotation when volvulus is present
- Division of Ladd's bands (bands from the cecum crossing over the duodenum)
- Repositioning of the cecum and its mesentery in the left upper quadrant while the small bowel is placed in the right abdomen
- Widening of the mesenteric base
- Performance of an incidental appendectomy, as the appendix is abnormally positioned in the left upper quadrant

If a volvulus is present, the surgeon will resect the necrotic bowel. If extensive necrosis is identified, the surgeon may confer with the family regarding options of care; they may elect to provide end-of-life care. If the viability of the bowel is questionable, a "second look" operation may be preformed to minimize the amount of bowel requiring resection.

The postoperative care will vary based on the intraoperative findings. Patients undergoing an elective operation will usually require nasogastric decompression until the resumption of bowel function. Once the pediatric patient has the nasogastric tube removed, the diet will be advanced from clear liquids to a general diet as tolerated. The patient should be encouraged to ambulate to promote clearance of pulmonary secretions and resolution of ileus. Intravenous pain management with opioids and NSAIDs should be transitioned to oral agents once clear liquids are tolerated.

For pediatric patients who require a "second look" operation or who have an extensive bowel resection, postoperative intensive care monitoring is essential. Management often entails mechanical ventilation, vasopressor therapy, and treatment of resultant coagulopathies and fluid/electrolyte abnormalities. Patients may also require chemical paralysis, as third spacing from resuscitation and bowel injury may make oxygenation and ventilation a challenge. Pain medication and sedation should be administered as indicated.

Patients with suspected malrotation may have been evaluated by a pediatric gastroenterologist; however, it is also recommended that surgical consultation be arranged. Pediatric patients diagnosed with volvulus *always* require urgent surgical consultation. Patients with extensive bowel necrosis or resection require postoperative care in the intensive care unit. A child with intestinal failure should be managed by a pediatric gastroenterologist or an intestinal rehabilitation team; however, if catastrophic bowel loss occurs, then referral to an intestinal transplant program is recommended.

Caregiver education regarding the need for surgery and recovery expectations for the child should be reviewed. Caregiver handouts are available from the American Pediatric Surgical Nurses Association website (www.apsna.org).

For children who undergo a Ladd procedure, it is imperative that caregivers be educated about the possibility of the child developing a postoperative volvulus. If their child were to become symptomatic with vomiting, they should seek immediate emergent care. Caregivers should also be informed that their child had an appendectomy as part of the Ladd procedure. The appendectomy was performed as their appendix was found on the left side of their abdomen rather than being found in the normal right lower quadrant position—a situation that may confuse the child's HCPs in the futureif the patient presents with abdominal pain.

Disposition and discharge planning

Outcomes for children following the Ladd procedure for malrotation are excellent. There are few potential complications aside from the potential for future bowel obstruction from adhesions—a risk associated with any abdominal surgery. Unfortunately, for children with volvulus, outcomes can vary dramatically, ranging from complete recovery to intestinal failure to death.

Pediatric patients who undergo a Ladd procedure for malrotation will follow up with the surgeon in 1 to 2 weeks. For children with a volvulus, the follow-up will depend on the associated morbidity. These patients often require prolonged hospitalization and may have many additional care needs at discharge. For those who experience intestinal failure, care may be transitioned to a gastroenterologist specializing in intestinal rehabilitation.

The prognosis for pediatric patients with malrotation is excellent. Once recovery occurs, they can resume all of their daily activities and routine health maintenance visits can continue. For children with intestinal failure, the prognosis depends on their ability to achieve intestinal adaptation by enteral nutrition with the goal of normal growth.

PYLORIC STENOSIS

Pathophysiology

In pyloric stenosis, the circumferential muscle of the pyloric sphincter becomes hypertrophied, resulting in elongation and obliteration of the pyloric channel. The muscular hypertrophy may be related to abnormal nerve innervation (deficiency of nerve terminals, peptide-containing nerve fibers, mRNA production of nitric oxide synthetase), increased insulin, and platelet-derived growth factors. Abnormal innervation leads to failure of pyloric muscular relaxation (Aspelund & Langer, 2007). Eventually, a high-grade gastric outlet obstruction develops, accompanied by compensatory dilation, hypertrophy, and hyperperistalsis of the stomach.

Epidemiology and etiology

The incidence of hypertrophic pyloric stenosis (HPS) is on the rise, with the disorder occurring at a rate of 2 to 5 cases per 1,000 live births (MacMahon, 2006). There is a 4:1 male predominance, with the disorder often diagnosed in the first-born male (MacMahon; O'Dowd, 2007). The etiology of HPS is unknown, although some evidence supports a genetic association, which may be coupled with environmental factors. To date, five HPS-related genetic loci have been identified (Chung, 2008). Other etiologies that have been hypothesized include congenital redundancy of the pyloric mucosa, abnormalities of enteric innervation, diminished levels of nitric oxide synthetase, elevated concentration of gastrin, and exposure to erythromycin (motilin agonist) prenatally or in the first 2 months of life (Chung).

Presentation

The hallmark symptom of HPS is nonbilious, projectile, and progressive emesis occurring 30 to 60 minutes after feeding, starting between 2 and 6 weeks of age, although symptoms can occur as late as 3 months after birth. Early in the course of the disorder, vomiting is intermittent. As gastric outlet obstruction develops further, however, vomiting becomes more continuous. Bilious emesis should raise concern for a bowel obstruction.

The infant may express persistent hunger with weight loss; dehydration may also be evident. In some patients, palpation of the hypertrophied pylorus in the midepigastrium, also known as the "olive sign," may be appreciated. Gastric peristalsis may be visible with feeding.

Differential diagnosis

Pylorospasm, gastroenteritis, feeding intolerance, milk allergy, overfeeding, and gastroesophageal reflux (GER) are all potential differential diagnoses when HPS is suspected. Pylorospasm—spasmodic contraction of the pylorus with poorly coordinated gastric emptying—is observed most commonly in neonates (Gilet et al., 2008). In these infants, variability in pyloric muscle measurements and fluid flow into the duodenum may be noted on ultrasound. Although gastroenteritis may be a consideration, patients with HPS do not have diarrhea or fever. The most common diagnosis for exclusion is GER. Infants with GER may also have weight loss, although projectile vomiting is an uncommon finding.

Plan of care

The gastric secretions of patients with HPS contain high concentrations of hydrochloric acid. With the progressive vomiting of HPS, patients become dehydrated, hypochloremic, hypokalemic, hyponatremic, and alkalotic. In an effort to retain sodium and water, the kidney excretes potassium and hydrogen ions, leading to paradoxical aciduria. An elevated unconjugated hyperbilirubinemia related to transient impairment of glucuronyl transferase activity may also be present; this imbalance usually resolves after surgery.

The preference of most surgeons is to confirm the diagnosis with an abdominal ultrasound. Ultrasound findings of a pylorus muscle wall thickness of 3 mm or more and a pyloric channel length of 14 mm or more are considered diagnostic for HPS (Figure 26-20). In addition, specific measurements apply to premature infants. An upper GI study may be of value if there are concurrent suspicions for malrotation and GER. A "string sign" (elongated and thickened pyloric channel), "beak sign" (filling of the proximal pylorus), or "double shoulder sign" (thickened pylorus compressing the antrum of the stomach) may be noted when HPS is present.

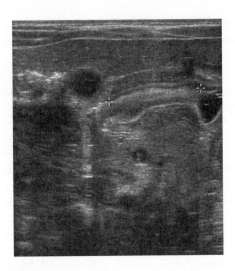

FIGURE 26-20

Ultrasound of an Infant with Pyloric Stenosis. The length of the pylorus is marked (2.2 cm).

Source: Courtesy of Sarah Martin and Kelly Finkbeiner.

Although operative intervention is indicated, correction of HPS is not an emergent procedure. Prior to administration of anesthesia, infants should be hemodynamically stable with age-appropriate vital signs, normal electrolytes, and a urine output of at least 1 mL/kg/hr. Bicarbonate levels should be less than 30 mEq/L, because infants with metabolic alkalosis are at high risk for developing respiratory depression under anesthesia. Intravenous fluids (rehydration may be indicated) and electrolyte supplementation as needed should be administered. An orogastric or nasogastric tube may be considered for persistent vomiting; however, some surgeons prefer not to place a nasogastric tube because it may stimulate GI tract secretions.

The Ramstedt pyloromyotomy (open procedure) is the most common surgical procedure performed for HPS; it involves the extramucosal splitting of the hypertrophied pylorus. More recently, minimally invasive procedures have become more common due to their r ability to reduce hospital stays (Hall et al., 2009; St. Peter & Ostlie, 2008).

Caregiver teaching handouts are available from the American Pediatric Surgical Nurses Association website (www.apsna.org).

Diagnosis and discharge planning

A variety of postoperative feeding regimens are used in patients with HPS, such as the pyloric regimen (Table 26-31) or delayed ad lib feeds. Breastfeeding is considered safe and appropriate. Postoperative vomiting is common and occurs due to gastric distention and atony. The majority of infants tolerate ad lib feeds (volume of at least 60 mL) within 24 to 48 hours of the operation. Persistent vomiting beyond

TABLE 26-31

Pyloric Regimen		
Feeding Interval	**Formula**	**Breastmilk**
Initial feed	Pedialyte 15 mL	Pedialyte 15 mL
1 hour later	Pedialyte 30 mL	Pedialyte 30 mL
2 hours later	Half-strength formula 30 mL	Breastfeed 2 minutes
2 hours later	Full-strength formula 30 mL	Breastfeed 2 minutes
3 hours later	Full-strength formula 45 mL	Breastfeed 5 minutes
3 hours later	Full-strength formula 60 mL	Breastfeed 7 minutes
3 hours later	Ad lib feeds	Ad lib feeds

72 to 96 hours post surgery may occur in infants with an incomplete pyloromyotomy; an upper GI series may be valuable to determine whether this condition is present.

Given that the surgical patient's wounds are usually infiltrated with local anesthetic, typically only acetaminophen is prescribed for pain control. The wounds should be assessed for infection and incisional hernias. Gastric mucosal tears or duodenal perforation are life-threatening complications.

When the infant has tolerated 60 mL for at least in two consecutive feedings without emesis, the child is usually ready for discharge. Caregiver education should include calling or returning for rectal temperature greater than 101.5°F (38.6°C), persistent emesis, abdominal pain, or any signs or symptoms of wound infection.

Usual follow-up takes place with the pediatric surgeon in 2 weeks. Follow-up should be arranged with the primary care provider in 1 week for wound evaluation and a weight check. Many centers are moving toward phone follow-up and seeing infants only if a problem is suspected.

> **Critical Thinking**
> A toxic child with bilious emesis requires emergent surgical consultation. If volvulus is suspected, operative intervention should proceed without additional diagnostic testing to optimize bowel salvage.

LIVER FAILURE

Barbara V. Wise

PATHOPHYSIOLOGY

Acute liver failure (ALF) is characterized by sudden loss of metabolic and synthetic liver function that, if untreated, leads to encephalopathy and multiple organ dysfunction. Local tissue injury occurs to the hepatocytes from exposure to an outside agent. During the acute injury, there is an increase in the number of inflammatory cells, accompanied by proliferation of the periportal ductules. Regeneration of liver cells starts within 1 week of injury, but complete recovery, with proliferation of normal liver and ductal cells, occurs over several weeks (Kozer et al., 2006).

EPIDEMIOLOGY AND ETIOLOGY

The etiology of pediatric ALF includes infections, toxins (18%), metabolic disorders (7%), autoimmune disease, infiltrative disease, acute hepatitis (6%), and ischemia; nevertheless, for the majority of patients (47%), the cause is undetermined (Lee et al., 2008b; Murray et al., 2008). Acetaminophen overdose accounts for 13% of children diagnosed with ALF (James et al., 2008). Worldwide, viral hepatitis A and B are the most frequent cause of ALF; in the United States, hepatitis accounts for only 15% to 20% of ALF incidence (Ciocca et al., 2008; Lee et al., 2005b; Murray et al., 2008; Stravitz & Kramer, 2009).

PRESENTATION

ALF is characterized by sudden onset of symptoms, including jaundice, a change in mental status with lethargy or hallucinations, ascites, easy bruising, and vomiting (Lee et al., 2005b). The history should elicit information about recent exposure to infectious agents and a list of prescription and over-the-counter drugs. Family history of α_1-antitrypsin, Wilson's disease, or galactosemia should also be elicited. Past medical history may indicate developmental delay, seizures, or growth failure. Findings on physical examination will vary by etiology, but may reveal hepatomegaly with or without splenomegaly, ascites, petechiae, Kayser-Fleisher rings (Wilson's disease), and fector hepaticus (sweet breath).

ALF associated with acetaminophen ingestion is evidenced by a hyperacute biochemical response with elevated alanine aminotransferase (ALT) level (median > 4,000 IU/L) and elevated bilirubin level (median > 4.5 ng/dL). The most serious complication is cerebral edema that leads to hepatic encephalopathy (HE), coma, and eventually death. The presenting clinical features include nausea, vomiting, and anorexia. In a severe acetaminophen overdose, hypoglycemia and lactic acidosis are found as part of the laboratory evaluation (Murray et al., 2008). The physical examination reveals hepatomegaly and tenderness on palpation. Jaundice and encephalopathy are late findings, presenting on days three to five after the ingestion.

Children with ALF are at risk for bacterial and viral infections. The most common pathogens for infection are *Staphylococcus aureus* and *Streptococcus* species; and sites of infection include the lungs, urinary tract, and catheter-related bloodstream infection. Signs and symptoms are nonspecific, such as tachycardia, intestinal bleeding, decreased urine output, and change in mental status. Fever may not be present (Squires, 2008; Stravitz & Kramer, 2009).

In contrast to the findings seen with adults, HE presents as a late, subtle symptom in children with ALF, but is present in 80% of patients (Novelli et al., 2008). Infants with HE are difficult to assess, as they typically present with nonspecific symptoms such as irritability and inconsolable crying. Children may present with an altered mental status, complaints of increased sleeping, elevated ammonia level, and poor school performance. Caregivers often state that their HE-affected children are not "acting" like themselves. When HE progresses to stage 3 or 4, the infant and child becomes more somnolent or combative, and may or may not respond to painful stimuli (Squires, 2008). A complete neurological examination and electroencephalograph (EEG) are obtained to classify the stage of HE, which ranges from 0 to 5 (Table 26-32).

DIFFERENTIAL DIAGNOSIS

The differential diagnoses for ALF include acutely decompensated chronic liver failure and sepsis. Table 26-33 lists potential causes of ALF.

PLAN OF CARE

Diagnosis of ALF is established when no known chronic liver failure etiology is present and there is biochemical indication of liver injury with coagulopathy (prothrombin time > 15 seconds, INR ≥ 1.5) not corrected by vitamin K supplementation. Risk factors that predict the need for liver transplantation or death are as follows: total

bilirubin ≥ 5 mg/dL, INR ≥ 2.55, and presence of hepatic encephalopathy (Squires et al., 2006).

General management of ALF is determined by the specific etiology. Three variables guide the management of ALF:

- Early identification of causes that require supportive or intensive care
- Monitoring for multiple organ dysfunction to improve chances of spontaneous recovery
- Assessment of the need for transplantation

Acetaminophen is primarily metabolized in the liver through two pathways—glucuronidation and sulfation. Children have a diminished capacity for glucuronidation, so that ingestion of a large dose of acetaminophen results in cell death when the metabolite exceeds the liver's ability to metabolize *N*-acetyl-*p*-benzoquinonemine. Acetaminophen is a dose-related toxin. To prevent hepatic injury, the cumulative dose of acetaminophen should not exceed 75 mg/kg/day. Unintentional ingestion is usually found in younger children (6 months to 11 years of age); other possible causes of acetaminophen overdose include using adult formulations in young children, administering

TABLE 26-32

Stages of Hepatic Encephalopathy		
Stage	**Clinical Findings**	**Neurologic Examination**
Grade 1	Crying, confused, mood changes	Difficult to test
Grade 2	Drowsy, inappropriate behavior, inattention to task	Tremor, apraxia
Grade 3	Stupor, obeys commands, combative	Difficult to test
Grade 4	Comatose but arousable	Decerebrate or decorticate
Grade 4a or 5	Deep coma	Decerebrate or decorticate

TABLE 26-33

Etiology of Acute Liver Failure		
Infection	**Medications and Toxins**	**Metabolic/ Immune**
Herpes simplex	Acetaminophen	Galactosemia
Echo virus	Valproic acid	Tyrosinemia
Adenovirus	Isoniazid	Fatty acid defects
Parvovirus	Amiodarone	Mitochondrial defects
Enterovirus	Phenobarbital	Wilson's disease
Hepatitis A, B, C, D, and E	Carbamazepine	Natural killer (NK) cell dysfunction
Human herpes virus 6 (HHV-6)	Minocycline/ tetracycline	Urea-cycle disorder
Epstein-Barr virus	Methotrexate	Autoimmune disorders: Chediak-Higashi syndrome
Yellow fever	Cyclophosphamide	Neonatal hemochromatosis
Parmyoxovirus	Vitamin A toxicity	Hemagophagocytic lymphohistiocytosis
Escherichia coli sepsis	Mushroom poisoning	
	Ecstasy	
	Phenytonin	
	Ephedra	
	Lichen alkaloid	

combination OTC products that include acetaminophen, and the misconception on the part of caregivers that acetaminophen is nontoxic.

Initial therapy to manage ALF after acetaminophen overdose involves administration of the antidote, *N*-acetylcysteine. Treatment should begin as rapidly as possible, usually within 8 hours of ingestion, at 300 mg/kg in 21 hours (see Chapter 37). Spontaneous recovery from ALF is more likely following acetaminophen overdose than ALF deriving from many other causes.

Lee et al. (2009) examined the administration of *N*-acetylcysteine antidote in 173 patients with ALF, not associated with acetaminophen ingestion, comparing patients receiving *N*-acetylcysteine to placebo. Survival at 21 days was not significantly different for the two groups; however, transplant-free survival at 1 year and outcomes for those patients who received liver transplants were improved in the experimental group. Similar findings have been reported in several large case studies (Cochran & Losek, 2007; Kortsalidoudaki et al., 2008).

Infectious complications account for 11% to 20% of the morbidity associated with ALF. These complications are managed by maintaining aseptic technique when handling invasive lines, obtaining daily blood cultures, and administering broad-spectrum antibiotics with evidence of infection. Changes in blood pressure or heart rate indicate infection or increasing cerebral edema. Some centers administer prophylactic antimicrobials and antifungal agents to patients awaiting transplantation because infection is a contraindication for surgery. In a combined pediatric and adult study, patients receiving prophylactic antibiotics were compared with those receiving no prophylaxis. Findings indicated that 58% of patients in the control group developed a bacterial infection (Salmerón et al., 1992). Center-specific guidelines, in consultation with infectious disease specialists, should be used to manage children with ALF (Cochran & Losek, 2007).

The primary objective in managing HE is to prevent brain edema and increased intracranial pressure (ICP). Early consultation with neurosurgery is indicated in patients with ALF. Excessive stimulation should be avoided. Restraints may be necessary if the patient is combative and confused. Frequent monitoring of ammonia levels is required, given that the liver is unable to detoxify ammonia in ALF. Periodic neurological examinations should be performed to monitor for increased ICP. Intravenous fluids are administered at 85% to 90% of maintenance levels, with strict monitoring of intake and output. Medications that affect mental status may need to be discontinued or temporarily withdrawn to allow for an accurate assessment of the patient's cognition. Other strategies based on adult experience involve the administration of lactulose or neomycin for bowel decontamination to reduce ammonia production by intestinal flora. No pediatric studies, however, have been completed to evaluate the effectiveness of these medications

in the prevention of HE (Cochran & Losek, 2007; Squires, 2008). Mannitol is an osmotic therapy administered to decrease brain edema by lowering cerebrospinal fluid volume and brain water content, thereby resulting in improved cerebral perfusion. Direct ICP monitoring and selective intubation may be required in children with encephalopathy, although this therapy remains controversial (Leonis & Balistreri, 2008b; Stravitz & Kramer, 2009).

Another option in the management of HE is a bioartificial liver support system—that is, an apparatus that uses an extracorporeal device to remove the protein-bound and water-soluble toxins, thereby providing a bridge to transplantation. The cells for the bioartificial systems are derived from porcine hepatocytes, immortalized human cells, and hepatic tumor cells (Debray et al., 2006). Limited Phase I and II clinical trials have been performed to evaluate the efficacy of bioartificial and artificial liver support systems. The results of these studies appear promising, with improvement in both clinical and biochemical parameters being noted by researchers (Novelli et al., 2008). However, several adverse events were reported, including infection, disseminated intravascular coagulation, and allergic reactions. A Cochrane Review included 12 trials comparing artificial or bioartificial support systems with standard medical therapy and found no significant effect on outcomes of ALF; mortality in acute-on-chronic liver failure was somewhat improved. Of note, the support systems markedly improved HE (Liu et al., 2004; McKenzie et al., 2008).

Bleeding is a rare complication of ALF, occurring in fewer than 5% of patients. Children with adequate platelets are unlikely to experience an episode of acute bleeding. Gastrointestinal bleeds can usually be prevented by administration of acid-reducing agents. Administration of vitamin K, however, is unlikely to prevent bleeding in ALF. Children with esophageal varices may be stabilized with administration of crystalloids, packed red blood cells, fresh frozen plasma (FFP), and cryoprecipitates. Factor VII is the first factor depleted in ALF; it is administered to promote formation of a stable clot. The advantage of using recombinant factor VII compared with FFP is that the former approach limits the patient's exposure to infectious agents and uses a relatively small dose volume to normalize prothrombin time (Cochran & Losek, 2007). If the bleeding continues, an infusion of octreotide may be administered to decrease portal venous pressure.

When the child is hemodynamically stable, an endoscopic evaluation is performed to identify the source of bleeding. In severe bleeding, a Sengstaken-Blakemore tube is inserted to provide balloon tamponade. This measure will temporarily control bleeding until a definitive surgical or interventional radiologic procedure is performed. Sclerotherapy may be required to eliminate a bleeding variceal lesion (Leonis & Balistreri, 2008a). This treatment has been shown to be effective in eliminating esophageal varices and reducing the incidence of bleeding varices

(Cochran & Losek, 2007; Howard et al., 1988; Stravitz & Kramer, 2009).

Children with repeated episodes of bleeding may benefit from placement of a distal portorenal shunt. Efforts to prevent rebleeding with a shunt are more efficacious in children with extrahepatic obstruction compared to those with intrahepatic disease (Stravitz & Kramer, 2009).

DISPOSITION AND DISCHARGE PLANNING

Approximately 13% of patients referred for liver transplantation are diagnosed with ALF of unknown etiology. Clinical and laboratory parameters that predict poor outcomes in children with ALF include PT greater than 50 seconds, time to onset of HE of more than 7 days, elevated liver function studies (ALT ≤ 2,384 IU/L, bilirubin > 17.4 mg/dL), and younger age (less than 10 years). In addition, development of multiple organ dysfunction is a poor prognostic indicator. Several factors contribute to the high rates of pretransplant mortality associated with ALF: late referral to a transplant center, long wait times on the list, and medical conditions that signal deterioration of the patient's condition, such as brain stem herniation, kidney dysfunction, and infection (Lee et al., 2005b). Overall survival for ALF with and without liver transplantation is 61% (Lee et al.). Survival rates for ALF without liver transplantation are highest in children with acetaminophen overdose (94%), while survival rates for patients with ALF caused by metabolic disease, unknown causes, or other drug toxins are 44%, 43%, and 41% respectively (Baliga et al., 2004; Squires, 2008).

PANCREATITIS

Jennifer Bevacqua

PATHOPHYSIOLOGY

Pancreatitis is broadly divided into two categories—acute and chronic—and its severity ranges from mild to severe.

Acute pancreatitis is characterized by abdominal pain (or a surrogate symptom, such as irritability or listlessness), along with an elevation in serum pancreatic enzymes. It results from inflammation due to insult or injury, with the inflammation sometimes extending to peripancreatic tissue. In some patients, additional systemic effects are noted. A noxious, inciting event triggers alterations in the acinar cells, most likely activation of intracellular trypsinogen and other digestive enzymes. These enzymes then autodigest the gland and further activate enzyme precursors, resulting in additional damage (Lowe & Greer, 2008; Radhakrishnan & Sutphen, 2006). The subsequent events in the development of acute pancreatitis are outlined in Figure 26-21.

The histopathology varies depending on the cause of the pancreatitis.

Chronic pancreatitis may be classified into three histologic subcategories: chronic calcific pancreatitis, chronic obstructive pancreatitis, and chronic inflammatory pancreatitis. The calcific and inflammatory types involve irreversible scarring of the acinar and ductal cells (postacute recurrent pancreatitis), eventually leading to gland fibrosis as well as exocrine and endocrine dysfunction. Chronic obstructive pancreatitis may be reversible if the obstruction is relieved prior to the development of scarring and fibrosis. In chronic pancreatitis, the gland is infiltrated with lymphocytes, plasma cells, and macrophages, whereas acute pancreatitis involves neutrophilic infiltration (Radhakrishnan & Sutphen, 2006).

Severe acute pancreatitis (SAP) is defined as acute pancreatitis associated with either local complications (e.g., peripancreatic fluid collection, necrosis, abscess, pseudocyst) or systemic complications (e.g., organ dysfunction). This type of pancreatitis may result from bacterial translocation in the gut, leading to abscess formation or sepsis. The subcategories of necrotic and hemorrhagic pancreatitis generally belong to the acute pancreatitis category, whereas familial and tropical (related to malnutrition) belong to the chronic pancreatitis category (Nathens et al., 2004; Radhakrishnan & Sutphen, 2006).

EPIDEMIOLOGY AND ETIOLOGY

Although pancreatitis is not common in children, its incidence in this population is reportedly increasing. Recent studies report increases in incidence between 1.5- and 22-fold over a 4- to 11-year period. This trend is attributed to the following factors: a higher level of awareness of pancreatitis; more intense investigation of symptoms; increased survival of children with complicated systemic illnesses; changes in referral patterns; true increase in incidence; and/ or a combination of these factors. While this disorder may be rare, higher mortality rates in children with pancreatitis are associated with younger age, male gender, chemotherapy, and bone marrow transplantation (Lopez, 2002; Lowe & Greer, 2008; Nydegger et al., 2006; Salvatore et al., 2006; Sanchez-Ramirez et al., 2007; Werlin et al., 2003).

Pancreatitis in adults is predominantly attributable to biliary tract pathology (e.g., gallstones) and alcohol abuse, whereas the etiologies for pancreatitis in pediatric patients are vast and varied. Complications of pancreatitis in adults can be fatal; in contrast, in pediatric patients, fatalities generally are linked to a systemic illness and not pancreatitis alone. Table 26-34 lists the etiologies of acute pancreatitis. Traumatic pancreatitis accounts for approximately 10% to 25% of all cases; another 20% to 35% are classified as idiopathic. More than 200 pharmaceuticals, illicit drugs, and toxins have been associated with pancreatitis, although,

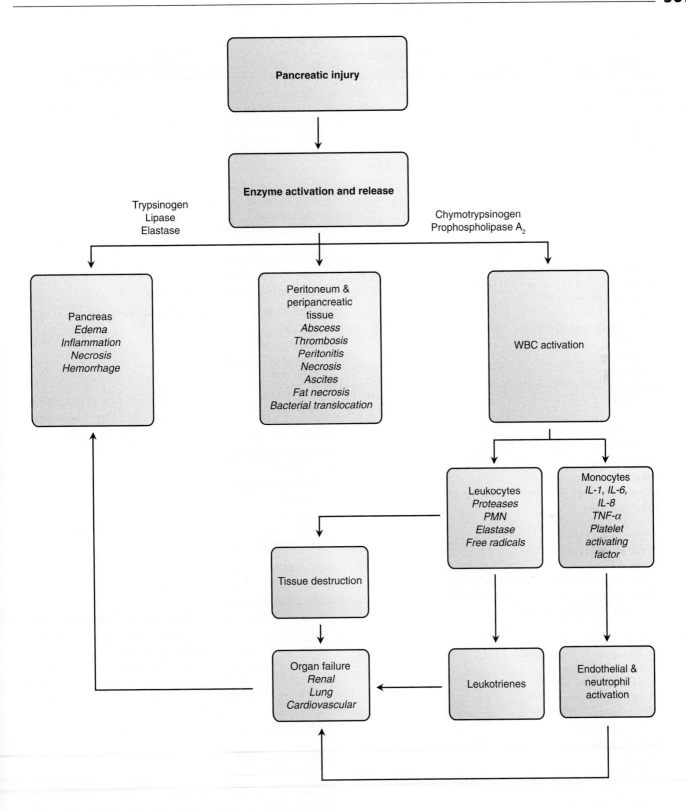

Note: White blood cells (WBC), polymorphonuclear neutrophil (PMN), interleukin (IL), tumor necrosis factor (TNF).

FIGURE 26-21

Pathophysiology of Pancreatitis.

Source: Used with permission. Copyright Elsevier©. Modified from Radhakrishnan, K. & Sutphen, J. (2006). Pancreatitis. In Wyllie, R., Hyams, J. & Kay, M. (Eds.). *Pediatric Gastrointestinal and Liver Disease* (3rd ed., pp. 1043–1062). Philadelphia: Elsevier Saunders.

TABLE 26-34

Etiologies of Acute Pancreatitis

Infectious
- Mycoplasma
- Typhoid fever
- Leptospira
- Verotoxin-producing *E. coli*
- Mumps
- Coxsackie B virus
- Echovirus
- Influenza A and B
- Varicella
- Rubeola
- Rubella
- Hepatitis A and B
- Human immunodeficiency virus (HIV)
- Epstein-Barr virus (EBV)
- Measles
- Cytomegalovirus (CMV)
- Ascariasis
- Malaria
- *Clonarcis sinensis*
- *Cryptosporidium*
- *Varicella*
- *Yersinia*
- *Salmonella*
- Disseminated herpes simplex virus (HSV)

Systemic disease
- Shock, peritonitis, sepsis
- Cerebral vascular accident
- Cerebral palsy
- Anorexia nervosa, bulimia
- Pheochromocytoma
- Fetal alcohol syndrome
- Submersion injury
- Systemic inflammatory response syndrome
- Inflammatory, vasculitis, collagen disorders
  - Henoch-Schönlein purpura
  - Hemolytic uremic syndrome
  - Kawasaki disease
  - Inflammatory bowel disease
  - Reye's syndrome
  - Systemic lupus erythematosus
  - Polyarteritis nodosa
- Transplantation (bone marrow; solid organ)
- Diabetes mellitus

Mechanical/structural
- Trauma
- Duodenal ulcer perforation
- Congenital anomalies
  - Pancreas divisum
  - Choledochal cyst
  - Stenosis of the pancreatic duct or ampulla of Vater
  - Anomalous pancreaticobiliary union
  - Annular pancreas
  - Caroli's disease

TABLE 26-34

Etiologies of Acute Pancreatitis *(Continued)*

- Obstruction
  - Intrinsic obstruction from stones, sludge or stricture
  - Sphincter of Oddi dysfunction
  - Mass effect from tumors or hematoma
  - Enteric duplication cyst
  - Duodenal web

Metabolic
- Hyperlipidemia: types I, IV, and V
- Hypercalcemia
- Hyperparathyroidism
- Kidney disease
- Refeeding syndrome
- Inborn error of metabolism

Drugs and toxins (see Table 26-35)

Post endoscopic retrograde cholangiopancreatography (ECRP)

Malignancy
- Acute lymphoblastic leukemia
- Acute myeloid leukemia
- Brain tumor

Postoperative
- Cardiovascular
- Orthopedic
- Fundoplication

Hereditary pancreatitis
- Trypsinogen gene mutation
- SPINK gene mutation
- Cystic fibrosis

Idiopathic

Source: Nydegger et al., 2006.

valproic acid is the most common agent from these groups (Table 26-35). Etiologies of chronic pancreatitis are summarized in Table 26-36.

In children younger than 3 years of age, acute pancreatitis is most commonly associated with multiple organ disease. Although idiopathic pancreatitis is possible in this age group, it is unlikely. An exhaustive evaluation is recommended in infants and toddlers with pancreatitis of uncertain origin (Kandula & Lowe, 2008; Lopez, 2002; Lowe & Greer, 2008; Pietzak & Thomas, 2000; Radhakrishnan & Sutphen, 2006; Werlin et al., 2003).

PRESENTATION

Symptoms of acute pancreatitis typically include fever, abdominal pain, nausea, vomiting, and anorexia. Of note, signs and symptoms of pancreatitis may often be nonspecific, requiring a high index of suspicion for diagnosis. Uncommon presenting signs and symptoms are back pain, dyspnea, altered level of consciousness, kidney failure, hypotension, ascites, pleural effusions, and fluid retention. In young or nonverbal children, irritability or listlessness

TABLE 26-35

Medications and Toxins Associated with Pancreatitis in Children

Anticoagulants
Calcium
Oncologic agents
- Azathioprine
- 6-Mercaptopurine
- l-Asparaginase
- Cisplatin
- Cytarabine
- Cyclophosphamide
- Methotrexate
Antiepileptic agents
- Valproic acid
- Carbamazepine
- Fosphenytoin
Anti-infectives
- Sulfonamides
- Metronidazole
- Erythromycin
- Nitrofurantoin
- Tetracycline
- Pentamidine
- Isoniazid
- Penicillin
Antihypertensives
- Methyldopa
- Enalapril
- Clonidine
- Procainamide
Diuretics
- Furosemide
- Chlorothiazides

Anti-inflammatory agents
- Mesalamine
- Nonsteroidal anti-inflammatory drugs
- Corticosteroids
- Indomethacin
Hormonal
- Estrogens
Acid blockers
- Cimetidine
- Ranitidine
Pain relievers
- Acetaminophen
- Salicylates
Opiates
Drugs of abuse
- Ethyl alcohol
- Methyl alcohol
- Amphetamines
- Heroin
- Cocaine
Toxins
- Organophosphates
- Spider venom
- Scorpion venom

Sources: Pietzak, & Thomas, 2000; Radhakrishnan & Sutphen, 2006; Werlin et al., 2003.

TABLE 26-36

Etiologies of Chronic Pancreatitis

Congenital ductal anomalies
- Pancreas divisum
- Choledochal cyst
- Stricture
Trauma
- Acquired stricture or other long-standing obstruction
Sclerosing cholangitis
Idiopathic fibrosing cholangitis
Hereditary disorder
- Cystic fibrosis
- Cationic trypsinogen gene mutation
- SPINK-1 mutation
- Possibly other gene mutations yet to be identified
Tropical pancreatitis
Metabolic disorders
- Hyperlipidemias
- Partial lipodystrophy
- Hypercalcemia
- Organic acidemias
Autoimmune disorder
Wilson's disease
Hemochromatosis
Idiopathic

Source: Nydegger et al., 2006.

may serve as a surrogate for verbalization of abdominal pain. If developmentally able, the child may localize abdominal pain to the epigastric or left upper abdominal quadrant and may complain of back pain. The pain and vomiting often worsen after eating (Kandula & Lowe, 2008).

The physical examination may reveal abdominal tenderness upon palpation, diminished bowel sounds, and abdominal distention. The patient may also have jaundice and tachycardia. Cullen's sign (bruising around the umbilicus) and Grey-Turner's sign (flank bruising) may be noted in older children and adults, but are uncommon in young children. These signs indicate intra-abdominal or retroperitoneal bleeding and are most commonly associated with traumatic pancreatitis. Patients with SAP may experience local or systemic complications such as shock, ascites, pleural effusions, and metabolic disturbances (Nydegger et al., 2006; Radhakrishnan & Sutphen, 2006).

Chronic pancreatitis usually results from serial episodes of acute pancreatitis. A history of acute pancreatitis accompanied by abdominal pain is common. Nevertheless, in some patients, chronic abdominal pain (without acute episodes) may be the only manifestation. On rare occasions, these patients may present with diabetes, malabsorption, or obstructive jaundice of unknown etiology (Radhakrishnan & Sutphen, 2006). Physical examination findings replicate those of acute pancreatitis.

DIFFERENTIAL DIAGNOSIS

The signs and symptoms of acute pancreatitis may be vague or nonspecific in a child. Consequently, the HCP must have a high index of suspicion for pancreatitis in the setting of abdominal pain. Viral gastroenteritis is a common misdiagnosis (Lowe & Greer, 2008). Other differential diagnoses to consider include cholecystitis, peptic or duodenal ulcer disease, pneumonia, appendicitis, hepatitis, trauma, and foreign body ingestion. A diagnostic algorithm for identifying pancreatitis is presented in Figure 26-22.

PLAN OF CARE

Amylase and lipase are commonly used biochemical tests in the diagnosis of pancreatitis. Amylase is an enzyme produced in both the salivary glands and the pancreas.

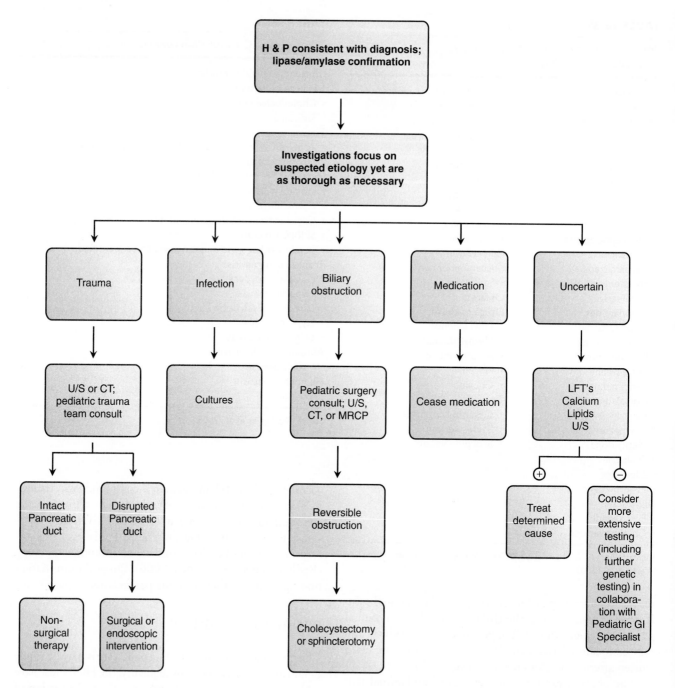

Note: History and physical examination (H & P), ultrasound (US), computed tomography (CT), magnetic resonance cholangiopancreatography (MRCP), liver function tests (LFT's), gastrointestinal (GI).

FIGURE 26-22

A Diagnostic Algorithm for Acute or Recurrent Pancreatitis.

Source: Used with permission. Copyright © Wiley-Blackwell Publishing. Nydegger, A., Couper, R., & Oliver, M. (2006). Childhood pancreatitis. *Journal of Gastroenterology and Hepatology, 21*(3), 499–509.

It converts starch to sugar. Of note, the ovaries, intestines, and skeletal muscles also produce small amounts of amylase; kidney damage or disease may lead to hyperamylasemia due to the kidney's reduced clearance of this enzyme. Consequently, hyperamylasemia is not related to pancreatitis alone. Although fractionation of the enzyme is possible to measure for pancreatic origin, it is uncommonly done and no evidence supports its use over conventional measurement of amylase and lipase in tandem as a means of assessing for pancreatitis (Fischbach, 2004).

Normal values of amylase vary according to the method of testing; check with your laboratory for reference ranges. Serum amylase levels greater than threefold normal levels should prompt consideration of pancreatitis (Nydegger et al., 2006). The sensitivity and specificity of serum amylase, in children, range from 75% to 92% and 20% to 60%, respectively (Pietzak & Thomas, 2000). Most importantly, developmental patterns of expression need to be considered: Amylase levels are very low for the first 2 months of life and most of the activity is of salivary origin and children up to 2 years of age have virtually no pancreatic amylase. Adult levels may not be reached until the later school-age or adolescent years (Fischbach, 2004; Lowe & Greer, 2008). In children with hyperamylasemia but normal lipase and urinary amylase–creatinine clearance ratio, the diagnosis of macroamylasemia should be considered. Macroamylasemia is a benign condition, found in 1% of the population, in which amylase binds to immunoglobulins that are too large to pass through normal glomerular filtration.

Lipase is a glycoprotein that, in the presence of bile salts and colipase, changes fats to fatty acids and glycerol. A threefold increase in serum lipase provides better sensitivity and specificity than amylase in the diagnosis of pancreatitis. Lipase levels remain elevated for 7 to 10 days, whereas amylase levels generally clear more quickly (Fischbach, 2004; Nydegger et al., 2006; Radhakrishnan & Sutphen, 2006).

Age-appropriate values and variances should be considered. Young patients may not be able to express lipase above a diagnostic threshold, yet may still have other evidence of pancreatitis. Some patients may be able to mount a selective elevation of either amylase or lipase at presentation, but not both. For these reasons, obtaining both tests is recommended for pediatric patients with suspected pancreatitis (Lowe & Greer, 2008).

No other tests have proven superior to serum amylase and lipase in the diagnosis of pancreatitis. Severity of pancreatitis in adults has been successfully measured by C-reactive protein (CRP), phospholipase A, trypsinogen activation peptide (TAP), IL-6 and IL-8, trypsinogen 2, SPINK-1, and TNF-α receptor. Hypocalcemia, transient hypoglycemia, hyperbilirubinemia (possibly due to obstruction of pancreatic duct), increased liver function tests, and hypoalbuminemia may also be found in conjunction with pancreatitis (Radhakrishnan & Sutphen, 2006).

Conventional radiography has limited utility in providing diagnostic information. Nevertheless, certain "soft" signs may be seen on radiograph in a patient with pancreatitis, such as a sentinel loop of distended bowel adjacent to the pancreas or calcifications in the pancreas (Radhakrishnan & Sutphen, 2006).

Ultrasound is the imaging study of choice in suspected pancreatitis, as it delineates pancreatic characteristics well (Lowe & Greer, 2008). On ultrasound, acute or chronic pancreatitis may appear as diffuse or local pancreatic enlargement, poorly defined borders, decreased or irregular echogenicity, dilated ducts, or pancreatic pseudocyst. Pseudocysts, phlegmons, and abscesses can be drained via ultrasound-guided technique. In addition to examination of the pancreas, the gallbladder can be evaluated for outflow obstruction due to sludge or stones, which may be an etiology for the pancreatitis. Overlying bowel gas may obscure the view of the pancreas and should prompt repeat ultrasound or other imaging. Additionally, although not rigorously studied in children, endoscopic ultrasound allows a highly detailed study of the pancreatic duct and parenchyma (Lowe & Greer; Nydegger et al., 2006; Radhakrishnan & Sutphen, 2006; Stringer, 2005).

Computed tomography of the abdomen offers more detail than ultrasound. To enhance compliance (thereby improving study quality) and reduce fear associated with CT scanning, sedation should be considered in any patient younger than 8 years of age. In pancreatitis, findings on contrast-enhanced CT may include enlargement of the pancreas, hemorrhage, necrosis, details of traumatic injury, or pseudocyst. As with ultrasound, interventions such as abscess, phlegmon, or pseudocyst drainage can be guided by CT. Abdominal CT should be considered when ultrasound study is inadequate, the patient is having a difficult or prolonged course of disease, or the diagnosis is ambiguous (Lowe & Greer, 2008; Radhakrishnan & Sutphen, 2006).

Magnetic resonance cholangiopancreatography (MRCP) is a noninvasive study that helps in diagnosis of congenital or acquired structural abnormalities. This technique also avoids the use of ionizing radiation. As with CT, sedation should be considered in young children undergoing this imaging study. MRCP does not reveal the details of small, peripheral ducts well; thus it may not identify early phases of chronic pancreatitis (Lowe & Greer, 2008; Nydegger et al., 2006; Radhakrishnan & Sutphen, 2006).

Endoscopic retrograde cholangiopancreatography (ERCP) is an invasive procedure that is used to visualize anatomy, perform manometry of the sphincter of Oddi, and perform therapeutic maneuvers when indicated (i.e., gallstone extraction, sphincterotomy). Sedation is required for any patient undergoing this procedure. Because ERCP may exacerbate inflammation, its use should be avoided during an acute attack of pancreatitis (Stringer, 2005).

Grading systems for pancreatitis based on ERCP results have been used for adults, but a corresponding system for pediatric patients has not yet been defined. There is a 5% complication rate from ERCP in children, with potential problems including pancreatitis, cholangitis, pain, perforation, ileus, and fever (Radhakrishnan & Sutphen, 2006).

The mainstay of treatment for mild acute pancreatitis is supportive in nature: intravenous fluid resuscitation, pain management, management of metabolic complications, pancreatic rest, and monitoring for complications. Generous fluid resuscitation may prevent pancreatic microcirculation and systemic hypovolemia. There is no role for prophylactic antibiotics in mild disease. Likewise, nasogastric decompression is rarely needed unless the patient develops severe nausea or vomiting or there is concern for aspiration in association with a paralytic ileus.

Pancreatitis can cause significant abdominal and back pain. Analgesia may be accomplished with fentanyl. Meperidine is used for pain relief in some centers, but this agent is not an opioid of choice due to the accumulation of normeperidine and its adverse effects (Taketomo et al., 2010). Morphine is controversial for this indication because it may increase sphincter of Oddi pressure (Radhakrishnan & Sutphen, 2006). A patient-controlled analgesia (PCA) pump may be considered.

Traditional wisdom implies no enteral feeding proximal to the jejunum; however, more recent studies suggest enteral feedings may be safe and improve survival outcomes (Ioannidis et al., 2008). Jejunal or more distal feedings result in negligible increases in enzyme, bicarbonate, and volume output from the pancreas, allowing the pancreas to rest. Nasojejunal or parenteral nutrition are options in pancreatitis, with nasojejunal feedings having clear advantages in adult patients—namely, fewer infections, less likelihood of surgical intervention, and decreased length of hospital stay (Marik & Zaloga, 2004). No evidence exists on when to restart oral feedings; recommendations include restarting them when pain and vomiting have subsided and enzyme levels are declining (Lowe & Greer, 2008; Radhakrishnan & Sutphen, 2006). Some centers use low-fat diets in patients with recent pancreatitis, although there is no evidence to support this therapy.

Treatment of SAP includes monitoring for and addressing complications while providing supportive care—intravenous fluid resuscitation, pain management, management of metabolic complications, and pancreatic rest. Admission to a tertiary children's hospital and possibly a pediatric critical care unit should be considered. Local pancreatic problems such as sepsis, pulmonary complications, acute kidney failure, and metabolic alterations (hyperglycemia, acidosis, hypocalcemia) are some possible complications that may require treatment. As with therapy for mild, acute pancreatitis, nasogastric decompression is indicated if the patient develops severe nausea or vomiting or there is concern for aspiration in association with paralytic ileus. Pain may be significant and should be managed accordingly.

Severe acute pancreatitis does not preclude enteral feedings. Nasojejunal feedings are superior to parenteral nutrition and can be used safely in these patients. Evidence and considerations in advancing feedings are as previously described for treatment of mild acute pancreatitis.

No evidence exists regarding the use of prophylactic antibiotics in pediatric patients with severe acute pancreatitis. In a consensus statement published by the Society for Critical Care Medicine regarding severe acute pancreatitis in adults, the use of routine prophylactic systemic antibacterial or antifungal agents in patients with necrotizing pancreatitis was not recommended (Nathens et al., 2004). Nevertheless, several pediatric authors contend that prophylaxis may play a role in younger patients. Prophylactic broad-spectrum antibiotics when pancreatic necrosis is present or infection is suspected or known is recommended (Nydegger et al., 2006; Radhakrishnan & Sutphen, 2006; Stringer, 2005). To date, additional therapies such as medications to suppress pancreatic secretion (glucagons, somatostatins, octreotide), antiproteases, and antioxidants have not proven to confer significant benefits in the reduction of severe acute pancreatitis.

The mainstays of treatment of chronic pancreatitis are medical. If possible, the offending agent should be removed or the etiology reversed. Ensure that all investigations for a root cause have been exhausted. Medical treatment includes pain management, nutritional support, and occasionally islet cell autotransplantation. The last technique involves resection of the pancreas, with islet cells then being reinfused into the patient's liver. Flare-ups should be treated in the same approach as acute pancreatitis. Pain may significantly affect the patient's quality of life. Nevertheless, in late-stage chronic pancreatitis, pain is often negligible because the gland has "burned out." A chronic pain management team consultation is valuable in determining and managing the pain relief regimen. Pain associated with eating may be mitigated by the addition of pancreatic enzyme supplementation to the patient's diet (Nydegger et al., 2006; Radhakrishnan & Sutphen, 2006).

Nutritional support is important to prevent malnutrition and maintain growth. Nasojejunal feeding can offer adequate caloric support while minimizing pancreatic stimulation. Enteral feeding should be continued until the patient is able to tolerate oral feedings (as evidenced by no pain or vomiting). Fecal fat loss estimation and fluid and electrolyte replacement may be required. As well as providing a high-caloric diet with adequate protein and fat supplementation, HCPs should ensure that multivitamins (especially fat-soluble vitamins) are carefully added to the patient's diet. Antioxidant therapy may be beneficial in certain subgroups (Nydegger et al., 2006).

Besides pain, malnourishment, and hormone dysfunction, other chronic or recurrent problems may occur with chronic pancreatitis. Diabetes mellitus may be seen in as many as 25% of patients with long-standing chronic pancreatitis (Radhakrishnan & Sutphen, 2006). Conversely, because chronic pancreatitis involves decreased glucagon secretion, it may result in hypoglycemic episodes.

Surgical options depend on the etiology of pancreatitis. Surgical intervention is uncommon in nontraumatic acute pancreatitis in the pediatric population. However, once the acute episode has resolved, correction of an underlying lesion may be necessary to prevent recurrence. Surgical intervention for acute pancreatitis is limited to the following procedures:

- Cholecystectomy or cholecystostomy for biliary stone disease
- Choledochal cyst excision
- Pseudocyst drainage or excision
- Sphincterotomy for pancreatic divisum
- Debridement for severe necrotizing pancreatitis (Stringer, 2005)

For most patients, surgery is delayed until the acute event has passed. With infected pancreatic necrosis, early surgery is associated with a high mortality in adults, thus supporting the implementation of early antimicrobial therapy with surgical intervention to follow.

In chronic pancreatitis, surgery can be useful in some circumstances, although it is considered only after medical management has failed. For a dilated main pancreatic duct, the following procedures may be considered:

- Lateral longitudinal pancreaticojejunostomy (modified Puestow procedure)
- Distal pancreatectomy with caudal Roux-en-Y pancreaticojejunostomy (DuVal procedure)
- Longitudinal pancreaticojejunostomy with anterior resection of the pancreatic head (Frey procedure)

A partial pancreatectomy or ductal stent may be used to treat unremitting symptoms of chronic pancreatitis. An anomaly such as pancreas divisum may be surgically treated by transduodenal sphincteroplasty, endoscopic sphincterotomy, or longitudinal pancreaticojejunostomy (Stringer, 2005).

Complications of acute and chronic pancreatitis can be local, be systemic, or affect only certain organs (Table 26-37). A pseudocyst is one of the more commonly seen complications. Such cysts may present with pain, nausea, vomiting, or jaundice after an episode of pancreatitis or the patient may be asymptomatic. If the patient is asymptomatic, close follow-up is required to monitor for associated risks such as infection, hemorrhage, and rupture of the pseudocyst.

The patient (if developmentally able) and caregivers should be educated on the definition, etiology, and pathophysiology of pancreatitis. The therapeutic management plan should be explained and mutually agreed upon. Expectations of outcomes, possible complications, and long-term considerations should be clearly delineated, with

TABLE 26-37

Complications of Acute and Chronic Pancreatitis

Local

Pseudocyst
Abscess
Necrosis
Pancreatic ductal strictures or fibrosis
Pancreatic calculi, fistula
Hemorrhage
Adenocarcinoma

Systemic

Multiple organ dysfunction
Thrombosis

Cardiovascular

Shock
Fluid loss/sequestration
Bleeding
Pericarditis
Pericardial effusion
Myocardial depression

Respiratory

Pleural effusion
Acute respiratory distress syndrome

Renal

Acute kidney failure
Hypovolemia
Shock
Renal vessel thrombosis

Hematologic

Disseminated intravascular coagulation
Hemolysis
Thrombocytopenia

Metabolic

Exocrine insufficiency
Hypocalcemia
Acidosis
Hyperlipidemia
Hyperkalemia
Hyperglycemia/hypoglycemia
Diabetes mellitus

Gastrointestinal

Jaundice
Ileus
Ascites
Hemorrhage
Stress ulcers
Obstruction (biliary or bowel)

(Continued)

TABLE 26-37

**Complications of Acute and Chronic Pancreatitis
(Continued)**

Gastrointestinal

Bowel infarction
Hepatic or portal vein thrombosis
Hepatorenal syndrome
Splenic hematoma

Neurological

Decreased mental status
Encephalopathy

Sources: Nydegger et al., 2006; Pietzak & Thomas, 2000;
Radhakrishnan & Sutphen, 2006.

written information being provided for the family to review. While the patient remains hospitalized, the plan should be reviewed daily with the patient and family. Patients should be advised to avoid smoking and alcohol, as practices these may lead to exacerbation of the pancreatitis (Nydegger et al., 2006).

DISPOSITION AND DISCHARGE PLANNING

Counsel the patient and family about how to recognize symptoms of reoccurrence and when to seek medical care (increasing abdominal pain, nausea, vomiting, anorexia, and back pain). In nonverbal patients, families should seek medical care for surrogate signs of illness such as irritability or listlessness. Follow-up with the primary care provider, gastroenterology, or surgery teams may be necessary. An interim history, physical examination, and repeat diagnostic study will be necessary to ensure resolution of the pancreatitis.

SUPERIOR MESENTERIC ARTERY SYNDROME

Pamela Ruppel

PATHOPHYSIOLOGY

The superior mesenteric artery (SMA) normally branches off the aorta at an acute angle, travels in the root of the mesentery, and crosses over the duodenum usually just to the right of midline. In SMA syndrome (SMAS), the artery obstructs the duodenum as it crosses over it, leading to dilatation of the proximal duodenum and stomach. The third or transverse portion of the duodenum is the most immobile portion of the GI tract. It lies between the SMA anteriorly and the aorta and spine posteriorly, and is held in a fixed position by the ligament of Treitz. The angle between the SMA and the aorta has been calculated

at between 25 and 60 degrees but can be greatly reduced in SMAS (Waseem & Salvatore, 2004).

EPIDEMIOLOGY AND ETIOLOGY

Superior mesenteric artery syndrome (also known as Wilkie syndrome) is a rare condition. Its precise incidence is unknown, and the syndrome is diagnosed in less than 0.3% of upper GI barium studies. SMAS affects females more commonly than males. Any condition that decreases the angle between the aorta and the SMA predisposes the affected individual to compression of the portion of the duodenum that lies between these two vessels. Many of these conditions are associated with rapid weight loss. Spinal fusion surgery for scoliosis and anorexia nervosa are two such predisposing conditions. In spinal surgery, the angle is acutely changed with the repositioning of the spine and there is often an accompanying rapid weight loss following the procedure. In anorexia nervosa, SAMS may occur due to the induced weight loss and change in distribution of fat. This syndrome may also occur in conjunction with cancer treatment and associated weight loss, pancreatitis, peptic ulcer, bariatric surgery, and various other intra-abdominal inflammatory conditions.

Patients with neurologic injury may be prone to developing SMAS. Individuals with spastic syndromes such as cerebral palsy, quadriplegics, and paraplegics are considered to be at higher risk for this condition due to hyperextension of the spine with increased lumbar lordosis, prolonged supine positioning, or increasing flaccidity of abdominal musculature even with the absence of significant weight loss (Biank & Werlin, 2006).

PRESENTATION

The classic symptoms of SMAS are epigastric fullness and bloating after meals, bilious vomiting, and midabdominal pain that may be relieved by the prone or knee–chest position. This initial history is usually nonspecific and intermittent, with increasing frequency of symptoms being noted over time. Patients themselves may alter their eating habits to relieve their symptoms by eating smaller meals and mostly liquids. They may develop a fear of eating that may lead to weight loss and a resultant worsening of symptoms. A delay in diagnosis is common (Smith et al., 2009). Fluid and electrolyte losses can be significant, and bilious vomiting predisposes a patient to acidosis and dehydration.

DIFFERENTIAL DIAGNOSIS

SMAS with consequent megaduodenum must be differentiated from other disorders that may cause similar duodenal dilatation, including myotonic dystrophy, systemic lupus erythematosus, scleroderma, myxedema, amyloidosis, and chronic idiopathic intestinal pseudo-obstruction (Waseem & Salvatore, 2004).

PLAN OF CARE

The diagnosis of SMAS can be made with an upper GI barium study. An abdominal radiograph of the kidneys, ureters, and bladder (KUB) may reveal a dilatation in the small bowel but is not diagnostic of the syndrome. A contrast-enhanced spiral CT scan allows visualization of the vascular compression of the duodenum and excludes other pathologic conditions. It is useful in evaluation of intra-abdominal and retroperitoneal fat. Magnetic resonance angiography (MRA) is equivalent to CT scanning in evaluating the exact angle between the SMA and the aorta; this imaging technique does not expose the patient to radiation and may soon become the gold standard for diagnosis of SMAS (Lippl et al., 2002). Endoscopy is of minor diagnostic value, as patients are generally NPO prior to endoscopy and may not have the characteristic liquid stasis of duodenal contents present (Lippl et al.). The upper GI series reveals characteristic dilatation of the first and second portions of the duodenum. There is abrupt compression of the duodenal mucosal folds, a back-and-forth movement of barium proximal to the obstruction site, and a delay in gastroduodenal transit of 4 to 6 hours. In addition, an abrupt cutoff of contrast material at the third portion of the duodenum is usually observed (Waseem & Salvatore, 2004).

Therapeutic management for SMAS varies; optimal management requires reversal of the causative factor when possible. Initial care involves decompression with a nasogastric tube, intravenous fluids, and electrolyte replacement. Conservative treatment focuses on bypassing the area of obstruction with a jejunostomy tube and providing enteral feedings until weight is gained, the angle between the aorta and SMA is increased, and the obstruction and retroperistalsis resolve. Prokinetic medications such as metoclopramide have been used with some success in this disorder. Positioning of the patient on the left side or in the knee–chest position after meals often helps relieve symptoms. A liquid diet is initially indicated if feeding by mouth is preferred and generally small, frequent high-calorie supplements are recommended. Solid food is introduced after the patient has transitioned to a full liquid, then soft food diet. Parenteral nutrition may be used to halt weight loss and malnutrition associated with the syndrome if the patient is unable to tolerate an enteral diet.

Surgical treatment is recommended if conservative treatment fails, or if preferred by the patient. Although several surgical techniques may be used to relieve obstruction, the most commonly employed approach is the transposition of the third part of the duodenum anteriorly to the SMA (Waseem & Salvatore, 2004). Duodenojejunostomy, gastrojejunostomy, and resection (or lysis) of the ligament of Treitz are other surgical methods for relieving the profound dilatation and stasis of the proximal small bowel (Biank & Werlin, 2006).

Consultations with various subspecialties promote a comprehensive therapeutic management and are best provided by an interprofessional team that includes consultants from gastroenterology, surgery, nutrition, and psychology. If long-term hospitalization is required, child life specialists and a rehabilitative team may become involved in the patient's illness management.

Patients and family education involves discussion of therapies and nutritional support. Treatment plans must also include consideration of the psychological aspects of the syndrome. If acute weight loss is associated with an eating disorder, this problem must be managed as well as the syndrome (Merrett et al., 2009). SMAS is a chronic problem, often with a delayed diagnosis; consequently, patients are prone to developing anxiety and depression. Some patients even become anxious with a return to a normal diet after resolution of SMAS.

DISPOSITION AND DISCHARGE PLANNING

The expected outcome of SMAS is excellent (Biank & Werlin, 2006). With increase in patient weight and fat distribution through high-calorie feedings, resolution of compression of the proximal duodenum is usually successful. Surgical therapy is curative but reserved for those patients who cannot be managed medically.

Recurrence of SMAS is rare, but should be suspected in patients with resolution of SMAS who later redevelop symptoms. Chronic idiopathic pseudo-obstruction, gastroparesis, and other diseases that result in hypoactive gut motility cannot be ruled out without a thorough evaluation. Radiographic studies should be repeated on patients with recurrence of symptoms. Patients with anorexia nervosa and bulimia nervosa must be monitored closely by medical and psychological specialists to prevent recurrence of disease states and complications related to this disorder. Those individuals who have neurological injury and recurrent SMAS often require surgical correction (Biank & Werlin, 2006).

TYPHLITIS

Riza V. Mauricio

PATHOPHYSIOLOGY

Typhlitis has been known by many terms, including necrotizing colitis, neutropenic colitis, and ileocecal syndrome. Common findings are inflammation of the ascending colon, terminal ileum, and cecum. Most pathology originates in the cecum; thus, the term typhlitis which is derived from the Greek word *typhlon*, meaning "cecum." In this condition, mucosal wall injury from cytotoxic therapy and intramural infection leads to mucosal wall thickening, ischemia, ulceration, hemorrhage, and ultimately perforation (Abu-Hilal & Jones, 2008; Hobson et al., 2005; King, 2002; Mullassery et al., 2009; Schlatter et al., 2002).

EPIDEMIOLOGY AND ETIOLOGY

Typhlitis is a life-threatening disorder. Although its exact incidence is unknown, in a 1990 postmortem review of 191 leukemic children the rate was found to be 10%. In this investigation, other associated comorbidities were lymphoblastic lymphoma (relapse), induction chemotherapy, bone marrow hypoplasia (secondary to chemotherapy), and aplastic anemia.

In another study the overall incidence rate of typhlitis in children with cancer was 5%. Seventy-six percent of the affected patients were being treated for hematologic malignancies. Typhlitis was reported in15% of all patients with Burkitt's lymphoma, 12% with acute myeloblastic leukemia, and 5% with acute lymphocytic leukemia. Profound neutropenia in the presence of impaired immune function secondary to cytotoxic therapy for malignancy was the most common predisposing condition.

Coinfection has been reported with bacterial, fungal, or viral agents and is often polymicrobial, though, *Clostridium septicum* is the most frequently identified pathogen (Abu-Hilal & Jones, 2008; Hobson et al., 2005; Katz et al., 1990; King, 2002; King et al., 1984; Moran et al., 2009; Schlatter et al., 2002).

PRESENTATION

Historically, patients with typhlitis have often received a cytotoxic agent or stem cell transplant, or experienced mucositis in the previous 2 weeks. During the same period, they commonly develop profound neutropenia and granulocytopenia. The classic triad of symptoms for typhlitis is fever, right lower quadrant pain, and vomiting. Abdominal pain may be described as diffuse or periumbilical, confounding the diagnosis. Other signs and symptoms that have been reported include watery or bloody diarrhea, abdominal distention, and poor appetite (Hobson et al., 2005; Katz et al., 1990; Mullassery et al., 2009; Schlatter et al., 2002).

The findings during physical examination vary depending on the severity of disease. Tenderness on palpation to the right lower quadrant and absent bowel sounds are common. Tympany during percussion, mass palpated at the right lower quadrant, peritoneal signs (guarding, abdominal wall rigidity, rebound tenderness), diffuse abdominal and periumbilical tenderness, and hypotension have all been reported (Abu-Hilal & Jones, 2008; Haut, 2008; Hobson et al., 2005; King, 2002; Lee et al., 2008; Mullassery et al., 2009; Schlatter et al., 2002).

DIFFERENTIAL DIAGNOSIS

Conditions that may mimic typhlitis include: acute appendicitis, pseudomembranous colitis, ischemic colitis, obstructive ileus, and bowel obstruction.

PLAN OF CARE

Survival depends on early suspicion in at-risk pediatric patients. Beyond a platelet count, there are no diagnostic laboratory studies for typhlitis. Nevertheless, tests supportive to care should be obtained, such as complete blood counts and coagulation panels. Blood and stool cultures to identify coinfection should be obtained, although they are positive in fewer than 25% of patients. An association between typhlitis and hypokalemia, hyperbilirubinemia, and hypoalbuminemia has been reported. It has been postulated that these imbalances may be related to comorbidities such as loss of protein and electrolytes in the stool, inadequate oral intake, and kidney insufficiency. Moran et al. (2009) report that absolute levels of hypokalemia and hypoalbuminemia are not helpful to define disease severity; however, a rise over time is associated with disease progression.

Plain abdominal radiographs are highly sensitive to the presence of typhlitis. Computed tomography and ultrasound are also used as imaging modalities in patients, but do not have greater sensitivity than radiography. They may prove useful, however, for serial evaluation of comorbidities such as abscess formation. At diagnosis, the CT scan of the abdomen and pelvis may show circumferential thickening of the cecum with edema and inflammation of the adjacent mesenteric fat. The ultrasound may identify absent peristalsis of the right lower quadrant, thickened hypoechoic bowel walls, fluid around bowel loops, free fluid in the pelvis, or bowel wall air (Abu-Hilal & Jones, 2008; Hobson et al., 2005; Moran et al., 2009; Schlatter et al., 2002).

The majority of patients with typhlitis can be managed successfully with supportive care consisting of bowel rest, abdominal decompression, broad-spectrum antimicrobial therapy, granulocyte colony-stimulating factor (GCSF), intravenous fluids for hydration, parenteral nutrition, and pain management (Hobson et al., 2005; Mullassery et al., 2009). Surgery is indicated when the patient has persistent bleeding, bowel perforation, or clinical deterioration suggesting bowel necrosis.

Patients with typhlitis frequently receive care from hematology/oncology specialists. Additional specialist support from infectious diseases, pediatric surgery, nutrition, pain service, and critical care services may be useful depending on the severity of the disease at presentation.

Patient and family teaching regarding the etiology of the disease, its morbidity and mortality if untreated, and the disease trajectory will be useful to enhance their understanding of the need for prolonged hospitalization and supportive management. Child life services and spiritual support may be valuable for family coping.

DISPOSITION AND DISCHARGE PLANNING

In the 1980s, mortality from typhlitis was reported to be as high as 50% to 100%. More recently, due to early recognition and supportive management, survival has been reported to be 100%. Moran et al. (2009) report a mean hospitalization length of stay for typhlitis of 17 days, ranging from 16 days for patients with mild disease to 33 days for patients with severe disease. Continuation of care at home may be considered with demonstration of bowel and immune function recovery (Abu-Hilal & Jones, 2008; Avci et al., 2008; Moran et al., 2009; Shamberger et al., 1986).

> **Critical Thinking**
> Fever, vomiting, and right lower quadrant abdominal pain in a patient with neutropenia are suggestive of typhlitis.

REFERENCES

1. Abad-Sinden, A., & Sutphen, J. (2003). Nutritional management of the pediatric short bowel syndrome. *Practical Gastroenterology, 27*(12), 28–46.

2. Abi-Hanna, A., & Lake, A. (1998). Constipation and encopresis in childhood. *Pediatrics in Review, 19*, 1–23.

3. Abu-Hilal, M., & Jones, J. (2008). Typhlitis: Is it in immunocompromised patients? *Medical Science Monitor, 14*(8), CS67–CS70.

4. Adëback, P., Nemeth, A., & Fischler, B. (2003). Cognitive and emotional outcome after pediatric liver transplantation. *Pediatric Transplantation, 7*, 385–389.

5. Agency for Healthcare Research and Quality (AHRQ). (2004). *Preventable hospitalizations: A window into primary and preventive care, 2000.* HCUP Fact Book No. 5. AHRQ Publication No. 04-0056.

6. A-Kader, H. H., & Ghishan, F. K. (2006). Abnormalities of hepatic protein metabolism. In R. Wyllie & J. S. Hyams (Eds.), *Pediatric gastrointestinal and liver disease* (pp. 899–902). Netherlands: Saunders.

7. Alhashimi, D., Al-Hashimi, H., & Fedorowicz, Z. (2009). Antiemetics for reducing vomiting related to acute gastroenteritis in children and adolescents. *Cochrane Database of Systematic Reviews, 2.* Art.No. CD005506. doi: 10.1002/14651858.CD005506.pub4

8. Allen, S., Ignacio, R., Falcome, R., Alonso, M., Brown, R., Garcia, V., et al. (2006). The effect of a right-sided aortic arch on outcome in children with esophageal atresia and tracheoesophageal fistula. *Journal of Pediatric Surgery, 41*(3), 479–483.

9. American Academy of Pediatrics (AAP). (2004). Statement of endorsement: Managing acute gastroenteritis among children: oral rehydration, maintenance, and nutritional therapy. *Pediatrics, 11*, 507.

10. American Academy of Pediatrics (AAP), Subcommittee on Hyperbilirubinemia. (2004). Clinical practice guideline: Management of hyperbilirubinemia in the newborn infant 35 or more weeks of gestation. *Pediatrics, 114*, 297–316.

11. American Academy of Pediatrics (AAP). (2009a). Section 2: Recommendations for care of children in special circumstances. In L. Pickering, C. Baker, D. Kimberlin, & S. Long (Eds.), *Red book: 2009 report of the Committee on Infectious Diseases* (28th ed., pp. 105– 162). Elk Grove Village, IL: Author.

12. American Academy of Pediatrics (AAP), Committee of Infectious Diseases. (2009b). Prevention of rotavirus disease: Updated guidelines for use of rotavirus vaccine. *Pediatrics, 123*, 1412–1420.

13. American Gastroenterological Association (AGA). (2003). Medical position statement: Short bowel syndrome and intestinal transplantation. *Gastroenterology, 124*, 1105–1110.

14. American Pediatric Surgical Association. (2009). Retrieved from http://www.eapsa.org/AM/Template.cfm?Section=Resources& CONTENTID=1567&TEMPLATE=/CM/ContentDisplay.cfm

15. Applebaum, H., Lee, S., & Paupong, D. (2006). Duodenal atresia and stenosis-annular pancreas. In J. Grosfeld, J. O'Neill, E. Fonkalsrud, & A. Coran (Eds.), *Pediatric surgery* (6th ed., Vol. 2, pp. 1260–1276). Philadelphia, PA: Mosby.

16. Applegate, K., Anderson, J., & Klatte, E. (2006). Intestinal malrotation in children: A problem-solving approach the upper gastrointestinal series. *Radiographics, 26*(5), 1485–1500.

17. Aspelund, G., & Langer, J. (2007). Current management of hypertrophic pyloric stenosis. *Seminars in Pediatric Surgery, 16*, 27–33.

18. Avci, Z., Alioglu, B., Anuk, D., Yilmaz Ozbek, O., Azap, O. K., & Ozbek, N. (2008). Double invasive fungal infections and typhlitis in children with acute lymphoblastic leukemia. *Pediatric Hematology and Oncology, 25*, 99–106.

19. Bailey, K., Wales, P., & Gerstle, J. (2007). Laparoscopic versus open reduction of intussusception in children: A single-institution comparative experience. *Journal of Pediatric Surgery, 42*, 845–848.

20. Baker, S., Liptak, G., Colletti, R., Croffie, J., DiLorenzo, C., Ector, W., et al. (2006). Evaluation and treatment of constipation in infants and children: Recommendations of North American Society for Pediatric Gastroenterology, Hepatology and Nutrition. *Journal of Pediatric Gastroenterology, 43*(3), e1–e13.

21. Baliga, P., Alvarez, S., Lindblad, A., Zeng, L., & SPLIT (2004). Posttransplant survival in pediatric fulminant hepatic failure: The SPLIT experience. *Liver Transplantation, 10*(11), 1364–1371.

22. Balistreri, W., Bezerra, J., & Ryckman, F. (2007). Biliary atresia and other disorders of the extrahepatic bile duct. In F. Suchy, R. Sokol, & W. Balistreri. (Eds.), *Liver disease in children* (3rd ed. pp. 247–269). New York: Cambridge University Press.

23. Barnes, G., & Townley, R. (1973). Duodenal mucosal damage in 31 infants with gastroenteritis. *Archives of Disease in Childhood, 48*, 343.

24. Barshes, N., Chang, I., Karpen, S., Carter, B., & Goss, J. (2006). Impact of pretransplant growth retardation in pediatric liver transplant. *Journal of Pediatric Gastroenterology Nutrition, 43*, 89–94.

25. Bassett, M. D., & Murray, K. F. (2008). Biliary atresia: Recent progress. *Journal of Clinical Gastroenterology, 42*, 720–729.

26. Beasley, S. (2005). Esophageal atresia and tracheoesophageal fistula. In K. Oldham, P. Colombani, R. Foglia, & M. Skinner (Eds.), *Principles and practice of pediatric surgery* (Vol.2, pp. 1039–1052). Philadelphia, PA: Lippincott Williams & Wilkins.

27. Bekker, J., Ploem, S., & de Jong, K. (2009). Early hepatic artery thrombosis after liver transplantation: A systematic review of the incidence, outcome and risk factors. *American Journal of Transplantation, 9*, 746–757.

28. Berg, C., Steffick, D., Edwards, E., Heimbach, J., Magee, J., Washburn, W., et al. (2009). Liver and intestine transplantation in the United States 1998–2007. *American Journal of Transplantation, 9*(Pt 2), 907–932.

29. Bhutta, Z. (2007). Acute gastroenteritis in children. In R. Kliegman, R. Behrman, H. Jenson, & B. Stanton (Eds.), *Nelson textbook of pediatrics* (18th ed., pp. 1605–1621) Philadelphia, PA: Saunders/Elsevier.

30. Biank, V., & Werlin, S. (2006). Superior mesenteric artery syndrome in children: A 20-year experience. *Journal of Pediatric Gastroenterology and Nutrition, 42*, 522–525.

31. Bickell, N., Aufses, A., Rojas, M., & Bodian, C. (2006). How time affects the risk of rupture in appendicitis. *Journal of the American College of Surgeons, 202*(3), 401–406.

32. Bitterman, R., & Zich, D. (2006). Acute gastroenteritis. In J. Marx, R. Hockberger, & R. Walls (Eds.), *Rosen's emergency medicine: Concepts and clinical practice* (6th ed., Vol. 2, pp. 1460–1490). Philadelphia, PA: Mosby/Elsevier.

33. Blackburn, S. (2007). *Maternal, fetal, and neonatal physiology: A clinical perspective.* St. Louis: Saunders.

34. Bond, L. R., Hatty, S. R., Horn, M. E. C., Dick, M., Meire, H. B., & Bellingham, A. J. (1987). Gallstones in sickle cell disease in the United Kingdom. *British Medical Journal, 295*, 234–236.

35. Borowitz, S., Cox, D., Sheen, J., & Sutphen, J. (2005). Treatment of childhood constipation by primary care physicians: Efficacy and predictors of outcomes. *Pediatrics, 115*, 873–877.

36. Bradshaw, W. (2009). Necrotizing enterocolitis: Etiology, presentation, management and outcomes. *Journal of Perinatal Neonatal Nursing, 23*(1), 87–94.

37. Bucuvalas, J., & Alonso, E. (2008.) Long-term outcomes after liver transplantation in children. *Current Opinion in Organ Transplant, 13*, 247–251.

38. Bucuvalas, J., Alonso, E., Magee, J., Talwalker, J., Hanto, D., & Doo, E. (2008). Improving long-term outcomes after liver transplantation in children. *American Journal of Transplantation, 8*, 2506–2513.

39. Bundy, D., Byerley, J., Liles, E., Perrin E., Katznelson, J., & Rise, H. (2007). Does this child have appendicitis? *Journal of the American Medical Association, 298*(4), 438–451.

40. Byrne, A., Goeghegan, T., Govender, P., Lyburn, I., Colhoun, E., & Torreggiani, W. (2005). The imaging of intussusception. *Clinical Radiology, 60*, 39–46.

41. Campbell, A., & Herold, B. (2004). Strategies for the prevention of cytomegalovirus infection and disease in pediatric liver transplantation recipients. *Pediatric Transplantation, 8*, 619–627.

42. Campbell, K., Yazigi, N., Ryckman, F., Alonso, M., Tiao, G., Balistreri, W., et al. (2006). High prevalence of renal dysfunction in long-term survivors after pediatric liver transplantation. *Journal of Pediatrics, 148*, 475–80.

43. Centers for Disease Control and Prevention (CDC). (2003). Managing acute gastroenteritis among children: Oral rehydration, maintenance, and nutritional therapy. *Morbidity and Mortality Weekly Report, 52* (No. RR-16), 1–16.

44. Centers for Disease Control and Prevention (CDC). (2009). Prevention of rotavirus gastroenteritis among infants and children: Recommendations of the Advisory Committee on Immunization Practices (ACIP). *Morbidity and Mortality Weekly Report, 58* (No. RR-2), 1–25.

45. Chang, C., & Shiano, T. (2007), Review article: Drug hepatotoxicity. *Alimentary Pharmacology and Therapeutics, 25*, 1135–1151.

46. Chang, Y., Kong, M., Hsia, S., Wu, C., Lai, M., Yan, D., et al. (2007). Usefulness of ultrasonography in acute appendicitis in early childhood. *Journal of Pediatric Gastroenterology and Nutrition, 44*(5), 592–595.

47. Chardot, C. (2006). Biliary atresia. *Orphanet Journal of Rare Diseases, 1*(28). doi: 10.1186/1750-1172-1-28.

48. Chen, X., Milkovich, S., Stool, D., van As, A., Reilly, J., & Rider, G. (2006). Pediatric coin ingestion and aspiration. *International Journal of Pediatric Otorhinolaryngology, 70*, 325–329.

49. Chua, J., Chui, C., & Jacobsen, A. S. (2006). Role of surgery in the era of highly successful air enema reduction of intussusception. *Asian Journal of Surgery, 29*, 267–273.

50. Chung, E. (2008). Infantile hypertrophic pyloric stensosis: Genes and environment. *Archives of Disease in Childhood, 93*, 1003–1004.

51. Ciocca, M., Ramonet, M., Cuarterolo, M., Lopez, S., Cernadas, C., & Alvarez, F. (2008). Prognostic factors in paediatric acute liver failure. *Archives of Disease in Childhood, 93*, 48–51.

52. Cochran, J., & Losek, J. (2007). Acute liver failure in children. *Pediatric Emergency Care, 23*(2), 129–135.

53. Coliste, A., Lucia, O., Cozzi, D., Briganti, V., Morini, F., Spagnol, L., et al. (2008). Prenatal diagnosis of duodenal obstruction selects cases with a higher risk of maternal–foetal complications and demands in utero transfer to a tertiary centre. *Fetal Diagnosis and Therapy, 24*(4), 478–482.

54. Colomb, V., & Goulet, O. (2009). Nutrition support after intestinal transplantation: How important is enteral feeding? *Current Opinion in Clinical Nutrition and Metabolic Care, 12*, 186–189.

55. Coughlin, E. (2003). Assessment and management of constipation in pediatric primary care. *Pediatric Nursing, 29*(4), 296–301.

56. Dasgupta, R., & Langer, J. C. (2007). Evaluation and management of persistent problems after surgery for Hirschsprung disease in a child. *Journal of Pediatric Gastroenterology and Nutrition, 46*, 13–19.

57. Davis, A., Rosenthal P., & Glidden D. (2009). Pediatric liver retransplantation: Outcomes and prognostic scoring tool. *Liver Transplantation, 15*, 199–207.

58. Debray, D., Yousef, N., & Durand, P. (2006). New management options for end stage chronic liver disease and acute liver failure: Potential for pediatric patients. *Paediatric Drug, 8*(1), 1–13.

59. Delghani, N., & Ludemann, J. (2008). Ingested foreign bodies in children: BC Children's Hospital emergency room protocol. *British Columbia Medical Journal, 50*(5), 257–262.

60. DeRusso, P., Ye, W., Shepherd, R., Haber, B., Shneider, B., Whitington, P., et al. (2007). Growth failure and outcomes in infants with biliary atresia: A report from the Biliary Atresia Research Consortium. *Hepatology, 46*, 1632–1638.

61. Dew, M., Dabbs, A., & Myaskovosky L. (2009). Meta-analysis of medical regimen adherence outcomes in pediatric solid organ transplantation. *Transplantation, 88*(5), 736–746.

62. Dilliway, G. (2001). Constipation in infant and children. *Practitioner, 245*, 761–763.

63. Ein, S. H., & Daneman, A. (2006). Intussusception. In J. L. Grosfeld, J. A. O'Neil, E. W. Fonkalsrud, & A. G. Coran (Eds.), *Pediatric surgery* (6th ed., Vol. 2, pp. 1514–1550). Philadelphia, PA: Mosby Elsevier.

64. Encinas, J., Luis, A., Avila, L., Hernandez, F., Sarria, J., Gamez, M., et al. (2006). Nutritional status after intestinal transplantation children. *European Journal of Pediatric Surgery, 16*, 403–406.

65. Everly, M., Bloom, R., Tsai, D., & Trofe, J. (2007). Posttransplant lymphoproliferative disorder. *Annals of Pharmacotherapy, 41*, 1850–1858.

66. Fagerman, L. E., & Farber, L. D. (2007). Intussusception. In N. Browne, L. M. Flanigan, C. A. McComiskey, & P. Piper (Eds.), *Nursing care of the pediatric surgical patient* (pp. 289–299). Sudbury, MA: Jones and Bartlett.

67. Finder, J. (2007). Pulmonary disorders. In B. Zitelli & H. Davis, (Eds.), *Atlas of pediatric physical diagnosis* (5th ed., pp. 597–622). St. Louis, MO: Mosby.

68. Fischbach, F. (2004). *A manual of laboratory and diagnostic tests* (7th ed.). Philadelphia: Lippincott, Williams, & Wilkins.

69. Friday, J. (2006). Update on appendicitis: Diagnosis and presurgical management. *Current Opinion in Pediatrics, 18*(33), 234–238.

70. Fraser, J. D., Aguayo, P., Sharp, S. W., Ostlie, D. J., & St. Peter, S. D. (2009). The role of laparoscopy in the management of malrotation. *Journal of Surgical Research, 156*, 80–82.

71. Friesen, C. A., & Roberts, C. C. (1989). Cholelithiasis: Clinical characteristics in children. *Clinical Pediatrics, 28*(7), 294–298.

72. Gallagher, P. (2000). Disorders of erythrocyte metabolism and shape. In R. Christensen (Ed.), *Hematologic problems of the neonate* (pp. 209–237). Philadelphia: W. B. Saunders.

73. Gangemi, A., Tzvetanov, I., Beatty, E., Oberholzer, J., Testa, G., Sankary, H., et al. (2009). Lessons learned in pediatric small bowel and liver transplantation from living-related donors. *Transplantation, 87*(7), 1027–1030.

74. Gedicke, M., Gopal, M., & Spicer, R. (2007). A gasless abdomen does not exclude distal tracheoesophageal fistula: The value of a repeat x-ray. *Journal of Pediatric Surgery, 42*(3), 576–577.

75. Gilet, A. G., Dunkin, J., & Cohen, H. L. (2008). Pylorospasm (simulating hypertrophic pyloric stenosis) with secondary gastroesophageal reflux. *Ultrasound Quarterly, 24*(2), 93–96.

76. Gilger, M. (2006). Diseases of the gallbladder. In R. Wyllie & J. Hyams (Eds.), *Pedatric gastrointestinal and liver disease* (3rd ed.). Pp. 987–1001. Philadelphia: Saunders Elsevier.

77. Gilmour, S., Adkins, R., Liddell, G., Jhangri, G., & Robertson, C. (2009). Assessment of psychoeducational outcomes after pediatric liver transplantation. *American Journal of Transplantation, 9,* 294–300.

78. Ginsberg, G. (1995). Management of ingested foreign objects and food bolus impactions. *Gastrointestinal Endoscopy, 41*(1), 33–38.

79. Goldin, A., Sawin, R., Garrison, M., Zerr, D., & Christakis, D. (2007). Aminoglycoside-based triple-antibiotic therapy versus monotherapy for children with ruptured appendicitis. *Pediatrics, 119*(5), 905–911.

80. Gopal, M., & Woodward, M. (2007). Potential hazards of contrast study diagnosis of esophageal atresia, *Journal of Pediatric Surgery, 42*(6), E9–E10.

81. Greenspan, L., Gitelman, S., Leung, M., Glidden, D., & Mathias, R. (2004). Increased incidence of post-transplant diabetes mellitus in children. *Pediatric Nephrology, 17,* 1–5.

82. Grosfeld, J. (2005). Intussusception then and now: A historical vignette. *Journal of the American College of Surgeons, 201*(6), 830–833.

83. Guerrant, R., Van Gilder, T., Steiner, T., Thielman, N., Slutsker, L., Tauxe, R., et al. (2001). Practice guidelines for the management of infectious diarrhea. *Clinical Infectious Diseases, 32*(3), 331–351.

84. Gura, K. M., Lee, S., Valim, C., Zhou, J., Kim, S., Modi, B. P., et al. (2008). Safety and efficacy of a fish-oil–based fat emulsion in the treatment of parenteral nutrition–associated liver disease. *Pediatrics, 121*(3), 678–686.

85. Hall, N., Pacilli, M., Eaton, S., Reblock, K., Gaines, B., Pastor, A., et al. (2009). Recovery after open versus laparoscopic pyloromyotomy for pyloric stenosis: A double-blind multicentre randomized controlled trial. *Lancet, 373,* 390–398.

86. Harambat, J., Ranchin, B., Dubourg, L., Liutkus, A., Hadj-Haissen, A., Rivet, C., et al. (2008). Renal function in pediatric liver transplantation: A long-term follow-up study. *Transplantation, 86*(8), 1028–1034.

87. Haricharan, R., Proklova, L., Aprahamian, C., Morgan, T., Harmon, C., Barnhart, D., et al. (2008a). Laparoscopic cholecystectomy for biliary dyskinesia in children provides durable symptom relief. *Journal of Pediatric Surgery, 43,* 1060–1064.

88. Haricharan, R., Seo, J., Kelly, D., Mroczek-Musulman, E., Aprahamian, C., Morgan, T., et al. (2008b). Older age at diagnosis of Hirschsprung disease decreases risk of postoperative enterocolitis, but resection of additional ganglionated bowel does not. *Journal of Pediatric Surgery, 43,* 1115–1123.

89. Harmon, C., & Coran, A. (2006). Congenital anomalies of the esophagus, In J. Grosfeld, J. O'Neill, E. Fonkalsrud, & A. Coran (Eds.), *Pediatric surgery* (6th ed., Vol. 2, pp. 1051–1075). Philadelphia, PA: Mosby.

90. Harris, N., Ferry, J., & Swerdlow, S. (1997). Posttransplant lymphoproliferative disorders: Summary of the Society of Hematopathology workshop. *Seminars in Diagnostic Pathology, 14,* 8–14.

91. Hauser, G., Kaufman, S., Matsumoto, C., & Fishbein, T. (2008). Pediatric intestinal and multivisceral transplantation: A new challenge for the pediatric intensivist. *Intensive Care Medicine, 34,* 1570–1579.

92. Haut, C. (2008). Typhlitis in the pediatric patient. *Journal of Infusion Nursing, 31*(5), 270–272.

93. Heubi, J. E. (2007). Diseases of the gallbladder in infancy, childhood, and adolescence. In F. Suchy, R. Sokol, & W. Balistreri (Eds.), *Liver disease in children* (pp. 346–365). New York: Cambridge University Press.

94. Heyman, M. (2006). Lactose intolerance in infants, children, and adolescents. *Pediatrics, 118*(3), 1279–1286.

95. Hill, J., & Voight, R. (2000). Foreign bodies. In K. Ashcroft, J. P. Murphy, R. J. Sharp, D. L. Sigalet, & C. L. Snyder (Eds.), *Pediatric surgery* (3rd ed., pp. 146–151). Philadelphia: W. B. Saunders.

96. Hobson, M., Carney, D., Molik, K., Vik, T., Scherer, L. III, Rouse, T., et al. (2005). Appendicitis in childhood hematologic malignancies: Analysis and comparison with typhlitis. *Journal of Pediatric Surgery, 40,* 214–220.

97. Holcomb, G., & Holcomb, G. (1990). Cholelithiasis in infants, children, and adolescents. *Pediatrics in Review, 11*(9), 268–274.

98. Howard, E., Stringer, M., & Mowat, A. (1988). Assessment of injection sclerotherapy in the management of 152 children with esophageal varices. *British Journal of Surgery, 75,* 404–408.

99. Hryhorczuk, A., & Strouse, P. (2009). Validation of US as a first-line diagnostic test for assessment of pediatric ileocolic intussusception. *Pediatric Radiology, 39,* 1075–1079.

100. Imamoglu, M., Sarihan, H., Sari, A., & Ahmetoglu, A. (2002). Acute acalculous cholecystis in children: Diagnosis and treatment. *Journal of Pediatric Surgery, 37*(1), 36–39.

101. Ioannidis, O., Lavrentieva, A., & Botsios, D. (2008). Nutrition support in acute pancreatitis. *Journal of the Pancreas, 9*(4), 375–390.

102. James, L., Capparelli, E., Letzig, L., Roberts, D., Hinson, J., Kearns, G., et al. (2008). Acetaminophen-associated hepatic injury: Evaluation of acetaminophen protein adducts in children and adolescents with acetaminophen overdose. *Nature, 84*(6), 684–690.

103. Jen, H., & Shew, S. (2009). The impact of hospital type and experience on the operative utilization in pediatric intussusceptions: a nationwide study. *Journal of Pediatric Surgery, 44,* 241–246.

104. Kaechele, V., Wabitsch, M., Thiere, D., Kessler, A. L., Haenle, M. M., Mayer, H., et al. (2006). Prevalence of gallbladder stone disease in obese children and adolescents: Influence of the degree of obesity, sex, and pubertal development. *Journal of Pediatric Gastroenterology and Nutrition, 42,* 66–70.

105. Kaiser, A., Applegate, K., & Ladd, A. (2007). Current success in the treatment of intussusception in children. *Surgery, 142*(4), 469–477.

106. Kamath, B., Spinner, N., & Piccoli, D. (2007). Alagille syndrome. In F. J. Suchy, R. J. Sokol, & W. F. Balistreri (Eds.), *Liver disease in children* (pp. 326–345). New York: Cambridge University Press.

107. Kandula, L., & Lowe, M. (2008). Etiology and outcome of acute pancreatitis in infants and toddlers. *Journal of Pediatrics, 152*(1), 106–110.

108. Kapfer, S., & Rappold, J. (2004). Intestinal malrotation: Not just the pediatric surgeon's problem. *Journal of the American College of Surgeons, 199,* 628–635.

109. Kapur, R. (2009). Practical pathology and genetics of Hirschsprung's disease. *Seminars in Pediatric Surgery, 18,* 212–223.

110. Kato, T., Tzakis, A., Selvaggio, G., Gaynor, J., David, A., Bussotti, A., et al. (2006). Intestinal and multivisceral transplantation in children. *Annals of Surgery, 243*(6), 756–766.

111. Katz, J., Wagner, M., Gresik, M., Mahoney, D., & Fernbach, D. (1990). Typhlitis: An 18-year experience and postmortem review. *Cancer, 65*(4), 1041–1047.

112. Kenner, C., & Lott, J. W. (2003). Assessment and management of the gastrointestinal system. *Comprehensive neonatal nursing,* (3rd ed.). Philadelphia: W. B. Saunders.

113. Kharbanda, A., et al. (2005). A clinical decision rule to identify children at low risk for appendicitis. *Pediatrics, 116*(3), 709–716.

114. King, A., Rampling, A., Wight, D., & Warren, R. (1984). Neutropenic enterocolitis due to *Clostridium septicum* infection. *Journal of Clinical Pathology, 37*(3), 335–343.

115. King, N. (2002). Nursing care of the child with neutropenic enterocolitis. *Journal of Pediatric Oncology Nursing, 19*(6), 198–204.

116. Kiser, T., MacLaren, R., & Fish, D. (2009). Treatment of hepatorenal syndrome. *Pharmacotherapy, 29,* 1196–1211.

117. Klar, M. (2007). Hirschsprung's disease. In N. Browne, L. M. Flanigan, C. A. McComiskey, & P. Pieper (Eds.), *Nursing care of the pediatric surgical patient* (2nd ed., pp. 289–299). Sudbury, MA: Jones and Bartlett.

118. Kling, K., Lau, H., & Colombani, P. (2004). Biliary complications of living related pediatric liver transplant patients. *Pediatric Transplantation, 8,* 178–184.

119. Kortsalioudaki, C., Taylor, M., Cheeseman, P., Bansal, S., Mieli-Vergani, G., & Dhawan, A. (2008). Safety and efficacy of *N*-acetylcysteine in children with non–acetaminophen-induced acute liver failure. *Liver Transplantation, 14,* 25–30.

120. Kosmach-Park, B., & De Angelis, M. (2008). Intestine transplantation. In L. Ohler & S. Cupples (Eds.), *Core curriculum for transplant nurses* (pp. 455–511). St. Louis: Mosby.

121. Kotton, C. (2008). Update on infectious disease in pediatric solid organ transplantation. *Current Opinion in Organ Transplantation, 13,* 500–505.

122. Kovesi, T., & Rubin, S. (2004). Long-term complications of congenital esophageal atresia and/or tracheoesophageal fistula, *Chest, 126*(3), 915–925.

123. Kozer, E., Greenberg, R., Zimmerman, D., & Berkovitch, M. (2006). Repeated supratherapeutic doses of paracetamol in children: A literature review and suggested clinical approach. *Acta Paediatrica, 95,* 1165–1171.

124. Kwok, M., Kim, M., & Gorelick, M. (2004). Evidence-based approach to the diagnosis of appendicitis in children. *Pediatric Emergency Care, 20*(10), 690–698.

125. Lampl, B., Levin, T., Berdon, W., & Cowles, R. (2009). Malrotation and midgut volvulus: A historical review and current controversies in diagnosis and management. *Pediatric Radiology, 39,* 359–366.

126. Lee, J., Lim, G., Ah Im, S., Chung, N., & Hahn, S. (2008a). Gastrointestinal complications following hematopoietic stem cell transplantation in children. *Korean Journal of Radiology, 9*(5), 449–457.

127. Lee, T., Savoldo, B., Rooney, C., et al. (2005a). Quantitative EBV viral loads and immunosuppression alterations can decrease PTLD incidence in pediatric liver transplant recipients. *American Journal of Transplantation, 5,* 2222–2228.

128. Lee, W., Hynan, L., Rossaro, L., Fontana, R., Stravitz, R., Larson, A., et al. (2009). Intravenous *N*-acetylcysteine improves transplant-free survival in early stage non-acetaminophen acute liver failure. *Gastroenterology, 137*(3), 856–864.

129. Lee, W., McKiernan, P., & Kelly, D. (2005b). Etiology, outcome and prognostic indicators of childhood fulminant hepatic failure in the United Kingdom. *Journal of Pediatric Gastroenterology and Nutrition, 40,* 575–581.

130. Lee, W., Squires, R., Nyberg, S., et al. (2008b). Acute liver failure: Summary of a workshop. *Hepatology, 47,* 1401–1415.

131. Leonis, M., & Balistreri, W. (2008a). Evaluation and management of end-stage liver disease in children. *Gastroenterology, 134,* 1741–1751.

132. Leonis, M., & Balistreri, W. (2008b). Is there a "NAC" to treating acute liver failure in children? *Liver Transplantation, 14,* 7–8.

133. Limbos, M. (2005). Approach to the child with constipation. In L. Osborn, T. DeWitt, L. First, & J. Zenel (Eds.), *Pediatrics* (pp. 1347–1364). Philadelphia: Elsevier.

134. Lippl, F., Hannig, C., Weib, W., Allescher, H., Classen, M., & Kurjak, M. (2002). Superior mesenteric artery syndrome: Diagnosis and treatment from the gastroenterologist's view. *Journal of Gastroenterology, 37,* 640–643.

135. Liu, J., Gluud, L., Als-Nielsen, B., & Gluud, C. (2004). Artificial and bioartificial support systems for liver failure. *Cochrane Database of Systematic Reviews, 1,* CD003628. doi: 10.1002/14651858.CD003628. pub2

136. Livingston, E., & Passaro, E. (1990). Postoperative ileus. *Digestive Diseases and Sciences, 35,* 121–132.

137. Lopez, M. (2002). The changing incidence of acute pancreatitis in children: A single-institution perspective. *Journal of Pediatrics, 140*(5), 622–624.

138. Lorijn, F., Reitsma, J., Voskuijl, W., Aronson, D., Ten Kate, F., Smets, A., et al. (2005). Diagnosis of Hirschsprung's disease: A prospective comparative accuracy study of common tests. *Journal of Pediatrics, 146,* 787–792.

139. Louie, M., & Bradin, S. (2009). Foreign body ingestion and aspiration. *Pediatrics in Review, 30,* 295–301.

140. Lowe, M., & Greer, J. (2008). Pancreatitis in children and adolescents. *Current Gastroenterology Reports, 10*(2), 128–135.

141. MacMahon, B. (2006). The continuing enigma of pyloric stenosis of infancy: A review. *Epidemiology, 17,* 195–201.

142. Madan, R., Tan, M., Fernandez-Sesma, A., Moran, T., Emre, S., Campbell, A., et al. (2008). A prospective comparative study of immune response to inactivated influenza vaccine in pediatric liver transplant recipients and their healthy siblings. *Clinical Infectious Disease, 46,* 712–718.

143. Maisels, M. (2009). Neonatal hyperbilirubinemia and kernicterus: Not gone but sometimes forgotten. *Early Human Development, 85,* 727–732.

144. Maisels, M., Bhutani, V., Bogen, D., Newman, T., Stark, A., & Watchko, J. (2009). Hyperbilirubinemia in the newborn infant ≥ 35 weeks' gestation: An update with clarifications. *Pediatrics, 124,* 1193–1198.

145. Marik, P., & Zaloga, G. (2004). Meta-analysis of parenteral nutrition versus enteral nutrition in patients with acute pancreatitis. *British Medical Journal, 328*(7453), 1407.

146. Maron, D., & Fry, R. (2008). New therapies in the treatment of postoperative ileus after gastrointestinal surgery. *American Journal of Therapeutics, 15,* 59–65.

147. Mattei, P., & Rombeau, J. (2006). Review of the pathophysiology and management of postoperative ileus. *World Journal of Surgery, 30,* 1382–1391.

148. McDiarmid, S., Merion, R., Dykstra D., & Harper, A. (2004). Selection of pediatric candidates under the PELD system. *Liver Transplantation, 10,* S23–S30.

149. McGuire, B., Rosenthal, P., Brown, C., Busch, A., Calcatero, S., Claria, R., et al. (2009). Long-term management of the liver transplant patient: Recommendations for the primary care doctor. *American Journal of Transplantation, 9,* 1988–2003.

150. McKenzie, T., Lillegard, M., & Nyberg, S. (2008). Artificial and bioartificial liver support. *Seminars in Liver Disease, 28*(2), 210–217.

151. Merrett, N., Wilson, R., Cosman, P., & Biankin, A. (2009). Superior mesenteric artery syndrome: Diagnosis and treatment strategies. *Journal of Gastrointestinal Surgery, 13*(2), 287–292.

152. Metcalfe, M. S., Wemyss-Hoden, S. A., & Maddern, G. J. (2003). Management dilemmas with choledochal cysts. *Archives of Surgery, 138,* 333–339.

153. Miele-Vergani, G., & Hadzic, N. (2006). Biliary atresia and neonatal disorders of the bile ducts. In R. Wyllie & J. S. Hyams (Eds.), *Pediatric gastroenterology and liver disease* (pp. 869–881). Netherlands: Saunders.

154. Millar, A. J. (2008). Surgical disorders of the liver and bile ducts and portal hypertension. In D. Kelly (Ed.), *Disease of the liver and biliary system in children* (pp. 433–474). Oxford, UK: Wiley-Blackwell.

155. Millar, A., Rode, H., & Cywes, S. (2005). Intestinal atresia and stenosis. In K. Ashcraft, G. Holcomb, & J. Murphy (Eds.), *Pediatric surgery* (4th ed., pp. 416–436). Philadelphia, PA: Elsevier Saunders.

156. Møller, S., Henriksen, J., & Bendtsen, F. (2008). Pathogenic background for treatment of ascites and hepatorenal syndrome. *Hepatology International, 2,* 416–428.

157. Montgomery, D., & Fernando, N. (2008). Management of constipation and encorporesis in children. *Journal of Pediatric Health Care, 22*(3), 199–207.

158. Moran, H., Yaniv, I., Ashkenazi, S., Schwartz, M., Fisher, S., & Levy, I. (2009). Risk factors for typhlitis in pediatric patients with cancer. *Journal of Pediatric Hematology and Oncology, 31*(9), 630–634.

159. Morrow, S., & Newman, K. (2007). Current management of appendicitis. *Seminars in Pediatric Surgery, 16*(1), 34–40.

160. Mullassery, D., Bader, A., Battersby, A. J., Mohammad, Z., Jones, E. L., Parmar, C., et al. (2009). Diagnosis, incidence, and outcomes of suspected typhlitis in oncology patients: Experience in a tertiary pediatric surgical center in the United Kingdom. *Journal of Pediatric Surgery, 44*, 381–385.

161. Murray, K., Hadzic, N., Wirth, S., Bassett, M., & Kelly, D. (2008). Drug-related hepatotoxicity and acute liver failure. *Journal of Pediatric Gastroenterology and Nutrition, 74*, 395–405.

162. Mustafawi, A., & Hassan M., (2008). Congenital duodenal obstruction in children: A decade's experience. *European Journal of Pediatric Surgery, 18*(2), 93–97.

163. Nasr, A., & Langer, J. (2007). Evolution of the technique in the transanal pull-through for Hirschbsprung's disease. Effect on outcome. *Journal of Pediatric Surgery, 42*, 36–40.

164. Nathens, A., Curtis, J., Beale, R., Cook, D., Moreno, R., Romand, J., et al. (2004). Management of the critically ill patient with severe acute pancreatitis. *Critical Care Medicine, 32*(12), 2524–2536.

165. Ng, V. (2006). Neonatal hepatitis. In R. Wyllie & J. S. Hyams (Eds.), *Pediatric gastroenterology and liver disease* (pp. 851–881). Netherlands: Saunders.

166. Ng, V., Fecteau, A., Magee, J., Bucuvalas, J., Alonso, E., McDiamid, S., et al. (2008). Outcomes of 5-year survivors of pediatric liver transplantation: Report on 461 children from a North American multicenter registry. *Pediatrics, 122*, e1128–e1135.

167. Nicholson, L., & Preston, D. (2007, March). Dysfunctional elimination syndrome. *Advance for Nurse Practitioners*, pp. 27–32.

168. Novelli, G., Rossi, M., Morabito, F., Pugliese, F., Ruberto, F., Perrella, S., et al. (2008). Pediatric acute liver failure with molecular adsorbent recirculating system treatment. *Transplantation Proceedings, 40*, 1921–1924.

169. Nowicki, D. (2000). Esophageal defects. In B. Wise, C. McKenna, G. Garvin, & B. Harmon (Eds.), *Nursing care of the general pediatric surgical patient* (pp. 165–166). Gaithersburg, MD:Aspen.

170. Nydegger, A., Couper, R., & Oliver, M. (2006). Childhood pancreatitis. *Journal of Gastroenterology and Hepatology, 21*(3), 499–509.

171. O'Dowd, K. (2007). Hypertrophic pyloric stenosis. In N. T. Browne, L. M. Flanigan, C. A. McComiskey, & P. Pieper (Eds.), *Nursing care of the pediatric surgical patient* (pp. 317–324). Sudbury, MA: Jones and Bartlett.

172. O'Neill, J., Grosfeld, J., Fonkalsrud, E., Coran, A., & Caldamone, A. (2003a). Appendicitis. In J. ONeill, J. Grosfeld, E. Fonkalsrud, A. Coran, & A. Caldamone (Eds.), *Principles of pediatric surgery* (2nd ed., pp. 565–572). St. Louis, MO: Mosby.

173. O'Neill, J., Grosfeld, J., et al., (2003b). Duodenal obstruction. In J. O'Neill, J. Grosfeld, E. Fonkalsrud, A. Coran, & A. Caldamone (Eds.), *Principles of pediatric surgery* (2nd ed., p. 471). St. Louis, MO: Mosby.

174. Ostrow, J. D. (1984). The etiology of pigment gallstones. *Hepatology, 4*(5), 215S–222S.

175. Palasciano, G., Portincasa, P., Vinciguerra, V., Velardi, A., Tardi, S., Baldassarre, G., et al. (1989). Gallstone prevalence and gallbladder volume in children and adolescents: An epidemiological ultrasonographic survey and relationship to body mass index. *American Journal of Gastroenterology, 84*(11), 1378–1392.

176. Pascher, A., Kohler, S., Neuhaus, P., & Pratschke, J. (2008). Present status and future perspective of intestinal transplantation. *European Society of Organ Transplantation, 21*, 401–414.

177. Perlmutter, D. (2007). α1-Antitrypsin deficiency. In F. J. Suchy, R. J. Sokol, & W. F. Balistreri (Eds.), *Liver disease in children* (pp. 545–571). New York: Cambridge University Press.

178. Person, B., & Wexner, S. (2006). The management of postoperative ileus. *Current Problems in Surgery, 43*(1), 12–65.

179. Petersen, C. (2006). Pathogenesis and treatment opportunities for biliary atresia. *Clinics in Liver Disease, 10*, 73–88.

180. Pietzak, M., & Thomas, D. (2000). Pancreatitis in childhood. *Pediatrics in Review, 21*(12), 406–412.

181. Piper, H., Alesbury, J., Waterford, S., Zurakowski, D. & Jaksic, T. (2008). Intestinal atresias: Factors affecting clinical outcomes. *Journal of Pediatric Surgery, 43*(7), 1244–1248.

182. Pirenne, J., & Kawai, M. (2009). Intestinal transplantation: Evolution in immunosuppressant protocols. *Current Opinion in Organ Transplantation, 14*, 250–255.

183. Poki, H. O., Holland, A. J. A., & Pitkin, J. (2005). Double bubble, double trouble. *Pediatric Surgery International, 21*(6), 428–431.

184. Polson, J. (2010). Hepatotoxicity due to antibiotics. *Clinics in Liver Disease, 11*, 1–10.

185. Pratap, A., Gupta, D., Shakya, V., Adhikary, S., Tiwari, A., Shrestha, P., et al. (2007). Analysis of problems, complications, avoidance and management with transanal pull-through for Hirschsprung disease. *Journal of Pediatric Surgery, 42*, 1869–1876.

186. Quiros-Tejeira, R. E., Ament, M. E., Heyman, M. B., Martin, M. G., Rosenthal, P., Hall, T. R., et al. (1999). Variable morbidity in Alagille syndrome: A review of 43 cases. *Journal of Pediatric Gastroenterology and Nutrition, 29*(4), 431–437.

187. Radhakrishnan, K., & Sutphen, J. (2006). Pancreatitis. In R. Wyllie, J. Hyams, & M. Kay (Eds.), *Pediatric gastrointestinal and liver disease* (3rd ed., pp. 1043–1062). Philadelphia: Elsevier Saunders.

188. Rescorla, F. (1997). Cholelithiasis, cholecystitis, and common bile duct stones. *Current Opinion in Pediatrics, 9*, 276–282.

189. Reyes, J., Mazariegos, G., Bond, G., Green, M., Dvorchik, I., Kosmach-Park, B., et al. (2002). Pediatric intestinal transplantation: Historical notes, principles and controversies. *Pediatric Transplantation, 6*, 193–207.

190. Rosen, C., Buuonomo, C., Andrade, R., & Nurko, S. (2004). Incidence of spinal cord lesions in patients with retractable constipation. *Journal of Pediatrics, 143*, 409–411.

191. Rovner, A. J., Schall, J. L., Jawad, A. F., Piccoli, D. A., Stallings V. A., Mulberg, A. E., et al. (2002). Rethinking growth failure in Alagille syndrome: The role of dietary intake and steatorrhea. *Journal of Pediatric Gastroenterology and Nutrition, 35*(4), 495–502.

192. Rudolph, C., Mazur, L., Liptak, G., Baker, R., Boyle, J., Colletti, R., et al. (2001). Guidelines for evaluation and treatment of gastroesophageal reflux in infants and children: Recommendation of the North American Society for Pediatric Gastroenterology and Nutrition. *Journal of Pediatric Gastroenterology, 32*(suppl 2), S1–S32.

193. Salmerón, J., Tito, L., Rimola, A., Mas, A., Navasa, M., Llach, J., et al. (1992). Selective intestinal decontamination in the prevention of bacterial infections with acute liver failure. *Journal of Hepatology, 14*, 280–285.

194. Salvatore, M., Goldberg, R., Hadigan, C., Stark, P., & Wilson, I. (2006). Acute pancreatitis in the pediatric population: A large population-based study. *Journal of Pediatric Gastroenterology & Nutrition, 43*, E73.

195. Sanchez-Ramirez, C., Larrosa-Haro, A., Flores-Martinez, S., Sanchez-Corona, J., Villa-Gomez, A., & Macias-Rosales, R. (2007). Acute and recurrent pancreatitis in children: Etiological factors. *Acta Paediatrica, 96*(4), 534–537.

196. Sarwal, M. (2008). Out with the old, in with the new: Immunosuppression minimization in children. *Current Opinion in Organ Transplantation, 12*, 513–521.

197. Sauer, C. J. E., Langer, J. C., & Wales, P. W. (2005). The versatility of the umbilical incision in the management of Hirschsprung's disease. *Journal of Pediatric Surgery, 40*, 385–389.

198. Schlatter, M., Snyder, K., & Freyer, D. (2002). Successful nonoperative management of typhlitis in pediatric oncology patients. *Journal of Pediatric Surgery, 37*(8), 1151–1155.

199. Schmitt, B. (2007). *American Academy of Pediatrics Pediatric Telephone Protocols* (7th ed.). Elk Grove Village, IL: American Academy of Pediatrics.

200. Schunk, J. (2006). Foreign body-ingestion/aspiration. In G. Fleisher, S. Ludwig, & F. Henretig (Eds.), *Textbook of pediatric emergency medicine* (5th ed., pp. 307–314). Philadelphia: Lippincott Williams & Wilkins.

201. Scolapio, J. (2003). Nutritional disorders and their treatment in diseases of the gastrointestinal tract. In S. L. Friedman, K. R. McQuaid, & J. H. Grendell (Eds.), *Current diagnosis and treatment in gastroenterology* (pp. 192–200). New York: Lange/McGraw-Hill.

202. Seef, L. (2007). Herbal hepatotoxicity. *Clinics in Liver Disease, 11,* 577–596.

203. Selvaggi, G., & Tzakis, A. (2009). Small bowel transplantation: Technical advances/updates. *Current Opinion in Transplantation, 14,* 262–266.

204. Shamberger, R., Weinstein, H., Delorey, H., & Levey, R. (1986). The medical and surgical management of typhlitis in children with acute myelogenous leukemia. *Cancer, 57,* 603–609.

205. Shapiro, S. (2008). Hyperbilirubinemia and the risk for brain injury. In J. Perlman (Ed.), *Neurology: Neonatology questions and controversies* (pp. 195–209). Philadelphia: Saunders Elsevier.

206. Shemesh, E. (2004). Non-adherence to medications following liver transplantation. *Pediatric Transplantation, 8,* 600–605.

207. Shepherd, R., Turmelle, Y., Nadler, M., Lowell, J., Narkewicz, M., McDiarmid, S., et al. (2008). Risk factors for rejection and infection in pediatric liver transplantation. *American Journal of Transplantation, 8,* 396–403.

208. Sherman, P., Hassall, E., Fagundes-Neto, U., Gold, B., Kato, S., Koletzka, S., et al. (2009). A global, evidence-based consensus on the definition of gastroesophageal reflux disease in the pediatric population. *American Journal of Gastroenterology, 104,* 1278–1295.

209. Siegel, M. (2008). Practical CT techniques. In M. Siegel (Ed.), *Pediatric body CT* (2nd ed., pp. 1–21) Philadelphia: Lippincott Williams & Wilkins.

210. Singh, R., Cameron, B., Walton, J., Farrokhyar, F., Borenstein, S., & Fitzgerald, B. (2007). Postoperative Hirschsprung's enterocolitis after minimally invasive Swenson procedure. *Journal of Pediatric Surgery, 42,* 885–889.

211. Smink, D., Findelstein, J., Garcia Pena, B., Shannon, M., Taylor, G., & Fishman, S. (2004). Diagnosis of acute appendicitis in children using a clinical practice guideline, *Journal of Pediatric Surgery, 39*(3), 458–463.

212. Smith, B., Hakin-Zargar, M., & Thomson, J. (2009). Low body weight index: A risk factor for superior mesenteric artery syndrome in adolescents undergoing spinal fusion for scoliosis. *Journal of Spinal Disorders and Surgical Techniques, 22*(2), 144–148.

213. Spitz, L. (2005). Esophageal atresia and tracheoesophageal malformations. In K. Ashcroft, G. Holcomb, & A. Murphy (Eds.), *Pediatric surgery* (4th ed., pp. 352–367). Philadelphia, PA: Elsevier.

214. Squires, R. (2008). Acute liver failure in children. *Seminars in Liver Disease, 28*(2), 153–166.

215. Squires, R., Schneider, B., Bucuvalas, J., Alonso, E., Sokol, R., Narkewicz, M., et al. (2006). Acute liver failure in children: They really are not just small adults. *Journal of Pediatrics, 148,* 652–658.

216. Stowkowski, L. (2006). Fundamentals of phototherapy for neonatal jaundice. *Advances in Neonatal Care, 6,* 303–312.

217. St. Peter, S., & Ostlie, D. (2008). Pyloric stenosis: From a retrospective analysis to a prospective clinical trial—the impact of surgical outcomes. *Current Opinion in Pediatrics, 20,* 311–314.

218. St. Peter, S. D., Tsao, K., Spilde, T. L., Holcomb, G. W. 3rd, Sharp, S. W., Murphy, J. P., et al. (2008). Single daily dosing ceftriaxone and metronidazole vs standard triple antibiotic regimen for perforated appendicitis in children: A prospective randomized trial. *Journal of Pediatric Surgery. 43*(6), 981–985.

219. Stravitz, R., & Kramer, D. (2009). Management of acute liver failure. *Gastroenterology and Hepatology, 6,* 542–553.

220. Stringer, M. (2005). Pancreatitis and pancreatic trauma. *Seminars in Pediatric Surgery, 14*(4), 239–246.

221. Stuber, M., Shemesh, E., Seacord, D., Washington, J. III, Hellemann, G., McDiarmid, S., et al. (2008). Evaluating non-adherence to immunosuppressant medications in pediatric liver transplant recipients. *Pediatric Transplantation, 12,* 284–288.

222. Sudan, D. (2009). Advances in the nontransplant medical and surgical management of intestinal failure. *Current Opinion in Organ Transplantation, 14,* 274–279.

223. Sudan, D., DiBaise, J., Torres, C., Thompson, J., Raynor, S., Gilroy, R., et al. (2005). A multidisciplinary approach to the treatment of intestinal failure. *Journal of Gastrointestinal Surgery, 9*(1), 165–177.

224. Tabata, M., & Nakayama, F. (1981). Bacteria and gallstones: Etiological significance. *Digestive Diseases and Sciences, 26*(3), 218–224.

225. Taketomo, C., Hodding, J., & Kraus, D. (2010). *Pediatric dosage handbook* (16th ed.). Hudson, OH: Lexi-Comp.

226. Tandeter, H. (2009). Hypothesis: Hexitols in chewing gum may play a role in reducing postoperative ileus. *Medical Hypotheses, 72,* 39–40.

227. Taylor, R., Franck, L., Gibson, F., Donaldson, N., & Dhawan, A. (2009). Study of the factors affecting health-related quality of life in adolescents after liver transplantation. *American Journal of Transplantation, 9,* 1179–1188.

228. Teitelbaum, D., & Coran, A. (2006). Hirschsprung's disease and related neuromuscular disorders of the intestine. In J. L. Grosfeld, J. A. O'Neill, A. G. Coran, & E. W. Fonkalsrud (Eds.), *Pediatric surgery* (6th ed., Vol. 2, pp. 1514–1550). Philadelphia: Mosby Elsevier.

229. The, N. S., Honein, M. A., Caton, A. R., Moore, C., Siega-Riz, A. M., Druschel, C., et al. (2007). Risk factors for isolated biliary atresia, national birth defects prevention study, 1997–2002. *American Journal of Medical Genetics Part A, 143A,* 2274–2284.

230. Thomas, D., Greer, F., & Committee on Nutrition. (2010). Clinical report_probiotics and prebiotics in pediatrics. *Pediatrics, 126*(6), 1217–1231.

231. Thompson, J. (2001). The management of chronic constipation in children. *Community Practitioner, 74*(1), 29–30.

232. Tieder, J., Robertson, A., & Garrison, M. (2009). Pediatric hospital adherence to the standard of care for acute gastroenteritis. *Pediatrics, 124* (6), e1081–e1087. Retrieved from http://pediatrics.aappublications.org/cgi/content/abstract/124/6/e1081

233. Tredger, J., Brown, N., & Dhawan, A. (2006). Immunosuppression in pediatric solid organ transplantation: Opportunities, risks, and management. *Pediatric Transplantation, 10,* 879–892.

234. Tsakayannis, D., Kozakewich, H. P. W., & Lillehei, C. (1996). Acalculous cholecystitis in children. *Journal of Pediatric Surgery, 31*(1), 127–131.

235. Turban, S., Thuluvath, P., & Atta, G. (2007). Hepatorenal syndrome. *World Journal of Gastroenterology, 13*(30), 4046–4055.

236. Ueda, M., Egawa, H., Ogawa, K., Uryvhara, K., Fujimoto, Y., Kasahara, M., et al. (2005). Portal vein complications in the long-term course after pediatric living donor living transplantation. *Transplantation Proceedings, 37,* 1138–1140.

237. United Network for Organ Sharing (UNOS). (2009). Retrieved from http://www.optn.transplant.hrsa.org

238. Vandenplas, Y., Rudolph, C., Di Lorenzo, C., Hassall, E., Liptak, G., Mazur, L., et al. (2009). Pediatric gastroesophageal reflux clinical practice guidelines: Joint recommendations of the North American Society for Pediatric Gastroenterology, Hepatology, and Nutrition (NASPGHAN) and the European Society for Pediatric Gastroenterology, Hepatology, and Nutrition (ESPGHAN). *Journal of Pediatric Gastroenterology and Nutrition, 49*(4), 498–547.

239. Venkat, V., Nick, T., Wang, Y., & Bucuvalas, J. (2008). An objective measure to identify pediatric liver transplant recipients at risk for late allograft rejection related to non-adherence. *Pediatric Transplantation, 12,* 67–72.

240. Vincenti, F., & Kirk, A. (2008). What's new in the pipeline? *American Journal of Transplantation, 8,* 1972–1981.

241. Waltzman, M. (2006). Management of esophageal coins. *Current Opinion in Pediatrics, 18,* 571–574.

242. Waseem, M., & Salvatore, C. (2004). Abdominal pain: An uncommon cause. *Pediatric Emergency Care, 20*(8), 531–533.

243. Watson, M., Venick, R., Kaldas, F., Rastogi, A., Gordon, S., Colargelo, J.,et al. (2008). Renal function impacts outcomes after intestinal transplantation. *Transplantation, 86*(1), 117–122.

244. Weinberg, A., Horflen, S., Kaufman, S., Jesser, R., Devoll-Zabrocki, A., Fleckten, B., et al. (2006). Safety and immunogenicity of varicella-zoster virus vaccine in pediatric liver and intestine transplant recipients. *American Journal of Transplantation, 6,* 565–568.

245. Werlin, S., Kugathasan, S., & Frautschy, B. (2003). Pancreatitis in children. *Journal of Pediatric Gastroenterology & Nutrition, 37*(5), 591–595.

246. Wilhelmi, I., Roman, E., & Sanchez-Fauquier, A. (2003). Viruses causing gastroenteritis. *Clinical Microbiology & Infection, 9*(4), 247–262.

247. Wong, R., DeSandre, G., Sibley, E., & Stevenson, D. (2006). Neonatal jaundice and liver disease. In R. Martin, A. Fanaroff, & M. Walsh (Eds.), *Fanaroff and Martin's neonatal–perinatal medicine: Diseases of the fetus and infant* (pp. 1419–1465). Philadelphia: Mosby Elsevier.

248. Yardeni, D., Hirschi, R., Drongowski, R., Teitelbaum, D., Geiger, J., & Coran, A. (2004). Delayed versus immediate surgery in acute appendicitis: Do we need to operate during the night? *Journal of Pediatric Surgery, 39*(3), 464–469.

249. Zeinali, F., Stulberg, J., & Delaney, C. (2009). Pharmacological management of postoperative ileus. *Canadian Journal of Surgery, 52*(2), 153–157.

250. Zhang, S., Bai, Y., Wang, W., & Wang, W. (2005). Clinical outcome in children after transanal 1-stage endocrectal pull-through operation for Hirschsprung's disease. *Journal of Pediatric Surgery, 40,* 1307–1311.

Genetic and Metabolic Disorders

PHYSIOLOGY AND DIAGNOSTICS

Sarah Pihl

ORGANIZATION AND STRUCTURE OF THE HUMAN GENOME

The most important components of the human genome are the two types of nucleotide bases that compose the genetic code—namely, the purines (adenine and guanine) and the pyrimidines (cytosine and thymine) (Williams & Burns, 2009). These bases form long chains by 5' to 3' phosphodiester bonding (Figure 27-1). Further stability is added by hydrogen bonds that form between the complementary bases. Purines form two hydrogen bonds and pyrimidines form three hydrogen bonds; these varied bonding patterns, in turn, give DNA its characteristic double-stranded helix shape (Nussbaum et al., 2007). The sequence of the

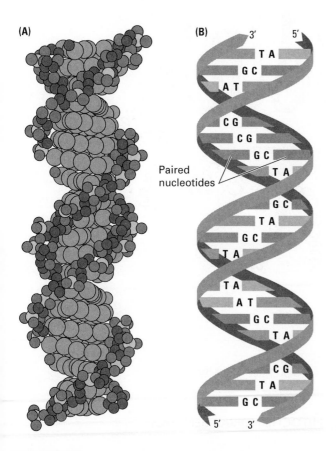

FIGURE 27-1

Molecular Structure of a DNA Double Helix a. A space-filling model in which each atom is depicted as a sphere. b. A diagram highlighting 5' to 3' bonding.

Source: Hartl, D. & Jones, E. (2006). *Essential Genetics: A Genomics Perspective.* Sudbury, MA: Jones and Bartlett Publishers.

bases constitutes the genetic code or genome. Within this code are genes, or sequences, found at specific locations in the genome. Not all sequences contain genes. A propensity of gene clustering is referred to as a "gene-rich" region on the chromosomes, whereas as region where genes are sparse is referred to as a "gene-poor" region or "gene desert" (Nussbaum et al., 2007).

Genes are typically preceded on the 5' end by a regulatory region called a promoter. Specifically, the cellular machinery that performs transcription and translation recognizes these promoters. Also located near the promoter region are enhancers and silencers. Enhancers increase transcription, whereas silencers decrease rates of transcription (Nussbaum et al., 2007).

As a gene is transcribed, not all copied components of the sequence will be utilized. Segments of the gene called introns are spliced out of the transcribed material prior to translation. Exons, or the retained regions, serve as the blueprint for the protein that is to be synthesized (Korf, 2007a).

During cell division, the genetic material is arranged in a larger, rod-shaped form called a chromosome. Histones, chromatin, and other proteins help the DNA organize itself into this condensed form (Nussbaum et al., 2007) (Figure 27-2). Humans have 46 chromosomes, arranged into 23 pairs of homologous chromosomes. Twenty-two of these pairs are autosomes, and one pair represents the sex chromosomes.

Function

Cell division occurs as mitosis or meiosis. Prior to either division process, the DNA is replicated.

During *mitosis*, the chromosomes are separated and yield two daughter cells with the same number of chromosomes as the original cell—that is, diploid cells (Nussbaum et al., 2007). Mitotic division is important in normal growth and differentiation of tissues.

Meiosis occurs in the reproductive organs and requires two cycles. The chromosomes are separated twice, yielding four cells, each with one-half the number of chromosomes of the original cell—that is, haploid cells (Nussbaum et al., 2007). In meiosis I, recombination occurs when sections of homologous chromosomes are exchanged. In meiosis II, the chromosomes are fully separated into the four daughter cells.

Transcription is the process by which the DNA template is copied into RNA as the first step in protein synthesis (Korf, 2007a). RNA uses the pyrimidine uracil instead of thymine and is single stranded. During transcription, the gene sequence is copied in the 5' to 3' direction, including introns and exons. The RNA is processed in the nucleus, the introns are removed, and other modifications are made until the final template for protein synthesis is produced (Korf).

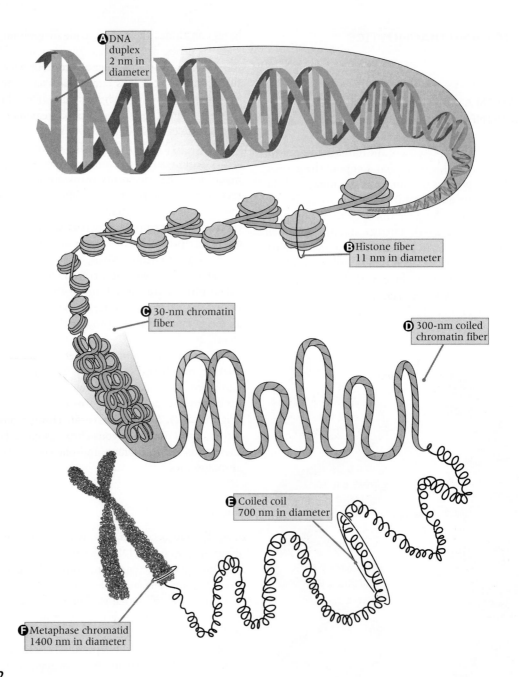

FIGURE 27-2

Levels of Condensation of DNA into a Metaphase Chromosome.

Source: Hartl, D. & Jones, E. (2006). *Essential Genetics: A Genomics Perspective.* Sudbury, MA: Jones and Bartlett Publishers.

This messenger RNA (mRNA) then migrates through the cytoplasm to the ribosomes, where translation occurs (Figure 27-3).

Translation is the process of constructing a protein by arranging amino acids according to the mRNA sequence (Nussbaum et al., 2007). Every three bases constitute a group known as a triplet or codon, which correlates to a specific amino acid or stop sequence. Joining of amino acids continues until a stop codon is reached, which terminates the translation process.

MITOCHONDRIAL GENETICS

The majority of cellular function is guided by the information contained within the human genome. A small portion is controlled by the genes contained on a small, circular strand of DNA within the mitochondria. Mitochondria are inherited only from the mother (Nussbaum et al., 2007). Mutations in mitochondrial DNA (mtDNA) can result in disorders such as Leber's hereditary optic neuropathy and myoclonic epilepsy with ragged-red fibers.

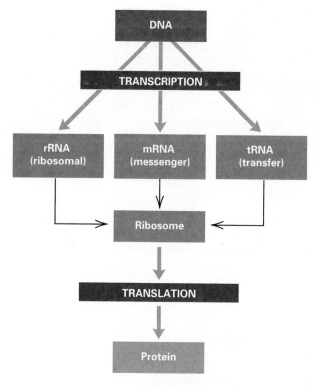

FIGURE 27-3

Processes of Transcription and Translation.

Source: Hartl, D. & Jones, E. (2006). *Essential Genetics: A Genomics Perspective.* Sudbury, MA: Jones and Bartlett Publishers.

SINGLE-GENE DISORDERS

Single-gene disorders are caused by individual genes containing mutations. A *gene mutation* is called "dominant" if the inheritance of a single allele from one parent yields a phenotypic change or produces disorder (Nussbaum et al., 2007). An example of a disorder with an *autosomal dominant* inheritance pattern is Huntington disease (Figures 27-4 and 27-5): All persons who inherit the mutation develop disease. By comparison, in an *autosomal recessive* inheritance pattern (Figure 27-6), an individual must inherit a gene mutation from both parents in order to exhibit the disorder (Nussbaum et al., 2007): Cystic fibrosis is a classic example of this inheritance pattern. If an individual inherits one mutation, typically he or she does not express any disease or phenotypic changes. However, that person is at risk for passing the gene along to his or her offspring and is known as a *carrier.* Consanguineous couples—those sharing a common relative—are at increased risk for having children with autosomal recessive disorders (Nussbaum et al.).

In X-linked recessive disorders, females classically are carriers and all males who inherit the gene exhibit disease. This outcome occurs because females have two X chromosomes, whereas males have an X chromosome and a Y chromosome (Nussbaum et al., 2007). Hemophilia A follows an X-linked recessive inheritance pattern, for example. Most genes expressed from the X chromosome

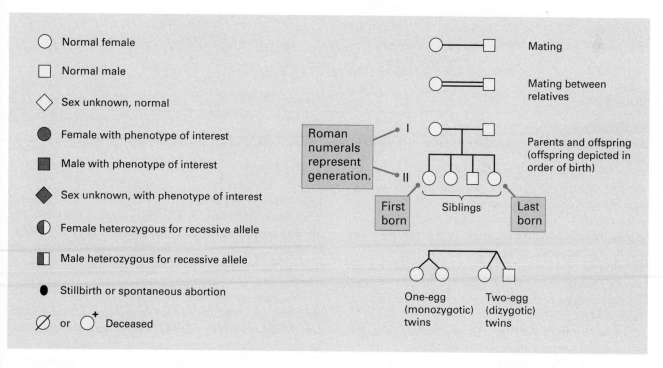

FIGURE 27-4

Human Pedigree.

Source: Hartl, D. & Jones, E. (2006). *Essential Genetics: A Genomics Perspective.* Sudbury, MA: Jones and Bartlett Publishers.

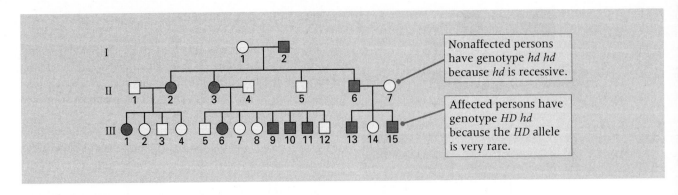

FIGURE 27-5

Autosomal Dominant Inheritance Pattern in Huntington Disease.

Source: Hartl, D. & Jones, E. (2006). *Essential Genetics: A Genomics Perspective.* Sudbury, MA: Jones and Bartlett Publishers.

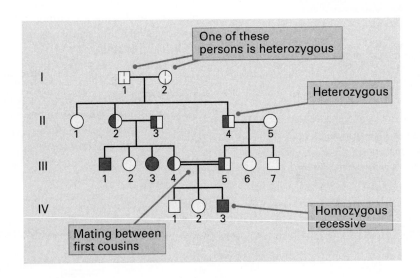

FIGURE 27-6

Autosomal Recessive Inheritance Pattern.

Source: Hartl, D. & Jones, E. (2006). *Essential Genetics: A Genomics Perspective.* Sudbury, MA: Jones and Bartlett Publishers.

come from the one chromosome; the other X chromosome is inactivated. Some disease patterns suggest an X-linked dominant pattern, such as Aicardi syndrome and Rett syndrome. This pattern lacks male-to-male transmission, so that only females are affected in these diseases (Nussbaum et al.). In some X-linked dominant disorders, however, the gene mutation is lethal to males (Table 27-1).

Frequently the same single-gene mutation will produce varying severity of disease and phenotype in different persons. These differences result from interactions between the genotype, cellular function, and environment. *Penetrance* is the number of individuals with a gene disorder who exhibit symptoms of that disease. *Expressivity* is the variation in expression in the individuals who have the gene disorder (Nussbaum et al., 2007). Additional processes also cause variations in phenotypic expression, including mosaicism, imprinting, uniparental disomy, and X-inactivation.

Mosaicism is the presence in an individual of two or more cell lines typically derived from the same original cell line (Williams & Burns, 2009). This pattern can also occur in the reproductive organs and may be passed on to the individual's offspring. Diagnosing mosaicism requires testing of the individual's blood and performing an epidermal skin biopsy.

TABLE 27-1

Inheritance Patterns

Autosomal Dominant	Autosomal Recessive
• One gene with mutation needed	• Two genes with mutation needed
• De novo mutation or affected parent	• Parents carriers for mutation
• Occurs in each generation	• May skip generations

X-Linked Dominant	X-Linked Recessive
• Females affected	• Males affected
• Lethal to males	• Mother and daughters may be carriers
• Inherited from mother	

Imprinting involves the expression of genes only from one specific parent, as a result of inhibition of gene expression through either methylation of cytosine or changes in histones (Nussbaum et al., 2007). The silencing of these genes can result in the expression of a gene disorder on the other chromosome (Robin, 2007).

Uniparental disomy (UPD)—a defect related to imprinting—occurs when both homologous chromosomes are derived from one parent (Williams & Burns, 2009). The lack of genetic material from the other parent can result in disease if the chromosome has regions that are imprinted. UPD can be caused by incomplete separation during meiosis or by a trisomy rescue, in which the cell loses one of the extra chromosomes so as to regain the correct number for viability (Nussbaum et al., 2007). An example of this type of disorder is Beckwith-Weidemann syndrome, which is caused by UPD of chromosome 11.

X-inactivation is a different gene silencing process that effectively turns off a majority of the genes found on the X chromosome. This random process helps regulate the amount of gene expression from the X chromosome (Robin, 2007). If a mutation exists in the active X chromosome, however, disease pathology may occur.

Gene mutations on a molecular level can produce profound disease through relatively small changes in the genetic code. The various types of changes include deletions, insertions, point mutations, and expansions. Segments affected may be small, involving only a single base, or large, removing the entire gene.

Deletions and *insertions* result in abnormal protein synthesis. *Point mutations* are single-base substitutions that may or may not result in changes to protein synthesis. Silent, missense, and nonsense types of point mutations are differentiated according to the change in protein synthesis that results from the mutation (Nussbaum et al., 2007). A silent mutation is a base substitution that does not change the associated amino acid or function of the protein. By comparison, missense mutations result in a different amino acid from the codon and a change in protein function. Premature termination of protein synthesis is the result of nonsense mutations, which change a functioning codon into a stop codon.

Diseases caused by *gene expansion* are attributable to repetitive unstable gene segments. As the gene is passed down through generations of a family, the numbers of repeats increases until the unstable region can no longer participate in gene expression (Nussbaum et al., 2007). When that happens, a disease such as fragile X syndrome occurs.

CHROMOSOMAL DISORDERS

Chromosomal disorders are defined as changes in structure or number of chromosomes that result in disease. These changes can occur during crossing over and cell division.

Aneuploidy is an abnormal number of chromosomes. Two of the most common types are monosomy and trisomy. Individuals with monosomies lack one of a pair of chromosomes. Those with trisomies have an additional, or third, chromosome, instead of the usual pair. Down syndrome (trisomy 21) and Turner syndrome (45,X) are examples of aneuploidy-caused diseases.

During recombination in meiosis, rearrangements of unbalanced or balanced chromosomal material may occur, taking the form of deletions, duplications, inversions, or insertions. With *deletions*, chromosomal material is lacking. With *duplications*, extra chromosomal material is present. *Inversions* rearrange chromosome structure. Translocations between chromosomes are more varied and material is switched between different chromosomes (Nussbaum et al., 2007). If the translocation is balanced, disease is not always present. Conversely, unbalanced translocations produce disease. Robertsonian translocations occur when two chromosomes fuse at the centromeres. This reciprocal translocation occurs primarily in chromosomes with centromeres near the end, such as chromosomes 14 and 21; the majority of chromosomal material is retained in such a case, resulting in a trisomy (Nussbaum et al.). *Insertions* are a rare type of translocation where material from a chromosome is inserted into another chromosome.

MULTIFACTORIAL DISORDERS

Multifactorial disorders are quickly becoming the predominant disease group in medicine today. These disorders do not follow the same inheritance patterns as single-gene or chromosomal disorders, but rather incorporate two or more genes and environmental factors (Robin, 2007). They have a propensity to occur in clusters within families who share genetics and environmental conditions. Examples of multifactorial disorders include heart disease and diabetes. Risk and prevention for these disorders currently depends on modification of environmental factors.

DIAGNOSTIC STUDIES

A genetic consult should be obtained to guide targeted testing for specific disorders and genetic evaluations of patients (Korf, 2007b). Indications for such testing include a strong family history, multiple congenital anomalies, developmental delay or regression, fertility and pregnancy problems, advanced maternal age, at-risk ethnicity (e.g., Ashkenazi Jew), and abnormal laboratory values (Table 27-2). The use of a human pedigree provides structure for genetic analysis (Figure 27-4).

Establishing the carrier status in individuals at risk of genetic disorders is important, especially for their offspring. Certain populations are at higher risk for some disorders than others. The information obtained from carrier testing will allow families to prepare for having a child with certain needs or explore alternative fertility choices. Sickle cell disease, Tay-Sachs disease, and cystic fibrosis are examples of genetic diseases where genetic counseling and testing may establish carrier status and have clinical utility, or may provide important information that will guide medical care.

Carrier testing can sometimes establish an individual's risk for diseases such as breast cancer. Individuals with the *BRCA1* and *BRCA2* mutations, for example, have a higher risk of developing breast cancer than those without these mutations (Nussbaum et al., 2007). Knowledge of carrier status can provide a patient with information to be factored into important healthcare decisions.

Cytogenetic testing

Karyotyping is a type of cytogenetic analysis that uses a microscope to examine stained chromosomes. The staining allows for analysis of each chromosome's unique

TABLE 27-2

Indications for Genetic Testing

- Family history
- Multiple congenital anomalies
- Development delay or regression
- Fertility problems or multiple miscarriages
- Advanced maternal age
- At-risk ethnicity
- Consanguinity
- Previous child with genetic disease
- Abnormal laboratory values

banding pattern and assessment for structural abnormalities. Structural chromosomal disorders make up a large portion of the genetic disorders identified today, however, some microdeletions and molecular mutations are not easily identified with karyotype analysis (Williams & Burns, 2009). In such cases, fluorescent in situ hybridization (FISH) analysis is a better diagnostic study for detecting microdeletions. FISH analysis requires the targeting of a specific region of the chromosome for review; consequently, a presumptive disorder must be selected for this test to be utilized (Descartes & Carroll, 2007). This test involves using small DNA probes that have been labeled with a fluorescent material. Patient samples are prepared with the target DNA probe and a control probe. If the microdeletion is present, then the number of target copies viewed will be abnormal. FISH technology is useful for diagnosing disorders such as Williams syndrome and 22q11 deletion syndrome (DiGeorge syndrome).

Molecular testing

A more sensitive form of chromosome analysis is comparative genome hybridization (CGH) or microarray technology. This process involves comparison of the patient's genome with a normal genome. The technology allows for comparison of the quantity of genomic material and may diagnose microdeletions and duplications. CGH will not detect translocations and should be used in conjunction with traditional karyotyping for this reason (Nussbaum et al., 2007).

When considering a disorder that has a known molecular genetic etiology, gene sequencing may provide a highly specific diagnosis, such as Noonan syndrome. The information obtained from this technology will include the type and location of the mutation, the amino acid that is being substituted, or termination of the sequence, if present.

Methylation analysis shows the particular methylation pattern of a gene (Nussbaum et al., 2007). This kind of analysis is used for diagnosis of imprinting defects in disorders such as Prader-Willi and Angelman syndromes. Test results may suggest UPD, and further analysis of chromosome markers will confirm a UPD diagnosis.

Southern blot analysis is used for diagnosis of gene expansion disorders. Examination of the number of repeats is possible through the separation of the DNA into specific fragments (Nussbaum et al., 2007).

Newborn screening—a national testing program—assesses neonates for numerous genetic disorders, particularly those that are metabolic in nature (Williams & Burns, 2009). With this type of testing, the blood samples collected from the neonate are placed on filter paper and then examined via tandem mass spectrometry for metabolites. A positive result on a newborn screen is not diagnostic, but requires follow-up testing for confirmatory diagnosis (Table 27-3).

TABLE 27-3

Testing Options		
Testing	**Analysis**	**Test**
Initial Evaluation		
	Structure	Karyotype
	Quantity	Comparative genome hybridization (CGH)
Targeted Evaluation		
	Microdeletion	Fluorescent in situ hybridization (FISH)
	Gene mutation	Sequencing
	Imprinting	Methylation
	Uniparental disomy (UPD)	Chromosome marker analysis
	Gene expansion	Southern blot analysis

PRENATAL TESTING

Molecular testing may be indicated in the prenatal period. Samples of fetal tissue may be obtained by amniocentesis or chorionic villi sampling (CVS). Amniocentesis, or sampling of amniotic fluid, is typically performed between gestational weeks 15 or 16. CVS sampling may occur in the tenth and twelfth weeks of the gestation. This early testing provides families with the opportunity to consider multiple treatment options if a diagnosis of a genetic disorder is confirmed.

Routine prenatal care incorporates aspects of genetic testing with laboratory sample analysis and ultrasound to assess for congenital malformations that have a link to genetic disorders. Maternal serum alpha-fetoprotein (MSAFP) is tested with a sample of maternal blood. Elevated levels of MSAFP are associated with neural tube defects and genitourinary abnormalities (Nussbaum et al., 2007). During prenatal ultrasounds, fetal structures are examined. Increased measurement of nuchal translucency (nuchal fold scan) is suggestive of a trisomy disorder (Nussbaum et al.).

GENETIC COUNSELING

Families may be referred to genetic counselors during prenatal care or following the initiation of a genetic consult (Williams & Burns, 2009). These specialty-trained and accredited HCPs provide education and education programs, assist in decision-making processes, and provide support group information.

INBORN ERRORS OF METABOLISM

Keli Hansen and Elizabeth Murphy Waibel

PATHOPHYSIOLOGY

Inborn errors of metabolism (IEM) refer to a group of congenital disorders that result in abnormalities in the synthesis or catabolism of proteins, carbohydrates, or fats. Most are due to a defect in an enzyme or transport protein. They cause an interference with everyday cell processing, specifically with the body's metabolic processes, resulting in either an inability to completely generate a metabolic end product or a buildup of toxic substances (Kamboj, 2008).

IEM can be divided into three groups. Group 1 includes disorders that result in accumulation of toxic compounds. Group 2 encompasses disorders of energy metabolism—that is, mitochondrial and cytoplasmic defects. Group 3 consists of derangements of the synthesis or the catabolism of complex molecules (Saudubray et al., 2006).

EPIDEMIOLOGY AND ETIOLOGY

More than 500 IEMs have been identified by researchers (Kamboj, 2008). The incidence of IEM varies widely, from 1 in 1,400 to 1 in 200,000 live births (Kwon & Tsai, 2007). Early identification with newborn screening is the key to preventing disease progression. Tandem mass spectrometry, the newest method for newborn screening, allows for earlier diagnosis (Raghuveer et al., 2006).

A review of cases from 1969 to 1996 in British Columbia, Canada, provides an estimate of incidence rates (Table 27-4).

Group 1 disorders

Group 1 consists of errors of amino acid catabolism (phenylketonuria, maple syrup urine disease, homocystinuria, tyrosinemia), organic acidurias (methylmalonic, propionic, isovaleric), urea-cycle disorders, sugar intolerances, metal intoxication, and porphyrias.

TABLE 27-4

Inborn Errors of Metabolism: Incidence Rates per 100,000 Births
• Amino acid disorders (excluding phenylketonuria): 7.6 Phenylketonuria: 7.5
• Organic acidemias: 3.7
• Urea-cycle diseases: 1.9
• Glycogen storage diseases: 2.3
• Lysosomal storage diseases: 7.6 Peroxisomal disorders: 3.5
• Mitochondrial diseases: 3.2

Source: Applegarth et al., 2000.

One of the most common IEM is a Group 1 amino acid disorder, phenylketonuria (PKU). Patients with PKU lack the enzyme phenylalanine hydroxylase, which is required to break down phenylalanine. Generally, neonatal screening tests for this disease. If it is not detected then, the infant may present with developmental delay, seizures, and a musty odor to the urine.

Another common IEM in Group 1 is galactosemia, a disorder of carbohydrate metabolism. It is detected early in most infants in the United States through newborn screening (Horslen, 2004). The onset of symptoms—vomiting, diarrhea, lethargy, and hypotonia—can occur within hours of milk ingestion. Ongoing galactose ingestion leads to hemolysis, jaundice, liver disease, lactic acidosis, and renal tubular acidosis. Chronic exposure to galactose can lead to failure-to-thrive, hepatomegaly, splenomegaly, cirrhosis, and cataracts.

Group 1 disorders include six known urea-cycle disorders, each of which is due to a missing enzyme in the cycle. The urea cycle is comprised of a series of biochemical reactions by which ammonia is detoxified. Defects result in an accumulation of ammonia, which is highly neurotoxic. A complete lack of the necessary enzyme results in onset of symptoms within the first 24 hours of life; these symptoms include irritability, vomiting, lethargy, hypotonia, and seizures. A partial enzyme deficiency results in onset of symptoms in later childhood or adulthood. These presentations may be triggered by a stressor or illness and are generally behavioral in nature, but can also be manifested as vomiting, lethargy, or delirium (Summar, 2005).

Group 2 disorders

Mitochondrial defects include lactic acidemias, respiratory chain disorders, and fatty acid oxidation defects. Cytoplasmic energy defects include disorders of glycolysis, glycogen metabolism, and hyperinsulinism. The mitochondrial defects are more severe than the cytoplasmic disorders.

Medium chain acyl-CoA dehydrogenase deficiency is an example of a Group 2 mitochondrial fatty acid oxidation defect. Fatty acid oxidation defects are caused by the deletion of a specific enzyme required to break down fats, which results in the buildup of fatty acids and a decrease in cell energy metabolism. Most children present with hypoglycemia, which in severe cases may be fatal. Hypoglycemia is most often seen after periods of illness and subsequent fasting. Other symptoms at presentation may include lethargy, hypotonia, failure-to-thrive, persistent vomiting, and hepatomegaly.

Group 3 disorders

Group 3 disorders include lysosomal storage disorders, peroxisomal disorders, and disorders of intracellular trafficking and processing (α_1-antitrypsin, congenital disorders of glycosylation, errors of cholesterol synthesis).

An example of a Group 3 disorder is lysosomal storage disease. Approximately 40 different lysosomal storage diseases are known to be related to defects in lysomal function (Winchester et al., 2000). The most common of which are Tay-Sachs, Gaucher, and Fabry diseases. Their symptoms vary among the different diseases, but can include developmental delay, movement disorders, seizures, hepatosplenomegaly, and bony abnormalities.

PRESENTATION

Inborn errors of metabolism, especially in the newborn period, can easily mimic other diseases or infections. The most common presentations are feeding intolerance, a history of vomiting, and altered mental status. As previously described, additional presentations may include failure-to-thrive and neurological deterioration. The relative rarity of these disorders, combined with the fact that presenting symptoms are nonspecific, poses a unique challenge for the health care professional (HCP) who must determine when they should be considered in the differential diagnosis. *An IEM should be considered in the differential diagnosis whenever a previously healthy newborn presents to the emergency department as acutely ill with any of the aforementioned symptoms* (Calvo et al., 2000; Kwon & Tsai, 2007). Determination of the exact diagnosis is not necessary; a high index of suspicion is enough (Kwon & Tsai). The exact diagnosis may take days or even months to confirm (Clay & Hainline, 2007).

The time range between birth and onset of symptoms may be hours to months and provides a clue to the inborn error. For example, urea-cycle disorders and organic acidemias usually present within 12 to 72 hours after birth. Maple syrup urine disease tends to present later in the first week of life. Inborn errors of metabolism that affect the liver, such as neonatal hemochromatosis, may present within the first week of life. Examples of IEM that present after the first week of life include galactosemia, tyrosinemia, and α_1-antitrypsin. Mitochondrial disorders may present at any time.

Evaluation for IEM includes an extensive history, focusing on any prior illnesses or episodes of decompensation, a detailed dietary history including introduction of new foods related to onset of symptoms, and a family history of metabolic disease or members with similar presentations. Consanguinity in parents or grandparents and a family history of early infant death without a known cause are also potential indicators of an IEM (Cleary & Green, 2005).

Specific physical examination findings may be strongly suggestive of an IEM. Neurological symptoms, such as ataxia, lethargy, seizures, and encephalopathy, or liver symptoms, such as hepatosplenomegaly or cholestatic jaundice, may lead the HCP to suspect an IEM. In addition, certain disorders of fatty oxidation may impair myocardial function resulting in cardiomyopathy. In older children with neurologic delays, it is important to consider an undiagnosed IEM (Cleary & Green, 2005). Maple syrup urine disease is characterized by urine that smells like burnt sugar. Methylmalonic and proprionic acidemias have a characteristic ketotic odor (Kwon & Tsai, 2007).

DIFFERENTIAL DIAGNOSIS

The range of IEM involves almost all body systems, and the specific differential diagnosis depends on the presenting symptoms. Infectious, neurologic, and toxicologic etiologies should all be considered as differential diagnoses (Kwon & Tsai, 2007). Table 27-5 provides a summary of IEM based on symptoms at presentation.

PLAN OF CARE

In general, diagnostic studies should include a complete blood count (CBC), electrolytes, glucose, ammonia, blood gas, uric acid, lactate, acyl carnitine profile, plasma, and urine amino acids; in addition, measurements of urine organic acids should be obtained if there is a suspicion of an IEM. Specific laboratory values may help narrow a diagnosis. For example, respiratory alkalosis with hyperammonemia is noted with urea-cycle disorders, whereas hyperammonemia with acidosis is noted in organic acidemias. Lactic acidosis is characteristic of mitochondrial disorders, glycogen storage diseases, disorders of gluconeogenesis and pyruvate metabolism, and fatty acid oxidation disorders. Abnormalities in the acyl carnitine profile, amino acid

TABLE 27-5

Differential Diagnosis for Inborn Errors of Metabolism	
Presenting Symptoms	**Differential Diagnosis**
Lethargy	Sepsis, liver failure, cardiac disease, pulmonary disease
Poor feeding	Food sensitivity, cardiac or pulmonary disease
Vomiting	Gastroenteritis, sepsis, mechanical obstruction, CNS disease, increased intracranial pressure, overfeeding
Respiratory distress	Pulmonary process, infection, cardiac process
Jaundice	Normal neonatal jaundice, liver failure, cystic fibrosis, hepatitis
Seizures	CNS disease, intracranial hemorrhage, electrolyte imbalances, hypoglycemia
Coma	Hyperammonemia, shock
Congestive heart failure	Cardiac defect, cardiomyopathy
Hypotonia	Neurological impairment

profile, and urine organic acids also are indicative of various types of IEM (Kamboj, 2008).

In the emergency setting, when there is a suspicion of metabolic disorder, immediate intervention may prevent long-term sequelae, and even a fatal outcome. Therapeutic management goals are twofold: (1) Remove toxic metabolites (halt any oral intake) and (2) prevent further catabolism by administering parenteral fluid with D_{10} at 1½ times the maintenance level as soon as possible (Kwon & Tsai, 2007). If possible, blood samples should be obtained prior to administration of glucose containing intravenous fluids, as the addition of glucose can alter the results of an organic acid profile, potentially masking the diagnosis (Calvo et al., 2000).

Occasionally it is not possible to control the metabolic abnormalities in this manner, and further steps may be required. Initial control of hyperammonemia can be attempted with sodium benzoate and sodium phenyl butyrate, which prevents ammonia accumulation. If these medications are not effective, hemodialysis is the preferred method of toxic metabolite removal, as it has the highest clearance rate and may also correct acidosis. In a patient who has a rising ammonia level or who has severe hyperammonemia, hemodialysis should be initiated immediately (Leonard & Morris, 2006).

Concurrent treatment for other presenting laboratory abnormalities should be addressed, such as shock, hypoglycemia, electrolyte imbalances, and metabolic acidosis. Additional therapies such as vitamin cocktails, specific therapeutic medications, and specialized diets may be implemented by the metabolic specialist.

Consultation with a genetic and/or metabolic specialist is essential in managing IEM once diagnosed, as therapy is disease specific. The treatment alternatives include limiting the intake of a compound that cannot be metabolized, supplementing a deficient substance, stimulating a different metabolic pathway, providing a cofactor to activate residual enzyme activity, supplying the deficient enzyme, transplanting an organ that supplies the deficient enzyme, and providing gene therapy (Kamboj, 2008). For example, treatment of urea-cycle disorders involves a low-protein diet, medications to aid in the excretion of ammonia, and amino acid supplements.

Caregivers must understand how stressors such as fever, surgery, illness, or accident cause metabolites such as ammonia and amino acid levels to rise. It is common for patients to be hospitalized during these times to stabilize their metabolic profiles.

DISPOSITION AND DISCHARGE PLANNING

Patients already diagnosed with IEM must be treated emergently upon presentation to the emergency department, as delays in their care may lead to significant morbidity or mortality. Clinical pathways should be designed for patients with IEM that expedite triage, initiate the administration

of parenteral glucose, and inform the genetics service of the patient's presence (Zand et al., 2008). Patients are followed by metabolic specialists and should be discharged only with an established follow-up appointment with the metabolic specialist. Serial lab tests and appointments with the nutritionist are also required to maintain steady growth and well-being. Flagging patients with IEM in the hospital system and providing families with letters describing the child's IEM and therapeutic management (Emergency Information Form) can prevent delays in life-saving care. Prognosis depends on the severity of presentation, response to therapy, and comorbidities.

OVERVIEW OF SELECTED GENETIC SYNDROMES

Sarah Pihl

22Q11.2 DELETION SYNDROME (DIGEORGE SYNDROME)

Epidemiology and etiology

The 22q11.2 deletion syndrome encompasses varied disorders including DiGeorge syndrome, velo-cardio-facial syndrome, and conotruncal anomaly face syndrome. The region affected by this mutation is inherited in an autosomal dominant fashion, and approximately 93% of those persons diagnosed with the syndrome have a de novo deletion (McDonald-McGinn et al., 2005).

Presentation

The phenotype of these pediatric patients typically includes cardiac outflow tract abnormalities, dysmorphic features, cleft palate, thymus and parathyroid aplasia or hypoplasia, and velopharyngeal insufficiency (McDonald-McGinn et al., 2005). Affected children typically exhibit mental retardation and growth delay (Thomas & Graham, 1997).

Differential diagnosis

Smith-Lemli-Opitz syndrome, Alagille syndrome, and VACTERL syndrome should be included in the differential diagnosis (McDonald-McGinn et al., 2005).

Diagnostic studies

Fluorescent in situ hybridization (FISH) or comparative genome hybridization (CGH) analysis for a deletion at chromosome 22q11.2 confirms the diagnosis (Thomas & Graham, 1997).

Therapeutic management

Management for 22q11.2 deletion syndrome includes surgical correction of the heart defect and cleft palate.

Frequent otitis media and respiratory tract infections are common (McDonald-McGinn et al., 2005). Annual hearing screenings should be performed to monitor for conductive hearing loss (Thomas & Graham, 1997). Children may have immune dysfunction due to thymus aplasia; thus avoidance of live vaccines and aggressive treatment of infection are recommended (McDonald-McGinn et al.). Rarely, complete absence of T-cell function occurs, so that patients need to be managed aggressively due to the risk of overwhelming infection. Therapeutic options include thymus transplantation, intravenous immunoglobulin infusion, and prophylactic antibiotics (Thomas & Graham).

Hypocalcemia in the newborn period may contribute to seizures. Oral calcium supplementation is the most common treatment, with the imbalance typically resolving by the time the child reaches 1 year of age (Perez & Sullivan, 2002). Speech therapy and early intervention programs during early childhood may aid with language development. Many children are diagnosed with a learning disability in late childhood (Thomas & Graham, 1997).

Speech therapy may prevent the hypernasal speech that many children affected by 22q11.2 deletion syndrome develop and help with any feeding difficulties or language delays. Physical therapy may aid with motor delay (McDonald-McGinn et al., 2005). Initial evaluation of the kidneys by ultrasound should be done to screen for renal anomalies. Cervical spine films should be obtained at approximately 4 years of age to assess for abnormality (McDonald-McGinn et al.).

ANGELMAN SYNDROME

Epidemiology and etiology

Angelman syndrome is caused by a maternal chromosome *SNRPN* deletion, unipaternal disomy (UPD), or imprinting defects in the paternal chromosome (Nussbaum et al., 2007). Abnormal methylation patterns are found in 78% of affected children. Approximately 68% of patients have a deletion in the *SNRPN* gene in chromosome 15q11.2-q13. *UBE3A* abnormalities account for 11% of children with this syndrome (Williams et al., 2008).

Presentation

Children with Angelman syndrome have dysmorphic features, short stature, and severe mental retardation. Gait ataxia, scoliosis, and inappropriately happy demeanor are common findings. Nighttime wakefulness and seizures occur in some children (Williams et al., 2008).

Differential diagnosis

Cerebral palsy, Rett syndrome, and idiopathic static encephalopathy should be included in the differential diagnosis (Williams et al., 2008).

Diagnostic studies

FISH or CGH analysis will assess for deletion of *SNRPN* gene. Methylation studies or imprinting analysis is the next step in diagnosis (Nussbaum et al., 2007). If the methylation studies are normal, sequencing of the gene *UBE3A* is the next diagnostic strategy (Williams et al., 2008).

Therapeutic management

Physical, occupational, and speech therapy may aid in accomplishing milestones, aiding communication, and mitigating feeding difficulties. Antiepileptic agents should be used for managing seizures, and sedatives are helpful in treating nighttime wakefulness (Williams et al., 2008).

CHARGE SYNDROME

Epidemiology and etiology

CHARGE syndrome is caused by a mutation in the *CDH7* gene located on chromosome 8 in 70% of affected children. It is typically a de novo mutation, but is inherited in an autosomal dominant pattern (Lalani et al., 2009).

Presentation

The acronym CHARGE comes from the typical constellation of anomalies associated with the syndrome: coloboma, heart defects, atresia of the choanae, retardation of growth and development, genital anomalies, and ear anomalies (Nussbaum et al., 2007).

Differential diagnosis

VACTERL syndrome, 22q11.2 deletion syndrome, Joubert syndrome, and prenatal exposure to isotretinoin (Accutane) should be included in the differential diagnosis (Lalani et al., 2009).

Diagnostic studies

The clinical diagnostic criteria are divided into major and minor exclusion criteria. Major criteria include coloboma, cranial nerve anomalies (which may present as swallowing difficulties or facial palsy), and outer, middle, and inner ear anomalies. Gene sequencing will support the clinical diagnosis (Lalani et al., 2009).

Therapeutic management

The management of patients with CHARGE syndrome requires many specialty services. Surgical correction of heart defects and choanal atresia is required (Nussbaum et al., 2007). Patients should be evaluated for kidney anomalies and hearing loss. Many patients suffer from feeding difficulties and gastroesophageal reflux. Children with CHARGE syndrome typically have delayed puberty and will require hormone therapy (Lalani et al., 2009).

CYSTIC FIBROSIS

Epidemiology and etiology

Cystic fibrosis is an autosomal recessive disease that affects the function of chloride channels (Boat & Acton, 2007). This dysfunction results in thick, viscous secretions that cause organ dysfunction of the lungs, pancreas, biliary tract, and sweat glands. The gene mutation is located in the *CFTR* gene (Nussbaum et al., 2007).

Presentation

Many children with cystic fibrosis present with poor growth due to chronic lung dysfunction or malabsorption. Others present with meconium ileus or nasal polyps. Frequent pulmonary infections, chronic cough, shortness of breath, and frequent, greasy stools are other symptoms of the disorder (Montgomery & Howenstine, 2009).

Differential diagnosis

Primary ciliary dyskinesia and celiac disease should be included in the differential diagnosis (Montgomery & Howenstine, 2009).

Diagnostic studies

Screening for cystic fibrosis is part of the newborn screening process in most states. The disease is diagnosed with a sweat test that assesses the amount of chloride excreted. A result of 60 mmol/L or greater is definitive for the disease (Montgomery & Howenstine, 2009). Additionally, testing for the *CTFR* mutation may be performed (Nussbaum et al., 2007).

Therapeutic management

Pediatric patients with cystic fibrosis are susceptible to pulmonary infections throughout life. Daily management involves pancreatic enzyme supplementation, bronchodilators, airway clearance techniques, and, for some patients, inhaled antibiotics (Nussbaum et al., 2007). Lung transplant is not curative, but is used to treat severe lung disease. Life expectancy for persons with cystic fibrosis rose to 37.4 years in 2008 (Montgomery & Howenstine, 2009). The reader is encouraged to reference http://ghr.nlm.nih.gov/condition/cystic-fibrosis for more information.

DOWN SYNDROME (TRISOMY 21)

Epidemiology and etiology

Down syndrome, or trisomy 21, is caused by a trisomy event or a Robertsonian translocation (Descartes & Carroll, 2007). Frequently, the Robertsonian translocation occurs between chromosomes 14 and 21. This disorder is a common cause of mental retardation (Nussbaum et al., 2007).

Presentation

Infants with Down syndrome are notably hypotonic. The neck and overall stature are short. Typical facial features include broad nasal bridge, low-set ears, epicanthal folds, brushfield spots (irises), and an open mouth with a protruding tongue (Van Cleve & Cohen, 2006). Hands have a characteristic simian crease (Nussbaum et al., 2007). Many children with Down syndrome have a cardiac defect, such as atrioventricular septal defect, ventricular septal defect (VSD), or tetralogy of Fallot. Gastrointestinal abnormalities typically include duodenal atresia, Hirschsprung's disease, and tracheoesophageal fistula. Hypothyroidism is common. The level of mental retardation in affected individuals varies. In addition, some patients with Down syndrome will have atlantoaxial instability secondary to laxity in the transverse ligament and poor muscle tone (Nussbaum et al.).

Differential diagnosis

Zellweger syndrome and trisomy 18 should be included in the differential diagnosis.

Diagnostic studies

A karyptype or CGH analysis will confirm the diagnosis (Nussbaum et al., 2007).

Therapeutic management

Management of children with Down syndrome is comprehensive and requires the services of an interprofessional team. Cardiac and gastrointestinal abnormalities should be corrected surgically. Children should be monitored for thyroid dysfunction and obstructive sleep apnea. Notably, children with this disorder are prone to chronic ear infections and hearing loss. Evaluation for atlantoaxial instability may be required prior to their participation in certain sports that are more strongly associated with cervical injury. The Special Olympics website is an excellent resource for screening and sport restriction guidelines (http://info.specialolympics.org/Special+Olympics+Public+Website/English/Coach/Coaching_Guides/Basics+of+Special+Olympics/Down+Syndrome+and+Restrictions+Based+on+Atlantoaxial+Instability.htm).

FRAGILE X SYNDROME

Epidemiology and etiology

Fragile X is the most common inherited form of mental retardation. It is caused by gene expansion in the *FMR1* gene on the X chromosome, a mutation that is inherited in an X-linked pattern. As the number of CGG repeats increases, the region becomes unstable and no longer participates in gene expression (Visootsak et al., 2005). This disorder typically becomes evident with repeats of 200 or more copies. Fragile X syndrome causes 3% to 6% of mental retardation incidence in the United States (Nussbaum et al., 2007).

Presentation

The pediatric patient who is affected by fragile X syndrome has moderate mental retardation and developmental delay. Mainly males are affected in this way, with females having milder mental retardation (Nussbaum et al., 2007). The facial appearance becomes more distinctive after puberty, characterized by a long face and large jaw, forehead, and ears (Visootsak et al., 2005). Some children develop seizures.

Differential diagnosis

Autism spectrum disorders have mental retardation and behavior findings in common with fragile X syndrome (Hagerman et al., 2009).

Diagnostic studies

Southern blot analysis will test for expansion of the *FMR1* gene (Nussbaum et al., 2007).

Therapeutic management

Management of children with fragile X syndrome involves behavioral therapy, educational intervention, and medical management of seizures (Hagerman et al., 2009).

MARFAN SYNDROME

Epidemiology and etiology

Marfan syndrome is caused by a mutation in the *FBN1* gene, which is expressed as dysfunction in connective tissues. It is an autosomal dominant disorder, although approximately 25% of affected children have a de novo mutation (Nussbaum et al., 2007).

Presentation

Affected pediatric patients are typically tall and thin. Displacement of the lens, or ectopia lentis, often occurs before the age of 10. Aortic root dilation and mitral valve prolapse are the more common cardiac complications (Dietz, 2009). Children may develop scoliosis, pectus excavatum, or pectus carinatum (Nussbaum et al., 2007). Approximately 60% have dural ectasia, an enlargement of the dura at the lumbosacral level. It is typically asymptomatic; however, some children complain of back and leg pain (Dietz).

Differential diagnosis

Loeys-Dietz syndrome, Stickler syndrome, and Ehlers-Danlos syndrome should be considered in the differential diagnosis (Dietz, 2009).

Diagnostic studies

Clinical diagnosis remains the standard and requires four major criteria: aortic root dilation, ectopia lentis, dural ectasia, and skeletal findings (Robinson & Fitzpatrick, 2007). Gene sequencing will support the diagnosis (Nussbaum et al., 2007).

Therapeutic management

Patients with Marfan syndrome need to be monitored for problems involving their ocular, cardiac, and skeletal systems. Annual echocardiographs are recommended, and patients may require cardiac medications such as beta blockers, calcium-channel blockers, and angiotensin-receptor blockers specific to their defect. Surgery to repair a dilated aorta or dysfunctional valve may be required (Dietz, 2009). Pediatric patients should be instructed to avoid contact sports and strenuous activities due to the strain that these activities place on the aorta (American Academy of Pediatrics, 1996). Scoliosis and pectus excavatum is often treated with bracing and surgery if severe (Nussbaum et al., 2007). Dura ectasia may be serially evaluated with magnetic resonance imaging (MRI) and pain control initiated in symptomatic children (Dietz). Pregnancy in patients with Marfan syndrome should be closely followed because the increased strain on the aorta that pregnancy incurs (Nussbaum et al.).

NOONAN SYNDROME

Epidemiology and etiology

Four genes are strongly associated with Noonan syndrome: *PTPN11, KRAS, SOS1,* and *RAF1.* A defect in the *PTPN11* gene is the most common mutation; it is found in 50% of affected children (Allanson, 2008). This mutation may be inherited in an autosomal dominant pattern, although it is typically a de novo mutation (Noonan, 1994).

Presentation

Children affected by Noonan syndrome have short stature, developmental delay, and cardiac defects (Descartes & Carroll, 2007). They have characteristic facial features such as a tall forehead, hypertelorism, low-set ears, and a short neck with low hairline. Approximately 30% of children will have a coagulation defect (Allanson, 2008).

Differential diagnosis

Turner syndrome, Costello syndrome, and cardiofaciocutaneous syndrome should be included in the differential diagnosis (Allanson, 2008).

Diagnostic studies

Diagnosis is based on the clinical findings. Gene sequencing of *PTPN11, KRAS, SOS1*, and *RAF1* will provide supportive results (Allanson, 2008).

Therapeutic management

Pulmonic stenosis is the major cardiac defect associated with Noonan syndrome and requires surgical correction. Children should have coagulation studies performed, and therapeutic management should include correction of associated defects. Early intervention therapies may help with developmental delay. Some pediatric patients have had success with growth hormone replacement therapy (Allanson, 2008).

PHENYLKETONURIA

Epidemiology and etiology

Phenylketonuria (PKU) is caused by a mutation in the *PAH* gene. This mutation results in a deficiency of phenylalanine hydroxylase activity and disrupts the liver's ability to break down phenylalanine. The disorder follows an autosomal recessive inheritance pattern (Nussbaum et al., 2007).

Presentation

Progressive mental retardation is the classic presentation of PKU (Rezvani, 2007). It is caused by brain damage as phenylalanine (Phe) builds up in the body (Williams, Mamotte, & Burnett, 2008).

Diagnostic studies

PKU testing is part of newborn screening in the United States, with its presence being detected through assay analysis. Plasma Phe levels greater than 1,200 µmol/L also support the diagnosis (Williams et al., 2008).

Therapeutic management

Therapy is lifelong and begins at birth (Nussbaum et al., 2007). Care should be provided by PKU specialists. Notably, the infant diet should consist of a Phe-free formula. A plan of formula feeding and breastfeeding is encouraged. Dietary restrictions are significant and focus on limiting the amount of protein and reducing Phe levels. Levels are monitored weekly for those younger than 1 year of age with a Phe goal of 2–6 mg/dL (120–360 µmol/L) (Rezvani, 2007; Williams et al., 2008). Sapropterin dihydrochloride (Kuvan) may be used to reduce the level of phenylalanine in the blood and has enabled some patients to liberalize their protein intake (Williams et al., 2008). Review the 2000 PKU consensus statement at http://consensus.nih.gov/2000/2000Phenyl ketonuria113PDF.pdf for more details.

PRADER-WILLI SYNDROME

Epidemiology and etiology

The cause in Prader-Willi syndrome is a paternal chromosome *SNRPN* deletion, maternal UPD, or imprinting defect in the maternal chromosome (Nussbaum et al., 2007). Abnormal methylation patterns are found in 99% of affected children. Approximately 70% of these children have a deletion in the *SNRPN* gene in chromosome 15q11.2-q13 (Cassidy & Schwartz, 2009).

Presentation

The phenotype for Prader-Willi Syndrome is comprised of severe hypotonia, feeding difficulties, mental retardation, and dysmorphic features (Chen et al., 2007). As the child grows, the hypotonia persists and the feeding difficulties improve (Nussbaum et al., 2007). Eventually, children develop hyperphagia and are at risk for morbid obesity. Characteristic behaviors include obsessive–compulsive disorder, stubbornness, and manipulation (Cassidy & Schwartz, 2009).

Differential diagnosis

Craniopharyngioma, fragile X syndrome, Bardet-Beidl syndrome, and Cohen syndrome should be included in the differential diagnosis (Cassidy & Schwartz, 2009).

Diagnostic studies

FISH or CGH analysis tests for deletion of the *SNRPN* gene. If there is no deletion, methylation and UPD analysis will provide final diagnosis (Cassidy & Schwartz, 2009).

Therapeutic management

Management options for affected children include growth hormone replacement to ensure adequate height and muscle mass (Chen et al., 2007). Sex hormone treatment may aid in full development of secondary sex characteristics. Cryptorchidism may be treated surgically if it remains a problem. Many pediatric patients with Prader-Willi syndrome benefit from behavioral interventions such as group home living, externally controlled diet, and exercise programs (Nussbaum et al., 2007). Serotonin reuptake inhibitors have proven helpful in treatment of behavioral problems, especially obsessive–compulsive behaviors (Cassidy & Schwartz, 2009).

RETT SYNDROME

Epidemiology and etiology

Rett syndrome is frequently caused by an X-linked dominant mutation in the *MECP2* gene. Dysfunction in this gene is thought to cause abnormal gene activation (Nussbaum et al., 2007).

Presentation

The classic presentation is a young girl who develops normally until 6 to 18 months of age, at which time her developmental progress first slows, and then regresses. Many caregivers note a loss of motor skills and speech. Head circumference growth slows, and microcephaly may develop. Varying degrees of spasticity and ataxia may be present. Repetitive hand wringing is common (Weaving et al., 2005). Children reach a state of stabilization at early school age, but then eventually progress to severe mental retardation. Later in life, seizures and breathing irregularities may present. Scoliosis is common (Nussbaum et al., 2007).

Differential diagnosis

Angelman syndrome, autism spectrum disorders, and cerebral palsy should be considered in the differential diagnosis (Nussbaum et al., 2007).

Diagnostic studies

Clinical diagnosis is based on features and behaviors associated with the syndrome. Gene sequencing of *MECP2* will provide support of the diagnosis (Weaving et al., 2005).

Therapeutic management

The care provided for patients with Rett syndrome is often limited to supportive therapy (Weaving et al., 2005). Pharmacologic therapy may be of some use for motor difficulties, breathing disturbances, or seizures; nevertheless, seizures may be very difficult to control. Early intervention therapies may provide additional help to improve motor skills and preserve mobility (Nussbaum et al., 2007).

TRISOMY 13

Epidemiology and etiology

Trisomy 13, also known as Patau syndrome, is a chromosomal disorder caused by an extra chromosome 13 (Nussbaum et al., 2007).

Presentation

Infants with trisomy 13 have severe central nervous system anomalies. Many also have a cleft lip and palate, polydactyly, and rocker-bottom feet (Descartes & Carroll, 2007). Cardiac defects—in particular, ventricular septal defects—are common. Trisomy 13 is often termed a "lethal anomaly," as many of those children affected by this disorder die within the first months of life. However, with supportive care, others may now expect a longer life span, albeit with significant abnormalities (Nussbaum et al., 2007).

Differential diagnosis

Meckel–Gruber syndrome, Smith-Lemli-Opitz syndrome, and trisomy 18 should be included in the differential diagnosis (Nussbaum et al., 2007).

Diagnostic studies

A karyotype or CGH analysis will provide definitive diagnosis (Nussbaum et al., 2007).

Therapeutic management

Surgical correction of cardiac defects may improve survival time. Hospice care may be provided to enhance comfort for those with shortened life spans.

TRISOMY 18

Epidemiology and etiology

Trisomy 18, also known as Edwards syndrome, is a chromosomal disorder caused by an extra chromosome 18 (Nussbaum et al., 2007).

Presentation

Persons who are affected by trisomy 18 have mental retardation, low-set ears, rocker-bottom feet; and hypertonia. A characteristic clenched fist is observed, with the second and fifth fingers overlapping the third and fourth digits

(Nussbaum et al., 2007). As with trisomy 13, cardiac defects are common, including ventricular septal defects (VSD), atrial septal defects (ASD), and coarctation of the aorta (COA) (Nussbaum et al.). Infants with trisomy 18 also have a poor survival rate; however, a small percentage live beyond the first year of life and will have severe handicaps (Descartes & Carroll, 2007).

Differential diagnosis

Pena-Shokeir syndrome and trisomy 13 should be included in the differential diagnosis (Nussbaum et al., 2007).

Diagnostic studies

A karyotype or CGH analysis will provide a definitive diagnosis (Nussbaum et al., 2007).

Therapeutic management

Surgical correction of cardiac defects may improve survival time. Hospice care may be provided to enhance comfort for those with shortened life spans.

TURNER SYNDROME

Epidemiology and etiology

Turner syndrome is a chromosomal disorder resulting from a lack of a second sex chromosome as noted by a typical karyotype of 45,X. The loss of the sex chromosome typically occurs early in the reproductive process during the formation of the gamete (i.e., when egg and sperm meet) (Nussbaum et al., 2007).

Presentation

Cystic hygroma on prenatal ultrasound is often the first abnormality noted. Newborn lymphedema is common. Characteristic features include short stature, a webbed neck, and a broad chest (Nussbaum et al., 2007). Cardiac defects are typical, with as many as 50% of affected children having a bicuspid aortic valve. Coarctation of the aorta is the second most common cardiac finding (Doswell et al., 2006). Most patients exhibit problems with infertility, and some may not present for evaluation until there is a delay in puberty or amenorrhea (Rapaport, 2007). Kidney anomalies are common—for example, horseshoe-shaped kidneys or double collecting systems—although most of these defects do not interfere with renal function (Doswell et al.).

Differential diagnosis

Noonan syndrome and XY gonadal agenesis syndrome should be considered in the differential diagnosis (Noonan, 1994).

Diagnostic studies

A karyotype or CGH analysis will confirm diagnosis. These tests may also be done prenatally (Nussbaum et al., 2007).

Therapeutic management

The patient's cardiac and kidney anatomy should be evaluated with an echocardiograph and renal ultrasound. Surgical management for COA is usually required, and evaluation by a pediatric cardiologist is recommended for those patients with bicuspid aortic valve. Affected children are at risk for aortic root dilation and valvular disease (Nussbaum et al., 2007).

If an individual with Turner syndrome falls below the fifth percentile on the growth curve, an endocrine consultation is warranted. In such patients, growth hormone replacement therapy may be appropriate. Timing, dose, and duration of therapy determine the success of this treatment. Many patients gain approximately 4 inches of additional height with the use of growth hormone replacement therapy. Estrogen therapy to support the development of secondary sex characteristics should not be started until growth hormone treatment nears completion, as growth hormone decreases the effectiveness of estrogen therapy (Nussbaum et al., 2007). Progesterone therapy may be initiated to aid in the onset of menstruation. Estrogen therapy is typically a long-term treatment for these pediatric patients to help maintain normal sexual function and reduce the risk of osteoporosis (Hjerrild et al., 2008).

VACTERL/VATER ASSOCIATION

Epidemiology and etiology

To date, no specific gene has been identified as causing VACTERL association, although mouse models involving a mutation in the *SHH* gene produce a similar phenotype to the disorder (Kim et al., 2001). Other research has suggested that this condition is an autosomal dominant disorder. There is also a higher incidence of VACTERL association in the children of diabetic mothers.

Presentation

VACTERL association is named after its common features: vertebral anomalies, imperforate anus or anal atresia, cardiac defects, tracheoesophageal fistula or esophageal atresia, renal anomalies, and limb anomalies. Ventricular and atrial septal defects and tetralogy of Fallot are the most commonly observed cardiac abnormalities (Miller & Kolon, 2001).

Differential diagnosis

Trisomy 13, trisomy 18, PHAVER syndrome, and Townes syndrome should be included in the differential diagnosis (Shaw-Smith, 2006).

Diagnostic studies

VACTERL or VATER association is diagnosed clinically by the presence of three or more of the primary features (Miller & Kolon, 2001).

Therapeutic management

Cardiac and gastrointestinal malformations should be managed surgically (Orenstein et al., 2007). If vertebral anomalies are present, the child should be monitored for scoliosis. A renal evaluation and monitoring of kidney function may aid in prevention of kidney failure (Miller & Kolon, 2001).

WILLIAMS SYNDROME

Epidemiology and etiology

A deletion in the *WBSCR* gene at 7q11.23 is responsible for Williams syndrome. This syndrome is inherited in an autosomal dominant manner, but de novo mutations are common (Morris, 2006).

Presentation

Affected children often have a cardiac defect, most commonly supravalvular aortic stenosis (Bernstein, 2007). They are usually short, with a distinctive facial appearance of broad brow, full lips, wide mouth, short nose, and a stellate iris pattern (Morris, 2006). Mental retardation, feeding difficulties, and a distinctive personality are typical (Kaplan, 2002). Patients are excessively social but may suffer from anxiety. Some children also have hypercalciuria (Kaplan).

Differential diagnosis

Noonan syndrome, Smith-Magenis syndrome, 22q11.2 deletion syndrome, and fetal alcohol syndrome are other syndromes with similar features (Morris, 2006).

Diagnostic studies

FISH analysis is the primary diagnostic test. Approximately 99% of children with Williams syndrome have the previously mentioned deletion in the *WBSCR* gene (Morris, 2006).

Therapeutic management

Heart defects should be evaluated by a pediatric cardiologist and may require surgical intervention. Early intervention programs and behavioral counseling are helpful in managing disabilities and behavior problems (Morris, 2006). If hypercalciuria is present, the child's calcium intake should be restricted and serum calcium levels monitored. Consultation with a kidney specialist is warranted. Patients should avoid vitamin supplementation due to their abnormal calcium and vitamin D metabolism. Monitoring for diabetes, thyroid function, cataracts, and other cardiac conditions such as mitral valve prolapse is necessary (Morris).

REFERENCES

1. Allanson, J. (2008). Noonan syndrome. *GeneReviews*. Retrieved from http://www.ncbi.nlm.nih.gov/bookshelf/br.fcgi?book=gene&part=noonan
2. American Academy of Pediatrics (AAP). (1996). Committee on Genetics: Health supervision for children with Marfan syndrome. *Pediatrics, 98*(5), 978–982.
3. Applegarth, D., Toone J., & Lowry, R. (2000). Incidence of inborn errors of metabolism in British Columbia, 1969–1996. *Pediatrics, 105*(1), e10.
4. Bernstein, D. (2007). Peripheral pulmonary stenosis. In R. Kliegman, R. Behrman, H. Jenson, & B. Stanton (Eds.), *Nelson textbook of pediatrics* (p. 1897). Philadelphia: Saunders-Elsevier.
5. Boat, T., & Acton, J. (2007). Cystic fibrosis. In R. Kliegman, R. Behrman, H. Jenson, & B. Stanton (Eds.), *Nelson textbook of pediatrics* (pp. 1803–1817). Philadelphia: Saunders-Elsevier.
6. Calvo, M., Artuch, R., Macia, E., Luaces, C., Vilaseca, M., Pou, J., et al. (2000). Diagnostic approach to inborn errors of metabolism in an emergency unit. *Pediatric Emergency Care, 16*(6), 405–408.
7. Cassidy, S., & Schwartz, S. (2009). Prader-Willi syndrome. *GeneReviews*. Retrieved from http://www.ncbi.nlm.nih.gov/bookshelf/br.fcgi?book=gene&part=pws
8. Chen, C., Visootsak, J., Dills, S., & Graham, J. (2007). Prader-Willi syndrome: An update for the primary pediatrician. *Clinical Pediatrics, 46*(7), 580–591.
9. Clay, A., & Hainline, B. (2007). Hyperammonemia in the ICU. *Chest, 132*(4), 1368–1378.
10. Cleary, M., & Green, A. (2005). Developmental delay: When to suspect and how to investigate for an inborn error of metabolism. *Archives of Diseases in Childhood, 90*, 1128–1132.
11. Descartes, M., & Carroll, A. (2007). Cytogenetics. In R. Kliegman, R. Behrman, H. Jenson, & B. Stanton (Eds.), *Nelson textbook of pediatrics* (pp. 502–517). Philadelphia: Saunders-Elsevier.
12. Dietz, H. (2009). Marfan syndrome. *GeneReviews*. Retrieved from http://www.ncbi.nlm.nih.gov/bookshelf/br.fcgi?book=gene&part=marfan
13. Doswell, B., Visootsak, J., Brady, A., & Graham, J. (2006). Turner syndrome: An update and review for the primary pediatrician. *Clinical Pediatrics, 45*(4), 301–313.
14. Hagerman, R., Berry-Kravis, E., Kaufman, W., Ono, M., Tartaglia, N., Lachiewicz, A., et al. (2009). Advances in the treatment of fragile X syndrome. *Pediatrics, 123*(1), 378–390.
15. Hjerrild, B., Mortensen, K., & Gravholt, C. (2008). Turner syndrome and clinical treatment. *British Medical Bulletin, 86*, 77–93.
16. Horslen, S. (2004). Carbohydrate metabolism. In W. Walker, O. Goulet, R. Kleinman, P. Sherman, B. Shneider, & I. Sanderson (Eds.), *Pediatric gastrointestinal disease: Pathophysiology, diagnosis, management* (4th ed., Vol. 2, pp. 1257–1274). Hamilton: BC Decker.
17. Kamboj, M. (2008). Clinical approaches to the diagnoses of inborn errors of metabolism. *Pediatric Clinics of North America, 55*(5), 1113–1117.
18. Kaplan, P. (2002). Williams syndrome: Does early diagnosis matter? *Clinical Pediatrics, 47*(4), 277–280.
19. Kim, J., Kim, P., & Hui, C. (2001). The VACTERL association: Lessons from the Sonic Hedgehog pathway. *Clinical Genetics, 59*, 306–315.

20. Korf, B. (2007a). The human genome. In R. Kliegman, R. Behrman, H. Jenson, & B. Stanton (Eds.), *Nelson textbook of pediatrics* (pp. 487–492). Philadelphia: Saunders-Elsevier.

21. Korf, B. (2007b). Integration of genetics into pediatric practice. In R. Kliegman, R. Behrman, H. Jenson, & B. Stanton (Eds.), *Nelson textbook of pediatrics* (pp. 522–527). Philadelphia: Saunders-Elsevier.

22. Kwon, K., & Tsai, V. (2007). Metabolic emergencies. *Emergency Medicine Clinics of North America, 25*(4), 1041–1060.

23. Lalani, S., Hefner, M., Belmont, J., & Davenport, S. (2009). CHARGE syndrome. *GeneReviews.* Retrieved from http://www.ncbi.nlm.nih.gov/bookshelf/br.fcgi?book=gene&part=charge

24. Leonard, J., & Morris, A. (2006). Diagnosis and early management of inborn errors of metabolism presenting around the time of birth. *Acta Paediatrica, 95*(1), 6–14.

25. McDonald-McGinn, D., Emanuel, B., & Zackai, E. (2005). 22q11.2 deletion syndrome. *GeneReviews.* Retrieved from http://www.ncbi.nlm.nih.gov/bookshelf/br.fcgi?book=gene&part=gr_22q11deletion

26. Miller, O., & Kolon, T. (2001). Prenatal diagnosis of VACTERL association. *Journal of Urology, 166*, 2389–2391.

27. Montgomery, G., & Howenstine, M. (2009). Cystic fibrosis. *Pediatrics in Review, 30*, 302–310.

28. Morris, C. (2006). Williams syndrome. *GeneReviews.* Retrieved from http://www.ncbi.nlm.nih.gov/bookshelf/br.fcgi?book=gene&part=williams

29. Noonan, J. (1994). Noonan syndrome: An update and review for the primary pediatrician. *Clinical Pediatrics, 33*(9), 548–555.

30. Nussbaum, R., McInnes, R., & Willard, H. (Eds.). (2007). *Thompson & Thompson: Genetics in medicine* (7th ed.). Philadelphia: Saunders Elsevier.

31. Orenstein, S., Peters, J., Khan, S., Youssef, N., & Hussain, S. Z. (2007). Congenital anomalies: Esophageal atresia and tracheoesophageal fistula. In R. Kliegman, R. Behrman, H. Jenson, & B. Stanton (Eds.), *Nelson textbook of pediatrics* (pp. 1543–1544). Philadelphia: Saunders-Elsevier.

32. Perez, E., & Sullivan, K. (2002). Chromosome 22q11.2 deletion syndrome (DiGeorge and velocardiofacial syndromes). *Current Opinion in Pediatrics, 14*, 678–683.

33. Raghuveer, T., Garg, U., & Graf, W. (2006). Inborn errors of metabolism in infancy and early childhood: An update. *American Family Physician, 73*(11), 1981–1990.

34. Rapaport, R. (2007). Hypergonadotropic hypogonadism in the female (primary hypogonadism). In R. Kliegman, R. Behrman, H. Jenson, & B. Stanton (Eds.), *Nelson textbook of pediatrics* (pp. 2386–2389). Philadelphia: Saunders-Elsevier.

35. Rezvani, I. (2007). Phenylalanine. In R. Kliegman, R. Behrman, H. Jenson, & B. Stanton (Eds.), *Nelson textbook of pediatrics* (pp. 529–532). Philadelphia: Saunders-Elsevier.

36. Robin, N. H. (2007). Patterns of genetic transmission. In R. Kliegman, R. Behrman, H. Jenson, & B. Stanton (Eds.), *Nelson textbook of pediatrics* (pp. 492–502). Philadelphia: Saunders-Elsevier.

37. Robinson, L., & Fitzpatrick, E. (2007). Marfan syndrome. In R. Kliegman, R. Behrman, H. Jenson, & B. Stanton (Eds.), *Nelson textbook of pediatrics* (pp. 2890–2893). Philadelphia: Saunders-Elsevier.

38. Saudubray, J., Sedel, F., & Walter, J. (2006). Clinical approach to treatable inborn metabolic diseases: An introduction. *Journal of Inherited Metabolic Diseases, 29*, 261–274.

39. Shaw–Smith, C. (2006). Oesophageal atresia, tracheo-oesophageal fistula, and the VACTERL association: Review of genetics and epidemiology. *Journal of Medical Genetics, 43*, 545–554.

40. Summar, M. (2005). Urea cycle disorders overview. In R. Pagon, T. Bird, C. Dolan, & K. Stephens (Eds.), *GeneReviews.* Seattle: University of Washington. Retrieved from http://www.ncbi.nlm.nih.gov/pubmed/20301396

41. Thomas, J., & Graham, J. (1997). Chromosome 22q11 deletion syndrome: An update and review for the primary pediatrician. *Clinical Pediatrics, 36*(5), 253–266.

42. Van Cleve, S., & Cohen, W. (2006). Part I: Clinical practice guidelines for children with Down syndrome from birth to 12 years. *Journal of Pediatric Health Care, 20*, 47–54.

43. Visootsak, J., Warren, S., Anido, A., & Graham, J. (2005). Fragile X syndrome: An update and review for the primary pediatrician. *Clinical Pediatrics, 44*(5), 371–381.

44. Weaving, L., Ellaway, C., Gécz, J., & Christodoulou, J. (2005). Rett syndrome: Clinical review and genetic update. *Journal of Medical Genetics, 42*, 1–7.

45. Williams, C., Dagli, A., & Driscoll, D. (2008). Angelman syndrome. *GeneReviews.* Retrieved from http://www.ncbi.nlm.nih.gov/bookshelf/br.fcgi?book=gene&part=angelman

46. Williams, J., & Burns, C. (2009). Genetic disorders. In C. Burns, A. Dunn, M. Brady, N. Starr, & C. Blosser (Eds.), *Pediatric primary care* (pp. 1111–1133). St. Louis: Saunders Elsevier.

47. Williams, R., Mamotte, C., & Burnett, J. (2008). Phenylketonuria: An inborn error of phenylalanine metabolism. *Clinical Biochemist Reviews, 29*, 31–41.

48. Winchester, B., Vellodi, A., & Young, E. (2000). The molecular basis of lysosomal storage diseases and their treatment. *Biochemical Society Transactions, 28*(2), 150–154.

49. Zand, D., Brown, K., Lichter-Konecki, U., Campbell, J., Salehi, V., & Chamberlain, J. (2008). Effectiveness of a clinical pathway for the emergency treatment of patients with inborn errors of metabolism. *Pediatrics, 122*, 1191–1195.

Hematologic and Oncologic Disorders

PHYSIOLOGY AND DIAGNOSTICS

Leonard A. Valentino

BLOOD PHYSIOLOGY

Blood is considered the vital humor for human life. It consists of the plasma (55%) and formed elements (45%), including cellular components and platelets (Alkire & Collingwood, 1990). Plasma is mostly water (90%), with 7% to 8% soluble proteins (albumin to maintain the osmotic pressure of blood, globulins, coagulation proteins), 1% electrolytes, and 1% other components. The principal function of the blood is to facilitate the delivery of oxygen and nutrients to the tissues so that aerobic function may occur (Martin, 1995). Tissues such as the heart and brain are oxygen-supply-dependent organs; in contrast, the organs of the splanchnic area, kidneys, skin, and resting muscle are oxygen-supply-independent organs (Bryan-Brown, 1988).

Oxygen is carried by hemoglobin, an iron-containing tetrameric protein composed of four globin molecules: two alpha-globin chains and two beta-globin chains (Perutz, 1969). The alpha- and beta-globin chains are composed of 141 and 146 amino acids, respectively. Each globin chain contains one heme molecule—a porphyrin ring composed of four pyrrole molecules linked together with an iron ion held tightly at the center of the molecule (Perutz, 1979). In adult hemoglobin (hemoglobin A), there are two alpha and two beta chains; in the fetus, the two alpha chains are paired with two gamma chains to make fetal hemoglobin (Oski & Gottlieb, 1971).

Other functions of blood include the transport of electrolytes (e.g., sodium), nutrients (e.g., glucose), and waste products (e.g., urea nitrogen), as well as maintenance of immune surveillance for danger signals (Gallucci & Matzinger, 2001; Matzinger, 1994; Pedra et al., 2009). To accomplish these tasks, blood must be maintained in a fluid state. The hemostatic system is vital to this role monitoring for breaches in vascular integrity (Smyth et al., 2009; Tanaka et al., 2009). The role of platelets, circulating factors promoting and regulating coagulation, and vascular components including subendothelial collagen and tissue factor are critical to this function (Butenas et al., 2009; Smith, 2009). It is also clear that these functional roles of blood, coagulation and immunity, cannot be easily separated and should be viewed as inextricably linked (Delvaeye & Conway, 2009).

Erythropoiesis and hemoglobin synthesis

Erythropoiesis, the production of red blood cells, involves not only cell proliferation but also differentiation. It is regulated by a network of signal transduction proteins and stimulatory and inhibitory cytokines (Nienhuis & Benz, 1977a, 1977b, 1977c; Ratajczak, 1994). Key to this process is hemoglobin synthesis, which follows the orderly process of eukaryotic protein biosynthesis. Transcription of the globin messenger ribonucleic acid (mRNA) is followed by translation of the globin polypeptide chains during the process of red cell development (Schmidt, 1972; Schweet et al., 1964; Weatherall & Clegg, 1969). During red cell maturation, the nucleus is extruded, following which globin biosynthesis ceases, resulting in a finite life span for the polypeptide chains (Smith, 1980). Structurally abnormal hemoglobins may be the result of single nucleotide base substitutions, leading to amino acid replacement or chain termination variants; nucleotide deletions or insertions, leading to deletion and frameshift mutations; and nonhomologous crossing over, leading to the production of fused globin chains (Forget, 1979). The thalassemia syndromes, which are characterized by absent or decreased synthesis of alpha- or beta-globin chains may be due to globin gene deletions, defect in globin gene transcription, or mRNA processing or stability (Forget).

Hemoglobin function, effects, and role in oxygen delivery

Oxygen delivery is the key function of the blood and can be expressed as the product of the blood flow (Q) and oxygen content of the blood ($QO_2 = Q \times O_2$ content). When QO_2 falls below a critical threshold, tissue O_2 uptake (VO_2) is limited by QO_2.

Hemoglobin carries oxygen in the blood, and its content can be assessed by measuring P_{50}, the partial pressure of oxygen at which the hemoglobin is 50% saturated. Normal P_{50} is 26 mmHg at 37°C (98.6°F) and a plasma pH of 7.40 (Figure 28-1).

Oxygen is taken up by hemoglobin in the lungs, where the partial pressure is high, and then released to the tissues, where the partial pressure is low. The affinity of hemoglobin for oxygen is regulated by chemical factors as well as the presence of oxygen. In the lungs, where the oxygen levels are high, hemoglobin has a higher affinity for oxygen, and this affinity increases disproportionately with each molecule of oxygen bound to it, a process known as cooperativity. Regulators of P_{50} include 2,3-diphosphoglycerate (2,3-DPG), the intracellular red cell and extracellular pH, and the proportions of adult and fetal hemoglobin or other variants present in the red cells (Aberman & Hew, 1985). As the concentration of protons (decreasing pH) or carbon dioxide increases, the affinity of hemoglobin for oxygen decreases, resulting in unloading of oxygen in hypoxic tissues, the so-called *Bohr effect* (Bucci & Fronticelli, 1981). The oxygen affinity of blood may be increased (reduced P_{50}) or decreased (increased P_{50}) due to amino acid substitutions (Novy et al., 1967), or reduced by increasing concentrations of 2,3-DPG or alkalosis (Bohr effect).

TRANSFUSION PHYSIOLOGY

Transfusion of blood may have been first attempted in 1492, as a means to treat the dying Pope Innocent VIII, who was in a coma. The first successful transfusion was administered, however, by Dr. Jean-Baptiste Denys on

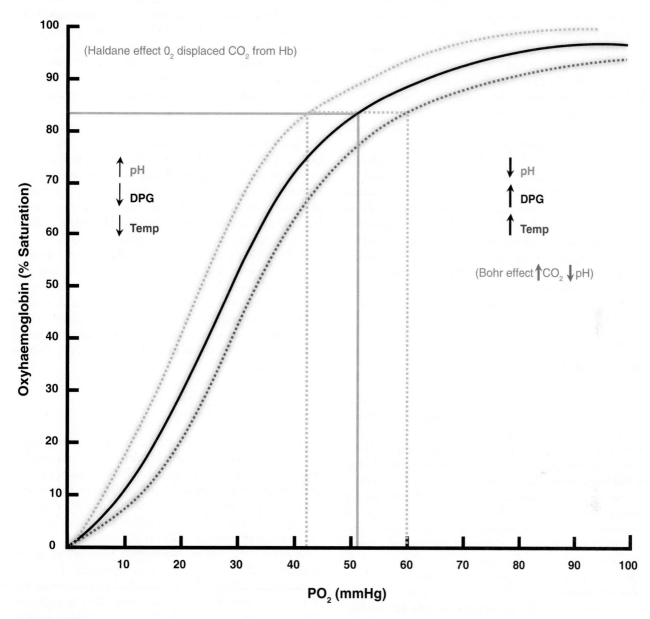

FIGURE 28-1

Oxyhemoglobin Dissociation Curve.

June 15, 1667, when blood from a sheep was transfused into a young boy. The modern age of transfusion began in 1901, when Landsteiner discovered the human blood groups—A, B, AB, and O (Kulkarni & Gera, 1999). Pretransfusion testing to determine the ABO and Rh blood type is now routinely performed (Table 28-1).

Serologic "reverse" typing is not performed in infants younger than 4 months of age, however, as all antibodies present are maternal in origin. Due to the complexity of neonatal transfusion, typically only group O blood is transfused into neonates and young infants. The guidelines for transfusion of red blood cells vary, but typically neonates with symptomatic anemia and hemoglobin values

TABLE 28-1

Blood Groups			
Blood Group Designation	**Red Blood Cell Antigen Expression**	**Serum Antibody Present**	**Donor Selection**
A	A	Anti-B	A or O
B	B	Anti-A	B or O
AB	A and B	None	Either A or B or AB or O
O	Neither A nor B	Anti-A and anti-B	O only

less than 7 gm/dL, those with hemoglobin values less than 10 gm/dL and in need of supplemental oxygen therapy, and those requiring ventilatory support with hemoglobin values less than 12 gm/dL are transfused with packed red blood cells. Most infants can tolerate volumes of packed red blood cells in the range of 10 to 20 mL per kg body weight. The hematocrit of stored red blood cells varies from 55% to 75%; hence, the expected increase in the hemoglobin concentration following administration of a transfusion should be approximately 2 gm/dL per 10 mL/kg transfused.

When possible, blood stored for less than 5 days should be used, as its potassium concentration is lower and its 2,3-DPG concentration higher. In addition, care should be taken to consider the impact of the storage medium used to collect the blood. For example, CPD-A contains 2,000 mg dextrose, 17.3 mg adenine, 1,660 mg trisodium citrate, 206 mg citric acid, and 140 mg monobasic sodium phosphate per 63 mL. The risk of electrolyte disturbances following transfusion, including hypocalcemia, must be considered whenever a transfusion is contemplated (Roseff et al., 2002).

BONE MARROW PHYSIOLOGY

Constituting approximately 4% of the total body weight, the bone marrow is a remarkably flexible organ found within the hollow cavity of primarily the flat and long bones. The color of the marrow varies depending on the fat content. Red marrow is hematopoietically active, producing red and white blood cells and platelets, whereas yellow marrow contains a predominance of fat. Within the marrow are a variety of stromal cells, including osteoblasts, osteoclasts, fibroblasts, macrophages, adipocytes, and endothelial cells. Macrophages are abundant within red marrow and serve as a source of iron for erythropoiesis.

Bone marrow contains three types of stem cells. Those of the hematopoietic system give rise to erythrocytes, leukocytes, and platelets. Mesenchymal stem cells differentiate into osteoblasts, chondrocytes, and myocytes. Endothelial stem cells are the basis of blood vessels.

Marrow cells are retained within the marrow space due to a combination of adhesive receptors and the endothelial barrier restricting passage of cells into the vessels within the marrow cavity (Alkire & Collingwood, 1990; Bianco et al., 1999; Hays, 1990).

CELL-BASED COAGULATION

Coagulation normally occurs on the surface of fibroblasts and activated monocytes; pathologically (Roberts et al.,

2006), it takes place on tumor and other cells. Tissue factor (TF) is the main initiator of coagulation (Nemerson, 1987, 1992; Nemerson & Pitlick, 1972) and functions in a cell-based model of thrombin generation. Activated monocytes provide a source of TF, whereas platelets are a source of phospholipids for thrombin generation. Monocytes are activated by various stimuli, including thrombin and cytokines, and they express cell-bound TF.

Zymogen factor VII (FVII) and its activated enzyme FVIIa are bound by TF, a process that results in the activation of FX to FXa and FIX to FIXa. FXa remains on the surface of the TF-bearing cell and, in the presence of FVa, converts a small amount of prothrombin to thrombin on the surface of the TF cell. This small amount of thrombin, which is not sufficient to convert fibrinogen to fibrin is, however, sufficient to activate platelets, FVIII, FV, and FXI. Following platelet activation, phospholipid-docking sites are exposed and binding of FVIIIa, FVa, and FXa occurs. FIXa, which is activated by TF-FVIIa, translocates to the platelet surface and converts FX to FXa. A burst of thrombin generation occurs after FXIa enhances FIXa generation on the activated platelet, thereby leading to greater production of FXa (Monroe & Hoffman, 2006; Roberts et al., 2006).

FIBRINOLYTIC SYSTEM

Activation of the coagulation mechanism generates thrombin, which in turn activates platelets, stimulates production of thrombin activatable fibrinolysis inhibitor (TAFI), and converts fibrinogen to fibrin, resulting in a thrombus. TAFI circulates in plasma as an inactive precursor; its conversion in the active enzyme (TAFIa) occurs via the action of thrombin or plasmin (Miljic et al., 2010).

Plasmin, the major fibrinolytic protease, is generated from the circulating plasma zymogen, known as plasminogen (PLG). PLG is converted to plasmin by one of two activators: tissue PLG activator (tPA) or urokinase (uPA) (Cesarman-Maus & Hajjar, 2005). Plasmin, in turn, cleaves both of its positive regulators, transforming tPA and uPA from single-chain peptides into more active two-chain polypeptides.

Although the major substrate for plasmin is fibrin within the thrombus, it may also bind circulating fibrin and fibrinogen. Fibrin degradation is enhanced by binding both PLG and tPA on its surface, a process that serves to localize the fibrinolytic mechanism to the site of the thrombus (Cesarman-Maus & Hajjar, 2005). TAFI downregulates the fibrinolytic mechanism and is considered to be the molecular link between coagulation and fibrinolysis (Miljic et al., 2010).

ANEMIA

Audrey Taylor and Leonard Valentino

APLASTIC ANEMIA

Pathophysiology

Aplastic anemia (AA) is a life-threatening disease of bone marrow failure. It is characterized by a reduction, absence, or severe dysplasia of the bone marrow hematopoietic elements. The causative injury in AA is thought to be a direct injury to the pluripotent stem cells. Results of bone marrow aspirate are remarkable for an absence of hematopoietic elements and an increase in fat cells, plasma cells, and mast cells. Decreased production of hematopoietic stem cells ultimately results in peripheral pancytopenia and bone marrow aplasia. In acquired AA, glycoprotein A—a transmembrane linker protein—is absent in approximately 20% of patients, as indicated by the absence of CD 55 and CD 59 (Bakhshi, 2009).

Aplastic anemia may be either congenital (20%) or acquired (80%). Three phases of AA have been identified: onset of disease, recovery, and late disease. The onset of the disease generally occurs when the immune system becomes activated in response to an initiating event (e.g., viral infection, drug exposure). During the recovery phase, stem cells begin to reproduce. A relapse of pancytopenia can cause the occurrence of late disease years after the initial onset of disease (Bakhshi, 2009).

Epidemiology and etiology

Aplastic anemia is a rare disorder. Its annual incidence in the United States is approximately 0.6 to 6.1 cases per 1 million population. The annual incidence internationally is approximately 2 cases per 1 million population in Europe and 4 to 14 cases per 1 million population in Asia. The incidence of AA usually peaks during three age periods, 2–5 years, 20–25 years, and after 60 years. The prevalence is roughly equal among males and females (Bakhshi, 2009).

Acquired AA may be caused by idiopathic, constitutional, or iatrogenic factors. Patients who present with idiopathic AA may have a history of recent exposure to drugs, chemicals, ionizing radiation, or viruses. Patients who present with iatrogenic AA often report a history of exposure to drugs or radiation. Affected individuals who have been exposed to drugs, chemicals, or radiation typically have transient marrow failure. Exposure to drugs or chemicals account for approximately 11% to 20% of all cases. Patients with constitutional AA have a congenital or genetic predisposition to bone marrow failure (Bakhshi, 2009).

Presentation

Patients typically seek medical attention when they become symptomatic with increased morbidity and mortality attributed to infections and bleeding. Symptom severity depends on the level of pancytopenia. Patients may present either with an insidious onset or after a chronic course. For most individuals, the history is remarkable for mucosal/gingival bleeding, headaches, fatigue, easy bruising, rash, fever, mucosal ulcerations, and recurrent viral infections. Physical examination findings may include pallor, tachycardia, petechial rash, purpura, ecchymoses, or jaundice (Bakhshi, 2009; Lieberman et al., 2009; Shimamura, 2009).

Differential diagnosis

Several disorders may present with pancytopenia and bone marrow suppression and must be distinguished from AA. These conditions include viral infections, drug exposures, toxic exposures, myelodysplastic syndromes, and congenital abnormalities.

Plan of care

A comprehensive diagnostic evaluation is required to confirm the diagnosis of AA. Diagnostic studies include a complete blood cell count (CBC) with differential, reticulocyte count, peripheral blood smear, and bone marrow aspirate (BMA) and biopsy. CBC results reveal pancytopenia. Reticulocytes are absent or severely depressed. Peripheral blood smears are instrumental in distinguishing aplasia from infiltrative and dysplastic causes. Results of BMA and biopsy are remarkable for reduction or absence of hematopoietic elements (Guinan, 2009).

Obtaining a successful outcome depends on several factors: the patient's age at the time of diagnosis, the availability of a histocompatible family donor, the level of organ destruction, the capacity for tissue regeneration, the ability to develop a therapeutic regimen that will control a misdirected and extraordinarily potent immune response, and the patient's level of commitment.

Therapeutic management consists of transfusions of red blood cells (RBCs) and platelets, antibiotic therapy, surgery, and bone marrow transplantation (BMT) or immunosuppressive therapy for patients who are unable to receive a BMT. Prior to undergoing immunosuppressive therapy or bone marrow transplant, patients typically have a central venous catheter placed by a surgeon or interventional radiologist to facilitate care.

Patients who have severe anemia will receive blood transfusion therapy with nonrelated, irradiated, leukoreduced, and cytomegalovirus (CMV)-negative RBCs.

Fevers are managed with empiric antibiotic therapy offering Gram-negative and staphylococcal coverage. Once the diagnosis of AA has been confirmed, patients who qualify will undergo a BMT with either an HLA-matched sibling or unrelated donor (Bakhshi, 2009). Immunosuppressive therapy is the treatment of choice if a histocompatible donor is not available for the patient.

Upon presentation, patients need to be referred to a hematologist, BMT specialist, social worker, dietician, and surgeon for consultation. An interprofessional team approach is critical for patients and their family members during this time to review the disease process, develop an individualized treatment plan, and identify resources and barriers. Patient and family education is critical to ensure that all involved fully understand the course of the disease, the level of commitment required to manage it, the side effects of the various treatment modalities, and the importance of returning to the clinic for follow-up visits.

Disposition and discharge planning

Patient outcomes for AA have significantly improved secondary to enhanced supportive care and BMT (Myers & Davies, 2009). The five-year survival rates for patients receiving immunosuppressive therapy and BMT are 75% and 90 %, respectively. Patients who undergo immunosuppressant therapy are at risk of late disease (Bakshi, 2009; Pack-Mabien & Haynes, 2009).

Patients will require intensive monitoring for rejection and infections, typically in an intensive care unit, following BMT and during immunosuppressive therapy. Outpatient care entails multiple follow-up clinic visits to monitor patients closely for complications (e.g., bleeding, infection), to take blood counts, and to monitor side effects of medications and overall well-being.

DIAMOND-BLACKFAN ANEMIA

Pathophysiology

Diamond-Blackfan anemia (DBA) is a rare congenital hypoplastic anemia resulting in constitutional bone marrow failure. Its inheritance is thought to occur in an autosomal dominant manner. The definitive cause is unknown; however, it is hypothesized that faulty ribosome biogenesis resulting in proapoptotic erythropoiesis leads to marrow failure. Mutations in genes that encode ribosomal proteins have been identified in most patients with DBA (Lipton & Ellis, 2009).

Patients present with severe normochromic macrocytic anemia, leucopenia, thrombocytopenia, and an inadequate reticulocyte response. Bone marrow aspirate reveals a reduction in all erythroid precursors, but normal granulocytic and megakaryocytic cell lines. There is also a 5% to 25% increase in fetal hemoglobin levels (Lipton & Ellis, 2009; Vlachos et al., 2008).

Epidemiology and etiology

DBA is a very rare inherited disease that affects approximately 600 to 700 people worldwide. Recent research has determined that the mutation for DBA is on chromosome 19, which encodes for a ribosomal protein (RP), known as RPS19 (Lipton & Ellis, 2009; Vlachos et al., 2008).

Presentation

In DBA, the patient history is remarkable for pallor and dyspnea during feeding, and hypotonia. Other clinical findings may include irregular heartbeat, fatigue, irritability, fainting episodes, physical defects, short statue, and failure-to-thrive. The physical defects vary, but may include craniofacial, hands and upper limbs, cardiac, or genitourinary abnormalities (Lipton & Ellis, 2009).

Differential diagnosis

Other diseases to consider that may present with similar characteristics include parvovirus B19 erythroblastopenia, Fanconi's anemia, transitory erythroblastopenia, autoimmune erythrobastopenia, and congenital dyserythropoieses (Lipton & Ellis, 2009).

Plan of care

Diagnosis occurs by age 2 years. The initial diagnostic evaluation to confirm the diagnosis includes CBC, adenosine deaminase activity, and bone marrow biopsy. Treatment depends on the degree of anemia. Therapeutic management includes steroid therapy, frequent blood transfusions, or bone marrow transplant (Myers & Davies, 2009). Follow-up with a hematologist, BMT specialist, and endocrinologist (if needed) is recommended (Lipton & Ellis, 2009; Vlachos et al., 2008).

Disposition and discharge planning

Approximately 20% to 30% of children with DBA have a spontaneous recovery. In addition, 60% to 70% of children have a favorable response following steroid treatment. Unfortunately, lifelong steroid therapy and frequent transfusion may cause adverse consequences. Adverse events secondary to prolonged steroid use include diabetes mellitus, glaucoma, osteopenia, and hypertension. Hemosiderosis is an adverse event that may occur as a result of frequent transfusions (Lipton & Ellis, 2009; Vlachos et al., 2008).

BETA THALASSEMIA

Pathophysiology

Beta thalassemia (β-thalassemia) is due to decreased or absent production of one or more beta-globin chains of hemoglobin, which results in a relative excess number of alpha-globin chains. Patients who are homozygous for this disease are unable to synthesize the beta chains, while those who are heterozygous are able to produce some chains. Intramedullary hemolysis, hemolytic anemia, and ineffective erythropoiesis are all factors that are thought to be responsible for the anemia associated with beta thalassemia. Peripheral hemolysis is both intracorpuscular and extravascular. A decrease in hemoglobin production causes hypochromia and microcytosis. Grossly abnormal RBC shapes may also be noted, including the presence of target cells, teardrop cells (dacrocytes), fragmented forms, echinocytes, and RBC inclusions in the peripheral blood (Muncie & Campbell, 2009).

Epidemiology and etiology

Beta thalassemia affects equal numbers of males and females. Its incidence is approximately 4.4 cases per 10,000 live births. The prevalence is increased among persons of Mediterranean, African, or Southeast Asian descent. More than 150 mutations in the beta-globin gene have been identified in affected individuals (Muncie & Campbell, 2009).

Presentation

Beta thalassemia is usually diagnosed during infancy. Children may present with pallor, irritability, growth retardation, abdominal enlargement (hepatosplenomegaly), and jaundice.

Differential diagnosis

Other disorders with a clinical presentation similar to that for beta thalassemia include iron-deficiency anemia, sideroblastic anemia, and anemia of chronic disease.

Plan of care

Laboratory data to confirm the diagnosis include a CBC with differential blood counts and reticulocyte count, serum ferritin, a peripheral smear, and hemoglobin electrophoresis. Absence of hemoglobin A, consisting of two alpha and two beta chains, is the hallmark of severe, homozygous beta thalassemia (also known as B⁰ thalassemia); lesser decreases in beta chain synthesis result in B⁺ thalassemia. In both forms, the level of hemoglobin A, which consists of two delta chains paired with two alpha chains, is elevated due to the impaired beta chain production. Fetal hemoglobin may also be increased.

Therapeutic management of beta thalassemia varies with the extent of disease. Iron supplements are ineffective in the management of microcytosis and should be avoided. Treatments that have been found to be effective include hypertransfusion to suppress the abnormal erythropoiesis, splenectomy to reduce hemolysis, iron chelation to reduce iron overload, and supportive care (Porter, 2009). Hydroxyurea may also be considered (Ehsani et al., 2009), and stem cell transplantation may be curative (Persons, 2009).

Disposition and discharge planning

Patients with beta thalassemia will require lifelong monitoring and possibly transfusions. Consultative services are needed both initially and on an ongoing basis with a hematologist and a social worker. Future consultative services may be provided by cardiology, endocrinology, child life, and psychology specialists.

G6PD DEFICIENCY

Pathophysiology

Hemolytic anemias can be categorized as inherited or acquired, and as due to intrinsic red cell disorders or disorders that are external to the red cells. Glucose-6-phosphate dehydrogenase (G6PD) deficiency is a hemolytic anemia in which the patient has virtually no anemia and almost no hemolysis in the absence of an exogenous challenge.

The metabolic integrity of RBCs depends on the activity of G6PD; thus G6PD-deficient RBCs are susceptible to oxidative damage and hemolysis. G6PD is the first enzyme in the hexose monophosphate shunt. This enzyme is required for the production of the reduced form of nicotinamide adenine dinucleotide phosphate (NADPH). NADPH is crucial in preventing oxidant damage. As a carrier of oxygen, the RBCs are particularly susceptible to oxidative damage. Reactive oxygen radicals damage the RBC membrane and hemoglobin, resulting in hemolysis of the red blood cell.

The gene controlling G6PD expression is found on the long arm of the X chromosome; hence, it is inherited in an X-linked fashion. As a consequence, mutations in G6PD follow the typical Mendelian X-linked inheritance pattern, and severe G6PD deficiency is much more common in males than in females. Rarely, females are affected with G6PD deficiency as the result of X chromosome inactivation or double heterozygosity (Jaffe, 1970; Sullivan & Glader, 1980).

Epidemiology and etiology

Three forms of G6PD deficiency have been described. In the first variant, the G6PD activity is less than 10% of normal, which results in a severe neonatal jaundice or a congenital nonspherocytic hemolytic anemia. In the second form, the G6PD activity is typically less than 30% of the normal range, which results in an asymptomatic steady state; individuals who carry this mutation are at risk for neonatal jaundice, acute hemolytic anemia, and favism. In the third class, the enzyme activity is greater than 85% of the normal reference range, which results in no clinical manifestation and is considered the "wild type" disease. Two isoforms of G6PD, known as G6PD-A and G6PD-B, fall into this last classification, with G6PD-B being considered the wild-type allele.

There is a high prevalence of G6PD in many populations in the tropical and subtropical parts of the world (Allison, 2009). Affecting individuals on five continents and more than 500 million people worldwide, this disorder has been hypothesized to be related to malaria exposure (Nkhoma et al., 2009).

Presentation

The clinical findings of classic G6PD deficiency are related to acute hemolytic anemia. Neonatal jaundice may also be observed (Watchko, 2009). Children with G6PD deficiency are clinically and hematologically normal for the majority of their lifetime and are considered to be in a steady state. Acute exacerbations may occur with ingestion of fava beans, resulting in favism; during the course of infection; or upon exposure to certain oxidative drugs, including antimalarials, sulfa-containing medications, some analgesics such as aspirin, and quinolones and certain other antimicrobials (Frank, 2005; Watchko).

Within 24 to 48 hours of an oxidative challenge, the patient's body temperature will often rise, accompanied by nausea, abdominal pain, diarrhea, and occasionally vomiting. A remarkable dark brown or even black discoloration of the urine is present within 6 to 24 hours after exposure. Jaundice may develop along with pallor and tachycardia. Rarely, hypovolemic shock or heart failure may ensue. Hepatosplenomegaly leads to abdominal distention and tenderness.

Neonatal jaundice related to G6PD deficiency has a peak incidence between the second and third days of life. Although intensely jaundiced, the infant is rarely severely anemic. It is estimated that approximately one-half of all newborns with mild jaundice may be G6PD deficient and more than three-fourths of those with severe hyperbilirubinemia may be deficient in the enzyme. For example, approximately 20% of newborns requiring phototherapy are deficient in G6PD.

Differential diagnosis

The differential diagnosis for anemia with jaundice and hemolysis is broad in scope. It includes exposure to toxins (e.g., lead), infections (e.g., malaria), disorders of hemoglobin synthesis such as beta thalassemia, and other hemolytic anemias.

Plan of care

The laboratory diagnosis of G6PD deficiency depends on measurement of enzyme activity within the RBCs (Frank, 2005; Minucci et al., 2009). It should be noted that G6PD is an age-related enzyme and its activity decreases as red blood cells age. Any condition involving reticulocytosis will result in an increase in G6PD activity, a factor that may result in a misdiagnosis after an acute hemolytic episode when the older, G6PD-deficient cells have been destroyed and the marrow response results in an outpouring of young reticulocytes into the peripheral blood replete with G6PD activity (Al-Sweedan et al., 2009; Frank; Mason et al., 2007).

Laboratory findings during an acute exacerbation consist of a severe anemia with hemoglobin values as low as 2.5 gm/dL. Prior blood counts are normal without anemia in the absence of oxidative stress. A marked variation in the size of the RBCs is possible, resulting in an increase in the RBC distribution width (RDW). Large polychromatic cells with spherocytic morphology may be observed as well as markedly irregularly shaped cells known as poikilocytes. The reticulocyte count increases and may reach levels as high as 30%. Inclusions within the reticulocytes and RBCs are usually present, are 1 to 3 microns in diameter, and occur near the red cell membrane. Heinz bodies may be easily recognized with methyl violet staining; these elements consist of denatured hemoglobin and are a manifestation of the oxidative injury to the hemoglobin. As the RBCs circulate through the spleen, Heinz bodies are removed, resulting in the classic "bite cells." Due to the hemolysis and generation of free hemoglobin, the serum haptoglobin is reduced. Hemoglobinemia and hemoglobinuria may also be present. The white blood cell (WBC) count may be elevated. Typically, there are no changes in the platelet count. The unconjugated bilirubin is elevated, but the liver enzymes are usually normal (Minucci et al., 2009).

Blood transfusion is usually indicated if a child is hemodynamically unstable or the hemoglobin level declines to less than 7 gm/dL. If the hemoglobin is less than 9 gm/dL and there is evidence of persistent brisk hemolysis with hemoglobinuria, blood transfusion may also be indicated. Dialysis may be required for acute kidney failure.

The management of hyperbilirubinemia and neonatal jaundice related to G6PD deficiency does not differ from that recommended for other causes. In mild cases, no treatment is necessary. For management of more significant increases in the bilirubin, phototherapy and hydration are usually sufficient. In severe cases, an exchange transfusion may be beneficial (Watchko, 2009).

Disposition and discharge planning

A small minority of children with G6PD deficiency have a chronic hemolytic anemia in the absence of an exogenous oxidative stress. These individuals typically have extremely low enzyme activity, defined as less than 10% of the normal reference range. They are invariably males who initially present with unexplained jaundice in the neonatal period.

The clinical course of acute hemolysis due to G6PD deficiency is usually self-limited and tends to resolve spontaneously. The hemoglobin level may return to the normal range in 3 to 6 weeks barring an iron deficiency. Rarely, kidney failure results from massive hemoglobinuria (Elyassi & Rowshan, 2009; Frank, 2005).

Once the diagnosis of G6PD deficiency has been established, patient and family education and counseling focus on the avoidance of oxidative stress. Typically, no other specific treatment is necessary.

SICKLE CELL ANEMIA

Pathophysiology

Hemoglobin S is the result of a single amino acid substitution at position 6 of the beta chain, in which a valine is present instead of a glutamic acid residue—a defect that leads to precipitation of the hemoglobin upon deoxygenation. This change in the hemoglobin structure results in the conversion of the biconcave discoid shape of the red blood cell to that of a sickle form. Sickled RBCs are more prone to hemolysis. Hence, the pathophysiology of sickle cell anemia is directly related to the polymerization of hemoglobin.

The secondary effects of this pathophysiology result in the clinical expression of the disease. As the sickle cells are deoxygenated and filled with polymerized hemoglobin, they become less deformable. Membranes become rigid, resulting in irreversibly sickled cells, which are more adhesive to the endothelium and lead to many of the clinical manifestations of the disease, including vaso-occlusive pain crisis and intrapulmonary thrombosis. The RBC life span is shortened in homozygous sickle cell disease (hemoglobin SS disease), to approximately 8 to 21 days.

Epidemiology and etiology

The sickle gene may have a protective effect against falciparum malaria; hence, the frequency of the sickle gene in a population parallels the incidence of malaria in the population. Approximately 8% of African Americans carry the sickle gene. In certain areas of Africa, where malaria is endemic, the prevalence is much higher (Meremikwu, 2009; Roseff, 2009).

Many genetic modifiers of sickle cell disease are known to exist, including G6PD deficiency in which the common G6PD A variant is associated with increased septic complications and a more severe anemia. Conversely, individuals who are homozygous for hemoglobin SS and who co-inherit alpha thalassemia may have a less severe phenotype. The effect of the alpha thalassemia decreases the cellular content of the hemoglobin S that delays the time needed for hemoglobin S polymerization. As a consequence, these individuals tend to have less significant laboratory abnormalities and a clinical phenotype that is not significantly different from that of individuals without alpha thalassemia.

The presence of alpha thalassemia does not protect children with hemoglobin SS disease from stroke. However, increasing the concentration of hemoglobin F reduces hemoglobin S polymerization, which in turn brings about a more prolonged survival of these cells. Increased levels of hemoglobin F (typically greater than 4%) are associated with reduced frequency of pain crisis and decreases in mortality.

Other sickle syndromes may occur including SC disease, SO-Arab, SD-Los Angeles, S Korle Bu, and hemoglobin C-Harlem. Sickle beta thalassemia results when mutations causing beta thalassemia and heterozygous sickle cell disease are co-inherited, producing a severe phenotype that is indistinguishable from that associated with hemoglobin SS disease (Meremikwu, 2009; Pack-Mabien & Haynes, 2009; Roseff, 2009).

Presentation

Clinical manifestations of sickle cell disease are extremely variable. Some patients may be asymptomatic, while others experience frequent painful episodes. Most individuals with homozygous SS disease fall between these extremes. The classic manifestation of sickle cell disease is the vaso-occlusive sickle crisis, in which children present with pain. Three-fourths of all children with sickle cell disease will present with hand–foot syndrome, consisting of painful and swelling of the hands and feet (dactylitis), in the first year of life. They may refuse to bear weight, be irritable, or have a fever. They may even appear septic. By approximately 4 years of age, 50% of patients will have experienced at least one acute pain crisis.

Older children may report rapid onset of a deep, throbbing pain. Rarely, local tenderness, erythema, warmth, and swelling may be present. These symptoms are thought to be due to bone marrow ischemia that leads to frank infarction of the bone marrow and to acute inflammatory infiltrates. The hands and feet are involved in young children; in older children, adolescents, and young adults, the lumbosacral spine, knee, shoulder, elbow, and femur are most frequently involved. Less often, the sternum, ribs, clavicles, calcaneus, iliac crest, mandible, and zygoma may be involved.

Acute chest syndrome is an acute illness characterized by the presence of chest pain, fever, and respiratory symptoms accompanied by a new pulmonary infiltrate on chest radiograph (CXR) from ischemia or infarction of a lung segment. Severe, acute abdominal pain may be the result of mesenteric vessel sickling or vertebral disease with nerve root compression. Patients may present with guarding, abdominal tenderness, fever, and leukocytosis—all common signs for other acute abdominal emergencies. Acute infarction of the brain can result in stroke, a complication that occurs in approximately 7% of children with sickle cell disease. The incidence of stroke is estimated to be 0.7% per year during the first 20 years of life, with the highest incidence noted in children between 5 and 10 years of age. Priapism may occur in males of all ages, with most patients reporting at least one episode.

Splenic sequestration is one of the leading causes of death in children with sickle cell anemia. Children with hemoglobin SS disease will typically undergo autosplenectomy. Those who do not are at risk for a sudden, rapid, and massive enlargement of the spleen due to trapping of sickle red blood cells. A distended abdomen with left-sided abdominal pain, vomiting, and shock may be indicative of splenic sequestration crisis. Profound hypotension with cardiac decompensation may be present, along with hemoglobin concentrations as low as 2 gm/dL. This complication may occur as early as 8 weeks of age. In the normal state, a patient with sickle cell anemia can compensate for the decreased RBC survival by increasing the bone marrow output by as much as sixfold to eightfold. Any temporary reduction in bone marrow activity due to intercurrent viral or bacterial infection may cause the hemoglobin and hematocrit to fall precipitously, however. Those patients experiencing aplastic crisis will exhibit extreme pallor and fatigue but no jaundice; laboratory evidence will prove the presence of severe anemia without reticulocytosis.

Infection is the most common cause of death in children with sickle cell anemia and sepsis or meningitis may occur in as many as 15% of children younger than five years of age, with an associated mortality of approximately 30%. The presence of pneumococcal sepsis is approximately 400 times greater in children with sickle cell disease compared to children without the disease. The increased risk of this form of sepsis reflects the functional asplenia that occurs in patients with sickle cell anemia (Booth et al., 2009; Field et al., 2009; Khatib et al., 2009; Pack-Mabien & Haynes, 2009; Roseff, 2009).

Differential diagnosis

Patients may first be diagnosed with osteomyelitis due to symptoms of extremity infection. Except for the presence of bacteremia, no laboratory tests can differentiate acute infection from a painful crisis. Other patients may confuse the initial symptoms of sickle cell disease with a traumatic injury. Acute chest syndrome mimics pneumonia, pulmonary embolism, and altitude illness (pulmonary syndromes).

Plan of care

The laboratory findings in sickle cell anemia are primarily related to hemolysis. The hemoglobin concentration may be decreased to a value as low as 7 gm/dL, though it typically remains between 8 and 9 gm/dL. The mean corpuscular volume (MCV) and other RBC indices are normal, but the reticulocyte count is frequently elevated to 4% to 10%. The serum bilirubin is elevated and the heptoglobin decreased. Other laboratory parameters indicative of hemolysis, such as an elevated LDH, are also present.

Most painful crises may be treated at home with increased fluid intake and oral analgesics. When these measures prove inadequate, hospitalization may be necessary to ensure more aggressive hydration and analgesia. Health care professionals (HCPs) should take care to avoid over-hydration due to the risk of volume overload and cardiac failure.

Oxygen therapy is of little use unless the patient is hypoxic. Continuous oxygen inhalation can suppress erythropoiesis and reduce reticulocyte counts, prolonging the painful crisis.

Analgesics—frequently opioid medications—should be given in doses sufficient to control the severe pain for any patient in crisis. Many patients with sickle cell disease report being undertreated for their pain. Hypoventilation due to the sedation associated with opioid analgesics should be avoided. Monitoring of the oxygen saturation and aggressive use of incentive spirometry may be useful. Nonsteroidal anti-inflammatory drugs (NSAIDs) may be helpful in some patients.

Hydroxyurea increases hemoglobin F levels and may be effective in decreasing the frequency of recurrent pain crises (Charache et al., 1979). Butyric acid analogs may also increase hemoglobin F production. It is estimated that an increase in the hemoglobin F concentration from 4% to 16% may decrease vaso-occlusive crisis by 50% (Hoppe et al., 2000; Olivieri & Vichinsky, 1998; Scott et al., 1996). A long-term follow-up study of patients taking hydroxyurea revealed a 40% reduction in mortality in patients who were compliant with the therapy (Steinberg et al., 2003).

Transfusions to improve the oxygen carrying capacity and decrease the proportion of erythrocytes that carry hemoglobin S may be beneficial, but are not typically used to treat chronic anemia or acute pain crisis. Common indications for transfusion therapy are stroke or recurrent acute chest syndrome. Care should be taken not to increase the hemoglobin concentration beyond 10 to 11 gm/dL. Episodic transfusion may be useful in the management of priapism that is unresponsive to medical therapy (Jesus & Dekermacher, 2009).

Correction of the underlying genetic defect with stem cell transplantation has been performed successfully in some patients with sickle cell disease (Bolanos-Meade & Brodsky, 2009; Persons, 2009).

Disposition and discharge planning

Routine health maintenance is the key to reducing the morbidity of sickle cell disease. Monitoring of the steady state blood count and baseline physical findings are useful in identifying acute exacerbations. Routine immunizations, including *Haemophilus influenzae* and conjugated pneumococcal vaccines, are essential to reducing the risk of life-threatening infection. Prophylactic penicillin should be given to all children younger than 5 years of age, and 1 mg per day of folic acid is recommended. Although iron deficiency is rare, because of the hemolysis-induced increased absorption of gastrointestinal iron, iron supplements may be necessary if iron deficiency is documented.

Transcranial Doppler examination may be able to identify those individuals at risk for stroke. Specifically, children with internal carotid or middle cerebral blood flow greater than 200 cm/sec may benefit from prophylactic maintenance RBC transfusions. Although the ideal age range and frequency for transcranial Doppler examination has not been determined, it is recommended every 6 months for patients between 2 and 16 years of age when the risk of stroke is highest (Adams et al., 1998; Tsivgoulis et al., 2009). Routine ophthalmologic examination should be started at school age, and repeated every few years due to the risk for retinopathy. Regular dental care may also reduce the risk for infection. Birth control options should be discussed with adolescent girls with sickle cell disease.

Due to the risk of iron overload with chronic transfusion therapy, care must be taken to limit transfusions unless clinically indicated (King et al., 2008). The incidence of transfusion-related complications such as infection, RBC sensitization, and iron overload may be reduced or avoided with this strategy. It is estimated that 7% to 20% of multiply transfused children with sickle cell disease are allo-immunized due to not only the numbers of transfusions given, but also to racial differences between common donor and recipient erythrocyte phenotypes (Vichinsky et al., 1990).

For patients with sickle cell disease who require surgery, a simple transfusion is recommended. In a study comparing the benefits of simple transfusion to exchange transfusion, there was no significant difference between the two groups in morbidity. Therefore, a simple transfusion designed to raise the preoperative hemoglobin level to 10 gm/dL should be administered to all patients with hemoglobin SS disease.

COAGULATION DISORDERS

DISSEMINATED INTRAVASCULAR COAGULATION

Kristen Osborn

Pathophysiology

Disseminated intravascular coagulation (DIC), also called consumptive coagulopathy or defibrination syndrome, is an acquired, life-threatening complication that results from a variety of disease processes (Dressler, 2004). It involves uncontrolled, intravascular coagulation and consumption of coagulation factors and platelets, and results in concurrent thrombosis and hemorrhage. Intravascular thrombosis results when excessive fibrinogen and platelets are deposited in the microvascular system (Mansen & McCance, 2006). This may lead to significant hemorrhage, multiple organ failure due to tissue ischemia and necrosis, capillary leakage, and edema, and may ultimately result in an increased mortality and morbidity (Kruger, 2006). DIC may occur as either an acute or a chronic process. In acute DIC, the sudden, rapid release of an abundance of procoagulant into circulation causes the rapid depletion of coagulation factors and results in bleeding. In chronic DIC, smaller amounts of procoagulant are released over a longer period of time, allowing the body to partially compensate for the irregularity (Kusuma & Schulz, 2009).

Epidemiology and etiology

DIC is a malfunction of the normal, adaptive coagulation mechanism in the body. The disorder is triggered by a systemic or localized injury to tissues in the body and may result from single or multiple underlying conditions (Kenet et al., 2008). DIC is recognized as a significant medical complication, as it greatly increases mortality risk beyond that associated with the underlying disorders (Kusuma & Schulz, 2009). Additionally, treatment of the underlying causes may not lead to the resolution of DIC.

Common causes of DIC include infection, trauma, malignancies, toxic or immunologic reactions, pregnancy complications, vascular irregularities, and liver failure (Dressler, 2004). Infection is the most common cause of DIC, occurring in as many as 35% of patients. Gram-negative sepsis is the most prevalent infectious trigger, but Gram-positive bacteria, viruses, fungal infections, and parasites have also been implicated in this disorder. Significant trauma, such as penetrating brain injuries, burns, and severe pancreatitis, may also result in DIC. Additionally, certain solid tumors and hematologic malignancies cause white blood cells to release tissue factor, thereby increasing the likelihood of DIC (Toh, 2006).

Presentation

Although DIC often follows no predictable pattern, in many patients diffuse bleeding is the initial presenting symptom. Bleeding may occur abruptly from surgical incisions or venipuncture sites, but may also be manifested as hematuria or melena. In addition, patients may display ecchymoses, purpura, and petechiae (Dressler, 2004).

The other major component of DIC, thrombosis, is not as easily observed but causes significant damage. Capillaries become blocked by small clots, leading to tissue ischemia, necrosis, and ultimately organ failure. Blockages may occur in virtually any vessel in the body, are commonly manifested by cyanosis of large areas of skin, and may eventually result in purpura fulminans (Dressler, 2009). Additionally, respiratory difficulties, abdominal pain, kidney failure, confusion, and seizures may become evident (Toh, 2006).

Differential diagnosis

Liver disease may produce coagulation abnormalities and clinical manifestations similar to those in DIC. However, the two may be distinguished based on measurement of factor activity. In liver disease, factor VII is significantly decreased and factor VIII may be normal or increased. In DIC, factor VII is only mildly decreased and factor VIII is decreased as well (Kruger, 2006).

Other conditions are also important to consider when evaluating any patient with thrombocytopenia, prolonged clotting times, and the presence of schistocytes. Idiopathic thrombocytopenic purpura (ITP) is associated with a recent viral infection and platelet autoantibodies. Hemolytic uremic syndrome (HUS) is commonly associated with symptoms such as abdominal pain, vomiting, kidney abnormalities, and anemia. In addition to thrombocytopenia, thrombotic thrombocytopenic purpura (TTP) involves anemia, kidney abnormalities, fever, and neurologic changes (Kruger, 2006).

Plan of care

Because the presentation of DIC can vary dramatically, several studies are necessary to confirm its diagnosis. Routinely available coagulation studies provide necessary diagnostic information. However, HCPs must realize that DIC is a rapidly evolving process. Changes occur quickly and patients must be monitored closely. Laboratory results may differ depending on the length of time for which patients have been experiencing clinical symptoms of DIC. In most cases, a diagnosis may be established based on clinical manifestations along with a platelet count, fibrinogen level, prothrombin time or International Normalized Ratio (INR), activated partial thromboplastin time, and a D-dimer test. The D-dimer test is the most specific study used to establish the diagnosis (Toh, 2006). The most common finding is a low platelet count, and most patients have a prolonged prothrombin time. In addition, providers may note schistocytes (RBC fragments) on a blood smear (Kruger, 2006).

Initially, the most effective treatment for acute DIC is to remove or correct the causative agent. Resolution of DIC will not occur without effective treatment of the underlying disorder (Kruger, 2006).

Next, homeostasis must be restored by correcting the complications associated with DIC. Clinical management of shock, hypoxia, and acidosis require aggressive support measures to restore vascular stasis and maintain blood volume. Fluid replacement, oxygen supplementation, and close monitoring of patient vital signs are essential (Toh & Dennis, 2003). Additionally, transfusion with platelets, cryoprecipitate, or fresh frozen plasma (FFP) may be recommended. Although controversial and not based on evidence from randomized clinical trials, the utilization of these products depends on the location and severity of hemorrhage and as prophylaxis for necessary procedures (Stewart, 2001). Administration of 10 to 15 mL/kg of FFP in a child usually increases procoagulant activity by 10% to 15%. Cryoprecipitate is equally effective as a rich source of fibrinogen. It is dosed as one bag per 3 kg body weight in infants and one bag per 6 kg body weight in older children.

Health care professionals should also consider administration of vitamin K as part of the effort to restore hemostasis, because many critically ill children, even those not experiencing DIC, become vitamin K deficient. Infants should be given 1 mg of parenteral vitamin K and adolescents should receive 2.5 to 10 mg (Barkin & Rosen, 2003a).

Other medications used to stabilize hemostasis in patients with DIC are controversial and not widely recommended. Aprotinin, a bovine pancreatic trypsin inhibitor, is a protein administered parenterally to reduce bleeding by slowing down fibrinolysis. Because results with this medication have been mixed, it is not routinely used. Heparin, a medication used to inhibit thrombin generation, is sometimes administered as a continuous intravenous infusion. It is administered in a dose of 5 to 10 units/kg/hr, without a loading dose bolus. Heparin has not been proven effective in the management of DIC in randomized clinical trials in certain patients. Antithrombin III is an α_2-globulin that inactivates certain clotting factor and inhibits coagulation. It is most often used in patients with DIC caused by sepsis.

Families must be informed that the management of DIC is complex and the effectiveness of therapies often uncertain. Additionally, prognosis is highly variable and based on multiple factors (Toh, 2006).

Disposition and discharge planning

Due to the introduction of new therapies and earlier recognition of systemic abnormalities in patients with DIC, the prognosis for many patients with this disorder has improved over the last several years. Follow-up is based on the underlying disorder and the severity of the clinical manifestations (Levi, 2007). Vital signs, including central venous pressure, should be monitored closely for signs of fluid overload or shock. Strict measurement of fluid intake and output must be maintained. Restoration of organ perfusion may be evidenced by normal blood pressure, urine output, and cardiac output. Platelet counts and monitoring of coagulation factors may be beneficial in the ongoing management of DIC (Dressler, 2004).

HEMOLYTIC UREMIC SYNDROME

Kristen Osborn

Pathophysiology

Hemolytic uremic syndrome (HUS) refers to a disorder originating in the microcirculation, which is characterized by hemolytic anemia, thrombocytopenia, and acute kidney failure. In the majority of HUS diagnoses, bacterial verotoxins are absorbed by intestinal mucosa and cause extensive damage to erythrocytes and endothelial cells (Elliott & Robins-Browne, 2005). This process produces swelling of the endothelial cells, especially in the glomerular arterioles in the kidneys. In turn, the damaged vessels release clotting factors that precipitate fibrin clot formation. The body then seeks to destroy these fibrin clots through fibrinolysis, which diminishes the population of circulating platelets and leads to thrombocytopenia. The massive swelling and thromboses lead to a decrease in glomerular filtration, hematuria, proteinuria, and oliguria. Children with HUS may require dialysis due to their impaired kidney function. Additionally, the swollen vessels damage the circulating erythrocytes themselves. Filtration of the damaged erythrocytes by the spleen, in turn, leads to a hemolytic anemia. Other organs, such as the brain, liver, and heart, may also become involved in the pathological process (Huether, 2006).

Two types of hemolytic uremic syndrome are distinguished. D+HUS, also called postdiarrheal or epidemic HUS, is usually seen in previously healthy children and preceded by an episode of acute gastroenteritis. D-HUS, also known as atypical or sporadic HUS, is less common but usually more severe than D+HUS. These cases may begin in the neonatal period, may have a familial link, and may recur (Zeng & Sadler, 2006).

Epidemiology and etiology

HUS is the most common cause of acute kidney failure in children. It occurs most often in children younger than 4 years of age and affects equal numbers of males and females. The mean age of onset is approximately 2 years (Zeng & Sadler, 2006). Cases of epidemic HUS tend to peak in the summer months. The most common cause of D+HUS is infection with *Escherichia coli* O157:H7, which produces a potent Shiga toxin (Razzaq, 2006). Other causes include infection with *Shigella dysenteriae*, *Citrobacter freundii*, and other *E. coli* subtypes, all of which produce Shiga toxins. Kidney failure is reported to occur in 50% to 70% of patients with D+HUS, although the majority of patients recover (Zeng & Sadler).

D-HUS, or atypical HUS, may have several causes. Approximately 10% to 20% of patients with D-HUS have inherited factor H deficiency. Other patients have membrane cofactor protein mutations. Both factor H deficiency and membrane cofactor protein mutations inhibit complement activation. D-HUS is also associated with *Streptococcus pneumoniae* infection and use of certain medications, such as cyclosporine and tacrolimus. This type of HUS tends to have a less favorable outcome. Almost one-half of all patients with D-HUS develop end-stage renal disease (ESRD), and approximately 25% die during the acute phase of their illness. Some patients develop irreversible brain damage. This disorder may occur at any age, but is more common in adulthood (Zeng & Sadler, 2006).

Presentation

Most cases of D+HUS have an incubation period of 3 to 5 days and present as a previously healthy child with abdominal pain, watery, nonbloody diarrhea, and fever. The disease progresses to hemorrhagic colitis within 5 to 7 days after the inception of diarrhea (Corrigan & Boineau, 2001). Kidney involvement ranges from mild to severe. Patients may also display signs of a normochromic, normocytic anemia and thrombocytopenia, including pallor, jaundice, weakness, petechiae, ecchymoses, hematuria, and hematemesis. Clinical manifestations may include hepatomegaly, splenomegaly, hypertension, and oliguria that may progress to anuria. Some patients also develop fluid overload, cardiovascular changes, edema, and central nervous system symptoms such as irritability, personality changes, drowsiness, tremors, and seizures. Pancreatic insufficiency develops in a small percentage of patients, usually manifested as diabetes mellitus (Barkin & Rosen, 2003b).

Differential diagnosis

Other diagnoses with findings similar to those noted in HUS include thrombotic thrombocytopenic purpura, disseminated intravascular coagulation, preeclampsia/eclampsia, systemic lupus erythematosus, and hemolytic transfusion reactions. Patients with artificial cardiac valves or intracardiac patches may also display similar symptoms (Zeng & Sadler, 2006).

Plan of care

Diagnostic findings in HUS include elevated blood urea nitrogen (BUN), creatinine, bilirubin, and potassium levels.

Reticulocytosis and abnormalities in RBC morphology (schistocytes and helmet cells) are also evident. Hemoglobin, hematocrit, and platelet counts are often low. Coagulation testing is normal. Stool cultures may be positive if a bacterial pathogen is the causative agent. Serum samples for ELISA testing should be obtained both at diagnosis and 2 weeks later to identify the presence of antibodies to the Shiga toxin *E. coli* serotypes (Razzaq, 2006).

Management of patients with D+HUS is largely supportive in nature. The primary goals of therapy include reversing kidney failure, addressing fluid/electrolyte imbalances and nutritional deficiencies, correcting anemia, and controlling hypertension. Approximately one-half of all patients with D+HUS require temporary hemodialysis to manage azotemia, fluid overload, and electrolyte imbalances. Dialysis is also recommended when BUN is greater than 100 mg/dL, even in the absence of fluid overload. Additionally, 75% of patients require RBC transfusion to correct symptomatic anemia. The goal of nutritional support is to maintain adequate caloric intake and may be accomplished orally if it does not cause abdominal pain or an increase in diarrhea. Hypertension must be corrected to prevent the development of congestive heart failure and encephalopathy. Oral nifedipine, a short-acting calcium-channel blocker, is recommended unless oral administration is not possible; in the latter scenario, intravenous nicardipine or nitroprusside should be considered (Corrigan & Boineau, 2001).

In patients with atypical HUS (D-HUS), management is more complex, with no well-established treatment norms. Plasmapheresis may be considered for patients with factor H deficiency, especially if neurologic symptoms are present. Although plasma exchange may temporarily alleviate symptoms of kidney involvement, it has not been shown to prevent progression to ESRD or recurrence (Camp-Sorrell, 2008). Poorer long-term prognosis for these patients may be predicted by the evidence of renal cortical necrosis on kidney biopsy performed during the acute phase of the disease.

Disposition and discharge planning

Mortality rates in D+HUS range from 3% to 5%. Overall, the prognosis for patients with D+HUS is much better than that for patients with D-HUS. A small percentage of patients develop ESRD and require lifelong dialysis. Some patients with D-HUS require kidney transplantation. However, recurrence rates still range from 8% to 30% with graft loss after transplantation.

Long-term complications are uncommon but may include proteinuria, decreased glomerular filtration, and hypertension (Fiorino et al., 2006). Such complications may initially resolve, only to recur up to one year later. For this reason, patients with both types of HUS require long-term follow-up. Blood pressures and urinalysis should be monitored for signs of long-term complications or relapse (Barkin & Rosen, 2003b).

HEMOPHILIA

Audrey Taylor, Leonard Valentino, and Kristen Osborn

Pathophysiology

Hemophilia is an X-linked recessive bleeding disorder whose inheritance follows typical Mendelian X-linked genetics. It is caused by deficient or defective factor VIII (hemophilia A) or factor IX (hemophilia B). Hemophilia is a disorder of "secondary hemostasis," meaning that fibrin clot formation is too unstable to adequately stop bleeding. When injury to a vessel occurs, both the intrinsic and extrinsic pathways of the clotting cascade are activated to stabilize the platelet plug so that bleeding may be contained. When one of the factors in either of the pathways is defective or deficient, such stabilization cannot adequately occur.

Factor VIII and factor IX play key roles in this process by assisting in the formation of a fibrin clot. In patients with either form of hemophilia, the defect in these factors prevents secondary hemostasis by causing the fibrin clot to become jelly-like and unstable, leading to delayed clotting and spontaneous bleeding (Ragni, 2006). The severity of bleeding depends on the residual level of factor VIII or factor IX in the plasma (Stephensen et al., 2009).

Epidemiology and etiology

Hemophilia A and B are the most common inherited bleeding disorders. First recognized in biblical times, introduction of the term *hemophilia* was ascribed to Schönlein in the late 1820s. The differentiation between two types of hemophilia, A and B, was not made until 1952 with the description of bleeding in a young English boy named Christmas. Hemophilia B is now often referred to as "Christmas disease" (Mannucci & Tuddenham, 2001). The incidence of hemophilia A is 1 in 5,000 male births and that of hemophilia B is 1 in 30,000 male births; 80% to 85% of all hemophilia is due to factor VIII deficiency (Pipe & Valentino, 2007; Sharathkumar & Pipe, 2008). There is neither a racial nor an ethnic predilection for hemophilia. There appears to be a higher incidence of this disease in the second and third decades of life, but this is likely due to delayed onset of bleeding symptoms in patients with milder disease. Although hemophilia is an X-linked recessive bleeding disorder, females may rarely be affected, as in the case of an affected father and a carrier mother or another genetic mutation (Ragni, 2006).

Individuals with less than 1% of the normal factor VIII or factor IX activity have severe disease and experience bleeding with minimal or no trauma; in these patients, unprovoked muscle and joint bleeding may occur between one and six times per month (Pipe & Valentino, 2007). Individuals with 1% to 5% of the normal factor VIII or factor IX activity are classified as having moderately severe disease and typically bleed with trauma or surgery. Those with more than 5% factor VIII or factor IX activity have mild hemophilia and usually bleed only with significant hemostatic challenges, such as those occurring with surgery or trauma.

Presentation

The majority of patients with hemophilia are diagnosed at birth due to a family history. One-third of patients with hemophilia have no family history and are determined to be a result of a new mutation. In 30% to 50% of patients, the earliest presenting symptoms of hemophilia are bleeding during or immediately following circumcision and/or subdural or periosteal bleeds during delivery, especially with vacuum extraction. In 1% to 2% of infants, perinatal intracranial hemorrhage occurs. Other neonatal symptoms may include cephalohematoma and excessive bleeding from puncture sites or the umbilical stump. Consequently, when there is a family history of hemophilia, birth trauma from forceps and vacuum extraction must be avoided (Kulkarni et al., 2009; Price et al., 2007; Stephensen et al., 2009).

In early childhood, as the child becomes more mobile, bruising and bleeding are likely to become more frequent. Oral bleeding, especially from a torn frenulum or with eruption of deciduous teeth, is common due to the instability of the jelly-like clots that form. Additionally, once mobility increases, the likelihood for resultant muscle (hematomas) and joint (hemarthroses) bleeds also increases. Patients with hemarthrosis will usually note an aura of tingling or warmth, followed by the onset of pain and decreased range of motion, as the joint capsule becomes distended. The majority of joint hemorrhages occur in the ankles, knees, and elbows (Stephensen et al., 2009). Both hematomas and hemathroses may lead to long-term complications for patients with hemophilia, such as pain, swelling, and decreased range of motion of affected joints. Bleeding after trauma or during surgery or other medical or dental procedures is also common. Some patients experience more serious bleeding complications such as intracranial or retroperitoneal hemorrhage or bleeding after surgical procedures (Price et al., 2007).

Differential diagnosis

Any disease or medical condition that affects fibrin clot formation must be considered in the list of differential diagnoses for hemophilia. This list should include von Willebrand disease, lupus erythematosus, factor XII deficiency, vitamin K deficiency, liver disease, DIC, and use of medications, such as heparin or warfarin (Ragni, 2006).

Plan of care

Diagnostic studies include a complete blood count, blood smear, prothrombin time (PT) and INR, partial thromboplastin time (PTT, also known as activated partial thromboplastin time [aPTT]), fibrinogen, and bleeding time. Hemophilia is suspected when the PTT is prolonged in the presence of a normal PT and platelet count. In addition, the bleeding time and fibrinogen concentration or thrombin time are normal. Assays for the activity of factor VIII or factor IX should be performed to confirm the deficiency and allow for classification of the type of hemophilia. The presence of an antibody inhibiting either factor VIII or factor IX activity may be excluded by performing a mixing study in which normal plasma in an equal volume is mixed with the patient's plasma and incubated for 30 to 60 minutes, then performing a PTT. When a deficiency of the factor VIII or factor IX is present, the PTT will correct into the normal range. In contrast, in the presence of an antibody inhibiting factor VIII or factor IX activity, this mixing procedure will not correct the PTT (Bhargava, 1981; Goodeve, 1998; Preston, 1998).

Prompt institution of coagulation factor replacement therapy minimizes the morbidity from hemorrhage. In general, patients experiencing major bleeding of any kind should receive 100% replacement intravenously; with minor bleeds in the joints or muscles, 50% to 60% replacement; and with mucocutaneous bleeding, 30% to 50% replacement (Tcheng, 2005).

Initial dosing for hemarthrosis in patients with factor VIII deficiency may be 25–50 units/kg of factor VIII concentrate, followed by 20 units/kg on the next day, with additional doses administered based on the treatment response. Similarly, bleeding in patients with hemophilia IX deficiency may be treated with 40–80 units/kg of factor IX concentrate, followed by 20 units/kg the following day, with subsequent treatments depending on the response to the initial therapy (Mannucci & Tuddenham, 2001; Pipe & Valentino, 2007). The dose of factor VIII concentrate may also be calculated based on the following formula:

Does of factor VIII in units = desired rise in plasma factor VIII activity × patient's body weight in kilograms × correction factors of 0.5

The correction factor is necessary because factor VIII is bound by von Willebrand factor and remains in the intravascular compartment. Calculation of the dose of factor IX concentrate is performed by multiplying the desired rise in factor IX activity times the patient's body weight in kilograms. Maintenance dosing of factor concentrates is based on the half-life of factor VIII (8–12 hours) and factor IX (12–24 hours). Maintenance dosing is recommended after surgical or invasive procedures (Ragni, 2006).

Episodic treatment for hemarthroses may result in reductions in pain and swelling. Unfortunately, such therapy does not prevent the long-term complications due to the bleeding, and the development of arthritis will ensue. Therefore, patients with severe hemophilia are frequently treated with prophylactic infusions of factor VIII or factor IX concentrates to prevent bleeding into the joints and other tissues (Coppola et al., 2009; Ljung, 2009; Mancuso et al., 2009; Valentino, 2004). Joint aspiration is usually avoided unless the patient has hip hemarthrosis, as this problem is associated with avascular necrosis of the femoral head. When a patient experiences joint bleeding, supportive care may be used to reduce the symptoms; it includes the application of ice, a compressive dressing, resting the joint, and elevating it.

The diagnosis of intramuscular hematoma is often difficult due to the deep nature of these hemorrhages and the vague symptoms elicited. Similar treatment recommendations may be used for patients with hemophilia A or B as for patients with hemarthrosis. Muscle hemorrhage should be considered severe when due to hemarthrosis, with the possibility of developing contractures, muscle atrophy, or pseudotumor formation. The development of iliopsoas hemorrhage is particularly dangerous and may result in severe morbidity (Valentino et al., 2006).

Bleeding into the central nervous system, into and around the airway, and into the peritoneal cavity may be life-threatening. Treatment of life-threatening hemorrhage usually seeks to maintain near-normal levels of the clotting factor for a minimum of 14 days with longer durations of prophylaxis administered to ensure resolution of the hemorrhage. After intracranial hemorrhage, the patient should be treated with prophylaxis for at least 6 to 12 months (Bladen et al., 2009; Fischer et al., 2008).

Less serious bleeding, such as from exfoliation of a deciduous tooth or a torn frenulum, may be treated with 20 unit/kg of factor VIII concentrate or 40 unit/kg of factor IX concentrate, along with administration of an antifibrinolytic medication such as aminocaproic acid. Dosing for aminocaproic acid is 50 mg/kg by mouth every 6 hours for 7 to 10 days (Ragani, 2006). If the bleeding comes from a tooth that has loosened but not completely exfoliated, that tooth should be removed promptly to minimize bleeding. Epistaxis is usually managed with topical pressure and petroleum gauze packing.

Patients with mild to moderate hemophilia A may be treated with desmopressin acetate (DDAVP), an agent that may be administered either parenterally or intranasally. It is *not* appropriate for patients with severe hemophilia A or patients with hemophilia B. Parenteral DDAVP may be administered at a dose of 0.3 mcg/kg for three doses. If bleeding does not respond, supplemental factor VIII concentrate should be given. Intranasal DDAVP may be dosed at 150 mcg in one nostril for patients weighing less than 50 kg. In patients weighing 50 kg or more, it may be dosed at 300 mcg.

For patients with severe hemophilia A or B, administration of exogenous factor VIII or factor IX concentrates may result in allo-immunization and the development of antibodies that inhibit the function of the infused factor concentrates. Inhibitors do not develop in all patients and are believed to be influenced by genetics, immune disturbances, environmental factors, and treatment-related variables. It is estimated that 30% of patients with severe hemophilia A and 2% to 5% of patients with severe hemophilia B develop inhibitors as some point in their lives. The median age for inhibitor development is 2 years and may occur after a median of 9 treatment days. Inhibitors are two times more likely to develop in African American patients (Ragani, 2006). Patients who develop these inhibitory antibodies are at particular risk for severe morbidity and mortality (Ananyeva et al., 2009; Astermark, 2009; Santagostino et al., 2009; Verbruggen, 2009).

Bleeding in the presence of an inhibitory antibody is difficult to control. The treatment requires administration of drugs that bypass the necessity for the factor VIII or factor IX activity (Pruthi et al., 2007; Valentino, 2010). The bleeding manifestations in these patients are identical to those in patients without inhibitory antibodies. However, the complications are more frequent due to the inability to successfully control hemorrhage. Inhibitory antibodies may be suspected when the patient has unabated bleeding despite the administration of adequate doses of factor concentrate.

Hemophilia patients with inhibitory antibodies against factor VIII may be treated with high doses of factor VIII or factor IX concentrates when the concentration of the inhibitory antibody is less than 5 Bethesda units/mL. Individuals with inhibitory antibody concentrations exceeding this level require a bypassing agent to control hemorrhage. In this scenario, recombinant activated factor VII or activated prothrombin complex concentrates are often administered. Although prothrombin complex concentrates are available, they are used less frequently.

The goal of therapy for patients with inhibitory antibodies is eradication of the antibody, which may be accomplished via immune tolerance induction therapy (Ingerslev, 2000; Kempton & White, 2009). This treatment involves administration of very large doses of factor VIII in an effort to tolerize the patient against the exogenous factor. The success rate for this therapy varies but is approximately 50% to 70%.

Any type of surgical or invasive procedure in hemophilia patients requires special preparation. Patients should avoid the use of NSAIDs and products containing aspirin for 1 to 2 weeks prior to the scheduled procedure. All patients should receive recombinant clotting factor concentrate to achieve 100% replacement immediately preceding such procedures. Dosing for factor VIII concentrate is initially recommended at 50 units/kg parenterally, with a maintenance dose of 25 units/kg. Factor IX is dosed initially at 75–100 units/kg, with a maintenance dose of 35–50 units/kg. In addition, prior to scheduling procedures, patients should be assessed for the presence of any inhibitors that might affect the efficacy of factor replacement therapy. Postoperative administration of factor concentrate at maintenance dosages should be continued for at least 3 weeks or until no further bleeding symptoms remain (Ragni, 2006).

The team of HCPs for a patient with hemophilia often includes a hematologist, physical therapist, complemental therapy specialist, and social worker. Specialists from other disciplines, such as orthopedics and dental professionals, may be consulted as needed (Price et al., 2007). Patient and family education, long-term treatment recommendations, and medical management of complications are best provided by a hemophilia treatment center (HTC); HTCs offer patients an interprofessional approach to care.

Disposition and discharge planning

Patients with severe hemophilia A and B frequently suffer from multiple disease complications. These may include life-threatening bleeding episodes, bone destruction from hemarthroses, compartment syndrome, infections such as hepatitis B and C from factor replacement, allergic reactions to clotting factor concentrate, thromboses, end-stage liver disease, and neurologic sequelae if intracranial hemorrhage occurs. The newer recombinant factor replacement concentrates are increasing in popularity for prophylactic treatment, a trend that has reduced many of the life-threatening bleeding episodes for patients. To prevent unexpected bleeding episodes, patients with hemophilia must avoid use of medications that inhibit platelets or coagulation factors, such as NSAIDs, aspirin, anticoagulants, and certain antibiotics. Additionally, if a central venous catheter access device is required for factor administration, infection or blood clots may develop (Ragni, 2006).

All patients, regardless of the type or severity of their disease, should have an annual evaluation at an HTC. This assessment includes testing for infectious diseases and other bloodborne pathogens. Vaccination for hepatitis A and B is recommended. Additionally, patients are encouraged to exercise and maintain a healthy weight to increase muscle strength and protect their joints (Centers for Disease Control and Prevention [CDC], 2010). Contact sports are generally contraindicated for patients with hemophilia, although patients may participate in other sports after a thorough physical therapy evaluation and discussion regarding requirements for protective equipment (Philpott et al., 2010).

HENOCH-SCHÖNLEIN PURPURA

Kristen Osborn

Pathophysiology

Henoch-Schönlein purpura (HSP) is an acute, systematic, immune complex-mediated vasculitis affecting the small vessels. Also referred to as anaphylactoid purpura, this disorder tends to be mild and self-limiting. HSP is classified as a nongranulomatous small-vessel vasculitis and is considered the most common vasculitis of childhood.

The specific pathogenesis of HSP is not completely understood. Immunoglobulin A (IgA) immune complexes are deposited in the small vessels of the renal glomeruli, the skin, and the gastrointestinal (GI) tract and cause petechiae, palpable purpura, GI hemorrhage, and glomerulonephritis (Roberts et al., 2007).

Epidemiology and etiology

Most cases of HSP are precipitated by upper respiratory infection, medication, or some other environmental trigger. Infectious agents linked to the development of HSP include Group A *Streptococcus*, parvovirus B19, *Bartonella henslae*, *Helicobacter pylori*, *Haemophilus parainfluenzae*, Coxsackie virus, adenovirus, mycoplasma, Epstein-Barr virus, hepatitis A and B viruses, *Varicella*, *Campylobacter*, and methicillin-resistant *Staphylococcus aureus* (MRSA). As many as 50% of patients who develop HSP have evidence of antistreptolysin O (ASO) antibodies, providing information that Group A *streptococcus* appears to be the most prevalent causative agent (Reamy et al., 2009; Tizard & Hamilton-Ayres, 2008).

The incidence of HSP ranges from 10 to 20 per 100,000 children, although it is believed that this estimate is low because many cases are not reported to public health agencies. HSP may be seen in all ages, but appears to be more common in young children. Seventy-five percent of patients are younger than 10 years of age, with the majority of cases occurring between 2 and 8 years of age. The disease is less common in African American children as compared to Caucasian or Asian children, and is seen more often in the winter, autumn, and spring than in the summer months. Both male and female predominance has been reported, although most sources state that males are affected twice as often as females (Eleftheriou et al., 2009; Roberts et al., 2007).

Presentation

The presentation of HSP may either be acute or insidious. Most patients report that an upper respiratory infection precedes the development of HSP and experience a prodrome of fever and fatigue, followed by the appearance of the classic rash of nonblanching, palpable, purpuric lesions. The disease usually presents with a tetrad of symptoms—rash, polyarthralgias, abdominal pain, and kidney disease. These symptoms may occur in any sequence (Reamy et al., 2009).

The nonpruritic rash begins as erythematous papules or wheals that progress to a combination of petechiae and purpura greater than 10 mm in diameter. The HSP rash is most commonly seen in dependent areas of the body that are subject to pressure and the extensor surface of the extremities; it commonly spares the trunk. The lesions, which may ultimately evolve to ecchymoses, gradually fade over approximately 10 days (Tizard & Hamilton-Ayres, 2008).

Between 50% and 75% of patients with HSP experience diffuse, colicky abdominal pain, often referred to as bowel angina. Some patients develop vomiting or melena. The majority of patients experience some degree of transitory arthritis or arthralgia. The joints most commonly affected are those of the lower extremities—that is, the knees, hips, ankles, and feet. Patients report symptoms of pain and swelling with decreased range of motion of the affected joints.

HSP also affects the renal system, where it is manifested as hematuria, proteinuria, and hypertension, and may progress to nephrotic syndrome and kidney failure (Barkin & Rosen, 2003b). Renal symptoms develop weeks to months after the initial presentation and affect between 20% and 60% of patients. The kidney lesions specific to HSP show a focal and proliferative glomerulonephritis on biopsy (Ballinger, 2003).

Differential diagnosis

Because HSP is believed to be somewhat autoimmune in nature, other autoimmune conditions must be considered when constructing the differential diagnosis list. IgA nephritis should be considered as an alternative diagnosis, as should other forms of vasculitis, systemic lupus erythematosus, acute hemorrhagic edema of infancy, and septicemia (Barkin & Rosen, 2003b).

Plan of care

Relatively few diagnostic studies are useful in the diagnosis of HSP. Therefore, the diagnosis is usually based on clinical features. Renal function testing at baseline may be beneficial for monitoring kidney disease. Other tests and imaging studies may be ordered to identify complications or progression of kidney disease. Clotting function is usually normal, and the platelet count may be normal or elevated. The presence of IgA complexes in the blood, skin, or glomeruli of patients may help to confirm a diagnosis of HSP.

In 1990, the American College of Rheumatology developed criteria for the diagnosis of HSP. These criteria include palpable purpura, age less than or equal to 20 years at diagnosis, bowel angina, and granulocytes in the walls of arterioles and vessels (Reamy et al., 2009).

HSP spontaneously resolves in more than 90% of patients; therefore, symptomatic management of systemic complications is the treatment of choice. In most patients, the only long-term complication is kidney disease. Medications are targeted at alleviating the patient's discomfort from clinical manifestations. Acetaminophen or NSAIDs are helpful in the management of arthritic discomfort, although NSAIDs may aggravate GI symptoms and should be avoided in patients with kidney disease. Rest and activity limitation

are encouraged to decrease the development of purpuric lesions. Some patients may be managed on an outpatient basis, but many will require hospitalization to monitor and control kidney function. Many HCPs recommend steroid administration for patients with kidney disease or other significant symptoms. The recommended treatment regimen is oral prednisone at 1–2 mg/kg/day for 2 weeks. Plasma exchange, high-dose intravenous immunoglobulin, and immunosuppressants, such as cyclophosphamide, have also shown to be effective therapies for HSP. If ESRD develops, kidney transplant may be necessary. Patients and families should be taught to monitor for signs of blood in the urine and evidence of hypertension. Additionally, families should return for follow-up if symptoms recur (Reamy et al., 2009; Roberts et al., 2007).

Disposition and discharge planning

Henoch-Schönlein purpura is usually a mild, self-limiting disease. Most cases resolve within 4 weeks without significant long-term complications. Renal impairment is the only serious complication reported, though renal involvement may range from mild to severe. The majority of patients with renal impairment present only with isolated hematuria or proteinuria; others experience acute nephritis or nephritic syndrome. A small percentage of patients will have persistent hypertension requiring long-term management. Orchitis and scrotal swelling have been reported in approximately 35% of male patients and may progress to testicular torsion. Table 28-2 lists complications associated with HSP. Recurrences are relatively common within the first 6 months of illness and are more common in children with evidence of kidney disease.

At the time of diagnosis, a baseline urinalysis and blood pressure should be obtained. Follow-up care for patients with resolving HSP should include urinalysis, blood pressure, BUN, and creatinine measurement to monitor for progression of renal impairment. For patients without significant kidney disease, including those with mild proteinuria or hematuria, monthly urinalysis should be performed for the first 6 months. If renal impairment is severe, patients should be referred to a nephrologist (Tizard & Hamilton-Ayres, 2008).

IMMUNE THROMBOCYTOPENIC PURPURA

Kristen Osborn

Pathophysiology

Immune thrombocytopenic purpura (ITP), formerly known as idiopathic thrombocytopenic purpura, is an acquired autoimmune disorder that results in accelerated platelet destruction by IgG, IgA, or IgM autoantibodies.

TABLE 28-2

Complications of Henoch-Schönlein Purpura	
Renal	**Gastrointestinal**
Acute or chronic kidney failure	Bowel infarction or perforation
Glomerulonephritis	Cholecystitis
Hematuria	Gallbladder sludge
Hemorrhagic cystitis	Intestinal colic
Hypertension	Intussusception
Nephritis	Pancreatitis
Nephrotic syndrome	
Proteinuria	
Ureteral obstruction	
Cardiopulmonary	**Central Nervous System**
Alveolar hemorrhage	Aphasia
Interstitial infiltrate	Cerebral hemorrhage
Myocarditis	Cerebral vasculitis
Pulmonary effusion	Neuropathy
	Seizures
Other	
Arthralgias	
Elevated liver transaminase levels	
Epistaxis	
Myositis	
Orchitis	
Parotitis	
Scrotal swelling	
Testicular torsion	
Uveitis	

Platelets become coated with autoantibody and are removed from the circulation by the spleen. These antibodies also affect platelet development by the bone marrow, causing a decrease in platelet production. Characteristic bone marrow findings in ITP include an increase in megakaryocytes or immature platelets (Jin & Bussel, 2006).

Epidemiology and etiology

ITP is a common acquired bleeding disorder in children, with an incidence of approximately 4 to 8 cases per 100,000 population per year. The acute form of the illness is the most prevalent form, although a small percentage of pediatric patients progress to the chronic form of the disorder. The condition presents in healthy children and is often precipitated by a viral illness. The peak age for presentation in children is between 2 and 6 years of age. ITP incidence is equally distributed between male and female patients until adolescence, when the incidence increases in females. It is more common in the spring.

ITP is associated with a variety of viral illnesses, including measles, mumps, chickenpox, infectious mononucleosis,

and the common cold. There is also limited evidence of an association between *Helicobacter pylori* infection and hepatitis C exposure and the development of ITP. These links are controversial and require further research for confirmation.

In most patients, acute ITP will improve spontaneously within 6 months even without treatment (Jin & Bussel, 2006).

Presentation

Most patients with diagnosed with ITP are previously healthy, well-appearing children who present with an acute onset of petechiae or purpura, easy bruising, and spontaneous bleeding of the skin and mucous membranes. Clinical manifestations vary from patient to patient, however, and are often influenced by the degree of thrombocytopenia. The spectrum of bleeding may range from common symptoms such as bruising, petechiae, and epistaxis, to rarer symptoms such as gingival bleeding, menorrhagia, hematuria, GI bleeding, and intracranial hemorrhage. Severity is also affected by patient age and the presence of comorbid conditions (Jin & Bussel, 2006).

Physical examination findings are commonly nonspecific and may include the bleeding symptoms as described previously. Hepatosplenomegaly, lymphadenopathy, or other signs of malignancy are not expected on physical examination.

Differential diagnosis

The initial diagnosis of ITP is usually established with the identification of thrombocytopenia on a complete blood count. Most pediatric patients with ITP have a benign medical history and physical examination. HCPs should consider other causes of thrombocytopenia such as medications or other autoimmune diseases, which are often revealed during a family history. Other findings, such as hearing loss, immunodeficiency, kidney disease, or any signs of systemic illness, should direct providers toward etiologies other than ITP (Jin & Bussel, 2006).

Plan of care

Diagnostic studies are necessary to confirm a diagnosis of ITP and are usually indicated in a patient who displays an isolated, but significant episode of thrombocytopenia without other significant symptoms. A complete blood count will most likely reveal a platelet count of 100,000 platelet/mm^3 or less, with normal red and white blood cell counts, and a normal differential. A peripheral blood smear may reveal the presence of giant platelets. The diagnosis is confirmed by performing a bone marrow aspirate to evaluate for malignant conditions. The bone marrow examination produces a normocellular result with the presence of increased megakaryocytes. Upon careful consideration of history, physical examination, and laboratory findings, a diagnosis of ITP may be confirmed (Jin & Bussel, 2006).

Treatment of ITP is based on whether the condition is acute or chronic. Although most cases of ITP will resolve spontaneously without treatment, pharmacologic management remains the mainstay of therapy. First-line treatment for patients with acute ITP consists of oral corticosteroids. Initial dosing is from 2 to 4 mg/kg/day, with the dose being tapered off as the platelet count begins to return to normal. Patients may remain on steroids from weeks to months, depending on their response to therapy. Other medical therapies include intravenous immunoglobulin (IVIG) and anti-D immunoglobulin (WinRho-D). Although both IVIG and WinRho-D produce a more rapid increase in platelet count, their side effects must be considered when this treatment is suggested. IVIG is dosed at 1 gm/kg/day and is administered parenterally over 4 to 6 hours for 2 consecutive days. WinRho-D is administered at 50 mg/kg as a single parenteral dose over 3 to 5 minutes. Patients receiving either IVIG or WinRho-D must be carefully monitored for signs of allergic reaction, including fever, chills, headache, and hemolytic anemia (Jin & Bussel, 2006).

Chronic ITP, which is defined as thrombocytopenia lasting 6 months or longer, is more challenging to manage. Options for treatment include regular administration of either IVIG or WinRho-D or splenectomy. Some studies have examined the use of immunosuppressive agents for the management of chronic ITP, although this regimen is not supported in children. Most commonly, laparoscopic splenectomy is recommended and proves successful in raising the platelet count in 60% to 80% of patients. Because postsplenectomy patients are at risk for sepsis from encapsulated organisms (*Streptococcus pneumoniae, Haemophilus influenzae, Neisseria meningitides*), it is recommended to delay surgery until patients are 5 years of age or older. These patients must be appropriately immunized with pneumococcal and meningococcal vaccines prior to the procedure. Additionally, patients receiving a splenectomy should be placed on prophylactic penicillin after the procedure to prevent septicemia (Jin & Bussel, 2006).

Supportive care for all patients with ITP includes measures to prevent bleeding. Medications that enhance bleeding should be avoided, such as aspirin products and NSAIDs. Immunizations or other injections should be delayed until platelet counts are relatively normal. If injections are unavoidable, pressure should be applied to the puncture site for at least 5 to 10 minutes to avoid hematoma development. Patients and families should be educated to avoid activities that may result in a bleeding episode, such as exercise and sports participation. To prevent intracranial hemorrhage, some experts recommend protective equipment for the heads of toddlers who are extremely active. It is imperative to teach caregivers to recognize the signs of bleeding and to know who to contact in case of an emergency (Jin & Bussel, 2006).

Disposition and discharge planning

At least 80% of patients with ITP improve spontaneously within 6 to 12 months of their diagnosis. In all patients, the prevention of bleeding should be the HCP's primary concern until recovery occurs. Other than bleeding, however, relatively few long-term complications are associated with ITP. The most serious complication is intraventricular hemorrhage (IVH). The risk of neurologic sequelae after IVH is high, which is why head injury precautions are suggested. Most patients with acute ITP demonstrate an increase in platelet count 1 to 2 weeks after beginning treatment, but the majority completely have recovered by 6 months. Platelet counts should be monitored regularly early in the course, with subsequent testing being scheduled based on the response to treatment. The severity of thrombocytopenia will determine the frequency with which platelet counts are needed. Chronic ITP, although monitored similarly to the acute disease, requires a longer-term commitment and usually results in splenectomy (Jin & Bussel, 2006).

PLATELET FUNCTION DISORDERS

Kristen Osborn

Pathophysiology

In platelet function disorders, platelet numbers are adequate, but the platelets themselves are dysfunctional. These disorders are classified as either acquired or hereditary (Table 28-3). Most hereditary platelet function disorders are relatively rare (Bennett, 2006). This section reviews acquired platelet function disorders caused by medications, the most common of which is heparin-induced thrombocytopenia (HIT). This severe adverse drug reaction is considered a life-threatening complication of heparin therapy. HIT is an immune-mediated antibody reaction to platelet factor 4 (PF4) and heparin (Arepally & Ortel, 2006). Although significant thrombocytopenia occurs as a result of the immune-mediated response, patients remain at high risk for clotting (Baroletti & Goldhaber, 2006).

Epidemiology and etiology

Despite the fact that risk factors for HIT have been identified, it remains unclear why some patients develop HIT and others do not. Risk factors for the development of HIT include female gender, being a postoperative orthopedic patient, longer duration of heparin administration, and use of unfractionated heparin as opposed to low-molecular-weight heparin. HIT occurs in 1% to 3% of patients who receive unfractionated heparin for 5 days or longer. It is relatively uncommon in the pediatric population (Warkentin et al., 2006).

TABLE 28-3

Platelet Function Disorders

Acquired

Medications	Diseases
Anesthetics	Aplastic anemia
Anticoagulants	Chronic kidney disease
Antidepressants	Ehlers-Danlos syndrome
Antihistamines	Heart bypass surgery
Aspirin	Leukemia
Some antibiotics	Marfan syndrome
Certain cardiac drugs	Osteogenesis imperfecta
Nonsteroidal anti-inflammatory drugs	
Ticlopidine	

Hereditary

Disorders of Platelet Adhesion

Bernard-Soulier syndrome

Disorders of Platelet Aggregation

Glanzmann thrombasthenia
Hermansky-Pudlak syndrome
Chediak-Higashi syndrome

Disorders of Platelet Secretion

Gray platelet syndrome (alpha granule deficiency)
Dense granule deficiency (delta storage pool deficiency)
Quebec platelet disorder

Disorders of Platelet Procoagulant Activity

Scott syndrome

Combined Abnormalities of Platelet Number and Function

May-Hegglin anomaly
Alport syndrome
Wiskott-Aldrich syndrome

Presentation

Patients with HIT are relatively variable in presentation, although most have significant thrombocytopenia that develops acutely between days 5 and 10 of heparin therapy. This disorder may also develop during a repeat course of heparin if the previous course occurred less than 30 days prior to the current course. Most patients experience approximately a 50% drop in platelet count (Warkentin, 2005). Additionally, thromboses may occur. Symptoms of a new-onset blood clot may be indicative of HIT. Other physical examination findings include heparin-induced skin lesions, which appear as necrotic lesions at the site of heparin injection. Rarely, acute systemic reactions, including hemodynamic instability,

respiratory distress, neurologic complications, and severe inflammation, may occur. Occasionally, delayed-onset HIT may occur after a patient has already stopped heparin therapy (Warkentin et al., 2006)

Differential diagnosis

Other causes of thrombocytopenia and thromboses, such as bacterial infection, medications, and bone marrow disease, should be excluded as part of the diagnostic process (Arepally & Ortel, 2006).

Plan of care

Confirming the HIT diagnosis may be challenging due to the variability and complexity of underlying conditions. Diagnostic studies include testing for the presence of HIT antibodies either by serologic or functional assays, or both (Arepally & Ortel, 2006).

Initial management of a patient with HIT involves the discontinuation of heparin therapy from all sources. Even in the absence of thromboses, immediate supplemental, nonheparin anticoagulant therapy must be initiated to prevent subsequent thrombotic events. When selecting a replacement therapy, several factors must be considered, such as medication availability, clinical manifestations, and the acuity of the patient. Many sources recommend the use of direct thrombin inhibitors (DTIs) in patients with HIT, as thrombin generation is an important component of the development of thromboses in this disorder. There are currently three commercially available medications approved by the U.S. Food and Drug Administration (FDA) for the management of HIT: argatroban, lepirudin, and bivalirudin. Coumadin should not be used in patients with a platelet count less than 150,000/mm³ to prevent the development of venous limb gangrene. Platelet transfusions are contraindicated because the addition of platelets into circulation will increase the likelihood of thrombosis development. The duration of anticoagulant therapy depends on the presence or absence of thromboses, but is routinely continued for 4 or more weeks (Baroletti & Goldhaber, 2006; Shantsila et al., 2009; Warkentin, 2005).

Disposition and discharge planning

The prognosis for a patient with HIT is usually determined by the severity of thrombotic complications. Anticoagulant therapy reduces the likelihood of death from thrombotic events, it does not affect the mortality associated with any underlying conditions. HIT is typically a self-limited disorder that does not require long-term management. Complications of HIT include pulmonary embolism, limb amputation secondary to limb ischemic syndromes (venous limb gangrene), adrenal hemorrhagic necrosis, and development of DIC. Patients should avoid future heparin exposure due to the risk of the development of repeated episodes of HIT. Follow-up for patients with HIT usually involves supportive care for sequelae from HIT induced thromboses (Warkentin et al., 2006).

THROMBOEMBOLIC DISORDERS

Kristen Osborn

Pathophysiology

A thrombus is a blood clot that is attached to the lining of a blood vessel. Once it breaks loose and is released into circulation, it becomes known as a thromboembolism. Thrombi may be found in both arterial and venous circulation. An embolus is a cluster of a variety of materials that is circulating in the bloodstream. Emboli may be made of air, amniotic fluid, bacteria, fat, or other foreign materials. An embolism causes obstruction of a blood vessel. An arterial thromboembolism is a vascular obstruction from a blood clot in an artery. A venous thromboembolism is located in a vein (Brashers, 2006). A combination of three factors, known as Virchow's triad—blood abnormalities, alteration of blood flow, and disruption of the vessel wall—leads to thrombus formation (Francis & Kaplan, 2006).

Thrombus development occurs when the clotting cascade is activated. Notably, conditions such as infection, inflammation, injury, roughening of the endothelium, and blood pooling within blood vessels predispose patients to the development of thrombi. Additional risk factors include the use of central venous catheters (CVCs) and parenteral nutrition. Fortunately, pediatric patients do not have as many acquired risk factors as their adult counterparts.

Arterial thrombosis is most often associated with roughening of the tunica intima by atherosclerosis or infection. Venous thrombosis occurs more commonly from conditions that reduce blood flow or from inflammation. Commonly, venous thrombi are manifested as deep vein thrombosis (DVT) or pulmonary embolism (PE) in children (Brashers, 2006; Francis & Kaplan, 2006; Parasuraman & Goldhaber, 2006).

Epidemiology and etiology

Fortunately, thromboembolic disease is not a common occurrence in pediatric patients, although its incidence has increased in the last 10 years. Most children who experience thromboembolic events have serious underlying medical conditions such as congenital heart disease, nephritic syndrome, systemic lupus erythematosus, or cancer; are postoperative; or have experienced a major trauma (Tormene et al., 2006). Pediatric patients at the highest risk for the development of DVT or PE are infants younger than 1 year of age and adolescents.

The single greatest risk factor for arterial or venous thrombosis in infants and children is the presence of a CVC. The incidence of thrombosis due to the presence of CVCs reflects the location of the line, the length of time the line has been in place, and the patient's underlying medical condition; this incidence varies from 10% to 50% of all patients who have a CVC. The incidence of thromboses in neonates is approximately 2.4 per 1,000 intensive care patients, with the majority of non-CVC-related cases involving renal vein thrombosis (RVT).

Other predisposing factors for thrombus formation in children include trauma, especially to the leg or pelvic area; immobilization; congestive heart failure; pregnancy; use of contraceptives; inherited or acquired coagulation protein abnormalities (protein C, protein S, and factor V Leiden deficiencies); and osteomyelitis. Cerebral thromboses resulting in stroke are most commonly seen in children with cardiac disease (Barkin & Rosen, 2003a; Revel-Vilk & Kenet, 2005.

Presentation

The presentation of any thrombotic event is based on the location of the thrombus. The majority of thromboses in children occur in the upper venous system, which predisposes these patients to the development of pulmonary embolism. Often, the clinical presentation in children is subtle and overlooked due to the presence of symptoms from underlying disease. If symptoms of thrombosis do occur, they may include swelling, pain, and discoloration near the site of the clot. Catheter-related symptoms may include sepsis and loss of patency of the line. Additional findings are variable, based on age and underlying condition, but may include thrombocytopenia, abdominal or inguinal pain, superior vena cava syndrome, chylothorax, and chylopericardium (Francis & Kaplan, 2006).

Peripheral arterial occlusion is commonly a result of atherosclerosis. This outcome is uncommon in children, but its rates are likely to increase due to the rising rates of obesity, hypercholesterolemia, type 2 diabetes, and physical inactivity in the pediatric population. Under normal circumstances, 70% of an artery has to be blocked for symptoms to occur. Such symptoms may include pain, coldness, numbness, and intermittent claudication in the affected limb. If a sudden blockage occurs in the lower aorta, iliac, or renal arteries, symptoms are much more sudden and severe (Francis & Kaplan, 2006; Nowak-Göttl et al., 2004).

Deep vein thrombosis of a lower extremity may present as leg pain of variable severity and swelling, often in the calf, which develops over one or several days. The site may also be warm and tender to the touch or completely asymptomatic. Superficial venous thrombosis presents as a painful area that runs along the course of a superficial vein and is not usually as serious as DVT (Francis & Kaplan, 2006).

Pulmonary embolism is usually associated with dyspnea, cough, hemoptysis, pleuritic pain, and anxiety. Physical examination also may reveal tachypnea, tachycardia, and an increased second heart sound. Arterial thrombi may lodge in the vessels of the heart or the brain. The presenting symptoms depend on the site of the clot (Brashers, 2006).

Differential diagnosis

In the majority of pediatric patients, a combination of factors influences thrombus formation. History may reveal hereditary prothrombic conditions, an early age of onset, and recurrent episodes of thromboembolism, recurrent spontaneous abortions, or thrombosis during pregnancy (Albisetti et al., 2007; Dietrich & Hertweck, 2008).

Plan of care

Before a diagnosis of thromboembolism is considered, the HCP must establish the pretest probability for emboli, as only 25% of patients suspected of having an embolus are ultimately confirmed to have this diagnosis. The presence of risk factors must be examined. Additionally, a combination of physical examination findings and diagnostic studies should be considered. The most commonly used diagnostic test in children is venous Doppler ultrasound—an imaging technology that is relatively sensitive and specific, yet noninvasive (Parasuraman & Goldhaber, 2006). Almost all patients with a thrombosis will have an elevated D-dimer level. A normal level may rule out thrombosis especially if a patient's risk is low. If the diagnosis remains unclear after ultrasound and D-dimer measurement, angiography or venography—which are considered the studies of choice for diagnosis—may be considered (Tormene et al., 2006). Computed tomography (CT) and magnetic resonance imaging (MRI) may be useful in disease of the larger vessels, but have not been validated in pediatric patients. For patients who are suspected of having a pulmonary embolism, a ventilation–perfusion lung scan should be performed. A negative lung scan is effective in ruling out a diagnosis of PE (Francis & Kaplan, 2006).

Patients who present with symptoms of an acute DVT or PE need immediate treatment for symptom relief as well as to prevent disease progression or recurrence. Supportive measures may include pain relief, elevation of the affected extremity, and removal of the CVC, if indicated.

Anticoagulant therapy is the hallmark of treatment. In patients with arterial disease, either unfractionated heparin or low-molecular-weight heparin (LMWH) is used. Unfractionated heparin is administered as a continuous intravenous infusion. Initially, patients should be bolused at 50 units/kg. The maintenance dose, 10–15 units/kg/hr parenterally, should be continued for 7 to 10 days. As a patient is weaned off heparin therapy, warfarin should be administered simultaneously. A loading dose of warfarin should be administered at 0.2 mg/kg, up to a maximum dose of 10 mg. The dose is then titrated based on laboratory results with the goal of maintaining the INR within the range of 2–3. The usual maintenance dose is 0.1 mg/kg/day by mouth. The goal of therapy is to maintain the PT at two times the control value. Therapy should be continued for 4 to 6 weeks to prevent recurrence of thromboses.

Use of LMWH for anticoagulation is becoming more prevalent in pediatric patients, as this type of heparin may be administered subcutaneously and eliminates the need for PT/PTT frequent monitoring. The recommended dose of LMWH in pediatric patients is 1.5 mg/kg subcutaneously (SQ) every 12 hours in infants aged 2 months and younger and 1 mg/kg SQ every 12 hours in children older than 2 months of age. For prophylaxis of DVT in these children, LMWH should be administered at 0.75 mg/kg and 0.5 mg/kg, respectively.

Fibrinolytics are reserved for the patients with the most severe disease and the largest thromboses. The newer antithrombotic drugs are not considered routine therapy in pediatric patients because there is not enough evidence currently available to support their use. Occasionally, surgical intervention for clot removal may be necessary (Francis & Kaplan, 2006; Parasuraman & Goldhaber, 2006; Yang et al., 2009).

Consultation with hematology, vascular surgery, cardiothoracic surgery, orthopedic surgery, pulmonology, and critical care specialists may be required for children with thromboembolism. Patient and family education must include education regarding signs and symptoms of bleeding and recurrence of clot formation.

Disposition and discharge planning

Children with thromboembolic events are usually treated for 3 to 6 months. Longer-term, prophylactic anticoagulant therapy may be necessary in patients who have multiple risk factors for recurrence of disease. Follow-up for children on anticoagulant therapy is based on the response to treatment and the duration of use of anticoagulant medications. The patient's PT, PTT, and INR should be monitored closely while on anticoagulation. In addition, if patients receiving LMWH use a subcutaneous catheter for administration of the medication, the catheter site should be assessed frequently (Francis & Kaplan, 2006).

VON WILLEBRAND DISEASE

Kristen Osborn

Pathophysiology

Von Willebrand disease (VWD) is classified as an autosomal dominant bleeding disorder. It causes a defect in the concentration, structure, or function of von Willebrand factor (Sadler et al., 2006). The gene that codes for this disease is located on the distal short arm of chromosome

12, although incomplete penetrance and variable expressivity have been reported (Armstrong & Konkle, 2006; Goodeve & James, 2009). Von Willebrand factor (VWF) is a plasma glycoprotein composed of multimers that cause platelet adhesion and act as a carrier protein for factor VIII. It is produced by endothelial cells and megakaryocytes and binds to connective tissue and platelets in areas of injury, helping to stabilize clots (Sadler et al.).

Three types of von Willebrand disease have been identified. Types 1 and 3 are caused by an insufficient quantity of VWF, whereas type 2 results from structural abnormalities in circulating VWF (Armstrong & Konkle, 2006). VWD type 2 is divided into four subtypes: type 2A, type 2B, type 2M, and type 2N (Sadler et al., 2006).

Epidemiology and etiology

VWD is the most common inherited bleeding disorder. Its incidence is estimated to be as high as 1% of the general population, although only 1 in 1,000 people has symptoms severe enough to require treatment (Armstrong & Konkle, 2006). Approximately 70% to 80% of patients have type 1 VWD; 15% to 20% are classified as having type 2 disease (Journeycake & Buchanan, 2003). Type 3 VWD is extremely rare and follows an autosomal recessive inheritance pattern. It is difficult to define the incidence and prevalence of VWD precisely because many mild cases go undiagnosed (Armstrong & Konkle).

Presentation

Providers should inquire about a family history of excessive bleeding. In many instances, although a diagnosis of a specific bleeding disorder may not have been made, there is evidence of a familial bleeding tendency. Excessive bruising, heavy menstrual bleeding, recurrent nosebleeds, and bleeding after minor procedures should lead the HCP to suspect VWD.

Clinical manifestations of VWD vary significantly and are based on the type of genetic mutation that the patient possesses. In general, VWD is a mild bleeding disorder and in some patients does not produce any symptoms of bleeding. Patients with type 1 VWD report symptoms such as mild mucocutaneous bleeding; ecchymoses and hematomas; prolonged, recurrent nosebleeds; postoperative bleeding; hematuria; and menorrhagia, with excessive bruising and heavy menstrual cycles being the most common. In patients with types 2 and 3, bleeding is more serious, tends to occur earlier, and may mimic hemophilia (Armstrong & Konkle, 2006).

Differential diagnosis

Several disease states have an effect on plasma VWF and factor VIII levels. Hypothyroidism reduces the circulating levels of VWF in plasma. Contraceptives containing estrogen may conversely increase those levels. Other factors, such as exercise, stress, inflammation, and pregnancy have the ability to increase plasma levels of VWF by one to three times of baseline levels (Armstrong & Konkle, 2006).

Plan of care

To confirm diagnostic suspicion, many institutions combine the necessary tests into a von Willebrand profile. The elements of this profile usually include a CBC, aPTT, PT, bleeding time, ristocetin cofactor, VWF antigen, and factor VIII level (Goodeve & James, 2009). Diagnosis is based on family history, bleeding symptoms, and laboratory data. Normal ristocetin cofactor and VWF antigen levels range from 50 to 200 IU/dL. Any patient with a value of 30 IU/dL or less should receive a diagnosis of VWD (Table 28-4). Further testing, including VWF multimers, gene sequencing, and antibody assays, may be necessary to determine the specific type of disease (National Heart, Lung, and Blood Institute [NHLBI], 2007).

Therapeutic management should be tailored based on the severity of bleeding symptoms and the patient's response to treatment. The primary goal is to maintain adequate hemostasis, which may include cessation of bleeding episodes or necessitate prophylaxis prior to medical procedures (Armstrong & Konkle, 2006).

First-line treatment for mild bleeding episodes consists of intravenous or intranasal DDAVP (NHLBI, 2007). DDAVP works by causing endothelial cells to release VWF, thereby promoting platelet adhesion. Its peak effect should occur in 30 to 60 minutes after administration and lasts for 6 to 12 hours. Many patients respond well to once-daily dosing (Armstrong & Konkle, 2006).

If a patient has an inadequate response to DDAVP, replacement with VWF concentrate should be considered. Dosing of VWF concentrate is based on ristocetin cofactor (RCo) and factor VIII (FVIII) units. For prophylaxis

TABLE 28-4

Laboratory Findings in Von Willebrand Disease	
Lab Test	**Possible Findings**
Complete blood count (CBC)	Normal, microcytic anemia, thrombocytopenia
Activated partial thromboplastin time (aPTT)	Normal or prolonged
Prothrombin time (PT)	Normal
Bleeding time	Normal to slightly prolonged (nonspecific finding)
Ristcetin cofactor	Low
Von Willebrand factor antigen	Low
Factor VIII level	Low or normal

during minor procedures, the goal is to achieve RCo and FVIII activity levels of 30 IU/dL. It is preferred to aim for activity levels of ≥ 50 IU/dL. This dose should be maintained for 1 to 5 days after the procedure.

For oral surgery, many patients benefit from administration of antifibrinolytics such as aminocaproic acid in combination with DDAVP (NHLBI, 2007). Topical agents, such as micronized collagen (Avitene), fibrin sealant, and Gelfoam or Surgicel soaked in topical thrombin, may be applied directly to the bleeding site in the nasal or oral cavity. Patients with more severe bleeding, including GI bleeding, may benefit from platelet transfusions. Menorrhagia, the most common presenting symptom in women, may be managed with the use of estrogen-containing contraceptives. Additionally, use of DDAVP and administration of antifibrinolytic agents during the first few days of the menstrual cycle have been shown to decrease menstrual blood flow (Armstrong & Konkle, 2006).

Disposition and discharge planning

Von Willebrand disease is generally a mild bleeding disorder; thus there are relatively few significant complications from this condition. Morbidity and mortality for patients with VWD are low, and prognosis is generally good. Recommendations for specific patient follow-up are based on the type of VWD. All patients, regardless of the type of their disease, should have a baseline evaluation of serum iron and ferritin levels to assess for iron deficiency. Women with menorrhagia require thorough gynecologic evaluations. Patients with type 3 VWD have the most severe clinical manifestations and generally require more comprehensive maintenance plans. These patients may require joint and muscle evaluation by a physical therapist. Additionally, any patient who received clotting factor concentrates prior to 1985 should be screened for hepatitis B and C and human immunodeficiency virus (Goodeve & James, 2009).

ONCOLOGIC DISORDERS

BONE MARROW TRANSPLANT AND GRAFT-VERSUS-HOST DISEASE

Jessica L. Diver

Bone marrow transplant

Bone marrow transplant (BMT) is the process of replacing absent, diseased, or damaged hematopoietic stem cells with healthy ones. For some pediatric patients, the indication for BMT is to *rescue* marrow that is disease free, as these patients would not recover with bone marrow suppression caused by high-dose chemotherapy and/or radiation. For other patients, BMT is used to replace diseased or

damaged cells with the healthy cells of another individual. This type of transplant may also prevent recurrence of disease through a proposed graft-versus-leukemia effect. Key concepts in bone marrow transplant are summarized in Table 28-5.

Types of bone marrow transplant
Autologous bone marrow transplant. In an autologous transplant, the patient receives his or her own cells following a preparative regimen of high-dose chemotherapy. This type of transplant is commonly used in solid tumor treatment and should be thought of as a rescue following otherwise toxic doses of chemotherapy. Such rescue therapy allows the patient to overcome the dose-limiting toxicity

TABLE 28-5

Key Concepts in Bone Marrow Transplantation	
Acute graft-versus-host disease (aGVHD)	An inflammatory process in which the donor cells attack host organs such as the skin, liver, and gastrointestinal tract, typically occurring in the 30–100 days post transplant
Allogeneic transplant	Infusion of stem cells from a donor other than the recipient; may include siblings, cord blood units or unrelated donors
Autologous transplant	Infusion of previously collected recipient cells into the pediatric patient
Chronic graft-versus-host disease (cGVHD)	A late complication of transplant resembling an autoimmune process and affecting the musculoskeletal system, mucous membranes, pulmonary system, or gastrointestinal tract, typically presenting more than 100 days post transplant
Hematopoietic stem cells	Cells that mature into red blood cells, white blood cells, and platelets
Preparative regimen	Chemotherapy, radiotherapy, and/or immunosuppression used in the days preceding transplant to eradicate tumor cells, myeloablate the patient, and immunosuppress the patient prior to infusion of stem cells
Syngeneic transplant	Stem cell transplant from an identical twin
Veno-occlusive disease (VOD)	A complication of transplant resulting in hyperbilirubinemia, weight gain, ascites, fluid retention, and hepatomegaly with right upper quadrant pain

of bone marrow suppression. The risks associated with an autologous BMT are associated with the toxicities of high-dose chemotherapy and tend to occur in the period surrounding the transplant, continuing until hematologic recovery is achieved.

Allogeneic bone marrow transplant. Allogeneic transplantation is the infusion of donor cells into a recipient. This type of transplant is indicated for patients with hematologic malignancies, immunodeficiencies, and certain genetic diseases (Table 28-6). Allogeneic donors may be a relative of the patient or an unrelated donor identified on the donor registry. A syngeneic transplant is an allogeneic transplant from an identical twin. An allogeneic transplant poses a greater risk to the patient for post-transplant complications, including graft-versus-host disease (GVHD). Pediatric patients undergoing an allogeneic transplant generally require more medications, prolonged isolation, and frequent monitoring as compared to autologous recipients.

Sources of hematopoeitic stem cells
Bone marrow harvest. Hematopoeitic stem cells are collected from marrow in the operating room. In most cases, the marrow is obtained from bilateral posterior iliac crests. The patient is placed under general anesthesia while large-bore aspirate needles are introduced and advanced until a sufficient number of stem cells are collected. A maximum of 20 mL/kg (of donor weight) of bone marrow is aspirated, although this maximum volume is not necessarily required to obtain an adequate cell dose. This technique can be used for either allogeneic or autologous collections. Its risks include those associated with general anesthesia, along with postoperative pain.

TABLE 28-6

Indications for Allogeneic Hematopoietic Stem Cell Transplantation	
Malignant	**Nonmalignant**
Myelodysplastic syndrome	Bone marrow failure
Leukemia	• Severe aplastic anemia
• Acute myelogenous	• Fanconi anemia
leukemia (AML)	• Diamond-Blackfan anemia
• Acute lymphoblastic	Hemoglobinopathies
leukemia (ALL)	• Sickle cell disease
• Juvenile myelomonocytic	• Proxysmal nocturnal
leukemia	hemoglobinuria Thalassemia
• Secondary leukemias	Immunodeficiencies
Lymphoma	• Severe combined
	immunodeficiency syndrome
	(SCIDS)
	• Wiskott-Aldrich syndrome
	• Leukocyte adhesion deficiency
	Inborn errors of metabolism
	• Adrenoleukodystrophy
	• Mucopolysaccharoidoses

Stem cell collection. Although stem cells are most concentrated in the marrow, they are found throughout the body's systemic circulation. Peripheral blood stem cell collection is performed utilizing an apheresis machine, in which the stem cells are separated as they filter through a centrifuge and the rest of the blood is returned to the patient. To stimulate the stem cells in the peripheral circulation, these patients are usually "primed" using growth colony-stimulating factor (GCSF). Chemotherapy can also be utilized to "prime" the blood for autologous collections. This method can be used for both autologous and allogeneic collections; its risks include those associated with GCSF side effects, such as bone pain (Taketomo et al., 2010). Additionally, the donor may require temporary central venous catheter (CVC) access if peripheral veins are not suitable for collection.

When umbilical cord blood is used as the source of the stem cells, the stem cells are collected from the umbilical cord and placenta immediately after delivery of an infant. This method of collection poses no risk to the donor. Umbilical cord blood transplants are advantageous as they offer decreased risk of viral disease transmission. Additionally, transplant centers are able to obtain the cord immediately upon request, in contrast to live allogeneic donors who require an evaluation and time-consuming evaluation. The disadvantages of using umbilical cord blood units include the limited number of cells they contain, which makes the cell dose insufficient for larger pediatric patients and some adults, as well as the prolonged time to engraftment.

Preparative regimen. Chemotherapy, radiation, and immunotherapy are used to prepare the bone marrow for transplant. This preparation involves eradication of any existing malignant cells, creation of space in the bone marrow for the new cells, and recipient immunosuppression to decrease the risk of rejection.

Chemotherapy, consisting of various combinations of drugs or single agents, depending on the disease, is administered in the days leading up to the infusion of stem cells. Chemotherapy can be used for myeloablation ("make space") and as an immunosuppressant. Patients with hematologic malignancies may receive preparative regimens utilizing busulfan to myeloablate and fludarabine to immunosuppress the host. Preparative regimens commonly used for Hodgkin's disease (HD) include CBV (cyclophosphamide, carmustine, etoposide) and BEAM (carmustine, etoposide, cytarabine, cyclophosphamide) (Gordon & Baker, 2006). Transplants for solid tumors such as neuroblastoma may include high-dose therapy with carboplatin, etoposide, and melphalan or cyclophosphamide and thiotepa. Patients with bone marrow failure will not require a regimen that is completely myeloablative, and patients with immunodeficiency who do not have T, B, or NK cells do not require complete immunosuppression.

Radiation therapy is indicated for treatment of malignancy and immunosuppression. Local-control irradiation is used in patients with central nervous system (CNS) involvement and those with solid tumors. Total-body irradiation is administered to patients who are receiving unrelated transplants as treatment of disease and for immunosuppression, thereby decreasing their risk for graft failure and graft-versus-host disease (GVHD) (Fisher & Abramovitz, 2006). Immunosuppression can also be achieved using an agent such as antithymocyte globulin, which binds with circulating T lymphocytes (Norville, 2008).

Complications of the preparative regimen. A number of complications are associated with the preparative regimen for BMT. Each of these complications and risks should be explained in full detail to the child's caregivers and in age-appropriate terms to the pediatric patient. It is essential that the HCPs who care for pediatric patients undergoing BMT are aware of these potential complications, and intervene accordingly. Three common complications associated with preparative regimens that are relevant to all BMT types are mucositis, pancytopenia, and veno-occlusive disease.

Mucositis. Mucositis is the destruction of mucosal cells throughout the gastrointestinal tract. In addition to mouth sores, pediatric patients may experience ulcerations from their esophagus to their rectum, causing severe pain, anorexia, bleeding, and increased risk for infection. Patients with mucositis may also experience nausea, vomiting, and diarrhea. Diligent oral care may help decrease the severity of these complications, and mouth rinses such as sodium chloride and those containing lidocaine may be used to prevent infection and reduce pain. Pediatric patients with mucositis may also require continuous opioid infusions and, depending on the duration of the mucositis, nutrition support may be required. Mucositis resolves upon engraftment—that is, the onset of cell production in the recipient, which varies based on the type of hematopoietic stem cells administered (Aquino & Sandler, 2006).

Pancytopenia. Pancytopenia is a result of marrow suppression. Decreased production of white blood cells, red blood cells, and platelets occurs approximately 7 to 10 days after the initiation of the preparative regimen. Low numbers of WBCs—specifically, neutrophils—increase the patient's risk for infection. The greatest risk for infection occurs when the patient's absolute neutrophil count (ANC) is less than 500 mm^3. WBCs are the first of the cell lines to recover, and their restoration will indicate the beginning of engraftment. Decreased RBC production causes anemia and may necessitate blood transfusions when the hemoglobin level is less than 7 to 8 gm/dL. Thrombocytopenia, or decreased platelet count (less than 100,000/mm^3), persists longer than neutropenia; during this period, the pediatric patient may experience bleeding and require platelet transfusions. Many pediatric centers maintain platelet counts between 10,000 and 20,000/mm^3 while the child remains an inpatient and in the absence of other factors

such as sepsis, severe mucositis, or active bleeding (Aquino & Sandler, 2006).

Veno-occlusive disease. Veno-occlusive disease (VOD) or sinusoidal obstructive syndrome (SOS) classically presents as elevated bilirubin (serum bilirubin ≥ 2.0 mg/dL), weight gain of 5% or greater of total body weight, and painful hepatomegaly. The peak incidence of VOD occurs between days 7 to 21 following the infusion of stem cells. This complication is the result of obstruction of blood flow through already narrow or fibrotic vessels in the liver. Multiple criteria for the diagnosis of VOD have been proposed, including the guidelines developed by the Center for International Blood and Marrow Stem Cell Transplant Research (CIBMTR), Hopkins Criteria, and Seattle Criteria. Diagnosis is made when reversal of hepatic blood flow is documented on ultrasound. Treatment for VOD includes supportive care; fluid restriction for patients with decreased urine output; diuretics such as furosemide, chlorothiazide, and spironolactone; and respiratory support as indicated.

Infusion of stem cells. The day of transplant is known as "Day 0," signifying the completion of the preparative regimen and days of rest and the beginning of counting positive days. For example, Day +1 is the first day after stem cell infusion. Although this is a very significant day in the treatment of patients receiving stem cell transplants, the actual infusion of cells is rather anticlimactic and completed through a CVC, oftentimes in the patient's own room. Stem cells are pushed via syringe or dripped into the patient via blood tubing without the use of a pump to preserve the integrity of cells. Stem cells are not irradiated or filtered. The procedure for infusing stem cells depends on the type of product the patient is receiving.

Products that have been cryopreserved, such as cord blood units or autologous stem cells, are frozen and contain the preservative dimethyl sulfoxide (DMSO). DMSO is toxic to cells once the product is thawed, requiring the cells to be delivered to the bedside frozen in liquid nitrogen and thawed in a warm-water bath immediately prior to infusion. These products are infused rapidly, within 30 minutes of thawing. Patients may receive antiemetics, antihistamines, corticosteroids, antipyretics, and diuretics as indicated prior to the infusion of cryopreserved stem cells. Side effects of DMSO include bradycardia, tachycardia, hypertension, nausea, vomiting, and a "garlic-like odor" caused by excretion of the drug through the lungs (Fisher & Abramovitz, 2006).

Fresh products, such as those obtained from a donor within 48 hours of the transplant, do not contain a preservative. They do contain an anticoagulant that is added during the collection of cells. The infusion of fresh products is very similar to a blood transfusion, with the duration depending on the patient's condition and the volume to be infused. In some situations, incompatible blood products are infused. This practice may necessitate premedications such as antihistamines, corticosteroids, diuretics, and antipyretics in addition to alkylating intravenous fluids containing sodium bicarbonate to protect the kidneys from damage secondary to hemolysis. Incompatible products may also be RBC depleted or volume reduced. The risks of an allogeneic infusion are similar to those of a blood product transfusion, and side effects of hemolysis such as red-colored urine due to hemoglobinuria may occur (Fisher & Abramovitz, 2006).

Post-transplant complications. The pediatric patient undergoing BMT is at great risk for opportunistic infection. The increased risk in these patients results from the immunosuppression caused by the preparative regimen and medications to reduce the risk of graft failure and GVHD. Opportunistic infections occur in three phases; pre-engraftment (less than 30 days before BMT), post-engraftment (30–100 days post-transplant), and late phase (more than 100 days post-transplant). It is essential that the HCP assess for infection and conscientiously select appropriate therapies for the prophylaxis and treatment of opportunistic infections, balancing risk for resistance with required therapies (CDC, 2000).

Pre-engraftment infection. Pre-engraftment is the period in the transplant process when the patient is the most immunosuppressed and neutropenic. Complications of the preparative regimen such as mucositis and GVHD increase the patient's risk for infection in the pre-engraftment phase. Common pathogens causing infection during this phase include Gram-negative bacteria, due to the breakdown of mucosal barriers, and Gram-positive cocci, likely related to the presence and maintenance of CVCs. Fungal infections may also occur during the pre-engraftment phase and can be prevented with fungal prophylaxis such as fluconazole (CDC, 2000).

Post-engraftment infection. Upon neutrophil recovery, the pediatric stem-cell transplant recipient continues to experience increased risk of infection due to impaired humoral and cellular immunity. Common infections during the post-engraftment phase include cytomegalovirus, *Aspergillus*, and *Candida* species. The presence of GVHD increases the risk that bacterial infections might become translocated from the gastrointestinal system. Due to the risk of viral infection, prophylaxis with antiviral agents or aggressive treatment strategies are indicated upon evidence of reactivation. Additionally, prophylaxis for *Pneumocystis jirovecii* pneumonia (PJP) with trimethoprim–sulfamethoxazole is initiated during this phase (Bradfield et al., 2006; CDC, 2000).

Late-Phase infection. The major risk for opportunistic infections occurring beyond Day +100 relates to the presence of chronic graft-versus-host disease and the need for continued immunosuppression. Patients in this phase with cGVHD require prophylaxis for encapsulated organisms. Additional prophylaxis for molds and viral infections may also be required during this phase for patients who continue on immunosuppression regimens. PJP prophylaxis continues for patients with persistent risk factors (Bradfield et al., 2006; CDC, 2000).

Graft-versus-host disease

Graft-versus-host disease is one of the most serious complications of allogeneic hematopoietic stem cell transplant. GVHD is the result of the donor cells' immune response to the recipient's tissues. Two types of GVHD exist, which are characterized by the time since transplant and presentation of the disease. Acute graft-versus-host disease (aGVHD) tends to occur in the first 100 days post-transplant; it is the result of inflammation in the skin, liver, and gastrointestinal system. Chronic graft-versus-host disease (cGVHD) resembles an autoimmune process that commonly affects the musculoskeletal system, mucous membranes, skin, and respiratory systems. The HCP caring for patients with GVHD must be familiar with prophylactic regimens and be prepared to intervene at the onset of symptoms.

Acute graft-versus-host disease

Pathophysiology. The disease course for aGVHD is a three-step process: (1) conditioning-induced tissue damage phase, (2) donor lymphocyte activation phase, and (3) cellular and inflammatory effector phase. The first phase involves tissue damage secondary to the preparative regimen, which leads to cellular activation and increased expression of host antigens and adhesion molecules. In the second phase, the host antigen-presenting cells present recipient antigens to donor T cells, thereby leading to recognition of mismatched minor antigens and activation of donor T cells and cytokine production. Barrier organs including the skin and bowel have a significant presence of dendritic cells, making them a specific target for aGVHD. In the third phase, natural killer cells and cytotoxic T lymphocytes cause further tissue injury (Moore & Feig, 2006).

Epidemiology and etiology. Risk factors for aGVHD include the source of stem cells (reduced incidence of GVHD is reported in patients receiving umbilical cord blood transplants) and the degree of human leukocyte antigen (HLA) match (mismatched products are strongly correlated with incidence and severity of aGVHD). Increased donor age and use of a female donor for a male recipient have also been shown to increase the risk of aGVHD. Although the mechanism is not clearly defined, more intensive preparative regimens and advanced disease are also associated with increased risk for aGVHD. Acute GVHD severity—that is, severity that requires treatment—occurs in 30% to 50% of sibling donor transplant recipients and as many as 50% to 80% of matched-unrelated donor transplant recipients (Moore & Feig, 2006).

Presentation. Three major organ systems are affected by aGVHD—the skin, the liver, and the gastrointestinal tract. Staging of aGVHD and the grading system of the associated complications are summarized in Table 28-7 and Table 28-8.

Acute GVHD of the skin may present as generalized erythema or facial flushing, or may manifest as a maculopapular rash (Figure 28-2). In severe cases, the rash may progress to bullae formation and desquamation. Acute GVHD of the liver may present with jaundice. Gastrointestinal aGVHD often presents as diarrhea, but may also be evidenced as vomiting, abdominal pain/cramping, anorexia, bloody stools, mucosal sloughing, and ileus. Clinical grading of aGVHD is based on the stool volume in a 24-hr period and symptoms.

Differential diagnosis. Various diseases and disorders may present with similar symptomology:

- Drug interaction
- Drug toxicity
- Infection
- Hepatitis
- Malabsorption
- Severe mucositis
- Veno-occlusive disease

TABLE 28-7

Clinical Staging of Acute Graft-Versus-Host Disease		
Stage **Skin**	**Liver**	**Gastrointestinal**
I Maculopapular rash over more than 25% of body surface	Serum bilirubin: 2–3 mg/dL	Diarrhea 5–10 mL/kg/day or persistent nausea
II Maculopapular rash over 25% to 50% of body surface	Serum bilirubin: 3–6 mg/dL	Diarrhea > 10–15 mL/kg/day
III Maculopapular rash over 50% to 100% of body surface	Serum bilirubin: 6–15 mg/dL	Diarrhea > 15 mL/kg/day
IV Desquamation and bulla formation	Serum bilirubin: > 15 mg/dL	Pain ± ileus

Source: Adapted from Klein, 2006.

TABLE 28-8

Overall Grading of Acute Graft-Versus-Host Disease			
Overall Grade	**Skin**	**Gastrointestinal**	**Liver**
I	I–II	0	0
II	I–III	I	I
III	II–III	II–III	II–III
IV	II–IV	II–IV	II–IV

Source: Adapted from Klein, 2006.

Plan of care. Acute GVHD of the skin is confirmed by biopsy revealing apoptotic bodies, eosinophilic bodies, and lymphocytic infiltration. Hyperbilirubinemia and transaminitis occur in liver aGVHD. Liver biopsy demonstrating bile duct damage and lymphocytic infiltration confirms the diagnosis, although this evidence is often difficult to obtain due to associated coagulopathies. Endoscopy/colonoscopy with biopsy determines the pathological grade of gastrointestinal aGVHD and reveals the presence of lymphocytic infiltration with crypt cell necrosis (Moore & Feig, 2006).

Prophylaxis of GVHD begins prior to the infusion of donor stem cells. Primary goals to reduce the risk of GVHD include reducing the number or function of T cells and modulating cytokines. Prophylactic therapy includes

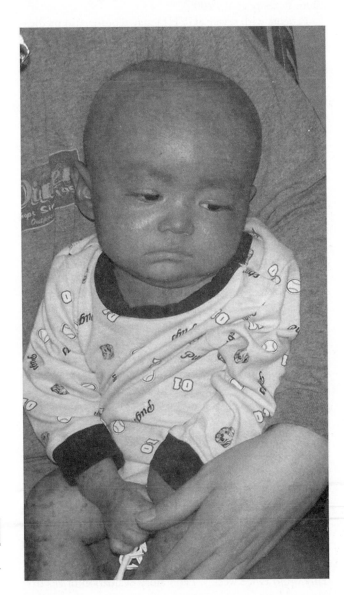

FIGURE 28-2

Skin: Graft-Versus-Host Disease (aGVHD). Generalized erythema of the face and maculopapular rash of the extremities.

Source: Courtesy of Jessica Lynne Diver.

a calcineurin inhibitor (tacrolimus or cyclosporine) and additional immunosuppressive agents. Side effects of calcineurin inhibitor medications include hypertension, nephrotoxicity, and hypomagnesemia (Taketomo et al., 2010). Additional nonspecific, cytotoxic agents such as methotrexate and steroids may also be used for prophylaxis and treatment of aGVHD. Treatment doses of steroids usually begin at 2 mg/kg to suppress the number and function of lymphocytes. Mycophenolate mofetil is a T-cell inhibitory agent used in the prophylaxis and treatment of GVHD. Second-line therapy for steroid-refractory GVHD may consist of antithymocyte globulin, monoclonal antibodies (daclizumab) and antitumor necrosis factor antibodies (etanercept) (Moore & Feig, 2006; Pczesny et al., 2009).

Patients with severe aGVHD may require pain medications to alleviate pain secondary to skin breakdown and abdominal pain and cramping. Bloody diarrhea may necessitate blood product transfusions. Pediatric patients with severe intestinal GVHD may need to be NPO (nothing by mouth) status and will require gradual reintroduction of one food at a time upon healing of the gastrointestinal tract. Consumption of certain dietary items, such as dairy products and acidic foods, may exacerbate symptoms of aGVHD.

The prevention and treatment of aGVHD predispose the patient to increased risk for infection. Fever in an immunocompromised host can precede sepsis and should be evaluated immediately. Many patients with aGVHD also retain their CVCs post-transplant, further increasing their risk for infection.

Depending on the acuity of the patient's presentation, the therapeutic management plan, and the patient's response to therapy, various subspecialties may be consulted. Consultations may include, but are not limited to, the following subspecialties: critical care, infectious diseases, dermatology, gastroenterology, hepatology, nutrition, rehabilitation team, child life, and other supportive services.

Patients may present at variable times post-transplant with symptoms of aGVHD. It is essential that the patient and the caregivers understand the signs and symptoms of aGVHD and be well educated about indications to call the HCP. Diarrhea, vomiting, and anorexia, for example, may indicate developing aGVHD. The caregiver and family should observe for skin rashes or facial flushing, in addition to yellowing of the skin or sclera and dark urine.

Disposition and discharge planning.

Patients with aGVHD require frequent follow-up with their HCPs, initially up to twice weekly. Laboratory evaluation of electrolytes and liver function tests as well as a CBC and screening tests for infection should be assessed routinely. Side effects of calcineurin inhibitors may require the patient to be discharged with antihypertensive medication and magnesium supplementation. Patients with severe intestinal GVHD

may require nutritional support at home. Home care nursing services may be required to ensure home therapies are available and comfortably performed by the caregiver. The caregiver of a child with intestinal GVHD requires education and support prior to discharge, especially when the patient's diet is restricted. Review of the complex medication regimen should occur prior to discharge and at each follow-up appointment to ensure compliance and accurate dosing.

Chronic graft-versus-host disease

Pathophysiology. Chronic graft-versus-host disease is a complex complication of allogeneic stem cell transplant that is not yet fully understood. This complication, which resembles an autoimmune disease, is the result of alloreactivity of donor T lymphocytes against recipient cells. Many factors, including the role of antigen-presenting cells, cytokine polymorphisms, and Th_1/Th_2 responses play a role in the development of cGVHD (Jacobsohn et al., 2006).

Epidemiology and etiology. Risk factors for the development of cGVHD are related to the donor source (reduced risk for cGVHD with sibling-donor transplants) and the ages of the donor and recipient. Additionally, nonmalignant diseases as an indication for transplant and use of cyclosporine with methotrexate have been associated with decreased risk for cGVHD. The incidence of cGVHD in patients receiving sibling-donor transplants is approximately 15%; the incidence is 46% in patients receiving matched-unrelated donor transplants (Jacobsohn et al., 2006).

Presentation. The pediatric patient with cGVHD may present with a variety of symptoms. Commonly affected organs include the skin, musculoskeletal system, liver, mucous membranes, and respiratory tract. Skin rash of cGVHD may present as randomly placed hypopigmented or hyperpigmented patches or as patchy erythema with roughness. Alopecia, brittle nails, and anhydrosis caused by sweat gland destruction may result from cGVHD.

The musculoskeletal system may manifest cGVHD signs and symptoms in the form of fasciitis, limited range of motion, and muscle cramps. Contractures of joints and sclerodermatic changes of overlying skin may be observed. It is essential that he HCP assess the joints closely, even in the absence of skin cGVHD, to assure that potentially debilitating disease is not overlooked (Figure 28-3 and Figure 28-4).

Mucous membranes such as the eyes and mouth may become dry and irritated. Ocular involvement in cGVHD occurs in as many as 35% to 40% of patients. Destruction of the lacrimal glands leads to dryness, photophobia, and burning. Complaints of difficulty swallowing, decreased secretions, and food sensitivity may indicate oral involvement. On assessment, the HCP may observe erythema with white plaques or lichenoid changes in the oral mucosa (Jacobsohn et al., 2006).

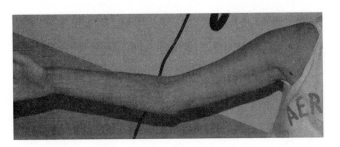

FIGURE 28-3

Skin and Musculoskeletal: Chronic Graft-Versus-Host Disease (cGVHD). Atrophy and sclerodermatic changes of the forearm.

Source: Courtesy of Jessica Lynne Diver.

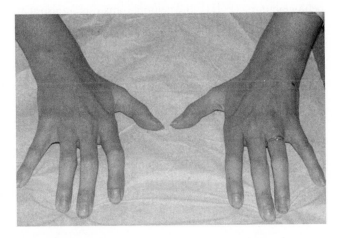

FIGURE 28-4

Musculoskeletal: Chronic Graft-Versus-Host Disease (cGVHD). Bilateral skeletal deformities and contractures of the digits.

Source: Courtesy of Jessica Lynne Diver.

Obstructive jaundice with elevated transaminases (specifically ALT and AST) may indicate cGVHD of the liver (Jacobsohn, et al., 2006).

An obstructive disease of the small airways called bronchiolitis obliterans is mediated by donor lymphocytes that target host epithelial cells. Bronchiolitis obliterans is a serious and late complication of cGVHD, with a 5-year survival rate estimated at 10%. Symptoms of bronchiolitis obliterans include cough and dyspnea. Patients also have changes on computed tomography (CT) scan that confirm air trapping and decreased performance in pulmonary function tests (Jacobsohn et al., 2006).

Differential diagnosis. Various diseases and disorders may present with symptomology similar to that of cGVHD:

- Drug reactions (antifungal agents, calcineurin inhibitors)
- Dyskeratosis congenital
- Pulmonary infection
- Rashes of childhood
- Viral infections (cytomegalovirus, Epstein-Barr virus, hepatitis)

Plan of care. Diagnostic studies for cGVHD include skin punch biopsy, liver biopsy to confirm the presence of portal fibrosis and bile duct dropout that may progress to cirrhosis and bridging necrosis, transaminases and bilirubin levels to evaluate for obstructive jaundice, and viral studies and chest CT to confirm the presence of bronchiolitis obliterans (Jacobsohn et al., 2006).

Immunosuppression is indicated for patients with active cGVHD, with steroids being the standard therapy. Regimens including mycophenolate mofetil, thalidomide, hydroxychloroquine, and pentostatin are also being studied for their role in the treatment of cGVHD. Extracorporeal photopheresis (ECP) has demonstrated efficacy in pediatric patients with steroid-refractory aGVHD and cGVHD. To perform apheresis, a CVC is required that exposes the autologous peripheral blood to ultraviolet light. In this treatment approach, the drug 8-methoxypsoralen is injected to sensitize cGVHD-causing cells; those cells are then exposed to ultraviolet A light, which inactivates them. Given the promising results with therapy cited in recent reports, ECP is likely to be adopted by more centers in the near future (Jacobsohn et al., 2006).

As described in the aGVHD section, immunosuppression places the pediatric patient at increased risk for opportunistic infections and their sequelae. Fever in these patients requires immediate attention from a HCP. Respiratory compromise may also require immediate intervention and stabilization while determining the cause of a patient's deterioration.

Depending on the acuity of the patient's presentation, the therapeutic management plan, and the patient's response to therapy, various subspecialties may be consulted. Consultations may include, but are not limited to, the following subspecialties: critical care, infectious diseases, dermatology, gastroenterology, hepatology, pulmonology, orthopedics, nutrition, rehabilitation team, child life, and other supportive services.

Patients may progress from aGVHD to cGVHD over time. Not surprisingly, the lack of improvement is frustrating for both patients and their families. It is essential that the patient and the caregivers understand signs and symptoms of the disease trajectory and be well educated about indications that warrant calling the HCP. Respiratory distress and jaundice, for example, may be signs of liver and pulmonary involvement.

Disposition and discharge planning. Patients with cGVHD require close follow-up with HCPs to assess progression of the disease and monitor for side effects associated with the therapeutic plan. Education for patients and caregivers should include signs and symptoms of cGVHD as well as other late effects of stem cell transplant. It is essential to educate the caregiver about routine follow-up care and to encourage compliance with the therapeutic plan and follow-up appointments with all indicated specialty services.

Chronic GVHD can be classified based on the type of onset; these classifications are also of prognostic value. Acute GVHD that merges into cGVHD is called progressive cGVHD. Quiescent cGVHD is the presentation of cGVHD after improvement of previous aGVHD episodes. In the absence of aGVHD, development of cGVHD is called de novo. De novo disease is associated with the best outcomes; quiescent disease has an intermediate prognosis; and progressive disease is associated with poor outcomes (Jacobsohn et al., 2006).

LEUKEMIA AND LYMPHOMA

Amy R. Newman

Leukemia

Pathophysiology. The hematopoietic (blood-forming) system arises from undifferentiated pluripotent stem cells. These stem cells proliferate and differentiate into two distinct cell lines: myeloid and lymphoid. Myeloid cells differentiate further into erythrocytes (red blood cells), monocytes, granulocytes, and thrombocytes (platelets). Lymphoid cells mature into either B or T cells. In leukemia, genetic abnormalities result in dysregulation of the hematopoietic development. Malignant stem cells lose their ability to differentiate into mature, properly functioning cells. These immature stem cells, called blasts, accumulate in the marrow spaces and can infiltrate other organs such as the thymus, spleen, liver, kidneys, and the central nervous system. Normal stem cell proliferation is limited, as both sufficient space and nutrients in the bone marrow are lacking; consequently, normal bone marrow function is limited or ceases altogether.

Epidemiology and etiology. Leukemia is a type of cancer that is characterized by an abnormal proliferation and accumulation of blood cells, usually leukocytes (white blood cells). The classification of childhood leukemia is based on the predominant cell line affected and the level at which cellular differentiation has been interrupted (acute or chronic). The three most common types of childhood leukemia are acute lymphoblastic leukemia (ALL), acute myelogenous leukemia (AML), and chronic myelogenous leukemia (CML).

ALL, which accounts for 75% of childhood leukemias, affects approximately 2,000 children each year in the United States (Pui, 2000). It occurs most frequently in children between the ages of 2 and 5 years, although it can be seen at any age, including in infants and young adults. Although no clear cause has been identified for ALL, several environmental and genetic associations have been suggested, including advanced maternal age, higher birth weight, paternal chemical exposure (pesticides, fungicides), ionizing radiation, and certain chemotherapeutic agents.

Inherited conditions associated with an increased risk of developing ALL include trisomy 21 (Down syndrome), Fanconi's anemia, ataxia telangiectasia, Klinefelter's syndrome, Shwachman-Diamond syndrome, and Bloom syndrome (Margolin et al., 2002; Tubergen & Bleyer, 2007).

AML accounts for 15% to 25% of leukemia in children. Its incidence is generally stable from birth until age 10, but then increases slightly during the adolescent years. Exposure to chemotherapeutic agents, such as alkylating agents, epipodophyllotoxins, and nitrosureas, as well as to ionizing radiation can increase the risk of developing AML. Children with trisomy 21, Diamond-Blackfan syndrome, Fanconi's anemia, Bloom syndrome, Kostmann syndrome, Li-Fraumeni syndrome, paroxysmal nocturnal hemoglobinuria (PNH), and neurofibromatosis are also at an increased risk of developing AML (Golub & Arceci, 2002).

CML, which accounts for 5% or fewer of childhood leukemias, is associated with a distinct chromosomal translocation, t(9;22), known as the Philadelphia (Ph+) chromosome. This disease is characterized initially by a chronic phase in which the white blood cell count is elevated, with granulocyte and granulocyte precursors appearing in the peripheral blood (Altman, 2002). Mild anemia and thrombocytosis may also be present. After a variable period of time (3 to 4 years without treatment), CML progresses to a more aggressive accelerated phase and then to a blast crisis (myeloid or lymphoid) that is similar to an acute leukemia.

Presentation. Presenting signs and symptoms reflect the degree of bone marrow infiltration with leukemic cells and the extent of extramedullary disease (Margolin et al., 2002). Pediatric patients with leukemia often present with nonspecific symptoms such as fevers, fatigue, anorexia, weight loss, and pain. Pain may be nonspecific, but is usually localized to bones or joints. In addition, caregivers may report persistent infections or adenopathy that has not responded to antibiotics. Physical examination reveals pallor, petechiae, hepatosplenomegaly, and adenopathy. Signs and symptoms of CNS involvement are rare, but can include headache, papilledema, retinal hemorrhages, cranial nerve palsies, and coma. Patients with acute leukemias who have a very high WBC count may develop leukostasis. The primary target organs in leukostasis are the lungs and CNS (Table 28-9).

Children with AML may present as more ill appearing than pediatric patients with ALL, secondary to more profound cytopenias. Heart failure may result from severe anemia. Due to their more severe thrombocytopenia, children with AML will typically report ecchymoses, petechiae, epistaxis, and gum bleeding. Patients with AML may also present with gum hypertrophy secondary to leukemic infiltration of the gingiva. Finally, pediatric patients may present with localized masses of leukemic cells called chloromas. Chloromas are most commonly found in the

TABLE 28-9

Hyperleukocytosis

- Hyperleukocytosis is an *oncologic emergency*.
- Leukemic patients presenting with white blood cell (WBC) counts greater than 100,000 cells/mm³ are at an increased risk of leukostasis and subsequent complications.
- Leukostasis is a clinicopathologic syndrome caused by sludging of circulating blasts in the tissue microvasculature. Intracerebral and pulmonary circulation are most often affected, but patients may also experience renal failure, cardiac failure, priapism, or dactylitis.
- Hyperleukocytosis is more clinically significant in patients with myeloid leukemias, with the most common complication being stroke.
- Patients with lymphoid leukemias present more often with hyperleukocytosis, but do not generally present with clinical changes until their WBC count is greater than 250,000 cells/mm³.
- Patients with pulmonary leukostasis may present with dyspnea, tachypnea, and hypoxemia, and can progress rapidly to respiratory failure.
- Impaired CNS circulation can result in headaches, seizures, and mental status changes.
- Emergent management is aimed at rapid reduction in the number of circulating WBCs.
  - Aggressive intravenous hydration should be initiated, and cytotoxic therapy initiated emergently in consultation with the oncology service.
  - Patients should be monitored closely for acute tumor lysis syndrome when therapy is started.
  - Controversy exists regarding the roles of leukapheresis and exchange transfusion in this setting. Both are generally reserved for those patients with a clinical presentation suggestive of leukostasis when the logistics of the procedure are easily and rapidly provided. Both procedures are not without potential complications, such as hypotension, symptomatic hypocalcemia, allergic reactions, catheter-related infections, and catheter-related thrombus.
  - Close monitoring of patients in the critical care setting is imperative, combined with careful ongoing pulmonary and neurologic assessments.

orbital or periorbital areas, but may be present in any site (including the CNS). Patients presenting with chloromas may exhibit ptosis or signs and symptoms consistent with spinal cord compression. Small nodules of leukemic cells—colorless to bluish/purplish in color—may also be found under the skin. Referred to as leukemia cutis, these nodules are more commonly seen in infants.

Pediatric patients with a specific subtype of AML (M3, acute promyelocytic leukemia [APL]) may present with a significant bleeding diathesis. Disseminated intravascular coagulation is often a result of the high level of thromboplastic activity in promyelocyte granules. Initiation of therapy in this setting can worsen DIC secondary to the breakdown of leukemic blasts and further release of thromboplastin.

Pediatric patients with CML may present quite differently from patients with either ALL or AML. Oftentimes they are asymptomatic, and laboratory abnormalities are discovered incidentally when routine blood work is performed. Alternatively, they may present with nonspecific, generalized symptoms such as fever, fatigue, weight loss, and anorexia. Splenomegaly may be present and may produce left upper quadrant pain. If patients present during blast crisis, they may also exhibit signs and symptoms similar to those of pediatric patients with ALL or AML.

Differential diagnosis. Diagnoses that may present with alterations in complete blood cell count include, but are not limited to, the following conditions:

- Infection
- Rheumatoid arthritis
- Bone marrow failure due to aplastic anemia or myelofibrosis
- Immune thrombocytopenia
- Congenital or acquired neutropenia
- Metastases from malignant solid tumors such as neuroblastoma or rhabdomysarcoma

Plan of care. CBC will generally reveal anemia, thrombocytopenia, and alterations in the number of WBCs. Blasts, other immature WBCs, and nucleated RBCs may be observed in the peripheral blood smear. A bone marrow aspiration alone is usually sufficient to evaluate for leukemia or other causes of bone marrow failure. Leukemias are diagnosed when bone marrow evaluation demonstrates more than 25% blasts in the marrow space. Blasts are further characterized morphologically, immunophenotypically, and immunohistochemically, thereby distinguishing the different leukemic subtypes. Samples of bone marrow are also analyzed for cytogenetic abnormalities.

Metabolic studies are obtained to determine baseline renal and hepatic function as well as to ascertain the patient's risk of developing acute tumor lysis syndrome (ATLS). A chest radiograph is obtained to evaluate for the presence of a mediastinal mass, which may compromise the pediatric patient's airway. A lumbar puncture (LP) is performed; if blasts are found and the patient's cerebrospinal fluid (CSF) leukocyte count is elevated, management of overt CNS leukemia requires a modified therapeutic management plan.

Most pediatric patients who present with leukemia are clinically stable and can be safely transitioned from the emergency department to the acute care unit. Prompt involvement of the oncology service is imperative to move swiftly in making the diagnosis. Initial management is aimed at identifying and managing any life-threatening complications, such as sepsis, DIC, ATLS, hyperleukocytosis, and leukostasis. After evaluation of hematologic and metabolic laboratory values, patients should be started on aggressive intravenous hydration. Transfusions of packed RBCs and platelets may be indicated if the patient is severely anemic or thrombocytopenic. It is recommended that a platelet count greater than 80,000 cells/mm³ be established prior to undertaking the initial LP so as to minimize the risk of introducing blasts into the CNS. Occasionally patients may require transfusions of FFP or cryoprecipitate to correct coagulation disorders. Patients presenting with fever and neutropenia secondary to the presumed leukemia should be empirically started on broad-spectrum antimicrobial agents. Patients presenting with WBC counts greater than 100,000 cells/mm³ or evidence of ATLS require intensive hydration and recombinant urate oxidase (rasburicase). If ATLS is already present, patients may need to be admitted to the intensive care unit for close monitoring.

Treatment of ALL.   Pediatric patients with ALL are initially divided into two categories—standard risk and high risk—based on their WBC count and their age at presentation. Children ages 1 to 9 years old with a WBC count of less than 50,000 cells/mm³ are considered to be at standard risk. Infants younger than 1 year of age and children 10 years of age or older or with a WBC count of greater than 50,000 cells/mm³ are considered to be at higher risk. This kind of risk stratification helps determine the intensity of therapy that children require to obtain and maintain complete remission. Initial treatment approaches are based on these risk groups, and results of cytogenetic testing are used to further classify patients (Table 28-10).

The rapidity of response to initial therapy and the amount of leukemia in the bone marrow after induction therapy (minimal residual disease [MRD]) have also been identified as important indicators of prognosis. A complete remission is generally defined as follows:

- The absence of leukemic cells in the peripheral blood with the return of normal blood counts
- Fewer than 5% blasts in a normal bone marrow environment
- No other evidence of disease in other areas of the body (Margolin et al., 2002)

Patients who have not achieved a complete remission after 4 to 6 weeks of therapy are at a higher risk of relapse and shortened long-term survival.

Pediatric patients with ALL are generally treated for 2.5 to 3.5 years depending on their risk group status and gender. Treatment is divided into three phases: induction, consolidation, and maintenance.

The first 4 to 6 weeks constitutes *induction*. The goal of induction therapy is to produce a complete remission. Bone marrow evaluation is performed after the initial 4 weeks of treatment. If complete remission has been attained, the patient will proceed to the consolidation phase. If complete remission has not been attained, the induction phase may be extended.

Consolidation uses more intensive doses of chemotherapy. The goals of consolidation therapy are to rapidly decrease the number of residual leukemic cells (minimizing the chance of mutation to resistance) and to treat cells that are already resistant to lower doses of chemotherapy. Consolidation therapy typically comprises multiple agents given at varying schedules and dose intensities depending on the pediatric patient's risk group features.

Following consolidation, patients proceed to *maintenance* therapy, which is the longest phase of treatment—lasting from 2 to 3 years, depending on the patient's gender and risk group. The backbone of maintenance therapy is mercaptopurine and methotrexate given continuously throughout maintenance with intermittent doses of IV vincristine and glucocorticoids.

In addition, all pediatric patients with ALL receive CNS-directed therapy. The CNS is considered a sanctuary site for leukemic cells, as the blood–brain barrier protects the CNS from therapeutic levels of many of the chemotherapeutic agents that are administered systemically. This CNS "prophylaxis" generally consists of intrathecal (IT) administration of methotrexate. In most modern protocols, CNS radiation is limited to patients with the highest risk of developing CNS disease (T-cell ALL) and those with overt CNS involvement at diagnosis. Emergency radiation may be required for patients with retinal leukemia at diagnosis or during treatment.

Treatment of AML.   Treatment for patients with AML is considerably different than treatment for patients with ALL. Initial strategies were modeled after ALL therapy,

TABLE 28-10

Common Chromosomal Abnormalities in Childhood Leukemia and Associated Prognosis		
	Good	**Poor**
Acute lymphoblastic leukemia (ALL)	Trisomies 4, 10, and 17	t(9;22) (Philadelphia chromosome)
	t(12;21) (TEL/AML 1 fusion)	Rearrangement of *MLL* gene on chromosome 11q23
	Hyperdiploidy (51–65 chromosomes or DNA index ≥ 1.16)	Severe hypodiploidy (< 44 chromosomes)
Acute myelogenous leukemia (AML)	Inv(16)/t(16;16)	Monosomy 5
	t(8;21)	Deletion of 5q
		Monosomy 7
		FLT3-ITD with high allelic ratio

but outcomes were poor (Clark et al., 2009). Instead, a model consisting of shorter, more intensified therapy was found to be more successful with AML. Recently, investigators have started to stratify patients with AML into risk groups, identifying those patients at highest risk for relapse. Risk stratification for AML is based on response to therapy and the cytogenetic characteristics of the patient's leukemic clone.

Treatment for AML consists of four to six cycles of chemotherapy. The first two cycles are called "induction," and similar to induction in ALL, aim to induce remission. Induction generally incorporates three or more chemotherapeutic agents, and results in prolonged (3 to 6 weeks), profound marrow hypoplasia. During this time, patients are at high risk for infection and bleeding. With this intensive induction regimen, 85% of patients will achieve remission (Golub & Arceci, 2002).

As with ALL, patients with AML require continued treatment to maintain remission. Post-remission therapy can include ongoing chemotherapy or allogeneic hematopoietic stem cell transplant (HSCT). Lower-risk patients are treated with chemotherapy. Higher-risk patients may receive HSCT if a well-matched related or unrelated donor is available. The benefits of transplant versus continued chemotherapy are currently under investigation by multiple centers. CNS treatment and prophylaxis are also required. Patients receive intrathecal cytarabine with most cycles of chemotherapy, but do not generally require radiation therapy. Chloromas are managed with chemotherapy unless the patient has an incomplete response or neurologic compromise, such as vision loss or spinal cord compression, becomes evident. In such situations, emergency radiation may be required.

The intensification of therapy for pediatric patients with AML, in addition to the disease process itself, puts these children at high risk for developing life-threatening complications. Improved supportive care has resulted in reduced treatment and disease-related mortality. Necessary supportive therapies include transfusion support to minimize hemorrhage, liberal use of antimicrobials to prevent or treat infections, and either parenteral or enteral nutrition to maintain optimal health status. Skillful interprofessional teamwork is required to provide optimal supportive care.

Treatment of CML.   Pediatric patients with CML are treated quite differently from those with either ALL or AML. Historically, children were treated with single-agent chemotherapy, including agents such as busulfan and hydroxyurea. This resulted in stabilization or reduction of WBC counts, but not eradication of the Ph+ chromosome. Use of interferon-alpha (IFN-α) improved rates of remission compared to the hydroxyurea regimen, however, and patients who were treated with this approach were found to remain in cytogenetic remission (absence of Ph+ chromosome) for more extended periods of time. However, most patients eventually developed progressive

disease. In addition, the side effects of IFN-α (e.g., fever, chills, fatigue, malaise, myalgias, depression, neurologic symptoms) caused many patients to discontinue therapy.

Recently, molecularly targeted therapy has revolutionized the way CML is treated. Imatinib mesylate—an orally administered tyrosine kinase inhibitor—targets the BCR-ABL fusion protein. This agent induces a high rate of cytogenetic remission, with minimal side effects. Following promising results in pediatric and adult trials, imatinib mesylate has become the treatment of choice for chronic-phase CML. Patients with a complete hematologic response within 3 to 6 months, a complete cytogenetic response within 6 to 12 months, and a complete molecular response within 12 to 18 months have a greater than 90% rate of long-term leukemia-free survival. At this time, imatinib mesylate is continued indefinitely; investigation of the possible cessation of treatment is in progress (Suttorp, 2008).

Patients with CML who present with symptoms of leukostasis require emergent treatment with one or more of the following interventions: leukapheresis, chemotherapy, and aggressive IV hydration, allopurinol, or recombinant urate oxidase. Hyperleukocytosis is considered an oncologic emergency that requires urgent intervention (Table 28-9).

HSCT is the only known curative therapy for CML; its 1-year survival rate ranges from 60% to 80%, and its 10-year disease-free survival rate is 50% (Clark et al., 2009). Previously, HSCT either from a family or unrelated donor was the recommended therapy for patients with chronic-phase CML. In the era of imatinib mesylate, and given the potential morbidity and mortality associated with HSCT, the role of such transplants has become less clear. Indications for and the timing of HSCT in CML patients are currently being debated.

Patients and families are often overwhelmed with the diagnosis of leukemia. Initial education is aimed at helping them understand the diagnosis, the urgency of starting therapy, therapeutic plan options, and required supportive care. Interprofessional team members, including physicians, nurses, social workers, and child life specialists, are employed to provide individualized education to each child and his or her family.

Disposition and discharge planning.   Criteria for initial discharge for ALL patients include initiation of chemotherapy, no evidence of ongoing tumor lysis, absence of complications related to the disease or treatment (e.g., infection, mouth sores, persistent vomiting), and completion of basic new-diagnosis teaching. Essentials of new-diagnosis teaching include the basics of the disease, potential complications, and—most importantly—occasions on which to seek medical attention. Signs and symptoms for which patients and families are prompted to call include fevers, chills, persistent nausea or vomiting, poor oral intake, pain, bleeding, and mouth sores. Close follow-up generally in a pediatric oncology clinic is required initially one to two times per week.

The discharge criteria for patients with CML are somewhat different from those for patients with ALL, as normalization of blood counts in the former population may take considerably longer. Once the diagnosis has been established and imatinib mesylate therapy started, patients may be discharged if they do not require frequent transfusions or other symptom management and initial education has been completed. Patients are followed initially once or twice weekly, with close monitoring of blood counts and intermittent reevaluations of bone marrow status.

Pediatric patients with AML require prolonged hospitalizations. Due to the aggressive nature of the disease and the required therapy, patients receive initial treatment on an inpatient basis and remain hospitalized until recovery of blood counts. This process may take up to 30 to 40 days. At this time, if patients are free of infection and other complications, they may be discharged to home until the start of the next treatment. Oftentimes these patients remain hospitalized for months at a time secondary to treatment-related complications and infection.

Prognosis varies considerably among the different leukemias and risk groups. Overall event-free survival for children with ALL is 80%. Children with lower-risk ALL have survival rates as high as 95%. Overall event-free survival for children with AML is 50% to 70% (Horner et al., 2009). Children with lower-risk AML have survival rates of 70% to 80%. Patients with CML require prolonged therapy, but those with complete remission may have long-term event-free survival greater than 90% (Suttorp, 2008).

Lymphoma

Pathophysiology. Lymphomas are a heterogeneous group of neoplasms in which the lymphocyte is the malignant cell of origin. Two broad categories of lymphomas have been defined: Hodgkin lymphoma (HL) and non-Hodgkin lymphoma (NHL). NHL results from malignant proliferation of lymphocytes of T-, B-, or indeterminant-cell origin. In this type of disease, abnormal cells rapidly multiply, spreading in a random, diffuse, unpredictable, and aggressive pattern, forming masses or tumors at one or multiple sites within the body. In contrast, HL spreads more slowly and in a more orderly fashion. The characteristic binucleated cells of HL ("Reed-Sternberg cells") have the appearance of an "owl's eye." Although HL usually spreads to adjacent lymph nodes, hematogenous spread can also occur with disease involving the liver, spleen, bone, bone marrow, lungs, or brain.

Epidemiology and etiology. Lymphoma is the third most common type of cancer in children in the United States (Cairo et al., 2005). HL has four subtypes: lymphocyte predominant, nodular sclerosing, mixed cellularity, and lymphocyte depleted. This group of lymphomas typically affects adolescents and young adults between the ages of 15 and 35 and adults who are more than 50 years old. HL accounts for 5% of cancers in children and adolescents younger than the age of 15 years. Males are affected more frequently than females in children younger than 10 years. In adolescence, males and females are affected equally. The Epstein-Barr virus (EBV) is believed to play a role in the development of HL, and children with immunodeficient states, either congenital or acquired, are at an increased risk of developing HL (Cairo & Bradley, 2007).

NHL accounts for approximately 6% of all childhood cancers. Three main types of NHL are described in the child and adolescent population: lymphoblastic lymphoma (LBL); mature B-cell lymphoma, including Burkitt lymphoma (BL), diffuse large B-cell lymphoma (DLBCL), and primary mediastinal large B-cell lymphoma; and anaplastic large cell lymphoma (ALCL). NHL affects males more often than females, and the risk of developing NHL increases steadily with age. Most patients present between the ages of 5 and 15 years old. EBV is thought to play a role in the development of BL, and patients with preexisting immunodeficient states are at an increased risk of developing NHL. It is likely that geographic, immunologic, viral, and genetic factors play important roles in the etiology of NHL (Magrath, 2002).

Presentation. Pediatric patients with HL typically present with an enlarged lymph node or grouping of lymph nodes. Patients with significant mediastinal adenopathy may present with signs and symptoms of superior vena cava (SVC) syndrome, such as cough, shortness of breath, orthopnea, and distended neck veins. Patients may report systemic symptoms, including fatigue, anorexia, weight loss, and pruritis. *B symptoms* (unexplained fevers above 38°C [100°F], unexplained weight loss of 10% within 6 months prior to diagnosis, drenching night sweats) may also be present; if so, they portend a poorer prognosis. On physical examination, patients will have painless swelling of a lymph node region, typically in the supraclavicular or cervical lymph node chains. The affected nodes are firmer than inflammatory nodes, may feel rubbery, and are not typically warm, tender, or erythematous on exam. Hepatosplenomegaly may also be present.

Pediatric patients with NHL present with a variety of signs and symptoms depending on the disease site involved. NHL of the abdomen may present as a palpable mass accompanied by pain, nausea, and vomiting. Patients may also describe a change in bowel habits or hematochezia. Patients with involvement of the mediastinum typically present with symptoms consistent with SVC syndrome (Table 28-11 and Figure 28-5). Patients may also describe dysphagia and chest pain (Figure 28-6 and Figure 28-7). NHL of the head and neck may result in facial swelling, snoring, and rhinorrhea as well as edema of the neck or

TABLE 28-11

Management of Mediastinal Tumors: Superior Vena Cava Syndrome

- Patients with mediastinal tumors can present with significant airway compromise and symptoms consistent with SVC syndrome.
- SVC syndrome refers to a collection of signs and symptoms that occur when the SVC is compressed by external pressure, obstructing venous drainage to the right side of the heart.
- SVC syndrome can result from enlarged lymph nodes or tumor compressing the SVC, invasion of the SVC by tumor. or an internal obstruction.
- SVC syndrome is most commonly seen in patients presenting with non-Hodgkin lymphoma, particularly lymphoblastic or large cell subtypes; Hodgkin lymphoma; and T-cell leukemias.
- Patients may present with orthopnea; symptoms of tracheal compression such as cough, dyspnea, air hunger and wheezing; anxiety due to hypoxia; headache; facial swelling; dizziness; and pallor.
- Imaging may reveal pericardial or pleural effusions, which can lead to cardiac tamponade and low-output heart failure.
- *Emergent management* is aimed at maintaining the airway and supporting circulation and perfusion.
  - Intubation is avoided as it may cause further narrowing of the trachea secondary to irritation and/or swelling of the tracheal mucosa; therefore, the initial challenge is to maintain the airway while obtaining a diagnosis.
- Compression of the SVC, trachea, or main stem bronchus places patients at increased risk of significant complications related to anesthesia, including death.
- Consultation with anesthesia is imperative, and collaboration with the oncology team should occur to determine the best option for making a tissue diagnosis.
- Diagnostic studies:
  - Pulmonary function tests should be obtained to evaluate the peak expiratory flow rate (PEFR).
  - Echocardiogram should be performed to evaluate heart function.
  - The least invasive means of obtaining tissue should then be pursued. This can include bone marrow aspirate with a local anesthetic, computed tomography (CT)–guided biopsy of a prominent lymph node, or aspiration of pleural fluid.
- Prompt initiation of therapy, including chemotherapy or radiation therapy, should follow. If tissue diagnosis is not possible, treatment is based on the diagnosis that is clinically most probable.
- Close ongoing evaluation of the airway in the critical care environment is necessary until reduction or stabilization of the airway is achieved.

supraclavicular region. Infrequently, patients will have CNS involvement, presenting with headache, vomiting, lethargy, or irritability. Patients may report systemic symptoms such as fatigue, fever, malaise, weight loss, anorexia, and night sweats.

NHL of the head and neck can lead to cervical lymphadenopathy, jaw swelling, unilateral tonsillar involvement,

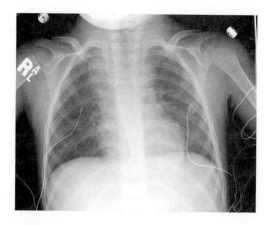

FIGURE 28-5

Chest radiograph of 3-year-old male presenting with Superior Vena Cava Syndrome (SVCS) and anterior mediastinal mass.

Source: Courtesy of Amy R. Newman.

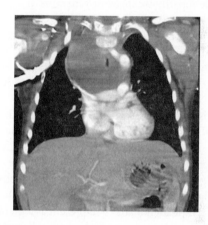

FIGURE 28-6

Computed Tomography (CT) coronal view depicting anterior mediastinal mass.

Source: Courtesy of Amy R. Newman.

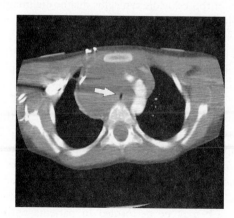

FIGURE 28-7

Axial images of same mass demonstrating > 50% reduction in tracheal diameter.

Source: Courtesy of Amy R. Newman.

nasal obstruction, cranial nerve palsies, and papilledema, depending on the site of disease. Signs of SVC syndrome may be present. Lung examination may reveal diminished breath sounds as well as wheezing, stridor, or crackles. Heart examination may elicit a pericardial rub or muffled heart sounds if a pericardial effusion is present. The abdomen may appear distended, hepatosplenomegaly may be present, and a mass may be palpable. Pallor or petechiae may result from early bone marrow involvement.

Differential diagnosis. Many different diseases may present with enlarged lymph nodes. Given this fact, the HCP should consider the following questions when listing likely diagnoses:

- Is the mass a node?
- What are the characteristics of the node (e.g., consistency, tenderness, erythema, matted)?
- Is the adenopathy localized or generalized?
- Are there other systemic signs of disease?

Thorough physical examination, review of laboratory findings, and evaluation of radiographic studies are important to differentiate lymphomas from other disease processes. The most common nonmalignant alternative diagnosis is infection. Patients who present with signs and symptoms suggesting lymphoma should also be evaluated for EBV, toxoplasmosis, cytomegalovirus (CMV), and mycobacterial infections. Findings may also be suggestive of the diagnosis of systemic lupus erythematosus. Finally, other malignant diseases should be excluded. Occasionally abnormal lymphadenopathy will present as a metastatic site from another primary tumor such as nasopharyngeal carcinoma or other soft-tissue sarcomas.

Plan of care. Occasionally, HL or NHL will be found incidentally when a patient has chest radiographs (CXR) for other purposes. More typically, diagnostic imaging will be obtained when a patient presents with persistent adenopathy or a palpable mass. Computed tomography scan of the affected area will generally be performed first. Often, CT scans will reveal pathologic enlargement of lymph nodes warranting further imaging to "stage" the patient. Staging involves determining the size of the tumor/mass and the extent to which the cancer has spread within the body (typically stages I to IV) (Table 28-12 and Table 28-13). It is important to predict survival and direct treatment. Oftentimes staging will include additional CTs of the neck, chest, abdomen, and pelvis; bone scans (if the patient presents with bone pain); and bone marrow aspirates and biopsies. LP may be performed in patients with symptoms concerning for CNS involvement. Positron emission tomography (PET) scans may also be obtained. PET scans use a radiolabeled isotope to identify areas of the body with high metabolic activity believed to be consistent with tumor activity.

TABLE 28-12

Ann Arbor Staging Classification for Hodgkin Lymphoma

Stage	Description
I	Involvement of a single lymph node region or a single extralymphatic organ or site
II	Involvement of two or more lymph node regions on the same side of the diaphragm or Localized contiguous involvement of only one extralymphatic organ or site and its regional lymph node(s) on the same side of the diaphragm
III	Involvement of lymph node regions on both sides of the diaphragm, which may also be accompanied by involvement of the spleen or by localized contiguous involvement of an extralymphatic organ or site, or both
IV	Diffuse or disseminated involvement of one or more extralymphatic organs or tissues, with or without associated lymph node involvement

Source: Used with permission from Carbone, P., et al. (1971). Report of the Committee on Hodgkin's Disease Staging Classification. *Cancer Research,* 31, 1860–1861.

TABLE 28-13

St. Jude Staging System for Pediatric Non-Hodgkin Lymphoma

Stage	Definition
I	A single tumor (extranodal) or involvement of the same anatomic area (nodal), with the exclusion of the mediastinum and abdomen
II	A single tumor (extranodal) with regional lymph node involvement Two or more nodal areas on the same side of the diaphragm Two single (extranodal) tumors on the same side of the diaphragm A primary GI tract tumor, with or without involvement of associated mesenteric lymph nodes, completely resectable
III	Two single tumors (extranodal) on opposite sides of the diaphragm Two or more nodal areas above and below the diaphragm Any primary intrathoracic tumor Extensive primary intra-abdominal disease (unresectable) Any paraspinal or epidural tumor, whether or not other sites are involved
IV	Any of the preceding findings with initial involvement of the CNS, bone marrow, or both

Source: Used with permission. Copyright© Elsevier. Murphy, S. (1980). Classification, staging and end results of treatment of childhood non-Hodgkin's lymphomas: Dissimilarities from lymphomas in adults. *Seminars in Oncology,* 7, 332–339.

Once staging and infectious disease testing are complete, a sample of the tumor needs to be obtained. In collaboration with the oncology team, radiology and surgical services should be consulted to determine the least invasive procedure that can yield the necessary specimen. Once a piece or section of the tumor has been removed, pathologists review the morphology of the sample and apply immunohistochemical stains, flow cytometry, and cytogenetic analysis to it to make an accurate diagnosis.

Patients with HL often present with painless lymph node swelling in the supraclavicular or cervical lymph nodes. The initial CXR will reveal the extent of disease within the chest and determine whether a mediastinal mass is present that may compromise the patient's airway. CT scan of the chest is performed to determine the degree to which the trachea and bronchi are constricted. Initial management focuses on maintaining the airway and working with the anesthesia, oncology, and surgical services to determine the best approach to obtain tissue for diagnosis. CT scan may also reveal pleural or pericardial effusions that require immediate intervention. Until a diagnosis is made and treatment is initiated, patients may require close observation for airway compromise in the pediatric intensive care setting.

Treatment of HL has evolved considerably over the past 40 years. Initial therapies have traditionally included high-dose radiation therapy to involved lymph node regions and chemotherapy. Unfortunately, patients were found to have significant late effects secondary to radiation therapy, including musculoskeletal abnormalities, an increased risk of secondary malignancies, infertility, and an increased risk of cardiovascular disease (Hodgson et al., 2007). Intensification of chemotherapy has allowed radiation doses to be reduced and radiation fields to be reduced in size, thereby minimizing the exposure of normal tissues to the effects of radiation therapy.

Patients are currently stratified into risk categories (low-risk, intermediate-risk, high-risk) based on the extent of lymph node and organ involvement, the absence or presence of B symptoms, and the presence of bulky nodal disease. Doses, combinations of different chemotherapeutic agents, and length of therapy are selected based on a patient's risk group category, with intermediate- and high-risk patients requiring more intensive chemotherapy. Several cycles of chemotherapy are administered, followed by repeat imaging to evaluate the patient's response to treatment. Patients who experience a reduction in the size of their tumors after the initial cycles of chemotherapy are deemed early responders. Early response to therapy is believed to be a good prognostic sign. Current clinic trials are aimed at identifying whether this subset of patients can be treated without radiation or with reduced radiation doses (Schwartz, 2003). In the absence of participation in a clinical trial, the current standard of care for all patients is to receive multiagent chemotherapy with low-dose involved-field radiation therapy, typically after the completion of all chemotherapy.

Due to the rapid growth of tumor cells, patients with NHL often present emergently. Depending on the site of disease, they may have acute respiratory failure, SVC syndrome, ileus and acute abdomen, anuria, cranial nerve palsies, or paraplegia (Reiter & Ferrando, 2009). In patients with mediastinal adenopathy, close monitoring of the airway is imperative. Surgical services should be consulted to evaluate the role of surgery in patients with abdominal and paraspinal tumors. Although most patients can be managed with chemotherapy alone, the possible use of surgery or radiation should be considered. Aggressive hydration and close monitoring of hematologic and metabolic laboratory values should be implemented, as patients can be at high risk of developing ATLS. Once therapy has been initiated, airway patency improved, and the risk of ATLS lowered, patients may be transitioned from the intensive care environment to an acute care unit.

Improved understanding of the biology of NHL over the last several decades has allowed researchers to better classify and treat the disease. Therapeutic management plans are based on the type of NHL and the extent of tumor involvement at presentation. Currently, multiagent, combination chemotherapy is the cornerstone of treatment for all NHLs.

Therapy for patients with LBL is similar to therapy for patients with ALL, with treatment lasting 2 to 3 years. Patients with overt CNS disease at the time of presentation will receive intrathecal (IT) chemotherapy throughout the course of their treatment as well as chemotherapeutic agents, such as intravenous (IV) high-dose methotrexate (which crosses the blood–brain barrier) and cranial radiation. Patients without overt CNS disease at diagnosis will be treated with IT chemotherapy and IV high-dose methotrexate without cranial radiation. Chemotherapy for mature B-cell lymphomas is given for 4 to 7 days; these cycles are typically repeated every 21 days. Patients receive 2 to 8 cycles of chemotherapy depending on the stage of their disease and their response to therapy. Therapy is very intense and can lead to severe toxicities, such as myelosuppression, mucositis, and typhlitis. Patients with CNS involvement are treated with triple-agent IT chemotherapy and IV high-dose methotrexate. The role of cranial radiation in this population is less clear. Treatment for ALCL is generally limited to two to three cycles of combination chemotherapy. CNS involvement and relapse are rare in this subgroup of patients; for this reason, CNS-directed therapies are limited to steroids and IV methotrexate. Although NHLs are radiosensitive tumors, the response to chemotherapy is generally rapid and robust, limiting the role of irradiation in this patient population (Reiter & Ferrando, 2009).

Patients presenting with suspicion of HL and NHL will require immediate consultation by oncology. Depending on their presenting symptoms and diagnostic findings, a number of specialty consultations may also be required, such as: critical care, pulmonology, surgical services, cardiothoracic surgery, neurology, neurosurgery, immunology, and infectious diseases. Consultations with a rehabilitation team, psychologists, and child life are often introduced early in the course of treatment to ensure the best physical and psychological outcomes.

Patients and families are initially educated on the disease process itself and the work-up required to make a final diagnosis. Education regarding the required treatment quickly ensues, focusing on chemotherapy combinations, side effects of chemotherapy, and the role of radiation therapy in the setting of HL. Additional education regarding the emergent management of ATLS and SVC syndrome should be included.

Disposition and discharge planning. Once the patient's disease status is deemed stable and his or her hematologic and metabolic laboratory values have improved, discharge is anticipated. Essentials of new-diagnosis teaching include understanding the basics of the disease, potential complications, and—most importantly—occasions at which to seek medical attention. Signs and symptoms for which patients and families are prompted to call HCPs include fevers, chills, persistent nausea or vomiting with subsequent poor oral intake, pain, bleeding, and mouth sores. Close follow-up, generally in a pediatric oncology clinic, is recommended. Depending on the frequency of their treatments, patients are typically seen once weekly following treatment and monitored closely for toxicities related to therapy and an appropriate disease response. Diagnostic imaging is repeated at set time intervals to monitor the patient's response to therapy.

Overall survival rates for patients with HL are excellent, approximately 90% (Reiter & Ferrando, 2009). Overall survival for patients with NHL has improved dramatically over the past 30 years. Patients with localized disease (stages I and II) have a greater than 95% chance of survival. Patients with advanced-stage disease (stages III and IV with bone marrow and CNS involvement) have an 80% to 90% overall survival rate. Several subgroups of patients, including those with BL with both bone marrow and CNS involvement, patients with primary mediastinal DLBCL, and those with systemic ALCL, have survival rates in the range of 50% to 70% (Cairo et al., 2005).

SOLID MASS TUMORS

Central Nervous System Tumors

Paul M. Kent and Jennifer Misasi

Pathophysiology. Pediatric tumors of the central nervous system represent a clonal expansion of cells with acquired alterations in the genes that normally regulate cell growth and development. Such tumors include a wide range of pathologic categories, with each tumor being uniquely different in histologic diagnosis, the degree of anaplasia, the initial location, and the dissemination within and beyond the CNS.

Medulloblastomas have a classic phenotypic appearance composed of sheets of small rounds cells with little cytoplasm and frequent mitosis on microscopy. *Ependymomas* have proven more difficult to consistently grade histologically. The World Health Organization (WHO) classification places ependymal cell tumors into three categories: grade I—myxopapillary or subependymoma; grade II—cellular, papillary, tanycytic, or ependymoma; and grade III—anaplastic (Rorke et al., 1985). *Low-grade gliomas* are astrocytic, olidroglial, mixed, or benign neuroepithelial. *High-grade gliomas* include anaplastic, mixed, oligodendrogliomas, and glioblastoma multiforme (Pizzo & Poplack, 2001).

Epidemiology and etiology. Central nervous system tumors are the most common solid tumors in pediatric patients. They account for approximately 17% of all childhood malignancies in persons younger than 20 years of age. Approximately 2,200 cases are newly diagnosed each year. Ten percent of children in the general population have some sort of inherited disorder that places them at risk for developing CNS tumors. The peak incidence of these solid masses occurs within the first decade of life (Baggott et al., 2002).

Presentation. Due to the heterogeneity of this group of tumors, patients' symptoms and disease presentation will depend on the location of the tumor (Table 28-14 and Figure 28-8). The *supratentorial* region contains the cerebral hemispheres (cerebrum) and the ventricles, while the *infratentorial* region (often referred to as the "posterior fossa") is composed of the cerebellum, medulla, pons, and brain stem. The presentation also depends on the pediatric patient's age, developmental stage, and tumor histology. Commonly observed symptoms include progressive irritability, listlessness, and vomiting. Pediatric patients who have supratentorial tumors frequently have seizures and complain of morning headaches. Those with infratentorial tumors experience diplopia, gait disturbances, nystagmus, and weakness. Unexplained vomiting without signs of gastroenteritis, infection, or anorexia is a "red flag" for a pediatric patient with a CNS tumor.

Differential diagnosis. Several disorders and diseases have symptoms or presenting characteristics similar to those of CNS tumors and should be included in the differential diagnosis:

- Benign tumors
- Gastroenteritis
- Hemorrhage
- Infection
- Intracranial hypertension
- Migraine
- Trauma

TABLE 28-14

Types and Locations of Central Nervous System Tumors

Tumor	Presenting Signs and Symptoms	Standard Treatment	Location
Medulloblastoma	↑ Intracranial pressure, vomiting, headache, blurred vision	Surgery, radiation, and chemotherapy	Infratentorial in the posterior fossa
Primitive neuroectodermal tumor (PNET)	Visual disturbances, seizures, paralysis, emotional lability	Surgery, radiation, and chemotherapy	Supratentorial, in the cerebrum
Ependymoma	Headache, vomiting	Surgery ± radiation	Supratentorial, hemispheric
Craniopharyngioma	Headache, nausea, vomiting, ↑ intracranial pressure	Surgery, radiation, and chemotherapy	Supratentorial, midline
Pineal tumor	Headache, nausea, vomiting, papilledema, precocious puberty	Surgery, radiation, and chemotherapy	Supratentorial, midline
Astrocytoma	Headache, vomiting ataxia, hemiparesis, irritability—related to tumor location	Surgery, radiation, and chemotherapy	Infratentorial in the frontal, temporal, or parietal region

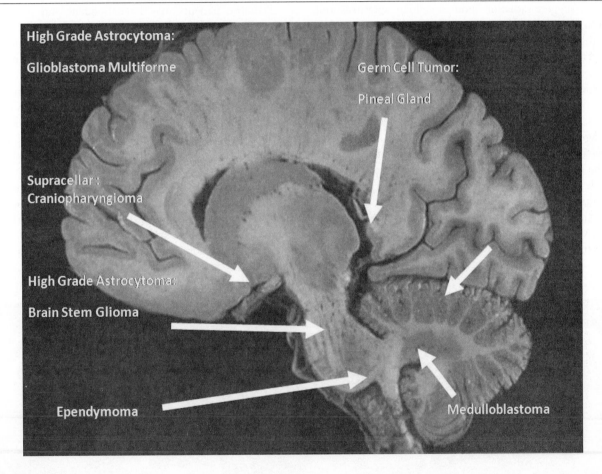

FIGURE 28-8

Central Nervous System Tumors.

Source: Courtesy of Paul M. Kent.

Plan of Care. Computed tomography and magnetic resonance imaging are the diagnostic studies most commonly used to diagnose CNS system tumors. The initial CT (without contrast) is performed to quickly evaluate for emergent pathology such as expanding mass, herniation, or bleeding. It is usually followed by a CT with IV contrast, MRI and magnetic resonance angiography (MRA), or both. These imaging studies provide information about the location, size, and make-up of the tumor (vascular, multiple, necrosis) and are often helpful in narrowing the differential diagnosis (Figure 28-9).

The therapeutic plan for CNS tumors consists of surgical resection, chemotherapy, and local radiation therapy. Complete resection of the tumor is the primary goal; however, resection may not be practical if the tumor resides in a critical location such as the brain stem. The degree of resection achieved affects patient survival. The combination of chemotherapy and radiation increases survival for patients with high-risk medulloblastomas, although the use of radiation significantly increases the long-term toxicity risk. Radiation poses an acceptable risk to developing neuronal structures in infants and children younger than 3 years of age. Postmortem examination of 34 children's brains after they had undergone radiation therapy demonstrated demyelination, focal necrosis, cortical atrophy, endothelial proliferation, and telangiectatic vascular proliferation with vascular thickening (Oi et al., 1990). These findings suggest radiation induces cellular apoptosis and produces structural defects in the surviving neurons that may directly suppress neural and cognitive development. Given these undesirable effects, high-dose chemotherapy and stem cell transplant are often the primary treatment strategies for CNS tumors in younger pediatric patients.

Consultation will often include a number of subspecialties. The patient's acuity level at time of presentation or diagnosis will dictate the care setting and subspecialty involvement. An interprofessional team is required to care for the pediatric patient with a CNS tumor; members may include professionals from pediatric oncology, neurology, neurosurgery, radiation oncology, critical care, child life, rehabilitation service, nutrition, and social and spiritual services. Additional consultants may be introduced if therapy elicits unmanageable symptoms.

The diagnosis of a CNS tumor may be overwhelming for both the patient and the family. Understanding the disease process requires understanding the symptoms related to the tumor and tumor progression, goals of care, management plan, and use of technology (central venous catheters). Side effects of therapy may affect the disposition of the patient within the hospital setting. Preparing and reassuring the patient, caregivers, and family members will provide them with insight into the global care plan.

Disposition and discharge planning. Depending on the histology of the tumor, the five-year survival rate ranges from 55% to 75% (Pollack, 1994). Factors affecting survival include the location of the tumor, the extent of surgical resection, the presence of metastasis at diagnosis, the histological subtype, the age of the child at diagnosis, and the initial response to therapy.

Pediatric patients may have frequent and prolonged hospitalizations depending on their tumor type and sequelae. Discharge plans will be coordinated by the interprofessional team. The family must understand when to seek medical attention from the oncologist and when to call for emergency assistance. In addition, the family should be provided with guidelines regarding when to be seen in the clinic, when to go to the emergency department, and how to problem-solve issues at home. Family meetings and a designated "go to" HCP are necessary to empower a family to care for a critically ill pediatric patient at home.

Follow-up appointments in the pediatric oncology clinic should be scheduled prior to the patient's discharge home. Home care nursing care may be required for the initial transition to home and should also be arranged, along with delivery of home equipment, before the patient leaves

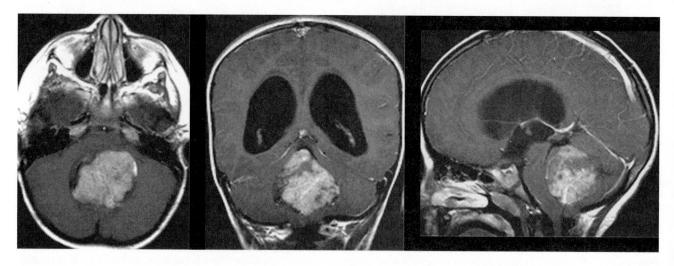

FIGURE 28-9

Axial, Coronal, and Sagittal MRI Images of a Child with Medulloblastoma.

Source: Carroll, W., & Finlay, J. (2010). *Cancer in Children and Adolescents.* Sudbury, MA: Jones and Bartlett Publishers.

the hospital setting. Years of therapy-related complications may ensue, and appropriate follow-up with subspecialties services will be required.

Retinoblastoma

Paul M. Kent and Jennifer Misasi

Pathophysiology. Retinoblastoma arises from the embryonic retinal cells in one or both eyes. It can extend as a nodular mass/tumor into the vitreous humor (Figure 28-10). Microscopic findings provide information that determines the degree of differentiation. "Flexner-Wintersteiner" rosettes (spoke-and-wheel cell formation on microscopy), necrosis, and calicification are characteristic findings. The identification of the oncogene *RB1* has led to the ability to identify which cases are inherited, thereby permitting genetic screening of family members for this gene.

Epidemiology and etiology. Retinoblastoma is an infrequent malignancy in childhood, accounting for only 1% to 3% of all childhood cancers. It is often present at birth, with two-thirds of affected children being diagnosed by age 2 years and 95% by age 5 years (Young et al., 1999). Bilateral disease is diagnosed at an earlier age than unilateral disease and is associated with the familial, inherited form. Metastasis is common, especially to the orbit, brain (pineal gland), and regional lymph nodes. Bone marrow infiltration is rare.

Presentation. Diagnosis usually occurs within the first 2 years of life. Children with a positive family history of retinoblastoma are often diagnosed before development of any clinical symptoms due to early screening. The most common signs are leukocoria, the "white eye" in photographs (Figure 28-11), and strabismus (Figure 28-12). Other less common symptoms are glaucoma; a painful, red eye; and orbital cellulitis.

Differential diagnosis. Most commonly diagnosed are the nonmalignant disorders of pseudoretinoblastomas—namely, endophthalmitis, persistent hyperplastic primary vitreous, and Coat's disease (exudative retinitis). All of these disorders may present with retinal detachment and retrolenticular fibrosis.

Plan of care. Diagnosis is made via a detailed fundoscopic examination conducted by an ophthalmologist. For best results, the ophthalmic examination is performed under general anesthesia. Other diagnostic studies that will aid in the determination of tumor extension and metastasis are CT and MRI. CT is useful to identify calcifications; MRI will differentiate retinoblastoma from Coat's disease. If metastasis is noted, then further biopsies and lumbar puncture are required.

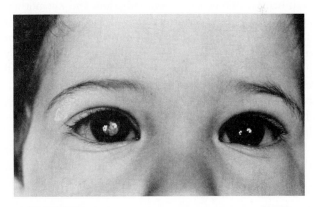

FIGURE 28-11

Retinoblastoma-Leukocoria of the Left Eye.

Source: © National Cancer Institute/Photo Researchers, Inc.

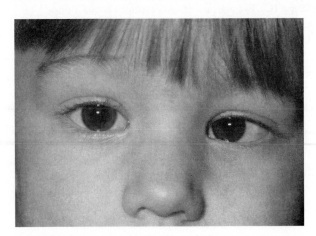

FIGURE 28-12

Retinoblastoma-Strabismus.

Source: © Dr. P. Masazzi/Photo Researchers, Inc.

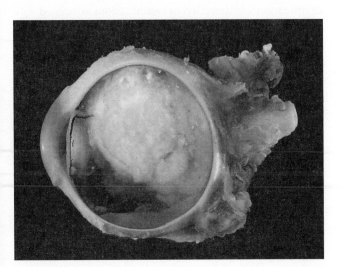

FIGURE 28-10

Cross-Section of an Eye with Retinoblastoma.

Source: Carroll, W. & Finlay, J. (2010). *Cancer in Children and Adolescents.* Sudbury, MA: Jones and Bartlett Publishers.

Classification and staging systems for retinoblastoma have evolved over time. The Reese-Ellsworth classification for retinoblastoma, published in 1963, was once the most commonly used system to predict outcomes after radiation therapy. However, as therapy evolved, it became less useful. In 2006, the International Classification of Retinoblastoma was developed; it focused on tumor seeding (Shields, 2006). The most recently proposed staging system—the International Retinoblastoma Staging System—incorporates key elements from both of the earlier classification systems while adding new elements of progression (Table 28-15) (Chantada et al., 2008).

Therapeutic management is based on the classification group, which explains the search for an effective staging system. The therapies utilized follow the guidelines developed by the Children's Oncology Group (COG) Clinical Trials Organization, in association with the National Cancer Institute (NCI). The goal of therapy is to prevent tumor extension and preserve vision. Modalities that may be incorporated into the therapeutic plan include enucleation, cryotherapy, photocoagulation, radiation, and chemotherapy. Enucleation is performed only if there is significant concern for tumor invasion in the optic nerve, choroids, or orbit, and there is no hope of salvaging vision. Cryotherapy is useful for managing equatorial and peripheral small retinoblastomas. Photocoagulation is used to treat small posterior retinoblastomas. Radiation therapy is used when diffuse vitreous seeding is observed, and chemotherapy is indicated in advanced metastatic disease.

Provision of care by an interprofessional team allows for the best outcomes in pediatric patients with retinoblastomas.

TABLE 28-15

International retinoblastoma staging system.

Stage 0. Patients treated conservatively

Stage I. Eye enucleated, completely resected histologically

Stage II. Eye enucleated, microscopic residual tumor

Stage III. Regional extension
    a. Overt orbital disease
    b. Preauricular or cervical lymph node extension

Stage IV. Metastatic disease
    a. **Hematogenous metastasis**
       (without CNS involvement)
      1. Single lesion
      2. Multiple lesions
    b. **CNS extension** (with or without any other site of regional or metastatic disease)
      1. Prechiasmatic lesion
      2. CNS mass
      3. Leptomeningeal and CSF disease

Source: Chantada G, Doz F, Antonelli CBG et al. A proposal for an international retinoblastoma staging system. *Pediatr Blood Cancer* 2008; 50(3): 733.

The team may include members from the following subspecialties: oncology, ophthalmology, radiation, genetics, neurology, neurosurgery, plastic surgery, prosthetics, rehabilitation services, nutrition, child life, and social and spiritual services.

The diagnosis of retinoblastoma and the possibility of blindness can be overwhelming for the patient and family. Understanding the disease process, symptoms related to the tumor and tumor progression, goals of care, management plan, use of technology (central venous catheters), and side effects of therapy will allow caregivers and family members to care for their child. As part of the therapy and educational plan, families will also need genetic counseling and screening.

Disposition and discharge planning. Secondary malignancies diagnosed later in life are common, especially in infants who received aggressive radiation therapy. These malignancies may include osteogenic sarcoma, soft-tissue sarcomas, and melanomas (Rodriguez-Galindo & Meadows, 2010). The orbital structure may be deformed secondary to enucleation contraction or radiation therapy. Vision may be impaired or lost, especially in bilateral eye disease. Children of retinoblastoma survivors have an increased risk of retinoblastoma. Extension of the tumor into the CNS is associated with an extremely poor prognosis.

Pediatric patients may have frequent and prolonged hospitalizations based on tumor extension and sequelae. Discharge should be coordinated by the interprofessional team. The families must know when to seek medical attention from the oncologist or emergency department team, and how to problem-solve issues at home. Family meetings and a designated "go to" HCP are necessary to empower a family who is taking a pediatric patient with retinoblastoma home. Follow-up in the pediatric oncology clinic involves examination and detection of complications associated with therapy, such as orbital contraction (requiring surgical repair or prosthesis), vision loss, and secondary malignancies.

Ewing sarcoma

Paul M. Kent and Jennifer Misasi

Pathophysiology. Studies suggest that Ewing sarcoma (EWS) originates from neuronal and epithelial cells. Degrees of neural differentiation can be determined with the use of diagnostic studies such as stains for S-100 protein, immunohistochemistry, or electron microscopy. Ninety-five percent of individuals with EWS have a t(11;22) or t(21;22) chromosomal translocation, which results in the fusion of the *EWS* gene on chromosome 22 with the *FLI1* gene on chromosome 11 or the *ERG* gene on chromosome 21. The protein product that results from this fusion leads to the creation of a chimeric protein that induces malignant transformation (Arndt & Crist, 1999).

Epidemiology and etiology. There are 2.1 diagnosed cases of EWS per 1 million population, and EWS is the second most common bone malignancy in childhood following osteosarcoma (Ries et al., 1999). The Ewing family of tumors (EWS and primitive neuroectodermal tumor) may arise in any bone or soft tissue, but frequently occurs in the flat bones, particularly the pelvis. Its peak incidence occurs during adolescence. EWS is extremely uncommon in children of African and Asian descent, for unknown reasons. In contrast to osteosarcoma, EWS does not appear to be caused by exposure to radiation, nor has it been associated with familial cancer syndromes or tumor suppressor genes (Ries et al.).

Presentation. The most common initial complaint is pain or swelling in a bone or joint, frequently thought initially to be due to a sports-related injury. This pain may have an acute onset, or it may develop over several months; it may have either a constant or intermittent characteristic. Fevers, night sweats, and weight loss are common (especially with metastases) and can lead to an initial diagnosis of osteomyelitis. Over time, a palpable mass may be appreciated. Twenty-five percent of patients diagnosed with EWS have metastases at diagnosis. In those patients, 50% of the metastases are located in the lung, followed by bone (25%), and bone marrow (25%) (Arndt & Crist, 1999).

Differential diagnosis. The initial differential diagnosis may include tendonitis, osteomyelitis, or sepsis. Once radiographs have been obtained, the differential diagnosis may also include osteosarcoma, histiocytosis, or osteomyelitis. Biopsy reveals small, round, blue cells that may be confused with neuroblastoma, lymphoma, or rhabdomyosarcoma. Differentiation can be accomplished with immunohistochemistry and genetic testing such as cell-surface staining for CD99 and Fli-1, both of which are classic findings in EWS. Identification of the *EWS* gene translocation is critical to securing the correct diagnosis. A skilled bone pathologist is required to differentiate EWS from the other small, round, blue cell tumors of childhood.

Plan of care. Initial diagnostic studies include radiographs of the affected area, CBC, and blood cultures, as trauma and infection are often a part of the initial screening. Radiographs may reveal a classic *onion skinning* (lamellated periosteal reaction) or *Codman's triangle* (periosteal lysis from the bone) suggestive of malignancy. CT, MRI, or PET scanning may be used to identify the tumor location, tumor extension, and distant sites of metastasis (Figure 28-13). Definitive diagnosis is made through open biopsy, if possible, with the sample being sent fresh for cytogenetic and molecular genetic studies. The biopsy incision for bone tumors should be positioned

so that it can be incorporated into future surgical incisions for definitive care.

Several staging systems have been developed for adult sarcoma based on the histologic grade of the tumor, the location of the tumor, and the presence or absence of metastases. In pediatrics, however, EWS is always considered "high grade"; thus these patients are stratified according to the presence or absence of metastatic disease.

Pediatric, adolescent, and young adult patients thought to have sarcoma should be referred to a pediatric oncology center. These centers have the necessary specialists needed to assess the immunohistochemical and genetic features of the tumor and provide the expert interprofessional team required to deliver therapy. Tumor resection, local radiation therapy, and chemotherapy are the therapeutic management strategies of choice. Neoadjuvant (induction) chemotherapy allows for treatment of microscopic disease prior to tumor resection. The response to chemotherapy can be evaluated at the time of surgery. Radiation therapy or surgery can be used to achieve "local control" of the primary tumor. Tumor resection is usually preferred over radiation because it produces fewer long-term side effects, including the risk of secondary malignancies. Newer limb-salvage procedures avoid 90% to 95% of amputations for patients with EWS (Aksnes et al., 2008).

Provision of care by an interprofessional team allows for the best outcomes in pediatric patients with EWS. This team may include members from of the following

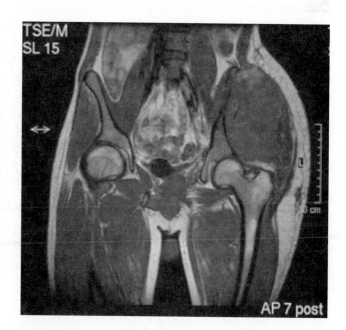

FIGURE 28-13

Ewing Sarcoma: Pelvic MRI.

specialties: oncology, orthopedics, radiation, genetics, plastic surgery, prosthetics, rehabilitation services, nutrition, psychologist, child life, and social and spiritual services.

The diagnosis of EWS can be overwhelming for both the patient and the family. Understanding the disease process, symptoms related to the tumor and tumor progression, goals of care, management plan, use of technology (central venous catheters), and side effects of therapy will allow caregivers and family members to care for their child both when in the hospital and at home.

Disposition and discharge planning. Chemotherapy has substantially improved the overall survival rate for patients with EWS. For localized disease, there is now a three-year survival rate of 80%. Patients with metastatic disease, axial or pelvic lesions, larger tumors, or relapse have a poorer prognosis (Grier et al., 2003).

Pediatric patients may have frequent and prolonged hospitalizations depending on their tumor type, location, and sequelae. Discharge plans should be coordinated by the interprofessional team. The family must understand when to seek medical attention by the oncologist, when to go to the emergency department, and how to problem-solve issues at home. Family meetings and a designated "go to" HCP are necessary to empower a family taking a pediatric patient with EWS home. Follow-up continues in the pediatric oncology clinic, where vigilant examinations assess for complications of therapy such as growth disturbance, cardiac toxicity, and secondary malignancies.

Osteosarcoma

Paul M. Kent and Jennifer Misasi

Pathophysiology. Osteosarcoma arises from a clonal proliferation of osteoblasts. The "new bone" formation has histological chaotic-looking spindle formation and necrosis. Inactivation of tumor suppressor pathways p53, MDM2, and RB is found in approximately 50% of patients (Arndt & Crist, 1999) as well as less well-characterized abnormalities such as loss of heterozygosity for chromosomes 3q, 13q, and 18q.

Epidemiology and etiology. Osteosarcoma is the most common bone malignancy in childhood, with approximately 250 new cases diagnosed every year. The peak incidence corresponds with the adolescent growth spurt (ages 12–15 years for girls and 15–19 years for boys), with no sex- or race-based predilection being noted. Ninety-five percent of cases arise spontaneously without any identifiable cause, with only 5% having a known risk factor such as: previous ionizing radiation, Paget's disease, hereditary retinoblastoma, Li-Fraumeni syndrome, enchondromatosis, hereditary multiple exostoses, or fibrous dysplasia

(Arndt & Crist, 1999). High-grade osteosarcoma accounts for 98% of osteosarcoma and can be classified into four subtypes: osteoblastic, fibroblastic, chondroblastic, and telangiectactic. However, these subtypes lack prognostic importance. Two subtypes are associated with a lower risk of metastasis and better prognosis—parosteal and periosteal osteosarcoma.

Presentation. The most common initial complaint is pain or swelling in a bone or joint, frequently thought initially to be due to a sports-related injury. Pain may be described as either constant or intermittent, and usually develops over several months. Osteosarcoma generally involves the metaphysis of long tubular bones, notably the distal femur or proximal tibia, where the fastest-growing growth plates are located. A local mass or pain may be present, sometimes with weakness in nearby joints. Systemic complaints may be noted with metastases.

Differential diagnosis. Radiographic evidence may mimic that associated with EWS, histiocytosis, lymphoma, or osteomyelitis. Initial biopsy will reveal sheets of osteoblasts and new bone formation, which can be confused with a healing fracture, osteoid osteoma, or a fibrous tumor.

Plan of care. Initial diagnostic studies include radiographs of the affected area, CBC, and blood cultures, as trauma and infection are often the initial considerations. Radiographs may reveal a *starburst* or *bone-in-bone* formation or a lytic lesion with cortical destruction and a *Codman's triangle* (periosteal lysis from the bone) suggestive of malignancy (Figure 28-14 and Figure 28-15). MRI is recommended for local evaluation of intramedullary involvement and tumor extension. Chest radiographs and CT may be performed to evaluate for lung metastases. Bone scan is used for evaluation of further bony involvement. The definitive diagnosis for osteosarcoma is made through open biopsy. The biopsy incision for bone tumors should be positioned so that it can be incorporated into future surgical incisions for definitive care.

The services of a skilled bone pathologist are needed to differentiate osteosarcoma from other bony diseases. A staging work-up must be completed once the diagnosis is determined. Several staging systems have been developed for adult sarcoma using the histologic grade of the tumor, the location of the tumor, and the presence or absence of metastases; in pediatric patients, osteosarcoma is stratified according to the presence or absence of metastatic disease.

Pediatric patients who are thought to have sarcoma should be referred to a pediatric oncology center. These centers have the facilities to assess the immunohistochemical and genetic features necessary to diagnosis the tumor and may provide the expert interprofessional team required to deliver comprehensive therapy.

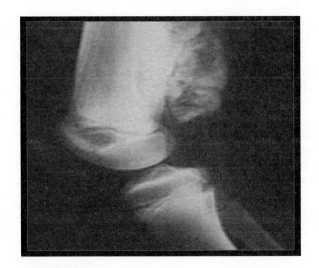

FIGURE 28-14

Osteosarcomas.

Source: Courtesy of Paul M. Kent.

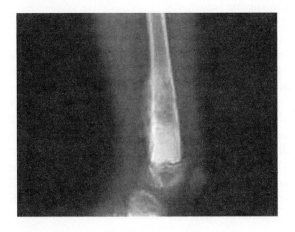

FIGURE 28-15

Sites of Metastases.

Source: Meyer, W., Cripe, T., & Stevens, M. (2010). In W. Carroll & J. Finlay, *Cancer in Children and Adolescents.* Sudbury, MA: Jones and Bartlett Publishers.

Tumor resection and chemotherapy are the therapeutic management of choice for osteosarcoma. Radiation therapy, due to poor sensitivity, is rarely used in treating patients with this type of sarcoma. Neoadjuvant (induction) chemotherapy allows treatment of microscopic disease prior to tumor resection, allowing for evaluation of therapy response at the time of surgery. Due to the toxic effects of the chemotherapy, a cardiac and audiology evaluation should be completed prior to therapy. Newer limb-salvage procedures are able to avoid 90% of amputations for those patients with osteosarcoma. Risk-based therapy is being studied in an effort to tailor the chemotherapy based on the percentage of "tumor necrosis" at time of resection. In one study, those patients with a "poor response" (defined as less than

90% necrosis at the time of surgery) will be randomized to receive or not receive more intense treatment, while those with a "good response" (90% or more necrosis) will be randomized to receive or not receive interferon therapy (Aksnes et al., 2008).

Provision of care by an interprofessional team allows for the best outcomes in pediatric patients with osteosarcoma. This team may include members from the following specialties: oncology, orthopedics, radiation, genetics, plastic surgery, prosthetics, rehabilitation services, nutrition, psychologist, child life, and social and spiritual services.

The diagnosis of osteosarcoma can be overwhelming for both the patient and the family. Providing the patient and family with education so that they may understand the disease process, possible tumor progression, the treatment and its side effects, and the use of technology allows them to make decisions and participate in the therapeutic plan while in the hospital and at home.

Disposition and Discharge Planning. Survival rates depend on the presence or absence of metastases at diagnosis and the response to neoadjuvant chemotherapy. Fifteen percent of patients with osteosarcoma achieve cure with surgery alone, whereas multiagent chemotherapy in combination with surgery has improved cure rates from 60% to 80% in other patients. Depending on the degree of necrosis at the time of surgery, patients with nonmetastatic osteosarcoma (70% of cases) have cure rates in the range of 65% to 75%. More than 25% of pediatric patients with osteosarcoma have metastases at the time of diagnosis that are located in the lung and bones. Patients with isolated lung nodules can achieve cure with aggressive surgical resection, whereas those with multiple lung nodules or bone metastases have a poorer prognosis (Ward et al., 1994).

Few patients with osteosarcoma who relapse will survive. The exceptions are those individuals with isolated lung nodules that occur after completion of therapy and those who are 3 years post (initial) surgical resection. This subgroup has been reported to have achieved long-term disease control.

For those patients who relapse and for whom complete resection of all disease is not possible, new treatments are desperately needed. Experimental therapies include activation of the immune system to eradicate cancer cells using interferon or muramyl tripeptide phosphatidylethanolamine; inhibition of growth factors such as insulin-like growth factor -1 receptor blockage; blockage of neo-angiogenesis with "antiangiogenic drugs," and prevention of bone resorption with bisphosphonates. These therapies appear promising, but as yet have unproven efficacy. Notably, stem cell therapies have not proven effective for osteosarcoma.

Pediatric patients with osteosarcoma may have frequent and prolonged hospitalizations based on tumor type, location, and sequelae. Discharge plans should be coordinated by the interprofessional team. The patient and caregivers must have the instructions that describe when to seek medical attention from the oncologist, when to go to the emergency department, and how to problem-solve issues at home. Family meetings and a designated "go to" HCP are necessary to empower a family taking a pediatric patient home. Follow-up in the pediatric oncology clinic involves vigilant examination to monitor complications of therapy such as growth disturbance, cardiac toxicity, and secondary malignancies. Physical therapy will be required to regain function in the affected limb or prosthesis.

Rhabdomyosarcoma

Paul M. Kent and Jennifer Misasi

Pathophysiology. Rhabdomyosarcoma (RMS) is the most common of the "soft-tissue sarcomas" in children. It is one of the small, round, blue cell tumors of childhood thought to arise from primitive mesenchymal cells, which normally mature into striated muscle. The etiology of such disease is unclear; however, dysregulation of gene expression in these cells is thought to result in several different types of soft-tissue sarcomas. In RMS, for example, it results in neo-angiogenesis, autocrine growth, evasion of apoptosis, immortalization, metastasis and invasion, and resistance to growth inhibition (Meyer et al., 2010).

Epidemiology and etiology. Rhabdomyosarcoma is the third most common solid tumor malignancy in childhood, accounting for 350 new cases per year. Almost two-thirds of all cases occur in children 10 years of age or younger. Males and persons of African American descent have slightly higher incidence rates. Pediatric patients with the RB mutation for retinoblastoma, neurofibromatosis-type 1, and a variety of congenital anomalies are at increased risk (Wexler & Helman, 1997).

The most common variant of RMS is the embryonal form. It can develop in any body site, although it has a predilection for the head, neck, orbits, and genitourinary system. It is most common in children between ages 1 and 8 years.

The botryoid subtype of the embryonal variant is the form most commonly seen in infants. It arises from the bladder or vagina.

The alveolar variant usually develops in the extremities or bone marrow and is characterized by a translocation between the long arm of chromosome 2 or chromosome 1 and the long arm of chromosome 13 [(t(2;13), t(1;13)]. This form of RMS is most commonly seen in adolescents and young adults (Arndt & Crist, 1999; Meyer et al., 2010).

Presentation. RBS is a very heterogeneous cancer; thus the presenting symptoms and physical examination findings will vary according to the anatomic presentation of the primary tumor, metastases, and age of the pediatric patient. Tumors of the orbit usually grow rapidly and are detected early due to the obvious physical changes they produce. Parameningeal head and neck tumors may present with epistaxis, sinusitis, nasal obstruction, visible masses, facial nerve palsy, drainage from the affected ear, and conductive hearing loss. Genitourinary tumors may present with urinary retention, straining to void, hematuria, or unexplained vaginal bleeding secondary to tumor invasion or obstruction. Extremity tumors are often tender, palpated masses that are firm and fixed to palpation.

Differential Diagnosis. Several disorders and diseases have symptoms or presenting characteristics similar to those seen with RMS:

- Benign tumors (desmoid)
- Fibrosarcoma
- Infection
- Lymphoma
- Organizing hematoma
- Soft-tissue Ewing sarcoma

Plan of care. Initial diagnostic studies may include radiographs of the affected area and chest. CT, MRI, PET scans, and ultrasounds may be used to identify location, tumor extension, and distant sites of metastasis such as the head and neck, chest, abdomen and pelvis, and extremities. Bone marrow aspiration is recommended. Definitive diagnosis is made through open biopsy.

The grouping and staging of the findings determine the therapy to be used and the patient's prognosis (Table 28-16 and Table 28-17). Pediatric patients thought to have RMS

TABLE 28-16

Rhabdomyosarcoma Grouping Classification			
Group I	**Group II**	**Group III**	**Group IV**
All of the tumor is removed at surgery; no lymph node involvement	A: tumor removed at surgery; microscopic disease B: spread to lymph nodes; all removed at surgery C: spread to lymph nodes; removed at surgery; microscopic disease	Tumor was removed and visible cells are seen; no metastatic sites	Metastatic at diagnosis

Source: Baggott et al., 2002.

TABLE 28-17

Rhabdomyosarcoma Staging Classification			
Stage 1	**Stage 2**	**Stage 3**	**Stage 4**
Cancer is any size, not spread to lymph nodes and in favorable sites such as the eye, gallbladder, head and neck, near testes or vagina	Cancer found in any one area not included in Stage 1, not spread to lymph nodes, and is 5 centimeters or smaller	Cancer found in any one area not included in Stage 1, is 5 centimeters or smaller with lymph node spread, or is 5 centimeters or larger with possible lymph node involvement	Tumor is any size, spread to lymph nodes and other metastatic sites (bone, lung, bone marrow)

Source: Baggott et al., 2002.

should be referred to a pediatric oncology center. These centers have the facilities to assess the immune histochemical and genetic features of the tumor, which aids with establishing the diagnosis, and they may provide the expert interprofessional team required to deliver therapy. A multimodal approach is taken to optimally treat patients diagnosed with RMS. Tumor resection, local radiation therapy, and chemotherapy are all used. Chemotherapy is based on the stage of the cancer.

Provision of care by an interprofessional team allows for the best outcomes in pediatric patients with RMS. This team may include members from the following specialties: oncology, ophthalmology, radiation, genetics, plastic surgery, prosthetics, rehabilitation services, nutrition, psychologist, child life, and social and spiritual services.

The diagnosis of RMS can be overwhelming for both the patient and the family. Understanding the disease process, symptoms related to the tumor and tumor progression, goals of care, management plan, use of technology, and side effects of therapy will allow caregivers and family members to care for their child while in the hospital and at home.

Disposition and discharge planning. Survival rates for RMS have increased significantly over the past 50 years. The prognosis reflects the age of the patient, the location of the tumor and its group/stage, and the pathology (Meyer et al., 2010) (Figure 28-16). For example, patients with embryonal tumors in Group I or II, or Group II stage 1, have a 93% survival rate. By comparison, those with alveolar tumors in Group IV stage 4 have a less than 30% survival rate. The prognosis for patients who experience relapse is poor (Meyer et al.).

Pediatric patients may have frequent and prolonged hospitalizations depending on their tumor type, location,

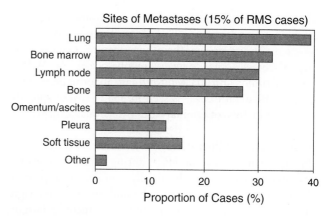

FIGURE 28-16

Survival Rates.

Source: Baggott et al., 2002.

and sequelae. Tumor excision may impair body functions, requiring extensive support services. Discharge plans should be coordinated by the interprofessional team. The patient and caregivers must have the instructions that describe when to seek medical attention of the oncologist, when to go to the emergency department, and how to problem-solve issues at home. Family meetings and a designated "go to" HCP are necessary to empower a family taking a pediatric patient home. Follow-up in the pediatric oncology clinic involves vigilant examination to monitor for complications associated with therapy, such as recurrence or secondary malignancy.

Wilms' tumor

Paul M. Kent and Jennifer Misasi

Pathophysiology. Wilms' tumor (nephroblastoma) arises in pluripotent embryonic renal precursor cells. Although most Wilms' tumors have no genetic abnormalities, the gene *WT1* at chromosome 11p13 is responsible for normal genitourinary and sexual development and has been implicated in tumor genesis. Wilms' tumor has a classic "triphasic histology," consisting of blastemal cells, which are undifferentiated small blue cells; stromal cells, which are immature spindle cells; and epithelial cells, which make up the glomeruli and tubules.

Epidemiology and etiology. Wilms' tumor is the second most common abdominal malignancy in childhood, after neuroblastoma, and the most common renal tumor, accounting for 6% of all childhood cancers. This type of tumor is rare in infancy; rather, it presents most frequently at the age of 2 to 3 years, with 80% of all Wilms' tumors being diagnosed before age 5 years. Approximately 1% to 3% of Wilms' tumor patients have a familial associations, and 10% to 17% have a genetic syndrome or congenital abnormality such as Denys-Drash syndrome (congenital nephrotic syndrome with kidney failure), Beckwith-Wiedemann syndrome (hemihypertrophy, macroglossia, hypoglycemia, organomegaly, omphalocele), or WAGR (Wilms' tumor, aniridia, genitourinary abnormalities, retardation). Bilateral disease is seen in 5% to 6% of sporadic cases and in 16% of familial cases (Matsumaga, 1981).

Presentation. Wilms' tumor is often found by the caregiver during a bath or by the HCP during a health screening and maintenance visit. It usually consists of a painless flank mass that does not cross the midline. Systemic signs and symptoms are common and may include fatigue, pain, fever, and hematuria. Physical examination findings may include aniridia, macroglossia, hypertension (from renal artery compression), abdominal obstruction, IVC thrombus, or genitourinary abnormalities. Laboratory disorders include acquired von Willebrand disease (8%) and polycythemia (from erythropoietin secretion) (Grundy et al., 2010).

Differential diagnosis. Several disorders and diseases have symptoms or presenting characteristics similar to those seen with Wilms' tumor:

- Cystic kidney disease
- Gastrointestinal malformation
- Germ cell tumor
- Hepatoblastoma
- Infection
- Lymphoma
- Neuroblastoma

Plan of care. Initial diagnostic studies include CBC, basic metabolic, coagulation panels, urinalysis, and calcium. The coagulation studies will be pertinent to identify pediatric patients with acquired von Willebrand disease prior to surgical resection. Imaging studies include renal and abdominal ultrasounds and CT (with contrast) of the chest, abdomen, and pelvis. The ultrasound is especially useful to identify tumor extension into the inferior vena cava with obstruction. The chest CT evaluates for pulmonary metastases. The abdominal CT is useful to identify tumor extension, IVC thrombus, and bilateral disease. The "claw sign" (a splayed-open kidney with tumor emerging from it) may be noted. Bone scans are used to further stage the patient.

Children thought to have Wilms' tumor should be referred to a pediatric oncology center. Such centers have the facilities needed to assess the immunohistochemical and genetic features of the tumor. The center's HCPs may also establish the diagnosis and provide the expert interprofessional team required to deliver therapy.

Therapeutic management consists of a multimodal approach (as with all other childhood cancers) and often includes nephrectomy, radiation therapy, and chemotherapy. Therapy is based on the stage determined by CT and bone scans. Surgical biopsy of the tumor is contraindicated, as it increases the risk of "tumor spillage"—an event that advances the patient to stage II–III, requiring abdominal radiation as treatment. Chemotherapy is used preoperatively for patients with stage III and IV tumors and those who cannot have a complete resection. Radiation is delivered to the abdominal tumor bed if the patient has stage II or III disease and to the lungs for those patients with pulmonary metastases.

Provision of care by an interprofessional team allows for the best outcomes in pediatric patients with Wilms' tumor. This team may include members from the following specialties: pediatric oncology, pediatric surgery, pediatric nephrology, radiation oncology, nutrition, child life, and social and spiritual services.

The diagnosis of Wilms' tumor can be overwhelming for both the patient and the family. Understanding the disease process, symptoms related to the tumor and tumor progression, goals of care, management plan, use of technology, and side effects of therapy will allow caregivers and family members to care for their child while in the hospital and at home.

Disposition and discharge planning. The three-year survival rate for patients with stage I or II disease is more than 95%. The survival rate for those with stage III or IV disease, with favorable histology, approaches 85%. Patients with unfavorable or anaplastic histology have a poor prognosis. Approximately 10% to 15% of patients with Wilms' tumors have metastatic disease at diagnosis, with metastases most commonly noted in the lung and liver (Breslow et al., 1995). Patients with the nephrectomy and flank irradiation may be at risk for late-onset kidney failure; this risk is increased for those with WAGR syndrome (Breslow et al., 2000).

Pediatric patients may have frequent and prolonged hospitalizations depending on their tumor type, location, and sequelae. Tumor excision may impair body functions, requiring extensive support services. Discharge plans should be coordinated by the interprofessional team. The patient and caregivers must have the instructions that describe when to seek medical attention of the oncologist, when to go to the emergency department, and how to problem-solve issues at home. Family meetings and a designated "go to" HCP are necessary to empower a family taking a pediatric patient home. Follow-up in the pediatric oncology clinic involves vigilant examination to monitor for complications associated with therapy, such as recurrence or secondary malignancy. Follow-up care includes imaging studies every 3 months for 2 to 5 years; those patients with the various syndromes associated with Wilms' tumors should be followed until age 7 years (Grundy et al., 2010).

Neuroblastoma

Amy R. Newman

Pathophysiology. The diagnosis of neuroblastoma encompasses a heterogeneous grouping of tumors for which the biology of the tumor largely dictates the clinical behavior (Park et al., 2008). Neuroblastomas belong to the small, round, blue cell neoplasms of childhood. Arising from primordial neural crest cells, the two predominant cell types in these neoplasms are neuroblasts and Schwann cells.

Neuroblasts are pluripotent cells that arise in the neural crest, then migrate to the dorsal aorta and form various components of the sympathetic nervous system. These components include the sympathetic ganglia, the chromaffin cells of the adrenal medulla, and the paraganglia. What causes the persistence of embryonal cells that develop into neuroblastic tumors is unclear. Genes that dictate neural cell development and differentiation may be mutated, lost, or amplified, causing uncontrolled cellular proliferation and lack of programmed cell death. The origin of Schwann cells is controversial, but a common pluripotent stem cell is believed to be the origin of both neuroblasts and Schwann cells (Shusterman & George, 2009).

The degree of cellular differentiation and maturation exhibited by the different neuroblastic tumors determines their histopathologic subtype. Neuroblastic tumor subtypes include neuroblastoma, ganglioneuroblastoma, and ganglioneuroma, with neuroblastoma representing the most undifferentiated, least mature malignant subtype (Park et al., 2008).

Epidemiology and etiology. Neuroblastoma, a neoplasm of the sympathetic nervous system, is the most common type of extracranial solid tumor in childhood. It accounts for 7% to 10% of all malignancies in children younger than 15 years of age, and is the most frequently diagnosed malignancy during infancy (Maris et al., 2007). In the United States, 650 cases are diagnosed each year, and such tumors account for 15% of all deaths from childhood cancer. A slightly increased incidence is seen in Caucasian infants compared to other races and in males compared to females (Shusterman & George, 2009). The incidence of neuroblastoma peaks between the ages of 0 and 4, with the median age of diagnosis being 23 months (Park et al., 2008).

The cause of neuroblastoma remains largely unknown. Embryonal origin and young age of onset suggest that prenatal and perinatal exposures may be important (Shusterman & George, 2009). Suggested environmental factors include paternal exposure to electromagnetic fields and prenatal exposure to alcohol, pesticides, and certain medications. A potential relationship is believed to exist between neuroblastoma and assisted pregnancies. None of these suggested relationships has been confirmed in independent studies, however.

Neuroblastoma has been noted to occur in patients with other neural crest disorders, such as Hirschsprung's disease, neurofibromatosis type 1, and congenital hypoventilation syndrome. Familial history has been identified in 1% to 2% of cases (Park et al., 2008).

Presentation. Neuroblastomas can develop anywhere within the sympathetic nervous system, although most primary tumors are found within the chest, abdomen, or pelvis. The clinical presentation is quite variable and depends on the location of the primary tumor, the presence of metastases, and any concomitant paraneoplastic syndromes. Approximately 40% of patients present with localized disease—that is, a primary tumor with no evidence of distant metastases. Some degree of lymph node involvement surrounding the tumor may be present. Sixty-five percent of patients present with tumors in the abdomen, with at least 50% of tumors arising from the adrenal medulla. Many children are asymptomatic, and tumors are often found incidentally when imaging is performed for some other purpose.

Physical examination findings may include abdominal tenderness, distention, and hepatomegaly. Large abdominal or pelvic masses may also alter venous and lymphatic return of the lower extremities, leading to lower-extremity and scrotal edema. Occasionally, abdominal tumors spontaneously hemorrhage, resulting in an increase in the size of the mass with an accompanying increase in the patient's pain and abdominal distention (Shusterman & George, 2009). Tumors of the upper thoracic spine can be associated with mechanical obstruction, resulting in superior vena cava syndrome (SVCS). Approximately 5% to 15% of tumors present in the paraspinal region, with the tumor extending into the neural foramina, which results in spinal cord compression. Such patients may report motor weakness, pain, sensory loss, or difficulty with defecation/urination (Maris et al., 2007). Children with cervical masses may exhibit symptoms of Horner's syndrome, including unilateral ptosis, myosis, and anhydrosis. Other, less frequently observed presenting findings include diarrhea (due to increased secretion of vasoactive intestinal peptide), hypertension, and flushing (due to increased secretion of catecholamines), skin nodules, and hypotonia.

Patients with widely disseminated disease often present as ill appearing, exhibiting signs and symptoms consistent with systemic involvement, such as fever, pain, and irritability. Metastatic sites may include bone, bone marrow, and the liver. If bone or bone marrow involvement has occurred, patients may report generalized pain, fatigue, weakness, and more frequent infections. Physical examination may reveal pallor and bruising. Tumor infiltration of the periorbital bones can result in proptosis and periorbital ecchymoses—classic signs of metastatic neuroblastoma that are referred to as "raccoon eyes." Infants younger than 1 year of age may present with localized tumors, plus skin, liver, or bone marrow involvement.

A small percentage of patients with neuroblastoma (2%–4%) will present with signs and symptoms consistent with opsoclonus-myoclonus ataxia (OMA) syndrome. Conversely, as many as 50% of children who present with OMA syndrome are found to have neuroblastoma. Signs and symptoms of OMA syndrome include myoclonic jerking and random eye movements, with or without cerebellar ataxia. Such patients generally have small primary (thoracic) tumors that are easily resected, and they rarely require additional therapeutic interventions. Unfortunately, surgical resection frequently does not result in cessation of psychomotor or neurologic deficits, prompting the addition of glucocorticoids, intravenous immunoglobulin, or other chemotherapy agents to the therapeutic regimen (Maris et al., 2007; Rothenberg et al., 2009).

Differential diagnosis. Differential diagnosis is based on the child's clinical presentation, including the location of the primary tumor site and the presence of metastases. Differential diagnosis of masses found in the abdomen includes Wilms' tumor, hepatoblastoma, non-Hodgkin lymphoma (NHL), germ cell tumors, and soft-tissue sarcomas (rhabdomyosarcoma as well as non-rhabdomyosarcoma). Lymphomas, germ cell tumors, and infection should be considered in children presenting with a mediastinal mass. Paraspinal masses can include the previously mentioned diagnoses as well as desmoid tumors, epidermoid tumors, and teratomas. Once a biopsy is performed, immunohistological staining will be performed to discriminate amongst other small, round, blue cell tumors (rhabdomyosarcoma, NHL, Ewing's sarcoma family of tumors, and leukemias).

Plan of care. Children presenting with a mass or other signs and symptoms of malignancy undergo a complete laboratory and radiographic evaluation. HCPs should obtain a CBC to evaluate for bone marrow dysfunction, which is suggestive of the presence of bone marrow disease. Bilateral bone marrow aspirates and biopsies are performed to detect the presence of tumor cells in the bone marrow environment. A complete chemistry panel and serum ferritin should also be obtained. Elevations of lactate dehydrogenase (LDH) and ferritin are nonspecific findings, but often suggest that the patient has more aggressive, high-risk disease. Abnormal liver function tests suggest the presence of liver involvement. In addition, urine is evaluated for elevated catecholamine metabolites, including vanillylmandelic acid (VMA) and homovanillic acid (HVA).

If a mass is found or suspected on plain radiograph, a CT scan or MRI is performed to better evaluate the primary tumor site. The CT scan aids in determining the size of the tumor, invasion of other local structures, and lymph node involvement; such imaging will also aid in the determination of the potential surgical resectability of the tumor. MRI is the preferred imaging modality for intracranial and paraspinal masses. In addition, ^{99}mTc-diphosphonate scintigraphy (bone scan) is performed to evaluate for the presence of bony metastases. Sensitivity and specificity for detecting bony metastases as well as occult soft-tissue disease are enhanced through the use of metaiodobenzylguanidine (MIBG) scintigraphy. Ninety percent of neuroblastomas exhibit increased uptake of MIBG at primary tumor and metastatic sites, so this technology is a more specific method of disease evaluation than bone scintigraphy (Maris et al., 2007).

Biopsy of tissue from the primary tumor or a metastatic site is necessary to make the final diagnosis, which is based on the presence of characteristic histopathologic features of tumor tissue or the presence of tumor cells in the bone marrow accompanied by raised concentrations of urinary catecholamines (Maris et al., 2007). Specific biologic features of the tumor, such as the presence of *MYCN* oncogene amplification, DNA ploidy, and determination of Shimada histology, are examined with this kind of analysis.

The extent of disease at presentation, in addition to the initial surgical management of the tumor, determines the patient's stage according to the International Neuroblastoma Staging System (INSS) (Table 28-18). Patient stage, age, and the biologic features of the tumor determine the patient's risk of recurrence, and treatment is tailored to risk level. Favorable biologic characteristics include nonamplification of the *MYCN* oncogene, a DNA index of greater than 1, and favorable Shimada classification. Patients with localized, *MYCN*-nonamplified tumors that can be grossly resected have 95% cure rates with surgery alone. If unfavorable biologic features are present, patients may require chemotherapy to reduce their risk of recurrence. Patients with more locally invasive disease that is unresectable upon presentation require moderately intensive chemotherapy to reduce tumor burden and facilitate subsequent surgical resection of the tumor.

If initial biopsy of more locally invasive tumors reveals unfavorable biologic features, patients are treated as "high risk," similar to patients with metastatic tumors. Patients with metastatic disease at presentation generally have a poor prognosis; therefore, they are treated with aggressive multimodal therapy. Such therapy is divided into four phases: induction, local control, consolidation, and maintenance.

Induction consists of four to seven cycles of intensive multiagent chemotherapy. The goal of induction chemotherapy is to reduce the overall disease burden, shrink the primary tumor, and eradicate sites of metastatic disease. Seventy to eighty percent of patients have a significant response to initial chemotherapy (Esiashvili et al., 2009).

TABLE 28-18

International Neuroblastoma Staging System

Stage	Definitions
I	Localized tumor with complete gross excision, with or without microscopic residual disease; representative ipsilateral lymph nodes negative for tumor microscopically (nodes attached to and removed with the tumor may be positive).
2A	Localized tumor with incomplete gross excision; representative ipsilateral nonadherent lymph nodes negative for tumor microscopically.
2B	Localized tumor with or without complete gross excision, with ipsilateral nonadherent lymph nodes positive for tumor. Enlarged contralateral lymph nodes must be negative microscopically.
3	Unresectable unilateral tumor infiltrating across the midline (defined as the vertebral column), with or without regional lymph node involvement; or localized unilateral tumor with contralateral regional lymph node involvement; or midline tumor with bilateral extension by infiltration (unresectable) or by lymph node involvement.
4	Any primary tumor with dissemination to distant lymph nodes, bone, bone marrow, liver, skin, and/or other organs (except as defined for Stage 4S).
4S	Localized primary tumor (as defined for Stage I, 2A, or 2B), with dissemination limited to the skin, liver, and/or bone marrow (limited to infants younger than I year of age).

Source: Reprinted with permission. © 2008 American Society of Clinical Oncology. All rights reserved. Brodeur, G., et al. (1993). Revisions of the international criteria for neuroblastoma diagnosis, staging, and response to treatment. *Journal of Clinical Oncology, 11*(8), 1466–1477.

Induction chemotherapy is followed by surgical resection of the primary tumor site, with or without subsequent irradiation (local control). The goal of consolidation therapy is to eliminate any remaining tumor cells; this phase consists of myeloablative chemotherapy followed by autologous stem cell rescue. Once they have recovered from the toxicities associated with high-dose chemotherapy with stem cell rescue, patients undergo external-beam radiation therapy to the primary tumor and any major metastatic sites.

Finally, patients commence with maintenance therapy, which aims to eliminate any minimal residual disease. Historically, maintenance consisted of retinoids, which are believed to induce terminal differentiation of neuroblastoma cells. Current pediatric clinical trials are exploring the use of immunotherapy in addition to retinoids to reduce the incidence of recurrence in high-risk patients.

Patients with an incidental finding of a mass in the chest or abdomen, who are asymptomatic, can safely be admitted to an acute care setting. Prompt staging and consultation with pediatric oncology and general surgery are imperative so that plans for surgical resection or biopsy of primary or metastatic sites may be arranged.

Patients with orbital, mediastinal, spinal cord, or extensive abdominal disease often present more emergently. In all of these patients, the process of obtaining a diagnosis and initiation of chemotherapy should be expedited.

Patients with orbital involvement should be promptly evaluated by an ophthalmologist to assess their visual acuity and visual fields. Due to the high risk of SVCS in patients with mediastinal disease, ongoing monitoring of respiratory and cardiac function is critical. Spinal cord compression with resultant loss of motor function, loss of sensation, and bowel/bladder dysfunction represents an oncologic emergency.

Immediate consultation with neurosurgery, pediatric oncology, and radiation oncology specialists is imperative, as prompt treatment is critical to ensure maintenance or return of normal neurologic functioning.

The optimal treatment strategies for such patients are the subject of debate. When patients have minimal symptoms, chemotherapy usually provides excellent relief. When patients have acute or severe neurologic symptoms, one has only a short time (24 hours) before neurologic damage becomes permanent. Surgical intervention in this setting is preferred, but can result in long-term complications related to major scoliotic deformities. When surgery is not feasible, a combination of chemotherapy, irradiation, and corticosteroid treatment (to reduce edema) is an alternative (De Bernardi et al., 2001).

Extensive abdominal disease and a rapidly enlarging tumor or liver can result in hemodynamic compromise secondary to hemorrhage, impaired venous return, and ineffective respiratory effort. Young infants younger than 2 months of age have been found to be particularly sensitive to this phenomenon, and should be monitored closely for respiratory failure and hemodynamic collapse.

Patients with high-risk disease who are undergoing intensive therapy are at a high risk of treatment-related morbidity. Multiagent chemotherapy results in profound myelosuppression, which often requires the patient's admission to the hospital for treatment of febrile neutropenia, mucositis, and colitis. Nutritional status becomes significantly compromised, and nutritional support in the form of either parenteral or enteral nutrition is often required. These risk factors require astute observation and ongoing evaluation of such patients when they present to the acute care environment, including monitoring closely for signs and symptoms of pending sepsis. Similarly, when patients are hospitalized following myeloablative chemotherapy with stem cell rescue, their risk of infection, mucositis, and other end-organ toxicities is quite high. Aggressive supportive care, including antimicrobial agents, transfusion support, pain management, and oral care, is critical to optimize the patient's health status. Finally, immunotherapy is accompanied by multiple infusion-related complications, including anaphylaxis, severe hypotension, and capillary leak syndrome. Patients must be monitored closely in an acute care environment by HCPs who are familiar with management strategies aimed at avoiding or quickly managing such side effects.

Patients and families are generally shocked and fearful when presented with a cancer diagnosis, particularly if the child has been previously healthy. Initial education is directed at reviewing the child's potential diagnosis, required evaluation, and need for surgical intervention. Ongoing information regarding the patient's status is critical, as it may take several days for the diagnosis to be confirmed. Child life specialists, where available, should be engaged as soon as possible to help the child understand and process, the diagnosis, and the necessary interventions in a manner that is developmentally appropriate. Once the diagnosis and treatment plan have been established, details should be explained to the patient and family. These details include the side effects of chemotherapeutic medications, the timing of any additional surgeries, the management of potential toxicities, and the need for ongoing follow-up with the pediatric oncology group.

Disposition and discharge planning. Neuroblastomas display a wide variety of clinical behaviors, ranging from spontaneous regression to very aggressive, rapid growth and spread. Consequently, overall survival rates for patients with these neoplasms is equally varied. Patient age, stage of disease, and biologic features of the tumor are all strong prognostic factors. Infants younger than the age of 18 months generally have more favorable biologic features, portending an improved prognosis. The overall cure rate for patients with stage 1 and 2 disease is more than 90%, for patients with stage 3 disease is 60%, and for patients with stage 4 disease is 40% to 50% (Shusterman & George, 2009). The population of 4S (special) patients represents a unique subgroup of infants who have disseminated disease, but paradoxically have a favorable prognosis and a high rate of spontaneous regression (70%). Overall cure rates are estimated at 90% in 4S patients.

The initial hospitalization of a child with neuroblastoma can last for several weeks. Generally, the first portion of the hospitalization encompasses the diagnostic evaluation, including potential surgical resection or biopsy. This period is closely followed by the initiation of chemotherapy, with subsequent management of any related toxicities. During this time, intensive education continues, ensuring that patients and families are knowledgeable about the disease and its management.

Prior to discharge, patients must have recovered from any surgical complications, have completed initial therapies, and be free of toxicities, such as infection, mucositis, or persistent nausea and vomiting. The intensity of prescribed chemotherapy for neuroblastoma patients generally requires weekly follow-up in the outpatient pediatric oncology clinic.

Critical Thinking

Unexplained vomiting without signs of gastroenteritis, infection, or anorexia is a particularly common "red flag" for a pediatric patient with a central nervous system tumor.

TUMOR LYSIS SYNDROME

Jennifer R. Madden

Pathophysiology

"Tumor lysis syndrome (TLS or acute tumor lysis syndrome [ATLS]) is characterized by a group of metabolic derangements caused by massive and abrupt release of cellular components into the blood after the rapid lysis of malignant cells" (Coiffier et al., 2008, p. 2767). In this disorder, the body becomes overwhelmed by the sudden load of intracellular metabolites, which results in hyperuricemia, hyperphosphatemia, hypocalcemia, and hyperkalemia.

Hyperuricemia occurs as a result of nucleic acid catabolism, principally catabolism of purine. The purine catabolism pathway involves the enzyme xanthine oxidase, which catabolizes hypoxanthine first into xanthine and then into uric acid. When present in the body in excessive amounts, uric acid can become deposited in and obstruct the renal tubules, leading to kidney insufficiency. Malignant cells have elevated levels of phosphorus; therefore extensive lysis leads to a sudden increase in serum phosphorus levels. A consequence of hyperphosphatemia is increased calcium precipitation in the kidneys, and with concurrent kidney insufficiency secondary hypocalcemia occurs. Potassium is another by-product of cell lysis and can also be exacerbated by kidney insufficiency.

Prevention of these events is key to management of TLS. Once they are evident, however, interfering with purine catabolism, maintaining kidney function, and preventing the secondary effects of electrolyte dysfunction are the goals of therapy (Coiffier et al., 2008).

Epidemiology and etiology

Age and gender preferences for TLS are unknown. Instead, patients are deemed to be at intermediate and high risk for TLS based on tumor-related and preexisting clinical factors.

- *Tumor-related factors.* The tumors at highest risk for leading to TLS in pediatric patients have high growth rates or sensitivity to chemotherapy—specifically, non-Hodgkin lymphoma (especially Burkitt), acute lymphoblastic leukemia (ALL), and acute myelogenous leukemia (AML). TLS in solid tumors is rare. Patients with elevated lactate dehydrogenase (LDH) levels are also at increased risk for developing TLS.
- *Preexisting clinical factors.* Uremia/hyperuricemia; oliguria, anuria, or acidic urine; dehydration; and kidney insufficiency/failure exacerbate the effects of the excess metabolites in the system (Bercovitz et al., 2009; Coiffier et al., 2008).

Tumor lysis syndrome is classified as either laboratory TLS (LTLS) or clinical TLS (CTLS). This designation is used to differentiate those patients who have life-threatening problems from those who require little or no therapy. Laboratory TLS—the more common type of TLS—includes alterations by 25% from baseline of at least two of the following measurements: serum calcium, phosphorus, potassium, and uric acid. Clinical TLS includes LTLS and one or more of the following: kidney insufficiency, cardiac dysrhythmia, seizures (Coiffier et al., 2008; Tosi et al., 2008). The incidence of LTLS in patients with high-grade non-Hodgkin lymphoma ranges from 17% to 42%, while the incidence of CTLS ranges from 3% to 6% (Coiffier et al.).

Presentation

TLS most commonly occurs shortly after the initiation of therapy (within 2 days); thus the HCP should maintain a high index of suspicion in pediatric patients with cancers who are considered to be at high or intermediate risk of developing this syndrome. In addition, a history of massive tumor burden or symptoms of superior vena cava or tracheal obstruction is of importance. Other symptoms of TLS are listed in Table 28-19 (Coiffier et al., 2008; Colen, 2008).

Physical examination findings may include the following:

- Skin: cool, diaphoretic, pale, or mottled, or decreased or irregular pulses
- Lungs: tachypnea, crackles, decreased breath sounds, or tracheal shift
- Abdomen: ascites or hepatomegaly
- Musculoskeletal: muscle spasm or tetany
- Neurologic: paresthesias, weakness, mental status changes, seizures, or Chvostek's and Trousseau's signs (Table 28-20)

Differential diagnosis

Metabolic causes of electrolyte derangement and kidney insufficiency should be considered such as dehydration,

TABLE 28-19

Symptoms of Tumor Lysis Syndrome
• Anorexia
• Cardiac arrhythmias
• Congestive heart failure
• Diarrhea
• Edema
• Fluid overload
• Hematuria
• Lethargy
• Muscle cramps
• Nausea
• Oliguria
• Seizures
• Sudden death
• Syncope
• Tetany
• Vomiting

TABLE 28-20

Signs of Hypocalcemia	
Chvostek's sign	Tap on the facial nerve located anterior to the ear lobe and below the zygomatic arch. A positive sign is twitching or contraction of the facial muscles.
Trousseau's sign	Inflate a blood pressure cuff above systolic pressure on the upper arm for several minutes. A positive sign is carpopedal spasm, wrist/metacarpophalangeal/thumb flexion, and hyperextension of the fingers.

abdominal/pelvic masses, and drug nephrotoxicity from chemotherapeutic agents and other medications (Coiffier et al., 2008).

Plan of care

A serum comprehensive metabolic panel that includes calcium, phosphorus, potassium, uric acid, and creatinine measurements should be monitored every 6 hours for 24 to 48 hours to follow the metabolic load from TLS and kidney function. Urinalysis is recommended every 12 hours. Serum LDH should be examined at least every 24 hours.

The goal of therapeutic management is to prevent kidney failure in those patients considered to be at intermediate or high risk for TLS-induced hyperuricemia. This determination is based on the recommendations of the Expert Panel for the Management of Pediatric and Adult Tumor Lysis Syndrome, which has identified several risk categories; low, intermediate, and high (Coiffier et al., 2008).

Based on case reports and clinical examples, the Expert Panel recommends observation and close monitoring for *low-risk patients*—those with cancers who are unlikely to develop TLS (Coiffier et al., 2008).

For *intermediate-risk patients*, the therapeutic plan recommendation from the Expert Panel includes vigorous hydration and allopurinol for prevention of hyperuricemia. Hydration promotes the clearance of uric acid through the kidney. Allopurinol blocks the conversion of hypoxanthine and xanthine to uric acid. The HCP should administer D_5 0.25NS intravenous fluid (initially without additional potassium, calcium, or phosphorus) at a rate of 2 to 3 $L/m^2/day$ (200 mL/kg/day for those patients who weigh 10 kg or less) if the patient's cardiac and kidney function can withstand this treatment. Monitor urine output closely and maintain it in the range of 80 to 100 $mL/m^2/hr$ (4–6 mL/kg/hr for those who weigh 10 kg or less). Urine specific gravity should be 1.010 or less (Coiffier et al., 2008). Allopurinol should be started before induction therapy, and should continue until laboratory values have returned to low risk levels. This agent is contraindicated in those patients with a preexisting allergy to the medication or any signs of allergic response upon administration. The oral pediatric dose of allopurinol is 50 to 100 mg/m^2 every 8 hours (maximum dose of 300 $mg/m^2/day$) or 10 mg/kg/day divided every 8 hours (maximum dose of 800 mg/day). IV administration is 200 to 400 $mg/m^2/day$ divided into one to three doses (maximum dose of 600 mg/day) for patients who are unable to take oral medication. The dosing is adjusted based on the patient's kidney function.

Based on the results of at least one well-designed, randomized study, recombinant urate oxidase (rasburicase) is recommended in intermediate-risk patients if hyperuricemia results despite administration of allopurinol. Rasburicase decreases uric acid by converting it to allantoin, which is more water soluble and more easily excreted by the kidney than uric acid (Coiffier et al., 2008).

The Expert Panel makes no recommendation regarding alkalinization for those patients receiving allopurinol, as there is no evidence to support this practice's efficacy. Alkalinization may also increase the patient's risk of developing calcium phosphate crystals in the kidney; therefore, it is indicated only for those individuals with metabolic acidosis. Alkalinization is not required in those receiving rasburicase (Coiffier et al., 2008).

For *high-risk patients*, the Expert Panel recommends aggressive therapy, admission to an intensive care unit (or similarly monitored setting), and consultation with a kidney specialist for potential dialysis therapy. Induction therapy should be held, if possible, until TLS therapy has been initiated. Hydration (as in intermediate-risk patients) and administration of recombinant urate oxidase (rasburicase) are recommended. Rasburicase is contraindicated in patients with G6PD deficiency and in those who are pregnant or lactating. Recommended dosing is 0.1 to 0.2 mg/kg/day

administered in 50 mL of diluent over 30 minutes. The duration of therapy is 1 to 7 days based on therapeutic goals to reduce uric acid levels. Because rasburicase can interfere with uric acid in blood samples, these samples should be placed on ice until analyzed (Coiffier et al., 2008). Patients should be monitored for hypersensitivity reactions—specifically, for anaphylaxis and methemoglobinemia.

Additional therapeutic management goals are to treat hyperphosphatemia, hyperkalemia, and hypocalcemia.

Hyperphosphatemia. Asymptomatic patients should be treated with hydration and phosphate-binding agents. Phosphate-binding agents include aluminum hydroxide and calcium carbonate. If the patient is symptomatic, dialysis or hemofiltration may be indicated (Coiffier et al., 2008).

Hyperkalemia. Avoid external sources of potassium while the patient is at risk of this imbalance, and continuously monitor the patient for life-threatening dysrhythmias. Verify elevated levels of serum potassium with an electrocardiograph (ECG) and repeat these levels to rule out hemolysis as the cause. If the patient is asymptomatic, potassium-binding resins may be administered orally. Diuretics such as furosemide to increase kidney excretion of potassium may also be administered. If patients develop life-threatening dysrhythmias, therapies may include IV insulin (which increases cell uptake of potassium) and glucose (which treats the resultant hypoglycemia), calcium chloride or gluconate (which stabilizes the myocardium), or sodium bicarbonate (which increases cell uptake of potassium) (Bercovitz et al., 2009; Coiffier et al., 2008). Patients who do not respond to potassium-lowering strategies are at risk for kidney failure and should be considered early as candidates for dialysis. Patients at high risk for TLS should be prepared for dialysis prior to the administration of cytotoxic chemotherapeutic agents.

Hypocalcemia. If the patient is asymptomatic, no therapy is usually indicated. Symptomatic patients are treated with calcium chloride or gluconate.

The acuity of the pediatric patient presenting with TLS may dictate the involvement of specialty consultants, such as those from nephrology, critical care, cardiology, and nutrition, in the patient's care. Additional interprofessional team members may include child life, social work, rehabilitation, and surgical services specialists.

With the diagnosis of TLS comes discussion of the patient's prognosis, treatment planning, and complications of therapy. Tumor lysis syndrome is a complication that is often predictable; thus preventive measures can be implemented. These steps may include admission or transfer to the intensive care unit and/or dialysis, both of which increase patient and family stress. Providing families with ongoing, repetitive education that focuses on the cancer diagnosis, its management, and the complication risk will help them in times of highest stress. Families may also benefit from the services of social workers, psychologists, child life specialists, and spiritual advisors.

Disposition and discharge planning

Patients with TLS should be monitored closely for at least 24 to 48 hours after the initiation of induction therapy (Coiffier et al., 2008). Follow-up of the patient's serum electrolytes and hematologic studies, medication titration, and kidney therapies are commonly coordinated by the oncology service. Outcomes for patients with TLS depend on resolution of the metabolic derangements. Long-term kidney complications are related to the severity of kidney injury.

LONG-TERM EFFECTS OF CANCER THERAPY

Barbara A. Lockart

Cancer is no longer an incurable disease for a majority of pediatric patients. Advances in the delivery of radiation therapy, combination chemotherapy agents, blood product use, growth factors, and hematopoietic cell transplants have greatly improved the survival rates for childhood and adolescent cancers. Surveillance, Epidemiology, and End Results (SEER) data from 1975 to 2006 report that the 5-year survival rate in 1975 was 58%, but increased to 80% in 2006. Treatment modalities and survival rates are vastly different for the 4-year-old child who is diagnosed with standard-risk pre-B acute lymphoblastic leukemia (ALL) when compared to the 15-year-old adolescent with high-risk pre-B ALL. The greatest strides have come in improving outcomes for acute leukemias and lymphomas (Horner et al., 2009). For many patients with childhood cancers, the focus is not only on curing the disease, but also on minimizing adverse, lifelong effects of treatment.

Long-term and late effects

For many pediatric patients, diagnosis of a malignancy means the beginning of a chronic illness, not a terminal illness. Chemotherapy and radiation have the potential to have long-term, lasting effects on the health and well-being of the survivor. "Complications, disabilities or adverse outcomes that are persistent and are the result of the disease process, the treatment, or both, are generally referred to as 'late-effects'" (Meadows, 2003, p. 117). Most pediatric oncologists define survivorship as the patient being 5 years post diagnosis with a minimum of 2 years free of cancer treatment (Meadows).

As early as 1975, cancer treatment was recognized as having the potential to negatively impact the health of a survivor. D'Angio (1975) stated that "the child cured of cancer must be followed for life, not so much because late recurrence of disease is feared as to permit early detection of the delayed consequences of radio- and chemotherapy" (p. 868).

A current treatment challenge in caring for pediatric patients with cancer is maximizing the potential for achieving and maintaining a cure while minimizing the risk of chronic health care issues that might negatively impact the survivor's quality of life. The majority of survivors of childhood cancer will be affected by at least one late effect during their lifetime; moreover, more than 25% of survivors experience a late effect determined to be severe or life threatening (Geenen et al., 2007; Oeffinger et al., 2006).

Survivors face psychosocial and financial challenges as well as physical late effects. Neurocognitive late effects may not become evident for years. Twenty-three percent of survivors require special education services compared to 8% of their siblings. Additionally, survivors are less likely than their siblings to graduate from high school (Mitby et al., 2003). Many survivors report challenges obtaining insurance. Given their complex health screening needs, this difficulty may result in suboptimal health for the survivor population (Fish & Ginsberg, 2009).

Cancer survivors may be affected by either a long-term effect of treatment or a late effect of treatment. Long-term effects occur during treatment and continue once treatment is completed. These effects may or may not resolve over time. An example is amputation. In contrast, late effects may occur months to years after treatment is completed. Cardiomyopathy and breast cancer (occurring in the radiation field) are considered late effects of treatment that may present 15 to 20 years after treatment is completed.

Late effects are the result of treatment, disease specifics, complications during treatment, and individual host factors such as gender, age at time of treatment, and genetic make-up. Any organ system in the body may be affected. As cancer survivors age, the full impact of treatment effects are realized; however, the costs associated with their lifelong care have yet to be fully recognized.

Pediatric patients receiving care for late effects may be influenced by numerous factors, including access to health care, insurance limitations, and understanding by both survivor and HCP about the individual's unique health care needs. Care may be provided in an oncology clinic, a clinic dedicated to late effects, a community HCP's office, or an adult oncology center.

Long-term care

To provide appropriate care for survivors, the HCP must be aware of the pediatric patient's previous therapeutic management. Therapy has evolved over time; as a consequence, therapies vary depending on the type of cancer.

Given the risk of numerous late effects from radiation, including endocrine disorders and secondary malignancies, the HCP must be aware of whether this modality was used in the patient's therapeutic management. Survivors who received a blood transfusion prior to 1993 should be screened for hepatitis C; those who received larger radiation fields for a Wilms' tumor should be screened for scoliosis (Children's Oncology Group [COG], 2008).

The age at which the survivor was treated also influences the likelihood of development of late effects. Radiation received prior to completion of linear growth will adversely affect adult height. Adolescents who receive such therapy once growth is nearly complete do not experience the same loss of linear growth as younger children do.

Gender also influences development of late effects. Females are more likely than males to experience late effects secondary to treatment. These adverse effects of treatment are noted in both physical and psychosocial functioning of female survivors (Armstrong et al., 2007).

Patients may not recall the details of their treatment, particularly if they were very young when diagnosed. Loss or lack of personal record-keeping of the complex care received may also mean that comprehensive information on the patient history is unavailable (Kadan-Lottick et al., 2002). Providing health care for survivors of childhood cancers is also challenging in that the caregivers become less involved as the survivor ages.

Evidence-based guidelines

The Children's Oncology Group (2008) has developed evidence-based guidelines for monitoring and managing patients for the late effects of therapy. The goals include monitoring for potential late effects, counseling the survivor on health maintenance, and providing information about current research on survivorship issues. These guidelines are predicated on data from the Childhood Cancer Survivor Study (CCSS), an ongoing study monitoring survivors of childhood cancer for treatment morbidity and mortality.

Although it is not possible to make generalizations about the health care needs of cancer survivors, certain populations of cancer survivors receive more intensive treatment and, therefore, are at higher risk for late effects of treatment. Combination of treatment modalities to manage pediatric patients also has the potential to compound the effects of therapy. For example, patients who receive both anthracyclines and radiation to the chest are at a higher risk for developing cardiotoxicity than patients who receive anthracyclines alone (Oeffinger & Hudson, 2004).

Commonly seen acute systemic late effects

A number of acute late effects have been diagnosed in survivors of pediatric cancer. The systemic findings are described here and summarized in Table 28-21.

Cardiovascular Late Effects. Cardiovascular complications are commonly reported following treatment with anthryacline and radiation to the chest, spine, head, or neck. There is a relationship between the dosage of anthracyclines and radiation received and the likelihood of developing late effects (COG, 2008). Patients who were

TABLE 28-21

Systemic Late Effects of Childhood Cancer Therapy	
Late Effect	**Risk Factors**
Cardiovascular	
Cardiomyopathy Arrhythmia Congestive heart failure	Agents: doxorubicin, daunorubicin, epirubicin, idarubicin, mitoxanthrone Radiation: chest, mediastinum, axilla, thoracic spine, whole abdomen or upper abdominal areas Age: younger than 5 years at time of treatment Gender: female Race: African descent Dose: high dose confers higher risk of developing late effect
Cerebrovascular Stroke/moyamoya	Radiation: neck, cranium
Pulmonary	
Pulmonary fibrosis Lung cancer Pneumonia	Radiation: chest, lung Chemotherapy agents: bleomycin, busulfan, cyclophosphamide, carmustine, lomustine Surgery: chest, lung
Endocrine	
Hypopituitarism	Radiation: whole brain, pituitary region, total body Surgery: removal of pituitary gland

(Continued)

TABLE 28-21

Systemic Late Effects of Childhood Cancer Therapy *(Continued)*

Late Effect	Risk Factors
Endocrine	
Hyperthyroidism	Radiation: neck, cervical spine, supraclavicular, whole brain, total body, mantle, minimantle
Thyroid nodules	Radiation: neck, cervical spine, supraclavicular, whole brain, total body, mantle, minimantle Gender: female Age: younger age at time of treatment
Gonad failure	Radiation: abdomen, pelvis, whole brain, pituitary region, total body Surgery: oophorectomy, hysterectomy, orchiectomy Chemotherapy agents: alkylating agents
Growth hormone failure	Radiation: whole brain, orbit, ear, infratemporal, nasopharyngeal, total body Surgery: suprasellar region
Neurologic	
Stroke Moyamoya	Radiation: cranium, neck, chest Preexisting condition: Down syndrome, neurofibromatosis I Age: younger than 4 years at time of treatment
Carotid artery disease	Radiation: neck
Gastrointestinal	
Liver dysfunction	Radiation: abdomen Chemotherapy: methotrexate
Hepatic fibrosis	Radiation: abdomen Preexisting conditions: hepatitis, veno-occlusive disease
Bowel obstruction	Radiation: abdomen, pelvic, spine Surgery: abdomen
Hepatitis B	Supportive care: blood transfusion prior to 1972
Hepatitis C	Supportive care: blood transfusion prior to 1993
Esophageal stricture	Radiation: esophagus Contributing factor: chronic graft-versus-host disease
Musculoskeletal	
Osteonecrosis	Radiation: gonadal, bone Medication: dexamethasone, prednisone Age: older than 10 years at time of treatment
Osteoporosis/osteopenia	Radiation: cranium, total body Chemotherapy: methotrexate Medication: dexamethasone, prednisone Contributing factors: growth hormone deficiency, hyperthyroidism, gonadal failure
Kidney/Genitourinary	
Bladder dysfunction	Radiation: pelvis Chemotherapy: cyclophosphamide, ifosfamide Surgery: total or partial cystectomy Supportive care: mesna not used with cyclophosphamide or ifosfamide infusions
Renal dysfunction	Radiation: kidney Chemotherapy: ifosfamide (higher doses increase risk of dysfunction) Surgery: nephrectomy Age: younger age at time of treatment Contributing factors: history of kidney dysfunction, use of other kidney toxic therapies, immunosuppression for chronic graft-versus-host disease

(Continued)

TABLE 28-21

Systemic Late Effects of Childhood Cancer Therapy *(Continued)*	
Late Effect	**Risk Factors**
Immunologic	
Asplenia	Radiation: spleen
	Surgery: splenectomy
	Medications: immunosuppression to manage graft- versus-host disease
	Contributing factor: graft-versus-host disease
Chronic infections	Medications: immunosuppression to manage graft-versus-host disease
Hypogammaglobulinemia	Contributing factors: CD4 T-cell dysfunction
IgA deficiency	

treated for relapsed disease are also more likely to develop cardiovascular complications (Diller et al., 2009). These late effects include cardiomyopathy, cardiac arrhythmias, valvular abnormalities, angina, and stroke (Diller et al.).

Pulmonary late effects. Pulmonary late effects may be found following radiation therapy to either the chest or lung fields. Pulmonary fibrosis, lung cancer, and other chronic lung conditions such as oxygen dependency and recurrent pneumonia have been reported. These health conditions may not become acutely problematic until 20 to 25 years post therapy (Diller et al., 2009). Survivors post hematopoietic cell transplant often develop pulmonary complications secondary to the combination of total-body radiation and conditioning agents used to prepare for the transplant.

Endocrine late effects. Late effects to the endocrine and metabolic system vary from thyroid dysfunction to obesity as a result of radiation to either the brain or the organ system producing the affected hormone. For example, patients with Hodgkin lymphoma who receive radiation to the neck are at greater risk for developing hypothyroidism than their siblings. Hypothyroidism is more common than hyperthyroidism among those patients with a late effect of thyroid dysfunction (Diller et al., 2009). Hypopituitarism may be attributed to radiation or to surgical removal of the pituitary gland (COG, 2008). Lack of cortisol in these survivors may necessitate stress doses of steroids during an acute illness.

Neurologic late effects. Survivors are at risk for a variety of neurological consequences of treatment for childhood cancer. Long-term effects such as cataracts from cranial radiation or steroid use, or hearing loss from cranial radiation or chemotherapy may become progressively worse as the survivor ages. Due to the combined effects of neurosurgery, chemotherapy agents, and radiation, survivors of CNS tumors are at high risk for developing neurological late effects. Treatment consisting of cranial, neck, and chest radiation places survivors at risk for seizure disorders and strokes (Diller et al., 2009; Jordan & Duffner, 2009; Packer et al., 2003).

Gastrointestinal late effects. Gastrointestinal late effects may result from radiation therapy, chemotherapy, surgery, or supportive care received during such therapy. Bowel obstructions have been reported in adult survivors of childhood cancer and carry a significant risk of mortality. Adhesions and strictures are more common in patients who had both abdominal surgery and radiation to the abdominal area. Survivors who received blood transfusions prior to 1993 are at risk for hepatitis C (COG, 2008; Kenney et al., 2010; Oeffinger & Hudson, 2004).

Musculoskeletal late effects. Seven percent of survivors of childhood cancers report osteonecrosis, osteoporosis, or osteopenia. These conditions have significant consequences for the overall function and well-being of the survivor. Potential complications from these effects include fractures, pain, and decreased mobility. For example, 5.9% of survivors of ALL report having fractures as a late effect (Haddy et al., 2009). Factors influencing musculoskeletal disorders are depend on the patient's age at the time of diagnosis and the type of therapy received. Estrogen deficiency contributes to the development of osteopenia or osteoporosis; however, unlike in the general population, gender is not a factor in the development of either condition (COG, 2008).

Kidney/Genitourinary late effects. Both chemotherapy and radiation therapy to the kidneys or bladder may cause long-term complications, including hypertension, electrolyte abnormalities, and growth disturbances. Radiated areas do not show normal growth, especially in younger children. A survivor whose bladder was radiated as a child is at risk for decreased bladder function and capacity. Use of chemotherapy agents such as cyclophosphamide and ifosfamide is associated with hemorrhagic cystis, renal tubular acidosis, Fanconi's syndrome, and other kidney toxicities. The combination of chemotherapeutic agents with either kidney toxic agents or radiation to the kidney increases the risk of late effects (COG, 2008; Oeffinger & Hudson, 2004).

Immunologic late effects. For most survivors of childhood cancer, their immune function returns to normal after treatment. Nevertheless, two patient populations are at increased risk for continued immune dysfunction: hematopoietic cell transplant survivors and patients without a spleen. For hematopoietic cell transplant survivors with chronic graft-versus-host disease (GVHD) who are treated with prolonged immunosuppression, the risk of immune dysfunction is even higher (COG, 2008). Splenectomy was routinely performed as part of stage identification for patients with Hodgkin lymphoma until the 1980s. Although this procedure is no longer routinely done, there remains a subset of survivors who are asplenic due to either abdominal radiation or splenectomy, or as a sequela to GVHD following hematopoietic cell transplant. Chronic conditions such as sinusitis or bronchitis have the potential to become life-threatening illnesses in this population (COG; Oeffinger & Hudson, 2004).

Relapse of primary diagnosis

Most pediatric oncologists define survivorship as beginning when the patient is 5 years post diagnosis and a minimum of 2 years post treatment, at which point relapse is usually considered unlikely. While it is true that the risk of relapse decreases over time, relapse remains a possibility throughout a survivor's lifetime. Relapse was the leading cause of death in the CCSS group, for example. Of those survivors who relapsed, only 50% survived. Survivors of CNS tumors and Ewing sarcoma had the highest risk of a relapse (Armstrong et al., 2009; Mertens et al., 2008; Robison et al., 2005; Wasilewski-Masker et al., 2009).

Secondary malignancy

The risk of a secondary malignancy in survivors of childhood cancer reflects various treatment-related factors, lifestyle choices, and genetic influences. The impact and interrelationship of these risk factors is not yet fully understood, however radiation and several classes of chemotherapeutic agents are known carcinogens. Monitoring and screening for secondary malignancies should, therefore, be based on the treatment received, any predisposing factors such as family history, and the same risk factors seen in the general population (Hudson et al., 2009) (Table 28-22).

Pregnancy and birth defects

Results from the research in the CCSS group demonstrate that female survivors of childhood cancer have a lower overall pregnancy rate than their siblings, although for many survivors their fertility remains intact (Green et al., 2009a, 2009b; Mueller et al., 2009). Treatment with alkylating agents, radiation, or surgery to the sex organs or brain is associated with an increased risk of infertility in both males

TABLE 28-22

Secondary Malignancies	
Late Effect	**Risk Factors**
Secondary malignancy	Radiation: any Chemotherapy: alkylating agents, epipodophyllotoxins Age: young age at time of original diagnosis Gender: female Contributing factors: chronic graft-versus-host disease Genetic predisposition (hereditary cancer syndromes), environmental factors (smoking, sun exposure), diagnosis of Ewing sarcoma, Hodgkin lymphoma, bilateral retinoblastoma

and females (Pallat & Hutter, 2008). Numerous variables influence the risk of infertility, including age at the time of treatment, doses received, and gender. It has been reported that males are more sensitive to the effects of alkylating agents than females (Agarwal & Chang, 2007; Brannigan, 2007; COG, 2008).

In a female cancer survivor, the combination of pregnancy and treatment with cardiotoxic therapy may cause congestive heart failure or cardiomyopathy. Any survivor who received these treatments should have her cardiac function monitored during pregnancy. Cardiology service consult for these patients is recommended.

There is no increased risk of birth defects noted in the offspring of either male or female survivors of childhood cancers (COG, 2008). Radiation to the pelvis, abdomen, spine, or total body is related to lower-birth-weight babies and more spontaneous miscarriages (Green et al., 2002). Chemotherapy, surgery, and radiation should be considered when evaluating the health of a pregnant cancer survivor. Optimal care of the pregnant survivor includes conversation between the HCP and treating oncology team, and referral to a high-risk obstetrics team.

Healthcare team

Survivors of childhood cancer have unique healthcare needs that stretch across the life span and may require health care from a variety of pediatric and adult subspecialists. As survivors live longer, their cancer-related healthcare needs will become more evident, and late effects may require various subspecialty consultations and therapeutic plans. The cancer survivor's health maintenance must be tailored to the specific treatment received, cancer type, genetics, and other lifestyle choices such as smoking, sunbathing, and alcohol consumption. Establishing an HCP team to ensure comprehensive care is essential to promote optimal health. The best care is provided by an interprofessional team that includes social and educational support systems as well as subspecialists needed to manage late effects.

REFERENCES

1. Aberman, A., & Hew, E. (1985). Clarification of the effects of changes in P50 on oxygen transport. *Acute Care, 11*(3–4), 216–221.

2. Adams, R., McKie, V., Hsu, L., Files, B., Vichinsky, E., Pegelow, C., et al. (1998). Prevention of a first stroke by transfusions in children with sickle cell anemia and abnormal results on transcranial Doppler ultrasonography. *New England Journal of Medicine, 339*(1), 5–11.

3. Agarwal, S. K., & Chang, R. J. (2007). Fertility management for women with cancer. *Cancer Treatment Research, 138*, 15–27.

4. Aksnes, L., Bauer, H., Jebsen, N., Folleras, G., Allert, C., Haugen, G., et al. (2008). Limb-sparing surgery preserves more function than amputation: A Scandinavian sarcoma group study of 118 patients. *Journal of Bone and Joint Surgery, British Volume, 90-B*(6), 786–794.

5. Albisetti, M., Moeller, A., Waldvogel, K., Bernet-Buettiker, V., Cannizzaro, V., Anagnostopoulos, A., et al. (2006). Congenital prothrombotic disorders in children with peripheral venous and arterial thromboses. *Acta Haematologica, 117*, 149–155.

6. Alkire, K., & Collingwood, J. (1990). Physiology of blood and bone marrow. *Seminars in Oncology Nursing, 6*(2), 99–108.

7. Allison, A. (2009). Genetic control of resistance to human malaria. *Current Opinion in Immunology, 21*(5), 499–505.

8. Al-Sweedan, S., Jdaitawi, H., Khriesat, W., Khader, Y., & Al-Rimawi, H. (2009). Predictors of severe hemolysis in patients with glucose-6-phosphate dehydrogenase deficiency following exposure to oxidant stresses. *Hematology/Oncology and Stem Cell Therapy, 2*(2), 354–357.

9. Altman, A. (2002). Chronic leukemias of childhood. In P. A. Pizzo & D. G. Poplack (Eds.), *Principles and practice of pediatric oncology* (4th ed., pp. 591–614). Philadelphia: Lippincott Williams & Wilkins.

10. Ananyeva, N., Lee, T., Jain, N., Shima, M., & Saenko, E. (2009). Inhibitors in hemophilia A: Advances in elucidation of inhibitory mechanisms and in inhibitor management with bypassing agents. *Seminars in Thrombosis and Hemostasis, 35*(8), 735–751.

11. Aquino, V., & Sandler, E. (2006). Supportive care of the pediatric hematopoietic stem-cell transplant patient. In R. Klein (Ed.), *Pediatric hematopoietic stem cell transplantation* (pp. 1–26). New York: Informa Healthcare USA.

12. Arepally, G., & Ortel, T. (2006). Heparin-induced thrombocytopenia. *New England Journal of Medicine, 355*(8), 809–817.

13. Armstrong, E., & Konkle, B. (2006). Von Willebrand disease. In N. Young, S. Gerson, & K. High, *Clinical hematology* (pp. 830–841). St. Louis: Mosby.

14. Armstrong, G., Liu, O., Yasiu, Y., Neglia, J., Leisenring, W., Robison, L., & Mertens, A. (2009). Late mortality among 5-year survivors of childhood cancer: A summary from the childhood cancer survivor study. *American Society of Clinical Oncology, 27*(14), 2328–2338.

15. Armstrong, G., Sklar, C., Hudson, M., & Robison, L. (2007). Long-term health status among survivors of childhood cancer: Does sex matter? *Journal of Clinical Oncology, 25*(28), 4477–4489.

16. Arndt, C., & Crist, W. (1999). Common musculoskeletal tumors of childhood and adolescence. *New England Journal of Medicine, 341*(5), 342–352.

17. Astermark, J. (2009). Inhibitor development: Patient-determined risk factors. *Haemophilia, 16*(102), 66–70.

18. Baggott, C., Kelly, K., Fochtman, D., & Foley, G. (2002). *Nursing care of children and adolescents with cancer* (3rd ed.). Philadelphia: W. B. Saunders.

19. Bakhsi, S. (2009). Aplastic anemia. *eMedicine Hematology.* Retrieved from http://emedicine.medscape.com

20. Ballinger, S. (2003). Henoch-Schönlein purpura. *Current Opinion in Rheumatology, 15*, 591–594.

21. Barkin, R., & Rosen, P. (2003a). Hematologic disorders. In R. Barkin & P. Rosen, *Emergency pediatrics* (pp. 694–696, 709–711). St. Louis: Mosby.

22. Barkin, R., & Rosen, P. (2003b). Renal disorders. In R. Barkin & P. Rosen, *Emergency pediatrics* (pp. 819–824). St. Louis: Mosby.

23. Baroletti, S., & Goldhaber, S. (2006). Heparin-induced thrombocytopenia. *Circulation, 114*, 355–356.

24. Bennett, J. (2006). Inherited and acquired disorders of platelet function. In N. Young, S. Gerson, & K. High, *Clinical hematology* (pp. 767–780). St. Louis: Mosby.

25. Bercovitz, R., Greffe, B., & Hunger, S. (2009). Acute tumor lysis syndrome in a 7-month-old with hepatoblastoma. *Current Opinion in Pediatrics* [Epub ahead of print].

26. Bhargava, M. (1981). Factor VIII deficiency diseases: An approach to laboratory diagnosis and management. *Indian Pediatrics, 18*(11), 787–791.

27. Bianco, P., Riminucci, M., Kuznetsov, S., & Robey, P. (1999). Multipotential cells in the bone marrow stroma: Regulation in the context of organ physiology. *Critical Reviews in Eukaryotic Gene Expression, 9*(2), 159–173.

28. Bladen, M., Khair, K., Liesner, R., & Main, E. (2009). Long-term consequences of intracranial haemorrhage in children with haemophilia. *Haemophilia, 15*(1), 184–192.

29. Bolanos-Meade, J., & Brodsky, R. (2009). Blood and marrow transplantation for sickle cell disease: Overcoming barriers to success. *Current Opinion in Oncology, 21*(2), 158–161.

30. Booth, C., Inusa, B., & Obaro, S. (2009). Infection in sickle cell disease: A review. *International Journal of Infectious Diseases, 14*(1), e2–e12.

31. Bradfield, S., Neudorf, S., Rubin, E., & Sandler, E. (2006). Prevention and treatment of infectious disease. In R. Klein (Ed.), *Pediatric hematopoietic stem cell transplantation* (pp. 27–63). New York: Informa Healthcare USA.

32. Brannigan, R. (2007). Fertility preservation in adult male cancer patients. In T. Woodruff & K. Snyder (Eds.), *Oncofertility: Fertility preservation for cancer survivors* (pp. 28–49). New York: Springer.

33. Brashers, V. (2006). Alterations in cardiovascular function. In K. McCance & S. Huether, *Pathophysiology: The basis for disease in adults and children* (pp. 1096–1100). St. Louis: Elsevier Mosby.

34. Breslow, N., Takahima, J., Ritchey, M., Strong, L., & Green, D. (2000). Renal failure in the Deny-Drash and Wilms tumor-aniridia syndromes. *Cancer Research, 60*(15), 4030–4032.

35. Breslow, N., Takahima, J., Whitton, J., Mokfneff, J., B'Angio, G., & Green, D. (1995). Second malignant neoplasms following treatment for Wilm's tumor: A report from the national Wilm's Tumor Study Group. *Journal of Clinical Oncology, 13*, 1851–1859.

36. Bryan-Brown, C. (1988). Blood flow to organs: Parameters for function and survival in critical illness. *Critical Care Medicine, 16*(2), 170–178.

37. Bucci, E., & Fronticelli, C. (1981). Measurement of the Bohr effect: Dependence on pH of oxygen affinity of hemoglobin. *Methods in Enzymology, 76*, 523–533.

38. Butenas, S., Orfeo, T., & Mann, K. (2009). Tissue factor in coagulation: Which? Where? When? *Arteriosclerosis, Thrombosis, and Vascular Biology, 29*(12), 1989–1996.

39. Cairo, M., & Bradley, M. (1997). Lymphoma. In R. M. Kliegman, R. E. Behrman, H. B. Jenson, & B. F. Stanton (Eds.), *Nelson textbook of pediatrics* (18th ed., Chapter 496). Retrieved from http://www.mdconsult.com/

40. Cairo, M., Raetz, E., Lim, M., Davenport, V., & Perkins, S. (2005). Childhood and adolescent non-Hodgkin lymphoma: New insights in biology and critical challenges for the future. *Pediatric Blood & Cancer, 45*, 753–769.

41. Camp-Sorrell, D. (2008). Hemolytic uremic syndrome. *Oncology Nursing Forum, 35*(4), 593–596.

42. Centers for Disease Control and Prevention (CDC). (2000). Guidelines for preventing opportunistic infections among hematopoieitic stem cell transplant recipients. Retrieved from http://www.cdc.gov/mmwr/preview/mmwrhtml/rr4910a1.htm

43. Centers for Disease Control and Prevention. (2010). Information for People with Hemophilia. Retrieved from http://www.cdc.gov/ncbddd/hemophilia/people.html

44. Cesarman-Maus, G., & Hajjar, K. (2005). Molecular mechanisms of fibrinolysis. *British Journal of Haematology, 129*(3), 307–321.

45. Chantada, G., Doz, F., Antoneli, C., Grundy, R., Clare Stannard, F., Dunkel, I., et al. (2008). A proposal for an international retinoblastoma staging system. *Pediatric Blood & Cancer, 50*(3), 733.

46. Charache, S., Scott, S., & Charache, P. (1979). Acute chest syndrome in adults with sickle cell anemia: Microbiology, treatment, and prevention. *Archives of Internal Medicine, 139*(1), 67–69.

47. Children's Oncology Group (COG). (2008). *Long-term follow-up guidelines for survivors of childhood, adolescent and young adult cancers.* Arcadia, CA: Author.

48. Clark, J., Berman, J., & Look, A. (2009). Myeloid leukemia, myelodysplasia, and myeloproliferative disease in children. In S. H. Orkin, D. E. Fisher, A. T. Look, S. E. Lux, D. Ginsburg, & D. G. Nathan (Eds.), *Oncology of infancy and childhood* (pp. 331–402). Philadelphia: Saunders Elsevier.

49. Coiffier, B., Altman, A., Piu, C., Younes, A., & Cairo, M. (2008). Guidelines for the management of pediatric and adult tumor lysis syndrome: An evidence-based review. *Journal of Clinical Oncology, 26*(16), 2767–2778.

50. Colen, F. N. (2008). Oncologic emergencies: Superior vena cava syndrome, tumor lysis syndrome, and spinal cord compression. *Journal of Emergency Nursing, 34*(6), 535–537.

51. Coppola, A., Franchini, M., & Tagliaferri, A. (2009). Prophylaxis in people with haemophilia. *Thrombosis and Haemostasis, 101*(4), 674–681.

52. Corrigan, J., & Boineau, F. (2001). Hemolytic-uremic syndrome. *Pediatrics in Review, 22*(11), 365–369.

53. D'Angio, G. (1975). Pediatric cancer in perspective: Cure is not enough. *Cancer, 35*, 866–870.

54. De Bernardi, B., Pianca, C., Pistamiglio, P., Veneselli, E., Viscardi, E., Pession, A., et al. (2001). Neuroblastoma with symptomatic cord compression at diagnosis: Treatment and results with 76 cases. *J Clin Oncol., 19*, 183–190.

55. Delvaeye, M., & Conway, E. (2009). Coagulation and innate immune responses: Can we view them separately? *Blood, 114*(12), 2367–2374.

56. Dietrich, J., & Hertweck, S. (2008). Thrombophilias in adolescents: The past, present, and future. *Current Opinion in Obstetrics and Gynecology, 20*, 269–274.

57. Diller, L., Chow, E., Gurney, J., Hudson, M., Kadin-Lottick, N., Kawashima, T., et al. (2009). Chronic disease in the Childhood Cancer Survivor Study cohort: A review of published findings. *Journal of Clinical Oncology, 27*(14), 2339–2355.

58. Dressler, D. (2004). DIC: Coping with a coagulation crisis. *Nursing, 34*(5), 58–62.

59. Dressler, D. (2009). Death by clot: Acute coronary syndromes, ischemic stroke, pulmonary embolism, and disseminated intravascular coagulation. *AACN Advanced Critical Care, 20*(2), 166–176.

60. Ehsani, M., Hedayati-Asl, A., Bagheri, A., Zeinali, S., & Rashidi, P. (2009). Hydroxyurea-induced hematological response in transfusion-independent beta-thalassemia intermedia: Case series and review of literature. *Pediatric Hematology and Oncology, 26*(8), 560–56.

61. Eleftheriou, D., Dillon, M., & Brogan, P. (2009). Advances in childhood vasculitis. *Current Opinion in Rheumatology, 21*, 411–418.

62. Elliott, E., & Robins-Browne, R. (2005). Hemolytic uremic syndrome. *Current Problems in Pediatric and Adolescent Health Care, 35*, 310–330.

63. Elyassi, A., & Rowshan, H. (2009). Perioperative management of the glucose-6-phosphate dehydrogenase deficient patient: A review of literature. *Anesthesia Progress, 56*(3), 86–91.

64. Esiashvili, N., Anderson, C., & Katzenstein, H. (2009). Neuroblastoma. *Current Problems in Cancer, 33*(6), 333–360.

65. Field, J., Knight-Perry, J., & Debaun, M. (2009). Acute pain in children and adults with sickle cell disease: Management in the absence of evidence-based guidelines. *Current Opinion in Hematology, 16*(3), 173–178.

66. Fiorino, E., Raffaelli, R., & Adam, H. (2006). Hemolytic-uremic syndrome. *Pediatrics in Review, 27*, 398–399.

67. Fischer, K., Valentino, L., Ljung, R., & Blanchette, V. (2008). Prophylaxis for severe haemophilia: Clinical challenges in the absence as well as in the presence of inhibitors. *Haemophilia, 14*(suppl 3), 196–201.

68. Fish, J., & Ginsberg, J. (2009). Health insurance for survivors of childhood cancer: A pre-existing problem. *Pediatric Blood & Cancer, 53*, 928–930.

69. Fisher, V., & Abramovitz, L. (2006). Appendix: A brief overview of hematopoietic stem cell transplantation. In R. Klein (Ed.), *Pediatric hematopoietic stem cell transplantation* (pp. 601–624). New York: Informa Healthcare USA.

70. Forget, B. (1979). Molecular genetics of human hemoglobin synthesis. *Annals of Internal Medicine, 91*(4), 605–616.

71. Francis, C., & Kaplan, K. (2006). Venous and arterial thrombosis. In N. Young, S. Gerson, & K. High, *Clinical hematology* (pp. 1089–1105). St. Louis: Mosby.

72. Frank, J. (2005). Diagnosis and management of G6PD deficiency. *American Family Physician, 72*(7), 1277–1282.

73. Gallucci, S., & Matzinger, P. (2001). Danger signals: SOS to the immune system. *Current Opinion in Immunology, 13*(1), 114–119.

74. Geenen, M., Cardous-Ubbink, M., Kremer, L., van den Bos, C., Heinen, R., Jaspers, M., et al. (2007). Medical assessment of adverse health outcomes in long-term survivors of childhood cancer. *American Medical Association, 297*(24), 2705–2715.

75. Golub, T., & Arceci, R. (2002). Acute myelogenous leukemia. In P. A. Pizzo & D. G. Poplack (Eds.), *Principles and practice of pediatric oncology* (4th ed., pp. 545–589). Philadelphia: Lippincott Williams & Wilkins.

76. Goodeve, A. (1998). Laboratory methods for the genetic diagnosis of bleeding disorders. *Clinical and Laboratory Haematology, 20*(1), 3–19.

77. Goodeve, A., & James, P. (2009). Von Willebrand disease. *NIH Gene Reviews.* Retrieved June 2, 2010, from www.ncbi.nlm.nih.gov/bookshelf

78. Gordon, B., & Baker, K. S. (2006). Hematopoietic stem-cell transplantation for children with hodgkin's and non-Hodgkin's lymphoma. In R. Klein (Ed.), *Pediatric hematopoietic stem cell transplantation* (pp. 529–554). New York: Informa Healthcare USA.

79. Green, D., Kawashima, T., Stovall, M., Leisenring, W., Sklar, C., Mertens, A., et al. (2009a). Fertility of female survivors of childhood cancer: A report from the Childhood Cancer Survivor Study. *Journal of Clinical Oncology, 27*, 2677–2685.

80. Green, D., Kawashima, T., Stovall, M., Leisenring, W., Sklar, C., Mertens, A., et al. (2009b). Fertility of male survivors of childhood cancer: A report from the Childhood Cancer Survivor Study. *Journal of Clinical Oncology, 27*, 1–9.

81. Green, D., Whitton, J., Stovall, M., Mertens, A., Donaldson, S., Ruymann, F., et al. (2002). Pregnancy outcome of female survivors of childhood cancer: A report from the Childhood Cancer Survivor Study. *American Journal of Obstetrics and Gynecology, 187*(4), 1070–1080.

82. Grier, H., Krailo, M., Tarbell, N., Link, M., Fryer, C., Pritchard, D., et al. (2003). Addition of ifosfamide and etoposide to standard chemotherapy for Ewing's sarcoma and primitive neuroectodermal tumor of bone. *New England Journal of Medicine, 348*(8), 694–701.

83. Grundy, P., Dome, J., Katappurakat, J., Perlman, E., & Ritchey, M. (2010). Renal tumors. In W. Carroll & J. Finlay (Eds.), *Cancer in children and adolescents* (pp. 329–337). Sudbury, MA: Jones and Bartlett.

84. Guinan, E. (2009). Acquired aplastic anemia in childhood. *Hematology/ Oncology Clinics of North America, 23*(2), 171–191.

85. Haddy, T., Mosher, R., & Reaman, G. (2009). Late effects in long-term survivors after treatment for childhood acute leukemia. *Clinical Pediatrics, 48*(6), 601–608.

86. Hays, K. (1990). Physiology of normal bone marrow. *Seminars in Oncology Nursing, 6*(1), 3–8.

87. Hodgson, D., Hudson, M., & Constine, L. (2007). Pediatric Hodgkin lymphoma: Maximizing efficacy and minimizing toxicity. *Seminars in Radiation Oncology, 17*, 230–242.

88. Hoppe, C., Vichinsky, E., Quirolo, K., van Warmerdam, J., Allen, K., & Styles, L. (2000). Use of hydroxyurea in children ages 2 to 5 years with sickle cell disease. *Journal of Pediatric Hematology and Oncology, 22*(4), 330–334.

89. Horner, M. J., Ries, L. A. G., Krapacho, M., Neyman, N., Aminou R., Howlader, N., et al. (Eds.), (2009). *SEER cancer statistics review, 1975–2006.* Bethesda, MA: National Cancer Institute. Retrieved from http://seer.cancer.gov/csr/1975_2006/

90. Hudson, M., Mulrooney, D., Bowers, C., Sklar, C., Green D., Donaldson, S., et al. (2009). High risk populations identified in Childhood Cancer Survivor Study investigations: Implications for risk-base surveillance. *Journal of Clinical Oncology, 27*(14), 2405–2414.

91. Huether, S. (2006). Alterations of renal and urinary tract function in children. In K. McCance & S. Huether, *Pathophysiology: The basis for disease in adults and children* (p. 1343). St. Louis: Elsevier Mosby.

92. Ingerslev, J. (2000). Hemophilia: Strategies for the treatment of inhibitor patients. *Haematologica, 85*(10 suppl), 15–20.

93. Jacobsohn, D., Vogelsang, G., & Schultz, K. (2006). Chronic graft-vs.-host disease in children. In R. Klein (Ed.), *Pediatric hematopoietic stem cell transplantation* (pp. 85–109). New York: Informa Healthcare USA.

94. Jaffe, E. (1970). Hereditary hemolytic disorders and enzymatic deficiencies of human erythrocytes. *Blood, 35*(1), 116–134.

95. Jesus, L., & Dekermacher, S. (2009). Priapism in children: Review of pathophysiology and treatment. *Jornal de Pediatria (Rio), 85*(3), 194–200.

96. Jin, D., & Bussel, J. (2006). Immune, posttransfusional, and neonatal thrombocytopenia. In N. Young, S. Gerson, & K. High, *Clinical hematology* (pp. 781–788). St. Louis: Mosby.

97. Jordan, L., & Duffner, P. (2009). Early-onset stroke and cerebrovascular disease in adult survivors of childhood cancer. *Neurology, 73*, 1–2.

98. Journeycake, J., & Buchanan, G. (2003). Coagulation disorders. *Pediatrics in Review, 24*(3), 83–91.

99. Kadan-Lottick, N. S., Robison, L. L., Gurney, J. G., Neglia, J. P., Yasui, Y., Hayashi, R., et al. (2002). Childhood cancer survivors' knowledge about their past diagnosis and treatment. *American Medical Association, 287*(14), 1832–1839.

100. Kempton, C., & White, G. (2009). How we treat a hemophilia A patient with a factor VIII inhibitor. *Blood, 113*(1), 11–17.

101. Kenet, G., Strauss, T., Kaplinski, C., & Paret, G. (2008). Hemostasis and thrombosis in critically ill children. *Seminars in Thrombosis and Hemostasis, 34*(5), 451–458.

102. Kenney, L. B., Nancarrow, C. M., Najita, J., Vrooman, L. M., Rothwell, M., Recklitis, C., et al. (2010). Health status of the oldest adult survivors of cancer during childhood. *Cancer, 116*(2), 497–505.

103. Khatib, R., Rabah, R., & Samaik, S. (2009). The spleen in the sickling disorders: An update. *Pediatric Radiology, 39*(1), 17–22.

104. King, A., Noetzel, M., White, D., McKinstry, R., & Debaun, M. (2008). Blood transfusion therapy is feasible in a clinical trial setting in children with sickle cell disease and silent cerebral infarcts. *Pediatric Blood & Cancer, 50*(3), 599–602.

105. Klein, R. (Ed.). (2006). *Pediatric hematopoietic stem cell transplantation.* New York: Informa Healthcare USA.

106. Kruger, D. (2006). Acute systemic disseminated intravascular coagulation: Managing a complex medical condition. *Journal of the American Academy of Physician Assistants, 18*(5), 28–32.

107. Kulkarni, R., & Gera, R. (1999). Pediatric transfusion therapy: Practical considerations. *Indian Journal of Pediatrics, 66*(3), 307–317.

108. Kulkarni, R., Soucie, J., Lusher, J., Presley, R., Shapiro, A., Gill, J., et al. (2009). Sites of initial bleeding episodes, mode of delivery and age of diagnosis in babies with haemophilia diagnosed before the age of 2 years: A report from the Centers for Disease Control and Prevention's (CDC) Universal Data Collection (UDC) project. *Haemophilia, 15*(6), 1281–1290.

109. Kusuma, B., & Schulz, T. (2009). Acute disseminated intravascular coagulation. *Hospital Physician, 16*(3), 35–40.

110. Levi, M. (2007). Disseminated intravascular coagulation. *Critical Care Medicine, 35*(9), 2191–2195.

111. Lieberman, L., Kirby, M., Ozolins, L., Mosko, J., & Friedman, J. (2009). Initial presentation of unscreened children with sickle cell disease: The Toronto experience. *Pediatric Blood & Cancer, 53*(3), 397–400.

112. Lipton, J., & Ellis, S. (2009). Diamond-Blackfan anemia: Diagnosis, treatment, and molecular pathogenesis. *Hematology/Oncology Clinics of North America, 23*(2), 261–282.

113. Ljung, R. (2009). Prophylactic therapy in haemophilia. *Blood Reviews, 23*(6), 267–274.

114. Magrath, I. (2002). Malignant non-Hodgkin's lymphomas in children. In P. A. Pizzo & D. G. Poplack (Eds.), *Principles and practice of pediatric oncology* (4th ed., pp. 661–731). Philadelphia: Lippincott Williams & Wilkins.

115. Mancuso, M., Graca, L., Auerswald, G., & Santagostino, E. (2009). Haemophilia care in children: Benefits of early prophylaxis for inhibitor prevention. *Haemophilia, 15* (suppl 1), 8–14.

116. Mannucci, P., & Tuddenham, E. (2001). The hemophilias: From royal genes to gene therapy. *New England Journal of Medicine, 344*(23), 1773–1779.

117. Mansen, T., & McCance, K. (2006). Alterations of leukocyte, lymphoid, and hemostatic function. In K. McCance & S. Huether, *Pathophysiology: The basis for disease in adults and children* (pp. 986–991). St. Louis: Elsevier Mosby.

118. Margolin, J., Steuber, C., & Poplack, D. (2002). Acute lymphoblastic leukemia. In P. Pizzo & D. Poplack (Eds.), *Principles and practice of pediatric oncology* (4th ed., pp. 489–544). Philadelphia: Lippincott Williams & Wilkins.

119. Maris, J., Hogarty, M., Bagatell, R., & Cohn, S. (2007). Neuroblastoma. *Lancet, 369*(9579), 2106–2120.

120. Martin, J. (1995). Red blood cell physiology. *Biomedical Instrument Technology, 29*(2), 150–151.

121. Mason, P., Bautista, J., et al & Gilsanz, F. (2007). G6PD deficiency: The genotype–phenotype association. *Blood Reviews, 21*(5), 267–283.

122. Matsumaga, E. (1981). Genetics of Wilms' tumor. *Human Genetics, 57*, 231–246.

123. Matzinger, P. (1994). Tolerance, danger, and the extended family. *Annual Review of Immunology, 12*, 991–1045.

124. Meadows, A. T. (2003). Pediatric cancer survivors: Past history and future challenges. *Current Problems in Cancer, 27*, 112–126.

125. Meremikwu, M. (2009). Sickle cell disease. clinicalevidence.bmj.com/ceweb/conditions/bly/2402/2402_I6.jsp *Clin Evid* (Online),7,2009. pii: 2402.

126. Mertens, A., Liu, O., Neglia, J., Wasilewski, K., Leisenring, W., Armstrong, G. T., et al. (2008). Cause-specific late mortality among 5-year survivors of childhood cancer: The Childhood Cancer Survivor Study. *Journal of the National Cancer Institute, 100*(19), 1368–1379.

127. Meyer, W., Cripe, T., & Stevens, M. (2010). Soft-tissue sarcoma. In W. Carroll & J. Finlay (Eds.), *Cancer in children and adolescents* (pp. 341–351). Sudbury, MA: Jones and Bartlett.

128. Miljic, P., Heylen, E., Willemse, J., Djordjevic, V., Radojkovic, D., Colovic, M., et al. (2010). Thrombin activatable fibrinolysis inhibitor (TAFI): A molecular link between coagulation and fibrinolysis. *Srpski Arhiv za Celokupno Lekarstvo, 138*(suppl 1), 74–78.

129. Minucci, A., Giardina, B., Zuppi, C., & Capoluongo, E. (2009). Glucose-6-phosphate dehydrogenase laboratory assay: How, when, and why? *IUBMB Life, 61*(1), 27–34.

130. Mitby, P. A., Robison, L. L., Whitton, J. A., Zevon, M. A., Gibbs, I. C., Tersak, J. M., et al. (2003). Utilization of special education services and educational attainment among long-term survivors of childhood cancer: A report from the Childhood Cancer Survivor Study. *Cancer, 97*(4), 1115–1126.

131. Monroe, D., & Hoffman, M. (2006). What does it take to make the perfect clot? *Arteriosclerosis, Thrombosis, and Vascular Biology, 26*(1), 41–48.

132. Moore, T., & Feig, S. (2006). Acute graft-vs.-host disease. In R. Klein (Ed.), *Pediatric hematopoietic stem cell transplantation* (pp. 65–84). New York: Informa Healthcare USA.

133. Mueller, B., Chos, E., Kaminen, A., Daling, J., Fraser, A., Wiggins, C., et al. (2009). Pregnancy outcomes in female childhood and adolescent cancer survivors. *Archives of Pediatrics & Adolescent Medicine, 163*(10), 879–886.

134. Muncie, H. Jr., & Campbell, J. (2009). Alpha and beta thalassemia. *American Family Physician, 80*(4), 339–344.

135. Myers, K., & Davies, S. (2009). Hematopoietic stem cell transplantation for bone marrow failure syndromes in children. *Biology of Blood and Marrow Transplantation, 15*(3), 279–292.

136. National Heart, Lung, and Blood Institute. (2007). The diagnosis, evaluation, and management of von willebrand disease. Retrieved from http://www.nhlbi.nih.gov/guidelines/vwd/

137. Nemerson, Y. (1987). Tissue factor and the initiation of blood coagulation. *Advances in Experimental Medicine and Biology, 214,* 83–94.

138. Nemerson, Y. (1992). The tissue factor pathway of blood coagulation. *Seminars in Hematology, 29*(3), 170–176.

139. Nemerson, Y., & Pitlick, F. (1972). The tissue factor pathway of blood coagulation. *Progress in Hemostasis and Thrombosis, 1,* 1–37.

140. Nienhuis, A., & Benz, E. (1977a). Regulation of hemoglobin synthesis during the development of the red cell (first of three parts). *New England Journal of Medicine, 297*(24), 1318–1328.

141. Nienhuis, A., & Benz, E. (1977b). Regulation of hemoglobin synthesis during the development of the red cell (second of three parts). *New England Journal of Medicine, 297*(25), 1371–1381.

142. Nienhuis, A., & Benz, E. (1977c). Regulation of hemoglobin synthesis during the development of the red cell (third of three parts). *New England Journal of Medicine, 297*(26), 1430–1436.

143. Nkhoma, E., Poole, C., Vannappagari, V., Hall, S., & Beutler, E. (2009). The global prevalence of glucose-6-phosphate dehydrogenase deficiency: A systematic review and meta-analysis. *Blood Cells, Molecules, and Diseases, 42*(3), 267–278.

144. Norville, R. (2008). Hematopoietic stem cell transplantation. In N. E. Kline (Ed.), *Essentials of pediatric oncology nursing* (3rd ed, pp. 98–108). Glenview, IL: Association of Pediatric Oncology Nurses.

145. Novy, M., Edwards, M., & Metcalfe, J. (1967). Hemoglobin Yakina. II. High blood oxygen affinity associated with compensatory erythrocytosis and normal hemodynamics. *Journal of Clinical Investigation, 46*(11), 1848–1854.

146. Nowak-Göttl, U., Duering, C., Kempf-Bielack, B., & Sträter, R. (2004). Thromboembolic diseases in neonates and children. *Pathophysiology of Haemostasis and Thrombosis, 33,* 269–274.

147. Oeffinger, K., & Hudson, M. (2004). Long-term complications following childhood and adolescent cancer: Foundations for providing risk-based health care for survivors. *A Cancer Journal for Clinicians, 54,* 208–236.

148. Oeffinger, K., Mertens, A., Sklar, C., Kawashima, T., Hudson, M., Meadows, A., et al. (2006). Chronic health conditions in adult survivors of childhood cancer. *New England Journal of Medicine, 355,* 1572–1582.

149. Oi, S., Kokunai, T., Iiichi, A., Matsumoto, S., & Raimondi, A. (1990). Radiation-induced brain damage in children: Histological analysis of sequential tissue changes in 34 autopsy cases. *Neurologica Medico-Chirurgica, 30*(1), 36–42.

150. Olivieri, N., & Vichinsky, E. (1998). Hydroxyurea in children with sickle cell disease: Impact on splenic function and compliance with therapy. *Journal of Pediatric Hematology and Oncology, 20*(1), 26–31.

151. Oski, F., & Gottlieb, A. (1971). The interrelationships between red blood cell metabolites, hemoglobin, and the oxygen-equilibrium curve. *Progress in Hematology, 7,* 33–67.

152. Pack-Mabien, A., & Haynes, J. (2009). A primary care provider's guide to preventive and acute care management of adults and children with sickle cell disease. *Journal of the American Academy of Nurse Practitioners, 21*(5), 250–257.

153. Packer, R. J., Gurney, J. G., Punyko, J. A., Donaldson, S. S., Inskip, P. D., Stovall, M., et al. (2003). Long-term neurologic and neurosensory sequelae in adult survivors of a childhood brain tumor: Childhood Cancer Survivor Study. *Journal of Clinical Oncology, 21*(17), 3255–3261.

154. Paczensy, S., Choi, S., & Ferrara, L. (2009). Acute graft-vs.-host disease: New treatment strategies. *Current Opinion in Hematology, 16,* 427–436.

155. Pallat, M., & Hutter, J. (2008). The Committee on Bioethics, Section on Hematology/Oncology and Section on Surgery: Preservation of fertility in pediatric and adolescent patients with cancer. *Pediatrics, 121*(5), e1461–e1469.

156. Parasuraman, S., & Goldhaber, S. (2006). Venous thromboembolism in children. *Circulation, 113,* e12–e16.

157. Park, J., Eggert, A., & Caron, H. (2008). Neuroblastoma: Biology, prognosis, and treatment. *Pediatric Clinics of North America, 55*(1), 97–120.

158. Pedra, J., Cassel, S., & Sutterwala, F. (2009). Sensing pathogens and danger signals by the inflammasome. *Current Opinion in Immunology, 21*(1), 10–16.

159. Persons, D. (2009). Hematopoietic stem cell gene transfer for the treatment of hemoglobin disorders. *Hematology/American Society for Hematology Education Program,* 690–697.

160. Perutz, M. (1969). Structure and function of hemoglobin. *Harvey Lectures, 63,* 213–261.

161. Perutz, M. (1979). Regulation of oxygen affinity of hemoglobin: Influence of structure of the globin on the heme iron. *Annual Review of Biochemistry, 48,* 327–386.

162. Philpott, J., Houghton, K., & Luke, A. (2010). Physical activity recommendations for children with specific chronic health conditions: Juvenile idiopathic arthritis, hemophilia, asthma, and cystic fibrosis. *Clinical Journal of Sports Medicine, 20*(3), 167–172.

163. Pipe, S., & Valentino, L. (2007). Optimizing outcomes for patients with severe haemophilia A. *Haemophilia, 13*(suppl 4), 1–16.

164. Pizzo, P., & Poplack, D. (2006). *Principles and practice of pediatric oncology* (5th ed.). Philadelphia: Lippincott, Williams, & Wilkins.

165. Pollack, I. (1994). Brain tumors in children. *New England Journal of Medicine, 331,* 1500–1507.

166. Porter, J. (2009). Optimizing iron chelation strategies in beta-thalassaemia major. *Blood Reviews, 23*(suppl 1), S3–S7.

167. Preston, F. (1998). Laboratory diagnosis of hereditary bleeding disorders: External quality assessment. *Haemophilia, 4*(suppl 2), 12–18.

168. Price, V., Hawes, S., & Chan, A. (2007). A practical approach to hemophilia care in children. *Paediatrics & Child Health, 12*(5), 381–383.

169. Pruthi, R., Mathew, P., Valentino, L., Sumner, M., Seremetis, S., Hoots, W., et al. (2007). Haemostatic efficacy and safety of bolus and continuous infusion of recombinant factor VIIa are comparable in haemophilia patients with inhibitors undergoing major surgery: Results from an open-label, randomized, multicenter trial. *Thrombosis and Haemostasis, 98*(4), 726–732.

170. Pui, C. H. (2000). Acute lymphoblastic leukemia in children. *Current Opinions in Oncology, 12,* 3–12.

171. Ragni, M. (2006). The hemophilias: Factor VIII and factor IX deficiencies. In N. Young, S. Gerson, & K. High, *Clinical hematology* (pp. 814–829). St. Louis: Mosby.

172. Ratajczak, M. (1994). "Molecular mechanisms of regulating human erythropoiesis": Theoretic basis: New treatment strategies. *Acta Haematologica Polonica, 25*(2 suppl 1), 41–49.

173. Razzaq, S. (2006). Hemolytic uremic syndrome: An emerging health risk. *American Family Physician, 74*(6), 991–996.

174. Reamy, B., Williams, P., & Lindsay, T. (2009). Henoch-Schönlein purpura. *American Family Physician, 80*(7), 697–704.

175. Reiter, A., & Ferrando, A. (2009). Malignant lymphomas and lymphadenopathies. In S. H. Orkin, D. E. Fisher, A. T. Look, S. E. Lux, D. Ginsburg, & D. G. Nathan (Eds.), *Oncology of infancy and childhood* (pp. 417–505). Philadelphia: Saunders Elsevier.

176. Revel-Vilk, S., & Kenet, G. (2005). Thrombophilia in children with venous thromboembolic disease. *Thrombosis Research, 118,* 59–65.

177. Ries, L., Smith, M., Gurney, J., Linet, M., Tamra, T., Young, J., et al. (Eds.). (1999). *Cancer incidence and survival among children and adolescents: United States SEER Program 1975–1995.* NIH Pub. No. 99-4649. Bethesda, MD: National Cancer Institute, SEER Program, pp. 100–110.

178. Roberts, H., Hoffman, M., & Monroe, D. (2006). A cell-based model of thrombin generation. *Seminars in Thrombosis and Hemostasis, 32*(suppl 1), 32–38.

179. Roberts, P., Waller, T., Brinker, T., Riffe, I., Sayre, J., & Bratton, R. (2007). Henoch-Schönlein purpura: A review article. *Southern Medical Journal, 100*(8), 821–824.

180. Robison, L., Green, D., Hudson, M., Meadows, A., Mertens, A., Sklar, C., et al. (2005). Long-term outcomes of adult survivors of childhood cancer. *American Cancer Society, 104*(11), 2557–2564.

181. Rodriguez-Gallindo, C., & Meadows, A. (2010). Retinoblastoma. In W. Carroll & J. Finlay (Eds.), *Cancer in children and adolescents* (pp. 437–454). Sudbury, MA: Jones and Bartlett.

182. Rorke, L., Gilles, F., Davis, R., & Becker, L. (1985). Revision of the World Health Organization classification of brain tumors for childhood brain tumors. *Cancer, 56,* 1869–1886.

183. Roseff, S. (2009). Sickle cell disease: A review. *Immunohematology, 25*(2), 67–74.

184. Roseff, S., Luban, N., & Manno, C. (2002). Guidelines for assessing appropriateness of pediatric transfusion. *Transfusion, 42*(11), 1398–1413.

185. Rothenberg, A., Berdon, W., D'Angio, G., Yamashiro, D., & Cowles, R. (2009). The association between neuroblastoma and opsoclonus-myoclonus syndrome: A historical review. *Pediatric Radiology, 39*(7), 723–726.

186. Sadler, J., Budde, U., Eikenboom, C., Favaloro, E., Hill, G., Holmberg, L., et al. (2006). Update on the pathophysiology and classification of von Willebrand disease: A report of the Subcommittee on von Willebrand Factor. *Journal of Thrombosis and Haemostasis, 4,* 2103–2114.

187. Santagostino, E., Morfini, M., Auerswald, G., Benson, G., Salek, S., Lambert, T., et al. (2009). Paediatric haemophilia with inhibitors: Existing management options, treatment gaps and unmet needs. *Haemophilia, 15*(5), 983–989.

188. Schmidt, B. (1972). Genetic aspects of hemoglobin synthesis. *Angewandte Chemie International Edition, 11*(7), 576–583.

189. Schwartz, C. (2003). The management of Hodgkin disease in the young child. *Current Opinion in Pediatrics, 15,* 10–16.

190. Schweet, R., Arlinghaus, R., Shaeffer, J., & Williamson, A. (1964). Studies on hemoglobin synthesis. *Medicine (Baltimore), 43,* 731–745.

191. Scott, J., Hillery, C., Brown, E., Misiewicz, V., & Labotka, R. (1996). Hydroxyurea therapy in children severely affected with sickle cell disease. *Journal of Pediatrics, 128*(6), 820–828.

192. Shantsila, E., Lip, G., & Chong, B. (2009). Heparin-induced thrombocytopenia. *Chest, 135,* 1651–1664.

193. Sharathkumar, A., & Pipe, S. (2008). Bleeding disorders. *Pediatrics in Review, 29*(4), 121–130.

194. Shields, C. (2006). The International Classification of Retinoblastoma predicts chemoreduction success. *Ophthalmology, 113,* 2276–2280.

195. Shimamura, A. (2009). Clinical approach to marrow failure. *Hematology/American Society for Hematology Education Program,* 329–337.

196. Shusterman, S., & George, R. (2009). Neuroblastoma. In S. H. Orkin, D. E. Fisher, A. T. Look, S. E. Lux, D. Ginsburg, & D. G. Nathan (Eds.), *Oncology of infancy and childhood* (pp. 509–540). Philadelphia: Saunders Elsevier.

197. Smith, D. (1980). The molecular biology of mammalian hemoglobin synthesis. *Annals of Clinical and Laboratory Science, 10*(2), 116–122.

198. Smith, S. (2009). The cell-based model of coagulation. *Journal of Veterinary Emergency and Critical Care (San Antonio), 19*(1), 3–10.

199. Smyth, S., McEver, R., Weyrich, A., Morrell, C., Hoffman, M., Arepally, G., et al. (2009). Platelet functions beyond hemostasis. *Journal of Thrombosis and Hemostasis, 7*(11), 1759–1766.

200. Steinberg, M., Barton, F., Castro, O., Pegelow, C., Ballas, S., Kutler, P., et al. (2003). Effect of hydroxyurea on mortality and morbidity in adult sickle cell anemia: Fisks and benefits up to 9 years of treatment. *Journal of the American Medical Society, 289*(13), 1645–1651.

201. Stephensen, D., Tait, R., Brodie, N., Collins, R., Cheal, R., Keeling, D., et al. (2009). Changing patterns of bleeding in patients with severe haemophilia A. *Haemophilia, 15*(6), 1210–1214.

202. Stewart, C. (2001). Disseminated intravascular coagulation. *Australian Critical Care, 14*(2), 71–75.

203. Sullivan, D., & Glader, B. (1980). Erythrocyte enzyme disorders in children. *Pediatric Clinics of North America, 27*(2), 449–462.

204. Suttorp, M. (2008). Innovative approaches of targeted therapy for CML of childhood in combination with paediatric haematopoietic SCT. *Bone Marrow Transplantation, 42,* S40–S46.

205. Taketomo, C., Hodding, J., & Kraus, D. (2010). *Pediatric dosage handbook.* Hudson, OH: Lexi-Comp.

206. Tanaka, K., Key, N., & Levy, J. (2009). Blood coagulation: Hemostasis and thrombin regulation. *Anesthesia and Analgesia, 108*(5), 1433–1446.

207. Tcheng, W. (2004). Bleeding disorders and coagulopathies. In L. Osborn, T. DeWitt, L. First, & J. Zenel (Eds.), *Pediatrics* (pp. 705–712). Philadelphia: Elsevier Mosby.

208. Tizard, E., & Hamilton-Ayres, M. (2008). Henoch-Schönlein purpura. *Archives of Disease in Childhood: Education & Practice Edition, 93,* 1–8.

209. Toh, C. (2006). Disseminated intravascular coagulation. In N. Young, S. Gerson, & K. High, *Clinical hematology* (pp. 1134–1143). St. Louis: Mosby.

210. Toh, C., & Dennis, M. (2003). Disseminated intravascular coagulation: Old disease, new hope. *British Medical Journal, 327,* 974–977.

211. Tormene, D., Gavasso, S., Rosetto, V., & Simioni, P. (2006). Thrombosis and thrombophilia in children: A systematic review. *Seminars in Thrombosis and Hemostasis, 32,* 724–728.

212. Tosi, P., Barosi, G., Lazzaro, C., Lise, V., Marchetti, M., Morra, E., et al. (2008). Consensus conference on the management of tumor lysis syndrome. *Haematologica, 93*(12), 1877–1885.

213. Tsivgoulis, G., Alexandrov, A., & Sloan, M. (2009). Advances in transcranial Doppler ultrasonography. *Current Neurology and Neuroscience Reports, 9*(1), 46–54.

214. Tubergen, D., & Bleyer, A. (2007). The leukemias. In R. M. Kliegman, R. E. Behrman, H. B. Jenson, & B. F. Stanton (Eds.), *Nelson textbook of pediatrics* (18th ed., Chapter 495). Philadephia: Elsevier.

215. Valentino, L. (2004). Secondary prophylaxis therapy: What are the benefits, limitations and unknowns? *Haemophilia, 10*(2), 147–157.

216. Valentino, L. (2010). Assessing the benefits of FEIBA prophylaxis in haemophilia patients with inhibitors. *Haemophilia, 16*(2), 263–271.

217. Valentino, L., Martinowitz, U., Doobs, H., & Murali, P. (2006). Surgical excision of a giant pelvic pseudotumour in a patient with haemophilia A. *Haemophilia, 12*(5), 541–544.

218. Verbruggen, B. (2009). Diagnosis and quantification of factor VIII inhibitors. *Haemophilia, 16*(102), 20–24.

219. Vichinsky, E., Earles, A., Johnson, R., Hoag, S., Williams, A., & Lubin, B. (1990). Alloimmunization in sickle cell anemia and transfusion of racially unmatched blood. *New England Journal of Medicine, 322*(23), 1617–1621.

220. Vlachos, A., Ball, S., Dahl, N., Alter, B., Sheth, S., Ramenghi, V., et al. (2008). Diagnosing and treating Diamond-Blackfan anaemia: Results of an international clinical consensus conference. *British Journal of Haematology, 142*(6), 859–876.

221. Ward, W., Mikaelian, K., Dorey, F., Mirra, J., Sassoon, A., Holmes, E., et al. (1994). Pulmonary metastases of stage IIB extremity osteosarcoma and subsequent pulmonary metastases. *Journal of Clinical Oncology, 12,* 1849–1858.

222. Warkentin, T. (2005). Heparin-induced thrombocytopenia. *Disease-a-Month, 51,* 141–149.

223. Warkentin, T., Poncz, M., & Cines, D. (2006). Heparin-induced thrombocytopenia. In N. Young, S. Gerson, & K. High, *Clinical hematology* (pp. 887–899). St. Louis: Mosby.

224. Wasilewski-Masker, K., Liu, O., Yasiu, Y., Leisenring, W., Meacham, L., Hammond, S., et al. (2009). Late recurrence in pediatric cancer: A report from the Childhood Cancer Survivor Study. *Journal of the National Cancer Institute, 101,* 1–12.

225. Watchko, J. (2009). Identification of neonates at risk for hazardous hyperbilirubinemia: Emerging clinical insights. *Pediatric Clinics of North America, 56*(3), 671–687.

226. Weatherall, D., & Clegg, J. (1969). The control of human hemoglobin synthesis and function in health and disease. *Progress in Hematology, 6,* 261–304.

227. Wexler, L., & Helman, L. (1997). Rhabdomyosarcoma and the undifferentiated sarcomas. In P. Pizzo & D. Poplack (Eds.), *Principles and practice of pediatric oncology* (3rd ed., pp. 799–829). Philadelphia: Lippincott-Raven.

228. Yang, J., Parades, N., & Chan, A. (2009). Antithrombotic therapy in children with venous thromboembolism. *Hämostaseologie, 1,* 80–86.

229. Young, J., Smith, M., Roffers, S., Liff, J., & Bunin, G. (1999). Retinoblastoma. In L. Ries, M. Smith, J. Gurney, M. Linet, T. Tamra, J. Young, & G. Bunin (Eds.), *Cancer incidence and survival among children and adolescents: United States SEER Program 1975–1995.* NIH Pub. No. 99-4649. Bethesda MD: National Cancer Institute, SEER Program.

230. Zeng, X., & Sadler, J. (2006). Thrombotic thrombocytopenic purpura and hemolytic-uremic syndrome. In N. Young, S. Gerson, & K. High, *Clinical hematology* (pp. 809–813). St. Louis: Mosby.

Immunologic and Rheumatologic Disorders

PHYSIOLOGY AND DIAGNOSTICS

Kenneth Quinto, Lori Broderick, and Johanna Chang

PHYSIOLOGY

Smooth functioning of the immune system depends on the following features:

- *Diversity* allows the adaptive immune system to respond to a large variety of antigens.
- *Specificity* enables distinct antigens to elicit specific immune responses.
- *Memory* provides an enhanced response to repeated exposures to the same antigens.
- *Clonal expansion* quickly increases the number of antigen-specific lymphocytes to keep pace with quickly dividing microbes.
- *Specialization* generates optimal responses based on the type of microbe.
- *Contraction* and *homeostasis* enable the immune response to respond to newly encountered antigens.
- *Nonreactivity to self* prevents injury to health host cells during the immune response (Abbas et al., 2007).

The main effector cells of the adaptive immune response are composed mainly of three cell types:

- *B lymphocytes* are the cells involved with antibody production. After appropriate stimulation, B lymphocytes are able to produce all four classes of antibodies (immunoglobulins), including IgA, IgE, IgM, and IgG. These cells are essential in the production of protective antibodies elicited by vaccines.
- *T lymphocytes* are classically separated into two main subsets, CD4+ helper T lymphocytes and CD8+ cytotoxic T lymphocytes. Whereas B lymphocytes produce antibodies to help protect the body against invasion by extracellular microbes, CD8+ cytotoxic T lymphocytes destroy host cells that have been infected with intracellular microbes. CD4+ T lymphocytes are not directly involved with microbial elimination, but do play a vital role in activation of the adaptive and innate immune system by inducing B-lymphocyte differentiation for antibody production and activating macrophages for enhanced phagocytosis and elimination of microbes (LaRosa & Orange, 2008).
- *Natural killer* (NK) *cells* are cytotoxic lymphocytes that must receive an activating signal. Activation may occur by interferons, cytokines, and other receptors such as Fc.

The adaptive immune system employs different strategies to combat different types of microbes (Adelman et al., 2002). Antibodies secreted by B lymphocytes bind to extracellular microbes to enhance ingestion and destruction by phagocytes. Antibodies also prevent extracellular microbes from further infecting host cells. CD8+ T lymphocytes destroy host cells infected with intracellular microbes to eliminate the infection. Natural killer cells transfer granzymes into targeted cells, such as viruses, resulting in cell destruction through apoptosis rather than lysis.

DIAGNOSTICS

As described in the prior section, several layers exist to protect the host from perceived danger and pathogens such as from viruses, bacteria, and fungi. Sometimes, however, the host mistakenly perceives host antigens as pathogenic, leading to immunologic dysfunction. This section focuses on diagnostic testing and evaluation of suspected immunologic disorders.

As with any clinical question, the evaluation of a pediatric patient with suspected immunodeficiency requires a thorough history with delineation of prior infections, complete physical examination, and review of any prior diagnostic studies. Because disorders of the immune system may present in many different age groups and may be associated with delays in diagnosis, a given patient may have undergone a significant number of prior evaluations whose results may aid in diagnosis. Particular attention to chronologic patterns of infection or apparent flares of disease and correlation with symptoms or laboratory results can be highly suggestive of defects in specific aspects of the immune response.

Cellular evaluation

A cursory evaluation of the immune system may consist of a complete blood count (CBC) and quantitative immunoglobulins (QIgs) to identify the existing major components. The presence or absence of one or more components of the immune system may quickly narrow the list of differential diagnoses. The health care professional (HCP) may then pursue additional testing focused on the specific defect.

T cells represent approximately 75% of the lymphocyte population in the peripheral blood. As such, a CBC from which the absolute lymphocyte count may be calculated is a critical first test. Given their majority presence in the circulating cells, a substantial decrease in the number of lymphocytes may be due to a T-cell deficiency, whereas one would not expect a B- or NK-cell deficiency to have such a dramatic effect on the total number of lymphocytes due to their smaller contributing numbers. T-cell deficiency may be seen in DiGeorge syndrome as well as in conditions resulting from combined T- and B-cell deficiencies such as severe combined immunodeficiency (SCID) and Wiskott-Aldrich syndrome.

Establishment of a T-cell sector, while important, does not rule out a T-lymphocyte-based deficit. Instead, additional functional assays are required to determine whether those cells may be active participants in host immunity.

Careful evaluation of T-cell function is important not only for determining its role in the cellular immune response, but also for delineating its role as a contributing factor to the humoral immune response. Functional assays for T cells include analysis of delayed-type hypersensitivity reactions, proliferative assays, and cytotoxicity assays. Type IV (cell-mediated, antibody-independent) hypersensitivity reactions are mediated by T cells that have been sensitized to an antigen—that is, by T cells that are capable of responding to an antigen that they have previously encountered, leading to a predominantly Th_1-type cytokine cascade and local immune response. HCPs have taken advantage of this natural response and used it as a measure of cell-mediated immunity and T-cell functionality using a common antigen, generally derived from *Candida* or the tuberculin protein (Gordon et al., 1980). During testing, candidal antigens are injected into the dermis, with subsequent measurements of erythema and induration being made at 24, 48, and 72 hours post injection. These measurements may reveal a positive response, or in vivo activity of cell-mediated immunity. Conversely, a lack of erythema or induration is described as anergy, and may be indicative of a T-cell defect. The HCP should be wary, however: In the presence of an overwhelming immune response within the host, the test may be falsely negative and further correlation is required.

B-cell functionality may be initially evaluated by quantitative immunoglobulin, specifically titers of IgA, IgG, and IgM. As previously noted, plasma cells are derived from B cells, and are the only cells in the body capable of producing and secreting immunoglobulin. Thus most antibody deficiencies are related to defects in B-cell development and function. Immunoglobulin production may be interrupted at any developmental stage, thereby making evaluation of each class of immunoglobulin crucial for a thorough immunologic evaluation. The titers of each class of immunoglobulin, both individually and in comparison to one another, can be instructive, not only in diagnosis, but also in prediction of risk of future infections. For example, IgA is protective against mucosal infections, and a selective deficiency of this immunoglobulin may be seen in patients with recurrent pneumonias and other respiratory tract infections (Morell et al., 1986). Care must be taken in the interpretation of these values, however, as titers change with patient age. Additionally, because immunoglobulins, along with albumin, form a substantial portion of the circulating protein, any protein-losing enteropathy or overall protein loss may concomitantly reduce immunoglobulin titers. Other sources of potential loss should be examined during the course of the immunologic evaluation.

The remaining subclasses of immunoglobulins—specifically, IgE and IgD—are traditionally evaluated separately from IgA, IgG, and IgM. IgE is frequently used in evaluation of atopy, but plays an important role in the pathogenesis of parasitic infections as well. While normally present in very low titers compared to the other subclasses

of immunoglobulin, great heterogeneity in IgE levels occurs between individuals, especially nonatopic individuals, and levels also vary with age. Significant elevations may be seen in hyper-IgE syndrome and Wiskott-Aldrich syndrome (Ozcan et al., 2008). In contrast, IgD is infrequently measured during the evaluation of a patient with suspected immunodeficiency. Its levels vary widely between individuals, and several studies have demonstrated that there is no appreciable relationship between the circulating levels of IgD and the occurrence of immunoglobulin or antibody deficiencies (Hiemstra et al., 1989; Litzman et al., 1997). The one exception may be as part of the evaluation for the periodic fever disorders, specifically, hyper-IgD syndrome (HIDS), in which IgD levels are elevated.

The ability of B cells to respond to antigen challenge may be further evaluated by functional antibodies or immunization titers, most commonly tetanus and pneumococcal titers. These titers are selected for their prevalence in the immunized population as well as for the antigen responses that they induce, which is dependent on both the host and the antigen. The pneumococcal vaccine targets the polysaccharide capsule to promote opsonization and subsequent phagocytosis. The ability of the host to generate antibodies to tetanus (a protein), requires both the cellular and humoral arms of the immune system. Given that this interaction is choreographed by multiple cell types, cytokine production, and cellular differentiation, the inability to generate a response—such as to a booster vaccination—points to an immunological defect. The challenge lies in the possibility that titers may not specifically identify the source of the defect, whether in antigen presentation or processing, cytokine production, or cellular proliferation (Schauer et al., 2003).

In addition, these titers must be interpreted with respect to the patient's age, as immunoglobulin levels do not remain constant through infancy, childhood, and adulthood (Fosarelli et al., 1985; Jolliff et al., 1982). The utility of further delineation of immunoglobulin subclasses may be useful in specific cases of recurrent infections to encapsulated organisms such as *Pneumococcus*. In children older than 3 years of age, exposure to polysaccharides present in the pneumococcal capsule generates production of IgG_2. In contrast, in infants and younger children, the antibody response almost uniformly consists of IgG_1, similar to the antibodies produced in response to protein antigens (Rodrigo et al., 2000; Uddin et al., 2006). This distinction is important not only in the interpretation of immunoglobulin titers in different age groups, but may also be representative of a specific deficiency of the IgG_2 subclass and should be considered in certain clinical settings of recurrent pneumococcal infections (Uddin et al.).

Patients presenting with recurrent infections may also be evaluated for defects in neutrophil killing. The oxidative abilities of neutrophils—also known as respiratory burst—can be measured by a measure of NADPH oxidase function. In this assay, peripheral blood cells are activated in the presence of the nitroblue tetrazolium (NBT) dye, which forms a dark blue precipitate in cells producing superoxide; those cells can then be visualized under a microscope (Bogomolski-Yahalom & Matzner, 1995; Dahlgren & Karlsson, 1999). Although the NBT test is both a qualitative and quantitative test to diagnose chronic granulomatous disease (CGD) and other disorders of neutrophil reduction ability, it is technically difficult, requiring the services of experienced technicians. For this reason, other methods have become more common (Dahlgren & Karlsson). The preferred method for diagnosis is currently dihydrorhodamine (DHR), a flow cytometric assay that quantifies neutrophil oxidative capacity through the analysis of DHR to rhodamine (O'Gorman & Corrochano, 1995).

Complement and cryoglobulins

Complement describes a family of circulating proteins that act together to promote opsonization, bacteriolysis, and phagocytosis of microorganisms (Pettigrew et al., 1999). Deficiency of each component of the classical and alternate pathways is quite rare, accounting for fewer than 1% of patients with primary immunodeficiency. However, in patients with recurrent infections, notably infections caused by encapsulated bacteria such as *Neisseria*, the evaluation of the complement system should not be ignored. The primary screening test for deficiencies in the complement pathway is the total hemolytic complement assay, or CH50. This assay combines patient serum with red blood cells from sheep that have been coated with rabbit-antisheep antibodies to examine the ability of the serum proteins to lyse the sheep erythrocytes. To generate a normal CH50 value, the complement pathway must be intact (Pettigrew et al.; Wen et al., 2004). Importantly, this test does not provide quantitative data on any individual component, as the concentration of a single protein may be significantly decreased without affecting the end value.

Cryoglobulins are immunoglobulins that precipitate as serum is cooled below core body temperature. These precipitates can be seen in a multitude of diseases, including the vasculitides, chronic infections, or autoimmune disorders (Kallemuchikkal & Gorevic, 1999). The HCP must take care in the interpretation of cryoglobulin studies, especially in the intensive care setting, as administration of heparin may induce the formation of precipitatable complexes between fibronectin, fibrin, and fibrinogen, leading to a false-positive test. Further characterization of the precipitate may be required to identify the components.

Advanced testing for specific diseases

Once an immunologic defect is clinically suspected, further testing may be employed to better characterize the nature of the defect. Flow cytometry and genetic analysis are becoming more widely used to phenotypically characterize cellular populations and as markers of functionality (O'Gorman & Scholl, 2002). Briefly, flow cytometry evaluates cell-surface antigens, or cluster of differentiation (CD) markers, expressed by cells using fluorochrome-labeled antibodies; working in a high-throughput fashion, it examines thousands of cells within a sample population per minute. This technology may be used in initial evaluations as an alternative means to quantify leukocyte populations. For example, in DiGeorge syndrome and SCID, the number of T cells, as evaluated by CD3 positivity, will be absent. Additionally, specific cell markers may be used to further delineate cells within a population. In leukocyte adhesion deficiency (LAD) syndromes, flow cytometry is used to assess the presence of the $\beta2$ integrins CD11 subclasses/CD18 on leukocytes and myeloid cells (Fischer et al., 1988). The use of flow cytometry for functional analysis is exemplified, as previously described, by its application in evaluating for NAPDH oxidase capacity of neutrophils in suspected CGD.

The Human Genome Project has led to the identification of multiple genetic defects present in immunodeficiencies. For some conditions, the link between the genetic defect and clinical symptomatology is obvious, as in CGD, in which defects in the neutrophil NADPH oxidase protein complex leads to impaired phagocytosis. For others, the link is not as clear. Nevertheless, for many of the immunodeficiencies, genetic testing is employed not only for diagnosis, but also for genetic counseling of parents with respect to risk to future offspring.

ANAPHYLAXIS

Ronald M. Ferdman

PATHOPHYSIOLOGY

The principal pathophysiologic event in anaphylaxis is the activation of mast cells, and to a lesser extent, basophils. Although mast cells are activated primarily by IgE-mediated mechanisms, several other non-IgE-mediated activation pathways exist. IgE-mediated reactions were historically labeled as "anaphylactic," while non-IgE-mediated reactions were termed "anaphylactoid." More recent nomenclature is "immunologic" and "non-immunologic" anaphylaxis. It is impossible to clinically distinguish between these reactions based on symptoms, therefore the single term "anaphylaxis" is used (Kemp et al., 2008).

Antigen-specific IgE is produced in genetically susceptible individuals in response to exposure to any variety of allergens. Specific IgE binds to high-affinity IgE receptors, $F_c\varepsilon RI$, on the surface of mast cells; and is available to bind to allergen. Allergen reexposure via antigen-presenting cells causes aggregation of receptor-bound IgE, and this cross-linking sets off a series of intracellular signals that very rapidly lead to mast cell activation. Several non-IgE-mediated immunologic mechanisms for mast cell activation have been described. Activation of the complement system generates complement split products, including C_{3a} and C_{5a} (anaphylatoxins), which can bind to complement receptors on the mast cell surface. Other mechanisms, including immune complexes, IgG, IgM, neuropeptides such as substance P, and T-cell activation, have also been reported to activate mast cells, but their clinical roles in causing anaphylaxis in humans remain unclear (Simons, 2008).

Many cases of anaphylaxis have non-immunologic causes. Certain chemicals appear to cause direct non-receptor-mediated mast cell activation, including radiocontrast media, components of insect venom, opiate analgesics, and vancomycin. Nonsteroidal anti-inflammatory drugs (NSAIDs) may induce anaphylactoid syndromes via inhibition of the cyclo-oxygenase enzyme, thereby shifting eicosonoid metabolism toward production of leukotrienes, while angiotensin-converting enzyme (ACE) inhibitors increase concentrations of bradykinin through effects on the kinin–kallikrien forming system. Physical factors, such as exercise and exposure to cold temperatures, can also cause mast cell activation and anaphylaxis through as-yet-unidentified mechanisms.

Whatever the mechanism, mast cell and basophil activation results in production and release of mediators that have potent actions on a variety of target organs. Some mediators are preformed and are released immediately; others must be generated de novo and are released within hours after mast cell activation.

Preformed mediators are stored within intracellular granules. The most important preformed mediator is histamine; other preformed mediators include proteases (e.g., tryptase, carboxypeptidase, and chymase) and proteoglycans (e.g., heparin and condroitin sulfate) (Brown, 2007; Lemon-Mule et al., 2008; Ogawa & Grant, 2007; Simons, 2008).

At the same time that degranulation and release of preformed mediators are occurring, newly formed mast-cell-derived mediators are generated and released over the next several hours. Important newly generated mediators include arachidonic acid and other lipid mediators (platelet-activating factor [PAF], leukotriene C_4, and prostaglandin D_2), and cytokines (IL-4, IL-5, IL-13, TNF-α, eotaxin, others). Many of these molecules, especially the lipid mediators, have similar and perhaps even more potent actions than histamine and serve to enhance the allergic reaction.

The various de novo mediators and cytokines recruit and activate other inflammatory cells, including eosinophils, basophils, neutrophils, and T lymphocytes. Newly recruited inflammatory cells generate their own cadre of inflammatory products and are in part responsible for initiating and propagating the late-phase allergic reaction. Biphasic reactions may also occur via non-mast cell mechanisms, specifically through TNF-α induced PAF production (Pushparaj et al., 2009) and IL-33 (a T-cell product) (Vadas et al., 2008), which have been implicated as important mediators in anaphylactic shock. A recent study suggested that individuals who had lower levels of PAF acetylhydrolase, the enzyme that inactivates PAF, were more likely to experience severe and even fatal anaphylaxis. Mast cell mediators also can activate the complement system, the kinin–kallikrien contact system, and the coagulation system (Simons et al., 2007). Disseminated intravascular coagulation (DIC) has been reported with such activation, and was responsible for 8% of deaths in a study of fatal anaphylaxis over a 10-year period in the United Kingdom (Pumphrey, 2004).

Both the preformed and newly formed mediators affect a number of vital target organs—most importantly, the vasculature, heart, and lungs. Effects on the vascular endothelium include vasodilatation and increased vascular permeability, leading to both distributive and hypovolemic hypotension and shock. In particular, histamine can affect the heart directly and can cause vasospasm of coronary arteries. This mediator also has direct inotropic and chronotropic effects on the myocardium, and it can shorten diastole through effects on the sinoatrial node. By comparison, PAF decreases coronary blood flow and delays atrioventricular conduction. These combined effects can add a component of cardiogenic shock to the reaction via low venous return, poor cardiac output, and myocardial ischemia. Laryngeal edema occurs as a result of increased vascular permeability in the larynx. Histamine and the lipid mediators stimulate bronchial smooth muscle contraction, resulting in bronchospasm. They also increase both the production and the viscosity of mucus. Together with bronchospasm, this effect can result in significant bronchiolar mucus plugging. Pulmonary vasospasm may lead to decreased left ventricular filling and add a component of obstructive shock to the anaphylactic cascade.

Many of the non-life-threatening manifestations of anaphylaxis, such as flushing, pruritus, urticaria/angioedema, rhinorrhea, sneezing, conjunctivitis, and headache are mostly histamine mediated, although prostaglandins and leukotrienes are also involved. These mediators cause uterine cramping and gastrointestinal (GI) symptoms through smooth muscle contraction and increased intestinal vasculature permeability.

EPIDEMIOLOGY AND ETIOLOGY

Anaphylaxis occurs across all age groups and all populations, yet its exact incidence is unknown. Considering that the clinical entity of anaphylaxis has been known for more than 100 years, there are relatively few studies published on its epidemiology. Those studies that do exist report wide variations in the incidence and prevalence of anaphylaxis. Methods of study have included retrospective review of hospital admissions and emergency department visits, searches of computer-linked medical databases, patient questionnaires, and analysis of self-injectable epinephrine prescription patterns (Clark & Carmargo, 2007; Lieberman et al., 2006). Part of the variation in incidence estimates stems from the lack of consistent diagnostic criteria for anaphylaxis used both by clinicians and by investigators (Campbell et al., 2008; Pongracic & Kim, 2007). Other confounders include small sample sizes and the practice of focusing on specific populations or etiologies.

A recent working group of the American College of Allergy, Asthma, and Immunology (ACAAI) on the epidemiology of anaphylaxis estimated that the overall lifetime prevalence for anaphylaxis in all ages is between 0.5% and 2% (50 to 200 cases per 100,000) (Lieberman et al., 2006). Authorities agree that even the higher range may be an underestimate due to factors such as under-recognition, under-diagnosis, and under-prescribing of self-injectable epinephrine. Indeed, one study that reviewed literature regarding the incidence of just four major causes of anaphylaxis (food, drug, latex, and insect stings) estimated the frequency of anaphylaxis in the general U.S. population to be between 1.2% and 15% (Neugat et al., 2001). Approximately 100,000 episodes occur each year in the United States, approximately two-thirds are new cases, and an estimated 1% are fatal (Neugat et al.).

Despite the difficulties estimating the true prevalence of anaphylaxis, it appears certain that its incidence has increased steadily over the last several decades, as has the incidence of other allergic conditions such as asthma,

allergic rhinitis, and eczema. A recent study found that the annual incidence of anaphylaxis in Minnesota increased from 21 cases per 100,000 person-years during 1983–1987 to 48 cases per 100,000 person-years during 1990–2000 (Leiberman et al., 2006). Similar dramatic increases in incidence have been reported from other areas of the Unites States as well as from Western Europe and Australia (Liew et al., 2009; Muraro et al., 2007; Roberts, 2007; Simons & Sampson, 2008).

The epidemiologic data in infants are even more sparse than those in adults. Anaphylaxis has been described in infants as young as 1 month of age and fatal results have been reported (Simons, 2007). Some reports suggest that the incidence of anaphylaxis in children is the same as the incidence in adults, whereas others cite pediatric incidences as low as 0.19 case per 100,000 population. In a survey of French school children, researchers estimated that 1 in 1,000 has a personalized anaphylaxis emergency plan. In another study, more than 5% of boys 12 to 17 months of age in Canada received a prescription for epinephrine. Some evidence also indicates that the rate of occurrence of anaphylaxis is increasing in children (Simons & Sampson, 2008).

The list of reported causes of anaphylaxis is almost endless (Lieberman et al., 2005; Oswalt & Kemp, 2007). Nevertheless, some common etiologic agents and classes of allergens have been identified as causing the majority of reactions. To simplify the various causes, they can be classified into IgE-mediated, non-IgE-immune-mediated and non-immune-mediated causes (Table 29-1). There is some overlap in these classes: For example, different antibiotics may cause anaphylaxis through one of each of the three mechanisms, while radiocontrast media (RCM) may work through several different mechanisms simultaneously.

IgE-mediated causes

Foods are the most common cause of anaphylaxis in pediatric patients, accounting for more than 50% of cases in some series (Lieberman et al., 2005; Webb & Lieberman, 2006). Foods also account for a large proportion of these reactions in older children and adults. The most commonly implicated foods in young children are peanuts, cow's milk, egg, and (less commonly) soy and wheat. In older children, tree nuts and seafood, especially shellfish, are important causes. Virtually any food can cause anaphylaxis, but these seven—peanuts, egg, milk, wheat, soy, tree nuts, and seafood—account for at least 90% of cases in the United States. Moreover, peanuts and tree nuts are responsible for the vast majority of fatalities (Clark et al., 2004; Lieberman et al., 2005).

Exposure to foods can occur by direct ingestion, or indirectly through human breastmilk. It is not uncommon for caregivers to report reactions the first time a food is consumed by an infant. Primary sensitization can occur in utero, through breastmilk, or through accidental exposure

TABLE 29-1

Causes of Anaphylaxis

IgE-Mediated Causes

Food (most common: milk, egg, peanuts, tree nuts, shellfish, seafood, wheat, soybean)

Drug and other medicinal products
- Antibiotics (most common: penicillin, cephalosporin)
- Nonsteroidal anti-inflammatory drugs (NSAIDs)
- Latex
- Biologic proteins (insulin, hormones, chemotherapeutic)
- Anesthetic agents
- Allergen immunotherapy

Insects
- Stinging insects—Hymenoptera (bees, wasps, hornets, yellow jackets, fire ants)
- Biting insects—bed bugs, kissing bugs

Animal danders

Non-IgE-Mediated Causes

Immune complex
- Blood, blood products
- Immunoglobulin
- Protamine
- Radiocontrast media (RCM)

Direct mast cell release
- Vancomycin
- Opioids
- Muscle relaxants
- RCM

Arachidonic acid pathway alteration
- NSAIDs

Contact kinin–kallikrien system activation
- Hemodialysis membranes
- RCM

Physical stimuli
- Exercise
- Exercise plus food
- Cold

that can cause allergic reactions, antibiotics—primarily penicillins—remain the most common class of drugs causing anaphylaxis in children. Cephalosporins are the next most common cause. Anaphylaxis to non-beta-lactam antibiotics (e.g., macrolides, sulfonamides, and quinolones) does occur, albeit less frequently. In older adolescents and adults, NSAIDs are the class of drugs that cause the most anaphylaxis. Allergies to NSAIDs are typically agent specific, but some individuals may cross-react to the entire class. While NSAIDs may react via IgE, a more common mechanism is through aberration of the arachidonic acid pathway.

Latex is a relatively uncommon cause of anaphylaxis in the general population. This etiology is more common in high-risk groups such as patients with myelomeningocele, congenital urologic malformations, and pediatric patients who required multiple surgeries (Chiu & Kelly, 2005).

Allergen immunotherapy ("allergy shots") has been reported to cause anaphylaxis at a rate of approximately 1 per 2 million injections (Bukantz et al., 2008).

Stinging insect venom-induced anaphylaxis is more common in adults but can occur at any age, and in children may account for as many as 5% of cases. The most common causative insect stings are from the order *Hymenoptera*—specifically, the families *adpidae* (honeybee, bumble bee), *vespidae* (wasp, yellow jacket, hornet), and *apidae* (fire ant). Bed bug (*Cimicoidae*) infestations are making a resurgence in the United States, and the painless bites of bed bugs and kissing bugs (*Triatominae*) can be a cause of nocturnal anaphylaxis. Anaphylaxis from other insects, including spiders, mosquitoes, and flies, is extremely rare (Chiu & Kelly, 2005).

Vaccine allergic reactions are rare, occurring in approximately 1 patient for every 1,000,000 doses (Bohlke et al., 2003). Allergy to gelatin, a common preservative in some vaccines, is the most common cause of anaphylaxis to vaccines. Egg-allergic patients may have reactions to the egg-containing vaccines for influenza and yellow fever. It is also possible to have a reaction to other vaccine ingredients, such as preservatives, antibacterials, and even the immunizing component itself. Many other biologic proteins such as insulin, hormones, and chemotherapy may cause anaphylaxis. Exquisitely sensitive patients may develop anaphylaxis through contact with animal danders such as those from horses and cats.

Non-IgE-immune-mediated and non-immune-mediated causes

Non-IgE immune mechanisms include immune complex formation, activation of the complement system, and perhaps IgG-mediated pathways. Causes of anaphylaxis for these patients include blood and blood products, immunoglobulin, and protamine. Vancomycin, opioids, and muscle relaxants cause direct mast cell histamine release. Disturbance in the arachidonic acid pathway is the major

(crawling, putting food in mouth, from siblings or adult caregivers). Anaphylaxis resulting from food additives is very rare.

Anisakiasis is a parasitic infection caused by ingesting undercooked saltwater fish infected with *Anisakis simplex*. However, allergic reactions to this parasite can occur hours after the fish is consumed, when larval nematodes penetrate the gastric mucosa. Allergy tests to the fish will be negative, but IgE can be detected against anisakiasis (Daschner et al., 2000). In contrast, rupture or leak of hydatid cysts from tapeworms of *Echinococcus* species can result in sudden anaphylaxis (Vuitton, 2004).

Drug reactions account for approximately 5% to 15% of cases of anaphylaxis. Of the multiple medications cause of aspirin and NSAID reactions. Activation of the contact kinin–kallikrien forming system may be the pathway of reactions to dialysis membranes. Radiocontrast media may cause direct mast cell release, but may also work through immune complex formation, through activation of the contact system, or perhaps even through interaction with the F_c portion of mast-cell-bound immunoglobulin.

Certain physical stimuli may trigger anaphylactic reactions through poorly understood mechanisms. The most common physical stimuli reported are exercise and cold. Urticaria is a more common reaction to cold, but it can progress to anaphylaxis for large exposures, such as rapid cold-water immersion (Fernando, 2009).

In exercise-induced anaphylaxis, the onset of symptoms is associated with physical exertion. In a subset of patients, exercise-induced anaphylaxis is food dependent, with symptoms developing only if exercise takes place within a few hours of eating, and sometimes only if a specific food is eaten before exercise. In these patients, exercise alone or eating the food alone is not sufficient to cause anaphylaxis—only the combination of exercise and food produces this disorder. Symptoms may occur at any stage of exercise, and rarely shortly after exercise ceases. Early symptoms include a feeling of warmth, flushing, pruritus, urticaria, and fatigue. With continued exercise angioedema, GI symptoms, laryngeal, and hypotension/collapse may ensue. Bronchospasm occurs less commonly in exercised-induced anaphylaxis compared to other causes of anaphylaxis. Headache is not an uncommon complaint and can persist for hours to days after attacks. If the anaphylactic reaction is associated with food, the food must usually be ingested within minutes to hours before exercise. Occasionally, co-triggers such as NSAIDs, alcoholic beverages, temperature extremes, seasonal allergen exposure, and timing of menstrual cycle may influence the degree of symptoms experienced.

Exercise-induced anaphylaxis is most common in female adolescents and young adults. Its diagnosis is based on clinical evidence and is made by associating symptoms with exercise and excluding other diagnoses. IgE plays a role in food-associated exercise-induced anaphylaxis, so skin tests can help identify or confirm suspected food allergies. A positive exercise challenge can rule in the diagnosis, but may not rule it out because it may be difficult to reproduce all of the various circumstances associated with normal exercise (Beaudouin et al., 2006; Romano et al., 2001).

Intraoperative anaphylaxis is estimated to occur in 1 in 3,500 to 20,000 general anesthetic administrations, with mortality estimated to be as high as 6% (Bleasel et al., 2009; Chacko & Ledford, 2007; Dewachter & Mouton-Faivre, 2008). It is difficult to recognize intraoperative anaphylaxis due to the multiple physiologic changes that often occur during surgery; in addition, other non-allergic surgical complications can present with similar symptoms. It is also difficult to differentiate between immune and non-immune mechanisms from the pharmacologic reactions of the large variety of medications that are administered near simultaneously during surgical procedures. The most common causes of anaphylaxis related to anesthesia are muscle relaxants, induction agents or hypnotics, colloids (Dextran, mannitol, hydroxyethyl starch), and protamine. Other less common causes include isosulfran blue dye, gelatin solution used for hemostasis, chlorhexidine, ethylene oxide, streptokinase, methylmethacrylate, and chymopapain. Latex, antibiotics, and opioids, if used during the procedure, are among the most common causes of intraoperative anaphylaxis. True anaphylaxis to local anesthetics has been reported, but is rare. Most local anesthetic reactions are thought to be vasovagal.

Idiopathic anaphylaxis accounts for a large proportions of cases, at least a quarter to one-half of all cases in most reported series. Idiopathic anaphylaxis, especially recurrent episodes are more common in adults than children. Obviously, idiopathic anaphylaxis is a diagnosis of exclusion (Greenberger, 2007).

PRESENTATION

The clinical manifestations of anaphylaxis are widespread and varied, and can affect multiple organ systems either individually or in combination (Kemp, 2007; Lieberman et al., 2005; Ogawa & Grant, 2007; Sampson et al., 2006). The skin is affected in approximately 90% of patients, and dermatologic manifestations may include urticaria, angioedema, pruritus, and flushing. Urticaria can appear on any skin surface. Angioedema can occur not only on skin, but also on mucosal surfaces as well such as the mouth, lips, tongue, and other areas of the oropharyngeal or GI tract.

Both the upper and lower respiratory tracts can be affected by anaphylaxis. Respiratory symptoms are especially common, occurring in 70% of patients. Ocular symptoms include conjunctival erythema, lacrimation, and itching. Nasal manifestations may consist of sneezing, rhinorrhea, and congestion. Upper airway edema, including tongue and uvular swelling, and especially laryngeal edema, can cause complete airway obstruction and suffocation. Symptoms of early laryngeal edema include a sensation of "tightness" or a "lump" in the throat, a staccato cough, stridor, recurrent clearing of the throat, dysphonia such as hoarseness or a high-pitched voice, and pooling of saliva with difficulty swallowing. Lower respiratory symptoms are caused by bronchoconstriction and increased production of mucus; they consist of coughing, wheezing, and dyspnea. Respiratory tract involvement is life threatening and is the most common cause of death in children with anaphylaxis.

Cardiac manifestations occur in approximately 20% of patients, but can be fatal, and include hypotension, tachycardia, and shock. Paradoxical bradycardia has been described in anaphylaxis. Hypotension, poor perfusion, and hypoxia can result in end-organ dysfunction, leading to problems such as incontinence, confusion, dizziness, syncope, collapse, and seizures. Hypotension and shock are responsible for a large proportion of deaths in adults, but are less common in children. Nevertheless, hypotension may be missed if the initial blood pressure measurement is made after epinephrine is administered. Arrhythmias occur rarely in anaphylaxis, but may either result from direct effects on the myocardium and conduction system or as a complication of medical management.

Gastrointestinal symptoms are more common than realized, occurring in approximately 30% of patients who experience anaphylaxis. It is not uncommon for GI symptoms to be the only manifestation, or to precede other symptoms, especially in children with food-allergic reactions. Symptoms include cramping, abdominal pain, nausea, vomiting, and diarrhea. Some patients describe having a metallic taste in their mouths. Uterine contraction may occur in women, sometimes manifested as back or abdominal pain. Direct central nervous system (CNS) involvement is rare, but many individuals experience a severe anxiety often described as a "sense of impending doom."

Although any or all of these symptoms may occur during allergic reactions, it is rare that a single individual will experience all possible symptoms. Until recently, no clinical consensus existed regarding which symptoms were sufficient to make the diagnosis of anaphylaxis. In 2006, a symposium focusing on the definition and management of anaphylaxis, sponsored by the National Institute of Allergy and Infectious Disease (NIAID) and the Food Allergy and Anaphylaxis Network (FAAN), brought together experts from multiple medical, academic, governmental, and lay organizations to develop a clinical criteria for the definition of anaphylaxis (Table 29-2) (Sampson et al., 2006).

It is important to note that patients may have allergic reactions that consist of a single, but nevertheless life-threatening symptom that does not meet the current clinical definition of anaphylaxis. For example, isolated severe bronchospasm in the absence of any other symptom does not meet the criteria for "anaphylaxis," yet may result in death from airway obstruction and hypoxemia. Patients who meet this definition will require the same therapeutic management as patients with anaphylaxis in terms of avoidance and need for self-injectable epinephrine (Sicherer & Simons, 2007).

Fatalities are caused primarily by respiratory compromise and cardiovascular collapse. In children, death due to respiratory failure is more common. The average interval between onset of symptoms and fatality varies depending on the antigen, with the longest interval being for foods (25 to 35 minutes or more), and the shortest being for insect stings and drugs (5 to 20 minutes) (Pumphrey, 2004). Rarely does the onset of the anaphylactic reaction occur more than 1 hr after exposure to the allergen, but exceptions do occur—thus late onset, several hours after exposure, can be seen especially, with food allergies.

Most of the acute manifestations of anaphylaxis resolve fairly quickly. However, both protracted and biphasic patterns can be seen. In protracted reactions, symptoms may

TABLE 29-2

Clinical Criteria for Diagnosing Anaphylaxis

Anaphylaxis is highly likely when *any one* of the following three criteria are met:

Criterion 1. Acute onset of an illness (within minutes to several hours) with involvement of the skin, mucosal tissue, or both (e.g., generalized hives, pruritus or flushing, swollen lips/tongue/uvula), even in the absence of a known or suspected trigger AND at least one of the following:
- Respiratory compromise (e.g., dyspnea, wheeze/bronchospasm, stridor, reduced PEF, hypoxemia)
- Reduced BP or associated symptoms of end-organ dysfunction (e.g., collapse, syncope, incontinence)

Criterion 2. Two or more of the following that occur rapidly (minutes to several hours) after exposure to a likely allergen for that patient:
- Involvement of the skin or mucosal tissue (e.g., generalized hives, pruritus or flushing, swollen lips/tongue/uvula)
- Respiratory compromise (e.g., dyspnea, wheeze/bronchospasm, stridor, reduced PER, hypoxemia)
- Reduced BP or associated symptoms of end-organ dysfunction (e.g., collapse, syncope, incontinence)
- Persistent gastrointestinal symptoms (e.g., crampy abdominal pain, vomiting)

Criterion 3. Reduced BP rapidly (minutes to several hours) after exposure to a known allergen for that patient
- Infants and children: low systolic BP (age specific) or greater than 30% decrease from baseline BP
- Adults: systolic BP of less than 90 mmHg or greater than 30% decrease from that person's baseline BP

Note: Peak expiratory flow (PEF); blood pressure (BP).

*Low systolic blood pressure for children is defined as less than 70 mmHg from 1 month to 1 year of age; less than (70 mmHg + [2 × age in years]) from 1 to 10 years of age; and less than 90 mmHg for 11 to 17 years of age.

Source: Adapted with permission from Sampson, H., Munoz-Furlong, A., Campbell, R., et al. (2006). Second symposium on the definition and management of anaphylaxis: Summary report: Second National Institute of Allergy and Infectious Disease/Food Allergy and Anaphylaxis Network Symposium. *Journal of Allergy and Clinical Immunology, 117,* 391–397.

persist for hours and even for days. Oral exposures and a slower onset of the primary reaction may be associated with a higher likelihood of a protracted reaction, whereas insect venom reactions rarely are protracted. Biphasic reactions occur in as many as 25% of patients (Kemp et al., 2008). In biphasic reactions, a second reaction occurs several hours after the resolution of the primary reaction, even in the absence of re-exposure to the antigen. Most biphasic reactions occur within 8 hours of the initial reaction, but the onset of the second reaction can range from 1 to 72 hours later. The second reaction typically occurs at the same or a lesser magnitude than the primary reaction, but a more severe reaction is seen in approximately 10% of patients, and as many as 40% of affected individuals require additional therapeutic management. It is not possible to predict which individuals will develop a biphasic reaction, but this course is more likely to be seen in conjunction with food allergies. Patients with very severe primary reactions, those who require more than one dose of epinephrine, and those who had a delay in administration or inadequate dosing of epinephrine may also be more likely to have a biphasic reaction (Ellis & Day, 2007; Jarvinen et al., 2008; Mehr et al., 2009; Sampson et al., 2006).

The diagnosis of anaphylaxis in infants can present additional challenges. Some of the symptoms of anaphylaxis—such as the feeling of warmth, itching or tingling, throat, and chest tightness, dyspnea, nausea, and pain—cannot be communicated by infants. Some symptoms of anaphylaxis may potentially be confused with normal infant behaviors, such as drooling, crying, and postprandial drowsiness. Other symptoms may be attributed to less serious conditions such as emesis from gastroesophageal reflux or pain from colic. Sometimes the signs of anaphylaxis in infants are obvious, but other times may be confused with other, more common serious conditions, such as respiratory distress due to croup, asthma or bronchiolitis, or rapid unresponsiveness from seizures or sepsis. Hypotension may go undetected in infants if blood pressure is not measured correctly or promptly. In infants, anaphylaxis may be the first clinical manifestation of sensitization to a trigger, and caregivers may not realize what the symptoms represent if they are unaware of the sensitization. Allergic reactions may occur the seemingly first time the infant eats a food, but prior exposures may have been unknown, or sensitization may have occurred in utero or via breastfeeding (Muraro et al., 2007; Simons, 2007).

DIFFERENTIAL DIAGNOSIS

The differential diagnosis of anaphylaxis is broad and varies with the patient's age (Table 29-3). One of the most common conditions that mimics anaphylaxis is

TABLE 29-3

Differential Diagnoses for Anaphylaxis

Anxiety or Psychiatric

Vasovagal

Panic attack

Hyperventilation

Hysteria

Munchausen or Munchausen syndrome by proxy (child maltreatment)

Flush Syndromes

Carcinoid tumor

Pheochromocytoma

Neural crest tumor

Thyroid medullary carcinoma

Disorders of Excess Histamine

Exogenous: scombroid poisoning

Endogenous: mastocytosis, mast cell leukemia, basophil leukemia

Other Shock Conditions

Cardiogenic shock

Hypovolemic shock

Septic shock

Other Conditions Causing Sudden Collapse

Pulmonary embolism, myocardial infarction, stroke

Hypoglycemia

Inborn errors of metabolism

Seizure disorder

Acute poisoning

Sudden infant death syndrome (SIDS)

Disorders Causing Single Symptoms

Dermatologic: acute urticaria and angioedema, hereditary angioedema (HAE)

Lower respiratory: acute asthma

Upper respiratory: vocal cord dysfunction, foreign body aspiration, epiglottitis, croup, HAE, tracheomalacia, laryngeal web, vascular rings

Gastrointestinal: pyloric stenosis, malrotation, intussusception, HAE

Foods and Medications

Foods: sulfites, ethanol

Medications: vancomycin, niacin, dystonic reactions (antipsychotics, antidepressants, anti-Parkinsonian)

vasovagal reaction. Symptoms of vasovagal reactions include pallor, diaphoresis, nausea, vomiting, hypotension, bradycardia, and, if severe, syncope. Anaphylactic symptoms, in contrast to vasovagal reaction symptoms, include flushing (instead of pallor) and tachycardia (instead of bradycardia, although bradycardia can occur in anaphylaxis). Other anaphylactic symptoms not seen in vasovagal reactions are urticaria, angioedema, itching, respiratory, and GI symptoms. Symptoms of other anxiety-related disorders, such as panic attacks and hyperventilation, can include the sensation of breathlessness, globus, tachycardia, and even syncope, but are not associated with angioedema, urticaria, or hypotension (Kemp, 2007; Leiberman et al., 2005; Oswalt & Kemp, 2007).

Many conditions may present with a single symptom of anaphylaxis. Urticaria and angioedema may be isolated problems or early symptoms of anaphylaxis, for example, and patients who experience these conditions should be evaluated to determine whether other organ systems are involved. Both acute urticaria and angioedema are most commonly caused by reactions to any variety of allergens. In adults, isolated angioedema not uncommonly occurs with use of ACE inhibitors, and much more rarely can occur with malignancies. Hereditary angioedema (HAE) is a fairly rare autosomal dominant condition caused by deficient or dysfunctional C_1-esterase inhibitor. Although it is a congenital deficiency, most patients develop angioedema initially in adolescence. This angioedema may occur in the extremities; in the bowel wall, leading to severe abdominal pain; or in the tongue and larynx, potentially leading to suffocation. In patients with HAE, complement C_4 levels remain low even between acute attacks—a fact that can be used as a screening test (Zuraw, 2008).

Isolated lower respiratory symptoms can occur with acute asthma attacks, but similar symptoms may also occur during anaphylaxis. Patients who experience such symptoms should be evaluated for concurrent symptoms of upper airway edema, skin, GI, and cardiovascular involvement. A potential cause of isolated upper airway symptoms is vocal cord dysfunction. This condition results from paradoxical adduction of vocal cords during inspiration, can mimic laryngeal edema, and may present with cough, stridor, and wheezing, but patients will not have other manifestations of anaphylaxis (Noyes & Kemp, 2007). Tracheal foreign-body aspiration may cause acute onset of respiratory distress in young children, but also should not have any associated nonrespiratory symptoms. Epiglottitis is another cause of upper airway obstruction, although it is now a rare infection since the introduction of the *Haemophilus influenzae* vaccine; when it does occur, epiglottitis is associated with fever.

Any condition that results in acute shock or collapse can be mistaken for anaphylaxis—for example, septic, hypovolemic, or cardiogenic shock. Myocardial infarction, pulmonary embolism, and strokes are rare in the pediatric age

group. Hypoglycemia, seizures, and acute poisoning may present with collapse. Acute dystonic reactions can present with tongue swelling and chest tightness, and should be suspected in patients treated with antipsychotic, antidepressant, and antiemetic drugs. Sulfites, although less commonly used in restaurants today, can still be found in dried fruits, meats, and wines; these chemicals can cause asthma-like symptoms, flushing, and urticaria in susceptible individuals.

Scombroid poisoning can almost exactly mimic anaphylaxis. In certain fish, such as tuna, mackerel, mahi mahi, anchovy, and herring, endogenous histidine is converted to histamine by bacterial enzymes if the fish is not properly refrigerated. Scombroid poisoning is essentially histamine poisoning. It results in flushing, headaches, nausea, vomiting, diarrhea, and hypotension. This condition should be suspected if several people develop similar symptoms after eating the same fish meal. Also, patients with scombroid poisoning often describe the fish as having a "metallic taste." Allergy tests to the implicated fish will be negative if scombroid poisoning is the true etiology (Chegini & Meltcalfe, 2005).

Many different conditions may cause flushing, but fortunately most are very rare in children. These etiologies include carcinoid, gastrointestinal tumors that produce VIP or substance P; pheochromocytomas; and medullary cancer of the thyroid. Flushing can occur as a result of use of certain medications such as vancomycin, anti-Parkinsonian drugs, and niacin. Consumption of alcohol alone can cause flushing, but may also exacerbate flushing when used concomitantly with certain drugs.

Disorders of histamine excess are caused by the overproduction of endogenous histamine due the abnormal proliferation of histamine containing cells. Mastocytosis is a disorder characterized by abnormal mast cell proliferation. It can be either systemic, with mast cells accumulating in multiple organ systems, or isolated to a single organ, usually the skin. Although exaggerated histamine release can occur from typical IgE-mediated triggers, it may result also from non-IgE-related triggers such as local trauma, RCM, nonallergenic insect venom components, and several medications. In these scenarios, the patient's symptoms may be indistinguishable from the histamine-induced symptoms of anaphylaxis. Affected patients may have elevated tryptase and histamine levels at baseline, as well as specific organ dysfunction due to infiltrating mast cells. Mast cell and basophil leukemia may also be associated with excessive histamine production (Butterfield, 2006).

In infants, the differential should include congenital conditions. Anatomical airway obstruction from laryngeal webs, vascular rings, or tracheomalacia can present with rapid respiratory decompensation, especially in association with acute respiratory infections. Pyloric stenosis, malrotation, and intussusception can present with acute GI symptoms and even shock. A multitude of metabolic disorders can also present with collapse or shock in infants. Child maltreatment and Munchausen's syndrome by proxy should always be considered in cases of rapid onset of unexplained symptoms. Sudden infant death syndrome (SIDS) is a diagnosis of exclusion (Simons, 2007).

PLAN OF CARE

The diagnosis of anaphylaxis is made clinically, and an accurate medical history is the key to its prompt recognition and therapeutic management (Lieberman et al., 2005). Patterns of symptoms consistent with anaphylaxis should be queried, including those related to the specific major organ systems typically involved: upper and lower respiratory tract, skin, GI tract, cardiovascular, and central nervous system. Triggers should be sought, and a complete history of all foods eaten, medications, insect bites, physical activity, and environment prior to onset of the reaction should be reviewed, with specific inquiry into common triggers, such as nuts and seafood. For repeated reactions, keeping a symptom diary can be helpful.

Tolerance of a certain food or medication in the past does not mean that a new allergy to that agent has not developed. Occasionally, a patient may experience a period of relative hyposensitivity that lasts for several days after a significant reaction, during which the patient may come into contact with the allergen and have less or even no symptoms; this may lead to a false assumption that the individual is not allergic to that allergen. For most of these patients, however, re-exposure to the same allergen will cause some type of allergic reaction, although subsequent reactions may be of equal, lesser, or greater severity. The more common scenario is one in which a person is inadvertently exposed to an allergen to which he or she was previously known to be allergic, rather than developing an allergy to a new unrelated allergen. In highly allergic individuals, especially those allergic to nuts and seafood, even trace exposures may result in significant symptoms. Some individuals may become symptomatic if they smell or inhale airborne particles released during cooking, and even small amounts of cross-contamination from shared cooking utensils can result in significant allergic reactions.

There are no highly sensitive laboratory tests available for the diagnosis of anaphylaxis, but laboratory testing is rarely needed to make the diagnosis. Of the multiple mast cell and basophil mediators, commercially available testing exists for only tryptase and histamine. Histamine and tryptase levels do not necessarily correlate with each other, and only one but not the other may be elevated (Lieberman et al., 2005; Simons et al., 2007). Assays for other mast-cell-derived products, specifically β-tryptase (which is more selective for mast cell activation), proteases, and prostaglandin metabolites, may be available in the future.

With tryptase testing, blood tryptase levels should be obtained within 1 to 2 hours but no more than 6 hours after onset of symptoms. A comparison baseline level can be checked 24 hours after resolution of symptoms, or on a preexisting frozen specimen if available. While elevated tryptase levels support the diagnosis of anaphylaxis, a normal level does not rule out anaphylaxis. Tryptase levels are less likely to be elevated in food anaphylaxis compared to other triggers.

Histamine has a short half-life and samples are difficult to collect and handle, making tests targeting histamine less clinically useful in diagnosing anaphylaxis. Plasma histamine can be assayed, but levels should obtained within 10 to 15 minutes but no more than 60 minutes after onset of symptoms and frozen immediately. The histamine metabolite *N*-methylhistamine is more stable, and 24-hr urine collections of *N*-methylhistamine and histamine may be elevated in anaphylaxis. Just as with tryptase, normal histamine levels do not exclude the diagnosis of anaphylaxis.

Other tests may be helpful to aid in the differential diagnosis of anaphylaxis. Pheochromocytomas can result in elevations of blood and urine metanephrines and urinary catecholamines, vanillylmandelic acid (VMA), and homovanillic acid (HMA) levels. Serum serotonin and urinary 5-hydroxyindolacetic acids (5-HIAA) levels are elevated in carcinoid syndrome. Neural crest tumors, certain gastrointestinal tumors, and thyroid carcinomas may secrete various vasoactive mediators and produce elevated levels of urinary VMA, HMA, and serum vasoactive intestinal peptide (VIP), among other substances. None of these vasoactive mediators should be elevated in anaphylaxis (Lieberman et al., 2005).

Allergy testing, whether by skin testing or by measurement of allergen-specific IgE levels in the blood, can be useful to confirm sensitivity to clinically suspected triggers. For non-IgE-mediated triggers, there are no proven laboratory tests that can confirm a causal role. Challenge testing is rarely done to confirm sensitivity, owing to the high inherent risk of triggering another anaphylactic reaction. Sometimes a challenge test can be used to prove that an allergen is not a cause of anaphylaxis in low-risk situations where testing results and clinical history are unclear. Such challenge testing should be performed only by experienced practitioners and only in locations where adequate personnel and equipment are available to treat anaphylactic reactions (Simons et al., 2007).

As with all medical emergencies, the first step in the therapeutic management of anaphylaxis is to assess the patient's airway, breathing, and circulation (ABCs), as well as adequacy of mentation, and must be monitored continually until the reaction has subsided. Patients should be placed in a recumbent position with their legs elevated. In severe cases of anaphylaxis, as much as 50% of intravascular fluid may shift to the extravascular space within 10 minutes. There have been reports of sudden death due to "empty ventricle syndrome" as a result of inadequate venous return and cardiac filling in patients who maintained an upright or sitting posture (Lieberman et al., 2005; Muraro et al., 2007).

The cornerstone of therapeutic management of anaphylaxis is epinephrine, which should be administered simultaneously with the previously mentioned measures. Immediate administration of epinephrine is vital, and delays in its administration have been associated with poor outcomes and death (Kemp, 2008; Sicherer & Simons, 2007). It is unnecessary to wait for the development of potentially life-threatening symptoms (respiratory or cardiac) before epinephrine is administered; this medication should ideally be given at the onset of milder symptoms such as pruritus, urticaria, and angioedema alone. There is *no* absolute contraindication to the use of epinephrine in anaphylaxis. Most subsequent therapeutic interventions depend on the initial response to epinephrine. Poor response or development of adverse effects to epinephrine indicates the need to initiate additional therapies. Anywhere from 16% to 36% of patients will need two or more doses of epinephrine to treat anaphylaxis (Kemp et al., 2008; Sicherer & Simons, 2007).

The preferred route of administration of epinephrine is intramuscularly (IM). Care must be taken to select a needle of sufficient length to avoid subcutaneous delivery, which is not as effective as IM. For most young children, a ½-inch needle is sufficient; however, for obese patients, especially adolescent females, a ¾-inch needle may be necessary. The best location for injection is the lateral thigh, into the vastus lateralis muscle. Studies in children at risk for anaphylaxis showed time to peak plasma epinephrine concentration was 8 ± 2 minutes after injection of 0.3 mg of epinephrine from an EpiPen® intramuscularly in the vastus lateralis, compared to 34 ± 14 minutes after injection of 0.01 mg/kg epinephrine subcutaneously into the deltoid.

Intravenous (IV) administration of epinephrine is effective, but is not preferred over IM injection due to the time and difficulty needed to start an IV line and mix the medication. In addition, there is an increased risk of cardiac arrhythmia with IV administration compared to IM administration. The use of IV epinephrine is usually reserved for patients in cardiac arrest or with profound hypotension that has failed to respond to previous doses of IM epinephrine and fluid resuscitation.

For IM administration, the 1:1,000 concentration of epinephrine is used. The dose is 0.01 mg per kg of body weight (0.01 mL per kg of body weight). The maximum dose is usually 0.3 mg, but doses up to 0.5 mg can be used in very large patients or in severe or nonresponsive cases. The first dose should be administered as soon as possible, and doses can repeated every 5 minutes, or even more frequently if clinically indicated.

For patients with severe hypotension who are unresponsive to IM epinephrine, or in case of cardiac arrest, IV epinephrine may be used instead of IM epinephrine.

The dose of IV epinephrine in terms of mg/kg body weight is equivalent to the IM dose, but care must be taken in that the IV concentration is 1:10,000; thus the dose calculated by volume is 0.1 mL/kg, to a maximum of 3 to 5 mL.

In cases where it is impossible to place an intravenous line, both the intraosseous and endotracheal routes may be used to administer epinephrine. In general, inhaled epinephrine (from inhalers or nebulizers) has less systemic bioavailability and is not as effective as epinephrine delivered by the other routes (Simons et al., 2000). There are currently no commercially available oral preparations of epinephrine.

While tachycardia is the rule in anaphylaxis, paradoxical bradycardia can also be seen. Atropine can be used to treat bradycardia, but only after epinephrine is tried (Kemp et al., 2008; Lieberman et al., 2005; Muraro et al., 2007; Sicherer & Simons, 2007).

Supplemental oxygen should be administered in most patients until adequate oxygen saturation is demonstrated, and in all patients with respiratory symptoms. Adequate respiration should be confirmed, and an artificial airway should be established and maintained if needed. At least one large-bore IV catheter should be placed in case fluid resuscitation is required. Actual hypotension, or clinical signs of hypotension, such as dizziness, light-headedness, or syncope, should initially be treated with boluses of normal saline. It is not uncommon to need 30 to 40 mL/kg or more for children with severe anaphylaxis. Refractory hypotension can be treated with IV dopamine or norepinephrine continuous infusions (Lieberman et al., 2005; Muraro et al., 2007). Some case reports describe refractory hypotension responding to IV vasopressin (Sampson et al., 2006).

Second-line therapies are started after administration of adequate epinephrine, fluids, and assurance of adequate airway, breathing, and circulation. H_1 antihistamines, the most common being diphenhydramine, are usually administered next (Sheikh et al., 2007). The dose of diphenhydramine is 1 mg/kg body weight, to a maximum of 50 mg per dose. Diphenhydramine may be administered through the oral, IV, or IM route. While the dose of diphenhydramine is the same for both the parenteral and oral forms, parenteral dosing will lead to both a more rapid and higher serum level, because oral diphenhydramine has only 40% to 60% oral bioavailability. Oral dosing can be used for patients with milder anaphylactic reactions; if this route of administration is used, note that liquid diphenhydramine is more rapidly absorbed than either the tablet or capsule form.

Glucocorticoids can also be administered orally or IV. Unlike diphenhydramine, most have nearly 100% oral bioavailability, so IV administration may be reserved for those patients who are unable to take oral medications. The dose of oral prednisone is 0.5 to 1 mg/kg, and that for IV methylprednisolone is 1 to 2 mg/kg. Glucocorticoids can be given IM, but this route has no advantage over the IV route; indeed, use of the IM route may cause atrophy at the site of injection and increase the risk for acute avascular necrosis of the hip joint if the steroids are administered in the thigh. Glucocorticoids are recommended in most cases of significant anaphylaxis, as they may decrease the incidence of biphasic or protracted reactions.

Inhaled short-acting beta-agonists, such as albuterol, may be added for relief of wheezing, especially in patients with preexisting asthma. For refractory bronchospasm not responsive to epinephrine and inhaled albuterol, IV aminophylline and isoproterenol have been suggested as potential additional therapies. H$_2$ antihistamines are often added in severe cases, although data regarding their efficacy are lacking. H$_2$ antihistamines can be helpful to protect patients against stress- and steroid-induced gastritis (Lieberman et al., 2005; Muraro et al., 2007).

None of the second-line agents is a substitute for epinephrine. Epinephrine is the drug of choice and should always be given first, with selected second-line agents being administered next as needed.

Special circumstances

Certain situations can decrease the efficacy or increase the possible toxicity of epinephrine. Epinephrine works to reverse the symptoms of anaphylaxis through both α-adrenergic and β-adrenergic actions. Patients being treated with β-adrenergic blockers may be resistant to the β-adrenergic effects of epinephrine, and continued doses of epinephrine can lead to unopposed α-adrenergic vasoconstrictor effects, worsening both blood pressure and perfusion. Significant β-blocking effects can be seen with any form of β-blocker, even eye drops (Kemp et al., 2008).

In the rare pediatric patient being treated with β-adrenergic blocker medications, epinephrine is still the first drug of choice for the therapeutic management of anaphylaxis. However, if clinical improvement is not seen after the first one or two doses, caution with additional doses is needed to avoid paradoxical α-adrenergic-mediated effects. In these patients, therapeutic management with glucagon can be attempted, although this approach has not been studied specifically in anaphylaxis. Glucagon reverses refractory hypotension and bronchospasm by increasing cAMP levels through non-β-receptor mechanisms. This medication can be used as adjunctive therapeutic management for β-blocked patients who do not respond to epinephrine. The recommended dosage for glucagon is 1 to 5 mg (20–30 mcg/kg, up to maximum dose of 1 mg in children) IV over 5 minutes, followed by a 5 to 15 mcg/min infusion titrated to clinical effect (Sampson et al., 2006).

A normal compensatory response to hypotension occurs through the ACE pathway. As a consequence, patients treated with ACE inhibitors may have exaggerated symptoms and not respond as expected to epinephrine.

Tricyclic antidepressants impair epinephrine metabolism, so their use can lead to increased plasma and tissue concentrations of epinephrine. Cocaine and amphetamines sensitize the myocardium to effects of epinephrine, such that increased cardiac toxicity may occur. Certain clinical conditions, such as untreated hyperthyroidism, hypertension, peripheral vascular disease, and ischemic heart disease, can also increase the risk of toxicity of epinephrine, although most of these conditions are rare in children (Kemp et al., 2008; Meuller, 2007). However, none of these situations is an absolute contraindication to the use of epinephrine in anaphylaxis.

DISPOSITION AND DISCHARGE PLANNING

No exact guidelines have been developed regarding how long a period of monitoring is necessary after resolution of an anaphylactic reaction. Patients with milder symptoms, who have rapid resolution of symptoms, and who received only one dose of epinephrine, may require only 6 to 8 hours of observation. For patients with severe anaphylaxis, involving any life-threatening manifestation such as hypotension or respiratory compromise, at least a 24-hr observation period is recommended to monitor for biphasic reactions. Prolonged monitoring is also indicated for patients who require two or more doses of epinephrine. In general, food-associated anaphylactic reactions require a longer observation period than reactions associated with insect stings or drug use. In patients with underlying cardiopulmonary disease, including asthma, and in those who live distant from emergency medical care, longer observation periods should be considered. Protracted reactions may persist for several days and require multiple daily doses of epinephrine or even a continuous epinephrine infusion. These patients need to be observed at least 24 hours after their last dose of epinephrine (Kemp, 2007; Lieberman et al., 2005; Oswalt & Kemp, 2007; Tole & Lieberman, 2007).

Once a person has experienced an anaphylactic reaction, subsequent management consists of measures to reduce the risk of occurrence of future reactions and to reduce risk of harm from future unavoidable exposures to the inciting agent. At the initial follow-up visit, a thorough history and physical examination, along with appropriate diagnostic tests, are indicated to confirm the diagnosis and cause of the anaphylactic reaction. An assessment for risk of future reactions should be made. For example, a patient with intraoperative anaphylaxis would be at a low risk for future reactions outside of the operating room, while a patient with peanut anaphylaxis may be at risk every day. Referral to an allergist for evaluation and education is recommended (Muraro et al., 2007; Simons et al., 2007).

The importance of avoidance of the trigger cannot be overstated. In patients who have developed anaphylaxis, that allergen must be avoided in all quantities, in all forms, and potentially for the rest of their lives. In highly sensitized individuals, even minute traces of allergen can cause allergic reactions. In general, most reactions are stereotypical—that is, future reactions are usually similar to previous reactions. Also, in general, the higher the allergy test level, the more severe the reaction. Nevertheless, exceptions to these patterns are not uncommon. Patients may have more severe reactions with future exposures than they had with initial exposures, and individuals with relatively low allergy test levels may nevertheless have severe reactions. It is not possible in clinical practice to reliably estimate how much allergen will be necessary to trigger a reaction, or how severe the reaction will be upon subsequent exposures to an allergen.

Given these caveats, once a patient has had an anaphylactic reaction, the goal is for "zero" exposure in the future. Until proven otherwise, all potentially cross-reacting agents should be avoided. For example, patients who are allergic to shrimp should avoid other shellfish until they are proven to be safe. Children who are allergic to cow's milk are likely to also be allergic to goat's milk; likewise, patients who are allergic to hen eggs are likely to be allergic to duck eggs. Patients who are allergic to latex need to be warned about possible cross-reactions with foods such as avocado, banana, and kiwi (Lieberman et al., 2005).

While complete avoidance may be possible for patients who are allergic to prescribed medications, it is quite challenging for those who react to foods, over-the-counter medications, insect stings, and other commonly encountered allergens. Families must develop the habits that make accidental re-exposures less likely. For example, in children who are allergic to peanuts, the entire household should become peanut free and no peanut-containing products should be brought into the house. Family members must read the ingredients of all foods and medications, even those considered unlikely to contain the trigger. Ingredients should be reviewed even in products they have safely purchased in the past, as the ingredient lists for those products may change. Allergy warnings, such as statements regarding the possibility of contamination due to shared processing, should be noted. Foods without exact ingredient lists should not be used.

Extra precautions need to be taken when eating outside of the home. Allergic individuals should eat only in restaurants where they are certain their food is free of any ingredients to which they are allergic and prepared in a manner to avoid cross-contamination. In schools, all appropriate staff members—teachers, aides, nurses, cafeteria staff—need to be educated regarding each child's allergies, and they should be supplied with a list of permitted and restricted foods. Rules against sharing of food and classroom projects that use food ingredients should be established. Extra precautions need to be taken on holidays or for class birthday parties where candy and pastries may be brought in from outside the school. These precautions need to extend to out-of-classroom activities and field trips as well.

Initially, young children need to be protected against accidental exposures by their parents and other adult caregivers. As they grow, they should receive age- and development-stage-appropriate education so that they will learn the skills necessary to protect them in any environment they enter (Lieberman et al., 2005; Simons et al., 2007).

Management of any underlying pulmonary (especially asthma) and cardiac disease should be optimized. Any contributing factors, including environmental conditions (temperature, humidity, pollen season), changes in health status prior to the attack (viral infections, stress, fatigue), and menstrual status, should be identified and mitigated if possible. Co-triggers such as alcohol, NSAIDs, and opioids should be addressed and avoided. Any medication that either increases the risk or severity of anaphylactic reaction or interferes with the therapeutic management of anaphylaxis should be stopped or changed if at all possible. These drugs include β-blockers, ACE inhibitors, monoamine oxidase (MAO) inhibitors, and tricyclic antidepressants (Lieberman et al., 2005; Simons, 2008; Simons et al., 2007).

In addition to strict avoidance of the allergen, patients must be prepared to treat anaphylaxis if accidental exposure occurs. As emphasized earlier, epinephrine is the drug of choice to treat anaphylactic reactions, yet multiple studies have shown under-prescription by HCPs and underusage of self-injectable epinephrine by patients and families (Campbell et al., 2008; Krugman et al., 2006; Pongracic & Kim, 2007; Sicherer et al., 2000). Self-injectable epinephrine should be prescribed for all patients who have had an anaphylaxis experience, whether or not a specific trigger has been identified. Also, self-injectable epinephrine should be prescribed for "at risk" patients. An at-risk patient is one who may have not had a full anaphylactic reaction, but who has certain features that nevertheless put him or her at risk for a life-threatening reaction. At-risk individuals included those who have had reactions to trace levels of allergen, those in whom repeated exposure is very likely, and those who have had non-life-threatening reactions to high-risk allergens such as nuts, shellfish, or insect venom. Patients who have asthma or who are being treated with β-blockers or ACE inhibitors can also be considered at risk. Teenagers with food allergies are considered an at-risk group unto themselves. Lastly, patients who live in remote areas with poor medical access or those who had ambiguous initial reactions can also be considered at risk (Sicherer & Simons, 2007; Simons et al., 2007).

Self-injectable epinephrine is available in two dosages: 0.15 mg for patients weighing 15 kg or less, and 0.3 mg for those weighing 30 kg or more. Fortunately, anaphylaxis is uncommon in very young children, but there will be patients weighing less than 15 kg for whom 0.15 mg is too high a dose. Similarly, there is also no fixed dose available for children in the weight range between 15 kg and 30 kg, so the HCP needs to choose whichever dose, 0.15 mg or 0.3 mg, is closer to the patient's weight. A reasonable approach is to use the 0.15 mg dose for children weighing

20 kg or less, and the 0.3 mg dose for those weighing more than 20 kg (Sicherer & Simons, 2007).

It is important that parents, all adult caregivers, and the child, when age appropriate, learn how and when to administer epinephrine to the at-risk child. They should also know how to properly store the units to maintain their potencies, and keep track of expiration dates to assure an effective dose is available at all times. Both of the available brands of self-injectable epinephrine available in the United States come with trainer units that can be dispensed to families to allow them to practice and to teach others proper self-injectable epinephrine technique.

Anywhere from 18% to 35% of patients who experience anaphylaxis require more than one dose of epinephrine (Ellis & Day, 2007; Jarvinen et al., 2008; Mehr et al., 2009; Oren et al., 2007; Tole & Lieberman, 2007). Therefore, patients should be instructed to seek immediate emergency medical care, even if they have had an excellent response to epinephrine, for monitoring and further therapeutic management if necessary. Most patients should be prescribed at least two doses of epinephrine in case a second dose is needed prior to arrival of emergency medical care. All patients who have experienced a biphasic reaction in the past, and any patient who lives far from medical care or who is traveling, will need additional doses. Most school-age children will need an epinephrine unit that can be kept at school.

Patients need to be instructed to carry a self-injectable epinephrine unit with them at all times since accidental contact, especially with foods and insect stings, cannot be predicted. If children are old enough to go out without their caregivers, they should always have at least one friend who knows about their allergies and the epinephrine in case the patient is unable to treat himself or herself.

Unintentional injection of epinephrine into a finger or thumb has the potential to cause severe hypoxic injury from constriction of end arterioles in the digits. Symptoms may include local pain or numbness, pallor, cyanosis, hypothermia, paresthesia, weakened pulse, and potentially necrosis. The rate of occurrence of unintentional injections is unknown, but reports of such events are increasing. There are no accepted recommendations for therapeutic management. Fortunately, most injuries improve with observation and local warming, and they rarely cause permanent harm. Many additional antidotes have been reported, the most common being topical application of nitroglycerin paste and local injection of phentolamine and/or lidocaine. Nevertheless, the decision to treat an accidental epinephrine injection needs to be made on a case-by-case basis (Simons et al., 2009).

A written personalized anaphylaxis emergency plan should be supplied to the family, school, and other caregivers. The information in this plan should include specific delineation of the triggers that need to be avoided, symptoms and signs of anaphylaxis, the need to promptly administer epinephrine and other medications, and circumstances in which to summon emergency rescue and family members (Choo & Sheikh, 2007; Nurastov et al., 2008). A medical identification bracelet or necklace should be considered in all patients who have anaphylaxis, especially school-age and older children who may have reactions away from their caregivers.

Specific therapeutic managements do exist for selected triggers. Most of these should be administered by an experienced allergist and in locations prepared to treat anaphylaxis. It has been well proven in multiple controlled studies that anaphylaxis from Hymenoptera venom stings can almost entirely be prevented with allergen immunotherapy. Allergen vaccination is typically given over a 3- to 5-year period, and can result in long-lasting protection (Chiu & Kelly, 2005). Unfortunately, there is currently no routinely available protocol for allergen desensitization to specific foods. Multiple successful protocols have been recently reported in the research setting, however, and will likely become clinically available in the near future (Plaut et al., 2009).

If a child has an anaphylactic sensitivity to a medication that is absolutely necessary and for which no adequate substitute exists, several options are available. For medications needed urgently and for the short term, such as antibiotics or chemotherapeutic drugs, rapid desensitization may be attempted. Several variations have been proposed, but in general the first dose administered is in the range of 1/10,000th or less of the therapeutic dose. Incremental doubling doses are given every 15 to 20 minutes until the therapeutic dose is reached, usually over approximately 4 to 6 hours. If possible, the oral form of the medication is preferred due to its association with a lower incidence of severe reactions, but most patients require the IV form. The desensitized state will be maintained as long as the medication is administered continually but will be lost if the drug is stopped for more than two to three half-lives, in which case the desensitization procedure needs to be repeated. For medications that are needed daily for long periods of time, such as NSAIDs or prophylactic antibiotics, slow oral desensitization over several days or weeks can be attempted. If this effort proves successful, the desensitized state can be maintained for as long as the drug is taken regularly. For drugs that cause anaphylaxis through non-IgE mechanisms, anaphylaxis can sometimes be avoided if the drug is given very slowly, as in the case of vancomycin.

Pretreatment with a combination of H_1 and H_2 antihistamines and glucocorticoids can block anaphylactic reactions to RCM and many biologic proteins. It is generally not possible to avoid IgE-mediated anaphylactic reactions with pretreatment (Lieberman et al., 2007; Simons et al., 2007).

IMMUNODEFICIENCIES

Brenda Reid

PRIMARY IMMUNODEFICIENCIES

Pathophysiology

Primary immunodeficiency diseases (PIDs) are a genetically heterogeneous group of disorders that affect distinct components of both the innate and adaptive immune system, such as neutrophils, macrophages, dendritic cells, complement, proteins, natural killer cells, and T and B lymphocytes. More than 120 distinct genes have been identified that account for the more than 150 known forms of PID. The genetic defects in the adaptive immune system may affect the function or numbers of the cells of the humoral (B-lymphocyte) immune system, the cellular (T-lymphocyte) immune

system, or both. Defects in the innate immune system affect phagocyte or complement function (Geha et al., 2007).

Epidemiology and etiology

The major hallmark of any primary immunodeficiency is susceptibility to infection (Cooper et al., 2003). The types of infections and clinical manifestations that occur in the various PIDs depend on the genetic defect (Table 29-4). Although PID is usually diagnosed in childhood, patients may present at any age. The incidence of PID is estimated to be 1 per 10,000 individuals, except for selective IgA deficiency, which affects approximately 1 per 500 people. Patients with IgA deficiency are mainly asymptomatic, and usually do not have an increased risk of infections (Lederman, 2000).

Approximately, three-fourths of PIDs are caused by a humoral (B lymphocyte) or combined humoral and cellular abnormalities (B lymphocyte and T lymphocyte). Inheritance of PID may be X-linked, autosomal recessive, or autosomal dominant depending on the disease. PID affects both males and females (Stiehm et al., 2004). The genetic mutation may be de novo with no prior family history (Lederman, 2000) (Table 29-5). Risk factors for immunodeficiency include a family history of immunodeficiency, early infant deaths, parental consanguinity, autoimmunity, and increased incidence of lymphoid malignancy in family members (Lavine & Roifman, 2008).

TABLE 29-4

Infections Associated with Subtypes of PI Deficiencies			
Type	**Types of Infections**	**Organisms**	**Other Features**
Humoral (B cell)	Sinopulmonary, otitis media, gastrointestinal, cellulitis, meningitis, osteomyelitis	Encapsulated bacteria: *Haemophilus*, pneumococci, streptococci Parasites: *Giardia lamblia*, *Cryptosporidium* Virus: enterovirus	Autoimmunity, GI problems including malabsorption
Cellular (T cell or combined T and B cell)	Pulmonary, gastrointestinal, skin	Fungal: *Candida* species, *Pneumocystis jirovecii* Viral: CMV, EBV, RSV, parainfluenza, adenovirus, viral GI disease *Mycobacterium* species	Failure-to-thrive, oral thrush, skin: rashes, dermatitis, postvaccination disease from live viral vaccines
Phagocytic disorders	Severe skin and visceral infections by common pathogens	Bacteria: *Staphylococcus aureus*, *Pseudomonas* species, *Serratia* species, *Klebsiella* species Fungi: *Candida*, *Nocardia*, *Aspergillus*	Granuloma formation, including granulomatous enteritis, poor wound healing, abscesses oral cavity infections, anorectal infections
Complement disorders	Meningitis, septicemia	*Neiserria* infections: meningococcal, pneumococcal	Rheumatoid disorders: lupus-like syndrome, angioedema

Note: Cytomegalovirus (CMV), Epstein-Barr virus (EBV), respiratory syncytial virus (RSV).

Source: Stiehm et al., 2004.

TABLE 29-5

Genetics of Primary Immunodeficiencies

Type	Age of Onset	Laboratory Findings	Associated Findings	Inheritance	Genetics
Humoral					
Agammaglobulinemia	After 6 months of age	Absent IgG, IgA, and IgM Absent antibody responses Absent B cells	Absence of tonsils and lymph nodes	XL AR	*Bruton's tyrosine kinase** *Mutations in μ heavy chain, λ5, Igα, Igβ, BLNK*
Common variable immune deficiency	Any age peak in second decade	Low IgG, ± IgA and IgM Absent antibody responses to vaccines Normal to ↑ numbers of B cells ± Autoimmune cytopenias	Autoimmunity lymphoproliferative and granulomatous diseases Lymph nodes present to increased Hepatomegaly Splenomegaly	10% have positive family history AR or AD	Alterations in *TACI, BAFFR, Msh5* may act as contributors Unknown
Hyper-IgM	After 6 months of age to older	Very low IgG and IgA, ↑ IgM B cell numbers normal to increased	Neutropenia Autoimmunity	XL AR	*CD40 ligand** *CD40, AICDA, UNG*†
Specific antibody deficiency with normal IgG level and normal B cells	Any age	Normal IgG Inability to produce antibody responses to vaccines	Autoimmunity Lymph nodes normal to ↑ Hepatomegaly Splenomegaly ↑ Association in syndromes	AR or AD	Unknown
Transient hypogammaglobulinemia of infancy	After 6 months to 4–5 years	Low IgG and IgA Specific antibodies to vaccines present	Normal lymphoid tissue	Variable	Unknown
Cellular					
SCID	Before 6 months of age	Markedly ↓ T cells ↑ or ↓ B cells B cells§ ↓ NK cells or normal ↓ IgG, IgA, and IgM	Absent lymphoid tissue Absent thymic shadow on x-ray	XL AR	*γc, JAK3, IL7Rα, CD45, CD3γ, CD3ε, CD3ς, RAG ½, Artemis, ADA, Omenn syndrome, CD8, Zap 70, MHC Class I and II, CD25, STAT 5b, and* unknown
Wiscott-Aldrich syndrome	Birth to 1 year of age	T cells progressively ↓ B cells normal ↓ IgM, ± ↑ IgA, IgE ↓ Polysaccharide	↓ Small platelets Lymphopenia Eczema Lymphoma Autoimmunity	XL	*WASP*
Ataxia telangiectasia	Before 3 years of age	↓ IgA, IgE and IgG subclasses Variable antibody deficiency ↑ Alpha fetoprotein Chromosomal instability	Ataxia Telangiectasia Radiation sensitivity ↑ Frequency of malignancy	AR	*ATM*

(Continued)

TABLE 29-5

Genetics of Primary Immunodeficiencies (Continued)

Type	Age of Onset	Laboratory Findings	Associated Findings	Inheritance	Genetics
Cellular (Continued)					
DiGeorge anomaly	Birth to any age	T cell ↓ or normal B cell normal Immunoglobulins normal or ↓ ↓ Calcium, PTH	Heart defects Abnormal facies Autoimmunity	De novo AD	Deletion in chromosome *22q11* or *10p*
Innate Defects					
IRAK4 deficiency	Infancy	Lymphocytes and monocytes Toll and IL-1 receptor Signaling IRAK 4 pathway abnormal	Invasive bacterial infections	AR	*IRAK4*
WHIM syndrome	Any age	Neutropenia Lymphopenia Hypogammaglobulinemia ↓ B cell numbers	Warts Human papillomavirus infections	AD	*CXCR4*
Other					
Hyper-IgE (Job's syndrome)	Any age	Normal T and B cells ↑ IgE Staphyloccus aureus infections	Thickened skin Pneumatoceles Eczema Nail candidiasis Broad nasal tip Delayed shedding of primary teeth Hypermobility of joints	De novo AD	*STAT3* *TYK2*
Chronic mucocutaneous candidiasis	Any age	T and B cell numbers normal Impaired DTH to *Candida* antigens Normal antibodies	Skin and nail changes Autoimmunity	AD AR Sporadic	*AIRE* Unknown
Chronic granulomatous disease	After 6 months of age May present older	Abnormal killing; faulty oxidative burst via NBT or flow cytometry testing Granuloma on x-ray	GI abnormalities Abscesses	De novo XL AR	*CYBB*: electron transport protein (gp91phox)* *CYBA*: electron transport protein (p22phox)†
Complement deficiencies	Any age	Absent CH50 ± Absent alternate pathway Absent specific complement component	Autoimmunity Angioedema	AR AD	C_1 inhibitor‡ C_2, C_8, C_{1q}, C_{1r}, C_{1s}, C_{4A}, C_{4B}, C_3, C_5, C_6, C_7, $C_{8\alpha}$, $C_{8\beta}$, C_9, factors I, H, D, MBP, MASP2, ITGB2, MCP** Properidin*

Note: X-Linked (XL/*), autosomal recessive (AR/†), autosomal dominant (AD/‡), depends on specific genetic defect (§), increased (↑), decreased (↓).
Source: Adapted from Geha et al., 2007.

History

Patients with PID present with recurrent or unusual infections. These infections may be persistent or due to unusual microorganisms that rarely cause problems in healthy people. The warning signs of immunodeficiency are listed in Figure 29-1 (Jeffrey Modell Foundation, 2009). However, not all patients present with infections; some may present with autoimmune diseases or even lymphoid malignancy (Lavine & Roifman, 2008).

History and physical examination should begin with a detailed pregnancy and birth history to identify maternal risk factors, length of gestation, birth weight, and neonatal problems, such as delayed separation of the umbilical cord, jaundice, and respiratory problems. Assessment of growth and development is essential, and height, weight, and head circumference should be plotted over time to evaluate for evidence of failure-to-thrive or poor growth. Development should be assessed to identify any motor (fine or gross),

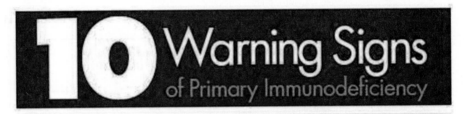

FIGURE 29-1

10 Warning Signs of Primary Immunodeficiency.

Source: Courtesy of Jeffrey Modell Foundation, 2009 and the CDC.

language, cognitive, social, or emotional delays. Chronic disease and some of the syndromes associated with PID, such as ataxia telangiectasia or DiGeorge syndrome, can lead to delay in attaining developmental milestones (Stiehm et al., 2004).

The immunization history should be reviewed, paying close attention to any adverse effects from vaccination. Complications from live viral vaccines, such as acquiring vaccine strain disease, suggest a cellular problem. Failure to develop antibodies to vaccination suggests a humoral deficiency. It is essential to know the vaccination history when assessing antibody function, as inadequate immunization may account for lack of specific vaccine antibody response, rather than an inability to produce antibodies due to an underlying immune problem (Stiehm et al., 2004).

A detailed history of all current and past medications should be completed. Immunosuppressive medications or previous history of immunoglobulin therapy may influence immune evaluation tests. Documentation of other illnesses, including the severity of childhood diseases such as chickenpox, previous hospitalizations, days of school or work absences, and a detailed immune system review including problems such as allergies, anaphylaxis, arthritis, or autoimmunity, is necessary (Stiehm et al., 2004).

Family history should focus on family members with similar diseases, recurrent infections, unexplained death, or autoimmune diseases. Identifying consanguinity and ethnicity is necessary, as certain PIDs are more common in particular ethnic populations (e.g., SCID in Navajo patients). History of infectious illnesses, such as tuberculosis, in other family members that may cause illness in the PID-affected patient should be obtained. Similarly, social history may reveal exposures to potentially harmful agents. Determination of attendance at school or daycare programs can help to identify the risk of exposure to respiratory pathogens (Stiehm et al., 2004).

The infection history may offer insights into the component of the immune system that is most likely affected (see Table 29-4). For example, infections with Gram-negative organisms, viruses, protozoa, fungi, or mycobacteria are more common in patients with cellular immunodeficiencies. Patients with humoral immunodeficiencies are prone to infections with Gram-positive encapsulated organisms and *Mycoplasma* species. Individuals with innate defects are predisposed to staphylococcal and Gram-negative infections, particularly those involving *Klebsiella* and *Serratia marcescens*; by comparison, recurrent neisserial infections are hallmarks of complement deficiencies (Lederman, 2000). The infection history should focus on the age of onset, duration, frequency, sites, organisms, treatment, and response to therapy (Stiehm et al., 2004).

Physical examination of patients suspected of having PIDs begins with an assessment of the patient's appearance, demeanor, and level of activity. These factors are suggestive of the patient's overall state of health. Vital signs including oxygen saturation, if cardiac or respiratory symptoms are present, should be measured. Characteristic facial features or skeletal anomalies are part of certain syndromes associated with PID, such as DiGeorge syndrome, hyper-IgE syndrome, and cartilage hair hypoplasia. Careful physical examination will uncover these changes. In addition, close attention to the patient's nutritional state, looking for signs of muscle wasting or atrophy from failure-to-thrive, is an essential part of the assessment. Evaluation of potential sites of infection, such as the ears, chest, skin, and joints, is imperative. A detailed assessment of immune organs, such as the tonsils, lymphoid tissue, and spleen, is also of primary importance. Lymphoid tissue should be assessed for size; in PID, this tissue may be either absent, small, or enlarged. The size of lymphoid tissue aids in specific diagnosis of PID. For example, the absence of lymphoid tissue should lead the HCP to suspect a form of SCID or X-linked agammaglobulinemia (Stiehm et al., 2004).

Early diagnosis of PID is important so that appropriate therapy may be instituted before there is end-organ damage occurs. For patients with antibody deficiency, early institution of gammaglobulin therapy can prevent the development of pulmonary complications from repeated lung infections (Wood et al., 2007). Severe forms of immunodeficiency, such as SCID, should be viewed as a medical emergency. Furthermore, early diagnosis is essential for making genetic information available to the families of affected individuals, so that other family members who might potentially be affected by the same defect may be identified and treated (Lederman, 2000).

Differential diagnosis

In the evaluation of PID, the HCP should consider non-immune causes of recurrent infections, such as increased exposure to pathogens at daycare programs or from older siblings at home. These children have normal growth and development, respond quickly to appropriate treatment, recover completely, and appear healthy between infections. They have a normal physical examination and laboratory evaluation (Stiehm et al., 2004).

Atopic disease may also be mistaken for recurrent upper respiratory infections. In these circumstances, children may have coughing and wheezing following viral respiratory tract infections. Such symptoms are frequently misdiagnosed as pneumonia rather than asthma. Children with atopic disease are also more likely to develop sinusitis, otitis media, and rhinitis due to their inflamed respiratory tissues. They have normal growth and development, and may have characteristic features on examination, such as allergic shiners (Stiehm et al., 2004).

As part of the diagnostic process, it is important to consider secondary causes of immunodeficiency, such as underlying chronic disease, medications, burns, malignancy, and infectious diseases (including HIV) that may account for the child's infections. Secondary immunodeficiencies may present in very similar manner to primary immunodeficiencies—that is, with failure-to-thrive and a sickly appearance. In secondary immunodeficiency, susceptibility to infections may be due to structural anomalies, inadequate clearance of secretions, obstruction, cardiovascular problems, a foreign body, resistant organisms, or continuous reinfection due to environmental exposures (Jaffe et al., 2001).

Plan of care

Evaluation of PID should focus on the component of the immune system that is most likely to be involved based on the initial history. Initial screening tests should include a complete blood count and differential. If lymphopenia is noted from the absolute lymphocyte count, a significant immune problem should be suspected. The CBC will also identify the presence of anemia, thrombocytopenia, or neutropenia, which may be associated with certain immunodeficiencies, such as common variable immune deficiency (CVID) (Lederman, 2000).

Quantitative immunoglobulins (IgG, IgA, IgM, IgE) and total protein and albumin (adjusted to the patient age) should also be measured. This kind of testing will identify patients with hypogammaglobulinemia. The total protein and albumin measurements will help to rule out a secondary loss of protein due to primary kidney or gastrointestinal disease as a cause of the low immunoglobulins. Evaluation of IgE will identify allergy or syndromes associated with elevated IgE, such as hyper-IgE syndrome. Evaluation for antibody deficiency includes measurement of specific antibody titers to vaccinations to evaluate the function of the IgG. If specific antibody titers are absent at initial evaluation, then challenging the patient with both protein and polysaccharide vaccines may be warranted (Lederman, 2000). As part of this assessment it is necessary to evaluate antibody production over time, as some patients will be able to initially respond to vaccination, but will not be able to sustain the antibody response. In young children with hypogammaglobulinemia, a transient form of hypogammaglobulinemia that will eventually normalize should be considered. Although difficult to predict at presentation, the pattern that patients follow assists in diagnosis. Invasive infections and low antibody levels at presentation are significant in predicting a more permanent antibody deficiency (Dalal & Roifman, 2001).

Complement activity may be evaluated by measuring the patient's total hemolytic complement (CH50); this assessment is warranted in patients who present with recurrent sepsis from pneumococcal or neisserial organisms. A normal CH50 excludes nearly all hereditary complement deficiencies. In patients with low but not absent CH50 and C_3, evaluation of the alternate complement pathway may be warranted (Stiehm et al., 2004).

Evaluation of phagocytic cells includes measurement of the absolute neutrophil count to rule out congenital agranulocytosis or cyclic neutropenia. To evaluate for chronic granulomatous disease (CGD—the most common phagocytic function disorder), a nitroblue tetrazolium (NBT) dye test measuring the oxidative metabolic response of neutrophils should be performed (Lederman, 2000).

Diagnosis of cellular immunodeficiencies starts with a total lymphocyte count and immunophenotyping of the absolute numbers of subsets of T and B lymphocytes to determine which of the subsets are abnormal. The results of immunophenotyping will aid the HCP in deciding which genetic defects to sequence (Lavine & Roifman, 2008).

The function of immune cells may be evaluated by performing delayed-type hypersensitivity (DTH) skin tests. A standardized panel of antigens prepared for DTH testing should be used. The presence of one or more positive delayed-type skin tests is generally indicative of intact cell-mediated immunity. Note that these tests are useful only in children older than 1 to 2 years, as even normal children are usually unresponsive to DTH testing in infancy (Lederman, 2000).

In specialized laboratories, lymphocyte function can be assessed by examining the patient's responses to mitogens (nonspecific immune stimulators) and selected antigens, which rely on immunological memory for infections that the patient has previously undergone. New testing methods, such as T-lymphocyte receptor excision circle measurement (TREC), can quantify the thymic gland's output of lymphocytes. Measurement of metabolic enzymes such as adenosine deaminase (ADA) or purine nucleoside phosphorylase (PNP) may be indicated in patients suspected of having SCID (Lavine & Roifman, 2008).

Other diagnostic tests may include radiological imaging of suspected sites of infection and skeletal radiographs to evaluate for associated skeletal abnormalities. Pulmonary function testing to evaluate lung function may be indicated. Once PID has been confirmed, genetic analysis to confirm the genetic abnormality should be performed (Lederman, 2000).

Specific therapy depends on the underlying PID (Table 29-6). All PIDs require immediate treatment of the presenting infection with antibiotic, antiviral, or antifungal agents. Management of associated symptoms, such as hypocalcemia in microdeletion 22q11 syndrome, and associated autoimmune symptoms is essential. To prevent further infections, HCPs may provide patients with suspected PID with leukocyte-poor, virus-free blood transfusions and deliver postexposure infectious prophylaxis for chickenpox with Varicella zoster immune globulin. Similarly, live viral vaccines should be avoided to prevent vaccine strain infections in PID-affected patients (Stiehm et al., 2004).

For some PIDs, complement deficiencies and prophylactic antibiotics may be the only preventive infection treatment offered. Other types of PID may require prophylaxis

TABLE 29-6

Management of Patients with Primary Immunodeficiency

Primary Immunodeficiency Disorder	Treatment Options
Humoral	Antibiotics
	Immunoglobulin (IVIG or SCIG)
Cellular	BMT*
	Experimental gene therapy[†]
	Immunoglobulin
	Antibiotic prophylaxis
	Antifungal prophylaxis
Phagocytic	Antibiotic prophylaxis
	Antifungal prophylaxis
	Gamma-interferon
	BMT if severe clinical course*
	Experimental gene therapy[†]
Complement	Antibiotic prophylaxis
	Pneumococcal and meningococcal vaccines

Note: Intravenous immunoglobulin (IVIG), subcutaneous immunoglobulin (SCIG), bone marrow transplant (BMT).

*Option for patients with SCID, CD40 ligand deficiency, Wiscott-Aldrich syndrome, or CGD.

[†]Available for patients with ADA-deficient SCID, γcSCID, or CGD.

Source: Adapted from Buckley, 2008.

with antibiotic, antifungal, or antiviral agents. Prophylaxis may also be considered during the diagnostic phase of all PID to prevent further infections (Lederman, 2000).

If antibody deficiency is present, treatment with immunoglobulin therapy is required for the remainder of the patient's life. The goal of immunoglobulin therapy is to replace the antibodies that the patient cannot produce. Patients may opt to receive this therapy by either the intravenous or subcutaneous route of administration. Intravenous infusions are usually given at a dose of 400 to 600 mg/kg every 3 to 4 weeks. Subcutaneous infusions are usually calculated at 120% of the patient's IV dose divided into a several times-a-week schedule (Berger, 2008). Once immunoglobulin therapy is initiated, patients require ongoing monitoring of their IgG levels to ensure that they are adequately replaced (Lederman, 2000).

Bone marrow transplant (BMT) may be the only treatment option for patients with SCID: Without a functional immune system, the child will not survive. BMT is also considered for patients with Wiscott-Aldrich syndrome, chronic granulomatous disease, and forms of combined immune deficiency (Cooper et al., 2003). The goal of BMT in PID is to replace the defective immune system with one from a healthy donor. In centers specializing in BMT for PID, cure may be attained in as many as 95% of patients, depending on the condition of the patient at the time of BMT and the available donor source. To maximize the opportunity for success with BMT and normal life span, it is imperative that PIDs are recognized early, so that patients receive BMT when they are in optimal condition (Slatter & Gennery, 2008).

Another treatment option for severe forms of PID is gene therapy. This treatment is currently available only under research protocols for ADA deficiency, X-linked SCID, and CGD. Enzyme replacement therapy is an option for patients with ADA deficiency (Lederman, 2000).

Disposition and discharge planning

Prior to initiation of therapy, patients with PID and their families require education regarding the diagnosis and proposed treatment plan. These materials should include information about medications and their potential side effects, proposed duration of therapy, required laboratory monitoring, and plans for follow-up. Referral of families for genetic counseling is an essential part of the management of PID, and children with PID will need to be re-referred as they reach adulthood (Buckley, 2008).

Immunoglobulin therapy is associated with specific concerns, including the need for informed consent/permission to treatment with a blood product, education regarding lifelong therapy, treatment protocols for infusion specific to the chosen route of administration, monitoring of lot numbers and dates of infusion, and potential reactions and risks of treatment (Wood et al., 2007). The family needs a plan for reporting and managing gammaglobulin adverse reactions, as many reactions may occur once the patient is discharged home (Garcia-Lloret et al., 2008). Many families will eventually be able to manage this treatment in the home setting, either independently or with the assistance of a home care agency (Bhole et al., 2008).

The lifelong nature of the treatment for PID poses unique challenges when it comes to health insurance. Many of the treatments are extremely expensive, such as gammaglobulin and BMT, and the cost of these therapies combined with the need for lifelong treatment makes adequate health insurance coverage essential. HCPs need to be aware of individual coverage and work with the patient and family to ensure ongoing treatment is available (Buckley, 2008).

School personnel need education about the child's particular disease, management of infections, vaccine restrictions, prescribed therapy, and precautionary measures that can minimize infection in the school. Caregivers and HCPs should be familiar with the laws in their area that allow for equal access to education for patients with chronic diseases as well as programs that may assist families financially to facilitate the child's school attendance (Buckley, 2008).

Discharge planning should also focus on life management issues related to living with PID. Challenges of living with these diseases can cause significant stress for the patient and family, and HCPs should be vigilant for signs of more serious psychological concerns. Learning effective coping strategies can assist families to deal with the chronicity of PID. Establishing a good support system through family members, friends, health care team members, and peers affected with PID can facilitate coping. Support organizations for patients with PID are available as a resource for families (Buckley, 2008).

SECONDARY IMMUNODEFICIENCY: HUMAN IMMUNODEFICIENCY VIRUS (HIV)

Pathophysiology

The HIV virus is a lenitivirus in the retrovirus family. Infection occurs when the virus enters the body and binds to CD4 receptors on host T lymphocytes. Through a complex process of specific HIV glycoprotein binding to host T-lymphocyte CD4 receptor and chemokine coreceptor 5 (CCR5) coreceptors, HIV fuses its envelope with the lymphocyte cell membrane and enters the host cell. Within 5 days after exposure, the infected cells make their way to the lymph nodes and eventually to the peripheral blood, where viral replication rapidly ensues. The time between infection and antibody response is known as the "window period." Seroconversion to HIV antibody positivity may occur as early as 10 to 14 days after infection, but usually occurs 3 to 4 weeks after the initial contact. Nearly all patients seroconvert with 6 months of infection. HIV infection is a lifelong, as the virus infects long-lived memory T cells (Simpkins et al., 2009).

The pathogenesis of HIV relates to the effect of HIV replication on the immune responses of the patient. The HIV viral burden directly and indirectly mediates CD4+ T-cell destruction in the thymus, bone marrow, lymphoid organs, and nervous system. The end result is failure of T-cell production and eventual immune suppression of both the cellular and humoral arms of the immune system (Calles et al., 2009). The polyclonal activation of B lymphocytes results in increased immunoglobulin production. Despite the high levels of IgG, most pediatric patients have poorly functioning antibody, impaired neutrophil function, leucopenia, abnormal cytokine production, and splenic dysfunction, which collectively lead to increased susceptibility to bacterial infections (Moylett & Shearer, 2006).

Epidemiology and etiology

An estimated 33 million people worldwide are living with HIV infection. Most reside in developing countries, with approximately two-thirds living in sub-Saharan Africa. The annual rate of new HIV infections is believed to have peaked at more than 3 million in the late 1990s. Approximately 14% of these infections occur in children older than 14 years of age; 10,000 are infected with HIV/AIDS and of those 100 die annually in the United States

Moylett & Shearer, 2006). Since the 1990s, the pediatric burden of HIV infection has largely shifted from very young children to the adolescent age group. This change is attributed to children who acquired HIV perinatally now surviving into adolescence, and the increasing number of new cases in the 13- to 24-year age group, in whomtransmission is from sexual contact and contact with infected blood (Aggarwal & Rein, 2003).

Presentation

The history should be carefully obtained to elicit possible exposures to the HIV virus. Viral transmission of HIV infection may occur through sexual intercourse, exposure to contaminated blood, or perinatal transmission. The Centers for Disease Control and Prevention (CDC, 2008) defines the clinical stages of HIV infection as not symptomatic, mildly symptomatic, moderately symptomatic, and severely symptomatic (Table 29-7).

Infants acquiring HIV via the maternal–fetal transmission route rarely manifest the acute viral syndrome of HIV, and are usually asymptomatic. Infrequently, infection acquired in utero may present in a similar manner to any other congenitally acquired viral infection: growth retardation, skin rash, lymphadenopathy, hepatosplenomegaly, and cytopenias (Havens et al., 2009).

The older HIV patient presents with the acute viral syndrome. Symptoms at the time of infection may include fever, fatigue, headache, myalgias, arthralgias, pharyngitis, lymphadenopathy, oral and genital ulcers, nausea, diarrhea, rash, aseptic meningitis, weight loss, thrush, or peripheral neuropathies. These symptoms generally occur within days to up to 10 weeks of the initial infection (Aggarwal & Rein, 2003).

Advances in management of HIV infection have dramatically decreased the incidence of opportunistic infections and other infectious complications (Table 29-7). Differences between the clinical entities of HIV in children and adults have been noted, however. Untreated children have a more rapidly progressive course, and *Pneumocystis jirovecii* infection and encephalopathy occur early in patients who experience rapid progression. Children also have a higher incidence of bacteremia and lymphocytic interstitial pneumonitis (LIP). Conversely, they seldom develop Kaposi sarcoma, toxoplasmosis, cryptococcosis, and CMV infections (Moylett & Shearer, 2006).

Failure-to-thrive or wasting may indicate HIV infection. Assessment of development should focus on developmental milestones, as delays—particularly impairment in the development of expressive language—may indicate HIV encephalopathy. Similarly, loss of previously attained milestones may indicate a CNS insult due to progressive HIV or opportunistic infection. In older children, behavioral abnormalities, such as loss of concentration or memory, may indicate HIV encephalopathy (Moylett & Shearer, 2006).

TABLE 29-7

HIV Clinical Classification System

Category N: Not Symptomatic

Children with no signs or symptoms considered to be the result of HIV infection or who have only one of the conditions listed in category A

Category A: Mildly Symptomatic

Children with two or more of the following conditions but none of the conditions listed in categories B or C:
- Lymphadenopathy (> 0.5 cm at more than two sites; bilateral + one site)
- Hepatomegaly
- Splenomegaly
- Dermatitis
- Parotitis
- Recurrent or persistent upper respiratory infection, sinusitis, or otitis media

Category B: Moderately Symptomatic

Children who have symptomatic conditions attributed to HIV infection, other than those listed for category A or category C; examples of conditions in clinical category B include, but are not limited to, the following:
- Anemia (< 8 mg/dL), neutropenia (< 1,000/mm^3), or thrombocytopenia (< 100,000/mm^3) persisting ≥ 30 days
- Bacterial meningitis, pneumonia, or sepsis (single episode)
- Candidiasis, oropharyngeal (i.e., thrush) persisting > 2 months in children aged > 6 months of age
- Cardiomyopathy
- Cytomegalovirus infections with onset before 1 month of age
- Diarrhea, recurrent or chronic
- Hepatitis
- Herpes simplex virus stomatitis, recurrent (i.e., more than two episodes within 1 year)
- Herpes simplex virus bronchitis, pneumonitis, or esophagitis with onset before 1 month of age
- Herpes zoster (i.e., shingles) involving at least two distinct episodes or more than one dermatome
- Leiomyosarcoma
- Lymphoid interstitial pneumonia or pulmonary lymphoid hyperplasia complex
- Nephropathy
- Nocardiosis
- Fever lasting > 1 month
- Toxoplasmosis with onset before 1 month of age
- Varicella, disseminated (i.e., complicated chickenpox)

Category C: Severely Symptomatic

Children who have any condition listed in the 1987 surveillance case definition for AIDS, with the exception of lymphoid interstitial pneumonia (which is a category B condition)

Source: Centers for Disease Control and Prevention, 2008.

Few physical findings are specific to HIV infection; rather, many findings in patients are caused by opportunistic infections. Assessment starts with evaluation of height, weight, and head circumference. These measurements should be performed over time to evaluate for failure-to-thrive and signs of encephalopathy, which is evidenced by loss in head circumference. Attention should also focus on changes in fat distribution that may indicate the lipid abnormalities and insulin resistance that has been described in HIV (Moylett & Shearer, 2006).

Parotid enlargement, tonsillar hypertrophy, and aphthous ulcers are findings on the head and neck examination that are suggestive of HIV infection. The oral pharynx should be examined for signs of oral candidiasis (thrush)—a common infection found in children with HIV. If oral candidiasis is found, consideration should be given to the presence of candidal esophagitis, which may cause feeding difficulties or retrosternal pain. The eyes should be examined for signs of CMV retinitis (Moylett & Shearer, 2006).

Evaluation of the pulmonary system is important to look for signs of lung disease from infection or LIP. Cardiac examination should focus on the presence of cardiomyopathy or congestive heart failure. In the abdominal examination, hepatomegaly and splenomegaly, are common findings in pediatric HIV (Moylett & Shearer, 2006).

Close examination of the lymphoid system is imperative. HIV-related findings include generalized cervical, axillary, or inguinal lymphadenopathy. Lymphadenopathy may be the first sign of infection during the asymptomatic phase of HIV, but may regress during periods of well-controlled disease or in end-stage AIDS. New nodes in patients on antiretroviral therapy may indicate that the disease has progressed, and that treatment failure has occurred. A new single large node is suspicious for lymphoma (Moylett & Shearer, 2006).

Neurological changes are common findings in HIV-infected patients, derived from both opportunistic infections and associated encephalopathy. Motor development delay, hypotonia, hypertonia, and pyramidal tract signs may indicate progressive HIV encephalopathy or opportunistic CNS infection. Spastic diplegia and oral motor dysfunction are early signs of encephalopathy, whereas acquired microcephaly and cerebral atrophy are later signs that suggest a poor prognosis. Ischemic and hemorrhagic strokes may occur in pediatric HIV, but they are usually related to infection or other mechanisms rather than hypercoagulable states (Moylett & Shearer, 2006).

Several skin findings are associated with HIV infection, including HIV dermatitis. An erythematous and papular rash, it is found in approximately 25% of children with this disease. Bleeding or bruising may be observed on the skin and mucous membranes of children with associated immune thrombocytopenia. Infectious rashes are also seen, such as vesicular lesions in dermatomal distribution from reactivation of herpes zoster, and candidal dermatitis that is unresponsive to the usual therapy (Moylett & Shearer, 2006).

Other physical findings may include digital clubbing from chronic lung disease and edema. Non-pitting edema is related to hypoalbuminemia caused by HIV nephropathy or malnutrition. Pitting edema suggests congestive heart failure (Moylett & Shearer, 2006).

Differential diagnosis

The differential diagnoses for HIV should include primary immunodeficiency disorders, many of which present in a similar manner. Of note, patients with severe combined immunodeficiency experience opportunistic infections and failure-to-thrive, and present at a similar age to patients with perinatally acquired HIV infection; patients with common variable immune deficiency typically have lymphadenopathy and associated lymphopenia (Stiehm et al., 2004).

Cancer should also be considered in the differential diagnosis for HIV. Undiagnosed cancer states may be associated with symptoms similar to the acute viral syndrome associated with HIV. Moreover, the chemotherapeutic agents used to treat cancer can render the patient susceptible to opportunistic infections. Other diseases requiring significant immunosuppressive medications should also be considered as potential causes of the symptoms (Simpkins et al., 2009).

Finally, consideration should be given to other infections that may present in a similar clinical manner. These infections include tuberculosis, Epstein-Barr virus, cytomegalovirus, and cryptococcal infections. They should be considered in the differential diagnosis in the absence of HIV antibody detection (Simpkins et al., 2009).

Plan of care

Several laboratory tests have been approved for screening and diagnosing HIV infection. All require informed consent/permission from the patient or caregiver prior to initiating testing. The choice of test depends on the patient's age and clinical indication (Table 29-8). Most commercially available tests detect HIV antibody. For patients older than 18 months of age, the confirmed presence of antibody is considered diagnostic of HIV infection. There are also newer rapid tests that detect antibody in blood or saliva and provide an antibody result in approximately 20 minutes. Positive antibody results from these tests should be confirmed by standard antibody tests (Simpkins et al., 2009).

Specific HIV viral detection using DNA or RNA polymerase chain reaction (PCR) is necessary when antibody testing is nondiagnostic. HIV DNA or RNA PCR is necessary for infants born to HIV-positive mothers, who will test positive due to maternal transfer of antibodies across the placenta, to confirm HIV infection. HIV PCR testing is also necessary for older children with symptoms of acute retroviral syndrome, as they may not have detectable viral antibodies. A definitive diagnosis of HIV infection requires

TABLE 29-8

HIV Screening and Diagnostic Testing		
Who	**What**	**Where**
HIV-exposed newborns	DNA PCR	Optional at birth; 2 to 3 weeks, 1 to 2 months, at or after 4 months
	Antibody	Optional after 12 months to confirm seronegativity
Children of HIV-positive mother	Antibody*	No maximum age
Adolescents	Antibody	Single screen at or after age 13 years; repeat annually if sexually active or injecting drugs
Clinical suspicion	Antibody†	Any age if clinical presentation is suggestive of underlying HIV infection

*Use infant testing algorithm if antibody positive and younger than 18 months of age.

†Use additional HIV RNA testing if clinical presentation is suggestive of acute retroviral syndrome.

Source: Simpkins et al., 2009.

that two different specimens test positive using appropriate techniques based on the patient age and the clinical situation (Simpkins et al., 2009).

Following antibody detection, further testing is indicated to determine the stage of HIV disease and to assist with treatment decisions. The CD4 T-cell count is a reliable indicator of the patient's current risk for opportunistic infections. CD4 counts will vary over time, and serial counts are usually a better measure of any significant changes. After seroconversion, CD4 counts tend to decrease and continue to decline over time (Moylett & Shearer, 2006).

Measurement of the viral load is a surrogate marker for the viral replication rate—most of the viral replication occurs in the lymph nodes rather than in the peripheral blood. The rate of progression to AIDS and death is related to the viral load: Patients with high viral loads are at greater risk to die from AIDS than those with undetectable viral loads (Brichard & Van der Linden, 2009).

Measurement of CBC and differential enables the HCPs to identify those patients with thrombocytopenia (which affects 10% of patients at the time of diagnosis), anemia (20% of patients at diagnosis), and neutropenia (10% of patients with early disease; 50% of patients with AIDS). Kidney, liver, and pancreatic function tests should be performed to detect impairment as a result of medication, HIV, or opportunistic infections. Amylase levels should

be evaluated to detect parotitis. Measurement of immunoglobulin levels over time can detect both hypergammaglobulinemia, which is associated with disease progression, and hypogammaglobulinemia, which is associated with poor prognosis (Brichard & Van der Linden, 2009).

Brain computed tomography (CT) scans demonstrate the presence of white matter degeneration, atrophy, and calcifications of the basal ganglia associated with progressive HIV encephalopathy. Evaluation of the kidneys for HIV nephropathy by ultrasound, renal CT, renal scintigraphy, or renal gallium scanning should be performed. Abdominal ultrasound will identify the calcifications in the liver, spleen, or kidneys observed in *P. jirovecii* pneumonia (formerly known as *P. carinii* pneumonia [PCP]), *Mycobacterium avium* complex (MAC), *Bartonella,* and *Histoplasma* infections. Abdominal CT scanning will identify the mesenteric adenopathy found in MAC infections (Moylett & Shearer, 2006).

The goal of anti-HIV antiretroviral therapy is to maximize the quality and longevity of the patient's life by achieving complete suppression of viral replication, preservation, or restoration of immunologic function and prevention of or improvement in clinical disease (Table 29-9). Recommendations on when to initiate therapy are more aggressive in infants and children because of the more rapid progression of the disease in the pediatric population and the differing ranges of normal

TABLE 29-9

Recommended Antiretroviral Regimens for Initial Therapy for HIV Infection in Children	
Non-nucleoside Reverse Transcriptase Inhibitor-Based Regimens	
Preferred regimen	Children ≥ 3 years: two NRTIs plus efavirenz*
Alternative	Children < 3 years or who cannot swallow capsules: two NRTIs plus nevirapine*
	Two NRTIs plus nevirapine (children ≥ 3 years)
Protease Inhibitor-Based Regimens	
Preferred regimen	Two NRTIs plus lopinavir/ritonavir
Alternative	Two NRTIs plus nelfinavir (children > 2 years)
Use in special circumstances	One or two NRTIs plus nelfinavir plus (efavirenz [children ≥ 3 years] or nevirapine)
	Zidovudine plus lamivudine plus abacavir
	Two NRTIs plus low-dose ritonavir plus (indinavir or fosamprenavir or saquinavir), only in adolescents who can receive adult doses
Two-Drug NRTI Backbone Options (for Use in Combination with Additional Drugs	
Preferred	Zidovudine plus (lamivudine or didanosine or emtricitabine)
	Didanosine plus (lamivudine or emtricitabine)
Alternative	Abacavir plus (zidovudine or lamifudine or emtricitabine or Stavudine)
	Stavudine plus (lamivudine or emtricitabine)
Use in special circumstances	Stavudine plus didanosine

*Efavirenz is currently available only in capsule form; nevirapine would be the preferred non-nucleoside reverse transcriptase inhibitor (NNRTI) for children younger than 3 years of age or who require a liquid formulation. Amprenavir should not be administered to children younger than 4 years of age.

Source: National Institute of Health, 2009.

TABLE 29-10

Indications for Initiation of Antiretroviral Therapy		
Age	**Criteria**	**Recommendation**
< 12 months	Regardless of clinical signs and symptoms, immune status or viral load	Treat
1 to < 5 years	AIDS or significant HIV-related signs and symptoms[a]	Treat
	CD4 < 25% regardless of symptoms or HIV RNA level[b]	Treat
	Asymptomatic or mild symptoms[c] and CD4 ≥ 25% and HIV RNA ≥ 100,000 copies/mL	Defer[d]
	Asymptomatic or mild symptoms[c] and CD4 ≥ 25% and HIV RNA < 100,000 copies/mL	
≥ 5 years	AIDS or significant HIV-related signs and symptoms[a]	Treat
	CD4 < 350 cells/mm³ [e]	Treat
	Asymptomatic or mild symptoms[c] and CD4 ≥ 350 cells/mm³ and HIV RNA ≥ 100,000 copies/mL	Consider
	Asymptomatic or mild symptoms[c] and CD4 ≥ 350 cells/mm³ and HIV RNA < 100,000 copies/mL	Defer[d]

[a]CDC clinical categories C and B (except for the following category B conditions: single episode of serious bacterial infection or lymphoid interstitial pneumonitis).

[b]The data supporting this recommendation are stronger for patients with a CD4 percentage less than 20% than for those with a CD4 percentage between 20% and 24%.

[c]CDC clinical category A or N or the following category B conditions: single episode of serious bacterial infection or lymphoid interstitial pneumonitis.

[d]Clinical and laboratory data should be reevaluated every 3 to 4 months.

[e]The data supporting this recommendation are stronger for patients with a CD4 count less than 200 cells/mm³ than for those with CD4 counts between 200 and 350 cells/mm³.

Source: National Institute of Health, 2009.

CD4 counts by age. Current NIH treatment guidelines are outlined in Table 29-10. In clinical trials, early institution of antiretroviral therapy in infants younger than 1 year of age has been shown to reduce infant mortality by 76% and HIV progression by 75%. Children older than 1 year of age have less risk of disease progression; in these patients, treatment is initiated based on significant signs and symptoms (Brichard & Van der Linden, 2009) (Table 29-8). Important issues to consider when selecting drugs for HIV treatment include the age, weight, and pubertal stage of the patient; the baseline HIV resistance pattern; the patient's likelihood of developing resistance to selected drugs; the likelihood of pregnancy while the patient is taking the selected drugs; and the ease of administration of the drugs (e.g., formulation, schedule, food restrictions) (Simpkins et al., 2009).

Primary prevention of opportunistic infections, for which drugs are selected based on patient age and CDC guidelines, is recommended. The most common opportunistic infection is PCP, and cotimoxazole is recommended as prophylaxis for all HIV-exposed infants until HIV infection is excluded, for all HIV-exposed infants younger than 1 year of age, and for all children and adolescents older than 1 year of age whose CD4 values fall into the severe immunosuppression category. Primary prevention of MAC infections by using azithromycin or clarithromycin is recommended for the following groups:

- Children older than 6 years of age with CD4 counts < 50 cells/mm³
- Children 2 to 5 years of age with CD4 counts < 76 cells/mm³
- Children 1 to 2 years of age with CD4 counts < 500 cells/mm³
- Children younger than 1 year of age with CD4 counts < 750 cells/mm³

Toxoplasmosis is less common in children, but its prevention is recommended for HIV-infected children who are seropositive for *Toxoplasma* immunoglobulin G and have severe immunosuppression, defined as follows:

- CD4 counts < 15% for children younger than 6 years of age
- CD4 counts < 100 cells/mm³ for children younger than 6 years of age (CDC, 2009)

The immunization schedule for children with HIV infection is the same as that for their healthy peers, albeit with some exceptions. Severely symptomatic patients with CD4 percentages less than 15% or CD4 counts of less than 200 cells/mm³ should not receive live viral vaccines due to the risk of vaccine-acquired disease. Children with higher CD4 counts should receive measles/mumps/rubella (MMR) and Varicella vaccines separately, not as the combined MMR-V, as the higher titer of Varicella in this vaccine has not been tested for safety in HIV-infected children. In addition, HIV children older than 6 months of age should receive annual influenza vaccination with killed injectable formulations of the influenza vaccine as well as pneumococcal polysaccharide immunization (Simpkins et al., 2009).

Learning of a new diagnosis of HIV infection in oneself or one's child is devastating for most people. HCPs should offer hope and reassurance about the availability of effective treatments that can improve the quality of life and length of survival for people living with HIV. Referral to an HIV specialist will allow prompt access to specific medical care and psychosocial supports (Simpkins et al., 2009). The management of HIV infection in children poses unique challenges. The interprofessional health care team treating the pediatric patient should include HIV specialists, nurses, nutritionists, rehabilitative services (if long-term hospitalization is necessary), social workers, and psychologists. Attention to the complex services needed will provide the optimal support to patients with this rapidly evolving disease (Simpkins et al.).

Disposition and discharge planning

A concern upon diagnosis of a child with HIV is that other family members may be infected. HIV screening should be recommended and offered to all immediate family members with unknown HIV status. Screening should extend to other sexual partners and all siblings regardless of age, as infected children may remain asymptomatic into adolescence (Havens et al., 2009).

Disclosure of the HIV diagnosis to children poses unique concerns. Consideration should be given to the child's abilities to comprehend the diagnosis and the ability of caregivers to cope with stress of the diagnosis, access support, discuss other stigmatizing secrets that may be related to the disclosure of a diagnosis of HIV, and cope with disclosing the diagnosis to others. Exploration of sources of support for both children and caregivers is imperative, and clinicians should encourage ongoing open communication about health, illness, and living issues (Wiener et al., 2007).

Factors that lead to increased need for social and psychological support services include poverty, substance abuse, depression, social isolation, lack of health care, unemployment, homelessness, domestic violence, and fear of loss of support services, all due to the diagnosis. Immigrant families may have additional concerns, as they often bring their experiences of living with HIV from their home countries and will need education about the services available to them in the United States (Havens et al., 2009).

Health teaching about antiviral and prophylactic medications is necessary. Emphasis should be placed on the side effects of medications and the importance of adherence to treatment. HIV treatment is unique in its requirement for 90% to 100% adherence to the drug regimen to avoid the development of viral resistance and the loss of efficacy of antiviral drugs (Simpkins et al., 2009).

Discharge planning should also address transmission risk. This teaching offers an opportunity to review strategies for prevention of HIV transmission with parents or adolescent patients. Although HIV infection is not a reason to exclude children from school or sports, consideration should be given to the risk of viral transmission in high-impact sports, such as boxing (Simpkins et al., 2009).

Addressing the need for advanced care planning is also important. Parents infected with HIV should plan for the care of their dependent children. HIV-infected adolescents should identify a substitute decision maker for health issues in the event that they become unable to make their own decisions. Despite advances in care, some patients continue to experience medical complications that lead to death. Integrating palliative care with HIV-specific care can reduce distress by managing specific physical and emotional symptoms, encouraging clear communication, and promoting effective decision making (Simpkins et al., 2009).

JUVENILE IDIOPATHIC ARTHRITIS

Johanna Chang

PATHOPHYSIOLOGY

Juvenile idiopathic arthritis (JIA) is an autoimmune disease with genetic and environmental components. The complex genetic inheritance of the various forms of JIA suggests a non-Mendelian inheritance pattern that reflects the interaction of both major histocompatibility complex (MHC) and non-MHC genes. Oligoarticular disease has been associated with human leukocyte antigen-A2 (HLA-A2), HLA-DRB1*11, and HLA-DRB1*08. Rheumatoid factor (RF)-positive polyarticular JIA has been associated with HLA-DR4, similar to adults with rheumatoid arthritis. In enthesitis-related arthritis (ERA), 76% of patients are HLA-B27 positive (Ravelli & Martini, 2007).

Immune dysregulation clearly plays a role in the pathogenesis of JIA. Specific immunodeficiencies, including Wiskott-Aldrich syndrome, Good's syndrome, Nezelof's syndrome, selective immunoglobulin A (IgA) deficiency, hypogammaglobulinemia, and immunoglobulin G (IgG) subclass deficiencies are strongly associated with chronic arthritis. Levels of circulating immune complexes, which often contain rheumatoid factor and immunoglobulin M (IgM), have been shown to reflect arthritis activity in polyarticular JIA, and high levels of interleukin-1 (IL-1) and interleukin-6 (IL-6) are found in systemic JIA. Tumor necrosis factor alpha (TNF-α) appears to also play an important role in polyarticular disease. Studies have suggested that the imbalance between type 1 (Th$_1$) and type 2 (Th$_2$) helper T cells may be the leading causes of increased inflammation (Cassidy & Petty, 2005d).

Hormonal factors may also be implicated in the disease pathway. Differences in sex ratio and characteristic pre- or post-adolescent peaks in incidence of types of childhood arthritis have spurred research into hormone differences in patients with JIA. The results of these studies suggest that low androgen levels in prepubertal patients and high prolactin levels may be implicated in disease pathogenesis (Chikanza, 1999; Da Silva et al., 1993).

EPIDEMIOLOGY AND ETIOLOGY

The incidence of JIA ranges from 1 to 22 patients per 100,000 population, while the prevalence ranges from 8 to 150 patients per 100,000 population (Weiss & Ilowite, 2005). The age of onset and presentation vary for each JIA subtype. JIA has been described in patients of all races and from all geographic areas, although the variable incidence and prevalence of the disease throughout the world likely reflects both environmental and other multifactorial inheritance patterns.

Infection can cause transient arthritis and may be linked to autoimmune disease. Arthritis after viral infections is common and usually self-limited. Post-vaccination arthritis has been described after immunization with the measles/mumps/rubella (MMR) vaccine. Pediatric patients with JIA have been found to have positive parvovirus B19 IgM antibodies compared to normal healthy controls, a development that is thought to occur secondary to molecular mimicry, as there is no consistent evidence for an association of any viral infection with JIA (Oguz et al., 2002). Studies have implicated highly conserved bacterial heat shock proteins as potential arthritis triggers.

Classifications

JIA is a chronic arthritis of childhood that is also known by several other terms, including "juvenile chronic arthritis" (JCA) and "juvenile rheumatoid arthritis" (JRA). This phenotypically diverse disease is characterized by objective arthritis in one or more joints for a minimum of 6 weeks in a patient 16 years of age or younger, after other types of childhood arthritis have been excluded. Many institutions prefer to classify childhood arthritis using the 1997 criteria proposed by the International League of Associations for Rheumatology (ILAR) (Table 29-11).

PRESENTATION

Many patients with a new diagnosis of JIA report a history of minor physical trauma to an extremity. Joint microtrauma in the context of benign hypermobility and congenital pain insensitivity, for example, may predispose an individual to joint inflammation. The initiation of chronic inflammation

TABLE 29-11

International League Against Rheumatism Classification of Juvenile Idiopathic Arthritis	
Category	**Subcategories**
Systemic	
Oligoarthritis	1. Persistent
	2. Extended
Polyarthritis	1. Rheumatoid factor negative
	2. Rheumatoid factor positive
Psoriatic arthritis	
Enthesitis-related arthritis	
Undifferentiated arthritis	1. Fits no other category
	2. Fits more than one category

Source: Adapted from Petty et al., 2004.

has also been thought to be associated with trauma given that weight-bearing joints are more frequently affected than non-weight-bearing joints.

Diagnosis of juvenile idiopathic arthritis is a diagnosis of exclusion, and other diseases with similar presentation must first be considered, including septic arthritis and malignancy. The onset type of disease is determined by the course of the disease during the first 6 months and includes differentiation of disease as polyarticular, oligoarticular, systemic, enthesitis related, psoriatic, or undifferentiated.

Diagnosis of JIA depends largely on patient history and physical examination. A history of morning stiffness lasting at least 15 minutes that improves later in the day and responds to heat (warm shower) or NSAIDs is suggestive of active synovitis. Arthritis is defined clinically as the presence of joint swelling accompanied by warmth or tenderness or limitation of motion with tenderness on motion.

Oligoarticular JIA

Oligoarticular JIA is the most common form of JIA, affecting 50% to 60% of patients with JIA. Pediatric patients with oligoarticular JIA have arthritis in few than five joints for at least 6 weeks. Oligoarticular JIA is divided into *persistent* oligoarticular JIA and *extended* oligoarticular JIA. Patients who initially present with arthritis in fewer than five joints but then progress to have involvement of more than four joints after a period of 6 months are diagnosed with extended oligoarticular JIA. Approximately 50% of patients with oligoarticular JIA will develop extended disease, and 30% will develop extended disease within the first 2 years (Weiss & Ilowite, 2005). Involvement of the ankle or wrist joints and presence of a high erythrocyte sedimentation rate (ESR) are predictors for extended oligoarticular JIA.

Patients with a diagnosis of psoriasis, a family history of psoriasis, a positive HLA-B27, or a positive rheumatoid factor are excluded from the diagnosis of oligoarticular JIA. The peak age of onset is between 1 and 5 years, and females are affected more than males (female-to-male ratio of 4:1). The most frequently affected joints are the knees, ankles, and wrists. Patients with antinuclear antibody (ANA)-positive oligoarticular JIA are in the highest risk category for anterior uveitis, which is almost always asymptomatic, and require frequent ophthalmologic exams for early detection to prevent long-term sequelae of uveitis, such as blindness.

Physical examination findings of *active* arthritis include joint swelling or warmth and pain on motion of a joint. Physical examination findings of *chronic* arthritis include joint contractures and bone asymmetry, such as leg-length discrepancy and mandibular asymmetry. Bone asymmetry occurs because increased inflammation leads to increased blood flow to the growth plate, resulting in accelerated growth. Patients with uveitis can exhibit physical signs of eye damage, including synechiae and cataract (Cassidy & Petty, 2005c; Goldmuntz & White, 2006; Ravelli & Martini, 2007).

Polyarticular JIA

Children with polyarticular JIA have arthritis in *five or more* joints for at least 6 weeks. Polyarticular JIA affects 30% to 55% of all patients with JIA. Patients with polyarticular JIA are further classified based on presence of rheumatoid factor—a finding that is more similar to adult rheumatoid arthritis. Patients with a positive RF or anticyclic citrullinated protein (CCP) antibody tend to have more erosive disease and a chronic course progressing into adulthood. The peak age of onset for polyarticular JIA is biphasic, and the disease typically affects females more than males (female-to-male ratio of 5:1). Children with polyarticular JIA often present with symmetric arthritis involving the small joints of the hands, although arthritis of larger joints such as the knee or ankle can also accompany small joint disease.

Physical examination findings of *active* arthritis include joint swelling or warmth and pain on motion of a joint. Physical examination findings of *chronic* arthritis include joint contractures and bone asymmetry, such as leg-length discrepancy and mandibular asymmetry, as well as signs of erosive disease such as Boutonniere and swan-neck deformities. Patients with polyarticular JIA may occasionally develop rheumatoid nodules, which are typically firm, mobile, and nontender and usually appear over pressure points and tendon sheaths. Uveitis affects approximately 5% of patients with polyarticular disease (Cassidy & Petty, 2005a, 2005b; Goldmuntz & White, 2006; Ravelli & Martini, 2007).

Systemic JIA

Patients with systemic JIA may be part of a different disease spectrum and usually present with high inflammatory markers, including a fever accompanied by rash. Systemic JIA affects 4% to 17% of all patients with JIA (Ravelli & Martini, 2007). This type of JIA does not have a peak age of onset, and it affects males and females equally. Its diagnosis requires the presence of arthritis with a minimum of 2 weeks of daily quotidian fevers accompanied by a typical evanescent, nonfixed, erythematous rash; lymphadenopathy; hepatomegaly or splenomegaly; or serositis.

Physical examination findings include an erythematous, evanescent rash that characteristically appears during fever; hepatomegaly; splenomegaly; serositis; and arthritis. Although patients with systemic JIA often present with symmetric, polyarticular arthritis, some may not present with arthritis until later in the disease course.

Approximately 10% of children with systemic JIA develop a life-threatening complication known as macrophage-activating syndrome (MAS) or secondary hemophagocytic histiocytosis (HLH). Triggers include viral illness and the addition or change of medication. Clinically, patients appear severely ill with persistent fever that can be accompanied by rash, hepatosplenomegaly, lymphadenopathy, liver failure, and neurologic changes. A bone marrow biopsy demonstrating phagocytosis of other hematopoietic cells by macrophages or histiocytes is diagnostic (Cassidy & Petty, 2005d; Ravelli & Martini, 2007).

Enthesitis-related arthritis (ERA)

Patients with ERA typically have arthritis of both small and large joints with involvement of the hips, sacroiliac joints (SI), and lower back, as well as enthesitis, or inflammation at the region of tendon insertions. The population diagnosed with ERA includes patients with arthritis secondary to inflammatory bowel disease (IBD), reactive arthritis, or ankylosing spondylitis. Patients with ERA account for 3% to 11% of all patients with JIA and 13% of all patients with a rheumatologic condition (Ravelli & Martini, 2007). ERA mainly affects male patients older than the age of 6 years, although it typically involves older patients who are in their preteen or adolescent years. Although this form of JIA is strongly associated with uveitis, the uveitis differs from the asymptomatic uveitis of oligoarticular and polyarticular JIA due to its painful symptomatology. Most patients have a positive HLA-B27; 82% to 95% of patients with ankylosing spondylitis are HLA-B27 positive.

Physical examination findings include tenderness on palpation of the 2, 6, or 10 o'clock positions on the patella, the tibial tuberosity, the attachment of the Achilles tendon, or the plantar fascia (enthesitis); abnormalities in the contour of the spine when the patient is in the standing and fully flexed position; a Schober test measurement of less than 6 cm; pain with direct pressure over the SI joints or with compression of the pelvis; and decreased thoracic excursion (less than 5 cm) (Cassidy & Petty, 2005b; Goldmuntz & White, 2006; Ravelli & Martini, 2007).

Psoriatic arthritis

Psoriatic arthritis is characterized by swelling of the digits ("dactylitis") and is usually accompanied by a diagnosis of psoriasis in the patient or in a first-degree family member. This diagnosis is made when patients with chronic arthritis and definite psoriasis or chronic arthritis meet two of the following criteria: dactylitis, nail pitting or onycholysis, or a family history of psoriasis. Psoriatic arthritis can occur before, during, or after dermatologic manifestations. This disease affects 2% to 11% of all patients with JIA (Ravelli & Martini, 2007). The age of onset is typically during the preschool years or in middle to late childhood. Psoriatic arthritis is slightly more common in girls, with a female-to-male ratio of 2.5:1. This form of JIA is highly correlated with anterior uveitis; 15% to 20% patients with psoriatic arthritis have an asymptomatic chronic uveitis, while a very low percentage develop a painful symptomatic uveitis similar to that seen in patients with ERA.

Physical examination findings include dactylitis, which is present in 50% of patients; nail pitting, which is present in 75% of patients; and skin findings consistent with psoriasis (Cassidy & Petty, 2005a; Goldmuntz & White, 2006; Ravelli & Martini, 2007).

Undifferentiated arthritis

Patients who do not satisfy the inclusion criteria for any of the six ILAR classifications or who meet criteria for more than one of the six ILAR classifications can be included in the category of undifferentiated arthritis. Patients with undifferentiated arthritis must have objective arthritis for a minimum of 6 weeks (Cassidy & Petty, 2005a; Goldmuntz & White, 2006).

DIFFERENTIAL DIAGNOSIS

The differential diagnoses for suspected JIA can be divided into three major categories: monoarthritis, polyarthritis, and other causes of prolonged fever and rash (Cassidy & Petty, 2005d; Goldmuntz & White, 2006) (Table 29-12). Preliminary investigations for evaluation of limb pain may be useful to narrow the differential diagnosis (Table 29-13).

TABLE 29-12

Differential Diagnoses for Juvenile Idiopathic Arthritis

Type of Arthritis	Differential Diagnosis
Monoarthritis	Infection: septic arthritis, post-infectious arthritis, Lyme disease, post-*Streptococcus* arthritis
	Mechanical: fracture, benign hypermobility, slipped capital femoral epiphysis, Legg-Calvé-Perthes, osteochondritis dissecans
	Malignancy: bone and synovial membrane tumors
Polyarthritis (acute: within 72 hours)	Infection: septic arthritis, acute rheumatic fever, toxic synovitis
	Malignancy: leukemia, neuroblastoma
	Hematologic: sickle cell crisis (dactylitis), hemophilia
	Mechanical: trauma, fracture
Polyarthritis (chronic: more than 4 weeks)	Infection: viral (parvovirus), bacterial (Lyme disease, rubella, tuberculosis), acute rheumatic fever, fungal
	Pigmented villonodular synovitis
	Connective tissue disease: systemic lupus erythematosus, sarcoidosis, dermatomyositis, inflammatory bowel disease; vasculitis
Fever and rash (suspected systemic JIA)	Periodic fever syndromes: periodic fever, aphthous ulcers, pharyngitis, adenopathy (PFAPA); familial Mediterranean fever; hyper-IgD syndrome
	Infection: differs from JIA by presence of positive blood cultures/antibodies, persistent fevers and rash
	Malignancy (leukemia, neuroblastoma): differs from systemic JIA by presence of nonquotidian fevers, bone pain
	Other rhematologic diseases: • Chronic infantile neurologic cutaneous and articular syndrome (CINCA)/neonatal-onset multi-inflammatory disease (NOMID): differs from systemic JIA by presence of fixed rash, undulating fevers, neurologic symptoms • Kawasaki disease: differs by presence of fixed rash, mucocutaneous disease, coronary artery dilation • Lupus: differs by constant fevers, presence of positive antinuclear antibody and double-stranded DNA, cytopenias

TABLE 29-13

Initial Evaluation for Suspected Juvenile Idiopathic Arthritis

Labs	Imaging	Consults
CBC with differential • Monitor for signs of infection (high WBC, left shift)	Plain films • Quick, no sedation needed • Not very sensitive for osteomyelitis	Orthopedic surgery • If osteomyelitis or septic arthritis is suspected; if radiographs suggest mechanical causes such as Legg-Calvé-Perthes or SCFE • Joint aspiration may be helpful
Blood smear • May be useful when considering malignancy	CT/MRI • Very sensitive for bone and soft-tissue disease • Younger children may require sedation	Rheumatologist • If rheumatologic illness is suspected
• Erythrocyte sedimentation rate High ESR in context of low CRP is common in active rheumatologic diseases	Bone scan • Sensitive for osteomyelitis, may be helpful in suspected malignancy	Ophthalmologist • Slit lamp eye exam may be helpful; presence of uveitis may be indicative of rheumatologic disease
• C-reactive protein may be elevated in inflammatory diseases		Hematologist • Bone marrow aspiration may be needed
Blood culture • Especially if child is febrile		

Note: Complete blood count (CBC), white blood cell count (WBC), slipped capital femoral epiphysis (SCFE), computed tomography (CT), magnetic resonance imaging (MRI).

One of the most important diagnoses to evaluate for in the context of possible JIA is infection, such as osteomyelitis or septic arthritis. Patients with osteomyelitis may have point tenderness, which is often not present in JIA. The most commonly affected bone in osteomyelitis is the femur, followed by the tibia, humerus, fibula, radius, calcaneus, and ilium. Pediatric patients with infection often appear very ill or even toxic. A definitive diagnosis of septic arthritis may be made after joint aspiration and analysis of the synovial fluid, which is characteristically cloudy or turbid with a high white cell count and positive Gram stain (50% of cases). Positive cultures from synovial fluid are noted 70% of the time, while a positive blood culture occurs 40% to 50% of the time (Tse & Laxer, 2006). Complaints of severe pain and inability to ambulate are not typical of JIA, and these patients should be evaluated carefully for other diseases, including infection. If infection is suspected, prompt treatment with empiric antibiotics may be warranted.

In cases of suspected systemic JIA, the differential diagnosis for fever and rash needs to be carefully considered. Leukemia can closely mimic systemic JIA; notably, 15% of children with leukemia present with arthritis, fevers, and rash (Goldmuntz & White, 2006).

PLAN OF CARE

Patients with rheumatologic disease such as JIA can have inflammatory and autoimmune components. As a consequence, markers of inflammation may be helpful to evaluate for disease activity and response to therapy. Autoantibodies can also be identified and in some cases are used to characterize disease.

Patients with JIA typically have elevated markers of inflammation, including platelets, ESR, and C-reactive protein (CRP). Patients with rheumatologic disease can have a normal CRP in the context of an elevated ESR, which may be indicative of disease activity.

The antinuclear antibody (ANA) consists of immunoglobulins directed against structures within the cell, such as DNA, ribonuclear proteins, and histones. It is found in various autoimmune diseases, including systemic lupus erythematosus, mixed connective tissue disease, scleroderma, Sjogren syndrome, and JIA. However, it can also be present in patients with infections or malignancy. Approximately 10% of the population tests positive for low-titer ANA but are asymptomatic. The presence of ANA is important to determine in patients with JIA to assess their risk of developing uveitis.

Rheumatoid factor (RF) is an uncommon autoantibody in children and should not be used as a screening test for rheumatic disease in pediatric patients. The main indication for obtaining a RF is to classify patients with polyarticular JIA; patients with polyarticular JIA and high-titer RF are more likely to have erosive joint disease and a prolonged disease course. Low titers of RF can be seen in patients with infection or malignancy; this finding is noted to occur in fewer than 5% of healthy children. By comparison, a positive RF test is seen in 5% to 10% of patients with JIA. Some literature supports the contention that the presence of CCP is more prognostic of erosive joint disease than the presence of RF; consequently, many rheumatologists also test for the anti-CCP in addition to RF in patients with polyarticular JIA.

In systemic JIA, widespread inflammation typically leads to marked elevations in ESR, CRP, white blood cell count, platelets, ferritin, and D-dimer. Elevation in transaminases may also be seen, although severe liver dysfunction is atypical. Anemia with hemoglobin in the range of 7 to 10 gm/dL is also common. Macrophage-activating syndrome (MAS) is characterized by a precipitous drop is ESR and white blood cell and platelet counts. Coagulopathy, including DIC, can occur.

HLA-B27 is one of the histocompatibility genes important in transplantation; it is also associated with seronegative (or RF-negative) spondyloarthropathies. It occurs in as many as 90% of patients with ankylosing spondylitis, 25% to 50% of patients with IBD, 50% to 75% of patients with reactive arthritis, and fewer than 25% of patients with psoriatic arthritis. Fewer than 20% of patients who test positive for HLA-B27 develop the most severe form of ERA, ankylosing spondylitis (Cassidy & Petty, 2005d; Szer et al., 2006).

Imaging is an important modality to support the diagnosis of JIA and monitor disease progression. Radiographs may be used to evaluate for fractures. Early changes seen on radiographs include periarticular soft-tissue swelling and widening of the joint space secondary to accumulation of intra-articular fluid or synovial hypertrophy. Osteopenia is also commonly seen. Later changes include joint-space narrowing, erosions, subluxation, and joint fusion. Radiographs should be obtained of all active joints prior to treatment initiation and then repeated every 6 to 12 months to monitor for disease progression.

Magnetic resonance imaging (MRI) is more sensitive for detection of erosions, which are not usually appreciated on radiographs before 2 years of active disease. MRI is also the most sensitive imaging modality for suspected inflammation of the temporomandibular joint and sacroiliac joint. Contrast with MRI can be used to accurately diagnose synovitis. Ultrasound is highly sensitive for the presence of fluid and can be useful in identifying the accumulation of intra-articular fluid as well as tenosynovitis, or inflammation of the tendon sheaths, which can be associated with arthritis (Cassidy & Petty, 2005d; Tse & Laxer, 2006; Wallace, 2006).

The goals of JIA therapy are pain and disease control, and prevention of damage and disability. Most of the damage in patients with arthritis is secondary to polyarticular and systemic JIA and occurs within 2 years. MAS, however, is a life-threatening disease that requires immediate treatment, including supportive therapy and administration of high-dose steroids, cyclosporine, etoposide, or rituximab.

Several medications are used to treat JIA (Table 29-14). NSAIDs, such as ibuprofen and naprosyn, are considered first-line therapy. The average time to symptomatic improvement from NSAID therapy is 1 month; however, 25% of children do not demonstrate clinical improvement until 8 to 12 weeks of treatment. NSAIDs are generally well tolerated, with the most common adverse effects being abdominal pain and anorexia. Pediatric patients experiencing significant gastritis can benefit from using antacids, histamine-2 blockers, proton-pump inhibitors, or switching to a cyclo-oxygenase 2 (COX-2) inhibitor. Patients maintained on NSAIDs often have biannual monitoring for kidney or hepatic dysfunction.

If significant synovitis involving multiple joints persists for 3 to 6 months, or if radiologic evidence of destructive disease is present, many rheumatologists also initiate treatment with nonbiologic disease-modifying antirheumatic drugs (DMARDs), which include methotrexate, sulfasalazine, leflunomide, azathioprine, hydroxychloroquine, cyclosporine, thalidomide, and tacrolimus. Methotrexate is the most commonly prescribed DMARD for JIA. Approximately 70% of children have a favorable clinical response to this medication. Clinical response may not become evident until 4 to 6 weeks after therapy has been initiated, however, and may not be maximal until the patient has received 3 to 6 months of treatment. Higher doses of methotrexate may be given via the subcutaneous route—a strategy that may be used if oral methotrexate therapy is not successful. Concomitant use of daily folic acid is helpful to decrease the frequency and severity of methotrexate adverse effects, which include oral ulcers, decreased appetite, and nausea. Diagnostic studies monitoring for bone marrow suppression and kidney and hepatic toxicity are usually obtained every 6 to 8 weeks in patients treated with methotrexate.

If significant synovitis persists despite the addition of nonbiologic DMARDs to the therapeutic regimen, many rheumatologists then consider additional treatment with biologic agents, including TNF-α inhibitors such as etanercept, infliximab, or adalimumab. Administration of TNF-α inhibitors is associated reactivation of tuberculosis; therefore, patients who will be treated with these medications should demonstrate a negative PPD (tuberculin) test prior to starting anti-TNF therapy. Both etanercept, a TNF-receptor blocker, and adalimumab, a humanized monoclonal antibody, are given as weekly subcutaneous injections; infliximab, a monoclonal antibody, is given as a several-hr intravenous infusion, usually on a monthly basis. Other biologic agents used for treatment of JIA include anakinra, which inhibits IL-1; abatacept (CTLA4-Ig), which blocks signal transduction between B and T cells; and rituximab (anti-CD20 antibody), which depletes antibody-producing lymphocytes. Patients on biologic treatment need to be monitored carefully for bone marrow suppression and signs of infection (Cassidy & Petty, 2005d; Szer et al., 2006).

TABLE 29-14

Commonly Used Medications for the Treatment of Juvenile Idiopathic Arthritis

	Medication	Indication	Mechanism	Dose	Toxicity
NSAIDs	Naproxen, ibuprofen, indomethacin, sulindac, celecoxib	First line for JIA	COX-1, COX-2 inhibition.	Variable; naproxen: 10 mg/kg/dose BID; ibuprofen 10 mg/kg/dose TID; indomethacin 1–3 mg/kg/day divided BID	Gastritis, hepatotoxicity, kidney toxicity, coagulation suppression
DMARDs	Methotrexate	JIA, SLE	Antimetabolite (folate analog). Suppresses inflammatory cytokine production, inhibits DHFR, inhibits lymphocyte proliferation in high doses.	0.5–1 mg/kg/dose (up to 20 mg PO or 25 mg SQ) every week	GI (pain, N/V, ulceration), hepatotoxicity (fibrosis), malignancy
	Sulfasalazine	ERAs, JIA	Antibacterial/anti-inflammatory. Unclear.	30–50 mg/kg/day divided BID–TID	Watch for sulfa allergies; GI toxicity; monitor white blood cell count
	Hydroxychloroquine	SLE, other connective tissue disease	Multiple. Inhibits phospholipid function and binds DNA.	6 mg/kg/day up to 400 mg PO daily	Retinal hyperpigmentation (retinal exam 1–2 times/year)
Glucocorticoids	Methylprednisolone, prednisone, prednisolone	When you need quick, effective, anti-inflammatory effect (used in virtually all inflammatory conditions)	Induce transcription of anti-inflammatory and immunomodulatory genes. Suppress inflammatory cytokine production. At high doses IV, it blocks cell signaling and depletes lymphocyte numbers.	Low dose (5–10 mg/day), medium dose (1–2 mg/kg/day), high dose (30 mg/kg/dose pulses, up to 1 gm)	Hypertension (especially with pulses); atrophy of skin; impaired wound healing; body fluid retention; decreased body growth; hypernatremia, hypokalemia; peptic ulcer disease; liver function tests abnormal (mild); at risk of infection; muscle weakness; osteopenia/osteoporosis; glaucoma; cataracts; depression; euphoria
Cytotoxic Agents	Thalidomide	SoJIA	Inhibits cytokine secretions and T-cell proliferation		Extremely teratogenic, can cause peripheral neuropathy
	Cyclophosphamide	SLE (severe LN or CNS involvement); severe vasculitis	Alkylating agent, depletes T and B cells	1 mg/kg/day, 10 mg/kg/dose every 2 weeks, 500–750 mg/m²/dose Every 4–8 weeks	Hemorrhagic cystitis (void every 2 hours with infusion, MESNA); must be dose adjusted for kidney insufficiency; fertility concerns; pancytopenia; malignancy
	Mycophenylate mofetil (Cellcept, Myfortic)	SLE	Inhibits de novo synthesis of guanine (T and B cells cannot salvage). Inhibits T and B cells.	Goal dose 600 mg/m² BID; may need to start at lower dose and titrate upward as tolerated	GI toxicity (diarrhea); pancytopenia

(Continued)

TABLE 29-14

	Commonly Used Medications for the Treatment of Juvenile Idiopathic Arthritis *(Continued)*				
	Medication	**Indication**	**Mechanism**	**Dose**	**Toxicity**
Cytotoxic Agents	Azathioprine	SLE	Purine analog; metabolized to 6-MP. Inhibits T cells.	0.5–2.5 mg/kg/day	Check TMPT enzyme to make sure medication can be metabolized; pancytopenia. Can check 6-MMPN and 6-TGN levels
	Cyclosporine	SLE	Calcineurin inhibitor (translocation of NF-AT). Blocks transcription of T-cell genes.	3–5 mg/kg/day	Grapefruit juice increases levels; pancytopenia, can check levels; is kidney toxic
Biologic Agents	TNF-alpha inhibitors: etanercept, infliximab, adalimumab	Spondyloarthropathy, JIA, uveitis when first and second-line medications are ineffective	Competitively inhibit TNF-alpha receptors; TNF causes inflammation, T- and B-cell signaling, and T-cell proliferation.	Variable	CHF (especially infliximab); must check PPD prior to starting medication (TB activation); malignancy; demyelinating disease; development of ANA/autoimmunity
	IL-1 receptor antagonist (IL-1ra): anakinra (Kineret)	SoJIA	A recombinant form of the natural IL-1 receptor antagonist. Blocks cell signaling by IL-1-alpha and beta.	1–3 mg/kg/day	Immunosuppression; very painful injection
	CTLa-4 Ig (abatacept/Orencia)	JIA, SLE	A fully human, soluble fusion protein, which works by selectively modulating a co-stimulatory signal that is required for full T-cell activation.	10 mg/kg/dose up to 500 mg IV every 2–4 weeks	
	Rituximab	SLE, JIA, TTP	Anti-CD20 Ab; targets pre-B and mature B cells, but not plasma or stem cells.	375 mg/m² every week × 4 doses or 500 mg/m² every 2 weeks × 2 doses	Try to immunize with pneumococcal and meningococcal vaccines prior to starting medication; can be hypotensive with infusion, must run slowly, especially first dose

Note: Oral (PO), subcutaneous (SQ), intravenous (IV), three times a day (TID), twice a day (BID), nausea/vomiting (N/V), gastrointestinal (GI), central nervous system (CNS), congestive heart failure (CHF), purified protein derivative (PPD), systemic lupus erythematosus (SLE), juvenile idiopathic arthritis (JIA), systemic JIA (SoJIA), 6-mercaptopurine (6-MP), thiopurine methyltransferase (TPMT), 6-methylmercaptopurine ribonucleotide (6-MMPN), 6-thioguanine nucleotide (6-TGN), tumor necrosis factor (TNF), antinuclear antibody (ANA), thrombotic thrombocytopenic purpura (TTP).

Steroids have never been proven to be disease modifying and produce serious toxic side effects with their long-term use. Nevertheless, these agents are very effective in reducing inflammation and are often used in patients with JIA. Low doses (5–15 mg/day) are helpful in patients with severe polyarticular JIA and ERA. In patients with systemic JIA and those with severe uveitis, moderate to high doses (more than 1 mg/kg/day) are used to control the underlying inflammation. The toxicities of steroids include immunosuppression, hypertension, diabetes, cataracts, osteoporosis, avascular necrosis, and obesity (Cassidy & Petty, 2005d; Szer et al., 2006).

Intra-articular steroid (IAS) injections are rapid acting and help to provide symptomatic relief while patients are waiting for systemic medications to take effect. This therapy can be substituted for NSAIDs when used to treat patients with monoarticular or oligoarticular arthritis. Although IAS injections are rarely curative, the rapid pain relief can encourage normal activity and prevent the formation of joint contractures (Cassidy & Petty, 2005b, 2005c, 2005d; Szer et al., 2006).

Autologous stem cell transplant (ASCT) may be considered if all other therapies fail. ASCT has been performed in Europe many years, although protocols are not yet standardized. In a recent study, 34 patients with JIA ranging in age from 12 to 60 months underwent ASCT. At time of follow-up, 18 patients (53%) had reached drug-free remission, 6 patients (18%) had achieved a partial response, 7 patients (21%) had no response, and 3 patients died. All 3 deaths occurred in patients with systemic JIA who developed MAS and infection. Two patients later relapsed and required immunosuppressive treatment complicated by infection; they also died. Recent changes in protocol include less T-cell depletion in stem cell preparations, exclusion of patients with systemic JIA with fever or evidence of MAS at the time of conditioning, and increased monitoring for development of MAS. Since these changes in the protocol have been implemented, there have been no further reports of transplant-related deaths (De Kleer et al., 2004; Wulffratt et al., 2005).

Patients with a suspected septic arthritis should be hospitalized and receive an immediate consultation from orthopedic surgery. Orthopedic surgery specialists may also have a role in caring for children with severe disease leading to joint contractures, bone growth discrepancy, or joint replacement. Many children will benefit from occupational therapy and physical therapy to improve or regain fine and gross motor skills and range of motion. In addition, a physical therapist can be helpful in evaluating for appropriate footwear and can assist in providing appropriate insoles for children with leg-length discrepancy secondary to arthritis. Occupational therapists may be able to provide splints to maintain appropriate joint positions to decrease the likelihood of forming joint contractures.

Children with JIA are at risk for uveitis and require regular ophthalmology visits depending on the subtype and duration of disease (Table 29-15). Treatment of uveitis typically includes topical steroids to decrease inflammation and mydriatic agents to decrease eye pressures, which may become elevated as a response to topical steroids.

The care of a child with a chronic disease requires good patient and family education. Treatment programs should be family centered and ideally involve an interprofessional team consisting of a pediatric rheumatologist, advanced practice nurse, social worker, physical and occupational therapist, and psychologist. Consultation with a psychiatrist or nutritionist may also be helpful. Children should be encouraged to maintain regular school attendance and engage in appropriate physical activity, including non-weight-bearing exercises such as swimming, which can be modified depending on the disease activity of each child. Patients should also continue to follow up with their primary care provider to ensure that they receive appropriate vaccines and health supervision. Children on immunosuppressive regimens should receive only inactivated vaccines and are recommended to receive the influenza vaccine annually. These children are at high risk for infection, and families are often asked to call their primary care provider or pediatric rheumatologist in the event that a patient develops a fever or any other signs of infection. Educational information may be found at www.arthritisfoundation.org.

DISPOSITION AND DISCHARGE PLANNING

Patients with JIA are typically not hospitalized, with the exception of children with systemic JIA, who often receive

TABLE 29-15

Frequency of Ophthalmologic Examination in Patients with Juvenile Idiopathic Arthritis					
High Risk		**Medium Risk**		**Low Risk**	
Oligoarticular or polyarticular onset + younger than 7 years at JIA onset + ANA positive	Frequency: every 3 months	• Oligoarticular or polyarticular onset + younger than 7 years at JIA onset + ANA negative **OR** • Oligoarticular or polyarticular onset + younger than 7 years at JIA onset + ANA negative or positive	Frequency: every 6 months	Systemic JIA	Frequency: every 12 months

Note: Juvenile idiopathic arthritis (JIA), antinuclear antibody (ANA).

a diagnosis after a prolonged hospitalization to evaluate for other causes of fever of unknown origin.

Although the mortality rate for JIA is low, with an assumed overall rate of less than 1.5% (Minden et al., 2002), most patients with JIA have some long-term persistence of disease activity. A recent study showed that only 40% to 60% of patients had inactive or disease remission at follow-up after 10 years (Oen, 2002). Over the past decade, however, there has been a notable decrease in the number of patients with serious functional debility—now estimated at 2.5% to 10% of the total patient population. Predictors of poor outcome include greater severity of arthritis, evolution to extended arthritis, symmetrical disease, wrist or hip involvement, presence of RF, persistent active disease, and presence of erosions on radiographs. Structural changes secondary to arthritis are common; a recent study found that more than one-half of the patients with JIA had changes in body function and structure at the time of follow-up during adolescence and adulthood (Minden et al.).

Children with oligoarticular JIA tend to have less bone damage and the best outcomes. Many will go into remission, with studies showing remission rates ranging from 3% to 75%, although approximately one-third to one-half will have polyarticular extension of disease (Guillaume et al., 2000). One study demonstrated that only 12% of patients with extended oligoarticular JIA achieved remission, compared to 75% of patients with persistent oligoarticular JIA (Minden et al., 2002). Patients with extended oligoarticular JIA have 20% to 30% chance of uveitis with the sequela of blindness if the disease goes unrecognized and untreated. Recent studies suggest that as many as 15% of children with uveitis ultimately develop significant visual impairment, with 10% suffering blindness in at least one eye (Goldmuntz & White, 2006).

Patients with polyarticular JIA have a more guarded outcome with higher risk of potential damage. Prognosis is worse in the context of positive RF, small joint or hip involvement, or presence of erosive disease. Patients with polyarticular JIA who have not gone into remission by age 16 are likely to have a more chronic course.

The prognosis is also guarded for patients with systemic JIA. Although 50% will recover without problems, the one-half will have a more unremitting course that can lead to substantial joint damage. Predictors of poor prognosis include age younger than 6 years at diagnosis; disease duration greater than 5 years; more than 6 months of sustained fevers; treatment with corticosteroids; or platelet level greater than 600,000 unit/L. Significant morbidity and mortality can occur in patients with systemic JIA who develop MAS.

For all patients with arthritis, local growth disturbances, such as severe limb-length discrepancy and micrognathia, may require surgical consultation and management (Cassidy & Petty, 2005a, 2005b, 2005c, 2005d).

> **Critical Thinking**
>
> It is very rare to have musculoskeletal sprain resulting in acute swelling in children younger than 3 years of age. Be wary about referring these patients to orthopedics but instead consider a referral to rheumatology specialists, as children do not get ligament or meniscal tears like older teens and adults.

SYSTEMIC LUPUS ERYTHEMATOSUS

Johanna Chang and Joyce Hsu

PATHOPHYSIOLOGY

The pathophysiology of systemic lupus erythematosus (SLE) is not fully completely understood. SLE is a multisystem inflammatory autoimmune disease characterized by autoantibodies to nuclear and cellular components. The triggers to antibody formation are unknown but may include environmental factors such as UVB radiation, viral infections, and industrial chemicals. Immune dysregulation (including abnormal B- and T-lymphocyte function), neutrophil abnormalities, abnormal formation and deposition of immune complexes, and aberrant apoptosis are likely involved in SLE pathogenesis.

Definition and criteria

SLE is characterized by the presence of autoantibodies, especially antinuclear antibodies (ANA). Diagnosis of SLE is based on the American College of Rheumatology (ACR) criteria, which were last revised in 1997 (Table 29-16). The presence of four criteria has a sensitivity of 96% and a specificity of 100% in childhood lupus. Fifty percent of patients who do not initially meet all of the SLE diagnostic criteria, but who are followed by a rheumatologist, will eventually meet the diagnostic criteria (Benseler & Silverman, 2007; Cassidy et al., 2005).

EPIDEMIOLOGY AND ETIOLOGY

The estimated annual incidence of SLE in children in the United States is 0.6 per 100,000 population. There is a female predilection for this disease: In children, the female-to-male ratio is 4:1, and this ratio increases to 9:1 in adults. Although population studies have not confirmed a racial predisposition for SLE, higher frequency and increased severity of disease have been noted in non-Caucasian populations. In particular, Asians, Native Americans, African Americans, and Hispanics tend to have a higher incidence of SLE and may have more severe disease (Cassidy et al., 2005; Stichweh et al., 2004). Pediatric patients account for approximately 15% of 20% of all patients with SLE. In the pediatric population, this disease usually presents more aggressively, and with more renal involvement, than in adult-onset SLE.

A connective tissue disease other than SLE occurs in 1 of 10 families of patients with SLE, and a case-control study showed that 10% of patients with SLE had a first-degree relative with SLE. Certain HLA haplotypes may increase susceptibility to SLE: HLA-DR2 and HLA-DR3 increase risk of development of SLE by twofold to threefold in Caucasians, and the presence of HLA-DR2 and DR7 in African Americans is associated with SLE. Complement deficiencies in C_{1q}, C_{1r}, C_{1s}, C_4, and C_2 are associated with lupus-like syndromes. Lupus has also been associated with chronic granulomatous disease and IgA deficiency. Sex hormones appear to have a significant effect in SLE development; as noted earlier, in childhood, the ratio of females to males with SLE is 4:1, increasing to 9:1 in adolescence. Males with Klinefelter's syndrome have relative deficiency of androgens and have an increased frequency of SLE (Cassidy et al., 2005; Klein-Gitelman et al., 2002; Stichweh et al., 2004).

Several medications may induce a lupus-like syndrome. Many patients, for example, test positive for ANA against histones (antihistone antibodies). Although antiepileptic drugs are the most common cause of drug-induced SLE in childhood, several other medications—such as isoniazid, minocycline, and hydralazine—have been identified as affecting this disease's development. The clinical symptoms of drug-induced lupus usually resolve after discontinuation of the offending agent (Cassidy et al., 2005).

PRESENTATION

The presentation of SLE in childhood varies. Of note, although this section focuses on systemic lupus erythematosus, an isolated dermatologic lupus—also known as discoid lupus—occurs rarely in the pediatric population. The most common disease manifestations of SLE are malar rash, arthritis, and the presence of constitutional symptoms (fever, fatigue, and weight loss) (Hiraki et al., 2008). These same symptoms are commonly observed with disease flares (Table 29-17).

Approximately 20% to 70% of pediatric SLE patients have involvement of the central nervous system and peripheral nervous system, referred to as neuropsychiatric lupus. Symptoms include headache (typically severe, lasting more than 24 hours, and refractory to standard analgesic treatment), psychosis, cognitive dysfunction, seizure, movement disorders, and cranial and peripheral neuropathies. Lupus nephritis, which affects 29% to 80% of pediatric patients, typically manifests during the first year of diagnosis and is more severe compared to kidney disease in adult patients with SLE.

TABLE 29-16

American College of Rheumatology Criteria for Classification of Systemic Lupus Erythematosus

1. Malar rash
2. Presence of discoid lupus rash
3. Photosensitivity
4. Oral or nasal mucocutaneous ulcerations
5. Arthritis
6. Nephritis
   a. Proteinuria > 0.5 gm/day
   b. Cellular casts
7. Encephalopathy
   a. Seizures
   b. Psychosis
8. Pleuritis or pericarditis
9. Cytopenia
10. Positive immunoserology
    a. Positive test for double-stranded DNA (dsDNA) antibodies
    b. Positive test for anti-Smith (anti-Sm) antibodies
    c. Positive findings for antiphospholipid antibodies as shown by
       i. Positive test for IgG or IgM anticardiolipin antibodies
       ii. Positive test for lupus anticoagulant
       iii. False-positive serologic test for syphilis for at least 6 months
    d. Positive test for antinuclear antibody (ANA)

Source: Adapted from Cassidy et al., 2005.

TABLE 29-17

Presentation of Systemic Lupus Erythematosus	
System	**Presentation**
Cardiovascular	• Hypertension • Pericarditis (most common cardiac manifestation—occurs in 30% of children with SLE) • Myocarditis • Coronary artery disease • Valvular disease (Libman-Sacks endocarditis—less common in children) • Raynaud's phenomenon
Dermatologic	• Malar rash sparing nasolabial folds (occurs in one-third to one-half of children at disease onset) • Photosensitive rash (rash on sun-exposed areas) • Alopecia • Oral ulcer (classically, painless ulceration on the hard palate) • Nasal ulcer • Periungual erythema • Livedo reticularis (associated with antiphospholipids) • Discoid lesions (more common in Asians)
Endocrine	• Autoimmune thyroid disease • Rarely, hypoparathyroidism or hyperparathyroidism, juvenile-onset type 1 diabetes, Addison's disease

(Continued)

TABLE 29-17

Presentation of Systemic Lupus Erythematosus (Continued)	
System	**Presentation**
Gastrointestinal	• Pancreatitis • Protein-losing enteropathy • Fatty infiltration of the liver secondary to steroid therapy • Autoimmune hepatitis • Lupus-anticoagulant-associated Budd-Chiari syndrome
Hematologic	• Leukopenia • Thrombocytopenia, idiopathic thrombocytopenic purpura • Evan's syndrome • Hemolytic anemia • Thrombotic thrombocytopenic purpura • Thromboembolism • Menorrhagia • Secondary APLS • Catastrophic APLS (CAPS) • Functional asplenia
Musculoskeletal	• Arthritis (typically nonerosive) of bilateral small joints of hands, wrists, elbows, shoulders, knees, and ankles • Myalgia
Neurological	• Recurrent headache • Depression • Cognitive disorder • Psychosis • Seizure disorder
Oncologic	• Increased risk of lymphoma
Ophthalmologic	• Cotton-wool spots • Uveitis • Keratoconjunctivitis sicca (secondary to Sjogren syndrome)
Pulmonary	• Pleural effusions • Pleuritis • Pneumonitis • Pulmonary hemorrhage • Pulmonary hypertension (rarely)
Renal	• Most common symptom—present in 75% of children with SLE • Microscopic hematuria • Proteinuria, nephrotic syndrome

Note: Antiphospholipid antibodies (APLS), catastrophic antiphospholipid antibody syndrome (CAPS).

Source: Adapted from Cassidy et al., 2005.

Coagulation abnormalities occur frequently in patients with pediatric lupus. Approximately one-third of patients test positive for lupus anticoagulant and are at increased risk for thrombotic events. Patients who experience coagulopathy secondary to the presence of antiphospholipid antibodies can rarely develop catastrophic antiphospholipid antibody syndrome (CAPS), which is characterized by microangiopathic changes with thrombosis in multiple organs and

TABLE 29-18

Differential Diagnoses for Systemic Lupus Erythematosus		
Disease Category	**Common Features**	**Differences**
Other autoimmune diseases (mixed connective tissue disease, drug-induced lupus, autoimmune hepatitis, Evan's syndrome, primary antiphospholipid antibody syndrome, primary Sjogren syndrome)	Fever, cytopenia, fatigue, rash	Lack of specific autoantibodies (dsDNA, Smith, histone), specific features unique to specific diseases (e.g., Gottron's papules in juvenile dermatomyositis [JDMS])
Malignancy	Fever, cytopenia, fatigue, pain, lymphadenopathy, hepatosplenomegaly	Night pain, bone tenderness, night sweats, normal complement, no urinary changes
Systemic vasculitis	Fever, fatigue, rash	Nodules, calf pain, positive anti-neutrophilic cytoplasmic antibodies (ANCA), bruits
Systemic juvenile idiopathic arthritis	Arthritis, fatigue, fever, rash, lymphadenopathy, marked anemia	Lack of specific autoantibodies, normal complements, no major organ dysfunction
Systemic viral infection	Fever, lymphadenopathy, hepatosplenomegaly, cytopenias	Lack of specific autoantibodies, normal complements

Source: Adapted from Cassidy et al., 2005.

can present with multiple organ dysfunction (Benseler & Silverman, 2007; Klein-Gitelman et al., 2002).

DIFFERENTIAL DIAGNOSIS

Lupus may resemble other disease states (Table 29-18). For this reason, differential diagnoses may only be determined by physical examination findings and diagnostic studies.

PLAN OF CARE

A number of diagnostic studies contribute to the diagnosis of SLE (Table 29-19). ANA is the most common autoantibody present in SLE-affected patients; and is present in 98% of the pediatric patients with this disease. Ten to fifteen

TABLE 29-19

Diagnostic Studies for Systemic Lupus Erythematosus

Diagnostic Study	Rationale
CBC with differential	Check for cytopenia Consider checking Coombs test for hemolytic anemia
ESR, CRP	Look for markers of inflammation
ANA with titer, ENA panel (SS-A, SS-B, RNP, anti-Smith), dsDNA	Serologies sensitive and/or specific to SLE
Coagulation panel (PT/PTT/INR), DRVVT, anti-cardiolipin IgM/IgG, B-2 glycoprotein antibodies	Check for hematologic abnormalities secondary to a lupus anticoagulant
C_3, C_4	Check for inflammatory consumption secondary to SLE
Liver function panel	Check for autoimmune hepatitis
BUN, creatinine, urine analysis	Check for lupus nephritis
TSH, free T_4, anti-TPO, anti-thyroglobulin	Check for autoimmune thyroiditis
Fasting lipid panel	Monitor for dyslipoproteinemia

Note: Complete blood count (CBC), erythrocyte sedimentation rate (ESR), C-reactive protein (CRP), antinuclear antibody (ANA), extractable nuclear antigen (ENA), Sjogren syndrome (SS), anti-ribonucleoprotein (RNP), dsDNA (anti-double-stranded DNA), PT (prothrombin time), PTT (partial thromboplastin time), INR (International Normalized Ratio), DRVVT (dilute Russell viper venom time), IG (immunoglobulin), BUN (blood urea nitrogen), TSH (thyroid-stimulating hormone), TPO (thyroid peroxidase).

Source: Adapted from Cassidy et al., 2005.

percent of healthy children have a positive ANA test, a rate that may increase nonspecifically with infections. An ANA value of 1:320 is considered high titer and should be further characterized with an extractable nuclear antigen panel if symptoms suggestive of SLE exist. The most specific antibodies for SLE include ANA, anti-double-stranded DNA (dsDNA), and anti-Smith antibodies, all of which are part of the ACR diagnostic criteria. The dsDNA level correlates with lupus nephritis and may be followed over time.

Given the amount of inflammation they experience, patients with SLE often have a high erythrocyte sedimentation rate (ESR). Complement components such as C_3 and C_4 are consumed by the circulating immune complexes, and their concentrations often fall to low levels in active disease.

Patients with SLE often present with hematologic abnormalities. The anemia of SLE may be either hemolytic in nature or the anemia of chronic disease. Leukopenia, especially lymphopenia, is common. Thrombocytopenia can also be present. Cytopenias usually resolve with SLE treatment. Development of thrombotic thrombocytopenic purpura (TTP) is considered an emergency that requires hospitalization of the patient and aggressive treatment.

Coagulation abnormalities in patients with SLE can be due to either the presence of antiphospholipid (APL) antibodies, such as a lupus anticoagulant or anticardiolipin antibodies, or circulating immune complexes. APL antibodies and the lupus anticoagulant are measured in a number of ways and must be present on at least two occasions, 12 weeks apart, to meet the ACR diagnostic criteria.

More than 60% of patients with SLE have kidney disease. Urinalyses in patients with active SLE nephritis often show proteinuria, hematuria, pyuria, or the presence of urinary casts. The International Society of Nephrology/Renal Pathology Society (ISN/RPS) classification is, therefore, based on renal biopsies. Once performed, the activity and chronicity of kidney involvement will guide treatment options. Patients who manifest symptoms of neuropsychiatric lupus may need further diagnostic evaluation to exclude non-SLE causes of CNS disease, such as infection. Lumbar puncture to examine the cerebrospinal fluid (CSF) cell count, protein, and culture, along with brain imaging, may be warranted. Patients with neuropsychiatric lupus may demonstrate elevated opening pressures accompanied by an elevated CSF protein count and cell count. Secondary autoimmune thyroid disease is also possible in patients, and periodic evaluation of anti-thyroglobulin and antithyroid peroxidase (TPO) antibodies via thyroid function studies should be obtained (Benseler & Silverman, 2007; Cassidy et al., 2005).

Radiologic studies may provide further information on the organs affected by SLE. Chest radiographs may indicate signs of serositis, including cardiomegaly, secondary to pericarditis and pleural effusion. A cardiac echocardiograph may evaluate for cardiac function, presence of valvular disease, and evidence of pulmonary hypertension. Pulmonary function tests, with measurement of carbon monoxide diffusing capacity, may be useful to monitor for pulmonary fibrosis. Joint radiographs and magnetic resonance imaging may demonstrate characteristics of arthritis (typically nonerosive), bony abnormalities, and soft-tissue swelling. A kidney ultrasound may be required if nephritis is present, and an abdominal ultrasound is required with abnormal liver function tests. A head MRI and magnetic resonance angiogram are recommended if concerns of lupus cerebritis arise. Given that 10% of patients with pediatric lupus develop avascular necrosis, many rheumatologists order a bone density scan to evaluate the bone health of patients who are taking a chronic course of corticosteroids (Benseler & Silverman, 2007; Cassidy et al., 2005).

Treatment for pediatric patients with SLE is based on whether the disease is considered mild, moderate, or severe. Most lupus therapies provided for children have been extrapolated from adult clinical trial data; therefore, they may not be completely applicable. Patients with childhood-onset SLE require treatment with high-dose corticosteroids and other immunosuppressive agents more often than adults.

Children with mild lupus do not have kidney or other major organ system involvement. They may have rashes, arthralgias or arthritis, leukopenia, anemia, fever, and fatigue. Treatment for mild disease involves NSAIDs, low-dose corticosteroids (prednisone 0.5 mg/kg/day), and disease-modifying agents such as hydroxychloroquine and low-dose methotrexate (0.5 mg/kg/week). Patients with APL antibody syndrome may require prophylaxis with aspirin or other anticoagulation.

In moderate lupus, patients have mild disease with mild organ system involvement, such as minor pericarditis, pneumonitis, hemolytic anemia, thrombocytopenia, mild renal disease, and mild CNS disease. Treatment includes medium-dose corticosteroids (prednisone 1–2 mg/kg/day), hydroxychloroquine, low-dose methotrexate, azathioprine, and mycophenolate mofetil (MMF).

Severe lupus is characterized by life-threatening organ system abnormalities, such as severe hemolytic anemia, CNS disease, lupus nephritis, and lupus crisis. Treatment is aggressive in these patients, and consists of high-dose intravenous corticosteroids (2–3 mg/kg/day or pulse dose 30 mg/kg/day) in combination with immunosuppressive agents such as cyclophosphamide, azathrioprine, metho-trexate, cyclosporine, MMF, or rituximab. In certain situations, plasmapheresis, intravenous immune globulin (IVIG), and anticoagulation may be required as stabilization therapy. Dialysis and kidney transplant have been used in patients with end-stage renal disease.

Patients with neuropsychiatric lupus are typically treated with immunosuppressive medications such as high-dose steroids in conjunction with cyclophosphamide or azathioprine. They may also require treatment with antidepressants or psychotropic medication.

Management is directed at preventing permanent organ system damage through the use of medications: for chronic maintenance, to treat acute flares, and to prevent long-term side effects. Although steroids are the mainstay of treatment, they are used sparingly due to their own morbidities. Occasionally, steroid-induced diabetes may occur, requiring short-term treatment with insulin. Additionally, significant complications may arise from use of aggressive immunosuppressive medications, such as severe infections, bone marrow toxicity, infertility, and secondary malignancy. General supportive care is also important—for example, use of sun block, appropriate vaccinations, infection control, adequate nutrition with good calcium/vitamin D supplementation, and exercise (Cassidy et al., 2005; Klein-Gitelman et al., 2002).

Given that lupus nephritis is the most common morbidity in pediatric patients with SLE, consultation with a nephrologist is often helpful. A nephrologist may manage hypertension secondary to renal damage or steroid-induced hypertension, or perform a kidney biopsy to provide necessary diagnostic and prognostic information. If the patient develops APL syndrome, consultation with a hematologist for appropriate management may be considered. A nutritionist may suggest an appropriate diet, especially in patients with severe lupus nephritis leading to kidney failure. Patients with long-standing illness may benefit

from rehabilitation therapy. In patients with neuropsychiatric lupus, an interprofessional team approach involving a neurologist, a psychologist, and a psychiatrist is best.

The diagnosis of SLE is difficult for patients and families, as it requires the adoption of a new lifestyle and the need to take multiple medications daily. Compliance with the therapeutic plan can be difficult for adolescents, who may subsequently experience severe consequences and poor outcomes. Patients and families need to learn to monitor for signs of disease recurrence.

Given that patients with SLE usually take one or more immunosuppressive medications, patients and their families also need to learn to identify the signs of possible infection, such as fever, rash, headache, and prolonged nausea/vomiting or diarrhea. Patients exhibiting any physical signs concerning for possible lupus flare or infection are usually asked to call their primary rheumatologist for advice, see their primary care provider, or go to an acute care facility for evaluation. Patients with severe infection may need to be hospitalized for parenteral antibiotics and steroids.

DISPOSITION AND DISCHARGE PLANNING

The natural history of lupus is characterized by a variable and largely unpredictable clinical course, punctuated by periods of flare and quiescence. Untreated SLE often results in progressive deterioration and has a significant mortality rate. However, earlier and more accurate diagnosis and better approaches to treatment have dramatically improved survival in pediatric patients with SLE over the last 20 years. For lupus patients diagnosed since 2000, the 5-year survival rate approaches 100%, and the 10-year survival rate is close to 90%. Nevertheless, cumulate organ damage is common in patients with pediatric-onset SLE, with the frequency of damage ranging from 50.5% to 61%. Outcomes tend to be worse in patients with proliferative renal disease or CNS disease, and both are the leading causes of death in patients with SLE if they occur as a result of infections (Benseler & Silverman, 2007; Ravelli et al., 2005).

Discharge instructions for patients who are newly diagnosed with SLE should incorporate both detailed written and verbal instructions. The following information is a component of preparation for discharge and follow-up:

- List of medications, reasons for those medications, dosages, and side effects
- Symptoms of flare and education on when to seek medical attention
- Phone numbers to call or instructions to see the primary care provider or go to the acute care center in the event of possible infection or concerning symptoms
- Supplies
  - If the patient has kidney disease and signs of hypertension, the patient may need a blood pressure cuff and teaching.

- If the patient is on high-dose steroids and has signs of steroid-induced diabetes, the patient may need diabetes teaching, supplies, and teaching.
- Appointments with pertinent subspecialists (pediatric rheumatologists, nephrologists, hematologists, primary care provider).

Routine follow-up care for patients with SLE includes once- or twice-yearly visits with an ophthalmologist, as well as periodic screening of antibodies, complement elements, thyroid function, and lipid panels. An echocardiograph, pulmonary function tests, and DEXA scan may be indicated yearly.

VASCULITIS

Regina Mosier

PATHOPHYSIOLOGY

Vasculitis can be the result of conditions or diseases such as autoimmune disorders and drug reactions (Miller & Pachman, 2007). All vasculitic disorders are characterized by necrosis and inflammation of the blood vessels (Singh & Dass, 2002). Although the exact pathophysiology of vasculitides is unknown, clinical evidence points to an infectious agent (Ozen, 2002). The possibility that the condition is caused by clones of toxic shock syndrome toxin-producing bacteria such as staphylococci or pyrogenic exotoxin-producing streptococci is being studied (Brogan & Dillon, 2000). Small-vessel vasculitis may also be characterized by immune involvement of small blood vessels in association with antineutrophil cytoplasm antibodies (ANCA); however, how these factors interact in the pathophysiology remains unclear (Yalcindag & Sundel, 2002).

EPIDEMIOLOGY AND ETIOLOGY

Vasculitis is uncommon in children, with two specific exceptions—Kawasaki disease (KD) and Henoch-Schönlein purpura (HSP). General vasculitis has an incidence of 50 per 100,000 pediatric patients per year (Rowley et al., 2009).

Differentiating between the specific diagnoses when presented with a patient who has a vasculitic disorder depends on symptomatology, laboratory findings, and the exclusion of all other diagnoses. Many other disease processes can imitate systemic vasculitis—namely, bacterial endocarditis, Lyme disease, hypertensive arteriopathy, effects of vasoconstrictive drugs, thoracic outlet syndrome, and cholesterol embolism. All vasculitic diseases have the vague findings of malaise, fever, and pain (Table 29-20).

Classification

Classification of vascular diseases can be broken into groupings based on the size and location of the blood vessels affected. Two notable classifications are the Chapel Hill nomenclature criteria (CHCC) and the American College of Rheumatology (ACR) criteria (Ozen, 2005), though neither has been validated in children. The following disorders are organized in the CHCC format due to its more inclusive nature (Ozen, 2002).

TABLE 29-20

Differential Diagnoses for Vascular Diseases	
Differential Diagnosis	**Criteria**
Takayasu arteritis	Patient younger than 40 years of age at diagnosis
	Claudication of extremities
	Reduced brachial pulse
	Difference in blood pressure between right and left arms greater than 10 mmHg
	Bruising above subclavian artery and/or aorta
	Arteriographic pathology
	At least three criteria must be present for diagnosis.
Kawasaki disease	Fever of unknown origin for at least 5 days
	Changes at extremities such as plantar or palmar erythema, edema of wrist, or periungually (with desquamation during reconvalescence)
	Changes at mucous membranes such as cheilitis, pharyngitis, and glossitis
	Polymorphous exanthema
	Acute nonsuppurative lymphadenopathy (at least 1 lymph node larger than 1 cm in diameter)
	Besides fever, four of the other criteria must be positive for diagnosis.

(Continued)

TABLE 29-20

Differential Diagnoses for Vascular Diseases *(Continued)*	
Differential Diagnosis	**Criteria**
Wegener disease	Inflammation of nose or mouth (ulcerative features)
	Pulmonary infiltrations on chest radiograph
	Abnormal urinalysis (more than 5 red blood cells per high-power field or red cell casts in sediment)
	Histology: granulomatous inflammation with fibrinoid necrosis
	At least two of these four criteria must be present for diagnosis.
Churg-Strauss syndrome	Asthma
	Eosinophilia (more than 10% in blood cell count)
	History of any allergy
	Changes in paranasal sinuses
	Mononeuropathy/polyneuropathy
	Lung nonfixed infiltrates on chest radiograph
	Biopsy
	At least four of these six criteria must be present for diagnosis.
Behçet's disease	Recurrent genital ulcers
	Ocular lesions (anterior or posterior uveitis, retinal vasculitis)
	Skin lesions (erythema nodosum, pseudofolliculitis, acne-like lesions)
	Pathergy test positivity (appears within 24 hours, maximizes in 48 hours, 1- to 2-mm elevated lesion)
Polyarterites nodosa	**Major Criteria** Kidney involvement Musculoskeletal findings
	Minor Criteria Cutaneous findings Cardiac involvement Lung involvement Acute-phase reactants Gastrointestinal involvement Peripheral neuropathy Central nervous system disease Hypertension Constitutional symptoms Presence of HbsAg
	Five of the criteria with one major criteria must be present for the diagnosis.
	or
	Weight loss greater than 4 kg
	Livedo reticularis
	Testicular pain or tenderness
	Myalgia, muscular weakness, leg tenderness
	Mononeuropathy/polyneuropathy
	Diastolic blood pressure greater than 90 mmHg
	Elevated azotemia (greater than 0 mg/dL) or creatininemia (less than 1.5 mg/dL)
	Serum Australia antigen
	HBsAg positivity
	Arteriographic abnormalities
	Biopsy of small or medium-sized arteries containing
	polymorphonucleate granulocytes
	At three presenting factors out of the 10 must be present for the diagnosis.

LARGE-VESSEL VASCULITIS

Takayasu arteritis

Takayasu arteritis (TA), also known as "pulseless disease," primarily affects the aorta and its branches and can result in vessel stenosis or occlusion (Kim & Dedeoglu, 2005; Rigante, 2006). First identified by Migito Takayasu in 1908, it is the most common cause of giant-cell or large-vessel vasculitis in young patients and occurs most frequently in females aged 15 to 30 years who are living in Eastern countries (Rigante; Singh & Dass, 2002). In Japanese patients, TA has been frequently identified with the haplotype A24 B52 DR2. This disease has also been linked to *Mycobacterium* tuberculosis (TB). When TA is associated with TB infection, it is thought that a large-vessel hypersensitivity response leads to an autoimmune reaction, resulting in TA (Singh & Dass).

Presentation.   Signs and symptoms of TA include malaise, fever, nocturnal sweating, elevations in acute inflammatory markers, weight loss, visual abnormalities, headache, dysarthria, and arthralgias. Physical examination findings may include the following:

- Upper-extremity systolic blood pressure variance (10 mmHg)
- Subclavian artery or abdominal aorta bruit
- Decreased or absent brachial artery pulse
- Normochromic, normocytic anemia (present in 50% of affected children)

With vessel stenosis or occlusion, decreased brachial artery pulse, stroke, dysarthria, visual abnormalities, hypertension, and heart failure may also result.

Plan of care.   Radiographic studies may show calcification or widening of the aorta or other affected arteries. Doppler imaging and magnetic resonance imaging may be useful for greater clarification of vessel changes. Biopsy of affected vessels may note loss of muscle and elastic tissues in arterial walls. Immunofluorescence may be remarkable for elevated IgG, IgM, and properden levels (Singh & Dass, 2002).

Therapeutic management of TA relies primarily on steroids, especially in the acute phase of the illness. Cytotoxic drugs, including cyclophosphamide, azathioprine, and methotrexate, and anti-TNF agents have also been used in these patients with some success (Kim & Dedeoglu, 2005). Narrowing or occlusion of vessels may require surgical correction (Rigante, 2006).

Disease identification may be delayed due to the infrequency of this diagnosis in the pediatric population and lowered suspicion for its presence. Consultation with cardiology, cardiovascular surgery, immunology, hematology, or critical care medicine may be of benefit.

MEDIUM-VESSEL VASCULITIS

Kawasaki disease

Kawasaki disease (KD) is a medium muscular artery, acute, self-limiting, multisystemic vasculitic syndrome occurring primarily in pediatric patients younger than 2 years of age. It has also been referred to as mucutaneous lymph node syndrome. Its incidence ranges from 9.1 to 32.5 per 100,000 population per year. The male-to-female ratio is 1.5:1, and 85% of cases occur in children younger than 5 years of age. KD has a greater prevalence in Japan. It is hypothesized that environmental factors such as infectious agents and genetic factors influence its distribution (Ozen, 2002). In particular, the haplotype A24 B52 DR2 has been identified with high frequency in Japanese patients with KD.

Presentation.   Kawasaki disease presents with an *acute phase* lasting 1 to 2 weeks, a *subacute phase* in the third and fourth weeks, and a final *convalescent phase* from the fourth through eighth weeks of the disease course (Rigante, 2006). Clinical criteria for classical KD consist of fever that persists for 5 or more days plus at least four of the principal symptoms listed in Table 29-21. Approximately 10% of patients will have a fever and fewer than four clinical criteria; this variant is referred to as *incomplete Kawasaki disease* (Kim & Dedeoglu, 2005).

Plan of care

There are no diagnostic studies specific for KD. Those useful to measure inflammation are erythrocyte sedimentation rate and C-reactive protein. The ESR is usually 40 to 100 mm/hr, while the CRP concentration may be greater than 3 mg/dL (Freeman & Shulman, 2006). Other findings may include neutrophil leucocytosis, normocytic anemia, eosinophilia, hypoalbuminemia, hypokalemia, and elevated fibrinogen and liver transaminase levels (Rigante, 2006). In some patients, chest radiographs may show peribronchial cuffing or increased interstitial markings and abdominal ultrasonography may show gallbladder hydrops. Abnormalities in the coronary arteries may appear within the first 10 days of the child developing a fever; consequently, serial echocardiography should be performed with suspected, indeterminate, and definitive KD. Echocardiography may also reveal decreased ventricular function, mild valvular regurgitation, or pericardial effusion (Freeman & Shulman). Young infants should be evaluated with echocardiography if they have fever lasting 7 or more days with laboratory evidence of systemic inflammation (Freeman & Shulman).

Therapeutic management of KD starts with intravenous immunoglobulin (2 gm/kg) and high-dose acetylsalicylic acid (ASA [aspirin]) consisting of 80 to 100 mg/kg/day divided into four doses. The ASA dose is decreased to 3 to 5 mg/kg/day (single dose) after the patient has been

TABLE 29-21

Diagnostic Criteria for Kawasaki Disease		
Fever for 5 days	**Classic Clinical Criteria**	**Other Clinical and Laboratory Findings**
Plus four of the five principal symptoms or More than four symptoms and coronary vessel involvement	Bilateral conjunctival congestion	Cardiovascular: heart murmur, gallop rhythm, muffled heart sounds, ECG changes, enlarged heart on CXR, angina pectoris, or myocardial infarction
	Changes in lips and mouth (reddened, strawberry tongue; dry cracked lips; oral erythema)	Gastrointestinal tract: diarrhea, nausea, vomiting, and abdominal pain
	Polymorphous skin rash	Joints: pain, swelling
	Changes in periphery (reddening of palms and soles, indurative edema)	Skin: redness and crusting, small pustules, transverse furrows of the finger nails
	Acute cervical lymphadenopathy (larger than 1 cm)	Respiratory: cough, rhinorrhea
		Leukocytosis with neutrophilia and immature forms, elevated ESR, elevated CRP, anemia, abnormal plasma lipids, hypoalbuminemia, hyponatremia, thrombocytosis after week 1, sterile pyuria, elevated serum transaminases, elevated serum gamma glutamyl transpeptidase, pleocytosis of cerebrospinal fluid, leukocytosis in synovial fluid

Note: Electrocardiograph (ECG), chest radiograph (CXR), C-reactive protein (CRP), erythrocyte sedimentation rate (ESR).

afebrile for 48 to 72 hours. It is then continued for 6 to 8 weeks to capitalize on its antiplatelet effect. If coronary abnormalities are present, however, ASA therapy continues indefinitely and is based on the risk level as outlined by the American Heart Association (Freeman & Schulman, 2006):

- *Risk level I:* normal coronary arteries. ASA is needed only for the first 6 to 8 weeks, as previously noted, and no invasive cardiac studies are required. Families of these patients should receive counseling every 5 years because of the ongoing increased risk of myocardial ischemia, infarction, and sudden death. Patients with KD have long-term endothelial dysfunction and abnormally high lipid profiles.
- *Risk level II:* transient coronary artery ectasia or dilation that resolves by 8 weeks after the acute phase of the disease. All of the recommendations are the same as those for risk level I patients, except that counseling should occur every 3 years (instead of every 5).
- *Risk level III:* small to medium (3–6 mm or *z* score of 3–7) coronary artery aneurysms. Administer ASA therapy until regression of disease occurs. Physical activity is limited for the first 8 weeks for patients younger than 10 years of age. A cardiac stress test should be done every 2 years and before any sports participation for those patients who are older than 10 years of age. Patients should not engage in high-impact sports

while on antiplatelet therapy. Echocardiography and electrocardiography are recommended on a yearly basis. Angiography is recommended if any abnormalities are found on the stress test.
- *Risk level IV:* large (more than 6 mm) aneurysms and coronary arteries with multiple complex aneurysms without any obstruction. Administer ASA on a long-term basis, along with warfarin or low-molecular-weight heparin. Yearly cardiac stress tests are recommended. Patients should not engage in high-impact sports. Echocardiography and electrocardiography should be performed every 6 months, and cardiac catheterization every 6 to 12 months. Counseling should include atherosclerosis risk factors and reproductive issues for women of child-bearing age.
- *Risk level V:* obstruction of the coronary artery aneurysms on angiography. All of the recommendations are the same as those for risk level IV patients, except that β-adrenergic blocking agents should also be administered to decrease the myocardial workload (Freeman & Shulman, 2006).

Infectious diseases and cardiology services should be consulted for initial and ongoing management of patients with KD. Those patients with significant respiratory, cardiovascular, or neurological involvement should be considered for transfer to a pediatric intensive care unit (PICU) for care and stabilization.

Patient and family education is based on the patient's risk level (as previously described), medications, and long-term follow-up needs.

The risk of coronary dilation is decreased by 3% in patients who are older than one year of age if they receive IVIG within 10 days of their presenting symptoms. Approximately 50% of patients who develop coronary aneurysms will experience regression of the dilation; 80% will experience resolution within 5 years. Monitoring continues well after 5 years, given that myointimal proliferation can lead to stenosis of the coronary artery over time. This blockage is most common with large aneurysms and at the entrance or exit of vessels (Freeman & Shulman, 2006).

The mortality rate for KD is 1.25%, with death most likely to occur in the first year of disease onset. Thrombosis that results in a myocardial infarction is the main cause of death in patients with KD. Coronary artery grafts, angioplasty, stents, and cardiac transplantation have been used with some success in those patients with severe coronary involvement.

Polyarterites nodosa

Polyarterites nodosa (PAN), first noted by Kussmaul and Maier more than 100 years ago, is a multisystem disease that affects the arteries of small and medium-sized vessels. The most commonly involved organs are the skin, joints, kidneys, gastrointestinal tract, and peripheral nerves. PAN is a very rare disease in children and may not be diagnosed until found during postmortem evaluation. It affects males and females equally, with the peak age of 9 to 11 years. Although PAN's etiology is unknown, the disease has been associated with hepatitis B virus and streptococcal infection (Singh & Dass, 2002).

Presentation. Diagnosis of PAN is difficult due to this disease's nonspecific signs and symptoms. The initial symptoms include fever, malaise, and weight loss. The typical presentation (85% of patients) is notable for kidney and other visceral involvement with localized lesions in arterial bifurcations. This can lead to the characteristic finding of fibrinoid necrosis of vessel walls with occlusions (Rigante, 2006). Fifty percent of those patients presenting with PAN have skin involvement such as purpura, nodules, ulcerations, and gangrene. Magnetic resonance imaging may be negative for aneurysms even when they are actually present; consequently, cerebral angiography is recommended for patients suspected of having PAN.

Plan of care. Vessel biopsy may be useful for diagnosis; however, it may not show fibrinoid necrosis. Tests for the autoantibody MPO-ANCA are negative in those individuals with medium-sized vessel PAN and positive in those with small-vessel disease (Oomura et al., 2006). Fifteen percent of patients with PAN test positive for ANCA; most have an elevated ESR, and 30% test positive for HBsAg (Rigante, 2006; Singh & Dass, 2002).

Therapeutic management with long-term glucocorticoids is recommended. Long-term outcomes, however, may be improved with the addition of cytotoxic therapy. Cyclophosphamide—the most commonly used agent—may be administered for as long as 1 to 2 years after the disease is in remission. Monitoring of serial ESR and CRP levels throughout therapy is recommended. Relapse is common, although its incidence is lower in children than in adults. Mortality rates in children are also lower. If PAN is left untreated, it has a 5-year survival rate of less than 15% (Singh & Dass, 2002).

SMALL-VESSEL VASCULITIS

Wegener granulomatosis

Wegener granulomatosis (WG) is characterized by immune involvement of small blood vessels in association with antineutrophil cytoplasm antibodies (ANCA). How these factors interact in the pathophysiology is unclear (Yalcindag & Sundel, 2001). WG is extremely rare in children.

Presentation. Clinical findings for WG are related to the location of the necrotizing granulomatous vasculitis, which most often affects the upper and lower respiratory tracts and kidneys. Pediatric patients have a higher occurrence of subglottic stenosis and nasal abnormalities compared to adults. Nasal findings include mucosal ulcerations and recurring nose bleeds (Rigante, 2006).

Plan of care. Diagnostic studies for WG consist of enzyme-linked immunosorbent assays with an indirect immunofluorescence of peripheral blood neutrophils and ANCA.

Therapeutic management includes immunosuppressant agents such as steroids, cyclophosphamide, and azathioprine. It is directed based on a comprehensive plan developed by specialists in hematology/oncology, cardiology, immunology, otolaryngology, and pulmonology.

WG causes significant morbidity and mortality, often leads to relapses, and has a high risk for chronic organ damage even with aggressive therapy. Long-term follow-up is necessary to monitor for relapse (Rigante, 2006.) Prognosis may be improved if therapy is initiated before the development of kidney failure (Yalcindag & Sundel, 2001).

Churg-strauss syndrome

Churg-Strauss syndrome (CSS) is a small-vessel vasculopathy in which patients test positive for ANCA. First described in 1951, it is associated with a combination of findings, much like all of the other vasculopathies, but is singled out by its association with allergic symptoms and asthma (Rigante, 2006). CSS is rare in both pediatric and adult populations, but with awareness has come increasing detection of this disease. The vasculitis is characterized by hypereosinophilia. The resulting eosinophilic clusters promote the development of inflammatory nodules (granulomatosis) that involve the blood vessels of several other systems—pulmonary, gastrointestinal, and peripheral nerves. In addition, these clusters may affect the heart, kidneys, and dermis.

Presentation.   CSS may present early on with nasal polyps and allergic rhinitis, which then develops into unrelenting sinus allergies. New-onset or worsening asthma is another cardinal feature and may be the initial presenting symptom. Pulmonary infiltrates have been reported in one-third of all patients. Dermal nodules have been appreciated on pressure point areas. As the disorder progresses, symptoms of neuropathy or mononeuritis multiplex occur, producing severe tingling, numbness, and "shooting" pains in the hands and feet. Associated muscle wasting and loss of extremity strength have been noted as well.

Plan of care.   In addition to a detailed history and physical examination, rheumatologic and immunologic studies, liver and kidney functions, chest radiograph (CXR) and other diagnostic imaging studies, nerve conduction tests, and tissue biopsies (lung, skin, nerve) may be performed to aid in the diagnosis of CSS. Definitive diagnosis is based on a tissue biopsy that confirms the presence of peripheral eosinophilia. Series of CXRs may demonstrate transient pulmonary infiltrates, and sinus radiographs and imaging will likely show parasinus abnormalities.

The goal of therapy is to place the patient in remission as quickly and as safely as possible. The treatment for CSS consists of infliximab or etanercept with plasmapheresis and immunoglobulin supplementation. Prednisone may be administered for 1 month and cyclophosphamide for 6 months. This combination has had some success in inducing remission (Rigante, 2006). Therapeutic management is based on a comprehensive plan developed by HCPs from multiple subspecialties, including hematology/oncology, cardiology, rheumatology, immunology, gastroenterology, nephrology, dermatology, and pulmonology.

ALL VESSELS

Behçet's disease

The classic findings in Behçet's disease are the presence of recurrent oral aphthous ulcerations (at least 3 times in 12 months). Also common are eye symptoms such as iridocyclitis, hypopyon, vitreitis, retinal vasculitis, and macular edema. Other nonspecific symptoms include genital ulcers, skin lesions, and vascular, neurological, and articular disease (Rigante, 2006).

Behçet's disease specifically affects young adult males. Its prevalence is especially high in countries of the Middle East, Far East, and those bordering the Mediterranean Sea, including Italy, Greece, Turkey, Israel, Saudi Arabia, Iran, China, Korea, and Japan (Rigante, 2006). There is an association of the HLA-B51 haplotype with this disease.

Pathergy testing may be useful, although diagnosis is usually based on history and physical examination. In this testing, the patient's forearm is punctured with a sterile needle; the puncture site is then examined in 24 hours. When Behçet's disease is present, a red lesion should appear by 24 hours; it should then measure its largest diameter, with an elevation of 1 to 2 mm, by 48 hours.

The choice for treating Behçet's disease depends on the clinical picture and the need to alleviate symptoms. Initial therapy starts with steroids, although the long-term treatment consists of immunosuppression with drugs such as cyclosporine, cyclophosphamide, and chlorambucil (Rigante, 2006). Therapeutic management is based on a comprehensive plan developed by HCPs from multiple subspecialties, such as hematology/oncology, cardiology, ophthalmology, immunology, gastroenterology, nephrology, dermatology, and pulmonology.

The prognosis for patients with anterior uveitis in Behçet's disease is usually good, with little vision loss. In contrast, patients with posterior inflammation of the eye usually experience some degree of visual loss (Rigante, 2006).

REFERENCES

1. Abbas, A., Lichtman, A., & Pillai S. (2007). *Cellular and molecular immunology.* Philadelphia: Saunders Elsevier.
2. Adelman, D., Casale, T., & Corren, J. (2002). *Manual of allergy and immunology.* Philadelphia: Lippincott Williams & Wilkins.
3. Aggarwal, M., & Rein, J. (2003). Acute human immunodeficiency virus syndrome in an adolescent. *Pediatrics, 112,* 323–324.
4. Beaudouin, E., Renaudin, J., Morisset, M., Codreanu, F., Kanny, G., & Moneret-Vautrin, D. (2006). Food-dependent exercise-induced anaphylaxis: Update and current data. *European Annals of Allergy and Clinical Immunology, 38,* 45–51.
5. Benseler, S., & Silverman, E. (2007). Systemic lupus erythematosus. *Rheumatic Disease Clinics of North America, 33,* 471–498.
6. Berger, M. (2008). Subcutaneous administration of IgG. *Immunology and Allergy Clinics of North America, 28*(4), 779–802.
7. Bhole, M., Burton, J., & Chapel, H. (2008). Self-infusion programmes for immunoglobulin replacement at home: Feasibility, safety and efficacy. *Immunology and Allergy Clinics of North America, 28*(4), 821–832.
8. Bleasel, K., Donnan, G., & Unglik, G. A. (2009). General anesthetic allergy testing. *Current Allergy and Asthma Reports, 9,* 50–56.
9. Bogomolski-Yahalom, V., & Matzner, Y. (1995). Disorders of neutrophil function. *Blood Reviews, 9*(3), 183–19.
10. Bohlke, K., Davis, R., Maarcy, S., Braun, M., DeStefano, F., & Black, S., et al. (2003). Risk of anaphylaxis after vaccination of children and adolescents. *Pediatrics, 112,* 815–820.
11. Brichard, B., & Van der Linden, D. (2009). Clinical practice treatment of HIV infection in children. *European Journal of Pediatrics, 168,* 387–392.

12. Brogan, P., & Dillon, M. (2000). Vasculitis from the pediatric perspective. *Current Rheumatology Reports, 2*, 411–416.

13. Brown, S. (2007). The pathophysiology of shock in anaphylaxis. *Immunology and Allergy Clinics of North America, 27*, 165–175.

14. Buckley, R. (2008). Immune Deficiency Foundation diagnostic and clinical care guidelines for primary immunodeficiency diseases. Retrieved from http://www.primaryimmune.org/publications

15. Bukantz, S., Bagg, A., & Lockey, R. (2008). Adverse effects and fatalities associated with subcutaneous allergen immunotherapy. *Clinical Allergy and Immunology, 21*, 455–468.

16. Butterfield, J. (2006). Systemic mastocytosis: Clinical manifestations and differential diagnosis. *Immunology and Allergy Clinics of North America, 26*, 487–514.

17. Calles, N., Evans, D., & Terlonge, D. (2009). Pathophysiology of the human immunodeficiency virus. Retrieved from www.scribd.com

18. Campbell, R., Luke, A., Weaver, A., St. Sauver, J., Bergstralh, E., Li, J., et al. (2008). Prescriptions for self-injectable epinephrine and follow-up referral in emergency department patients presenting with anaphylaxis. *Annals of Allergy, Asthma, and Immunology, 101*, 631–636.

19. Cassidy, J., & Petty, R. (2005a). Chronic arthritis in childhood. In J. Cassidy, R. Petty, R. Laxer, & C. Lindsley (Eds.), *Textbook of pediatric rheumatology* (5th ed., pp. 206–260). Philadelphia: Saunders Elsevier.

20. Cassidy, J., & Petty, R. (2005b). Polyarthritis. In J. Cassidy, R. Petty, R. Laxer, & C. Lindsley (Eds.), *Textbook of pediatric rheumatology* (5th ed., pp. 261–273). Philadelphia: Saunders Elsevier.

21. Cassidy, J., & Petty, R. (2005c). Oligoarthritis. In J. Cassidy, R. Petty, R. Laxer, & C. Lindsley (Eds.), *Textbook of pediatric rheumatology* (5th ed., pp. 274–290). Philadelphia: Saunders Elsevier.

22. Cassidy, J., & Petty, R. (2005d). Systemic arthritis. In J. Cassidy, R. Petty, R. Laxer, & C. Lindsley (Eds.), *Textbook of pediatric rheumatology* (5th ed., pp. 291–303). Philadelphia: Saunders Elsevier.

23. Cassidy, J., Petty, R., Laxer, R., & Lindsley, C. (2005). *Textbook of pediatric rheumatology* (5th ed.). Philadelphia: Elsevier Saunders.

24. Centers for Disease Control and Prevention (CDC). (2008). Revised surveillance case definitions for HIV infections among adults, adolescents, and children aged < 18 months and for HIV infection and AIDS among children aged 18 months to < 13 years—United States. Retrieved from http://www.cdc.gov

25. Centers for Disease Control and Prevention (CDC). (2009). Guidelines for the prevention and treatment of opportunistic infections among HIV exposed and infected children. Retrieved from http://www.cdc.gov

26. Chacko, T., & Ledford, D. (2007). Peri-anesthetic anaphylaxis. *Immunology and Allergy Clinics of North America, 27*, 213–230.

27. Chegini, S., & Metcalfe, D. (2005). Contemporary issues in food allergy: Seafood toxin-induced disease in the differential diagnosis of allergic reactions. *Allergy and Asthma Proceedings, 26*, 183–190.

28. Chikanza, I. (1999). Prolactin and neuroimmunomodulation: In vitro and in vivo observations. *Annals of the New York Academy of Sciences, 876*, 119–130.

29. Chiu, A., & Kelly, K. (2005). Anaphylaxis: Drug allergy, insect sting and latex. *Immunology and Allergy Clinics of North America, 25*, 389–405.

30. Choo, K., & Sheikh, A. (2007). Action plans for the long-term management of anaphylaxis: Systematic review of effectiveness. *Clinical and Experimental Allergy, 37*, 1090–1094.

31. Clark, S., Bock, S., Gaeta, T., Brenner, B., Cydulka, R., & Camargo, C. (2004). Multicenter study of emergency department visits for food allergies. *Journal of Allergy and Clinical Immunology, 113*, 347–352.

32. Clark, S., & Carmargo, C. (2007). Epidemiology of anaphylaxis. *Immunology and Allergy Clinics of North America, 27*, 145–163.

33. Cooper, M., Pommering, T., & Koranyi, M. (2003). Primary immunodeficiencies. *American Family Physician, 68*, 2001–2008, 2011.

34. Dahlgren, C., & Karlsson, A. (1999). Respiratory burst in human neutrophils. *Journal of Immunological Methods, 232*(1–2), 3–14.

35. Dalal, I., & Roifman, C. (2001). Hypogammaglobulinemia of infancy. *Immunology and Allergy Clinics of North America, 21*(1), 129–139.

36. Daschner, A., Alonso-Gomez, A., Cabanos, R., Suarez-de-Parga, J., & López-Serrano, M. (2000). Gastroallergic anisakiasis: Borderline between food allergy and parasitic disease: Clinical and allergologic evaluation of 20 patients with confirmed acute parasitism by Anisakis simplex. *Journal of Allergy and Clinical Immunology, 105*, 176–181.

37. Da Silva, J., Peers, S., Perretti, M., & Willoughby, D. (1993). Sex steroids affect glucocorticoid response to chronic inflammation and to interleukin-1. *Journal of Endocrinology, 136*(3), 389–397.

38. De Kleer, I., Brinkman, D., Ferster, A., Abinum, M., Quartier, P., Van Der Net, J., et al. (2004). Autologous stem cell transplantation for refractory juvenile idiopathic arthritis: Analysis of clinical effects, mortality, and transplant related morbidity. *Annals of Rheumatic Diseases, 63*(10), 1318–1326.

39. Dewachter, P., & Mouton-Faivre, C. (2008). What investigation after an anaphylactic reaction during anaesthesia? *Current Opinion in Anesthesiology, 21*, 363–368.

40. Ellis, A., & Day, J. (2007). Incidence and characteristics of biphasic anaphylaxis: Prospective evaluation of 103 patients. *Annals of Allergy, Asthma, and Immunology, 98*, 64–69.

41. Fernando, S. (2009). Cold-induced anaphylaxis. *Journal of Pediatrics, 154*, 148.

42. Fischer, A., Lisowska-Grospierre, B., Anderson, D., & Springer, T. (1988). Leukocyte adhesion deficiency: Molecular basis and functional consequences. *Immunodeficiency Reviews, 1*(1), 39–54.

43. Fosarelli, P., Winkelstein, J., DeAngelis, C., & Mellits, E. D. (1985). Serum immunoglobulins in the first year of life. *Clinical Pediatrics, 24*(2), 84–88.

44. Freeman, A., & Shulman, S. (2006). Kawasaki disease: Summary of the American Heart Association Guidelines. Retrieved March 31, 2009, from www.aafp.org/afp

45. Garcia-Lloret, M., McGhee, S., & Chatila, T. (2008). Immunoglobulin replacement therapy in children. *Immunology and Allergy Clinics of North America, 28*(4), 833–859.

46. Geha, R., Notarangelo, L., Casanova, J., Chapel, H., Conley, M., Fischer, A., et al. (2007). Primary immunodeficiency diseases: An update from the International Union of Immunological Societies Primary Immunodeficiency Diseases Classification Committee. *Journal of Allergy and Clinical Immunology, 120*(4), 776–794.

47. Goldmuntz, E., & White, P. (2006). Juvenile idiopathic arthritis: A review for the pediatrician. *Pediatrics Reviews, 27*(4), e24–32.

48. Gordon, E., Krouse, H., Kinney, J., Stieh, E., & Klaustermeyer, W. (1980). Delayed cutaneous hypersensitivity in normals: Choice of antigens and comparison to in vitro assays of cell-mediated immunity. *Journal of Allergy and Clinical Immunology, 72*(5), 487–494.

49. Greenberger, P. (2007). Idiopathic anaphylaxis. *Immunology and Allergy Clinics of North America, 27*, 273–293.

50. Guillaume, S., Prieur, A., Coste, J., & Job-Deslandre, C. (2000). Long-term outcome and prognosis in oligoarticular-onset juvenile idiopathic arthritis. *Arthritis and Rheumatism, 43*, 1858–1865.

51. Havens, P., Mofenson, L., & Committee on Pediatric AIDS. (2009). Evaluation and management of an infant exposed to HIV-1 in the United States. *Pediatrics, 123*, 175–187.

52. Hiemstra, I., Vossen, J., van der Meer, J., Weemaes, C., Out, T., & Zegers, B. (1989). Clinical and immunological studies in patients with an increased serum IgD level. *Journal of Clinical Immunology, 9*(5), 393–400.

53. Hiraki, L., Benseler, S., Tyrrell, P., Herbert, D., Harvey, E., & Silverman, E. (2008). Clinical and laboratory characteristics and long-term outcome of pediatric systemic lupus erythematosus. *Journal of Pediatrics, 152*(4), 550–556.

54. Jaffe, E., Lejtenyi, C., Noya, F., & Mazer, B. (2001). Secondary hypogammaglobulinemia. *Immunology and Allergy Clinics of North America, 21*(1), 141–163.

55. Jarvinen, K., Sicherer, S., Sampson, H., & Nowak-Wegrzyn, A. (2008). Use of multiple doses of epinephrine in food-induced anaphylaxis in children. *Journal of Allergy and Clinical Immunology, 122*, 133–138.

56. Jeffrey Modell Foundation. (2009). 10 warning signs of immunodeficiency. Retrieved from http://www.info4pi.org/aboutpi

57. Jolliff, C., Cost, K., Stivrins, P., Grossman, P., Nolte, C., Franco, S., et al. (1982). Reference intervals for serum IgG, IgA, IgM, C3 and C4 as determined by rate nephelometry. *Clinical Chemistry, 28*(1), 126–128.

58. Kallemuchikkal, U., & Gorevic, P. (1999). Evaluation of cryoglobulins. *Archives of Pathology and Laboratory Medicine, 123,* 119–125.

59. Kemp, S. (2007). Office approach to anaphylaxis: Sooner better than later. *American Journal of Medicine, 120,* 664–668.

60. Kemp, S., Lockey, R., & Simons, F. (2008). Epinephrine: The drug of choice for anaphylaxis. A statement of the World Allergy Organization. *Allergy, 63,* 1061–1070.

61. Kim, S., & Dedeoglu, F. (2005). Update on pediatric vasculitis. *Current Opinion in Pediatrics, 17,* 695–702.

62. Klein-Gitelman, M., Reiff, A., & Silverman, E. (2002). Systemic lupus erythematosus in childhood. *Rheumatic Disease Clinics of North America, 28*(3), 561–577.

63. Krugman, S., Chiaramonte, D., & Matsui, E. (2006). Diagnosis and management of food-induced anaphylaxis: A national survey of pediatricians. *Pediatrics, 118,* e554–e560.

64. LaRosa, D., & Orange, J. (2008). Lymphocytes. *Journal of Allergy and Clinical Immunology. 121*(2 suppl 2), S364–S369.

65. Lavine, E., & Roifman, C. (2008). Primary immunodeficiency. In F. Lang (Ed.), *Encyclopedia of molecular mechanisms of disease* (p. 2). Germany: Springer.

66. Lederman, H. (2000). The clinical presentation of primary immunodeficiencies. Retrieved from http://www.primaryimmune.org/publications

67. Lemon-Mule, H., Nowak-Wegrzyn, A., Berin, C., & Knight, A. (2008). Pathophysiology of food-induced anaphylaxis. *Current Allergy and Asthma Reports, 8,* 201–208.

68. Lieberman, P., Camargo, C., Bohlke, K., Jick, H., Miller, R., Sheikh, A., et al. (2006). Epidemiology of anaphylaxis: Findings of the American College of Allergy, Asthma and Immunology Epidemiology of Anaphylaxis Working Group. *Annals of Allergy, Asthma, and Immunology, 97,* 596–602.

69. Lieberman, P., Kemp, S., Oppenheimer, J., Land, D., Bernstein, I., & Nicklas, R. (Eds.). (2005). The diagnosis and management of anaphylaxis: An updated practice parameter. *Journal of Allergy and Clinical Immunology, 115,* S483–S523.

70. Liew, W., Williamson, E., & Tang, M. (2009). Anaphylaxis fatalities and admissions in Australia. *Journal of Allergy and Clinical Immunology, 123,* 434–442.

71. Litzman, J., Ward, A., Wild, G., Znojil, V., & Morgan, G. (1997). Serum IgD levels in children under investigation for and with defined immunodeficiency. *International Archives of Allergy and Immunology, 114*(1), 54–58.

72. Mehr, S., Liew, W., Tey, D., & Tang, M. (2009). Clinical predictors for biphasic reactions in children presenting anaphylaxis. *Clinical and Experimental Allergy, 39,* 1390–1396.

73. Meuller, U. (2007). Cardiovascular disease and anaphylaxis. *Current Opinion in Allergy and Clinical Immunology, 7,* 337–341.

74. Miller, M., & Pachman, L. (2007). Vasculitis syndromes. In R. Kliegman et al. (Eds.), *Nelson textbook of pediatrics* (18th ed., pp. 1684–1687). New York: Saunders.

75. Minden, K., Niewerth, M., Listing, J., Biedermann, T., Bollow, M., Schontube, M., et al. (2002). Long-term outcome in patients with juvenile idiopathic arthritis. *Arthritis and Rheumatism, 46*(9), 2392–2401.

76. Morell, A., Muehlheim, E., Schaad, U., Skvaril, F., & Rossi, E. (1986). Susceptibility to infections in children with selective IgA- and IgA-IgG subclass deficiency. *European Journal of Pediatrics, 145,* 199–203.

77. Moylett, E., & Shearer, W. (2006). Pediatric human immunodeficiency virus infection. In J. A. McMillan, R. D. Feigin, C. DeAngelis, & M. D. Jones (Eds.), *Oski's pediatrics: Principles in practice* (4th ed., pp. 942–952). Philadelphia: Lippincott Williams & Wilkins.

78. Muraro, A., Roberts, G., Clark, A., Eigenmann, P., Halken, S., Lack, G., et al. (2007). The management of anaphylaxis in childhood: Position paper of the European Academy of Allergology and Clinical Immunology. *Allergy, 62,* 857–871.

79. National Institute of Health. (2009). HIV/AIDS. Retrieved from http://www.health.nih.gov

80. Neugat, A., Ghatak, A., & Miller, R. (2001). Anaphylaxis in the United States: An investigation into its epidemiology. *Archives of Internal Medicine, 161,* 15–21.

81. Noyes, B., & Kemp, J. (2007). Vocal cord dysfunction in children. *Paediatric Respiratory Reviews, 8,* 155–163.

82. Nurastov, U., Worth, A., & Sheikh, A. (2008). Anaphylaxis management plans for the acute and long-term management of anaphylaxis: a systemic survey. *Journal of Allergy and Clinical Immunology, 122,* 353–361.

83. Oen, K. (2002). Long-term outcomes and predictors of outcomes for patients with juvenile idiopathic arthritis. *Best Practice & Research: Clinical Rheumatology, 16,* 347–360.

84. Ogawa, Y., & Grant, J. A. (2007). Mediators of anaphylaxis. *Immunology and Allergy Clinics of North America, 27,* 249–260.

85. O'Gorman, M., & Corrochano, V. (1995). Rapid whole-blood flow cytometry assay for diagnosis of chronic granulomatous disease. *Clinical and Diagnostic Laboratory Immunology, 2*(2), 227–232.

86. O'Gorman, M., & Scholl, P. (2002). Role of flow cytometry in the diagnostic evaluation of primary immunodeficiency disease. *Clinical and Applied Immunology Reviews, 2*(6), 321–335.

87. Oguz, F., Akdeniz, C., Unuvar, E., Kucukbasmaci, O., & Sidal, M. (2002). Parvovirus B19 in the acute arthropathies and juvenile rheumatoid arthritis. *Journal of Paediatrics and Child Health, 38*(4), 358–362.

88. Oomura, M., Yamawaki, T., Naritomi, H., Terai, T., & Shigeno, K. (2006). Polyarteritis nodosa in association with subarachnoid hemorrhage. *Internal Medicine 45*(9), 655–658.

89. Oren, E., Banajeri, A., Clark, S., & Camargo, C. (2007). Food-induced anaphylaxis and repeated epinephrine treatments. *Annals of Allergy, Asthma, and Immunology, 99,* 429–432.

90. Oswalt, M., & Kemp, S. (2007). Anaphylaxis: Office management and prevention. *Immunology and Allergy Clinics of North America, 27,* 177–191.

91. Ozcan, E., Notarangelo, L., & Geha, R. (2008). Primary immune deficiencies with aberrant IgE production. *Journal of Allergy and Clinical Immunology, 122*(6), 1054–62.

92. Ozen, S. (2002). The spectrum of vasculitis in children. *Best Practice & Research: Clinical Rheumatology, 16,* 411–425.

93. Ozen, S. (2005). Problems in classifying vasculitis in children. *Pediatric Nephrology, 20,* 1214–1218.

94. Pettigrew, H., Teuber, S., & Gershwin, M. (2009). Clinical significance of complement deficiencies. *Annals of the New York Academy of Science, 1173,* 108–123.

95. Petty, R., Southwood, T., Manners, P., Baum, J., Glass, D., Goldenberg, J., et al. (2004). International League of Associations for Rheumatology classification of juvenile idiopathic arthritis: Second revision. *Journal of Rheumatology, 31*(2), 390–392.

96. Plaut, M., Sawyer, R., & Fenton, M. (2009). Summary of the 2008 National Institute of Allergy and Infectious Diseases–US Food and Drug Administration Workshop on Food Allergy Clinical Trial Design. *Journal of Allergy and Clinical Immunology, 124,* 671–678.

97. Pongracic, J., & Kim, J. (2007). Update on epinephrine for the treatment of anaphylaxis. *Current Opinion in Pediatrics, 19,* 94–98.

98. Pumphrey, R. (2004). Fatal anaphylaxis in the UK, 1992–2001. *Novartis Foundation Symposium, 257,* 116–128.

99. Pushparaj, P., Tay, H., H'ng, S., Pitman, N., Xu, D., McKenzie, A., et al. (2009). The cytokine interleukin-33 mediates anaphylactic shock. *Proceedings of the National Academy of Science, 106,* 9773–9778.

100. Ravelli, A., & Martini, A. (2007). Juvenile idiopathic arthritis. *Lancet, 369,* 767–778.

101. Ravelli, A., Ruperto, N., & Martini A. (2005). Outcome in juvenile onset systemic lupus erythematosus. *Current Opinion in Rheumatology, 17*(5), 568–573.

102. Rigante, D. (2006). Clinical review of vasculitic syndromes in the pediatric age. *European Review for Medical and Pharmacological Sciences, 10,* 337–345.

103. Roberts, G. (2007). Anaphylaxis to foods. *Pediatric Allergy and Immunology, 18*, 543–548.

104. Rodrigo, M., Vendrell, M., Cruz, M., Miravitlles, M., Pascual, C., Morell, F., et al. (2000). Utility of the antibody response to a conjugated *Haemophilus influenzae* type B vaccine for diagnosis of primary humoral immunodeficiency. *American Journal of Respiratory Critical Care Medicine, 162*, 1462–1465.

105. Romano, A., Di Fonso, M., Giuffreda, F., Papa, G., Artesani, M., Viola, M., et al. (2001). Food-dependent exercise-induced anaphylaxis: Clinical and laboratory findings in 54 subjects. *International Archives of Allergy and Immunology, 125*, 264–272.

106. Rowley, A., Ozen, S., Sundel, R., & Saulsbury, F. (2009). *A clinician's pearls and myths in rheumatology.* London: Springer.

107. Sampson, H., Munoz-Furlong, A., Campbell, R., Adkinson, N., Bock, S., Branum, A., et al. (2006). Second symposium on the definition and management of anaphylaxis: Summary report—Second National Institute of Allergy and Infectious Disease/Food Allergy and Anaphylaxis Network Symposium. *Journal of Allergy and Clinical Immunology, 117*, 391–397.

108. Schauer, U., Stemberg, F., Rieger, C., Buttner, W., Borte, M., Schubert, S., et al. (2003). Levels of antibodies specific to tetanus toxoid, *Haemophilus influenzae* type b, and pneumococcal capsular polysaccharide in healthy children and adults. *Clinical and Diagnostic Laboratory Immunology, 10*(2), 202–207.

109. Sheikh, A., ten Broek, V., Brown, S., & Simons, F. (2007). H$_1$-antihistamines for the treatment of anaphylaxis: Cochrane systematic review. *Allergy, 62*, 830–837.

110. Sicherer, S., Forman, J., & Noone, S. (2000). Use assessment of self-administered epinephrine among food-allergic children and pediatricians. *Pediatrics, 105*, 359–362.

111. Sicherer, S., & Simons, F. (2007). Self-injectable epinephrine for first-aid management of anaphylaxis. *Pediatrics, 119*, 638–646.

112. Simons, F. (2007). Anaphylaxis in infants: Can recognition and management be improved? *Journal of Allergy and Clinical Immunology, 120*, 537–540.

113. Simons, F. (2008). Anaphylaxis. *Journal of Allergy and Clinical Immunology, 121*, S402–S407.

114. Simons, F., & Sampson, H. (2008). Anaphylaxis epidemic: Fact or fiction? *Journal of Allergy and Clinical Immunology, 122*, 1166–1168.

115. Simons, F., Frew, A., Ansotegui, I., Bochner, B., Golden, D., Finkelman, F., et al. (2007). Risk assessment in anaphylaxis: Current and future approaches. *Journal of Allergy and Clinical Immunology, 120*, S2–S24.

116. Simons, F., Gu, X., Johnston, L., & Simons, K. (2000). Can epinephrine inhalations be substituted for epinephrine injection in children at risk for systemic anaphylaxis? *Pediatrics, 106*, 1040–1044.

117. Simons, F., Lieberman, P., Reed, E., & Edwards, E. (2009). Hazards of unintentional injection of epinephrine from autoinjectors: A systematic review. *Annals of Allergy, Asthma, and Immunology, 102*, 282–287.

118. Simpkins, K., Siberry, G., & Hutton, N. (2009). Thinking about HIV infection. *Pediatrics in Review, 30*, 337–349.

119. Singh, S., & Dass, R. (2002). Clinical approach to vasculitides. *Indian Journal of Pediatrics, 69*, 881–888.

120. Slatter, M., & Gennery, A. (2008). Clinical immunology review series: An approach to the child with recurrent infections in childhood. *Clinical and Experimental Immunology, 152*, 389–396.

121. Stichweh, D., Arce, E., & Pascual, V. (2004). Update on Pediatric systemic lupus erythematosus. *Current Opinion in Rheumatology, 16*(5), 577–587.

122. Stiehm, E., Ochs, H., & Winkelstein, J. (2004). Immunodeficiency disorders: General considerations. In E. R. Stiehm, H. D. Ochs, & J. A. Winkelstein (Eds.), *Immunologic disorders in infants and children* (5th ed., pp. 289–345). Philadelphia: Elsevier Saunders.

123. Szer, I., Kiura, Y., Malleson, P., & Southwood, T. R. (Eds.). (2006). *Arthritis in children and adolescents.* London: Oxford University Press.

124. Tole, J., & Lieberman, P. (2007). Biphasic anaphylaxis: Review of incidence, clinical predictors, and observation recommendations. *Immunology and Allergy Clinics of North America, 27*, 309–326.

125. Tse, S., & Laxer, R. (2006). Approach to acute limb pain in childhood. *Pediatrics in Review, 27*, 170–180.

126. Uddin, S., Borrow, R., Haeney, M., Moran, A., Warrington, R., Balmer, P., et al. (2006). Total and serotype-specific pneumococcal antibody titres in children with normal and abnormal humoral immunity. *Vaccine, 24*(27–28), 5637–5644.

127. Vadas, P., Gold, M., Perelman, B., Liss, G., Lack, G., Blyth, T., et al. (2008). Platelet-activating factor, PAF acetylhydrolase, and severe anaphylaxis. *New England Journal of Medicine, 358*, 28–35.

128. Vuitton, D. (2004). Echinococcosis and allergy. *Clinical Reviews in Allergy and Immunology, 26*, 93–104.

129. Wallace, C. (2006). Current management of juvenile idiopathic arthritis. *Best Practice and Research Clinical Rheumatology, 20*(2), 279–300.

130. Webb, L., & Lieberman, P. (2006). Anaphylaxis: A review of 601 cases. *Annals of Allergy, Asthma, and Immunology, 97*, 39–43.

131. Weiss, J., & Ilowite, N. (2005). Juvenile idiopathic arthritis. *Pediatric Clinics of North America, 52*, 413–442.

132. Wen, L., Atkinson, J., & Giclas, P. (2004). Clinical and laboratory evaluation of complement deficiency. *Journal of Allergy and Clinical Immunology, 113*(4), 585–593.

133. Wiener, L., Mellins, C., Marhefka, S., & Battles, H. (2007). Disclosure of an HIV diagnosis to children: History, current research and future directions. *Journal of Behavioral Pediatrics, 28* (2), 155–166.

134. Wood, P., Stamworth, S., Burton, J., Jones, A., Peckham, D., Green, T., et al. (2007). Recognition, clinical diagnosis and management of patients with primary antibody deficiencies: A systematic review. *Clinical and Experimental Immunology, 148*, 410–423.

135. Wulffraat, N., Vastert, B., & Tyndall, A. (2005). Treatment of refractory autoimmune diseases with autologous stem cell transplantation: Focus on juvenile idiopathic arthritis. *Bone Marrow Transplantation, 35*(suppl 1), S27–S29.

136. Yalcindag, A., & Sundel, R. (2002). Vasculitis in childhood. *Current Opinion in Rheumatology, 13*, 422–427.

137. Zuraw, B. (2008). Hereditary angioedema. *New England Journal of Medicine, 359*, 1027–1036.

Infectious Disorders

FEVER

Valerie Ebert

FEVER IN A NEONATE

Pathophysiology

A fever in a neonate (FIN) is defined as a neonate, aged birth to 28 days, with a fever derived as a rectal temperature of ≥ 38°C (100.4°F). Neonates are at higher risk of developing a serious bacterial infection (SBI) due to their immune function. In the third trimester of pregnancy, a transfer of maternal IgG across the placenta to the fetus occurs; this transfer and that of endogenous fetal IgG production leads to high levels of IgG in the newborn at birth. At birth, neonates have no preexisting immunologic memory or well-functioning adaptive immunity (Marodi, 2006). The adaptive immune system in a neonate is naive, with no prior exposure to pathogens. The innate immune system in neonates is also impaired. While they have normal levels of B and T cells, the function of these cells are less efficient (Marodi). Also, the cytotoxic activity of their natural killer cells is decreased when compared to adult natural killer cells (Lewis, 1998).

Given that the neonate's immune system is vulnerable to pathogenic organisms, it is necessary to perform a complete evaluation when a neonate develops a fever. The rapid development of the immune system in the first 3 months of life reduces newborns' susceptibility to a SBI and, therefore, decreases the requirements of testing and procedures recommended in the older pediatric patient with a fever.

Epidemiology and etiology

In febrile neonates with a temperature of 38°C (100.4° F) or higher, there is a 12% incidence of a SBI (Ishimine, 2006). A fever documented at home should be treated in the same way as a fever documented in a health care setting. The two most common bacterial infections are urinary tract infections (UTI) and occult bacteremia (Ishimine, 2006). In neonates with bacteremia, approximately 25% will develop meningitis (Klein, 2000). Viral infections are the most common cause of fever. Nevertheless, given the neonate's diminished immune system function and increased chance of becoming infected with virulent organisms, more serious causes of fever must be excluded.

Presentation

The evaluation of the neonate with a fever requires a thorough history. In addition to questions regarding symptom development, a comprehensive prenatal history is necessary. It is especially important to obtain information about maternal infections, fever, group B *Streptococcus* (GBS)

status, and any infection requiring antibiotic therapy. The history should also include the neonate's delivery mode, any complications, any prolonged rupture of membranes, and the postdelivery state. Review of postnatal care and any complications that may have occurred in the nursery may also provide insight into potential exposures.

The physical examination begins with an assessment of the ABCs (airway, breathing, and circulation) and the patient's vital signs (temperature, heart rate, respiratory rate, blood pressure, pulse oximetry). A factor to consider is the limited amount of information that can be obtained from the physical examination of a neonate, as behavioral responses are limited at this age (Ishimine, 2006). One of the most important aspects of the physical examination in a neonate is the child's appearance, including whether he or she appears toxic or nontoxic. A toxic infant may have lethargy or decreased activity, irritability or inconsolability, decreased tone, or poor perfusion. However, neonates may also present appearing nontoxic yet still have an SBI (Baraff, 2000).

The examination should be performed by completely undressing the patient to allow for a thorough assessment of the skin and evaluation of rashes. Assessment of localizing signs or symptoms may aid in diagnosis. While signs of meningitis are nonspecific at this age, a bulging fontanel and nuchal rigidity may be present. Despite a thorough examination, in many neonates there are no specific or localizing symptoms.

Differential diagnosis

SBI in the neonate are caused by a distinctive set of organisms. The most common organisms causing an SBI, including bacteremia, meningitis, UTI, and pneumonia, in a neonate including the following pathogens:

- Group B *Streptococcus*
- *Escherichia coli*
- *Listeria monocytogenes*
- *Staphylococcus aureus*
- *Enterococcus* species
- Herpes simplex virus (HSV)
- Cytomegalovirus (CMV)
- Varicella-zoster virus
- Respiratory syncytial virus (RSV)
- *Candida* species

Plan of care

Several diagnostic studies are recommended in all neonates with a fever. Often referred to as a *full septic work-up*, these studies include: a complete blood count (CBC) with manual differential, a urinalysis (UA), a urine culture obtained from a suprapubic or catheter specimen, a blood culture, and a lumbar puncture with cerebrospinal fluid (CSF) study (Baraff, 2008). In this age group, a normal white blood cell (WBC) count cannot be used to exclude an SBI. If there is CSF pleocytosis, a sample of CSF should be sent for HSV polymerase chain reaction (PCR) assessment. Recent research has indicated that HSV PCR testing can save 17 lives per 10,000 neonates; it is a cost-effective strategy if reserved for neonates with CSF pleocytosis (Caviness et al., 2008).

Often these diagnostic studies fail to establish an etiology, as the source of the neonate's fever is often a viral infection. This has led many researchers to recommend expanding viral testing in febrile neonates. For example, testing of blood and CSF for enterovirus via PCR can decrease the length of time a neonate is hospitalized and on empiric antibiotics (Robinson et al., 2002).

A chest radiograph is indicated if any upper airway or pulmonary signs are noted on presentation. Neonates presenting with nasal congestion should be evaluated for RSV; parainfluenza 1, 2 and 3; and influenza A and B. If the neonate is positive for RSV, all diagnostic studies are still required, as the child's risk for an SBI does not change (Ishimine, 2006).

The therapeutic plan may be individualized for each patient and will depend on the diagnostic study findings. If the laboratory evaluation is negative, the neonate will require admission to a pediatric unit and should be hemodynamically monitored. Increasing the level of care is recommended if at any time the neonate appears toxic or his or her condition deteriorates.

If the child is nontoxic in appearance, the health care professional (HCP) may wait until all laboratory studies are collected before starting empiric antibiotics. Currently recommended empiric antibiotic courses in the neonate with fever are ampicillin and gentamicin *or* ampicillin and cefotaxime. Until results of the CSF examination are obtained, meningitis dosing of these antibiotics should be used. In most neonates, acyclovir is not recommended as part of the empiric regimen; however, it may be added to the empiric regimen if there is CSF pleocytosis, prolonged rupture of membranes, primary maternal HSV infection, fetal scalp electrode use, mucocutaneous lesion, or seizures (Ishimine, 2006).

If the laboratory evaluation suggests a UTI, all studies—including the lumbar puncture—still should be performed. The neonate should be admitted to the hospital and parenteral antibiotics (ampicillin and gentamicin) started. The patient may be discharged home on oral antibiotics once results of the culture and susceptibilities are available, and if the neonate is afebrile and feeding well. It is recommended that the neonate be treated with antibiotics for a total of 14 days. Radiographic evaluation including a renal ultrasound and voiding cysto-urethrogram (VCUG) will need to be performed; these studies may be completed on an outpatient or inpatient basis once the patient is afebrile.

If CSF pleocytosis is present, the neonate should be admitted to the hospital and administered empiric antibiotics dosed at meningitis levels. Although most neonates with CSF pleocytosis have viral meningitis, transfer to the intensive care unit should be considered in all neonates with meningitis. Parenteral acyclovir is also recommended empirically while awaiting the results of cerebrospinal fluid for HSV via PCR. CSF.

Specialist care is generally not required during the initial evaluation of a nontoxic neonate with fever. However, it is recommended that an infectious diseases specialist be consulted whenever meningitis is suspected. An infectious diseases specialist may direct management as to appropriate antibiotic therapy and additional diagnostic studies. Critical care specialists should be involved in the care of all toxic-appearing neonates.

Once it has been established that a neonate has a fever, the necessary procedures and tests are extensive and can be both intimidating and upsetting to parents. It is important that caregivers receive information on all procedures their child is about to undergo; be educated about the necessity for hospital admission, visiting policies, and access to lactation services if breastfeeding; and receive emotional, social, and spiritual support.

Disposition and discharge planning

If cultures are negative after 48 to 72 hours and the neonate is stable and afebrile, the patient may be discharged home without antibiotics. Close follow-up after discharge is necessary, as there is the possibility of cultures being identified with a pathogen as a result of either a true organism or a contamination. Therefore, follow-up with the primary care provider is recommended within 48 hours of discharge.

The majority of neonates with fever will have no identifiable source, and the fever will be attributed to a presumptive viral infection. Only 12% of neonates presenting to the emergency department with a fever will have an SBI (Ishimine, 2006). Given the advances in intensive care and antibiotics, neonatal meningitis now has a 10% to 20% mortality rate (Heath et al., 2003).

The immature neonatal immune system makes vaccinations shortly after birth impractical. The HCP, however, should advise families to use good hand washing techniques and careful hygiene with diaper changes. Exposure to close contacts who have been immunized with Tdap, influenza, and H1N1 is recommended. Also, all live-vaccinated children and adults should avoid contact with the neonate initially until their HCP says it is safe to interact.

FEVER WITHOUT A SOURCE

Pathophysiology

Young infants have decreased immunologic function and are more likely to be infected with virulent organisms than older children and adults (Ishimine, 2006). The younger the pediatric patient, the more at risk he or she for developing an SBI. This is why the pediatric patient with a *fever without a source* (FWS) is classified into one of the following categories: neonate (previously described), young infant, and older infant and toddler (Table 30-1). The majority of pediatric patients who develop FWS will have a self-limiting viral illness. It can be difficult to differentiate between the pediatric patient in the early stages of an SBI and the pediatric patient with a common viral illness; thus many studies have been done and recommendations made based on the risks and benefits of invasive laboratory tests and the judicious use of antibiotics.

Epidemiology and etiology

The epidemiology of SBI has changed dramatically with the widespread use of vaccines to prevent *Haemophilus influenzae* type b and *Streptococcus pneumoniae*. *H. influenzae* type b conjugate vaccination (Hib) has reduced the incidence of invasive infection by 90% in the industrialized world (Waddle & Jhaveri). The pneumococcal conjugate vaccine (PCV 7) has decreased the incidence of pneumococcal bacteremia by 66% and reduced invasive *S. pneumoniae* disease from 51.1 to 98.2 cases per 100,000 person years in children younger than 1 year of age (Waddle & Jhaveri). Immunization greatly affects the risk of occult infection; consequently, the diagnostic practices differ in the young infant age group (29–90 days) and in the older infant and toddler age group (3–36 months).

Three SBIs that can cause fever with no clinical symptoms are bacteremia, UTI, and pneumonia. In young infants who present with a fever ≥ 38°C (100.4°F) without a source, there is a 6% to 10% prevalence of an SBI; 5% will have bacteremia (Bachur & Harper, 2001; Powell, 2007). The incidence of occult UTI in febrile infants younger than 12 months of age is also 5% (Baraff, 2008). Viral infections can be confirmed in 40% to 60% of young infants with a fever (Powell), and a confirmed viral infection lowers the risk of an SBI (Byington et al., 2004).

Among older immunized infants and toddlers, UTIs are a common cause of fever, with an overall prevalence of 2% to 5% (Ishimine, 2006). The prevalence is greater in certain groups, including females and uncircumcised males. The incidence of occult bacteremia ranges from

0.25% to 0.9% (Hertz et al., 2006; Stoll & Rubin, 2004); before the widespread use of Hib and PCV 7 vaccines, this incidence was in the range of 2% to 6% (Baraff, 2000).

Presentation

When FWS is present, the HCP should evaluate whether the previously healthy patient is appears well or is toxic in appearance. If the child is toxic in appearance, regardless of age, he or she should be admitted to the hospital, started on empiric antibiotics, and subjected to a full diagnostic evaluation.

If the child is well appearing, the extent of the diagnostic evaluation and use of empiric antibiotics depends on both the patient's age and the results of preliminary laboratory studies.

- In the young infant, the physical examination cannot be relied upon, and a more extensive diagnostic study is required.
- In the older infant and toddler population, a higher fever is used for definition because the incidence of occult bacteremia increases with temperature (Ishimine, 2006). Most infections can be identified for this age group through history and physical examination.

Differential diagnosis

Serious bacterial infections that may not be identified through history and physical examination include occult bacteremia, UTI, and occult pneumonia. The most common bacterial pathogens are listed in Table 30-2.

Plan of care

The diagnostic studies for the toxic-appearing pediatric patient of any age include the following tests:

- CBC
- Urinalysis (UA) and urine culture
- Blood culture
- Lumbar puncture (LP)

TABLE 30-1

Definitions of Fever			
	Neonate	**Young Infant**	**Older Infant and Toddler**
Age	0–28 days	29–90 days	3–36 months
Fever (rectal temperature)	≥ 38°C (100.4°F)	≥ 38°C (100.4°F)	≥ 39°C (102.2°F)

TABLE 30-2

Common Bacterial Pathogens	
Young infant	Group B *streptococcus, Listeria monocytogenes, Salmonella, Escherichia coli, Neisseria meningitides, Streptococcus pneumoniae, Haemophilus influenza type b, Staphylococcus aureus*
Older infant and toddler	*Salmonella, Neisseria meningitides, Streptococcus pneumonia*

There are no standardized practice parameters for the well-appearing young infant. The three most common management strategies for FWS in the young infant, known as the Boston, Rochester, and Philadelphia criteria, are summarized in Table 30-3.

Common diagnostic studies include CBC, catheter-obtained UA and culture, and blood culture. If the young infant has diarrhea, a stool specimen for white blood cells is recommended, and a chest radiograph (CXR) should be obtained if the patient has symptoms of a respiratory illness (Ishimine, 2006).

The most controversial aspect of the evaluation in the well-appearing young infant is the debate over the necessity for a lumbar puncture. The incidence of meningitis is low in febrile infants—4.1 per 1,000 patients (Ishimine, 2006). A normal CBC and physical examination do not preclude a diagnosis of meningitis in this age group. For this reason,

a lumbar puncture should be strongly considered (Boston and Philadelphia criteria). Caregivers need to be involved in this decision-making process; however, the HCP must be aware that caregivers often choose the option that will limit testing and treatments (Baraff, 2008). If the decision is made to not perform the lumbar puncture, then consider using the Rochester criteria and not administering antibiotics. If the patient's clinical status deteriorates and a lumbar puncture becomes necessary, the prior use of antibiotics may prevent the growth and identification of the bacteria in the CSF culture.

The well-appearing older infant and toddler requires less evaluation than the young infant because the physical examination is more informative, the patient may be able to communicate some of his or her symptoms, and the patient is more likely to have received the previously noted immunizations. Laboratory studies are indicated based on clinical

TABLE 30-3

Criteria for the Management of Fever in the Young Infant			
Rochester Criteria			
		Laboratory Parameters	**Plan**
Low risk	• Well appearing • Term • No prior antibiotics, including perinatal • No hospitalization • No underlying disease	• WBC: 5,000–15,000/µL • Bands: ≤ 1,500/µL • UA: < 10 WBCs/hpf • Stool: < 5 WBCs/hpf	Discharge home with follow-up in 24 hours No antibiotics given
High risk	Ill appearing or well appearing and does not meet laboratory criteria	Does not meet above criteria	Admit and start empiric antibiotics
Boston Criteria			
Low risk	• Well appearing • No antibiotics or immunizations in prior 48 hours • No dehydration • No ear, soft-tissue, or bone infections	• WBC: < 20,000/µL • CSF: WBC < 10/µL • UA: < 10 WBCs/hpf • CXR: no infiltrate	Discharge home after injection of ceftriaxone (50 mg/kg) Follow-up in 24 hours
High risk	Ill appearing or well appearing and does not meet laboratory criteria	Does not meet above criteria	Admit and start empiric antibiotics
Philadelphia Criteria			
Low risk	• Well appearing • Unremarkable exam	• WBC: < 15,000/µL • Band/neutrophil ratio: < 0.2 • UA: < 10 WBCs/hpf and negative Gram stain • CSF: WBC < 8/µL and Gram stain negative • Stool: no blood and few or no WBCs on smear • CXR: no infiltrate	Discharge home with follow-up in 24 hours No antibiotics given
High risk	Ill appearing or well appearing and does not meet above criteria	Does not meet above criteria	Admit and start empiric antibiotics

Note: White blood count (WBC), urinalysis (UA), cerebrospinal fluid (CSF), chest radiograph (CXR).

Source: Baker et al., 1993; Baskin et al., 1992; Jaskiewicz et al., 1994.

presentation and findings. Diagnostic studies to exclude a serious occult infection are necessary only if a focal infection cannot be identified and if a viral cause of the fever is not suspected. Viruses are the most common cause of pneumonia in the 3- to 36-month age range (Baraff, 2008). A CXR is recommended in this age group if the patient has tachypnea, crackles, decreased breath sounds, or increased work of breathing. In the absence of these signs, a CXR should be considered if the pulse oximetry reading is less than 95%, the fever is 40°C (104°F) or greater, or if the WBC count is greater than 20,000/mm³ (Baraff).

Empiric therapeutic management for bacteremia in the young infant is designed to cover the organisms listed in Table 30-2. Consider administering parenteral ampicillin, ceftriaxone or cefotaxime, and vancomycin. In toxic-appearing older infants and toddlers, consider parenteral ceftriaxone or cefotaxime and vancomycin until culture susceptibilities are available. As previously noted, older infants and toddlers are at very low risk for occult bacteremia; consequently, if the well-appearing child has received three doses of the PCV 7 and Hib vaccines, no blood tests are recommended (Palazzi & Feigin, 2009). If the patient has received fewer than three doses of the PCV 7 vaccine, a CBC and blood culture should be collected, but the blood culture may be held until results of the CBC are returned. If the WBC is 15,000/mm³ or higher, or if the absolute neutrophil count (ANC) is 10,000 or greater, the blood culture should be sent and ceftriaxone 50 mg/kg up to 1 gm given (Ishimine, 2006; Palazzi & Feigin). A subset of patients age 3 to 24 months, with fevers of 40°C (104°F) or greater, prolonged gastroenteritis, or a petechial rash are at increased risk for bacteremia (Ishimine; Palazzi & Feigin). If a blood culture is collected, the HCP can elect to either withhold antibiotics or give them, depending on the provider's assessment of risk. If antibiotics are selected, then consider ceftriaxone 50 mg/kg and follow up with the patient once the blood culture results are available.

Collection of urine for UA and culture in the well-appearing child with a fever and no identifiable source is recommended only in certain populations (Table 30-4). If the UA is suggestive of a UTI, the urine culture must still be performed to identify the organism and antimicrobial susceptibilities. If the child is toxic in appearance or is unable to take oral antibiotics, the patient should be admitted to the hospital for administration of parenteral antibiotics. If the older infant or toddler is not ill appearing and can take oral antibiotics, consider an injection of ceftriaxone and a prescription for a first- or third-generation cephalosporin. Follow-up in one to two days is important to reassess the patient and discuss the final results of the culture, including changing antibiotics based on susceptibilities if necessary.

Disposition and discharge planning

If the young infant was not admitted to the hospital, he or she must be re-evaluated within 24 hours and have all culture results followed until the final disposition. The older infant and toddler must also be followed and, if collected, his or her culture results reviewed when available. If the blood culture results are positive, the patient must be immediately re-evaluated. Admission to the hospital depends on which organism is growing, how the child appears, and if the fever is still present. If the patient is still febrile and the blood culture grew *S. pneumoniae*, the patient should be admitted to the hospital, a full diagnostic evaluation completed (including CSF studies), and parenteral antibiotics started (Ishmine, 2006). If the patient is afebrile and the blood culture is positive for *S. pneumoniae*, the blood culture should be repeated and the patient started on oral antibiotics (Bachur & Harper, 2000).

For *Neisseria meningitides, H. influenzae* type b, *S. aureus*, Gram-negative rods, and other pathogens, the patient should be admitted to the hospital and started on parenteral antibiotics (Ishimine, 2006). A lumbar puncture with CSF studies is necessary if meningitis is suspected or if *N. meningidis* or *H. influenzae* is reported on culture (Powell, 2007). If a contaminant is suspected, contact the microbiology laboratory

TABLE 30-4

Patients with Fever Without a Source Who Need Urinalysis and Urine Culture Collection		Girls	Boys: Uncircumcised	Boys: Circumcised
History of urinary tract infection		Yes	Yes	Yes
Age	6 months	Yes	Yes	Yes
	6 to 24 months	Yes	Yes	No
	Older than 24 months	No	No	No

Source: Baraff, 2008; Ishimine, 2006.

and/or infectious disease specialist for an impression of the likelihood of contamination. If the patient appears well, then he or she can be followed clinically until the organism is identified (Ishimine, 2006).

FEVER OF UNKNOWN ORIGIN

Pathophysiology

The definition of a fever of unknown origin (FUO) is an illness of more than 3 weeks' duration, with a fever of 38.3°C (101°F) or greater on most days, and without diagnosis after 1 week of intense investigation. The cause is often an uncommon presentation of a common disease (Long, 2005).

Epidemiology and etiology

Approximately one-third of all FUOs are caused by infection (Long & Edwards, 2008). Table 30-5 lists most common systemic infectious diseases associated with FUO in children in the United States (Powell, 2007). The next most frequent conditions are connective tissue diseases, which account for approximately 15% of diagnoses (Long & Edwards). Of these, juvenile rheumatoid arthritis (JRA) and systemic lupus erythematosus (SLE) are the most common (Powell). Another frequent cause of FUO is a neoplasm; this etiology accounts for 10% of diagnoses (Long & Edwards). Leukemia and lymphoma are the most common causes in this category. Hepatoma, neuroblastoma, and soft-tissue sarcomas account for the other frequently seen malignancies causing prolonged fevers (Long & Edwards).

Other less common diagnoses for FUO include drug fever, factitious fever, familial dysautonomia, central nervous system (CNS) dysfunction, dehydration, and anhidrotic ectodermal dysplasia (Long & Edwards). Table 30-6 lists noninfectious diseases seen in patients with FUO.

Presentation

The initial evaluation includes a very detailed history and physical examination. The history should include specifics about the fever—when did it occur, how was the temperature taken, what was the highest temperature, how long did each fever last, and what were the associated symptoms. Comprehensive history includes questions concerning animal exposure, lifetime travel history, atypical food ingestion (e.g., game meat, dirt, raw foods), medication history, and family medical history. Predominant symptoms of an infectious etiology are fever and chills, night sweats, and weight loss with an intact appetite (Cunha, 2007). The predominant symptoms of patients with a rheumatic-inflammatory cause are arthralgias, myalgias, chest pain, and abdominal pain (Cunha). Patients with neoplasms may experience night sweats, decreased appetite, weight loss, and fatigue.

The physical examination should be inclusive and may need to be repeated several times for serial evaluation. Complete a full rectal exam and test for occult blood to assess for a pelvis abscess or tumor (Palazzi & Feigin, 2009).

TABLE 30-5

Systemic Infections Most Commonly Associated with Fever of Unknown Origin in Children
Salmonellosis
Tuberculosis
Rickettsial disease
Syphilis
Lyme disease
Cat-scratch disease
Atypical prolonged common viral diseases
Infectious mononucleosis
Cytomegalovirus infection
Viral hepatitis
Coccidioidomycosis
Histoplasmosis
Malaria
Toxoplasmosis

Source: Powell, 2007.

TABLE 30-6

Noninfectious Differential Diagnosis		
Connective Tissue Disease	**Malignancies**	**Miscellaneous**
Juvenile rheumatoid arthritis	Lymphoma	Drug fever
Systemic lupus erythematosis	Leukemia	Factitious fever
Inflammatory bowel disease	Neuroblastoma	Diabetes insipidus
Polyarteritis nodosa	Hepatoma	Familial dysautonomia
	Soft-tissue sarcoma	Kawasaki disease
		Hemophagocytic Lymphohistocytosis
		Sarcoidsis
		Pancreatitis
		Thyrotoxicosis
		Poisioning
		Reccurrent or relapsing fever
		CNS dysfunction

Source: Lorin, 1998; Powell, 2007.

It is best to conduct the exam while the child is febrile to better note his or her level of distress. If the patient appears acutely ill, the evaluation for FUO should be completed in the hospital; if not, it can be performed in the outpatient setting.

Differential diagnosis

The differential for FUO is extensive (see Tables 30-5 and 30-6). Less common causes to consider are external heat sources, Munchausen-by-proxy, malingering, or infection with human immunodeficiency virus (HIV).

Plan of care

Diagnostic studies should be directed by findings in the history and physical examination. A septic work-up is indicated if no discernable source for the fever is identified; it would include obtaining a CBC, blood culture, UA and culture, erythrocyte sedimentation rate (ESR), C-reactive protein (CRP), complete metabolic panel, CXR, and tuberculin skin testing (Miller et al., 1995; Powell, 2007). Testing for HIV may also be considered.

If no diagnosis can be made after the initial evaluation, repeat the history and physical examination and consider referral to a specialist (e.g., infectious diseases, rheumatology, and/or hematology) and admission to the hospital. As an inpatient, the child can be more closely observed, fever patterns documented, and further radiologic and laboratory tests performed. Additional diagnostic studies to consider include computed tomography (CT) of the abdomen, sinuses, chest, or mastoids. Bone marrow biopsy, radionuclide scans, serologies, or immunoglobulins may also be of value.

By definition, patients with FUO have been ill for sometime. This chronicity may instill in both caregivers and patients a high level of anxiety due to the lack of a definitive diagnosis and need for extensive testing. Provide the family with a rationale for all testing and hospitalization, if required, and specialty consultation. Child life specialists and social work may be valuable supports for the patient and family.

Disposition and discharge planning

In 10% to 20% patients with FUO, a diagnosis is never determined (Palazzi & Feigin, 2009). Close follow-up and further evaluation of any recurrent fevers is necessary. Recurrent FUO suggests a connective tissue origin. The longer a patient goes without a diagnosis, the less likely the source is to be infectious. Infectious causes of FUO usually resolve in one year even if medication is never given. Mortality rates for pediatric patients with a fever of unknown origin are 6% to 9%

(Palazzi & Feigin). If there is a final diagnosis for FUO, then follow-up will be tailored to the demands of the disease process identified.

FEVER AND NEUTROPENIA

Pathophysiology

Neutropenia is defined as an ANC of less than 500 neutrophils/mm^3, or less than 1,000 neutrophils/mm^3 and an anticipated decline to less than 500 neutrophils/mm^3 within a few days. Fever is defined as a single temperature of 38.3°C (101°F) or greater, or a temperature of 38°C (100.4°F) or greater for at least 1 hour (Hughes et al., 2002). Rectal temperatures are contraindicated in neutropenic patients because of the potential for bacterial translocation.

In children, cancer and cancer therapy are the primary causes of neutropenia and a resulting immunodeficient state. While other causes of neutropenia are possible, most treatment guidelines are based on clinical trials conducted with cancer patients. Cytotoxic chemotherapy weakens the patient's innate immune system not only by a reduction in the neutrophil count, but also through an impaired mucocutaneous barrier. This barrier can be broken down by mucositis, nasogastric tube erosion, or breakdown of skin integrity through venous access with central venous catheters (CVC). Organ obstructions and bowel perforations allow access of intestinal bacteria into the bloodstream (Koh & Pizzo, 2008).

Epidemiology and etiology

One-third of neutropenic patients will have a febrile episode if their ANC remains less than 500 neutrophils/mm^3 for longer than 7 days (Koh & Pizzo, 2008). In more than one-half of these episodes, a source for the fever is never identified (Hakim et al., 2009). Bacteremia is the most common microbiologically documented infection (Castagnola et al., 2007; Hakim et al.). Overall, Gram-positive bacteria account for 60% to 70% of infections; staphylococcal and streptococcal species predominate. Gram-negative organisms represent another significant source, with *Escherichia coli* and *Klebsiella* being the most commonly noted species (Hughes et al., 2002). While fungi are important to consider in the differential diagnosis, they are more frequently a cause of secondary infections; they are rarely a primary cause of fever (Koh & Pizzo). Viruses account for 5% to 8% of documented sources; however, as new diagnostic tests become available, viral etiologies are becoming a more commonly documented source of fever (Hakim et al.). Table 30-7 lists common pathogens infecting febrile neutropenic patients.

TABLE 30-7

Pathogens Most Commonly Found in Neutropenic Patients with Fever	
Category	**Organism**
Bacteria: Gram positive	*Staphylococcus* species:
	• Coagulase-positive (*S. aureus*)
	• Coagulase-negative (*S. epidermidis*)
	Streptococcal species: *Viridans group, S. pneumoniae, S. pyogenes*
	Enterococcus faecalis/faecium
	Corynebacterium species
Bacteria: Gram negative	*Escherichia coli*
	Klebsiella species
	Pseudomonas aeruginosa
	Enterobacter species
	Citrobacter species
	Proteus species
Fungi	*Candida* species (*C. albicans, C. tropicalis*, and others)
	Aspergillus species (*A. fumigates, A. flavus*)
Viruses	Herpes simplex virus
	Varicella-zoster virus
	Cytomegalovirus
	Parainfluenza virus

Source: Hakim et al., 2009; Hughes et al., 2002; Kannangara, 2006; Koh & Pizzo, 2008.

Presentation

A thorough history and physical examination are necessary to attempt to identify the presumed infectious source. In addition to a detailed history, include questions regarding chemotherapeutic agents received, use of steroids, antibiotic prophylaxis or other prior antibiotic use, and any procedures that may have been recently performed.

Patients with neutropenia may be unable to induce an inflammatory response, complicating the physical examination findings. For example, a patient with a skin infection may not have induration, erythema, or purulence. Therefore, particular attention should be paid to the skin, perirectal area, oropharynx, abdomen, lungs, sinuses, and all vascular access sites. If no source for the fever is immediately identified, repeat the physical examination daily.

Differential diagnosis

A fever in a neutropenic patient is not always due to an infectious cause. Consider allergic and hypersensitivity reactions to drugs and blood transfusions, graft-versus-host disease, thrombosis, and paraneoplastic fever in the differential diagnosis.

Plan of care

Diagnostic studies are an integral component of the initial evaluation of the febrile neutropenic patient. Blood should be obtained immediately, before antibiotic therapy is started, and sent for bacterial and fungal cultures. At least two cultures should be collected, including one from a peripheral site (Hughes et al., 2002). All lumens of CVCs should be sampled as potential source sites. Viral cultures are recommended during seasonal outbreaks (Koh & Pizzo, 2008). Further cultures are indicated if localizing symptoms are present at wound sites, surgical sites, or around CVCs. A chest radiograph is indicated if respiratory symptoms are present, and CSF testing is needed if a CNS infection is suspected.

The goal of therapeutic management is to provide antibiotic coverage for the most common pathogens infecting febrile neutropenic pediatric patients. Antibiotic therapy has reduced the mortality rate for febrile neutropenia caused by Gram-negative bacteria from 80% to 10–40% (Walsh et al., 2006b). The ideal empiric antibiotic coverage meets several requirements: It should be bactericidal, have few side effects, and limit the potential for emergence of resistant organisms. The institution's most commonly encountered pathogens and rates of antibiotic resistance also influence antibiotic selection, including information available regarding microbes isolated from other febrile neutropenic patients, especially methicillin-resistant *S. aureus* (MRSA).

A low-risk patient has no comorbidities; is not toxic appearing; has no signs of bacterial infection; and has an ANC of 100 cells/mm³ or more, an absolute monocyte count of 100 cells/mm³ or more, a normal CXR, neutropenia for fewer than 7 days, and evidence of bone marrow recovery (Hughes et al., 2002). For the uncomplicated, low-risk patient, antibiotic monotherapy is suitable, such as cefepime, ceftazidime, piperacillin/tazobactam, imipenem/cilastatin, or meropenem.

For a patient at high risk for a bacterial infection, or if antibiotic resistance is a concern, a multiple-antibiotic regimen is appropriate. The benefits of this regimen include a decrease in the emergence of antibiotic resistance and synergistic effects against Gram-negative bacilli; however, there is an increased risk for drug toxicity. The most common multiple-drug regimens include an aminoglycoside and an antipseudomonal β-lactam antibiotic, or an aminoglycoside and a carbapenem (Hughes et al., 2002).

Vancomycin is not part of a standard empiric antibiotic regimen, and its use should be limited to prevent the emergence of bacterial resistance. Vancomycin is indicated for patients being treated in institutions with high rates of resistance, and those with CVC infections, known colonization with resistant organisms, sepsis, or blood culture positive for Gram-positive bacteria prior to susceptibility testing (Hughes et al., 2002; Walsh et al., 2006b).

While oral antibiotics are used in low-risk adults with febrile neutropenia, their use has not yet been recommended for initial therapy in pediatric patients. New studies, however, are being conducted that may result in a change to this recommendation.

Antifungal agents are not usually required for initial therapy, as fungal infections are more common in patients with prolonged neutropenia (more than 10 days) and those with secondary infections. *Candida* species, followed by *Aspergillus* species, are the most common organisms of fungal infections in this population (Koh & Pizzo, 2008). Amphotericin B is the empiric antifungal agent most frequently used in practice. A liposomal formulation of amphotericin B is now in use that is well tolerated and produces similar therapeutic success. Favorable evidence for the use of echinocandin and capsofungin has led some experts to recommend using caspofungin instead of amphotericin B for empiric antifungal coverage (Garnock-Jones & Keam, 2009).

Antiviral agents are to be reserved for laboratory-documented or clinically apparent infections, such as skin or mucous membrane lesions caused by herpes simplex or varicella-zoster viruses. Recommended antiviral medications include acyclovir, valacyclovir, and famciclovir for infections caused by herpes simplex or varicella-zoster viruses. Ganciclovir or foscarnet is recommended for treatment of cytomegalovirus—a virus seen more often in patients who undergo bone marrow transplants (Hughes et al., 2002).

Granulocyte colony-stimulating factor (G-CSF) is used in the management of patients with neutropenia to decrease the duration of their neutropenia and is commonly included in many chemotherapy protocols. Some evidence indicates that the use of G-CSF in febrile neutropenic pediatric patients decreases the number of days of neutropenia (up to 9 days), and reduces the length of hospitalization (Ozkaynak et al., 2005). Its use has not been shown to decrease febrile neutropenic mortality, however, and current guidelines by the Infectious Diseases Society of America (IDSA) do not yet recommend this medication's routine use in febrile neutropenic patients (Hughes et al., 2002). Conditions in which use of G-CSF should be considered include delayed bone marrow recovery, sepsis, fungal infections, or other severe infections (Hughes et al.; Kannangara, 2006).

Antibiotic prophylaxis of afebrile neutropenic patients should be limited to trimethoprim–sulfamethoxazole for the prevention of *Pneumocystis jiroveci* infection. The use of other antimicrobials is not recommended due to the increased risk for microbial drug resistance. Antifungal prophylaxis is not recommended for all neutropenic patients; however, certain disease processes may predispose a patient to fungal infections, and prophylaxis is appropriate in those instances (Hughes et al., 2002).

The febrile neutropenic pediatric patient has most likely had previous hospitalizations, and given the original diagnosis, the patient and family have likely already experienced significant amounts of distress. It is important to keep families well informed of all planned procedures and the necessity for peripheral blood draws despite the presence of central venous access. Informing them of a planned timetable for administration of antibiotics is very helpful so that families can visualize an end point. Given that the neutropenic patient is especially susceptible to infection, families need to be educated on all the ways they can help reduce this risk. Neutropenic precautions may entail many lifestyle changes for the family. Child life specialists can help the patient cope with his or her hospitalization and the numerous procedures the patient may undergo.

Disposition and discharge planning

To determine the efficacy of the antibiotic regimen, it is recommended waiting 3 to 5 days before changing antibiotic therapy. Once a microbial source is identified, then antibiotic coverage should be adjusted as necessary to minimize side effects while maintaining broad-spectrum coverage to reduce breakthrough bacteremia. Antibiotics should be continued for at least 7 days, and until repeat cultures are negative and the patient is asymptomatic. CBC, serum creatinine, urea nitrogen, and transaminases studies should be repeated every 3 days to monitor for antibiotic drug toxicity (Hughes et al., 2002).

A low-risk patient who is afebrile for 48 hours or longer, has an ANC of 100 cells/mm³ or more, and in whom no source of infection has been identified can be changed to oral cefixime. A high-risk afebrile patient should continue with the parenteral antibiotic regimen. A low-risk patient who has taken 3 to 5 days of antibiotics, who has been afebrile for 48 hours, and who has an ANC of 500 cells/mm³ or more for two consecutive days may have his or her antibiotics stopped (Hughes et al., 2002). The low-risk patient who looks clinically well and who has been afebrile since day 3 to 5 of antibiotics, but whose ANC remains 500 cells/mm³ or less, may have his or her antibiotics stopped after day 7 of antibiotics and after 5 to 7 days of being afebrile. This patient must continue to be closely observed; if the fever returns, the patient's antibiotics should be restarted. Table 30-8 summarizes the management of low-risk patients. If the patient is considered to be at high risk, the ANC is 100 cells/mm³ or less, the patient has mucositis, or the patient is unstable, the antibiotics should be continued whether the patient is febrile or afebrile (Hughes et al.).

If the patient remains febrile during the first 3 to 5 days, then he or she may have a nonbacterial infection, an infection resistant to the antibiotic course, a slow response

TABLE 30-8

Management of Low-Risk Patients with Fever of Unknown Origin		
	ANC ≥ 500 cells/mm³	**ANC < 500 cells/mm³**
Afebrile		
After 48 hours	Change to oral antibiotic (cefixime)	Change to oral antibiotic if ANC ≥ 100 cells/mm³
Day 3 to 5 of antibiotics	Stop antibiotics	Stop antibiotics after afebrile for 5 to 7 days
Persistent Fevers		
After 3 days of fever	Reassess	Reassess
Day 3 to 5 of antibiotics (reassessment negative)	Stop antibiotics after ANC ≥ 500 cells/mm³ for 4 to 5 days	Continue antibiotics for 2 weeks

Note: Absolute neutrophil count (ANC).

Source: Hughes et al., 2002.

or subtherapeutic drug levels, a secondary infection, drug fever, or an infection in a poorly perfused location (Kannangara, 2006). After 3 days of persistent fevers, the patient should be reassessed, involving completion of a repeat physical examination, new blood cultures, CXR, inspection of CVCs, and diagnostic imaging of any suspected focus.

If by day 5 no source is identified and the patient remains febrile, then one of three choices is recommended by the IDSA: continue the current antibiotics if patient is clinically stable, change the antibiotics if progression of disease is suspected or drug toxicity is present, or begin empiric antifungal coverage (amphotericin B) if no resolution of the patient's neutropenia is expected in the next 5 to 7 days (Hughes et al., 2002). Other sources recommend empiric antifungal therapy if the fever persists for 5 or more days while the patient is taking antibiotics (Walsh et al., 2006b). If the patient is clinically well but continues to have fevers and no source of infection has been identified, antibiotics may be stopped after the ANC is 500 cells/mm³ or more for 4 to 5 days, but close monitoring should continue. Such a patient should also be reassessed with diagnostic studies directed at fungal, viral, or mycobacterial infections as a source for the persistent fever. The patient who continues to have fevers and an ANC of 500 cells/mm³ or less should be continued on antibiotics for 2 weeks; after reassessment, the antibiotics may be stopped if the patient is stable and there has been no further disease progression (Hughes et al.). All cultures must be reviewed until final disposition, and the patient should be re-evaluated immediately if growth is reported.

HEALTH CARE–ASSOCIATED INFECTIONS

Catherine O'Keefe

PATHOPHYSIOLOGY

Health care–associated infections (HAI), like any infectious disease, result from the interaction between a host, an agent, and the environment. The pediatric patient (*host*) carries a unique set of intrinsic physiologic characteristics into the hospital setting. Those persons with chronic illness or immunodeficiency (congenital or acquired) may have impaired immune response (Siegel & Grossman, 2008). Newborn and premature infants face additional challenges due to the innate deficiencies of their immune system, complications associated with congenital anomalies, and compromised skin and mucous membranes (Foglia et al., 2007a). Furthermore, the very premature infant is often subjected to a lengthy hospitalization (many months) with multiple invasive procedures and prolonged antibiotic therapy. In all age groups, within a very short time after admission, colonies of the surrounding bacterial *environment* can develop in the pediatric patient's skin, respiratory, or genitourinary tracts. *Agents* such as invasive devices and procedures, as well as prolonged antibiotic therapy, combine with the host and the environment to potentially produce an HAI.

EPIDEMIOLOGY AND ETIOLOGY

An HAI is defined as an infection that is not present upon admission but that develops within 48 hours of admission. Infections not present at discharge but apparent within 10 days after discharge are also classified as HAIs (Horan et al., 2008; Siegel & Grossman, 2008). HAIs are preventable, adverse events that result in significant morbidity and mortality among pediatric patients, particularly those in intensive care units (ICU). The most common pediatric HAI is a central line–associated bloodstream infection (CLA-BSI), followed by ventilator-associated pneumonia (VAP), and then surgical site infections (SSI).

In addition to the increased risks for the patient, HAIs impose a significant financial burden on the healthcare system. Children who develop a hospital-acquired BSI require an additional 14.6 ICU days and 21.1 hospital days and incur a 13% mortality rate (Slonim et al., 2001). The increased direct cost has been calculated at close to $40,000 (Elward et al., 2005). Pediatric patients with VAP also experience a longer ICU length of stay (13 days) and higher associated mortality (10.5%) (Srinivasan et al., 2009). The additional direct costs for VAP have been reported to exceed $50,000 (Brilli et al., 2008).

The National Healthcare Safety Network (NHSN) system of the Centers for Disease Control and Prevention (CDC) gathers device-associated and procedure-associated infection surveillance data from NHSN-participating facilities. Pediatric HAIs involving CLA-BSI, urinary catheter–associated urinary tract infections (CA-UTI), and VAP data for 2007 are summarized in Table 30-9 (Edwards et al., 2008). Data gathered and reported by the NHSN allow acute care facilities to analyze HAI trends as well as design effective quality improvement activities.

Certain groups of pediatric patients are higher risk of acquiring an HAI: neonates; older pediatric patients with transplants, burns, and neoplasms; and a patient of any age who requires mechanical ventilation. In addition, several chronic conditions affect the immune status of pediatric patients, making them more vulnerable to specific pathogens. For example, patients with humoral immune dysfunction have an impairment of the polyclonal B cells. These patients are more prone to infections due to Gram-positive (*Staphylococcus*, *Streptococcus*) and Gram-negative bacteria (*Escherichia coli*, *Klebsiella*). Patients with cell-mediated immune defects are more prone to infections with pathogens such as *Listeria monocytogenes*, *Candida* spp., herpes simplex virus, *Pneumocystis jirovecii*, *Streptococcus pneumoniae*, and *Coccidiodes immitis* (Muralidhar & Muralidhar, 2007).

Younger infants in neonatal ICUs and older infants and children in pediatric ICUs make up a special subset of the hospitalized pediatric population. Both of these intensive care settings have reported higher HAI rates than their adult counterparts. The incidence of HAIs among neonatal ICUs varies from 6% to 40%, depending on the definition being used (Newby, 2008). Some of the neonatal ICU data that are reported refer to "late onset" (when the child has reached 5 to 7 days of age); other data are based on the traditional time period of 48 hours from time of admission. Perinatal transmission of infection is generally not considered an HAI. The pediatric ICU prevalence of HAI has been reported to be as high as 6% to 12% (Banerjee et al., 2006).

TABLE 30-9

Health Care–Associated Infection Rates*			
Location	CLA-BSI	CA-UTI	VAP
Pediatric medical/surgical ICU	2.9	5.0	2.1
Neonatal ICU (Level III)	2.0–3.7†	1.0–4.7†	0.9–2.6†

Notes: Central line–associated bloodstream infections (CLA-BSI), urinary catheter–associated urinary tract infections (CA-UTI), ventilator-associated pneumonia (VAP), umbilical catheter–associated bloodstream infections (UCA-BSI).

*Rates are pooled per device days.

†Rates in the neonatal ICU are inversely related to birth weight.

Source: Adapted from Edwards et al., 2008.

Premature infants may be subjected to unique exogenous factors that place them at higher risk for HAIs. These issues include maternal infections contracted during the peripartal period, as well as peripartal procedures such as fetal scalp electrode monitoring, umbilical cannulation, invasive monitoring, and circumcisions.

The nature of the hospital environment and accompanying procedures and care activities lends itself to increased handling and more intimate contact between the pediatric patient and HCPs. Healthcare professionals who do not practice safe hygienic practices or who are ill may be a significant source of pediatric HAIs. Visitors to the hospitalized pediatric patient, if not properly screened for communicable disease, may also be a source of infection.

Pathogens associated with HAIs in pediatric settings are very different than those in adult settings. In recent years, respiratory syncytial viruses (RSV) and *Bordatella pertussis* have played a larger role in transmission in pediatric facilities (Forgie & Marrie, 2009); also, ICUs for patients of any age may harbor Gram-negative bacilli and multidrug-resistant organisms (MDRO) (Siegel & Grossman, 2008). The incidence of methicillin-resistant *Staphylococcus aureus* (MRSA) and vancomycin-resistant *Enterococcus* (VRE) continues to increase, particularly in those pediatric patients who are transferred from long-term care facilities. Bacteria responsible for pediatric VAP include *Pseudomonas aeruginosa*, *S. aureus*, and non-typable *Haemophilus influenzae* (Bigham et al., 2009; Zaoutis & Coffin, 2008). A recent study reported similar microbiology of pediatric VAP but also a 38% incidence of polymicrobial VAP (Srinivasan et al., 2009).

PRESENTATION

New-onset fever is common to most HAI presentations. In the premature infant or neonate, however, temperature instability or hypothermia may be a more common symptom of infection. Poor feeding or increased irritability can also be an early subtle sign of an HAI. Other risk factors to consider when obtaining the history include an immunocompromised host, mechanical ventilation, central venous catheters (CVC), arterial catheter use, urinary drainage catheter, packed red blood cell transfusion, extracorporeal membrane oxygenation (ECMO), dialysis, and parenteral nutrition (PN) (Elward & Fraser, 2006). Prolonged therapy increases risk.

The most common HAIs occur in blood, urine, respiratory tract, and surgical sites; thus clinical changes in these specific areas warrant close monitoring. For example, a mechanically ventilated patient with frequent oxygen desaturations or changes in the amount or character of sputum should be evaluated for VAP. Frequently, these patients will also have increased oxygen requirements or ventilator support. Purulent discharge, erythema, or dehiscence of a surgical site should lead the HCP to consider a health care–associated SSI; similarly, patients with prolonged indwelling bladder catheterization who present with abdominal or flank pain and an abnormal urinalysis should be considered at high risk for a CA-HAI.

DIFFERENTIAL DIAGNOSIS

When a mechanically ventilated patient presents with fever and deteriorating respiratory status, the following diagnoses should also be considered:

- Respiratory distress syndrome (RDS)
- Bronchopulmonary dysplasia (BPD)
- Atelectasis
- Aspiration
- Pulmonary hemorrhage
- Air leak syndrome (Baltimore, 2003; Klompas, 2007)

For a patient with a CVC or other invasive monitoring device who presents with temperature instability, poor feeding, and irritability, potential diagnoses should take into account the following considerations:

- Translocation of microbes from another site
- Blood and blood product transfusion-related infection
- Contaminated intravenous fluids or medications

Surgical site infections are primarily contracted during the operation. However, a small subset of pediatric SSIs may be caused by preoperative exposures. Patients with indwelling urinary catheters may experience asymptomatic bacteriuria or cystitis—conditions that are not considered true infections but that nevertheless require removal of the catheter (Zaoutis & Coffin, 2008).

PLAN OF CARE

Specimens for culture and susceptibilities should be obtained before starting antimicrobial therapy whenever possible. Wound aspirates are preferred over swabs to maximize pathogen yield. Blood samples for culture should be drawn peripherally as well as from any CVC lumens. Urine specimens should be obtained by urinary catheter or suprapubic aspiration. Sputum samples are not easily obtained from pediatric patients except when endotracheal or tracheal tubes are in place.

Other biologic markers of new-onset infection include the complete blood count and differential. The pediatric patient may exhibit neutropenia or leukocytosis depending on the pathogen responsible for the infection. Thrombocytosis, anemia, and elevated inflammatory markers, such as erythrocyte sedimentation rate and C-reactive protein may also be noted.

Radiographic changes are particularly useful for diagnosing VAP. To radiographically confirm the diagnosis of VAP, the CDC recommends that the mechanically ventilated patient have two serial chest radiographs with one or more of the following:

- New or progressive and persistent infiltrate
- Consolidation
- Cavitation
- Pneumatoceles (1 year of age or younger) (Horan et al., 2008)

Prevention is the key to therapeutic management of HAIs. Few formal studies have been conducted in the pediatric population; thus many of the recommended strategies to prevent HAI are based on adult data. To date, though, the most effective means of preventing the spread of pathogens from HCPs to patients remains good hand hygiene (Boyce & Pittet, 2002). Additional preventive measures to augment hand hygiene include the following steps: (1) decontamination of stethoscopes and mobile communication devices; (2) removal of wristwatches and rings (and other HCP personal objects that may come in patient contact); and (3) appropriate isolation of known or potentially contagious patients (Brady et al., 2009; Jeans et al., 2009; Lecat et al., 2008; Yildirim et al., 2008).

HAI-specific prevention "bundles" have also been developed by the CDC's Healthcare Infection Control Practices Committee (HICPAC) and adapted to pediatrics by the Institute for Healthcare Improvement (IHI) and the Child Health Corporation of America/National Initiative for Children's Healthcare Quality (CHCA/NICHQ). A prevention bundle is defined as a set of evidence-based "best practices" that individually improve care, but when practiced together result in significantly reduced infection rates (Siegel & Grossman, 2008).

The CHCA/NICHQ-developed bundle is aimed at preventing CLA-BSIs in the pediatric population. The CLA-BSI prevention bundle addresses three major categories: catheter insertion, access, and maintenance. Specific activities related to hand hygiene, dressings, sterile barrier, sterile technique, and skin preparation are detailed. A recent study conducted at 26 free-standing children's hospitals affiliated with CHCA demonstrated a statistically significant decrease in CLA-BSI infections with use of the bundle (Jeffries et al., 2009).

The VAP prevention bundle was first developed for adults and then modified to pediatrics by IHI. The pediatric version includes the following elements:

- Hand washing
- Elevation of the head of the bed by 30 to 45 degrees (if safe and practical)
- Measuring gastric residuals every 4 hours
- Thorough oral care every 2 hours

- Separate suction apparatus for oral and hypopharyngeal secretions
- Oral and hypopharyngeal suctioning before repositioning the patient or the endotracheal tube
- In-line endotracheal suctioning
- Appropriate equipment care, to include keeping all ventilatory equipment off the bed, and draining ventilator condensation frequently without opening the circuit (Curley et al., 2006; Foglia et al., 2007b)

Implementation of the pediatric VAP prevention bundle has successfully reduced the incidence of pneumonia in mechanically ventilated pediatric patients (Brilli et al., 2008; Curley et al., 2006). Details for the pediatric VAP prevention bundle can be accessed at www.nichq.org/pdf/VAP.pdf.

Surgical site infections can be diagnosed as long as 30 days after the surgical procedure or as long as one year after a surgical implant (Owens & Stoessel, 2008). The CDC has published SSI prevention bundles, and the IHI has provided the necessary pediatric modifications. The pediatric SSI prevention bundle focuses primarily on antibiotic prophylaxis and preoperative skin preparation. It is important to note the surgical wound class and duration of operation, as these factors influence the potential for an SSI (Owens & Stoessel).

Initial therapeutic management of pediatric CLA-BSIs is empirical, and local antimicrobial susceptibility patterns should be considered in the choice of therapy (Smith, 2008). Based on the pathogens most commonly associated with CLA-BSIs, the therapy should be broad and provide Gram-positive and Gram-negative bacteria coverage; it should also provide coverage for MDRO. Subsequent blood culture and susceptibility results should then be used to tailor the therapy and narrow the antibiotic spectrum. Removal of invasive devices is often considered in documented HAI. Limited or difficult venous access, however, makes removal of the CVC in the presence of a CLA-BSI a complicated decision in pediatrics. There is little evidence to guide the HCP in choosing whether to remove the catheter or whether to attempt to clear the bloodstream and CVC of infection with antimicrobials. In any event, persistent bacteremia while the patient is taking broad-spectrum antibiotics for a CLA-BSI does warrant serious concern, and CVC removal should be considered in this situation.

The initial therapeutic management of pediatric VAP is also empiric broad-spectrum antibiotic therapy. The choice of antimicrobials should take into account the presence of underlying disease, the patient's risk for MDRO, recent antimicrobial therapy, and the local antibiotic resistance patterns. If aspiration is a consideration, then antimicrobial coverage should include anaerobes (Foglia et al., 2007b). Targeted antibiotic therapy should be initiated when a pathogen has been isolated and the susceptibility pattern determined.

Surgical site infections are managed primarily by surgical drainage or debridement, with antibiotics being administered as a second-line therapy. Presumed postoperative pathogens are procedure and site specific. For example, genitourinary and abdominal wounds need broad-spectrum coverage that includes anaerobic bacteria, whereas skin infections do not (Coffin & Zaoutis, 2008).

Pediatric specialists are invaluable in the prevention and management of HAIs. Pediatric infectious disease specialists should be consulted for appropriate antibiotic management and monitoring recommendations. In addition, pediatric infectious diseases specialists often serve as hospital epidemiologists and in that capacity can implement appropriate infection control policies and procedures. Moreover, infection control practitioners serve as a resource to staff and families during times of change as well as for problem-solving unique situations. Other "organ-specific" pediatric specialists may be consulted as necessary. For example, pediatric pulmonary/respiratory personnel provide supportive care and recommendations regarding ventilatory support and readiness to wean from mechanical ventilation. Certified wound specialists should be consulted to evaluate and manage wounds complicated by infection.

The responsibility for prevention of HAIs lies primarily with the HCP. Patients should receive explanations of infection control practices within the context of their age and developmental level. Families should be enlisted as part of the team and be invested in maintaining a safe and hygienic environment. They should be empowered to question HCPs regarding hand washing when entering their child's room. All visitors should be properly screened for infectious diseases and instructed in appropriate hand hygiene isolation precautions.

DISPOSITION AND DISCHARGE PLANNING

Pediatric HAIs are a significant cause of morbidity and mortality with several national quality improvement organizations developing strategies to reduce this risk. The cost of HAIs is generally not reimbursable and the Centers for Medicare Services has proposed regulations for nonpayment for HAI (Anderson, 2007).

Pediatric patients who incur an HAI should be followed until evidence indicates that the infection has cleared. Blood culture results for the patient with a CLA-BSI should be obtained daily until they are negative. The first day of a negative blood culture should be considered the first day of effective therapy. For those patients with an SSI, the first day of effective therapy is when the infected site is effectively debrided or drained. The progress of a pediatric VAP can be monitored with serial chest radiographs, neutrophil count, and evaluation of inflammatory markers.

Patients with HAIs may be discharged when they are stable and appropriate antimicrobial therapy has been determined.

Discharge should be coordinated with home healthcare agencies if the patient is going home on parenteral antibiotic therapy. Appropriate drug levels (e.g., vancomycin, gentamicin) should be monitored. Adverse events associated with long-term antibiotic therapy can include bone marrow suppression, liver toxicity, and kidney dysfunction. Consequently, diagnostic studies to evaluate bone marrow, liver, and kidney function should be performed regularly.

FUNGAL INFECTIONS

Catherine O'Keefe

There are an estimated 250,000 fungal species in the world, yet only a few cause clinical illness in immunocompetent hosts: histoplasmosis, coccidioidomycosis, and blastomycosis (Kleiman, 2008a).

HISTOPLASMOSIS (*HISTOPLASMA CAPSULATUM*)

Pathophysiology

Histoplasmosis is caused by the dimorphic fungus *Histoplasma capsulatum* var. *capsulatum (H. capsulatum)*. Infection occurs when the mold spores are inhaled and migrate to the distal bronchioles and pulmonary alveoli, where they are phagocytized by alveolar macrophages. Once inside the macrophage, the mold converts to yeast. Within 1 to 3 weeks after inoculation, the immunocompetent host launches a specific cell-mediated immune response, in which sensitized T cells activate the macrophages to kill the yeast (Kauffman, 2009). The respiratory tract becomes inflamed and histopathologic changes occur. The subsequent lesions eventually become encapsulated, fibrotic, granulomatous, and sometimes calcified (American Academy of Pediatrics [AAP], 2009; Kleiman, 2008b).

H. capsulatum is an intracellular pathogen; thus it can survive in tissues in the latent form for years. If the previously infected immunocompetent host becomes immunocompromised, with weakened cell-mediated immunity, the pathogen may become reactivated and cause disease (Kauffman, 2009).

Epidemiology and etiology

Hyperendemic areas for *H. capsulatum* include the Mississippi, Ohio, and Missouri River valleys of the United States. Exposure typically is associated with the following activities:

- Cleaning, renovating, or excavating older homes or abandoned buildings (industrial settings and schools)
- Cutting firewood, tree stumps, and bird roosts
- Gardening
- Exploring barns, hollow trees, and caves

Mold growth in the soil is facilitated by bat, bird, and chicken droppings; dry and windy conditions contribute to its spread. Less than 5% of all persons who are infected with this pathogen become symptomatic (AAP, 2009). The intensity of illness depends on the size of the inoculum as well as the immune status of the host (AAP; Kauffman, 2009; Kleiman, 2008b). There is no person-to-person transmission. Reinfection is possible with large inoculums (AAP).

Presentation

The presentation of histoplasmosis varies widely, but can be categorized as either pulmonary or disseminated. Depending on the intensity of the exposure, pulmonary histoplasmosis can range from an influenza-like illness with mild respiratory symptoms to severe respiratory failure. Disseminated histoplasmosis can affect healthy children younger than the age of 2 or any pediatric patient with an impaired immune system. The overwhelming disseminated infection, which is referred to as progressive disseminated histoplasmosis (PDH), can be fatal if not treated.

A careful history of potential exposure to *H. capsulatum* is important for making this diagnosis. Spores may be carried on air currents for several miles; consequently, the environmental history should extend to areas beyond that of the home, school, and local play area. Review travel history for visits to hyperendemic areas. Exposure history should also include family members or other close contacts, particularly if they are exhibiting similar symptoms.

Symptomatic patients may experience prolonged weight loss, fatigue, and fever. Respiratory complaints of a persistent dry cough and substernal chest discomfort may also be reported. Many patients, however, will not have any abnormal findings. Pulmonary histoplasmosis can be severe, and may be complicated by acute respiratory distress syndrome, erythema multiforme, or joint symptoms such as polyarticular, symmetrical arthritis, and erythema nodosum (Kauffman, 2007).

Early signs of PDH may be prolonged fever and failure-to-thrive. Extrapulmonary sites of PDH may include the meninges, kidneys, heart, gastrointestinal (GI) tract, and reticuloendothelial system. Meningitis has been reported in 60% of infected infants (Kleiman, 2008b). Pericarditis is also not uncommon (Kauffman, 2007). With these complications in mind, a history of a malaise, headache, altered mental status, cranial nerve palsies, behavioral changes, ataxia, weakness, painful rash, myalgias, arthralgias, chest pain, or dyspnea should be elicited. Past medical history should also be reviewed for presence of risk factors for disseminated histoplasmosis, such as age (infants), acquired immunodeficiency syndrome (AIDS), hematologic malignancies, solid-organ transplant, hematopoietic stem cell transplant, immunosuppressive agents, and congenital T-cell deficiencies.

Physical examination findings may include the following conditions:

- Hepatosplenomegaly
- Lymphadenopathy
- Pallor and petechiae (in the presence of pancytopenia)
- Mucous membrane ulcers
- Skin ulcerations and nodules
- Molluscum-like papules (Kauffman, 2007)

Differential diagnosis

Symptomatic pulmonary histoplasmosis must first be differentiated from tuberculosis. Other diagnoses to consider are listed here (Kauffman, 2007; Kleiman, 2008b):

- Blastomycosis (overlapping endemic regions)
- Coccidioidomycosis
- Respiratory distress syndrome
- Pneumonia
- Lymphoma
- Septicemia
- Reticuloendothelial or primary GI tract neoplasm

Plan of care

There are several methods of confirming the diagnosis of histoplasmosis. Culture, histopathology, and antigen detection are the most useful when considering acute, diffuse pulmonary histoplasmosis and PDH in which the fungal burden may be high (Wheat, 2006). In chronic pulmonary histoplasmosis, cultures will usually be positive, but specimens must be obtained via bronchoscopy, either by direct tissue sampling or by bronchoalveolar lavage (BAL). The cultures may take as long as 4 weeks to grow (Wheat).

Antigen detection can be performed on most body fluids but has the highest sensitivity with urine when there is a heavy fungal load. Results are usually available within 24 to 48 hours. Antigen testing has proven useful in monitoring patient response to therapy. Note that positive antigen tests have also been reported in infections caused by other mycotic agents, such as blastomycosis and paracoccidioidomycosis (Kauffman, 2007; Wheat, 2006).

When milder pulmonary disease or any of the other subacute histoplasmosis syndromes are suspected, the serologic tests for antibodies are a more appropriate choice. The antibody assays entail complement fixation (CF) of both mold and yeast and immunodiffusion assay (ID). A single titer of 1:32 or greater is suggestive of histoplasmosis but not diagnostic; a fourfold rise in titer is required for definitive diagnosis. A positive ID is 80% sensitive but more specific than the CF assay (Kauffman, 2007). Nevertheless, false positives have been reported when patients are infected

by other mycotic infections. In addition, the antibody test will remain positive for many years after the acute infection and may be misleading when evaluating the patient with an atypical pulmonary presentation. Promising preliminary data suggest that amplification of the sample by polymerase chain reaction (PCR) may improve the accuracy of diagnosing histoplasmosis (Maubon et al., 2007).

Additional laboratory data that may contribute to the diagnosis of PDH include pancytopenia, progressive elevation of hepatic enzymes, and increased lactate dehydrogenase (LDH) and serum ferritin levels (Wheat et al., 2007). Radiographic evidence is consistent with the severity of respiratory involvement and can range from patchy infiltrates to lobar consolidation. Hilar adenopathy may also be observed. Complications of pulmonary histoplasmosis can include mediastinal granuloma and mediastinal fibrosis (Kauffman, 2009). Computerized tomography (CT) of the chest will confirm the presence of these abnormal findings and the extension to vital structures such as the bronchus, great vessels, and esophagus.

Treatment is not necessary for most infections, particularly for immunocompetent children who have acute histoplasmosis. The following indications require supportive care and antifungal therapy (AAP, 2009; Kauffman, 2007; Wheat, 2006; Wheat et al., 2007):

- Acute pulmonary histoplasmosis with diffuse infiltrates and moderate to severe symptoms
- PDH
- Chronic cavitary pulmonary histoplasmosis
- Central nervous system infections
- Acute infections in immunocompromised patients
- Serious illness after intense exposure
- Pulmonary disease with symptoms lasting more 4 weeks
- Granulomatous adenitis obstructing critical structures (e.g., bronchi, blood vessels, esophagus)

For the last two indications, the efficacy of antifungal agents is unknown, according to 2007 guidelines developed by the Infectious Diseases Society of America (IDSA).

Due to the insidious onset and often confusing early presentation of severe histoplasmosis, patients may not be diagnosed until an acute event occurs. The patient may present to the emergency department with acute cardiopulmonary failure or septic shock without an obvious etiology. In these emergent situations, patients require immediate resuscitation and stabilization in an intensive care setting. The decision to start empiric antifungal therapy should then be based on the index of suspicion for the diagnosis of severe pulmonary histoplasmosis or PDH.

Pharmacologic management depends on the extent and severity of disease as well as the immune capacity of the patient. Most recommendations for antifungal therapy are based on adult clinical trials and expert opinion (Kleiman, 2008b).

Amphotericin B is the first-line medication of choice, as it produces more rapid improvement than the azoles. The choice of which amphotericin B formulation to use depends on the site of the histoplasmosis infection as well as the kidney function of the patient. Amphotericin B (deoxycholate formulation) can be nephrotoxic but has better cerebrospinal fluid penetration if needed (AAP, 2009). If kidney toxicity is a concern, the lipid-associated formulations may be a better choice. Amphotericin B is dosed intravenously (IV) at 0.5 to 1.5 mg/kg infused over a 2-hour period once daily. Intrathecal dosing is 0.025 to 0.5 mg, given twice a week. Amphotericin B should be administered for 1 to 2 weeks, depending on the clinical response of the patient, with the patient then being transitioned to an oral azole (itraconazole 5–10 mg/kg/day, divided into two doses). Although the efficacy of itraconazole in children has not been well established, it appears to be well tolerated. The oral solution is absorbed at a higher rate (30%) than the capsule form (Wheat et al., 2007). Continued oral antifungal treatment may continue for 6 to 12 weeks or longer, depending on the initial severity of disease and the immune status of the patient. The reader is referred to the most cuurent edition of the *Red Book: Report of the Committee on Infectious Diseases*, which has an excellent reference table and explanatory text detailing the pharmacologic management of histoplasmosis (AAP).

Other manifestations of histoplasmosis such as pericarditis and rheumatologic findings do not require antifungal therapy. Pericarditis responds well to indomethacin, and rheumatologic symptoms can be managed with nonsteroidal anti-inflammatory medications (NSAIDs).

A pediatric infectious diseases specialist should be consulted if histoplasmosis is suspected, to assist in the diagnostic evaluation. Additional specialty services to be consulted may include rheumatology, pulmonology, cardiology, surgery, endocrine, renal, or gastroenterology, depending on the site-specific manifestations of the disease.

Patients and families should be advised of the long-term nature of the pharmacologic management and the need for diligent adherence to the medical regimen. Side effects of the medication therapy should be reviewed with both the caregivers and the patient (depending on the patient's level of understanding). Additional teaching should be specific to the clinical findings of the patient. For example, if granulomatous lesions remain in the lung after resolution of the acute infectious phase of the disease, caregivers should be forewarned that their child will always have an "abnormal" chest radiograph. Caregivers need to be aware of the possible source of the infection and know how to avoid future exposures.

Disposition and discharge planning

Most infections with histoplasmosis resolve spontaneously without treatment or negative sequelae. Unfortunately, mortality rates are high (7% to 23%) in disseminated disease, even with appropriate treatment. Chronic pulmonary infection can result in permanent lung damage.

Patients should be followed for the duration of therapy, which can last anywhere from several weeks to months. While on amphotericin B, the patient should have regular kidney function and electrolyte monitoring (BUN, creatinine, magnesium, potassium levels). Long-term itraconazole therapy requires regular liver function tests. Periodic evaluations every 3 to 6 months after discontinuation of antifungal therapy should be considered to monitor for relapse. Urine antigen levels can be used to monitor for suspected treatment failure or relapse.

Reactivation of the infection is possible if the patient experiences an intense exposure or alteration in his or her immune status. This event may occur years after the primary infection. Immunosuppressed individuals may require lifetime suppressive therapy to prevent relapse.

It is not practical to recommend complete avoidance of a ubiquitous pathogen such as *H. capsulatum,* particularly when 95% of immunocompetent individuals who are infected experience spontaneous resolution without negative sequelae. Nevertheless, pediatric patients who live in, or travel to, hyperendemic areas should attempt to avoid locations in which there is a significant disturbance of the soil or demolition of buildings. Caregivers should take special precaution to protect immunocompromised individuals (including healthy young infants) by avoiding intense exposure.

COCCIDIOIDOMYCOSIS (*COCCIDIOIDES IMMITIS* AND *COCCIDIOIDES POSADASII*)

Pathophysiology

Coccidioidomycosis is caused by dimorphic fungi that are spore-forming molds in soil. After inhalation, the spores germinate in the lungs, with subsequent cleavage and spread of endospores; these serve to exponentially increase the number of fungal elements in the host. Granulomatous inflammation then develops (Kleiman, 2008c). The inflammatory response is primarily neutrophilic and is dependent upon T-cell–mediated immunity to clear the organism from the host. Although the fungus is spread by lymphohematogenous dissemination, it rarely causes extrapulmonary infection.

Epidemiology and etiology

Both species that cause coccidioidomycosis—*Coccidioides immitis* and *Coccidioides posadasii*—are endemic in hot, arid regions of the southwestern United States—for example, southern California, Arizona, western and southern Texas, New Mexico, southern Nevada, and Utah. They can also be found in northern Mexico and certain areas of Central and South America. *C. posadasii* is the predominant species outside California.

Coccidioidomycosis, also known as San Joaquin Valley fever, is asymptomatic or mild in 95% of infections. However, it can cause life-threatening infection regardless of the host's immune status. Inhalation of just one spore can cause pulmonary infection; with high inoculum exposures, symptomatic disease is likely. Exposures have been reported during dust storms, seismic events, archaeological digs, recreational activities, and military training. The spores can be carried on dusty clothing or agricultural products as well. Person-to-person transmission does not occur, and infection is thought to provide lifelong immunity. Infection rates are the highest in the summer and early fall, and the rate of positive skin tests increases with the length of time the child lives in the endemic region (AAP, 2009; Kleiman, 2008c).

Coccidioidomycosis is a reportable disease to the CDC in fewer than 40 states. In 2007, 8,121 cases of coccidioidomycosis were reported in the United States, with the highest incidence occurring among persons older than 65 years of age; the incidence rate is 0.87 per 100,000 population in children younger than 1 year of age (Centers for Disease Control and Prevention [CDC], 2009d).

Presentation

Primary infection is asymptomatic or self-limited in 60% of patients, with fewer than 5% experiencing pulmonary complications, and fewer than 1% presenting with disseminated disease (Kleiman, 2008c). The risk of exposure may be determined by taking a careful history of travel or residence in an endemic area. Even a very brief visit to an endemic region should not be overlooked, given the low level of inoculum required for primary pulmonary infection. The incubation period typically is 10 to 16 days, but can range from 1 to 4 weeks.

In primary pulmonary coccidioidal infection, the patient may present with complaints of fever, malaise, mild respiratory distress, and a characteristic rash (erythema nodosum or erythema multiforme). Symptoms of extrapulmonary or disseminated disease can occur weeks, months, or a year after the initial infection.

Patients experiencing disseminated coccidioidomycosis may present with complaints of chronic illness, weight loss, and persistent fever. Extrapulmonary sites of dissemination may include skin, joints, and the CNS. As a consequence, the patient may present with complaints of painful rash or discrete lesions, arthralgias, arthritis, or signs of CNS problems such as headache, altered mental status, ataxia, lethargy, or confusion. Past medical history should be reviewed to determine the presence of risk factors for disseminated disease and poor outcomes, such as age, ethnicity, and immune status. Young infants and persons of Filipino or African descent have an increased risk of severe disease. T-cell dysfunction, solid-organ transplantation, and immunosuppression due to use of corticosteroids or antitumor necrosis factor (TNF) are also associated with higher risk.

The physical examination of a patient with *symptomatic* primary pulmonary infection is very similar to that of a patient with community-acquired pneumonia. Oftentimes, treatment is delayed because *Coccidioides* is not considered as a possible pathogen. In addition, children commonly present with a diffuse erythematous rash or morbilliform rash consistent with erythema multiforme. One to three weeks later, rheumatologic symptoms such as erythema nodosum and arthritis may appear—a complication more common in females (termed *valley fever* and *desert rheumatism*) (Kleiman, 2008c).

Potential extrapulmonary sites for disseminated coccidioidal infection include the skin, lymph nodes, bones, joints, and CNS (Parish & Blair, 2008). Skin lesions may present as papules, nodules, abscesses, verrucous plaques, or ulcers (Anstead & Graybill, 2006). Bone and joint involvement may be manifested in the form of knee, ankle, wrist, or spinal pain. Synovitis and osteomyelitis are the most common manifestations of osteoarticular disseminated coccidioidal infection. Persistent regional lymphadenopathy should be evaluated for the presence of fungal elements, as abscess formation is frequently present. Physical examination findings of disseminated coccidioidal CNS infection are similar to those of bacterial meningitis, with the exception of the slow onset common with *Coccidioides* infection. Hydrocephalus is often present at initial diagnosis in pediatric patients.

Differential diagnosis

The clinical picture of coccidioidomycosis must be distinguished from other diseases through a careful history, especially for patients who do not live in endemic areas. Other diagnoses to consider include the following conditions:

- Influenza
- Pneumonia
- Histoplasmosis
- Blastomycosis
- Pericarditis
- Septic arthritis
- Cryptococcosis
- Chlamydial and mycoplasmal infections (AAP, 2009; Kleiman, 2008c)

Plan of care

Diagnostic studies may be microbiologic, histopathologic, or serologic.

Microbiologic culture (sputum, tissue, broncheoalveolar lavage fluid, and other body fluids) is the most definitive and can be grown in approximately 5 to 7 days.

Special precautions must be taken by laboratory personnel when handling these specimens; therefore, the HCP indicate the possible presence of *Coccidioides* when ordering the culture.

Histopathologic (tissue obtained by biopsy) verification of *Coccidioides* spherules is confirmed by the presence of endospores. Specimens should be sent to the CDC, where special antibody staining is available, if there is any doubt in the histopathologic appearance (Anstead & Graybill, 2006).

Serology (serum or CSF) is the method relied upon most frequently; however, the sensitivity and specificity of the assays are low. The presence of coccidioidal-specific IgM may be detected in the first 1 to 3 weeks after primary infection. IgM can be detected using immunodiffusion (ID) or complement-fixing (CF) methods (Anstead & Graybill, 2006). Coccidioidal-specific IgG cannot be detected for several weeks after primary infection and may persist for several years after the primary infection resolves. The utility of nucleic amplification of coccidioidal DNA (PCR) in the diagnosis of *Coccidioides* has yet to be determined (Parish & Blair, 2008). Radiography and magnetic resonance imaging (MRI) may be necessary to determine the extent of pulmonary, osteoarticular, and CNS involvement.

Evidence-based treatment guidelines are limited due to insufficient clinical trial data. The most recent IDSA guidelines, which were published in 2005, are based on relatively weak evidence and rely heavily on expert clinical experience (AAP, 2009; Anstead & Graybill, 2006; Galgiani et al., 2005). The current management of *Coccidioides* primary infection depends in a large part on the severity of disease and presence of risk factors that may contribute to a complicated disease course. Mild infection usually does not require therapy and is self-limiting. Careful consideration should, however, be used for patients with the following conditions:

- Immunosuppression (e.g., AIDS, organ transplant recipients, high-dose corticosteroid or TNF inhibitor use)
- Diabetes mellitus
- Preexisting cardiopulmonary disease
- Filipino or African descent
- Severe primary infection: weight loss greater than 10% of total body weight; intense night sweats for more than 3 weeks; extensive infiltrates in one or both lungs; prominent or persistent hilar adenopathy; anticoccioidal CF antibody titer greater than 1:16; inability to engage in daily activities such as attending school; persistent symptoms for more than 2 months; or age greater than 55 years of age (Galgiani et al., 2005)

If treatment is deemed necessary, then the azole antifungal medications are considered first-line therapy. Itraconazole has demonstrated slightly better efficacy than other medications in the azole class, particularly in the treatment of skeletal coccidioidomycosis (Ampel, 2009). The reader is referred to the current edition *Red Book: Report of the Committee on Infectious Diseases*, which has an excellent reference table and explanatory text detailing the pharmacologic management of coccidioidomycosis (AAP, 2009). Duration of therapy is debatable and based on expert opinion. In many cases, 3 to 6 months of treatment is suggested; however, treatment may be required for as long as one year.

Treatment of coccidioidal meningitis is often augmented by parenteral amphotericin B to assure complete CNS penetration (Anstead & Graybill, 2006). Severe cases of meningeal infection may require ventricular–peritoneal shunting. Surgical drainage of infected sites may be necessary, although this step is uncommon in children.

A pediatric infectious diseases specialist should be consulted if coccidioidal infection is suspected, to assist in the diagnostic evaluation. Additional specialty services that might be consulted include rheumatology, pulmonology, surgery, orthopedics, or dermatology, depending on the site-specific manifestations of the disease.

The long-term nature of treatment needs to be emphasized to both patients and caregivers. If itraconazole is prescribed, it is best absorbed after consumption of a high-fat meal and with an acidic beverage. Caregivers should be warned of the side effects and possible adverse events associated with antifungal therapy. Relapse and recurrence rates should be thoroughly reviewed with both the caregivers and the patient.

Disposition and discharge planning

Primary coccidioidomycosis outcomes can range from uneventful healing to long-term CNS involvement (Anstead & Graybill, 2006). The severity of the primary infection as well as the presence of risk factors determines morbidity and mortality. Chronic pulmonary complications are rare in children. Calcified pulmonary granulomas can develop even in asymptomatic presentations with spontaneous resolution (Kleiman, 2008c).

Patients should be followed for the duration of therapy, which can be several weeks to months. While on amphotericin B, the patient should have regular kidney function and electrolyte monitoring (BUN, creatinine, magnesium, potassium levels). Long-term itraconazole therapy requires regular liver function tests. Patients should be evaluated every 3 to 6 months for as long as 2 years after the primary infection occurs to monitor for resolution, late relapse, or dissemination. Normal laboratory, radiographic (as applicable) and clinical presentation findings signal the recovery from infection.

Candidate vaccines for coccidioidomycosis are in development but are not anticipated in the near future. Prophylaxis is not recommended even in immunocompromised individuals. Areas with endemic infection should be avoided, especially areas near construction sites or other areas where the soil may be easily aerosolized.

BLASTOMYCOSIS (*BLASTOMYCES DERMATITIDIS*)

Pathophysiology

Blastomyces dermatitidis is a dimorphic fungus that produces conidia from the hyphae of the mycelial form at room temperature and in soil. Infection occurs after inhalation of the conidia into the lungs. Once the conidia reaches body temperature in the infected tissue, it is transformed into the yeast form. The yeast then germinate and are phagocytized by pulmonary macrophages, beginning suppurative inflammation (AAP, 2009). Most infection is preventing from spreading by the actions of T lymphocytes and lymphokine-activated macrophages. In more severe infections, however, lymphohematogenous spread distributes the infection to extrapulmonary sites. Both acute and chronic granulomatous changes can be present at the same time (Kleiman, 2008d).

Epidemiology and etiology

Blastomyces dermatides thrives in warm, moist, acidic environments. It is endemic throughout eastern North America: in the Mississippi, Ohio, and lower St. Lawrence River valleys; in the Lake Michigan basin; in several eastern U.S. states; in northern Ontario; and in bordering eastern Manitoba (Chapman et al., 2008). The infection affects children less frequently than adults. The most commonly affected sites are the lungs, skin, and bones. This infection's incidence in the pediatric population is as high as 2% to 11% (Walsh et al., 2006a). There is no person-to-person transmission, nor have any age-, gender-, or ethnicity-specific risk factors been defined.

Presentation

The range of symptoms associated with *B. dermatitidis* infection is broad. The pediatric patient with primary pulmonary infection may present with mild influenza-like illness (nonproductive cough) or fever, cough, and pleuritic pain progressing to respiratory failure (Kleiman, 2008d; McKinnell & Pappas, 2009). Additional symptomology may include headache, weight loss, abdominal pain, and night sweats (Walsh et al., 2006a). Painless cutaneous lesions represent a common form of extrapulmonary infection. It is important to elicit a careful history of travel to endemic regions in such cases, as the incubation period is approximately 30 to 45 days (AAP, 2009).

The respiratory examination findings in blastomycosis may be similar to those associated with pneumonia. Skin and oral mucous membrane lesions initially appear as nontender papules, which then develop into nodular, verrucous, or ulcerative lesions with purulent drainage. All types of lesions can be present at the same time. Osseous manifestations are similar to those of acute or subacute suppurative osteomyelitis and adjacent soft-tissue abscesses are common (Kleiman, 2008d).

Differential diagnosis

As with the other primary fungal pulmonary infections, tuberculosis is the primary differential diagnosis for blastomycosis. Other diagnoses to consider are these:

- Bacterial pneumonia
- Other mycotic infections
- Neoplasms
- Pyoderma gangrenosum or keratoacanthoma

Plan of care

Diagnosis is often delayed due to the low level of suspicion with this indolent and insidious disease. In addition, diagnosis has traditionally relied heavily on culture and histopathology. Sputum and bronchoscopic specimens have a high diagnostic yield in culture, but require 2 to 4 weeks to grow. Traditional serologic tests using complement fixation or immunodiffusion techniques are limited by low sensitivity and specificity and have been replaced by more sensitive rapid assays—specifically, radioimmunoassay and enzyme-linked immunosorbent assay (ELISA) (McKinnell & Pappas, 2009). Radiography may be necessary to fully evaluate pulmonary disease as well as end-organ or osseous involvement. Lytic lesions of the vertebrae, ribs, pelvis, or skull are highly suspicious of blastomycosis (Kleiman, 2008d). Additional nonspecific diagnostic findings include mild anemia, leukocytosis with mild bandemia, and an elevated ESR.

The pediatric patient may experience an acute pneumonia that spontaneously resolves before the diagnosis of blastomycosis is ever considered; thus no specific antifungal therapy may be required. At the other end of the disease spectrum is the patient whose pneumonia does not resolve with antibiotics and who progresses to severe respiratory or extrapulmonary infection. Antifungal therapy is warranted for patients with severe pulmonary or disseminated non-CNS disease, with CNS disease, or if immunocompromised (Chapman et al., 2008; Walsh et al., 2006a). Even so, some HCPs treat all infections in an effort to prevent extrapulmonary dissemination (Chapman et al.).

Antifungal therapy for severe blastomycosis consists of amphotericin B (deoxycholate), 0.7 to 1.0 mg/kg/day, or lipid formulation amphotericin B, 3 to 5 mg/kg/day, for 1 to 2 weeks or until clinical improvement is noted. A heavy burden of disseminated disease may require extended amphotericin B therapy. Although comparative clinical trials have not been conducted to demonstrate the superiority of one medication over another, clinical experience indicates that the lipid formulation of amphotericin B is efficacious and safer than amphotericin B (McKinnell & Pappas, 2009).

Treatment can be completed with oral itraconazole after improvement is noted, 10 mg/kg/day (maximum dose, 400 mg) for 12 months. The exception is CNS disease, which must be treated with amphotericin B for the full therapeutic course (Chapman et al., 2008). Mild to moderate disease can be treated with itraconazole (5 to 7 mg/kg/day) alone for 6 to 12 months. IDSA guidelines recommend measurement of serum itraconazole levels after two weeks (time to steady state). Although evidence-based therapeutic levels have not yet been identified, expert opinion recommends adjusting the dosage to maintain a medication level between 1.0 mcg/mL and 10 mcg/mL (Chapman et al.).

Adjuvant therapy may include surgical incision and drainage of abscesses and/or debridement of devitalized bone.

A pediatric infectious diseases specialist should be consulted if blastomycosis is suspected, to assist in the diagnostic evaluation. Additional specialty services that might be consulted include rheumatology, pulmonology, surgery, orthopedics, or dermatology, depending on the site-specific manifestations of the disease.

The long-term nature of treatment needs to be emphasized to both patients and caregivers. If itraconazole is prescribed, it is best absorbed after consumption of a high-fat meal and with an acidic beverage. Caregivers should be warned of the side effects and possible adverse events associated with antifungal therapy. Relapse and recurrence rates should be thoroughly reviewed with both the caregivers and the patient.

Disposition and discharge planning

Early and aggressive therapy is required in pediatric patients to avoid unnecessary relapses, particularly in patients with disseminated disease. Endogenous reactivation is possible.

Regular monitoring for adherence to the medication regimen and adverse events associated with long-term medication therapy is recommended. Patients should be evaluated every 3 to 6 months for as long as 2 years after the primary infection occurs to monitor for resolution, late relapse, or dissemination. Should the HCP wait and monitor the mildly ill patient, any evidence of extrapulmonary disease should be ruled out as well as scheduled long-term follow-up appointments.

The mortality rate with this infection is higher in immunocompromised individuals. In addition, acute respiratory distress syndrome due to blastomycosis has mortality rates reported to be as high as 50% to 89% (McKinnell & Pappas, 2009).

Currently, there is no human vaccine available to prevent blastomycosis. Immunocompromised individuals should avoid travel to hyperendemic regions and take precautions to avoid intense exposure.

> **Critical Thinking**
>
> Recent travel to fungal endemic regions should be considered when evaluating a pediatric patient with a respiratory illness whose presentation is consistent with community-acquired pneumonia but is not responding to traditional therapies.

OPPORTUNISTIC INFECTIONS

Catherine O'Keefe

The immunocompetent individual has an armamentarium of defenses against infection, including circulating neutrophils, natural killer (NK) cells, the complement system, skin and mucosal integrity, and cell-mediated and circulating immunoglobulins (de la Morena, 2008). In contrast, the immunoincompetent individual has limited defenses against infection due to an underlying immune defect or deficit. Opportunistic infections, by definition, occur in patients who have such an altered host defense response to pathogen exposure. In addition, any pathogen can potentially cause an opportunistic infection in a vulnerable patient. The pathogenesis of opportunistic infections is frequently mediated by the specific mechanism of the immune defect (Castagnola & Buratti, 2009).

The last two decades have seen a growing number of patients with primary and secondary immunodeficiencies who are at high risk for opportunistic infections. This phenomenon is largely due to increased recognition and diagnosis of primary immunodeficiencies as well as medical advances in chemotherapy, hematopoietic stem cell transplants, solid-organ transplants, intensive care of trauma–surgical patients, and the care of the extremely premature infant.

CANDIDAL INFECTIONS

Pathophysiology

Candida spp. are yeast-like fungi. These unicellular structures have a sterol-containing cytoplasmic membrane and reproduce by budding (Smith & Steinbach, 2008). They are ubiquitous organisms found on skin, mucous membranes, and the intestinal tract (AAP, 2009). *Candida* spp. are considered opportunistic mycoses that are not virulent enough to cause illness in a healthy, immunocompetent individual. Among the host defense mechanisms in the immunocompetent patient against *Candida* infection are the following:

- An intact skin and mucous membrane barrier
- Phagocytic cells
- Functioning complement pathways
- Sufficient number and variety of immunoglobulins

- Cell-mediated immunity
- Innate protective bacterial flora

In contrast, in the presence of primary or secondary immunodeficiencies in which immunity against yeast growth is ineffective, *Candida* spp. can result in serious life-threatening infections. Unique virulence factors also contribute to serious infections in certain individuals. For example, some *Candida* isolates can form a biofilm that provides a degree of protection against most fungicidal activity (Smith & Steinbach, 2008). Invasive candidiasis is the most serious *Candida* infection involving hematogenous spread to at least one normally sterile extravascular site: eye, CNS, heart, lung, kidney, liver, or spleen (Festekjian & Neely, 2009). *Candida* spp. have the potential to propagate and form abscesses in end organs, commonly referred to as "fungal balls."

Epidemiology and etiology

An increased incidence of invasive fungal infections in hospitalized patients has been observed over the past two decades (Zaoutis et al., 2009). This trend is likely due to the larger numbers of pediatric patients receiving hematopoietic stem cell transplants (HSCT), intensive medical–surgical therapies, cytotoxic chemotherapy, immunosuppressive therapies, and broad-spectrum antibiotics.

Candida spp. appear to be responsible for the majority of fungal infections, with incidence rates as high as 80% being noted (Fisher & Zaoutis, 2008). Recent advances in empiric antifungal therapy have markedly reduced the morbidity and mortality associated with fungal bloodstream infections and invasive disease. However, systemic candidiasis continues to be a source of significant mortality. Pediatric patients have a lower mortality rate from *Candida*-associated illness than adults; however, this rate is still reported in the 10% to 54% range (Festekjian & Neely, 2009). Mortality rates for pediatric cancer and bone marrow transplant patients are even higher, with a reported range of 56% to 80% (Fisher & Zaoutis). Beyond the cost in human suffering, invasive *Candida*-associated illness has been determined to increase length of hospital stay by 3 to 5 weeks, with a concomitant financial cost in excess of $100,000 (Festekjian & Neely; Moran et al., 2009).

More than 200 *Candida* species have been identified, although only 12 cause illness in pediatric patients: *C. albicans, C. parapsilosis, C. tropicalis, C. glabrata, C. krusei, C. lusitaniae, C. stellatoideae, C. kefyr, C. pseudotropicalis, C. dubliniensis, C. intermedia,* and *C. guillermondi* (Smith & Steinbach, 2008). *C. albicans* continues to be the most common infectious agent in children (Fisher & Zaoutis, 2008; Smith & Steinbach). In recent years, emerging epidemiologic trends have indicated a shift in the *Candida* species responsible for pediatric candidemia and invasive candidiasis. The

dominance of *C. albicans* is being challenged by an increase in non-*albicans Candida* species—specifically, *C. parapsilosis and C. tropicalis* (Arendrup et al., 2009; Fisher & Zaoutis; Moran et al., 2009; Neu et al., 2009). Attention to these epidemiologic trends is necessary to identify the emergence of *Candida* spp. resistant to fluconazole, which is the mainstay of therapy. Currently, *C. glabrata* and *C. krusei* have demonstrated decreasing sensitivity to fluconazole (Neu et al.).

Presentation

When *Candida* infection is suspected, the history should include careful attention to the presence of risk factors associated with candidemia and candidiasis. These include central venous catheters, premature birth, and underlying immune deficiency (Festekjian & Neely, 2009). In addition, the clinician should review recent medical care, including immunosuppressive therapy such as cytotoxic chemotherapy and chronic corticosteroid use.

Candidemia cannot be differentiated from bacteremia on the basis of signs and symptoms. As with any bloodstream infection, the clinical manifestations can be subtle and nonspecific, ranging from temperature instability, to hypotension, to respiratory distress or failure. Thus the patient with persistent fever, negative blood culture(s), and associated septic shock should be considered to have candidemia until proven otherwise. The HCP should also consider a fungal source in the presence of a persistent fever despite antimicrobial therapy (Smith & Steinbach, 2008). End-organ involvement will have a specific set of organ-specific signs and symptoms. For example, CNS infection may present with the typical meningeal signs of nuchal rigidity and altered mental status.

Differential diagnosis

Bloodstream and end-organ infections can be caused by a variety of pathogens. Therefore, the clinician should investigate bacterial, viral, and parasitic sources for fever and end-organ failure.

Plan of care

Timely diagnosis of candidemia and invasive candidiasis is critical to the appropriate management of the pediatric patient leading to improved outcomes. Acquired resistance in fungi is rare; therefore, species identification is the most useful in guiding therapy (Arendrup et al., 2009). Diagnostic techniques in the past have been time consuming, leading to a subsequent delay in treatment. This practice can have devastating outcomes.

Current diagnostics have improved the timeliness of species identification, which in turn has led to decreased use of broad-spectrum antifungals. Newer stains with microscopy have increased the sensitivity, specificity, and speed of species identification. Latex agglutination kits allow for rapid identification of *C. albicans, C. dubliniensis, C. krusei,* and *C. glabrata*. Newer diagnostic tests include antigen detection tests and polymerase chain reaction. Both technologies have potential for use in children but require further standardization before their widespread adoption for the pediatric population (Arendrup et al., 2009).

Traditionally, once candidemia was identified, a complete evaluation for evidence of end-organ involvement ensued. This effort included radiography, ultrasonography, CSF analysis, and/or dilated ophthalmologic examination. Some experts have questioned the necessity of this extensive evaluation (Festekjian & Neely, 2009). The most current IDSA clinical practice guidelines continue to recommend at the minimum a lumbar puncture and a dilated retinal examination for neonates (Pappas et al., 2009).

Therapeutic options should be guided by the underlying immune disorder, local epidemiologic data, and pediatric pharmacokinetics (Castagnola & Buratti, 2009; Fisher & Zaoutis, 2008). The most recent IDSA guidelines offer comprehensive recommendations for the management of patients who either have or are at risk for candidiasis. The use of a newer class of antifungal drugs, echinocandins, and the expanded-spectrum azoles are reviewed in detail in the guidelines, with supporting evidence for their use being presented (Pappas et al., 2009). The reader is referred to the published IDSA clinical practice guidelines for detailed drug selection, duration, and pediatric dosing considerations (Pappas et al.). A recent Cochrane review concluded that there were no reported differences in mortality or treatment efficacy among the various antifungal agents when used with children. However, less nephrotoxicity was noted with the lipid preparation of amphotericin B when compared with deoxycholate amphotericin B (Blyth et al., 2010).

Fluconazole prophylaxis against neonatal candidiasis in the extremely premature infant has been studied in several randomized trials (Bertini et al., 2005; Kaufman et al., 2001; Kaufman et al., 2005; Kicklighter et al., 2001; Manzoni et al., 2006; Manzoni et al., 2007). The neonatal dosage is 3 mg/kg/day, given twice weekly for 4 to 6 weeks. This routine and extended use of fluconazole have raised concern for emerging fluconazole resistance. Studies to date have allayed these fears (Healy et al., 2008; Manzoni et al., 2008). Nevertheless, caution should be exercised and the decision to implement a fluconazole prophylaxis protocol in the neonatal intensive care unit (NICU) should be based on the unit's candidiasis prevalence rate (Arendrup et al., 2009; Reed et al., 2010). IDSA clinical practice guidelines recommend antifungal prophylaxis for the following groups of pediatric patients: solid-organ transplant recipients; patients with chemotherapy-induced neutropenia for the duration of the neutropenia; and stem cell transplant recipients with neutropenia (Pappas et al., 2009).

A pediatric infectious diseases specialist should be consulted if candidiasis is suspected, to assist in the diagnostic evaluation and therapeutic management. Additional specialty services to be consulted may include pulmonology, surgery, neurosurgery, renal, ophthalmology, or dermatology depending on the site-specific manifestations of the disease.

The long-term nature of treatment needs to be emphasized to both patients and caregivers. Caregivers should be warned of the side effects and possible adverse events associated with long-term antifungal therapy.

Disposition and discharge planning

Regular monitoring for adherence to the medication regimen and adverse events associated with long-term medication therapy is recommended. Amphotericin B causes varying degrees of decreased kidney function, so patients receiving this therapy should be monitored for hyponatremia and hypokalemia.

PNEUMOCYSTIS JIROVECII (FORMERLY *CARINII*) PNEUMONIA

The classification and nomenclature of *Pneumocystis* has changed considerably since this organism was first described in 1909 as a member of the protozoan family and named *Pneumocystis carinii*. In 1988, *P. carinii* was reclassified as a fungus after ribosomal RNA sequencing revealed its homology to fungi. Since then, *Pneumocystis* has been found to possess unique genetic characteristics and strict host specificity in every mammal that has been studied. Eventually, the organism was renamed *P. jirovecii* to identify the form that uniquely affects humans (Catherinot et al., 2010; Krajicek et al., 2009). However, the clinical illness in humans continues to be referred to as *Pneumocystis carinii* pneumonia (PCP).

Pneumocystosis was first noted in the 1940s and 1950s in large cohorts of malnourished and premature infants with pneumonitis in Central and Eastern Europe. By the 1960s, an understanding of *Pneumocystis* as an opportunistic pathogen was reported in children with leukemia as well as in those with congenital immunodeficiencies (Catherinot et al., 2010). The acquired immune deficiency syndrome (AIDS) epidemic of the 1980s furthered the medical community's understanding of pneumocystosis as an opportunistic infection. *P. carinii* pneumonia became the AIDS-defining illness. Since the 1980s, the introduction of PCP prophylaxis and more effective antiretroviral therapy has contributed to a significant decline in PCP among HIV-infected individuals (CDC, 2009a; Gona et al., 2006). Even so, PCP continues to be the most common opportunistic infection among immunocompromised individuals (Catherinot et al.).

Pathophysiology

Pneumocystis can be seen microscopically in both trophic form and cysts. It has an affinity for alveolar tissue and attaches to the alveolar epithelium. The survival and proliferation of *Pneumocystis* depends on the alveolar fluid and surrounding cells, although this pathogen maintains an extracellular existence. Pulmonary gas exchange is impaired as the inflammatory process ensues. Pulmonary clearance of *Pneumocystis* requires functioning macrophages and adequate numbers of CD4+ T cells (CDC, 2009a).

Epidemiology and etiology

Pneumocystis is thought to be an airborne pathogen; however, the actual environmental source is uncertain. High seroprevalence rates of anti-*Pneumocystis* antibodies have been reported in healthy infants and adults, suggesting asymptomatic carriage of or colonization with *Pneumocystis* is possible (CDC, 2009a; Krajicek et al., 2009). The scientific community continues to debate the issue of latent reactivation of *Pneumocystis* infection, with the majority of reported studies arguing against it (Catherinot et al., 2010; Gigliotti & Wright, 2008).

The peak incidence of PCP in HIV-infected pediatric patients is 3 to 6 months of age. The widespread use of PCP prophylaxis and highly active antiretroviral therapy (HAART) has significantly reduced the frequency of *Pneumocystis* pneumonia in the HIV-infected population. In fact, the incidence of HIV-infected children with PCP has declined by 95% in the HAART era (CDC, 2009a). The CDC Pediatric Spectrum of Disease Project reported a decrease in PCP infection rates from 25 cases per 1,000 HIV-infected children in 1994 (pre-HAART era) to 6 cases in 2001 (HAART era) (CDC). PCP continues to be a significant global heath problem in developing countries, with 44% of all AIDS-related pediatric deaths in Africa being attributed to PCP (CDC).

Other populations at risk for PCP include patients with primary or secondary immunodeficiencies, including recent reports of individuals with autoimmune disorders receiving potent monoclonal antibody therapy (e.g., infliximab) (Krajicek et al., 2009). The single most important factor in determining risk for PCP is the cell-mediated immunity of the host (Gigliotti & Wright, 2008).

Mortality rates from PCP in the HIV-infected population have decreased to 10% to 20%, with non-HIV-infected individuals faring worse (30% to 50% mortality). This difference may occur because non-HIV-infected individuals experience a delay in the PCP diagnosis and treatment (CDC, 2009a).

Presentation

The HCP should obtain a careful medical history that includes a review of risk factors associated with PCP, while maintaining a high index of suspicion for this diagnosis in the immunocompromised patient. A sensitive social history may reveal behaviors that place the individual at risk for HIV infection. The pediatric patient may present with nonspecific symptoms such as a nonproductive cough, fever, weight loss, chills, and progressive dyspnea. In the HIV-infected individual, symptoms are progressive and may develop over several weeks. In contrast, the immunocompromised patient without HIV infection often presents more acutely with fulminant respiratory failure. The intensity of symptoms may correlate with a change in immunosuppressive therapy (Catherinot et al., 2010; Gigliotti & Wallace, 2008).

The physical examination findings are similarly nonspecific. The patient may have tachypnea, fever, mild crackles and rhonchi, chest discomfort, and increased respiratory effort progressing to severe respiratory distress (CDC, 2009a; Gigliotti & Wallace, 2008). Although rare (occurring in fewer than 2.5% of HIV-infected adults and children), *Pneumocystis* infection can cause extrapulmonary manifestations in almost any organ system (CDC).

Differential diagnosis

When PCP is suspected, the following differential diagnoses should be considered:

- Acute respiratory distress syndrome (ARDS)
- Cytomegalovirus
- Lymphocytic interstitial pneumonia (LIP)
- *Mycoplasma* infections
- Viral pneumonia
- Pulmonary embolism
- Tuberculosis
- *Mycobacterium avium* complex (MAC) infection
- Legionellosis

Plan of care

Pneumocystis cannot be sustained in culture. As a consequence, its microbiologic confirmation continues to depend on microscopy and specific stains of bronchoscopic alveolar lavage (BAL) or induced-sputum specimens. Fluorescein-labeled monoclonal anti-*Pneumocystis* antibodies stain is considered the study of choice for the diagnosis of PCP (Catherinot et al., 2010).

When PCP is found in a non-HIV-infected individual, the *Pneumocystis* load is typically lower and more difficult to detect. In those cases the sputum specimen is less useful than the BAL specimen. Sputum specimens are unreliable and difficult to obtain in young children; thus the bronchoscopic approach with BAL is the appropriate specimen collection for infants and children. Three consecutive morning nasogastric aspirates can be useful only if the aspirate is positive. Open lung biopsies may be required in atypical forms of PCP, such as granulomatous

Pneumocystis. PCR methods of diagnosis are still considered investigational (Catherinot et al., 2010). If the HIV status of an individual with PCP is unknown, then HIV testing should be performed.

PCP presents on a chest radiograph as bilateral, diffuse, reticular, or granular (ground glass) opacities; nevertheless, the CXR may be normal at the time of diagnosis in as many as 39% of patients (Catherinot et al., 2010). High-resolution CT of the chest will reveal similar "ground glass" opacities but is more sensitive for detection of PCP at an early stage (Demirkazik et al., 2008).

Treatment for PCP should begin promptly and consists of trimethoprim–sulfamethoxasole (TMP-SMX) in three or four divided doses for 21 days (CDC, 2009a). The dose for children (older than 2 months of age) is 15 to 20 mg/kg/day of the TMP component and 75 to 100 mg/kg/day of the SMX component. Initial therapy should be parenteral and can be switched to oral once the child has demonstrated a positive response to therapy (CDC). Alternative therapy for those who cannot tolerate TMP-SMX, or who have not shown a clinical response to this regimen in 5 to 7 days, may include parenteral pentamidine isethionate, atovaquone, dapsone plus TMP, or clindamycin plus primaquine. Only limited data are available on the use of these alternative drugs with children. The reader is referred to the most recent edition of *Red Book: Report of the Committee on Infectious Diseases* for dosing of the alternative drugs (AAP, 2009).

Adjunctive therapy with corticosteroids has been shown to be beneficial for HIV-infected adults with PCP. There are limited data on this treatment available for children, but most clinicians would agree that a 5-day burst of corticosteroids followed by 2 weeks of tapering doses is indicated in moderate to severe cases of PCP. Secondary prophylaxis (TMP-SMX) should be initiated at the conclusion of therapy and continue until the patient is no longer immunocompromised.

Primary prophylaxis is indicated for HIV-infected individuals in any of the following situations:

- CD4+ count < 500 cells/mm^3 or < 15% (1 to 5 years of age) or 200 cells/mm^3 (6 years of age or older)
- History of oropharyngeal candidiasis
- Previous episode of PCP

Prophylaxis should continue until the patient's CD4+ count is consistently above the age-specific cutoff point for a period of 3 months; it should be restarted if the CD4+ count falls below the age-specific cutoff point. Infants born to HIV-infected mothers should receive PCP prophylaxis beginning at 4 to 6 weeks of age, with this regimen continuing until definitive tests reveal the child to have a negative HIV status. Immunocompromised patients not infected with HIV should also receive primary prophylaxis.

The TMP-SMX prophylaxis dose for children 4 weeks of age or older is 150 mg/m^2/day TMP and 750 mg/m^2/day SMX, administered orally twice a day for 3 consecutive days per week. Alternatively, the TMP-SMX dose may be given as a single daily oral dose 7 days a week (Catherinot et al., 2010; CDC, 2009a).

A pediatric infectious diseases specialist should be consulted if PCP is suspected, to assist in the diagnostic evaluation, therapeutic management, and prophylaxis recommendations. Additional specialty services to be consulted may include pulmonary and critical care specialists, depending on the severity of the disease.

Adherence to medication regimen needs to be emphasized to both patients and caregivers. TMP-SMX is relatively safe. Adverse reactions tend to occur in the second week of therapy, and include a mild maculopapular rash, myelosuppression, mild gastrointestinal distress, hepatitis, and kidney disorders in the form of interstitial nephritis (AAP, 2009). Unless the reaction was life threatening, TMP-SMX can be restarted in incremental doses after the reaction subsides. If erythema multiforme, Stevens-Johnson syndrome, or urticarial rashes appear, TMP-SMX should be discontinued and not restarted. Caregivers should be warned of the side effects and possible adverse events associated with PCP prophylaxis or treatment drugs. Oral TMP-SMX may be given with water on an empty stomach. Relapse and recurrence rates should be thoroughly reviewed with both the caregivers and the patient.

Disposition and discharge planning

Regular monitoring for adherence to medication regimen and adverse events associated with long-term medication therapy is recommended. While on TMP/SMX patients should be evaluated at least monthly for evidence of bone marrow suppression. Regular monitoring of the CD4+ cell count will allow for timely resumption of PCP prophylaxis should that be necessary.

Immunocompromised individuals at risk for PCP and their caregivers should be counseled regarding the early signs of respiratory infection. Early and aggressive therapy is required in pediatric patients to avoid unnecessary respiratory complications. PCP recurrence is more common among individuals with HIV infection.

NONTUBERCULOUS *MYCOBACTERIUM* INFECTION

Pathophysiology

The modes of entry of *Mycobacterium avium* complex (MAC) into the human can include skin abrasions, inhalation, or ingestion. MAC invades and translocates across the mucosal epithelium and is carried to the lymph nodes by the lymphatic system. Hematogenous spread (dissemination) to distal organs occurs only in the presence of immunodeficiency. Cellular immunity against MAC appears to be critical to host immunity, with macrophage activation being necessary to eliminate intracellular MAC. Patients with a critically low CD4$^+$ T-cell count (e.g., those with AIDS) are at greatest risk for contracting disseminated MAC infection (Doncker et al., 2010).

Epidemiology and etiology

Several species of nontuberculous *Mycobacterium* (NTM) cause a wide spectrum of clinical syndromes. *Mycobacterium avium* complex consists of two related NTM species (*M. avium* and *M. intracellulare*) that can cause a variety of illnesses, including lymphadenitis, pulmonary, and disseminated infections (Wallace, 2008). This review is limited to disseminated MAC (DMAC), which almost always appears in the presence of impaired immunity.

NTM is a ubiquitous and opportunistic organism found widely distributed in the environment. Prior to the use of HAART, MAC was the second most common opportunistic infection among HIV-infected children. Since the introduction of HAART, its incidence has decreased from 1.3 to 1.8 episodes per 100 person-years (pre-HAART era) to 0.14 to 0.2 episode per 100 person-years (HAART era) (CDC, 2009a).

Presentation

Symptoms of disseminated MAC may be nonspecific and may have been present for weeks prior to the onset of acute illness (AAP, 2009). The history preceding onset of illness may not be helpful unless there is a precedent diagnosis of primary or secondary immunodeficiency to raise the HCP's suspicion for this infection.

The clinical manifestations experienced by the child with DMAC are similar to those noted in HIV-infected children with advanced immunosuppression. The range of symptoms associated with DMAC include persistent/recurrent fever, weight loss or failure to gain weight, night sweats, abdominal pain, fatigue, diarrhea, and hematologic deficiencies such as anemia and neutropenia (AAP, 2009; CDC, 2009a). Wallace (2008) describes skin lesions as a frequent early manifestation of DMAC, sometimes related to placement of central venous catheters.

DIFFERENTIAL DIAGNOSIS

As with the other primary pulmonary infections in the immunocompromised child, tuberculosis is the primary differential diagnosis for NTM infection. Other diagnoses to consider include:

- Bacterial pneumonia
- Primary mycotic infections
- Neoplasms

Plan of care

Definitive diagnosis is based on recovery of MAC from a normally sterile site—blood, bone marrow, liver, visceral lymph nodes, pleural fluid, middle ear fluid, or CSF (AAP, 2009; Cassidy et al., 2009; CDC, 2009a; Wallace, 2008). Biopsy specimens may also be obtained. MAC bacteremia is intermittent early in the illness and will likely require multiple samples to detect infection. Culture is critical not only to differentiate NTM from *M. tuberculosis,* but also to identify which NTM species is causing illness and to perform macrolide susceptibility testing (CDC). Cultures may take 1 to 2 weeks to turn positive. Laboratory personnel should be alerted to the possibility of NTM to assure proper culture media and drug susceptibility testing. NTM should always be tested for susceptibility to clarithromycin and azithromycin.

MAC has demonstrated resistance to many antimicrobial drugs but is fairly susceptible to macrolides, rifamycins, ethambutol, amikacin, streptomycin, and fluoroquinolones. Treatment usually requires a combination of two to three drugs given for several months. Monotherapy has been shown to result in emergence of high-level drug resistance. Initial empiric therapy begins with a minimum of two drugs: clarithromycin (15 mg/kg/day, every 12 hours) and ethambutol (15 to 25 mg/kg/day, once daily). Rifampin (10 to 20 mg/kg/day, once daily) can be added as a third drug, although experts disagree on the safety and tolerability of this three-drug regimen in children. The three-drug regimen should be chosen on a case-by-case basis and in consultation with a pediatric infectious diseases expert. Drug–drug interactions can occur between rifamycins, protease inhibitors (PIs), and efavirenz, resulting in increased clearance and toxicity. Rifamycins should be avoided if at all possible in HIV-infected children receiving PIs and efavirenz.

The initial response to therapy may take weeks to months to appear. Serial blood cultures should be obtained to determine the bacterial load. If a surgically inserted device such as central venous catheter, peritoneal dialysis catheter, or ventriculoperitoneal shunt has been found to be associated with the infection, then the device must be removed (Wallace, 2008). Therapy should continue for the lifetime of the patient or until the patient's immune system recovery occurs.

A pediatric infectious diseases specialist, preferably with experience in pediatric HIV infection, should be consulted if DMAC is suspected, to assist in the diagnostic evaluation and therapeutic management. Additional specialty services to be consulted may include hematology/oncology, pulmonology, GI, surgery, or dermatology, depending on the site-specific manifestations of the disease.

The long-term nature of treatment needs to be emphasized to both patients and caregivers. Caregivers should be warned of the side effects and possible adverse events associated with long-term antimicrobial therapy. Relapse and recurrence rates should be thoroughly reviewed with both the caregivers and the patient.

Disposition and discharge planning

Early and aggressive empiric therapy is required in pediatric patients to avoid unnecessary morbidity and mortality in the setting of NTM infection. Regular monitoring for adherence to the medication regimen and adverse events associated with long-term medication therapy is recommended. In particular, long-term ethambutol use has been associated with ocular toxicity. Children who are old enough should have a baseline ophthalmologic examination for visual acuity and color discrimination (CDC, 2009a). Patients and families should be counseled to contact their primary care provider if any visual changes are noted. Patients and families should be warned that rifampin may discolor urine, sweat, tears, or other body fluids to an orange-red color. Soft contact lenses may be permanently stained. Regular (at least monthly) monitoring of liver function, evidence of bone marrow suppression, and renal clearance is necessary while the patient remains on this drug regimen.

RESISTANT ORGANISMS

Alice Pong

PATHOPHYSIOLOGY

The pathophysiology of infections caused by antibiotic-resistant bacteria is similar to the pathophysiology of infections caused by antibiotic-susceptible organisms. Resistance to first-line antibiotics may lead to treatment delays; thus disease may be more extensive than might otherwise occur. Moreover, bacteria that acquire genes for drug resistance may also acquire genes for virulence factors that are absent in antibiotic-susceptible bacteria. For example, strains of community-acquired methicillin-resistant *Staphylococcus aureus* (CA-MRSA) are associated with virulence factors such as Panton Valentine leukocidin (PVL) (Diep & Otto, 2008).

Bacteria use three types of mechanisms to evade antibiotic activity (Leclerq, 2002; Livermore, 2000; Toltzis, 2004):

- Production of an enzyme or substrate that leads to a change in the antibiotic, rendering it less active
- Alteration of the target site of the antibiotic in the bacterial cell
- Changes in drug entry or active removal of the drug from the bacterial cell

Beta-lactamase enzymes that inactivate penicillin and other antibiotics with beta lactam rings in their chemical structure are examples of resistance occurring due to production of enzymes that alter antibiotic structures (Livermore, 2000; Toltzis, 2004). Aminoglycoside resistance is also mediated by modifying enzymes that lead to structural changes in these drugs (Toltzis). Alteration in the target site of the drug occurs in MRSA and drug-resistant *Streptococcus pneumoniae* (DRSP) when the penicillin-binding proteins, which serve as the binding site of beta lactam antibiotics, undergo mutations leading to decreased affinity of the drug to these sites (Chambers, 1999; Livermore). Resistance to macrolide and aminoglycoside antibiotics (that work by inhibiting ribosomal activity), develops when mutations cause changes in the ribosomal binding sites. Finally, some bacteria develop structures in the cell wall that either prohibit entry of the antibiotic into the cell (porin-channel mutations) or actively remove drug from the periplasmic space (efflux pumps).

EPIDEMIOLOGY AND ETIOLOGY

Antibiotic-resistant organisms can be acquired directly from contact with another infected or colonized person, transmitted via an intermediate person such as another HCP, or from contact with an object such as a piece of durable medical equipment. Pathogens can develop through selection of antibiotic-resistant organisms from the patient's endogenous bacterial flora. This may occur for patients on broadspectrum antibiotic therapy, especially if dosing is low relative to the minimum inhibitory concentration (MIC) of the drug needed to kill the bacteria.

Antibiotic-resistant organisms often colonize a susceptible host before infections develop. For example, colonization of the nares and other skin sites with MRSA is associated with an increased rate of recurrent infections (Davis et al., 2004). Patients on ventilator support are often colonized in their respiratory tract with bacteria before ventilator-associated pneumonia (VAP) develops. Antibiotic treatment used to treat colonization can contribute to selection of antibiotic-resistant organisms. Trauma or other disease processes associated with a breakdown in mucosal or skin barriers also allow colonizing organisms to more easily invade sterile sites.

Risk factors for becoming colonized and infected with antibiotic-resistant organisms include the following conditions:

- Prior antibiotic therapy
- Hospitalization
- Living in a chronic care facility (Graffunder & Venezia, 2002; Toltzis, 2004)

Local epidemiology of resistant organisms varies by geographic area and by patient population. Individual hospital epidemiology can differ considerably between different institutions even within the same geographic area. Hospital antibiograms are useful tools to determine which resistance patterns may be prevalent in a particular hospital and can be used as guides for empiric therapy.

In general, antibiotic-resistant organisms are not as prevalent in pediatric populations as in adult populations. Exceptions to this rule are DRSP and CA-MRSA. The prevalence of DRSP increased in the 1990s, when rates of penicillin resistance reached as high as 21.5% (Richter et al., 2009). Mutations in penicillin-binding proteins caused increased beta lactam resistance in DRSP. Concomitant resistance to macrolides and other antibiotic classes, as well as increasing beta-lactamase production in nontypable strains of nontypable *Haemophilus influenzae,* have created significant challenges for HCPs in treating bacterial upper respiratory infections such as otitis media and sinusitis (Block et al., 1995). Invasive pneumococcal disease such as pneumonia and meningitis from DRSP are also more difficult to treat; for this reason, vancomycin in conjunction with a beta lactam antibiotic is now standard empiric therapy for bacterial meningitis in children.

The introduction of the conjugated pneumococcal vaccine in 2000 has led to a significant decrease in pneumococcal disease in the United States in the last decade (Karnezis et al., 2009). Nevertheless, concern exists that over time a replacement of nonvaccine pneumococcal serotypes in respiratory flora such as serotype 19A will occur. These nonvaccine strains can also be multidrug resistant (Farrell et al., 2007; Karnezis et al.). Efforts continue toward creating pneumococcal vaccines to cover these newly resistant strains.

CA-MRSA was first identified as a problem in the late 1990s. Reports of otherwise healthy children with severe invasive MRSA infections were identified in several parts of the United States, including Illinois, Minnesota, and Texas (Frank et al., 1999; Herold et al., 1998; Sattler et al., 2002). These infections were seen in children without the traditional risk factors for MRSA infection such as hospitalization, chronic illness, and antibiotic therapy; other differences were also seen. These organisms appeared to be more susceptible to non-beta lactam classes of antibiotics such as clindamycin

and trimethoprim–sulfamethoxazole. They also seemed to cause primarily skin and soft-tissue infections. The recurrence rate of infections in children was also higher, which suggested prolonged colonization and increased invasiveness.

It is now known that these community-acquired strains of MRSA contain the same *mecA* gene carried by hospital-acquired MRSA. This gene encodes a penicillin-binding protein mutation that makes these bacteria resistant to all currently available beta lactam antibiotics (Ma et al.). The gene is packaged in a chromosome cassette (SCC mec IV) that is much smaller than the gene cassette (SCCmec I, II, III) associated with hospital-acquired MRSA (Ma et al.). The smaller gene cassette does not hold associated resistance genes for other antibiotic classes making a greater number of treatment options possible. Other virulence factors such as Panton Valentine leukocidin and arginine catabolic mobile element may increase the invasive potential and colonization potential that lead to recurrent infections (Diep & Otto, 2008).

Although resistance in Gram-negative bacilli is much more commonly seen in adult populations, pediatric infections with these organisms are still seen, particularly in patients in the critical care and oncology arenas (Toltzis, 2004). Examples of these organisms include extended spectrum beta-lactamase (ESBL) producing *Escherichia coli* and *Klebsiella pneumonia* and multidrug-resistant *Pseudomonas.* Table 30-10 lists resistant organisms that are commonly seen in the pediatric acute care population.

PRESENTATION

Infections caused by drug-resistant organisms usually present with the same symptoms as infections caused by drug-susceptible bacteria. The difference is that the patient may exhibit a poor response to standard therapy. Pediatric patients with otitis media secondary to DRSP often present with recurrent symptoms or no improvement of symptoms with standard amoxicillin doses, for example. Children with furunculosis secondary to MRSA do not respond to beta lactam antibiotics such as cephalexin. In situations where invasive disease is present, such as with meningitis or severe pneumonia, it is important to understand the resistance patterns that exist so that appropriate empiric antibiotic therapy can be started while awaiting culture results.

Patients who are already ill, such as those in the intensive care unit, may be colonized with resistant organisms prior to developing an infection. They may have other illnesses or be on therapy with immunosuppressive drugs that can alter disease presentation or have multiple sites of infection with different organisms. These patients may present with new clinical symptoms such as fever or increased respiratory secretions. These developments should prompt additional diagnostic testing, including bacterial cultures, to explore the possibility of infection.

TABLE 30-10

Summary of Resistant Organisms				
Organism	**Antibiotic Organism Is Resistant to**	**Mechanism**	**Most Common Type(s) of Infection**	**Treatment Options**
Drug-resistant *Streptococcus pneumoniae*	Beta lactams (penicillin, cephalosporins)	Penicillin-binding protein mutations	Otitis media Sinusitis Pneumonia Bacteremia	Vancomycin Clindamycin High-dose beta lactam Fluoroquinolones
Methicillin-resistant *Staphylococcus aureus* (MRSA)	Beta lactams	*mecA* gene (penicillin-binding protein mutation)	Skin and soft tissue Wounds Bacteremia Pneumonia Osteomyelitis Sepsis (less common)	Vancomycin Clindamycin* Trimethoprim–sulfamethoxazole Linezolid
Vancomycin-resistant enterococci (usually *E. faecium*)	Vancomycin Often also resistant to ampicillin	Van A, B, C gene mutations (altered target for vancomycin)	Urinary tract infection Intra-abdominal infection Nosocomial infection	Linezolid Daptomycin†
Haemophilus influenzae, nontypable	Ampicillin	Beta-lactamase	Otitis media Sinusitis	Amoxicillin–clavulanate Extended-spectrum cephalosporins
Extended-spectrum beta-lactamase (ESBL) producing *Escherichia coli* and *Klebsiella pneumoniae*	Extended-spectrum beta lactams	Extended-spectrum beta-lactamases	Urinary tract infections Nosocomial infections	Carbapenem (meropenem, imipenem)

* Organisms with inducible methylase gene may become resistant in high-inoculum infections.
† Not yet approved for children by the U.S. Food and Drug Administration.

DIFFERENTIAL DIAGNOSIS

The differential diagnosis of infection caused by antibiotic-resistant organisms includes situations where poor drug penetration exists. Cerebrospinal fluid concentrations of antibiotics are often much lower than serum concentrations. These concentrations often increase with inflammation, yet remain considerably lower than serum concentrations. As the MIC of the bacteria to the antibiotic increases, it may be that the lower levels present in the sequestered tissue are not high enough to kill the bacteria. In addition to CSF, bone and eye tissue are other areas where drug distribution may be poor. Abscesses and devitalized tissue can also be a source of ongoing clinical symptoms, as antibiotic penetration may not be sufficient in these regions. These sites often require surgical intervention and debridement to eliminate all of the infection.

Another factor that may confound a patient's response to therapy is the presence of foreign devices or material. Persistent positive blood cultures in patients with catheter-associated bloodstream infections may be present despite adequate antibiotic coverage and clinical improvement in the patient. Ventriculoperitoneal shunts, central venous catheters, and other implanted devices often require surgical removal before complete eradication of bacteria can be achieved.

Finally, failure to achieve clinical improvement in the treatment of infections may be related to relative subtherapeutic dosing of antibiotics. Standard doses of most antibiotics may not be enough to reach sites such as the central nervous system or other deep tissues. For example, antibiotic doses to treat CNS infections may be significantly higher than those used to treat other sites.

PLAN OF CARE

Bacterial cultures to identify pathogens and determine their associated antibiotic susceptibility profiles are critical in the management of all infectious processes, but are especially important when dealing with antibiotic-resistant pathogens. Identification of the pathogenic organism and knowledge of drug susceptibility allow the HCP to select the most active agent to treat a given infection. In situations where patients are critically ill and broad-spectrum antibiotics are given empirically, the cultures also allow narrowing of antibiotic coverage to decrease the promotion of additional antibiotic resistance. With drug-resistant organisms, additional antibiotic susceptibility testing may need to be requested from the microbiology laboratory.

Ideally, cultures should be obtained prior to starting antibiotic therapy; of course, in the acute care situation, this is not always possible. Cultures should still be obtained even if antibiotic therapy has been started, and they should be obtained from the primary site of infection whenever possible. Blood cultures should also be considered, particularly in acutely ill patients or when the primary site of infection may not be easy to culture, such as in deep tissue infections.

Empiric therapy of patients with infections involving antibiotic-resistant organisms should be guided by the most likely pathogens given the site of infection. Therapy should also be supported by local hospital and geographic epidemiology. For example, the prevalence of CA-MRSA in some communities has led to empiric therapy of skin and soft-tissue infections with non-beta lactam antibiotics such as clindamycin and vancomycin (Sattler et al., 2002). Increasing DRSP prevalence has led to a recommendation of high-dose amoxicillin (90 mg/kg/day) as the first-line therapy for most children with otitis media and risk factors for DRSP (Dowell et al., 1999); in contrast, in children with no risk factors or areas with little DRSP, standard antibiotic dosing of amoxicillin (40 to 50 mg/kg/day) is sufficient. Hospital antibiograms and surveillance reports that are published nationally and locally can be very helpful when HCPs are making decisions about the best therapy for a particular patient.

In addition to recognizing the most active antibiotic to use, it is important to understand the pharmacokinetics and pharmacodynamics of antibiotics and to know how to achieve the most effective, but safe dose (Drusano, 1998). Antimicrobials such as vancomycin, for which the therapeutic index may be narrow, require close monitoring of serum concentrations. In this situation, the area under the concentration curve/over the minimum inhibitory concentration (AUC/MIC) is theoretically the best pharmacokinetic parameter to use in targeting appropriate dosing (Rybak et al., 2009).

In summary, therapy should be directed at choosing the antibiotic(s) with the following characteristics:

- The best combination of efficacy against the infecting organism(s)
- The best pharmacokinetic profile to reach the site of infection
- The least likelihood of adverse effects for the patient

Removal of foreign devices and debridement of abscesses and devitalized tissue may also be necessary. Consultation with surgical specialties including orthopedics, otolaryngology, and general surgery is often needed to obtain cultures as well as to drain infected spaces that may not have adequate antibiotic concentrations.

Infectious diseases consultants can be helpful in the management of patients with antibiotic-resistant bacterial infections. They can facilitate interpretation of microbiology results and help to tailor antibiotic therapy. Communication with the microbiology laboratory is also important to assure appropriate susceptibility testing. Likewise, pharmacy consultations can be efficacious to determine the optimal dosing regimen for a patient.

Education of patients and families about drug-resistant organisms must be performed when these infections occur. Good hand washing practices should be encouraged to prevent additional infections. Fortunately, most of these organisms do not cause infections in otherwise healthy persons. In the case of CA-MRSA, although colonization may occur in multiple family members, most individuals will not develop active disease. Families should also be educated on the correlation between unnecessary antibiotic use and increasing antibiotic resistance.

DISPOSITION AND DISCHARGE PLANNING

Patients with infections caused by drug-resistant organisms are at risk for increased morbidity and, for hospitalized patients, increased length of stay (Cosgrove et al., 2005; Foglia et al., 2007a; Lautenbach et al., 2001; Toltzis, 2004). Patients often become colonized with resistant organisms placing them at higher risk for future infections, particularly if ongoing medical treatment is needed.

Repeat cultures from infected blood and other sterile sites are helpful to determine microbiologic cure in patients with infections caused by all organisms, even if they are not drug resistant. Although microbiologic resolution should be expected in sterile sites such as blood, colonization of skin and other nonsterile areas may persist even in the absence of disease. Repeat cultures of these areas obtained as surveillance for colonization of drug-resistant organisms is usually discouraged in patients who have recovered from their initial infection. The exception occurs in an outbreak situation, where ongoing transmission within the hospital is suspected and surveillance cultures are being performed to track transmission.

Prevention of infections by antibiotic-resistant organisms can be a challenge. Selection of antibiotic-resistant organisms can be decreased with the following practices:

- Appropriate antibiotic use
- Avoidance of unnecessary broad-spectrum therapy
- Minimizing the duration of antibiotic courses (Dellit et al., 2007)

Antimicrobial stewardship programs have increased in the last several years, with the goals of optimizing antibiotic use and decreasing rates of infection with resistant organisms (Dellit et al., 2007). Drug-resistant organisms can be spread in health care facilities via HCPs and fomite transmission on inanimate surfaces such as stethoscopes, stethoscope cloth sleeves, name badges, rings, and wristwatches. Recognition of HCP transmission is increasing. In 2007, hospitals in the United Kingdom adopted a physician's dress code that includes no long sleeves, jewelry, or neckties (Satter & Tanner, 2007). Appropriate isolation precautions for patients with antibiotic-resistant pathogens are important in the hospital environment and other health care facilities. Contact isolation of patients with most multidrug-resistant organisms is recommended by the CDC, with gloves and gowns being worn by HCP to prevent transmission of organisms between patients (Siegel et al., 2007).

Hand washing is the single most important infection prevention activity that HCPs and the general public can perform to decrease transmission of all infections. Alcohol-based hand sanitizers facilitate hand hygiene, are convenient, and in some cases may be superior to hand washing with soap and water as. In addition, these products provide for less irritation to the hands; the products stay on the hands longer; and they have been found to increase the antibacterial effect (CDC, 2002).

SEXUALLY TRANSMITTED INFECTIONS

Darcy Egging

PATHOPHYSIOLOGY

Adolescent females are physiologically at a higher risk of contracting a sexually transmitted infection (STI) than adult women due to their thinner cervical mucus and columnar epithelium, which makes them more susceptible to *Neisseria gonorrhoeae* and *Chlamydia trachomatis* (Mollen, 2009; Shafii et al., 2009).

EPIDEMIOLOGY AND ETIOLOGY

Adolescents have the highest rate of STI, largely because they are exploring their sexual potential at a time of burgeoning independence. Sixty-five percent of twelfth-grade females have had vaginal intercourse and 15% have had more than four partners, a factor that increases the risk of becoming infected with an STI (Biro, 2007; Eaton et al., 2008; Shafii et al., 2009).

PRESENTATION

In taking the history, a nonjudgmental approach may allow the adolescent to be open and honest (Fonseca & Greydanus,

2007; Mollen, 2009). When discussing sexuality and sexual risk behaviors, the HCP should interview the patient alone. Ensure confidentiality unless the information causes concern for the patient's safety—for example, suicidal ideation, or child maltreatment (Shafii et al., 2009). When asking questions pertaining to sex, be very specific—for example, "Have you had sex with a boy, a girl, or both?" Suggested topics for the sexual history interview are listed in Table 30-11. Physical examination findings for specific infections are described in the sections that follow. *Prepubescent children with symptoms of an STI should be evaluated for sexual assault by a trained sexual assault examiner* (see Chapter 36).

DIFFERENTIAL DIAGNOSIS

The differential diagnoses to consider with STIs include syphilis, molluscum contagiosum, seborrheic keratosis, herpes simplex virus (HSV), human papillomavirus (HPV), chancroid, gonorrhea, lymphogranuloma venereum (LGV), vaginitis, and urethritis.

PLAN OF CARE

The reader is encouraged to review the *Sexually Transmitted Diseases Treatment Guidelines 2010* published by the United States Centers for Disease Control and Prevention at http://www.cdc.gov/std/treatment/2010/STD-Treatment-2010-RR5912.pdf for more specific diagnostic study and therapeutic management information.

DISPOSITION AND DISCHARGE PLANNING

Instruct patients with risky sexual behaviors to use condoms to avert infection. If they are diagnosed with an STI, stress the following points:

- Follow the medication regimen.
- Follow-up with their primary care provider is needed to ensure that the therapy has been effective.
- Treatment of sexual partners is imperative.

TABLE 30-11

Topics for the Sexual History Interview

- Sexual orientation
- Sexual activity
- Sexual abuse
- Partners
- Previous sexually transmitted infection
- Pregnancy
- Condoms
- Contraception

Source: Shafii et al., 2009.

LYMPHOGRANULOMA VENEREUM

Lymphogranuloma Venereum is a rare disease in the United States; it is more commonly seen in Africa, Asia, South America, and the Caribbean. This infection is caused by *Chlamydia trachomatis* types L1, L2, and L3. Incubation is 3 to 30 days. The peak incidence is in persons aged 15 to 40 years, and is higher in males than in females (Frenkl & Potts, 2008; Mollen, 2009; Workowski & Berman, 2006).

Presentation

Diagnosis is usually made on clinical presentation. Patient usually present with painful unilateral lymphadenopathy, and they often describe a genital or rectal ulcer that recently resolved. The lymph nodes may become infected and produce abscesses that may fuse and break down, causing large sinuses. Women and homosexuals may present with proctocolitis and perirectal or deep iliac lymph-node enlargement if the primary lesion arises from the rectum or cervix.

Plan of care

The nucleic acid amplification test (NAAT) is the test of choice for all strains of *Chlamydia*. Other tests that may be considered are culture, direct immunofluorescence, genotyping; *Chlamydia* serology (which has a low sensitivity); and testing for other STIs, including syphilis, human papillomavirus virus (HPV), human immunodeficiency virus (HIV), genital *Chlamydia*, gonorrhea, and tricomoniasis.

Doxycycline 100 mg orally, 2 times per day for 21 days, is the treatment of choice. An alternative regimen is erythromycin base 500 mg orally, 4 times per day for 21 days. Azithromycin 1 gm orally, once weekly for 3 weeks, may be effective, although clinical data are lacking (Bayram & Malik, 2008; CDC, 2010b; Frenkl & Potts, 2008; Mollen, 2009; Workoski & Berman, 2006).

HUMAN PAPILLOMAVIRUS

Human papillomavirus is the most prevalent STI in patients less than 24 years of age with an estimated 4.6 million new HPV infections in persons age 15 to 24 years (Weinstock et al., 2004).

Presentation

Typically HPV is asymptomatic, but it may sometimes vary in presentation from benign genital warts to cancer. Genital warts (condylomata acuminata) may occur on the vulva, perianal area, vaginal walls, or cervix. They rarely occur in the throat and the condition is then called recurrent respiratory papillomatosis (RRP). They usually have a cauliflower-like appearance, but may also present as flat, popular, or keratotic warts. The warts are most common on the cervix of women and the prepuce of men (Bayram & Malik, 2008; Hollier & Workowski, 2008; Mollen, 2009; Trigg et al., 2008).

Various types of HPV are possible, each of which causes different symptoms. For example, types 6 and 11 cause genital warts, whereas types 16 and 18 are known to cause abnormal Papanicolaou (Pap) tests with precancerous changes and may lead to carcinoma in situ of the cervix. HPV-16 has been reported to cause 50% to 60% of all cervical cancers; HPV-8 causes 10% to 20% of these cancers (National Network for Immunization Information [NNII], 2007).

Plan of care

Diagnosis is usually made on visual inspection or on a Pap test as a high-grade dysplasia (Bayram & Malik, 2008; Trigg et al., 2008).

In the absence of genital warts, no treatment is recommended. HPV infections frequently resolve without intervention. For external warts, podofilox 0.5% solution or gel may be applied. The schedule is 2 times per day for 3 days, wait 4 days, and then repeat for 4 cycles. An alternative is imiquimod 5% cream applied daily 3 times per week for as long as 16 weeks. For severe infections, provider-administered therapy such as cryotherapy, podophyllin resin 10% to 25%, or trichloreacetic acid (TCA); surgical removal; intralesional interferon; or laser surgery may be considered. Regardless of which therapy is selected, only 60% to 80% of patients achieve resolution on the first treatment, and a 30% recurrence rate is common (Bayram & Malik, 2008; Frenkl & Potts, 2008; Mollen, 2009; Workoski & Berman, 2006).

Two vaccines are available to immunize patients against HPV. The first, known as HPV4, provides protection against HPV types 6, 11, 16 and 18. The second, known as HPV2, is a bivalent vaccine for HPV types 16 and 18. Routine vaccination has been recommended to start for females between the ages of 11 and 12 years (NNII, 2010).

HERPES SIMPLEX VIRUS

Two types of herpes simplex virus exist: HSV-1 and HSV-2. It is believed that the majority of people with genital herpes are infected with HSV-2, although it is difficult to distinguish between the two subtypes. As many as 50% of first-episode infections of genital herpes are caused by HSV-1; recurrences and subclinical shedding are more common with HSV-2 infection (Bayram & Malik, 2008; Frenkl & Potts, 2008; Mollen, 2009; Workoski & Berman, 2006).

Presentation

The clinical diagnosis of genital herpes is both insensitive and nonspecific. The classic painful, multiple vesicular or ulcerative lesions are absent in many infected persons. As many as 70% of people with HSV are asymptomatic. The lesions begin with vesicles that rupture, exposing an ulcer. The cervix and vagina may be involved with leucorrhea. Dysuria and inguinal adenopathy are often present (Bayram & Malik, 2008; Frenkl & Potts, 2008; Mollen, 2009; Workoski & Berman, 2006).

Plan of care

Diagnostic testing consists of viral culturing to identify whether the infection is caused by HSV-1 or HSV-2. Sensitivity for culture is only 70%, however, and it may take up to 5 days for results to become available. Polymerase chain reaction testing for HSV DNA has a greater sensitivity than viral cultures, but has not yet been approved by the U.S. Food and Drug Administration for genital HSV testing.

Type-specific HSV serological assays are available for individuals with a subclinical infection or a questionable history of the disease. The serological assays are not used for asymptomatic patients, however. These assays will differentiate between types 1 and 2. Type 2 HSV is almost always sexually acquired. HSV-1 is more difficult to interpret, as many individuals with the HSV-1 antibody may have oral HSV acquired during childhood. Type-specific HSV serologic assays may be useful in the following scenarios:

* Recurrent genital symptoms or atypical symptoms with negative HSV cultures
* Clinical diagnosis of genital herpes without laboratory confirmation
* A sexual partner with genital herpes

Consider HSV serologic testing in a comprehensive evaluation for STIs among persons with multiple sex partners and HIV infection (Bayram & Malik, 2008; Frenkl & Potts, 2008; Mollen, 2009; Workoski & Berman, 2006).

Therapeutic management is twofold, consisting of education and pharmacologic treatment. The two main goals of education counseling are to help the patient cope with the infection and to prevent spreading of the disease (Table 30-12). Pharmacologic therapy may be subdivided into first-episode and recurrent-episode treatments; these therapies are summarized in Table 30-13.

GONORRHEA

Gonorrhea is an STI caused by *Neisseria gonorrhoeae,* a Gram-negative diplococcus. It is the second most common STI in the United States. Women younger than the age of 25 years are at greatest risk of developing this infection. Other risk factors include new or multiple sexual partners, inconsistent use of condoms, and illicit drug use. Gonorrhea is the major cause of cervicitis and pelvic inflammatory disease (PID) in females, and urethritis in men. Untreated gonorrhea may result in infertility, ectopic pregnancy, and chronic pelvic pain (Bayram & Malik, 2008; CDC, 2007; Frenkl & Potts, 2008; Mollen, 2009; Workoski & Berman, 2006).

Presentation

Males typically present symptomatically, whereas females may remain asymptomatic until complications occur. Clinical presentation may be similar to urinary tract infection symptoms such as frequency, urgency, and burning with urination. Females may have inflammation of the bartholin

---

TABLE 30-12

Recommendations for Herpes Simplex Virus Counseling

* Persons who have genital herpes should be educated concerning the natural history of the disease, with emphasis on the potential for recurrent episodes, asymptomatic viral shedding, and the attendant risks of sexual transmission.

* Persons experiencing a first episode of genital herpes should be advised that suppressive therapy is available and is effective in preventing symptomatic recurrent episodes, and that episodic therapy sometimes is useful in shortening the duration of recurrent episodes.

* All persons with genital HSV infection should be encouraged to inform their current sexual partners that they have genital herpes and to inform future partners before initiating a sexual relationship.

* Sexual transmission of HSV can occur during asymptomatic periods. Asymptomatic viral shedding is more frequent with genital HSV-2 infection than with genital HSV-1 infection, and is most frequent during the first 12 months after acquiring HSV-2.

* All persons with genital herpes should remain abstinent from sexual activity with uninfected partners when lesions or prodromal symptoms are present.

* The risk of sexual transmission of HSV-2 can be decreased by the daily use of valacyclovir by the infected person.

* Recent studies indicate that latex condoms, when used consistently and correctly, may reduce the risk for genital herpes transmission.

* Sexual partners of HSV-infected persons should be advised that they might be infected even if they have no symptoms. Type-specific serologic testing of asymptomatic partners of persons with genital herpes is recommended to determine whether risk for HSV acquisition exists.

* Asymptomatic persons diagnosed with HSV-2 infection by type-specific serologic testing should receive the same counseling messages as persons with symptomatic infection. In addition, such persons should be taught about the clinical manifestations of genital herpes.

Source: Workowski & Berman, 2006.

TABLE 30-13

Therapeutic Options for Treatment of HSV Infection

Recommended Regimen for First-Episode HSV

Select one:

- Acyclovir 400 mg orally three times per day for 7–10 days **OR**
- Acyclovir 200 mg orally five times per day for 7–10 days **OR**
- Famciclovir 250 mg orally three times per day for 7–10 days **OR**
- Valacyclovir 1 gm orally twice a day for 7–10 days

Treatment may be extended as needed.

Recommended Regimen for Recurrent Episodes HSV

Select one:

- Acyclovir 400 mg orally three times a day for 5 days **OR**
- Acyclovir 800 mg orally twice a day for 5 days **OR**
- Acyclovir 800 mg orally three times a day for 2 days **OR**
- Famciclovir 125 mg orally twice daily for 5 days, **OR**
- Famciclovir 1 gm orally twice daily for 1 day **OR**
- Valacyclovir 500 mg orally twice a day for 3 days **OR**
- Valacyclovir 1 gm orally once a day for 5 days

Source: Bayram & Malik, 2008; Frenkl & Potts, 2008; Mollen, 2009; Workoski & Berman, 2006.

and skenes glands and a mucoid discharge from the cervix. Men often complain of penile discharge (Bayram & Malik, 2008; Frenkl & Potts, 2008; Mollen, 2009; Workoski & Berman, 2006).

Plan of care

Diagnostic studies consist of testing of endocervical, vaginal, male urethral, or urine specimens. Culture, nucleic acid hybridization tests, and NAAT are available for the detection of genitourinary infection with *N. gonorrhoeae*. Culture and nucleic acid hybridization tests require female endocervical or male urethral swab specimens. Additionally, when testing for gonorrhea, all patients should be tested for other STIs, including *Chlamydia*, syphilis, and HIV (Bayram & Malik, 2008; Frenkl & Potts, 2008; Mollen, 2009; Workoski & Berman, 2006).

Therapeutic management for uncomplicated gonococcal infections of the cervix, urethra, and rectum is Ceftriaxone 250 mg in a single intramuscular (IM) dose (CDC, 2010b).

CHLAMYDIA

Chlamydia infection, which is caused by *C. trachomatis*, is an STI often associated with gonorrhea. It is the leading cause of PID, which can lead to infertility and chronic pelvic pain (CDC, 2007)

Presentation

As many as 75% of all chlamydial infections are asymptomatic. In other patients, this infection may present as cervicitis, endometriosis, salpingitis, and PID.

Plan of care

The U.S. Preventive Services Task Force recommends routine *Chlamydia* screening for all women 25 years of age and younger who are sexually active. NAAT is the test of choice for all strains of *Chlamydia* (Bayram & Malik, 2008; Birnbaumer & Anderegg, 2010; Chiaradonna, 2007; Frenkl & Potts, 2008; Mollen, 2009; Workoski & Berman, 2006).

Therapeutic management consists of either azithromycin (1 gm orally once) or doxycycline (100 mg 2 times daily for 7 days). Clinical trials show that both azithromycin and doxycycline are equally efficacious; however, if compliance is a concern, then azithromycin is recommended. Sexual activity is to be withheld for a period of 7 days after azithromycin or during the entire course of treatment with doxycycline.

Alternative therapies include the following options (Bayram & Malik, 2008; Birnbaumer & Anderegg, 2010; CDC, 2010b; Chiaradonna, 2007; Frenkl & Potts, 2008; Mollen, 2009, Workoski & Berman, 2006):

- Erythromycin base 500 mg orally 4 times per day for 7 days **OR**
- Erythromycin ethylsuccinate 800 mg orally 4 times per day for 7 days **OR**
- Ofloxacin 300 mg orally 2 times per day for 7 days **OR**
- Levofloxacin 500 mg orally daily for 7 days

SYPHILIS

Syphilis is a systemic STI caused by the spirochete *Treponema pallidum*. This disease is less prevalent in the pediatric population; however, all pregnant women are highly encouraged to be tested for syphilis. Maternal–fetal transmission may result in premature labor, fetal demise, or congenital syphilis (Bayram & Malik, 2008; Trigg et al., 2008). In the adolescent population, syphilis is more commonly seen in the females and in individuals who are illicit drug users (Mollen, 2009).

Presentation

Syphilis progresses through three stages: *primary, secondary*, and *tertiary*. A preliminary stage of latent infection (either very early or late) may be detected by serology testing before the presence of symptoms.

Primary syphilis presents with an ulcer or chancre. This ulcerative area is usually seen in the anogenital area or mouth. Although there is often only a single lesion, multiple lesions may occur. The chancre is a painless ulcer, approximately 1 to 2 cm in diameter.

Secondary syphilis develops 4 to 10 weeks after primary infection and may present as myalgias, lymphadenopathy, influenza-like symptoms, or skin rash (usually on the soles of the feet and palms of hands). Due to these general symptoms, syphilis is known as the "great imitator" (Bayram & Malik, 2008; Birnbaumer & Anderegg, 2010; Frenkl & Potts, 2008; Mollen, 2009).

Tertiary syphilis occurs 2 to 19 years after initial symptoms in an untreated patient; this condition is rarely seen in the adolescent population. Symptoms usually involve the cardiovascular and nervous systems. Tertiary syphilis is rarely seen in the United States because of the implementation of prevention programs and antibiotics.

The diagnosis of syphilis should be considered in any sexually active patient with a genital ulcer or generalized rash (Bayram & Malik, 2008; Biggs & Williams, 2009; Birnbaumer & Anderegg, 2010; Frenkl & Potts, 2008; Mollen, 2009).

Infants and children suspected of syphilis infection should have CSF examination for neurosyphilis and exploration of medical records for congenital transmission (CDC, 2010b).

Plan of care

Diagnostic study of choice for latent, secondary, and tertiarty syphilis is serological testing. The two tests usually used are the Venereal Disease Research Laboratory (VDRL) and rapid plasma regain (RPR) test, both of which are classified nontreponemal tests. For definitive diagnosis, nontreponemal testing plus treponemal testing is necessary. Treponemal testing includes the fluorescent treponemal antibody, absorbed (FTA-Abs), and the *T. palladium* particular agglutination (TP-PA) tests. Many disorders may produce false-positive results in the nontreponemal testing, including Lyme disease, chlamydial infections, viral infections, narcotic addictions, sarcoidosis, lymphoma, and aging. Therefore, both study types are recommended when testing for syphilis (Bayram & Malik, 2008; Biggs & Williams, 2009; Birnbaumer & Anderegg, 2010; Frenkl & Potts, 2008; Mollen, 2009).

Therapeutic management for all stages of syphilis in adults is consists of benzathine penicillin G 2.4 million units, given once via the IM route. Alternative therapies include doxycycline orally 2 times per day for 14 days or tetracycline 500 mg 4 times per day for 14 days. Potentially effective therapy includes ceftriaxone 1 gm daily IM or IV for 10 days or azithromycin 2 gm orally once. Adolescents who are diagnosed with syphilis must be monitored closely and should be evaluated for HIV. Consider consultation with an infectious diseases specialist to ensure appropriate management of these patients (Biggs & Williams, 2009; Mollen, 2009).

VAGINITIS

Vaginitis is a common infection caused by *Candida albicans* (vulvovaginal candidiasis), *Trichomonas vaginalis* (a single-celled flagellated protozoan organism), and/or bacterial vaginosis (BV). BV is a polymicrobial clinical syndrome resulting from replacement of the normal H_2O_2-producing *Lactobacillus* sp. in the vagina with high concentrations of anaerobic bacteria (e.g., *Prevotella* sp., *Mobiluncus* sp.), *Gardnerella vaginalis*, and *Mycoplasma hominis*. Herpes simplex virus can also cause vaginitis. Patients who are more susceptible to vaginitis of any type include those who are currently taking corticosteroids, who are taking broad-spectrum antibiotics, who have a history of diabetes, or who are pregnant (Mollen, 2009).

Vulvovaginal candidiasis

Presentation.   Vulvovaginal candidiasis may present with a vaginal discharge that is cottage cheese-like in appearance, accompanied by intense vaginal irritation and itching. The thick, white discharge is present in only 20% to 60% of the patients with candidiasis; however, it is a strong predictor of the disease when it occurs. Vulvar and vaginal inflammation may also be present.

Plan of care.   Diagnosis is made by wet prep looking for hyphae, pseudohyphae, or budding yeast on a slide prepared with 10% potassium hydroxide (KOH). An estimated 50% of females with cultures that test positive for *Candida* have a negative wet prep (Bayram & Malik, 2008; Biggs & Williams, 2009; Mollen, 2009).

Table 30-14 summarizes the many therapeutic management options of vulvovaginal candidiasis.

Trichomonas vaginalis

Presentation.   Typical symptoms of *T. vaginalis* infection include vulvar irritation, dyspareunia (painful intercourse), dysuria, urinary frequency, vaginal odor, and vaginal discharge, which is frequently green/yellow in color.

Plan of care.   Diagnosis is made by observing motile trichomonads on a saline wet prep. Patients should also be evaluated for gonorrhea and vulvovaginal candidiasis, as coinfection is not uncommon.

Therapeutic management consists of metronidazole 2 gm orally, to be given in a single dose. An alternative regimen is metronidazole 500 mg orally, given 2 times per day for 7 days (Bayram & Malik, 2008; Biggs & Williams, 2009; CDC, 2010b; Mollen, 2009).

Bacterial vaginosis

Presentation.   BV is the most prevalent cause of vaginal discharge or malodor; however, more than 50% of women with

TABLE 30-14

Therapeutic Management Recommendations for Vulvovaginal Candidiasis

Recommended Regimens

Intravaginal Over-the-CounterAgents

Butoconazole 2% cream, 5 gm intravaginally for 3 days **OR**
Clotrimzaole 1% cream, 5 gm intravaginally for 7–14 days **OR**
Clotrimazole 2% cream, 5 gm intravaginally for 3 days **OR**
Miconazole 2% cream, 5 gm intravaginally for 7 days **OR**
Miconazole 4% cream, 5 gm intravaginally for 3 days **OR**
Miconazole 100 mg vaginal suppository, one suppository for 7 days **OR**
Miconazole 200 mg vaginal suppository, one suppository for 3 days **OR**
Miconazole 1,200 mg vaginal suppository, one suppository for 1 day **OR**
Ticonazole 6.5% ointment, 5 gm intravaginally in a single application **OR**

Oral Prescriptive Agent

Fluconazole 150 mg tablet, one tablet in a single dose

Source: CDC, 2010b.

BV are asymptomatic. The cause of the microbial alteration is not fully understood. BV is associated with having multiple sexual partners, a new sexual partner, douching, and lack of vaginal lactobacilli. It is unclear whether this infection results from a sexually transmitted pathogen. Women who have never been sexually active are rarely affected. Treatment of male sexual partners has not proven beneficial in preventing recurrent infection (Bayram & Malik, 2008; Biggs & Williams, 2009; CDC, 2010b; Mollen, 2009).

Plan of care.   Diagnosis of BV is made when three of the following four criteria are met (Bayram & Malik, 2008; Biggs & Williams, 2009; CDC, 2010b; Mollen, 2009):

- Homogeneous, thin, white discharge that smoothly coats the vaginal walls
- Presence of clue cells on microscopic examination
- pH of vaginal fluid > 4.5
- "Fishy" odor of vaginal discharge before or after addition of 10% KOH ("whiff test") (CDC, 2010b)

Therapeutic management is directed at relief of symptoms. Medications of choice are as follows:

- Metronidazole 500 mg orally, 2 times per day for 7 days **OR**
- Metronidazole gel 0.75%, one applicator intravaginally, once per day for 5 days **OR**
- Clindamycin cream 2%, one applicator intravaginally at bedtime for 7 days

Sexual partners do not need to be treated. Many HCPs recommend that patients treated with metronidazole avoid consuming alcohol for at least 24 hours following the completion of therapy to prevent nausea, headaches, and flushing (Bayram & Malik, 2008; Biggs & Williams, 2009; CDC, 2010b; Mollen, 2009).

PELVIC INFLAMMATORY DISEASE

PID is a polymicrobial infection of the upper female genital tract. This term is used to describe any combination of endometriosis, salpingitis, tubo-ovarian abscess, and pelvic peritonitis. The most common infectious organisms in PID are *N. gonorrhoeae* and *C. trachomatis*; organisms that are less frequently implicated are *G. vaginalis, H. influenzae,* and *Streptococcus* (Bayram & Malik, 2008; Biggs & Williams, 2009; CDC, 2010b; Crossman, 2006; Lareau & Beigi, 2008; Mollen, 2009; Song & Advincula, 2005).

Presentation

Diagnosis of PID may be difficult due to the variety of symptoms associated with this condition. Common symptoms that may be observed are abdominal pain, dyspareunia, vaginal discharge, and abnormal vaginal bleeding. Physical findings associated with PID include cervical motion tenderness, elevated temperature of more than 101°F (38.3°C), abnormal cervical or vaginal mucopurulent discharge, elevated erythrocyte sedimentation rate and C-reactive protein, and a positive cervical infection with *N. gonorrhoeae* or *C. trachomatis*.

Plan of care

The most specific criteria for diagnosing PID are as follows:

- Endometrial biopsy with histopathologic evidence of endometritis
- Transvaginal sonography or MRI showing thickened, fluid-filled tubes with or without free pelvic fluid or tubo-ovarian complex, or Doppler studies suggesting pelvic infection (e.g., tubal hyperemia)
- Laparoscopic abnormalities consistent with PID

A diagnostic evaluation that includes more extensive studies may be warranted when diagnosis is elusive or the extent of infection unknown. Endometrial biopsy may be considered in females undergoing laparoscopy who do not have visual evidence of salpingitis, as some female patients with PID have endometritis alone (Bayram & Malik, 2008; Biggs & Williams, 2009; CDC, 2010b; Mollen, 2009).

Therapeutic management consists of hospitalization and IV antibiotic therapy if any of the following conditions is present:

- Surgical emergency cannot be excluded
- Pregnancy
- Unresponsive clinically to oral antibiotic therapy
- Inability to comply with outpatient antibiotic regimen
- Severe illness, nausea, vomiting, or high fever
- Tubo-ovarian abscess

Many HCPs prefer to hospitalize adolescent females who are diagnosed with acute PID, regardless of illness severity, although controversy exists as to the best treatment. Younger women with mild to moderate acute PID have similar outcomes with either outpatient therapy or inpatient therapy. Further, clinical response to outpatient treatment is similar among younger and older women; thus the decision to hospitalize adolescents with acute PID should be based on the same criteria used for older women. Whether women in their later reproductive years will benefit from hospitalization for treatment of PID also is unclear, although women aged 35 years or older who are hospitalized with PID are more likely than younger women to have a complicated clinical course (Bayram & Malik, 2008; Biggs & Williams, 2009; CDC, 2010b; McWilliams et al., 2007; Mollen, 2009; Trigg et al., 2008).

Therapeutic management for patients with mild to moderate PID may be accomplished with either parenteral or oral antibiotic therapy, as evidence-based practice suggests that the two approaches offer similar clinical efficacy. Clinical experience should guide decisions regarding transition to oral therapy, which may be initiated within 24 hours of clinical improvement. Adolescent females who do not respond to oral therapy within 72 hours should be re-evaluated to confirm the diagnosis and the administration of parenteral therapy on either an outpatient or inpatient basis (Table 30-15). An oral therapy alternative to parenteral cephalosporin therapy is a fluoroquinolone (levofloxacin 500 mg orally once daily or ofloxacin 400 mg 2 times per day for 14 days), with or without metronidazole (500 mg orally 2 times per for 14 days). For those with positive gonorrhea studies:

- If the NAAT is positive, parenteral cephalosporin is recommended.
- If culture is positive, treatment should be based on results of antimicrobial susceptibility.

Although information regarding other outpatient regimens is limited, amoxicillin/clavulanic acid and doxycycline or azithromycin with metronidazole has demonstrated short-term clinical cure. No data have been published regarding the use of oral cephalosporins for the treatment

TABLE 30-15

Treatment for Pelvic Inflammatory Disease
Parenteral
Recommended Parenteral Regimen A
• Cefotetan 2 gm IV every 12 hours **OR**   • Cefoxitin 2 gm IV every 6 hours **PLUS** doxycycline 100 mg orally or IV every 12 hours
Recommended Parenteral Regimen B
Clindamycin 900 mg IV every 8 hours **PLUS** gentamicin loading dose IV or IM (2 mg/kg of body weight), followed by a maintenance dose (1.5 mg/kg) every 8 hours. Single daily dosing may be substituted with 3 to 5 mg/kg.
Alternative Parenteral Regimen
Ampicillin/sulbactam 3 gm IV every 6 hours **PLUS** doxycycline 100 mg orally or IV every 12 hours
Oral
• Ceftriaxone 250 mg IM in a single dose **PLUS** doxycycline 100 mg orally twice a day for 14 days, *with or without* metronidazole 500 mg orally twice a day for 14 days **OR**   • Cefoxitin 2 gm IM in a single dose and probenecid 1 gm orally administered concurrently in a single dose **PLUS** doxycycline 100 mg orally twice a day for 14 days, *with or without* metronidazole 500 mg orally twice a day for 14 days **OR**   • Other parenteral third-generation cephalosporin **PLUS** doxycycline 100 mg orally twice a day for 14 days, *with or without* metronidazole 500 mg orally twice a day for 14 days

Source: Bayram & Malik, 2008; Biggs & Williams, 2009; CDC, 2010b; Lareau & Beigi, 2008; Mollen, 2009; Trigg et al., 2008.

of PID (Bayram & Malik, 2008; Biggs & Williams, 2009; CDC, 2010b, Lareau & Beigi, 2008; Mollen, 2009; Trigg et al., 2008).

TUBO-OVARIAN ABSCESS

As many as 30% of patients with PID develop tubo-ovarian abscesses (TOA). Rupture rates are as high as 15% and are considered a surgical emergency. In this condition, the ovary becomes infected with purulent material from the fallopian tube.

Presentation

Clinical presentation is an ill-appearing female with severe abdominal pain with peritoneal signs on palpation and fever (Bayram & Malik, 2008; Biggs & Williams, 2009; CDC, 2010b; Lareau & Beigi, 2008; Mollen, 2009; Trigg et al., 2008).

Plan of care

Diagnostic studies may include ultrasound and MRI. Transvaginal ultrasound may be useful with a sexually active female (perforated hymen). Computed tomography of the abdomen and pelvis may also provide findings such as fluid or air level, kidney stones, appendicitis, or bowel obstruction or perforation. The preparation for CT should include both oral and IV contrast. MRI of the abdomen is suggested when the ultrasound is equivocal and provides more detail (Bayram & Malik, 2008; Biggs & Williams, 2009; Lareau & Beigi, 2008; Mollen, 2009; Trigg et al., 2008).

Therapeutic management includes hospitalization and parenteral therapy similar to the plan of care for PID. TOA may require aspiration or surgical excision. A ruptured TOA is a life-threatening condition and requires emergent surgery. Hysterectomy and bilateral salpingo-oophorectomy may be necessary in patients with overwhelming infection (Bayram & Malik, 2008; Biggs & Williams, 2009; Lareau & Beigi, 2008; Mollen, 2009; Trigg et al., 2008).

SYSTEMIC INFLAMMATORY RESPONSE SYNDROME AND SEPTIC SHOCK

Sylvia del Castillo, Alyssa Rake, and Elizabeth Farrington

In 1992, *systemic inflammatory response syndrome* (SIRS) was proposed as a term by the American College of Chest Physicians and the Society of Critical Care Medicine (SCCM) to describe the nonspecific inflammatory process that occurs in adults after trauma, infection, burns, pancreatitis, and other diseases (Bone et al., 1992a; Bone et al., 1992b). Sepsis was defined as SIRS associated with infection; septic shock (SS) was defined as sepsis with cardiovascular organ failure (Table 30-16).

The SIRS criteria were initially developed for use in adults, and it was not until 2005 that a consensus definition was published for SIRS in children. To meet the pediatric SIRS criteria, two of the following four elements must be present: (1) hyperthermia or hypothermia, (2) tachycardia or bradycardia, (3) tachypnea, and (4) high or low white blood cell count (Annane et al., 2003). Table 30-17 provides SIRS criteria for age-specific vital signs and laboratory values.

PATHOPHYSIOLOGY

In sepsis, toxins and superantigens associated with some Gram-positive bacteria activate the immune system to produce cytokines such as tumor necrosis factor alpha (TNF-α), and interleukin-1-beta (IL-1β) to initiate a cytokine cascade that results in fever and vasodilation. This cascade further promotes the production of other pro-inflammatory cytokines (IL-8, interferon-gamma), as well as anti-inflammatory cytokines (soluble TNF receptor, IL-1 receptor antagonist protein, IL-4, IL-10) that attempt to maintain an optimal immune system. However, uncontrolled inflammation

TABLE 30-16

Definitions of Systemic Inflammatory Response Syndrome, Infection, Sepsis, Severe Sepsis, and Septic Shock	
Systemic inflammatory response syndrome (SIRS)	The presence of at least two of the following four criteria, one of which must be abnormal temperature or leukocyte count: • Core temperature greater than 38°C (100.4°F) or less than 36°C (96.8°F); must be measured by rectal, bladder, oral, or central catheter probe. • Tachycardia defined as at least 2 standard deviations above normal for age in the absence of external stimulus, chronic drugs, or painful stimuli; or otherwise persistent elevation over a 0.5- to 4-hour time period **OR** for children younger than 1 year: bradycardia, defined as a mean heart rate less than the 10% percentile for age in the absence external vagal stimulus, beta blocker drugs, or congenital heart disease; or otherwise unexplained depression over a 0.5-hour time period. • Mean respiratory rate greater than 2 standard deviations above normal for age or mechanical ventilation for an acute process not related to underlying neuromuscular disease or receipt of general anesthesia. • Leukocyte count elevated or depressed for age (not secondary to chemotherapy-induced neutropenia) or more than 10% immature neutrophils.
Infection	A suspected or proven (by positive culture, tissue stain, or polymerase chain reaction test) infection caused by any pathogen **OR** a clinical syndrome associated with a high probability of infection. Evidence of infection includes positive findings on clinical exam, imaging or laboratory tests (e.g., white blood cells in a normally sterile body fluid, perforated viscus, chest radiograph consistent with pneumonia, petechial or purpuric rash, or purpuria fulminans).
Sepsis	SIRS in the presence of or as a result of suspected or proven infection.
Severe sepsis	Sepsis plus one of the following: cardiovascular organ dysfunction **OR** acute respiratory distress syndrome **OR** two or more other organ dysfunctions.
Septic shock	Sepsis and cardiovascular organ dysfunction.

TABLE 30-17

Systemic Inflammatory Response Syndrome Criteria for Age-Specific Vital Signs and Laboratory Variables					
	Heart Rate (beat/min)		**Respiratory Rate (breath/min)**	**Leukocyte Count (× 10³/mm)**	**Systolic Blood Pressure (mm Hg)**
Age Group	**Tachycardia**	**Bradycardia**			
0 days–1 week	> 180	< 100	> 50	> 34	< 72
1 week–1 month	> 180	< 100	> 40	> 19.5 or < 5	< 75
1 month–1 year	> 180	< 90	> 34	> 17.5 or < 5	< 100
2–5 years	> 140	NA	> 22	> 15.5 or < 5	< 94
6–12 years	> 130	NA	> 18	> 13.5 or < 4.5	< 105
13–18 years	> 110	NA	> 14	> 11 or < 4.5	< 117

Lower values correspond to the 5th percentile; upper values correspond to the 95th percentile.

Source: Used with permission from Nichols, D., Allen, M., Klein, N., & Peters, M. (2008). *Rogers' textbook of pediatric intensive care* (4th ed.) Philadelphia: Lippincott Williams & Wilkins, p. 1214.

and persistent infection can lead to SS and multiple organ dysfunction syndrome (MODS).

Pediatric patients demonstrate diverse hemodynamic profiles during SS: 58% have low cardiac indexes responsive to inotropic medications with or without vasodilators, 20% exhibit high cardiac indexes and low systemic vascular resistance (SVR) responsive to vasopressor therapy, and 22% present with both vascular and cardiac dysfunctions, necessitating the use of vasopressors and inotropic support (Ceneviva et al., 1998). The pediatric patient differs from the adult SS patient in that low cardiac output (CO), not low SVR, is associated with mortality. Seventy-eight percent of children show some degree of cardiac dysfunction on presentation after fluid resuscitation. Furthermore, approximately 50% of patients require a change in their vasopressor or inotropic management, or addition of another agent, emphasizing that the hemodynamic status in children can change rapidly. Lastly, a reduction in oxygen delivery, rather than a defect in oxygen extraction, can be the major determinant of oxygen consumption in children (Pollack et al., 1985).

The relative ability of infants and children to augment cardiac output through increased heart rate (HR), as seen in adults, is limited by their preexisting elevated HR, which precludes proportionate increases in HR without compromising diastolic filling time. In addition, in adults, ventricular dilation is a compensatory response used to maintain CO. However, the increased connective tissue content of the infant's heart, and diminished content of actin and myosin, limits the potential for acute ventricular dilation (Feltes et al., 1994).

Neonatal SS can be further complicated by the physiologic transition from the fetal circulation to the neonatal circulation. Sepsis-induced acidosis and hypoxia can increase peripheral vascular resistance (PVR), and thus arterial pressure, thereby maintaining the patency of the ductus arteriosus. This effect results in persistent

pulmonary hypertension (PPHN) of the newborn and persistent fetal circulation. The combination of neonatal SS and PPHN increases the workload on the right ventricle, leading to right ventricular failure, tricuspid regurgitation, and hepatomegaly. Therefore, therapies directed at reversing right ventricular failure, by reducing pulmonary artery pressures, are commonly needed in neonates with fluid-refractory septic shock and pulmonary hypertension.

EPIDEMIOLOGY AND ETIOLOGY

The incidence of pediatric severe sepsis in the United States has increased from more than 42,000 cases involving children younger than 19 years of age in 1995, to 47,700 cases in 1999. The increased incidence is influenced by the advances in medical technology that support the delivery and care of very-low-birth-weight (VLBW) infants, who make up a substantial part of this population (Watson & Carcillo, 2005; Watson et al., 2001). The World Health Organization (WHO) reported in 2004 that 1.6 million neonates die each year from infection, and as many as 60% of deaths in developing countries are due to communicable diseases. Despite controlling for gestational age, birth weight, acidosis, disseminated intravascular coagulation (DIC), and neutropenia, refractory shock remains the most important risk factor for mortality in infants in both developed and nondeveloped countries (Han et al., 2003). Severe sepsis causes more deaths in the United States than cancer, and has a reported total annual cost of approximately $4 billion (Watson et al.).

Although rates of severe sepsis are increasing, overall hospital mortality among children with underlying disease has decreased, declining from 12.8% in 1995 to 10.5% in 1999 (Watson & Carcillo, 2005). Children who were previously healthy and develop sepsis have better outcomes than those with chronic illness. Underlying disease, in combination with the age of the patient, prove to be important predictors of sepsis in the United States, as patients with underlying disease are estimated to account for 49% of the sepsis and septic shock population. Prematurity and VLBW are significant risk factors for sepsis that are not present in older children and adults. Other comorbidities associated with septic shock by age groups include chronic lung disease and congenital heart disease in the infant population, whereas neuromuscular diseases are seen in children between 1 and 9 years of age, and cancer is a more common comorbidity among adolescents (Watson & Carcillo, 2005).

Before the onset of puberty, male gender is a risk factor for sepsis and septic shock, with a male-to-female ratio of 1.7:1 being seen in the first year of life; this ratio decreases to 1.33:1 between 1 and 9 years of age. The exact cause of the differences is not known, and cannot be explained by differences in hormonal levels, as the level of testosterone in prepubescent children is quite low (Bindl et al., 2003; Watson et al., 2003). In adults, the same preferences are observed, with men having a higher incidence of sepsis and SS than women; however, there is no difference in mortality for the two genders (Wichmann et al., 2000). The mortality rate for pediatric patients with SS ranges between 6% and 15% in patients with associated chronic illnesses, whereas it is only 2% in previously healthy children (Carcillo, 2003; Kutko et al., 2003).

In addition to age, a number of comorbid conditions are associated with increased incidence of SS (Table 30-18). These comorbidities are present in as many as 40% of patients with septic shock (Balk, 2000; Han et al., 2003). The advancement of research and technology has allowed for more invasive procedures to be performed (e.g., three-stage palliative surgery for cyanotic congenital heart disease; small bowel, liver, pancreas, heart, lung, and bone marrow transplant) in the pediatric population, all of which increase the risk of sepsis.

Several environmental and genetic factors allow healthy and immunocompromised children to develop sepsis or septic shock. The site of the infection has been shown to have an important effect on the outcome of the patient,

TABLE 30-18

Risk Factors Associated with Septic Shock

Prematurity/very low birth weight

Compromised immune status
- Acquired immune deficiency syndrome
- Malignancy
- Transplantation procedures and recipients
- Use of cytotoxic and immunosuppressant agents
- Malnutrition
- Diabetes mellitus

Musculoskeletal or neurologic disease

Chromosomal or congenital disease

Increased number of resistant microorganisms

with pulmonary, GI, and CNS infections having higher mortality rates as compared to genitourinary tract, skin, and soft-tissue infections (Opal, 2005). The skin itself is an extremely important first line of defense in protecting the body against infection with any type of bacteria, although Gram-positive bacteria tend to be the most strongly associated bacteria with skin infections. Malnutrition and vitamin deficiencies can compromise the protective barrier that the skin and mucosal membranes provide, thereby leading to severe alterations in leukocyte chemotaxis, adherence, and phagocytic killing (Balk, 2000).

Microorganism load and intrinsic virulence are critical factors in determining the outcome of an invasive microbial infection (Cross et al., 1993; Opal & Chohen, 1999). Cohen et al. (2004) completed an extensive review of the microbiology of septic shock and demonstrated marked differences in mortality based on the identity of the infecting microorganism and the site of infection.

Virulence

Gram-positive bacteria. The more virulent Gram-positive bacteria include *Staphylococcus aureus* and *Streptococcus pyogenes*, which are associated with mortality rates as high as 40% in patients with pneumonia, bloodstream, GI, or CNS infections. By comparison, infections caused by *Streptococcus pneumoniae* and *Staphylococcus epidermidis* (coagulase-negative staphylococci [CONS]) have a mortality rate of 20% when they occur in the same sites. The structure of the cell wall of Gram-positive bacteria allows for production of exotoxins that function as superantigens. These superantigens do not interact in a typical manner with the immune system to produce a regulated inflammatory response, but rather cause massive activation of T cells, which results in overproduction of cytokines and symptoms of MODS. A classic example is toxic shock syndrome, which is produced by the toxic shock syndrome toxin 1 (TSST-1) of *S. aureus*.

Gram-negative bacteria. The development of broad-spectrum antibiotics has led to the emergence of more virulent strains of bacteria within the community and in the hospital setting, making health care–associated infections one of the more common causes of sepsis and septic shock (Richards et al., 1999). Infections with *Pseudomonas aeruginosa* have the highest incidence of mortality (30% to 80%) among infections involving the lungs, bloodstream, GI, or CNS, when compared to other Gram-negative bacteria such as *Escherichia coli, Acinetobacter* species, and *Bacteroides fragilis. Neisseria meninigitidis,* which is commonly associated with meningitis, may lead to systemic involvement and septic shock. In Gram-negative sepsis, endotoxin release is responsible for manifestations of SS: The higher the level of endotoxin found, the greater the incidence of MODS and possibility of death.

Fungus. Sepsis associated with a *Candida* species has an extremely poor prognosis when this pathogen is found in large concentrations of the serum, or in organs such as the eye, lung, or liver. *Candida* sepsis may be seen in immunocompromised or chronically ill patients with health care–associated infections who have had invasive devices or procedures, or have been on broad-spectrum antibiotic therapy or parenteral nutrition. The use of broad-spectrum antibiotic therapy suppresses normal protective flora, which then allows the *Candida* species to proliferate (Balk et al., 2004). The high mortality rate depends more heavily on the patient's immune status rather than on the actual organism involved (Opal, 2005).

PRESENTATION

A thorough history is vital to determine the etiology of patients who present in septic shock. In neonates, a detailed maternal and birth history in conjunction with onset and duration of symptoms should be elicited. Infants may have a history of poor feeding, irritability, emesis, or diarrhea, which may also lead to severe dehydration. There may or may not be a history of fever. Infants and immunosuppressed patients may be unable to maintain their core body temperature when septic; as a consequence, they may present with hypothermia. Older children will usually have a history of fever and illness prodrome. A patient with a history of oncologic disease or organ transplant is at increased risk of septic shock.

The physical examination is invaluable in establishing a diagnosis of septic shock within a reasonable amount of time. Indeed, studies have shown that delay in making the diagnosis and initiating treatment contribute to the development of peripheral vascular failure and organ dysfunction (Khilnani et al., 2008). Obtaining vital signs is imperative. Establishing the heart rate indicates the patient's ability to maintain cardiac output. One of the most telling signs of sepsis or SS in older patients who present with fever and tachycardia is persistent hypotension and tachycardia in spite of volume resuscitation. Blood pressure is maintained until severe cardiovascular compromise occurs; therefore, the HCP should not be reassured by normal blood pressure parameters.

Pertinent physical examination findings by systems are as follows:

- Neurologic: Irritability and lethargy may be seen in the neonate or older child; anxiety may be evident in an older child.
- Respiratory: Tachypnea may be seen as compensation for a metabolic acidosis. Nasal flaring, grunting, subcostal or suprasternal retractions, with or without crackles, or wheezes on auscultation may indicate a disease process of the lungs.

- Cardiovascular: Tachycardia is seen early. A gallop rhythm may indicate septic myocardial depression or myocarditis. Hepatomegaly and jugular venous distention from poor myocardial function may be seen.
  - *Warm shock*: warm extremities with bounding pulses, brisk capillary refill; widened pulse pressure as a result of decrease in diastolic blood pressure from peripheral vasodilatation; systolic blood pressure is usually maintained until severe cardiovascular compromise has occurred; will progress to cold shock if treatment is delayed.
  - *Cold shock*: more common than warm shock in the pediatric population; cool, mottled extremities with weak pulses and delayed capillary refill (more than 2 seconds).
- Renal: The patient will exhibit oliguria (urine output less than 1 mL/kg/hr).
- Skin: The presence and type of rash can help narrow the etiology and focus the treatment (Khilnanai et al., 2008).

The criteria for diagnosis of MODS are defined as involvement of two or more systems (Table 30-19).

A presenting sign in sepsis may be a rash, which can begin as nonspecific maculopapular and progress to petechiae and purpura. Petechiae can appear as macules or papules and are nonblanching. They are caused by intradermal hemorrhage and can coalesce or expand to larger purple ecchymosis or purpura.

DIFFERENTIAL DIAGNOSIS

The differential diagnosis for acute onset of fever and leukocytosis in the pediatric patient includes, but is not limited to, otitis media, urinary tract infection, upper respiratory tract infection, bronchiolitis, pneumonia, sepsis, and abscess. As more chronic or atypical causes for fever and leukocytosis, one should also consider collagen vascular disease (e.g., juvenile rheumatoid arthritis, systemic lupus erythematosus, vasculitis), and oncologic disorders such as leukemia, tuberculosis, and other atypical infections.

The differential diagnosis for a purpuric rash includes meningococcal disease, toxic shock syndrome from *Staphylococcus* or *Streptococcus*, disseminated intravascular coagulation, measles, Rocky Mountain spotted fever, Henoch-Schönlein purpura, idiopathic thrombocytopenic purpura/thrombotic thrombocytopenic purpura, Epstein-Barr virus, parvovirus, serum sickness, Kawasaki disease, and dengue fever.

The differential for hypotension—or, more specifically, shock—includes sepsis, hypovolemia, heart failure, pneumothorax, cardiac tamponade, neurogenically mediated anaphylaxis, and poisoning. Infectious etiologies of shock such as viremia and fungemia may be difficult

TABLE 30-19

Criteria for Diagnosis of Multiple Organ Dysfunction Syndrome

I. Cardiovascular

1. Systolic blood pressure (mmHg)
   - < 65 in infants
   - < 75 in children or < 85 in adolescents
2. Heart rate (beats/min)
   - < 50 or > 220 in infants
   - < 40 or > 200 in children
3. Continuous infusion of inotropic agents
4. Serum pH < 7.20 (with a normal $PaCO_2$)

II. Respiratory

1. Respiratory rate (breaths/min)
   - > 90 in infants
   - > 70 in children
2. PaO_2/FIO_2 ratio < 200 (in the absence of congenital heart disease)
3. Mechanical ventilation (> 24 hours in a postoperative patient)
4. $PaCO_2$ > 65 torr
5. PaO_2 < 40 torr (in the absence of congenital heart disease)

III. Neurologic

1. Glasgow Coma Scale score < 5
2. Fixed and dilated pupils

IV. Hematologic

1. Hemoglobin < 5 gm/dL
2. White blood cell count < 3,000/mm^3
3. Platelet count < 20,000/mm^3
4. Prothrombin time > 20 sec or activated partial thromboplastin time > 60 sec

V. Renal

1. Blood urea nitrogen > 100 mg/dL
2. Creatinine > 2.0 mg/dL (in the absence of preexisting renal disease)
3. Dialysis

VI. Gastrointestinal

1. Blood transfusions > 20 mL/kg in 24 hours because of hemorrhage

VII. Hepatic

1. Total bilirubin > 5 mg/dL and aspartate aminotransferase or lactate dehydrogenase > twice normal (without evidence of hemolysis)

Source: Used with permission from Kutko, M., Calarco, M. P., Flaherty, M., et al. (2003). Mortality rates in pediatric septic shock with and without multiple organ system failure. *Pediatric Critical Care Medicine, 4*(3), 333–337.

to distinguish from bacterial sepsis and should also be considered.

PLAN OF CARE

The initial diagnostic study includes a CBC, electrolytes, kidney function tests, liver function tests, and DIC panel. In evaluating the CBC, leukocytosis and a left shift on the differential classically lead the clinician to suspect bacterial infection, but these findings are not specific for bacterial infection (Baraff et al., 1993; Trautner et al., 2006). A low WBC count in sepsis may be seen in conjunction with a bacterial, fungal, or viral infection. Calculating an absolute neutrophil count (ANC) is helpful, as patients with overwhelming sepsis can become neutropenic. Electrolytes such as sodium, potassium, calcium, and magnesium are necessary for adequate cellular function; their levels are often low in septic states. Conversely, if there is acute kidney dysfunction, the same electrolytes may be elevated. Liver and kidney function should be evaluated. The presence of metabolic acidosis on arterial blood gas (ABG) analysis and an elevated lactate level are indicative of hypoperfusion. Compensatory respiratory alkalosis may occur as well. Disseminated intravascular coagulation may also present during sepsis.

To guide appropriate antibiotic therapy, it is prudent to send cultures as early as possible to identify the inciting organism. Blood and urine cultures are easily obtainable and should be sent during the initial evaluation. If the pediatric patient presents with any mental status change or altered level of consciousness, a lumbar puncture is indicated to screen for meningitis. Cerebrospinal fluid culture, cell counts, and chemistries should all be evaluated. If there is suspicion for pneumonia, ideally the HCP will obtain a respiratory culture, although this is difficult in a pediatric patient who is not intubated. Any abscess or other external source of infection should be aspirated and cultured.

A CXR should be performed if the patient has respiratory symptoms or there is concern for carditis. Acute-phase reactants such as C-reactive protein are often used to screen for bacterial infection or severity of illness. CRP is elevated under many inflammatory conditions and, although nonspecific for infection, its measurement has been shown to be a useful means to distinguish bacterial from other types of infection in pediatrics (Pulliam et al., 2001). Several other acute-phase reactants are also being studied and may prove useful in this context, such as procalcitonin and IL-6 (Hsaio & Baker, 2005).

Most patients should be sent to the emergency room for initial management and stabilization. If their shock is reversed quickly, they may be candidates to continue antibiotic and other supportive treatment on the inpatient unit. Conversely, if they remain unstable and need continued resuscitation or central monitoring, they should be admitted to an ICU.

The landmark study by Rivers et al. (2001) demonstrated a 33% reduction in mortality in adult patients with sepsis when they were aggressively treated within 6 hours of presentation with early fluid resuscitation, early red cell transfusion, and early inotropic therapy. Such goal-directed therapy has been advocated for patients who present in SS. The components of early goal-directed therapy include prompt resuscitation of poor perfusion through administration of intravenous fluids and appropriately targeted inotropic and/or vasopressor therapy, early empiric antimicrobial therapy, drainage of infection, and appropriate and continuous monitoring of the patient's hemodynamic status.

The pediatric task force of the Society of Critical Care Medicine published clinical practice parameters for goal-directed therapy in 2002 (Carcillo & Fields, 2002). The most recent 2005 Pediatric Advanced Life Support (PALS) guidelines also include management parameters in their Septic Shock Algorithm (American Heart Association, 2006). The 2008 Surviving Sepsis campaign addressed pediatric-specific guidelines, which incorporate similar guidelines into an algorithm to guide the HCP (Figure 30-1) (Dellinger et al., 2008).

In addition to goal-directed therapy, support of the airway and breathing is essential to optimize oxygen delivery. Supplemental oxygen should be administered to all patients presenting with signs of SS; endotracheal intubation may also be necessary. Given that goal-directed therapy includes aggressive fluid resuscitation, early and immediate vascular access is essential for adequate treatment of SS. Ideally, two peripheral intravenous catheters should be placed promptly. Intraosseous access should be considered in any patient in whom peripheral vascular access is not rapidly established. Although ideal, a central venous catheter is not required for initial fluid resuscitation.

All patients with SS suffer from some degree of hypovolemia due to a number of factors: increased insensible loses (e.g., through excessive sweating, fever, and increased respiratory rate); excessive fluid losses from diarrhea or vomiting; third spacing of fluid due to capillary leak; or diminished oral intake. Relative hypovolemia occurs due to systemic vasodilation.

No data exist to suggest that there is any difference in survival rates in pediatric patients who are resuscitated with colloids (blood products) versus crystalloid fluids. The choice of fluid is less important than the volume administered. Adequate volume is necessary to sustain cardiac preload, increase stroke volume, and improve oxygen delivery. Both crystalloids and colloids (specifically, packed red blood cells) have equivalent effects in improving stroke volume. In addition, both restore tissue perfusion to the same degree if they are titrated to the same level of filling pressure (Rackow et al., 1983).

It is recommended to push isotonic crystalloid fluid (normal saline or lactated Ringer's solution) in a 20 mL/kg bolus administered over 5 minutes. Immediate reassess the patient for signs of improved perfusion using clinical criteria such as reduction in heart rate, improvement of blood pressure, capillary refill, quality of pulses, and mental status. If the clinical signs of shock persist, another 20 mL/kg of isotonic fluid should be administered. A total of at least 60 mL/kg within the first 15 to 30 minutes of treatment may be necessary. Some children require as much as 200 mL/kg in the first hour (Vincent & Gerlach, 2004). Patients remaining in shock despite fluid resuscitation should receive inotropic support to help them attain normal blood pressure for age and a capillary refill time of less than 2 seconds. Every hour that goes by without implementing these therapies in associated with a 1.5-fold increased risk of mortality (Carcillo et al., 1991).

Patients who do not respond rapidly to initial fluid boluses or those with insufficient physiologic reserve should be considered for invasive hemodynamic monitoring. Invasive monitoring of central venous pressure (CVP) is instituted to ensure that the satisfactory right ventricular preload is present (normal CVP = 10–12 mmHg), and that oxygen-carrying capacity is optimized by transfusion of packed red blood cells (PRBC) to correct anemia (hemoglobin concentration > 10 gm/dL). Fluid-refractory shock is defined as the persistence of signs of shock after sufficient fluids have been administered to achieve a CVP of 8–12 mmHg, and/or signs of fluid overload as evidenced by new-onset crackles, increased work of breathing and hypoxemia from pulmonary edema, hepatomegaly, or a diminished mean arterial pressure. Diuretics, peritoneal dialysis, or renal replacement therapy are indicted for patients who develop signs and symptoms of fluid overload.

As much as 40% of CO may be required to support the work of breathing in the presence of respiratory distress. In this circumstance, an elective tracheal intubation followed by mechanical ventilation will assist in redistributing blood flow away from respiratory muscles and toward other vital organs. However, mechanical intubation is not without adverse effects. It is imperative that the patient receive adequate fluid resuscitation before the intubation, as the change from spontaneous breathing to positive-pressure ventilation will decrease the effective preload to the heart. Ventilation may reduce left ventricular afterload—an effect that may be beneficial in patients with low cardiac index (CI) and high SVR. In addition, it may provide an alternative method to alter acid–base balance. If sedatives and analgesics are used for intubation, choosing agents that do not cause further vasodilation (e.g., morphine) is critical. The SCCM recommends avoiding agents that will blunt endogenous catecholamine release, such as propofol, thiopental, benzodiazepines, and inhalational agents (Brierley et al., 2009). Some sources have recommended ketamine,

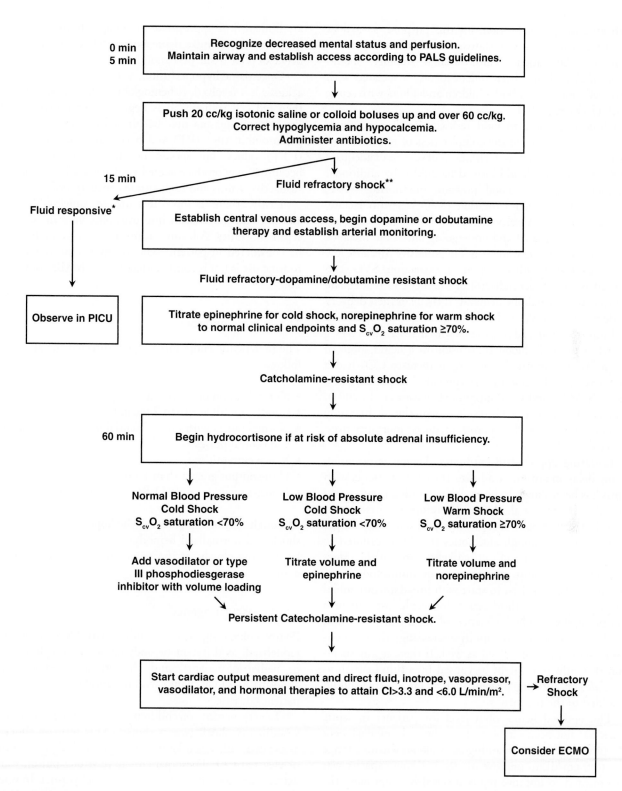

FIGURE 30-1

Approach to Pediatric Shock.

Note: Pediatric Advanced Life Support (PALS), pediatric intensive care unit (PICU), cardiac index (CI), extracorporeal membrane oxygenation (ECMO), *Normalization of blood pressure and tissue perfusion, **Hypotension, abnormal capillary refill or extremity coolness.

Source: Used with permission from Dellinger, R., Levy, M., Carlet, J., et al. (2008). Surviving Sepsis Campaign: international guidelines for management of severe sepsis and septic shock: 2008. *Critical Care Medicine, 36*(1), 315.

with atropine premedication, for this purpose, as it does not affect cardiovascular status. Etomidate, although it maintains the patient's cardiovascular stability, should be *avoided*, as it has been independently associated with increased mortality in both children and adults with septic shock (Jackson, 2005).

Clinical response to fluid resuscitation is a relatively insensitive indicator for the completeness of restoration of microvascular blood flow. Definitions of success of adequate fluid resuscitation should instead be guided by additional parameters: invasive blood pressure monitoring, CVP, mixed venous oxygen saturation (SVO_2), serum lactate, and urine output. An elevated serum lactate level suggests tissue is hypoperfused and undergoing anaerobic metabolism, even in patients who are not hypotensive. Because low CO is associated with increased O_2 extraction, SVO_2 can be used as an indirect indicator of whether CO is adequate to meet tissue metabolic demand. If tissue oxygen delivery is adequate, then SVO_2 should be greater than 70%. In a goal-directed study, adult patients who maintained a SVO_2 greater than 70% (blood transfusion to a hemoglobin of 10 gm/dL and inotropic support to increase CO) had a 40% reduction in mortality as compared to patients who had only MAP and CVP monitored (Rivers et al., 2001). When de Oliveria et al. (2008) later reproduced this study in children with SS, this approach reduced mortality from 39% to 12%.

Initiating appropriate antibiotic therapy is essential, as any delay in antibiotic administration in patients with sepsis has been shown to be associated with an increase in mortality (Kumar et al., 2006). Therefore, the first dose is given in the first hour of sepsis or septic shock (Dellinger et al., 2008). Although antibiotics should be tailored to each specific patient and to the likely source of the infection, prior infections, neutropenia, or immunodeficiencies, in general it is best to start with broad antimicrobial coverage, such as a third-generation cephalosporin or a fluoroquinolone. The incidence of methicillin-resistant *Staphylococcus aureus* is rapidly increasing; thus vancomycin should be considered as well. If there is any suspicion that infection might be caused by a fungus such as *Candida,* an antifungal agent such as fluconazole should be added to the regimen.

The optimal hemoglobin level for patients in septic shock has not been established. In the early management of sepsis in adults, maintaining hemoglobin within a range of 7 to 9 gm/dL to improve oxygen-carrying capacity was documented to improve sepsis survival by improving tissue perfusion (Zimmerman, 2004). Anemia in sepsis has been associated with increased mortality, as has the administration of blood (Finfer et al., 2004; Vincent & Gerlach, 2004). Therefore, the SCCM (1999) recommends that hemoglobin concentration be maintained within the range 8–10 gm/dL, with the understanding that there are limited data supporting this guideline. Given that pediatric data

are limited, it is appropriate to extrapolate from the adult literature to maximize tissue oxygen delivery if there is evidence of poor tissue perfusion.

Once tissue hypoperfusion, acute hemorrhage, or lactic acidosis has resolved, if hemoglobin is less than 7 gm/dL, then red cell transfusion is begun (Zimmerman, 2004). Fresh frozen plasma may be infused to correct abnormal prothrombin time (PT) and partial thromboplastin time (PTT) values, but should not be infused too quickly because it may produce acute hypotensive effects caused by vasoactive kinins and high citrate concentration.

Lastly, there is no literature to suggest that 5% albumin administration improves outcomes in regard to sepsis mortality. Albumin administration, may however, be considered in patients who are hypoalbuminemic. Its routine use is not recommended by SCCM (Brierley et al., 2009).

Therapeutic endpoints

The therapeutic endpoints for goal-directed therapy are as follows:

- Normalization of heart rate
- Capillary refill less than 2 seconds
- Normal pulses with no differential between peripheral and central pulses
- Warm extremities
- Urine output greater than 1 mL/kg/hr
- Normal mental status (Dellinger et al., 2008)

Although reassuring, patients who appear to have reversed shock and normalized hemodynamics should continue to be followed closely, as the potential for deterioration still exists.

Cardiovascular agents

Pharmacologic support in children with SS must be individualized, as different hemodynamic abnormalities exist in pediatric patients, and the primary hemodynamic abnormalities may change with time and progression of the patient's disease.

Twenty percent of children present with predominant vasodilatory shock (warm shock). This form of shock is associated with vasodilation and capillary leak, but normal or elevated CO. These patients have strong pulses, warm extremities, good capillary refill, and tachycardia. In warm shock, using a vasopressor to promote vasoconstriction would provide the greatest benefit; options include dopamine, norepinephrine, phenylephrine, or vasopressin.

Fifty-eight percent of children present with cold shock: or predominately a poor CO state. These patients have vasoconstriction, increased cardiac afterload, and a high SVR. Clinically, a poor CO state is manifested by weak pulses, cool extremities, slow capillary refill, and hepatic and pulmonary congestion. Using an inotrope with or without a vasodilator would be most beneficial in patients in cold shock (e.g., dobutamine, epinephrine, or milrinone). Careful assessment of clinical response is critical, as a combination of vasodilatory and cold shock with a low SVR and poor CO occurs in 22% of children.

Dopamine. The 2008 Surviving Sepsis guidelines suggest using dopamine as the first-line agent for inotropic support with fluid refractory septic shock (Dellinger et al., 2008). Dopamine has both direct and indirect effects on dopamine receptors, alpha receptors, and beta receptors on both the heart and the peripheral vasculature. One of the mechanisms of dopamine action is enhancement of endogenous catecholamine release. In severe septic states, presynaptic vacuoles may be depleted of norepinephrine, which may explain why dopamine may have diminished activity in patients with sepsis. In addition, infants younger than 6 months of age may not have developed their component of sympathetic innervations; therefore, they have reduced releasable stores of epinephrine (Brierley et al., 2009).

Recently obtained adult data have raised concerns about increased mortality with the use of dopamine. One possible explanation for this relationship is the ability of dopamine to reduce the release of hormones from the anterior pituitary gland, such as prolactin, through stimulation of the DA$_2$ receptor. This effect may reduce cell-mediated immunity and inhibition of thyrotropin-releasing hormone release, thereby worsening the impaired thyroid function known to occur in critical illness. For these reasons, some clinicians prefer to use low-dose norepinephrine as a first-line agent for fluid-refractory hypotensive hyperdynamic shock.

Dopamine should be started at 5 mcg/kg/min and titrated upward in increments of 2.5 mcg/kg/min every 3 to 5 minutes until the goal of improved perfusion and/or blood pressure is achieved. The maximum recommended dose of dopamine is 20 mcg/kg/min; higher doses may contribute to increased myocardial oxygen demand without yielding much improvement in vasopressor activity. Dopamine-resistant shock is diagnosed after titration of dopamine to 20 mcg/kg/min with the persistence of signs and symptoms of shock. Once this dose is reached, patient evaluation should be repeated. Measure hemoglobin and administer red cell transfusion to improve the hemoglobin to 8–10 gm/dL if needed, as this intervention may improve tissue oxygen. Measure CVP to assess intravascular volume status (the goal is 8 to 12 mmHg), and obtain a SVO$_2$ reading once the hemoglobin has been corrected. This value, along with the findings from the clinical examination, serves as a marker of cardiac output.

Dopamine-resistant shock. Dopamine-resistant shock commonly responds to norepinephrine or high-dose epinephrine, depending on the patient. Epinephrine is recommended for cold shock (0.05 to 0.3 mcg/kg/min), or norepinephrine (0.05 to 0.3 mcg/kg/min) can be titrated for warm shock to restore normal perfusion and blood pressure.

Norepinephrine is a directly acting agent that is naturally produced in the adrenal gland. A potent vasopressor, it redirects blood flow away from skeletal muscle to the splanchnic circulation, even in the presence of decreased cardiac output. Norepinephrine has been used extensively to elevate SVR in septic adults and children. If the patient's clinical state is characterized by low SVR (e.g., wide pulse pressure with diastolic blood pressure less than one-half of systolic blood pressure), then norepinephrine is recommended. Nearly 20% of children with volume-refractory SS have a low SVR (Ceneviva et al., 1998). Notably, among children who are intubated and receiving sedatives or analgesics, the incidence of low SVR may be even higher.

In patients with impaired contractility, the additional afterload imposed by norepinephrine may substantially compromise CO. In some patients with both impaired or marginal CO and decreased SVR, it may be necessary to support myocardial contractility through the addition of an agent such as dobutamine.

Epinephrine is a directly acting agent that is naturally produced in the adrenal gland. The principal stress hormone, it has widespread metabolic and hemodynamic effects in the body. Epinephrine exerts both inotropic and chronotropic effects. As with norepinephrine, epinephrine infusions may be started as low as 0.02 mcg/kg/min and titrated upward in 0.05 to 0.1 mcg/kg/min increments every 3 to 5 minutes to achieve the desired clinical response or until the dose reaches 2 mcg/kg/min (although higher doses have been used). Epinephrine is a reasonable choice for the treatment of patients with low CO and poor peripheral perfusion, because it increases HR and myocardial contractility (Bollaert et al., 1990). Depending on the dose, this agent may exert variable effects on SVR. At low doses (less than 0.3 mcg/kg/min), epinephrine exerts greater β$_2$-adrenergic receptor activation, resulting in vasodilation in skeletal muscle and cutaneous vascular beds, shunting blood flow away from the splanchnic circulation. At higher doses, α$_1$–adrenergic receptor activation becomes more prominent and may increase SVR and heart rate. For patients with markedly elevated SVR, epinephrine may be administered simultaneously with a vasodilator.

Epinephrine increases glucogenesis and glycogenolysis, resulting in elevated serum glucose concentrations. For this reason, all patients receiving epinephrine infusions should have their glucose levels monitored closely.

Dobutamine is a nonselective β$_2$-adrenergic agonist, so it leads to improved inotrophy (contractility), chronotrophy (increased HR), and some lusitophy (improved myocardial relaxation). The β$_2$-related activity can lead to peripheral vasodilation and must be considered prior to its use in a patient who may already be hypotensive. If hypotension is present, the patient should receive a combination of dobutamine plus another vasopressor therapy. Thus dobutamine may be considered in the patient who has signs and symptoms or laboratory values consistent with poor tissue perfusion, but has an adequate blood pressure to tolerate some degree of vasodilation. Dobutamine should be initiated at a rate of 2.5 mcg/kg/min and titrated in increments of 2.5 mcg/kg/min every 3 to 5 minutes to a maximum infusion rate of 20 mcg/kg/min. Careful attention to the patient's blood pressure is critical. Improved perfusion, decreased lactate, and an increased SVO_2 will help tailor the dose to the patient's unique circumstances.

Vasodilator medications are occasionally required in the treatment of septic pediatric patients who have markedly elevated SVR and normal or decreased CO. Vasodilators decrease SVR and improve cardiac output by decreasing ventricular afterload. Nitroglycerin (NTG) or nitroprusside (NTP) may be used for this indication. These agents have a short half-life; therefore, if hypotension occurs, they can be rapidly reversed by stopping the infusion. Both drugs can be infused at an initial rate of 0.5 mcg/kg/min and titrated in increments of 0.5 mcg/kg/min to a maximum infusion rate of 5 to 10 mcg/kg/min. If nitroprusside is used, the patient should be observed for sodium thiocyanate accumulation in the setting of kidney failure, and cyanide toxicity with hepatic failure or with prolonged infusions (more than 72 hours) of more than 3 mcg/kg/min. If the patient tolerates infusions of NTG or NTP, the HCP should consider switching to milrinone, a longer-acting agent.

Milrinone is a phosphodiesterase type III (PDE III) inhibitor that produces its hemodynamic effects by inhibiting the degradation of cyclic AMP in smooth muscle cells and cardiac myocytes. PDE III inhibitors work synergistically with catecholamines, which produce their hemodynamic effects by increasing the production of cyclic AMP. Milrinone is useful in the treatment of patients with diminished myocardial contractility and output, and decreased systemic resistance (Lindsay et al., 1998). The major concern with milrinone is the drug's long half-life (2 to 6 hours); once it is administered, it takes several hours to reach the desired steady state. To achieve the desired serum level more rapidly, a loading dose of 50 mcg/kg is recommended. This loading dose is administered over 10 to 30 minutes, but must be done with caution in patients with SS: Its administration may precipitate hypotension, requiring volume infusion or vasopressor infusion. Administering the loading dose over several hours may avoid this adverse effect. The (nonloading) infusion dose of milrinone is 0.25 to 0.75 mcg/kg/min.

Consulting with the critical care team early in the patient's presentation can ensure organ perfusion is maximized and sepsis guidelines are comprehensively applied. As SS may develop into a prolonged hospital course with a number of sequelae, specialty services such as infectious diseases, nephrology, gastroenterology/hepatology, cardiology,

pulmonary, oncology, and neurology may become an integral part of the interprofessional team. Nutrition, rehabilitation medicine, child life, social workers, and spiritual advisors are often essential to ensure optimal outcomes for patients with sepsis and septic shock.

Patient and family education should include discussions about the goals of therapy, supportive equipment and medication, interprofessional team approach, and ongoing health and safety of the family.

DISPOSITION AND DISCHARGE PLANNING

Sepsis, despite modern advancements in medicine, remains the most common cause of death in children. The risk of death increases as shock, multisystem involvement, and refractory shock develop (Han et al., 2003). Few studies have examined either short- or long-term outcomes in those pediatric patients who survive. In 2000, the average length of stay for a patient with sepsis aged 1 to 19 years was 19 days (Watson & Carcillo, 2005). Patients young than 1 year of age and premature or low-birth-weight infants have longer length of stays. If pediatric patients survive severe septic shock, they can sustain long-term organ damage such as neurologic damage, prolonged weakness, chronic kidney failure requiring dialysis, and even amputations. Many will require long-term hospitalization and rehabilitation.

In addition to ongoing efforts aimed at improving mortality, the prevention of sepsis is crucial. The incidence, and thus the mortality, of diseases attributable to some specific microbes have dramatically decreased with the help of vaccinations—for example, sepsis from *Haemophilus influenzae* type b and *Streptococcus pneumoniae*. The goal of decreasing mortality is associated with improving early treatment. In the United Kingdom, through extended education and distribution of guidelines for managing meningococcal disease in pediatric patients, the mortality rate has declined from 23% to 2% (Booy et al., 2001). The 2008 Surviving Sepsis guidelines contain sentinel approaches to reducing mortality and morbidity.

TRAVEL ORGANISMS AND PARASITES

John Leake

With the advent of modern air travel, hundreds of millions of individuals cross international borders each year. Many of these travelers lack appropriate knowledge concerning risk factors for tropical infection, vaccination, and malaria prophylaxis (Freedman, 1998; Ryan & Kain, 2000).

The diagnosis of infection in returning travelers can be challenging. Presenting symptoms and signs are often nonspecific. Patients may have sought medical care abroad, modifying "classic" disease manifestations, including the incubation period. Health care professionals lacking adequate tropical medicine training may not recognize disease features that would lead to diagnostic suspicion and appropriate testing and therapy. Further, global disease trends vary throughout the world and evolve over time. Consequently, it is important to stay up-to-date on epidemiologic trends relevant to areas from which a traveler has returned. Internet-based and other resources now make this task increasingly feasible.

When considering the cause of a travel-related infection, the astute HCP will keep the following elements in mind:

- Geographic distribution of illnesses with respect to itinerary
- Usual incubation period (time from initial infection to onset of symptoms)
- Season
- Activities (e.g., visiting friends and relatives, tourism, camping/backpacking) and duration in each area
- Pretravel immunizations administered, malaria medications taken, and compliance/possibility of missed doses
- The traveler's past medical history and immune status

As opposed to infections in developed countries, which tend to be caused by a single microbe, multiple infections (e.g., dengue fever and *Giardia* infection) are not uncommon in travelers, especially in longer-term travelers. Finally, considering "routine," non-travel-related causes of fever (e.g., sinusitis, pyelonephritis) may be useful.

MALARIA

Pathophysiology

Malaria is a systemic, mosquito-borne disease that is caused by protozoan parasites of the genus *Plasmodium*. Despite more than a century of study, the pathophysiology of malaria is still not completely understood. After infective sporozoites are injected during feeding by female mosquitoes of the genus *Anopheles*, they transit to the liver, where they give rise to tissue schizonts. Hepatic schizonts develop into merozoites, which then leave the liver and infect circulating erythrocytes. Two species, *P. vivax* and *P. ovale*, generate liver hypnozoites that may cause later relapses. Parasites in the blood trigger paroxysmal fever and other symptoms. Hemolysis, red blood cell (RBC) sequestration in the spleen and in the systemic microvasculature, and inflammation generated in response to infection are responsible for the pathophysiologic derangements associated with malaria (McIntosh et al., 2004).

Epidemiology and etiology

Four well-described *Plasmodium* protozoan species cause malaria: *P. falciparum, P. vivax, P. ovale,* and *P. malariae.* There is little *P. vivax* in Africa due to widespread fixation of a mutation that decreases expression of the erythrocyte Duffy blood receptor used by *P. vivax* to invade erythrocytes. During the past several years, a fifth species, *P. knowlesi*—a simian strain in Southeast Asia—has been shown to infect humans. Globally, however, infection with *P. falciparum* accounts for most severe malaria disease and death. The vast majority of persons returning to the United States infected with *P. falciparum* acquired their infection in sub-Saharan Africa during the previous 1 to 2 months. In recent years, a rise in severe disease due to *P. vivax* has also been reported in Indonesia and elsewhere (Rogerson & Carter, 2008).

The importance of malaria to global health cannot be overemphasized. Among febrile children in many health facilities where malaria is endemic, it is the presumed cause of the fever, prompting empiric treatment. It substantially diminishes many nations' gross national product (Hotez, 2008). Malaria has profoundly shaped the human genome, especially variations in RBC morphology and function (Kwiatkowsky, 2005). *Fever in a traveler returning from an endemic area is considered malaria until proven otherwise.* Each year, some 10 to 20 travelers returning home to the United States die of malaria; in many fatal cases, this diagnosis was never considered (CDC, 2009b).

Presentation

Once parasites reach the circulation and infect RBCs, fever and other symptoms commence, often but by no means invariably, with a cyclic 2- to 3-day periodicity (shorter with *P. knowlesi*). Chills, headache, malaise, cough, vomiting, diarrhea (especially in infants), and other systemic manifestations make malaria difficult to distinguish from many other tropical infections. The severe malaria spectrum includes cerebral malaria, in which the knobby protrusions of infected RBCs stick and block cerebral microvascular circulation, leading to progressive alterations in mental status, seizures, and cerebral edema; severe malarial anemia, with potential hypoxia and circulatory collapse; acute respiratory distress syndrome (ARDS), which may be confused with pneumonia; hypotension ("algid" malaria), sometimes accompanied by positive blood culture; and severe acute kidney insufficiency ("blackwater fever").

Differential diagnosis

Usual causes of bacterial sepsis include staphylococcus and Gram-negative bacteria (especially common in Africa), brucellosis, dengue, hepatitis, influenza, leptospirosis, typhoid, typhus, and other *Rickettsia*.

Plan of care

Thick and thin smears, ideally obtained during a fever spike, are the mainstay of diagnosis. Rapid diagnostic tests (RDTs) that identify conserved malarial antigens are increasingly used elsewhere and are now available in the United States (http://www.cdc.gov/malaria/diagnosis_treatment/diagnosis_rdt.htm). These tests may be especially useful where an expert in the microscopic diagnosis of malaria is lacking. PCR technology is highly sensitive and specific for malaria, but is not routinely available for clinical diagnosis in most areas.

Atovaquone–proguanil and chloroquine are the first-line treatment options for chloroquine-resistant and chloroquine-sensitive strains, respectively. There is widespread chloroquine resistance in most of the world (Kain et al., 2001). For severe disease, intravenous quinidine or artesunate (the latter available from the CDC) is recommended. Special attention should be paid to blood glucose and cardiac rhythm with IV quinidine administration, given its potential to cause hypoglycemia and long QT syndrome. Exchange transfusion should be considered when parasitemia reaches more than 5% to 0%. Corticosteroids are of little proven benefit and may worsen cerebral malaria (Warrell et al., 1982); additional proposed adjunctive therapies have yet to be widely evaluated.

Consultation with specialty services is based on the severity of presentation and the patient's response to therapy. Specialists from infectious diseases, along with those from neurology, gastroenterology, nutrition, critical care, and rehabilitation medicine services, may prove valuable as part of the interprofessional team.

Patient and family instructions must include the need to seek medical care rapidly for fever in endemic areas, regardless of malaria chemoprophylaxis; peridomestic mosquito control, including insecticide-treated bed nets; personal protective measures (e.g., long trousers and use of insecticide); and avoidance of mosquito bites at dawn and dusk.

Disposition and discharge planning

Follow-up with an infectious disease specialist is often warranted, especially if new fevers suggest relapse. Other specific follow-up (e.g., with neurology services) may be considered as needed.

Personal protective measures (use of insecticide-treated bed nets, protective clothing, and DEET- or picaridin-containing insect repellant) to prevent mosquito bites are recommended; even full compliance to chemoprophylactic regimens does not always prevent malaria. No effective vaccine is yet available for malaria, although several clinical trials are ongoing.

DENGUE

Pathophysiology

Infection with dengue virus causes a systemic febrile illness that is usually mild and self-limited (dengue fever); however, it may result in severe disease with bleeding, hemoconcentration, and third-spacing in the pleural or peritoneal cavity (dengue hemorrhagic fever [DHF]) with or without shock (dengue shock syndrome [DSS]) (Eddleston & Pierini, 1999). Not all apparently severe disease cases meet DHF/DSS criteria, however; thus additional novel case definitions have been proposed (Smith & Tambyah, 2007).

Increased vascular permeability and coagulopathy results from massive cytokine release during dengue infection; most patients with DHF/DSS have had prior infection with another dengue virus serotype. Antibody-dependent enhancement leading to more severe disease upon subsequent dengue infection has been proposed as an explanation for this phenomenon (Halstead, 2007).

Epidemiology and etiology

Dengue virus (*Flavividae* family) is the most important arboviral infection worldwide, with an estimated 50 to 100 million cases annually. Four serotypes (DEN 1, 2, 3, and 4) exist throughout the tropics. Virologic surveillance has shown that periodic introduction of new strains and serotypes sustains population-level transmission, and cocirculation of multiple serotypes increases the risk of DHF/DSS. Anthropophilic daytime-biting *Aedes aegypti* mosquitoes are the principal vectors in most areas; *A. albopictus* also transmits dengue viruses efficiently. Several interrelated factors are associated with the viability and size of *Aedes* populations, such as environmental (temperature, rainfall) and human behavioral factors (attention to removal of periurban and peridomestic water receptacles, such as used tires, plant containers, and undrained/untreated pools). Global incidence of dengue is perennially high in Southeast Asia, India, the Caribbean, and Central and South America.

Presentation

After an incubation period of approximately 3 to 14 days, clinical manifestations usually include one or more of the following: fever, headache (often "retro-orbital"), significant malaise, and moderate to severe musculoskeletal pain. A transient macular rash (first few days of illness) or maculopapular rash (days 3 to 6) is often present. Dengue is a leading cause of undifferentiated fever among young children in many tropical countries.

Differential diagnosis

Dengue should be considered among travelers returning from tropical areas who present with undifferentiated fever or fever with or without rash, arthralgia, hemorrhagic manifestations (petechiae, epistaxis, gastrointestinal bleeding), or encephalitis.

Plan of care

Diagnostic studies should include a complete blood count, which commonly reveals leukopenia with relative lymphocytosis and thrombocytopenia; a rising hematocrit and reduced platelet count should signal concern for imminent DHF. Serologic diagnosis in developed countries usually includes ELISA-based tests for antidengue IgM and IgG. Viral culture and PCR are not readily available for routine clinical diagnosis, although the virus may be cultured using mosquito cell lines.

The mainstay of severe dengue treatment consists of fluid and electrolyte monitoring, careful replacement of fluids to maintain circulating blood volume yet minimize extravascular fluid loss, correction of acidosis, and transfusion of blood, platelets, or fresh frozen plasma for severe hemorrhage. Salicylates should be avoided due to their interactions with platelet function and the potential increased risk of coagulopathy or Reye's syndrome.

Consultation with specialty services is based on the severity of presentation and the patient's response to therapy. Specialists from infectious diseases, along with those from neurology, critical care, and rehabilitation medicine, may prove valuable as members of the interprofessional team.

Patient and family education should consist of the admission and therapeutic management plan. The involvement of specialists and need for multiple diagnostic studies should be discussed as a component of the comprehensive plan of care. Long-term rehabilitation may also be indicated due to profound weakness, and discussion with the family should include support for the patient's continued care outside of the hospital environment.

Disposition and discharge planning

No specific follow-up is usually required for most pediatric patients, although profound weakness may last for several weeks during convalescence and patients may participate in rehabilitation on an outpatient basis.

Avoidance of daytime-biting mosquitoes is essential. Education should emphasize promptly seeking medical care if the patient develops severe systemic signs (especially nosebleeds or petechiae, severe abdominal pain, difficulty breathing, or altered mental status) during or after recent travel. Often in endemic areas, widespread public information is available (including public notices) regarding the epidemiologic situation during a given time period. Mosquito control activities may reduce transmission in some areas. Vaccine candidates against all four serotypes that cause dengue infection are being evaluated in clinical trials; it will be important to induce adequate protective immunity to each serotype given the potential risk of subsequent DHF.

JAPANESE ENCEPHALITIS (JE VIRUS)

Pathophysiology

In Japanese encephalitis, after the bite of infective mosquitoes, viremia with transit across the blood–brain barrier occurs. Lack of prior antibody (e.g., from vaccination), delayed production of antibody during acute infection, advanced age, and other risk factors (e.g., cysticercosis) that may disrupt the blood–brain barrier increase the disease progression within the central nervous system. It is likely that several as yet poorly understood viral and host factors contribute to disease outcome in the face of JE virus infection.

Epidemiology and etiology

Like dengue virus, JE virus is a mosquito-borne flavivirus. JE is the principal cause of encephalitis in East and Southeast Asia and the Indian subcontinent. Approximately 50,000 cases and 10,000 fatalities occur in Asia each year. *Culex* mosquitoes and birds (as with West Nile virus, a JE virus serogroup member) constitute the primary enzootic cycle. Amplification of virus occurs in domestic pigs; thus copresence of irrigated fields where mosquitoes breed and peridomestic pigs forage increases JE virus infection risk.

Presentation

Although most JE virus infections are subclinical, severe headache, meningeal signs, vomiting, decreased mental status, and seizures occur among symptomatic patients, with severe neurologic sequelae affecting a substantial proportion. Acute flaccid paralysis, respiratory muscle weakness, and Parkinsonian movement disorders are also possible.

Differential diagnosis

Enterovirus, herpes simplex virus (HSV), other mosquito-borne viruses (e.g., Western equine encephalomyelitis [WEE], St. Louis encephalitis [SLE], Eastern equine encephalitis [EEE]), and rabies make up the differential diagnoses.

Plan of care

Diagnostic studies typically include those aimed at peripheral and CSF leukocytosis. Serologic assays to detect IgM antibody directed against JE virus are the mainstay of diagnosis. Initially negative tests may need to be repeated later during the disease course. MRI often reveals signal changes in the basal ganglia, thalami, and brain stem. Hyponatremia, presumed to be due to syndrome of inappropriate antidiuretic hormone (SIADH), is commonly observed. Elevated CSF opening pressure and brain swelling may be seen at autopsy (Solomon, 2004).

Therapeutic management is supportive, with special attention being paid to control of intracranial pressure and seizures. Corticosteroids and interferon-alpha have not been shown to improve JE outcome.

Consultation with specialty services is based on the severity of presentation and the patient's response to therapy. Specialists from infectious diseases, along with those from neurology, critical care, and rehabilitation medicine, may prove valuable as members of the interprofessional team.

Patient and family education includes personal protective measures to prevent mosquito bites and vaccination if living in endemic areas or traveling there for prolonged stays.

Disposition and discharge planning

Careful follow-up is frequently required for a large proportion of JE survivors with neuropsychiatric sequelae.

Widespread incorporation of brain-derived JE vaccines into routine childhood immunization programs has dramatically decreased JE incidence in many Asian nations. Newer cell-culture–derived vaccines are available, although so far they are approved only for adults. Vaccination is recommended for travelers who will be staying in endemic areas for 1 month or longer, and for shorter-term travelers who will be staying in rural areas with high rates of transmission during peak or epidemic seasons. For more information, see the CDC's JE vaccine recommendations (http://www.cdc.gov/vaccines/recs/provisional/downloads/je-july2009-508.pdf).

TYPHOID

Pathophysiology

Typhoid fever results from infection with *Salmonella enterica* serotype *typhi,* a member of the *Enterobacteriaciae* family. Ingestion of an infective dose of more than 1,000 organisms and, in some persons, lack of sufficiently low gastric pH allow the bacteria to reach the small intestine, invade the blood through Peyer's patches, and survive within lymphoid tissues, the liver, and the spleen. From these intracellular locations, subsequent widespread bacteremia occurs with a few weeks, and circulating endotoxin triggers a systemic inflammatory response.

Epidemiology and etiology

Annual global estimates of typhoid are in the range of 15 million cases and 500,000 deaths (Parry et al., 2002). Endemic and epidemic disease occurs throughout the tropics. The Indian subcontinent is the location where most North American travelers, many of whom are visiting

friends and relatives for extended (more than 1 month) stays, acquire infection.

Presentation

Fever, headache, and malaise occur in nearly all patients, with the fever increasing dramatically in the second week of illness. A relative bradycardia is observed in some patients with high fever, but is not always present. Nearly all patients have some abdominal findings (pain, cramps, nausea, vomiting, diarrhea, or, not uncommonly, constipation). In addition, hepatomegaly and splenomegaly are common. Transient rose spots (blanching erythematous macules) are seen in a minority of patients. Confusion, apathy, delirium, obtundation, and (rarely) convulsions are manifestations of CNS involvement. Intestinal perforation is the most important life-threatening complication.

Differential diagnosis

Malaria, dengue, leptospirosis, influenza, bacterial gastroenteritis, entamoebiasis, tuberculosis, other causes of encephalitis, Epstein-Barr virus, toxoplasmosis, and visceral leishmaniasis should all be considered in the differential diagnosis.

Plan of care

Laboratory confirmation is most commonly achieved by blood culture; larger volumes increase the diagnostic yield. The bone marrow contains higher numbers of organisms than the blood does, so it is usually the best source for positive cultures. Stool cultures are positive in less than one-half of patients and often do not become positive until the second or third week of illness. Obtaining a culture of the organism (from whatever source) helps guide definitive antimicrobial therapy—an especially important consideration given the potential for antimicrobial resistance. Peripheral WBC may be normal or somewhat reduced (although there may be an increased percentage of immature neutrophils), and platelet counts are often reduced. Liver function tests may be elevated to 2 to 3 times normal. Serologic tests (e.g., Widal's test, agglutination reaction) are neither sensitive nor specific for typhoid, and as a rule are unhelpful in identifying patients in developed countries.

Therapeutic management for typhoid usually consists of ceftriaxone or ciprofloxacin as first-line treatment in most areas; patients who are unable or unlikely to absorb oral antibiotics should be treated intravenously until they improve. The widespread prevalence of nalidixic acid resistance may correlate with decreased ciprofloxacin efficacy. Azithromycin is also effective, as are beta lactams and sulfa derivatives for susceptible strains. Prompt surgical intervention may be life-saving for intestinal perforation.

Consultation with specialty services is based on the severity of presentation and the patient's response to therapy. Specialists from infectious diseases, along with those from neurology, gastroenterology/hepatology, nutrition, hematology, general surgery, critical care, and rehabilitation medicine, may prove valuable as members of the interprofessional team.

Patient and family education should consist of the admission and therapeutic management plan. The involvement of specialists and need for multiple diagnostic studies should be discussed as a component of the comprehensive plan of care.

Disposition and discharge planning

Close follow-up should be assured given the possibility of relapse, which occurs in approximately 10% of patients. Relapses are usually successfully treated with the same regimen as initially provided. Assurance that two to three stool cultures are negative will allow most patients to resume school and work attendance.

Vaccination for travelers, especially those visiting friends and relatives in highly endemic areas (e.g., the Indian subcontinent) for extended periods, is necessary, as are food and water precautions in endemic areas. The CDC website describes methods of water disinfection for travelers (http://wwwnc.cdc.gov/travel/yellowbook/2010/chapter-2/water-disinfection.aspx).

LEPTOSPIROSIS

Pathophysiology

After infection with pathogenic leptospires (*Leptospira interrogans* complex), symptomatic patients have either a self-limited febrile illness or a severe multisystem illness usually affecting the liver, kidneys, coagulation system, vascular endothelium, and, in *leptospirosis pulmonary syndrome*, bleeding into the lungs.

Epidemiology and etiology

Although precise incidence estimates are lacking, leptospirosis is the most common zoonotic infection worldwide (Bharti et al., 2003). In selected areas, it represents one of the most important causes of ICU admission, especially during predictable or sporadic periods of heavy rain. Exposure to the urine of infected mammals or marsupials (rats, wild or pet dogs, and other peridomestic or feral animals) is the source of infection. Walking or wading in infected fresh water or mud and exposure through occupational or recreational activities such as river rafting and adventure racing are common sources of infection. Walking barefoot with or without cuts on the skin is another common risk factor.

Presentation

A large subset of patients with infections are asymptomatic, being diagnosed only retrospectively (e.g., through population-level serosurveys). A wide variety of systemic manifestations may occur, however, usually becoming evident 2 to 20 days after infection. Fever, headache, painless conjunctival suffusion or hemorrhage, myalgias especially of bilateral gastrocnemus and soleus muscles, vomiting and abdominal pain, and a transient nonspecific or purpuric rash are frequent complaints. A small minority (5% to 10% in most places) of infected patients develop one or more of the classic triad of symptoms described as *Weil's disease*: hepatic insufficiency, kidney insufficiency, and hemorrhage. Not all of these symptoms may be present in severe leptospirosis in children. Hemoptysis and pulmonary hemorrhage, indicative of leptospirosis-associated severe pulmonary hemorrhagic syndrome (SPHS), are especially ominous. Since the mid-1990s, SPHS has become increasingly common in the Americas (Gouveia et al., 2008).

Differential diagnosis

Dengue (especially DHF mimicking Weil's disease), meningococcemia, typhoid, typhus, malaria, viral hemorrhagic fevers, viral hepatitides, and influenza should be considered in the differential diagnosis.

Although leptospires are unusual among spirochetes in their ability to be cultured using special media, serologic assays are the principal means of diagnostic confirmation in the tropics and in developed regions. ELISA-based and microscopic agglutination tests (MAT) using a panel of many serovars are used to identify leptospirosis. The latter are more sensitive and specific in most areas but are time-consuming and require special expertise. PCR and rapid diagnostic formats including dip-stick assays are available in many areas.

Therapeutic management of patients with suspected leptospirosis should not await serologic confirmation. Intravenous penicillin, ceftriaxone, and doxycycline are used in hospitals for treating patients with severe leptospirosis in endemic areas. Treatment with oral doxycycline or amoxicillin may be reasonable alternatives for less severely ill patients.

Consultation with specialty services is based on the severity of presentation and the patient's response to therapy. Specialists from infectious diseases, along with those from neurology, gastroenterology, nutrition, nephrology, hematology, pulmonology, critical care, and rehabilitation medicine, may prove valuable as members of the interprofessional team.

Patient and family education should focus on avoiding potentially contaminated fresh water sources during flooding, especially those near rodents and other zoonotic reservoirs; control of rodent populations; canine vaccination for pets; and control of stray dogs.

Disposition and discharge planning

Follow-up is generally based on the severity of the patient's illness and the possible sequelae of disease. Thus patients may be seen via follow-up with specialists or be scheduled to see their primary care provider as needed.

Education should highlight avoidance of potentially contaminated fresh water exposures, such as walking barefoot through flood waters. Careful observation for fevers and other symptoms after recreational activities such as white-water rafting is also essential. Once-weekly doxycycline may be highly effective as a preventive measure in selected high-risk settings (such as for military personnel performing jungle exercises, or emergency workers during flood relief activities).

> ### Critical Thinking
> Fever in a traveler returning from tropical regions should be considered to be caused by malaria until proven otherwise. When assessing the individual, consider the patient as if he or she had not traveled, and be aware of the possibility of multiple concomitant or sequential infections after a given trip abroad.

VECTOR-BORNE INFECTIONS

John Leake

Vector-borne diseases remain significant causes of illness and death in developed and developing countries, in spite of environmental control measures that have markedly reduced their incidence in many endemic areas. For example, Lyme disease is listed among the top reported U.S. infections (approximately 20,000 cases per year) and plague remains prevalent in approximately 40 countries. Several common features permit categorization of vector-borne diseases as a whole, despite their highly diverse human clinical presentations and vector ecologies:

- Hematophagous arthropod vectors sustain transmission among vertebrate hosts during feeding.
- Vector-borne diseases tend to show seasonality, often peaking during summertime months when climatic conditions favor abundant vector populations.
- Widened geographic distribution and expanded seasonal disease activity may become increasingly common with regional and global climate change.
- For clinical decisions in individual patients, a history of vector exposure is suggestive but only rarely excludes or rigorously supports the diagnosis.
- Benefit may be derived from early treatment to prevent life-threatening illness even prior to laboratory

confirmation, especially with Rocky Mountain spotted fever and plague.
- Common preventive measures may decrease risk of vector-borne diseases, such as insecticide use and personal protective measures to decrease arthropod bites, and environmental control measures to reduce mosquito and other vector populations.

MOSQUITO-BORNE DISEASES

Information on malaria, dengue, and Japanese encephalitis appears earlier in this chapter.

West nile virus

Pathophysiology.   After a period of viremia, the West Nile virus (WNV) gains access to the CNS. Toll-like receptor 3-mediated inflammation appears to facilitate viral transit across the blood–brain barrier (Wang et al., 2004). The basal ganglia, thalami, and other areas within the brain have been shown to contain viral antigen after infection with this pathogen, and viral damage to the anterior horn cells of the spinal cord may result in a polio-like acute flaccid paralysis. Immunosuppression in animal models results in prolonged viremia, decreased humoral responses, and increased pathology both within and outside the CNS.

Epidemiology and etiology.   A variety of medically important arthropod-borne viruses exist throughout the world. In North America, alphaviruses (Western and Eastern equine encephalitis viruses) and flaviviruses (St. Louis encephalitis) have caused sporadic disease in individual patients and modest summertime outbreaks for several decades. In 1999, WNV, which had hitherto been restricted to Africa and parts of Asia, was first detected in New York City. Within 5 years, it was established throughout North America in numerous mosquito and bird species, resulting in substantial disease activity in humans and horses.

The North American WNV outbreak has broadened the understanding of viral transmission (through transfusion, organ transplantation, congenital, and possible human milk routes) and ecology (numerous bird and mosquito species in a complex enzootic cycle of *Culex* mosquito and other vectors overlaid on bird habitats and migratory pathways). As one result of this greater understanding, blood donor screening and enhanced surveillance (in selected areas) for WNV are now performed in the United States and Canada.

Presentation.   Only about one in five WNV-infected persons develops symptoms. Most symptomatic WNV infection presents with abrupt fever, headache, malaise, myalgias, and weakness. Diarrhea and maculopapular rash are common. Approximately 1 of 150 infections results in neuroinvasive disease (encephalitis, meningitis, or acute flaccid paralysis resembling polio). Seizures and movement disorders occur, as in Japanese encephalitis infection; both flaviviruses often affect the thalami and basal ganglia, although WNV antigen can be widely found throughout the brain in experimental models. Age and underlying medical conditions (e.g., immunosuppression after transplantation or chemotherapy) are known risk factors for neuroinvasive disease (Arnold et al., 2005). Rarely, WNV infection results in Guillain-Barré syndrome, myocarditis or cardiac arrhythmias, pancreatitis, hepatitis, and eye disease (optic neuritis, uveitis, chorioretinitis).

Differential diagnosis. The differential diagnosis for WNV infection is broad and includes enterovirus, herpes simplex virus, alphaviral (Western and Eastern equine encephalitis viruses) or other arboviral encephalitis (e.g., St. Louis encephalitis virus), other viral causes of encephalitis (e.g., influenza, parainfluenza, and other respiratory viruses; parvovirus; others), leptospirosis, and community-acquired bacterial (e.g., meningococcal) meningitis (especially if treated with antibiotics before CSF samples are obtained).

Plan of care. Serologic assays detecting IgM and neutralizing antibodies in serum (and in neuroinvasive disease, CSF) support the diagnosis of WNV infection. Care should be exercised in interpreting single positive serologic results, however, as antibody may persist for more than a year (Roehrig et al., 2003). CSF antibody is believed to be more sensitive than PCR for diagnosis of WNV neuroinvasive disease. Nucleic acid amplification and immunohistochemistry may be of value to confirm the presence of WNV, especially in fatal cases.

Therapeutic management consists of supportive care. WNV-containing immunoglobulin preparations and other evaluated therapies (ribavirin, interferon) have yet to be considered of adequate benefit to warrant their use.

Consultation with specialty services is based on the severity of presentation and the patient's response to therapy. Specialists from infectious diseases, along with those from neurology, nutrition, critical care, and rehabilitation medicine, may prove valuable members of the interprofessional team.

Patient and family education should consist of the admission and therapeutic management plan. The involvement of specialists and need for multiple diagnostic studies should be discussed as a component of the comprehensive plan of care.

Disposition and discharge planning. Rehabilitation to improve weakness and sometimes movement and neuropsychiatric disorders may be an important part of the care (Arnold et al., 2005). Follow-up is planned as needed for weakness and neuropsychiatric sequelae.

Prevention. Avoidance of mosquito bites, especially in areas with reported or suspected WNV activity, is highly recommended (see the CDC recommendations at http://wwwnc.cdc.gov/travel/yellowbook/2010/chapter-2/protection-against-mosquitoes-ticks-insects-arthropods.aspx). Vaccine candidates are in development.

Other arboviruses

In addition to WNV, other medically important arboviruses found in North America include Western equine encephalitis virus (WEE), Eastern equine encephalitis virus (EEE), St. Louis encephalitis virus (SLE), Powassan (POW), LaCrosse (LAC), and Colorado tick fever virus (CTF). The location of exposure, patient age, seasonality, and other features may provide diagnostic clues for these illnesses, but the epidemiologic and clinical features of these arbovirus infections overlap with other infectious and noninfectious CNS conditions; thus specialized laboratory testing is necessary to confirm the etiologic agent. The microbiology, epidemiology, vector biology, and clinical features of most medically important arboviruses have been extensively reviewed elsewhere (Calisher, 1994).

TICK-BORNE ILLNESSES

Ixodid (hard-backed) ticks transmit more pathogens than any other invertebrate vector, second only to mosquitoes in causing vector-borne illness.

Lyme disease

Pathophysiology. *Ixodes* ticks acquire *Borrelia burgdorferi* during a blood meal from an infected small mammal (e.g., white-footed mouse). After inoculation of *Borrelia burgdorferi* spirochetes into the skin, the organism disseminates to numerous organs and adheres to a variety of human cells, presumably explaining the potential breadth of clinical symptoms. Outer surface proteins A, B, and C, along with flagellar and other proteins, trigger cell-mediated and humoral immune responses that usually protect against subsequent infection. Persons treated early during infection may have negative serologic results.

Epidemiology and etiology. In addition to spreading Lyme disease, *Ixodes* ticks may transmit anaplasmosis or babesiosis. Deer play a role in the tick life cycle but do not serve as infectious reservoirs. Lyme disease incidence peaks in summer and early fall along with maximal (especially nymphal deer) tick activity. New England and the Mid-Atlantic States, the upper Midwest, and northern California are major U.S. disease foci.

Presentation. The clinical Lyme disease spectrum includes three categories: early localized, early disseminated, or late disease. *Early localized disease*, the most common manifestation and one that usually precedes other stages when they occur, consists primarily of the erythema migrans rash. Rash occurs at recent tick bite sites, starting as an erythematous macule or papule that expands to more 5 cm, sometimes with a central unaffected zone referred to as a "target lesion" (Figure 30-2). Fever, headache, myalgia, and arthralgia are common in the first week of infection. Facial nerve palsy should be presumed to be due to Lyme disease until proven otherwise in endemic areas. Cardiac conduction abnormalities and CNS manifestations are sometimes serious complications that occur less commonly in pediatric patients.

Differential diagnosis. The differential diagnoses for Lyme disease include influenza, anaplasmosis, babesia, viral or (less likely) bacterial meningoencephalitis, acute disseminated encephalomyelitis, Bell's palsy, Rocky Mountain spotted fever, Epstein-Barr virus, pauciarticular juvenile rheumatoid arthritis (children), and reactive arthritis or Reiter's syndrome (adults).

Plan of care. Recognition of erythema migrans is usually sufficient for diagnosis in endemic areas. During the first month of infection, serologic assays are not ideally sensitive. Screening assays followed by confirmatory Western blot testing remain the diagnostic. The diagnostic test of choice. Serial serologic tests are generally not beneficial for predicting response to treatment.

For early localized disease, the therapeutic management in children aged 8 years and older is doxycycline 100 mg orally 3 times per day for 14 to 21 days; for children younger than 8 years of age and those intolerant of doxycycline, amoxicillin 50 mg/kg/day divided 3 times per day or cefuroxime 30 mg/kg/day divided 2 times per day for 14 to 21 days is acceptable. For early disseminated and late disease, treatment is as follows:

- For multiple erythema migrans, the same oral regimen as for early localized disease but for 21 days
- For isolated facial nerve palsy, the same oral regimen as for early localized disease but for 21 to 28 days
- For arthritis, the same oral regimen as for early localized disease but for 28 days

For persistent or recurrent arthritis, carditis, or meningitis/encephalitis, intravenous ceftriaxone 75 to 100 mg/kg/day (maximum of 2 gm daily) for 14 to 28 days, or penicillin 300,000 unit/kg/day in divided doses every 4 hours (maximum of 20 million unit/day) for 14 to 28 days, is recommended.

Consultation with specialty services is based on the severity of presentation and the patient's response to therapy. Specialists from infectious diseases, along with those from neurology, cardiology, rheumatology, critical care,

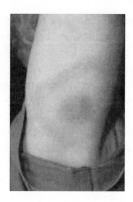

FIGURE 30-2

Lyme Disease – Target Lesion.
Source: Courtesy of CDC/James Gathany.

and rehabilitation medicine, may prove valuable members of the interprofessional team.

Patient and family education should consist of the admission and therapeutic management plan. The involvement of specialists and need for multiple diagnostic studies should be discussed as a component of the comprehensive plan of care.

Disposition and discharge planning. Extremely prolonged or multiple repeated courses of antibiotics are very rarely needed (Wormser et al., 2006). Follow-up is planned with specialty services as indicated based on the extent of the disease, such as cardiology, infectious diseases, neurology, and rheumatology.

A previously licensed vaccine for Lyme disease is no longer available due to low demand. Prevention consists of avoiding tick-infested areas, wearing protective clothing, using insect (especially DEET-containing) repellants applied to exposed skin and clothing as directed, inspecting children and pets for tick attachment, and removing ticks using proper technique. Prophylactic antibiotics are not recommended for asymptomatic tick bite exposure.

Tularemia

Pathophysiology. The causative agent of tularemia is *Francisella tularensis*, a Gram-negative coccobacillus. Once in the body, this organism replicates within macrophages and is transported to regional lymph nodes and the liver, spleen, and kidney. Multiple organ failure, sepsis, acute respiratory distress syndrome, and necrotizing granulomas in affected tissues are characteristics among fatal cases and animal models (Michell et al., 2006).

Epidemiology and etiology. Tularemia is primarily a tick-borne illness; *Dermacentor* and *Ixodes* ticks serve as its principal vectors. Rarely, disease may be due to ingestion of contaminated water, improperly cooked meat, or after exposure to infective aerosols (e.g., after mowing lawns near dead infective rabbit carcasses).

Presentation. Clinical manifestations comprise several syndromes, among which ulceroglandular and glandular tularemia are most frequent. Along with abrupt fever, chills, headache, and myalgias, ulceroglandular tularemia starts with a maculopapular lesion at the entry site, with subsequent slow-to-heal, painful lymphadenopathy with or without ulceration (ulceroglandular and glandular, respectively). Oculoglandular, oropharyngeal, intestinal, typhoidal, and pneumonic presentations are less common. Typhoidal and pneumonic tularemia are associated with the highest fatality rates (more than 30%) and may arise from progression after untreated ulceroglandular or glandular disease, or from inhalation of the aerosolized organisms. Fever, cough, dyspnea, chest pain/pleuritis, and hilar lymphanopathy are hallmarks of pneumonic tularemia (Goodman et al., 2005).

Differential diagnosis. Plague, cat-scratch disease, tuberculosis, brucellosis, bacterial pneumonia, and sepsis should be considered in the differential diagnosis for tularemia.

Plan of care. Serologic assays above a diagnostic cutoff value (usually greater than 1:128) or with a fourfold rise between acute and convalescent sera very strongly support diagnosis of acute infection; direct fluorescent-antibody assay (DFA) or PCR on a tissue specimen (e.g., ulcer aspirate) are used for conclusive disease confirmation. Blood, skin, ulcer, or respiratory tract cultures may permit growth in specialized (cysteine-enriched) media.

Aminoglycosides (especially streptomycin and gentamicin), ciprofloxacin, and doxycycline are active against most strains that cause tularemia. Resistance to beta lactams (penicillins, cephalosporins) is to be expected.

Consultation with specialty services is based on the severity of presentation and the patient's response to therapy. Specialists from infectious diseases, along with those from neurology, pulmonology, gastroenterology, nutrition, ophthalmology, critical care, and rehabilitation medicine, may prove valuable members of the interprofessional team.

Patient and family education should consist of the admission and therapeutic management plan. The involvement of specialists and need for multiple diagnostic studies should be discussed as a component of the comprehensive plan of care.

Disposition and discharge planning. Follow-up is generally based on the severity of the patient's illness and the possible sequelae of disease. Thus patients may be seen on follow-up with specialists or be scheduled to see their primary care provider as needed.

Arthropod-bite preventive measures and checking for tick bites, care in handling wild rabbits and other potentially infected carcasses, and vaccination for laboratory workers are recommended for disease prevention.

Rocky mountain spotted fever

Pathophysiology. Infection with *Rickettsia rickettsii*, an obligate intracellular Gram-negative coccobacillus, results in the systemic vasculitis associated with Rocky Mountain spotted fever (RMSF). The organisms localize to vascular endothelium in numerous sites.

Epidemiology and etiology. Transmission occurs after tick bite with *Dermacentor* (or rarely other) ticks, or very rarely after blood transfusion. Outdoor activity and pet ownership are risk factors; most disease occurs in the summertime. Lack of known recent tick bite should not discount the possibility of infection in endemic areas. In the United States, most cases occur in the Southeast and South Central states; disease occurs in selected areas throughout the Americas.

Presentation. After an incubation period of approximately one week (range of 2 to 14 days), fever, severe headache, and myalgia are usually present, often accompanied by vomiting and decreased appetite. On days 2 to 5 after onset of fever, most patients (approximately 80%) develop a characteristic rash on the wrists, ankles, palms, and soles, which may spread rapidly to the trunk. Thrombocytopenia is common and, less reliably, leukopenia or anemia; hyponatremia is frequently observed. Severe disease may variably manifest within the CNS, heart, lungs, intestinal tract, and kidneys.

Differential diagnosis. The differential diagnoses for consideration are meningococcemia, enterovirus, typhus, anaplasmosis, ehrlichiosis, typhoid, dengue, leptospirosis, Epstein-Barr virus, gastroenteritis, and pneumonia.

Plan of care. The diagnosis of RMSF is confirmed by serologic assays (especially immunofluorescent assay) measuring rickettsial group-specific antibodies, which often do not appear until days 7 to 10 of illness; serial antibody measurements are, therefore, appropriate. Immunohistochemistry or PCR may also be used to confirm RMSF from tissue specimens, including a rash site (ideally obtained before antibiotics or less than 24 hours after initiation of antibiotics).

For therapeutic management, doxycycline is favored for all patients of ages for 7 to 10 days, until fever has ceased for 72 hours, and until clinical disease has resolved; doxycycline is associated with better treatment outcomes, and there is low risk of dental staining given the treatment regimen required. Fluoroquinolones may be used but data on their effectiveness are limited. Chloramphenicol was the previous standard but is no longer recommended because of risks of serious adverse reactions. *Treatment should not await serologic confirmation in the appropriate epidemiologic and clinical setting.*

Consultation with specialty services is based on the severity of presentation and the patient's response to therapy. Specialists from infectious diseases, along with those from hematology, neurology, critical care, and rehabilitation medicine, may prove valuable as members of the interprofessional team.

Patient and family education should consist of the admission and therapeutic management plan. The involvement of specialists and need for multiple diagnostic studies should be discussed as a component of the comprehensive plan of care. Long-term rehabilitation may also be indicated, and discussion with the family should include support for continued care outside of the hospital environment.

Disposition and discharge planning. The illness may take several weeks to resolve. Disseminated intravascular coagulation (DIC) and the septic-shock-like picture leads to death in approximately 25% of untreated patients. Sequelae are most often related to CNS manifestations (hearing loss, weakness, peripheral neuropathy, incontinence, cerebellar and motor disorders) or limb amputation (Dantas-Torres, 2007).

Follow-up is planned with specialty services based on the extent of the patient's disease; services consulted may include infectious diseases, audiology, neurology, gastroenterology, hematology, and orthopedics. For all persons, it is important to use the same tick preventive measures as for Lyme disease.

Other tick-borne diseases

Several other medically important tick-borne infections are reported more rarely in the United States, and result from either sporadic endemic transmission or travel. Among these are the following conditions:

- Anaplasmosis (*A. phagocytophilum*)
- Ehrlichiosis (*E. chaffeensis, E. ewingii*)
- Babesiosis
- Tick-borne relapsing fever (*Borrelia hermsii, B. recurrentis*)
- Colorado tick fever
- Tick-borne encephalitis (especially after travel to northern or central Europe; a vaccine for this infection is available)

These conditions have been comprehensively reviewed elsewhere (Calisher, 1994; Goodman et al., 2005; Spach et al., 1993).

FLEA-BORNE ILLNESSES: PLAGUE

Pathophysiology. *Yersinia pestis*, a Gram negative coccobacillus, is the biologic agent of plague. After the bite of an infective flea, the organisms migrate to regional lymph nodes, where they survive phagocytosis by mononuclear cells and induce hemorrhagic necrosis resulting in the intensely swollen, painful nodes characteristic of bubonic plague. Dissemination may occur to other lymph nodes, liver, spleen, and elsewhere, with resultant hypotension. In pneumonic plague, the bacilli enter the lungs through inhalation or hematogenously. Meningitis can also occur.

Epidemiology and etiology. Plague is maintained in an enzootic cycle between in flea and rodent populations throughout a large rural area in the western United States; New Mexico, Arizona, and Colorado report the majority of cases. Numerous disease foci exist worldwide, especially in Madagascar and elsewhere in Africa.

Presentation. Like tularemia, plague presents as one of several classic syndromes. *Bubonic plague* is characterized by acute fever with a large, painful regional node (bubo) in the groin, axilla, or neck (Figure 30-3). Septicemic plague causes severe overwhelming sepsis with shock, DIC, and multiple organ failure. The diagnosis is more difficult in the rare subset of patients presenting without a bubo. Pneumonic plague presents with cough, dyspnea, chest pain, and sometimes hemoptysis; patients with pneumonic plague (but not other disease variants) can spread the disease via person-to-person contact. Septicemic and pneumonic disease forms are associated with high case fatality (25% to more than 50%).

Differential diagnosis. The differential diagnosis for plague includes tularemia, bacterial sepsis (e.g., meningococcemia),

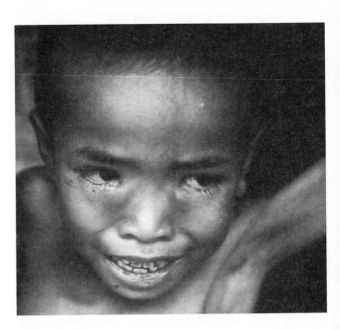

FIGURE 30-3

Axillary bubo.

Source: Courtesy of CDC.

cat-scratch disease, staphylococcal or streptococcal lymphadenitis, tuberculosis, and brucellosis.

Plan of care. Collection of lymph node (bubo) aspirate, blood culture, or another clinical specimen usually allows recovery of the organism in culture. Gram stains reveal characteristic pleomorphic bipolar "safety pin" morphology. Fluorescent antibody tests, serologic assays (among unvaccinated persons), PCR, and immunohistochemistry are sometimes used to confirm the diagnosis.

Streptomycin, gentamicin, doxycycline, and ciprofloxacin are the usual recommended therapies. Surgical drainage of lymph nodes may be warranted.

Consultation with specialty services is based on the severity of presentation and the patient's response to therapy. Specialists from infectious diseases, along with those from neurology, pulmonology, hematology, critical care, and rehabilitation medicine, may prove valuable members of the interprofessional team.

Patient and family education should consist of the admission and therapeutic management plan. The involvement of specialists and need for multiple diagnostic studies should be discussed as a component of the comprehensive plan of care. Long-term rehabilitation may also be indicated, and discussion with the family should include support for continued care outside of the hospital environment.

Disposition and discharge planning. Follow-up is generally based on the severity of the patient's illness and the possible sequelae of disease. Thus patients may be seen on follow-up with specialists or be scheduled to see their primary care provider as needed.

Avoidance of rodents and rodent fleas and vaccination for laboratory workers are recommended as preventive strategies.

VIRAL INFECTIONS

David Nathalang

ADENOVIRUS

Pathophysiology

Adenovirus is a double-stranded, non-enveloped DNA virus belonging to the Adenoviridae family; it has 51 serotypes. Initial attachment by the virus to the host cell membrane receptors is a relatively slow process, taking up to 6 hours, that is accomplished by a variety of viral surface proteins. After attachment, penetration of the host cell occurs rapidly by either endocytosis or direct invasion, and viral nucleic acid is released into the host cell. Viral proteins allow for control of the host cell functions and the synthesis of new virus, which are released after cell lysis (Lenaerts

et al., 2008). The incubation period with this type of infection is usually 2 to 14 days for respiratory illnesses and 3 to 10 days for gastroenteritis (AAP, 2009).

Epidemiology and etiology

Persons of all ages are susceptible to infection with adenovirus, and incidence is inversely related to age. Patients younger than 5 years tend to be at highest risk of infection, which is worsened when patients are grouped together, as seen with daycare programs or the overcrowding prevalent among lower -socioeconomic populations (AAP, 2009). Males are at slightly higher risk of infection compared to females (Cherry & Chen, 2009). Infections can occur sporadically throughout the year, especially with gastroenteritis, although respiratory disease epidemics usually occur between winter and early summer.

Close contact is usually necessary for effective spread of adenovirus, although this requirement varies with different serotypes. Transmission is typically accomplished by airborne virus-containing droplets that contact the mucous membranes of the nose and orophaynx; small-particle droplets may travel farther than larger-sized droplets and infect lower respiratory tract structures. Conjunctiva can be infected via droplet contact, direct contact with contaminated fingers, or contact with contaminated fluids; the last route is the primary mode of transmission causing epidemic keratoconjunctivits due to contaminated swimming pools. Gastrointestinal infection may be due to fecal–oral transmission or swallowed virus during a respiratory infection. Fomite spread is possible and is an important cause of nosocomial infections. Disinfection can be accomplished by immersion in 1% sodium hypochlorite solution for 10 minutes or steam autoclaving; adenovirus is resistant to alcohol, detergents, and chlorhexidine (Demmler, 2008). Transmission of adenovirus is also possible via transplanted tissue.

Presentation

The majority of infections are benign and self-limited, involving the respiratory tract, eyes, or GI system. Along with symptoms of the common cold, acute febrile pharyngitis and tonsillitis are common. Fever, exudative tonsillitis, and cervical lymphadenopathy usually last for 5 to 7 days, but may persist for as long as 2 weeks (Cherry & Chen, 2009). Pneumonia caused by adenovirus is usually acute, presenting with fever and cough. Crackles and sometimes wheezes can be heard on examination. More severe forms can be seen with serotypes 3, 7, and 21, which may result in tachypnea and dyspnea due to hypoxia or hypercarbia. Survivors can develop obliterative bronchiolitis, bronchiectasis, or hyperlucent lung syndrome, characterized by a decrease in pulmonary vasculature and decreased peripheral air entry. Besides pneumonia, adenovirus may cause bronchiolitis, a benign laryngotracheobronchitis, and a pertussis-like syndrome.

Ocular manifestations are commonly benign, such as follicular conjunctivitis characterized by an erythematous conjunctiva with itching, burning, increased lacrimation, and a foreign body sensation. Most episodes of conjunctivitis last for 10 days to 3 weeks without complication. In contrast to follicular conjunctivitis, epidemic keratoconjunctivitis may cause prolonged symptoms and usually results from exposure to a contaminated source, such as swimming pools, ophthalmic instruments, or hand contact. Photophobia, hyperemia, conjunctival edema, and lacrimation occur after an incubation period of 5 to 10 days, with some presentations mimicking bacterial periorbital cellulitis. After 7 to 10 days, painful, punctuate epithelial opacities develop on the corneal center, coinciding with resolution of the conjunctivitis. In some patients, these epithelial opacities heal with residual subepithelial infiltrates, and persistent vision changes can occur in severe cases. Conjunctivitis associated with fever and pharyngitis is the hallmark of pharyngoconjunctival fever.

Gastroenteritis typically affects pediatric patients younger than the age of 3 years predominantly with diarrhea, although concurrent abdominal pain and vomiting are possible. Gastroenteritis can be the primary illness or in association with other adenoviral infections. Both mesenteric lymphadenitis and appendicitis have been known to present with lower right quadrant pain, pharyngitis, and fever. Other possible GI manifestations include hepatitis and intussusception.

In immunocompromised patients, pneumonitis, gastroenteritis, hepatic failure, colitis, hemorrhagic cystitis, and meningoencephalitis are all possible manifestations (Lenaerts et al., 2008). Diarrhea and fever tend to be the initial clinical presentations. Severe disseminated disease with multiple organ involvement or sepsis-like presentations with cardiovascular compromise are also possible in either immunocompromised or very young patients.

In addition to those infections previously described, cardiac, neurologic, genitourinary, and systemic presentations may arise (Table 30-20).

Differential diagnosis

The following disorders and diseases may be evaluated in the presentation of adenovirus:

- Pharyngitis
  - Other viruses: influenza, Epstein-Barr virus (EBV), enterovirus
  - *Streptococcus pneumoniae*
- Pneumonia
  - Other viral lower respiratory infections: respiratory syncytial virus (RSV), influenza
  - Bacterial infections
- Conjunctivitis
  - Herpes virus
  - *Neisseria gonorrhoea*

TABLE 30-20

Summary of Adenoviral Infections

Respiratory	Common cold, nasopharyngitis, pharyngitis, tonsillitis, otitis media, pharyngoconjunctival fever, bronchitis, laryngotracheobronchitis, bronchiolitis, pertussis-like syndrome, pneumonia, pleural effusions, obliterative bronchiolitis, bronchiectasis, hyperlucent lung syndrome
Ocular	Follicular conjunctivitis, hemorrhagic conjunctivitis, pharyngoconjunctival fever, keratoconjunctivitis, oculogenital syndrome
Gastrointestinal	Gastroenteritis, mesenteric lymphadenitis, appendicitis, intussusception, hepatitis, hepatic failure, colitis
Skin	Erythematous maculopapular rash, Stevens-Johnson syndrome
Genitourinary	Hemorrhagic cystitis, nephritis, urethritis, cervicitis, genital lesions, orchitis, oculogenital syndrome, hemolytic-uremic syndrome, hemorrhagic fever with renal syndrome
Cardiac	Myocarditis, dilated cardiomyopathy, pericarditis
Neurologic	Meningitis, meningoencephalitis, encephalitis, transverse myelitis, Reye-like syndrome
Miscellaneous	Arthritis, thyroiditis, deafness, mononucleosis-like syndrome, Kawasaki-like syndrome

- Gastroenteritis
  - Other viral infections
  - Bacterial causes

Plan of care

With the exception of serotypes 40 and 41, adenovirus is readily identifiable by cell culture, with growth typically present after 3 to 5 days. Positive culture from blood, pleural fluid, pericardial fluid, or CSF is indicative of disseminated or severe disease. Due to the possibility of positive culture even without disease, however, results obtained from nasopharyngeal, throat, urine, or stool samples should be correlated with clinical symptoms.

Antigen identification by immunofluorescence, ELISA, or latex agglutination is used for rapid identification of virus or confirmation of culture results and can detect serotypes 40 and 41 (which do not grow well on culture). Viral nucleic acid can be detected by PCR or probe hybridization. PCR has also been used to quantify the viral load in immunocompromised patients serially, allowing for early detection of infection and measurement of treatment effectiveness.

Serologic diagnosis of adenoviral infection requires an increase in antibody titers between two serially collected specimens. In part due to the difficulty of obtaining a pre-illness or convalescent serum sample, serologic studies are not recommended for identification of acute infection; instead, they are typically reserved for epidemiologic studies.

Adenovirus infections are usually benign and self-limited. Thus therapeutic management is usually supportive in nature, involving fever control with acetaminophen, proper hydration, and rest during acute episodes. Severe lower respiratory infections may require supplemental oxygen and mechanical ventilation for hypoxia and hypercarbia. Overwhelming infection may cause cardiovascular compromise, necessitating the use of vasopressor and inotropic agents. Immunosuppression medications should be decreased or stopped if possible; the risks of acute rejection should be weighed against the benefit of decreased immunosuppression during an acute infection. Ophthalmology specialists should be consulted for patients with keratoconjunctivitis.

Although multiple antiviral agents have been used, none have show consistent success against the wide spectrum of adenovirus infections. Cidofovir has been successful in treatment of adenovirus infections in immunodeficient patients and patients with hemorrhagic cystitis and keratoconjunctivitis; hydration and probenicid should be employed simultaneously to avoid nephrotoxicity (Lenaerts et al., 2008). Ribavirin has been demonstrated to be effective against disseminated and other types of infection in immunocompromised patients; nevertheless, there is not enough evidence to support its regular use as a first-line agent (Echavarria, 2008). Anemia is the most common adverse effect of ribavirin treatment, but is reversible after discontinuation of the medication.

Contact precautions should be enforced for patients with conjunctivitis and for patients with gastroenteritis who are diapered or incontinent. Both contact and droplet precautions should be used for patients with respiratory infections requiring hospitalization.

Normal infection control emphasizing good hand hygiene should be enforced to limit viral transmission. Cover coughs to limit transmission by airborne droplets. Avoid finger-to-eye contact in the case of ocular involvement.

Patient and family education should include information regarding the majority of adenoviral infections are self-limited and benign. Supportive treatment, with fever control and rest, is the usual therapy. Proper hydration is essential in the care of gastroenteritis, and the patient or family should consult an HCP if symptoms are excessive, worsen, or persist.

Disposition and discharge planning

Typically follow-up is not required for most infections. Severe infections with possible sequelae should be followed by the appropriate specialist.

The prognosis with most adenoviral infections is usually good, although severe or complicated infections may be associated with permanent sequelae. Patients with keratoconjunctivitis may have persistent vision changes, and should be followed by an ophthalmologist, whereas patients who exhibit signs or symptoms of residual lung disease should be followed by a pulmonologist.

CYTOMEGALOVIRUS

Pathophysiology

Cytomegalovirus (CMV) is a double-stranded DNA of the Herpesviridae family. Its initial attachment to host cell membranes is accomplished via glycoproteins on the viral envelope. After fusion with the cell membrane, the viral genome is introduced into the host cell's nucleus, resulting in synthesis of viral proteins and viral protein assembly. Due to viral DNA and protein buildup over the next 20 hours, the size of the host cell increases greatly, causing the "cytomegaly" for which the virus is known, as well as large "owl's eye" intranuclear inclusions. Approximately 24 hours after the initial invasion, the virus acquires an envelope as it exits the nucleus and is released from the host cell. The virus then spreads by viremia to multiple organs, including the kidneys, lungs, liver, and brain. The incubation period of CMV is usually 3 to 12 weeks for CMV acquired by blood transfusion and 1 to 4 months for CMV acquired by tissue transplantation (AAP, 2009).

After the primary infection, CMV remains in a latent form within leukocytes and tissue. Reactivation of the virus may occur with immunodeficiency, like that seen with post-transplant immunosuppression or HIV infection. CMV may be responsible for suppression of the T-cell response to viral presence, explaining its ability to remain in the host after the primary infection ends (Demmler-Harrison, 2009).

Epidemiology and etiology

CMV infection is common and can be affected by host characteristics such as age, gender, and race. Although there is no seasonal increase in incidence of CMV, certain periods during life are associated with increased infection. Congenital CMV infection is seen in 0.2% to 2.2% of all live births, with 10% to 20% of affected infants presenting with some type of defect, including hearing loss, ocular damage, or cognitive or motor dysfunction (AAP, 2009). Close grouping of children, as seen with lower-socioeconomic populations and daycare programs, is a definite risk factor for CMV infection; it is one reason why children ages 1 to 3 years have the highest prevalence of active CMV infection. Another period of increased infection occurs during adolescence, when intimate contact and sexual activity are risk factors for transmission. The last period of increased infection is during childbearing.

Vertical transmission may occur during intrauterine life or perinatally. CMV can cross the placenta and infect the fetus before birth, leading to congenital defects. Perinatal infections can occur either during birth due to contact with CMV-saturated secretions during vaginal delivery or after birth due to ingestion of CMV-infected human milk or contact with contaminated saliva.

Horizontal transmission can occur from direct contact, by contact with contaminated secretions, or by fomite transmission. Direct contact is major cause of transmission within close groupings of children, resulting in the high rate of infection associated with daycare programs (Pass, 2008). Saliva, urine, seminal, and cervical secretions all can be infected with CMV, leading to higher incidences of infection seen with increased sexual activity. Fomites are a major source of infection in the hospital setting.

Latent CMV persists in blood products, so infection after transfusion is a possibility. The risk of infection can be reduced by processing blood products prior to transfusion. CMV can also be found in transplanted tissues such as bone marrow and solid organs; transmission via this method can lead to significant morbidity or mortality in an immunosuppressed recipient.

Presentation

Congenitally infected infants are usually healthy with no clinical symptoms at birth. However, CMV infection is associated with unilateral or bilateral hearing loss in some patients. Moreover, a subset of patients present with hearing loss later in life instead of presenting at birth; these complications may be missed by newborn hearing tests (Demmler-Harrison, 2009). Severely affected newborns can present with a variety of neurologic symptoms, such as microcephaly, seizures, and poor muscle tone. Some patients will have cytomegalic inclusion disease, classically associated with intrauterine growth retardation; hepatosplenomegaly; pneumonia; thrombocytopenia; and neurologic dysfunction presenting as microcephaly, chorioretinitis, or hearing loss. "Blueberry muffin" lesions—dark magenta-colored papules or nodules—may be seen as well, although they are usually associated with rubella-associated congenital infections.

Infection with CMV in older pediatric patients is common and usually remains asymptomatic. In other individuals, CMV may cause mononucleosis syndrome, which usually presents with prolonged fever and severe malaise, as well as a maculopapular or rubelliform rash, headaches, abdominal pain, and myalgias in some patients. Similar to EBV-caused mononucleosis, patients can have a morbilliform rash with ampicillin administration. Unlike EBV-caused mononucleosis, patients usually do not present with pharyngitis, tonsillitis, or splenomegaly. Rare complications include pneumonitis, myocarditis, splenic infarction,

adrenal insufficiency, and meningoencephalitis, among others.

Pneumonia is another possible presentation of CMV infection and is usually benign. In contrast, the interstitial pneumonitis seen in immunocompromised patients is associated with severe morbidity and mortality. This disease presents initially with fever and cough, progressing to hypoxia and respiratory embarrassment with concomitant diffuse interstitial infiltrates on chest radiographs. Patients with pneumonitis usually have a poor outcome, and the mortality in this population is high.

Gastrointestinal symptoms are usually characterized by self-limited episodes of dysphagia, abdominal pain, nausea, vomiting, diarrhea, and feeding intolerance, although hemorrhage is occasionally seen. Patients may present with severe dehydration or weight loss due to inadequate feeding or inability to compensate for fluid losses. Occasionally, a mild hepatitis with hepatomegaly is noted in some patients, but it usually does not progress to liver failure.

Neurological symptoms are often seen in congenital CMV infections and are associated with necrotizing encephalitis in those patients. Clinically, these patients present with microcephaly, cerebral palsy, seizures, and neurodevelopmental delay. In older patients, CMV infection can cause encephalitis and occasionally myelitis, which may present with an ascending paralysis similar to that seen in Guillain-Barré syndrome. Meningoencephalitis occasionally accompanies mononucleosis, causing photophobia, headache, and nuchal rigidity in affected patients. Risk of chorioretinitis is higher in newborns with symptomatic disease and is associated with white, perivascular infiltrates, hemorrhage, and necrosis. In neonates and infants, the only ocular findings may be failure to track and strabismus.

CMV is a significant cause of morbidity and mortality in immunocompromised patients, who may initially present with symptoms of nonspecific fever, malaise, and arthralgias. Pneumonia, retinitis, and GI illness tend to cause the most morbidity in this population. In patients who have received stem cell transplants, pneumonia is a common concern, in addition to GI disease (Pass, 2008). Retinitis may cause minimal, nonspecific symptoms initially, but can progress to vision changes and total blindness if severe; notably, retinitis is the most common CMV-associated disease in patients with AIDS (Gandhi & Khanna, 2004). Gastritis, hepatitis, gastroenteritis, and pancreatitis are all possible GI manifestations, while neurologic processes, such as encephalitis and painful neuropathies, can also occur. CMV infection after solid-organ transplant is more likely to involve the transplanted organ (Gandhi & Khanna); pneumonitis is seen in transplanted lungs, and hepatitis can occur in transplanted livers (Table 30-21).

TABLE 30-21

Summary of Cytomegalovirus Infections

Congenital	Hearing loss, microcephaly, seizures, hepatomegaly, hepatitis, splenomegaly, thrombocytopenia, hemolytic anemia, ascites, Dandy-Walker-like malformations, cognitive and motor deficiencies, chorioretinitis, optic atrophy, cytomegalic inclusion disease, growth retardation, pneumonia/pneumonitis, long bone osteitis, cutaneous vasculitis, sepsis-like syndrome, "blueberry muffin" lesions
Systemic	Mononucleosis
Pulmonary	Pneumonia, pneumonitis
Cardiac	Myocarditis, pericarditis
Neurologic	Meningoencephalitis, encephalitis, myelitis, peripheral neuropathy, polyradiculopathy, Guillain-Barré syndrome
Ocular	Chorioretinits, uveitis
Hearing	Sensorineural hearing loss, labyrinthitis, Ménière's syndrome
Gastrointestinal	Acute gastroenteritis, hepatitis, splenic infarction, ulcerative colitis, proctitis
Hematologic	Hemolytic anemia, thrombocytopenia
Musculoskeletal	Arthralgias, arthritis
Skin	Maculopapular rash, thrombocytopenia-associated petechia and purpura, ampicillin rash
Miscellaneous	Adrenal insufficiency

Differential diagnosis

The following disorders and diseases may be evaluated in the presentation of CMV:

- Congenital CMV infection
  - Other TORCH infections: toxoplasmosis, HSV, syphilis, rubella
  - HIV
  - Genetic or metabolic disorder
  - Intrauterine exposure to medications, toxins
- Mononucleosis
  - EBV
  - Hepatitis A or B
  - HIV
  - Rubella
  - Adenovirus
  - Herpesvirus 6, 7, or 8
- Pneumonia and pneumonitis
  - Other viral pneumonias: HSV, varicella-zoster, measles, RSV, influenza, adenovirus

- Bacterial pneumonia: *Streptococcus, Staphylococcus*
- Aspiration pneumonia
- Pulmonary hemorrhage
- Cardiac disease
  - Other viral causes: adenovirus, EBV
  - Congenital cardiac disease
- Gastrotenteritis
  - Other viruses: enterovirus, rotovirus, adenovirus
  - Bacteria: *Salmonella, Shigella, Campylobacter*
  - Parasitic disease: *Cryptosporidium, Giardia*
- Neurologic disease
  - Viral infections: toxoplasmosis, HSV, influenza
  - Bacterial infections: *Pneumococcus, Meningococcus*
  - Genetic or metabolic disorders: galactosemia, urea-cycle deficiencies, hypothyroidism

Plan of care

CMV can be isolated by cell culture from a variety of sources, including urine, saliva, naospharyngeal and sinus washings, bronchoalveolar lavage samples, conjunctiva, tears, middle ear fluid, human milk, peripheral blood, semen, cervical or vaginal secretions, CSF, amniotic fluid, or tissue biopsy. Most cultures grow within 1 to 2 weeks, although results can vary between 1 day to 6 weeks depending on the concentration of virus in the sample studied (Demmler-Harrison, 2009). Shell vial assay—a technique involving the preparation of samples with antigen detection via fluorescein-conjugated monoclonal antibody—can increase the speed with which identification can be made and is particularly reliable when used on samples obtained by bronchoalveolar lavage or urine.

Cytologic identification can be accomplished by visualization of type A Cowdry inclusions inside the nucleus of enlarged infected cells and is best done for urine, bronchoalveolar lavage, and biopsy samples. CMV antigens can also be detected by various types of assays, including immunofluorescent assays, latex agglutination assays, and enzyme immunoassays. CMV pp65 antigen can be detected in the white blood cells of patients; results can be obtained within 24 hours (AAP, 2009).

Detection of CMV DNA can be performed by PCR or DNA hybridization techniques. PCR is highly sensitive for CMV and has the added benefit of being able to quantify a patient's viral load. When this technology is used to detect CMV DNA in the CSF of a symptomatic newborn, the presence of CMV is correlated with higher morbidity.

Serologic testing can be performed by comparing antibody titers measured in the patient when symptomatic to titers measured when the patient is asymptomatic. A four-fold increase in paired specimens is considered diagnostic for infection. However, testing for seroconversion is usually clinically invaluable, as baseline titers must be obtained during convalescence. Moreover, development of increased IgM antibodies has been seen with reactivation of CMV.

Patients with mononucleosis will present with mild elevation of hepatic aminotransaminases, peripheral lymphocytosis, and elevated ESR, but will not have heterophil antibodies. Congenital CMV infection is best confirmed with a positive viral culture within 3 weeks of birth (Pass, 2008); PCR testing for viral nucleic acid is also possible. Prenatal testing, such as fetal ultrasound and amniocentesis, may be used for virus detection or to demonstrate evidence of CMV infection.

Fortunately, most CMV infections are either asymptomatic or benign. Nevertheless, a subset of patients, especially extremely young or immunocompromised patients, will be severely affected. In those patients, initial therapeutic management should target cardiovascular and respiratory compromise. Patients with hemodynamic instability should have fluids administered, with inotropic agents used as needed. Patients with respiratory issues should receive supplemental oxygen and may require positive-pressure ventilation. Standard isolation protocols should be employed.

Antiviral therapy is rarely used in immunocompetent patients with mild disease. For immunocompromised patients, induction with an antiviral agent for 2 to 3 weeks followed by a maintenance period lasting as long as needed—and indefinitely in the case of immunodeficiency—should be considered (Demmler-Harrison, 2009). Ganciclovir is the usual first-line antiviral agent used for CMV infection; it has been used for both induction and maintenance of CMV infections, and has shown some benefit when used for congenital infections. It may be associated with dose-related neutropenia, anemia, and thrombocytopenia (Biron, 2006). Valganciclovir is a prodrug of ganciclovir that can be taken orally; this route of administration leads to similar serum drug levels as IV ganciclovir (Biron). Foscarnet has been used for ganciclovir-resistant disease in immunocompromised patients, although its adverse effects profile, which includes medication-related kidney toxicity, limits its widespread usage. Cidofovir has not been well studied in children, but the literature shows favorable results in adult patients with HIV (AAP, 2009). This agent is also associated with nephrotoxicity, however. For CMV retinitis, fomivirsen can be used as an intraocular treatment.

Given that most transmission of CMV occurs via direct contact, contaminated fluids, or fomites, good hand hygiene and education are important to prevent infection. CMV-negative blood products should be administered to seronegative patients; if they are not available, blood products can be filtered to remove white blood cells, frozen in glycerol prior to administration, or have buffy coats removed to decrease the chance of CMV transmission (AAP, 2009). Prophylactic antiviral therapy is also a possible method of prevention.

Family education includes discussion of the risk of symptomatic congenital infections and hearing loss that may present later in life; normal newborn hearing screening will not detect hearing loss in these patients. As noted earlier, proper hand washing is important to prevent the spread of CMV. Pregnant patients should know their CMV serologic status and take steps to prevent primary CMV infection if they are seronegative.

Disposition and discharge planning

Most CMV infections are benign and self-limited. Congenital CMV infection is associated with significant long-term morbidity; hearing loss is the most common sequela of congenital infection and may progress in some patients (Demmler-Harrison, 2009). Retinitis may be reactivated in some patients later in life. Thus follow-up with specialists who include, but are not limited to, specialists in ophthalmology, otolaryngology, rehabilitative medicine, nutrition, and gastroenterology may be required to promote best care and quality of life.

EPSTEIN-BARR VIRUS

Pathophysiology

Epstein-Barr virus is a double-stranded DNA virus of the Herpesviridae family, with two major genotypes. Its initial invasion of nasopharyngeal epithelial cells results in its subsequent spread to local B cells. Glycoprotein gp350 allows attachment to B-cell CD21 surface receptors and penetration of the cell (Leach & Sumaya, 2009). Once inside the host cell, the virus's outer envelope is removed and the viral DNA gains entrance to the cytoplasm. Infection of B cells usually leads to rapid expression of viral proteins, accompanied by lysis of the host cell and release of newly created virus. Some B cells will not undergo rapid viral replication and lysis, but instead enter a latent phase resulting in immortalization of the cell with possible reactivation later. The typically incubation period is approximately 30 to 50 days (AAP, 2009).

During latent infection, EBV DNA remains in the cytoplasm in the form of plasmids. A limited number of viral proteins are produced, such as Epstein-Barr nuclear antigen-1 (EBNA-1) and latent membrane protein 1 and 2, which enable maintenance of viral plasmids, regulation of gene expression, upregulation of B-cell proliferation, and prevention of host cell apoptosis (programmed cell death) (Kutock & Wang, 2006). During this time, EBV evades the cellular immune system by a variety of mechanisms, particularly by the expression of a limited number of viral genes simultaneously, which decreases the risk of detection by cytotoxic T cells (Cohen, 2000). Failure to control EBV infection by the immune system can lead to uncontrolled proliferation of B cells and the spectrum of lymphoproliferative disease associated with EBV infection.

Epidemiology and etiology

Humans are the only known reservoir of EBV. Infections are widespread and not affected by season. Most affected children are infected by 6 years of age if they belong to a lower-socioeconomic group or live in a developing countries; infection typically occurs later in children of higher socioeconomic status or from industrialized countries (Katz, 2008). The incidence of infectious mononucleosis is between 50 and 100 cases per 100,000 population, and tends to be higher in 15- to 19-year-old youths (Leach & Sumaya, 2009). Immunocompromised patients, such as males with X-linked lymphoproliferative disease, are at higher risk of developing severe disease.

Close contact is usually required for transmission of EBV, and sharing of oral secretions is thought to play a major role in its spread. Additionally, virus can be shed either continuously or intermittently, even after the period of acute infection. Virus can also be shed in urine, cervical fluid, male reproductive fluid, and human milk. Occasionally, blood product transfusion can be the source of infection. Considering that the virus can remain viable in saliva for several hours outside of the body, fomites may be a source of infection, although the exact role of this mode of transmission is unknown.

Presentation

The majority of EBV infections are asymptomatic or nonspecific. EBV is the classic cause of infectious mononucleosis, a self-limited lymphoproliferative disease (Kutok & Wang, 2006), which usually presents with a prodrome of fatigue, possibly with fever, before starting the acute phase of infection characterized by an abrupt fever, sore throat, malaise, and fatigue. Symmetric lymphadenopathy, especially cervical, is common, as well as an exudative pharyngitis in the first week of illness. Splenomegaly caused by red pulp hyperplasia occurs in one-half of infected children, reaches its largest size by the end of the second week, and can lead to spleen rupture either spontaneously or due to trauma. Splenic rupture will present with left upper quadrant abdominal pain radiating to the top of the left shoulder pain (Kehr's sign), in addition to signs of hypovolemia, such as tachycardia, poor perfusion, and hypotension. Hepatomegaly is noted in more than one-half of patients with infectious mononucleosis and can occasionally cause jaundice. Patients treated with ampicillin or amoxicillin may develop a maculopapular, pruritic rash on the face, trunk, and extremities, known as an "ampicillin rash."

Symptoms may last for as long 3 to 4 weeks, with organomegaly persisting for as long as 3 months (Leach & Sumaya, 2009). In 10% of infectious mononucleosis patients, a chronic, active infection may occur, with symptoms lasting for a year or longer. In immunocompromised patients, disseminated disease may initially present similarly to IM and then progress to severe disease affecting multiple organ systems (Leach & Sumaya, 2009).

EBV infection has been associated with malignancy. Burkitt's lymphoma, a B-cell tumor, usually presents initially as a rapidly progressive jaw or abdominal mass in patients who live in central Africa and New Guinea, and as an abdominal mass in patients who live elsewhere. Hodgkin's lymphoma, also of B-cell origin, can cause cervical, supraclavicular, or mediastinal lymphadenopathy. Nasopharyngeal carcinomas, gastric carcinomas, non-Hodgkin's lymphomas, B-cell lymphomas, T-cell lymphomas, and other lymphoproliferative diseases, such as hemophagocytic lymphohistiocytosis, are also related to EBV infection. Solid-organ transplant recipients are at risk of post-transplantation lymphoproliferative disorder, which may initially present with vague symptoms of fever, malaise, and weight loss with associated lymphadenopathy, hepatosplenomegaly, or focal neurologic findings on examination (Leach & Sumaya, 2009). Patients with HIV have a higher likelihood of certain EBV-related diseases: non-Hodgkin's lymphoma, Hodgkin's lymphoma, oral hairy-cell leukoplakia, leimyosarcoma, body-cavity lymphoma, and lymphocytic interstitial pneumonitis (Leach & Sumaya).

EBV may also present as a variety of neurologic disorders, including meningitis with headache, fever, and nuchal rigidity, or as encephalitis associated with seizures, altered mental status, or coma. Airway obstruction, due to severe tonsillopharyngitis or neck abscess, is a known complication of EBV infection. Cardiac manifestations, including myocarditis and pericarditis, are possible but rare. Hematologic problems are also possible and include thrombocytopenia, neutropenia, pancytopenia, and anemia (Table 30-22).

Differential diagnosis

The following disorders and diseases may be evaluated in the presentation of EBV:

- Infectious mononucleosis
  - CMV
  - Toxoplasmosis
  - Adenovirus
  - Rubella
  - Hepatitis
  - Acute HIV
- Lymphoproliferative disorders
  - Sepsis
  - Other malignancies
  - Systemic connective tissue disorders

Plan of care

Atypical lymphocyte counts of more than 10% of the total leukocyte count are suggestive of EBV infection. Identification of EBV can be accomplished by isolation,

TABLE 30-22

Summary of Epstein-Barr Virus Infections

Systemic	Infectious mononucleosis, chronic active infectious mononucleosis
Cardiac	Mild electrocardiograph changes (ST and T wave), myocarditis, pericarditis
Respiratory	Tonsillopharyngitis, cervical and peritonsillar abscesses, pneumonia
Neurologic	Aseptic meningitis, meningoencephalitis, encephalitis, subacute sclerosing panencephalitis, cerebellitis/cerebellar ataxia, dysautonomia, Parkinson's-like syndrome, deafness, myelitis, optic neuritis, cranial nerve palsies, transverse myelitis, Guillain-Barré syndrome, peripheral neuropathy
Hematologic	Thrombocytopenia, neutropenia, aggamaglobulinemia, pancytopenia, hemolytic anemia, aplastic anemia
Gastrointestinal	Splenomegaly, hepatomegaly, hepatitis, pancreatitis, extrahepatic biliary obstruction
Genitourinary	Orchitis, genital ulcers
Oncologic	Burkitt's lymphoma, nasopharyngeal carcinoma, gastric carcinoma, Hodgkin's lymphoma, non-Hodgkin's lymphoma, undifferentiated B- and T-cell lymphomas, hemophagocytosis, lymphohistiocytosis, post-transplantation lymphoproliferative disorder, oral hairy-cell leukoplakia, leimyosarcoma, body-cavity lymphoma, lymphocytic interstitial pneumonitis
Miscellaneous	Orchitis, proctitis, arthritis, "Alice-in-Wonderland" syndrome

detection of viral antigen, detection of viral DNA and RNA, or serologic studies. Although direct identification by culture from either blood or oropharyngeal secretions is possible, this technique is labor intensive and not routinely performed in most laboratories. EBV infection can be inferred by demonstrating immortalization of B cells after exposure to the virus, but this step is not clinically practical due to the 6 to 8 weeks usually required to obtain results. Viral antigens (such as EBNA) can be detected by immunohistochemistry. Identification of viral nucleic acid is the most specific test for EBV and can be achieved by Southern blot, in situ hybridization, or PCR. Quantification of viral load by PCR has the added benefit of being able to estimate disease severity.

Testing for Paul-Bunnell heterophile antibodies can be performed by rapid assays such as the Monospot, Mono-Test, or Mono-Diff test. Heterophile antibodies can also be seen with other disease entities, such as CMV, measles, HIV, or drug reactions, however, and they may not be produced in patients younger than 4 years of age. When evaluating heterophile antibody–negative patients, testing for IgM and IgG to early antigen (EA), EBNA, or viral capsid antigen (VCA) is usually performed; this technique is a reliable method for determining whether an infection is acute, previous, or due to reactivation. With acute infection, patients will typically have high titers of IgM or IgG antibodies to VCA with or without antibodies to early antigen, but will not have antibodies to EBNA. In contrast, patients with previous infections will show mostly antibodies to EBNA, although they may still have antibodies to VCA and EA. Patients with reactivated infection will usually have both antibodies to VCA and antibodies to EBNA (Katz, 2008).

Therapeutic management for infectious mononucleosis usually involves rest, fluids, and antipyretics, though some patients may have more severe presentations. Fluid replacement may be required to counteract dehydration. Patients with mild upper airway obstruction will benefit from humidified air and elevation of the head, whereas patients with severe obstruction may need a nasopharyngeal airway, tonsillectomy, or tracheostomy. Any patient with infectious mononucleosis who presents with abdominal pain, signs of peritonitis, left shoulder pain, hypotension, or shock should be examined for splenic rupture. Patients with splenic rupture will need aggressive fluid and blood replacement via large-bore IV access and emergent surgical intervention.

Antiviral agents, such as acyclovir, are usually not effective against EBV infection, although acyclovir has been shown to reduce viral replication in the oropharynx (Katz, 2008). Short courses of steroids should be used in the case of severe complications such as impending upper airway obstruction from tonsillar inflammation, massive splenomegaly, myocarditis, thrombocytopenic purpura, hemolytic anemia, or onset of a hemophagocytic syndrome.

Treatment of EBV-related lymphomas and carcinomas will require chemotherapy or radiation, with possible surgical debulking performed under the guidance of a pediatric oncologist. Antiviral agents have demonstrated limited efficacy in the treatment of lymphoproliferative disease. Respiratory and cardiovascular support may be required for complications that are due to the disease or that arise during treatment. Patients who have received solid-organ transplants may require a decrease in their immunosuppressant regimen during periods of active disease.

Patients with infectious mononucleosis should be aware of regular shedding in saliva and should avoid practices that can increase the risk of transmission (e.g., kissing, sharing drinks). Patients with recent EBV infection should avoid donating blood or organs. Standard universal precautions should be sufficient to prevent EBV transmission in the hospital setting.

Patients with splenomegaly secondary to infectious mononucleosis should avoid any contact or wheeled sports and play until cleared for such activities by their HCP. Sudden abdominal pain that refers to the left shoulder should be emergently evaluated for possible splenic rupture.

Fatigue due to infectious mononucleosis usually persists for 1 month, but may last longer in some cases.

Disposition and discharge planning

Patients will need to follow up with their primary care provider to be cleared for contact and wheeled sports and play if they develop infectious mononucleosis-induced splenomegaly. Patients with EBV-related carcinomas or lymphoproliferative diseases should have regular follow-up with an oncologist, or any other specialist needed if complications arise.

The prognosis for infectious mononucleosis is usually excellent. The rare mortality associated with this disease is usually due to splenic rupture, hemorrhage, secondary infection, neurological complications, hepatic failure, or cardiac complications. Splenomegaly usually peaks at 2 to 3 weeks of illness and improves over the next 1 to 3 months (Leach & Sumaya, 2009). Patients may be cleared when they are asymptomatic and neither splenomegaly nor hepatomegaly is palpable on examination, which may be anywhere from 3 weeks to 6 months after the episode of infectious mononucleosis. The prognosis for the various EBV-related lymphoproliferative diseases depends on the disease type and the patient's immunologic status.

ENTEROVIRUS

Pathophysiology

Enteroviruses constitute a broad group of single-strand RNA viruses belonging to the Picornaviridae family, which includes 3 polioviruses, 24 group A coxsackieviruses, 6 group B coxsackieviruses, 34 echoviruses, and 5 new enteroviruses. Enterovirus usually enters via the nasopharynx or GI tract and attaches to host cell surface receptors. After passing through the cell membrane, the virus sheds its coat. Replication then ensues in the cytoplasm at a rapid rate, leading to spread of the virus to regional lymph nodes by the second day of infection. Virus enters the bloodstream around the third day, and an episode of minor viremia occurs, resulting in the distribution of virus to other areas of secondary infection, leading to symptomology. Virus continues to replicate in these areas of secondary infection and enters the bloodstream, producing an episode of major viremia lasting from the third to seventh days, with further seeding and disease at specific sites, such as the heart and CNS.

Poliovirus can invade the CNS during the episode of major viremia and continues to replicate within neural cells, especially the anterior horn cells in the spinal cord (Maldonado, 2008). The incubation period for nonparalytic poliomyelitis is 3 to 6 days and that for paralytic poliomyelitis is 7 to 21 days (AAP, 2009).

Epidemiology and etiology

Similar to the situation with EBV, humans are the only reservoir for enterovirus. Rates of infection are inversely related to age, with the highest incidence being noted in children younger than 1 year of age (Modlin, 2008). Infections are reported worldwide, and with the highest incidence occurring in the summer and early fall seasons. Overall, the incidence of poliovirus has dramatically decreased due to efforts of the World Health Assembly's eradication programs, but can still present in a population as an endemic. The risk of paralytic poliomyelitis increases with age and is currently 0.1% to 2% of the total number of cases (Cherry & Krogstad, 2009).

The majority of enterovirus infection is transmitted via the fecal–oral route, likely due to the fact that enterovirus is shed in feces for as long as 8 weeks after an acute infection. Infants requiring regular diaper changes are significant sources of infection. Respiratory secretions can contain shed virus for as long as 3 weeks after an acute infection. Fomite transmission is also a possibility, as enterovirus can survive on a surface for a prolonged period of time. Neonates can be infected either by crossing of the virus across the placenta or during birth by contact with virus-contaminated fluids and feces.

Presentation

Due to the large number of viruses classified as enteroviruses, a wide range of clinical presentations is possible. The majority of enteroviral infections are asymptomatic or feature a nonspecific febrile illness. Respiratory manifestations of enterovirus can range from febrile pharyngitis and the occasional common cold to more severe pneumonia. Pleurodynia, also known as Bornholm disease, is characterized by fever and paroxysms of sudden, severe chest pain lasting 15 to 30 minutes.

Gastrointestinal symptoms due to coxsackievirus and echovirus are also common, such as vomiting, diarrhea, and abdominal pain. Hand–foot–mouth disease caused by coxsackievirus A16 is usually seen in patients younger than 10 years of age. It often presents after a mild prodrome of fever and malaise with painful, intraoral ulcers on the tongue and buccal mucosa, as well as lesions on the hands and feet. Herpangina also presents with intraoral lesions, including painful, vesicular lesions on the soft palate, uvula, tonsils, and oropharynx; it lasts for 7 days, and is usually caused by group A coxsackievirus.

Pericarditis and myocarditis, mostly due to group B coxsackievirus, are serious disease entities that can present with symptoms of congestive heart failure, including tachypnea, tachycardia, shortness of breath, or hypotension if severe. Arrhythmias may also occur.

Coxsackievirus B5 and echovirus cause most cases of meningitis, which presents with fever, headaches, and neck stiffness, and which usually resolves without sequelae. Encephalitis, caused mostly by echovirus, can present with seizures, ataxia, or altered mental status. It may be life-threatening if the brain stem is involved.

Other possible manifestations of enterovirus infection include acute hemorrhagic conjunctivitis that presents with sudden eye pain associated with photophobia, blurred vision, erythema of the eye, and subconjunctival hemorrhages that usually resolve in 7 to 12 days. Neonatal patients can present with a sepsis-like illness or disseminated disease. Immunocompromised patients are at risk for chronic or severe illness, as well as meningoencephalitis, arthritis, and polymyositis (Table 30-23) (Cherry & Krogstad, 2009).

Most poliovirus infections are asymptomatic or present as pharyngitis with a low-grade fever (abortive poliomyelitis). As many as 5% of patients have aseptic meningitis presenting with nuchal rigidity, headache, and fever, which occurs after a period of fever, malaise, and headache. Patients with paralytic poliomyelitis also experience an initial illness characterized by fever and malaise, before being afflicted with asymmetric paralysis. This development may be preceded (by 12 to 24 hours) by changes in deep or superficial reflexes (Cherry & Krogstad, 2009). Weakness can occur suddenly or over hours, and usually peaks at 48 hours (Kidd et al., 1996); nevertheless, it may take as long as 5 days to become fully manifest (Cherry & Krogstad). The lower limbs are more likely to be affected by paralysis than the upper limbs, and weakness is usually more proximal than distal.

Bowel and bladder control can also be lost with poliovirus infections. Diaphragm and thoracic muscles can be affected in the spinal form of the disease, causing respiratory failure. In the bulbar form of poliomyelitis, respiratory failure occurs secondary to involvement of the brain stem's control of breathing or cranial nerve dysfunction (especially cranial nerve 10) causing airway compromise. Hypotension may also occur with injury to the medulla.

Differential diagnosis

The following disorders and diseases may be evaluated in the presentation of enterovirus:

- Bacterial causes of pharyngitis, pneumonia, pericarditis, meningitis, sepsis
- Other viruses for upper respiratory infection, GI infections, rashes, encephalitis, neonatal illness
- Hand–foot–mouth disease
  ○ Aphthous stomatitis
  ○ HSV infection
- Aseptic meningitis
  ○ Meningococcemia
  ○ *Pneumococcus*
- Paralytic disease
  ○ Guillain-Barré syndrome
  ○ Peripheral neuritis (toxic, herpes zoster)
  ○ Arbovirus
  ○ Rabies
  ○ Tetanus
  ○ Botulism
  ○ Tick paralysis
- Rash
  ○ Measles
  ○ Rubella
  ○ Roseola
- Myocarditis
  ○ Other cardiotropic viruses: adenovirus, influenza type a, mumps
- Paralytic poliomyelitis
  ○ Non-poliomyelitis enteroviruses (especially coxsackie A7, enterovirus 71)
  ○ Guillain-Barré syndrome
  ○ Infant botulism
  ○ West Nile encephalitis
  ○ Lyme disease

Plan of care

Detection of enterovirus infection is usually accomplished by isolation in cell culture. It is important to obtain samples

TABLE 30-23

Summary of Enterovirus Infections	
Respiratory	Common cold, pharyngitis, croup, bronchitis, bronchiolitis, pneumonia, pleurodynia (Bornholm disease)
Gastrointestinal	Herpangina, stomatitis, gastroenteritis, constipation, peritonitis, pseudoperitonitis, appendicitis, pseudo-obstruction, mesenteric adenitis, intussusception, hepatitis, pancreatitis
Cardiac	Pericarditis, myocarditis
Neurologic	Aseptic meningitis, encephalitis, meningoencephalitis, paralytic poliomyelitis, Guillain-Barré syndrome, transverse myelitis, cerebellar ataxia
Ocular	Acute hemorrhagic conjunctivitis, conjunctivitis, uveitis
Skin	Various exanthems, hand–foot–mouth disease, Stevens-Johnson syndrome
Renal	Nephritis, hemolytic uremic syndrome
Genitourinary	Orchitis, epididymitis
Hematologic	Acute infectious lymphocytosis
Musculoskeletal	Arthritis, myositis, myalgia
Systemic	Sepsis-like illness (neonates)
Miscellaneous	Parotitis

from several different sites or fluids simultaneously, such as nasopharynx, throat, rectum, stool, blood, urine, and CSF. Cultures from the stool, rectum, and throat typically have the highest sensitivity. For detection of poliovirus, multiple samples should be obtained, each 24 hours apart; fecal samples will have the highest yield. Note that many group A coxsackieviruses do not grow well in cell culture.

Detection of viral nucleic acid is accomplished by nucleic acid probes or PCR. Results from PCR tend to be available more quickly than those from culture, yet offer equal specificity. PCR can also detect enteroviruses that cannot grow on cell culture, but is unable to specify the type of enterovirus after detection.

Serologic detection of enterovirus is possible, but requires comparison of serum samples taken during acute infection and 2 to 4 weeks after infection. Due to the impracticality and insensitivity of serologic detection, other methods of detection are more commonly used.

No specific therapeutic management exists for enterovirus infections, although newer antiviral medications that specifically target enterovirus, such as pleconaril, which prevents viral attachment and uncoating, are being developed (Sawyer, 2001). Most therapies center on supportive measures for patient with complications. Patients with respiratory compromise will require supplemental oxygen and may require mechanical ventilation if their condition is severe. Dehydration may be significant in patients with gastroenteritis or those with decreased oral intake due to oral lesions, as seen with herpangina and hand–foot–mouth disease. Fluid replacement and electrolyte management are crucial in these patients, and analgesics are helpful in patients with painful oral lesions. Patients with cardiac manifestations should be evaluated by a cardiologist; an echocardiograph will be helpful to determine the severity of cardiac dysfunction. Inotropic support, diuretics, and afterload-reducing agents should be administered as needed while the patient is cared for in a critical care unit. Intravenous immunoglobulin has been used for meningoencephalitis in immunodeficient patients, in patients with myocarditis, and in patients with life-threatening presentations. Steroids have been employed in the past, but there is insufficient evidence to support their routine use as a treatment for enterovirus infection.

With paralytic poliomyelitis, respiratory compromise is the most common cause of mortality and morbidity. Signs of impending respiratory failure should be noted: deviated uvula or tongue, increased pharyngeal secretions, ineffective coughing, inability to tolerate liquids, shortened sentences, increased work of breathing, and tachypnea. Patients in severe respiratory distress or failure should receive immediate airway and ventilator support. Cardiovascular instability is a known complication of poliomyelitis, and should be supported with inotropic agents and administration of fluids as needed. Patients with bladder involvement will need catheterization or parasympathetic stimulants.

Given that most transmission of enterovirus infection occurs via contact with contaminated feces, secretions, or fomites, good hand hygiene and sanitary practices are essential to limit viral spread. In the hospital setting, both standard and contact precautions should be employed when caring for patients with these infections. Poliovirus vaccines—either the inactivated vaccine or the oral live-attenuated vaccine—are the primary method of prevention of poliovirus. The inactivated vaccine is the immunization of choice in the United States; vaccine-associated paralytic poliomyelitis from the use of oral, live-attenuated vaccine is no longer of concern (Maldonado, 2008).

Patient and family education includes discussion of vaccine-associated paralytic poliomyelitis as a possible adverse effect of the oral polio vaccine; this outcome does not occur with inactivated poliovirus vaccines. Patients admitted to the inpatient setting will require education about the therapeutic and diagnostic plan, interprofessional team members, and goals for rehabilitation.

Disposition and discharge planning

Usually no follow-up is needed for most enterovirus infections, although severe infections with possible sequelae should be followed by the appropriate specialist. Patients with paralytic poliomyelitis or encephalitis should be followed by a neurologist and a rehabilitation specialist if symptoms persist.

The prognosis for patients with enteroviral infections is usually good, with full recovery to baseline status being the norm. Patients who experience multiple episodes of myocarditis can develop dilated cardiomyopathy. The prognosis for patients with paralytic poliomyelitis depends on the severity of the muscle involvement. Prolonged paralysis is a possible sequela, and new neuromuscular symptoms can recur years later in some patients.

HERPES SIMPLEX VIRUS

Pathophysiology

Herpes simplex virus is a double-stranded DNA virus that usually invades the host through mucous membranes or skin, either intact or broken. After attachment to, and penetration of, the host cell membrane via various glycoproteins, the viral genome is released and transcription commences. As HSV spreads throughout the body, cellular damage initiates a localized inflammatory reaction resulting in the formation of the characteristic vesicles. The incubation period can be anywhere from 2 days to 2 weeks (AAP, 2009).

Latent infection occurs as the virus spreads from the site of invasion to nearby sensory nerve endings, even in the case of an asymptomatic primary infection. The virus migrates to sensory ganglia, where additional virus is synthesized.

The viral genome then remains in a static, suppressed state until it is reactivated by any number of triggers—for example, immunosuppression, stress, trauma, or infection. At that point, the virus travels back down the axon and is released. HSV-1 usually remains latent in the trigeminal ganglia, whereas HSV-2 usually infects the sacral ganglia, although any sensory ganglia can be latently infected.

HSV is believed to evade the immune system by using a variety of mechanisms during its latent stage. The virus can block the activity of major histocompatibility complex class I and class II proteins, thereby affecting the T-cell–mediated immune response, as well as prevent host cell apoptosis in response to viral invasion (Whitley & Roizman, 2001).

Epidemiology and etiology

HSV infections are ubiquitous and occur on a year-round basis. Humans are the only hosts for HSV, and patients with latent infections will intermittently shed virus. HSV type 1 (HSV-1) infections usually occur in childhood, especially in the daycare population. HSV type 2 (HSV-2) is usually transmitted sexually; the incidence of these infections is higher in the adolescent population and in patients with multiple sexual partners (Gutierrez & Arvin, 2009). Neonatal infection is seen in 1 per 3,000 to 1 per 20,000 live births; 20% of affected neonates present with disseminated disease, and approximately 30% present with CNS disease (AAP, 2009).

Both symptomatic and asymptomatic patients typically shed virus intermittently; patients with primary infections tend to have higher levels of shedding than patients with recurrent infections. Transmission is usually accomplished by direct contact with HSV lesions or exposure to contaminated secretions. Neonates typically become contaminated when they travel through the vaginal canal during childbirth; their risk of infection is higher with maternal primary infection than with maternal recurrent infection. Neonates may also become infected in utero. Virus is relatively unstable in the environment, so fomite transmission does not play a large role in spread of HSV.

Presentation

The most common presentation of HSV infection is gingivostomatitis; this sign is typically caused by HSV-1, but can also be caused by HSV-2. Multiple, grouped vesicles form on the lips, gingival, tongue, hard palate, and other oral mucous membranes, and can be accompanied by fever, submandibular lymphadenopathy, and malodorous breath (Gutierrez & Arvin, 2009). Lesions ulcerate over the next 5 days with occasional bleeding, before resolving over the next 7 days. Patients may present with dehydration secondary to poor oral intake. Recurrent infection, known as herpes labialis, will present with vesicles that progress to ulcers following a prodrome of pain, burning, or itching in the area.

The more common form in sexually active patients, genital herpes is usually caused by HSV-2, with symptoms often being the result of a recurrent infection. Vesicles start on the genital organs and perineum, progress to ulcerative lesions, and heal over the next 14 to 21 days. Lesions on the buttocks, groin, and thighs are also possible. In classic genital herpes, lesions will be accompanied by pain, itching, inguinal lymphadenopathy, and vaginal or urethral discharge. Occasionally, fever, malaise, myalgia, and headaches may also occur. Recurrent genital herpes presents with lesions that progress to crusted ulcers over 5 days, then heal over the next 9 to 11 days.

Other possible skin manifestations include eczema herpeticum, also known as Kaposi varicelliform eruption. Patients with eczema are often simultaneously infected with HSV, resulting in vesicular lesions in areas of dermatitis that can be widespread and severe. Painful, vesicular lesions on the distal fingers that appear purulent filled but have minimal discharge after incision are characteristic of herpetic whitlow. Athletes who participate in sports requiring close physical contact can also be infected by HSV, as seen with herpes gladiatorum in wrestlers and scrum-pox in rugby players.

Keratoconjunctivitis can occur from either primary or recurrent infection. This condition presents with corneal injection, watering, itching, and occasionally fever. Extension of the infection to the cornea is a serious complication that may be characterized by photophobia, vision changes, chemosis, and lacrimation. Retinitis is another possible result of an HSV infection; rarely, acute retinal necrosis is seen. Recurrent ocular infections may occasionally cause symptoms that are more severe than the initial infection.

Meningitis due to HSV is usually mild and unlikely to cause sequelae. Patients will often complain of headache and photophobia; nuchal rigidity will be noted on physical examination. In contrast, untreated HSV encephalitis is deadly. This complication usually presents with nonspecific fever, malaise, or irritability, which then progresses to altered mental status, seizures, or focal neurological findings, followed by coma and death. HSV-2 is associated with most cases of meningitis, whereas HSV-1 is the typical cause of encephalitis in this population.

Neonatal HSV infection can manifest as severe, rapidly progressing, disseminated disease. Pulmonary and hepatic complications may result in respiratory embarrassment, hepatomegaly, and hepatic dysfunction. Some neonatal infections involve the CNS, such that seizures are a possible manifestation. The majority of infected neonates have infections of their skin, eyes, and mouths, and achieve better outcomes compared to other HSV-infected patients (Whitley & Roizman, 2001).

In immunocompromised patients, HSV can cause severe, chronic, ulcerative skin lesions, which may involve large areas of skin (Gutierrez & Arvin, 2009). Single organs can be involved, as seen with tracheobronchitis, pneumonia, or esophagitis. Other patients present with disseminated disease with multiorgan involvement (Gutierrez & Arvin, 2009). Meningoencephalitis and hepatitis are also possible manifestations (Table 30-24).

Differential diagnosis

The following disorders and diseases may be evaluated in the presentation of HSV:

- Gingivostomatitis
  - Aphthous stomatitis
  - Stevens-Johnson syndrome
  - Herpangina
  - Hand–foot–mouth disease
  - Bacterial infection
  - Fungal infection
  - Other viral causes
- Genital herpes
  - Other sexually transmitted diseases
  - Fungal infection
  - Scabies
  - Lichen planus or sclerosis
  - Herpes zoster
  - Atopic dermatitis
- Keratoconjunctivitis
  - Scleritis
  - Iritis
  - Conjunctivitis
- Encephalitis
  - Other viral encephalitis
  - Bacterial infection, empyema, meningitis
  - Lyme disease

TABLE 30-24

Summary of Herpes Simplex Virus Infections	
Skin	Genital herpes/vulvovaginitis, eczema herpeticum, herpetic whitlow, herpes gladiatorum, scrum-pox, erythema multiforme
Gastrointestinal	Gingivostomatitis, recurrent herpes labialis, pharyngitis, esophagitis, hepatitis
Ocular	Keratoconjunctivitis, retinitis, acute retinal necrosis
Neurological	Meningitis, encephalitis, meningoencephalitis, Bell's palsy, atypical pain syndrome, trigeminal neuralgia, ascending myelitis, post-infectious encephalomyelitis
Respiratory	Tracheobronchitis, pneumonia
Systemic	Disseminated disease

- Protozoal infection
- Oncologic entities
- Vascular disease or malformation
- Cerebral infarction

Plan of care

Identification by cell culture is the study of choice for HSV detection. The best samples for this purpose are acquired from aspirated fluid or swabbing the bases of lesions, especially when lesions are in the vesicular form. In neonates, the conjunctiva, mouth, nasopharynx, and rectum should all be swabbed for virus, and blood, urine, stool, and CSF should also be tested. Viral growth can usually be detected in 2 to 3 days, although some samples may require as long as 7 days before growth is detectable. Addition of antibodies specific to HSV-1 or HSV-2 will increase the specificity of the test.

Direct immunofluorescent staining can be performed for rapid detection of virus on cell samples, but not on samples collected from CSF, tracheal aspirate, oropharyngeal, or bronchoalveolar lavage. Although immunofluorescent staining is sensitive (80% to 90% compared to culture), the results should still be confirmed with culture. HSV antigen can be detected by a variety of assays and by ELISA; glycoprotein G–specific assays have proven to be both sensitive and specific for HSV infection. Cytologic changes can be detected by either Papanicolaou staining or Tzank testing, although other forms of testing are more sensitive and specific for the diagnosis.

Detection of nucleic acid is possible with PCR, with this technology having been shown to be more sensitive than culture. PCR is an excellent method of detecting HSV in CSF, especially considering the difficulty associated with culturing HSV from CSF samples. Another advantage of PCR testing is its ability to detect asymptomatic shedding of virus.

Serologic testing can be used to determine primary HSV infection; however, its clinical value is marginal given the need to obtain samples during both the acute and convalescent phases of the illness. Production of IgM can occur with both primary and recurrent illness. Moreover, cross-reactivity between HSV-1 and HSV-2 antibodies means that most commercial test are unable to perform typing of HSV.

With HSV encephalitis, CSF typically shows a pleocytosis consisting primarily of lymphocytes (neutrophils earlier in the disease coarse), as well as an RBC count is excess of $1,000/mm^3$ owing to hemorrhagic necrosis (Prober, 2008). CSF samples should be sent if PCR testing is planned, as cultures are usually negative for HSV except in the neonatal patient. Electroencephalography will usually show HSV-related paroxysmal lateral epileptiform discharges (PLEDs)—that is, a background of slow activity with periodic, unilateral or bilateral focal spikes. Temporal lobe enhancement is typically seen on MRI.

Acyclovir is the usual first-line therapy for HSV infections. A nucleoside analogue, this agent acts as a competitive inhibitor for HSV DNA polymerase. Acyclovir is excreted by the kidney and can cause nephrotoxicity, neutropenia, and neurotoxicity. Valacyclovir is metabolized into acyclovir after ingestion and can achieve higher serum concentrations than oral acyclovir, which is known for its poor bioavailability. Famciclovir is another oral medication that can be used for the treatment of HSV. Valacyclovir and famciclovir are under study for approval by the U.S. Food and Drug Administration (FDA) for use in children. In patients with acyclovir-resistant virus, both foscarnet and cidofovir have been used as therapies.

Gingivostomatitis may be associated with dehydration due to a lack of oral intake. In patients who develop this complication, fluid replacement is necessary and parenteral nutrition may be required in severe cases. Pain control can and should be used to facilitate adequate intake. Acyclovir has been shown to be beneficial in treating gingivostomatitis in patients with primary infection. With recurrent herpes labialis, oral acyclovir has questionable effectiveness, although it has been used to decrease the overall number of recurrences (Prober, 2008).

Genital herpetic lesions should be kept clean and dry to promote wound healing and decrease the risk of infection. Burrow solution sitz baths or compress treatments can also be used for symptomatic relief, although prolonged soaking can impede healing. Acyclovir is recommended for treatment of lesions in patients with primary illness, and has been shown to decrease the total duration of illness if started within 6 days of onset of primary disease and 2 days of onset of recurrent disease (AAP, 2009). Intravenous acyclovir should be administered for severe cases. As with recurrent herpes labialis, acyclovir can be used for suppressive therapy for recurrent genital herpes.

Due to the high mortality and morbidity associated with HSV encephalitis, intravenous acyclovir should be started promptly in all patients suspected of having this disease. Patients should be admitted to the intensive care unit for close monitoring, cardiovascular and respiratory support as needed, seizure control, fluid replacement, and intracranial pressure monitoring (severe cases).

Immunocompromised patients with significant disease should also receive parenteral acyclovir; foscarnet should be considered if acyclovir resistance is encountered. Patients with any ocular manifestations of HSV infection should be urgently seen by an ophthalmologist, who may administer a variety of cycloplegic and anti-inflammatory agents in addition to intravenous acyclovir. Possible treatments include 1% trifluridine, 0.1% iododeoxyuridine, and 3% vidarabine. Steroids are generally contraindicated in patients with conjunctivitis.

Contact precautions are indicated for all patients in whom mucocutaneous lesions are present and in neonatal patients born to women with active genital herpes. Precautionary measures should especially be used for patients with eczema, severe rashes, abraded skin, or burns, as these areas can be sites of viral invasion. Condoms or abstinence can limit the rate of transmission during episodes of symptomatic genital herpes. Prophylactic acyclovir can be given to decrease the number of recurrent illness. Cesarean sections should be considered for women in labor with active genital lesions; use of fetal scalp monitors should be avoided in such circumstances.

Patient and family education includes discussion of the avoidance of topical analgesics with oral lesions to prevent the possibility of overdose with ingestion. Patients and families should understand that the type of HSV infection that causes oral lesions is not a sexually transmitted disease. Patients with difficulty swallowing due to oral lesions should not participate in daycare programs. Hydration is important during episodes of gingivostomatitis; appropriate pain control can improve oral intake.

Some patients may develop significant anxiety or depression after being newly diagnosed with genital herpes (Green & Wang, 2004). Emotional support and education can help limit the negative psychosocial impact of this diagnosis.

Disposition and discharge planning

No follow-up is needed for most infections, but severe infections with possible sequelae should be followed by the appropriate specialist. Patients with ocular involvement should be followed by an ophthalmologist.

Most HSV mucocutaneous lesions are not associated with significant morbidity. By comparison, secondary infection and dehydration can cause severe complications. Patients with HSV encephalitis usually survive with treatment, but may experience significant neurologic sequelae. Disseminated disease may is associated with significant morbidity and mortality. Patients with ocular manifestations of HSV infection can progress to blindness if not treated early.

INFLUENZA

Pathophysiology

Influenza is a single-stranded RNA virus belonging to the Orthomyxoviridae family. Three major types of influenza exist: A, B, and C. Epidemic disease is usually caused by types A and B.

Embedded in the surface membrane of the influenza virus are hemagglutinin (HA) and neuraminidase (NA) surface antigens, which play important roles in the attachment of virus to host cell membranes and the release of virus from infected cells, respectively. Different subtypes of these surface antigens account for the large variety of influenza strains. Influenza A and B have both HA and NA, whereas influenza C has only HA.

The initial invasion of the influenza virus typically takes place in the mucosal cells of the respiratory tract. Using HA surface antigen, the virus attaches to the host cell and gains entrance. Necrosis of the infected cell triggers an inflammatory response in the surrounding area, resulting in symptomology. The incubation period of influenza virus is usually 2 days, but can range anywhere from 1 to 7 days (AAP, 2009).

Changes in influenza surface antigens are responsible for epidemics of influenza due to the creation of de novo strains. As a consequence of this "antigenic drift," minor variations to the antigen enable proliferation of virus in the face of antibodies to previous strains, leading to seasonal epidemics. In contrast, "antigenic shift" occurs when major changes to viral surface antigens lead to the creation of a new subtype of antigen. When sections of genetic material mix between nonhuman and human viral strains while existing in the same host, or when primarily animal forms of influenza obtain the ability to infect humans, antigenic shift can cause epidemics and pandemics. For example, the pandemic (H1N1) 2009 influenza virus has properties associated with swine, avian, and human viruses (Mossad, 2009).

Epidemiology and etiology

Incidence of disease is highest in young children and the elderly. Children younger than the age of 4 years, and especially those younger than the age of 2 years, have the highest risk of developing infection requiring hospitalization (Coffin et al., 2006). Seasonal epidemics are seen during winter months (January, February), but can occur anytime from November to May in the United States. Incidence is increased in the summer months in countries in the southern hemisphere. Risk for mortality and morbidity is increased in patients with chronic lung disease, cardiac disease, kidney disease, malignancy, diabetes, neurologic disease, neuromuscular disease, or any other chronic condition.

The influenza virus is highly contagious, in part due to the low dosage required for infection, and in part due to the high concentration of virus in ejected secretions. Transmission most commonly takes place via aerosolized droplet from coughing and sneezing, although the virus can also be transmitted by direct contact. Fomites play a role in its transmission as well. The H1N1 virus is also spread by droplet, contact, or fomites, much like other strains of influenza.

Presentation

Classic influenza is characterized with sudden fever, headache, myalgia, and malaise, which is followed in 2 to 4 days by respiratory signs and symptoms, such as cough, sore throat, and nasal congestion. Ocular symptoms, tearing, photophobia, or pain can also occur simultaneously.

Pulmonary manifestations of influenza-associated illness vary. Influenza is a common cause of acute otitis media, which may present with high fever, rhinorhea, cough, and sore throat. Bronchiolitis and croup are other illnesses caused by influenza, although influenza-associated croup tends to be more severe than parainfluenza-associated croup. Severe infection can produce a progressive bronchopneumonia.

Encephalitis is a known neurological presentation of influenza and can be associated with seizures or mental status changes. Acute necrotizing encephalopathy secondary to influenza has also been documented. Febrile seizures, transverse myelitis, and Guillain-Barré syndrome are also possible. Reye's syndrome may be seen with administration of salicylate-containing medication during influenza illness; affected patients usually present with febrile convulsions that progress to lethargy and coma (Glezen, 2009). Fatty degeneration of the liver with cerebral edema is the hallmark of this disease.

Neonatal patients may present with a septic-like illness characterized by lethargy, shock, and apnea (Glezen, 2009). Immunocompromised patients typically have lower respiratory tract or neurological disease (Subbarao, 2008) (Table 30-25).

Infection with the avian influenza A virus (H5N1) in adults usually presents with a mild prodrome of fever and cough, when progresses first to pneumonia, then to acute respiratory distress syndrome (ARDS). Overall mortality with this variant has been estimated at 61%, although a milder illness is more commonly seen in children [Writing Committee of the Second World Health Organization

TABLE 30-25

Summary of Influenza Virus Infections	
Respiratory	Classic influenza, nonspecific upper respiratory illness, acute otitis media, croup, bronchiolitis, pneumonia, asthma exacerbations, adult respiratory distress syndrome (with avian flu), hemorrhagic bronchopneumonia (with H1N1)
Cardiac	Myocarditis, pericarditis
Gastrointestinal	Abdominal pain, nausea, vomiting, diarrhea, Reye's syndrome
Renal	Glomerulonephritis, acute kidney failure
Musculoskeletal	Myositis
Neurologic	Febrile seizures, encephalopathy, encephalitis, acute necrotizing encephalitis, transverse myelitis, Guillain-Barré syndrome, Reye syndrome
Systemic	Nonspecific febrile illness, sepsis-like picture in infants

Consultation on Clinical Aspects of Human Infection with Avian Influenza A (H5N1) Virus [WHO], 2008].

H1N1 infection usually presents with classic influenza symptoms; fever, headache, myalgias, cough, and sore throat. Complications of H1N1 infection are similar to other strains of influenza, including pneumonia, myocarditis, myositis, or even encephalitis. Severe disease with ARDS, shock, and organ failure is also possible (CDC, 2009c).

Differential diagnosis

The following disorders and diseases may be evaluated in the presentation of influenza:

- Other viral causes
  - RSV
  - Adenovirus
  - Influenza virus
  - Parainfluenza virus
- Bacterial infections

Plan of care

Viral culture is the study of choice for diagnosis of influenza, but can take up to 6 days for virus identification. Certain techniques, such as shell vial methods, can decrease the time required for detection. Specimens from patients collected in the first 3 days of their illness have the highest chance of growth in culture.

Rapid detection tests can identify the presence of influenza virus much more quickly than culture, with some yielding results within 30 minutes. The sensitivity and specificity vary for different tests, and further subtyping and characterization of the virus is not possible with these diagnostic tools. Immunoassays for viral antigens also exist, and can be used for the identification of influenza A antigen. The sensitivity of rapid detection tests and immunofluorescence assays to H1N1 is variable, with false-negative results often occurring (CDC, 2009c).

Viral nucleic acid can be detected by PCR, which has proven to be very sensitive compared to other detection methods. Offering even higher sensitivity and specificity than regular PCR, reverse transcriptase-PCR can be used to detect the presence of viral nucleic acid and is useful in the confirmation of H1N1 infection (CDC, 2009c).

As with other viruses, serologic testing can be performed to determine the existence of an influenza infection. A fourfold increase in antibody titers is considered sufficient for diagnosis. Because the samples need to be drawn over significant intervals, however, the clinical utility of serologic testing is marginal.

Patients with Reye's syndrome will have elevated serum aminotransferases, coupled with increased serum ammonia levels. Lumbar puncture will produce normal CSF findings.

The majority of influenza infections are treated with supportive care, although patients with severe respiratory involvement may need supplemental oxygen or even positive-pressure ventilation. In some cases, patients may benefit from early administration of an antiviral agent, especially if they have underlying chronic disease, are at risk for serious infection, or already have severe disease early in their course. In all cases where influenza is suspected, salicylate and salicylate-containing medications should be avoided due to the risk of Reye's syndrome. Standard and droplet precautions should be employed in hospitalized patients.

Influenza can be treated with two classes of antivirals: adamantanes and neuraminidase inhibitors. Adamantanes (i.e., amantidine, rimantadine) block attachment of the influenza virus to the host cell and release of viral RNA. They have been shown to decrease the total duration of illness if started within 48 hours of the onset. Both amantidine and rimantadine are effective against influenza A, although resistance is increasing; neither is effective against influenza B. CNS symptoms, such as anxiety or difficulty in concentrating, progressing to delirium, hallucinations, and seizures, are possible with both amantidine and rimantadine, especially in patients with kidney insufficiency.

Neuraminidase inhibitors (i.e., zanamivir, oseltamivir, peramivir) limit the number of new copies of the virus that are released from infected cells. They are effective against both influenza types A and B, and should be the first treatment option for H1N1 illness, as this strain is resistant to adamantanes (CDC, 2009c). Neuraminidase inhibitors can decrease the severity and overall duration of illness if started within the first 2 days of infection. Zanamivir—an inhaled agent—is effective for both treatment and prophylaxis of influenza, but may cause bronchospasm in certain patients; thus it should not be used in patients with reactive airway disease. Oseltamivir—an oral formulation—is the usual treatment for avian influenza A (WHO, 2008); its dosing should be adjusted in patients with kidney insufficiency. Peramivir is an intravenous formulation that has recently been granted an emergency use authorization by the FDA for the treatment of H1N1 under special circumstances (CDC). Empiric treatment with peramivir for H1N1 should be initiated in any patient who is hospitalized, has progressive or severe disease, or has risk factors for severe illness, such as age younger than 5 years, chronic lung disease, asthma, neurological disease, cardiac disease, hematologic disease, hepatic disease, kidney disease, metabolic disease, immunocompromise, or long-term aspirin use (CDC).

Inactivated influenza vaccine should be administered yearly, especially to those patients with chronic diseases who are at high risk for developing serious complications. Younger patients—those 6 months to 2 years of age—may need two doses of vaccine to achieve an adequate response.

Possible adverse effects of vaccination include mild fever, malaise, and myalgias. A live-attenuated influenza vaccine is now available and is administered via nasal spray. A vaccine to the H1N1 virus is also available. Prophylaxis with antiviral agents may also be considered in certain high-risk patients.

Patient and family education should include information about supportive care. Adequate fluid intake should be emphasized to prevent dehydration. Patients and families should be instructed to carefully read the ingredient lists of over-the-counter medications before taking any of these drugs, as some may contain salicylates.

Disposition and discharge planning

Follow-up is rarely needed for most patients with influenza infections. The exception is patients with severe infections who may experience possible sequelae; they should be followed by the appropriate specialist.

The prognosis is usually good in the case of uncomplicated disease. It is worse in patients with chronic diseases such as malignancies, diabetes, kidney disease, congenital heart disease, and chronic lung disease. Patients with bacterial superinfection are also at risk for severe disease and increased morbidity or mortality.

HUMAN METAPNEUMOVIRUS

Pathophysiology

Belonging to the Paramyxoviridae family, human metapneumovirus (hMPV) is a single-stranded RNA virus with two major types, A and B. Similar to RSV, hMPV typically invades via the epithelial cells of the respiratory tract. Its viral proteins enable the virus to enter host cells and replicate. A provoked inflammatory response may play a role in the production of patient symptomology. The usual incubation period for hMPV infection is 3 to 5 days (AAP, 2009). Epithelial cell necrosis and ciliary destruction have been noted in infected airways (Principi et al., 2006).

Epidemiology and etiology

Almost all patients with hMPV infection will have been infected by the age of 10 years (Principi et al., 2006). Patients younger than 2 years of age have a higher chance of infection (Cherry, 2009). The risk of severe disease that requires hospitalization appears to peak between 6 and 12 months of age (Williams & Crowe, 2008). Infections have a seasonal predilection for winter months that may extend into early spring, similar to RSV and influenza virus.

The exact method of transmission of hMPV has not been identified, although respiratory secretions, direct contact, and fomites are all possible modes of its spread.

Presentation

The majority of hMPV infections are respiratory in nature. Upper respiratory tract infections may be associated with rhinitis, pharyngitis, or otitis media. Most hospitalized patients who develop hMPV infections, however, present with lower respiratory tract infections, such as bronchiolitis and pneumonia. Bronchiolitis due to hMPV tends to be similar to RSV-associated bronchiolitis, making clinical differentiation between the two conditions difficult—both present with fever and cough that can progress to respiratory distress with crackles on examination. Human metapneumovirus is also a known cause of asthma exacerbations. Rare cases of encephalitis and encephalopathy have been documented in conjunction with hMPV infection. Immunocompromised patients are at higher risk of pneumonia and increased severity of illness. Simultaneous infection with RSV is associated with more severe disease. Table 30-26 lists other manifestations of hMPV infections.

Differential diagnosis

The following disorders and diseases may be evaluated in the presentation of human metapneumovirus:

- Respiratory illness
  - Other viral causes (adenovirus, rhinovirus)
  - Primary bacterial infection or superinfection
- Encephalitis
  - Other viral encephalitis
  - Bacterial infection, empyema, meningitis
  - Lyme disease
  - Protozoal infection
  - Oncologic entities
  - Vascular disease or malformation
  - Cerebral infarction

Plan of care

As with other viruses, isolation of hMPV by viral culture is possible, but the slow growth of the virus in medium limits this test's clinical usefulness. More rapid diagnosis

TABLE 30-26

Summary of Human Metapneumovirus Infections	
Respiratory	Mild upper respiratory infection, laryngitis, pharyngitis, otitis media, croup, bronchiolitis, pneumonia, asthma exacerbation
Ocular	Conjunctivitis
Neurologic	Encephalitis, encephalopathy
Systemic	Nonspecific febrile illness

can be made via immunofluorescence or by detection of viral nucleic acid via reverse transcriptase-PCR, which is currently the most commonly used method of diagnosis. Serologic testing, as with the detection of other viruses, has limited clinical utility.

Therapeutic management for hMPV infection primarily consists of supportive measures, which may extend to supplemental oxygen and mechanical ventilation in patients with severe disease. Bronchodilator treatment appears to help alleviate symptoms in some patients, but no controlled trials have been performed to support its use in all patients. Ribavirin has been shown to be effective in vitro and has been used in animal studies (Cherry, 2009). Standard and contact isolation precautions should be enforced for all hospitalized patients with hMPV infection. Normal infection control emphasizing good hand hygiene should be enforced to limit viral transmission.

Patient and family education regarding hMPV infections includes discussion about supportive care. Adequate fluid intake should be emphasized to prevent dehydration.

Disposition and discharge planning

The prognosis is usually good for patients with uncomplicated disease. Some patients may have some residual bronchial hyperreactivity, especially if there is a family history of asthma. In patients who experience respiratory sequelae, follow-up with a pulmonologist is recommended.

PARVOVIRUS B19

Pathophysiology

A non-enveloped, single-strand DNA virus of the Parvoviridae family, parvovirus B19 has a unique restriction: It can replicate only in actively dividing cells. Its initial invasion occurs via the respiratory tract. After an episode of viremia, erythrocyte precursor cells become infected. Replication of the virus leads to destruction of the host cell, effectively reducing the number of precursor cells available for erythrocyte production, and resulting in a decrease in reticulocytosis and anemia. Anemia can be especially severe in patients with chronic hemolytic anemia, who are more dependent on constant erythrocyte production. The usual incubation period for B19 infection is 4 to 14 days, but can be as long as 21 days (AAP, 2009).

The rash, arthritis, and arthralgias characterizing erythema infectiosum are possibly immune related, although the exact mechanism has not been defined (Cherry & Schulte, 2009). In the case of B19-associated hydrops fetalis with intrauterine infection, anemia leads to cardiac failure with resultant generalized edema. B19-caused myocarditis may be responsible for cardiac failure (Brown, 2008).

Epidemiology and etiology

Infection with parvovirus B19 is common, with one-half of all children being affected at some point by the age of 15 years. B19 replicates only in human erythrocyte precursors, and humans are the only known hosts for the virus. The incidence of B19 infection usually increases in winter and spring. Patients with diseases causing increased RBC destruction (e.g., sickle cell anemia, hereditary spherocytosis, G6PD deficiency, autoimmune hemolytic anemia) are at increased risk of experiencing transient aplastic crisis.

Most B19 infections are transmitted via respiratory secretions or transfusion with contaminated blood products. Transplacental transmission of the virus causing intrauterine infection is also a possibility.

Presentation

The classic illness associated with B19 infection is erythema infectiosum, also referred to as fifth disease. With this presentation, an intensely erythematous rash appears on the patient's cheeks accompanied by circumoral pallor approximately 1 week after a self-limited (2 to 3 days) illness characterized by fever, headache, myalgias, and malaise. The "slapped cheek" rash is followed in a few days by a maculopapular, lacy, pruritic rash that starts on the trunk and spreads to the extremities. The rash is self-limited, but may return weeks or months later. Arthralgias are usually noted in the knees, but are more common in adults than in children.

A transient aplastic crisis is often seen in patients with chronic hemoglobinopathies, hemolytic disease, or any other disease associated with increased RBC destruction or limited RBC production. This manifestation usually lasts 7 to 10 days and occurs with erythrocyte precursor lysis caused by viral replication. Patients will present with fatigue, pallor, and hypotension if the crisis is severe. Potential complications of transient aplastic crisis include congestive heart failure, stroke, and splenic sequestration (Young & Brown, 2004).

Perinatal transmission of B19 infection results in hydrops fetalis. Severe anemia leads to cardiac failure in the fetus, with resultant edema, ascites, and effusions. Intrauterine growth retardation and miscarriage are other possible outcomes of B19 infection in pregnant women.

Immunocompromised patients may be affected with chronic anemia due to pure RBC aplasia (Florea et al., 2007). Table 30-27 lists other B19-associated illnesses.

Differential diagnosis

The following disorders and diseases may be evaluated in the presentation of B19 infection:

TABLE 30-27

Summary of Parvovirus B19 Virus Infections

Hematologic	Transient aplastic crisis, thrombocytopenia, neutropenia pancytopenia, hemophagocytic syndrome, Diamond-Blackfan syndrome
Musculoskeletal	Juvenile rheumatoid arthritis, arthralgias, polyarthropathy syndrome
Skin	Papulopurpuric glove-and-socks syndrome, erythema multiforme, Henoch-Schönlein syndrome, petechial/purpuric rashes
Cardiac	Myocarditis
Respiratory	Pneumonia, acute respiratory distress syndrome
Gastrointestinal	Hepatitis
Renal	Glomerulosclerosis, nephrotic syndrome
Neurologic	Encephalitis, meningitis, meningoencephalitis, neuropathy, Guillain-Barré syndrome, carpal tunnel syndrome, stroke, transverse myelitis
Systemic	Erythema infectiosum, hydrops fetalis (neonates), intrauterine growth retardation (neonates), abortion

- Rash
  - Other viral exanthems (e.g., rubella)
  - Scarlet fever
- Anemia
  - Bacterial infection (e.g., *Streptococcus pneumoniae*)
  - Drug-induced bone marrow suppression (e.g., from use of chloramphenicol)

Plan of care

Although B19 is difficult to grow in culture, which limits the clinical utility of viral isolation by culture, other methods are available for detection of this pathogen. Viral nucleic acid can be detected by DNA hybridization or by PCR; the latter is more sensitive. Most detection of B19 infection; however, occurs via serologic testing. Identification of B19-specific IgM antibodies suggests acute or recent infection.

Therapeutic management is supportive in nature; no antiviral therapy specific for B19 is available. In the case of anemia, transfusion of red blood cells may be required. Intravenous immunoglobulin (IVIG) has been found to be effective in the treatment of chronic infections. Intrauterine RBC transfusions can be used to treat hydrops fetalis secondary to intrauterine infection. Immunosuppression may need to be withdrawn in the case of severe illness. Standard and contact precautions should be employed for hospitalized patients with B19 infection. Normal infection control emphasizing good hand hygiene should be enforced to limit viral transmission.

Patient and family education includes instruction to pregnant patients that they be followed closely for fetal complications of the infection.

Disposition/discharge planning

Follow-up is rarely needed for most patients with B19 infection. The exception is patients with severe infections who may experience possible sequelae; they should be followed by the appropriate specialist. The prognosis is usually good in the case of uncomplicated disease.

> **Critical Thinking**
> Bacterial superinfection may occur in patients with influenza or metapneumovirus, especially in the case of progressive or rapidly worsening disease in the face of appropriate antiviral therapy.

SELECTED INFECTIONS

CROUP

Mark D. Weber

Pathophysiology

Laryngotracheobronchitis (LTB), also referred to as "croup," is an infection that affects all portions of the subglottic airway—larynx, trachea, and bronchi. In response to the infectious pathogen, the mucosa of the subglottic airway may become edematous with subsequent epithelial necrosis. These airway changes result in a decrease in internal diameter, thereby increasing resistance to air flow and causing an increased work of breathing.

According to *Poiseuille's law,* airway resistance is inversely proportional to the forth power of the diameter:

$$\text{Resistance} = 8 \times \text{viscosity} \times \text{length}/\pi \times \text{radius}^4$$

As the internal diameter of the airway becomes smaller, there is a dramatic increase in airway resistance. When the diameter of a tube is decreased, the rate of flow through it increases—a phenomenon known as the *Venturi effect.* The increased flow leads to a decrease in the amount of outward pressure exerted on the wall of the trachea. The resulting negative intraluminal pressure may lead to airway collapse according to the *Bernoulli principle* (Figure 30-4).

Epidemiology and etiology

Croup accounts for as many as 90% of infectious airway obstructions. This disease primarily affects young children, with the typical age range for presentation being 6 months to 3 years (Stroud & Friedman, 2001). The prevalence of croup is higher in males than in females (1.4:1), and the peak incidence for the disease in North America occurs in late autumn.

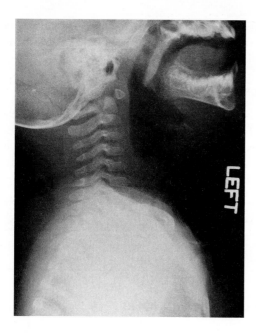

FIGURE 30-4

Lateral Neck Radiograph, Croup.

Source: Courtesy of Mark D. Weber.

TABLE 30-28

Westley Croup Score

Five component items make up the score:
- *Stridor:* (0) none; (1) with agitation only; (2) at rest
- *Retractions:* (0) none; (1) mild; (2) moderate; (3) severe
- *Air entry:* (0) normal; (1) mild decrease; (2) marked decrease
- *Cyanosis:* (0) none; (4) cyanosis with agitation; (5) cyanosis at rest
- *Level of consciousness:* (0) normal, including asleep; (5) disorientated

Total Score Ranging from 0 to 17 Points

Mild croup (0–2): occasional barking cough; no stridor at rest; none to mild suprasternal and/or intercostal retractions

Moderate croup (3–5): frequent barking cough; easily audible stridor at rest; suprasternal and intercostal retractions at rest; no or little distress or agitation

Severe croup (6–11): frequent barking cough; prominent inspiratory and occasionally expiratory stridor; marked retractions; decreased air entry on auscultation; significant distress and agitation

Source: Adapted from Westley et al., 1978.

Croup is most frequently caused by parainfluenza type 1 and 2, but occasionally may be caused by parainfluenza type 3. Respiratory syncytial virus and influenza types A and B have also been reported as the infectious agents in croup. Infrequently, LTB is a bacterial infection, with *Mycoplasma pneumoniae* being the most common causative agent.

Presentation

The most commonly noted symptoms with croup are a barking cough, hoarseness, and stridor. These symptoms frequently begin 12 to 48 hours after the start of a nonspecific upper respiratory infection. Stridor is a common finding due to the anatomical narrowing at the level of the cricoid. It may be present on inspiration or in a biphasic pattern that occurs on both inspiration and expiration. Symptoms may be more prominent at night. One hypothesis for this pattern is that it reflects a nighttime physiologic nadir of endogenous cortisol levels.

The duration of symptomology generally peaks in 48 hours and can last up to 1 week (Shah & Sharieff, 2007). In some patients, however, symptoms increase in severity and progress to respiratory failure. The pediatric patient with impending respiratory failure frequently demonstrates biphasic stridor, severe retractions, hypoxemia, and tachypnea. The Westley croup score provides HCPs with an objective measure of disease severity for therapeutic management decision-making purposes and evaluation comparisons (Table 30-28).

Differential diagnosis

Table 30-29 summarizes the differential diagnoses for croup.

Plan of care

Radiographic studies may provide some additional diagnostic information. For example, a lateral neck film may reveal haziness in the subglottic area with a normal-appearing supraglottic area (Figure 30-4). An anterior–posterior radiograph may also show narrowing of the subglottic area, referred to as the "steeple sign." (Figure 30-5). Although radiographs are frequently obtained, positive findings are seen in only 50% of cases (Stroud & Friedman, 2001).

Therapeutic management for mild to moderate croup is usually supportive. Humidified air has commonly been used as first-line treatment. The theory is that it provides a soothing vasoconstriction of airway mucosa. More recent data, however, suggest that inhaled moist air probably provides no benefit in emergency settings (Moore & Little, 2006). Antipyretics should be given to the febrile patient, as the reduction in body temperature they induce may result in reduced metabolic demand and work of breathing. Steroids may lead to a decrease in the permeability of the capillary endothelium and stabilization of the lysosomal membranes. One dose of oral dexamethasone (0.6 mg/kg) has been shown to result in faster resolution of croup symptoms and reduce risk for airway obstruction (Bjornson et al., 2004).

TABLE 30-29

Differential Diagnoses for Croup

- Epiglottitis
- Bacterial tracheitis
- Foreign body
- Anaphylaxis with angioedema
- Subglottic stenosis
- Laryngeal web
- Retropharyngeal/peritonsillar abscess

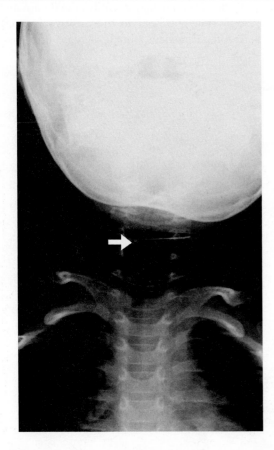

FIGURE 30-5

Lateral Neck Radiograph.

Source: Courtesy of David Paulk, Arcadia University.

TABLE 30-30

Croup: Indications for Hospital Admission

- Failure to improve after nebulized epinephrine or steroid administration
- Need for supplemental oxygen
- Toxic appearance
- Poor oral intake
- Recurrent emergency department visit within 24 hours
- Retractions at rest

The patient with moderate to severe croup will require more intensive management and closer monitoring (Table 30-30). The level of hypoxemia will determine the amount of supplemental oxygen required. Generally, blow-by oxygen is sufficient. For more significant airway edema, consider nebulized epinephrine administered at a dose of 0.5 mL of a 2.25% solution in 3 mL of normal saline. As the nebulized medication is inhaled into the airway, it will produce an alpha-adrenergic–mediated vasoconstriction of the mucosal vasculature. Improvements in air entry should be seen in 10 to 30 minutes. Because of the potential for postadministration rebound edema, patient monitoring is imperative for at least 4 hours when epinephrine is given. With severe croup, IV fluid administration will likely be required, as the child may have increased insensible fluid losses combined with a history of decreased oral intake. Consequently, dexamethasone dosing may be given via the IV route to facilitate its action.

If respiratory distress is progressing to respiratory failure, a trial of heliox may be initiated in an attempt to avert endotracheal intubation for airway support. Helium, when combined with oxygen at a ratio of 80% helium to 20% oxygen, has a threefold lower density than air. The density of a gas is proportional to its *Reynolds number*. A gas with a Reynolds number greater than 3,000 will promote turbulent flow. When the Reynolds number falls to less than 2,000, laminar flow is promoted. The administration of heliox is thought to decrease the Reynolds number of the inspired gas in patients with airway edema, thereby providing for improved laminar flow through the narrowed airway. The enhanced laminar flow, in turn, is hypothesized to improve airway mechanics and lead to reduced work of breathing, although a systematic review failed to support this effect (Vorwerk & Coats, 2008).

If the child progresses to respiratory failure, endotracheal intubation will be required. Upon intubation, anticipate the need for an endotracheal tube that is 0.5 to 1 size smaller due to the tracheal edema.

An otolaryngology consultation should be obtained for the patient who fails to improve with standard medical management or who has recurrent hospital admissions for croup. Children in this clinical situation will likely require a formal airway evaluation with endoscopy/bronchoscopy by either pulmonology or otolaryngology. The critical care team should be consulted for comprehensive care should the patient require any airway support or manipulation.

Family education can start by instructing the family on the basic management of croup at home. Simple measures may include humidified or cool night air. The family should be able to recognized signs of respiratory distress requiring care, such as tachypnea, retractions, and stridor. Any signs or distress or a history of decreased oral intactness warrants evaluation by the primary care provider (PCP).

Disposition and discharge planning

After initial treatment in the emergency department, the decision for discharge or hospital admission needs to be made. The best time for this evaluation is 4 hours after the last dose of nebulized epinephrine or steroids. This time frame will allow for the evaluation of any potential rebound edema. The child can be discharged to home if he or she does not have stridor at rest, has normal oxygen saturation on room air, and has the ability to take oral fluids. A 24-hour follow-up with the PCP should be arranged. The long-term prognosis for the child should be good as there are limited sequelae related to croup, although short-term complications related to rebound edema and clinical deterioration can occur.

EPIGLOTTITIS

Mark D. Weber

Pathophysiology

The epiglottis is a cartilaginous structure, located at the base of the tongue, that is covered with epithelium. In epiglottitis this structure undergoes a severe inflammatory process. The inflammation may affect the epiglottis and extend to the surrounding structures, including the aryepiglottic folds and the soft tissue of the arytenoids. As the inflammation progresses, a ball-valve effect forces the epiglottis posteriorly. These changes can progress to complete airway obstruction.

Epidemiology and etiology

Three fourths of all epiglottitis infections occur in children between the ages of 1 and 5 years. There is a slight male predominance in incidence (1.2:1). The severity of disease is often greater in children than that seen in adults (Mayo-Smith et al., 1995).

The incidence of epiglottitis has decreased dramatically in the United States since the introduction of the *Haemophilus influenzae* (Hib) vaccine, as *H. influenzae* type b was traditionally the most common causative agent (Acevedo et al., 2009). Other causative agents include *Staphylococcus aureus*, Group A *Streptococcus*, and *Streptococcus pneumoniae*. A preexisting viral infection or local tissue trauma may make the epithelium more susceptible to such bacterial infection.

Presentation

The onset of symptoms with epiglottitis can be sudden, with a rapid progression to total airway obstruction. The patient may appear toxic with fever of 38.8–40°C (101.8–104°F), severe sore throat, and dysphagia. Clinical signs of airway obstruction may be observed, such as muffled voice, drooling, and a tripod sitting position. The last sign represents the patient's attempt to maintain airway patency through neck extension and forward leaning with hands on knees (Figure 30-6).

Differential diagnosis

Table 30-31 summarizes the differential diagnoses for epiglottitis.

Plan of care

If epiglottitis is considered to be the etiology of the patient's symptoms, then initial management is to maintain airway patency. Agitation may lead to full airway obstruction, For this reason, all noxious stimuli such as taking oral or

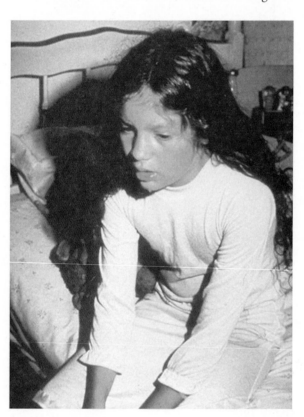

FIGURE 30-6

Tripod Sitting Position.

Source: Courtesy of the National EMSC Resource Alliance.

TABLE 30-31

Differential Diagnosis for Epiglottitis
• Pharyngitis
• Laryngitis
• Croup
• Uvulitis
• Inhaled foreign body
• Retropharyngeal/peritonsillar abscess

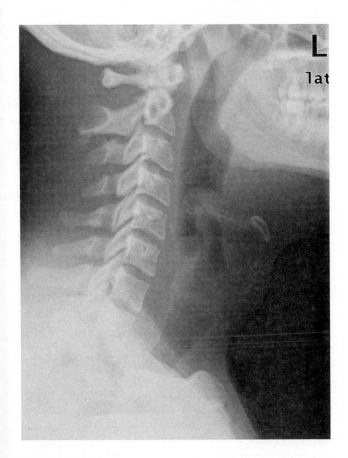

FIGURE 30-7

Lateral Neck Radiograph, Epiglottitis.

Source: Courtesy of Mark D. Weber.

rectal temperatures, examining the oropharynx, starting an intravenous line, or administering oxygen by face mask should be avoided, and the focus placed on keeping the patient calm. When the airway and patient are stabilized, a lateral neck radiograph may reveal an enlarged epiglottis and distention of the hypopharynx (the thumb sign) or postlingual triangle (Figure 30-7).

If full airway obstruction is imminent, endotracheal intubation is required. Intubation of the inflamed airway is extremely difficult and should be performed only by those skilled in this maneuver, such as a pediatric anesthesia or otolaryngology specialist. It is also best performed in the operating room. The intubation is frequently performed with the child sedated, but spontaneously breathing, should endotracheal intubation be too difficult to obtain. On occasion, the airway may need to be secured surgically. Direct laryngoscopy will reveal a beefy red, swollen epiglottis and aryepiglottic folds. Once the airway is secured, blood cultures and a surface culture swab of the epiglottis can be obtained.

In children, approximately 60% of blood cultures will reveal a positive organism (Mayo-Smith et al., 1995). Antimicrobial therapy is started empirically and can be tailored when culture and susceptibilities are available. A third-generation cephalosporin (Shah & Sharieff, 2007)

or vancomycin plus a third-generation cephalosporin is recommended if penicillin-resistant pneumococci or methicillin-resistant *S. aureus* is suspected. Treatment is usually continued for 7 to 10 days.

In those patients who require endotracheal intubation and mechanical ventilation, the average number of ventilated days is 3.5 (Shah et al., 2004). Extubation should be planned such that advanced airway equipment (e.g., flexible bronchoscope) is available, or the extubation is performed with an endotracheal tube exchanger in place.

When epiglottitis is suspected, immediate consultation with the pediatric anesthesia or otolaryngology service is indicated. Difficult airway equipment should be at the bedside and the critical care team available to ensure comprehensive care is initiated immediately. Consultation with infectious diseases specialists should be considered to ensure the best choice of antibiotic therapies.

Patient and family education focuses on the nature of the infection and disease course, intensive care management, and the goal of therapies.

Disposition and discharge planning

The patient should be evaluated by the PCP within 48 hours of discharge. Potential complications include deep neck space infections, vocal granulomas, and recurrent illness (Shah et al., 2004). Mortality has been reported to be as high as 12% in those patients for whom airway patency was not secured (Damm et al., 1996).

MENINGOCOCCEMIA

Lisa Sansalone

Pathophysiology

Meningococcemia is an infection caused by the presence of *Neisseria meningitidis,* a Gram-negative encapsulated diplococcus, in the bloodstream. The invasiveness of this pathogen is enhanced by the presence of its polysaccharide capsule, which resists destruction from phagocytosis (Pathan et al., 2003).

N. meningitidis infection initiates a cascade of multiple organ dysfunction that is characterized by small-vessel changes, pathologic vasoconstriction and vasodilation, loss of thromboresistance, and diffuse intravascular coagulation (Pathan et al., 2003). Invasion of endothelial cells and endotoxin release are major components in the pathogenesis of the disease process. Impaired organ perfusion leads to cardiac dysfunction, renal impairment, and gastrointestinal mucosal ischemia. Pulmonary involvement includes secondary complications such as pulmonary edema from volume resuscitation and hemorrhage from disseminated intravascular coagulation. Central nervous system involvement may include direct invasion of the meninges with meningitis and encephalitis, or it may result from impaired perfusion (Pathan et al., 2003). The host's death from meningococcemia may occur within hours of the onset of symptoms.

Epidemiology and etiology

Meningococcemia can be classified into two categories: chronic and acute. Chronic infection is characterized by fever lasting for more than one week without meningeal signs (Wood, 2007). The chronic form of meningococcemia is rare and can resemble other arthritis–dermatitis syndromes. Acute meningococcemia is much more common; it represents the fulminant infection. For the purpose of this section, only the acute form of meningococcemia will be addressed.

Approximately 1,400 to 2,800 cases of acute meningococcal disease are reported annually, with 30% of these cases being identified as meningococcemia. Meningitis and pneumonia account for the majority of the remaining pathologic infections. A preponderance of these cases (97%) are classified as sporadic; the other 3% are associated with outbreaks. Acute meningococcemia follows a seasonal pattern, with a peak noted in late winter and early spring (Kaplan et al., 2006).

Estimates of the mortality rate associated with meningococcemia range from 7% to 20%. The fatality rate is influenced by age and *Neisseria* serotype. Although 13 serotypes of *Neisseria* have been identified, only 5 are major pathogens that contribute to human disease. The most fatal strain (W-135 serotype) has a 21% mortality rate, with higher rates being found in children with interleukin-1 cluster polymorphisms. In addition, patients who present with shock, seizure, hypothermia, purpura fulminans, total WBC count less than $500/mm^3$, or total platelet count less than $100,000/mm^3$ have a poorer prognosis (Pathan et al., 2003). Older children are at an increased risk of death, and substantial long-term sequelae are reported in 11% to 19% of survivors of invasive meningococcal disease (Gardner, 2006; Kaplan et al., 2006).

Approximately 10% of the population has nasopharyngeal colonization with *Neisseria;* overcrowded conditions increase the carrier rate (Yazdankhah & Caugant, 2004). Bacterial transmission occurs via droplet spread on a person-to-person basis, thereby increasing the risk for epidemic outbreaks.

At-risk populations for infection are as follows: children younger than 4 years of age (excluding neonates who are younger than 6 months of age, who may be protected by passive maternal antibodies); overcrowded populations, including school children, adolescents in dormitories, and military personnel; and complement = deficient populations. Approximately 50% to 60% of complement-deficient patients have at least one episode of active meningococcemia in their lifetime and are at risk for recurrent infection, as they lack the ability to mount a bacteriolytic response to the pathogen that causes meningococcemia. The following complement deficiencies have been associated with higher risk of active infection from *N. meningitides:* systemic lupus erythematus, multiple myeloma, severe liver disease, enteropathies, HIV infection, functional and acquired asplenia, immunoglobulin deficiencies, and nephritic syndromes (Pathan et al., 2003).

Presentation

Meningococcemia initially mimics many acute viral processes, a factor that often results in delayed diagnosis. The HCP may elicit a recent history of upper respiratory symptoms, fever, headache, nausea, vomiting, myalgias, or arthralgias. Not all pediatric patients appear toxic on presentation. Most patients have nonspecific symptoms in the first 4 to 6 hours but become critically ill within 24 hours (Thompson et al., 2006).

Fifty percent of patients with acute meningococcal meningitis have cutaneous findings, including petechiae on extremities and trunk. Stellate purpura with a central gunmetal hue is considered highly suggestive of meningococcemia infection (Figure 30-8). In addition, pediatric patients with meningococcal meningitis may exhibit altered mental status, neck stiffness, irritability, cranial nerve palsies, gait disturbances, ataxia, nausea, vomiting, signs consistent with increased intracranial pressure, and seizures (Thompson et al., 2006). Patients with advanced acute infection may exhibit decreased peripheral and central perfusion, hypotension, tachycardia, fever or hypothermia, leucopenia, and thrombocytopenia (Pathan et al., 2003).

Differential diagnosis

Differential diagnoses for the cutaneous findings of purpura and petechiae include Henoch-Schönlein purpura (HSP),

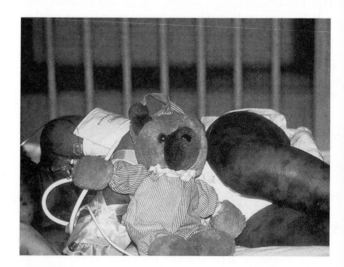

FIGURE 30-8

Meningicoccal Purpura.

Source: Courtesy of the National EMSC Resource Alliance.

idiopathic thrombocytopenic purpura (ITP), collagen vascular disease, erythema multiforme, hypersensitivity vasculitis, and neoplastic processes. Additional differential diagnoses include the following infectious etiologies:

- Bacterial sepsis from *Neisseria gonorrhoeae*, *Haemophilus influenzae*, and *Streptococcus pneumoniae*
- Endocarditis
- Rocky Mountain spotted fever
- Viral illnesses (including echo and coxsackieviruses)
- Toxic shock syndrome
- Leptospirosis

Plan of care

Isolation of the meningococcal organism from normally sterile body fluid such as blood, synovial, or CSF provides a definitive diagnosis. Laboratory studies for diagnosis and evaluation for multiple system organ involvement include blood, throat, and CSF cultures and analysis; complete blood count with differential; coagulation studies; liver function tests; and blood gases.

Blood cultures have almost 100% specificity and are positive 50% of the time with active infection. Throat culture swabs may also isolate *N. meningitidis* but have less specificity.

Lumbar puncture may be indicated for patients with suspected meningococcal meningitis. Spinal fluid reveals polymorphonuclear leukocytosis. Gram stain may be negative if there is no CSF involvement (Wood, 2007), and cultures may be sterile in patients treated with antibiotics. Nevertheless, the presence of pleocytosis is suggestive of meningococcal meningitis in the presence of sterile cultures. PCR testing may be performed on serum or spinal fluid to detect the presence of noncultivatable or slow-growing microorganisms that may be seen in patients who have been partially treated with antibiotics prior to obtaining culture specimen (Anderson et al., 2009).

CBC may reveal leukocytosis, with increased percentages of neutrophils and bands reflective of an acute bacterial infection. In addition, thrombocytopenia and anemia may be present in patients with more advanced states of infection. Coagulation studies may reflect the presence of disseminated intravascular coagulation, evidenced by decreased serum prothrombin and fibrinogen as well as prolonged D-dimer, fibrin degradation product, and activated partial thromboplastin time. Blood gases may reflect metabolic acidosis, with elevated lactate levels being seen in patients with decreased perfusion states (Wood, 2007).

Chest radiography is helpful in making the diagnosis, as 8% to 15% of patients with confirmed meningococcemia have clinical pneumonia. This finding has been associated with Group Y serotypes of the organism. Magnetic resonance imaging may be indicated for assessing tissue viability and osseus involvement from the disseminated intravascular coagulation seen with active infection.

Skin scraping or needle aspiration of skin lesions will yield positive culture and Gram stain findings in 50% of infected patients. Histologic findings include thrombi in dermal vessels composed of neutrophils, platelets, and fibrin. In addition, neutrophilic pustules may be reported (Anderson et al., 2009).

Immediate resuscitation for the patient with meningococcemia includes anticipation of multiple organ dysfunction. Early transfer to a tertiary care center allows for continued antibiotic therapy, availability of ventilator and vasopressor support, fluid management, and specialty consultation. Establishment of central venous access and placement of invasive arterial monitoring devices early in the course of treatment and resuscitation are recommended due to the increased vascular permeability associated with this disease, which typically necessitates interventions including volume expansion, intravenous fluids, and vasopressor agent support. Anticipate severe hypotension, decreased cardiac output, increased capillary permeability, and disseminated intravascular coagulation. Patients with meningococcal infection who have disseminated intravascular coagulation may need fresh frozen plasma, cryoprecipitate, factor VII, packed red blood cells, and platelet transfusions to prevent further complications of hemorrhage (Welch & Nadel, 2003).

Patients with refractory shock may respond to hydrocortisone (1 mg/kg every 6 hours) administered to treat adrenocortical insufficiency. In addition, high-dose dexamethasone has been shown to reduce hearing loss and other neurologic complications of meningitis caused by *H. influenzae* infection. While the efficacy and safety of dexamethasone has not been evaluated in the setting of meningococcal meningitis, some HCPs are using it in pediatric patients with clinical evidence of meningitis without shock (Welch & Nadel, 2003).

Droplet isolation should be instituted to decrease exposure of the health care staff to contaminated secretions from the patient with meningococcemia. These precautions may be lifted after the first 24 hours of appropriate antibiotic coverage.

Pharmacotherapeutic goals include eradication of bacteria, reduction of morbidity, and prevention of disease complications. Antibiotics should be initiated as soon as possible, without waiting for obtaining lab specimens or culture results. Broad-spectrum antibiotic coverage for a minimum of 5 to 7 days is recommended (Welch & Nadel, 2003). Penicillin G is the antibiotic of choice for susceptible isolates, to be dosed at 500,000 units/kg/day, divided every 4 hours. Given the presence of known penicillin-resistant strains in different regions of the world, third-generation cephalosporins are acceptable choices while cultures and susceptibilities are pending; dose cefotaxime at 200 mg/kg/day, divided every 8 hours, or ceftriaxone at 100 mg/kg/day, divided every 12 hours (Wood, 2007). HCPs should be aware that stable patients who receive intravenous antibiotics may become unstable secondary to cytokine release with antibiotic administration.

Because of this potential complication, patients should be closely monitored after the administration of antibiotics.

Surgical care and considerations include the possibility of extensive skin and muscle grafting for coverage of large defects and partial or full extremity amputation(s). A conservative approach to treatment is recommended until distinct lines of demarcation between viable and nonviable tissue are present. Long-term therapeutic management goals focus on limb and organ preservation. This effort may include repeated surgical revisions of extremities, dialysis for toxin clearance and kidney failure, and long-term seizure pharmacotherapy (Hart & Thompson, 2006).

Many experimental therapies are being studied to counteract effects of the cytokine release and complications of coagulation disorders, in hopes of decreasing the morbidity and mortality associated with these conditions. To dates, the usefulness of such studies' findings have been limited by population size considerations, confounding variables with multiple organ involvement, and the ethical implications of randomized controlled trials, which would withhold or delay treatments from patients with this aggressive disease process. Investigational treatments include protein C infusions, anti-endotoxin therapies, low-dose heparin infusions, steroid administration, tissue plasminogen activator therapy, antithrombin III infusions, and topical nitroglycerin. Plasmapheresis, which removes inflammatory mediators, is also under investigation for meningococcemia. Additional studies include shock management, corrective coagulopathy therapies, inflammatory response modulation, and neutralization of endotoxins (Anderson et al., 2009).

During the acute phase of illness, patients require the expertise of multiple pediatric specialists, including critical care specialists, infectious diseases specialists, neurologists, surgeons, plastic surgeons, dermatologists, and nephrologists. In addition, early involvement of rehabilitation, physical, occupational, and respiratory therapy services may be indicated if prolonged immobility is anticipated. Child life specialists are helpful for preparing children for numerous procedures, providing play therapy, and assisting with developmentally appropriate interventions. Psychiatric evaluation and long-term follow-up are warranted if prolonged illness, hospitalization, and disabilities exist. Profound body-image issues may arise with meningococcemia patients who require surgical treatments, amputations, and/or grafting (Garralda et al., 2009).

Family education and support includes antimicrobial prophylaxis, which is recommended for all close contacts in the home, school, workplace, and hospital to eradicate potential colonization after exposure. There is greater than a 1% transmission rate from exposure to a known infected source. Single-dose prophylaxis includes the following options:

- Ciprofloxacin 500 mg orally
- Ceftriaxone 125 mg IM for infants and children younger than 15 years of age
- Ceftriaxone 250 mg IM for children older than 15 years of age and adults (Gardner, 2006)

The alternative prophylaxis regimen uses rifampin:

- Rifampin for infants younger than 1 month: 5 mg/kg orally every 12 hours for 48 hours
- Rifampin for infants/children older than 1 month: 10 mg/kg orally every 12 hours for 48 hours (maximum, 600 mg)
- Rifampin for adults: 600 mg orally every 12 hours for 48 hours

Rifampin resistance is increasing and should only be used in consultation with infectious diseases experts (Fraser et al., 2006).

Early patient and caregiver teaching includes offering support while the results of diagnostic studies are pending and anticipation of complications and their resultant therapies. In addition, a lengthy intensive care stay may be expected based on response to therapies and multiple organ dysfunction. Long-term educational goals include preparation of patients and families for possible limb preservation surgeries, prosthesis referral, and psychosocial therapeutic interventions for the pediatric patient and caregivers (Garralda et al., 2009).

Disposition and discharge planning

Meningococcemia survivors may require long-term management of grafting and amputation sites. Patients and caregivers should anticipate referral to inpatient rehabilitation centers when the patient becomes medically stable. In addition, extensive extremity involvement may result in the loss of participation in activities of daily living, school, and extracurricular activities. For this reason, pediatric patients with permanent disabilities may benefit from aggressive psychotherapy. Referral to amputee programs with prosthetic capabilities is recommended. Patients with meningococcal meningitis will require auditory testing to rule out the possibility of hearing deficits associated with meningitis and antibiotic therapies (Welch & Nadel, 2003).

In the United States, the mortality rate for patients with acute meningococcemia remains approximately 10% despite the advent of modern therapeutic interventions. Mortality rates are highest in the adolescent and young adult age group. Most deaths occur within 48 hours of symptom onset. Poor prognostic indicators include extreme hyperpyrexia, shock, cutaneous findings, neurologic changes including seizures, leucopenia, thrombocytopenia, and hypothermia (Wood, 2007). Those patients who present with disseminated intravascular coagulation have a documented mortality rate exceeding 50% (Anderson et al., 2009). The most common sequelae of meningococcal infection include hearing loss, skin necrosis requiring grafting, amputations, deafness, seizures, and ataxia (Kaplan et al., 2006).

The MCV4 (Meningococcal Conjugate Vaccine 4) prevents infection from *N. meningitidis* serotypes A, C, Y, and W-135, which account for approximately 75% of the invasive meningococcal strains found in the United States. The W-135 strain is believed to be responsible for 70% of the infections in the United States (Pelton, 2009). There is currently no preventive measure available for serotype B, which is believed to account for most cases of meningococcemia in infants younger than 1 year of age. The MCV4 vaccine confers a longer duration of protection with similar efficacy than previously available vaccines. Ideally, the vaccine is administered as a single intramuscular injection when the child is between 11 and 12 years of age. If not previously administered, it is recommended that all adolescents receive immunization prior to high school entry. In addition, high-risk populations, such as individuals with functional asplenia and complement deficiency, should receive vaccination (CDC, 2005).

RETROPHARYNGEAL/PERITONSILLAR ABSCESS

Mark D. Weber

Pathophysiology

The retropharyngeal space extends from the base of the skull to the posterior mediastinum and is bound by the buccopharyngeal fascia anteriorly, the prevertebral fascia posteriorly, and the carotid sheaths laterally. It is filled with lymph node chains that drain the nasopharynx, adenoids, posterior nasal sinuses, and middle ear. Abscess formation in this space may occur following trauma to the pharynx or by a primary infection from any of the draining structures. Infection can be isolated to a single lymph node and extend to the abscess wall or rupture and spread purulent material throughout the retropharyngeal space (Roberson, 2004).

Peritonsillar abscess (PTA) is associated with pharyngitis or tonsillitis. Similar to what happens with some retropharyngeal abscesses (RPA), a local cellulitis may develop and progress first to phlegmon, then to abscess, although suppurative adenitis is the most common presentation. The location may be in the superior, middle, or inferior tonsillar poles, with the superior pole being most prevalent. RPA and PTA may extend to significantly obstruct the upper airway.

Epidemiology and etiology

Retropharyngeal abscesses occur most commonly in children ages 1 to 5 years (Craig & Schunk, 2003). Peritonsillar abscess is the most common deep neck infection in pediatric patients and is most often seen in adolescents (Schraff et al., 2001).

Infections are usually polymicrobial. Common pathogens are *Streptococcus pyogenes, Staphylococcus aureus,* and *Haemophilus* species. Resistant species such as methicillin-resistant *S. aureus* are becoming more common. Anaerobic bacteria such as *Fusobacteria, Bacteroides, Prevotella,* and *Veillonella* have also been implicated.

Presentation

The history associated with RPA may include endotracheal intubation, oral foreign object (pen, straw), dental procedure, or recent infection in any of the structures that drain into the retropharyngeal space. The PTA history should include symptoms or diagnosis of recent pharyngitis or snoring. The child with RPA or PTA will present with fever and complaints of a severe sore throat and dysphagia. Pain is usually unilateral. Trismus (decreased and painful range of neck motion), neck swelling, drooling, or a muffled ("hot potato") voice can be present in both PTA and RPA (McClay et al., 2003; Szuhay & Tewfik, 1998). Patients with RPA may have chest pain if mediastinal extension of the infection occurs; patients with PTA may have ear pain on the affected side.

On physical examination, tripod positioning with partial airway obstruction may be observed (Figure 30-9). The patient may be ill or toxic appearing and have associated dehydration due to poor oral intake and insensible losses. Anterior cervical lymphadenopathy may be appreciated. If the patient is able to tolerate an oral exam, the HCP may note lateral compression of the posterior pharynx, fluctuant mass (RPA), or swollen tonsil with uvula deviation (PTA).

Differential diagnosis

The differential diagnoses for RPA and PTA are listed in Table 30-32. Epiglottitis should also be considered if a patient presents with fever and signs of upper airway obstruction.

Plan of care

The PTA/RPA therapeutic plan begins with airway assessment, which includes supporting the patient's ventilation and oxygenation. Any airway compromise should be addressed before diagnostic studies are undertaken. Agitation of the patient may lead to complete airway obstruction, so noxious stimuli should be avoided. This includes taking oral temperatures, examining the oropharynx, starting an intravenous line,

TABLE 30-32

Differential Diagnoses for Retropharyngeal/Peritonsillar Abscess

- Epiglottitis
- Bacterial tracheitis
- Pharyngitis
- Esophagitis
- Sinusitis
- Torticollis

administering oxygen by face mask, or performing diagnostic studies. If the patient is a *stable and willing* participant, then obtaining a lateral neck radiograph may help differentiate RPA from epiglottitis. In RPA, there may be evidence of widening of the retropharyngeal space (Figure 30-9).

If complete airway obstruction is imminent, endotracheal intubation is required. Intubation of the obstructed airway is extremely difficult and should be performed only by those HCPs skilled in this maneuver, such as a pediatric anesthesia or otolaryngology specialist. It is also best performed in the operating room with difficult airway equipment readily available. The intubation is frequently performed with the child sedated but spontaneously breathing, and may require a smaller endotracheal tube due to oropharyngeal distortion as a result of mass effect.

Diagnostic studies for the evaluation of RPA/PTA include a complete blood count and differential. White blood counts are usually high. Blood cultures may be obtained but are rarely positive. In PTA, a throat culture should be performed to evaluate for group A *Streptococcus*. If a neck abscess is drained, the drainage should be sent for culture; both aerobic and anaerobic organisms may be

present. Computed tomography with IV contrast may be used as a diagnostic tool for both RPA and PTA; it may identify the extent of infection and differentiate abscess from cellulitis. Chest radiographs are also valuable in evaluating for mediastinal expansion in RPA. Consultation with otolaryngology and infectious diseases may be warranted.

Surgical drainage is required for airway compromise and may be considered if the abscess is larger than 2 cm or if the patient fails to respond to IV antibiotics within 24 hours (Roberson, 2004). Tonsillectomy is reserved for patients with PTA and recurrent tonsillitis and for those who fail to respond to other drainage techniques.

Empiric antimicrobial therapy is initiated to treat infection with both aerobic and anaerobic organisms. It should be tailored when culture and susceptibility results are available. Consider providing coverage (vancomycin, linezolid) for resistant organisms as community prevalence dictates. Initial management consists of IV antibiotics such as ampicillin–sulbactam or clindamycin. Once the patient is no longer febrile and improving, therapy can be changed to similar oral agents to complete the 14-day course.

Consultation with specialists depends on the severity of the patient's illness and the response to therapies. Infectious diseases, otolaryngology, pulmonology, and critical care services may be involved in the patient's comprehensive management plan.

Patient and family education focuses on the nature of the infection, disease course, and symptoms of recurrence.

Disposition and discharge planning

Prognosis is usually good if RPA is treated early. Severe and life-threatening complications include full airway obstruction, septicemia, and mediastinal extension. PTA, if severe and untreated, may also lead to airway obstruction or septicemia. Recurrent infection is not uncommon. Discharge can be anticipated once the patient is afebrile, able to take oral nutrition, and free of respiratory distress at rest. The patient should be evaluated by the primary care provider within 48 hours of discharge, and follow-up with specialists maybe indicated post discharge.

TOXIC SHOCK SYNDROME

Bradley Tilford

Toxic shock syndrome is a term used to describe two acute, toxin-mediated, multisystem febrile illnesses caused by *Staphylococcus aureus* and *Streptococcus pyogenes* (group A *Streptococcus* [GAS]). The illnesses share similar pathophysiology, but have important differences in clinical presentation, morbidity, and mortality. In this section, toxic shock syndrome caused by *Staphylococcus aureus* will be referred

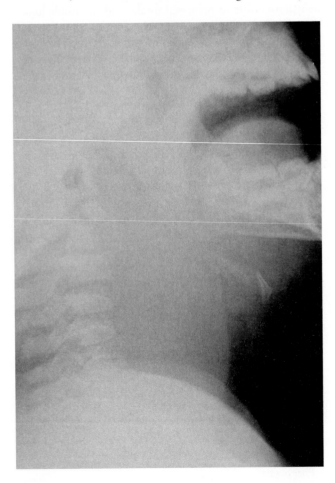

FIGURE 30-9

RPA.

Source: Courtesy of Karin-Reuter-Rice.

to as TSS, while STSS refers to the illness caused by *Streptococcus pyogenes.*

Pathophysiology

Some variants of *S. aureus* and GAS produce protein toxins capable of causing massive activation of the host cellular immune response. They act as superantigens by binding simultaneously to the MHC type II receptors on antigen-presenting cells and the T-cell receptors on helper T cells. While a typical antigen activates less than 1% of host T cells, superantigen binding may activate 20% to 30% of T cells. The activated T cells respond with a massive production of inflammatory cytokines, resulting in rash, fever, hypotension, and other characteristic features of the syndrome (Lappin & Ferguson, 2009; Lazar & Bogue, 2007).

Epidemiology and etiology

The clinical syndrome now known as toxic shock syndrome was first described in the late 1970s associated with colonization or localized infection from *S. aureus.* An epidemic of TSS occurred in menstruating women in 1980 and 1981 associated with the use of super-absorbent tampons and vaginal colonization with *S. aureus* (Lazar & Bogue, 2007). Menstrual TSS has an annual incidence of 1 case per 100,000 population, with a case fatality rate of 3.3% (Singhi et al., 2008).

Streptococcal toxic shock syndrome was described in the late 1980s associated with GAS infection. The annual incidence of invasive GAS infections is 1.5 to 5.2 cases per 100,000 population; 8% to 14% of these patients will develop STSS. The case fatality rate of STSS is 5% to 10% in children and 30% to 70% in adults (Singhi et al., 2008).

Presentation

Both TSS and STSS may begin with a nonspecific prodrome of lethargy, myalgia, sore throat, abdominal pain, diarrhea, and rash. Patients quickly develop fever and hypotension resulting in multiple organ dysfunction. TSS is typically associated with colonization, as *S. aureus* is recovered from the blood in only 10% of cases. In contrast, STSS is often associated with localized infection, and blood cultures are positive for GAS in more than 70% of cases (Lazar & Bogue, 2007). Diagnosis requires a high index of suspicion and is based on the characteristic clinical presentations. Case definitions from the CDC (1997, 2010a) are summarized in Table 30-33 and Table 30-34.

Differential diagnosis

The differential diagnosis of a child who presents with abrupt onset of fever, hypotension, and rash must include sepsis, acute viral infection, bacterial meningitis, meningococcemia, and, in endemic areas, Rocky Mountain spotted fever. Sepsis and acute viral infection resulting in hypotension are more common in patients with indwelling medical devices and in immunosuppressed patients. Meningococcemia presents with petechiae that quickly progresses to purpura. Kawasaki disease and scarlet fever may mimic some aspects of the presentation of toxic shock syndrome, but are not usually associated with hypotension (Singhi et al., 2008).

Plan of care

Essentials of management of toxic shock syndrome include aggressive hemodynamic and respiratory support, removal,

TABLE 30-33

Toxic Shock Syndrome: CDC Case Definition

Clinical Criteria

1. Fever: temperature ≥ 102.0°F (39°C)
2. Rash: diffuse macular erythroderma
3. Desquamation: 1–2 weeks after onset of illness, especially the palms and soles
4. Hypotension: SBP ≤ 90 mmHg or less than 5th percentile for age for patients younger than 16 years of age
5. Multisystem involvement (three or more of the following):
   a. Gastrointestinal: vomiting or diarrhea
   b. Muscular: severe myalgias or CK level at least twice the upper limit of normal
   c. Mucous membranes: hyperemia of the conjunctiva, oropharynx, or vagina
   d. Kidney: BUN or creatinine at least twice the upper limit of normal or urinary sediment with pyuria
   e. Liver: total bilirubin, AST or ALT at least twice the upper limit of normal
   f. Hematologic: platelets < 100,000/mm³
   g. Neurologic: altered mental status without focal neurologic signs in the absence of fever or hypotension

Laboratory Criteria

1. Negative results on blood, throat, or cerebrospinal fluid cultures (blood culture may be positive for *S. aureus*) if samples were obtained
2. No rise in serum titers to Rocky Mountain spotted fever, leptospirosis, or measles if obtained

Probable TSS Case: Fulfills four of the five clinical criteria and meets the laboratory criteria.

Confirmed TSS Case: Fulfills all five clinical criteria (unless the patient dies before desquamation) and meets the laboratory criteria.

Note: Systolic blood pressure (SBP), creatine kinase (CK), blood urea nitrogen (BUN), alanine transaminase (ALT), aspartate transaminase (AST).

Source: CDC, 1997.

TABLE 30-34

Streptococcal Toxic Shock Syndrome: CDC Case Definition

Clinical Criteria

1. Hypotension: SBP ≤ 90 mmHg or less than 5th percentile for age for patients younger than 16 years of age
2. Multisystem involvement (two or more of the following):
   a. Kidney: Creatinine ≥ 2 mg/dL for adults or 2 times the upper limit of normal for age
   b. Hematologic: Platelets ≤ 100,000/mm³ or evidence of disseminated intravascular coagulation
   c. Liver: ALT, AST, or total bilirubin at least twice the upper limit of normal for age
   d. Pulmonary: Acute respiratory distress syndrome
   e. Skin: Generalized erythematous macular rash that may desquamate
   f. Musculoskeletal: Necrotizing fasciitis, myositis, or gangrene

Laboratory Criteria

1. Isolation of group A *Streptococcus*

Probable STSS Case: Meets the clinical case definition, absence of another etiology for illness, and isolation of group A *Streptococcus* from a nonsterile site.

Confirmed STSS Case: Meets the clinical case definition with isolation of group A *Streptococcus* from a normally sterile site (e.g., blood, cerebrospinal fluid, joint, pleural, or pericardial fluid).

Note: Systolic blood pressure (SBP), alanine transaminase (ALT), aspartate transaminase (AST).

Source: CDC, 2010a.

or debridement of a localized site of infection if present, and antibiotic therapy directed at killing the causative organisms and neutralizing toxins.

Pediatric patients presenting with toxic shock should immediately receive supplemental oxygen and fluid resuscitation with isotonic crystalloids via a peripheral IV line. If an IV cannot be placed quickly, intraosseus access should be obtained. If shock persists despite administration of 40 to 60 mL/kg of isotonic fluid, then vasopressor and/or inotropic support should be started with dopamine, epinephrine, or similar agents. Inotropic support should not be delayed while waiting to obtain central venous access. If respiratory distress develops, additional support with noninvasive positive-pressure ventilation or mechanical ventilation may be necessary. The child will require care in a pediatric intensive care unit and should be transferred by a dedicated pediatric transport team if those resources are not available at the presenting hospital (Brierley et al., 2009).

Potential sites of *S. aureus* or GAS infection or colonization should be identified. Tampons, wound packing, and other foreign bodies should be removed if present. A pediatric surgeon should evaluate skin and soft tissue infections

for drainage or debridement. Failure to remove the source of *S. aureus* or GAS may result in continued toxin production and death (Singhi et al., 2008).

Broad-spectrum parenteral antibiotics should be initiated as soon as possible, preferably within the first hour of presentation. Blood and urine cultures should be obtained. Obtaining cultures of sputum or CSF may be considered, but antibiotic therapy should not be delayed while awaiting their results. When the source has been identified as *S. aureus* or GAS, then antibiotic therapy can be tailored to their susceptibilities. A reasonable starting antibiotic regimen is ceftriaxone and vancomycin. If the suspicion for toxic shock syndrome is high, then clindamycin should also be administered, as it may decrease bacterial toxin production. Clindamycin is effective against many isolates of community-acquired MRSA. Given that 60% to 80% of *S. aureus* strains isolated from the community are now identified as MRSA, it is prudent to start vancomycin at the initiation of antibiotic therapy. This agent may be discontinued after antibiotic sensitivities have been reviewed. With any life-threatening infection, consultation with a specialist in pediatric infectious diseases is advisable (Djillali et al., 2004; Lappin & Ferguson, 2009).

Intravenous pooled human immunoglobulins (IVIG) have been reported as being beneficial in some cases of toxic shock syndrome. Their effect is likely due to bacterial toxin neutralization and attenuation of the host's systemic inflammatory response. Further studies are needed to identify the optimal dosing and those patients who are most likely to benefit from IVIG, but it is reasonable to attempt this therapy in a patient with toxic shock syndrome who is refractory to aggressive intensive care support and parenteral antibiotics (Djillali et al., 2004; Lappin & Ferguson, 2009).

Consulting with the critical care team early in the patient's presentation can ensure organ perfusion is maximized. As toxic shock may develop into a long-term hospitalization with the possibility of sequelae, specialty services such as infectious disease, nephrology, cardiology, and pulmonary may become an active part of the interprofessional team. Nutrition, rehabilitation medicine, child life, social services, and spiritual advisors are often essential to ensure optimal outcomes.

Patient and family education should address the goals of therapy, supportive equipment and medication, the interprofessional team approach, and psychosocial support of the family.

Disposition and discharge planning

Patients with TSS or STSS are at risk for multiple organ dysfunction and may require vasopressor/inotropic support, mechanical ventilation, and dialysis, among other interventions. They should be cared for in a PICU setting until they have been stable off vasopressors/inotropes and are requiring no more than 2 to 4 liters of supplemental oxygen via nasal cannula for at least 24 hours. These patients will require an extended course of antibiotics, which may necessitate long-term venous access such as a peripherally inserted central venous catheter. Children with kidney failure may require continued care in the PICU, depending on the dialysis capability of the hospital. As with any child with severe illness requiring ICU care, evaluations by speech therapy, physical therapy, and occupational therapy should be considered, and some patients may benefit from inpatient rehabilitation.

TRACHEITIS

Mark D. Weber

Pathophysiology

Tracheitis is an invasive bacterial infection of the larynx, trachea, or bronchi. The invasion leads to an inflammatory process that causes adherent mucopurulent pseudomembranes to form inside the airways. These membranes or secretions may result in narrowing of the subglottic region and airway compromise. Respiratory failure may follow. Severe tracheitis can lead to complications such as subglottic stenosis, hypopharyngeal and esophageal stenosis, acute respiratory distress syndrome, and multiple organ dysfunction syndrome (Hopkins et al., 2006; Huang et al., 2009).

Epidemiology and etiology

Patients presenting with tracheitis range in age from 3 weeks to 16 years, with the mean age being 4 years. There is a male-to-female predominance with this disease of 2:1. Tracheitis is more frequently seen in the fall and winter seasons.

The pathogens that most commonly cause tracheitis are *Staphylococcus aureus* and community-acquired MRSA, although *Moraxella catarrhalis, Haemophilus influenzae* type b, *Klebsiella,* and *Pseudomonas aeruginosa* have also been reported as causative agents. Several anaerobes have also been implicated: *Peptostreptococcus, Bacterioides,* and *Prevotella.* Many patients will have an antecedent viral infection or trauma.

Presentation

The patient with tracheitis may have a prodrome of upper or lower respiratory infection, which is followed by fever, cough, stridor, and respiratory distress. The presentation may either be acute or subacute. The patient with an acute presentation may have a high fever, toxic appearance, elevated WBC count, stridor, bark-like cough, and hoarseness. The patient with a subacute presentation may have a several-day history of croup-like symptoms; tracheitis can be initially misdiagnosed as croup. For these patients, the diagnosis of tracheitis is considered later, when the patient does not respond to traditional croup therapies (Liston et al., 1983). Lower respiratory tract disease findings may be present and are usually associated with concurrent viral pathology.

Differential diagnosis

Table 30-35 lists the differential diagnoses for tracheitis.

Plan of care

If tracheitis is considered as the etiology of the patient's symptoms, then initial management focuses on maintaining airway patency. Secretions may be copious and tenacious. Agitation may lead to full airway obstruction, so noxious stimuli must be avoided during diagnostic study. Taking an oral or rectal temperature, examining the oropharynx, starting an IV line, and administering oxygen by face mask are *not* recommended unless the patient is a *willing* participant. If the patient is willing to participant, obtain a lateral neck radiograph, which may be useful to differentiate tracheitis from epiglottitis, croup, and retropharyngeal abscess. Airway narrowing or a hazy trachea from pseudomembrane formation may be evident (Figure 30-10).

If complete airway obstruction is imminent, endotracheal intubation is required. Intubation of the secretion-obstructed airway is extremely difficult and should be performed only by those HCPs skilled in the maneuver such as a pediatric anesthesia, critical care, or otolaryngology specialist. It may need to be performed in the operating room and difficult airway equipment should be readily available. The intubation is frequently performed with the child sedated but spontaneously breathing, should endotracheal intubation be too difficult to obtain. Fifty percent of patients require airway support, with those younger than the age of 4 years having the highest risk (Bernstein et al., 1998). If intubation is indicated, anticipate the need for a smaller endotracheal tube—0.5 to 1 size smaller. The time course for mechanical ventilation is usually 3 to 7 days. Positive-pressure ventilation can be complicated by the thick secretions and pseudomembranes associated with tracheitis. Also, air leak syndromes are not uncommon.

TABLE 30-35

Differential Diagnoses for Tracheitis
• Epiglottitis
• Croup
• Retropharyngeal/peritonsillar abscess
• Uvulitis
• Candidiasis

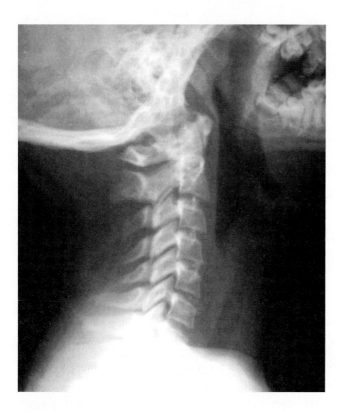

FIGURE 30-10

Differential Diagnosis for Tracheitis.

Source: Courtesy of Mark D. Weber.

As both bacterial (airway) and viral (lower respiratory tract) processes may be occurring at the same time, the WBC count and differential may not clearly be indicative of bacterial infection. Blood cultures are rarely positive. Tracheal aspirates should be cultured for both aerobic and anaerobic pathogens.

If endotracheal intubation is not required for airway support, then laryngotracheobronchoscopy may be considered for definitive diagnosis. This procedure allows for the visualization of purulent secretions (culture), an erythematous trachea, and pseudomembranes.

Empiric antimicrobial therapy is designed to treat the aforementioned aerobic and anaerobic organisms. It should be tailored when culture and susceptibility results are available. Consider providing coverage (vancomycin, linezolid) for resistant organisms as community prevalence dictates. Initial management consists of IV antibiotics such as ampicillin–sulbactam, clindamycin, or third-generation cephalosporins. Once the patient is no longer febrile and improving, then therapy can be changed to similar oral agents to complete the 10-day course.

Consultation with specialists will depend on the severity of the patient's illness and the response to therapies. Involvement of the infectious diseases, otolaryngology, pulmonology, and critical care services may be indicated based on the acuity of illness and therapeutic management plan.

Patient and family education focuses on the etiology of the infection, disease course, and symptoms of recurrence.

Disposition and discharge planning

Discharge can be anticipated once the patient is afebrile, able to take oral nutrition, and free of respiratory distress at rest. The patient should be evaluated by the primary care provider within 48 hours of discharge, as well as any specialty service that may have been involved in the patient's hospital plan of care. During follow-up assessment of the patient, air entry should be performed—laryngeal stenosis has been identified as a potential sequela to tracheitis (Huang et al., 2009).

TUBERCULOSIS

Catherine O'Keefe

Tuberculosis, while being considered an "ancient" disease, remains a significant global public health problem, with children bearing a heavy burden of disease. Because young children contribute little to the transmission of tuberculosis, however, they have not been designated as high priority in most national health programs (Swaminathan & Rehka, 2010). Table 30-36 defines key terms related to this disease.

Pathophysiology

Tuberculosis is caused by infection with one of the acid-fast bacilli (AFB) of the *Mycobacterium tuberculosis* complex (*M. tuberculosis, M. bovis, M. africanum*). The most common cause of tuberculosis is *M. tuberculosis*. Infection occurs when the host inhales the infectious airborne droplet

TABLE 30-36

Tuberculosis: Definitions of Terms

Latent Tuberculosis Infection (LTBI): occurs as the result of close contact with an infectious individual with no clinical evidence of disease.

Tuberculosis Disease: progression of infection to disease with discernible signs and symptoms and abnormal radiographic findings. It is further classified as:

• Pulmonary disease (PTB): limited to the pulmonary parenchyma

• Extrapulmonary disease (EPTB): lymphatic or hematogenous seeding of various highly vascular organs

Miliary Tuberculosis: disseminated disease involving a massive bacteremia and disease in two or more organs.

Multidrug-resistant (MDR) Tuberculosis:– tuberculosis infection or disease resistant to isoniazid and rifampin.

Extensively drug-resistant (XDR) Tuberculosis: tuberculosis infection or disease resistant to isoniazid and rifampin, at least one fluoroquinolone, and at least one of the following: amikacin, kanamycin, or capreomycin.

Source: AAP, 2009.

and the pathogen takes up residence in the alveoli of the lung. The tubercle bacilli are very slow growing and hardy; as a consequence, they are able to remain dormant for years before reactivation and presentation of disease. Nevertheless, hematogenous-lymphatic spread of *M. tuberculosis* allows the bacilli to invade other vascular organs of the body, with clinical disease often extending to extrapulmonary sites (EPTB) (Starke & Jacobs, 2008).

The pathogenicity of *M. tuberculosis* is influenced by a variety of host immune factors and *M. tuberculosis* virulence factors. These factors combine to determine the intensity of the local inflammatory response as well as the degree and severity of subsequent clinical disease (Rock et al., 2008). In the immunocompetent host, the local inflammatory response serves to contain the infection in the lung, with a granuloma eventually forming at the infection site. In instances of extremes of age or cell-mediated immune defects, the inflammatory response is not as efficient; in these patients, there is more potential for extensive infection and active clinical disease. Such is the case in HIV-infected individuals, which explains the high incidence of HIV-related tuberculosis disease.

Epidemiology and etiology

Person-to-person contact is required for transmission of *M. tuberculosis*. The mucous droplets containing tubercle bacilli are aerosolized when the infected individual coughs, sneezes, laughs, or sings (Starke & Jacobs, 2008). Infants and young children (younger than 10 years of age) with pulmonary tuberculosis have little ability to transmit disease. Pediatric patients typically have small lesions and a nonproductive or ineffective cough—factors that result in an insignificant expulsion of the tubercle bacilli (AAP, 2009).

An estimated 2 billion individuals worldwide have latent tuberculosis infection (LTBI), though specific data for children are lacking (Starke & Jacobs, 2008). Additionally, 8 to 10 million people annually are diagnosed with tuberculosis disease; among those are 1.3 million children younger than 15 years of age (Starke & Jacobs). Worldwide childhood mortality due to tuberculosis is estimated to approach 130,000 deaths per year, ranking this disease among the top 10 major causes of death of children (WHO, 2009).

Tuberculosis surveillance in the United States began in 1953, when an overall case rate of 52.6 cases per 100,000 population was reported. By 2008, this rate had dropped to 4.2 cases per 100,000 population, with children (younger than 15 years of age) having the lowest case rate—1.6 cases per 100,000 population, or 6% (CDC, 2009e). Approximately 20% of tuberculosis disease in the United States is extrapulmonary tuberculosis (EPTB). The most common extrapulmonary sites affected are lymphatic sites (40.4%), followed by pleural (19.8%), other (11.8%), bone/joint (11.3%), genitourinary (6.5%), meningeal (5.4%), and peritoneal (4.9%) sites. Children experience

a disproportionately higher incidence of lymphatic spread (12% of all cases) and meningeal spread (13% of all cases) (Peto et al., 2009)

Although the United States is experiencing its lowest case rate since 1953, the rate of decline in tuberculosis incidence has slowed since 2000. This trend is largely due to the increased tuberculosis rate among persons of foreign origin as compared to U.S.-born individuals—5% increase versus 62% decline, respectively (CDC, 2009e). The incidence of tuberculosis is strongly correlated with socioeconomic status, with the heaviest infection and disease burden found in developing countries that lack the resources needed to provide effective screening and treatment programs. Approximately 75% of the tuberculosis cases in children occur in 22 countries, primarily in Africa and Southeast Asia (WHO, 2009). The high incidence in these regions is likely due to crowding, malnutrition, lack of access to health care, and the high incidence of HIV in these countries (Swaminathan & Rehka, 2010). Coinfection with HIV and tuberculosis is common, and influences the age of infectious tuberculosis contacts. HIV tends to be an infection of young adults; thus persons with HIV-related tuberculosis—who are likely parents—are increasingly exposing their young children to tuberculosis (WHO).

Children typically contract tuberculosis from adults who have the disease yet may be undiagnosed or nonadherent to their medication regimen. The age group at highest risk for progression from infection to disease includes children younger than 2 years of age, with a somewhat smaller peak occurring during adolescence (Swaminathan & Rehka, 2010). Children with HIV infection are also at increased risk for progression from tuberculosis infection to disease (Starke & Jacobs, 2008).

Presentation

The presentation of tuberculosis varies widely, ranging from asymptomatic LTBI to pulmonary and extrapulmonary disease. Pulmonary parenchyma and intrathoracic lymph nodes are the most common sites for clinical disease among pediatric tuberculosis patients. Extrapulmonary tuberculosis disease may involve one or more body systems or sites. The most commonly affected areas are the lymphatics and the central nervous system, followed by pleural (6%), miliary (5%), and skeletal (4%) sites (Swaminathan & Rehka, 2010). Involvement of the abdominal viscera/gastrointestinal tract, genitourinary tract, and skin is rare in pediatrics. Age often influences the site of extrapulmonary tuberculosis. Specifically, infants and young children present more often with meningeal, disseminated, and lymphatic tuberculosis and adolescents with pleural, genitourinary, or peritoneal disease (Starke & Jacobs, 2008).

Most cases of pediatric tuberculosis are acquired in the home. Therefore, a detailed family and social history of potential exposure to *M. tuberculosis* is important in making the diagnosis. This investigation should include inquiry into all of the following issues:

- Personal travel or exposure to individuals who have traveled to endemic areas
- Personal experience or exposure to individuals who have resided in crowded environments such as jails, prisons, group homes, and homeless shelters
- Illicit IV drug users
- Family history of tuberculosis

Because many adult infectious contacts may be undiagnosed, it is important to ask about household members with a chronic cough that has not been treated or that has not responded to traditional treatment.

Past medical history should also be reviewed for the presence of risk factors for tuberculosis, such as defects in cell-mediated immunity, steroid therapy, cancer chemotherapy, and hematologic malignancies. In addition, a detailed history of previous tuberculosis diagnosis or treatment should be ascertained. Particular emphasis should be placed on determining whether the individual completed the prescribed medication regimen, as this information may provide clues about resistance patterns.

The child with LTBI is asymptomatic and is identified by exposure history, positive tuberculin skin test (TST), and a normal chest radiograph (CXR). Pediatric patients with pulmonary tuberculosis disease may or may not exhibit any respiratory or constitutional symptoms. It is only after careful screening and radiographic evaluation that the child may be diagnosed. Infants may experience a nonproductive cough and mild dyspnea. Children who are infected after 7 years of age have a greater chance of presenting with fever, anorexia, weight loss, night sweats, productive cough, chest pain, and hemoptysis (Starke & Jacobs, 2008). Progressive primary tuberculosis—a rare complication—is manifested as a toxic appearance, high fever, moderate to severe cough, night sweats, and abnormal or absent breath sounds over the affected area. In these patients, the radiographic findings are disproportionately abnormal. Pleural tuberculosis presents with fever, chest pain, shortness of breath, and decreased breath sounds over the affected pleural effusion or empyema. High fevers may persist for weeks into the treatment course (Starke & Jacobs).

Lymphatic tuberculosis is the most common manifestation of extrapulmonary tuberculosis. Tubercular cervical lymphadenitis or *scrofula* is most often reported, in addition to infection of the supraclavicular, tonsillar, and submandibular nodes. Clinical manifestations include unilateral, firm, discrete, matted lymphadenopathy (Khan et al., 2009; Starke & Jacobs, 2008). Typically, the patient does not exhibit any constitutional or other symptoms of tuberculosis. The focus for tubercular lymphadenitis is primarily pulmonary; however, in a small number of patients, the source is the mouth, tonsils, oropharynx, or head and neck tissues (Marais et al., 2006).

Central nervous system tuberculosis—that is tubercular meningitis (TBM)—represents the most severe complication of tuberculosis. Children younger than 2 years of age have a higher incidence of TBM (Rock et al., 2008). The presentation of TBM is insidious and can occur months after initial infection. Initially, the pediatric patient may have nonspecific findings such as fever, anorexia, weight loss, and subtle behavioral changes. Within 1 to 2 weeks, the child may present with vomiting, seizures, and altered sensorium. Physical examination findings may include nuchal rigidity, altered deep tendon reflexes, and cranial nerve palsies (most often the sixth cranial nerve). Focal neurologic deficits as well as hydrocephalus may be observed as a result of tuberculoma(s), tubercular brain abscess(es), or cerebral infarcts. Long-term neurologic deficits, coma, and death can occur. Timely diagnosis and treatment may or may not alter the course of TBM. Several staging criteria have been used over the years to provide prognostic indicators for neurodevelopmental outcomes of TBM; contemporary staging includes a combination of the well-known Glasgow Coma Scale (GCS) and degree of focal neurologic deficits (Rock et al.). A lower GCS score combined with multiple local neurologic deficits at the time of diagnosis and initiation of treatment heralds a poor neurodevelopmental prognosis.

Miliary tuberculosis has an indolent course marked by nonspecific symptoms such as malaise, anorexia, listlessness, weight loss, and low-grade fever. As the disease progresses, the presentation becomes consistent with the location of disseminated organisms. The most frequently affected distal organs are the lungs, spleen, liver, and bone marrow. Physical findings may include hepatomegaly, splenomegaly, severe respiratory distress, hypoxia, and pneumothorax (Starke & Jacobs, 2008).

Osteoarticular tuberculosis is most often seen in the large weight-bearing bones or joints. Vertebral bodies are the site most commonly affected, followed by the hip and the knee. Tubercular osteomyelitis can present either acutely or subacutely. Vertebral tuberculosis may go unrecognized for years, with the child eventually presenting with low-grade fever, irritability, generalized back pain, and refusal to walk. The lower thoracic or upper lumbar regions are most commonly involved with this form of the disease. Paraspinal abscess formation (Pott's disease) and bony destruction are possible. Extraspinal skeletal tuberculosis presents with persistent pain, swelling, and stiffness across the involved joint (Hosalker et al., 2009).

Differential diagnosis

Other diagnoses to consider will depend on the site-specific clinical manifestations of the disease, but include the following conditions:

- Actinomycosis
- Coccidiodomycosis
- Histoplasmosis

- Brucellosis
- Pneumonia
- Pleural effusion
- Bronchiectasis
- Lymphadenopathy
- Pericarditis
- Fever without a source
- Meningitis (aseptic or bacterial)
- Osteomyelitis
- Bone tumors/sarcomas
- Failure-to-thrive

Plan of care

Targeted screening, along with rapid diagnosis and treatment of LTBI and tuberculosis disease, make up the cornerstone of tuberculosis control. Diagnosing pediatric tuberculosis infection can be challenging, however. Children typically have a low bacillary load and *M. tuberculosis* is difficult to isolate.

The tuberculin skin test is the most widely used screening test for LTBI and tuberculosis disease; it is utilized to initially screen the child with known risk factors for either LTBI or tuberculosis disease. An experienced HCP should administer and interpret the TST to assure reliable results. Precise measurement of the palpable induration should be interpreted within the context of risk factors to determine a positive or negative TST. The *Red Book* provides the most up-to-date criteria for administration and interpretation of the TST (AAP, 2009). The TST is low in sensitivity, however, and a negative result should not be relied upon, particularly in infants and young children with a high index of suspicion for LTBI or tuberculosis disease (Chang & Leung, 2010). The TST also has low specificity in individuals who have received the bacilli Calmette-Guerin (BCG) vaccine, who have been exposed to non-tuberculous mycobacteria, or who are immunocompromised (Dodd et al., 2010).

If a TST is positive, the next step is a CXR. A positive TST with a normal CXR and no physical findings of disease is considered diagnostic for LTBI. A positive TST with an abnormal CXR should prompt more definitive diagnostic testing.

The definitive diagnosis of tuberculosis disease is made by the isolation of *M. tuberculosis* via culture. Several specimens are suitable for culture, though they vary in their diagnostic yield. Typically, sputum cannot be obtained from infants and young children. The alternative is to obtain gastric aspirates. Correct collection includes the placement of a nasogastric tube for morning aspiration of gastric contents before ambulation or eating. Gastric aspirates are best obtained in the hospital to assure accurate collection over three consecutive mornings. Other potentially infectious bodily fluids, including bronchial washings, cerebrospinal fluid, bone or joint aspirates, pleural fluid, and biopsies, may also be submitted for culture. Acid-fast bacillus (AFB) smear/stains can provide preliminary results

but are rarely helpful. Cultures can take up to 10 weeks for isolation of an organism. Unfortunately, only 70% of infants and fewer than 50% of children diagnosed with tuberculosis disease by clinical criteria have a positive *M. tuberculosis* culture.

Culture of *M. tuberculosis* can reveal the species involved and drug susceptibility pattern. This information is particularly important in areas where multidrug-resistant (MDR) and extensively drug-resistant (XDR) tuberculosis are prevalent. When it is impossible to obtain an isolate from the infant or child, every attempt should be made to identify the index case and obtain a culture and susceptibility.

Nucleic acid amplification by PCR has provided some future possibilities in the diagnosis of tuberculosis disease. The PCR technology's diagnostic utility in pediatric patients is limited by its varying degrees of sensitivity—95% in AFB smear positive cases and 40% to 70% sensitivity is AFB smear negative cases (Marais & Pai, 2007). Interferon-gamma release assays (IGRA) have been developed in hopes of increasing the precision of diagnosing LTBI and tuberculosis disease. Three products have been licensed by the FDA for this purpose—T-SPOT.*TB*, QuantiFERON-TB Gold, and QuantiFERON-TB Gold In-Tube—and have been found to have significantly greater specificity and higher positive predictive values than the TST (Bergamini et al., 2009). However, their clinical utility for use in children younger than 4 years of age has been limited by indeterminate results and low sensitivity (Bergamini et al., Lighter et al., 2009).

Given the difficulties in determining a definitive bacteriologic confirmation of tuberculosis disease, the clinician often must rely on clinical criteria for a presumptive diagnosis. These criteria include (1) close contact with a contagious source case, (2) positive TST result, and (3) CXR findings suggestive of pulmonary disease (Swaminathan & Rehka, 2010).

A CXR should always be obtained to evaluate for pulmonary disease. When chest radiographic findings are abnormal, CT scan or MRI is helpful to further define the nature of suspicious lesions. It bears repeating that a significant portion of children with confirmed pulmonary disease can have a normal CXR and a negative TST (Swaminathan & Rehka, 2010).

Due to the epidemiologic link between HIV and tuberculosis, the child who is suspected to have tuberculosis should also be tested for HIV. Furthermore, the child with HIV should be tested annually for tuberculosis.

The primary objective in treatment of tuberculosis infection and disease is to contain and reduce the *M. tuberculosis* load as rapidly as possible. Additional considerations include complete eradication of the organism, prevention of drug resistance, and avoidance of drug-related adverse events (Marais, 2008). Although infants and children are rarely contagious, they should be admitted to a room equipped with negative air flow, and all caregivers should wear respiratory-fitted masks (e.g., N95 masks) when caring for the patient. Special attention should be paid to the pediatric patient's visitors, as the index case is likely one of the child's family members. All visitors should be medically screened and excluded from the hospital setting unless they have been cleared for infection or disease. Consultation with the hospital infection prevention team is recommended.

Pharmacologic management is the mainstay of therapy and requires careful attention to the specific diagnosis. Refer to the current edition of the *Red Book: Report of the Committee on Infectious Diseases* (AAP, 2009) for additional reference tables and explanatory text detailing the pharmacologic management of LTBI and pulmonary tuberculosis. Similar guidelines are followed when managing EPTB but require expert infectious diseases consultation regarding choice of drug combinations, duration of therapy, and supportive measures. Steroids are used as an adjunctive therapy for tuberculous meningitis, and have been reported to reduce the mortality rate and the development of tuberculomas (Prasad & Singh, 2008; Shah, 2009). The most common steroid dosing regimens are dexamethasone 0.3 to 0.4 mg/kg/day for the first 2 weeks, then tapered for 2 weeks, or prednisolone 2 mg/kg/day for 2 weeks, followed by a taper for 2 weeks (Prasad & Singh). One study reported better outcomes with higher-dose steroid (prednisolone 4 mg/kg/day) for 1 week, followed by a taper of 2 mg/kg/day (Shah). Steroid therapy is appropriate only for non-HIV-infected patients.

A pediatric infectious diseases specialist should be consulted if tuberculosis infection or disease is suspected, to assist in the diagnostic evaluation and management. Additional specialty services to be consulted might include pulmonology, cardiology, surgery, neurology, endocrine, renal, ophthalmology, or gastroenterology, depending on the site-specific manifestations of the disease.

Patients and families should be advised of the long-term nature of the pharmacologic management and the need for diligent adherence to the medical regimen. Side effects of the medication therapy should be reviewed with both the caregivers and the patient (depending on the child's level of understanding). Additional teaching should be specific to the clinical findings of the patient and the projected long-term sequelae. Granulomatous lesions and hilar adenopathy often remain in the lung after resolution of the acute infectious phase of the disease, so caregivers should be forewarned that their child will always have an "abnormal" chest radiograph. Caregivers also need to be made aware of the possible source of the infection and learn how to avoid future exposures.

Disposition and discharge planning

Patients should be followed for the duration of therapy, which may be several months. In addition, arrangements should be made for follow-up with any specialty consultants who were involved in the child's care during hospitalization. The local or regional health department tuberculosis program should be involved in discharge planning. When nonadherence to the medication regimen is a concern, patients may require alternative pharmacologic dosing regimens that will allow for direct observed therapy (DOT) provided by a public health nurse.

The pediatric patient should be monitored regularly for drug-related adverse events as well as clinical response to therapy. Drug-related hepatitis is a concern with isoniazid (INH) and rifampin therapy. However, in an otherwise healthy infant or child, INH should hold no significant threat for untoward effects. In contrast, in patients with severe disease such as TBM or miliary tuberculosis, monthly monitoring of liver function is warranted. The patient and family should be advised to contact their clinician should any signs of hepatotoxicity such as vomiting, abdominal pain, or jaundice occur (AAP, 2009). Peripheral neuritis is a rare occurrence associated with INH therapy; however, this complication can be prevented with concomitant administration of pyridoxine. When rifampin is ordered, the patient and family should be warned that this drug will change the color of the child's urine to a deep orange-red color. In the case of pulmonary tuberculosis, a CXR should be performed following 2 months of therapy to evaluate the patient's response to the treatment (AAP).

Prevention and control of tuberculosis requires coordination between the healthcare team and the local health department. The diagnosis of a child with LTBI or tuberculosis disease usually heralds a source case within his or her household. Timely investigation and medical screening of all contacts serves to contain the infection and prevent further spread.

Critical Thinking

Pediatric patients with tuberculosis rarely present with obvious pulmonary symptoms; instead, most are diagnosed by contact tracing. When evaluating a patient with nonspecific diagnoses such as failure-to-thrive and fever without a source, always consider the diagnosis of tuberculosis, particularly in the presence of tuberculosis risk factors.

REFERENCES

1. Acevedo, J., Lander, L., Choi, S., & Shah, R. (2009). Airway management in pediatric epiglottitis: A national perspective. *Otolaryngology: Head and Neck Surgery, 140*, 548–551.

2. American Academy of Pediatrics (AAP). (2009). Pickering, L., Baker, C., Kimberlin, D., & Long, S. (Eds.), *Red Book: 2009 report of the Committee on Infectious Diseases* (28th edition). Elk Grove Village, IL: Author.

3. American College of Critical Care Medicine, Society of Critical Care Medicine. (1999). Practice parameters for hemodynamic support of sepsis in adult patients in sepsis. *Critical Care Medicine, 27*, 639–660.

4. American Heart Association (AHA). (2006). *Pediatric advanced life support provider manual 2005*, Dallas: Author. pp. 61–114.

5. Ampel, N. (2009). Coccidioidomycosis: A review of recent advances. *Clinics in Chest Medicine, 30*(2), 241–251.

6. Anderson, D. (2007). Underresourced hospital infection control and prevention programs: Penny wise, pound foolish? *Infection Control and Hospital Epidemiology, 28*(7), 767–773.

7. Anderson, M., Glode, M., & Smith, A. (2009). Meningococcal infections. In R. Feigin, J. Cherry, G. Demmler-Harrison, & S. Kaplan (Eds.), *Textbook of pediatric infectious diseases* (6th ed., Vol. 1, pp. 1350–1363). Philadelphia: Saunders.

8. Annane, D., Aegerter, P., Jars-Giuncestre, M. C., Guidet, B., & CUB-REA Network. (2003). Current epidemiology of septic shock. *American Journal of Respiratory Critical Care Medicine, 168,* 165–172.

9. Anstead, G., & Graybill, J. (2006). Coccidioidomycosis. *Infectious Disease Clinics of North America, 20,* 621–643.

10. Arendrup, M., Fisher, B., & Zaoutis, T. (2009). Invasive fungal infections in the paediatric and neonatal population: Diagnostic and management issues. *Clinical Microbiology and Infectious Diseases, 15,* 613–624.

11. Arnold, J., Revivo, G., Senac, M., & Leake, J. (2005). West Nile virus encephalitis with thalamic involvement in an immunocompromised child. *Pediatric Infectious Disease Journal, 24*(10), 932–934.

12. Bachur, R., & Harper, M. (2000). Reevaluation of outpatients with *Streptococcus pneumoniae* bacteremia. *Pediatrics, 105,* 502–509.

13. Bachur, R., & Harper, M. (2001). Predictive model for serious bacterial infections among infants younger than 3 months of age. *Pediatrics, 108,* 311–316.

14. Baker, M., Bell, L., & Avner, J. (1993). Outpatient management without antibiotics of fever in selected infants. *New England Journal of Medicine, 329,* 1437–1441.

15. Balk, R. (2000). Severe sepsis and septic shock: Definitions, epidemiology, and clinical manifestations. *Critical Care Clinics, 16*(2), 179–192.

16. Balk, R., Ely, E., & Goyette, R. (2004). *Sepsis handbook* (2nd ed.). Chicago: Society of Critical Care Medicine.

17. Baltimore, R. (2003). The difficulty of diagnosing VAP. *Pediatrics, 112*(6), 1420–1421.

18. Banerjee, S., Grohskopf, L., Sinkowitz-Cochran, R., Jarvis, W., National Nosocomial Infections Surveillance System, & Pediatric Prevention Network. (2006). Incidence of pediatric and neonatal intensive care unit–acquired infections. *Infection Control and Hospital Epidemiology, 27*(6), 561–570.

19. Baraff, L. (2000). Management of fever without a source in infants and children. *Annals of Emergency Medicine, 36*(6), 602–614.

20. Baraff, L. (2008). Management of infants and young children with fever without source. *Pediatric Annals, 37*(10), 673–679.

21. Baraff, L., Schriger, D., Bass, J. W., Fleisher, C., Britto, J., Morrison, A., et al. (1993). Practice guideline for the management of infants and children 0 to 36 months of age with fever without source. *Pediatrics, 92*(1), 1–12.

22. Baskin, M., O'Rourke, E., & Fleisher, G. (1992). Outpatient treatment of febrile infants 28 to 89 days of age with intramuscular administration of ceftriaxone. *Journal of Pediatrics, 120,* 22–27.

23. Bayram, J., & Malik, M. (2008). Gynecologic infections. In J. G. Adams (Ed.), *Emergency medicine* (pp. 1371–1388). Philadelphia: Saunders Elsevier.

24. Bergamini, B., Losi, M., Vaienti, F., D'Amico, R., Meccugni, B., Meacci, M., et al. (2009). Performance of commercial blood tests for the diagnosis of latent tuberculosis infection in children and adolescents. *Pediatrics, 123,* e419–e424.

25. Bernstein, T., Brilli, R., & Jacobs, B. (1998). Is bacterial tracheitis changing? A 14- month experience in a pediatric intensive care unit. *Clinical Infectious Diseases, 27*(3), 458–462.

26. Bertini, G., Perugi, S., Dani, C., Filippi, L., Pratesi, S., & Rubaltelli, F. (2005). Fluconazole prophylaxis prevents invasive fungal infection in high-risk, very low birth weight infants. *Journal of Pediatrics, 147,* 166–171.

27. Bharti, A., Nally, J., Ricaldi, J., Matthias M., Diaz M., Lovett M., et al. (2003). Leptospirosis: A zoonotic disease of global importance. *Lancet Infectious Diseases, 3*(12), 757–771.

28. Biggs, W., & Williams, R. (2009). Common gynecologic infections. *Primary Care Clinics Office Practice, 36,* 33–51.

29. Bigham, M., Amato, R., Bondurrant, P., Fridriksson, J., Krawczeski, C., Roake, J., et al. (2009). Ventilator-associated pneumonia in the pediatric intensive care unit: Characterizing the problem and implementing a sustainable solution. *Journal of Pediatrics, 154*(4), 582–587.

30. Bindl, L., Buderus, S., Dahlem, P., Demirakca, S., Goldner, M., Huth, R., et al. (2003). Gender-based differences in children with sepsis and ARDS: The ESPNIC ARDS Database Group. *Neonatal and Pediatric Intensive Care, 29,* 1770–1773.

31. Birnbaumer, D., & Anderegg, C. (2010). Sexually transmitted diseases. In J. A. Marx (Ed.), *Rosen's emergency medicine concepts and clinical practice* (7th ed., pp. 1282–1296). Philadelphia: Mosby Elsevier.

32. Biro, F. (2007). Editorial: Adolescents, sexual activity, and sexually transmitted infections. *Journal of Pediatric Adolescent Gynecology, 20,* 219–220.

33. Biron, K. (2006). Antiviral drugs for cytomegalovirus diseases. *Antiviral Research, 71,* 154–163.

34. Bjornson, C., Klassen, T., Williamsom, J., Brant, R., Mitton, C., Plint, A., et al. (2004). A randomized trial of a single dose of oral dexamethasone for mild croup. *New England Journal of Medicine, 23*(13), 1306–1313.

35. Block, S., Harrison, C., Hedrick, J., Tyler, R., Smith, R., Keegan, E., et al. (1995). Penicillin-resistant *Streptococcus pneumoniae* in acute otitis media: Risk factors, susceptibility patterns and antimicrobial management. *Pediatric Infectious Disease Journal, 14*(9), 751–759.

36. Blyth, C., Hale, K., Palasanthiran, P., O'Brien, T., & Bennett, M. (2010). Antifungal therapy in infants and children with proven, probable or suspected invasive fungal infections. *Cochrane Database of Systematic Reviews, 2.* doi: 10.1002/14651858.CD006343.pub2

37. Bollaert, P., Bauer, P., Audubert, G., Lambert, H., & Larcan, A. (1990). Effects of epinephrine on hemodynamics and oxygen metabolism is dopamine-resistant septic shock. *Chest, 98,* 949–953.

38. Bone, R., Balk, R., Cerra, F., Dellinger, R., Fein, A., Knaus, W., et al. (1992a). Definitions for sepsis and organ failure and guidelines for the use of innovative therapies in sepsis: The ACCP/SCCM Consensus Conference Committee, American College of Chest Physicians/Society of Critical Care Medicine. *Chest, 101,* 1644–1655.

39. Bone, R., Sprung, C., & Sibbald, W. (1992b). Definitions for sepsis and organ function. *Critical Care Medicine, 20,* 724–726.

40. Booy, R., Habibi, P., Nadel, S., de Munter, C., Britto, J., Morrison, A., et al. (2001). Reduction in case fatality rate from meningococcal disease associated with improved healthcare delivery. *Archives of Disease in Childhood, 85,* 386–390.

41. Boyce, J., & Pittet, D. (2002). Guidelines for hand hygiene in healthcare settings: Recommendations of the Healthcare Infection Control Practices Advisory Committee and HIPAC/SHEA/APIC/IDSA Hand Hygiene Task Force. *American Journal of Infection Control, 30,* S1–S46.

42. Brady, R., Verran, J., Damani, N., & Giba, A. (2009). Review of mobile communication devices as potential reservoirs of nosocomial pathogens. *Journal of Hospital Infection, 71,* 295–300.

43. Brierley, J., Carcillo, J., Choong, K., Cornell, T., DeCaen, A., Deymann, A., et al. (2009). Clinical practice parameters for hemodymanic support of pediatric and neonatal septic shock: 2007 update from the American College of Critical Care Medicine. *Critical Care Medicine, 37*(2), 666–688.

44. Brilli, R., Sparling, K., Lake, M., Butcher, J., Myers, S., Clark, M., et al. (2008). The business case for preventing ventilator-associated pneumonia in pediatric intensive care unit patients. *The Joint Commission Journal on Quality and Patient Safety, 34*(11), 629–638.

45. Brown, K. (2008). Human parvoviruses. In S. Long, L. Pickering, & C. Prober (Eds.), *Long's principles and practice of pediatric infectious diseases* (3rd ed.). Philadelphia: Saunders Elsevier.

46. Byington, C., Enriquez, R., Hoff, C., Tuohy, R., Taggart, E., Hillyard, D., et al. (2004). Serious bacterial infection in febrile infants 1 to 90 days old with and without viral infections. *Pediatrics, 113,* 1662–1666.

47. Calisher, C. (1994). Medically important arboviruses of the United States and Canada. *Clinical Microbiology Reviews, 7*(1), 89–116.

48. Carcillo, J. (2003). Pediatric septic shock and multiple organ failure. *Critical Care Clinics, 19,* 413–440.

49. Carcillo, J., Davis, A., & Zaritsky, A. (1991). Role of early fluid resuscitation in pediatric septic shock. *Journal of the American Medical Association, 266,* 1242–1245.

50. Carcillo, J., & Fields, A. (2002). Clinical practice parameters for hemodynamic support of pediatric and neonatal patients in septic shock. *Critical Care Medicine, 30*(6), 1365–1377.

51. Cassidy, P., Hedberg, K., Saulson, A., McNelly, E., & Winthrop, K. (2009). Nontuberculous mycobacterial disease prevalence and risk factors: A changing epidemiology. *Clinical Infectious Diseases, 49,* e124–e129.

52. Castagnola, E., & Buratti, S. (2009). Clinical aspects of invasive candidiasis in paediatric patients. *Drugs 2009, 69*(suppl 1), 45–50.

53. Castagnola, E., Fontana, V., Caviglia, I., Caruso, S., Faraci, M., Floredda, F., et al. (2007). A prospective study on the epidemiology of febrile episodes during chemotherapy-induced neutropenia in children with cancer or after hemopoietic stem cell transplantation. *Clinical Infectious Diseases, 45,* 1296–1304.

54. Catherinot, E., Lanternier, F., Bougnoux, M., Lecuit, M., Couderc, L. & Lortholary, O. (2010). Pneumocystis jirovecii pneumonia. *Infectious Disease Clinics North America, 24*(1), 107–138.

55. Caviness, A., Demmler, G., Swint, J., & Cantor, S. (2008). Cost-effectiveness analysis of herpes simplex virus testing and treatment strategies in febrile neonates. *Archives of Pediatric and Adolescent Medicine, 162*(7), 665–674.

56. Ceneviva, G., Paschall, J., Maffel, F., & Carcillo, J. (1998). Hemodynamic support in fluid refractory pediatric septic shock. *Pediatrics, 102,* e19.

57. Centers for Disease Control and Prevention (CDC). (1997). Case definitions for infectious conditions under public health surveillance. *Morbidity and Mortality Weekly Report, 46*(No. RR-10), 39–40.

58. Centers for Disease Control and Prevention (CDC). (2002). Guideline for hand hygiene in healthcare settings: Recommendation of the Healthcare Infection Control Advisory Committee and the HICPAC/SHEA/APIC/IDSA Hand Hygiene Task Force. *Morbidity and Mortality Weekly Report, 51*(RR-16).

59. Centers for Disease Control and Prevention (CDC). (2005). Prevention and control of meningococcal disease: Recommendations of the Advisory Committee on Immunization Practices (ACIP). *Morbidity and Mortality Weekly Report 2005, 54*(RR-7), 1–21.

60. Centers for Disease Control and Prevention (CDC). (2007). Summary of a review of the literature: Programs to promote *Chlamydia* screening. Infertility Prevention Social Marketing Campaign. Retrieved from http://www.cdc.gov/std/HealthComm/ChlamydiaLitReview2008.pdf

61. Centers for Disease Control and Prevention (CDC). (2009a). Guidelines for the prevention and treatment of opportunistic infections among HIV-exposed and HIV-infected children. *Morbidity and Mortality Weekly Report, 58*(RR-11), 1–248.

62. Centers for Disease Control and Prevention (CDC). (2009b). Malaria surveillance—United States, 2007. *Morbidity and Mortality Weekly Report, 58*(SS02), 1–16.

63. Centers for Disease Control and Prevention (CDC). (2009c). Recommendations for use of antiviral medications for the management of influenza in children and adolescent for the 2009–2010 season: Pediatric supplement for health care providers. Retrieved from http://cdc.gov/h1n1flu/recommendations_pediatric_supplement.htm

64. Centers for Disease Control and Prevention (CDC). (2009d). Summary of notifiable disease—United States, 2007. *Morbidity and Mortality Weekly Report, 56*(53), 22.

65. Centers for Disease Control and Prevention (CDC). (2009e). Tuberculosis surveillance: Morbidity trend tables. Retrieved from http://www.cdc.gov/tb/statistics/default.htm

66. Centers for Disease Control and Prevention (CDC). (2010a). Streptococcal toxic-shock syndrome (STSS). 2010. case definition. Retrieved from http://www.cdc.gov/ncphi/disss/nndss/casedef/streptococcalcurrent.htm

67. Centers for Disease Control and Prevention. (CDC). (2010b). Sexually transmitted diseases treatment guidelines. *Morbidity and Mortality Weekly Report (MMWR), 59*(R-12), 1–116.

68. Chambers, H. (1999). Penicillin-binding protein–mediated resistance in pneumococci and staphylococci. *Journal of Infectious Diseases, 179*(suppl 2), S353–S359.

69. Chang, K., & Leung, C. (2010). Systematic review of interferon gamma release assays in tuberculosis: Focus on likelihood ratios. *Thorax, 65,* 271–276.

70. Chapman, S., Dismukes, W., Proia, L., Bradsher, R., Pappas, P., Threlkeld, M., et al. (2008). Clinical practice guidelines for the management of bastomycosis: 2008 update by the Infectious Diseases Society of America. *Clinical Infectious Diseases, 46*(12), 1801–1812.

71. Cherry, J. (2009). Human metapneumovirus. In R. Feigin, J. Cherry, G. Demmler-Harrison, & S. Kaplan (Eds.), *Feigin and Cherry's textbook of pediatric infectious diseases* (6th ed.). Philadelphia: Saunders Elsevier.

72. Cherry, J., & Chen, T. (2009). Adenoviruses. In R. Feigin, J. Cherry, G. Demmler-Harrison, & S. Kaplan (Eds.), *Feigin and Cherry's textbook of pediatric infectious diseases* (6th ed.). Philadelphia: Saunders Elsevier.

73. Cherry, J., & Krogstad, P. (2009). Enteroviruses and parechoviruses. In R. Feigin, J. Cherry, G. Demmler-Harrison, & S. Kaplan (Eds.), *Feigin and Cherry's textbook of pediatric infectious diseases* (6th ed.). Philadelphia: Saunders Elsevier.

74. Cherry, J., & Schulte, D. (2009). Human parvovirus B19. In R. Feigin, J. Cherry, G. Demmler-Harrison, & S. Kaplan (Eds.), *Feigin and Cherry's textbook of pediatric infectious diseases* (6th ed.). Philadelphia: Saunders Elsevier.

75. Chiaradonna, C. (2007). The *Chlamydia* cascade: Enhanced STD prevention strategies for adolescents. *Journal of Pediatric Adolescent Gynecology, 21,* 233–241.

76. Coffin, S., & Zaoutis, T. (2008). Healthcare-associated infections. In S. Long, L. Pickering, & C. Prober (Eds.), *Principles and practice of pediatric infectious diseases* (3rd ed., pp. 577–587). Philadelphia: Elsevier.

77. Coffin, S., Zaoutis, T., Rosenquist, A., Heydon, K., Herrera, G., Bridges, C., et al. (2006). Incidence, complications, and risk factors for prolonged stay in children hospitalized with community-acquired influenza. *Pediatrics, 119*(4), 740–748.

78. Cohen, J. I. (2000). Epstein-Barr virus infection. *New England Journal of Medicine, 343*(7), 481–492.

79. Cohen, J., Cristofaro, P., Carlet, J., & Opal, S. (2004). A new system of classification of infection. *Critical Care Medicine, 32,* 1510–1526.

80. Cosgrove, S., Qi, Y., Kaye, K., Harbarth, S., Karchmer, A., & Carmeli, Y. (2005). The impact of methicillin resistance in *Staphylococcus aureus* bacteremia on patient outcomes: Mortality, length of stay, and hospital charges. *Infection Control and Hospital Epidemiology, 26*(2), 166–174.

81. Craig, F., & Schunk, J. (2003). Retropharyngeal abscess in children: Clinical presentation, utility of imaging and current management. *Pediatrics, 111*(6), 1394–1398.

82. Cross, A., Opal, S., & Sadoff, J. (1993). Choice of bacteria in animal sepsis. *Infectious Immunology, 61,* 2741–2747.

83. Crossman, S. (2006). The challenge of pelvic inflammatory disease. *American Family Physician, 73*(5), 859–864.

84. Cunha, B. (2007). Fever of unknown origin: Focused diagnostic approach based on clinical clues from the history, physical examination, and laboratory tests. *Infectious Disease Clinics of North America, 21,* 137–1187.

85. Curley, M., Schwalenstocker, E., Deshponde, J., Ganser, C., Bertoch, D., Brandon, J., et al. (2006). Tailoring the Institute of Health Care Improvement 100,000 Lives campaign to pediatric settings: The example of ventilator-associated pneumonia. *Pediatric Clinics of North America, 53*, 1231–1251.

86. Damm, M., Eckel, H., Jungehülsing, M., & Roth, B. (1996). Airway endoscopy in the interdisciplinary management of acute epiglottitis. *International Journal of Pediatric Otolaryngology, 38*(1), 41–51.

87. Dantas-Torres, F. (2007). Rocky Mountain spotted fever. *Lancet Infectious Diseases, 7*(11), 724–732.

88. Davis, K., Stewart, J., Crouch, H., Florez, C., & Hospenthal, D. (2004). Methicillin-resistant *Staphylococcus aureus* (MRSA) nares colonization at hospital admission and its effect on subsequent MRSA infection. *Clinical Infectious Diseases, 39*, 776–782.

89. de la Morena, M. (2008). Immunologic development and susceptibility to infection. In S. Long, L. Pickering, & C. Prober (Eds.), *Principles and practices of pediatric infectious diseases* (3rd ed., pp. 86–94). Philadelphia: Elsevier.

90. de Oliveria, C., de Oliveria, D., Gottschald, A., Moura, J., Costa, G., Ventura, P., et al. (2008). ACCM/PALS hemodynamic support guidelines for pediatric septic shock: An outcome comparison with and without monitoring central venous oxygen saturation. *Intensive Care Medicine, 34*, 1065–1075.

91. Dellinger, R., Levy, M., Carlet, J., Bion, J., Parker, M., Jaeschke, R., et al. (2008). Surviving Sepsis campaign: International guidelines for management of severe sepsis and septic shock: 2008. *Critical Care Medicine, 36*(1), 296–327.

92. Dellit, T., Owens, R., McGowan, J. Jr., Gerding, D., Weinstein, R., Burke, J., et al. (2007). Infectious Diseases Society of America and the Society of Healthcare Epidemiology of America guidelines for developing an institutional program to enhance antimicrobial stewardship. *Clinical Infectious Diseases, 44*, 159–177.

93. Demirkazik, F., Akin, A., Uzun, O., Akpinar, M., & Ariyurek, M. (2008). CT findings in immunocompromised patients with pulmonary infections. *Diagnostic and Interventional Radiology, 14*, 75–82.

94. Demmler, G. (2008). Adenoviruses. In S. Long, L. Pickering, & C. Prober (Eds.), *Long's principles and practice of pediatric infectious diseases* (3rd ed.). Philadelphia: Saunders Elsevier.

95. Demmler-Harrison, G. (2009). Cytomegalovirus. In R. Feigin, J. Cherry, G. Demmler-Harrison, & S. Kaplan (Eds.), *Feigin and Cherry's textbook of pediatric infectious diseases* (6th ed.). Philadelphia: Saunders Elsevier.

96. Diep, B., & Otto, M. (2008). The role of virulence determinants in community-associated MRSA pathogenesis. *Trends in Microbiology, 16*(8), 361–369.

97. Djillali, A., Clair, B., & Salomon, J. (2004). Managing toxic shock syndrome with antibiotics. *Expert Opinion in Pharmacotherapy, 5*, 1701–1710.

98. Dodd, P., Millington, K., Ghani, A., Mutsvangwa, J., Butterworth, A., Lalvani, A., et al. (2010). Interpreting tuberculin skin tests in a population with a high prevalence of HIV, tuberculosis, and non-specific tuberculin sensitivity. *American Journal of Epidemiology, 171*, 1037–1045.

99. Doncker, A., Balabanian, K., Bellanne-Chantelot, C., deGuibert, S., Revest, M., Bachelerie, F., et al. (2010). Two cases of disseminated *Mycobacte-rium avium* infection associated with a new immunodeficiency syndrome related to CXCR4 dysfunction. *Clinical Microbiology and Infectious Diseases.* doi: 10.1111/j.1469-0691.2010.03187.x

100. Dowell, S., Butler, J., Giebink, G., Jacobs, M., Jernigan, D., Musher, D., et al. (1999). Acute otitis media: Management and surveillance in an era of pneumococcal resistance: A report from the Drug-resistant *Streptococcus pneumoniae*. Therapeutic Working Group. *Pediatric Infectious Disease Journal, 18*(1), 1–9.

101. Drusano, G. (1998). Infection in the intensive care unit: β-lactamase-mediated resistance among Enterobacteriaceae and optimal antimicrobial dosing. *Clinical Infectious Diseases, 27*(suppl 1), S111–S116.

102. Eaton, D., Kann, L., Kinchen, S., Shanklin, S., Ross, J., Hawkins, J., et al. (2008). Youth Risk Behavior Surveillance—United States 2007. *Morbidity and Mortality Weekly Report, 57*(4), 1–131.

103. Echavarría, M. (2008). Adenoviruses in immunocompromised hosts. *Clinical Microbiology Reviews, 21*(4), 704–715.

104. Eddleston, M., & Pierini, S. (Eds.). (1999). *Oxford handbook of tropical medicine.* Oxford, UK: Oxford University Press.

105. Edwards, J., Peterson, K., Andrus, M., Dudeck, M., Pollock, D., Horon, T., et al. (2008). National Healthcare Safety Network (NHSN) report, data summary for 2006 through 2007. *American Journal of Infection Control, 36*(9), 609–626.

106. Elward, A., & Fraser, V. (2006). Risk factors for nosocomial primary bloodstream infection in pediatric intensive care unit patients: A 2-year prospective cohort study. *Infection Control and Hospital Epidemiology, 27*(6), 553–560.

107. Elward, A., Hollenbeak, C., Warren, D., & Fraser, V. (2005). Attributable cost of nosocomial primary bloodstream infection in pediatric intensive care unit patients. *Pediatrics, 115*(4), 868–872.

108. Farrell, D., Klugman, K., & Pichichero, M. (2007). Increased antimicrobial resistance among nonvaccine serotypes of *Streptococcus pneumoniae* in the pediatric population after the introduction of 7-valent pneumococcal vaccine in the United States. *Pediatric Infectious Disease Journal, 26*(2), 123–128.

109. Feltes, T., Pignatelli, R., Kleinert, S., & Mirascalo, M. (1994). Quantitated left ventricular systolic mechanisms in children with septic shock utilizing noninvasive wall stress analysis. *Critical Care Medicine, 22*, 1647–1658.

110. Festekjian, A., & Neely, M. (2009). Incidence and predictors of invasive candidiasis associated with candidaemia in children. *Mycoses.* doi: 10.1111/j.1439-0507.2009.01785.x

111. Finfer, S., Bellamo, R., Boyce, N., French, J., Myburgh, J., Norton, R., et al. (2004). A comparison of albumin and saline for fluid resuscitation in the intensive care unit. *New England Journal of Medicine, 350*, 2247–2256.

112. Fisher, B., & Zaoutis, T. (2008). Treatment of invasive candidiasis in immunocompromised pediatric patients. *Pediatric Drugs, 10*, 281–298.

113. Florea, A., Ionescu, D., & Melhem, M. (2007). Parvovirus B19 infection in the immunocompromised host. *Archives of Pathological Laboratory Medicine, 131*, 799–804.

114. Foglia, E., Fraser, V., & Elward, A. (2007). Effect of nosocomial infections due to antibiotic-resistant organisms on length of stay and mortality in the pediatric intensive care unit. *Infection Control and Hospital Epidemiology, 28*(3), 299–306.

115. Foglia, E., Meier, M., & Elward, A. (2007). Ventilator-associated pneumonia in neonatal and pediatric intensive care unit patients. *Clinical Microbiology Reviews, 20*(3), 409–425.

116. Fonseca, H., & Greydanus, D. (2007). Sexuality in the child, teen and young adult: Concepts for clinicians. *Primary Care: Clinical in Office Practice, 34*, 275–292.

117. Forgie, S., & Marrie, T. (2009). Healthcare-associated atypical pneumonia. *Seminars in Respiratory Critical Care Medicine, 30*(1), 67–85.

118. Frank, A., Marcinak, J., Mangat, P., & Schreckenberger, P. (1999). Community-acquired and clindamycin susceptible methicillin-resistant *Staphylococcus aureus* in children. *Pediatric Infectious Disease Journal, 18*(11), 993–1000.

119. Freedman, D. (Ed.). (1998). Travel medicine. *Infectious Disease Clinics of North America, 12*(2), 1–554.

120. Frenkl, T., & Potts, J. (2008). Sexually transmitted infections. *Urologic Clinics of North America, 35*, 33–46.

121. Fraser, A., Gafter-Gvili, F., Paul, M., & Leibovici, P. (2006). Antibiotics for preventing meningococcal infections. *Cochrane Database of Systemic Reviews 2006, 4*(CD004785).

122. Galgiani, J., et al. (2005). Treatment guidelines for coccidiodomycosis. *Clinical Infectious Diseases, 41*(9), 1217–1223.

123. Gandhi, M., & Khanna, R. (2004). Human cytomegalovirus: Clinical aspects, immune regulation, and emerging treatments. *Lancet Infectious Disease, 4,* 725–738.

124. Gardner, P. (2006). Prevention of meningococcal disease. *New England Journal of Medicine, 355*(14), 1466–1473.

125. Garnock-Jones, K., & Keam, S. (2009). Caspofungin: In pediatric patients with fungal infections. *Pediatric Drugs, 11*(4), 259–269.

126. Garralda, M., Gledhill, J., Nadel, S., Neasham, D., O'Connor, M., & Shears, D. (2009). Longer-term psychiatric adjustment of children and parents after meningococcal disease. *Pediatric Critical Care Medicine, 10*(6), 1–6.

127. Gigliotti, F., & Wright, T. (2008). *Pneumocystis jirovecii (P. carinii).* In S. Long, L. Pickering, & C. Prober (Eds.), *Principles and practices of pediatric infectious diseases* (3rd ed., pp. 1203–1206). Philadelphia: Elsevier.

128. Glezen, P. (2009). Influenza viruses. In R. Feigin, J. Cherry, G. Demmler-Harrison, & S. Kaplan (Eds.), *Feigin and Cherry's textbook of pediatric infectious diseases* (6th ed.). Philadelphia: Saunders Elsevier.

129. Gona, P., Van Dyke, R., Williams, P., Dankner, W., Chernoff, M., Nachman, S., et al. (2006). Incidence of opportunistic and other infections in HIV-infected children in the HAART era. *Journal of the American Medical Association, 296,* 292–300.

130. Goodman, J., Dennis, D., & Sonenshine, D. (Eds.). (2005). *Tick-borne diseases of humans.* Washington, DC: ASM Press.

131. Gouveia, E., Metcalf, J., de Carvalho, A., Aires, T., Villasboas-Bisneto, J., Queirroz, A., et al. (2008). Leptospirosis-associated severe pulmonary hemorrhagic syndrome, Salvador, Brazil. *Emerging Infectious Diseases, 14*(3), 505–508.

132. Graffunder, E., & Venezia, R. (2002). Risk factors associated with nosocomial methicillin-resistant *Staphylococcus aureus* (MRSA) infection including previous use of antimicrobials. *Journal of Antimicrobial Chemotherapy, 49,* 999–1005.

133. Green, J., & Wang, C. (2004). Psychosocial issues in genital herpes management. *Herpes, 11,* 60–62.

134. Gutierrez, K., & Arvin, A. (2009). Herpes simplex viruses 1 and 2. In R. Feigin, J. Cherry, G. Demmler-Harrison, & S. Kaplan (Eds.), *Feigin and Cherry's textbook of pediatric infectious diseases* (6th ed.). Philadelphia: Saunders Elsevier.

135. Hakim, H., Flynn, P., Knapp, K., Srivastava, D., & Gaur, P. (2009). Etiology and clinical course of febrile neutropenia in children with cancer. *Journal of Pediatric Hematology/Oncology, 31,* 623–629.

136. Halstead, S. (2007). Dengue. *Lancet, 370,* 1644–1652.

137. Han, Y., Carcillo, J., Dragotta, M., Bills, D., Watson, R., Westerman, M., et al. (2003). Early reversal of pediatric–neonatal septic shock by community physicians is associated with improved outcome. *Pediatrics, 112*(4), 793–799.

138. Hart, C., & Thompson, A. (2006). Meningococcal disease and its management in children. *British Medical Journal, 333*(7570), 685–690.

139. Healy, C., Campbell, J., Zaccaria, E., & Baker, C. (2008). Fluconazole prophylaxis in extremely low birth weight neonates reduces invasive candidiasis mortality rates without emergence of fluconazole-resistant *Candida* species. *Pediatrics, 121,* 703–710.

140. Heath, P., Yusoff, N., & Baker, C. (2003). Neonatal meningitis. *Archives of Disease in Childhood Fetal Neonatal Edition, 88,* F173–F178.

141. Herold, B., Immergluck, L., Maranan, M., Lauderdale, D., Gaskin, R., Boyle-Vavra, S., et al. (1998). Community-acquired methicillin-resistant *Staphylococcus aureus* in children with no identified predisposing risk. *Journal of the American Medical Association, 279*(8), 593–598.

142. Hertz, A., Greenhow, T., Alcantara, J., Hansen, J., Baxter, R., Black, S., et al. (2006). Changing epidemiology of outpatient bactermeia in 3- to 36-month old children after the introduction of the heptavalent-conjugated pneumococcal vaccine. *Pediatric Infectious Disease Journal, 25*(4), 293–300.

143. Hollier, L., & Workowski, K. (2008). Treatment of sexually transmitted infections in women. *Infectious Disease Clinics of North America, 22,* 665–691.

144. Hopkins, A., Lahiri, T., Salerno, R., & Heath, B. (2006). Changing epidemiology of life-threatening upper airway infections: The reemergence of bacterial tracheitis. *Pediatrics, 118,* 1418–1421.

145. Horan, T., Andrus, M., & Dudeck, M. A. (2008). CDC/NHSN surveillance definition of health care–associated infection and criteria for specific types of infections in the acute care setting. *American Journal of Infection Control, 36*(5), 309–332.

146. Hosalkar, H., Agrawal, N., Reddy, S., Sehgal, K., Fox, E., & Hill, R. (2009). Skeletal tuberculosis in children in the Western world: 18 new cases with a review of the literature. *Journal of Child Orthopedics, 3,* 319–324.

147. Hotez, P. (2008). *Forgotten people, forgotten diseases: The neglected tropical diseases and their impact on global health and development.* Washington, DC: ASM Press.

148. Hsiao, A., & Baker, D. (2005). Fever in the new millennium: A review of recent studies of markers in serious bacterial infection in febrile children. *Current Opinion in Pediatrics, 17,* 56–61.

149. Huang, Y., Peng, C., Chiu, N., Lee, K., Hung, H., Kao, H., et al. (2009). Bacterial tracheitis in pediatrics: 12 year experience at a medical center in Taiwan. *Pediatrics International, 51,* 110–113.

150. Hughes, W., Armstrong, D., Bodey, G., Bow, E., Brown, A., Calandra, T., et al. (2002). Guidelines for the use of antimicrobial agents in neutropenic patients with cancer. *Clinical Infectious Diseases, 34,* 730–751.

151. Ishimine, P. (2006). Fever without a source in children 0 to 36 months of age. *Pediatric Clinics of North America, 53,* 167–194.

152. Jackson, W. (2005). Should we use etomidate as an induction agent for endotracheal intubation with septic shock? A critical appraisal. *Chest, 127,* 1031–1038.

153. Jaskiewicz, J., McCarthy, C., & Richardson, A. (1994). Febrile infants at low risk for serious bacterial infection: An appraisal of the Rochester criteria and implications for management: Febrile Infant Collaborative Study Group. *Pediatrics, 94,* 390–396.

154. Jeans, A., Moore, J., Nicol, C., Bates, C., & Read, R. (2009). Wrist watch use and hospital-acquired infection. *Journal of Hospital Infection, 74*(1), 16–21.

155. Jeffries, H., Mason, W., Brewer, M., Oakes, K., Munoz, E., Gornick, W., et al. (2009). Prevention of central venous catheter-associated bloodstream infections in pediatric intensive care units: A performance improvement collaborative. *Infection Control and Hospital Epidemiology, 30*(9), 645–651.

156. Kain, K., Shanks, G., & Keystone, J. (2001). Malaria chemoprophylaxis in the age of drug resistance. I. Currently recommended drug regimens. *Clinical Infectious Diseases, 33*(2), 226–234.

157. Kannangara, S. (2006). Management of febrile neutropenia. *Community Oncology, 3,* 585–591.

158. Kaplan, S., Schutze, G., Leake, J., Barson, W., Halasa, N., Byington, C., et al. (2006). Multicenter surveillance of invasive meningococcal infections in children. *Pediatrics, 118*(4), e979–e984.

159. Karnezis, T., Smith, A., Whittier, S., Haddad, J. Jr., & Saiman, L. (2009). Antimicrobial resistance among isolates causing invasive pneumococcal disease before and after licensure of heptavalent conjugate pneumococcal vaccine. *PLos One, 4*(6), e5965.

160. Katz, B. (2008). Epstein-Barr infections (mononucleosis and lymphoproliferative disorders). In S. Long, L. Pickering, & C. Prober (Eds.), *Long's principles and practice of pediatric infectious diseases* (3rd ed.). Philadelphia: Saunders Elsevier.

161. Kauffman, C. (2007). Histoplasmosis: A clinical and laboratory update. *Clinical Microbiology Reviews, 20*(1), 115–132.

162. Kauffman, C. (2009). Histoplasmosis. *Clinics in Chest Medicine, 30*(2), 217–225.

163. Kaufman, D., Boyle, R., Hazen, R., Patrie, J., Robinson, M., & Donowitz, L. (2001). Fluconazole prophylaxis against fungal colonization and infection in preterm infants. *New England Journal of Medicine, 345,* 1660–1666.

164. Kaufman, D., Boyle, R., Hazen, K., Patrie, J., Robinson, M., & Grossman, L. (2005). Twice weekly fluconazole prophylaxis for

prevention of invasive *Candida* infection in high risk infants < 1000 grams birth weight. *Journal of Pediatrics, 147,* 172–179.

165. Khan, R., Harris, S., Verma, A., & Syed, A. (2009). Cervical lymphadenopathy: Scrofula revisited. *Journal of Laryngology & Otology, 123,* 764–767.

166. Khilnani, P., Deopujari, S., & Carcillo, J. (2008). Recent advances in sepsis and septic shock. *Indian Journal of Pediatrics, 75,* 821–830.

167. Kicklighter, S., Springer, C., Cox, T., Hulsey, T., & Tutner, R. (2001). Fluconazole for prophylaxis against candidal rectal colonization in the very low birth weight infant. *Pediatrics, 107,* 293–298.

168. Kidd, D., Williams, A., & Howard, R. (1996). Poliomyelitis. *Postgraduate Medical Journal, 72,* 641–647.

169. Kleiman, M. (2008a). Classification of fungi. In S. Long, L. Pickering, & C. Prober (Eds.), *Principles and practice of pediatric infectious diseases* (3rd ed., pp. 1170–1172). Philadelphia: Elsevier.

170. Kleiman, M. (2008b). *Histoplasma capsulatum* (histoplasmosis). In S. Long, L. Pickering, & C. Prober (Eds.), *Principles and practice of pediatric infectious diseases* (3rd ed., pp. 1197–1202). Philadelphia: Elsevier.

171. Kleiman, M. (2008c). *Coccidiodes immitis* and *Coccidiodes posadasii* (coccidioidomycosis). In S. Long, L. Pickering, & C. Prober (Eds.), *Principles and practice of pediatric infectious diseases* (3rd ed., pp. 1213–1218). Philadelphia: Elsevier.

172. Kleiman, M. (2008d). *Blastomyces dermatitidis* (blastomycosis). In S. Long, L. Pickering, & C. Prober (Eds.), *Principles and practice of pediatric infectious diseases* (3rd ed., pp. 1207–1212). Philadelphia: Elsevier.

173. Klein, J. (2000). Bacterial meningitis and sepsis. In J. Remington & J. Klein (Eds.), *Infectious diseases of the fetus and newborn infant* (pp. 943–998). Philadelphia: WB Saunders.

174. Klompas, M. (2007). Does this patient have ventilator-associated pneumonia? *Journal of the American Medical Association, 297*(14), 1583–1593.

175. Koh, A., & Pizzo, P. (2008). Fever and granulocytopenia. In S. Long, L. Pickering, & C. Prober (Eds.), *Principles and practice of pediatric infectious diseases* (3rd ed.). Philadelphia: Churchill Livingstone.

176. Krajicek, B., Thomas, C., & Limper, A. (2009). Pneumocystis pneumonia: Current concepts in pathogenesis, diagnosis, and treatment. *Clinics in Chest Medicine, 30*(2), 265–278.

177. Kumar, A., Roberts, D., Wood, K., Light, B., Parrillo, J., Sharma, S., et al. (2006). Duration of hypotension before initiation of effective antimicrobial therapy is the critical determinant of survival in septic shock. *Critical Care Medicine, 34*(6), 1589–1596.

178. Kutko, M., Calarco, M., & Flaherty, M., Helmrich, R., Ushay, H., Pon, S., et al. (2003). Mortality rates in pediatric septic shock with and without multiple organ system failure. *Pediatric Critical Care Medicine, 4*(3), 333–337.

179. Kutok, J., & Wang, F. (2006). Spectrum of Epstein-Barr virus–associated diseases. *Annual Review of Pathology: Mechanisms of Disease, 1,* 375–404.

180. Kwiatkowsky, D. (2005). How malaria has affected the human genome and what human genetics can teach us about malaria. *American Journal of Human Genetics, 77*(2), 171–192.

181. Lappin, E., & Ferguson, A. (2009). Gram-positive toxic shock syndromes. *Lancet Infectious Disease, 9,* 281–290.

182. Lareau, S., & Beigi, R. (2008). Pelvic inflammatory disease and tubo-ovarian abscess. *Infectious Disease Clinics of North America, 22,* 693–708.

183. Lautenbach, E., Patel, J., Bilker, W., Edelstein, P., & Fishman, N. (2001). Extended-spectrum β-lactamase–producing *Escherichia coli* and *Klebsiella pneumoniae:* Risk factors for infection and impact of resistance on outcomes. *Clinical Infectious Diseases, 32,* 1162–1171.

184. Lazar, I., & Bogue, C. (2007). Infectious disease–associated syndromes. In D. S. Wheeler, H. Wong, & T. Shanley (Eds.), *Pediatric critical care medicine: Basic science and clinical evidence* (pp. 1511–1514). London: Springer-Verlag.

185. Leach, C., & Sumaya, C. (2009). Epstein-Barr virus. In R. Feigin, J. Cherry, G. Demmler-Harrison, & S. Kaplan (Eds.), *Feigin and Cherry's textbook of pediatric infectious diseases* (6th ed.). Philadelphia: Saunders Elsevier.

186. Lecat, P., Cropp, E., McCord, G., & Haller, N. (2009). Ethanol-based cleanser versus isopropyl alcohol to decontaminate stethoscopes. *American Journal of Infection Control, 37*(3), 241–243.

187. Leclerq, R. (2002). Mechanisms of resistance to macrolides and lincosamides: Nature of the resistance elements and their clinical implications. *Clinical Infectious Diseases, 34,* 482–492.

188. Lenaerts, L., De Clercq, E., & Naesens, L. (2008). Clinical features and treatment of adenovirus infections. *Reviews in Medical Virology, 18,* 357–374.

189. Lewis, D. (1998). Cellular immunity of the human fetus and neonate. *Immunology and Allergy Clinics of North America, 18*(2), 291.

190. Lighter, J., Rigaud, M., Eduardo, R., Peng, C-H., & Pollack, H. (2009). Latent tuberculosis diagnosis in children by using the QuantiFERON-TB Gold In-Tube test. *Pediatrics, 123,* 30–37.

191. Lindsay, C., Barton, P., Lawless, S., Kitchen, L., Zorka, A., Garcia, J., et al. (1998). Pharmacokinetics and pharmacodynamics of milrinone lactate in pediatric patients with septic shock. *Journal of Pediatrics, 132,* 329–334.

192. Liston, S., Gehrz, R. C., Siegel, L. G., & Tilelli, J. (1983). Bacterial tracheitis. *American Journal of Diseases of Children, 137*(8), 764–767.

193. Livermore, D. (2000). Antibiotic resistance in staphylococci. *International Journal of Antimicrobial Agents, 16,* S3–S10.

194. Long, S. (2005). Distinguishing among prolonged, recurrent, and periodic fever syndromes: Approach of a pediatric infectious diseases specialist. *Pediatric Clinics of North America, 52,* 811–835.

195. Long, S., & Edwards, K. (2008). Prolonged, recurrent and periodic fever syndromes. In S. Long, L. Pickering, & C. Prober (Eds.), *Principles and practice of pediatric infectious diseases* (3rd ed.). Philadelphia: Churchill Livingstone.

196. Ma, X., Ito, T., Tiensasitorn, C., Jamklang, M., Chongtrakool, P., Boyle-Vavra, S., et al. (2002). Novel type of staphylococcal cassette chromosome *mec* identified in community-acquired methicillin-resistant *Staphylococcus aureus* strains. *Antimicrobial Agents and Chemotherapy, 46*(4), 1147–1152.

197. Maldonado, Y. (2008). Polioviruses. In S. Long, L. Pickering, & C. Prober (Eds.), *Long's principles and practice of pediatric infectious diseases* (3rd ed.). Philadelphia: Saunders Elsevier.

198. Manzoni, P., Arisio, R., Mostert, M., Leonessa, M., Farina, D., Latino, M., et al. (2006). Prophylactic fluconazole is effective in preventing fungal colonization and fungal systemic infections in preterm neonates: A single center, 6 year, retrospective cohort study. *Pediatrics, 117,* e22–e32.

199. Manzoni, P., Stolfi, I., Pugni, L., Decembrino, L., Magnami, C., Vetrano, G., et al. (2007). A multicenter, randomized trial of prophylactic fluconazole in preterm infants. *New England Journal of Medicine, 356,* 2483–2495.

200. Manzoni, P., Leonessa, M., Galletto, P., Latino, M., Arisio, R., Maule, M., et al. (2008). Routine use of fluconazole prophylaxis in a neonatal intensive care unit does not select natively fluconazole-resistant *Candida* subspecies. *Pediatric Infectious Disease Journal, 27,* 731–737.

201. Marais, B. (2008). Tuberculosis in children. *Pediatric Pulmonology, 43,* 322–329.

202. Marais, B., & Pai, M. (2007). Recent advances in the diagnosis of childhood tuberculosis. *Archives of Diseases in Childhood, 92,* 446–452.

203. Marais, B., Wright, C., Schaaf, H., Gie, R., Hesseling, A., Enarson, D., et al. (2006). Tuberculous lymphadenitis as a cause of persistent cervical lymphadenopathy in children from a tuberculosis-endemic area. *Pediatric Infectious Disease Journal, 25,* 142–146.

204. Marodi, L. (2006). Neonatal innate immunity to infectious agents. *Infection and Immunity, 74*(4), 1999–2006.

205. Maubon, D., Simon, S., & Aznar, C. (2007). Histoplasmosis diagnosis using a polymerase chain reaction method: Application on human samples in French Guiana, South America. *Diagnostic Microbiology and Infectious Disease, 58*(4), 441–444.

206. Mayo-Smith, M., Spinale, J., Donskey, C., Yukawa, M., Li, R., & Schiffman, F. (1995). Acute epiglottitis: An 18 year experience in Rhode Island. *Chest, 108*(6), 1640–1647.

207. McClay, J., Murray, A., & Booth, T. (2003). Intravenous antibiotic therapy for deep neck abscesses defined by computed tomography. *Archives of Otolaryngology Head and Neck Surgery, 129*(11), 1207–1212.

208. McIntosh, C., Beeson, J., & March, K. (2004). Clinical features and pathogenesis of severe malaria. *Trends in Parasitology, 20*(12), 597–603.

209. McKinnell, J., & Pappas, P. (2009). Blastomycosis: New insights into diagnosis, prevention, and treatment. *Clinics in Chest Medicine, 30*(2), 227–239.

210. McWilliams, G., Hill, M., & Dietrich, C. (2007). Gynecologic emergencies. *Surgical Clinics of North America, 88*, 265–283.

211. Michell, S., Griffin, K., & Titball, R. (2006). Tularemia pathogenesis and immunity. In B. Anderson, H. Friedman, & M. Bendinelli (Eds.), *Microoganisms and bioterrorism* (pp. 121–137). New York: Springer.

212. Miller, M., Szer, I., Yogev, R., & Bernstein, B. (1995). Fever of unknown origin. *Pediatric Clinics of North America, 42*, 999–1015.

213. Modlin, J. (2008). Enteroviruses: Coxsackieviruses, echoviruses, and newer enteroviruses. In S. Long, L. Pickering, & C. Prober (Eds.), *Long's principles and practice of pediatric infectious diseases* (3rd ed.). Philadelphia: Saunders Elsevier.

214. Mollen, C. (2009). Sexually transmitted infections. In J. M. Baren, S. G. Rothrock, J. A. Brennan, & L. Brown (Eds.), *Pediatric emergency medicine* (pp. 543–559). Philadelphia: Saunders Elsevier.

215. Moore, M., & Little, P. (2006). Humidified air inhalation for treating croup. *Cochrane Database of Systematic Reviews, 3*(CD002870).

216. Moran, C., Spalding, J., Benjamin, D., & Reed, S. (2009). *Candida albicans* and non-*albicans* bloodstream infections in adult and pediatric patients: Comparison of mortality and costs. *Pediatric Infectious Disease Journal, 28*, 433–435.

217. Mossad, S. (2009). The resurgence of swine-origin influenza A (H1N1). *Cleveland Clinic Journal of Medicine, 76*(6), 337–343.

218. Muralidhar, V., & Muralidhar, S. (2007). *Hospital acquired infections.* Kent, UK: Anshan.

219. National Network for Immunization Information (NNII). (2007, February 1). Human papilloma virus. Retrieved from http://www.immunizationinfo.org/issues/hpv-vaccines/human-papillomaviruses-hpvs

220. National Network for Immunization Information (NNII). (2010, March 31). Human papilloma virus: Understanding the disease. Retrieved from http://www.immunizationinfo.org/vaccines/human-papillomavirus-hpv

221. Neu, N., Malik, M., Lunding, A., Whittier, S., Alba, L., Kubin, C., et al. (2009). Epidemiology of candidemia at Children's Hospital, 2002–2006. *Pediatric Infectious Disease Journal, 28*, 806–809.

222. Newby, J. (2008). Nosocomial infection in neonates: Inevitable or preventable? *Journal of Perinatal and Neonatal Nursing, 22*(3), 221–227.

223. Opal, M. (2005). Concept of PIRO as a new conceptual framework to understand sepsis. *Pediatric Critical Care Medicine, 6*(3 suppl), S55–S60.

224. Opal, M., & Chohen, J. (1999). Clinical Gram-positive sepsis: Does it fundamentally differ from Gram-negative bacterial sepsis. *Critical Care Medicine, 27*, 1608–1616.

225. Owens, C., & Stoessel, K. (2008). Surgical site infections: Epidemiology, microbiology and prevention. *Journal of Hospital Infection, 70*(S2), 3–10.

226. Ozkaynak, M., Krailo, M., Chen, Z., & Feusner, J. (2005). Randomized comparison of antibiotics with and without granulocyte colony-stimulating factor in children with chemotherapy-induced febrile neutropenia: A report from the Children's Oncology Group. *Pediatric Blood Cancer, 45*, 274.

227. Palazzi, P., & Feigin, R. (2009). Fever without source and fever of unknown origin. In R. Feigin, J. Cherry, G. Demmler-Harrison, & S. Kaplan (Eds.), *Feigin and Cherry's textbook of pediatric infectious diseases* (6th ed., pp. 854–860). Philadelphia: Saunders.

228. Pappas, P., Kauffman, C., Andes, D., Benjamin, D., Calandra, T., Edwards, J., et al. (2009). Clinical practice guidelines for the management of candidiasis: 2009 update by the Infectious Diseases Society of America. *Clinical Infectious Diseases, 48*, 503–535.

229. Parish, J., & Blair, J. (2008). Coccidioidomycosis. *Mayo Clinic Proceedings, 83*(3), 343–349.

230. Parry, C., Hien, T., Dougan, G., White, N., & Farrar, J. (2002). Typhoid fever. *New England Journal of Medicine, 347*(22), 1770–1782.

231. Pass, R. (2008). Cytomegalovirus. In S. Long, L. Pickering, & C. Prober (Eds.), *Long's principles and practice of pediatric infectious diseases* (3rd ed.). Philadelphia: Saunders Elsevier.

232. Pathan, N., Faust, S., & Levin, M. (2003). Pathophyisiology of meningococcal meningitis and septicemia. *Archives of Disease in Childhood, 88*(7), 601–607.

233. Pelton, S. (2009). Prevention of invasive meningococcal disease in the United States. *Pediatric Infectious Disease Journal, 28*(4), 329–332.

234. Peto, H., Pratt, R., Harrington, T., LoBue, P., & Armstrong, L. (2009). Epidemiology of extrapulmonary tuberculosis in the United States, 1993–2006. *Clinical Infectious Diseases, 49*, 1350–1357.

235. Pollack, M., Fields, A., & Ruttimann, U. (1985). Distributions of cardiopulmonary variables in pediatric survivors and nonsurvivors of septic shock. *Critical Care Medicine, 13*, 454–459.

236. Powell, K. (2007). Fever without a focus. In R. Kliegman, R. Behrman, H. Jenson, & B. Stanton (Eds.), *Nelson textbook of pediatrics* (18th ed., pp. 1087–1093). Philadelphia: Saunders Elsevier.

237. Prasad, K., & Singh, M. (2008). Corticosteroids for managing tuberculous meningitis. *Cochrane Database of Systematic Reviews, 1*, CD002244.

238. Principi, N., Bosis, S., & Esposito, S. (2006). Human metapneumovirus in paediatric patients. *Clinical Microbiology and Infection, 12*(4), 301–308.

239. Prober, C. (2008). Herpes simplex virus. In S. Long, L. Pickering, & C. Prober (Eds.), *Long's principles and practice of pediatric infectious diseases* (3rd ed.). Philadelphia: Saunders Elsevier.

240. Pulliam, P., Attia, M., & Cronan, K. (2001). C-reactive protein in febrile children 1 to months of age with clinically undetectable serious bacterial infection. *Pediatrics, 108*, 1275–1279.

241. Rackow, E., Falk, J., Fein, I., Siegel, J., Packman, M., Haupt, M., et al. (1983). Fluid resuscitation in circulatory shock: A comparison of the cardiorespiratory effects of albumin, hetastarch, and saline solutions in patients with hypovolemic and septic shock. *Critical Care Medicine, 11*, 839–850.

242. Reed, B., Caudle, K., & Rodgers, P. (2010). Prophylaxis in high risk neonates. *Annals of Pharmacotherpy, 44*(1), 178–184.

243. Richards, M., Edwards, J., & Culver, D. (1999). Nosocomial infections in medical intensive care units in the United States: National Nosocomial Infections Surveillance System. *Critical Care Medicine, 27*(5), 887–892.

244. Richter, S., Heilmann, K., Dohrn, C., Riahi, F., Beekmann, S., & Doern, G. (2009). Changing epidemiology of antimicrobial-resistant *Streptococcus pneumoniae* in the United States, 2004–5. *Clinical Infectious Diseases, 48*(1), e23–e33.

245. Rivers, E., Nguyen, B., Havstad, S., Ressler, J., Muzzin, A., Knoblich, B., et al. (2001). Early Goal Directed Therapy Collaborative Group: Early goal-directed therapy in the treatment of severe sepsis and septic shock. *New England Journal of Medicine, 345*(19), 1368–1377.

246. Roberson, D. (2004). Pediatric retorpharyngeal abscess. *Clinical Pediatric Emergency Medicine, 5*, 37–40.

247. Robinson, C., Willis, M., Meagher, A., Gieseker, K., Rotbart, H., & Glodé, M. (2002). Impact of rapid polymerase chain reaction results on management of pediatric patients with enteroviral meningitis. *Pediatric Infectious Disease Journal, 21*(4), 283–286.

248. Rock, R., Olin, M., Baker, C., Molitor, T., & Peterson, P. (2008). Central nervous system tuberculosis: Pathogenesis and clinical aspects. *Clinical Microbiology Reviews, 21,* 243–261.

249. Roehrig, J., Nash, D., Maldin, B., Labowitz, A., Martin, D., Lanciotti, R., et al. (2003). Persistence of virus-reactive serum immunoglobulin m antibody in confirmed West Nile virus encephalitis cases. *Emerging Infectious Diseases, 9*(3), 376–379.

250. Rogerson, S., & Carter, R. (2008). Severe vivax malaria: Newly recognised or rediscovered? *PLoS Medicine, 5*(6), e136. doi:10.1371/journal.pmed.0050136

251. Ryan, E., & Kain, K. C. (2000). Health advice and immunization for travelers. *New England Journal of Medicine, 342,* 1716–1725.

252. Rybak, M., Lomaestro, B., Rotscahfer, J., Moellering, R., Craig, W., Billeter, M., et al. (2009). Vancomycin therapeutic guidelines: A summary of consensus recommendations from the Infectious Diseases Society of America and American Society of Health-System Pharmacists, and the Society of Infectious Diseases Pharmacists. *Clinical Infectious Diseases, 49*(3), 325–327.

253. Satter, R., & Tanner, L. (2007, September 17). U.K. hospitals issue doctor's dress code. Associated Press. Retrieved from http://www.usatoday.com/news/health/2007-09-17-472598993_x.htm

254. Sattler, C., Mason, E. Jr., & Kaplan, S. (2002). Prospective comparison of risk factors and demographic and clinical characteristics of community-acquired, methicillin-resistant versus methicillin-susceptible *Staphylococcus aureus* infection in children. *Pediatric Infectious Disease Journal, 21*(10), 910–916.

255. Sawyer, M. (2001). Enterovirus infections: Diagnosis and treatment. *Current Opinion in Pediatrics, 13,* 65–69.

256. Schraff, S., McGinn, J., & Derkay, C. (2001). Peritonsillar abscess in children: A 10-year review of diagnosis and management. *International Journal of Pediatric Otorhinolaryngology, 57*(3), 213–218.

257. Shafii, T., Bernstein, T., & Burstein, G. (2009). The adolescent sexual health visit. *Obstetrical Gynecological Clinics of North America, 36,* 99–117.

258. Shah, I. (2009). Steroid therapy in children with tuberculous meningitis. *Scandinavian Journal of Infectious Diseases.* doi: 10.1080/00365540902856552

259. Shah, R., Roberson, D., & Jones, D. (2004). Epiglottitis in the *Haemophilus influenzae* type B vaccine era: Changing trends. *Laryngoscope, 114*(3), 557–560.

260. Shah, S., & Sharieff, G. (2007). Pediatric respiratory infections. *Emergency Medicine Clinics of North America, 25,* 961–979.

261. Siegel, J., & Grossman, L. (2008). Pediatric infection prevention and control. In S. Long, L. Pickering, & C. Prober (Eds.), *Principles and practice of pediatric infectious diseases* (3rd ed., pp. 9–23). Philadelphia: Elsevier.

262. Siegel, J., Rhinehart, E., Jackson, M., Chiarello, L., & Healthcare Infection Control Practices Advisory Committee. (2007). Guidelines for isolation precautions: Preventing transmission of infectious agents in healthcare settings. Retrieved from http://www.cdc.gov/ncidod/dhap/pdf/isolation2007.pdf

263. Singhi, S., Jayashree, M., Straumanis, J., & Kotloff, K. (2008). Toxin-related diseases. In D. Nichols (Ed.), *Rogers' textbook of pediatric critical care* (4th ed., pp. 1460–1465). Philadelphia: Lippincott Williams & Wilkins.

264. Slonim, A., Kurtines, H., Sprague, B., & Singh, N. (2001). The costs associated with nosocomial bloodstream infections in the pediatric intensive care unit. *Pediatric Critical Care Medicine, 2*(2), 170–174.

265. Smith, A., & Tambyah, P. (2007). Severe dengue virus infection in travelers. *Journal of Infectious Diseases, 195*(8), 1081–1083.

266. Smith, M. (2008). Catheter-related bloodstream infections in children. *American Journal of Infection Control, 36*(10), S173. e1–S173.e3.

267. Smith, P., & Steinbach, W. (2008). *Candida* species. In S. Long, L. Pickering, & C. Prober (Eds.), *Principles and practices of pediatric infectious diseases* (3rd ed., pp. 1172–1178). Philadelphia: Elsevier.

268. Solomon, T. (2004). Flavivirus encephalitis. *New England Journal of Medicine, 351,* 370–378.

269. Song, A., & Advincula, A. (2005). Adolescent chronic pelvic pain. *Journal of Pediatric and Adolescent Gynecology, 18,* 371–377.

270. Spach, D., Liles, W., Campbell, G., Quick, R., Anderson, D., & Fritsche, T. (1993). Tick-borne diseases in the United States. *New England Journal of Medicine, 329,* 936–947.

271. Srinivasan, R., Asselin, J., Gildengorin, G., & Wiener-Kronish, J. (2009). A prospective study of ventilator-associated pneumonia in children. *Pediatrics, 123*(4), 1108–1115.

272. Starke, J., & Jacobs, R. (2008). *Mycobacterium* tuberculosis. In S. Long, L. Pickering, & C. Prober (Eds.), *Principles and practice of pediatric infectious diseases* (3rd ed., pp. 770–788). Philadelphia: Elsevier.

273. Stoll, M., & Rubin, L. (2004). Incidence of occult bacteremia among highly febrile young children in the era of the pneumococcal conjugate vaccine: A study from a Children's Hospital Emergency Department and Urgent Care Center. *Archives of Pediatric and Adolescent Medicine, 158,* 671–675.

274. Stroud, R., & Friedman, N. (2001). An update on inflammatory disorders of the pediatric airway: Epiglottitis, croup, and tracheitis. *American Journal of Otolaryngology, 22*(4), 268–275.

275. Subbarao, K. (2008). Influenza. In S. Long, L. Pickering, & C. Prober (Eds.), *Long's principles and practice of pediatric infectious diseases* (3rd ed.). Philadelphia: Saunders Elsevier.

276. Swaminathan, S., & Rehka, B. (2010). Pediatric tuberculosis: Global overview and challenges. *Clinical Infectious Diseases, 50(S3),* S184–S194.

277. Szuhay, G., & Tewfik, T. (1998). Peritonsillar abscess or cellulitis? A clinical comparative paediatric study. *Journal of Otolaryngology, 27*(4), 206–212.

278. Thompson, M., Ninis, N., Perera, R., Mayon-White, R., Phillips, C., Bailey, L., et al. (2006). Clinical recognition of meningococcal disease in children and adolescents. *Lancet, 367*(9508), 397–403.

279. Toltzis, P. (2004). Antibiotic-resistant Gram-negative bacteria in hospitalized children. *Clinical Laboratory Medicine, 24,* 363–380.

280. Trautner, B., Caviness, A., Gerlacher, G., Demmler, G., & Macias, C. (2006). Prospective evaluation of the risk of serious bacterial infection in children who present to the emergency department with hyperpyrexia (temperature of 106 degrees F or higher). *Pediatrics, 118*(1), 34–40.

281. Trigg, B., Kerndt, P., & Aynalem, G. (2008). Sexually transmitted infections and pelvic inflammatory disease in women. *Medical Clinics of North America, 92,* 1083–1113.

282. Vincent, J., & Gerlach, H. (2004). Fluid resuscitation in severe sepsis and septic shock: An evidence-based review. *Critical Care Medicine, 32*(11 suppl), S451–S454.

283. Vorwerk, C., & Coats, T. (2008). Use of helium–oxygen mixtures in the treatment of croup: A systematic review. *Emergency Medical Journal, 25,* 547–550.

284. Waddle, E., & Jhaveri, R. (2009). Outcomes of febrile children without localizing signs after pneumococcal conjugate vaccine. *Archives of Disease in Childhood, 94,* 144–147.

285. Wallace, R. (2008). *Mycobacterium* species. In S. Long, L. Pickering, & C. Prober (Eds.), *Principles and practices of pediatric infectious diseases* (3rd ed., pp. 778–792). Philadelphia: Elsevier.

286. Walsh, C., Morris, S., Brophy, J., Hiraki, L., Richardson, S., & Allen, U. (2006). Disseminated blastomycosis in an infant. *Pediatric Infectious Disease Journal, 25*(7), 656–658.

287. Walsh, T., Roilides, E., Groll, A., Gonzales, C., & Pizzo, P. (2006). Infectious complications in pediatric cancer patients. In P. Pizzo &

D. Poplack (Eds.), *Principles and practice in pediatric oncology* (5th ed., pp. 1269–1299). Philadelphia: Lippincott Williams & Wilkins.

288. Wang, T., Town, T., Alexopoulou, L., Anderson, J., Fikrig, E., & Flavell, R. (2004). Toll-like receptor 3 mediates West Nile virus entry into the brain causing lethal encephalitis. *Nature Medicine, 10,* 1366–1373.

289. Warrell, D., Looareesuwan, S., Warrell, M., Kasemsarn, P., Intaraprasert, R., Bunnag, D., et al. (1982). Dexamethasone proves deleterious in cerebral malaria: A double-blind trial in 100 comatose patients. *New England Journal of Medicine, 306,* 313–319.

290. Watson, R., & Carcillo, J. (2005). Scope and epidemiology of pediatric sepsis. *Pediatric Critical Care Medicine, 6*(3 suppl), S3–S5.

291. Watson, R., Carcillo, J., Linde-Zwirble, W., Clermont, G., Lidicker, J., & Angus, D. (2003). The epidemiology of severe sepsis in newborns, infants, and children in the U.S. *American Journal of Respiratory Critical Care Medicine, 167,* 695–701.

292. Watson, R., Linde-Zwirbe, W., Lidicker, J., et al. (2001). The increasing burden of severe sepsis in U.S. children. *Critical Care Medicine, 29*(suppl), A8.

293. Weinstock, H., Berman, S., & Cates, W. (2004). Sexually trasmitted diseases among American youth: Incidence and prevalence estimates, 2000. *Perspectives Sexual Reproductive Health, 36,* 6–10.

294. Welch, S., & Nadel, S. (2003). Treatment of meningococcal infection. *Archives of Disease in Childhood, 88*(7), 608–614.

295. Westley, C., Cotton, E., & Brooks, J. (1978). Nebulized racemic epinephrine by IPPB for the treatment of croup. *American Journal Disease Children, 132,* 484–487.

296. Wheat, F., Freifeld, A., Kleiman, M., Baddley, J., McKinsey, D., Loyd, J., et al. (2007). Clinical practice guidelines for the management of the patients with histoplasmosis: 2007 update by the Infectious Diseases Society of America. *Clinical Infectious Diseases, 45*(7), 807–825.

297. Wheat, L. (2006). Histoplasmosis: A review for clinicians from nonendemic areas. *Mycoses, 49*(4), 274–282.

298. Whitley, R., & Roizman, B. (2001). Herpes simplex infections. *Lancet, 357,* 1513–1518.

299. Wichmann, M., Inthorn, D., Andress, H., & Schildberg, F. (2000). Incidence and mortality of severe sepsis in surgical intensive care patients: The influence of patient gender on disease process and outcome. *Intensive Care Medicine, 26,* 167–172.

300. Williams, J., & Crowe, J. Jr. (2008). Human metapneumovirus. In S. Long, L. Pickering, & C. Prober (Eds.), *Long's principles and practice of pediatric infectious diseases* (3rd ed.). Philadelphia: Saunders Elsevier.

301. Wood, C. (2007). *Neisseria meningitides* (meningococcus). In R. Kliegman (Ed.), *Nelson textbook of pediatrics* (18th ed.). Philadelphia: Saunders.

302. Workowski, K., & Berman, S. (2006). Sexually transmitted diseases treatment guideline. *Morbidity and Mortality Weekly Report, 55*(11), 1–100.

303. World Health Organization (WHO). (2004). *The world health report 2004: Changing history.* Retrieved from http://www.who.int/whr/2004/en/

304. World Health Organization (WHO). (2009). Global tuberculosis control—epidemiology, strategy, financing. Retrieved from http://www.who.int/tb/publications/global_report/2009/ev/index.html

305. Wormser, G., Dattwyler, R., Shapiro, E., Halperin, J., Steere, A., Klempner, M., et al. (2006). The clinical assessment, treatment, and prevention of Lyme disease, human granulocytic anaplasmosis, and babesiosis: Clinical practice guidelines by the Infectious Diseases Society of America. *Clinical Infectious Diseases, 43*(9), 1089–1134.

306. Writing Committee of the Second World Health Organization Consultation on Clinical Aspects of Human Infection with Avian Influenza A (H5N1) Virus (WHO). (2008). Update on avian influenza (H5N1) virus on infection in humans. *New England Journal of Medicine, 358,* 261–273.

307. Yazdankhah, S., & Caugant, D. (2004). *Neisseria meningitides:* An overview of the carriage state. *Journal of Medical Microbiology, 53*(9), 821–832.

308. Yildirim, I., Ceyhan, M., Cengiz, A., Bagdat, A., Barin, C., Cutluk, T., et al. (2008). A prospective comparative study of the relationship between different types of ring and microbial hand colonization among pediatric intensive care unit nurses. *International Journal of Nursing Studies, 45,* 1572–1576.

309. Young, N., & Brown, K. (2004). Parvovirus B19. *New England Journal of Medicine, 350,* 586–597.

310. Zaoutis, T., & Coffn, S. (2008). Clinical syndromes of device-associated infections. In S. Long, L. Pickering, & C. Prober (Eds.), *Principles and practice of pediatric infectious diseases* (3rd ed., pp. 587–599). Philadelphia: Elsevier.

311. Zaoutis, T., Jafri, H., Huang, L., Locatelli, F., Barzilai, A., Ebell, W., et al. (2009). A prospective, multicenter study of caspofungin for the treatment of documented *Candida* or *Aspergillus* infections in pediatric patients. *Pediatrics, 123,* 877–884.

312. Zimmerman, J. (2004). Use of blood products in sepsis: An evidence based review. *Critical Care Medicine, 32*(11 suppl), S542–S547.

Kidney and Genitourinary Disorders

PHYSIOLOGY AND DIAGNOSTICS

Sara Jandeska

PHYSIOLOGY

Embryology

During the third week of gestation, often prior to diagnosis of pregnancy, nephrogenic structures begin their development. By the fifth week of gestation, the metanephros (embryologic kidney) has developed a blood supply with primitive glomeruli and a collecting system. Penetration of the ureteric bud of the mesonephric duct into the metanephros induces differentiation of fibroblastic tissue into tubules, while reciprocally the ureteric bud is stimulated to branch into a mature collecting system.

Nephron development is complete once the glomeruli feed into the proximal tubules. Nephronogenesis starts at the eighth week of gestation, and is completed by 34 weeks' gestation. The first nephrons develop at the corticomedullary junction. With increasing gestation, future nephrons are formed centripetally, with the last forming in the superficial cortex. Glomeruli form within the first 40 days of postnatal life in premature infants (Rodriguez et al., 2004).

Any insult during renal embryogenesis can decrease nephron mass. For example, congenital obstruction of the ureter (ureteropelvic junction, ureterovesicular junction) or urethra (posterior urethral valves) variably affects kidney development. In animal models, chronic unilateral ureteral obstruction prevents maturation of the entire nephron. Apoptosis (programmed cell death) of the distal tubules results in atrophy and dilatation of the collecting system, which appears as hydronephrosis. Relief of obstruction postnatally does not reverse injury sustained in utero. The onset, severity, and extent of obstruction determine the rate of decrease in kidney function, which is most evident when increased glomerular filtration is required during periods of rapid growth (e.g., during the first year of life, at 3 to 4 years of age, in adolescence).

Renal blood flow and glomerular flow rate

Renal blood flow. The renal blood flow in the fetal kidneys is less than 10% of cardiac output, supplying the most mature, corticomedullary nephrons. At birth, a rapid increase in cardiac output is accompanied by a decrease in renal vascular resistance, as mediated by local production of nitric oxide, prostaglandin, and kinins. Increases in glomerular flow rate (GFR) reflect increased renal blood flow as well as perfusion of less mature cortical glomeruli. The rate of increase in GFR depends on the gestational age. When it is corrected to match the body surface area,

children reach adult measurements by one year of age (Table 31-1).

Renal blood flow requires appropriate intravascular volume, directed by adequate cardiac output to the systemic circulation, with oxygenated blood. When renal arterial systolic pressures are within an appropriate range (for patient age), glomerular blood flow remains constant. Autoregulation occurs by multiple mechanisms. For example, the myogenic reflex occurs at the afferent renal arteriole in response to stretch. Under the control of an intact smooth-muscle layer, a constant intraglomerular blood flow is maintained when intravascular volume is within appropriate range.

Tubuloglomerular feedback requires an intact juxtaglomerular apparatus (JGA), a collection of epithelial cells within the distal convoluted tubule that is in contact with the afferent and efferent arterioles, which enables the JGA to sense the concentration of sodium ions (Na^+) in the ultrafiltrate (Figure 31-1). Decreases in sodium content stimulate renin secretion, thereby increasing total body sodium and intravascular volume. Renin is converted to angiotensin II (a potent vasoconstrictor) in the lung and to aldosterone (a mineralocorticoid) in the adrenal gland.

TABLE 31-1

Measured Glomerular Filtration Rate	
Age	**Mean GFR (mL/min/1.73 m²)**
Preterm Infants	
1–7 days	18.7 ± 5.5
8–14 days	35.4 ± 13.4
6–24 weeks	67.4 ± 16.6
Term Infants	
1–3 days	20.8 ± 5
4–14 days	36.8 ± 7.2
15–19 days	46.9 ± 12.5
1–3 months	85.3 ± 35.1
4–6 months	87.4 ± 22.3
7–12 months	96.2 ± 12.2
1–2 years	105.2 ± 17.3
Children	
3–4 years	111.2 ± 18.5
9–10 years	110 ± 21.6
16–34 years	112 ± 13

Source: Adapted from Schwartz & Furth, 2007. Courtesy of Dr. George Schwartz.

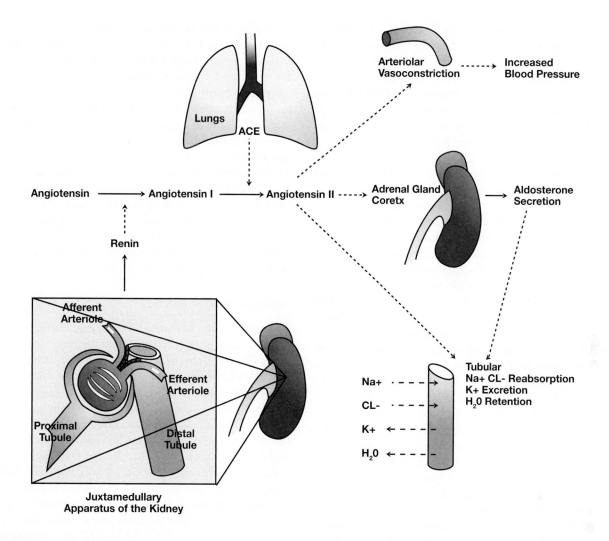

FIGURE 31-1

Juxtamedullary Apparatus of the Kidney.

Source: Courtesy of Mary Puchalski, NNP.

The JGA is also stimulated by via dopaminergic and sympathetic (α_1) pathways, resulting in a renin-mediated vasoconstriction of efferent arterioles, which in turn increases intraglomerular pressure and GFR.

Adequate perfusion of the glomeruli results from net intravascular pressures between the afferent and efferent arterioles. Maximally dilated afferent arterioles will promote blood flow; however, optimal pressure also requires elevated efferent arteriolar pressure, via angiotensin-mediated vasoconstriction. Prostaglandin inhibitor therapy (e.g., nonsteroidal anti-inflammatory drugs [NSAIDs]) for medical closure of patent ductus arteriosus frequently results in acute kidney failure due to inhibition of afferent arteriolar vasodilatation. Likewise, angiotensin-converting enzyme (ACE) inhibitors and angiotensin II receptor blockers affect intraglomerular pressure by decreasing efferent arteriolar tone. Use of these agents prior to delivery or during the neonatal period has been associated with acute kidney failure (Dutta & Narang, 2003; Sedman et al., 1995).

Glomerular flow rate. Kidney function is reflected by the patient's glomerular flow rate. Measuring clearance of inulin—a substance freely filtered at the glomerulus (without extrarenal excretion or tubular reuptake or secretion)—is the study of choice for assessing the GFR. This tedious process requires a steady state of serum inulin (by intravenous infusion) and accurate urine collection. For small children accurate urine collection can be difficult to obtain. Consequently. For these children, or for those individuals with bladder dysfunction, urinary catheterization may be required. Other methods to measure GFR include use of isotopes (DTPA, EDTA), which are injected intravenously and filtered by the kidney, with subsequent uptake and excretion monitored by nuclear imaging. GFR is calculated by a subtraction technique, as decreased isotope in kidney parenchyma is measured over time.

A more practical approach is to estimate GFR (eGFR) by use of serum creatinine. This substance is derived from skeletal muscle creatine, and converted into creatinine in the liver. It is freely filtered at the glomerulus and secreted by proximal tubular epithelium into the urine. Children with low muscle mass should appropriately have low measurements of serum creatinine, irrespective of age. Serum creatinine is elevated at birth, however, initially reflecting an equilibrium between maternal and fetal serum concentrations of creatinine. As renal blood flow and GFR increases, maturation of tubule function, which limits backlead of creatinine, results in decreased values of serum creatinine. Moreover, both the degree of prematurity (Table 31-1) and the birth weight affect the rate at which serum creatinine decreases. Notably, serum creatinine may be slow to reflect acute kidney injury in part due to low muscle mass. Normal serum creatinine for a full-term infant is in the range of 0.2 to 0.4 mg/dL at 1 month of age. Likewise, use of serum creatinine in children with chronic kidney disease may lead to overestimation of eGFR due to the relatively increased excretion of creatinine by tubular secretion.

In 1976, Schwartz and colleagues established an equation to estimate GFR using serum creatinine, patient height, and a constant:

$$\text{eGFR mL/min/1.73 m}^2 = (k)(\text{height})/\text{serum creatinine}$$

The constant k varies according to age and gender, with a value of 0.45 corresponding to term infants until 12 months of age, 0.55 for children and adolescent females, and 0.7 for adolescent males 12 to 17 years of age. Height is measured in centimeters and serum creatinine in mg/dL.

Since 2008, many clinical laboratories have abandoned the Jaffe reaction (a colorimetric reaction using sodium picrate upon which the Schwartz equation was based) to measure serum creatinine, and now use an isotope dilution method that results in improved specificity in measuring serum creatinine. Consequently, the Schwartz equation (using this newer method) was modified to use a k value of 0.413 for all ages and genders (Schwartz et al., 2009). Healthcare professionals (HCPs) should consult their hospital laboratory to determine which equation is appropriate for their patient population.

Another method, based on serum concentration of cystatin C (a proteinase inhibitor produced by nucleated cells), has been shown to measure GFR with accuracy superior to that of serum creatinine in children (Andersen et al., 2009). Cystatin C is freely filtered by the glomerulus and resorbed by proximal tubular epithelium. Serum levels are unaffected by patient anthropomorphics and inflammation. Cystatin C has the advantage of providing eGFR for populations who are unable to rely on serum creatinine (e.g., patients with hepatic failure, spina bifida, or malnutrition) and may detect kidney injury with increased sensitivity following chemotherapy (Zaffanello et al., 2007). At the current time, there is no universally accepted single cystatin C–based equation; published formulas are derived from linear regression analysis of measured GFR calculated by the clearance of a freely filterable exogenous marker (i.e., iohexol, iothalamate) for various patient populations (Bokenkamp et al., 1998; Grubb et al., 2005; Schwartz et al., 2009; Zappitelli et al., 2006).

Assessing tubular function

The glomerular basement membrane restricts passage of cells, large proteins (larger than 50 nm), and charged molecules from the bloodstream into the urinary space. Electrolytes, small proteins (albumin, immunoglobulin), and water are resorbed by the tubular epithelium and reenter the circulation—a process critical to maintain homeostasis.

Resorption of electrolytes predominantly occurs within the proximal convoluted tubules, using a sodium concentration gradient established by the epithelial sodium–potassium ATPase to maintain a low intracellular sodium concentration. Cotransporters for sodium and amino acids, phosphate, glucose, calcium, and potassium are unique to this part of the nephron. Transport of potassium in the ascending loop of Henle via the Na^+-K^+-$2Cl^-$ cotransporter requires return of potassium back into the lumen (by the renal outer medullary potassium channel [ROMK]), so as to permit further sodium chloride (NaCl) reuptake in the presence of potassium and to generate a positive voltage to drive calcium and magnesium into the interstitium. Calcium enters the medulla by a nonspecific paracellular mechanism, whereas magnesium enters by its novel paracellin channel.

Within the distal convoluted tubules, sodium is actively reclaimed via the epithelial sodium channel (ENaC), with its expression being controlled by aldosterone. The voltage gradient established by sodium uptake results in excretion of potassium ions via ROMK in the cortical collecting ducts and hydrogen ions via hydrogen ATPase.

Tubular function is determined by comparing the rate of excretion of an electrolyte with age-specific norms. The fractional excretion of an electrolyte requires simultaneous measurement in serum and urine, along with measurement of creatinine, to evaluate tubular function in the context of GFR.

Fractional excretion of sodium. The normal response of the JGA to decreased renal blood flow is renin secretion, so as to maximize total body water by increasing tubular reuptake of sodium. However, decreased glomerular function with serum chemistries showing an increase in blood urea nitrogen (BUN) and creatinine may also reflect parenchymal injury. To determine if kidney dysfunction is simply due to decreased renal blood flow, the fractional excretion of sodium (FeNa) is measured. In patients without a history of chronic kidney disease, the fractional excretion of sodium is less than 1% (in premature neonates, it can be as low as 4% at 28 weeks' gestational age) (Al-Dahhan et al., 1983). Fractional excretion greater than these values in an azotemic child is consistent with tubular damage; sequelae of prolonged decreased renal blood flow (i.e., acute tubular necrosis), primary intrinsic renal disease, or obstruction preventing urine output are some common etiologies of such abnormalities.

Expression of cotransporters, channels, and Na⁺-K⁺-ATPase is a developmental process. Consequently, the FeNa level is highest in premature infants, as high as 3% in full-term neonates (Trachtman, 2004), and less than 1% in infants by 2 months of age (Al-Dahhan et al., 1983). Reflecting these differences, formula for premature infants contains higher concentrations of sodium compared to formula for term infants, so as to prevent a net negative sodium balance and promote normal growth. FeNa can be used to assess the etiology of hyponatremia in this age group, to determine if infants have renal wasting of sodium, or to determine if they are not producing a maximally dilute urine (using urine and serum osmoles). Renal wasting of sodium may be due to pseudohypoaldosteronism following chronic tubular injury (e.g., bilateral hydronephrosis), true hypoaldosteronism (e.g., congenital adrenal hyperplasia), or excessive diuretic use.

Transtubular potassium gradient. Potassium is essential for cellular function, and maintenance of the proper levels requires an appropriate concentration gradient between the intracellular and extracellular compartments. Na-K-ATPase is primarily responsible for maintaining a high intracellular concentration of potassium; insulin and catecholamines direct potassium into the cell to a lesser degree. Movement of potassium is also influenced by changes in acid–base balance. Acidosis increases serum potassium, as hydrogen ions displace potassium ions from the intracellular compartment, and alkalosis is associated with decreases in serum potassium with reversed cation movement.

Urinary concentration requires a highly osmolar medullary interstitium, resulting from potassium accrual. Unlike most electrolytes, potassium is actively eliminated by the kidney at the distal nephron. This process requires aldosterone-directed function of the Na⁺-K⁺-ATPase to increase the intracellular potassium concentration, adequate delivery of sodium to the open epithelial sodium channel (ENaC), a voltage gradient established by sufficient sodium uptake, and transtubular passage of potassium through its channel into the lumen.

The transtubular potassium gradient (TTKG) is a calculated value, reflecting tubular secretion of potassium:

$$TTKG = \frac{\text{Urine potassium} \times \text{serum osm}}{\text{Serum potassium} \times \text{urine osm}}$$

Under hyperkalemic conditions, aldosterone is secreted and potassium is eliminated by the kidney. Simulataneous measurement of potassium and osmoles from serum and urine is required to determine the TTKG, because antidiuretic hormone (ADH)–mediated resorption of water affects the final concentration of potassium in urine.

Neonates do not excrete potassium as efficiently as older children, reflecting immaturity of Na⁺-K⁺-ATPase activity and poor sodium resorption distally. Lower TTKG ranges (2.5–5) have been documented among premature infants of less than 30 weeks' gestational age, with TTKG ranges increasing (8–14) at 3 weeks of age (more than 30 weeks' gestation) and in full-term infants (Nako et al., 1999). A TTKG of less than 5 in infants and less than 4 in children, under hyperkalemic conditions, indicates hypoaldosteronism or tubular dysfunction (pseudohypoaldosteronism) (Choi & Ziyadeh, 2008). The TTKG naturally decreases with age as the kidney gains a hypertonic medullary interstitium and the ability to produce concentrated urine.

Tubular reuptake of potassium occurs in the proximal tubules and thick ascending loops of Henle. Hypokalemia can result from deficient transporter activity or excessive distal secretion under aldosterone control. Maintaining the appropriate potassium balance requires adequate dietary intake without gastrointestinal losses. Intracellular movement of potassium due to metabolic alkalosis, insulin, or catecholamines commonly occurs in the pediatric patient. To determine if hypokalemia is due to kidney disease, the fractional excretion of potassium (FeK) is measured. The kidney is less able to reclaim potassium compared to other electrolytes; maximal reuptake of potassium is 10% to 15% under hypokalemic conditions.

Fractional excretion of magnesium. Reuptake of filtered magnesium (FeMg) requires intact paracellular uptake via its channel, paracellin-1, found within the thick ascending loop of Henle. Efficient magnesium movement into the medullary interstitium relies on a voltage gradient established by resorption of sodium chloride. Active reuptake occurs in the collecting ducts, possibly using a Na/Mg exchanger. As a consequence of this mechanism, medications associated with magnesium wasting are associated with natriuresis and general tubular epithelial cell damage—namely, loop and thiazide diuretics, calcineurin inhibitors, cisplatin, ifosfamide, amphotericin B, and aminoglycosides. Transient wasting of magnesium can occur following recovery from acute kidney injury. In addition, hypomagnesemia has been associated with hypokalemia due to kaliuresis.

Hypomagnesemia is associated with hypocalcemia, as magnesium is a cofactor required for parathyroid hormone secretion. Symptoms include tetany, seizure, and ventricular arrhythmia (i.e., premature ventricular complexes). Hypomagnesemia without hypocalcemia may result in muscle spasm due to a lowered threshold for nerve stimulation. Normal serum magnesium is greater than 2 mg/dL; hypoparathyroidism due to hypomagnesemia usually occurs when the serum level falls to less than 1 mg/dL (Agus, 1999).

Given that renal excretion of magnesium depends on the balance between dietary intake and gastrointestinal output, a 24-hour urine collection is required to assess tubular function. Approximately 30% of magnesium is bound to albumin and, therefore, is not filtered at the glomerulus. Calculating the FeMg value requires that the serum magnesium concentration be multiplied by 0.7:

$$FeMg = \frac{Urine\ magnesium \times Serum\ creatinine}{0.7 \times Serum\ magnesium \times Urine\ creatinine}$$

Under conditions of hypomagnesemia due to extrarenal losses, the fractional excretion of magnesium should be less than 2%.

Tubular reuptake of phosphate. Eighty percent of the filtered phosphate load is reabsorbed by the sodium–phosphate cotransporter (NPT) located in the apical brush border of the proximal convoluted tubules. Although three types of NPT have been identified, NPT2a is responsible for reclaiming the majority of filtered inorganic phosphate. Thus the efficacy of phosphate reuptake is dictated by the amount of NPT2a cotransporters present on the apical brush border of the proximal convoluted tubules. The body maintains an intracellular pool of NPT, and hypophosphatemia results in migration of these transporters to the cell surface. Counteracting this effect are parathyroid hormone (PTH) and FGF23, a phosphaturic factor under the control of the *PHEX* gene. Binding of PTH to its receptor stimulates endocytosis of NPT. FGF23 also promotes endocytosis of NPT.

Hypophosphatemia can result from transcellular shifts, poor dietary intake, and gastrointestinal or renal losses. Chronic renal losses of phosphate result in abnormal mineralization of bone (e.g., rickets) and hypophosphatemia. Normal serum phosphorus levels in neonates younger than 5 years of age are higher than those in older children and adults (5–7 mg/dL versus 3–5 mg/dL, respectively) due to decreased GFR and response to filtered PTH (to downregulate NPT). Under hypophosphatemic conditions, reuptake of phosphate occurs at a level greater than 95%. The tubular reuptake may be calculated using serum and urine phosphate and creatinine levels:

Tubular reuptake = 1 − (Urine phosphate × Serum creatinine/Serum phosphate × Urine creatinine) × 100

This expression may be used to determine the percentage of filtered phosphate that is resorbed by the proximal convoluted tubules.

Diseases characterized by hypophosphatemic rickets include the following three conditions: (1) X-linked hypophosphatemia, in which *PHEX* gene mutation results in unregulated FGF23 activity; (2) autosomal dominant hypophosphatemic rickets, associated with decreased degradation of FGF23; and (3) oncogenic osteomalacia, a rare finding associated with benign, vascular mesenchymal tumors or metastatic prostate cancer, secondary to paraneoplastic products of FGF and other phosphaturic factors.

DIAGNOSTICS

Hydronephrosis can result from either obstruction of urine flow or reflux of urine from the bladder into the kidney. Ultrasonography is the test of choice to diagnose hydronephrosis, which requires the evaluation of the renal calyces, pelvis, ureter, and bladder for dilatation; evidence of duplication of the collecting system; and diverticula. Abnormalities of the renal parenchyma, including cyst formation, echogenicity, loss of corticomedullary differentiation, and thinning of the cortex, can also be detected via this modality; such abnormalities may reflect either kidney injury or congenitally acquired disease.

Voiding cystourethrography (VCUG) involves placement of a bladder catheter and instillation of either contrast or radionuclide. Both tracers allow the diagnosis of reflux, but contrast allows assessment of the urethra, bladder, and ureters for anatomical abnormalities.

Obstruction of urine flow between the kidney and ureterovesicular junction can be assessed by diuretic renogram, a nuclear medicine study that uses either DTPA or MAG3 as the radiotracer. A small amount of tracer is injected intravenously, and radioactivity within the kidneys due to tracer uptake is measured. A dose of furosemide is provided, and radioactivity is measured within the kidneys at 3-minute intervals. If no obstruction of urine flow is present, a rapid diuresis occurs with a decrease in detected counts within the renal parenchyma. If obstruction exists, the curve generated by plotting time on the *x*-axis and counts on the *y*-axis shows a plateau instead of a rapid downward slope. Generally, a nonobstructive pattern shows a *t* ½ of less than 10 minutes, whereas an obstructive pattern results in a *t* ½ of more than 30 minutes. The glomerular filtration rate and renal blood flow can also be quantified using this technique.

Finally, for evaluation of parenchymal scarring, DMSA—an isotope that is freely filtered and resorbed by the renal tubules—is administered intravenously. Poor uptake of DMSA reflects tubular damage. Evaluation should occur at least 6 months following acute kidney injury (i.e., pyelonephritis), as regeneration and recovery of epithelial cell function is a slow process.

ACUTE DISORDERS OF THE MALE GENITALIA

Jane E. Kramer

BALANITIS

Pathophysiology

Inflammation of the glans penis, foreskin (prepuce), or both is referred to as balanitis, posthitis, or balanoposthitis, respectively. Irritants or trauma may induce swelling, erythema, or tenderness and provide a portal for infectious organisms.

Epidemiology and etiology

The peak incidence of balanitis and balanoposthitis is in early childhood, between the ages of 2 and 5 years (Schwartz & Rushton, 1996). Incidence varies depending on age and inclusion criteria, but generally ranges from 1.5% to 5.9%. Inattention to hygiene of the foreskin is the most common cause in childhood. Ammoniacal diaper dermatitis may be the cause of balanitis or balanoposthitis in infants. Other presumptive irritants include soaps, detergents, bubble baths, or clothing. *Staphylococcus*, coliforms, *Pseudomonas,* and *Candida* have been cultured form children with these conditions, but are typically not causative. Group A *Streptococcus* has been determined to be a potential pathogen (Leslie & Cain, 2006). Trauma (including masturbation or sexual abuse) may be implicated. Although controversial, phimosis may be a risk factor.

Presentation

Typical symptoms include crying or irritability in infants, and dysuria, itching, or pain in older children. Inability to void is very rare. Parents should be asked about circumcision, bathing routines, irritant exposure, urethral drainage, and previous episodes. Presence of a urethral discharge or signs of trauma should raise the possibility of sexual abuse. Teens with balanitis should be asked about sexual practices and the use of condoms as a potential irritant.

On examination, tenderness, redness, and swelling of the glans and/or foreskin are typically noted. Preputial exudates may be present. The presence of urethral discharge, assessed by milking the length of the urethra in a proximal-to-distal direction, is concerning for a sexually transmitted infection (STI). Streptococcal balanitis presents with a fiery red surface and a thin purulent exudate from under the foreskin. Phimosis, or a partially nonretractile foreskin, may be present in any patient with balanoposthitis.

Differential diagnosis

Paraphimosis, hair tourniquet, and insect bites may also present with a swollen, erythematous penis. STIs usually present as a urethral discharge or epididymitis. A rare condition in older children is balanitis xerotica obliterans, also referred to as lichen sclerosus et atrophicus of the glans penis, which presents as white atrophic plaques on the glans and foreskin.

Plan of care

Discharge from the urethra should be cultured for STIs or a nucleic acid amplification test (NAAT) should be performed. The latter may be obtained from urine or a urethral swab. If infection with group A *Streptococcus* is suspected, a culture of the exudate should be sent for identification.

Sitz baths and gentle cleaning of the foreskin and glans are the mainstays of therapy. If an irritant etiology is suspected, application of a 0.5% to 1% hydrocortisone cream twice daily is suggested. Some authors recommend irrigation by medical personnel using a small angiocatheter if there is pain or difficulty retracting the foreskin (Huang, 2009). If these measures are not effective, oral antibiotics to cover skin flora may be prescribed (Leslie & Cain, 2006). Although this approach and the use of topical antimicrobials are not evidence-based treatments, they are widely quoted in the literature. Streptococcal infection is treated with 10 days of oral therapy. If an STI is suspected, empiric therapy with intramuscular ceftriaxone 125 mg and oral azithromycin 1 gm may be used.

Referral to the urologist for circumcision is indicated for patients with recurrent episodes of balanitis or balanoposthitis or if true phimosis develops. Patients and caregivers should be informed that dysuria may be mitigated by voiding in a tub of warm water. Parents should also be advised to avoid forceful retraction of the foreskin in infants and young boys. Once the foreskin is retractable, gentle cleaning with water may be performed daily.

Disposition and discharge planning

Most cases of balanitis resolve completely with treatment. After resolution of the acute inflammation, the patient should be followed up by urology. Follow-up examination assesses for phimosis and any post-inflammatory scarring. Reinforcement of proper hygiene is important to prevent recurrences. Soaps, powders, and other potential irritants should be avoided.

EPIDIDYMITIS

Jane E. Kramer

Pathophysiology

Epididymitis is an inflammation or infection of the epididymis, often caused by ascending urinary tract or sexually transmitted organisms. Occasionally, systemic inflammatory conditions or viral infections are implicated. Other contributing factors include straining or lifting, which can lead to reflux of urine into the ejaculatory duct and vas deferens into the epididymis. Swelling, tenderness, and erythema of the hemiscrotum ensue. *Perhaps the most important feature of this condition is the need to distinguish it from testicular torsion to assure salvage of the testis.*

Epidemiology and etiology

Most cases involve sexually active adolescents, with *Chlamydia trachomatis* and *Neisseria gonorrhoea* being the most common pathogens. In younger children, ascending urinary tract infections with organisms such as *Escherichia coli* and other Gram-negative pathogens can involve the epididymis. Risk factors include genitourinary tract malformations, neurogenic bladder, or recent urethral instrumentation or catheterization. Systemic diseases such as Henoch-Schönlein purpura (HSP) or Kawasaki disease, trauma, and medications (amiodarone) may also cause epididymitis.

Once thought to be uncommon in prepubertal boys, a prospective study in Israel revealed an incidence of 1.2 patients per 1,000 boys annually (Somekh et al., 2004). A growing body of evidence supports a postinfectious etiology for epididymitis, traceable to bacterial or viral pathogens. Multiple studies have shown most prepubescent boys with epididymitis do not have pyuria or positive urine cultures and, that their condition resolves without antibiotic treatment (Trainor, 2009). Elevated titers to *Mycoplasma pneumoniae*, enterovirus, and adenovirus have been documented (Somekh et al.).

Presentation

The patient with epididymitis presents with acute scrotal pain. Historical features may also include dysuria, fever, and incontinence. Adolescents should be queried about their sexual activity. Unilateral scrotal pain and swelling increase over 1 to 2 days. Fever is not uncommon, and penile discharge may be present in patients with STIs. Physical examination of the genitalia reveals inflammation of the hemiscrotum. Early in the infection, the epididymis may be palpable and tender, but when inflammation spreads to the testis and scrotal wall, this becomes indistinguishable. A well-known finding, Prehn's sign (elevation of the scrotum relieves pain of epididymitis, but not of testicular torsion) is not reliable in children. The cremasteric reflex is preserved in epididymitis.

Differential diagnosis

Children presenting with acute scrotal pain should be considered potential surgical emergencies. It is crucial to differentiate epididymitis from torsion of the testicle, which can have a similar, although usually more acute, presentation. Delay of more than 6 hours in the diagnosis of torsion predicts a decreased salvage rate for the testicle. Also in the differential diagnosis for the acute scrotum are torsion of the appendix testicle, incarcerated inguinal hernia, varicocoele, tumor, orchitis, and trauma. Thus epididymitis is a diagnosis of exclusion.

Plan of care

Doppler ultrasound is the study of choice for evaluating acute scrotal pain. In epididymitis, blood flow to the testicle and epididymis are increased when compared to the contralateral side. Radionuclide scanning is an alternative imaging modality. Urinalysis and urine culture should be obtained; pyuria and bacteruria are both suggestive of epididymitis. If sexual activity or abuse are suspected, a urethral culture or a NAAT should be performed by urine specimen or a urethral swab.

Rest and scrotal support are recommended. Acetaminophen or ibuprofen is indicated to treat fever and/or provide analgesia. Use of antibiotics is not universal in children with epididymitis. If the history, physical examination, or urinalysis suggests a urinary tract infection, antimicrobial therapy covering coliform organisms, such as trimethoprim–sulfamethoxasole or a cephalosporin should be administered. Patients may need imaging studies to rule out an anatomic or neurologic abnormality causing the urinary tract infection. Some studies suggest that a well-appearing prepubescent boy may be observed, without antibiotics, pending a urine culture result. If an STI is suspected, the recommended treatment regimen is a single 250-mg dose of ceftriaxone intramuscularly plus doxycycline 100 mg orally twice daily for 10 days. A fluoroquinolone antibiotic is a viable alternative.

History and physical examination may not provide a definitive diagnosis of epididymitis. Imaging is also not 100% sensitive or specific. Urologic consultation should be sought if the history and physical examination findings are worrisome, even in the face of preserved flow on ultrasound. The possible causes of acute scrotal pain should be discussed with the patient or family. Ruling out torsion is crucial.

Disposition and discharge planning

Epididymitis is managed on an outpatient basis. Failure of symptoms to resolve within 3 days should prompt reevaluation and may require hospitalization of the child. Patients and their families should be informed of the various causes of this condition and the need for rest, pain management, and, in some cases, antibiotics. The prognosis for complete recovery is excellent and a follow-up visit with the primary care provider (PCP) or the urologist should be arranged.

PHIMOSIS

Jane E. Kramer

Pathophysiology

Inability to retract the foreskin over the head of the penis is referred to as phimosis. The foreskin is naturally adherent to the glans at the time of birth and cannot be retracted, a condition referred to as "physiologic phimosis." By the time they reach 3 years of age, 90% of males can retract the foreskin; this percentage increases yearly. Phimosis in later childhood may be either physiologic or pathologic as a result of inflammation and scarring of the foreskin.

Epidemiology and etiology

Recurrent episodes of balanoposthitis are the most common causes of pathologic phimosis. Forceful retraction of the foreskin and, rarely, a chronic dermatitis known as balanitis xerotica obliterans (BXO) are other potential causes. Problems and questions about the foreskin are common in pediatric practice.

Presentation

During physical examination, the HCP is unable to retract the foreskin. The attempt is typically painless. Epithelial "pearls" are sometimes visualized under the foreskin and do not require intervention.

Differential diagnosis

Penile adhesions may be confused with phimosis. If the foreskin is retracted behind the glans and left in that position, paraphimosis may result. In this condition, venous congestion and edema of the retracted foreskin cause pain and make it difficult to return the foreskin to its normal position. *Paraphimosis is a urologic emergency.*

Plan of care

Topical application of a mid- to high-potency corticosteroid cream (e.g., clobetasone butyrate 0.05% or betamethasone 0.05%) to the foreskin twice daily for 4 to 8 weeks has been shown in a number of studies to loosen the phimotic ring in as many as 85% of patients (Palmer & Palmer, 2008; Yang et al., 2005). The most appropriate age for use of this treatment is controversial, but it is often administered after age 3 years. Participation by the caregiver for its application will enhance efficacy.

Referral for surgical management with circumcision or a dorsal slit procedure is reserved for phimosis that is unresponsive to steroid application, voiding problems, or BXO. Good hygiene of the uncircumcised penis should be emphasized, along with the natural history of the foreskin, in which it begins to retract with time.

Disposition and discharge planning

Most cases of physiologic phimosis resolve with time, and urologic referral is not indicated. Follow-up with the PCP should be scheduled after a steroid trial. If symptoms persist, then a urology consult is warranted. Patients should seek medical attention if the phimosis obstructs urination or signs of infection such as of the urinary tract or skin are suspected.

PRIAPISM

Jane E. Kramer

Pathophysiology

Priapism is a pathologic condition of sustained, painful penile erection unassociated with sexual excitation. The corpora cavernosa become engorged, which creates a swollen and edematous shaft, and produces pain. In sickle cell disease, erythrocyte sickling, subsequent vascular sludging, and stasis in the erectile tissue of the corporal bodies lead to priapism. Ischemia ensues and may incite an inflammatory response leading to fibrosis and potentially to impotence.

Epidemiology and etiology

Many definitions of priapism include a duration of 4 hours, but this finding is not necessary for diagnosis. The most common cause in children is sickle cell anemia. Sickling in the corporal bodies may occur without symptomatic sickling in other organs. As many as 27.5% of male children with sickle cell disease develop priapism, which usually has its onset during sleep (Mantadakis et al., 1999). Priapism has been described as early as 3 years of age, and its frequency increases with age. Trauma, spinal cord injury, and leukemic infiltration of the penis are other etiologies in children, as is sildenafil ingestion (Wills et al., 2007). Recreational use of erectile dysfunction drugs, cocaine, marijuana, and ecstasy abuse have also been described as causes.

Presentation

Important historical features include sickle cell disease, trauma, or medication exposure. Information regarding the duration of the erection and prior episodes and their treatment should also be sought. The child presents with a painful erection of variable duration. Inspection reveals the extent of tumescence or rigidity and tenderness. Embarrassment may delay the presentation of prepubescent or pubescent males.

Differential diagnosis

An unwanted, painful erection lasting 30 minutes or more is diagnostic for priapism.

Plan of care

A complete blood count (CBC) should be obtained, and a hemoglobin electrophoresis if the sickle cell status is unknown. Warm sitz baths and pain medications may be used early in the episode. When the patient presents for acute care, he should be kept on nothing-by-mouth (NPO) status in case conscious sedation should be required. Intravenous hydration should be started, along with parenteral administration of analgesia such as morphine. A recent review of priapism in sickle cell disease suggests an oral dose of pseudoephedrine or phenylephrine may be considered (Rogers, 2005). If the episode is approaching or has lasted more than 4 hours, aspiration of blood from the corpora, and irrigation with saline, or more commonly, a dilute adrenergic solution (phenylephrine or epinephrine) is required. This procedure should be performed under local anesthesia and/or conscious sedation. When these measures fail to produce detumescence, surgical management in the form of a shunt is required. Other treatment approaches for the patient with sickle cell disease include red cell transfusion (not well supported in the literature), and exchange blood transfusion (which has been associated with central nervous system complications including stroke when used for this purpose).

Urgent urologic consultation is needed if the duration of the erection is approaching or exceeds 4 hours. Consultation with a pediatric hematologist for the patient with sickle cell disease is recommended. Patients and caregivers should be educated about priapism and the current treatment options. They should be advised of the possibility of recurrence, especially if the patient has sickle cell disease, and instructed to present for care within 4 hours during a prolonged episode.

Disposition and discharge planning

Children and adolescents with priapism are admitted to the hospital for treatment of the condition and the underlying etiology. Follow-up with the PCP or pediatric hematologist and with a urologist should be scheduled as needed.

The prognosis is extremely good unless prolonged episodes lead to devastating consequences of erectile dysfunction. Although controlled trials of these modalities are lacking, the use of hydroxyurea or chronic transfusion may be considered for prevention in a child or adolescent with sickle cell disease experiencing repeated episodes of priapism.

TESTICULAR TORSION

Anita Lall Kewalramani

Pathophysiology

Testicular torsion is caused by twisting of the spermatic cord, leading to obstruction of testicular blood flow and eventually testicular ischemia. The degree of ischemia depends on both the number of twists and the amount of time the torsion has been present. In general, there is a 4- to 8-hour window before irreversible injury to the testicle occurs (Bellinger, 2002; Gatti & Murphy, 2008). Testicular torsion is a *true* surgical emergency (Gatti & Murphy).

Two main types of testicular torsion are distinguished: extravaginal (antenatal) testicular torsion and intravaginal testicular torsion. Extravaginal torsion is torsion of the entire scrotal contents. It occurs perinatally during the descent of the testis, allowing the tunica and testis to spin on their vascular pedicles. Extravaginal torsion usually presents at birth with a firm, nontender mass high in the scrotum (Bellinger, 2002; Gatti & Murphy, 2008). If a scrotal mass is present at birth, surgical exploration of the contralateral testis should occur to ensure that a "bell-clapper" deformity is not present, which would predispose the solitary testis to torsion later in life.

Intravaginal torsion may occur at any age. In most cases, it is caused by a congenital malformation of the processus vaginalis, where the tunica vaginalis covers the testicle, epididymis, and spermatic cord (Ringdahl & Teauge, 2006). This malformation, which is known as the "bell-clapper" deformity, results in abnormal fixation; the testicle and the epididymis hang freely in the scrotum, allowing them to twist within the tunica vaginalis. The bell-clapper deformity is usually bilateral (Gatti & Murphy, 2008).

Epidemiology and etiology

Testicular torsion occurs in approximately 1 in 4,000 males younger than the age of 25 years. Of these cases, 90% are due to intravaginal torsion (Ringdahl & Teague, 2006). While testicular torsion can occur at any age, it is most common in adolescence (Chan et al., 2009).

The cause of testicular torsion is usually unknown, and it typically occurs without any precipitating events. Possible predisposing factors include trauma, testicular tumor, testicles with horizontal lie, a history of cryptorchidism, and increasing testicular volume (Ringdahl & Teauge, 2006). Rapid growth and increasing vascularity of the testicle occurs during puberty, and is believed to be the reason for increasing incidence of testicular torsion in adolescents (Gatti & Murphy, 2008).

Presentation

The classic presentation of testicular torsion is the sudden onset of severe unilateral testicular pain, usually with swelling of the scrotum. Many patients will also have lower abdominal pain, nausea, and vomiting. Boys with testicular torsion rarely complain of dysuria. The pain of testicular torsion is usually unrelenting (Gatti & Murphy, 2008).

A complete physical examination should be performed, including assessment of the abdomen, inguinal area, and scrotum. Physical examination findings for testicular torsion include absence of the cremasteric reflex, affected testicle higher in the scrotum, varying location of the epididymis, or transverse lie of the testicle (Gatti & Murphy, 2008; Ringdahl & Teague, 2006). Due to the venous congestion of testicular torsion, the affected testicle may appear larger than the contralateral one (Ringdahl & Teague).

Differential diagnosis

The differential diagnosis for an acutely painful and swollen scrotum includes testicular torsion, torsion of the appendix testis, epididymitis, orchitis, hernia, or trauma. It is very difficult to differentiate testicular torsion from torsion of the appendix testis, epididymitis, or orchitis based on history alone; performing a thorough physical examination is a vital component of the diagnostic process (Ringdahl & Teauge, 2006). A history of scrotal trauma can also mask the diagnosis of testicular torsion. Severe pain lasting for more than an hour after the traumatic incident should be fully evaluated for torsion (Ringdahl & Teauge).

Plan of care

Diagnosis of testicular torsion is based on history, physical examination, and diagnostic studies. Laboratory studies are typically performed only when the diagnosis is in question. Urinalysis is typically unremarkable; a CBC with differential may demonstrate an elevated white blood cell count (but is nonspecific); C-reactive protein (CRP) may be elevated as an acute-phase reactant. If the diagnosis of testicular torsion is questionable, color Doppler ultrasound should be performed. In patients with testicular torsion, the affected testis will have decreased or absent blood flow as compared to the contralateral side. The torsed testis will also appear enlarged on ultrasound (Gatti & Murphy, 2008; Ringdahl & Teague, 2006).

When the history and physical findings are consistent with testicular torsion, and pain has been present for less than 6 hours, no further diagnostic studies are needed; surgical exploration should begin immediately (Ringdahl & Teague, 2006). Manual detorsion may be attempted (in a medial-to-lateral rotation) prior to surgery. This procedure is performed in an attempt to decrease the degree of ischemia to the affected testicle (Gatti & Murphy, 2008). The goal of surgery is to salvage the testicle. If the testicle cannot be salvaged, the testicle is resected by performing an orchiectomy. In contrast, if the testicle is detorsed successfully, then an orchiopexy is performed by suturing the testicle within the scrotum so that it may no longer twist. During surgical exploration, the contralateral testis is also fixed to the scrotal wall with nonabsorbable suture, to prevent future torsion.

Intravenous fluids and NPO status should begin immediately to prepare the patient for the operating room. Preoperative antibiotics may be administered, with the urologist/surgeon determining the postoperative need for continued antimicrobial therapy. To treat their pain, patients may receive analgesia preoperatively and postoperatively; and for nausea they may receive antiemetics. Postoperative recovery care involves following hemodynamics, pain management, and wound care.

Consultation with urology or general surgery upon patient presentation will facilitate prompt diagnosis and treatment. Patient and family education involves discussion of the emergent operative plan and possible loss of the testicle. Patients may benefit from child life involvement and social/spiritual support.

Disposition and discharge planning

Postoperative follow-up should be scheduled with the urologist or general surgeon within 1 week of discharge. Patients may be placed on restricted activity until cleared by the surgeon for a return to normal activity. Patients who had excision of a nonviable testicle may be scheduled 6 months from date of surgery for implantation of a prosthetic testicle.

The prognosis for testicular torsion is very good if there is no excessive delay in seeking treatment. Studies have shown that if exploration is performed within 4 to 6 hours of symptom onset, salvage rates may approach 90%;

however, these rates drop dramatically to 50% at 12 hours after symptom onset and to almost 10% after 24 hours (Davenport, 1996).

DIALYSIS AND RENAL REPLACEMENT THERAPY

Sara Jandeska

Dialysis—a medical procedure designed to substitute native kidney function—is used acutely in the pediatric intensive care unit. Dialysis involves the removal of electrolytes, toxins, and free water using the bloodstream or peritoneal cavity (a potential space). This process uses both diffusion and convection to remove solutes and water by interfacing the patient's blood with a dialysis solution. A semipermeable membrane separates these two compartments. Maximal flow of solutes across this membrane requires sufficient surface area for molecular transport. In hemodialysis, blood is circulated through a filter consisting of hundreds of porous lumens that are bathed in dialysis fluid. Peritoneal dialysis, in contrast, uses the patient's peritoneal membrane, a permeable surface containing thousands of capillaries.

Diffusion requires a concentration gradient between fluids. In this process, substances move from an area of a high concentration to an area of a low concentration. The rate of solute movement depends on the particle size, charge, and degree to which solutes are protein bound. *Osmosis* refers to flow of water down its concentration gradient. Movement of solutes from blood into dialysis fluid will decrease the concentration of water within the dialysis fluid, thereby promoting flow of water from the intravascular space into the dialytic space.

Convection occurs when the movement of water carries small solutes across the membrane, a process called solvent drag. When *ultrafiltration* is required, a volume of fluid is removed during a dialysis session. During hemodialysis, a hydrostatic pressure is created within the filter to force a prescribed volume of free water from the intravascular space into the dialysis fluid. Ultrafiltration during peritoneal dialysis increases in accordance with the osmolarity of the prescribed dialysis solution.

Dialysis is prescribed when medical interventions fail to manage disease resulting from kidney injury. As described in Table 31-2, kidney dysfunction results in electrolyte imbalance, anasarca, and accumulation of uremic toxins. Managing metabolic acidosis with alkali, restricting the use of potassium and phosphate, and limiting protein intake are required. Fluid restriction can also prevent a patient from receiving adequate nutrition—a significant problem for infants. Alternatively, dialysis can be used to clear a harmful substance from the bloodstream, provided that it

TABLE 31-2

Indications for Prescribing Dialysis	
Hypervolemia	Manifests as anasarca, hypertension, respiratory or heart failure, and hyponatremia
Electrolyte abnormalities	Hyperkalemia, acidosis, hyperphosphatemia, hypocalcemia
Azotemia/uremia	Can present with confusion, bradycardia, platelet dysfunction, and pericardial tamponade, or without symptoms
Removal of toxic substances	Medications, poisons, ammonia
Malnutrition	Decreased caloric intake secondary to volume restriction, increased metabolic demands, net catabolic state, malabsorption

is not protein bound, in patients who have otherwise normal kidney function.

MODES OF DIALYSIS

Hemodialysis

Acute hemodialysis requires a catheter to be placed in a large vein, usually the internal jugular, subclavian, or femoral vein. An uncuffed catheter is used to limit vessel damage (e.g., stenosis) and is meant for temporary, inpatient use. The catheter actually consists of two lumens. The "arterial" side draws blood out of the vein into the dialysis machine (Figure 31-2); the "venous" side returns the blood to the patient. Note that the holes on the "arterial" side are proximal to those on the "venous" side. If the lines were attached to opposite ports, recirculation of blood would occur, with decreased efficacy in clearance. Femoral catheter placement is problematic, as hip flexion distorts the lumen and renders the catheter unusable.

In hemodialysis, blood and dialysis fluid enter into a filter in a countercurrent fashion. The patient's blood enters at the top of the filter, and flow is divided among hundreds of hollow lumens running in parallel. The blood exits at the bottom of the filter and is returned to the patient. The dialysis fluid travels in a direction opposite to that of the blood flow, remaining outside the lumens and bathing the membranes. The countercurrent flow maximizes the concentration gradient between the blood and dialysis fluid, optimizing clearance of unwanted substances. For pediatric patients, blood flow is typically 150 to 350 mL/min and dialysis fluid flows at 500 mL/hr.

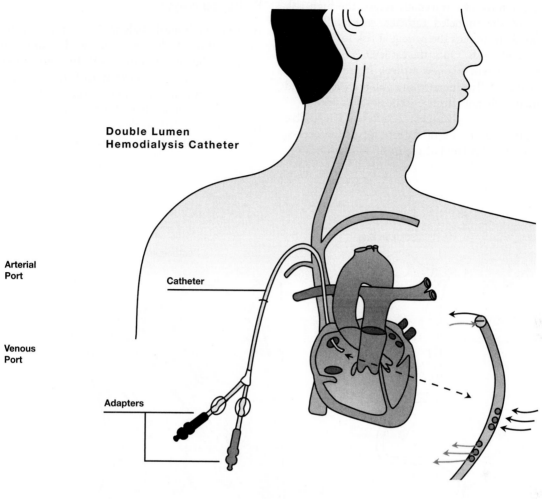

Double Lumen Hemodialysis Catheter

Arterial Port

Catheter

Venous Port

Adapters

FIGURE 31-2

Hemodialysis Catheter Placement.

Source: Courtesy of Medical Components Incorporated.

Dialysis efficiently removes osmotically active solutes. Equilibration of free water between the intracellular and intravascular compartments results in movement of free water into tissues. *Disequilibrium syndrome* is caused by dialysis-induced cerebral edema, presenting as nausea, headache, confusion, and seizure. Initial hemodialysis sessions should be short and run at a low blood flow rate without ultrafiltration. Mannitol—an osmotic agent that is poorly cleared by dialysis—can be prescribed prior to the procedure to avoid the potential for disequilibrium.

Too-rapid removal of fluid from the intravascular space may result in hypotension and shock. With this condition, tachycardia may precede nausea, crampy abdominal pain, and emesis. Treatment of symptoms includes small boluses of 5% dextrose, a decrease in the rate of ultrafiltration, and if shock occurs, administration of large saline boluses and

discontinuation of dialysis. In patients with chronic kidney disease, baroreceptor dysfunction resulting in bradycardia may require atropine or epinephrine to improve perfusion.

Patients who require hemodialysis following hospital discharge will require a tunneled hemodialysis catheter, if recovery of kidney function is anticipated, or internal vascular access (i.e., arteriovenous [AV] fistula or graft), if the patient is diagnosed with end-stage kidney disease. The tunnel creates traction within the subcutaneous tissues, allowing for maintenance of the proper placement of the catheter tip within the superior vena cava–right atrial junction. The insertion site should be cleaned every 2 to 3 days under aseptic conditions, and covered by a dry gauze and transparent dressing. The ports require a high-concentration (i.e., 5,000–10,000 units/mL) heparin lock using the volume listed on the port hub.

As with any form of intravenous access, the high risk of infection of the tunneled catheter, surrounding tissues, and bloodstream puts the patient at risk for cellulitis, endocarditis, and sepsis. Once the catheter is infected, its removal and placement of a new catheter in another vessel are usually required. Treatment with antibiotic "locks" and infusions are usually not effective strategies for cure.

Long-term catheter placement results in irreversible stenosis, limiting future use of the site for fistula access, and increasing the likelihood of aneurysm formation.

Peritoneal dialysis

In acute peritoneal dialysis (PD), the surgeon places a catheter through the abdominal wall, with its tip coiled in the right abdomen (Figure 31-3). In contrast to the hemodialysis catheter, the Tenckhoff catheter is a flexible, Silastic catheter consisting of a single lumen with multiple holes within the distal one-half of the internal portion of the tubing. Peritoneal dialysis fluid flows into the patient through the inflow port, dwells within the peritoneal space for a

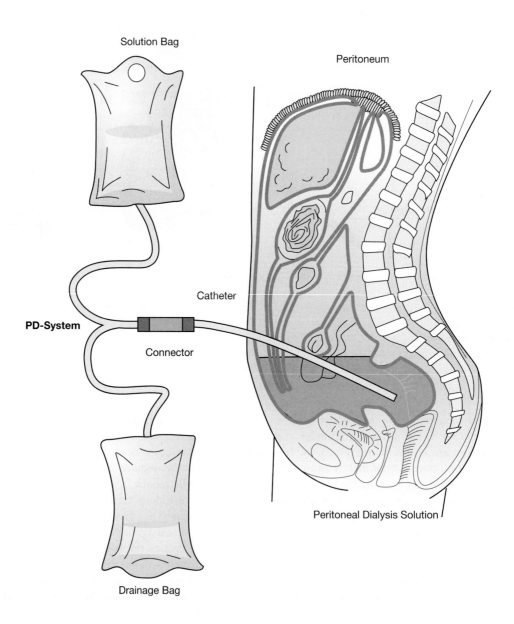

FIGURE 31-3

Peritoneal Dialysis Catheter Placement and Infusion of Dialysis Fluid into the Peritoneum.

Source: Courtesy of Medical Components Incorporated.

prescribed period of time, and then drains into a collection bag through the outflow port.

The PD fluid is hyperosmotic to serum, containing a high concentration of carbohydrate (glucose, icodextrin) to promote ultrafiltration as well as sodium, chloride, calcium, magnesium, and alkali (lactate, bicarbonate). The type of dialysis fluid prescribed varies by its concentration of carbohydrate, described as a percentage (i.e., 1.5%, 2.5%, 4.25%). The higher the percent carbohydrate in solution, the greater the volume of fluid removed during dialysis. Of note, fluid removal occurs initially from the intravascular space, and requires movement of extravascular fluid into the intravascular space to prevent shock.

The prescription for PD includes a fill volume, dwell time, number of cycles, and type of PD. The volume of PD fluid instilled into the peritoneal space is usually between 20 and 40 mL/kg/cycle. Ideally, the peritoneal lining will have healed around the PD catheter before a patient is dialyzed; healing takes approximately 2 weeks after insertion of the catheter. If PD is required quickly, a small volume of fluid (10 mL/kg/cycle) is used to avoid leakage around the catheter insertion site.

Patients may be dialyzed either solely during sleep (continuous cycling peritoneal dialysis [CCPD]) or throughout a 24-hour period (continuous ambulatory peritoneal dialysis [CAPD]), although some patients on CCPD may have a midday exchange to improve fluid removal. CAPD is used to maximize clearance, with fluid continuously moving within the intraperitoneal space. With this technique, however, the weight of the fluid limits the fill volume. Patients average 6 to 8 cycles of fluid, with dwell times of 3 to 4 hours each. In CCPD, which occurs during sleep, 8 to 10 cycles with dwell times of 30 to 45 minutes each are required. An automated machine instills and drains fluid at the bedside, calculating the net gains or losses of fluids at each cycle.

Traditionally, the peritoneal space is completely drained at the end of each cycle. An alternative method, known as tidal PD, drains a portion of the fluid instilled—a maneuver used to reduce pain from stretching the peritoneal membrane. Some patients on CCPD will receive a "last fill," consisting of a small volume of fluid placed after a course of CCPD is complete. To avoid overfilling the peritoneum, minimum fill and drain volumes are set on the automated cycler so as to detect any catheter malfunction or excessive fluid absorption by the patient across the peritoneal lining.

The most common complication of PD is peritonitis, usually due to passage of skin flora into the peritoneal space. Bacteria may gain direct entry to the peritoneum through the catheter, if it is used under unsterile conditions, or subcutaneously down the tissue plane surrounding the catheter. Similar to the hemodialysis catheter, the PD catheter insertion site requires regular cleaning under aseptic conditions. The end of the catheter contains an adapter that uses sterile tubing to connect to the cycler.

When not in use, the adapter is sealed by a sterile cap; thus HCPs should use sterile gloves when handling it. Less frequently, peritonitis occurs from migration of gut flora into the peritoneal space. Drained dialysis fluid appears cloudy, sometimes occurring before symptoms of peritonitis: abdominal pain (especially when fluid is instilled or drained), fever, nausea, emesis, diarrhea, and shock. Inflammation of the peritoneal space causes massive loss of fluid and protein. Treatment with intraperitoneal vancomycin or cefazolin with ceftazidime every 4 to 6 hours is standard therapy until identification and susceptibilities of a cultured organism are available.

The peritoneum is a potential space, normally occupied by a trace fluid that contains few macrophages and lymphocytes. Chronic noxious stimuli, such as high-osmolar peritoneal fluid, a plastic dialysis catheter, or infection, will promote a reparative process at the cellular level, resulting in scar formation in this region. Fibrotic tissue is nonfunctional and limits the surface area available for dialysis. Conversely, the peritoneal membrane can lose its selectivity for molecular transport, permitting significant loss of protein.

Hemodialysis versus peritoneal dialysis

The decision to dialyze a patient using the bloodstream or the peritoneum depends on the patient size, the urgency of correcting the identified defect, and existing anatomic restrictions. Hemodialysis can correct electrolyte imbalances, remove toxins, and clear free water more efficiently than peritoneal dialysis. However, a pediatric patient requires at least a 7 French double-lumen hemodialysis catheter to achieve an appropriate blood flow rate. Some nephrologists will place the catheter into the femoral vein due to constraints imposed by the length, which could advance into the right heart. In small pediatric patients, blood flow from the arterial port can draw the catheter against the wall of the vessel, preventing access to the circulation. In addition to these technical difficulties, hemodialysis can result in hypotension as blood is removed by the circuit (avoided in children weighing less than 10 kg by priming the circuit with the appropriate blood volume) and cytokines are released as blood interfaces with the dialysis membrane.

CONTINUOUS RENAL REPLACEMENT THERAPY

Many pediatric intensive care units use continuous renal replacement therapy (CRRT) instead of intermittent hemodialysis to manage fluid and electrolyte imbalances in this hemodynamically less stable population. CRRT relies on a hemodialysis catheter (identical to one used during acute intermittent hemodialysis) to provide dialysis and/or ultrafiltration for days at a time, using a machine designed specifically for this purpose (e.g., Prismaflex, Prisma, Aquarius). CRRT is the generic terminology; a patient is prescribed a regimen such as continuous venovenous hemofiltration (CVVH), continuous venovenous hemodialysis (CVVHD), or continuous venovenous hemodiafiltration (CVVHDF).

Unlike machines used for intermittent hemodialysis, CRRT machines contain software that enables intensive care nurses to manage this procedure. These devices have a user-friendly format and include safety features to prevent excessive patient fluid removal, entrance of air into the patient circulation, and inappropriate net fluid gains.

The machine used for CRRT appears different than that used for intermittent hemodialysis because it carries anticoagulant and replacement fluid, in addition to the dialysis fluid and effluent bag (waste products). To prevent clotting within the dialysis circuit, most nephrologists include sodium citrate in the fluid, which combines with calcium ion to render clotting factors inactive. The patient receives a continuous infusion of calcium (external to the circuit), enabling him or her to maintain normocalcemia. Alternatively, in patients receiving therapeutic heparin (e.g., those on extracorporeal life support), maintaining the ACT in the 180 to 220 msec range can maintain the circuit.

Replacement fluid limits the increase in viscosity within the hemodialysis filter while ultrafiltration occurs. Prior to the introduction of this option, nephrologists prescribed slow intermittent ultrafiltration (SCUF), where losses of free water decrease blood flow within the filter and sometimes lead to clot formation. The alternative, hemofiltration (CVVH), prescribes ultrafiltration but avoids increases in viscosity by instilling fluid prefilter, with this equivalent volume removed postfilter (automatically by the machine), to avoid net fluid gains.

HEMATURIA

Tresa E. Zielinski

PATHOPHYSIOLOGY

Hematuria is the presence of blood, ranging from microscopic to gross, in the urine. Microscopic hematuria is the presence of red blood cells (RBCs) that are not visible to the naked eye, whereas gross hematuria will change the color of the urine. Microscopic hematuria is defined by the presence of more than 5 RBCs per high-powered field (hpf). To identify this condition, microscopic analysis is the preferred method over routine urine strip testing, as the latter technique can produce false-positive results (Bergstein et al., 2005; Brenner, 1996; Diven & Travis, 2000). Both gross and microscopic blood can be concerning and indicate the need for further testing to evaluate its origin.

Hematuria can originate anywhere from the glomerular capillaries to the distal urethra. Glomerular hematuria derives from a breach in the integrity of the glomerular capillary wall, which is sensitive to injury and hypoxia; erythrocytes may appear dysmorphic (Fogazzi et al., 2008). Urinary tract abnormalities are more likely associated with normomorphic erythrocytes on examination (Fogazzi et al.). Blood may also be introduced to the urine from exogenous sources such as menses. Concurrent proteinuria can be helpful in differentiating between glomerular versus tubular injury, as it is more closely associated with glomerular disease (Massry & Glassock, 2001). Rarely is hematuria, by itself, an emergent situation; however, it may be an indicator of a more critical underlying kidney problem (Meyers, 2004).

EPIDEMIOLOGY AND ETIOLOGY

Asymptomatic hematuria in children is relatively common. The incidence of microscopic hematuria has been reported as ranging between 0.14% and 2% in children age 6–15 years depending on the number of collected specimens. The incidence of gross hematuria is estimated at 1.3 case per 1,000 population. For most patients, the etiology is unknown. For those with an identified cause, hypercalciuria is most common etiology, followed by postinfectious glomerulonenephritis. In a small number of patients, a structural abnormality or kidney disease leads to hematuria (Bergstein et al., 2005; Meyers, 2004).

PRESENTATION

In the history, the HCP should ask about family members with kidney disease. Historical questions should include all of the following:

- Has there been recent trauma?
- Is the patient menstruating?
- Is there a pattern to the hematuria—persistent, intermittent, or recurrent?
- Are there signs of infection, such as frequency, dysuria, or flank pain?
- Is the hematuria worse after exercise?
- Has there been recent pharyngitis?
- Does the child bruise easily or have a known coagulopathy?

The physical examination may reveal peripheral or periorbital edema or ascitis (fluid overload), pallor (a sign of anemia), hypertension, or abnormal hearing. Hypertension is a red flag that the etiology may be renal in origin (Bergstein et al., 2005; Brenner, 1996; Patel & Bissler, 2001; Schrier, 2001). Measure the child's weight and height, and compare these data to previous recordings. Either growth retardation or recent rapid weight gain may be a sign of kidney disease.

DIFFERENTIAL DIAGNOSIS

Differential diagnoses can be classified into glomerular (including primary, multisystem, infectious, or hereditary), vascular and tubulointerstitial disease (hypersensitivity, hereditary, vascular, papillary necrosis, and trauma) and urinary tract diseases (trauma, calculi, carcinoma, and structural defects). Other potential causes of hematuria include malignancy, excessive exercise, presence of a foreign body, and menstrual contaminant.

PLAN OF CARE

Diagnostic studies are specific to findings during the history and physical examination. Most patients should start with microscopic evaluation of the urine for RBCs and RBC casts and measurements to identify proteinuria. If these tests are positive, or if there is also a history of edema and hypertension, then further evaluation of kidney function is warranted. These tests include measurements of electrolytes, bicarbonate, blood urea nitrogen (BUN), creatinine, glucose, total and ionized calcium, albumin, phosphorus, an estimated glomerular filtration rate (eGFR), CBC and differential, protein–creatinine ratio, complement C3, and antistreptolysin O titer. If the results are negative, then consider ordering a CT scan if there is a history of trauma, urine culture and ultrasound if there are signs of infection, or ultrasound if there is suspicion of nephrolithiasis or structural abnormality (Meyers, 2004; Patel & Bissler, 2001; Tan, 2009).

Kidney biopsies are the most definitive way to diagnose disease in this organ; they are performed when diagnosis is required to determine a treatable disease, direct therapy, or determine prognosis (Brenner, 1996). Kidney biopsy should be performed only when the patient is clinically stable and when other diagnostic tests are inconclusive; a biopsy is not necessary in an asymptomatic child. Kidney biopsy requires patient sedation and may cause hematuria (Bergstein et al., 2005). Additional testing may be indicated based on preliminary results, including cholesterol levels, vitamin D, parathyroid hormone, urine electrolytes, antineutrophil cytoplasmic antibodies (ANCA), antinuclear antibody (ANA), and anti-double-stranded DNA antibody (Glassock, 2001; Patel & Bissler, 2001; Tan, 2009).

Hematuria alone does not require treatment; however, the underlying etiology may. Patients may need care to treat hypertension, fluid overload, bone demineralization, acidosis, hyperkalemia, or infection. Anemia is an extremely rare occurrence related to hematuria. Hypocalcemia is usually

related to hyperphosphatemia and is amenable to treatment with vitamin D and phosphate binders (Bergstein et al., 2005; Diven & Travis, 2000).

DISPOSITION AND DISCHARGE PLANNING

Consultation considerations include kidney disease specialists and urologists pending the etiology of the hematuria. Long-term follow-up may be required. The patient and family should be informed about the importance of good hydration and possibility of recurrence of gross hematuria with intercurrent illnesses. If hypertension is present, families should be taught to monitor the blood pressure in the home so as to evaluate the effectiveness of the treatment and allow medications to be adjusted if necessary.

HYPERTENSION

Tresa E. Zielinski

PATHOPHYSIOLOGY

The diagnosis of hypertension requires systolic or diastolic blood pressure (BP) measurements exceeding the 95th percentile for gender, age, and height on three occasions, typically taken in an outpatient clinic setting. The National High Blood Pressure Education Program Working Group on High Blood Pressure in Children and Adolescents published tables appropriate for the pediatric outpatient population, with recommendations for evaluation and treatment for pediatric hypertension; a free copy of these guidelines can be downloaded from U.S. Department of Health and Human Services' website.

Elevated blood pressure is classified as prehypertension, stage 1 hypertension, or stage 2 hypertension. All children and adults with a BP higher than 120/80 mmHg or between the 90th and 95th percentiles for gender, age, and height should be classified as having prehypertension. Such patients should have their blood pressure rechecked within 6 months to confirm this diagnosis. Stage 1 hypertension (BP between the 95th and 99th percentiles, plus 5 mmHg) is reevaluated on repeated visits (three separate measures within 1 month) to confirm. Those patients with stage 2 hypertension (greater than the 99th percentile, plus 5 mmHg) should be referred for evaluation within 1 week or sooner if symptomatic.

EPIDEMIOLOGY AND ETIOLOGY

Primary hypertension is strongly associated with a family history of hypertension and cardiovascular disease. It usually presents with measurements consistent with prehypertension or stage 1 hypertension. *Secondary hypertension* is more common in children than in adults, as a sequela of an underlying condition; in particular, more than one-half of pediatric cases are attributed to kidney disease (Lande & Flynn, 2009; Tan, 2009). Hypertension commonly results in end-organ damage. Left ventricular hypertrophy (LVH) is most common; however, hypertensive encephalopathy, stroke, and congestive heart failure have also been reported (HHS, 2005).

PRESENTATION

All children older than the age of 3 years should have blood pressure measured at every health care visit. This type of screening is also recommended for those younger than 3 years of age with a history of prematurity, congenital heart disease (repaired or unrepaired), kidney disease, transplant, malignancy, evidence of elevated intracranial pressure, recurrent urinary tract infections (UTIs), hematuria, or proteinuria (U.S. Department of Health and human Services [HHS], 2005).

It is most important to ensure that the blood pressure has been measured correctly when diagnosing hypertension (Flynn & Daniels, 2006; Lande & Flynn, 2009; Tan, 2009). Use the upper right extremity with an appropriate-sized cuff. Blood pressures should be measured after 5 minutes of rest either in a seated position with the feet touching the floor or in a supine position with the right arm supported at the level of the heart. Auscultation is the preferred method unless the child has an arterial line. Oscillometric devices vary in their accuracy and must be routinely validated. If an elevated BP is noted using an oscillometric device, that finding should be confirmed by auscultation before documenting that the patient has hypertension (HHS, 2005).

Once an elevated blood pressure has been documented, the history and physical examination can be tailored to explore for underlying causes and associated symptoms; see Table 31-3 and Table 31-4.

DIFFERENTIAL DIAGNOSIS

The list of differential diagnoses for elevated BP is extensive. Table 31-5 and Table 31-6 summarize these potential etiologies for consideration. Hypertension can also be

TABLE 31-3

History Clues for Hypertension	
Family history	Cardiovascular disease (myocardial infarction, stroke) • Primary hypertension Deafness • Congenital or familiar kidney disease Dyslipidemia • Primary hypertension Endocrine disorders • Familial endocrinopathies

TABLE 31-3

History Clues for Hypertension *(Continued)*	
	Hypertension • Primary hypertension Kidney disease • Congenital or familiar kidney disease Sleep apnea • Primary hypertension
Patient history	Chest pain • Cardiovascular disease Diaphoresis • Endocrinopathies • Cardiovascular disease, especially in infants Dyspnea on exertion • Cardiovascular disease Edema • Cardiovascular disease • Kidney disease Enuresis • Kidney vascular disease • Kidney scarring Growth failure • Endocrinopathies • Kidney disease Heat or cold intolerance • Endocrinopathies Heart palpations • Cardiovascular disease • Arrhythmias Headaches • Primary hypertension Hematuria • Kidney vascular disease • Kidney scarring Joint pain or swelling • Rheumatologic disorders Myalgias • Rheumatologic disorders Neonatal hypovolemia/shock • Kidney vascular disease • Kidney scarring Recurrent rashes • Rheumatologic disorders Snoring/sleep disorders • Primary hypertension Umbilical artery catheterization • Kidney vascular disease • Kidney scarring Urinary tract infections (recurrent) • Kidney vascular disease • Kidney scarring Weight or appetite changes • Endocrinopathies

Source: U.S. Department of Health and Human Services, National Institutes of Health, & National Heart, Lung, and Blood Institute. (2005). The fourth report on the diagnosis, evaluation, and treatment of high blood pressure in children and adolescents. Retrieved from http://www.nhlbi.nih.gov/health/prof/heart/hbp/hbp_ped.pdf

TABLE 31-4

Physical Examination Clues to Hypertension	
Height, weight, and body mass index (BMI)	• < 25: normal • 25–29.9: overweight • 30–39.9: obese • 40+: markedly obese
Head and neck	Elfin faces • Williams syndrome Moon faces • Cushing syndrome Thyroid enlargement • Hyperthyroidism Webbed neck • Turner syndrome Tonsillar hypertrophy • Sleep disordered breathing, sleep apnea
Eyes	Retinal changes • Suggestive of severe hypertension and secondary etiology Papilledema • Intracranial hypertension
Skin	Acne, hirsutism, striae • Cushing syndrome • Steroid use Café-au-lait spots or neurofibromas • Neurofibramatosis Ash leaf spots or adenoma sebaceum • Tuberous sclerosis Rash • Secondary kidney disease • Lupus erythematosus • Henoch-Schönlein purpura Acanthrosis nigricans • Type 2 diabetes
Chest	Murmur • Coarctation of the aorta Apical heave • Left ventricular hypertrophy
Abdomen	Abdominal bruit • Renovascular disease Mass • Hydronephrosis • Polycystic kidney disease • Kidney tumors • Neuroblastoma
Extremities	Pulse • Lower extremity < upper extremity suggests coarctation of the aorta Traction/casts • Orthopedic manipulation Asymmetry of limbs • Beckwith-Weideman syndrome Arthritis • Henoch-Schönlein purpura • Collagen vascular disease • Lupus erythematosus

TABLE 31-4

Physical Examination Clues to Hypertension (Continued)	
Neurologic	Muscle weakness • Liddle syndrome • Hyperaldosteronism Ascending paralysis • Guillain-Barré syndrome Diminished pain response • Familial dysautonomia
Genitalia	Ambiguous/virilization • Adrenal hyperplasia Advanced puberty • Intracranial tumors

Source: U.S. Department of Health and Human Services, National Institutes of Health, & National Heart, Lung, and Blood Institute. (2005). The fourth report on the diagnosis, evaluation, and treatment of high blood pressure in children and adolescents. Retrieved from http://www.nhlbi.nih.gov/health/prof/heart/hbp/hbp_ped.pdf

TABLE 31-5

Etiology of Hypertension in Children	
1–6 years of age	• Renal parenchymal disease • Renal vascular disease • Endocrine causes • Coarctation of the aorta • Essential hypertension
6–12 years of age	• Renal parenchymal disease • Essential hypertension • Renal vascular disease • Endocrine causes • Coarctation of the aorta • Iatrogenic illness
12–18 years of age	• Essential hypertension • Iatrogenic illness • Renal parenchymal disease • Renal vascular disease • Endocrine causes • Coarctation of the aorta

iatrogenic, related to "white coat syndrome" (anxiety with HCPs), or be a side effect of therapy such as medications.

PLAN OF CARE

Most patients with elevated blood pressure are asymptomatic. Moreover, they may not have a history suggestive of an underlying cause. Diagnostic studies may provide additional information in this regard. An evaluation and treatment algorithm for hypertension has been developed by HHS (Figure 31-5).

A CBC, kidney function studies (sodium, potassium, chloride, bicarbonate, BUN, creatinine, albumin, calcium,

TABLE 31-6

Other Etiologies of Hypertension in Children

Kidney disease	• Parenchymal disease
	• Pyelonephritis
	• Congenital abnormalities
	• Reflux nephropathy
	• Acute glomerulonephritis
	• Henoch-Schönlein purpura
	• Kidney trauma
	• Hydronephrosis
	• Hemolytic uremic syndrome
	• Kidney stones
	• Nephrotic syndrome
	• Wilms' tumor
	• Hypoplastic kidney
	• Polycystic kidney disease
	• Vascular
	• Renal vein thrombosis
	• Renal artery hypoplasia
	• Midaortic syndrome
	• Arteritis
	• Neurofibromatosis
Adrenal gland	• Cushing syndrome (overproduction of cortisol)
	• Hyperaldosteronism
	• Tumors—most common in adults
	• Congenital adrenal hyperplasia
	• Pheochromocytoma
Drugs	• Corticosteroids
	• Nonsteroidal anti-inflammatory drugs
	• Cox-2 inhibitors
	• Weight-loss medications
	• Nicotine
	• Cocaine
	• Amphetamines
	• Pseudoephedrine
	• Oral contraceptives (estrogen component)
	• Migraine medications
	• Caffeine
	• Epinephrine
	• Phenylephrine
	• Terbutaline
Sleep apnea	• Poor correlation in children
Stress, anxiety	
Coarctation of the aorta	• Classically hypertensive in upper extremities and diminished femoral pulses; low or unobtainable systolic pressures in the lower extremities
Endocrine disorders	• Hyperthyroidism
	• Primary hyperparathyroidism
	• Diabetes mellitus
	• Hypocalcaemia
Pregnancy	• Preeclampsia
	• Fluid overload
Metabolic syndrome	Three or more of the following:
	• Elevated serum triglyceride levels
	• Low serum high-density lipoprotein cholesterol
	• Impaired glucose tolerance
	• Hypertension

phosphorus), urinalysis, urine culture, renal ultrasound, fasting lipid panel, fasting glucose, echocardiograph, and retinal examination are recommended for all patients with confirmed BP greater than the 95th percentile. Fasting lipid panel and fasting glucose measurements should be also be obtained for overweight children with confirmed BP in the 90th to 94th percentiles, those with a family history of hypertension or cardiovascular disease, or those with chronic kidney disease. Pediatric patients with comorbidities such as diabetes or kidney disease and confirmed BP in the 90th to 94th percentiles should have an echocardiograph and retinal examination. A drug screen and sleep history and/or polysomnography can be completed as needed. These studies test for identifiable causes, comorbidities, and target-organ damage. Further studies may be considered as indicated, including plasma rennin tests and imaging studies such as renal scan, Doppler flow studies, and three-dimensional computed tomography (HHS, 2005).

Basic lifestyle changes are recommended as part of therapeutic management for all levels of hypertension. These changes include the following actions:

- Weight reduction if overweight
- Regular physical activity
- Diet modification

Consultation with specialists in pediatric hypertension are appropriate for those patients with stage 2 hypertension or for any child with prehypertension or stage 1 hypertension with comorbidities or target-organ damage.

In the past, few choices for pharmacologic therapy of hypertension were approved for use in children. However, more antihypertensive agents and medications have now been studied in children since the passage of the 1997 U.S. Food and Drug Administration Modernization Act of 1997 (FDA, 1997) and 2002 Best Pharmaceuticals for Children Act (FDA, 2002) (Flynn & Daniels, 2006; Lande & Flynn, 2009). Recommendations from *The Fourth Report on the Diagnosis, Evaluation, and Treatment of High Blood Pressure in Children and Adolescents* (2005) include the following guidelines:

- Antihypertensive therapy is indicated for children with symptomatic hypertension, secondary hypertension, target-organ damage, and diabetes, or for those children who are not responsive to lifestyle changes.
- Single pharmacologic agents should be maximized prior to adding other therapeutic agents to the medication regimen.
- The goal is reduction of the child's BP to less than the 95th percentile, or to the 90th percentile for children with comorbidities.

When prescribing pharmaceutical interventions, it is important to start the medication at the lowest recommended dose and monitor the child carefully for effectiveness and

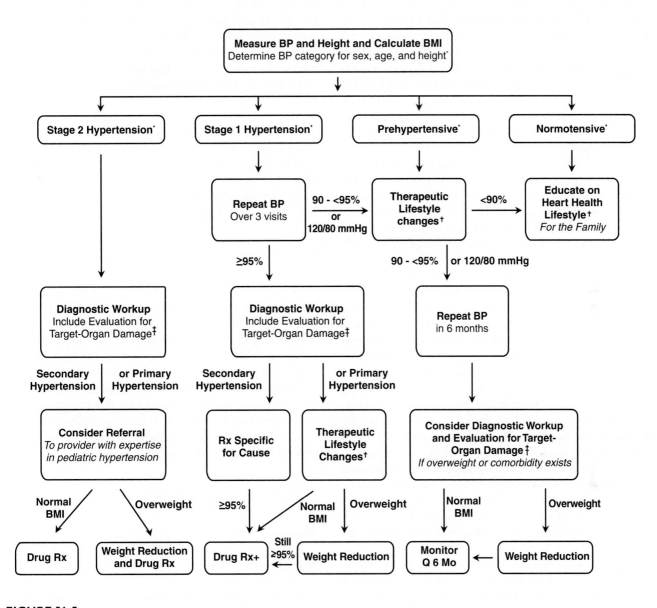

FIGURE 31-5

Evaluation and Treatment Algorithm for Hypertension in Pediatric Patients.

Note: Body mass index (BMI), blood pressure (BP), prescription (Rx), every (Q), diet modification and physical activity (†), especially if younger, very high BP, little or no family history, diabetic, or other risk factors (‡).

Source: U.S. Department of Health and Human Services National Institutes of Health National Heart, Lung, and Blood Institute. (2005). The Fourth Report on the Diagnosis, Evaluation, and Treatment of High Blood Pressure in Children and Adolescents. Retrieved from http://www.nhlbi.nih.gov/health/prof/heart/hbp/hbp_ped.pdf.

side effects. If BP goals have not been met, then dosing may slowly be increased either to the highest recommended dose or until adverse side effects are noted. A second drug from another class should then be added and increased in the same fashion until BP goals are met.

Angiotensin-converting enzyme (ACE) inhibitors and angiotensin II receptor blockers (ARBs) are the agents most commonly used to treat hypertension. ACE inhibitors block the conversion of angiotensin I to angiotensin II, a potent vasoconstrictor and a contributor to endothelial dysfunction. Through this mechanism, aldosterone secretion is reduced and natriuresis increased. ARBs decrease intraglomerular pressure by decreasing efferent arteriolar tone. These drugs are renoprotective, as they reduce microalbuminuria—an important precursor to diabetic nephropathy—in patients with diabetes. Due to the decrease in glomerular filtration ACE inhibitors and ARBs should be used with caution in patients with kidney dysfunction, as they increase the risk of hyperkalemia. Both ACE inhibitors and ARBs have been studied in children older than the age of 6 years and are FDA approved for use in this population (Flynn & Daniels, 2006). These agents should be used with extreme caution in children who are volume depleted, have excessive output, have bilateral renovascular hypertension, are pregnant, or have hyperkalemia.

Diuretic therapies such as thiazides, loop, and potassium-sparing agents can be used for hypertension that is believed to be related to fluid overload. These medications can also be used as complementary therapy with other antihypertensive agents. Potassium-sparing diuretics should be used with caution in patients on ACE inhibitors or ARBs due to the high risk for hyperkalemia (HHS, 2005).

Calcium-channel blockers reduce blood pressure by relaxing arteriolar smooth muscle. This may be the desired class of antihypertensive agents for use in the asthmatic patient, but are contraindicated in the patient with sick sinus syndrome. Other vasodilators, such as hydralazine and minoxidil, are usually reserved for patients resistant to other therapies due to their less favorable side-effect profile.

Peripheral alpha$_1$ antagonists and centrally acting alpha$_2$ agonists may cause orthostatic hypotension; alpha$_2$ agonists and beta$_1$ blockers decrease cardiac output by decreasing the heart rate. Both classes should be used with caution in ambulatory patients. Beta blockers are contraindicated in patients with heart block, asthma, or pregnancy; they should be used only with extreme caution in diabetic patients, as they decrease ability to identify a hypoglycemic event. Beta blockers and calcium-channel blockers may be the drugs of choice for children who have concurrent migraines.

Children with hypertension and end-organ dysfunction are considered to have hyptertensive crisis. Most patients with hypertensive crisis have underlying kidney dysfunction. Hypertensive encephalopathy may develop and can be further exacerbated by adverse effects of antihypertensive medications. Intravenous preparations of beta blocker (esmolol), alpha and beta blocker (labetolol), calcium-channel blocker (nicardipine), or vasodilator (hydralazine, nitroprusside) agents should be used for hypertensive emergencies. The agent selection should be based on criteria such as patient condition, underlying cause, cardiac function, neurologic status, and end-organ perfusion. Rapid acting agents such as labetalol, nicardipine, and nifedipine are useful agents for immediate blood pressure reduction. Monitor vital signs, neurologic assessment, fluid balance, and end-organ perfusion closely during therapy. Overcorrection may result in hypoperfusion, autodysregulation,

and cerebral ischemia. In the first 6–12 hours, controlled reduction of blood pressure should be no more than 25% to 33% of goal reduction. Gradual reduction, thereafter, should continue over the next 48–72 hours as needed. Patient management should occur in a pediatric intensive care unit to allow for the close monitoring that is needed (Fivush et al., 1997; Groshong, 1996; Hiren & Mitsnefes, 2005; Yiu et al., 2004).

Consultation with a kidney specialist or cardiologist will promote a comprehensive approach to diagnosis and therapy of the pediatric patient with asymptomatic hypertension. If the patient is expected to receive inpatient care, additional specialists such as critical care and neurology should be consulted. Family and patient education will depend on the etiology and treatment regimen.

DISPOSITION AND DISCHARGE PLANNING

Hypertension is a complex symptom. Patients may be asymptomatic and not understand the significance of this "silent killer." Education regarding the impact of hypertension on target organs may need to be repeated frequently. Follow-up with the PCP is required to reinforce lifestyle changes and monitor blood pressure, electrolytes, and pharmacologic side effects. Nutritional guidance may be indicated for those patients who have difficulty modifying their diet. Subspecialist care, such as from cardiology, nephrology, and ophthalmology services, may be warranted for patients with target-organ damage.

KIDNEY INSUFFICIENCY

Bonnie Kitchen

PATHOPHYSIOLOGY

Acute renal failure (ARF), also known as acute kidney failure, is a complex, multifactorial process and a potentially life-threatening condition with significant morbidity and mortality. Acute renal failure occurs when there is an abrupt and sustained loss of the kidney's ability to secrete water, regulate electrolyte balance, regulate acid–base balance, and eliminate waste products (Ghani et al., 2009). The decline in the glomerular filtration rate increases the blood concentrations of both urea and creatinine.

Renal vasoconstriction has been considered the primary component in the pathogenesis of ARF. In AFR, the renal epithelium is damaged, resulting in the release of vasoactive compounds, such as angiotensin, prostaglandins, endothelin and nitric oxide. These substances increase cortical vascular resistance, thereby decreasing renal blood flow and leading to tubular damage. The vasoactive compounds decrease GFR by constricting the afferent and efferent arterioles, which results in decreased urine output. Vasoconstriction, while an important component of ARF, is not the only causative factor.

Chronic renal failure (CRF), also known as chronic kidney disease (CKD), is defined as the presence of structural or functional kidney damage for longer than 3 months based on abnormalities in the kidney biopsy, imaging, or blood or urine samples; or a GFR of less than 60 mL/min/1.73 m^2 in children older than 3 months (Miller & MacDonald, 2006). Chronic kidney disease is divided into five stages, where stage 1 is normal GFR with known kidney damage and stage 5 is end-stage renal disease (ESRD) (Table 31-7).

EPIDEMIOLOGY AND ETIOLOGY

No consensus exists on the precise definitions of acute and chronic renal failure; as a consequence, it is difficult to ascertain prevalence rates (Zappitelli, 2008). For ARF, the incidence appears to be less than 1% based on those patients who require renal replacement therapy (RRT) (Zappitelli). The incidence of ARF in hospitalized children is reportedly increasing at 0.8 case per 100,000 children (Andreoli, 2008). Among neonates who have undergone cardiac surgery, have a patent ductus arteriosus, had a very low birth weight, had a low APGAR score, or had intrauterine exposure to nonsteroidal anti-inflammatory agents (NSAIDs) or antibiotics, estimates of incidence range from 8% to 24%. Acute renal failure is also reported in 1% to 3% of all neonatal admissions to intensive care units. In older children, ARF has an estimated incidence of 4 cases per 100,000 children. In preschool children, hemolytic uremic syndrome (HUS) accounts for 50% of children with ARF. Acute renal failure in school-age children is more commonly caused by glomerulonephritis.

The etiology of ARF can be classified as pre-renal, intrinsic renal disease, and post-renal (Table 31-8). Pre-renal disease is caused by decreased blood flow to the kidney. Intrinsic renal disease is an etiology that occurs within the kidney itself, and post-renal disease is caused by obstruction to the flow of urine from the kidney. Although these are separate entities, they are not mutually exclusive; thus one cause may precipitate further progression of the disease. The pre-renal form of ARF is the most common form in pediatrics.

The mortality rates in children with ARF differ in various studies, depending on the underlying disease

TABLE 31-7

Stages of Chronic Kidney Disease	
Stage	Glomerular Filtration Rate (mL/min/1.73 m^2)
1	90
2	60–89
3	30–59
4	15–29
5	< 15

TABLE 31-8

Causes of Renal Failure		
Pre-renal Failure	Intrinsic Renal Failure	Post-renal Failure
Hypovolemia	Kidney/Vessel Diseases	Obstruction
Gastroenteritis	Acute glomerulonephritis	Posterior urethral valves
Gastrointestinal damage	Acute tubular necrosis	Occluded urinary catheter
Diabetes ketoacidosis	Bilateral pyelonephritis	Neurogenic bladder
Hypoproteinuria	Hemolytic uremic syndrome	Surgical accident
Hemorrhage	Interstitial nephritis	Nephrolithiasis
Third space losses	Cortical or medullary necrosis	Ureterocele
	Vasculitis	Tumors
	Hypercalcemia	Trauma
	Hyperphosphatemia	
	Hyperuricemia	
Peripheral vasodilatation	Myoglobinuria	
Impaired cardiac output	Hemoglobinuria	
Bilateral renal vessel occlusion	Intratubular obstructions	
Medications	Iatrogenic factors	
Prostaglandin synthetase inhibitors		
Angiotensin-converting enzyme (ACE) inhibitors		
Cyclosporin A		
Diuretics		
Hepatorenal syndrome		

process. The highest mortality rates occur in pediatric patients with multiple organ dysfunction, with the majority of these cases being attributable to sepsis (Ghani et al., 2009). Tumor lysis syndrome accounts for approximately 12.5% of all pediatric patients with ARF. Although the mortality rates in children with ARF in the intensive care units remain high, complete recovery of kidney function may occur. When pre-renal causes are related to hypovolemia, restoration of intravascular volume most often reverses the failure.

Chronic kidney disease in children has a different etiology than the corresponding disease in adults. Congenital and urologic anomalies represent the largest cause of CKD in children (Warady & Chadha, 2007). Of these defects, obstructive uropathy is the most prevalent cause of CKD, with aplastic/hypoplastic/dysplastic kidney, reflex nephrology, and polycystic kidney disease being less prevalent (Miller & MacDonald, 2006). Diabetic nephropathy and hypertension are rarely the cause of CRF in children. Glomerular diseases represent the major cause of CRF in older children, with focal segmental glomerulosclerosis accounting for 8.7% of these patients (Warady & Chadha). Systemic immunologic diseases, renal infarctions, and hemolytic uremic syndrome are the other acquired causes of CKD (Miller & MacDonald).

Chronic renal failure is often unpredictable when the disease is in its early stages. The progression is influenced by both the underlying etiology and the presence of risk factors such as obesity, hypertension, proteinuria, genetics, age, race, and gender. Despite the complicating factors, progression to ESRD is inversely proportional to the rate of creatinine clearance. If chronic renal failure is recognized and treated early, kidney function deterioration may be delayed, and outcomes improved (Goldstein & Devarajan, 2008). Unfortunately, CKD is associated with multisystem sequelae, such as anemia, bone disease, growth failure, metabolic acidosis, malnutrition, hyperparathyroidism, insulin resistance, and immunologic dysfunction.

Epidemiologic data on CKD are derived from children receiving RTT and those with ESRD (Warady & Chadha, 2007). The incidence of ESRD in the pediatric population has increased since 1980; today the incidence is 1.5 patients per 100,000 children and the prevalence rate is 8.2 patients per 100,000 children (Miller & MacDonald, 2006). Since 1990, the incidence has increased by 32% (Warady & Chadha). Patients who are younger than 20 years of age account for less than 2% of the total ESRD population (Warady & Chadha). The number of children who are asymptomatic in the early stages of CKD is likely underreported, as the vast majority of these patients have yet to be diagnosed. The number of children with all stages of CRF may be 50 times higher than the currently reported number (Warady & Chadha).

CKD has different geographic incidence and prevalence rates. Males with CKD predominate over females, with males accounting for 64% of all patients. CKD also has a notable racial distribution, with Caucasians representing 64% of all patients, African Americans 19%, and Hispanics 14%, according to the North American Pediatric Renal Transplant Cooperative Study (Warady et al., 1997).

PRESENTATION

The clinical presentation of children with renal insufficiency differs depending on the acuity or chronicity of the disease. Some children may exhibit a variety of symptoms, such as hematuria, hypertension, and edema; other children will be asymptomatic (Table 31-9). The clinical presentation may be slow and insidious and present as growth failure. Clinical markers of kidney damage are evident in both acute and chronic renal failure (Table 31-10).

TABLE 31-9

Presenting Symptoms in Acute and Chronic Renal Failure

- Poor appetite
- Growth/height retardation
- Abdominal pain
- Edema
- Oliguria
- Hematuria
- Proteinuria
- Anuria
- Hypertension
- Rash
- Fever
- Arthralgias
- Electrolyte abnormalities

TABLE 31-10

Findings that May be Associated With Kidney Damage

- Elevated serum creatinine
- Elevated blood urea nitrogen (BUN)
- Hypoalbuminemia
- Serum sodium abnormalities
- Serum potassium abnormalities
- Serum phosphorus elevation
- Metabolic acidosis
- Proteinuria
- Hematuria
- Echogenic kidneys on ultrasound
- Small kidneys on ultrasound
- Absence of one kidney
- Hydronephrosis
- Urinary obstruction
- Renal artery stenosis
- Nephrocalcinosis
- Cystic kidneys
- Kidney scarring on imaging

The evaluation for renal failure should start with a complete and thorough history. A detailed nutritional history should include food preferences as well as daily fluid intake and voiding patterns. Gross or microscopic hematuria may be reported. Urinary tract infection with or without urgency, dysuria, frequency, and incontinence should be further explored. The developmental history should address milestones, growth parameters, and sensory abilities. A medication history may include present and previous medications, chemotherapeutic agents, over-the-counter medications, and traditional or cultural remedies. A past medical history should include prematurity, previous urologic conditions and procedures, recent surgeries, recent trauma, and other underlying medical problems. Family history should also include first-degree relatives with hypertension, kidney disease, and metabolic disorders.

The comprehensive physical examination should include careful attention to the patient's heart rate, blood pressure, height, and weight, as these data can be abnormal in kidney diseases. In children with a single kidney, oliguria or anuria may be seen due to an obstruction.

DIFFERENTIAL DIAGNOSIS

Differential diagnoses in acute and chronic kidney failure may be evident or require investigation. Table 31-11 provides a detailed list of diagnoses.

PLAN OF CARE

Given the complexity of the pathology for acute and chronic renal failure, an interprofessional team approach may provide the best outcomes. Because volume depletion is the most common cause of acute renal failure, fluid volume must be restored (Andreoli, 2008). Accurately assessing the percentage of dehydration and fully replenishing the body's fluid stores are of paramount importance.

TABLE 31-11

Differential Diagnoses for Acute and Chronic Renal Failure

- Acute dehydration
- Acute tubular necrosis
- Glomerulonephritis
- Hemolytic uremic syndrome
- Hepatorenal syndrome
- Intrinsic renal disease
- Obstructive uropathy
- Postoperative complication of organ transplantation
- Postoperative nephropathy
- Renal ischemia
- Renal vein thrombosis
- Sepsis

Ongoing replacement to compensate for persistent losses should be calculated and delivered via appropriate intravascular fluids. Urinary losses can be replaced on a milliliter-for-milliliter basis. Insensible losses should also be taken into account. Meticulous attention to fluid and electrolyte balance is necessary in the management of intrinsic kidney failure. Frequent weights, blood pressure, accurate recording of intake and output, and physical examination findings are important to determine the amount of ongoing therapy.

Caution is needed when severe kidney hypoperfusion is evident, as overly aggressive hydration may lead to fluid overload and pulmonary edema with respiratory compromise (Zappitelli, 2008). Calculating the fractional excretion of sodium may be helpful to guide hydration in simple kidney hypoperfusion versus acute tubular necrosis.

Hyponatremia is often appreciated with volume depletion. Note that children are at risk for seizure activity with a serum sodium level of less than 125 mEq/L. An infusion of hypertonic saline solution should be considered in such patients to lessen this risk (Andreoli, 2008).

Hyperkalemia is a potentially life-threatening electrolyte abnormality associated with both acute and chronic renal failure. Sodium bicarbonate, glucose, insulin, calcium chloride, sodium polystyrene, and albuterol are medications that can reduce the serum potassium level or stabilize the cardiac membrane. Sodium bicarbonate, albuterol, glucose, and insulin all shift potassium into the cells, while sodium polystyrene exchanges sodium for potassium in the colonic mucosa. Emergent dialysis is necessary if the serum potassium level exceeds 6 to 7 mEq/L and electrocardiography (ECG) shows tall, peaked T waves; prolongation of the P-R interval; flattening of P waves; or widening of the QRS complex. Continued hyperkalemia will result in ventricular tachycardia or ventricular fibrillation.

Chronic metabolic acidosis (defined as a bicarbonate level of less than 22 mEq/L) is a result of bicarbonate wasting and retention of acids by the kidney. In chronic kidney disease, it contributes to bone disease by causing the body to release calcium in an attempt to buffer the acidosis. Acidosis also causes a resistance to growth hormone and insulin-like growth factors. Bicarbonate dosing at 2 mEq/kg daily can correct this acidotic state (Miller & MacDonald, 2006).

Hyperphosphatemia is found in both acute and chronic renal failure. The inability of the kidney to excrete phosphorus leads to persistently increasing serum levels. When patients develop this imbalance, oral calcium carbonate should be delivered with meals, to bind the nutritional phosphorus and prevent gastrointestinal absorption. Limiting daily phosphorus intake is also important to decrease the phosphorus retention and its subsequent hyperparathyroidism and renal osteodystrophy. Limiting the potassium intake in daily foods is also necessary until kidney function is restored. In infancy, special formulas with low phosphorus and potassium, such as Similac PM 60/40, are available and should be initiated as soon as possible.

Guidelines for nutrition calories based on age should be strictly adhered to, as anorexia is common and malnutrition can occur rapidly in conjunction with renal failure. Protein malnutrition is common in children with chronic kidney disease due to anorexia and vomiting. Nutrition is particularly important given its major contribution to growth and development (Miller & MacDonald, 2006). According to the CARI guidelines (Voss et al., 2007), the daily intake of protein for children should be more than 0.75 gm/kg ideal body weight. Protein intake of 144% of the World Health Organization recommendations may be necessary for children who are receiving peritoneal dialysis.

Hypertension is common in the setting of renal failure, so blood pressure should be monitored closely. Normal values based on gender and height should be the target goal for all children in kidney failure. Hypertension should be treated with oral agents unless encephalopathy or seizure activity is present, in which case intravenous medications should be started rapidly. ACE inhibitors should be avoided or used cautiously in children with renal failure.

Medications should be adjusted based on the degree of renal failure in both acute and chronic renal failure. Many sources are available to assist the HCP with medication adjustments based on the GFR. *It is important to calculate the GFR. Equally important is to appreciate the percentage rise in the serum creatinine rather than the total level, because even a mild increase in the serum creatinine may indicate a decrease of as much as 50% of kidney function.*

Anemia is a significant problem with a complex array of causes in children with chronic kidney disease (Koshy & Geary, 2008). Despite the fact that it is a common complication, the etiology of the anemia needs to be investigated through measurement of hemoglobin, hematocrit, red blood cell indices, reticulocyte count, and iron parameters, and testing of the stool for occult blood (Miller & MacDonald, 2006). Iron deficiency and erythropoietin (EPO) deficiencies are the leading cause of anemia in CKD patients. However, chronic inflammation, chronic blood loss, vitamin deficiencies, hyperparathyroidism, hemaglobinopathies, and adverse effects of medications may also contribute to anemia. The correction of anemia has been associated with better exercise tolerance, physical performance, school attendance, and improved quality of life (Koshy & Geary).

The iron metabolic pathway is altered in CKD, such that iron delivery to the bone marrow is reduced, leading to anemia. Iron stores quickly become depleted—a deficiency that can be corrected with iron supplementation. Calculation of the serum transferrin saturation (dividing serum iron by total iron-binding capacity and multiplying by 100) provides a good indicator of iron stores (Koshy & Geary, 2008). If the iron stores are low, iron supplementation should be maximized. Iron repletion should begin at the onset of the anemia. Elemental iron should be delivered in doses of 2 to 3 mg/kg (up to 6 mg/kg), with a goal of ferritin level at least 100 ng/mL and a transferrin saturation of 20%. Iron should not be administered with calcium binders, as this combination decreases gastrointestinal absorption of iron.

The lack of EPO in an anemic patient with renal failure reflects the poor renal function and GFR. To correct this deficiency, recombinant EPO should be started at 80 to 120 units/kg weekly by subcutaneous or intravenous injection, with the dose being adjusted to reach a desired hemoglobin level of 11 to 12 gm/dL (Miller & MacDonald, 2006).

Healthy development of a skeletal and vascular system is crucial in the growing child and adolescent. Children with chronic renal failure have a dysregulation of mineral metabolism with subsequent alterations in growth and bone remodeling as well as cardiovascular calcifications that often present early in the course of the illness (Wesseling et al., 2008). Growth retardation has always been a notable finding in children with chronic kidney disease. Malnutrition, persistent metabolic acidosis, end-organ growth hormone resistance, and renal bone disease may all compromise growth. Even with correction of malnutrition and acidosis, children with CKD tend to grow poorly. As kidney disease progresses, growth failure worsens. Growth hormone (rhGH) is recommended if the child has a GFR less than 75 mL/min/1.73 m^2, his or her weight is less than 2 standard deviations below the norm for age, and his or her height is below the 25th percentile for age; no stimulation test for growth hormone is required. The recommended dose of rhGH is 0.05 mg/kg per day, for 6 days per week. Once a child reaches the 50th percentile in height velocity, rhGH dosing should be held. If a reduction in growth velocity occurs, the rhGH therapy may be reinstituted.

Renal osteodystrophy occurs from abnormal interaction of phosphorus, poor calcium absorption, and reduced renal activation of vitamin D (Miller & MacDonald, 2006). In children with CKD, these metabolic events occur early on in the disease. As the GFR declines, these problems become notably worse. The untreated hyperparathyroidism produces bone disease and places the child at risk for fractures and deformities. Treatment of renal osteodystrophy includes the active form of vitamin D supplements, calcium supplements, restriction of dietary phosphorus, and the use of phosphate binders. Although used as the standard of care, calcium-based phosphorus binders have been associated with increased risk of cardiovascular calcifications.

Consultation with the nephrology service is recommended whenever a patient presents with ARF or CKD. The nephrologist may prepare the patient for adjunctive renal support. Invasive renal therapies are designed to maximize kidney function and recovery. Renal replacement therapy by peritoneal dialysis or hemodialysis is an important and effective modality for children with ESRD. Peritoneal dialysis is an efficient and easy way to provide RTT to children. Hemodialysis is the most efficient but obtrusive way to deliver this therapy.

Caregivers of children with CKD have reported a lower quality of life, higher levels of anxiety, and maladaptive behaviors (Tong et al., 2008). Practicing effective communication, listening to caregiver concerns, and providing feedback in a supportive manner are ways that the HCP can help promote a healthier lifestyle for all family members.

DISPOSITION AND DISCHARGE PLANNING

Children with acute renal failure are at higher risk for long-term progressive loss of kidney function (Bunchman, 2008). After resolution of ARF, careful and routine monitoring of blood pressure, serum creatinine levels, and urine for protein should be performed. Families and HCPs need to be alert for early signs of kidney disease, with prompt referral to a specialist.

Families need to be taught about and fully understand the dietary modifications needed to provide a renal-friendly diet. The patient's energy intake should match that of healthy children of the same age. Monitoring of growth is important, and the child may need an adjunct to feeding such as a nasogastric or gastrostomy tube. Fluid restriction parameters need to be provided, and signs of dehydration and methods to prevent dehydration described. Medication administration, the rationale for medication choices, and side effects should be explained. A list of nephrotoxic drugs should be provided to caregivers.

Children with renal disease from urologic or congenital anomalies are at higher risk for infections. Good hand washing, clean technique with urethral catheterizations, prophylactic antimicrobial therapy, and constipation prevention are all effective strategies to reduce the risk of infection. Extensive education should be provided to multiple caregivers regarding peritoneal and hemodialysis. This education should be conducted by a HCP who specializes in renal replacement therapy.

KIDNEY TRANSPLANTATION

Tresa E. Zielinski

INDICATIONS

The recommendation for kidney transplant may be made for patients with either impending or actual kidney failure and is based on the etiology, expected trajectory of disease progression, and comorbidities. The etiology of kidney failure in children is different than that in adults, in that congenital, urologic, and hereditary disorders account for the greater portion of pediatric disease. An evaluation for a kidney transplant may begin when a patient has stage 3 chronic kidney disease (CKD); estimated creatinine clearance rate less than 60 mL/min/1.73m². If circumstances allow, transplantation before the patient requires dialysis

is preferred to avoid comorbidity and increased mortality (Kidney Disease Improving Global Outcomes, 2009).

CONTRAINDICATIONS

The few absolute contraindications to pediatric renal transplantation include malignancy, chronic illness with short life expectancy, and severe brain damage. Kidney transplantation should be delayed if a patient has active disease resulting in renal failure or comorbid infection (Kahan & Ponticelli, 2000; Lapoint Rudow et al., 2006). For some patients with severe developmental delay, multiple organ dysfunction, or poor long-term prognosis, transplantation may not be advisable. In these circumstances, the patient and family should be given options of dialysis, nonescalation of therapy, or withdrawal of care. Although medicine and technology may support the ability to transplant an organ, transplantation may not be in the best interest for all patients. Final decisions to pursue transplantation are made jointly by the patient, family, and healthcare team.

EVALUATION FOR TRANSPLANT

An interprofessional team should care for transplant patients and their families. Members of this team should include specialists from nephrology, transplant surgery, nursing, psychology, social work, nutrition, and a financial coordinator/discharge planner. In addition, child life therapy and spiritual support are essential to help families and patients cope with this emotionally and physically taxing situation.

The evaluation for transplant starts with laboratory studies (Table 31-12) and radiologic imaging, including ultrasound, echocardiogram, and angiograms as indicated (Tajani et al., 2000). ECGs and cardiac catheterizations are

TABLE 31-12

Kidney Transplant Evaluation: Laboratory Testing
• ABO typing (verified twice)
• Human leukocyte antigen (HLA) typing
• Renal function panel
• Complete blood count with differential
• Ionized calcium
• Serum beta$_2$ microglobulin
• Urinalysis (with protein-to-creatinine ratio when indicated)
• Lipids
• Vitamin D profile
• Parathyroid hormone
• Cytomegalovirus immunoglobulins G and M (IgG and IgM)
• Epstein-Barr virus IgG and IgM
• Varicella, measles, mumps, rubella, BK virus IgG
• HIV
• Hepatitis profile and hepatitis B surface antibody
• Preliminary and/or final cross-match

routinely performed in adult kidney failure patients; they are not usually required for pediatric patients.

Evaluation for sensitization, anti-human leukocyte antigen (HLA) antibodies, and panel reactive antibody (PRA) are completed to help determine which donor antigens should be avoided to prevent rejection and to determine the likelihood of matching the patient with an antigenically compatible organ (Tajani et al., 2000). With patients who are highly sensitized (resulting from blood product transfusions, previous transplants, or pregnancies), transplantation can be more difficult and rejection is more common (Jordan et al., 2006; Tajani et al.).

Urinary tract abnormalities should be evaluated and corrected prior to transplantation. Although nephrectomy is rarely required prior to transplant, patients with chronic urinary tract infections or recalcitrant hypertension might benefit from this procedure. Nephrectomies are routinely recommended for patients with Denys-Drash syndrome, as this condition has a high association with Wilms' tumor (Kasiske, 2001). Patients with disorders such as Eagle-Barrett syndrome (prune-belly syndrome), posterior urethral valves (PUV), or neurogenic bladder (e.g., some patients with spina bifida) usually require urodynamic testing to assess bladder fitness. The bladder may need augmentation to provide an adequate urinary reservoir.

A psychosocial evaluation is required by the Centers for Medicare and Medicaid Services (CMS) prior to listing the patient for transplant (HHS, 2007). This evaluation should include, but not be limited to, barriers to transplantation, the family's ability to adhere to post-transplant medical management and follow-up, readiness for transplantation, and any religious, psychosocial, or family preexisting conceptions of transplantation (Lapoint Rudow et al., 2006; Tajani et al., 2000). Coping mechanisms and ability to negotiate adverse outcomes should also be evaluated. Adequate resources must be identified for the family. The transplant team should discuss the patient's prognosis and quality of life both with and without transplant. Transplantation may need to be postponed based on information learned in this discussion so as to help the family prepare for the transplantation or to help the family identify that transplantation is not the best option for their child.

A financial evaluation is performed so that families will have information about their insurance coverage and the additional out-of-pocket expenses to be incurred. If no insurance is available or if out-of-pocket costs are prohibitive, other means of financial support may be identified. Dialysis and kidney transplantation are two of a few instances for which children are qualified for Medicare coverage. Discharge planners, financial planners, or social work team members can help the family apply for coverage under the appropriate Medicare sections (A, B, D). For many patients with insurance, the application to Medicare is mandatory.

DONOR SELECTION

In kidney transplantation, two donor options are possible: living or deceased donors. In most cases, a live donor is preferred unless there is a high suspicion of recurrent disease such as with focal segmental glomerulonephritis (FSGS) or hemolytic uremic syndrome (HUS) (Lapoint Rudow et al., 2006). Due to the highly effective immunosuppressants that are available today, the matching of a kidney is less important and the focus with a live donor is on that person's overall health. Live donors must be at least 18 years of age (age of consent) except in the case of an identical twin donor. In these highly unusual cases, donation may be considered with ethics consultation.

Donation from a deceased patient is common in children. Currently in the United States under the Share 35 allocation policy (HHS, 2008a), organs from deceased donors younger than the age of 35 are preferentially given to children active on the United Network for Organ Sharing (UNOS) waiting list prior to their eighteenth birthday. However, a kidney from a deceased donor may be preferred over that from a living donor if there is significant risk of bad graft or patient outcome (Tajani et al., 2000).

OUTCOMES FOR RECIPIENTS OF ORGANS FROM LIVE VERSUS DECEASED DONORS

Living-donated kidneys have superior graft and patient survival at 1, 5, and 10 years versus organs from deceased donors, most notably with the passing of time (HHS, 2008b). One possible etiology for this difference is the increase in warm and cold ischemic times and the higher rate of acute rejection with deceased donor kidneys.

Graft survival rates at 1 and 5 years for a deceased-donor organ are 91% and 69%, respectively, versus 91% and 86%, respectively, for a living-donated kidney. The survival rates for deceased-donor kidney recipients are 96% at 1 year and 82% at 5 years; the corresponding rates for living-donor kidney recipients are 98% and 91%, respectively. Although these data have been collected largely from adults, the same differences are observed with children and should be discussed with families.

PREPARATION FOR TRANSPLANT

In preparation for transplantation, the goal is to achieve optimal health given the patient's current disease state. This effort includes review of immunization history and attempts to achieve immunity to those viruses that require a live vaccine, such as measles, mumps, rubella, and varicella, prior to initiating immunosuppressive therapy (Lapoint Rudow et al., 2006; Tajani et al., 2000). Time considerations, reimbursement, and disease state should be taken into consideration when trying to achieve pretransplant immunity.

Optimization of physical health by treating the side effects of CKD such as anemia, growth, oral aversion, hypophosphate levels, hyperparathyroidism, and proteinuria should be ongoing prior to transplantation. Good nutrition is essential for healing after surgery and should be optimized at all phases of care. In some patients, parenteral nutrition may be required given the high metabolic requirements of kidney failure or the severe dietary restrictions related to the disorder. Varying degrees of protein, phosphorus, potassium, and sodium restriction are common prior to transplantation. Patients' dietary restrictions should be personalized to their biochemical deficiencies. Sodium restriction is the *only* absolute requirement and should be considered part of a heart-healthy diet, rather than simply a restriction. Patients should take in no more than 2 grams of sodium per day.

For a child to be listed for a deceased-donor transplant, two separate ABO blood type samples and HLA typing must first be verified (HHS, 2007). A PRA and serum sample are then sent each month to the Organ Procurement Organization (OPO). It is not uncommon to list the patient for a deceased-donor organ while continuing to investigate live-donor options. When an organ becomes available, a cross-match is performed by mixing the recipient's serum with the donor's cells. A negative cross-match is desired, as it indicates that an accelerated acute rejection episode is unlikely (Kasiske, 2001).

With a live-donor kidney transplant, two samples to identify blood type must be verified, and a PRA is explored to help determine which antigens may need to be avoided (Jordan et al., 2006; Tajani et al., 2000). An initial cross-match occurs prior to full evaluation of a donor, after verification of compatibility with the donor's blood type. If the cross-match is negative, a team dedicated to donor evaluation completes a full assessment to ensure that there is no conflict of interest. If the donor passes the evaluation, a final cross-match is performed to verify the negative results prior to scheduling the transplant.

Regardless of whether the transplant comes from a deceased or live donor, the recipient requires immunosuppressive agents to prevent rejection after transplantation (except for identical-twin transplant). For many patients, this therapy may begin just prior to the operation. Induction therapy, provided intraoperatively, may include interleukin-2 (IL-2) receptor inhibitors such as basiliximab (Simulect) or daclizumab (Zenapax). Thymoglobulin, alemtuzumab (Campath), and rituximab (Rituxan) may be used for induction in highly sensitized patients, ABO-incompatible donors, and patients who have undergone prior transplants (Jordan et al., 2006; Montgomery, 2010). Induction therapy also includes an abbreviated course of IV steroids. Steroids may be required in some patients with a history of systemic disease that led to failure of their native kidneys. These patients will require steroids as part of maintenance therapy, because prior disease increases the risk of rejection.

As an integral part of maintenance therapy, calcineurin inhibitors are the mainstay of immunosuppressive protocols. Their administration is usually accompanied by use of a second agent such as an antiproliferative agent (mycophenolate mofitil) or a mTOR inhibitor (Rapamune) (Tredger et al., 2006). Calcineurin inhibitors are nephrotoxic, so their levels should be monitored closely. Other side effects of immunosuppressive agents include leucopenia, thrombocytopenia, and anemia. Each agent should be watched closely based on its side-effect profile and doses adjusted or complications treated as necessary.

POSTOPERATIVE CARE

On the day of transplant, the patient's blood pressure must be monitored closely. In many cases, the donor is an adult and the kidney is preconditioned to higher perfusion pressures. Under those circumstances, the pediatric patient's blood pressure should be titrated up using volume, whenever possible, to maintain a central venous pressure (CVP) between 8 and 10 mmHg. If fluid overload or pulmonary edema becomes a concern, judicious use of inotropic support may be required, as vasoconstrictive therapy increases the risk for graft clotting at the anastamosis. The goal for the first 24 hours is to maintain euvolemia. All fluid removed or voided must be replaced to maintain hemodynamics. It is common for patients to develop high-output kidney failure in the immediate postoperative period, and the patient can quickly become unstable if the fluid balance is not closely monitored (Lapoint Rudow et al., 2006). Conversely, a patient may be anuric, requiring that only insensible losses be replaced. Accurate intake and output are critical in the first few hours to days post transplant.

Body weight measurement is vital for the child with kidney disease and remains so after a transplant. The weight is used in conjunction with the blood pressure, CVP, and pain assessment to appropriately assess and manage hypertension or hypotension.

Immediate postoperative labs include a renal function panel, CBC with differential, ionized calcium, serum beta$_2$ microglobulin, and ABG. Clotting times should be obtained if indicated. Basic chemistries and ionized calcium should be repeated every 4 to 8 hours as indicated and daily CBCs followed.

The length of stay following kidney transplant is brief. Most patients who receive transplants are discharged within a week; thus patient and family teaching should begin immediately regarding medications, indications, and dosing plans. Health maintenance with daily weights and every-12-hour blood pressure measurements and temperatures should be reviewed for discharge planning.

Poor initial graft function is noted more commonly with deceased-donor transplants. This problem can be an indication of acute tubular nephritis (ATN) with poor blood pressure control, whether hypertensive or hypotensive. Doppler ultrasound can be helpful in evaluating perfusion and obstruction. Dialysis may be required in the first few weeks post transplant, but is commonly a temporary adjunct in transplant recipients. It is more likely to be needed with a deceased-donor transplant (HHS, 2008a; Lapoint Rudow et al., 2006).

TRANSPLANT REJECTION

Rejection must always be considered in the differential diagnosis for patients after kidney transplant regardless of the problem. The presentation of rejection varies, but may include hypertension, proteinuria, oliguria, fever, or nonfunction. Definitive diagnosis of this condition is made by kidney biopsy.

Rejection is graded based on the Banff criteria, a histologic classification scheme that describes the type and severity of immune-mediated damage of the transplanted kidney. Generally, rejection can be categorized as cellular or vascular. *Vascular rejection* usually has poorer outcomes and arises from antibody-mediated damage to the endothelium. *Cellular rejection* is due to lymphocytic invasion into the tubular epithelium; it usually responds to high-dose steroids and occasionally thymoglobulin. Vascular rejection, which can result in irreversible damage despite treatment, often requires aggressive means to remove offending antibodies and/or B cells (e.g., IVIG, plasmapheresis, and rituximab). Table 31-13 outlines the timing, cause, treatment, histology,

TABLE 31-13

Kidney Transplant Rejection	
Hyperacute	
Timing	Minutes to hours after transplant/revascularization; after the blood flow has been restored to the transplanted kidney
Cause	Presence of preformed antibodies against donor antigen(s) present on the epithelium
Treatment	*Not* amenable to pharmacologic intervention
Histology	Glomerular and vascular thrombosis; antibody, platelet, and fibrin deposits
Signs and symptoms	Necrosis after reperfusion in the operating room; organ death
Accelerated, Acute	
Timing	3–5 days
Cause	Disruption of the vascular layer and interstitial hemorrhage; kidney is grossly tense due to hemorrhage; possible parenchymal tears associated with pain, tenderness, and swelling; possible life-threatening hemorrhage
Treatment	Polyclonal antilymphocyte antibodies that bind to and remove lymphocytes that are causing graft injury; plasmapheresis can remove the antidonor antibodies; pharmacotherapy with cyclophosphamide may dampen antibody production

TABLE 31-13

Kidney Transplant Rejection *(Continued)*	
Accelerated, Acute *(Continued)*	
Histology	Cellular and humoral rejection plus hemorrhage
Signs and symptoms	After initial decrease in serum creatinine, a plateau or rise; oliguria, hypertension, edema, proteinuria
Acute	
Cellular	
Timing	5–90 days
Cause	Initiated by alloantigen-specific T cells
Treatment	If mild, steroid bolus for 3 days; if moderate to severe, may also require antilymphocyte antibodies (thymoglobulin, ATGAM, OKT3)
Histology	Lymphocyte infiltrates; tubulitis—lymphocyte infiltrates below the tubular basement membrane with arteritis/endothelialitis if moderate to severe
Signs and symptoms	Rise in serum creatinine; oliguria, hypertension, edema, proteinuria
Humoral	
Timing	5–30 days
Cause	Antibody mediated
Treatment	Usually refractory to steroid therapy alone; see the treatment for accelerated, acute rejection; may respond to rituximab (anti-CD 20 monoclonal antibody)
Histology	Endothelialitis (arteritis)
Signs and Symptoms	Oliguria
Chronic	
Timing	More than 60 days
Cause	Transforming growth factor-beta (TGF-ß); may be related to previous episodes of acute rejection, although it can be seen on biopsy in patients who have never experienced any episodes of acute rejection, especially if intermittent medication noncompliance has been problematic
Treatment	May be amenable to treatment with antiproliferative agents such as rapamycin
Histology	Vascular smooth-muscle cell proliferation; obliterative intimal fibrosis of arteries (transplant arteriopathy); duplication of glomerular basement membranes (chronic transplant glomerulopathy); the hallmark is tubular atrophy
Signs and symptoms	Gradual decrease in renal function, hypertension, proteinuria, and edema

and signs and symptoms of the various types of rejection. Table 31-14 provides an example of a recommended rejection protocol; however, each patient must be considered individually.

TABLE 31-14

Protocol for Treatment of Biopsy-Proven Acute Kidney Transplant Rejection Based on Banff 97 Diagnostic Criteria

Ia: 3- to 5-day pulse methylprednisolone 10 mg/kg (not to exceed 500 mg) IV q day

Ib: 3- to 5-day pulse methylprednisolone 10 mg/kg (not to exceed 500 mg) IV q day plus
7–10 days of thymoglobulin IV based on response

First dose:
1. Methylprednisolone 10 mg/kg IV over 60 minutes
2. Tylenol 325–650 mg PO
3. Benadryl 1 mg/kg PO or IV
4. Thymoglobulin 1.5 mg/kg IV into a central vein over 6 hours; start 1 hour after steroids completed

Second dose:
1. Same
2. Same
3. May omit if no reaction to first dose of thymoglobulin
4. Thymoglobulin 1.5 mg/kg IV into a central vein over 4 hours

Third and subsequent doses:
1. Optional
2. Omit
3. Omit
4. Thymoglobulin 1.5 mg/kg IV into a central vein over 4 hours

A course of thymoglobulin is 7–10 doses, with the dose adjusted downward for leukopenia or thrombocytopenia:

ANC > 2,000	100% full dose
1,500–2,000	75% full dose
1,000–1,500	50% full dose
500–1,000	25% full dose

Thymoglobulin is packaged in 25-mg vials and is very expensive; try to order to the nearest number divisible by 25.

IIa: Same as Ib plus start oral prednisone 1 mg/kg PO daily (dose not to exceed 30 mg/day)

IIb: Same as IIb plus start oral prednisone 1 mg/kg PO BID

III: Same as IIb

C4d (+) staining of peritubular capillaries: start weekly rituximab 375 mg/m² and send HLA antibody-specific titers to donor antigens and any other antigens to which the patient may be sensitized.

Consider plasmapheresis if titers are high or not responding to rituximab.

This protocol should be used as a guideline only and may be altered at the discretion of the kidney transplant team.

Note: Intravenous (IV), by mouth (PO), twice daily (BID).

NEPHROLITHIASIS

Bonnie Kitchen

PATHOPHYSIOLOGY

Nephrolithiasis is a complex interaction of heredity, physical processes, and the environment. The event in stone formation is supersaturation, where the urinary solute exceeds its solubility product and crystallization of solutes occurs. When a solute is added to a solvent, it dissolves until an equilibrium status is achieved and no further dissolution takes place. In normal urine, naturally occurring inhibitors prevent the supersaturation point from being reached. In some instances, specific stone-forming substances are present and act as a complexor, an inhibitor, or both. Urinary solutes can exceed equilibrium and the solvent can become saturated. Crystallization then occurs and a stone is initiated. After initiation, growth of the stone is encouraged by the nuclei that are exposed to other crystals, cells, or casts, which results in crystal aggregation.

Supersaturation of lithogenic ions and crystallization of compounds in the urine are the major factors driving stone formation. Other factors that influence stone formation include urinary volume, pH, and urinary ions that act as promoters or inhibitors of lithogenesis.

EPIDEMIOLOGY AND ETIOLOGY

Nephrolithiasis is an uncommon disease in the pediatric population; however, its incidence has been increasing in the last few decades (Mohkam et al., 2007)—a trend that may be attributed to changes in dietary habits and the sedentary lifestyle seen in the past century (Reddy et al., 2005). The incidence of pediatric stone disease varies geographically. In the United States, it ranges from 1 patient in 1,000 hospital admissions to 1 patient in 7,600 hospital admissions (Nicoletta & Lande, 2006). Children older than 10 years of age have a 109 per 100,000 incidence rate (Mohkam et al.). The overall incidence could conceivably be higher, as the rates reported include only hospitalized children. This incidence rate is not nationally standardized, with populations in the southeastern United States and southern California having a higher incidence than populations in other parts of the country. Internationally, countries such as Turkey, Pakistan, Thailand, South Asia, South Africa, and some parts of South America report a prevalence as high as 0.8% (Dogan & Tekgul, 2007). In Europe, the reported incidence ranges from 0.13 to 0.94 case per 1,000 hospitalizations. Bladder stones occur in fewer than 10% of pediatric cases of nephrocalcinosis and are associated with urinary tract anomalies (Nicoletta & Lande).

In the pediatric population, Caucasians have a higher incidence of stone formation as compared to African

Americans and Asians. Although some debate persists, the majority of the literature describes boys and girls as being equally affected (Dogan & Tekgul, 2007). The mean age at presentation is 5.2 years for boys and 6.9 years for girls (Reddy et al., 2005). Children who require a ketogenic diet for seizure management have a nephrolithiasis occurrence rate of 5% to 7% (Vining, 2008).

Nephrolithiasis has traditionally been predominantly infectious in nature; however, in recent years, metabolic causes have emerged as the predominant factor in stone formation (Cameron et al., 2005). Seventy-five percent of children with nephrolithiasis have a predisposition to stone formation. More than 50% of patients have an identifiable metabolic risk factor (Nicoletta & Lande, 2006). Urinary tract anomalies account for 32% of patients, and 4% are infectious in nature. Often, children with stone formation have more than one predisposing factor, and structural, metabolic, and infectious factors may coexist (Davis & Avner, 2007c).

Types of stones

Hypercalciuria is the most common metabolic factor for the formation of stones in children in Western society (Schwaderer et al., 2008), accounting for 50% to 97% of children with identified metabolic pathologies (Cameron et al., 2005) and 53% to 81% of children with calcium stones. Hypercalciuria is defined as a calcium excretion of more than 4 mg/kg/day (5 mg/kg/day in infants) or a urinary calcium-to-creatinine ratio greater than 0.21:1. These measurements may vary according to age and ethnicity; for example, African Americans are less affected than Caucasian children, as they have a lower calcium excretion. Children with Beckwith-Wiedemann syndrome and cystic fibrosis have a higher prevalence of hypercalciuria. Urine volume and urine citrate content can also alter the stone formation.

Supersaturation measurements of calcium oxalate and phosphate should be performed to assess the propensity for forming stones. Children with a history of calcium oxalate stones generally secrete a higher fraction of dietary calcium in their urine. Twenty percent of children with hypercalciuria without nephrolithiasis will develop stones within 5 years.

Hypercalciuria occurs due to disturbances in one or more of three organ systems: increased gastrointestinal calcium absorption, imbalance of bone formation and reabsorption, or renal losses (Cameron et al., 2005). Absorptive hypercalciuria is the most common cause of excessive urinary calcium. With this condition, overly aggressive vitamin D supplementation or excessive ingestion of calcium-containing foods leads to increased intestinal absorption of calcium. Increased intestinal absorption causes a corresponding increase in serum calcium level and a subsequent decrease in serum parathyroid hormone level. Three types of absorptive hypercalciuria are known:

- Type I occurs without calcium load. It is uncommon and is the most severe form of absorptive hypercalciuria.
- Type II occurs with a high calcium intake orally, and is the most common form of absorptive hypercalciuria.
- Type III is rare and is characterized by an underlying kidney defect that causes excessive urinary phosphate excretion causing hypophosphatemia. The low serum phosphate levels stimulate vitamin D, which then increases calcium and phosphate absorption in the intestines. The absorbed calcium is excreted in the urine, causing the hypercalciuria.

Hyperoxaluria accounts for fewer than 2% to 3% of children with stone disease (Santos-Victoriano et al., 1998). Oxalate is an end product of normal metabolism and is excreted through the kidneys. Primary hyperoxaluria has three different presentations characterized by: (1) a rare infantile form with early nephrocalcinosis and rapid kidney failure; (2) a rare late onset form with occasional stone passage in late adulthood; and (3) the most common form with recurrent stone formation and progression to kidney failure (Cochat & Basmaison, 2000).

In type 1 (an autosomal recessive disorder), the liver has decreased alanine glyoxylate aminotransferase activity and allows the accumulation of glyoxylate. Glyoxylate is metabolized to oxalate and glycolate. The filtered oxalate may then either form calculi in the lumens of the kidneys or result in parenchymal precipitation of oxalate, which may produce kidney damage and failure (Cameron et al., 2005). Recurrent stones, nephrocalcinosis, renal insufficiency, and deposition of oxalate in the liver, eyes, and bone marrow are the characteristics of type 1 hyperoxaluria. The incidence rate for this form is 0.12 per 10 million children per year, with approximately 50% of affected children being diagnosed prior to 10 years of age. End-stage renal disease occurs in 50% of these individuals before the age of 25 years (Cochat & Basmaison, 2000).

Type 2 primary hyperoxaluria is a rare condition in which there is a deficiency of glyoxylate reductase; it typically causes nephrolithiasis only. Hyperoxaluria may also be the result of increased intestinal absorption secondary to bowel disease. In this situation, calcium in the intestines binds with oxalate, and both are excreted. Malabsorptive conditions increase the fatty acids in the lumen; these increased fatty acids then complex with calcium, and excess oxalate is absorbed. Ingestion of foods with a high oxalate content and ingestion of increased amounts of ascorbic acid are other causes of hyperoxaluria (Cameron et al., 2005).

Hyperuricosuria is found in 10% to 20% of children with a metabolic cause for nephrolithiasis. Uric acid is a weak acid that has a propensity to form stones in an acidic urine. Uric acid enhances calcium oxalate precipitation by lowering the solubility of this compound (Cameron et al., 2005). Idiopathic hyperuricosuria has a familial tendency and follows an autosominal dominant pattern. Children of

Italian or Jewish descent are more commonly affected and tend to have a more severe form of the disease (Nicoletta & Lande, 2006). Uric acid may result from an inborn error of metabolism—specifically, an error in purine metabolism.

PRESENTATION

Nephrolithiasis in the pediatric population is significantly different from the corresponding condition in adults. The evaluation for any child with suspected nephrolithiasis should start with a complete and thorough history. A detailed nutritional history should include food preferences; diets with large amounts of chocolate, nuts, strawberries, and vitamin supplements; special diets such as the ketogenic diet; and daily fluid intake. A medication history should include previously used as well as currently used medications, chemotherapeutic agents, over-the-counter medications, and traditional or cultural remedies. The medical history should include prematurity, previous urologic conditions and procedures, recent immobilization, recent surgery, recent trauma, and other clinical disorders such as previous urinary tract infection (UTI). The family history may indicate nephrolithiasis. Twenty percent to 50% of patients have a family history of stone disease. Family history should also include first-degree relatives with arthritis, gout, and renal diseases.

The physical examination should include careful attention to blood pressure, height, and weight, as these measurements can be abnormal in kidney diseases. The classic presentation of debilitating flank pain is less common in pediatric patients; 94% of affected adolescents have flank pain, whereas children age 0 to 5 do not (Nicoletta & Lande, 2006). Pain is the most common clinical symptom; it is typically described as nonspecific, dull, or sharp, and can be reported as abdominal pain or flank pain. Pain can be stationary, or it can radiate to the scrotum or labia with obstruction from a calculus. In children with a single kidney, oliguria or anuria may be seen due to an obstruction. Pediatric patients with bladder stones are often asymptomatic. Gross or microscopic hematuria may also be a primary presenting symptom, occurring in 30% to 90% of children with stone disease (Santos-Victoriano et al., 1998). Urinary tract infection with or without urgency, dysuria, frequency, and incontinence are seen in 20% to 50% of children with nephrolithiasis. Infants may present with colic-like symptoms; intermittent crying, poor feeding, irritability, and abdominal pain.

DIFFERENTIAL DIAGNOSIS

The differential diagnoses for abdominal or flank pain comprise a broad group, including surgical emergencies such as appendicitis, ovarian torsion, and ectopic pregnancy. Other diagnoses to consider are urinary tract infection, pancreatitis, and pyelonephritis.

PLAN OF CARE

A urinalysis in imperative in suspected nephrolithiasis, as it provides valuable information for making the diagnosis. The urinalysis should include the pH, microscopic evaluation for blood, white blood cells, and casts. A urine culture should be obtained to evaluate for acute or chronic urinary tract infection. Serum electrolytes, BUN, and serum creatinine are obtained to evaluate kidney function. A CBC is helpful in providing additional support for an infectious process (leukocytosis) or a chronic process (anemia). Additional laboratory studies include calcium, phosphorus, magnesium, and parathyroid hormone (PTH) levels to help determine the type of stone.

A 24-hour urine collection is important to evaluate the patient for other metabolic abnormalities as well as to measure volume and test pH, calcium, uric acid, creatinine, sodium, oxalate, citrate, and cystine levels. In younger children, a 24-hour sample may be difficult to obtain, and standards based on a single specimen have not been developed. Given that hypercalciuria is the most common pathology of kidney stones, the calcium excretion rate is an important measurement. An excellent screening test for this purpose is the calcium-to-creatinine ratio on a spot urine check. The normal ratio in children is less than 0.2 (Dogan & Tekgul, 2007). If the calcium-to-creatinine ratio is elevated, it should be measured monthly for 2 months.

The complete 24-hour urine evaluation is best performed 6 weeks after the passage of the stone. A metabolic evaluation should be performed on all pediatric patients after a first episode of nephrolithiasis, as more than 40% of children have an identifiable predisposition toward this disease. This study should be performed while the child is at home on a normal diet and free of infection (Gillespie & Stapleton, 2004).

If the stone is recovered, it should be sent to a laboratory that can evaluate its chemical analysis (Santos-Victoriano et al., 1998). Calcium oxalate stones account for 45% to 65% of pediatric stone disease; calcium phosphate account for 14% to 30%; and uric acid, struvite, and cystine stones account for 5% to 10% (Cameron et al., 2005).

During the acute phase of care, an abdominal flat plate radiograph may allow for visualization of calcium and uric acid stones, as they are radiolucent. Approximately 90% of urinary calculi are calcified to some degree. Intravenous pyelography has been replaced by ultrasonography. Ultrasound has been shown to be as accurate in diagnosing stones as plain films without the use of radiation and contrast agents. In particular, ultrasonography is helpful to reveal nephrolithiasis and associated obstruction or nephrocalcinosis (Gillespie & Stapleton, 2004). The study of choice is the helical CT scan, which has 96% to 98% sensitivity and specificity and does not require contrast. CT imaging has a greater potential to identify small stones and ureteral stones, detect obstruction, and evaluate for hydronephrosis; it can also identify alternative diagnoses when a stone is not found to be present (Nicoletta & Lande, 2006).

The initial medical management is directed at hydration, pain control, and treatment of concurrent infection (Santos-Victoriano et al., 1998). Increased fluid intake consisting of 1.5 to 2 times the maintenance requirements is the initial therapy for all types of stones. Increasing the daily fluid requirements dilutes stone-forming compounds, making them less likely to precipitate. This increased fluid intake increases the output by 2 to 3 times normal or more than 2 liters per day in adolescents, thereby promoting stone passage. Stones ranging from 2 to 6 mm have spontaneously passed in young children. This process is painful, and patients may require narcotic analgesia.

Hypercalciuria

Children with hypercalciuria should have an increased fluid intake on a lifelong basis, not just in the initial management of nephrolithiasis. The oral intake goal should be at least the required daily maintenance fluids (Santos-Victoriano et al., 1998) to promote urinary flow (Dogan & Tekgul, 2007). Carbonated beverages should be avoided and are not appropriate oral fluids.

Reducing dietary sodium and calcium to the recommended daily allowance is first-line management for hypercalciuria (Nicoletta & Lande, 2006). Dietary sodium restriction may help to reduce urinary calcium losses. Calcium should not be restricted to less than the daily-recommended allowance for adequate bone and growth, however. Because children with hypercalciuria tend to have a lower bone density, they should be monitored for this condition periodically (Schwaderer et al., 2008).

High protein consumption increases endogenous acid production, which leads to metabolic acidosis, which increases calcium reabsorption of the bone, which in turn increases urinary calcium excretion (Gillespie & Stapleton, 2004; Nicoletta & Lande., 2006). Children should still receive 100% of the daily recommended dietary allowance of protein for maximal growth and development.

Vitamin C and D supplements should be avoided and consumption of citrus juices should be limited, as they are converted into oxalate in the body. Potassium depletion can increase urinary excretion of calcium, so efforts to increase dietary potassium should be made. Potassium supplements may be necessary if the child is receiving diuretic therapy (Santos-Victoriano et al., 1998). A low oxalate diet (40–50 mg per day) may be beneficial, as most stones are made up of calcium oxalate.

Thiazide diuretics—chlorothiazide or hydrochlorothiazide—may be administered to decrease urinary calcium excretion (Gillespie et al., 2004). These diuretics stimulate calcium reabsorption in the distal tubules, thereby decreasing urinary calcium excretion. one adverse side effect of these medications is hypokalemia, which needs to be avoided.

Children with nephrolithiasis who are on a ketogenic diet for seizure control should be followed by an interprofessional team to manage these dietary restrictions.

Hyperoxaluria

Treatment for hyperoxaluria is complex and difficult, and should be followed by a nephrologist. Treatment includes high fluid intake as well as calcium oxalate crystallization inhibitor and pyridoxine as soon as the diagnosis is made (Cochat & Basmaison, 2000). Calcium oxalate crystallization inhibitors—potassium citrate or sodium citrate—are dosed at 100 to 150 mg/kg/day. Ten percent to 40% of children receiving pyridoxine are sensitive to the effects; thus treatment should begin at 3 mg/kg/day, with gradual increases to 15 mg/kg/day. Restricting consumption of foods with a high oxalate content has minimal effects on the disease; however, avoiding high-oxalate foods is still recommended (Gillespie et al., 2004). Calcium should not be restricted, as this limitation can further decrease calcium in the intestines by increasing calcium absorption. Vitamin C and D supplements should be avoided, as these substances are metabolized to oxalate (Nicoletta & Lande, 2006).

Dialysis is unsuitable for hyperoxylaturia, as it cannot sufficiently clear such large amounts of oxalate. Combined liver–kidney transplantation remains the only definitive treatment.

Medications may be associated with nephrolithiasis. A study by Mohkam et al. (2007) suggested that ceftriaxone may cause nephrolithiasis. Furosemide has also been associated with kidney stone formation in patients, especially in preterm infants. Other medications associated with nephrolithiasis include steroids, chemotherapeutic agents, protease inhibitors, supplemental vitamin D, enteral formulas, and parenteral nutrition high in calcium (Reddy et al., 2005). In any children receiving these medications and formulas, consideration of their hydration status is imperative.

Operative intervention for nephrolithiasis is at the discretion of the nephrologist and urologist, the patient, and the family. The most commonly performed treatment for kidney stone removal is extracorporeal shock wave lithotripsy (ESWL). With this technology, ultrasonic waves are focused on the stone, which breaks into tiny particles that can be passed more readily, and with less pain, in the urine. Holmium laser lithotripsy relies on pulse laser light, which is focused on the stone and breaks it into smaller fragments so that they may be passed painlessly through the urine.

Ureteroscopy (URS) may be indicated for patients with significant obstruction. In this procedure, the stone is broken or removed using instrumentation passed through an ureteroscope. A stent is placed temporarily to hold the ureter open for healing or until the stone has been passed. URS is often preferable to ESWL for stones in the mid- and lower ureter.

Consultation with the nephrology and/or urology service is suggested so that the patient and family may receive follow-up care on an outpatient basis. Specific diet, medications, and home care management are best planned with the nephrologist and the nutritionist.

Patient and family education should include information about the diagnosis and the plan of care. Instructions on diet and medications should be provided in both written and verbal formats. Teaching is directed toward signs and symptoms of obstruction as well as pain escalation, and patients and families are informed when they should seek treatment.

DISPOSITION AND DISCHARGE PLANNING

In a study by Schwarz and Dwyer (2006), children with stones had a 36% recurrence rate in the initial follow-up and a 29% recurrence rate at the 9-year contact. Families should be knowledgeable about the symptoms of future stones. Patients should follow up with their PCP and nephrology and/or urology specialists as indicated.

NEPHROTIC SYNDROME

Andrea Lynne Parker

PATHOPHYSIOLOGY

Nephrotic syndrome (NS) is a kidney filtration disorder wherein too much protein is filtered out of the blood. This phenomenon results in proteinuria, edema due to shifts in oncotic pressure from hypoalbuminemia, and hyperlipidemia.

Within each glomeruli of the kidney there are basement membrane epitheal cells called podocytes, which have foot processes that interlock. These interlocking foot processes create the 40-nm space known as the glomerular slit diaphragm. The glomerular slit diaphragm, along with the fenestrated endothelium and basement membrane, acts as a site of filtration within the glomerulus. Healthy podocytes contain negatively charged proteins, such as podocalyxin, podoplanin, and podoendin, which help to repel negatively charged proteins, such as albumin, thereby preventing filtration of protein (Lane & Kaskel, 2009). Proteins give the podocyte its structure and keep them from adhering to each other (Lane & Kaskel).

In patients with NS, the podocyte foot processes are missing, fused together, or damaged. Injury to the podocyte causes disruption of its negatively charged proteins, which collapses the podocyte structure, causes inability to maintain necessary spacing between podocytes, and disables the negatively changed protein barrier (Lane & Kaskel, 2009). Negatively charged proteins are then free to move across the filtration membrane into the urine. The level of protein in the urine is often directly correlated with the severity of podocyte malfunction or injury (Baum, 2008).

Edema occurs when plasma oncotic pressure drops due to the loss of circulating albumin, causing fluid to shift into the interstitial space, which further depletes intravascular volume. This fluid shift stimulates the rennin–angiotensin–aldosterone cycle to retain more sodium and thus more water. Hyperlipidemia results from two metabolic processes: (1) increased synthesis of lipoproteins in the liver in response to intravascular protein loss and (2) decreased lipid catabolism in response to a loss of lipoprotein lipase, an enzyme necessary for lipid breakdown.

EPIDEMIOLOGY AND ETIOLOGY

The etiology of NS is unknown. Although it may be caused by an underlying glomerular disorder, the vast majority (90%) of affected children have idiopathic nephrotic syndrome (INS) (Davis & Avner, 2007b). Preexisting conditions that can trigger INS, along with differential diagnoses, are listed in Table 31-15.

TABLE 31-15

Causes of Childhood Nephrotic Syndrome
Genetic Disorders
Nephrotic Syndrome Typical
Finnish-type congenital nephritic syndrome
Focal segmental glomerulosclerosis
Diffuse mesangial sclerosis
Denys-Drash syndrome
Schimke immuno-osseous dysplasia
Proteinuria with or without Nephrotic Syndrome
Nail-patella syndrome
Alport syndrome
Multisystem Syndromes with or without Nephrotic Syndrome
Galloway-Mowat syndrome
Charcot-Marie-Tooth disease
Jeune syndrome
Cockayne syndrome
Laurence-Moon-Biedl-Bardet syndrome
Metabolic Disorders with or without Nephrotic Syndrome
Alagille syndrome
α_1-Antitryspin deficiency
Fabry disease
Glutaric academia
Glycogen storage disease
Hurler syndrome
Lipoprotein disorders
Mitochondrial disorders
Sickle cell disease

(Continued)

TABLE 31-15

Causes of Childhood Nephrotic Syndrome *(Continued)*

Idiopathic Nephrotic Syndrome

Minimal change disease
Focal segmental glomerulosclerosis
Membranoproliferative glomerulonephritis
Membranous nephropathy

Secondary Causes

Infections

Hepatitis B and C
HIV-I
Malaria
Syphilis
Toxoplasmosis
Parvovirus B19

Drugs

Penicillamine
Gold
Nonsteroidal anti-inflammatory drugs
Pamidronate
Interferon
Mercury
Heroin
Lithium

Immunologic or Allergic Disorders

T-cell or cytokine dysfunction
Systemic lupus erythamatosus
Henoch-Schönlein purpura
Type I diabetes mellitus
Amyloidosis
Castleman disease
Kimura disease
Bee sting
Food allergens

Associated with Malignant Disease

Lymphoma
Leukemia

Glomerular Hyperfiltration

Oligomeganephronia
Morbid obesity
Adaption to nephron reduction

INS is further categorized as either minimal change NS (MCNS—occurring 60% to 85% of affected children), focal segmental glomerulosclerosis (FSGS), mesangial proliferative, membranoproliferative glomerulonephritis, and membranous nephropathy (Del Rio & Kaskel, 2008). These differentiations and diagnoses are made through renal biopsy.

Although NS may present at any age, congenital nephrotic syndrome (CNS) presents within the first 3 months of life, is caused by specific genetic defects, and requires kidney transplantation (Jalanko). NS presenting within months 4 to 12 of life is considered infantile NS; NS presenting after a child reaches 1 year of age is classified as childhood NS (Jalanko). Occurrence of NS is most common while children are between 2 and 8 years of age (Copelovitch, 2008).

NS is a disease process that primarily affects the pediatric population; children are 15 times more likely to develop NS than adults. The reported incidence is 2 to 3 patients per 100,000 children per year (Davis & Avner). According to Gipson et al. (2009). NS prevalence is 16 patients per 100,000 children. Males are nearly twice as likely to develop NS as females (Davis & Avner). Children of Asian, Arabian, Indian, and African American descent have a higher incidence of idiopathic NS than children of European descent (McKinney et al., 2001). African American and Hispanic children have a higher risk of steroid-resistant NS and FSGS (Eddy & Symons, 2003).

NS generally falls into two treatment categories: (1) steroid-sensitive nephritic syndrome (SSNS), which goes into remission after initial treatment with steroids, and (2) steroid-resistant nephritic syndrome (SRNS), which does not go into remission after the initial course of steroids. Although NS is considered to be a relapsing/remitting disease process, 95% of pediatric patients presenting with NS achieve remission after initial treatment (Gipson et al., 2009). Common childhood illnesses and infections may trigger a relapse, at which point steroid treatment is reinitiated.

Research continues into the etiology of NS. Currently, investigators are focusing on immune system dysfunction such as disordered T-cell regulation and allergic reactions, given that NS is responsive to immunosuppressive therapy and patients generally have high levels of IgE (Lane & Kaskel, 2009). Mutations of the *NPHS1* and *NPHS2* (podocin) and *WT1* genes have been found in cases of steroid-resistant NS (Davis & Avner, 2007b; Hodson & Alexander, 2008). The mutation of structural podocyte-associated proteins such as nephrin, podocin, and alpha-actinin-4 as well as the CD2AP gene have been linked to steroid-resistant NS that has progressed to focal segmental glomerulosclerosis (Del Rio & Kaskel, 2008). Researchers theorize that NS may be caused by a specific factor (possibly a cytokine) that alters permeability and filtration; such a factor may potentially be the link between immune system dysfunction and podocyte injury leading to proteinuria (Lane & Kaskel).

PRESENTATION

Patients typically present to a PCP or health care center with a chief complaint of edema—most notably, periorbital edema. This sign may often be confused with an allergic process that is unresponsive to initial allergy management. Further care is usually sought out when patients progress to more generalized edema, especially of dependent structures, such as the scrotum, feet, and abdomen. Urine is described as frothy or foamy.

Additional signs and symptoms may include sudden increase in weight secondary to interstitial fluid shifts and water retention. A complete set of vital signs may reveal hypertension. Due to low serum albumin, ascites, and an impaired immune system, patients with NS are at higher risk of spontaneous bacterial peritonitis and may present with fever, severe abdominal pain, peritoneal signs, and possible sepsis (Gipson et al., 2009). *Streptococcus pneumoniae* and Gram-negative organisms are the mostly likely causes of bacterial peritonitis in children with NS (Gipson et al.).

DIFFERENTIAL DIAGNOSIS

The differential diagnosis for NS includes conditions that may cause generalized edema, such as congestive heart failure and acute kidney failure (see Table 31-15).

PLAN OF CARE

A urine dipstick is the quickest way to determine if there is gross proteinuria in the urine; however, this test does not provide a measurement of the amount of protein lost. The 24-hour urine collection remains the study of choice for determining loss of protein. Protein loss consistent with NS is considered to be at least 4 gm/day in older children and adults and 40 mg/m²/hr or 50 mg/kg/day in young children (Baum, 2008). Given that a 24-hour urine collection may be difficult to obtain in a young child, checking the protein-to-creatinine ratio (Pr/Cr) of the first morning urine is often used to estimate protein excretion. Normal levels are less than 0.2 mg protein/1 mg creatinine in children older than 2 years of age, and less than 0.5 mg protein/1 mg creatinine in children age 6 months to 2 years (Hogg et al., 2000). While a Pr/Cr ratio of 2 or more is consistent with NS (Quigley, 2008), any child with an abnormal urinalysis and elevated Pr/Cr ratio needs further evaluation (Hogg et al.).

The evaluation of proteinuria includes a complete history and physical examination, blood pressure measurement, and studies that include a CBC with differential, complete metabolic panel, serum albumin, creatinine, and cholesterol levels. Serum C3/C4 complement, antinuclear antibody, hepatitis B and C, and HIV tests are recommended to differentiate NS from systemic lupus erythematosus, lymphoma, and other conditions that might present similarly to NS.

Immunological studies of IgG, IgM, and IgE may be helpful in diagnosing NS. IgG will be decreased, while IgM will be increased (Roy et al., 2009). An IgG:IgM ratio greater than 3 has been seen in patients with SSNS, with lower ratios seen in SRNS (Roy et al.). IgE levels are higher in patients with INS.

Renal biopsy is recommended for children age 12 years and older, as they are more likely to have a diagnosis of FSGS rather than MCNS and, therefore, are at greater risk for progressive kidney failure (Gipson et al., 2009). In NS, renal biopsy will reveal effacement of the podocytes including flattening, retraction of the foot processes, and a decrease in the number of slit diaphragms (Lane & Kaskel, 2009). Renal biopsy in patients with FSGS reveals multilayered cell injury and sclerosis of the glomeruli caused by accumulation of proteins and compensatory hypertrophy (Alpers, 2010).

Management starts with consultation with a pediatric nephrologist. The first-line treatment for NS is high-dose steroids—either prednisone or prednisolone—at 2 mg/kg/day or 60 mg/m²/day (maximum dose 80 mg/day), given in one to three divided doses, for 6 weeks. Treatment continues until the patient is in remission, which is typically achieved within 4 to 6 weeks of starting treatment (Hogg et al., 2000). Remission is defined as having 3 consecutive days with zero-trace protein via urine dipstick or a urine Pr/Cr ration of less than 0.2 (Gipson et al., 2009). Once proteinuria resolves, the patient is transitioned to a maintenance dose of 2 mg/kg or 40 mg/m² every other morning, with gradual tapering to occur over an additional 6 weeks (Hogg et al.). Studies suggest that patients receiving a longer period of initial treatment, consisting of 6 weeks of high-dose steroids and 6 weeks of maintenance, have a higher rate of long remission than patients receiving an initial treatment of 4 weeks of high-dose steroids and 4 weeks of maintenance.

Relapse is defined as a recurrence of urine Pr/Cr ratio to 2 or greater, or urine protein to 2 or greater, for three of five consecutive days after initial remission. Frequently relapsing NS is defined as two or more relapses within the first 6 months of initial treatment, or four or more relapses in a 12-month period. Treatment for initial or infrequent relapses consists of prednisone 2 mg/kg day until the urine is free of protein for three consecutive days, followed by 1.5 mg/kg of prednisone every other day for 4 weeks (Gipson et al., 2009).

Patients who do not go into remission after initial treatment or have frequent relapses are considered steroid resistant. Cytotoxic medications such as cyclophosphamide or chlorambucil are added to the treatment regimen for these patients, and have been shown to produce sustained remissions (Gipson et al., 2009). Cyclosporine A is an alternative therapy, but the NS relapse rate is high once this medication is discontinued (Bagga & Mantan, 2005). Other treatment options include levamisole, mycophenolate mofetil, sirolimus, and tacrolimus; these medications are usually given in combination with high-dose methylprednisolone to induce remission (Gipson et al.).

Supportive therapies include the use of angiotensin-converting enzyme type I inhibitors (ACEIs) or angiotensin type II receptor blockers. These medications decrease hypertension and exert renoprotective effects by reducing hydrostatic pressure within the glomerular capillary and inhibiting cytokine release and inflammation. Statins are used to control hypercholesterolemia when diet alone is not successful. Restriction of dietary sodium to 1,500 to 2,000 mg per day is recommended to control edema caused by water retention. Severe edema may require treatment with 25% albumin and diuretics. During administration of 25% albumin, patients should be monitored for hypertension, pulmonary edema, and congestive heart failure from rapid expansion of intravascular volume. Furosemide or other diuretics can cause electrolyte imbalances such as hypokalemia and hyponatremia and deplete intravascular volume, putting patients at higher risk for acute kidney failure. Over-the-counter antacids or H_2 blockers can also be used to protect gastric mucosa from prolonged steroid use.

If NS is suspected as a new diagnosis, consultation with a pediatric nephrologist is highly recommended prior to starting treatment. If the patient has been previously diagnosed with NS, the nephrologist should be consulted prior to making changes to the patient's treatment regimen.

Family teaching needs to include current information about the NS disease process, the process of monitoring of proteinuria at home, and common childhood illnesses and infections that may trigger a relapse, such as otitis media and sinusitis. It is very important for patients with NS to receive immunizations, especially pneumococcal vaccines to prevent bacterial peritonitis, and yearly influenza vaccinations. Patients should avoid live viral vaccines while they are on steroid therapy.

Patients and family need to be aware of the side effects of long-term steroid use, such as appetite stimulation, bone demineralization, cushingoid appearance, mood changes, decreased immune function, growth retardation, night sweats, hypertension, and cataracts. Rare but serious side effects include pseudotumor cerebri, depression, steroid psychosis, and steroid-induced diabetes. Teaching should also address the importance of tapering steroid use after extended therapy. Patients should be encouraged to maintain physical activity and avoid bed rest to prevent blood clot formation.

DISPOSITION AND DISCHARGE PLANNING

Based on the severity of their initial presentation and the existence of other comorbidities, patients with the first episode of NS may need to be admitted to the hospital for the initiation of steroid treatment and management of edema. Discharge planning should include a follow-up appointment with the PCP and pediatric nephrologist within a week of discharge. Patients should be followed monthly by a pediatric nephrologist during initial therapy or exacerbations, with greater time between visits during remission.

The outcome for NS patients depends on the response to initial steroid treatment. Ninety-five percent of patients with INS achieve remission after 12 weeks of initial treatment. An infrequent relapse rate of 49% is expected within 24 months, and a frequent relapse rate of 29% is expected with INS (Gipson et al., 2009). Patients with more frequently relapsing NS or SRNS are at higher risk for developing complications from long-term treatment regimens and progression to end-stage kidney disease or kidney failure.

Complications from NS include obesity and delayed bone growth from prolonged steroid use; dyslipidemia leading to increased risk of cardiovascular disease; higher risk of infections from immunosuppressive therapies; and thromboembolism from loss of antithrombin III factor in the urine, increased fibrinogen, and platelet hyperaggregability due to volume depletion.

Children with biopsy-proven MCNS have a 25% chance of relapse after puberty (Kyrieleis et al., 2009). The mortality rate is less than 1% (Copelovitch, 2008). Long-term extrarenal complications include osteoporosis, hypertension, and decreased visual acuity from cataracts and myopia. Males treated with immunosuppressive therapy are at risk for decreased sperm count and motility. Prognosis for more severe forms of NS, including SRNS and FSGS, is more difficult to determine.

PELVIC PAIN

Darcy Egging

PATHOPHYSIOLOGY

Puberty has been described as the period of newly developed sexual reproductive capacity. It begins at approximately age 10 years and can extend beyond 16 years of age (Greydanus et al., 2009). The average age of menarche in the United States is 12 to 13 years (Schwab & Posner, 2008). Normal menstrual cycles are between 21 and 45 days. Normal bleeding length is between 3 and 7 days, with blood loss averaging 20 to 40 mL (Greydanus et al.; Schwab & Posner). It takes approximately 5 years for the adolescent female to develop regular menstrual cycles (Quint & Sifuentes, 2004). Many of the conditions that cause pelvic pain are related to the menstrual cycle.

The hypothalamus is responsible for the secretion of hormones that stimulate puberty and regulate the menstrual cycle. Gonadotropin-releasing hormone (GnRH) triggers sexual development and normal sexual physiology for both males and females. GnRH stimulates the pituitary to release both follicle-stimulating hormone (FSH) and luteinizing hormone (LH). FSH stimulates follicular production and estrogen, while LH stimulates the corpus luteum and progesterone. Any dysfunction in the hypothalamus, pituitary, or ovaries may lead to menstrual difficulties (Dangal, 2005; Greydanus et al., 2009; Kimball, 2009). FSH levels rise several days prior to menstruation, causing a new follicle to develop. This developing follicle releases estrogen, which in turn causes the endometrium to become thicker, preparing the uterus for possible pregnancy. The surge in LH triggers ovulation. If a pregnancy does not occur, then the progesterone level drops and menstruation begins (Dangal; Munden, 2007).

EPIDEMIOLOGY AND ETIOLOGY

In the general population, an estimated 16% of individuals will have chronic pelvic pain. In the adolescent population, 3% to 5% of all visits to PCPs are for abdominal complaints (Song & Advincula, 2005).

PRESENTATION

A detailed history is required for all patients presenting with pelvic pain. Adolescents should be interviewed outside the presence of their parent or caregiver, if at all possible, to allow for free sharing of information between the patient and HCP. The HCP should be nonjudgmental and supportive (Hickey & Balen, 2003). Ascertain the pain history—its description, onset, quality, and anything that makes the pain better or worse. Determine associated signs or symptoms such as nausea, vomiting, or weight gain or loss (Forcier, 2009). In addition, find out the date of the last menstrual period (LMP). Is there vaginal discharge/bleeding? Are there symptoms of urinary tract infection? Is the patient sexually active, and if so, with how many partners and of which sex? If sexually active, which method of contraception (if any) is used? Past medical history should include the number of past sexual partners, pregnancies, sexually transmitted infections (STIs), dysmenorrhea, dyspareunia, age at menarche, length and regularity of menstrual cycles, and any systemic diseases (Schwab & Posner, 2008).

The physical examination should focus on the patient's chief complaint. If the complaint involves any gynecological problem, visualization of the genital area is necessary, a bimanual examination is essential, and if considering pregnancy or STI, a speculum examination is standard practice (Goodman & Uphold, 2003; Schwab & Posner, 2008). If the patient is virginal, a speculum examination may be withheld unless assessing for trauma.

DIFFERENTIAL DIAGNOSIS

The differential diagnoses for pelvic pain are broad and listed in Table 31-16 (Forcier, 2009; Schwab & Posner, 2008).

TABLE 31-16

Differential Diagnosis for Female Adolescent Pelvic Pain		
System	**Acute**	**Chronic**
Gynecological	Pregnant: • Normal, ectopic, miscarriage Nonpregnant: • Pelvic inflammatory disease (PID) • Tubo-ovarian abscess • Ovarian torsion • Ovarian cyst rupture • Mittelschmerz	Dysmenorrhea Endometriosis PID Adhesions
Gastrointestinal	Gastroenteritis, appendicitis, perforation, bowel obstruction, diverticulitis, Meckel's diverticulum	Irritable bowel disease Constipation
Urological	Kidney stone, urinary tract infection, pyelonephritis	
Musculoskeletal	Fascitis, arthritis	
Other	Psychosomatic, abdominal migraines, trauma	

MENSTRUAL DISORDERS

Dysmenorrhea

Dysmenorrhea is defined as pelvic pain during menstruation. A common problem, it affects 40% to 90% of all adolescent females. Because dysmenorrhea is a subjective finding, it is difficult to quantify the exact number of females who are affected monthly by this condition. Dysmenorrhea significantly contributes to females' absence from school and work (Dangal, 2005; Forcier, 2009; Harel, 2008; Mannix, 2008; Schwab & Posner, 2008).

Dysmenorrhea is classified as either primary or secondary. In primary dysmenorrheal, there is no pelvic pathology. If there is pelvic pathology, such as endometriosis, the condition is classified as secondary dysmenorrhea (Forcier, 2009; Schwab & Posner, 2008; Song & Advincula, 2005).

Primary dysmenorrhea is associated with prostaglandins, which are produced by the endothelium. Primary dysmenorrhea is usually first noted 6 to 12 months after menarche and is more prevalent with age. Symptoms can range from mild to severe. Pain is usually intermittent (crampy/colicky), dull pain that is located in the lower abdomen or back and can spread down the thighs. Patients may also complain of nausea, vomiting, headache, diarrhea, and fatigue. The pain can begin several hours prior to menses and usually improves in approximately 2 days. A vaginal examination should be performed if the patient is sexually active. It will be normal in primary dysmenorrhea. Secondary dysmenorrhea is uncommon in adolescence (Dangal, 2005; Forcier, 2009; Harel, 2008; Schwab & Posner, 2008; Song & Advincula, 2005).

Therapeutic management for dysmenorrhea consists of NSAIDs and oral contraceptives. NSAIDs inhibit prostaglandin synthesis and are usually considered the first-line treatment. Song and Advincula (2005) report that in a meta-analysis of 63 randomized controlled trials, NSAIDs were significantly more effective in controlling pain versus placebo. These medications are reportedly more effective if started 24 to 48 hours prior to menses. If a particular NSAID does not control symptoms; it is reasonable to try another. Oral contraceptives suppress ovulation and decrease prostaglandin release. Dosing is usually limited to 3 to 6 months, unless continued use for contraception is desired (Dangal, 2005; Forcier, 2009; Harel, 2008; Schwab & Posner, 2008; Song & Advincula, 2005).

Nonpharmacologic treatment for dysmenorrhea consists of exercise, rest, heat, or acupuncture (French, 2005).

Menorrhagia

Menorrhagia is defined as excessive bleeding (more than 80 mL), prolonged bleeding for more than 7 days, or abnormal uterine bleeding. As many as 14% of all females of reproductive age report having menorrhagia.

The most common causes of menorrhagia are anovulatory cycles and sexually transmitted infections. In an anovulatory cycle, the second one-half of the normal menstrual cycle does not occur. As a consequence, the endometrial lining continues to form with no opposition to the estrogen. Eventually irregular sloughing of the endometrial lining occurs. Coagulation disorders are the second most common cause of menorrhagia; thus the American College of Obstetricians and Gynecologists (ACOG) guidelines recommend screening for coagulation disorders and anemia for all patients presenting with menorrhagia. One study showed that 13% of all patients with abnormal uterine bleeding had von Willebrand disease (Apgar et al., 2007; Casablanca, 2008; Dangal, 2005; Harlow & Campbell, 2004; Kulp et al., 2008; Schwab & Posner, 2008).

Blood loss is a very subjective sign that is difficult to measure. To estimate this loss, the HCP, while taking the history, should ask about the number of pads used per day, the amount of blood on each pad, and the presence of blood clots. Are the pads so saturated that there is overflow to clothing or bedding? Other symptoms of blood loss may include fatigue, shortness of breath, pelvic pain, or pallor. Severe anemia and hypovolemic shock have been reported in patients with severe disease (Apgar et al., 2007; Schwab & Posner, 2008).

Diagnostic study and therapeutic management of menorrhagia depend on the severity of bleeding. A CBC, coagulation panel, type and screen (heavy bleeding), speculum examination, and pregnancy testing are standard means of assessment. If a specific coagulopathy is suspected, then further testing is indicated. If the patient is hemorrhaging, vaginal packing may be necessary. When the patient is stable, an abdominal ultrasound should be ordered. Further testing, such as endometrial biopsy and hysteroscopy, may be considered. An endometrial biopsy is ordered when evaluating patients for endometrial cancer; it is well tolerated and usually performed in the outpatient office. Hysteroscopy is not as readily performed, as it requires cervical dilation (Apgar et al., 2007; Dangal, 2005; Schwab & Posner, 2008).

Treatment is directed at restoring the normal uterine lining using oral contraceptives, progesterone, or both. Depending on the degree of bleeding and anemia, the patient may require blood transfusion or iron supplements (Apgar et al., 2007). Surgical options are not usually recommended for adolescents.

Premenstrual syndrome

Premenstrual syndrome (PMS) is a complex grouping of symptoms that occur during the second phase of the menstrual cycle. Most women of reproductive age will experience PMS; 3% to 8% will have severe enough symptoms to be classified as having premenstrual dysphoric disorder (PMDD) (Dangal, 2005; Nur et al., 2007; Schwab & Posner, 2008).

The etiology of PMS is unknown. Researchers, however, speculate that a decrease in serotonin leads to the psychological symptoms of PMDD. Heredity may also play a role in PMDD expression (Dangal, 2005; Nur et al., 2007; Schwab & Posner, 2008; Steiner, 2000).

Symptoms of PMS include headache, nausea, weight gain, breast tenderness, mood swings, bloating, food cravings, and fatigue. Pelvic pain is usually not a characteristic of PMS unless some other underlying condition is present. Behavioral symptoms include nervousness, irritability, anxiety, and depression. Table 31-17 summarizes the criteria for PMDD diagnosis (Steiner, 2000).

Therapeutic management consists of rest; exercise; decreased caffeine, sugar, and salt intake; and avoidance of alcohol and stress. If depression or anxiety is part of the symptomology, selective serotonin reuptake inhibitors (SSRIs) and anxiolytics have been prescribed with good results (Dangal, 2005; Nur et al., 2007; Schwab & Posner; 2008, Steiner, 2000).

Endometriosis

Endometriosis is the presence of endometrial gland and stroma-like tissue outside the uterine cavity. In adolescent

TABLE 31-17

Research Criteria for Premenstrual Dysphoric Disorder

Menstrual cycle disruption: five symptoms during the luteal phase that are absent postmenses, including a least one of the criteria marked with an asterisk:

1. *Markedly depressed mood, feelings of hopelessness, or self-deprecating thoughts
2. *Marked anxiety, tension
3. *Marked affective lability
4. *Persistent and marked anger or irritability
5. Decreased interest in usual activities
6. Difficulty in concentrating
7. Lethargy, easy fatigability, or marked lack of energy
8. Marked change in appetite, overeating, or specific food cravings
9. Hypersomnia or insomnia
10. A subjective sense of being overwhelmed or out of control
11. Other physical symptoms, such as breast tenderness or swelling, headaches, joint or muscle pain, a sensation of bloating, or weight gain

Menstrual cycle disruption markedly interferes with activities and relationships. It is not related to another disorder that persists beyond the previously described time period.

Criteria are confirmed during at least two consecutive menstrual cycles.

Source: American Psychiatric Association, 2000.

TABLE 31-18

Presenting Symptoms of Endometriosis in Adolescents

Cyclic and acyclic pain
Dysmenorrhea
Deep dyspareunia
Irregular menses
Gastrointestinal pain/nausea
Urinary symptoms
Vaginal discharge
Dyschezia (pain with defecation)

Source: Song & Advincula, 2005.

assessing markers such as C-reactive protein and cancer antigen 125 (CA-125) to assess the level of inflammation; however, these tests are not specific to endometriosis. Laparoscopy with biopsy is the only confirmatory test for endometriosis, but is reserved for those individuals with chronic pain who do not improve with standard treatments (Ballard et al., 2008; Greydanus et al., 2009; Ozawa et al., 2006; Riley et al., 2007; Song & Advincula, 2005; Templeman, 2009).

Therapeutic management of endometriosis is similar to that for menorrhagia and dysmenorrhea, and includes NSAIDs and oral contraceptives. Medroxyprogesterone acetate (Provera or Depo-Provera) has also been recommended. Medroxyprogesterone use may lead to bone density loss due to decreased serum estrogen, especially within the first 2 years of use. It has yet to be determined if this effect will lead to a greater incidence of osteoporosis later on in life (Wooltorton, 2005). It is not recommended to use GnRH agonists in adolescents with endometriosis due to the loss of bone density these agents cause.

Intrauterine devices have not been approved by the U.S. Food and Drug Administration for treatment of adolescent endometriosis; however, there is support for their use by ACOG. Laparoscopy is standard therapy and should be performed by a gynecologist who is familiar with adolescent endometriosis, as the presentation in young patients is much different than that in adults (Greydanus et al., 2009; Templeman, 2009).

OVARIAN DISORDERS

Ovarian cysts

Although cyst development in adolescents usually occurs after the onset of menses, cysts can also develop in prepuberty. They may be found incidental to other testing, and require no treatment (Templeman, 2004). Two types of cysts are distinguished: functional and hemorrhagic (corpus luteum). In the adolescent, functional ovarian cysts are common and usually asymptomatic. They develop during the first one-half of the menstrual cycle. Hemorrhagic, or

females who undergo laparoscopy for chronic pelvic pain, its incidence ranges from 40% to 65%. The etiology of endometriosis remains unclear; however, an association with endometrial tissue refluxed from the oviducts during menstruation has been suggested. Most women have this retrograde menstruation to some degree, so further study is required. Endometriosis is a progressive disease; consequently, symptoms worsen over time. There may also be a genetic predisposition to the condition (Ballard et al., 2008; Boyle & Torrealday, 2008; Cadogan et al., 2009; Greydanus et al., 2009; Ozawa et al., 2006; Riley et al., 2007; Song & Advincula, 2005; Templeman, 2009).

The hallmark symptom of endometriosis is painful menses; other findings include dyspareunia, pelvic mass, and infertility (Table 31-18). Endometriosis should be considered in adolescents with dysmenorrhea who do not respond to NSAIDs or oral contraceptives.

Diagnosis of endometriosis begins with a complete history and review of symptoms. The pelvic examination may normal, or there may be tenderness if the examination is performed during the later stages of the menstrual cycle. Diagnostic testing includes culture for STI, CBC for anemia, urinalysis for UTI, and pregnancy test. Ultrasound imaging may show scattered cysts, and MRI may reveal anomalies of the reproductive system. Some HCPs suggest corpus luteum, cysts differ from functional cysts in that they are usually seen after ovulation and during the second one-half of the menstrual cycle (Cadogan et al., 2009). Both types of cysts commonly resolve without treatment in 1 to 3 months (Forcier, 2009). Individuals with ovarian cysts are predisposed toward ovarian torsion (Anders, 2009).

Ovarian cysts can cause pain if they grow large enough to displace tissue internally. This pain is usually unilateral, dull, or colicky in nature. A ruptured ovarian cyst will present with acute onset of unilateral pelvic pain. This pain may mimic appendicitis, ovarian torsion, ectopic pregnancy, or pelvic inflammatory disease (PID) (McWilliams et al., 2008).

Pregnancy testing is standard in case of a cyst. The diagnosis of ovarian cysts is usually determined using transvaginal ultrasound (Jain, 2008). If a large amount of free fluid is seen on the ultrasound, a CBC may be considered to evaluate for anemia. Consider obtaining creatinine levels for those patients receiving contrast as part of a CT scan of the abdomen and pelvis (Bauman & Cloutier, 2008; McWilliams et al., 2008).

Therapeutic management usually consists of supportive care and serial examinations. Oral contraceptives may be prescribed to prevent ovulation or further cyst formation. These medications do not help in the resolution or reabsorbtion of existing cysts, however (Bauman & Cloutier, 2008). If the pain does not improve or if a cyst increases in size, a cystectomy is recommended (Shapiro et al., 2009). Free fluid from a ruptured ovarian cyst is usually reabsorbed and no further treatment is necessary. Surgical intervention is rare (Bauman & Cloutier, 2008; Cadogan et al., 2009; McWilliams et al., 2008).

Mittelschmerz

A ruptured functional cyst in midcycle is called mittelschmerz (Bauman & Cloutier, 2008; Cadogan et al., 2009). When a cyst ruptures, it releases a small amount of fluid, causing peritoneal irritation and sharp pain that usually lasts approximately 24 hours (Forcier, 2009). Mittelschmerz is a benign condition and is self-resolving. Other, more serious conditions must be considered prior to making this diagnosis (Bauman & Cloutier). Treatment consists of NSAIDs and patient and family information.

Ovarian (adnexal) torsion

Ovarian torsion (also known as adnexal torsion) is twisting of the ovary on its pedicle (Akata, 2008). This condition can occur at any age but peaks in adolescence (Bauman & Cloutier, 2008).

The ovary is suspended in the pelvis and is supported by the suspensory ligament of the ovary and the proper ovarian ligament. The ovary hangs below the fallopian tube within the broad ligament (mesovarium). Within this structure are the arteries and veins of the ovaries. When an ovarian torsion occurs, there is a twisting of the mesovarium (Anders, 2009; Bertolotto et al., 2008; Hiller et al., 2007; Scout et al., 2007). When the ovary's center of gravity is altered—for example, by the presence of a cyst—the ovary may tip, causing twisting and compromising the blood flow to the ovary, leading to ischemia. This ischemia causes the acute onset of severe pain (Bauman & Cloutier, 2008).

Ovarian torsion is a true surgical emergency. It is estimated to account for approximately 3% of all gynecological emergencies (Jain, 2008; Scout et al., 2007). Ovarian torsion is more common on the right side (Anders, 2009; Bauman & Cloutier, 2008).

Acute onset of abdominal pain is the hallmark symptom of torsion. The differential diagnosis is similar to that for ovarian cyst. In particular, ovarian torsion should be considered if the patient has a history of fallopian tube pathology (Bertolotto et al., 2008).

Diagnosis of ovarian torsion can be difficult. Diagnostic testing includes CBC for anemia, urinalysis for UTI, and pregnancy test. Color flow Doppler ultrasound is considered to be the definitive test for diagnosing ovarian torsion. False-negative results are possible depending on the amount of torsion. CT scans and MRI are reserved for patients who have nondefinitive findings and when symptoms are intermittent (Akata, 2008; Bertolotto et al., 2008; Hiller et al., 2007; Scout et al., 2007). Many issues must be considered when deciding which test is most appropriate.

Treatment of ovarian torsion consists of surgical consultation and laparoscopy. Ovarian salvage may be possible up to 24 hours after the onset of pain (Bauman & Cloutier, 2008).

Critical Thinking

Pregnancy should always be considered for the patient with pelvic pain. Ovarian disorders may be surgical emergencies, whereas menstrual problems tend to be more chronic in nature.

PYELONEPHRITIS AND NEPHRITIS

Andrea Lynne Parker

PATHOPHYSIOLOGY

Pyelonephritis

Pyelonephritis is a bacterial infection of the upper urinary tract that occurs from an ascending infection from within the bladder. Urinary stasis, infrequency of voiding, incomplete voiding, obstruction of urinary flow, and reflux of urine back into the kidneys are all mechanisms by which bacteria from a lower urinary tract infection can ascend, leading to pyelonephritis.

After filtration, urine passes through the collecting tubules, where water and substrates are reabsorbed. The concentrated urine then leaves the kidney via the renal pelvis and passes down the ureters into the bladder. Pyelonephritis affects the collecting tubules, interstitium, and renal pelvis structures, causing inflammation and scarring. On microscopic examination, hallmarks of acute pyelonephritis include areas of patchy interstitial suppurative inflammation, intratubular collections of neutrophils, and tubular necrosis (Alpers, 2010). After treatment, the neutrophilic infiltrate is replaced by macrophages, plasma cells, and lymphocytes. Acute areas of inflammation within the kidney are replaced with scar tissue made up of tubular atrophy, interstitial fibrosis, and lymphocytic infiltrate. This scarring reflects injury from inflammation, fibrosis, and damage to the underlying calyx and pelvis of the kidney.

Acute bacterial and chronic pyelonephritis can lead to tubulointerstitial nephritis (TIN), an inflammation that affects the interstitium and renal tubules of the kidney. TIN can be either acute or chronic. Its histological characteristics include interstitial edema, leukocytic infiltration, and focal tubular necrosis (Alpers, 2010). This disorder is characterized by major dysfunction of the collecting tubules, leading to inability to concentrate urine, salt wasting, and metabolic acidosis.

Nephritis

Nephritis is defined as inflammation within the kidney. This general term is often used interchangeably with the more specific term of glomerulonephritis (GN) unless otherwise specified.

GN is an inflammatory process that occurs within the gomeruli, resulting in glomerular injury. It can be either chronic or acute. Each kidney contains approximately 1 million glomeruli, which act as the primary sites of blood filtration. In GN, deposits of immunoglobulins, complement, and cell-mediated immune reactions with the glomeruli lead to inflammation and injury (Alpers, 2010). Antibody-associated injury can occur in either of two ways: by reaction of antibody with fixed antigens within the glomerulus or from the deposition of antigen–antibody complexes in the glomerulus. Research has supported the theory that cytotoxic antibodies directly target glomerular cell components, causing injury. On microscopic examination, glomerular injury presents as enlarged, hypercellular glomeruli caused by diffuse infiltration of leukocytes (both neutrophils and monocytes), diffuse proliferation of endothelial and mesangial cells, and formation of crescents in severe cases (Alpers).

Diseases that present as GN are classified into three categories: primary (wherein the kidney is the primary organ affected), secondary (caused by diseases that affect multiple organs), and hereditary. Examples of these three categories of GN follow:

- *Primary GN:* acute poststreptococcal glomerulonephritis (APSGN), rapidly progressive (crescentic) GN, membranous glomerulopathy, IgA nephropathy, membranoproliferative GN, and chronic GN
- *Secondary GN:* systemic lupus erythematosus (SLE), diabetes mellitus, amyloidosis, Goodpasture syndrome, microscopic polyarteritis/polyangitis, Wegner granulomatosis, Henoch-Schönlein purpura (HSP), and bacterial endocarditis
- *Hereditary GN:* Alport syndrome, thin basement membrane disease, Fabry disease

The topic of nephritis/glomerulonephritis is broad and encompasses many disease processes. For the purposes of this section, the focus will be on the diagnosis, treatment, and management of APSGN.

EPIDEMIOLOGY AND ETIOLOGY

Pyelonephritis

The pathogens most often isolated in urine cultures from infants and young children with pyelonephritis are normal bowel flora, including *Escherichia coli, Klebsiella* spp., *Proteus* spp., *Pseudomonas aeruginosa, Enterococcus* spp., *Serratia* spp., and *Staphylococcus aureus* (Prelog et al., 2007). Females have a higher rate of infection with *E. coli*, while males are more affected by other Gram-negative bacteria, such as *Klebsiella* spp., *Proteus* spp., *P. aeruginosa,* and *Enterobacter aerogenes* (Kanellopoulos et al., 2006).

Within the first year of life, uncircumcised males have the highest rates of urinary tract infection), followed by circumcised males, and then females (Shah & Upadhyay, 2005). Uncircumcised males are also at higher risk for developing pyelonephritis (Shah & Upadhyay).

There is equal distribution of incidence among ethnicities.

Approximately 5% to 10% of infants become bacteremic from pyelonephritis (Blackstone & Shaw, 2008). Bacteremia is found in 23% of patients younger than 2 months of age (Tuchman & Meyers, 2008). Although mortality is uncommon, children with acute pyelonephritis will have some degree of acute renal parenchymal injury.

TIN is diagnosed only by renal biopsy, therefore, its incidence is likely underreported. This disorder is thought to arise following a humoral and cell-mediated immune response that can be triggered by bacterial, viral, or fungal infections; hypersensitivity reactions to medications; autoimmune disorders; metabolic disease; and genetic conditions. Damage to renal tubules from acute infection is reversible, but chronic TIN can progress to end-stage renal disease.

Nephritis

Acute poststreptococcal glomerulonephritis (APSGN) is the most common form of primary nephritis/glomerulonephritis. It most often follows a pharyngeal or skin (pyoderma) infection with group A beta-hemolytic *Streptococcus*. APSGN is most commonly seen in children 5 to 15 years of age, with males more frequently affected than females, and with an equal ethnic distribution (Sethna & Meyers, 2008).

Secondary GN nephritis occurs as a complication of a preexisting systemic disease process. The preexisting disease leaves patients susceptible to glomerular injury. These conditions include bacterial endocarditis, ventriculoatrial shunts, syphilis, hepatitis B and C, candidiasis, SLE, and HSP. Parasitic infections such as malaria, schistosomiasis, leishmaniasis, filariasis, hydatid disease, trypanosomiasis, and toxoplasmosis can also induce secondary nephritis (Davis & Avner, 2007a).

Hereditary GN is a manifestation of a genetically determined disease process.

PRESENTATION

Pyelonephritis

Pyelonephritis presents as a UTI with high fever. In young children, it is usually the first indicator of a urinary obstructive process, such as vesicoureteral reflux or hydronephrosis. Any UTI accompanied by fever should be considered to be pyelonephritis until proven otherwise.

History should include duration of illness or recent diagnosis of UTI by another HCP. Assess the patient history for constipation and toileting habits. Inquire about any past history of UTI or structural anomalies as well as any family history of kidney dysfunction.

Patients presenting with pyelonephritis are ill appearing. They may be uncomfortable and lethargic. They will most likely have a fever greater than 38°C (100.4°F), with temperatures exceeding 39°C (102.2°F) being common. In conjunction with fever, pediatric patients may be tachycardiac, tachypneic, and dehydrated. Abdominal, suprapubic, and costovertebral pain may be present, although younger patients and infants may not be able to verbalize the locus of pain. Patients who have had a kidney transplant may not complain of pain in the transplanted kidney secondary to denervation. Urine samples may have a strong or unusual smell. Infants may present with nonspecific symptoms such as poor feeding, vomiting, irritability, and jaundice. Blood pressure is usually normal; hypertension may indicate more significant renal obstruction or disease, and hypotension is a very concerning sign of urosepsis or shock. Patients with TIN will often present with maculopapular rash, joint pain with flexion and extension, or very rarely, uveitis.

Nephritis

Patients with GN will often have a history of recent throat infection; APGSN usually develops within 1 to 2 weeks after streptococcal pharyngitis and within 3 to 6 weeks after streptococcal pyoderma (Davis & Avner, 2007a). Some patients may have evidence of skin infection. Urine output is decreased and dark in color. Patients will often complain of fatigue and headache. A rash, especially on the buttocks and posterior legs, along with arthralgia and weight loss are indicators of secondary GN.

Pediatric patients with APGSN present with elevated blood pressure, edema, and other symptoms of fluid overload or congestive heart failure, such as tachypnea, dyspnea, hepatic congestion, and gallop rhythm. These symptoms are evidence of decreased glomerular filtration and decreased urine formation. Patients may also present with signs and symptoms of their underlying disease process, such as vasculitis, butterfly rash for SLE, or lower extremity petechiae for HSP.

DIFFERENTIAL DIAGNOSIS

The differential diagnoses for both pyelonephritis (Table 31-19) and nephritis (Table 31-20) are extensive, with many similarities. Infants presenting with fever, irritability, and lethargy should receive a full sepsis evaluation.

TABLE 31-19

Differential Diagnoses for Pyelonephritis
Abdominal abscess
Abdominal aortic aneurysm
Acute abdomen
Appendicitis
Balanitis
Cervicitis
Chlamydial genitourinary infections
Cystic kidney disease
Cystitis
Diverticulitis
Ectopic pregnancy
Endometritis
Enterococcus faecalis infection
Epididymitis
Escherichia coli infection
Gonococcal infection
Haemophilus influenzae infection
Infective endocarditis
Interstitial cystitis
Klebsiella infection
Lower-lobe pneumonia
Nephritis, interstitial
Nephrolithiasis

(Continued)

TABLE 31-19

Differential Diagnoses for Pyelonephritis *(Continued)*

Oophoritis
Pancreatitis, acute and chronic
Papillary necrosis
Pelvic inflammatory disease
Postvaccination
Pregnancy
Proteus infection
Pseudomonas aeruginosa infection
Renal corticomedullary abscess
Renal vein thrombosis
Salpingitis
Splenic abscess
Splenic infarct
Staphylococcal infection
Streptococcus groups A, B and D infections
Struvite and staghorn calculi
Trauma
Tuberculosis
Ureaplasma infection
Ureteropelvic junction obstruction
Urethritis
Urinary tract infection
Urinary tract obstruction
Vesicoureteral reflux
Vesicovaginal and ureterovaginal fistula
Viral illness
Vulvovaginitis

TABLE 31-20

Differential Diagnoses for Nephritis

Acute poststreptococcal glomerulonephritis
Anti-GAM antibody disease
Antiphospholipid antibody syndrome
Bacterial endocarditis
Cryoglobulinemia
Escherichia coli infection
Goodpasture syndrome
Hematuria
Hemolytic-uremic syndrome
Hemorrhagic fever with renal failure syndrome
Henoch-Schönlein purpura
Hepatorenal syndrome
Hypercalcemia
Hypersensitivity vasculitis
Hypertension
IgA nephropathy
Immune complex disease
Medullary sponge kidney
Membranoproliferative glomerulonephritis—types 1, 2, and 3
Mitochondrial myopathy, encephalopathy, lactic acidosis, and stroke (MELAS) syndrome
Multicystic kidney disease
Nephrotic syndrome
Oliguria
Polycystic kidney disease
Polyarteritis nodosa group
Proteinuria
Pyelonephritis
Renal cortical necrosis
Rhabdomyolysis
Sarcoidosis
Shunt nephritis
Systemic lupus erythematosus
Systemic sclerosis
Tumor lysis syndrome
Ureteropelvic junction obstruction
Uric acid stones
Urinary tract infection
Urolithiasis
Wegener vasculitis
Wilms tumor
Wilson disease
Xanthinuria
Other considerations: Takayasu disease

PLAN OF CARE

Pyelonephritis

Basic evaluation for pyelonephritis includes urinalysis and culture with sensitivities (crucial for effective antimicrobial therapy), basic chemistry panel, CBC with differential, blood culture, CRP, and ESR. Urinalysis can rapidly detect infection with measurement of leukocyte esterase and nitrites. Urine culture will reveal new or continued UTI and guide antimicrobial therapy. Chemistry panel will reveal basic kidney function through BUN and creatinine, with elevations in each indicating a decrease in function. The WBC count will be high. A positive blood culture indicates bacteremia; CRP and ESR will be elevated, indicating an inflammatory process.

Children younger than 5 years of age should receive renal ultrasound and contrast voiding cysto-urethrogram (VCUG) to evaluate for any obstructive process within the urinary tract after first UTI or pyelonephritis. Children younger than 5 years of age with repeated UTIs are at greatest risk for developing substantial renal scarring. Children older than 5 years of age with repeated UTIs or pyelonephritis should receive these studies as well.

As patients with pyelonephritis are ill appearing on presentation, inpatient admission for administration of IV broad-spectrum antibiotics and hydration is warranted. Children younger than 3 months of age, those with a septic appearance, or patients who are not able to tolerate oral medications should be admitted for inpatient treatment. Third-generation cephalosporins such as ceftriaxone, or combination therapy with an aminoglycoside and penicillin, are given for 3 to 4 days intravenously, with 10 to 14 days of oral antibiotics continuing after discharge (Craig & Hodson, 2004; Shah & Upadhyay, 2005). Effective oral medications in this population include cefixime, ceftibuten, and amoxicillin/clavulanic acid (Hodson et al., 2007). The selection of an oral medication should be based on the results of culture and susceptibilities. Early intervention is key to preventing long-term kidney damage and scarring from inflammation, which could lead to chronic renal insufficiency and end-stage renal disease.

Pyelonephritis can be managed by the PCP, if the patient is not septic and can tolerate oral medications, with referral to a pediatric urologist for renal ultrasound and VCUG being made as part of follow-up care. Patients and family members will require teaching on the importance of continued oral antibiotic prophylaxis, the signs and symptoms of a UTI, and the need to seek treatment for suspected UTI.

Nephritis

Diagnostic evaluation for nephritis includes an electrolyte panel, creatinine, BUN, CBC with differential, urinalysis with urine culture and sensitivities, and throat culture. Crenated erythrocytes and erythrocyte casts seen on urinalysis are a hallmark of this disease (Sethna & Meyers, 2008). Proteinuria may also be present as a sign of glomerular injury. Throat cultures are positive for group A beta-hemolytic *Streptococcus* in 15% to 20% of patients with APSGN (Sethna & Meyers). If APSGN is suspected, a serum antistreptolysin-O (ASO) titer should be checked; it will be positive in 60% of patients with APSGN (Sethna & Meyers). If the pediatric patient has not had a recent throat or skin infection to trigger APSGN, then autoimmune panels such as serum complement levels (C3, C4), lupus serologies, anti-DNAase B, perinuclear antineutrophil antibody (P-ANCA), cellular antineutrophil cytoplasmic antibody (C-ANCA), and IgA are useful for evaluation of systemic disease. Low serum C3 levels are indicative of secondary GN. Abnormal results of these tests warrant further investigation for immunological disorders.

While supportive care is the mainstay of treatment for pediatric patients with APSGN, a 10-day course of a penicillin antibiotic is initiated to help prevent spread of nephritogenic organisms (Davis & Avner, 2007a) and will provide antibiotic coverage should the patient have a positive throat culture. APSGN is typically self-limiting, with 95% of patients recovering kidney function after treatment with penicillin (Davis & Avner). If complications such as hypertension or acute renal insufficiency develop, treatment consists of fluid and sodium-restricted diet,

diuretics such as furosemide, calcium-channel antagonists, vasodilators, or ACE inhibitors (Sethna & Meyers, 2008). Exacerbations of secondary forms of GN are treated with immunosuppressive therapy consisting of corticosteroids (prednisone) and cyclophosphamide to counteract the inflammatory process (Sethna & Meyers). Children who are septic, have electrolyte abnormalities, or are unable to tolerate oral medications or fluids should be admitted for inpatient management.

Patients with GN can also be managed by their PCP but should be referred to a pediatric nephrologist when hypertension and low urine output persist after treatment with antibiotics. Patients with secondary forms of GN will need follow-up with their respective specialists, who may refer them to a pediatric nephrologist if one is not already a part of the patient's care team.

If the HCP is concerned that a patient may have GN secondary to an immunological disease, repeat serum studies and referral to, or consultation with, a pediatric rheumatologist are warranted. HCPs may reassure patients and family members that APSGN is self-limiting and that full recovery is expected. Caregivers should monitor for decreased urine output and gross blood in the urine following completion of the antibiotic course, as these conditions may be signs of continued glomerular injury, and told to seek further treatment from the PCP or specialist if these signs are noted.

DISPOSITION AND DISCHARGE PLANNING

Pyelonephritis

Children younger than 5 years of age with febrile UTI should receive oral antibiotic prophylaxis, such as trimethoprim–sulfamethoxazole or nitrofurantoin, until cleared of any structural anomalies by a pediatric urologist. Follow-up with the PCP within 1 week of discharge should be arranged. At that time a repeat urinalysis and culture should be obtained to assess for continued infection after antibiotic therapy.

Outcomes depend on the severity of scarring to the kidney. Early antibiotic treatment of pyelonephritis is the best way to halt inflammation and scarring. Early detection and correction of structural defects also provides the patient with the best chance to retain kidney function. Repeated episodes of UTI and pyelonephritis, as well as delayed diagnosis of structural defect, put the patient at risk for significant renal impairment, which could lead to chronic renal insufficiency and end-stage renal disease.

Nephritis

Patients with APSGN should follow up with their PCP within 1 week of discharge. A repeat urinalysis to assess for hematuria should be completed. If it is positive, the patient should be referred to a pediatric nephrologist or rheumatologist for evaluation immunological studies. Monitoring the patient for signs of continued renal involvement, such as hypertension, renal insufficiency, or hematuria, is part of the long-term follow-up plan. Should symptoms of renal sequelae develop, a referral to a pediatric nephrologist is warranted. Patients with secondary nephritis should follow up with the specialist. Outcomes for APSGN are generally good, with complete return of kidney function being typical. Outcomes for secondary and hereditary forms of GN depend on the severity of the underlying disease.

RENAL TUBULAR ACIDOSIS

Cathy Haut, Bonnie Kitchen, and Sara Jandeska

PATHOPHYSIOLOGY

The kidney maintains normal serum acid–base balance by excreting hydrogen ion and reclaiming bicarbonate along the nephron. A healthy adult generates 70 mEq of H^+ daily from breakdown of amino acids derived from diet and muscle mass. Children generate 3 to 5 mEq/kg of H^+ per day; failure to eliminate this load results in metabolic acidosis. Secretion of H^+ via its ATPase occurs in the accessory cells of the collecting duct. To create maximally acidotic urine, proximal and distal nephron functions are required. Ammoniagenesis in the proximal tubular epithelial cell releases ammonia (NH_3) into the tubular lumen, where it binds with H^+ to create ammonium ion (NH_4^+). Ammonium ions accumulate within the medullary interstitium via the Na^+-K^+-2Cl cotransporter (by posing as K^+) in the thin ascending loop of Henle. Ammonia is secreted by an unknown mechanism into the distal tubular lumen, where it binds to H^+. In addition, an adequate concentration of sodium (more than 25 mEq/L) is required distally for sufficient uptake (created by the Na^+-K^+-ATPase under aldosterone control). A voltage gradient is created, promoting H^+ secretion.

Bicarbonate is filtered and, under a reaction catalyzed by carbonic anhydrase, reacts with H^+ in the lumen of the proximal convoluted tubule to produce carbon dioxide and water. Carbon dioxide freely passes into the tubular epithelial cell, where it reacts with carbonic anhydrase II to produce H^+ and bicarbonate. Bicarbonate is then transported into the bloodstream via a basolateral bicarbonate–chloride antiporter, while H^+ reenters the tubular lumen via a Na^+-H^+ exchanger (NHE3). RTA is a hyperchloremic metabolic acidosis with a normal to moderately decreased glomerular filtration rate and normal anion gap. There are three common types of RTA:

- Type I RTA (distal): decrease in acid excretion
- Type II RTA (proximal): failure of bicarbonate reabsorption with decreased ammonium absorption
- Type IV RTA: aldosterone deficiency or impairment of its effects, resulting in reduced potassium excretion, hyperkalemia, and acidosis

Aldosterone sufficiency is necessary for sodium reabsorption and potassium excretion in the distal nephrons; thus type IV is the only RTA presentation with hyperkalemia (Karet, 2009). Type III RTA is a rare form of the disorder, has characteristics of combined distal and proximal RTA, and is a result of inherited carbonic anhydrase II deficiency.

EPIDEMIOLOGY AND ETIOLOGY

RTA is a relatively uncommon clinical syndrome characterized by an inherited, acquired, or combination of defects in the renal tubules; the disorder results in failure to maintain a normal serum bicarbonate level despite consumption of a regular diet and normal metabolism and acid production (Herrin, 2004).

RTA is associated with many different etiologies. Type I RTA can be idiopathic; can result from tubulointerstitial conditions such as kidney transplantation, pyelonephritis, and obstructive uropathy; or can result from conditions associated with nephrocalcinosis such as hyperthyroidism or primary hyperparathyroidism. Type I RTA is also associated with growth deficiency and genetic problems such as Ehlers-Danlos syndrome, Marfan syndrome, and Wilson disease (Sharma et al., 2007). Both chronic hepatitis and Sjogren's syndrome (a chronic disorder involving dry mouth, dry eyes, and lymphocytic infiltration of exocrine glands, linked to autoimmune diseases such as systemic lupus erythematosus) have been reported to have an association with type I RTA. Sporadic autosomal dominant or recessive transmission with deafness, specifically sensorineural hearing loss, has also been reported. Medications or toxins that can cause type I RTA include amphotericin B, nonsteroidal analgesics, ifosfamide, lithium, and cyclosporine (an antirejection drug commonly used following kidney transplant). Hypergammaglobulinemic states can also result in type I RTA.

Type II RTA—the most common form of RTA in children—can occur without any related disease and is often associated with more generalized proximal tubular dysfunction and Fanconi syndrome (Katzir et al., 2008). In newborns, type II RTA may be considered an aspect of renal immaturity (Lurn, 2009). Dysproteinemic states and calcium-related conditions predispose patients to development of RTA. Hereditary disorders responsible for RTA include galactosemia, Wilson disease, glycogen storage disease type I, and Lowe syndrome. Type II RTA with

Fanconi syndrome occurs with several autosomal recessive disorders. Fanconi syndrome is a more generalized dysfunction of the proximal tubules, but also results in RTA, characterized by impaired reabsorption of bicarbonate, phosphate, amino acids, glucose, and uric acid (Hsu et al., 2005). Other causes of type II RTA include malignancy, nephritic syndrome, and chronic renal vein thrombosis.

Type IV RTA results from deficiency or resistance to aldosterone. It may occur in disease states such as Addison disease and diabetic neuropathy, or in hereditary disease such as pseudohypoaldosteronism types 1 and 2 (also known as Gordon syndrome). Angiotensin 1-converting enzyme inhibition (from medications such as captopril) and decreased response to aldosterone (as in obstructive uropathies or from potassium-sparing diuretics) may contribute to the etiology of this problem.

PRESENTATION

In many cases, RTA presentation is asymptomatic, but findings can differentiate between types. Type I RTA in children is linked to multiple genetic disorders, including sensorineural hearing loss and nephrocalcinosis. In addition to the characteristics of the associated hereditary disorders, its clinical presentation typically includes failure-to-thrive or short stature, anorexia, vomiting, and dehydration (Lurn, 2009). Type II RTA presents in infants with failure-to-thrive, hyperchloremic acidosis with hypokalemia, and rarely nephrocalcinosis. Hypertension may be found in children with type IV RTA who have underlying genetic disorders such as Gordon syndrome, renal parenchymal disease, or mineralocorticoid dysfunction (Bagga & Sinha, 2007). Other presentations of RTA include polyuria, polydipsia, a preference for savory foods, hypokalemia, refractory rickets, and metabolic acidosis that is not otherwise explained (Bagga & Sinha). Rickets or osteomalacia may indicate the presence of Fanconi syndrome, an associative problem with type II RTA.

The physical examination of an infant or child with suspected RTA may include failure-to-thrive (weight and height less than the 25th percentile), bossing forehead, and an abnormal eye examination (e.g., cataracts). Signs of rickets such as healing chest lesions, bowing of the lower extremities, and widening of the epiphysis of the wrists may be observed. An abdominal examination may reveal hepatosplenomegaly or enlarged kidneys.

DIFFERENTIAL DIAGNOSIS

Vomiting, diarrhea, or use of medications that cause diarrhea resulting in gastrointestinal electrolyte losses should be considered first in the differential diagnosis, as they are more common than RTA. Any extrarenal process that can result in metabolic acidosis, such as tube drainage of intestinal or pancreatic secretions or bile, must be evaluated prior to assuming RTA. Other differential diagnoses for RTA include renal acidosis as an effect of early kidney insufficiency, diabetic ketoacidosis, acid loads from parenteral nutrition or administration of ammonium chloride, and dilution acidosis (hyperchloremia) related to the rapid administration of normal saline (Andreeff, 2009). Acetazolamide and, to a lesser extent, topiramate inhibit carbonic anhydrase and produce a type II RTA when used chronically. When a metabolic acidosis is identified, the presence of a respiratory alkalosis should be determined, to ensure that renal compensation is not occurring.

PLAN OF CARE

RTA presents with metabolic acidosis and a normal anion gap. Anion gap represents the difference of unmeasured cations and anions in plasma and is calculated as follows:

$$\text{Anion gap} = [Na^+ + K^+] - [Cl^- + HCO_3^-] \textbf{ OR}$$
$$[Na^+] - [Cl^- + HCO_3^-]$$

Normal values are in the range of 8 to 16 mEq/L. Serum and urine electrolytes should be obtained. Findings of hyperchloremic metabolic acidosis, metabolic alkalosis with or without hypokalemia, hyponatremia with hyperkalemia, and hypercalciuria with normal serum calcium are often indicative of RTA (Bagga et al., 2005; Brown, 2010).

Calculating the fractional excretion (FE) of bicarbonate (HCO_3^-) and obtaining a urine pH are helpful in determining the type of RTA involved. The calculation for FE is as follows:

$$\text{FE } HCO_3^- = (CO_2[\text{ urine }] \times \text{Creatinine [serum]})/$$
$$(HCO_3^- [\text{serum}] \times \text{Creatinine [urine]})$$

If the FE HCO_3^- is more than 1% combined with an acidotic state or more than 5% combined with a normal serum HCO_3^-, proximal RTA is possible (Andreeff, 2009).

Type I RTA is confirmed by a urine pH of more than 5 during systemic acidosis. Type II RTA is diagnosed by measurement of urine pH and fractional HCO_3^- excretion during a HCO_3^- infusion. In type II disease, the urine pH will rise above 7.5 and the fractional excretion of HCO_3^- is more than 15% during the administration of HCO_3^-. Type IV RTA is confirmed by calculating a transtubular potassium concentration and urine anion gap:

$$\text{Urine anion gap} = [Na^+ + K^+] - Cl^-$$

If the potassium is elevated and the urine pH is less than 5.5 (transtubular gradient less than 5), type IV is likely (Andreeff, 2009).

In addition to determining the urine pH, urine for glucose and protein should be measured. Hypercalciuria may be evaluated by the calculation of a calcium-to-creatinine ratio. A 24-hour urine sample for citrate, calcium, potassium, and oxalate levels should also be obtained, as hypercalciuria and hypocitraturia are risk factors for nephrolithiasis and nephrocalcinosis.

Imaging studies may also be of diagnostic value in the evaluation of RTA. Long bone or wrist films assist in the evaluation of rickets, and ultrasound of the kidneys can diagnose renal dysplasia, hydronephrosis, nephrolithiasis, and nephrocalcinosis. Ultrasound is especially important in children with type IV RTA, as aldosterone unresponsiveness is a more common problem than deficiency and indicates the possibility of obstructive uropathy and parenchymal disease (Bagga & Sinha, 2007). Genetic or chromosomal evaluation is warranted for all children with RTA, regardless of type.

Emergency or inpatient treatment of an infant or child with hyperchloremic, non-anion gap acidosis seeks to replace bicarbonate, which can be administered intravenously. In the severely dehydrated child, slow rehydration and electrolyte replacement are important to avoid cardiac, renal, and neurological sequelae. When replacing bicarbonate, caution should be used because of the potential for side effects such as fluid overload, hypokalemia, hypercapnia (as a result of the decreased respiratory drive with increased bicarbonate serum levels), and tissue hypoxia. In addition, appropriate dilutions and rates of administration of intravenous bicarbonate should be used, especially in neonates, to avoid complications such as intraventricular hemorrhage (Taketomo et al., 2010).

Alkali therapy decreases growth retardation associated with RTA in children (Sharma et al., 2009). For outpatients, alkali is given as sodium bicarbonate or citrate after meals. In type I RTA, the initial dose of alkali is 2 mEq/kg/day, in two to three divided doses, increased slowly every few days until plasma bicarbonate levels are normal. In type II RTA, dosing ranges from 2 mEq/kg/day to 20 mEq/kg/day (Andreeff, 2009; Taketomo et al., 2010). Hydrochlorthiazide, or the addition of a potassium-sparing diuretic, may be helpful to correct acidosis while limiting alkali administration. In some patients, potassium supplements are necessary. Dietary restriction of sodium and potassium may be warranted, especially in hyperkalemic, type IV RTA. Diuretics may be administered to decrease calcium secretion in children with type IV RTA who have symptomatic hypercalciuria. In children with rickets or hypophosphatemia, vitamin D and phosphate supplements are important and may improve the acidification process.

Early consultation with a nephrologist is indicated to prevent long-term renal complications, especially nephrolithiasis and renal tubular scarring. Genetic or endocrine referral may also be helpful depending on the etiology and type of RTA. A dietician or nutritionist can provide assistance with assessment and management of weight gain and growth. In addition, because nutrition plays such an important part in early development, referral to a developmental specialist may be warranted.

Based on the patient's age and type of RTA, care is individualized. Thus no one set of educational instructions should be used. Patients and caregivers must be made aware of the side effects of bicarbonate therapy and of the potential complications from this treatment. If children become ill with a viral disease causing vomiting or diarrhea, they will require closer observation, additional fluid therapy, and perhaps adjustments to RTA treatment during the period of illness. Preparation for surgical procedures may also warrant additional preparation. Finally, families should made aware for the potential for progressive kidney disease as a result of untreated or incompletely treated RTA.

Regular follow-up with electrolyte evaluation is important as well as growth and development evaluations with the PCP. In addition, genetic counseling for further pregnancies is important.

A child with a chronic illness is often a challenge for financial and psychosocial reasons. Support is important for families to help them maintain optimal wellness for their child with RTA.

DISPOSITION AND DISCHARGE PLANNING

Clinical outcomes following hospitalization or new diagnosis may vary depending on the type of RTA and the age of the child. A neonate or young infant with type I RTA and no underlying disease process will do well and not need long-term treatment. A child with a more complicated illness or a genetic syndrome will require follow-up directed at supporting the underlying problems as well as management of the RTA. An interprofessional approach provides for the best outcomes.

RTA, especially types II and IV, is usually chronic. Thus children should be followed into adulthood and evaluated in terms of growth, stature, and kidney function. Infants or children diagnosed with type I RTA should have a hearing screen to identify any sensorineural hearing loss. Because type I RTA in older children may be associated with systemic lupus erythematosus, Sjogren's syndrome, or chronic hepatitis, appropriate evaluation for these problems is warranted (Bagga & Sinha, 2007).

Caution and protective therapies should be used when prescribing or administering drugs that can affect tubular function in the individual with RTA. Overall, the patient's prognosis depends on the underlying disease. The prognosis for type II RTA in infancy is excellent if the illness is related to renal immaturity. Type I RTA is usually permanent; nevertheless, if it is not caused by a significant tubular disorder and renal damage is prevented, prognosis is good. Children with severe systemic illness, which often includes type IV RTA and Fanconi syndrome, may experience significant morbidity (Dell & Avner, 2007).

URINARY TRACT INFECTION

Cathy Haut

PATHOPHYSIOLOGY

Urinary tract infection (UTI) starts when bacteria or fungus ascend the periurethral area and infiltrate bladder mucosa, causing a local inflammatory response; migration of this infection to the kidney is termed pyelonephritis. The invasion of pathogenic microorganisms, or their elements, into the systemic circulation results in a complex pro-inflammatory release of cytokines, which damage organ function either directly or indirectly via secondary mediators. Cytokines, such as tumor necrosis factor (TNF-α), interleukin-1 (IL-1), and interleukin-6 (IL-6), are peptides released from monocytes, macrophages, and epithelial cells in reaction to the infectious process, which in turn regulate the host response (Wagenlehner et al., 2007). If a child develops urosepsis as a result of a UTI, septic shock and multisystem organ failure may occur. Very little is known about the significance of the immune response, or the interaction of the host pathogen and environment, to predicting the ultimate outcome of the illness (Chang & Shortliffe, 2006; Wagenlehner et al.).

Vesicoureteral reflux (VUR) is an obstructive renal process caused by failure of the normal flap valve mechanism in the ureterovesical junction; this defect allows the reflux of urine from the bladder into the ureters and renal pelvis. Primary VUR results from congenital anomalies such as ureteral duplication, ureterocele with duplication, ureteral ectopia, and paraureteral diverticula. Secondary VUR occurs as a consequence of increased intravesical pressure or inflammatory processes such as neurogenic bladder, bladder outlet obstruction, foreign body or clinical cystitis. VUR is graded using the International Reflux Grading scale:

- Grade I: reflux into the ureter
- Grade II: reflux to the ureter, renal pelvis, and calyces
- Grade III: reflux to the ureter and collecting system with mild dilation of ureter and pelvis; calyces are mildly blunted
- Grade IV: reflux with dilation of the ureter and moderate blunting of renal calyces
- Grade V: reflux with severe dilation of ureter and pelvis; severe blunting of renal calyces

Approximately 80% of patients with VUR improve over time; grades I, II, and III typically resolve or improve within 3 years following diagnosis (Elder, 2007; Lum, 2007). Children with grades IV and V reflux and older

children with persistent VUR are less likely to have disease resolution (Elder, 2007).

EPIDEMIOLOGY AND ETIOLOGY

UTI is the term used to describe a bacterial or fungal infection of any part of the urinary tract (kidney, bladder, ureter, urethra). Urinary tract symptoms account for 5% to 14% of all pediatric emergency department visits (Freedman, 2005). Predisposition to or risk factors for UTI related to both age and gender; other risk factors include circumcision status; urinary tract structural abnormalities; immunocompromised status; fecal and perineal colonization; and in older children, sexual activity (Chang & Shortliffe, 2006).

UTI affects an estimated 7% of females and 2% of males younger than the age of 6 years (Bauer & Kogan, 2008). Typically, uncircumcised male infants have higher incidence of UTI in the first 3 months of life, and females younger than 12 months of age have the highest baseline rate (Shaikh et al., 2008).

Dysfunctional voiding or elimination is another significant risk factor for UTI (Shaikh & Hoberman, 2007). Genetic predisposition may be a factor in prevalence rates. Approximately 35% of siblings of children with VUR also have VUR (Elder, 2007).

UTIs are among the most common serious bacterial infections in children. The most significant issue is to identify those patients at risk for resultant kidney damage. UTIs in children following kidney transplant are a concern for graft failure (Dharnidharka et al., 2007).

UTIs in otherwise healthy children may be indicative of urinary tract abnormalities. Vesicoureteral reflux is the most common pathologic finding in young children after a UTI (Garin et al., 2006; Venhola et al., 2006). The relationship between UTI, renal scarring, and VUR is unclear, as is the progression of uncomplicated UTI to pyelonephritis, but some evidence suggests that recurrent UTI with pyelonephritis is linked to renal scarring (Fitzgerald et al., 2009). Research has also shown that early treatment of UTI results in decreased kidney involvement, but not decreased renal scar formation (Doganis et al., 2007).

Uropathogens for UTI include bacteria of enteric origin, such as Gram-negative *Escherichia coli, Pseudomonas aeruginosa,* and *Klebsiella* species and Gram-positive organisms such as group B *Streptococcus, Staphylococcus aureus,* and group D *Streptococcus.* Other pathogens that have been identified in UTIs include *Chlamydia trachomatis* and *Candida, Serratia,* and *Enterococcus* species (Chang & Shortliffe, 2006; Prelog et al., 2007).

Acute UTI is one of the most common indications for hospital admission of infants and children. The incidence of pediatric hospitalization for UTI is estimated to be greater than 45,000 children per year, bringing to annual costs more $180 million (Conway & Keren, 2009; Hellerstein, 2006). Outcomes of hospitalization vary, as length of stay (LOS), consistency of practice patterns, and completion of diagnostic procedures are not evidence based in all institutions.

PRESENTATION

Symptoms of UTI vary, with the presentation ranging from few or no symptoms to fulminating febrile illness, often dependent on age—young infants and children are at highest risk for systemic disease. Symptoms in infants and young children include failure-to-thrive, fever, irritability, lethargy, asymptomatic jaundice, and oliguria or polyuria. Children between the ages of 2 and 5 years may present with fever and abdominal pain, whereas older children may have the more classic symptoms of dysuria, urinary frequency, urgency, and pain. In children who are post kidney transplant, immunotherapy and denervation of the donor kidney will obscure the most common findings of UTI.

The HCP's review of systems in the setting of suspected UTI includes a history of previous UTI or febrile illness with unknown etiology, structural abnormalities, frequent bubble baths, initiation of toilet training for females, sexual activity in adolescents, and the possibility of child maltreatment.

Physical examination includes inspection of the sacral region in all children for dimples, pits, or a sacral fat pad, as these signs can indicate a neurogenic bladder. In males, the scrotum is examined for epididymitis. In children older than 5 years, costovertebral angle and suprapubic tenderness are assessed (Chang & Shortliffe, 2006). Gastrointestinal and respiratory symptoms can also be initial signs associated with UTI. The presence of other symptoms, such as lethargy or anorexia, cannot exclude UTI, especially in young febrile infants.

Neonates and infants differ in their presentation of UTI as compared to older children. Approximately 12% to 28% of children younger than 3 months of age with febrile illness will have serious illness—either UTI or occult bacteremia (Ishimine, 2007). Typically symptoms for infants are nonspecific, including poor feeding, diarrhea, failure-to-thrive, vomiting, mild jaundice, lethargy, fever, or hypothermia. Guidelines for evaluation of this age group include laboratory analysis of blood, urine, and cerebrospinal fluid.

DIFFERENTIAL DIAGNOSIS

Differential diagnoses for UTI symptoms in neonates, infants, and young children include UTI, bacteremia, meningitis, and viral infection. Immunization against *Haemophilis influenzae* and *Streptococcus pneumoniae* has increased the frequency of infants with febrile illness being diagnosed with UTI versus occult bacteremia (Shaikh & Hoberman, 2007). In older children, the differential diagnoses include UTI, vulvovaginitis, STI, vaginal foreign body, child maltreatment, abdominal disease or process, and urinary calculi.

PLAN OF CARE

The American Academy of Pediatrics (AAP, 1999) has published practice parameters for UTIs, including guidelines for diagnosis, treatment, and follow-up imaging studies. During the past decade, however, there has been discussion regarding the most appropriate guidelines for imaging patients with UTI and the value these studies have to improve outcomes in these individuals. The AAP guidelines are now more than 10 years old, and newer guidelines can be expected to be introduced in the near future.

Early, rapid diagnosis is the key to successful outcomes in managing a child with a UTI. Results of urinalysis—including dipstick for leukocyte esterase and nitrites, presence of more than five white blood cells or bacteria viewed per high-powered microscope field of the spun urinary sediment, and urine culture indicating organism and susceptibility—provide the basis for initiating treatment (Bauer & Kogan, 2008). A culture result of more than 100,000 cfu/mL is the traditional definition of a significant UTI, but interpretation of such findings must consider the method of urine collection and clinical presentation.

Historically, symptoms have been used to distinguish between lower and upper urinary tract infection. New diagnostic markers do exist, but need additional study to prove their worth in practice. Increased procalcitonin (PCT)—a polypeptide marker for biologic disease—has demonstrated pyelonephritis in children with febrile UTI and may be helpful in identifying the extent of renal scarring (Bauer & Kogan, 2008; Hellerstein, 2006). Urinalysis, C-reactive protein, and erythrocyte sedimentation rate are predictors of infection with febrile illness; however, they are not reliable indicators of pyelonephritis in the febrile child with UTI.

Imaging studies are important in the diagnosis of anatomic or structural abnormalities in children with UTI. The AAP guidelines (1999) state that infants and young children 2 months to 2 years of age with UTIs who do not demonstrate the expected clinical response within 2 days of antibiotic therapy should have prompt ultrasonography, and either voiding cystourethrography (VCUG) or radionuclide cystography should then be performed at the earliest convenient time. Young children 2 months to 2 years of age who demonstrate the expected response to therapy should have a sonogram and either a VCUG or radionuclide cystography at the earliest convenient time.

Ultrasonography can be used to identify kidney abnormalities such as size and shape, duplication anomalies, hydronephrosis, or hydroureters. Bladder evaluation is also possible, which may show thickening or abnormalities such as bladder diverticula or ureteroceles (Bauer & Kogan, 2008). Ultrasonography is noninvasive and does not involve radiation, which has benefits in the assessment of the child who does not respond promptly to therapy or the young child with a first, febrile UTI (Hellerstein, 2006). Doppler ultrasonography can be utilized to detect small areas of inflammation and to assist in the diagnosis of pyelonephritis.

VCUG is diagnostic of VUR, which is the causative factor in 50% of children with UTI (Bauer & Kogan, 2008; Garin et al., 2006). Dimercaptosuccinic acid scintigraphy scan (DMSA) is a nuclear medicine radio scan that is also used for evaluation of acute inflammation and kidney scarring (Bauer & Kogan; Smith, 2008). Scans can be used in the acute setting, but initial findings may resolve on follow-up. Thus, to determine the presence and extent of scarring or renal damage, the scan should be completed several months after the child's acute infection is first noted (Bauer & Kogan).

Guidelines for hospitalization for children with UTI include the inability to tolerate oral medications or maintain hydration, significant underlying medical conditions that may complicate management of the UTI, inadequate response to outpatient therapy, and suspicion of sepsis and septic shock (Shaikh & Hoberman, 2007). Recent research has indicated that children with febrile disease respond to oral antibiotics similarly to parenteral therapy and that young infants can be effectively managed with outpatient intravenous therapy (Chang & Shortliffe, 2006; Dore-Bergeron et al., 2009). Children who present with, or develop, urosepsis are best managed in an intensive care unit.

Urosepsis can present as febrile illness in a young infant or child, or it can manifest as a nosocomial infection in the intensive care unit. This infection results in significant morbidity and mortality if not treated promptly and appropriately. Treatment requires management of all critical issues, appropriate antimicrobial therapy, and control or removal of mitigating factors (Wagenlehner et al., 2007). It is extremely important to address stabilizing mechanisms in these children, in addition to providing broad-spectrum antimicrobial therapy.

The choice of the appropriate antibiotic and the length of treatment depend on the patient's age, severity of illness, associated or underlying disorders, infectious organisms, and local resistance patterns. Of key importance is beginning therapy in a timely manner. Delay in treatment of UTI in young infants may result in kidney involvement (Doganis et al., 2007). Recommended therapy for uncomplicated UTI is 7 to 10 days; complicated UTI is 14 days. Nevertheless, there is little difference between the two therapeutic durations related to bacteriuria at the end of treatment or the recurrence of UTI within 15 months

of treatment (Hodson et al., 2009). For sexually mature adolescents, a 3-day course of ciprofloxacin or levofloxacin may be indicated (AAP, 1999; Pong & Bradley, 2005). If sepsis is suspected, bacteremia is confirmed, the child is immunocompromised, or the child is younger than 3 months of age, 14 days of therapy is recommended, with initial therapy being delivered via the parenteral route (Pong & Bradley; AAP). There are very few clinical trials that support the dosing of antibiotics for either complicated or uncomplicated UTI. Multiple antibiotics have been successful in eliminating organisms, determination of specific therapy is based on resistance patterns and culture results.

Education for UTI involves a description of the problem, specific risk factors, and planned testing and treatment. Using the terms "cystitis" and "pyelonephritis" is appropriate in the discussion of infection. Caregivers should be instructed to offer plenty of fluids, give all medication, and administer antipyretics for fever control. Symptoms of recurrent UTI should be reviewed, such as painful urination, frequency, back or stomach pain, visible blood in the urine or foul-smelling urine, and gastrointestinal complaints such as vomiting, diarrhea, or anorexia. Young children may refuse to urinate or begin to have wetting accidents after toilet training is complete. In addition to describing symptoms, caregivers should be provided with the signs and symptoms of impending problems, such as dehydration, persistent fever, or swelling around the eyes or other body parts.

Information on prevention of future UTIs for families includes changing diapers often, changing underwear daily, and encouraging children to urinate often. It is helpful for females to wipe from front to back with careful cleansing after bowel movements. Showers are preferable for older children rather than baths and bubble bath; shampoo or perfumed soaps should be kept out of bath water. Fluid intake, restriction of caffeine-containing beverages, and prevention of constipation are other factors that help to prevent UTI in children. Sexually active adolescents should urinate as soon after intercourse as possible.

DISPOSITION AND DISCHARGE PLANNING

Once a child has improved clinically, is tolerating oral fluids, and is able to take oral antibiotics, discharge from the hospital is warranted. Imaging studies can be completed in the hospital if indicated. Follow-up after hospitalization or illness with UTI continues to be problematic, with less than one-half of all children with a first febrile UTI receiving the screening tests recommended by the AAP practice parameters (Cohen et al., 2005). Approximately 8% to 30% of children with UTI will experience reinfection, often within the first 6 months following the initial UTI (Shaikh & Hoberman, 2007). The AAP (1999) recommends continuing antibiotic therapy, or prophylactic treatment, until imaging studies are complete for children between the ages of 2 months and 2 years with a first UTI.

Despite UTI recurrence for children with VUR, controversy persists regarding appropriate follow-up imaging as well as the utility of antibiotic prophylaxis. Monitoring children with recurrent UTI and with higher-grade VUR is important to address the risk for and prevent additional kidney damage. Therapy for children with VUR requires continued research, as some recent studies recommend early surgical intervention, while others recommend observation without antibiotic prophylaxis (Bauer & Kogan, 2008). A recent meta-analysis examining the efficacy of surgery and medical treatment for VUR indicated that both of these approaches have equal efficacy (Venhola et al., 2009).

Discharge planning for the child with UTI involves adherence to current practice guidelines and ensuring that children with UTI have appropriate treatment and diagnostic testing. Review of imaging results, attention to VUR grading, and repeated urine cultures documenting therapy success are important components of the discharge and follow-up process. Ultimately, evidence-based protocols will emerge to better guide providers in managing children with UTI and modifying risks for development of further renal involvement.

REFERENCES

1. Agus, Z. (1999). Hypomagnesemia. *Journal of the American Society of Nephrology, 10*, 1616–1622.

2. Akata, D. (2008). Ovarian torsion and its mimics. *Ultrasound Clinics, 3*, 451–460.

3. Al-Dahhan, J., Haycock, G., Chantler, C., & Stimmler, L. (1983). Sodium homeostasis in term and preterm neonates. *Archives of Disease in Childhood, 58*, 335–342.

4. Alpers, C. (2010). Nephrotic syndrome. In V. Kumar, A. K. Abbas, N. Fausto, & J. C. Aster (Eds.), *Robbins and Cotran pathologic basis of disease* (8th ed.). Philadelphia: Saunders Elsevier.

5. American Academy of Pediatrics (AAP), Committee on Quality Improvement, Subcommittee on Urinary Tract Infection. (1999). Practice parameter: The diagnosis, treatment and evaluation of the initial urinary tract infection in febrile infants and young children. *Pediatrics, 103*(4), 843–852.

6. American Psychiatric Association. (2000). *Diagnostic and statistical manual of mental disorders* (4th ed., Text Revision, pp. 771-781). Washington, DC: Author.

7. Anders, J. (2009). Ovarian torsion in the pediatric emergency department: Making the diagnosis and importance of advocacy. *Clinical Pediatric Emergency Medicine, 10*, 31–37.

8. Andersen, T., Eskild-Jensen, A., Fokiaer, J., & Brochner-Mortensen, J. (2009). Measuring glomerular filtration rate in children: Can cystatin C replace established methods? A review. *Pediatric Nerphology, 24*, 929–941.

9. Andreeff, K. (2009). Renal tubular acidosis. In R. M. Perkins, J. D. Swift, D. A. Newton, & N. G. Anas (Eds.), *Pediatric hospital medicine: Textbook of inpatient management* (2nd ed., pp. 374–377). Philadelphia: Lippincott, Williams and Wilkins.

10. Andreoli, S. (2008). Management of acute kidney injury in children: A guide for pediatricians. *Pediatric Drugs, 10*(6), 379–390.

11. Apgar, B., Kaufman, A., George-Nwogu, U., & Kittendorf, A. (2007). Treatment of menorrhagia. *American Family Physician, 75*(12), 1813–1819.

12. Bagga, A., Bajpai, A., & Menon, S. (2005). Approach to renal tubular acidosis. *Indian Journal of Pediatrics, 72*, 771–776.

13. Bagga, A., & Mantan, M. (2005). Nephrotic syndrome in children. *Indian Journal of Medical Research, 122*(1), 13–28.

14. Bagga, A., & Sinha, A. (2007). Evaluation of renal tubular acidosis. *Indian Journal of Pediatrics, 7*, 679–686.

15. Ballard, K., Seaman, H., de Vriea, C., & Wright, J. (2008). Can symptomatology help in the diagnosis of endometriosis? Findings from a national care control study. Part 1. *Obstetrics and Gynecology Clinics of North America, 115*, 1382–1391.

16. Bauer, R., & Kogan, B. (2008). New developments in the diagnosis and management of pediatric UTI's. *Urology Clinics of North America, 35*, 47–58.

17. Baum, M. (2008). Pediatric glomerular diseases. *Current Opinion in Pediatrics, 20*, 137–139.

18. Bauman, B. H., & Cloutier, R. L. (2008). Ovarian Disorders. In J. M. Baren, S. G. Rothrock, J. A. Brennan, & L. Brown (Eds.)., *Pediatric Emergency Medicine* (pp. 689–691). Philadelphia: Saunders Elsevier.

19. Bellinger, M. (2002). Torsion of the spermatic cord. In B. Zitelli, & H. Davis (Eds.), *Atlas of pediatric physical diagnosis* (4th ed., pp. 495–496). Philadelphia: Mosby.

20. Bergstein, J., Leiser, J., & Andreoli, S. (2005). The clinical significance of asymptomatic gross and microscopic hematuria in children. *Archives of Pediatric and Adolescent Medicine, 159*, 353–355.

21. Bertolotto, M., Serafini, G., Toma, P., Zappetti, R., & Migaleddu, V. (2008). Adnexal torsion. *Ultrasound Clinics, 3*, 109–119.

22. Blackstone, M., & Shaw, K. (2008). Urinary tract infection. In M. Schwartz et al. (Eds.), *5-minute pediatric consult* (5th ed.). Philadelphia: Lippincott, Williams, & Wilkins.

23. Bokenkamp, A., Domanetzki, M., Zinck, R., Schumann, G., Byrd, D., & Brodehl, J. (1998). Cystatin C: A new marker of glomerular filtration rate in children independent of age and height. *Pediatrics, 101*, 875–881.

24. Boyle, K., & Torrealday, S. (2008). Benign gynecologic conditions. *Surgical Clinics of North America, 88*, 245–264.

25. Brenner, B. (Ed.). (1996). *The kidney*. Philadelphia: W. B. Saunders.

26. Brown, A. (2010). Renal tubular acidosis. *Dimensions of Critical Care Nursing, 29*(3), 112–119.

27. Bunchman, T. (2008). Treatment of acute kidney injury in children: From conservative management to renal replacement therapy. *Nature Clinical Practice Nephrology, 4*(9), 510–514.

28. Cadogan, M., Yazdani, A., & Taylor J. (2009). Pelvic pain. In P. Cameron, G. Jelinek., A. Kelly, L. Murray, & A. Brown (Eds.), *Textbook of adult emergency medicine* (3rd ed., pp. 603–607). Edinburgh: Elsevier.

29. Cameron, M., Sakhaee, K., & Moe, O. (2005). Nephrolithiasis in children. *Pediatric Nephrology, 20*(11), 1587–1592.

30. Casablanca, Y. (2008). Management of dsyfunctional uterine bleeding. *Obstetrics and Gynecology Clinics of North America, 35*, 219–234.

31. Chan, J., Knoll, J., Depowski, P., Williams, R., & Schober, J. (2009). Mesorchial testicular torsion: Case report and a review of the literature. *Urology, 73*(1), 83–86.

32. Chang, S., & Shortliffe, L. (2006). Pediatric urinary tract infections. *Pediatric Clinics of North America, 53*, 379–400.

33. Choi, M., & Ziyadeh, F. (2008). The utility of the transtubular potassium gradient in the evaluation of hyperkalemia. *Journal of the American Society of Nephrology, 19*, 424–426.

34. Cochat, P., & Basmaison, O. (2000). Current approaches to the management of primary hyperoxaluria. *Archives of Disease in Childhood, 82*, 470–473.

35. Cohen, A., Rivara, F., Davis, R., & Christakis, D. (2005). Compliance with guidelines for the medical care of first urinary tract infections in infants: A population based study. *Pediatrics, 115*, 1474–1478.

36. Conway, P., & Keren, R. (2009). Factors associated with variability of outcomes for children hospitalized with urinary tract infection. *Journal of Pediatrics, 154,* 789–796.

37. Copelovitch, L. (2008). Nephrotic syndrome. In M. Schwartz et al. (Eds.), *5-minute pediatric consult* (5th ed.). Philadelphia: Lippincott, Williams, & Wilkins.

38. Craig, J., & Hodson, E. (2004). Treatment of acute pyelonephritis in children. *British Medical Journal, 328,* 179–180.

39. Dangal, G. (2005). Menstrual disorders in adolescents. *Internet Journal of Gynecology and Obstetrics, 4*(1). Retrieved from http://www.ispub.com/journal/the_internet_journal_of_gynecology_and_obstetrics/volume_4_number_1_19/article_printable/menstrual_disorders_in_adolescents.html

40. Davenport, M. (1996). ABC of general surgery in children: Acute problems of the scrotum. *British Medical Journal, 312*(7028), 435–437.

41. Davis, I., & Avner, E. (2007a). Glomerular disease. In R. Kliegman, R. Behrman, H. Jenson, & B. Stanton (Eds.), *Nelson textbook of pediatrics* (18th ed.). Philadelphia: Saunders Elsevier.

42. Davis, I., & Avner, E. (2007b). Nephrotic syndrome. In R. Kliegman, R. Behrman, H. Jenson, & B. Stanton (Eds.), *Nelson textbook of pediatrics* (18th ed.). Philadelphia: Saunders Elsevier.

43. Davis, I., & Avner, E. (2007c). Upper Urinary Tract Causes of Hematuria. In R. Kliegman, R. Behrman, H. Jenson, & B. Stanton (Eds.), *Nelson textbook of pediatrics* (18th ed.). Philadelphia: Saunders Elsevier.

44. Del Rio, M., & Kaskel, F. (2008). Evaluation and management of steroid-unresponsive nephritic syndrome. *Current Opinion in Pediatrics, 20,* 151–156.

45. Dell, K., & Avner, E. (2007). Renal tubular acidosis. In R. M. Kliegman, R. E. Behrman, H. B. Jenson, & B. Stanton (Eds.), *Nelson textbook of pediatrics* (18th ed., pp. 2197–2200). Philadelphia: Saunders.

46. Dharnidharka, V., Agodoa, L., & Abbott, K. (2007). Effects of urinary tract infection on outcomes after renal transplantation in children. *Clinical Journal of the American Society of Nephrology, 2,* 100–106.

47. Diven, S., & Travis, L. (2000). A practical approach to hematuria in children. *Pediatric Nephrology, 14,* 65–72.

48. Dogan, H., & Tekgul, S. (2007). Management of pediatric stone disease. *Current Urology Reports, 8*(2), 163–173.

49. Doganis, D., Siafras, K., Mavrikou, M., Issaris, G., Martirosova, A., Perperidis, G., et al. (2007). Does early treatment of urinary tract infection prevent renal damage? *Pediatrics, 120,* e922–e928.

50. Dore-Bergeron, M., Gauthier, M., Chevalier, I., McManus, B., Tapiero, B., & Lebrun, S. (2009). Urinary tract infections in 1–3 month old infants: Ambulatory treatment with intravenous antibiotics. *Pediatrics, 124,* 16–22.

51. Dutta, S., & Narang, A. (2003). Enalapril-induced acute renal failure in a newborn infant. *Pediatric Nephrology, 18,* 570–572.

52. Eddy, A., & Symons, J. (2003). Nephrotic syndrome in childhood. *Lancet, 362,* 629–639.

53. Elder, J. (2007). Urologic disorders in infants and children. In R. M. Kliegman, R. E. Behrman, H. B. Jenson, & B. F. Stanton (Eds.), *Nelson textbook of pediatrics* (17th ed., pp. 2223–2231). Philadelphia: W. B. Saunders.

54. Fitzgerald, A., Lee, C. W., & Mori, R. (2009). Antibiotics for treating uncomplicated urinary tract infections in children (Protocol). *Cochran Collaboration (reprint), 2,* 1–10.

55. Fivush, B., Neu, A., & Furth, S. (1997). Acute hypertensive crises in children: emergencies and urgencies. *Current Opinion in Pediatrics, 9,* 233–236.

56. Flynn, J., & Daniels, S. (2006). Pharmacologic treatment of hypertesion in children and adolescents. *Journal of Pediatrics, 149,* 746–754.

57. Fogazzi, G., Edefoni, A., Garigali, G., Giani, M., Zolin, A., Raimondi, S., et al. (2008). Urine erythrocyte morphology in patients with microscopic haematuria caused by glomerulonephropathy. *Pediatric Nephrology, 23,* 1093–1100.

58. Forcier, M. (2009). Emergency department evaluation of acute pelvic pain in the adolescent female. *Clinical Pediatric Emergency Medicine, 10,* 20–30.

59. Freedman, A. (2005). Urologic diseases in North America project: Trends in resource utilization for urinary tract infections in children. *Journal of Urology, 173*(3), 949–954.

60. French, L. (2005). Dysmenorrhea. *American Family Physician, 71*(2), 285–291.

61. Garin, E., Olavarria, F., Nieto, V., Valenciano, B., Campos, A., & Young, L. (2006). Clinical significance of primary vesicoureteral reflux and urinary antibiotic prophylaxis after acute pyelonephritis: A multicenter, randomized, controlled study. *Pediatrics, 117*(3), 626–632.

62. Gatti, J., & Murphy, J. (2008). Acute testicular disorders. *Pediatrics in Review, 29*(7), 235–241.

63. Ghani, A., Al Helal, B., & Hussain, N. (2009). Acute renal failure in pediatric patients: Etiology and predictors of outcome. *Saudi Journal of Kidney Diseases and Transplantation, 20*(1), 69–76.

64. Gillespie, R., & Stapleton, F. (2004). Nephrolithiasis in Children. *Pediatrics in Review, 25*(4), 131–139.

65. Gipson, D., Massengill, S., Yao, L., Nagaraj, S., Smoyer, W., Mahan, J., et al. (2009). Management of childhood onset nephrotic syndrome. *Pediatrics, 124*(2), 747–757.

66. Glassock, R. (2001). Hematuria and proteinuria. In A. Greenberg (Ed.), *Primer on kidney disease* (pp. 38–46). San Diego: Acedemic Press.

67. Goldstein, S., & Devarajan, P. (2008). Progression from acute kidney injury to chronic kidney disease: A pediatric perspective. *Advances in Chronic Kidney Disease, 15*(3), 278–283.

68. Goodman, J., & Uphold, C. (2003). Metabolic and endocrine problems. In C. Uphold & M. Graham (Eds.), *Clinical guidelines in family practice* (4th ed., pp. 208–212). Gainesville, FL: Barmarrae Books.

69. Greydanus, D., Omar, H., Tsitsika, A., & Patel, D. (2009). Menstrual disorders in adolescent females: Current concepts. *Disease-a-Month, 55,* 45–113.

70. Groshong, T. (1996). Hypertensive crisis in children. *Pediatric Annals, 25*(7), 368–371, 375–376.

71. Grubb, A., Nyman, U., Bjork, J., Lindstrom, V., Rippe, B., Sterner, G., et al. (2005). Simple cystatin C-based prediction equations for glomerular filtration rate compared with the modification of diet in renal disease prediction equation for adults and the Schwartz and the Counahan-Barratt prediction equations for children. *Clinical Chemistry, 51*(8), 1420–1431.

72. Harel, Z. (2008). Dysmenorrhea in adolescents. *Annals of the New York Academy of Sciences, 1135,* 185–195.

73. Harlow, S., & Campbell, O. (2004). Epidemiology of menstrual disorders in developing countries: A systematic review. *BJOG: An International Journal of Obstetrics and Gynaecology, 111,* 6–16.

74. Hellerstein, S. (2006). Acute urinary tract infections: Evaluation and treatment. *Current Opinion in Pediatrics, 18,* 134–138.

75. Herrin, J. (2004). Renal tubular acidosis. In E. Avner, W. Harmon, & P. Wiandet (Eds.), *Pediatric nephrology* (5th ed.). Philadelphia: Lippincott, Williams and Wilkins.

76. Hickey, M., & Balen A. (2003). Menstrual disorders in adolescence: Investigation and management. *Human Reproduction Update, 9*(5), 493–504.

77. Hiller, N., Appelbaum, L., Simanovsky, N., Lev-Segi, A., Aharon, D., & Sella. T. (2007). CT features of adnexal torsion. *American Journal of Radiology, 189,* 124–129.

78. Hiren, P., & Mitsnefes, M. (2005). Advances in the pathogenesis and management of hypertensive crisis. *Nephrology, 17*(2), 210–214.

79. Hodson, E., & Alexander, S. (2008). Evaluation and management of steroid-sensitive nephritic syndrome. *Current Opinion in Pediatrics, 20,* 145–150.

80. Hodson, E., Willis, N., & Criag, J. (2007). Antibiotics for acute pyelonephritis in children. *Cochrane Database of Systematic Reviews 2007, 4,* CD003772. doi: 10.1002/14651858.CD003772.pub3

81. Hodson, M., Craig, J., Martin, S., & Moyer, V. (2009). Short versus standard duration oral antibiotic therapy for acute urinary tract infection in children. *Cochran Collaboration Review*, 1–33.

82. Hogg, R., Portman, R., Milliner, D., Lemley, K., Eddy, A. & Ingelfinger, J. (2000). Evaluation and management of proteinuria and nephrotic syndrome in children: Recommendations from a pediatric nephrology panel established at the National Kidney Foundation Conference on proteinuria, albuminuria, risk, assessment, detection and elimination (PARADE). *Pediatrics*, *105*, 1242–1249.

83. Hsu, S., Tsai, I., & Tsau, Y. (2005). Comparison of growth in primary Fanconi syndrome and proximal renal tubular acidosis. *Pediatric Nephrology*, *20*, 460–464.

84. Huang, C. (2009). Problems of the foreskin and glans penis. *Clinical Pediatric Emergency Medicine*, *10*, 56–59.

85. Ishimine, P. (2007). The evolving approach to the young child who has fever and no obvious source. *Emergency Medicine Clinics of North America*, *25*, 1087–1115.

86. Jain, K. (2008). Gynecologic causes of acute pelvic pain: Ultrasound imaging. *Ultrasound Clinics*, *3*, 1–12.

87. Jalanko, H. (2009). Congenital nephrotic syndrome. *Pediatric Nephrology*, *24*(11), 2121– 2128.

88. Jordan, S., Vo, A., Peng, A., Toyoda, M., & Tyan, D. (2006). Intravenous gammaglobulin (IVIG): A noval approach to improve transplant rates and outcomes in highly HLA-sensitized patients. *American Journal of Transplantation*, *6*, 459–466.

89. Kahan, B., & Ponticelli, C. (Eds.). (2000). *Principles and practice of renal transplantation*. London: Martin Dunitz.

90. Kanellopoulos, T., Salakos, C., Spiliopoulou, I., Ellina, A., Nikolakopoulou, N., & Papanastasiou, D. (2006). First urinary tract infection in neonates, infants and young children: A comparative study. *Pediatric Nephrology*, *21*, 1131–1137.

91. Karet, F. (2009). Mechanisms in hyperkalemic renal tubular acidosis. *Journal of the American Society of Nephrology*, *20*, 251–254.

92. Kasiske, B. (2001). In A. Greenberg (Ed.), *Primer on kidney disease*. San Diego: Academic Press.

93. Katzir, Z., Dinour, D., Reznik-Wolf, H., Nissenkorn, A., & Holtzman, E. (2008). Familial pure proximal tubular acidosis. *Nephrology Dialysis Transplantation*, *23*, 1211–1215.

94. Kidney Disease Improving Global Outcomes. (2009). KDIGO clinical guideline for the care of kidney transplant Recipients. *American Journal of Transplantation*, *3*(9 suppl), 1–65.

95. Kimball, J. (2009). Hormones of the reproductive system: Females. Retrieved from http://users.rcn.com/jkimball.ma.ultranet/Biology Pages/S/SexHormones.html

96. Koshy, S., & Geary, D. (2008). Anemia in children with chronic kidney disease. *Pediatric Nephrology*, *23*, 209–219.

97. Kulp, J., Mwangi, C., & Loveless, M. (2008). Screening for coagulation disorders in adolescents with abnormal uterine bleeding. *Journal of Pediatric and Adolescent Gynecology*, *21*, 27–30.

98. Kyrieleis, H., Lowik, M., Pronk, I., Cruysberg, H., Kremer, J., Oyen, W., et al. (2009). Long-term outcome of biopsy proven, frequently relapsing minimal change nephrotic syndrome in children. *Clinical Journal of the American Society of Nephrology*, *4*(10), 1593–1600.

99. Lande, M., & Flynn, J. (2009). Treatment of hypertension in children and adolescents. *Pediatric Nephrology*, *24*, 1939–1949.

100. Lane, J., & Kaskel, F. (2009). Pediatric nephrotic syndrome: From the simple to the complex. *Seminars in Nephrology*, *29*(4), 389–398.

101. Lapoint Rudow, D., Ohler, L., & Shafer, T. (Eds.). (2006). *A clinician's guide to donation and transplantation*. Lenexa, KS: Applied Measurement Professionals.

102. Leslie, J., & Cain, M. (2006). Pediatric urologic emergencies and urgencies. *Pediatric Clinics of North America*, *53*(3), 513–527.

103. Lum, G. (2007). Kidney and urinary tract. In W. W. Hay, M. J. Levin, J. M. Sondheimer, & R. R. Deterding (Eds.), *Current diagnosis and treatment in pediatrics* (18th ed., p. 706). New York: McGraw-Hill.

104. Lurn, G. (2009). Kidney and urinary tract. In W. W. Hay, M. J. Levin, J. M. Sondheimer, & R. R. Deterding (Eds.), *Current pediatric diagnosis and treatment* (19th ed., pp. 667–669). Philadelphia: McGraw-Hill, Lange.

105. Mannix, L. (2008). Menstrual-related pain conditions: Dysmenorrhea and migraine. *Journal of Women's Health*, *17*(5), 879–891.

106. Mantadakis, E., Cavender, J., Rogers, Z., Ewalt, D., & Buchanan, G. R. (1999). Prevalance of priapism in children and adolescents with sickle cell anemia. *Journal of Pediatric Hematology/Oncology*, *21*(6), 518–522.

107. Massry, S., & Glassock, R. (Eds.). (2001). *Massry and Glassock's textbook of nephrology*. Philadelphia: Lippincott, Williams, & Wilkins.

108. McKinney, P., Feltbower, R., Brocklebank, J., & Fitzpatrick, M. (2001). Time trends and ethnic patterns of childhood nephrotic syndrome. *Pediatric Nephrology*, *16*(12), 1040–1044.

109. McWilliams, G., Hill, M., & Dietrich, C. (2008). Gynecologic emergencies. *Surgical Clinics of North America*, *88*, 265–283.

110. Meyers, K. (2004). Evaluation of hematuria in children. *Urologic Clinics of North America*, *31*, 559–573.

111. Miller, D., & MacDonald, D. (2006). Management of pediatric patients with chronic kidney disease. *Pediatric Nursing*, *32*(2), 128–134.

112. Mohkam, M., Karimi, A., Gharib, A., Daneshmand, H., Khatami, A., Ghojevand, N., et al. (2007). Ceftriaxone associated nephrolithiasis: A prospective study in 284 children. *Pediatric Nephrology*, *22*, 690–694.

113. Montgomery, R. (2010). Renal transplantation across HLA and ABO antibody barriers: Integrating paired donation into desensitization protocols. *American Journal of Transplantation*, *10*, 49–57.

114. Munden, J. (2007). Reproductive system. In J. Munden (Ed.). *Professional guide to pathophysiology* (2nd ed., pp. 656–690). Philadelphia: Lippincott, Williams, & Wilkins.

115. Nako, Y., Ohki, Y., Harigaya, A., Tomomasa, T., & Morikawa, A. (1999). Transtubular potassium concentration grandient in preterm neonates. *Pediatric Nephrology*, *13*, 880–885.

116. National High Blood Pressure Education Program on High Blood Pressure in Children and Adolescents. (2004). The fourth report on the diagnosis, evaluation, and treatment of high blood pressure in children and adolescents. *Pediatrics*, *2*(114 suppl 4), 555–576.

117. Nicoletta, J., & Lande, M. (2006). Medical evaluation and treatment of urolithiasis. *Pediatric Clinics of North America*, *53*, 479–491.

118. Nur, M., Romano, M., & Siqueira, L. (2007). Premenstrual dysphoric disorder in the adolescent female. *Journal of Pediatric and Adolescent Gynecology*, *20*, 201–204.

119. Ozawa, Y., Murakami, T., Terada, Y., Yaegashi, N., Okamura, K., Kuriyama, S., et al. (2006). Management of the pain associated with endometrosis: An update of the painful problems. *Tohoku Journal of Experimental Medicine*, *210*, 175–188.

120. Palmer, L., & Palmer, J. (2008). The efficacy of topical betamethasone for treating phimosis: A comparison of two treatment regimens. *Urology*, *72*, 68–71.

121. Patel, H., & Bissler, J. (2001). Hematuria in children. *Pediatric Clinics of North America*, *48*(6), 1519–1537.

122. Pong, A., & Bradley, J. (2005). Guidelines for the selection of antibacterial therapy in children. *Pediatric Clinics of North America*, *52*, 859–872.

123. Prelog, M., Schiefecker, D., Fille, M., Wurzner, R., Brunner, A., & Zimmerhackl, L. (2007). Febrile urinary tract infection: Ampicillin and trimethoprim insufficient as empirical mono-therapy. *Pediatric Nephrology*, *23*, 597–602.

124. Quigley, R. (2008). Evaluation of hematuria and proteinuria: How should a pediatrician proceed? *Current Opinion in Pediatrics*, *20*, 140–144.

125. Quint, E., & Sifuentes, M. (2004). Common gynecologic and urinary problems in the pediatric and adolescent female. In M. Pearlman, J. Tintinalli, & P. Dyne (Eds.), *Obstetric and*

gynecolocial emergencies: Diagnosis and management (pp. 350–368). New York: McGraw-Hill.

126. Reddy, P., Sheldon, C., & Minevich, E. (2005). Management of pediatric stones. Journal of Urology, 174(4), 1708-1710.

127. Riley, C., Moen, M., & Videm, V. (2007). Inflammatory markers in endometriosis: Reduced peritoneal neutrophil response in minimal endometriosis. *Acta Obstetricia et Gynecologica Scandinavica, 86,* 877–881.

128. Ringdahl, E., & Teauge, L. (2006). Testicular torsion. *American Family Physician, 74*(10), 1739–1743.

129. Rodriguez, M., Gomez, A., Abitbol, C., Chandar, J., Duara, S., & Zilleruelo, G. (2004). Histomorphometric analysis of postnatal glomerulogenesis in extremely preterm infants. *Pediatric and Developmental Pathology, 7,* 17–25.

130. Rogers, Z. (2005). Priapism in sickle cell disease. *Hematology/Oncology Clinics of North America, 19,* 917–928.

131. Roy, R., Roy, E., Rahman, M., & Hossain, M. (2009). Serum immunoglobulin G, M and IgG:IgM ratio as predictors for outcome of childhood nephritic syndrome. *World Journal of Pediatrics, 5*(2), 127–131.

132. Santos-Victoriano, M., Brouhard, B., & Cunningham, R. (1998). Renal stone disease in children. *Clinical Pediatrics, 37,* 583–599.

133. Schrier, R. (Ed.). (2001). *Diseases of the kidney and urinary tract* (Vol. III). Philadelphia: Lippincott, Williams, & Wilkins.

134. Schwab, S., & Posner, J. (2008). Menstrual disorders. In J. Baren, S. Rothrock, J. Brennan, & L. Brown (Eds.), *Pediatric emergency medicine* (pp. 683–688). Philadelphia: Saunders Elsevier.

135. Schwaderer, A., Cronin, R., Mahan, J., & Bates, C. (2008). Low bone density in children with hypercalciuria and/or nephrolithiasis. *Pediatric Nephrology, 23,* 2209–2214.

136. Schwartz, G., & Furth, S. (2007). Glomerular filtration rate measurement and estimation in chronic kidney disease. *Pediatric Nephrology, 22,* 1839–1848.

137. Schwartz, G., Haycock, G., Edemann, C., & Spitzer, A. (1976). A simple estimate of glomerular filtration rate in children derived from body length and plasma creatinine. *Pediatrics, 58*(2), 259–263.

138. Schwartz, G., Munoz, A., Schneider, M., Mak, R., Kaskel, F., Warady, B., et al. (2009). New equations to estimate GFR in children with CKD. *Journal of the American Society of Nephrology, 20,* 629–637.

139. Schwartz, R., & Rushton, H. (1996). Acute balanoposthitis in young boys. *Pediatric Infectious Disease Journal, 15*(2), 176–177.

140. Schwarz, R., & Dwyer, N. (2006). Pediatric kidney stones: Long-term outcomes., *Pediatric Urology, 67*(4), 812–816.

141. Scout, L., Baltarowich, O., & Lev-Toaff, A. (2007). Imaging of adnexal torsion. *Ultrasound Clinics, 2,* 311–325.

142. Sedman, A., Kershaw, D., & Bunchman, T. (1995). Recognition and management of angiotensin converting enzyme inhibitor fetopathy. *Pediatric Nephrology, 9*(3), 382–385.

143. Sethna, C., & Meyers, K. (2008). Glomerulonephritis. In M. W. Schwartz et al. (Eds.), *5-minute pediatric consult* (5th ed.). Philadelphia: Lippincott, Williams, & Wilkins.

144. Shah, G., & Upadhyay, J. (2005). Controversies in the diagnosis and management of urinary tract infections in children. *Pediatric Drugs, 7*(6), 339–346.

145. Shaikh, N., & Hoberman, A. (2007). Urinary tract infections in childhood. In L. B. Zaoutis, & V. W. Chiang (Eds.), *Comprehensive pediatric hospital medicine* (pp. 407–413). Philadelphia: Mosby/Elsevier.

146. Shaikh, N., Morone, N., Bost, J., & Farrell, M. (2008). Prevalence of urinary tract infection in childhood. *Pediatric Infectious Disease Journal, 27,* 402–408.

147. Shapiro, E., Kaye, J., & Palmer, L. (2009). Laparoscopic ovarian cystectomy in children. *Pediatric Urology, 73,* 526–528.

148. Sharma, A., Sharma, R., Kapoor, R., Kornecki, A., Sural, S., & Filler, G. (2007). Incomplete distal renal tubular acidosis affects growth in children. *Nephrology Dialysis Transplantation, 22,* 2879–2885.

149. Sharma, A., Singh, R., Yang, C., Singh, R., Kapoor, R., & Filler, G. (2009). Bicarbonate therapy improves growth in children with incomplete distal renal tubular acidosis. *Pediatric Nephrology, 24,* 1509–1516.

150. Smith, E. (2008). Pyelonephritis, renal scarring and reflux nephropathy: A pediatric urologist perspective. *Pediatric Radiology, 38*(1), S76–S82.

151. Somekh, E., Gorenstein, A., & Serour, F. (2004). Acute epididymitis in boys: Evidence of a post-infectious etiology. *Journal of Urology, 171,* 391–394.

152. Song, A., & Advincula, A. (2005). Mini-review: Adolescent chronic pelvic pain. *Journal of Pediatric and Adolescent Gynecology, 18,* 371–377.

153. Steiner, M. (2000). Premenstrual syndrome and premenstrual dysphoric disorder: Guidelines for management. *Journal of Psychiatry and Neuroscience, 25*(5), 459–468.

154. Tajani, A., Harmon, W., & Fine, R. (Eds.). (2000). *Pediatric solid organ transplantation.* Munksgaard, Copenhagen: Special-Trykkeriet Viborg a-s.

155. Taketomo, C., Hodding, J., & Kraus, D. (2010). *Pediatric dosage handbook* (16th ed.). Hudson, OH: Lexi-Comp.

156. Tan, J. (2009). Nephrology. In J. Custer & R. Rau (Eds.), *The Harriet Lane handbook.* Philadehia: Elsevier Mosby.

157. Templeman, C. (2009). Adolescent endometriosis. *Obstetrics and Gynecology Clinics of North America, 36,* 177–185.

158. Templeman, C. (2004). Ovarian cysts. *Journal of Pediatric and Adolescent Gynecology, 17*(4), 297–298.

159. Tong, A., Lowe, A., Sainsbury, P., & Craig, J. (2008). Experience of parents who have children with chronic kidney disease: A systematic review of qualitative studies. *Pediatrics, 121,* 349–360.

160. Trachtman, H. (2004). Sodium and Water. In E. Avner, W. Harmon, & P. Niaudet., *Pediatric Nephrology,* (5th ed.). Philadelphia: Lippincott, Williams, & Wilkins.

161. Trainor, J. (2009). Diagnosis and management of testicular torsion, torsion of the appendix testis, and epididymitis. *Clinical Pediatric Emergency Medicine, 10*(1), 38–44.

162. Tredger, J., Brown, N., & Dhawan, A. (2006). Immunosupppression in pediatric solid organ transplantation: Opportunities, risks, and management. *Pediatric Transplantation, 10,* 879–892.

163. Tuchman, S., & Meyers, K. (2008). Pyelonephritis. In M. W. Schwartz et al. (Eds.), *5-minute pediatric consult* (5th ed.). Philadelphia: Lippincott, Williams, & Wilkins.

164. U.S. Department of Health and Human Services (HHS), National Institutes of Health National Heart, Lung, and Blood Institute. (2005). The fourth report on the diagnosis, evaluation, and treatment of high blood pressure in children and adolescents. Retrieved from http://www.nhlbi.nih.gov/health/prof/heart/hbp/hbp_ped.pdf

165. U.S. Department of Health and Human Services (HHS). (2007). 42 CFR Parts 405, 482, 488, and 498 Medicare program; hospital conditions of participation: Requirements for approval and re-approval of transplant centers to perform organ transplants; final rule. Retrieved from http://www.cms.gov/CFCsAndCoPs/downloads/trancenter-reg2007.pdf

166. U.S. Department of Health and Human Services (HHS). (2008a). OPTN: Organ Procurement and Transplant Network. http://optn.transplant.hrsa.gov/. Retrieved from http://optn.transplant.hrsa.gov/PoliciesandBylaws2/policies/pdfs/policy_7.pdf

167. U.S. Department of Health and Human Services (HHS). (2008b). OPTN/SRTR annual report. Retrieved from http://www.ustransplant.org/annual_reports/current/iKI_Recipients_dialysis.htm?o=2&g=2&c=8

168. U.S. Food and Drug Administration (FDA). (2002). Best pharmaceuticals for children. Retrieved from http://www.fda.gov/Drugs/DevelopmentApprovalProcess/DevelopmentResources/ucm049876.htm

169. U.S. Food and Drug Administration (FDA). (1997). Food and Drug Administration Moderization Act of 1997. Retrieved from http://www.fda.gov/RegulatoryInformation/Legislation/FederalFoodDrugandCosmeticActFDCAct/SignificantAmendmentstotheFDCAct/FDAMA/FullTextofFDAMAlaw/default.htm

170. Venhola, M., Huttuten, N., & Uhari, M. (2009). Meta-analysis of vesicoureteral reflux and urinary tract infection in children. *Scandinavian Journal of Urology and Nephrology, 40,* 98–102.

171. Vining, E. (2008). Special Issue: Ketogenic Diet and Related Dietary Treatments. *Epilepsia, 49*(s8), 27–29.

172. Voss, D., Hodson, E., & Crompton, C. (2007). Nutrition and growth in kidney disease: CARI guidelines. *Australian Family Physician, 36*(3), 253–254.

173. Wagenlehner, F., Weidner, W., & Naber, K. (2007). Pharmacokinetic characteristics of antimicrobials and optimal treatment of urosepsis. *Clinical Pharmacokinetics, 46*(4), 291–305.

174. Warady, B., & Chadha, V. (2007). Chronic kidney disease in children: The global perspective. *Pediatric Nephrology, 22,* 1999–2009.

175. Warady, B., Hebert, D., Sullivan, E., Alexander, S., & Tejani, A. (1997). Renal transplantation, chronic dialysis and chronic renal insufficiency in children and adolescents: The 1995 annual report of the North American Pediatric Renal Transplant Cooperative Study. *Pediatric Nephrology, 11,* 49–64.

176. Wesseling, K., Bakkaloglu, S., & Salusky, I. (2008). Chronic kidney disease: Mineral and bone disorder in children. *Pediatric Nephrology, 23,* 195–207.

177. Wills, B., Albinson, C., Wahl, M., & Clifton, J. (2007). Sildenafil citrate ingestion and prolonged priapism and tachycardia in a pediatric patient. *Clinical Toxicology, 45,* 798–800.

178. Wooltorton, E. (2005). Medroxyprogesterone acetate (Depo-Provera) and bone mineral density loss. *Canadian Medical Association Journal, 172*(6), 746.

179. Yang, S., Tsai, Y., Wu, C., Lui, S., & Wang, C. (2005). Highly potent and moderately potent topical steroids are effective in treating phimosis: A prospective randomized study. *Journal of Urology, 173*(4), 1361–1363.

180. Yiu, V., Orrbine, E., Rosychuk, R., MacLaine, P., Goodyer, P., Girardin, C., et al. (2004). The safety and use of short-acting nifedipine in hospitalized hypertensive children. *Pediatric Nephrology, 19*(6), 644–650.

181. Zaffanello, M., Franchini, M., & Fanos, V. (2007). Review: Is serum cystatin-C a suitable marker of renal function in children? *Annals of Clinical and Laboratory Science, 37*(3), 233–240.

182. Zappitelli, M. (2008). Epidemiology and diagnosis of acute kidney injury. *Seminars in Nephrology, 28*(5), 436–446.

183. Zappitelli, M., Parvex, P., Joseph, L., Paradis, G., Grey, V., Lau, S., et al. (2006). Derivation and validation of cystatin C–based prediction equations for GFR in children. *American Journal of Kidney Diseases, 48*(2), 221–230.

Musculoskeletal Disorders

PHYSIOLOGY AND DIAGNOSTICS

Jeffrey M. Mjaanes

PHYSIOLOGY

Embryology

The musculoskeletal system consists primarily of bone, muscle, tendons, and ligaments. It serves to protect vital organs, allow for respiration, provide locomotion, and facilitate storage of nutrients. The skeleton is formed from mesoderm during prenatal development. Limb buds appear as early as the fourth week of the embryonic period; joints form by week 6, and the limbs rotate during week 7. Primary ossification centers of all major bones begin to appear between weeks 7 and 12 during the fetal period, and virtually all are formed by birth. Postnatal growth mainly occurs before the child reaches age 3 and during adolescence. During the first two years after birth, the average child's length approximately doubles and his or her weight almost triples. Growth then proceeds at a fairly steady rate until puberty, at which time a final growth increase occurs.

Bone development

Most bone forms by replacing a cartilage matrix through a process known as endochondral ossification. Bone growth usually begins at primary ossification centers from which the diaphysis, or shaft, of the bone develops. During childhood, bone also begins to develop at secondary ossification centers, called epiphyseal centers, which are located at the ends of what will eventually become the adult long bones. As both types of ossification centers expand, the cartilage matrices at the leading edges approximate one another. This region, which is called the physis, or growth plate, does not fuse until the adult length of the bone is attained.

Apophyses are secondary growth plates located at sites where muscle–tendon units attach to bone (e.g., tibial tuberosity). Unlike physes, apophyses do not contribute to the growth of long bones, yet the physes and apophyses are composed of similar growth cartilage. Three zones of cartilage exist in growth plates: a proliferative zone, a hypertrophic (maturation) zone, and a zone of provisional calcification. The hypertrophic zone, where the cartilage cells or chondrocytes begin to terminally differentiate, appears to be the most susceptible to injury.

Growth plates are quite sensitive to mechanical forces, especially traction and compression. Studies using animal models show that sustained traction minimally promotes growth, whereas sustained pressure inhibits growth

to a significant degree—as much as 40% (Stokes, 2002). This phenomenon is known as the Hueter-Volkmann Law. For example, septic arthritis increases pressure in a joint, adversely affecting growth; in Osgood-Schlatter disease, traction on the tibial apophysis leads to enhanced growth and protuberance of the tubercle.

BASIC TENETS AFFECTING BONE HEALING

The Hueter-Volkmann principle

In the late nineteenth century, German surgeons Carl Hueter and Richard von Volkmann developed a hypothesis to explain bone growth in response to stress. The Hueter-Volkmann principle states that compression forces inhibit growth and tensile forces stimulate growth. This theory may explain the pathophysiology behind many growth plate injuries and highlights the importance of rapid diagnosis and proper treatment of these injuries. In most physeal injuries, the cartilage–bone interface of the growth plate is damaged. In low grade (i.e., Salter-Harris Type I) injuries, the damage to the growth cartilage and, therefore, long-term adverse sequelae are minimal. By comparison, in higher-grade injuries (i.e., Salter-Harris IV or V), damage to the physis can be significant and the probability of growth arrest is high. A classic example is slipped capital femoral epiphysis (SCFE), where the proximal femoral physis sustains a compressive, shearing load (Gholve et al., 2009). A significant correlation exists between delayed diagnosis and increased slip severity (Rhame et al., 2006).

Wolff's law

Julius Wolff, a nineteenth-century German anatomist and surgeon, proposed a theory to explain how bone remodels after injury. Wolff's law states that bone in a healthy person or animal will adapt to the loads it experiences. Therefore, if the bone is placed under a certain amount of loading or stress, the bone will internally remodel to become stronger and resist the stress. An obvious example involves weight-bearing exercise that increases bone mineral density (Stewart et al., 2005). The converse is also true, however. If the load upon a bone is decreased, the bone in effect becomes weaker, as in the case of prolonged immobilization. In the case of treatment for lower extremity musculoskeletal conditions, Wolff's law forms the rationale behind the "weight bearing as tolerated" approach to many injuries. Unless an unstable fracture could become displaced with weight bearing, most patients are allowed to bear some weight on the injured extremity during rehabilitation to facilitate remodeling and healing.

PHYSIOLOGY OF MOVEMENT

Muscle develops under similar circumstances as bone in the growing child. Most muscle growth occurs during the first four years of life, and then again in a wave during adolescence. New muscle cells form at the ends of the muscle–tendon unit near the myotendinous junction. Skeletal muscles provide posture and movement. The muscles start to contract as stimulus of the muscles fiber reaches the motor neurons. This production leads to energy that stems from the hydrolysis of adenosine triphosphate (ATP), extends to adenosine diphosphate (ADP), then shifts to phosphate, and ultimately produces muscle contraction. As muscles relax, they break down acetylcholine through cholinesterase.

Similar to bone growth plates, this area is also susceptible to injury, especially in adults. Common conditions such as "tennis elbow" and "golfer's elbow" are actually wrist extensor and flexor tendinopathies, respectively. Interestingly, in the growing child, muscle–tendon units tend to be stronger than the bone's nearby growth plates. The physis and the apophysis are the "weak links" in the chain. Thus, when the growth plate fails to adequately adapt to the stresses to which it is subjected, injury often results. As a consequence, skeletally immature athletes may develop proximal humeral epiphysiolysis ("Little League shoulder"), for example, while skeletally mature athletes develop rotator cuff strain.

EVALUATION OF THE MUSCULOSKELETAL SYSTEM

History

Evaluating a musculoskeletal condition or injury in children includes a thorough and detailed history. The age of the child may determine the source and the accuracy of the information obtained. Older children and adolescents are usually able to describe the onset, symptoms, and contributing factors for their condition; thus the history may be obtained from them directly. With young children, the health care professional (HCP) often has to rely on the child's caregiver to provide historical data.

Important components of the history include the onset of symptoms and their chronology, the nature of the symptoms, contributing and ameliorating factors, and the presence of any associated symptoms. One should note if the onset was insidious or acute, if direct trauma occurred, and if the exact mechanism of injury is known. Pain should be assessed as well as the effects of the symptoms on the patient's activity level. Inquire about whether any treatments or remedies were tried previously and whether these interventions were beneficial. The etiology of joint and limb pain may not always be orthopedic in origin. Other conditions such as neoplasia, autoimmune disorders, and infections can manifest as musculoskeletal complaints. Therefore, the HCP should ask about the presence or absence of pertinent associated symptoms, such as fevers, chills, night sweats, night pain, and rashes or skin changes.

Cases of musculoskeletal injury in children, especially infants and toddlers, may be due to nonaccidental trauma and physical abuse. Thus the HCP may maintain a high index of suspicion when taking the history in cases of fractures, limp, and musculoskeletal pain in young children or those with mental or physical disabilities. Note the interaction between the caregiver and the child, identify any discrepancies in the history, and determine whether the injury in question is consistent with the mechanism described. All HCPs are mandated reporters and should notify authorities if any suspicion of child abuse exists.

A complete medical history also includes any pertinent facts from the patient's past medical, family, and social histories. For young children, the birth and developmental history are essential. Prior injuries or surgeries to the same joint or limb are important to note for all patients. For upper extremity complaints, the HCP should always ask about a history of cervical injuries or pain; for lower extremity issues, a history of cervical, thoracic, or lumbar conditions should be noted. Inquiry includes a family history of bone or joint diseases, autoimmune disorders, or endocrine disorders. The social history should be tailored to the age of the child. For older children, the HCP should note regular activity level, sports participation, and hand dominance.

Physical examination

Evaluating a musculoskeletal complaint includes performing a complete physical examination if the injury is chronic or nonfocal. Usually the HCP not only examines the affected body part but also the joints or segments located proximally and distally. The physical examination should be performed in an orderly, sequential fashion to ensure no portion is overlooked. Inspection, palpation, manipulation, and special testing are all essential components of the examination. Some HCPs may find it helpful to review the anatomy of the body part in question prior to beginning the physical examination.

The first part of the physical examination—inspection—is often done subconsciously as the HCP observes the child while obtaining the history. A conscious effort should be made to inspect the surface anatomy for any deformity, swelling, discoloration, and malalignment. If the child is ambulatory, the examiner should observe the child's gait for any abnormalities such as limp, pain, or inability to bear weight. A child's gait essentially represents the active motion that the child can achieve at the hip, knee, and ankle. Active range of motion is described as the extent of motion the patient can achieve at a joint on his or her own accord. The HCP should note the degree of motion achieved actively in all directions for the joint in question.

Next, the examiner proceeds to palpate the affected area. Notice is made of any swelling or induration, temperature change, or tenderness. The intensity should be light at first so as not to cause significant discomfort to the child. It is often helpful to wait and examine the suspected area of maximal tenderness last to limit the patient's pain and apprehension.

Manipulation of the affected area includes passive range of motion, muscle strength testing, sensory and reflex assessment, and stability testing. Passive range of motion is the range through which the examiner can move the joint. In an individual without a joint abnormality, the active and passive range of motion should be the same. Therefore, the HCP truly needs to perform passive motion testing only if the observed active range of motion of the joint in question is abnormal. Strength testing is basically resisted motion testing of a joint. Examining the strength of the major muscle groups associated with the joint or body part assesses for pain, weakness, and limitations. Sensory testing and assessment of deep tendon reflexes are useful if nerve pathology is possible. Neurologic testing is an essential component of a thorough examination in cases of fracture or dislocation where there is the potential of nerve injury. Stability testing usually refers to an assessment of the integrity of a ligament or the laxity of a joint after injury.

For each joint, special tests have been developed to assess specific structures, such as ligaments or tendons, for injury. Over the years, scores of special tests have been described in the medical literature. These tests vary by joint and body segment. Some, such as Lachman's test for anterior cruciate ligament stability in the knee, are well known and have been studied extensively (Reider, 2005).

During the physical examination, ensuring the patient's comfort and maintaining privacy are paramount. Older children and adolescents are comfortable with the exam but younger children are often apprehensive. The caregiver can be used to assist in calming the patient if the clinician finds this beneficial. The patient should be dressed in a manner to facilitate examination of the injured region. For older children, shorts for lower extremity evaluation are often sufficient. For examination of the back or upper extremity, a gown is usually provided. The area in question should be exposed for inspection and ease of access for palpation and manipulation.

DIAGNOSTICS

Imaging studies

Often, a complete history and thorough physical examination provide insufficient information for the HCP to make a proper diagnosis. Further evaluation may necessitate use of diagnostic imaging or laboratory analyses. Musculoskeletal imaging may include radiography, computed tomography (CT), magnetic resonance (MRI), and ultrasound. Each mode of imaging has unique characteristics and advantages.

Plain radiographs are often the first images obtained, as they are often readily available, are relatively inexpensive, and provide excellent detail of bony structures. Specialized views exist for most body parts, although anterior–posterior (AP) and lateral views are minimally required for screening purposes. In addition, oblique views are often helpful for assessing the foot, hand/fingers, elbow, and ankle. In the ankle, the oblique view is called the "mortise" view because it allows for visualization of the ankle, or mortise, joint surface. In the hip, the most common lateral view is called a "frog-leg" lateral; for this image, the patient's hip is maximally abducted. The true lateral view of the shoulder is termed the "axillary" view. Radiographs of the cervical spine often include lateral views in flexion and extension in cases of instability and an open-mouth, or odontoid, view to evaluate for fracture at the odontoid base.

If a fracture or significant abnormality is detected on basic screening radiographs, more specialized views can be obtained to further assess the injury. In particular, when growth plate injuries are suspected in children and adolescents, consider obtaining contralateral radiographs of the uninjured side for comparison purposes (Nnadi et al., 2002).

Computed tomography is superior to radiographs in providing fine bony detail. In children, CT scans are useful for evaluation of complex growth plate or physeal fractures. Such images are also often obtained in adolescents and adults in suspected scaphoid fractures of the wrist when plain radiographs are ambiguous. CT scans present a radiation risk that is significantly higher than that associated with conventional radiographs (Junnila & Cartwright, 2006).

Magnetic resonance imaging provides excellent soft-tissue and bone marrow contrast. MRI can detect radiographic occult fractures in weight-bearing bones such as the tibial plateau, the proximal femur, and the tarsal navicular. Physeal fractures are also usually well visualized with MRI. No radiation exposure is associated with MRI, but contraindications to its use include claustrophobia, pacemakers, and certain metallic surgical clips.

Ultrasonography is becoming popular in the musculoskeletal arena as an imaging modality. This technique is useful for identification of tendon and superficial ligament pathology, is noninvasive, and is relatively inexpensive. The value of sonography is highly operator dependent, however, and its exact role in evaluating acute pediatric musculoskeletal injuries remains unclear (Martin, 2005).

In addition to diagnostic imaging, laboratory testing may prove useful in the evaluation of some pediatric patients with acute musculoskeletal complaints. For most acute fractures or dislocations, laboratory tests are of limited benefit. Nevertheless, such testing can be important in the child with certain complaints such as limp, fever, and pain without obvious trauma. In these patients, non-orthopedic etiologies must be considered. Antinuclear antibody, rheumatoid factor, erythrocyte sedimentation rate, and complete blood count tests may be valuable screening tools for patients with possible rheumatologic or auto-immune conditions. A screening complete blood count with differential, sedimentation rate, and C-reactive protein (CRP) may be helpful in identifying infectious disorders, such as transient synovitis or septic arthritis in the acutely limping child. The majority of pediatric patients who present with acute musculoskeletal complaints will not require laboratory work-up.

COMPARTMENT SYNDROME

Summer Watkins and Prasad Gourineni

PATHOPHYSIOLOGY

Compartment syndrome is a pressure-related medical condition that compromises the tissue within a closed facial space (Shadgan et al., 2008). The affected area usually sustains an injury or insult that causes severe swelling, which in turn limits perfusion. This complication may also occur following the sequelae to injury, infection, or surgery.

Compartment syndrome is attributable to inadequate blood flow through the capillaries. This decrease in perfusion makes it impossible for the blood supply to meet the metabolic demands of the involved tissues. A transition to anaerobic metabolism with ischemia then leads to a build-up of lactic acid, loss of osmolar gradient, and leaky capillaries. This process stimulates neutrophil activation, free-radical generation, and intravascular coagulation; if left untreated, it may result in muscle and nerve damage that is both severe and permanent (Laine et al., 2010). Specifically, damage can include muscle necrosis with rhabdomyolysis, paralysis, and contractures. Loss of limb and even death have been associated with compartment syndrome. Early recognition, pressure reduction techniques, and surgical intervention are the cornerstones of treatment for this medical emergency.

EPIDEMIOLOGY AND ETIOLOGY

Many medical conditions can lead to compartment syndrome. In patients of all ages, the most common causes are acute high-impact trauma and long bone fractures (wrist, distal tibia). Other potential causes include crushing trauma, burns, bleeding disorders, venomous bites, abdominal surgery, intravenous (IV) or intraosseous (IO) infiltrates, thromboembolic events, and vascular reconstruction/cannulation. In the pediatric population, the most common causes are displaced supracondylar humerus fractures, distal tibia fractures, and IV infiltrates. In athletes, a transient compartment syndrome can develop with heavy training due to muscle hypertrophy and increased intracompartmental pressure with exercise (Kliegman et al., 2007).

Seeing compartment syndrome in clinical practice is relatively rare. The diagnosis, however, should be part of the differential diagnosis list for patients with the previously mentioned medical conditions.

PRESENTATION

Diagnosis of compartment syndrome is a medical emergency. Early signs of this condition include pain disproportionate to the injury, refusal to move the affected area, or pain with a passive stretch (Shadgan et al., 2008). Severe skin swelling and taughtness of the affected extremity or abdomen may be observed. Late signs are the classic "three P's": paralysis, pallor, and pulselessness. Within the pediatric population, subjective data can be difficult to assess. The pediatric patient who has been comfortable with oral narcotics but then starts to require increasing doses or use of IV narcotics should be evaluated immediately. The "three A's"—anxiety (increasing), agitation, and analgesic requirement—have been shown to precede the classic three P's symptoms in children by several hours (Noonan & McCarthy, 2010).

DIFFERENTIAL DIAGNOSIS

Patients may exhibit one or more of the symptoms commonly associated with compartment syndrome—pain, swelling, venous, or nerve injury—without having the full disorder. If there has been a portal for entry or history of systemic disease, then infections such as cellulitis, osteomyelitis, or synovitis should be considered. Reflex sympathetic dystrophy syndrome is a neurological complication of trauma that should also be considered, especially if the complaint of pain and perfusion changes occur late in the patient's recovery.

PLAN OF CARE

If compartment syndrome is suspected, therapeutic management must be initiated immediately. HCPs should use strategies to improve the patient's condition while seeking evaluation by surgical specialists. All binding devices such as casting or splints must be removed. Removing a hard cast can reduce compartment pressure by 40% to 60%, and releasing the underlying padding can reduce the pressure by an additional 10% (Halanski & Noonan, 2008).

Keeping the extremity at the level of the heart is important. Elevation or dangling the limb both can further restrict blood flow. Administer oxygen and provide pain medication. Also, correct any hypotension with isotonic saline.

Invasive devices that can measure the level of compartmental pressure are available. Examples of these diagnostic tools include the mercury manometer system, the arterial line system, and the Stryker intracompartmental pressure monitoring system. These devices can be useful if questions arise regarding the severity of the pressure in the affected area. Compartment pressures greater than 35 mmHg (as measured by the slit or wick catheter technique) or greater than 40 mmHg (as measured by the needle technique) may prompt surgical intervention (Table 32-1) (Canale & Beaty, 2007). Another calculation seeks to measure the difference

TABLE 32-1

Compartment Testing Technique	
Slit	The skin is opened and a catheter is placed into the compartment.
Wick	A catheter with a wick is placed in the compartment.
Needle	A straight or side-port needle is placed into the compartment.

Note: In all of these compartment syndrome measuring techniques, the inserted device is connected to a pressure measuring device to record the compartment pressure in millimeters of mercury (mmHg).

between the diastolic blood pressure and the intracompartmental pressure. If it is more than 30 mmHg, this finding is suggestive of compartmental syndrome with a sensitivity greater than 80% (Janzing & Broos, 2001).

Once the diagnosis of acute compartment syndrome is made, the definitive treatment is an incisional fasciotomy (Noonan & McCarthy, 2010). This procedure is usually performed by a surgeon at the bedside or in the operating room depending on the level of urgency. Proper anesthesia should be administered prior to the procedure. Ideally, the patient should have been fasting according to the medical facilities anesthesia guidelines. Preoperative antibiotics should also be administered to prevent surgical infection. Cefazolin is a broad-spectrum antibiotic that covers the most probable skin contaminants—including *Staphylococcus aureus*—associated with surgical site infection in orthopedic procedures. Postoperative care includes open wound care and pain control. Continued observation for complications such as infection or continued compartment syndrome is required. Family and patient teaching would include initial injury care as well as fasciotomy care.

DISPOSITION AND DISCHARGE PLANNING

In many patients with compartment syndrome, the open wound is closed within a few days or a skin graft is placed. With early identification and quick treatment, full recovery can be expected within 6 months for most patients (Bae et al., 2001).

Prevention is actually the best therapy, however. Early recognition is important because the risk for permanent injury increases with time. Patients can regain normal function if surgical fasciotomy is accomplished within the first 6 hours (Laine et al., 2010).

Recognizing which areas of the body are more prone to compartment syndrome and under which circumstances allows the HCP to work with families to monitor for the early signs after injury—that is, the three A's, rather than waiting for the three P's.

> **Critical Thinking**
> - Severe pain out of proportion to the injury is a key indicator of compartment syndrome.
> - The presence of a pulse does not rule out compartment syndrome.

GAIT DISTURBANCES

Summer Watkins and Prasad Gourineni

Gait disturbances in children are common. A child may present with complaint of a limp or gait concern to a primary care physician, to a pediatric specialist, or to the emergency department (ED). A gait disorder may have an acute onset, or it may emerge over time. Common symptoms are leg length discrepancy, muscle weakness, muscle spasticity, in-toeing, out-toeing, infection, or pain. Close inspection and evaluation is necessary to identify the cause and proper management for the underlying disorder. New-onset limp and joint pain is considered a medical emergency.

HIP DYSPLASIA

Developmental dysplasia of the hip (DDH) is a condition characterized by a subluxation of the femoral head within the hip joint. Both the acetabulum and the proximal head of the femur are underdeveloped. Hip subluxation is present in 1 child in 1,000 live births. Hip dislocation is seen in 1 child in 10,000 live births. Females have the condition more commonly than males, with the female-to-male ratio being 8:1. In the United States, DDH occurs in approximately 1.5% of newborns (Stevenson et al., 2009). This disorder is thought to be due to hormone-induced joint laxity. Other risk factors include breech presentation, multiple gestation, first pregnancy, oligohydramnios, and family history of hip problems (Stein-Zamir et al., 2008).

Presentation

The usual presentation of hip dysplasia is a dislocatable or dislocated hip during the newborn examination. The Barlow and Ortolani maneuvers can be useful in infants younger than 6 months of age. The Barlow maneuver is performed by attempting to dislocate the hip while putting the leg into adduction. The Ortolani maneuver relocates a dislocated hip when the leg is abducted. These techniques are done in one motion, one hip at a time. A clunk—not a click—is felt with a positive test.

Hip dislocation usually produces asymmetric skin folds and a positive Galeazzi sign, although these findings are not always reliable indicators. The Galeazzi sign is positive when there is a difference in the femur length when the hips and knees are flexed to 90 degrees. In a walking child, a waddling gait may be observed when both hips are affected and a Trendelenberg gait may be observed when there is only one dysplastic hip.

Differential diagnosis

Other diagnoses should be considered when evaluating a patient for hip dysplasia. A hip click without hip instability in a newborn is a common and benign finding. Trauma should be considered if there is pain with the examination or if the patient has a history of injury. A tumor, infection, or inflammation in the pelvic or hip region can cause an alteration in hip motion, pain, and an altered gait. All patients with hip spasticity are prone to developing dysplasia and should be followed closely for this condition.

Plan of care

In the newborn period, a positive Ortoloni or Barlow test is the only diagnostic test that is needed; however, this finding is not of value in the older infant or child. Ultrasound is the diagnostic study of choice after 6 weeks of age when hip instability is detected on examination or if there is a risk factor for DDH (Rosendahl et al., 2010). Pelvic radiographs after 6 months of age are the primary tool used for following the progression of this disorder (Figure 32-1).

Once dysplasia has been established in patients younger than 6 months of age, a Pavlik Harness is applied. This device holds the hips in abduction and the knees in flexion—a position that promotes positioning of the acetabulum in the femoral head. Proper application of the harness is important to avoid risk of nerve damage and avascular necrosis of the femoral head. Studies of the Pavlik Harness have shown hip reduction in approximately 80% of patients and an incidence of avascular

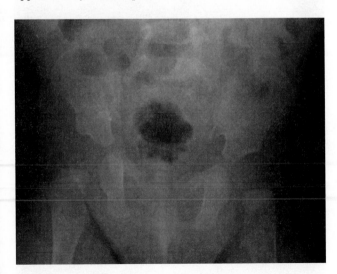

FIGURE 32-1

Bilateral Hip Dysplasia.

Source: Courtesy of Summer Watkins and Prasad Gourineni.

necrosis ranging from 0 to 22% (Kitoh et al., 2009). Residual dysplasia after 6 months may require additional bracing.

If the child presents with hip dislocation after 6 months of age, a closed reduction of the femur into the hip socket and spica cast placement are generally required. While the patient is under sedation or general anesthesia, the hip is properly positioned and then a spica cast is applied. The cast is generally worn for 6 to 12 weeks depending on the response.

If the patient presents with hip dislocation after 2 years of age, an open reduction and surgical placement of the femoral head within the acetabulum socket may be required. A spica cast is then placed for 6 to 12 weeks. This surgery is extensive and the patient requires an inpatient stay for postoperative for pain control, hemodynamic monitoring, and spica cast care education.

Disposition and discharge planning

Once the child is diagnosed with DDH, patient and family education focuses on the problem, complications, and management options. The need for bracing and casting can cause stress on the child and the family. Member of the interprofessional orthopedic team will help the family with daily concerns such as how to provide for car seat-belt safety and daily hygiene.

DISKITIS

Diskitis (also known as discitis) is inflammation, and often infection, of the intervertebral space. It is most often encountered in children younger than 5 years of age but may also be seen in older children and adolescents. An associated sequelae, osteomyelitis, is more common in children. Diskitis is typically caused by hematogenous seeding from a systemic infection that localizes in the lumbar spine. The most common infectious organism is *Staphylococcus aureus* (Lillie et al., 2008), but *Kingella kingae*, group A *streptococcus*, and *Escherichia coli* have also been noted as sources of infection.

Presentation

The usual presentation of diskitis includes back pain, fever, and fatigue. A limp, or refusal to walk or sit, may also be seen. Affected children tend to hold themselves in a straight, rigid position. Some older children may complain of abdominal pain. Pain with flexion of the spine can be tested by having the child bend over while standing. Minimal neurologic manifestations have been observed and

> **Critical Thinking**
> - Double diapering is not an adequate treatment for hip dysplasia; it does not provide adequate positioning to correct the deformity.
> - A hip click does not indicate dysplasia; it is a normal variation.
> - A hip ultrasound sooner than 6 weeks has a high incidence of false-positive results for dysplasia.

usually represent later sequelae. Lower extremity weakness has been reported as well.

Differential diagnosis

When evaluating a child with this presentation, other differential diagnoses should be evaluated. In particular, a spinal tumor can mimic an infectious process. Pain with a tumor is insidious, increases at night, and can cause focal neurological deficits such as loss of bowel and bladder control. Trauma, either acute or chronic, can cause disk bulging/herniation or fractures in the spine (spondylolysis/spondylolisthesis) in older children. The history in such a case generally includes a traumatic event or chronic high-impact activity.

Plan of care

Diagnostic studies that aid in the diagnosis of diskitis include a complete blood count (CBC) with differential, the inflammatory markers C-reactive protein (CRP) and erythrocyte sedimentation rate (ESR), and blood cultures. The ESR is a sensitive marker of pyogenic infection and is positive in more than 90% of patients with spinal infections (Carragee et al., 1997). Aspiration of the disk space is reserved for infections that are not responding to parenteral antibiotics; an organism is recovered from the site in only 50% to 60% of patients (Kliegman et al., 2007). The typical radiographic findings of disk space narrowing are commonly not appreciated until 2 to 3 weeks after the beginning of the infection (An & Seldomridge, 2006). A bone scan or MRI is more useful in the aid of diagnosis in the early stages.

Therapeutic management for diskitis includes activity restriction, pain control, immobilization with a spinal orthotics, and parenteral antibiotic therapy. If there is loculation of the infection on MRI or ultrasound, surgical incision and drainage are usually indicated. Parenteral antibiotics are administered for 4 to 6 weeks depending on the patient's response. A transition to oral therapy may also be considered once the fever has resolved for 72 hours.

If there is a positive blood or fluid culture, then susceptibility testing should be performed to direct antimicrobial therapy. Vancomycin 40 to 60 mg/kg/24 hours, divided, every 6 hours, is the recommended initial empirical therapy for new-onset diskitis caused by methicillin-resistant *Staphylococcus aureus* (MRSA) strains found within the community. If positive cultures are obtained, and the *S. aureus* is methicillin susceptible (MSSA), then therapy can be transitioned to nafcillin or oxacillin. If MRSA is reported, then therapy should be tailored based on the susceptibility pattern.

Disposition and discharge planning

Family teaching should include long-term antibiotic administration, activity restriction, and pain control. Social work or discharge planning staff will need to work with families to obtain parenteral therapy support at home. Follow-up with infectious diseases, orthopedics, and primary care

providers should be emphasized. Long-term outcome is universally favorable, although spontaneous fusion of the disk space may occur with more severe infections.

LEGG-CALVÉ-PERTHES DISEASE

Legg-Calvé-Perthes disease (LCPD) is a disorder that results from a temporary loss of blood supply to the proximal femoral epiphysis (Hoffmeister, 2008). The etiology of this condition is not well understood. Clotting abnormalities such as protein C and S deficiency and factor V Leiden mutation have been studied but have not been shown to have a significant correlation with LCPD (Glueck et al., 2007). Trauma, infection, inflammation, and acetabular retroversion have also been suggested as causes.

In LCPD, the arterial or venous blood supply has been temporarily blocked and the bone undergoes four stages of necrosis and repair. The initial stage begins with an ischemic event. Ossification is arrested and the bone becomes sclerotic. In the second stage, called the fragmentation stage, the bone is deformed or even fractured (Figure 32-2). In the third stage, called the healing stage or re-ossification stage, the old necrotic bone is reabsorbed and new bone is formed. The last stage is remodeling, when the residual deformity may be observed.

The typical age group affected by LCPD includes children between 4 and 8 years. This rare condition affects only 1 in 1,200 children. It is more common in boys (Hoffmeister, 2008).

Presentation

The usual presentation in a child with LCPD is persistent pain on the affected side. Pain may start in the hip and

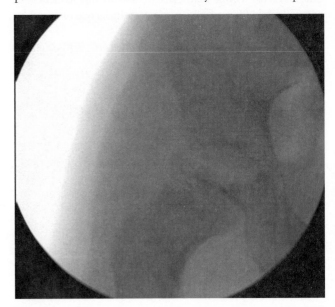

FIGURE 32-2

Legg-Calvé-Perthes Disease.

Source: Courtesy of Summer Watkins and Prasad Gourineni.

radiate to the thigh or knee, but is not usually severe and may be chronic in nature. A limp (abductor lurch or antalgic gait) may be seen or a leg length discrepancy may be measured. Limitation of internal rotation and abduction are usually confirmed on examination. Many patients with this condition have been noted to have delayed skeletal maturation and are often shorter than normal height for age.

Differential diagnosis

The possibility of septic hip or transient synovitis should be considered during diagnosis, although the range of motion is usually better for LCPD. Meyer's dysplasia—a mild dysplasia of the proximal femoral epiphysis—is a normal variation and is usually bilateral. This benign condition resolves over time.

Plan of care

Laboratory studies such as CBC, CRP, ESR, and blood cultures are usually normal in patients with LCPD; however, abnormal thyroid hormone levels and insulin-like growth factors have been noted in some children.

Diagnostic imaging includes radiographs of the hip or pelvis. Anterior–posterior and "frog-leg" views aid in tracking the progression of the disease. A bone scan or MRI can be useful in the early stages of the disease when radiographic changes are difficult to detect.

The goal of treatment is to keep the femoral head seated in the acetabulum and to promote good range of motion; thus the therapeutic management depends on the amount of epiphyseal involvement. Observation with normal activity is indicated for mild cases. Patients with more severe disease need activity restriction, physical therapy, and even bracing to hold the head of the femur in proper position to optimize its functional shape.

Disposition and discharge planning

Families need patience and dedication due to the potentially long treatment course. Their once-active child may now be restricted to quiet activities and range of motion exercises. In addition, patients may require immobilization with products such as orthotics or spica casting. Education on daily care for those children with prolonged immobilization is needed. Close follow-up by an orthopedic surgeon is necessary to monitor the progression of this disease and surgery may be beneficial. The outcomes of this disease are usually good. Proper treatment can reduce pain, promote good mobility, and prevent early development of arthritis.

SLIPPED CAPITAL FEMORAL EPIPHYSIS

Slipped capital femoral epiphysis (SCFE) is characterized by the separation of the growth plate in the proximal femoral head. The epiphysis begins to slip posteriorly and can progress into complete dissociation (Figure 32-3).

The epiphysis is at a great risk for developing avascular necrosis if the slip becomes unstable due to the fragile blood supply in this location. If left untreated, the morbidity with SCFE is high, with the disorder often leading to severe pain and limp.

The typical child with SCFE is between the ages of 12 and 15 years. Patients are most commonly African American or Hispanic males (Laine et al., 2010). SCFE is highly associated with obesity; more than 50% of affected patients rank above the 95th percentile for weight (Aronsson et al., 2006). The etiology of this condition is unknown but may be related to stresses on the physis from rapid growth. Genetic conditions such as Down syndrome have also been associated with SCFE.

SCFE is generally diagnosed as acute, chronic, or acute on chronic. *Acute* SCFE involves a sudden exacerbation within the past 3 weeks. There is usually radiological evidence of a shift in the femoral epiphysis without callus formation. *Chronic* SCFE features a gradual onset of symptoms over 3 weeks. Some remodeling of the bone is seen with imaging. *Acute on chronic* SCFE is seen when a patient has had symptoms for month or more that have been exacerbated with a minor injury.

Many HCPs find the classification of stable versus unstable SCFE to be more useful for treatment and prognostic purposes. With a *stable* slip, the patient can ambulate with or without crutches. A stable SCFE can rapidly progress into an unstable slip if left untreated or if a traumatic force is applied to the femoral head. With an *unstable* slip, the child is unable to ambulate even with crutches. A stable slip has a very low risk of complications. An acute, unstable, or severe presentation can lead to osteonecrosis of the head of the femur and chondrolysis of the hip joint (Loder et al., 1993).

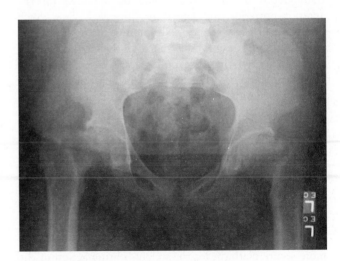

FIGURE 32-3

Bilateral Slipped Capital Femoral Epiphysis.

Source: Courtesy of Summer Watkins and Prasad Gourineni.

Presentation

The major symptom associated with SCFE is acute or chronic hip, thigh, or knee pain. Limited internal rotation and obligated external rotation of the hip are usually present on examination. A shortening of the affected leg and a Trendelenberg gait may be observed in patients with more severe disorders. In an acute, unstable SCFE, there is usually severe pain with a dramatic change in gait.

Differential diagnosis

When evaluating a child with hip pain, a variety of differential diagnoses should be considered. Trauma to the hip can cause a dislocation, a proximal femur fracture, or a pelvic fracture. Each of these disorders can resemble acute SCFE. SCFE can also precede a trauma or develop as result of a trauma; historical data along with radiological findings can be helpful to differentiate its etiology in these circumstances. A mass such as a cyst or tumor may result in joint pain or restricted motion. Hip impingement is an anatomical problem characterized by decreased joint mobility of the hip because of an abnormally shaped femoral neck or acetabulum. This distortion can cause cartilage tears and may progress in to arthritis. Septic arthritis should be considered emergently due to the risk of joint damage. An MRI should be considered whenever an abnormality is noted within the joint space. Hypothyroidism, hypopituitarism, and chronic kidney disease are all systemic disorders that have been shown to influence the progression of SCFE.

Plan of care

Radiographs of the pelvis should be obtained for the anterior–posterior and lateral or "frog-leg" view. Such imaging will allow good visualization of the femoral head of both hips. Posterior displacement of the femoral epiphysis can be seen on the lateral radiograph. The appearance of "ice cream slipping off a cone" may be appreciated. Other imaging modalities, such as CT or MRI, may be used when radiographic findings are unclear.

Once the patient is diagnosed with SCFE, strict non-weight-bearing status should be implemented until surgical intervention can be performed.

Therapeutic management consists of percutaneous pinning or in situ screw fixation of the femoral head through the growth plate. This intervention not only secures the femoral epiphysis to the head of the femur, but also promotes the closure of the growth plate. Both of these actions create a more secure platform for the weight-bearing action of the femur. For many patients, the nonaffected hip is pinned as a prophylactic measure, as there is a 30% to -40% chance of it being affected within 18 months if the growth plates are still open (Kliegman et al., 2007). For patients with more severe dysfunction, open osteotomy is performed to better align the affected hip into the socket, with internal fixation being used to secure the bones into place. This surgery can be complicated by avascular necrosis of the femoral head if the vessels are not carefully spared.

Disposition and discharge planning

Recovery for the percutaneous pinning or in situ screw fixation is generally well tolerated and most patients go home on the same day that the surgery is performed. Crutches are generally used for the first 2 to 3 weeks after surgery by those patients with stable SCFE. For those children with unstable SCFE, 6 to 8 weeks of protected ambulation with crutches may be required. Sports and vigorous activity should be avoided until closure of the growth plate is observed.

The recovery from open osteotomy is more complex than with the pinning/screw fixation technique. Patients who undergo the former procedure usually require inpatient admission for hemodynamic monitoring, pain medication administration, anterior hip precautions, and toe-touch gait training.

The treatment of a patient with a new diagnosis of SCFE often requires an interprofessional team approach. Physical therapists work on gait training, anterior hip precautions, and range of motion exercises. An orthopedic surgeon provides ongoing evaluation until the growth plates on both sides close. The primary care provider coordinates the overall care for comorbidities such as obesity or hypothyroidism.

TOXIC SYNOVITIS

Transient monoarticular synovitis, also known as toxic synovitis, is an inflammatory condition that primarily affects large joint spaces, usually the hip. Children between the ages of 3 and 8 years are most often affected, with the disorder typically involving only one joint. The exact cause of toxic synovitis is not completely understood, but studies suggest that it is a reaction to an acute or previous viral infection, trauma, or allergic reaction. Toxic synovitis as a reaction to arthritis in the hip joint has also been reported (Laine et al., 2010).

Presentation

The typical presentation consists of pain in the area of the affected joint, limping (antalgic) gait, and refusal to bear weight. Mild limitation of motion of the hip in abduction and internal rotation may be observed on physical examination. However, the child typically has some movement of the joint. Low-grade fever is commonly observed.

Differential diagnosis

Differential diagnoses to consider include more serious disorders such as septic arthritis, osteomyelitis, trauma, or a neoplastic lesion of the joint space. Septic arthritis is an orthopedic emergency in which the joint can be severely damaged by an infectious process. The child with this condition most often refuses to walk; has limited, if any, motion within the hip; has elevated inflammatory markers; and has a high fever.

Osteomylitis is a localized infection of the bone. The child may be toxic appearing, with high fever, have a positive blood culture, and have limited motion and pain of the affected extremity.

Trauma involving the joint space can be evaluated using good historical data and radiological imaging to look for a fracture or dislocation. Evaluation for a new lesion within the joint space includes a history of chronic onset and progression. An MRI or bone scan can be used to further assess this differ ential diagnosis.

Plan 3of care

Laboratory studies include CBC, CRP, and ESR. The inflammatory values may be mildly elevated, with a white blood cell (WBC) count exceeding 12,000 cells/mm^3 and an ESR of more than 40 mm/hr being common findings. Radiographs of the affected joint are taken to evaluate for bony abnormality. An ultrasound can be performed to evaluate the joint for fluid. If an effusion is found, the fluid can be aspirated for analysis of WBC count and culture, although findings are typically negative (Laine et al., 2010). Joint aspiration is usually performed by interventional radiology specialists under sedation using ultrasound. Usually 1 to 3 mL of fluid can be aspirated. An MRI or bone scan may be useful to evaluate for osteomyelitis or a bony lesion.

Once diagnosed, the patient with toxic synovitis is generally treated based on his or her symptoms. Rest of the affected joint and activity restriction are generally required until symptoms resolve. Nonsteroidal anti-inflammatory drugs (NSAIDs) such as ibuprofen may help reduce inflammation and aid in pain relief.

Disposition and discharge planning

The typical infection lasts a few days to a few weeks. No serious sequelae have been reported after resolution of toxic synovitis.

OSTEOMYELITIS

Katherine K. Shannon

PATHOPHYSIOLOGY

Osteomyelitis is an infection of the bone that may occur by hematogenous spread from bacteremia, local invasion from a contiguous infection, or direct inoculation from a sustained trauma or surgical procedure. The most common type of osteomyelitis in pediatric patients is hematogenous, as blood-borne organisms seed the metaphysis of the bone (Sonnen & Henry, 1996). The sharp vascular angles at the distal metaphysis predispose these vessels to thrombosis formation, focal necrosis, and bacterial seeding after any transient episode of bacteremia such as in an inner ear or respiratory tract infection (Frank et al., 2005). If osteomyelitis goes untreated, purulent material may extend through the cortex into the subperiosteal space. Once in the periosteal space, accumulation of purulent material increases and results in bone necrosis.

EPIDEMIOLOGY AND ETIOLOGY

One in 5,000 children younger than the age of 13 will develop osteomyelitis (Sonnen & Henry, 1996). Approximately 50% of infections occur in the first 5 years of life (Gutierrez, 2005). Males are twice as likely to be affected as females, and one-third of families report a history of blunt skeletal trauma (Frank et al., 2005). While any bone may be infected, the femur (23%) and the tibia (20%) are the most commonly affected sites (Gafur et al., 2008). Risk factors for osteomyelitis include sickle cell disease and other hemoglobinopathies, diabetes mellitus, chronic renal disease, rheumatoid arthritis, and conditions leading to immunocompromised status (Kocher et al., 2006).

The most common pathogen associated with osteomyelitis is *Staphylococcus aureus*, which accounts for 70% to 90% of acute osteomyelitis infections. Infections caused by community-acquired methicillin-resistant *S. aureus* (CA-MRSA) are becoming more prevalent, with incidence reported at some centers as high as 30% (Gafur et al., 2008). Other organisms implicated in osteomyelitis include group A hemolytic *Streptococcus*, *Streptococcus pyogenes*, *Streptococcus pneumoniae*, and *Kingella kingae* (Yagupsky, 2004). Group B β-hemolytic *Streptococcus* is classically associated with neonatal osteomyelitis. *Haemophilus influenzae* b has an extremely low incidence rate since the introduction of the *H. influenzae* b (Hib) vaccine (Howard et al., 1999).

PRESENTATION

The presenting history depends on the age of the child, the bone involved, and the severity of the infection.

Patients may have had a recent injury or infection, such as chickenpox, otitis media, or upper respiratory illness (Morrissy, 2001). The predominant feature of osteomyelitis is localized pain in the affected bone, described as constant and increasing in severity. If the upper extremity is involved, the patient may have stopped using the affected limb; if the infection is in the lower extremity, the child may limp or refuse to walk. Depending on the duration of symptoms, the patient may have high fever, chills, and vomiting (Tachdjian, 1997). Neonates, infants, and non-verbal patients may present with new onset of irritability, poor feeding, and change in sleep habits.

The predominant physical finding in osteomyelitis is discrete tenderness at the site of infection. The area may be edematous, erythematous, and warm to touch. The associated joint may have limited and painful range of motion (McCarthy, 2005). When the lower extremity is involved, the patient may have an antalgic gait (Morrissy, 2001). Depending on the duration of the infection, the child may also appear toxic.

DIFFERENTIAL DIAGNOSIS

Differential diagnoses for osteomyelitis include septic arthritis, toxic synovitis, cellulitis, rheumatic fever, fracture, and thrombophlebitis. Malignancies that may mimic osteomyelitis include osteosarcoma, Ewing sarcoma, leukemia, neuroblastoma, and Wilms' tumor (Kocher et al., 2006). In patients with sickle cell anemia, bone infarction should also be considered.

PLAN OF CARE

Initial serologic studies should include a CBC with differential, ESR, CRP, and blood cultures. The WBC is elevated (more than 12,000/μL) in 31% to 40% of children with acute hematogenous osteomyelitis (Song & Sloboda, 2001). The ESR and CRP—both of which are inflammatory markers—will be elevated (Gutierrez, 2005). The ESR rises slowly and typically becomes elevated (greater than 20 mm/hr) within 48 to 72 hours, whereas the CRP becomes elevated (greater than 10 mg/L) more quickly, within 6 hours of infection. The CRP also falls more quickly in response to effective management, making it a valuable marker for both identification of infection and response to treatment (Morrissy, 2001). Blood cultures are positive in 30% to 50% of patients with these types of infections (McCarthy, 2005), whereas direct bone aspiration for culture has a higher yield, identifying 48% to 85% of organisms (Song & Sloboda).

Plain radiographs should be obtained initially. This type of imaging can detect soft-tissue swelling in as early as 48 hours after symptoms begin; however, changes in the bone, such as bone destruction, cannot be detected via radiography for 7 to 10 days (Lazzarini et al., 2005).

Technetium-99m scintigraphy and MRI are both highly sensitive and specific in detecting uncomplicated acute hematogenous osteomyelitis in pediatric patients (Jaramillo et al., 1995). Because the entire skeleton may be imaged, scintigraphy is helpful in neonates and patients who are unable to verbalize the location of the pain, or if multifocal osteomyelitis is suspected (Connolly & Connolly, 2003). MRI is the imaging modality of choice when the patient has focal symptoms and the HCP has a strong suspicion of osteomyelitis. The high resolution is useful in differentiating between soft-tissue and bone infection (Copley, 2009). MRI is also the best option for detecting infections in the spine and pelvis and for planning surgical debridement when soft-tissue abscess is present.

Computerized tomography is useful in detecting abscess and areas of destruction (Pineda et al., 2006), whereas ultrasound is most useful in detecting intra-articular, soft-tissue, and subperiosteal fluid collections. Ultrasound has limited usefulness in patients with osteomyelitis as it lacks the inability to image cortical details of the bone (Song & Sloboda, 2001).

A diagnostic venous imaging study to evaluate deep vein thrombosis (DVT) should be considered in pediatric patients who are at high risk for DVT, have a longer duration of hospitalization, have more admissions to the intensive care unit, require more surgical procedures, or have an associated MRSA osteomyelitis (Hollmig et al., 2007).

Successful treatment of osteomyelitis requires appropriate antibiotic therapy and, possibly, surgical drainage. Patients often present to the emergency department owing to increasing bone pain, fever, or irritability. Most pediatric patients are hemodynamically stable and are admitted to an inpatient unit for antibiotic therapy and possible surgical debridement. Symptoms in neonates are vague, however, so diagnosis in this group may be delayed. As a consequence, neonates may be septic and hemodynamically unstable upon presentation, requiring resuscitation and intensive care unit admission (Gutierrez, 2005).

Intravenous antibiotics maximize bactericidal levels in the affected bone and prevent dissemination of disease; for this reason, they are considered first-line therapy for osteomyelitis. Placement of a percutaneous intravenous central catheter (PICC) is often necessary to accommodate long-term administration of parenteral antibiotics. The selection of antibiotic depends on the infectious organism identified from the cultures; it may also be made empirically based on known epidemiological trends in different age groups. Empiric antibiotics should, at a minimum, cover *S. aureus*, as this is the most common pathogen in all age groups. Antibiotics that provide coverage for *S. aureus* include oxacillin and first-generation cephalosporins such as cefazolin (Kocher et al., 2006). CA-MRSA infections are commonly treated with vancomycin, clindamycin, or linezolid (Saphyakhajon et al., 2008). Treatment of CA-MRSA poses a challenge as the bacteria are more invasive and less responsive to first-line therapy. Often patients with CA-MRSA infections require longer hospitalization and repeated surgical drainage (Saavedra-Lozano et al., 2008). In neonates, third-generation cephalosporins such as cefotaxime may be used, as they broaden the coverage to include group B *Streptococcus* and enteric Gram-negative bacilli (Frank et al., 2005).

Surgical intervention is indicated when there is presence of a large subperiosteal, soft-tissue or bone abscess; an area of necrotic bone; or failure to respond to antibiotic treatment (Morrissy, 2001; Song & Sloboda, 2001). Surgical debridement of the bone involves a periosteal incision and the creation of a window in the cortex to allow for drainage. A drain is often placed on a temporary basis, and the bone is immobilized in a well-padded cast or splint (Staheli, 2006). Surgical drains are removed after 24 to 72 hours, depending on surgeon preference.

To date, no established guidelines have been developed outlining the duration of antibiotic therapy for osteomyelitis. Therapy is dictated by the extent of infection, type of pathogen, abscess formation, response to treatment, and preference of the infectious disease specialist. Intravenous antibiotics are often given for 3 to 6 weeks before switching to oral agents (McCarthy, 2005); however, shorter courses of therapy have been studied. Peltola et al. (1997) found successful treatment of children with uncomplicated acute hematogenous osteomyelitis was achieved after a short course of high-dose intravenous antibiotic therapy followed by oral antibiotic therapy. Oral therapy began when the patient experienced a rapid fall in the CRP and an improvement in the clinical course. The average length of intravenous antibiotic therapy was 5 days, with a total antibiotic duration of 23 days. In a similar study, Jagodzinski et al. (2009) found effective management of acute osteomyelitis could be achieved in the majority of children after 3 to 5 days of intravenous therapy followed by 3 weeks of oral therapy. Neonates with osteomyelitis often need extended parenteral coverage; typically, they are not transitioned to oral antibiotics because intestinal absorption rates in this age group vary widely.

Once osteomyelitis is suspected, the HCP should consider consulting with members of the following specialties: orthopedics, infectious diseases, and occupational and physical therapy. Any patient presenting with hemodynamic instability should have a critical care consult. Patients may also benefit from incorporation of the following services in the therapeutic plan: nutrition, child life, social and spiritual support, and the rehabilitative team. In addition, symptoms or diagnosis of an osteomyelitis-associated DVT requires prompt consultation with specialists in hematology and critical care.

When the child is transitioned to oral antibiotics, caregivers need to be compliant with the medication regimen and to identify symptoms that might affect absorption of prescribed agents, such as vomiting and diarrhea. Intolerance of the oral medication or poor compliance with the medication regimen is an indication to resume intravenous therapy, as maintenance of therapeutic antibiotic levels is essential for effective management of osteomyelitis (Copley, 2009). If the child underwent surgical debridement, a cast or brace to maintain immobilization will be placed for 4 to 6 weeks, followed by protected weight bearing for 12 to 16 weeks. Caregivers will be responsible for assisting the child with activities of daily living as well as assessing the extremity for skin breakdown and impaired neurovascular function.

DISPOSITION AND DISCHARGE PLANNING

Through the development of effective antibiotic treatment, the mortality rate from osteomyelitis has been reduced from 50% to 1% (McCarthy, 2005). However, DVT has been recognized as a sequela to MRSA osteomyelitis. This condition is more common in children who are older than 8 years of age and had a concomitant CRP level greater than 6 mg/dL at presentation (Hollmig et al., 2007).

Discharge from the hospital may be considered when the child has a normal temperature and pulse range, has reduced pain with improved range of motion to the affected site, and has a decreased CRP (Kocher et al., 2006). Treatment may successfully be continued at home, so long as caregivers are able to reliably adhere to the antibiotic schedule. A child may sometimes be discharged home with a PICC line for continued IV antibiotic administration, and therefore will requires the assistance of a home health agency nurse to administer antibiotics and monitor the venous access device for catheter-related complications.

Follow-up is often with the primary care provider, infectious diseases specialist, and orthopedic surgeon. Close follow-up is necessary to monitor antibiotic compliance, assess response to therapy, and recognize complications. To assess for antibiotic-related complications such as neutropenia and changes in liver enzymes due to high doses of antibiotics, a CBC and liver function tests may be obtained (Song & Sloboda, 2001). Follow-up with the orthopedic specialist focuses on healing of the surgical site and bone repair and growth. Serial radiographs are obtained to assess for complications such as chronic osteomyelitis, pathological fracture, and physeal arrest. If the growth plate is involved, the patient is followed annually until he or she is skeletally mature.

Most children with acute hematogenous osteomyelitis will recover from the infection without sequelae. Complications such as bone abscess, septic arthritis, and bacteremia are usually associated with advanced infection. Long-term complications include limb-length discrepancy, abnormal gait, and recurrent infection (Kocher et al., 2006).

Recurrent and chronic osteomyelitis has been reported in 5% to 19% of cases (Frank et al., 2004; Gutierrez, 2005). Risk factors include inadequate antibiotic treatment, delay in diagnosis, and young age at the time of initial illness. Recurrent osteomyelitis may become chronic. In chronic osteomyelitis, a segment of the cortex becomes devascularized and forms a sequestrum, or dead bone. An involucrum, which is new bone with a limited vascular supply, may also form. Treatment involves several surgical procedures and long-term (4–6 months) antibiotic treatment (Staheli, 2006).

Appropriate diagnosis and treatment of bacterial infections such as otitis media may prevent bacterial seeding of the bone from a remote location. Wound care with consideration of prophylactic antibiotics may prevent soft-tissue infection from spreading to and seeding the bone. Adherence to *H. influenzae* type b vaccination schedule may maintain reduced rates of infection by this organism.

SEPTIC ARTHRITIS

Katherine K. Shannon

PATHOPHYSIOLOGY

Septic arthritis is an infection in the synovial space of the joint. Infection may invade the joint by hematogenous seeding of the synovial membrane, spread of an infection from the adjacent metaphyseal bone, or directly from traumatic or surgical contamination (Sonnen & Henry, 1996). Once bacteria enter the joint, an inflammatory response follows, resulting in the migration of leukocytes, primarily polymorphonuclear cells. The bacteria and leukocytes produce proteolytic enzymes that, in combination with increased intracapsular pressure, cause rapid destruction of the articular cartilage. Destruction of the cartilage may occur in as little as 6 hours (Kocher et al., 2006).

EPIDEMIOLOGY AND ETIOLOGY

The joints most often affected by septic arthritis are the hip (43%), knee (39%), elbow (8%), and ankle (4%) (Gafur et al., 2008). Osteomyelitis may lead to septic arthritis, especially in the hip, shoulder, elbow, and ankle, due to the intrarticular location of metaphyseal bone in these joints.

The peak incidence of septic arthritis is in children younger than 3 years of age. Males are affected twice as often as females (Frank et al., 2005). Risk factors include prematurity and immune compromised condition (Kocher et al., 2006). The most common infectious organism is *Staphylococcus aureus*; methicillin resistance to this pathogen (MRSA) is increasing (Gafur et al., 2008). *Kingella kingae* has been recognized more frequently, specifically in children younger than 4 years of age with history of an upper respiratory infection (Yagupskyk, 2004). Group B β-hemolytic *Streptococcus* is often found in neonates (McCarthy, 2005). Other organisms implicated in septic arthritis include group A *Streptococcus, Streptococcus pneumoniae, Klebsiella, Salmonella*, and *Neisseria gonorrhoeae*.

PRESENTATION

Children with septic arthritis complain of pain to the affected area. If the upper extremity is involved, the child may not use the extremity or have pain with dressing; in contrast, if the hip, knee, or ankle is involved, the child will limp or refuse to bear weight (Morrissy, 2001). Neonates may be irritable, be lethargic, refuse to eat, and fail to spontaneously move the affected limb (Gutierrez, 2005). Patients may have a history of recent illnesses, such as an upper respiratory or soft-tissue infection.

The joint involved is painful to palpation and likely erythematous, warm, and swollen. Range of motion is painful and limited. If the hip is affected, the patient may prefer to lie with the hip in external rotation, adduction, and mild flexion, as this position creates more space in the joint capsule. The child may appear ill, with a fever greater than 38°C (100°F) (Frank et al., 2005).

DIFFERENTIAL DIAGNOSIS

An important condition from which to differentiate septic arthritis of the hip is transient synovitis of the hip; the latter is a self-limited condition characterized by inflammation of the synovium of the hip joint. The therapeutic management for each of these diagnoses differs; thus an evidence-based algorithm was developed by Kocher et al. (2004) to differentiate the two. Diagnostic predictors include the following factors:

- History of fever
- Refusal to bear weight
- Erythrocyte sedimentation rate greater than 40 mm/hr
- White blood cell count greater than 12,000/μL

Kocher et al. (2004) reported that if all four of these criteria were met, there was a 93% chance the child had septic arthritis; the chance dropped to 73% if three were met, 35% if two were met, and 9.5% if only one was met.

Other diagnoses to consider when the hip is involved include fracture, slipped capital femoral epiphysis, Legg-Calvé-Perthes disease, and psoas abscess. Therefore, the differential diagnoses for a child with any painful joint should include osteomyelitis, post-streptococcal arthritis, juvenile rheumatoid arthritis, leukemia, Lyme disease, chondrolysis, and tuberculosis (Kocher et al., 2006).

PLAN OF CARE

Initial serological testing includes CBC with differential, ESR, CRP, and blood cultures. The WBC count may be elevated (more than 12,000/μL) in only 30% to 60% of patients (McCarthy, 2005). Both the ESR and the CRP will rise in response to bacterial infection. The ESR becomes elevated within 48 to 72 hours of infection, and is significantly higher (more than 50 mm/hr) in septic arthritis as compared to osteomyelitis (Morrissy, 2001). The CRP will begin to rise (more than 20 mg/L) 6 hours after infection, making this marker of greater value in early diagnosis of infection (Sucato et al., 1997). Serum blood cultures yield a pathogenic organism in 40% to 50% of infections, whereas aspiration of purulent material directly from the infected joint identifies a pathogen in 50% to 80% of patients with septic arthritis (McCarthy, 2005).

All patients with suspected septic arthritis should be assessed with radiographic studies, as the finding of joint space widening may indicate presence of an effusion (Jaramillo et al., 1995). Ultrasound is most useful in evaluating irritable joints, especially in the hip, as it shows distention of the joint capsule and joint effusion. If fluid is found in the joint, aspiration should be performed with ultrasound guidance (Jaramillo et al.). MRI may identify a joint effusion, but is most helpful in identifying an associated osteomyelitis abscess, which should be considered if the pediatric patient does not respond to antibiotic treatment within 48 hours of its initiation. Bone scans are indicated when infections are located in difficult-to-assess areas such as the ankle and the shoulder. Bone scans are especially beneficial for evaluating the neonate, as such patients may have several concurrent sites of infection (Kocher et al., 2006).

Children with septic arthritis usually present to the emergency department with joint pain and fever. Once septic arthritis is suspected, the orthopedic surgeon should be consulted for joint aspiration and possible surgical irrigation and drainage of the joint effusion. Indications for surgical irrigation and drainage are controversial for smaller joints, such as the wrist, as infections in these sites may resolve with antibiotics alone (Morrissy, 2001). For larger joints such as the knee and hip, irrigation should be performed emergently in the operating room due to the destructive nature of this condition. After irrigation of the joint, a drain is typically left in place until the drainage volume decreases. A splint or brace may be placed due to the risk of pathologic fracture.

Postoperatively, patients are admitted to the pediatric inpatient unit for monitoring of symptoms and antibiotic therapy. Physical therapy may be initiated to improve range of motion and muscle strength.

Parenteral antibiotic treatment is begun as soon as cultures are obtained. If prolonged delivery of IV antibiotics is anticipated, a peripherally inserted central venous catheter (PICC) is often placed. Infectious diseases specialists are typically consulted to guide antibiotic selection. Empiric antibiotics are selected based on the patient's age and clinical presentation, as well as on the community's pattern of antibiotic resistance. Cefazolin is often recommended, as it is effective against *S. aureus, Streptococcus pneumoniae*, and group A *Streptococcus*, which account for many of the infecting organisms (Kocher et al., 2006). Infants younger than 2 months of age should receive antibiotics that cover *S. aureus* and Gram-negative bacteria, such as nafcillin and cefotaxime. If the patient is allergic to penicillin, IV clindamycin may be used. If MRSA is the suspected pathogen, clindamycin, vancomycin, or linezolid is commonly used. *K. kingae* is sensitive to most penicillins and cephalosporins (Saphyakhajon et al., 2008).

There is no consensus for how long IV antibiotics should be given. Historically, IV antibiotics were administered for 3 to 6 weeks before patients were switched to oral agents (McCarthy, 2005), but more recent studies have found that when there is prompt improvement in the child's condition, shorter intravenous therapy may be considered (Ballock et al., 2009). Prospective studies by both Peltola et al. (2009) and Jagodzinski et al. (2009) suggest that a regimen consisting of 3 to 5 days of intravenous therapy followed by 2 to 3 weeks of oral antibiotics is safe, is cost-effective, and produces disease resolution in uncomplicated cases of septic arthritis. The decision to switch to oral antibiotics should consider the pediatric patient's clinical improvement, decline in CRP level (to less than 20 mg/L), and ability to tolerate the oral antibiotics.

Once septic arthritis is suspected, consultation with specialists from orthopedics, infectious diseases, and, later, occupational and physical therapy should be considered.

The decision to discharge the pediatric patient home relies on the caregiver's ability to reliably monitor the child's condition and adhere to the rigorous antibiotic regimen. Children sent home with PICC lines often require the skill of home health agency nurses to administer the medication and monitor the catheter for complications. Caregivers must protect the catheter from dislodgement and breakage, especially with young children. When oral antibiotics are initiated, caregivers must understand the importance of reporting vomiting and diarrhea, as both of these conditions affect drug absorption and may indicate a need to return to IV therapy. Depending on the site of infection, the patient's mobility may be limited, requiring physical therapy and caregiver assistance with activities of daily living.

DISPOSITION AND DISCHARGE PLANNING

Successful treatment of septic arthritis requires strict adherence to the often lengthy (2–3 weeks) oral medication regimen after intravenous therapy. Treatment failures are typically attributed to insufficient antibiotic duration (Copley, 2009). Complications include abnormal bone growth, unstable articulation of the joint, and decreased range of motion (Gutierrez, 2005).

Outpatient follow-up is often managed by the primary care provider and by infectious diseases and orthopedic specialists. The focus of follow-up is to identify lack of clinical, laboratory, or radiographic improvement and to recognize any treatment-related complications. Infectious diseases specialists often monitor CRP and ESR levels, as their declining levels direct treatment duration. CRP is expected to decline to less than 20 mg/L in 7 days and ESR to less than 25 mm/hr in 3 weeks (Kocher et al., 2006). Depending on the antibiotics used, laboratories studies such as a chemistry panel and CBC may be obtained to monitor for potential antibiotic-related complications such as neutropenia and liver abnormalities. Follow-up with the orthopedic surgeon involves obtaining radiographs of the affected joint to evaluate for bone repair and assess for complications such as unrecognized infectious foci, osteonecrosis, physeal arrest, pathologic fracture, and deformity.

Most children recover from septic arthritis without sequelae; however, complications occur in 10% to 25% of children (Gutierrez, 2005). Patients at higher risk for complications include those whose treatment is delayed more than 4 days, who are younger than 6 months of age, who have concurrent osteomyelitis of the femur, and who have septic dislocation of the hip joint (McCarthy, 2005). Most complications occur in the hip, with poor results noted in as many as 40% of children (McCarthy). Potential complications related to the hip include partial or complete destruction of the proximal femoral growth plate, osteonecrosis of the femoral head, trochanteric overgrowth, pseudoarthrosis of the femoral neck, complete dissolution of the femoral neck and head, progressive limb length discrepancy, varus or valgus alignment of the femoral head, unstable hip, and stiffness of the hip joint (McCarthy).

Identifying and treating skin or systemic infections early and adequately may reduce the exposure of infectious organisms into the bloodstream. Prompt treatment of osteomyelitis may prevent dissemination of infection to the joint. Neonates and premature infants are especially vulnerable to infection due to immature immune system; therefore, limiting invasive procedures, especially in neonatal intensive care units, may reduce their exposure to infecting organisms.

SPINAL FUSION

Mary Rodts

PATHOPHYSIOLOGY

Conceptually, a spinal fusion imitates a fracture of a bone. The surgeon creates an environment similar to a fracture by decorticating or removing the outer layer of the bone to mimic the need for bone healing. The bone graft then acts as a scaffold for bone remodeling. Bone remodeling proceeds through six phases: rest, activation, resorption, reversal, formation, and mineralization. Bone is constantly remodeling and is completely replaced between 3 and 6 months' time following mineralization of the bone (Sandhu, 2003).

EPIDEMIOLOGY AND ETIOLOGY

Spinal fusion, also termed spinal arthrodesis, describes the surgical procedure that joins one vertebra to an adjacent vertebra. The number of spinal fusions is increasing. In 1993, spinal fusion was the forty-first most frequently performed surgical procedure; in 2001, it was the nineteenth most common procedure. This increase is likely due to better imaging and surgical techniques. The age group experiencing the greatest increase in incidence is persons older than 40 years of age (Cowan et al., 2006).

Spinal deformity, trauma, degenerative conditions, tumors, and infections can all cause spinal instability. Some conditions—such as spinal fracture, tumor, and infection—require astute assessment to determine the degree of instability. Any spinal instability that renders the neural contents (spinal cord and nerves) at higher risk for injury may make spinal stabilization and fusion an urgent intervention.

Scoliosis, kyphosis, and spondylolisthesis are spinal deformities that sometimes require spinal fusion after there has been demonstrated progression of the spinal deformity despite conservative management. In most cases, these procedures are elective and may be scheduled at the convenience of the patient and family. Although degenerative conditions of the spine typically occur later in life, lumbar disk degeneration has also been seen in the late adolescent period, most commonly related to strenuous physical activity, post-traumatic injury, or congenital spinal deformity. Trauma, tumor, and infection can cause loss of bone integrity either by fracture, tumor invasion, or the infective process. When bone integrity is lost, the structural stability of the vertebra is often jeopardized.

TYPES OF SPINAL FUSION

The spinal column may be surgically fused from the posterior (Figure 32-4), posterolateral (Figure 32-5), or anterior approach (Figure 32-6). The surgical approach to be used is determined based on the diagnosis, location of pathology, and understanding of the biomechanical stability of the spinal column.

The majority of spinal deformity procedures are performed through a posterior approach. In some deformities, an anterior approach is proposed, as fewer segments require fusion, thereby leaving normal motion over more segments of the spine. In the case of a spinal tumor located in the vertebral body, an anterior approach is necessary to remove the

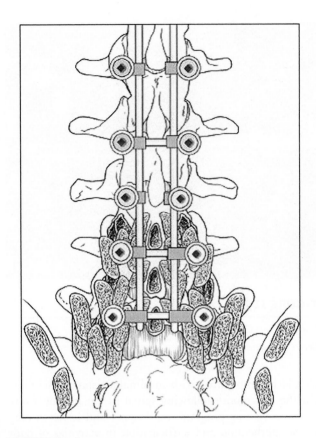

FIGURE 32-4

Posterior Spinal Fusion Demonstrating Placement of Bone Graft Material and Segmental Spinal Instrumentation.

Source: Courtesy of Mary Rodts.

tumor and stabilize the vertebra (Brady & Jackson, 2005). Hence, a tumor located in the posterior elements of the spinal column requires a posterior surgical approach. For the treatment of severe spinal deformity and problems that affect both columns of the spine, an anterior and posterior spinal fusion and stabilization may be required. In addition to the spinal fusion, spinal instrumentation consisting of rods, hooks, screws, and prosthetic devices is often required to achieve spinal stability. A combined anterior and posterior approach may be performed on the same surgical day, but this decision depends on the complexity of the deformity and the health of the patient.

Bone grafts may be autologous (usually from the patient's iliac crest), autogenous (from a cadaver donor), a combination of both types of bone, or a autologous or autogenous bone graft with bone morphogenic protein (BMP) to facilitate fusion healing (Dimar et al., 2006).

PLAN OF CARE

Radiologic studies useful to clarify diagnosis and determine surgical plan include plain radiographs, flexion/extension radiographs, hand film for bone age, CT scan, MRI, and

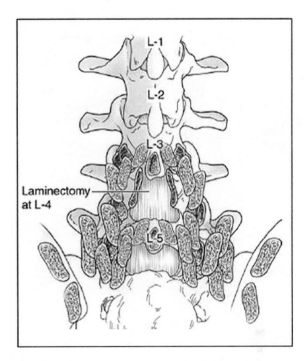

FIGURE 32-5

Posterolateral Spinal Fusion Demonstrating Lateral Placement of Bone Graft (Note the laminectomy, which prevents posterior fusion).

Source: Courtesy of Mary Rodts.

bone scans. Selection of the imaging modality is based on the patient's underlying pathology.

The management of the pediatric patient and young adult following spinal fusion includes assessment of respiratory compromise, spinal stability, hemodynamic stability, neurologic status, pain control, and readiness for rehabilitation.

Intraoperative history—such as blood loss, hypotension, respiratory stability, and kidney function—should be obtained, as these findings may alert staff to potential problems in the postoperative period. Most patients will not experience any adverse problems following spinal fusion. However, patients with large spinal deformities are at risk for increased blood loss due to increased operative time, respiratory changes due to thoracic rib cage alteration, and syndrome of inappropriate antidiuretic hormone secretion (SIADH) secondary to intraoperative volume replacement and spinal manipulation.

Following spinal fusion, the patient's neurolgic status must be evaluated and compared with the preoperative functional level. Any deterioration in sensation or strength should be documented and reported immediately to the surgeon. Neurologic assessment should be performed every 2 hours for the first 24 hours. If no deficit is seen, the neurologic assessment should be performed every shift until the patient is discharged.

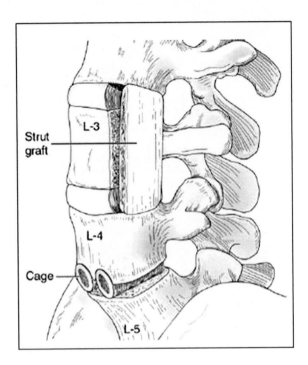

FIGURE 32-6

Anterior Spinal Fusion Demonstrating a Structural Allograft at the Proximal Level and an Implant with Bone Graft at the Distal Level.

Source: Courtesy of Mary Rodts.

Coordinated postoperative pain management is essential following spinal fusion. The use of narcotics with adjunctive muscle relaxants is typically needed for the first 2 to 4 weeks following surgery. The number of vertebrae fused will help dictate the length of time pain management will be needed. For a patient who has had a spinal fusion for deformity (which often encompasses between 4 and 14 vertebral levels), the level of pain postoperatively is significantly different than that for patient who has undergone a one-level spinal fusion.

Whether postoperative immobilization will be required is predicated on the stability of the spine following spinal fusion. Immobilization of the spine in a lumbosacral orthosis (LSO) (Figure 32-7) or a thoracolumbar orthosis (TLSO) will be necessary if the spinal column requires additional support until the spinal fusion solidifies. Spinal fusion most often occurs within 6 months of the surgical procedure. If spinal instrumentation has been used, postoperative immobilization may or may not be required; the decision on its usage is made by the spinal surgeon.

Resumption of physical activity following spinal fusion is important to prevent loss of muscle tone and strength postoperatively. The pediatric patient is progressed rapidly to sitting within the first 24 hours and to walking within 48 to 72 hours. Prior to patient discharge, the patient

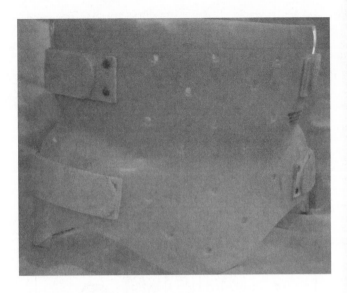

FIGURE 32-7

Lumbosacral Orthosis (LSO).

Source: Courtesy of Mary Rodts.

should be ambulatory with minimal assistance. Activities for the first month following spinal fusion include a progressive walking program, mild upper and lower extremity strengthening, and participation in activities of daily living.

Preoperative pulmonary consultation and pulmonary function testing (PFT) with arterial blood gases (ABG) should be obtained for any patient with a thoracic spinal deformity of greater that 65 degrees, a history of respiratory problems, or an underlying condition such as muscular dystrophy that may compromise pulmonary status. Neurologic consultation should be obtained if any neurologic deficits are present. Urology evaluation and urodynamic studies should be ordered if the patient has a history of urinary incontinence or urgency.

Patient education should occur prior to the elective spine fusion surgical procedure. The preoperative testing, surgical procedure, hospital course, and postoperative care should be explained in detail to both the child and the family. The patient undergoing a spinal fusion will do much better postoperatively if he or she has a thorough understanding of what is to be expected following the surgery. Equally important to the education of the patient is the development of the HCP–patient relationship that occurs during this time.

Activity following a spinal fusion is limited to allow fusion healing. No flexion, extension, or rotation of the spine should occur until the fusion has healed. This limitation is especially difficult for the pediatric patient, as it makes returning to usual childhood activities difficult. Alternative activities should be explored with the patient and family.

DISPOSITION AND DISCHARGE PLANNING

Plans for home care can be organized preoperatively to minimize anxiety over the patient going home after this type of procedure. If the patient is discharged to home, a companion for the first week is essential to assure post-procedure pain management, activity expectations, and resumption of normal activities. The majority of children will be ambulatory at the time of discharge and will not require a formal rehabilitation program. The decision regarding the necessity of a rehabilitation program is made based on diagnosis, preoperative activity level, and postoperative activity level. Patients who have neurologic compromise secondary to a diagnosis such as trauma, tumor, or infection may require a complete rehabilitation protocol. In conjunction with the rehabilitation specialists who will be overseeing the continued recovery period, a comprehensive rehabilitation plan should be developed. All HCPs who are involved with the care of the patient who undergoes spinal fusion must have not only an understanding of the diagnosis, but also familiarity with the type of surgery, surgical stabilization procedures, and postoperative restrictions that are necessary to ensure healing of the spinal fusion.

Adolescent patients undergoing spinal fusion have a good quality of life following surgery for scoliosis and spondylolisthesis. Patients with scoliosis have a slightly better long-term health-related quality of life than patients with spondylolisthesis. This difference reflects the degree of back pain in the patients undergoing surgery for spondylolisthesis (Helenius et al., 2008).

REFERENCES

1. An, H., & Seldomridge, J. (2006). Spinal infections: Diagnostic tests and imaging studies. *Clinical Orthopaedics and Related Research, 444*, 27–33.
2. Aronsson, D., Loder, R., Breur, G., & Weinstein, S. (2006). Slipped capital femoral epiphysis: Current concepts. *Journal of the American Academy of Orthopaedic Surgeons, 14*, 666–679.
3. Bae, D., Kadiyala, R., & Waters, P. (2001). Acute compartment syndrome in children: Contemporary diagnosis, treatment, and outcome. *Journal of Pediatric Orthopaedics, 21*, 680–688.
4. Ballock, T., Newton, P., Evans, S., Estabrook, M., Farnsworth, L., & Bradley, J. (2009). A comparison of early versus late conversion from intravenous to oral therapy in the treatment of septic arthritis. *Journal of Pediatric Orthopaedics, 29*(6), 636–642.
5. Brady, S., & Jackson, S. (2005). Anterior lumbar interbody fusion: Advances in spinal fusion technology. *AORN Journal, 82*(5), 817–823.
6. Canale, S., & Beaty, J. (2007). *Campbell's operative orthopaedics* (11th ed.). Philadelphia: Elsevier.
7. Carragee, E., Kim, D., Van Der Vlugt, T., & Vittum, D. (1997). The clinical use of erythrocyte sedimentation rate in pyogenic vertebral osteomyelitis. *Spine, 22*, 2089–2093.
8. Connolly, L., & Connolly, S. (2003). Skeletal scintigraphy in the multimodality assessment of young children with acute skeletal symptoms. *Clincal Nuclear Medicine, 28*(9), 746–754.
9. Copley, L. (2009). Pediatric musculoskeletal infection: Trends and antibiotic recommendations. *Journal of the American Academy of Orthopaedic Surgeons, 17*(10), 618–626.
10. Cowan, J., Dimick, J., Wainess, R., Upchurch, G., Chandler, W., & LaMarca, F. (2006). Changes in utilization of spinal fusion in the United States. *Neurosurgery, 58*(7), 15–19.
11. Dimar, J., Glassman, S., Burkus, K., & Carreon, L. (2006). Clinical outcomes and fusion success at 2 years of single-level instrumented posterolateral fusions with recombinant human bone morphogenetic protein-2/compression resistant matrix versus iliac crest bone graft. *Spine, 31*(22), 2534–2539.
12. Frank, G., Mahoney, H., & Eppes, S. (2005). Musculoskeletal infections in children. *Pediatric Clinics of North America, 5*(4), 1083–1106.
13. Gafur, O., Copley, L., Hollmig, S., Browne, R., Thornton, L., & Crawford, S. (2008). The impact of the current epidemioligy of pediatric musculoskeletal infection on evaluation and treatment guidelines. *Journal of Pediatric Orthopaedic, 28*(7), 777–785.
14. Gholve, P., Cameron, D., & Millis, M. (2009). Slipped capital femoral epiphysis update. *Current Opinions in Pediatrics, 21*(1), 39–45.
15. Glueck, C., Tracy, T., & Wang, P. (2007). Legg-Calvé-Perthes disease, venous and arterial thrombi, and the factor V Leiden mutation in a four-generation kindred. *Journal of Pediatric Orthopaedics, 27*(7), 834–837.
16. Gutierrez, K. (2005). Bone and joint infections in children. *Pediatric Clinics of North America, 52*(3), 779–794.
17. Halanski, M., & Noonan, K. J. (2008). Cast and splint immobilization. *Journal of the American Academy of Orthopaedic Surgeons, 16*(1), 30–40.
18. Helenius, I., Remes, V., Lamberg, T., Schlenzka, D., & Poussa, M. (2008). Long-term health-related quality of life after surgery for adolescent idiopathic scoliosis and spondylolisthesis. *Journal of Bone and Joint Surgery in America, 90*(6), 1231–1239.
19. Hoffmeister, E. (2008). Research sheds greater light on Legg-Calve-Perthes disease. *Lippincott's Bone and Joint Newsletter, 14*(1), 1–5.
20. Hollmig, S., Copley, L., Browne, R., Grande, L., & Wilson, P. (2007). Deep venous thrombosis associated with osteomyelitis in children. *Journal of Bone and Joint Surgery in America, 89*(7), 1517–1523.
21. Howard, A., Viskontas, D., & Sabbagh, C. (1999). Reduction in osteomyelitis and septic arthritis related to *Haemophilus influenzae* type B vaccine. *Journal of Pediatric Orthopaedics, 19*(6), 705–709.
22. Jagodzinski, N., Kanwar, R., Graham, K., & Bache, C. (2009). Prospective evaluation of a shortened regimen of treatment for acute osteomyelitis and septic arthritis in children. *Journal of Pediatric Orthopaedics, 29*(5), 518–525.
23. Janzing, H., & Broos, P. (2001). Routine monitoring of compartment pressure in patients with tibia fractures. *Injury, 32*(5), 415–421.
24. Jaramillo, D., Treves, S., Kasser, J., Harper, M., Sundel, R., & Laor, T. (1995). Osteomyelitis and septic arthritis in children: Appropriate use of imaging to guide treatment. *American Journal of Roetgenology, 165*(2), 399–403.
25. Junnila, J., & Cartwright, V. (2006). Chronic musculoskeletal pain in children: Part I. Initial evaluation. *American Family Physician, 74*(1), 115–122.
26. Kitoh, H., Kawasumi, M., & Ishiguro, N. (2009). Predictive factors for unsuccessful treatment of developmental dysplasia of the hip by the Pavlik Harness. *Journal of Pediatric Orthopaedics, 29*(6), 552–557.
27. Kliegman, R., Behrman, R., Jenson, H., & Stanton, B. (Eds.). (2007). *Nelson textbook of pediatrics* (18th ed.). Philadelphia: W. B. Saunders.
28. Kocher, M., Dolan, M., & Weinberg, J. (2006). Pediatric orthopaedic infections. In M. E. Abel, *Orthopaedic knowledge update: Pediatrics 3* (pp. 57–61). Rosemont, IL: American Academy of Orthopaedic Surgeons.
29. Kocher, M., Mandiga, R., Zurakowski, D., Barnewolt, C., & Kasser, J. (2004). Validation of a clinical prediction rule for the differentiation between septic arthritis and transient synovitis of the hip in children. *Journal of Bone and Joint Surgery, 86*-A(8), 1629–1635.

30. Laine, J., Kaiser, S., & Diab, M. (2010). High-risk pediatric orthopedic pitfalls. *Emergency Medicine Clinics of North America, 28*, 85–102.

31. Lazzarini, L., Mader, J., & Calhoun, J. (2005). Osteomyelitis in long bones. *Journal of Bone and Joint Surgery, 86-A*(10), 2305–2318.

32. Lillie, P., Thaker, H., Moss, P., Baruah, J., Cullen, L., Taylor, D., et al. (2008). Healthcare associated discitis in the era of antimicrobial resistance. *Journal of Clinical Rheumatology, 14*(4), 234–237.

33. Loder, R., Richards, B., Shapiro, P., Reznick, L., & Aronson, D. (1993). Acute slipped femoral epiphysis: The importance of physeal stability. *Journal of Bone and Joint Surgery, 75*(8), 1134–1140.

34. Martin, A. (2005). Investigating the limping child: The role of plain radiographs and ultrasound. *Radiography, 11*(2), 99–107.

35. McCarthy, J. (2005). Musculoskeletal infections in children: Basic treatment prinicples and recent advancements. In *AAOS instructional course lectures* (pp. 515–528). Chicago: American Association of Orthopaedic Surgeons.

36. Morrissy, R. (2001). Bone and joint sepsis. In R. Morrissy & S. Weinstein, *Lovell and Winter's pediatric orhopaedics* (5th ed., pp. 459–500). Philadelphia: Lippincott Williams & Wilkins.

37. Nnadi, C., Chawla, T., Redfern, A., Argent, J., Fairhurst (2002). Radiograph evaluation in children with acute hip pain. *Journal of Pediatric Orthopaedics, 22*(3), 342–344.

38. Noonan, K., & McCarthy, J. (2010). Compartment syndromes in the pediatric patient. *Journal of Pediatric Orthopedics, 2*(30), 96–101.

39. Peltola, H., Paäkkönen, M., Kallio, M., & Osteomyelitis–Septic Arthritis (OM-SA) Study Group. (2009). Prospective, randomized trial of 10 days versus 30 days of antimicrobial treatment, including short-term course o f parenteral therapy, for childhood septic arthritis. *Clinical Infectious Diseases, 49*(9), 1201–1210.

40. Peltola, H., Unkila-Kallio, L., Markku, J, & Fininish Study Group. (1997). Simplified treatment of acute staphylococcal osteomyelitis of childhood. *Pediatrics, 99*(6), 846–850.

41. Pineda, C., Vargas, A., & Rodriguez, A. (2006). Imaging of osteomyelitis: Current concepts. *Infectious Disease Clinics of North America, 20*(4), 789–825.

42. Reider, B. (2005). *The orthopaedic physical exam* (2nd ed.). Philadelphia: Saunders Elsevier.

43. Rhame, D., et al. (2006). Consequences of diagnostic delays in slipped capital femoral epiphysis. *Journal of Pediatric Orthopedics, 15*(2), 93–97.

44. Rosendahl, K., Dezateux, C., Fosse, K., et al. (2010). Immediate treatment versus sonographic surveillance for mild hip dysplasia in newborns. *Pediatrics, 125*(1), 9–16.

45. Saavedra-Lozano, J., Mejias, A., Ahmad, N., Peromingo, E., Ardura, M., Guillen, S., et al. (2008). Changing trends in actue osteomyelitis in children: Impact of methicillin-resistant *Staphylococcus aureus* infections. *Journal of Pediatric Orthopaedics, 28*(5), 569–575.

46. Sandhu, H. (2003). Physiology of bone. In R. DeWald (Ed.), *Spinal deformities: The comprehensive text* (pp. 116–120). New York: Thieme.

47. Saphyakhajon, P., Joshi, A., Huskins, W., Henry, N., & Boyce, T. (2008). Empiric antibiotic therapy for acute oseoarticular infections with suspected methicillin-resistant *Staphylococcus aureu* or *Kingella*. *Pediatric Infectious Disease Journal, 27*(8), 765–767.

48. Shadgan, B., Menon, M., O'Brien, P., & Reid, W. (2008). Diagnostic techniques in acute compartment syndrome of the leg. *Journal of Orthopaedic Trauma, 8*(22), 581–587.

49. Song, K., & Sloboda, J. (2001). Acute hematogenous osteomyelitis in children. *Journal of the American Academy of Orthopaedic Surgeons, 9*(3), 166–175.

50. Sonnen, G., & Henry, N. (1996). Pediatric bone and joint infections: Diagnosis and antimicrobial management. *Pediatric Clinics of North America, 43*(4), 933–947.

51. Staheli, L. (2006). Infection. In L. Staheli, *Practice of pediatric orthopaedics* (2nd ed.). Philadelphia: Lippincott, Williams & Wilkins.

52. Stein-Zamir, C., Volovik, I., Rishpon, S., & Sabi, R. (2008). Developmental dysplasia of the hip: Risk markers, clinical screening and outcome. *Pediatrics International, 50*, 341–345.

53. Stevenson, D., Mineau, G., Kerber, R., Biskochil, D., Schaefer, C., & Roach, J. (2009). Familial predisposition to developmental dysplasia of the hip. *Journal of Paediatric Orthopaedics, 29*(5), 463–466.

54. Stewart, K., Bacher, A., Hees, P., Tayback, M., Ouyang, P., & Jande Beur, S. (2005). Exercise effects on bone mineral density: Relationships to changes in fitness and fatness. *American Journal of Preventive Medicine, 28*(5), 453–460.

55. Stokes, I. (2002). Mechanical effects on skeletal growth. *Journal of Musculoskeletal and Neuronal Interactions, 2*(3), 277–280.

56. Sucato, D., Schwend, R., & Gillespie, R. (1997). Septic arthritis of the hip in children. *Journal of the American Academy of Orthopaedic Surgeons, 5*(5), 549–559.

57. Tachdjian, M. (1997). The hip. In M. Tachdjian, *Pediatric orthopedics: The art of diagnosis and principles of management*. Stamford, CT: Appleton & Lange.

58. Yagupskyk, P. (2004). *Kingella kingae*: From medical rarity to an emerging paediatric pathogen. *Lancet Infectious Disease, 4*(6), 358–367.

Neurologic Disorders

PHYSIOLOGY AND DIAGNOSTICS

Maureen A. Madden

ANATOMY AND PHYSIOLOGY

Principal components of the nervous system

The nervous system is broadly divided into two categories: the central nervous system (CNS) and the peripheral nervous system (PNS). The nerve cell, or neuron, is the conducting unit of the nervous system. Neurons generate and conduct impulses between and within the two systems. These signals are transmitted either as electrochemical waves traveling along thin fibers called axons or as chemicals released onto other cells. The neurons are held together and supported by specialized cells called glial cells, which aid in the function of the neurons.

Central nervous system

The CNS—the largest part of the nervous system—consists of the brain and the spinal cord. The brain plays a central role in the control of most bodily functions, including awareness, movement, sensation, thought, speech, and memory. The spinal cord is connected to the brain stem and runs through the spinal canal.

Principal parts of the brain. The brain is one of the largest organs of the body. It is divided into four major parts: the brain stem, the diencephalon, the cerebrum, and the cerebellum. The brain is protected by the bones of the cranial vault and the meninges. The cranial meninges and spinal meninges have the same structure. The meninges that protect the brain consist of the dura mater (outer layer), the arachnoid mater (middle layer), and the pia mater (inner layer) (Figure 33-1). The dura mater, as the outer, thicker layer, serves the role of a protective shield. The leptomeninges surround the brain and the spinal cord, further protecting them by housing the cerebrospinal fluid (CSF) that circulates through the subarachnoid space around the brain and spinal cord and through the ventricular system of the brain. The ventricular system consists of the cavities within the brain that connect to one another, the subarachnoid space, and the spinal cord's central canal.

The ventricular system consists of four ventricles in the brain (Figure 33-2 and Figure 33-3). Two lateral ventricles are found in each side, or hemisphere, of the cerebrum under the corpus callosum. The third ventricle is a slit between and inferior to the right and left sides of the thalamus, situated between the lateral ventricles. Each lateral ventricle connects with the third ventricle by a narrow opening called the foramen of Monroe or the interventricular foramen. The fourth ventricle, which lies between the cerebellum and the lower brain stem, connects with the third ventricle through the cerebral aqueduct known as the aqueduct of Sylvius. The fourth ventricle roof has three openings through which it connects with the subarachnoid space of the meninges; this arrangement allows

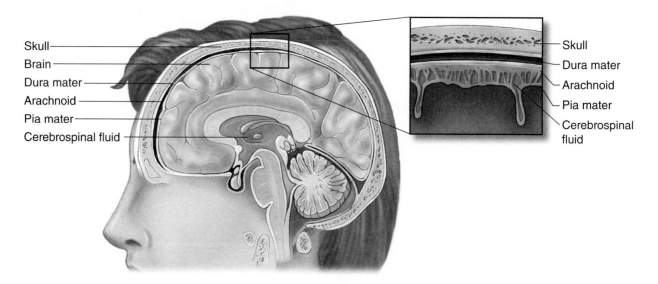

FIGURE 33-1

The Meninges.

Source: Pollak, A. (2011). *Critical Care Transport.* Jones and Bartlett Publishing.

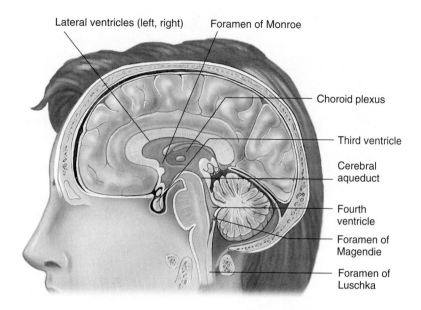

Lateral ventricles (left, right)

Foramen of Monroe

Choroid plexus

Third ventricle

Cerebral aqueduct

Fourth ventricle

Foramen of Magendie

Foramen of Luschka

FIGURE 33-2

Ventricles of the Brain.

Source: Pollak, A. (2011). *Critical Care Transport.* Jones and Bartlett Publishing.

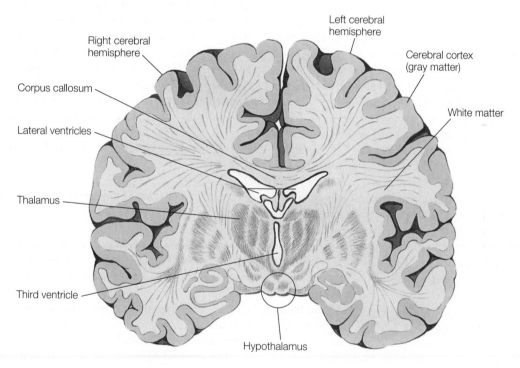

Left cerebral hemisphere

Right cerebral hemisphere

Cerebral cortex (gray matter)

Corpus callosum

White matter

Lateral ventricles

Thalamus

Third ventricle

Hypothalamus

FIGURE 33-3

Ventricles of the Brain: Cross-Section.

Source: Chiras, D. (2008). *Human Biology, 8th Ed.* Jones and Bartlett Publishers.

the CSF to circulate through the brain, spinal cord, and ventricles.

Structure and function of the brain stem.   The brain stem is composed of the medulla oblongata, the pons varolii, and the midbrain. A compact structure, it connects the brain to the spinal cord (Figure 33-4). The medulla oblongata is the lowest part of the brain stem and is interconnected with the cervical spinal cord. It contains all of the ascending and descending motor function (corticospinal)

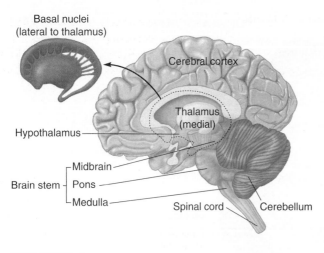

Basal nuclei
(lateral to thalamus)

Cerebral cortex

Thalamus
(medial)

Hypothalamus

Midbrain

Brain stem — Pons

Medulla

Spinal cord

Cerebellum

FIGURE 33-4

The Brain Stem.

Source: Pollak, A. (2011). *Critical Care Transport.* Jones and Bartlett Publishing.

tracts that connect the spinal cord to the various parts of the brain. These tracts make up the white matter of the medulla. Some of the motor tracts cross as they pass through the medulla. This crossing of the tracts, called "decussation of pyramids," explains why the cortex of the cerebrum motor areas controls skeletal muscle movements on the opposite side of the body. The medulla also contains an area of dispersed gray matter containing some white fibers called the "reticular formation," which functions in maintaining arousal and consciousness. The reticular system of the medulla contains three vital reflex centers that help to control involuntary actions, including many of the body's vital processes: the vasomotor center, which regulates the diameter of blood vessels; the cardiac centerm which regulates the force of contraction and heart rate; and the medullary rhythmicity area, which adjusts the rhythm of respiration.

The pons serves as a bridge between the midbrain and the medulla oblongata. Longitudinal fibers connect the spinal cord or medulla with the upper parts of the brain, and transverse fibers connect it with the cerebellum. The pneumotaxic and apneustic area in the pons helps control breathing. The pons also contains the nuclei and fibers of nerves that provide eye muscle control and facial muscle strength.

The midbrain, also called the mesencephalon, is located below the hypothalamus and contains the ventral cerebral peduncles that convey impulses from the cerebral cortex to the pons and spinal cord. It contains the dorsal tectum, a reflex center that controls the movement of the eyeballs and head in response to visual stimuli. Some cranial nerves responsible for eye muscle control also exit the midbrain.

Structure and function of the diencephalon. The diencephalon is located between the two cerebral hemispheres; it is superior to the midbrain and surrounds the third ventricle. The diencephalon is divided into two main areas: the thalamus and the hypothalamus. It also contains the optic tracts and optic chiasma, where optic nerves cross one another; the infundibulum, which attaches to the pituitary gland; the mamillary bodies, which are involved in memory and emotional responses to odor; and the pineal gland, an endocrine gland that secretes melatonin, which affects mood and behavior.

The thalamus integrates and relays sensory information to the cortex of the parietal, temporal, and occipital lobes. The superior aspect of the diencephalon, it lies medially to the basal ganglia. The thalamus plays an important role in interpretation of stimuli, thereby providing for conscious recognition of pain and temperature. It also has some awareness of crude pressure and touch.

The hypothalamus, which is located below the thalamus, is the inferior portion of the diencephalon. It regulates autonomic functions related to homeostasis, such as appetite, thirst, and body temperature. The hypothalamus controls and integrates the autonomic nervous system with the reception of sensory impulses from the internal organs. It acts as the intermediary between the nervous system and the endocrine system through the actions of the pituitary gland. The pituitary gland produces hormones that control many functions of the other endocrine glands—in particular, it regulates the production of hormones that have a role in growth, metabolism, sexual response, fluid and mineral balance, and the stress response. It is the hypothalamus that controls our feelings of rage and aggression.

Structure and function of the cerebrum. The largest part of the brain, the cerebrum controls voluntary actions, speech, senses, thought, and memory. Its surface is composed of gray matter and is referred to as the cerebral cortex. This outermost layer of the brain predominantly contains neuronal bodies—the body of the neurons that contains the cell nucleus. The gray matter actively participates in the storage and processing of information. The cells in the gray matter extend their axons to other areas of the brain. Beneath the cortex lies the cerebral white matter.

The cerebral hemispheres are separated into right and left sides by the longitudinal fissure. The cerebral cortex surface is composed of numerous folds called gyri, interspersed with intervening grooves or infoldings called sulci. The folds increase the surface area of the cortex, which contains motor areas for controlling muscular movements, sensory areas for interpreting sensory impulses, and associations with areas involved with emotional and intellectual processes. A mass of nerve fibers called the corpus callosum links the two cerebral hemispheres. Each hemisphere is divided into four lobes, which are named for the bones of the skull that lie upon them, and which are all interconnected (Figure 33-5).

The frontal lobes are located in the anterior portion of each hemisphere. They are responsible for voluntary muscular functions and, via their connections with other lobes, participate in the execution of sequential tasks, speech output, organizational skills, and aspects of mood, aggression, smell reception, memory, and motivation.

The parietal lobes are located behind the frontal lobes, in front of the occipital lobes, and are separated from these lobes by the central sulcus. They are responsible for evaluating sensory information of touch, pain, balance, spatial orientation, taste, and temperature.

The temporal lobes are located beneath the frontal and parietal lobes and separated from them by the lateral fissure. They process memory and evaluate hearing input and smell speech, and language functions. The temporal lobes are also a center for abstract thoughts and judgment decisions.

The occipital lobes form the back portion of each hemisphere. Their boundaries are not as distinct from the other lobes. The occipital lobes function in receiving and interpreting visual information.

Structure and function of the cerebellum.   The cerebellum, the second largest portion of the brain, is shaped like a butterfly. It is located beneath the cerebrum's occipital lobes and behind the brain stem's pons and medulla oblongata. The cerebellum consists of two partially separated hemispheres connected by the vermis, which is a centrally constricted structure. The cerebellum is composed of primarily white matter with a thin layer of gray matter on its surface called the cerebellar cortex. The cerebellum's primary function is as a reflex center to control equilibrium and coordination;

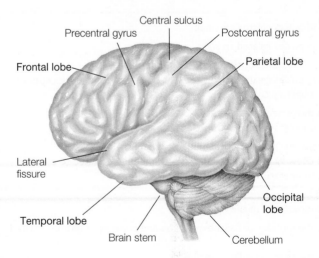

FIGURE 33-5

Lobes of the Brain.

Source: Chiras, D. (2008). *Human Biology, 8th Ed.* Jones and Bartlett Publishers.

it contributes to the generation of muscle tone, allowing for complex skeletal muscular movements and maintaining proper body posture and balance. Recently gathered evidence supports the cerebellum's role in diverse processes such as some types of memory and its influence on musical and mathematical skills.

Cranial nerves.   There are 12 pairs of cranial nerves of which 10 pairs originate from the brain stem. All 12 pairs exit the skull via various foramina of the skull. Cranial nerves may have only afferent or sensory function while others may have only efferent or motor function; and some mixed cranial nerves have both sensory and motor functions. The nomenclature for the cranial nerves is based on the order in which they originate from the brain, from the front to the back of the brain, using Roman numerals and names that indicate their function or distribution (Figure 33-6 and Table 33-1).

Peripheral nervous system

The PNS—the second major category of the nervous system—consists of all the nerves that connect the brain and spinal cord of the CNS with sensory receptors, muscles, and glands in the limbs and organs. The PNS is not protected by bone or the blood–brain barrier, so it is vulnerable to damage from toxins and mechanical injuries. This portion of the nervous system is divided into two subcategories: the afferent peripheral system and the efferent peripheral system. The afferent peripheral system (sensory neurons) consists of afferent or sensory neurons that convey information from receptors in the periphery of the body to the brain and spinal cord. The efferent peripheral system (motor neurons) consists of efferent or motor neurons that convey information from the brain and spinal cord to muscles and glands.

The efferent peripheral system is further subdivided into two categories: the somatic nervous system and the autonomic nervous system.

Somatic nervous system.   The somatic nervous system conducts impulses from the brain and spinal cord to skeletal muscle. It is responsible for coordinating body movements and for receiving external stimuli. This system is under conscious control and allows for regulation of activities. It causes a person to respond or react to changes in the external environment.

Autonomic nervous system.   The autonomic nervous system (ANS) functions in an automatic fashion without the involvement of conscious effort. It regulates the functions of the internal organs by controlling glands, cardiac muscle, and smooth muscle. The ANS maintains homeostasis by regulating heart rate and blood pressure, body temperature, and breathing. Motor impulses travel along peripheral nerve fibers that connect to the ganglia of the ANS outside

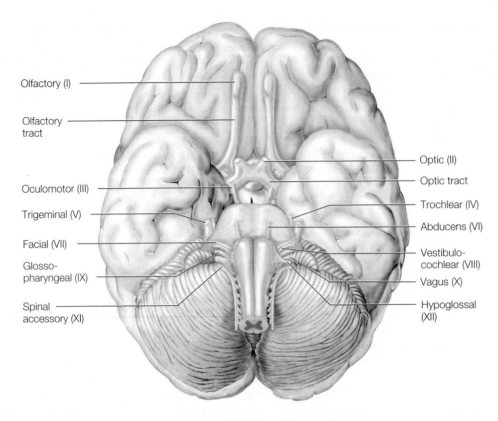

FIGURE 33-6

Cranial Nerves.

Source: Chiras, D. (2008). *Human Biology, 8th Ed.* Jones and Bartlett Publishers.

TABLE 33-1

Cranial Nerves and their Functions		
Cranial Nerve	**Function**	
Olfactory nerve (I)	Purely sensory	Conveys impulses related to smell
Optic nerve (II)	Purely sensory	Conveys impulses related to sight
Oculomotor nerve (III)	Mixed (mainly motor)	Controls movements of the eyeball and upper eyelid Conveys impulses related to muscle sense or position (proprioception) Controls pupillary constriction
Trochlear nerve (IV)	Mixed (mainly motor)	Controls movement of the eyeball Conveys impulses related to muscle sense
Trigeminal nerve (V)	Mixed	Three branches: maxillary, mandibular, and ophthalmic Controls chewing movements and delivers impulses related to touch, pain, and temperature in the teeth and facial area Optic area
Abducens nerve (VI)	Mixed (mainly motor)	Controls movement of the eyeball
Facial nerve (VII)	Mixed	Controls the muscles of facial expression and conveys sensations related to taste Controls the tear and salivary glands
Vestibulocochlear nerve (VIII)	Mixed (mostly sensory)	Transmits impulses related to equilibrium and hearing
Glossopharyngeal nerve (IX)	Mixed	Controls swallowing and senses taste Controls the salivary glands

(Continued)

TABLE 33-1

Cranial Nerves and their Functions *(Continued)*		
Cranial Nerve	**Function**	
Vagus nerve (X)	Mixed	Controls skeletal muscle movements in the pharynx, larynx, and palate
		Conveys impulses for sensations in the larynx, viscera, and ear
		Controls viscera in the thorax and abdomen
Accessory nerve (XI)	Mixed (mainly motor)	Helps control swallowing and movements of the head
Hypoglossal nerve (XII)	Mixed (mainly motor)	Controls muscles involved in speech and swallowing
		Sensory fibers conduct impulses for muscle sense

the CNS within cranial and spinal nerves. Receptors within various organs send sensory impulses to the brain and spinal cord.

The varied functions of the ANS are further subdivided into two parts: the sympathetic division and the parasympathetic division. The *sympathetic division* prepares the body for stressful situations by stimulating or speeding up activity; thus it involves energy expenditure. The systems fibers arise from the thoracic and lumbar regions of the spinal cord. The axons leave the spinal cord through the ventral roots of the spinal nerves, then leave the nerves, and finally enter a chain of paravertebral ganglia extending alongside the vertebral column. The sympathetic division uses acetylcholine in the preganglionic synapses as a neurotransmitter, where the impulse leaves the paravertebral ganglion to the postganglionic fiber. At the postganglionic fiber, the neurotransmitter norepinephrine is used at the synapses to transmit the impulse to the effector organ.

The *parasympathetic division* functions under normal nonstressful conditions. It also contributes to restoring the body to a restful state after a stressful experience, thereby balancing out the effects of the sympathetic division. The preganglionic fibers of the parasympathetic division arise from the brain stem and the sacral region of the spinal cord. The cranial and sacral nerves extend outward to ganglia located close to the viscera. The short postganglionic fibers transmit impulses to the muscles or glands within the viscera to generate an effect. They stimulate bodily activities such as digestion, urination, and defecation as well as restore or slow down other activities. Acetylcholine is the neurotransmitter used in the synapses at both the preganglionic and postganglionic fibers of the parasympathetic division.

THE SPINAL CORD: ANATOMY AND FUNCTION

The spinal cord begins as a continuation of the medulla oblongata. Its length ranges from approximately 16 to 18 inches, and its diameter varies at different areas where it is surrounded and protected by the bony vertebrae and intervertebral disks of fibrocartilage. The spinal cord is also protected by the spinal meninges. The outermost spinal meninx, called the dura mater, forms a tough outer tube of white fibrous connective tissue. The middle spinal meninx, called the arachnoid mater or spider layer, forms a delicate connective membranous tube on the interior aspect of the dura mater. The innermost layer of the transparent fibrous membrane of the pia mater forms a tube around and adheres to the surface of the spinal cord. Contained within the pia mater are numerous blood vessels and nerves (Figure 33-7).

The spinal cord is made up of a series of 31 segments, each giving rise to a pair of spinal nerves. A major function of the spinal cord is to convey sensory impulses from the periphery to the brain and then to conduct motor impulses from the brain to the periphery. The spinal cord contains both ascending and descending nerve tracts; the ascending nerve tracts carry sensory information from the periphery to the brain, while the descending nerve tracts conduct motor impulses from the brain to the muscles and glands. An additional function of the spinal cord is to provide a mechanism to integrate reflexes. Spinal nerves arise from the union of the dorsal and ventral roots of the spinal nerves.

Spinal nerves

Each spinal nerve pair is attached to an individual segment of the spinal cord via two pairs of roots. The posterior or dorsal root, or sensory root, contains only sensory nerve fibers. It conducts impulses from the periphery to the spinal cord. These fibers then extend into the posterior or dorsal gray horn of the spinal cord. The other root, the anterior or ventral root, attaches the spinal nerve to the cord at the anterior or ventral gray horn of the spinal cord. This motor root, which contains only motor nerve fibers, conducts impulses from the spinal cord to the periphery.

All of the spinal nerves are considered to be mixed nerves because they consist of both motor and sensory fibers. The spinal nerves are named and numbered based on the region and level of the spinal cord from which they emerge. Most exit the vertebral column between adjacent vertebrae. There are 8 pairs of cervical nerves, 12 pairs of thoracic nerves, 5 pairs of lumbar nerves, 5 pairs of sacral nerves, and a single pair of coccygeal nerves. The spinal nerves are numbered according to the order within the region, starting

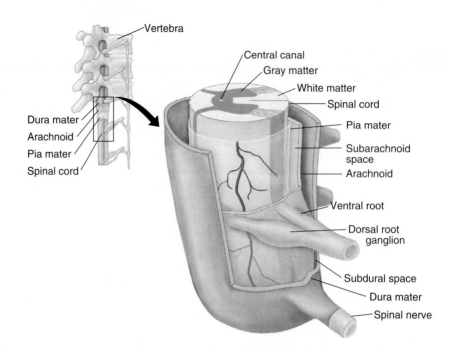

FIGURE 33-7

The Spinal Cord.

Source: Chiras, D. (2008). *Human Biology, 8th Ed.* Jones and Bartlett Publishers.

in a superior position (Figure 33-8): C1–C8 (cervical), T1–T12 (thoracic), L1–L5 (lumbar), S1–S5 (sacral), and Cx (coccygeal).

Classification of nerve cells. Nervous tissue consists of neurons (groupings of nerve cells) that transmit nerve impulses containing information, in the form of electrochemical changes. A nerve is a bundle of nerve cells or fibers. Other cells within nervous tissue, called neuroglia or glial cells, perform, support, and provide protection to the nerves. In addition, some other types of neuroglia cells do not conduct impulses. such as other neurons (Table 33-2).

Structure of a neuron. The nerve cell body contains a single nucleus that acts as the control center of the cell. The cytoplasm contains mitochondria, Golgi bodies, lysosomes, and a network of threads called neurofibrils that extend into the axon. The axon is referred to as the fiber of the cell. Within the cytoplasm of the cell body can be found an extensive network of rough endoplasmic reticulum, which has ribosomes attached.

Two types of nerve fibers are present on the nerve cell: dendrites and axons. Dendrites, which are short and branched, serve as the receptive areas of the neuron. A multipolar neuron will have multiple dendrites. In contrast, a nerve cell has only one axon; its long fiber or process begins as a single process, but may branch repeatedly and at its end has many fine extensions called axon terminals that make contact with the dendrites of other neurons. The large axons in the periphery are enclosed in fatty myelin sheaths produced by Schwann cells, a type of neuroglial cell that wraps tightly in layers around the axon.

Structural classification of neurons. Neurons are cells that conduct impulses from one part of the body to another. They may be classified by both structure and function. The structural classification consists of three types of cells:

- Multipolar neurons are neurons that have several dendrites and one axon.
- Bipolar neurons have one dendrite and one axon.
- Unipolar neurons have only one process extending from the cell body.

Most neurons in the brain and spinal cord are multipolar neurons. Bipolar neurons function as receptor cells in special sense organs. Unipolar neurons have only one process extending from the cell body, which then branches into a central aspect that functions as the axon and a peripheral branch that functions as the dendrite. These types of neurons make up the majority of the sensory neurons. The branch functioning as the axon enters the brain or spinal cord, whereas the dendrite branch connects to a peripheral part of the body.

Functional classification of neurons. Nerve cells receive input from receptors regarding changes in the environment. Receptors are the peripheral nerve endings of sensory nerves that respond to stimuli. Multiple types of receptors exist, each of which changes the energy of a stimulus

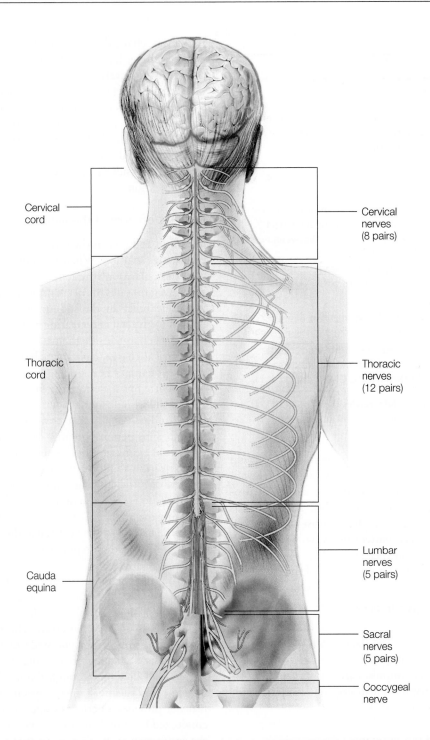

Cervical cord

Cervical nerves (8 pairs)

Thoracic cord

Thoracic nerves (12 pairs)

Lumbar nerves (5 pairs)

Cauda equina

Sacral nerves (5 pairs)

Coccygeal nerve

FIGURE 33-8

Spinal Nerves.

Source: Chiras, D. (2008). *Human Biology, 8th Ed.* Jones and Bartlett Publishers.

into nerve impulses. The first nerve cell that receives the impulse directly from a receptor is the sensory or afferent neuron; such neurons are of the unipolar type. These receptors make contact with only one end of the sensory neuron, thereby ensuring a one-way transmission of the impulse with the central process of the sensory neuron signaling to the spinal cord. From the sensory neuron, the impulse may pass through a number of multipolar-type neurons found in the spinal cord and brain. The sensory impulse is transmitted to the brain or spinal cord for interpretation. From the association of nerve cells or interneuron, the impulse is passed to the final nerve cell, the motor or efferent neuron. This multipolar neuron initiates the reaction—either muscular or glandular—to the original stimulus.

TABLE 33-2

Neuroglial Cells	
Name	**Function**
Astrocytes	Star-shaped cells that wrap around nerve cells to form the supporting network in the brain and spinal cord
	Attach neurons to their blood vessels, helping regulate nutrients and ions for nerve cells
Oligodendroglia	Have the appearance of small astrocytes
	Provide support by forming semi-rigid connective-like tissue rows between neurons of the brain and spinal cord
	Produce fatty myelin sheath on the neurons of the brain and spinal cord
Microglial cells	Small cells
	Protect the CNS by engulfing and destroying microbes (e.g., bacteria) and cellular debris
Ependymal cells	Line the ventricles of the brain
	Some produce CSF; others with cilia move the CSF through the CNS

Note: Central nervous system (CNS), cerebrospinal fluid (CSF).

In the nervous system, tissues are organized into several categories. The white matter comprises groups of myelinated axons from multiple neurons supported by the neuroglial cells. It forms nerve tracts in the CNS. The gray areas of the nervous system (gray matter) consist of nerve cell bodies and dendrites. Gray matter can also contain bundles of unmyelinated axons and their neuroglial. The cortex of the brain is the gray matter on the surface of the brain.

PHYSIOLOGY OF NERVE IMPULSES

The functional elements within the nervous system are the neurons. These cells are aligned in sequences to form circuits within which nerve impulses are transmitted electrochemically. Neurons require a neurotransmitter to transmit the impulse across the synapse.

Resting potential of the neuron

A neuron has the ability to produce a concentration of ions on either the inside or the outside of the cell membrane. Under normal circumstances, positively charged sodium ions are found in greater concentration outside the cell than inside it, whereas positively charged potassium ions are found in greater concentration inside the cell than outside it. The cell membrane, which serves as the barrier to the movement of these ions, is both semipermeable and selectively permeable. The electrolyte balance is maintained by the cell's sodium–potassium pump. The inside of the nerve fiber also houses negatively charged chloride ions and other negatively charged organic molecules. As a consequence, the nerve fiber has an electrical distribution such that the outside is positively charged while the inside is negatively charged. This electrical potential across the membrane, when a neuron is not actually transmitting, is known as the membrane resting potential. This potential represents the difference in electrical charge on either side of the member and is correlated with the difference in the concentration of ions on either side of the membrane, a condition referred to as polarization.

Action potential of the neuron

The fluid and ions in the intracellular space create a highly conductive solution. When a stimulus is applied to the neuron, the polarity of the ions is disrupted at that location. This event initiates the nerve impulse by triggering a change in permeability to the sodium ions, allowing sodium to enter into the cell and creating a change from a negative to a positive charge inside the nerve membrane. This reversal of electrical charge, called depolarization, creates the cell's action potential. The ions in the adjacent areas along the neuron attempt to restore the original polarity at the location of the stimulus. As repolarization occurs in the area of the stimulus, the adjacent areas themselves become depolarized. This action potential creates a wave-like progression, in one direction of the nerve fiber, of depolarization/repolarization along the length of the neuron. The stimuli must be of sufficient magnitude to conduct an impulse and, therefore, to create an action potential.

With the change in polarity, an impulse is conducted along the neuron to the next cell at the same amplitude and speed. This cell then repolarizes and returns to its resting potential membrane.

An unmyelinated nerve fiber conducts an impulse over its entire length, but the conduction is slower than that occurring along a myelinated fiber. A myelinated fiber, which is insulated by the myelin sheath, allows an action potential to jump from one node of Ranvier to the next as a means of rapidly conducting an impulse. Although ions cannot flow out through the myelin sheath of myelinated nerves, the break in the myelin sheath at the nodes of Ranvier provides a perfect escape route. Impulses are then conducted from node to node rather than continuing along the entire span of the axon, as in unmyelinated nerves. This type of conduction, called salutatory conduction, is advantageous because it increases the velocity of an impulse and conserves energy because the node simply needs to depolarize (not repolarize). The velocity of an impulse depends on both the thickness of the myelin and the distance between the nodes (Hickey, 2003).

Synapse

The junction between one neuron and the next at which an impulse is transmitted is called the synapse. Three anatomic structures are necessary for the impulse to be transmitted at the synapse: the presynaptic terminal, the synaptic cleft, and the postsynaptic membrane.

The presynaptic terminals are either inhibitory or excitatory in nature. When the terminal is excitatory, it secretes a substance into the synaptic cleft that simulates the effector neuron. Conversely, the inhibitory presynaptic terminal secretes a transmitter into the synaptic clef that inhibits the effector neuron. The excitatory or inhibitory transmitter secretions are released from the vesicles in the axon endings.

The synaptic cleft is the microscopic space located between the presynaptic terminal and the receptor area of the effector cell. The postsynaptic membrane is the part of the effector membrane that is proximal to the presynaptic terminal. When an action potential is created and moves over the presynaptic terminal, the membrane depolarizes, emptying some of the secretions from the presynaptic vesicles into the synaptic cleft. Depending on the type of transmitter substance secreted in the synaptic cleft, this change will result in either excitation or inhibition of the neuron (Hickey, 2003; Jenkins & Kochanek, 2007).

Neurotransmitters

Information is transmitted from one neuron to the next by a neurotransmitter. Such neurotransmitters may either excite, inhibit, or modify the response of another cerebral cell or cells. The presynaptic terminals of one neuron release a chemical that affects particular postsynaptic cells of another neuron. Each neuron generally releases the same transmitter at all of its separate terminals. To date, more than 30 neurotransmitters have been identified, including specific amines, catecholamines, amino acids, and polypeptides (Hickey, 2003; Johnston, 2006) (Table 33-3).

CEREBRAL BLOOD FLOW AND VASCULAR REACTIVITY

The cerebral circulation vascular reactivity is an important neuroprotective mechanism that allows the metabolic demands of the brain to be met via regulation of the cerebral blood flow through the adjustment of CNS vessel diameters to physiologic changes. The ability of the cerebrovascular system to react in this manner has limits, however; these constraints are defined physiologically as the upper and lower limits of autoregulation. Impairment of cerebral blood flow autoregulation is considered to be a potential factor in the development of secondary brain injury (Jenkins & Kochanek, 2007).

Perfusion pressure autoregulation of cerebral blood flow

The major cerebrovascular response to acute changes in perfusion pressure takes the form of pressure autoregulation. *Autoregulation* is the descriptive term applied to the mechanisms that link brain–blood flow with brain metabolism. The underlying concept of pressure autoregulation is that cerebral blood flow is maintained at a relatively constant rate over wide ranges of arterial blood pressure (Bruce, 1985). Local and global injuries can disrupt autoregulation, while arterial blood flow changes passively affect blood flow. Cerebral blood flow may be affected depending on the metabolic requirements at any given time, which create an increase or decrease in flow. The intimate and complex relationship between metabolism and blood flow is maintained in the absence of injury. When an injury damages the brain tissue, the autoregulatory mechanisms may be altered. Depending on the severity of the injury, the mechanisms may forever be disrupted (Johnston, 2006).

Blood–brain barrier development

The capillary endothelial blood–brain barrier (BBB) limits the movement of solutes, including drugs and proteins, between the blood and the brain. The BBB is a highly selective network of endothelial cells that make up the walls of capillaries and form the projections from the astrocytes located in close proximity to the neuron. The capillaries in the brain do not have pores between adjacent endothelial cells; as a consequence, the brain must transport molecules within cerebral capillaries through the endothelial cells via active transport, endocytosis, and exocytosis (Hickey, 2003). The presence of this barrier means that most medications are prevented from affecting the brain and spinal cord. The ability of any particular substance to move into the brain depends on the particle size, lipid solubility, chemical dissociation, and the protein-binding potential of the drug. The BBB is very permeable to water, oxygen, carbon dioxide, glucose, gases, and lipid-soluble compounds (Jenkins & Kochanek, 2007; Johnston, 2006).

Modified Monro-Kellie doctrine

The Monro-Kellie doctrine states that the cranial vault contains a fixed volume composed of three basic components: brain parenchyma (80%), blood (10%), and cerebrospinal fluid (10%). This vault is encased by the thick, inelastic dura mater and the semi-rigid cranium. The various components of the brain exist in a state of volume–pressure equilibrium, such that expansion of one induces a compensatory reduction in the volume of one or both of the others to maintain intracranial pressure (ICP). The Monro-Kellie equation is defined as follows:

Volume of the intracranial vault (constant) =
Volume of the brain + Volume of the CSF
+ Volume of the blood + (Volume of any mass lesion)

Cerebral perfusion pressure

As with all organs, the perfusion pressure of the brain is determined by the difference between the upstream and downstream pressures. In the brain, either the central

TABLE 33-3

Major Neurotransmitters		
Neurotransmitter	**Function**	**Pathway**
Cholinergic		
Acetylcholine	Nicotinic receptor: • Muscle contraction • Stimulate sympathetic and parasympathetic fibers Muscarinic: • Smooth muscle contraction • Memory and learning; regulation of breathing	Neuromuscular junction Preganglionic autonomic synapses Postganglionic parasympathetic fibers Basal forebrain to cortex; brain stem
Amino Acids		
Gamma-aminobutyric acid (GABA)	Inhibitory	Interneurons in cerebral cortex
Glutamate	Excitatory	Multiple pathways: intracortical, corticospinal, corticostriatal
Aspartate	Excitatory	
Glycine	Inhibitory	
Biogenic Amines		
Histamine	Excitatory	Hypothalamus
Serotonin 5-hydroxytryptamine (5-HT)	Inhibitory in pain pathways in spinal cord Regulation of sleep and attention	Midbrain to cerebral cortex
Epinephrine		Adrenal medulla; some CNS cells
Norepinephrine	Excitatory; alerting of cerebral cortex	Sympathetic nerves: pons to cerebral cortex, spinal cord
Dopamine	Inhibitory; regulation of movement and attention	Midbrain to basal ganglia and cerebral cortex
Puinergic		
Adenosine		CNS, Peripheral nerves
ATP		Sympathetic, sensory and enteric nerves
Gaseous		
Nitric oxide (NO)		CNS, Gastrointestinal tract

Note: Central nervous system (CNS).

Source: Adapted from Johnston, 2006.

venous pressure (CVP) or the ICP may provide the greater downstream pressure. Most commonly, the ICP is utilized in the determination of CPP. The CPP is used to assess the adequacy of cerebral perfusion because the cerebral blood flow is difficult to measure clinically. The normal range of CPP is 70 to 100 mmHg. The following equation describes cerebral perfusion pressure:

$$\text{Cerebral perfusion pressure (CPP)} =$$
$$\text{Mean arterial pressure (MAP)} - \text{ICP or CVP}$$

Glasgow coma scale

Certain aspects of a detailed neurologic exam cannot be assessed in young children due to their inability to follow commands or communicate verbally. Nevertheless, careful, serial assessment of the level of consciousness is the most important component of such an exam. Combative behavior may be appropriate for young children undergoing medical examinations and painful procedures, or it may be a sign of impaired neurologic function. A quiet child with eyes closed may simply be in a normal state of sleep or may have altered level of consciousness. The response to noxious stimuli by such a patient often provides clues to the degree of altered consciousness.

The Glasgow Coma Scale, Modified for Infants and Children, is the equivalent of the Glasgow Coma Scale (GCS) used to assess the mental state of adult patients. Given that many of the assessments for an adult patient would not be appropriate for infants, the pediatric version of the GSC has been slightly modified. The scale comprises three tests: eye, verbal, and motor responses. The three values are considered both separately and as a total score. The lowest possible score (the sum) is 3 (deep coma or death), while the highest is 15 (fully awake and aware person) (Table 33-4).

DIAGNOSTICS

Imaging studies

Computed tomography (CT) and magnetic resonance imaging (MRI) are noninvasive imaging techniques utilized in the diagnostic evaluation of the intracranial and intraspinal structures. These technologies are readily available and allow the nervous system to be imaged accurately, quickly, and safely. These noninvasive studies have largely replaced other invasive procedures for assessment of neurologic disorders (Table 33-5).

Computed tomography

Computed tomography scanning is a highly advanced diagnostic procedure for emergencies and for less emergent disorders. A noninvasive and rapid radiographic imaging technique, it uses conventional radiographic (x-ray) techniques to create cross-sectional pictures of the body, which are then enhanced by computer software.

CT images are generated by scanning an area in successive layers with x-ray beams that pass through the anatomic area from multiple directions. Detectors measure the degree of attenuation of the existing radiation. The computer then integrates this information and constructs the images in cross-section, which generates a three-dimensional image of the inside of an object from a large series of two-dimensional x-ray images taken around a single axis of rotation. The resulting cross-section, called a cut or slice, can vary in thickness. The data from a single CT imaging procedure, consisting of either multiple contiguous or one helical scan, can be viewed as images in the axial, coronal,

TABLE 33-4

Modified Glasgow Coma Scale and Glasgow Coma Scale Modified for Infants and Children				
Clinical Parameter	**Adult**	**Infants (Ages 0–12 Months)**	**Children (Ages 1–5 Years)**	**Score***
Eye opening	Open spontaneously	Open spontaneously	Open spontaneously	4
	Open in response to verbal stimuli	Open in response to verbal stimuli	Open in response to verbal stimuli	3
	Open in response to pain only	Open in response to pain only	Open in response to pain only	2
	No response	No response	No response	1
Best verbal response	Oriented	Coos and babbles	Oriented, appropriate	5
	Confused	Irritable cries	Confused	4
	Inappropriate words	Cries in response to pain	Inappropriate words	3
	Incomprehensible words or nonspecific sounds	Moans in response to pain	Incomprehensible words or nonspecific sounds	2
	No response	No response	No response	1
Best motor response†	Obeys	Moves spontaneously and purposefully	Obeys commands	6
	Localizes	Withdraws to touch	Localizes painful stimulus	5
	Withdraws	Withdraws in response to pain	Withdraws in response to pain	4
	Abnormal flexion	Responds to pain with decorticate posturing (abnormal flexion)	Responds to pain with decorticate posturing (abnormal flexion)	3
	Extensor response	Responds to pain with decerebrate posturing (abnormal extension)	Responds to pain with decerebrate posturing (abnormal extension)	2
	No response	No response	No response	1

* Score ≤ 12 suggests a severe head injury. Score < 8 suggests a need for endotracheal intubation and mechanical ventilation. Score ≤ 6 suggests a need for intracranial pressure monitoring.

† If the patient is intubated, unconscious, or preverbal, the most important part of this scale is motor response. This section should be carefully evaluated.

Sources: Adapted from Davis et al., 1987; James et al., 1985; Morray et al., 1984; Reilly et al., 1988; Teasdale & Jennett, 1974.

TABLE 33-5

Anatomic Imaging Techniques of the Nervous System: Indications	
Computed Tomography Scan	**Magnetic Resonance Imaging**
Detection and evaluation of acute intracranial bleeding	Small ischemic areas and stroke
Technique of choice for initial trauma evaluation	Delayed imaging for cerebral trauma
Initial evaluation for differentiation of acute ischemic stroke versus hemorrhagic stroke	Evaluation of ligamentous injuries
Initial 24 hours: evaluation of cerebral or cerebellar ischemic infarction	Evaluation of ischemic infarction after first 12 to 24 hours
Contrast study to evaluate tumors with enhancement	Smaller tumors esp. in posterior fossa
Evaluation of hydrocephalus	Spinal cord tumor or trauma
Detection of brain abscess	Intervertebral disk disease
Evaluate acute hemorrhage associated with arteriovenous malformation or cerebral aneurysm	Demyelinating, white matter, and other neurodegenerative diseases and conditions
Detection of abnormal calcification of cranial and vertebral bones	Epilepsy work-up
Imaging of bone structures	

Source: Adapted from Hickey, 2003.

or sagittal planes, depending on the diagnostic task. This creates detailed images of areas surrounded by bone and can show less dense tissues such as organs and blood vessels.

CT completely eliminates the superimposition of images of structures outside the area of interest. Its inherent high-contrast resolution can distinguish between tissues that differ in physical density by less than 1% (Gilman, 1998a, 1998b). Changes in tissue density, displacement and abnormalities of structures, and calcifications can be appreciated.

CT scans may be performed with or without radiocontrast media. Use of a radiopaque medium enhances image sharpness and areas of pathology that have resulted from breakdown of the blood–brain barrier. If anatomic image clarity is desired, iodinated radiopaque material is administered intravenously. Contraindications to contrast medium, which include pregnancy, allergy to shellfish or iodinated dye, unstable vital signs, or kidney function, must be considered prior to administration. Before any contrast medium is administered, blood urea nitrogen (BUN), creatinine levels, and occasionally creatinine clearance are checked to evaluate for adequate kidney function. Most protocols

require that the patient has no enteral food or liquids for 4 to 8 hours prior to the contrast-enhanced study. Patients need to be prepared for this procedure; specifically, they should be warned that they may experience flushing or a feeling of warmth, transient headache, a salty or metallic taste in the mouth, nausea, or vomiting with contrast medium administration. Intravenous or oral hydration is important to facilitate contrast medium clearance post procedure. Tubular necrosis and acute kidney failure can result from inadequate hydration or preexisting dysfunction (Hickey, 2003).

CT scanning of the head performed without contrast is most useful for assessing the following conditions:

- Ventricular size
- Hemorrhage
- Cerebral atrophy
- Large space-occupying lesions
- Congenital malformations of the brain
- Intracranial calcifications
- Areas of cerebral edema, infarction, and demyelination

CT scanning of the spine is most useful for assessing these conditions:

- The bones of the spine (vertebrae)
- Problems of the spine, such as tumors, fractures, deformities, infection, or spinal stenosis
- Herniated disks of the spine
- Compression fractures
- Congenital problems of the spine
- Problems seen during a standard x-ray
- Follow-up postoperative spinal surgery or therapy

In the detection of parenchymal, intraventricular, subdural, and epidural blood, CT scans and MRI have comparable utility. CT is more sensitive in detecting subarachnoid blood. In the evaluation of trauma, its fine bone detail makes CT scanning the modality of choice. A CT scan without contrast is used to evaluate presence of bleeding or hematoma when a cerebral aneurysm is suspected, and to screen candidates for bleeding prior to administration of thrombolytic therapy in ischemic stroke. Serial CT scans may be used to follow the evolution or resolution of cerebral hemorrhage or edema. In the spine, the bony structure of the vertebrae can be accurately defined using this imaging modality, as can the anatomy of the intervertebral disks and spinal cord (Hickey, 2003) (Table 33-6).

The advantages of CT imaging are many. This painless, widely available technique can be performed on both conscious and unconscious patients quickly. Sedation may be required for the pediatric patient due to the essential need to remain movement free throughout the procedure. CT scanning shows the anatomy of skull and vertebral bones well and is sensitive for detection of acute hemorrhage and

TABLE 33-6

Preferred Imaging Procedures for Neurologic Disorders	
Neurologic Disorder	**Imaging Procedure**
Cerebral or cerebellar ischemic infarction	CT in the first 12–24 hours; MRI after 12–24 hours (diffusion-weighted and perfusion-weighted MRI augments the findings, especially in the first 24 hours, and even before 8 hours)
Cerebral or cerebellar hemorrhage	CT in the first 24 hours; MRI after 24 hours; MRI and endovascular angiography for suspected arteriovenous malformation
Arteriovenous malformation	CT for acute hemorrhage; MRI and endovascular angiography as early as possible
Cerebral aneurysm	CT for acute subarachnoid hemorrhage; CT angiography or endovascular angiography to identify the aneurysm; TCD to detect vasospasm
Brain tumor	MRI without and with injection of contrast material
Head/cerebral trauma	CT initially; MRI after initial assessment and treatment
Multiple sclerosis	MRI without and with injection of contrast material
Meningitis or encephalitis	CT without and with injection of contrast material initially; MRI after initial assessment and treatment
Cerebral or cerebellar abscess	CT without and with injection of contrast material for initial diagnosis or, if the patient is stable, MRI instead of CT; MRI without and with injection of contrast material subsequently
Movement disorders	MRI; PET
Neonatal and development disorders	US in unstable premature neonates; otherwise, MRI
Epilepsy	MRI; PET; SPECT
Headache	CT in patients suspected of having structural disorders

Note: Computed tomography (CT), magnetic resonance imaging (MRI), positron emission tomography (PET), single-photon emission computed tomography (SPECT), transcranial Doppler (TCD), ultrasonography (US).

Source: Adapted from Gilman, 1998a.

calcifications. It is useful when other diagnostic techniques, such as MRI, are contraindicated.

CT scans use ionizing radiation exposure, which is a disadvantage in comparison to MRI. Other disadvantages include this technique's decreased sensitivity for detection of many common neurological diseases, lesions adjacent to bone, small soft-tissue lesions, posterior fossa lesions, and floor of the middle fossa lesions.

Magnetic resonance imaging. Magnetic resonance imaging is a noninvasive modality to image the brain and spinal cord. This technique appears to be free of biological risks, produces exquisite cross-section anatomic detail of the nervous system, and provides increased sensitivity in the detection of most intraxial lesions compared with CT imaging.

MRI applies a strong magnetic field to tissue protons. Protons within different body tissues will behave differently in the face of this force, as will protons within normal versus abnormal tissues of a similar type. The MRI technology takes advantage of the hydrogen atom and its differential distribution in tissues of the body. The generation of its signal intensity is detected, stored, and then analyzed by computer programs (Hickey, 2003).

Various radio frequency pulse sequences used in MRI scanning emphasize the different relaxation characteristics—termed T1 or T2 relaxation times—of

protons placed in a magnetic field. These components to the MR signal can be manipulated by varying the timing of the excitation, called pulse sequences. Depending on the weighting of the various components of the signal, images are of three general types: proton density, T1 weighted, or T2 weighted. The type of image needed depends on the type of tissue under study and the suspected pathology. The ability to manipulate pulse sequence and components enhances the usefulness of MRI.

MRI is particularly well suited for the study of neoplasms, cerebral edema, acute stroke, demyelination, degenerative diseases, and congenital anomalies, especially those affecting the posterior fossa and spinal cord. This imaging modality is capable of detecting small plaques in patients with multiple sclerosis and areas of localized gliosis in children with uncontrolled seizures. With the exception of calcification and mineralization, physiologic and pathologic tissue is better detected and delineated by MRI relative to CT.

The interpretation of MRI images depends on the choice of images, as previously noted. Initial evaluation for tumors needs to include all three types to be considered a complete study. Each type has distinct advantages and disadvantages in its ability to detect the presence of disease at certain tissue interfaces and its potential for false-positive information that should be evaluated in comparison to information obtained from the other sequences. In T1-weighted images,

CSF has signal intensity lower than the brain and fat has a signal intensity higher than the brain. Therefore, in this type of image, the CSF appears very dark, gray matter appears lighter, and white matter appears bright. In a T2-weighted image, in which the CSF signal is higher than the signal in the brain, CSF appears very bright and there is poor color discrimination between gray and white matter. Proton density images are "balanced," in that CSF is of intermediate signal intensity, similar to the signal intensity of the brain. Balanced imaging is useful in differentiating between CSF and an abnormal parenchymal signal near a CSF space, as pathological tissue will retain the "bright" signal seen on T2-weighted scans. Calcification generates a signal "void" because of the lack of mobile protons. Likewise, flow within structures generates a signal void because the excited protons leave the sectioned image plane before their signal can be registered (Michelson & Ashwal, 2007).

An MRI technique using fluid-attenuated inversion-recovery (FLAIR) is useful for detecting brain lesions because of its sensitive demonstration of lesions causing T2 prolongation against a suppressed CSF background. The superiority of FLAIR compared with T1-weighted images and T2-weighted images has been shown in many disorders, including stroke, multiple sclerosis, infections, and cerebral hemorrhage.

The contrast agent known as gadolinium-diethylenetri-amine penta-acetic acid (gadolinium-DTPA) is useful during MRI to highlight lesions associated with a disrupted blood–brain barrier. This medium alters the magnetic susceptibility of adjacent tissue, thereby providing information about the integrity of the BBB. Contrast-enhanced MRI scanning is unique in its ability to differentiate spinal cord tumors from adjacent edema and approaches the sensitivity of CT myelography in detecting intradural spinal metastatic disease (Michelson & Ashwal, 2007).

MRI studies are not obscured by bone; thus this imaging technique allows for detection of soft-tissue changes that are not detectable on CT scan. Areas poorly seen on CT scan, such as the posterior fossa and the spinal cord, can be more clearly defined by MRI. Thus MRI is especially beneficial in the following conditions:

- Ischemic and infracted areas
- Degenerative diseases
- Cerebral and spinal cord edema
- Hemorrhage
- Arteriovenous malformations
- Small tumors
- Congenital anomalies

MRI has several notable advantages:

- It provides detailed sagittal (right to left side); axial (top to bottom of the head), and coronal (front to back of the head) images for precise lesion assessment and location.

- MRI eliminates exposure risk because ionizing radiation is not used.
- It provides better differentiation than CT for water, iron, fat, and blood, by using physical and biochemical characteristics of the tissues imaged.
- A higher level of gray–white matter contrast is obtained with MRI compared with CT.
- MRI can detect soft-tissue changes not seen on radiographs, such as small tumors along cranial nerves and other tumors as small as 0.3 mm.
- It provides higher-resolution detail of the posterior fossa, skull base, and orbits compared with CT scan.

Disadvantages of MRI include the need to exclude a number of patients who could be adversely affected by the procedure because the strong magnetic field can move or dislodge metallic material and cause injury to body tissue. In the last few years, new MRI-compatible materials for neurological and orthopedic equipment have become available. It is imperative to screen patients accurately for the presence of any devices that are contraindications for MRI before scheduling the procedure (Hickey, 2003).

Physiologic imaging of metabolic function

Positron emission tomography (PET) and single photon emission computerized tomography (SPECT) use nuclear medicine technology to primarily evaluate the nervous system through cerebral metabolism and cerebral blood flow (CBF).

Positron emission tomography. PET scanning measures regional physiologic functions such as glucose uptake and metabolism, oxygen use, and CBF patterns. This type of imaging reveals the cellular-level metabolic changes occurring in an organ or tissue in real time and can be remarkably detailed. Its results are important and unique because disease processes often begin with functional changes at the cellular level. A PET scan can often detect these very early changes, whereas a CT scan or MRI may detect changes only later, as the disease begins to alter the structure of organs or tissues. Currently, neuroimaging PET scans are most commonly used to detect and provide understanding of brain disorders (including brain tumors, memory disorders, and seizures), cerebrovascular disease, cerebral trauma, and other CNS conditions (Hickey, 2003).

In PET, a very small dose of a radioactive chemical, called a radiotracer, is injected into the patient's bloodstream. Once inside the body, the radiotracer tag concentrates in the area of clinical interest and emits positrons. PET scans typically use glucose labeling. Glucose—the most common form of sugar in the body—is the brain's main source of energy. As cells consume chemically labeled glucose, positrons are emitted. Thus the PET scan reveals which areas of the body are burning the most sugar.

In the past, a major advantage of PET scanning was the clarity of images produced; today, however, functional MRI can create images with even more clarity. The disadvantages of the PET technology include its high expense, its limited availability for diagnostic purposes, and the necessity to produce the short-lived isotopes, which limits patient access to this imaging modality.

In preparation for a PET scan, no caffeine, alcohol, nicotine, or glucose should be consumed for 24 hours prior to the procedure. The patient cannot have any enteral intake for 6 to 12 hours before the procedure. In addition, the patient must be able to lie flat for the duration of the procedure, which typically lasts 2 to 3 hours. A venous access site is necessary to inject the radiotracer, with a second site required to access and draw samples for measurement of cerebral metabolic rates. Post procedure, the patient needs to have copious fluid intake to clear the isotope (Hickey, 2003).

Single photon emission CT.   Single photon emission computed tomography scans (SPECT) measure regional CBF and perfusion. This type of imaging can identify abnormalities in blood vessel tone or the ability of a vessel to dilate or constrict. The SPECT scan is based on the same principle as PET technology, except that only a single photon is emitted when the radioactive tag decays. The radioactive tracers used in SPECT are commercially prepared and do not require access to an online cyclotron, unlike PET. SPECT is useful to demonstrate hypoperfusion in focal and diffuse cerebral disorders such as dementia, seizures, stroke, and cerebral trauma; it has also been widely used as a confirmatory test for brain death (Hickey, 2003).

The major advantage of SPECT is its widespread availability within nuclear medicine departments. This technology detects cerebral perfusion changes and is helpful during acute events such as the following:

- Stroke
- Seizures
- Dementia
- Amnesia
- Trauma
- Neoplasms
- Brain death
- Persistent vegetative state (PVS)
- Psychiatric disorders (e.g., schizophrenia, depression)

The major disadvantages of SPECT are related to technical resolution concerns and this modality's high cost. The patient requires intravenous access for injection of the isotope, and the scan must be conducted within a 1 hour of its administration as the isotope decays in approximately 60 minutes. No special preparation or postprocedure care is necessary.

Cerebrospinal fluid and spinal procedures

Examination of the CSF is necessary to confirm the diagnosis of meningitis, encephalitis, and subarachnoid hemorrhage. This assessment is often helpful in evaluating demyelinating, degenerative, and collagen vascular diseases and for identifying the presence of malignant cells within the CSF. It is also the definitive diagnostic test for pseudotumor cerebri or benign intracranial hypertension.

Lumbar puncture.   Preparation of the patient is essential to complete a lumbar puncture (LP) procedure successfully. The indications for LP can be divided into diagnostic and therapeutic purposes. Diagnostic indications include the following conditions:

- Measurement of CSF pressure
- Examination of CSF for the presence of blood
- Evaluation of spinal dynamics for signs of blockage of CSF flow
- Collection of CSF for laboratory study
- Radiologic visualization of parts of the nervous system by injection of air, oxygen, or radiopaque material

Therapeutic indications for LP include these conditions:

- Introduction of spinal anesthesia
- Intrathecal injection of antibacterial, chemotherapeutic, or other drugs
- Removal of CSF in pseudotumor cerebri/benign intracranial hypertension

The contraindications to LP are relative and require careful judgment, weighing the risks against the potential benefits:

- Elevated intracranial pressure
- Signs and symptoms of impending cerebral herniation
- Skin infection at the site of the LP
- Thrombocytopenia
- Antiplatelet or anticoagulation therapy
- Critical illness (rare occasions)

In the presence of elevated ICP, whether due to a suspected lesion or mass of the brain or spinal cord or due to traumatic injury, transtentorial herniation or herniation of the cerebellar tonsils may potentially develop after the procedure is completed. For this reason, the patient must have a head CT and inspection of the eyes to evaluate for presence of papilledema prior to the procedure. Signs and symptoms of impending herniation include decerebrate or decorticate posturing, generalized tonic seizure, and abnormalities of pupillary size and reactivity. Pending herniation is also associated with respiratory abnormalities including hyperventilation, Cheyne-Stokes respiration, ataxic breathing, apnea, and respiratory arrest. Further stabilization and reduction of ICP must be achieved before LP may be considered as an assessment technique.

When there is a skin infection at the site of the LP and examination of the CSF is necessary, use of an alternative site such as ventricular or cistern magna tap may be indicated for the LP. A patient who is on antiplatelet or anticoagulation therapy, or who is thrombocytopenic, may have uncontrolled bleeding in the subarachnoid or subdural space; as a consequence, LP is contraindicated until platelet count improves or the effects of the anticlotting therapy are reversed. In circumstances where a patient's clinical condition is critical and an attempt at LP may produce cardiopulmonary arrest, the procedure should be deferred until the patient is stabilized and the LP may be performed safely under more controlled circumstances (Haslam, 2008).

Potential complications of LP include evidence of trauma to the tissues at the LP site with subsequent bleeding. It is important to determine whether the initial sample of CSF contains blood secondary to trauma or due to hemorrhage. If the tap was traumatic, CSF should clear progressively in successive samples. In contrast, if intracranial hemorrhage is present, successive samples of CSF will continue to be equally as discolored as the initial specimen obtained (Hickey, 2003).

Myelography. Myelography is performed to visualize the lumbar, thoracic, or cervical subarachnoid space or the entire spinal column as a diagnostic procedure for the following conditions:

- Spinal cord compression
- Spinal cord lesion (e.g., tumor, vascular abnormality)
- Vertebral bone displacement
- Intervertebral disk herniation
- Visualization of partial or complete obstruction of CSF or contrast medium

When a MRI is inconclusive, a myelogram may be performed. This procedure entails performing an LP with removal of approximately 10 mL of CSF. A water-soluble contrast medium is injected into the subarachnoid space, and radiographic films of the vertebral column and spinal cord are taken. The contrast medium will diffuse upward through the CSF and penetrate into the nerve root sleeves, nerve rootlets, and subarachnoid space. During this procedure, it is important to maintain the head at an elevation of approximately 30 degrees at all times to prevent upward dispersion of the contrast medium and entrance of the material into the cranial vault, which could result in seizures. The contrast medium may cause confusion, hallucinations, depression, hyperesthesia, chest pain, and arrhythmias.

Postprocedural care requires that the patient's head of bed continue to be elevated 30 degrees at all times for a total of 12 hours. The patient must be maintained on bed rest for 4 to 8 hours and kept quiet. The patient is monitored for symptoms of back pain, spasms, elevated temperature, difficulty voiding, nuchal rigidity, nausea, and vomiting. The patient should be well hydrated both before and after the procedure. No phenothiazine derivatives should be given to the patient for 48 hours post procedure due to the risk of seizures (Hickey, 2003).

Noninvasive cerebrovascular studies

Transcranial doppler. Transcranial Doppler (TCD) scanning uses the principles of Doppler technology to evaluate intracranial blood flow. With this approach, an ultrasound beam is sent through a thinning of the skull. The change in the pulsed wave resulting from basal cerebral arteries is then analyzed to provide information on the patency of vessels, flow velocity, turbulence, and directional flow of the moving column of blood in a major artery. TCD does not provide an actual image of the vessel or a measure of the CBF.

The TCD procedure is performed by placing a Doppler ultrasonic handheld probe on the skin over the thinned-skull area of the temporal bone. The sound waves reflect back the velocity of the blood flow and allow a graphic and audio recording of the flow. This test is noninvasive, does not require radiation or radioactive isotopes, and allows for serial studies to be conducted monitoring for changes over time. Moreover, no special preprocedure or postprocedure management is required for the patient.

TCD is utilized for the following purposes:

- Detection and monitoring of vasospasm with cerebral aneurysms
- Detection of intracranial stenosis and occlusion
- Evaluation of intracranial blood flow and collateral blood flow with extracranial stenosis
- Evaluation of vasomotor tone
- Monitoring the effect of thrombolytic agents on blood vessel in acute stoke
- Evaluation and monitoring of intracranial blood flow during surgery

Magnetic resonance angiography. Magnetic resonance angiogram (MRA) is a type of MRI scan that uses a magnetic field and pulses of radio wave energy to provide pictures of blood vessels inside the body. In many cases, this technology can provide information that cannot be obtained from other types of imaging studies.

MRA can find problems with the blood vessels that may be causing reduced blood flow, such as aneurysms, arteriovenous malformations (AVM), and occlusions. With MRA, both the blood flow and the condition of the blood vessel walls can be seen. This type of test is often used to look at the blood vessels that go to the brain, kidneys, and legs. The preparation and postprocedure care are similar to those with MRI (Hickey, 2003).

Cerebral blood flow studies. Xenon-133 is a radioactive tracer that is often used to assess cerebral perfusion and CBF. Its cerebral washout is proportional to CBF, which makes regional determination of CBF possible. Xenon-enhanced CT may be used with rapid sequential CT to quantify CBF. These studies of CBF are used to determine viability of cerebral tissue both globally and regionally. This technique may be used as a part of the criteria for determination of brain death.

Invasive cerebrovascular studies: cerebral angiography

Cerebral angiography is the diagnostic procedure of choice for aneurysms, AVMs, and other cerebrovascular abnormalities. This invasive imaging technique allows for the visualization of the lumen of blood vessels to determine their patency and identify narrowing (stenosis), vasospasm, thrombosis, or abnormalities such as aneurysm and displacement of vessels. Blood vessel displacement may be caused by space-occupying lesions such as hematomas, cysts, tumors, and abscesses.

With this technique, the patient receives a contrast medium, typically injected by the indirect route via catheterization of the carotid or vertebral arteries, using (most commonly) the femoral route or the brachial, subclavian, or axillary artery as a point of entry. Radiographic images are then taken at timed intervals, thereby providing for visualization of the intracranial and extracranial blood vessels.

Possible complications of cerebral angiography include the following issues:

- Allergic reaction to the contrast medium
- Seizures
- Stroke
- Pulmonary emboli
- Thrombosis
- Aphasia
- Visual deficits
- Carotid sinus sensitivity symptoms (hypotension, syncope, bradycardia)

Preparation for this procedure includes obtaining informed consent (parental permission) from the caregiver, with a full explanation of possible complications being given to the family. Most patients will require sedation because it is necessary to lie still during the procedure (Hickey, 2003). The age of the patient and his or her ability to cooperate will dictate the level of sedation required to complete the procedure. In anticipation of sedation, the patient should not have any liquids or solids for 4 to 8 hours prior to the procedure.

Postprocedure care includes the following measures:

- Bed rest for 8 hours
- Immobilization of the puncture site for 4 to 8 hours to prevent bleeding
- Frequent observation of the puncture site
- Monitoring of vital and neurological signs for a 24-hour period
- Serial assessment of pedal pulses in the affected leg if femoral puncture was performed
- Serial assessment of the color and temperature of the extremity containing the puncture site
- Forced fluids after contrast material is administered

Electroencephalography

An electroencephalograph (EEG) is a noninvasive diagnostic procedure that provides a continuous recording of spontaneous electrical activity of the brain waves using multiple reference electrodes placed on the scalp. The neuronal electrical signals from the cerebral cortex are recorded as a tracing on a graphic grid, which can then be interpreted by the HCP. The EEG provides complementary data to imaging studies such as MRI and CT scan. Its tracing documents the frequency, amplitude, and characteristics of the brain waves captured.

A variety of conditions may produce similar EEG changes, so the EEG is rarely specific to an individual cause. Even though pattern changes are nonspecific, some types are highly suggestive of specific conditions such as certain forms of epilepsy, herpes simplex encephalitis, and memory disorders. The EEG is also useful in follow-up observation of patients with altered levels of consciousness, in evaluation of subclinical seizure activity and control, and as an adjunct in the determination of brain death. For certain clinical conditions such as intractable seizures, continuous EEG monitoring with videotaping may be used to obtain continuous data about cerebral electrical activity and clinical activity, which can be correlated to determine whether the seizure or movement has an epileptogenic nature. Thus this technique is often helpful in determining specific areas of the brain that have an epileptogenic focus. Additionally, continuous EEG monitoring may be used for detection of seizure activity in patients with subclinical seizures.

Classification of brain waves. On the EEG, brain waves are classified according to the number of cycles per second or frequency and are recorded in hertz (Hz) units. The EEG has four frequency bands that are used in the interpretation of brain waves: delta (1–3 Hz), theta (4–7 Hz), alpha (8–12 Hz), and beta (13–20 Hz) (Haslam, 2008).

Delta rhythms are not normally present in an awake individual but are seen in slow-wave sleep states (stages 3 and 4 of sleep). Theta rhythms originate from the temporal lobes, although delta waves may also be seen in small amounts over the temporal region in normal adults.

Alpha rhythms are most prominent in the occipital leads. These waves can be blocked by opening of the eyes, mental effort, anxiety, apprehension, and sudden noise or touch.

Beta rhythms are most prominent in the frontal and central areas. Beta waves are triggered by opening of the eyes, mental activity, anxiety, or apprehension. These waves are prominent in patients who have received benzodiazepine and barbiturate medications. They may be altered by many factors, including age, state of alertness, eye closure or opening, drugs, and disease states. High-voltage slow and sharp waves are confined to the central regions during sleep in a normal EEG (Goldstein et al., 2007; Haslam, 2008).

Common EEG abnormalities. When an EEG contains epileptiform activities, abnormalities of amplitude, slowing of normal rhythms, or variations from age-specific patterns, it is considered to be abnormal. Abnormalities of waveforms include spikes and slow waves. *Spikes* are characteristically paroxysmal, sharp, and of high voltage; they are typically followed by a slow wave. Spikes and slow waves are associated with epilepsy but some normal patients may have this EEG finding (Haslam, 2008).

When physiologic activities that are not caused by cerebral activity but rather by motions such as eye movement or muscle contraction occur, the abnormal deflections captured on the graphic recording are considered to be *artifacts*.

Epileptiform activity appears as single or repetitive focal spikes on the graphic recording. These spikes can be divided into focal, multifocal, and generalized events. The EEG must be examined to differentiate the range of variations from a true form of epilepsy and abnormal activity related to cerebral lesions. Focal spikes are often associated with irritative lesions, including cysts, slow-growing tumors, and glial scar tissue (Haslam, 2008). Epileptiform activity may be exacerbated by activation procedures such as hyperventilation, photic stimulation, and sleep deprivation.

Slow waves are defined as waves in the 1 to 7 Hz range, and are further classified as either focal or diffuse abnormalities. *Focal* slow waves may be caused by a gray or white matter dysfunction that occurs in a circumscribed lesion such as a hematoma, tumor, infarction, or localized infectious process. The findings of a focal abnormality indicate a need for further diagnostic testing, such as MRI or CT scan. Generalized *diffuse* slow waves are usually seen with a metabolic, toxic, degenerative, inflammatory, widespread infectious etiology or a postictal condition. A pattern of diffuse slowing generally does not indicate a specific diagnosis but rather provides supportive diagnostic data (Hickey, 2003).

Electrocerebral silence or flat electroencephalography. When the graphic tracing has an absence of electrical activity, it is described as "flat." This state is indicative of absence of brain waves and is one finding associated with brain death.

Electromyography and nerve conduction velocity studies

Electromyography (EMG) and nerve conduction velocity studies (NCVS) are both types of electrophysiological studies. The EMG allows assessment of abnormalities in the neuromuscular system and is used in an attempt to differentiate between peripheral nerve injury or neuropathy or when it is unclear whether the primary problem is a myopathy or a neuropathy. This technology may also be used to differentiate among lesions of the anterior horn cell, root, plexus, and specific nerves and muscles. NCVS are conducted when nerve damage is suspected because of clinical symptoms of motor weakness or atrophy. Such studies are used in the diagnostic process for neuropathies. Both EMG and NCVS can be used to follow the progression of peripheral nerve disorders and their response to treatment (Hickey, 2003).

Evoked potentials. An evoked potential (EP) is a noninvasive technique in which a specific sensory stimulus is applied to the visual, auditory, or sensory system and the electrical response that follows from the central nervous system is recorded. The stimulus is repeated several times, with the patient's CNS being allowed to return to a resting state between stimuli. Each evoked response is measured. After a number of potentials have been recorded, a computer-generated average curve is calculated (Haslam, 2008; Hickey, 2003).

EPs are used for the following clinical applications:

- Diagnosis of lesions of the cerebral cortex, ascending pathways of the spinal cord, or thalamus
- Evaluation of the extent of CNS injury
- Diagnosis of neuromuscular disease
- Evaluation of comatose patients

EPs are separated into three categories based on the type of stimulus provided and the sensory system stimulated. The three afferent central pathways used in EPs are the visual, auditory, and somatosensory pathways.

Visual evoked potentials. In visual evoked potentials (VEPs), the retina is stimulated by checkerboard patterns and flashing lights, allowing the pathways to the occipital cortex to be evaluated. Each eye is tested separately, and its response is recorded with electrodes over the occipital region. If the patient wears eyeglasses, they should be worn during the procedure. The VEP test requires the cooperation of the patient during testing. VEPs are used in the diagnosis of optic neuropathies such as optic neuritis (often related to multiple sclerosis) and optic nerve lesions such as tumors.

Brain stem auditory evoked responses. Brain stem auditory evoked responses (BAERs) are used primarily to evaluate brain stem function. The stimuli provided (via headphones) include a series of clicks that vary in rate, intensity, and duration. Based on the site of origin, five wave formations are recorded: wave I from the acoustic nerve, wave II from the cochlear nucleus, wave III from the superior olivary complex, wave IV from the lateral lemniscus, and wave V from the inferior colliculus (Goldstein et al., 2007; Hickey, 2003).

Evoked potentials will be abnormal in patients with demyelinating diseases and brain stem abnormalities. BAERs are useful in diagnosing lesions in multiple sclerosis, acoustic neuroma, and lesions related to coma, as well as in evaluating hearing in infants and young children. BAER testing can be conducted on either alert or comatose patients.

Somatosensory evoked responses.   Somatosensory evoked responses (SSERs) measure peripheral nerve responses in the upper (median nerve) or lower (posterior tibial nerve) extremities. These responses are abnormal in many neurodegenerative disorders. SSERs are helpful in evaluating spinal cord function, sensory dysfunction associated with multiple sclerosis, and nerve root compression. This technique may also be used to monitor spinal cord function during operative procedures for conditions such as scoliosis, coarctation of the aorta repair, and myelomeningocele. SSER is the most accurate evoked potential utilized in the assessment of neurologic outcome in the patient who has suffered a neurologic insult (Hickey, 2003).

Intracranial pressure monitoring

A growing body of evidence-based data supports the theory that intracranial pressure monitoring in patients with severe traumatic brain injury (TBI) can positively affect their outcome. Therapeutic interventions directed at controlling abnormally elevated ICP have resulted in improved survival and neurologic outcomes. The major aim of monitoring and managing elevated ICP is to prevent cerebral ischemia.

Intracranial pressure can be monitored in a number of locations (intraventricular, intraparenchymal, subarachnoid/subdural, and epidural) and by different techniques. The most common methods of ICP monitoring use either an intraventricular catheter or an intraparenchymal catheter. The often preferred placement is an intraventricular catheter, because this system allows drainage of CSF; thus this setup provides a therapeutic option for increased ICP. The main disadvantages of ICP monitoring are the difficulty of placing the catheter, especially in patients with compressed ventricles; the increased risk of infection; and the possibility of malfunction of the catheter the smaller the ventricles become and/or the longer the catheter is in place.

The ultimate goal is to recognize elevated ICP and promptly treat it. Although an ICP greater than 20 mmHg often is the threshold for interventions, an increased cerebral perfusion pressure is also an indicator for therapeutic intervention (Goldstein et al., 2007).

ALTERED MENTAL STATUS

Jennifer J. Schoonover

PATHOPHYSIOLOGY

Mental status is the intellectual, emotional, psychological, and personality degree of competence shown by a person. It is a complex mix of level of consciousness, attention, memory, orientation, perception, thought process and content, insight, judgment, affect, mood, language, and higher cognitive function. An alteration in mental status occurs when dysfunction arises in any of these areas; it is symptom rather than a disorder.

Assessment of the content of the behavior directly measures the function of the cerebral hemispheres. Assessment of the level of consciousness, effects of stimuli, and the ability to move through the different phases of the sleep cycle measures the effectiveness of the ascending reticular activating system (ARAS). The relationship between these two functions has been described using the "light bulb switch" analogy: ARAS is the switch that stimulates function and cerebral hemispheres, and the bulb is the behavior. For example, to have a normal level of consciousness, the light bulb (cerebral hemisphere where content of behavior is displayed) must be functional and the switch (ARAS) must be turned on. If the light bulb is out, then there is a dysfunction with the bulb (cerebral hemisphere), the switch (ARAS), or both (Avner, 2006).

Brain stem reflexes—such as pupillary light reflexes (dilated pupils) or eye muscle movement reflexes (doll's eye test)—are lacking, the ARAS is not functioning properly and the cause is usually structural. When both the cerebral hemispheres are dysfunctional and the brain stem reflexes are intact, the cause is usually functional (infectious, metabolic, or toxic). The dysfunction or alteration at various levels may be evidenced by confusion, disorientation, delirium, lethargy, stupor, or coma. Patients may vacillate between these different levels.

ETIOLOGY

The incidence of altered mental status is unclear due to the nature of the illness and the underlying cause. The conditions that cause alterations in mental status may occur at any age, but may be more prevalent at certain times of life. For instance, the young infant may experience alterations in mental status due to infections of the brain or spinal cord, inborn errors of metabolism, congenital defect, or abusive head trauma. In childhood and adolescence, the incidence of toxic ingestions and accidental head trauma predominates as the etiology of altered mental status.

Structural causes include congenital or acquired defects such as hydrocephalus, brain or spinal cord tumors, cerebrovascular accidents (CVA), intracranial hemorrhage, and trauma to the brain or spinal cord. Functional causes include metabolic disorders, toxic ingestions, infections, seizures, electrolyte imbalances, prolonged hypoxemia, sleep deprivation, and psychiatric or behavioral illnesses.

PRESENTATION

Alterations in mental status may cause the individual to vacillate between three levels of alertness representing a spectrum of dysfunction: reduced, mixed, and hyper-alert. Reduced alertness may be associated with confusion, lethargy, stupor, or coma caused by either structural or functional disorders. The hyper-alert state is most often caused by functional disorders such as psychiatric or behavioral illnesses, hypoxemia, or toxic ingestions. In this state, the patient demonstrates signs of confusion with unclear thinking, restlessness, agitation, and delirium.

Historical inquiry can help to determine if the mental status changes are functional or structural in nature. Was the change sudden or gradual? Has it ever happened before? Was there a witnessed trauma? Does the patient have any associated symptoms such as seizures, fever, headache, weakness, numbness, dizziness, vomiting, diarrhea, or blurred or double vision? Does the patient admit to ingesting or inhaling any substances? Was the patient in a location where a substance could have been administered to him or her without that person's knowledge? What is the patient's access to prescription or other medications? What is the patient's proximity to radon, carbon monoxide, or lead? Is the patient taking any medication for any reason? Are there any underlying chronic illnesses? Past medical history such as brain or spinal tumor, seizure disorder, hypoglycemia or other metabolic disorder, hypertension, and liver or kidney disease may be related to the patient's present state. These are just some of the many questions that may narrow the differential diagnosis.

The results of the physical examination may be equally telling. Initial care seeks to ensure that the patient's airway, breathing, and circulation are stable. Respiratory failure, shock, and increased intracranial pressure may all cause mental status changes. With reduced alertness, maintenance of a patent airway may be difficult due to low muscle tone. An irregular respiratory rate or pattern may indicate increased intracranial pressure. Bruising, hematomas, hemotympanum, and retinal hemorrhages may indicate trauma. A fruity breath may be related to diabetic ketoacidosis or liver disease. A hypotonic patient with purpura may have overwhelming sepsis.

A thorough neurological assessment includes not only mental status, but pupillary size and reflex, deep tendon reflexes, muscle strength, cerebellar function, and if there is asymmetry of findings. Asymmetrical aspects of the examination and focal neurologic signs may indicate a structural cause, but the lack of focality does exclude it.

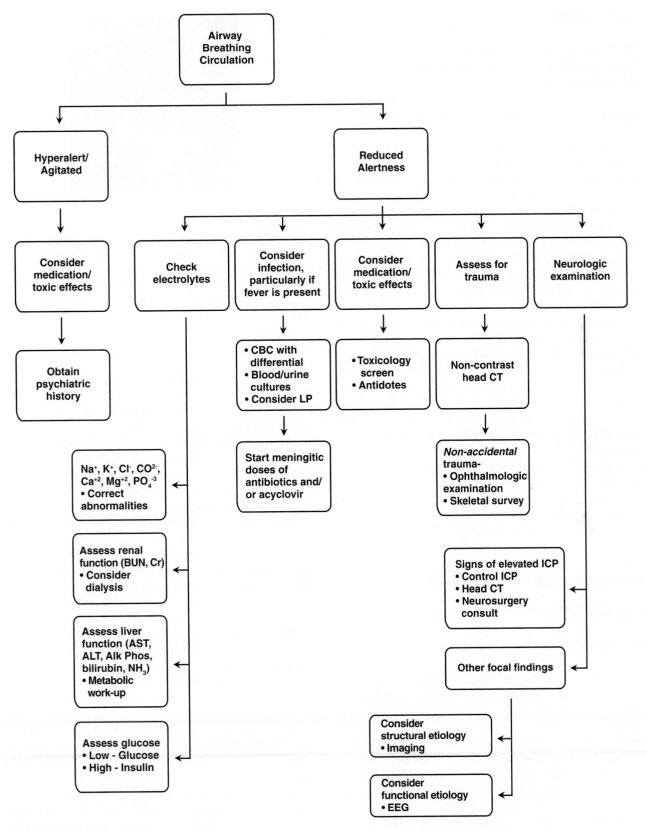

FIGURE 33-9

Algorithm for the Evaluation of Altered Mental Status.

Note: Complete blood count (CBC), blood urea nitrogen (BUN), aspartate aminotransferase (AST), alanine aminotransferase (ALT), alkaline phosphatate (Alk phos), electroencephalograph (EEG), intracranial pressure (ICP), computed tomography (CT), lumbar puncture (LP).

Source: Lehman R., & Mink, J. (2008). Altered Mental Status. *Clinical Pediatric Emergency Medicine, 9*(2), 68–75. Reprinted with permission from © Elsevier.

PLAN OF CARE

Evaluation for the underlying cause of the mental status change must be performed quickly, as many of the potential pathologies are life-threatening. Figure 33-9 provides an algorithm for initial evaluation. Management is then directed toward treating the underlying etiology. The evaluation of functional causes of reduced alertness starts with an evaluation of electrolytes, glucose, liver and kidney function, thyroid levels, and metabolic studies. If infection is suspected, then a CBC and differential, plus blood and urine cultures, are obtained. Cerebrospinal fluid analysis should be considered. The decision to perform a lumbar puncture should be based on the severity of illness and the presence of meningitic signs or symptoms.

If ingestion of a toxin is suspected as the etiology, a comprehensive toxicology screen is sent for analysis. For patients on medications for underlying chronic illnesses (e.g., seizures), testing for medication levels is warranted. If seizures are present, neuromonitoring via EEG may be beneficial. Psychological disorders may present similarly and are not easily differentiated without further study.

Diagnostic evaluation may also include radiological imaging. Most commonly, a non-contrast head CT scan is performed when evaluation is urgent. This imaging modality is valuable for identifying structural lesions, hematomas, and cerebral edema. The stable patient may be better imaged with MRI of the brain and/or spine.

Consultations with specialists are based on the known or suspected etiology, the need for assistance in diagnostic interpretation, or management expertise. The critical care service is consulted any time an altered level of consciousness threatens the patient's cardiovascular stability.

ARTERIOVENOUS MALFORMATION

Kelly Keefe Marcoux

PATHOPHYSIOLOGY

An intracranial arterious malformation (AVM) is a congenital malformation characterized by an abnormal persistent connection between arteries and veins in the brain without an interposed capillary bed. The capillaries fail to develop between arteries and veins during embryogenesis, usually around the third week of gestation. This defect results in abnormal shunting of blood, producing an enlargement of blood vessels that resemble a "bag of worms" (Figure 33-10). Gross visualization reveals dilated feeding arteries and a cluster of entangled vascular loops (referred to as the "core" or the "nidus") connected to vascular channels where the arterial blood is shunted and drains into large draining veins. AVMs may continue to change and grow postnatally, albeit only in relation to the prenatal

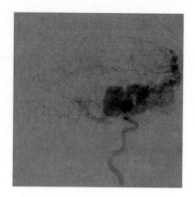

FIGURE 33-10

Angiogram of an Arteriovenous Malformation. The cerebral cartotid angiogram demonstrates a large right frontal AVM supplied by hypertrophied branches of the right anterior cerebral artery. There is venous drainage into the right superficial middle cerebral vein and the superior sagittal sinus.

Source: Courtesy of Kelly Keefe Marcoux.

malformation. Certain molecular biologic factors may also play an important role in development of an AVM, including basic fibroblast growth factor (bFGF) and vascular endothelial growth factor (VEGF).

AVMs are high-flow lesions that steal blood from healthy brain parenchyma adjacent to the AVM. The surrounding parenchyma may become persistently, slightly hypoxic, which leads to further angiogenesis—an effect referred to as the "steal phenomenon."

AVMs may be located in the cortex or deep within the brain parenchyma. They may range in size from 1 mm to greater than 10 cm, and can extend from the meninges through the parenchyma into the ventricles. There is often calcification within the AVM. These lesions are most commonly located supratentorially, and less commonly in the cerebellum, brain stem, thalamus, and basal ganglia. Smaller lesions (less than 2 cm) are more likely to bleed than larger ones, as are those located in the basal ganglia or thalamus (DiRocco et al., 2000).

A unique type of AVM, called the vein of Galen malformation (VOGM), accounts for approximately 30% of vascular malformations in children. This lesion is characterized by the persistence of the embryonic precursor to the vein of Galen and an abnormal shunt that is fed by extremely dilated arteries. VOGM are classified as either choroidal or mural based on their angioarchitecture.

AVMs are categorized via the Spetzler-Martin grading system, which is useful in predicting surgical morbidity, particularly for adults (Table 33-7). Under this system, the lesion is graded based on size, location relative to eloquent brain tissue, and pattern of venous drainage. Areas of the brain that are considered to be eloquent include language, visual, and sensorimotor areas, as well as the thalamus, hypothalamus, internal capsule, brain stem, cerebellar peduncles, and deep cerebellar nuclei. The size of a lesion is measured via angiography using the widest diameter of the nidus. The AVM is considered to have superficial drainage only if all drainage is from the cortical drainage system. The Spetzler-Martin grade is obtained by adding the three individual scores from each category. High-grade (grade 5) lesions are large, are located in eloquent areas of the brain, and have deep venous drainage; thus they are more difficult to resect. Low-grade (grade 1) lesions are small, are found in noneloquent brain areas, and have superficial venous drainage.

EPIDEMIOLOGY AND ETIOLOGY

Cerebral AVMs are uncommon lesions, occurring in only 0.5% to 1% of the pediatric population (DiRocco et al., 2000). Their etiology is unknown. These defects are present at birth, having been formed during the third week of gestation when capillaries fail to develop between certain cerebral arteries and veins. The majority of this malformations are located supratentorially and within the brain parenchyma. They are rarely familial, although some cerebral AVMs are associated with inherited disorders, such as von Hippel-Lindau syndrome, Osler-Weber-Rendu syndrome, Sturge-Weber disease, and neurofibromatosis.

Approximately 1 in 100,000 children has a cerebral AVM, but most remain asymptomatic during childhood. AVMs are the most common cause of nontraumatic intracranial hemorrhage in childhood and the most common cause of hemorrhagic stroke in infants.

TABLE 33-7

Spetzler-Martin Grading Scale for Arteriovenous Malformations	
Characteristics of AVM	**Points**
AVM Size	
Small (< 3cm)	1
Medium (3–6 cm)	2
Large (> 6 cm)	3
Location of AVM	
Noneloquent	0
Eloquent	1
Pattern of Venous Drainage	
Superficial only	0
Deep	1

Points are added together to determine the arteriovenous malformation (AVM) grade.

Source: Adapted from Spetzler & Martin, 1986.

PRESENTATION

AVMs usually become symptomatic between the second and fourth decades of life. The most common presentation in childhood is intraparenchymal hemorrhage, which occurs in 75% to 80% of children with this type of lesion (DiRocco et al., 2000). This presentation is associated with a high rate of morbidity and mortality. Alternatively, pediatric patients may present with focal neurological deficits related to the location of the AVM or due to the steal phenomenon in the adjacent brain tissue. Children may have complaints of periodic headaches. The most common and concerning presentation, however, is that of the child with an intracerebral hemorrhage. Although this is most often an intraparenchymal hemorrhage, it can also track into the subarachnoid space and intraventricular system. In this scenario, the pediatric patient is often otherwise healthy, may or may not have had periodic headaches, and presents acutely with severe headache, emesis, nuchal rigidity, and seizure activity (Table 33-8). A medical emergency, this condition and may rapidly progress to increased intracranial pressure and cerebral herniation if not managed aggressively.

An AVM may also present less dramatically, with focal neurological deficits or focal motor or complex partial seizure activity as well as generalized tonic–clonic seizures. Seizures may occur from an acute cerebral hemorrhage or an epileptogenic focus from a previous hemorrhage. Progressive neurologic deficits will vary depending on the intracerebral location of the AVM. Changes in behavior, headaches, nausea and vomiting, and hemiparesis may also be presenting symptoms.

Occasionally, an AVM may be discovered incidentally while assessing the patient for unrelated symptoms. When completing the physical examination, in addition to performing cranial nerve assessment, sensory and motor evaluation, mental status examination, cerebellar function, and reflexes, it is helpful to perform auscultation of the globes, temporal fossae, and the retroauricular or mastoid areas to assess for an intracranial bruit. The presence of a bruit may also be found in children with thyrotoxicosis, anemia, meningitis, and hydrocephalus. The bruit of an AVM is loud and harsh and accompanied by a thrill.

A choroidal VOGM has multiple arteriovenous fistulae and typically presents in the neonatal period, whereas

TABLE 33-8

Signs and Symptoms of Intracerebral Hemorrhage

- Severe headache
- Nausea and vomiting
- Altered level of consciousness
- Nuchal rigidity
- Focal neurological deficits
- Seizures—focal or generalized

a mural VOGM is characterized by a single arteriovenous fistula over the wall of the venous sac and commonly presents in infancy. VOGM usually presents differently than other AVMs in pediatric patients. Most commonly, this type of malformation presents in the neonatal period with an infant who has otherwise unexplained high-output cardiac failure, hydrocephalus, macrocephaly, and an audible intracranial bruit. If it presents in infancy, the infant may have hydrocephalus, macrocephaly, and cardiomegaly with or without cardiac failure. If it presents in older childhood or adolescence, the symptoms may include headaches and macrocephaly. Like other AVMs, the VOGM may present with intracerebral hemorrhage or subarachnoid bleeding.

Spinal AVMs are rare in childhood. These lesions are often associated with cutaneous angiomas such as Cobb's syndrome (port-wine–stained angiomas) and Osler-Weber-Rendu syndrome (hereditary hemorrhagic telangiectasia). Intracranial AVMs should be suspected in any child whose port-wine stain involves the cutaneous distribution of the trigeminal nerve.

DIFFERENTIAL DIAGNOSIS

The initial differential diagnosis in a pediatric patient presenting with an acute change in mental status includes any entity that may cause increased ICP, such as traumatic brain injury; brain tumor or neoplastic CNS metastasis; vascular etiologies; CNS infections (meningitis, encephalitis, abscess); hydrocephalus; metabolic disorders (diabetic ketoacidosis, hypoxic ischemic encephalopathy, sodium abnormalities, kidney failure); and status epilepticus. After CT scan reveals an intraparenchymal hemorrhage, the differential diagnosis becomes more focused, to include cerebral vascular etiologies such as arterial or venous infarctions, intracerebral hemorrhage, ruptured aneurysm, dural sinus thrombosis, subarachnoid hemorrhage, and VOGM or AVM.

PLAN OF CARE

CT scan of the brain without contrast is the initial diagnostic evaluation of the pediatric patient presenting with an acute change in neurologic status and possible intracranial hemorrhage. This imaging should be emergently performed and reviewed. If the child has an AVM, the CT scan will reveal hyperdense tubular structures with calcification around the AVM. If the AVM has bled, the primary lesion may be obscured by a hematoma (Figure 33-11). A CT scan is also invaluable to assess for hydrocephalus, cerebral edema with or without mass effect, and signs of cerebral herniation. In addition, CT angiography may be performed, if available, to provide better vascular detail (Figure 33-12).

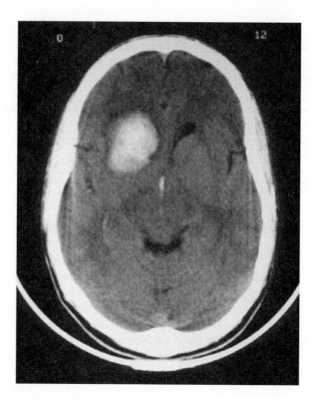

FIGURE 33-11

Computed Tomography (CT) of an Arteriovenous Malformation (AVM). Without contrast, the image reveals right frontal hemorrhage; the AVM is obscured by blood.

Source: Courtesy of Kelly Keefe Marcoux.

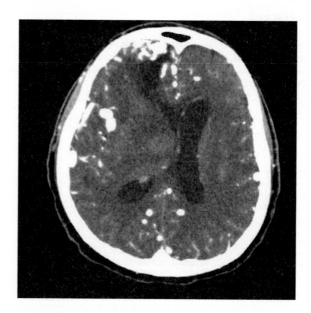

FIGURE 33-12

Computed Tomography Angiography (CTA) of Arteriovenous Malformation (AVM). The CTA reveals a large telangiectatic right frontal AVM with large draining veins. Note the hydrocephalus.

Source: Courtesy of Kelly Keefe Marcoux.

Once the patient is clinically stable or in a nonemergent setting, MRI and/or MRA should be performed to provide a more thorough evaluation of the AVM. An MRI with MRA will identify the architecture of the feeding vessels, nidus, and early draining veins; hemorrhage; presence and extent of associated hematomas; and vasospasm. However, it is important that the patient is stabilized before undergoing MRI due to the frequent need for sedation as well as the time required for an MRI.

The study of choice for diagnosis and evaluation of an AVM remains cerebral angiography. The angiogram of an AVM will reveal the dilated feeding arteries, the nidus, and the large draining veins (Figure 33-10). It delineates the morphology of the AVM, thereby allowing for grading based on the Spetzler-Martin criteria. Considerations with an angiogram include the need for general anesthesia, cannulization of the femoral artery (which may be challenging in infants and children due to their small vasculature), risk of significant blood loss due to low circulating blood volume, preexisting cardiac failure due to VOGM, and the cumulative amount of dye being given to small infants and children.

Laboratory evaluations that may be useful in the work-up of the child with an AVM include a CBC with differential, prothrombin time (PT) and activated partial thromboplastin time (aPTT), and blood type and cross-match. CSF analysis is not indicated in the diagnosis of an AVM. Furthermore, a lumbar puncture may be contraindicated if signs and symptoms of increased ICP are present due to expanding hematoma or cerebral herniation.

The goal of therapeutic management for an AVM is complete obliteration of the malformation. Infrequently, the lesion may be observed for changes over time. In the patient presenting with increased ICP, emergent management is indicated.

A ruptured AVM is a medical emergency due to the potential for increased ICP. The initial management is the same for any patient presenting with increased ICP—assessment and management of the airway, breathing, and circulation (ABCs); Glasgow Coma Scale score; cranial nerve function; and signs and symptoms of increased ICP. Once the patient's airway is secured and circulation is restored, methods to prevent or control increased ICP should be implemented. Initial methods to control increased ICP include maintaining the head in a midline position and the head of bed mildly elevated and in a midline position, maintaining normothermia and normocarbia, euvolemic osmolar therapy, CSF diversion, seizure prophylaxis, optimal cardiorespiratory support, adequate sedation and analgesia, and evacuation of hematoma as indicated. If the initial therapies fail to relieve the excess pressure, mild hyperventilation (PCO_2 in the range of 30–35 mmHg), moderate hypothermia, and barbiturate therapy should be considered.

In the critically ill child, emergent evacuation of the hemorrhage may be indicated. Otherwise, a multimodal treatment approach (surgery, endovascular embolization, steriotactic radiosurgery) is instituted to provide the best cure opportunity with minimal long-term complications (Dorfer et al., 2009). Most patients with AVMs (even those who are asymptomatic) should be treated due to the risk of future hemorrhage with potential catastrophic consequences. Children are at greater risk of initial hemorrhage compared to adults (Klimo et al., 2007).

For an AVM that is surgically accessible, microsurgery resection is the treatment of choice because it allows for complete obliteration of low-grade AVMs (grades I–III). Nevertheless, the significant morbidity and mortality risks of such surgery must be weighed against the current status of the AVM. Surgical resection and evacuation of a hematoma may be indicated in the immediate management of patient who has experienced intracerebral hemorrhage with associated progressive neurologic deficits. An angiogram may be done in the immediate postoperative phase to confirm complete obliteration of the AVM. A ventriculoperitoneal shunt (VPS) or an externalized ventricular drain (EVD) may be inserted if the child has hydrocephalus that is not relieved after the evacuation of the hemorrhage.

Endovascular embolization is often used as an adjunct to surgical resection. This technique may be indicated to decrease the size of the AVM nidus, which is helpful for radiosurgery, or to decrease the blood flow and occlude deep feeding arteries that control bleeding, which assists in the neurosurgical approach. The intra-arterial system is most commonly approached via the transfemoral route in pediatric patients. This allows access to the arterial system to embolize the AVM using *N*-butylcyanoacylate or other glue or coils. Embolization is beneficial in reducing the size of complex lesions and is sometimes performed in stages to decrease morbidity associated with the AVM and the procedures themselves.

Stereotactic radiosurgery is indicated for AVMs located deep within the parenchyma or in critical brain locations (e.g., basal ganglia, thalamus, brainstem). Radiosurgery delivers a relatively high dose of focused radiation precisely to the AVM. The irradiated vessels gradually occlude over time; on average, achievement of this effect may take two to four years. The annual risk of hemorrhage after radiosurgery is similar to risk of bleeding in an untreated AVM (Cohen-Gadol & Pollack, 2006). Patients who have undergone radiosurgery have also demonstrated decreased seizure activity. The disadvantage of radiosurgery includes the "time-to-obliteration interval," during which time AVM is still at risk of hemorrhage.

The following specialists are integral in the management of the child with an AVM: pediatric neurosurgeon, pediatric vascular neurosurgeon, pediatric neurologist, interventional neuroradiologist, neuroradiologist, and radiation oncologists. In addition, other members of the interprofessional team include pediatric intensivists, advanced practice nurses, nurses, neurodevelopmental specialists, neuropsychologists, physical and occupational therapists, speech therapists, and social workers.

The family of the child with an AVM should be informed of the possible prognosis of a cerebral AVM, particularly related to the location of the AVM, including, but not limited to, seizure activity, headaches, sensory and motor deficits, decline in school performance, and need for multiple hospitalizations and procedures. Information on available support groups should be provided for the patient and family.

DISPOSITION AND DISCHARGE PLANNING

There is a high risk of hemorrhage or rehemorrhage in a patient with a cerebral AVM, estimated to be approximately 2% to 4% annually (Hoh et al., 2000). Those patients at highest risk of hemorrhage are those who are young, have small AVMs, have had prior hemorrhage, have deep venous drainage, and have high-flow lesions (International RadioSurgery Association, 2009). In recent years, the accepted notion that children are at greater risk for subsequent hemorrhage than adults has been disputed (Fullerton et al., 2005). The greatest risk of rebleeding occurs in the first year after the initial hemorrhage, but decreases thereafter (DiRocco et al., 2000). Unique to pediatric patients is the recurrence of AVMs after total surgical resection, confirmed by postoperative angiogram (Ogilvy et al., 2001). It has been hypothesized that certain pathophysiological differences between pediatric and adult AVMs lead to recurrent AVMs in children, perhaps due to the relatively immature cerebral vasculature in children.

Outcomes are focused on prevention of further hemorrhage, prevention of seizures, and prevention of neurological deficits. Children who undergo complete surgical resection of an AVM reportedly have good outcomes with minimal morbidity (Kondziolka et al., 1992). If the pediatric patient has suffered an intracranial hemorrhage as a result of the AVM, neurological deficits may be present that require short- or long-term neurorehabilitative therapies. The GCS score may be used as an objective measure to determine the child's overall recovery of neurological function.

It is recommended that pediatric patients with cerebral AVMs undergo follow-up angiograms as they enter adulthood, if not before, to assess for recurrent AVM nidus or AVM growth, which may predispose them to ongoing risk of intracranial hemorrhage and potential catastrophic consequences. An AVM is considered to be recurrent if it is evident via angiogram in a patient whose previous posttreatment angiogram documented complete obliteration of the malformation. For patients with cerebral AVMs, there is a low threshold to perform a diagnostic studies (CT scan of brain, MRI/MRA) if they exhibit any change in neurological status, even a subtle one. Neuropsychological testing is particularly necessary for children who have received ionizing radiation.

Prognosis of an AVM greatly depends on the severity and location of the malformation. Children are more likely to have deep-seated lesions, located in the thalamus or basal ganglia, which make surgical resection more difficult. An AVM that hemorrhages is associated with increased morbidity and mortality. Ideally, a multimodality approach to obliteration of the malformation will help eliminate the risk of future intracranial bleeding and maintain or restore neurological function. Intensive neurorehabilitation is essential and geared toward restoring neurological function.

There is no prevention for development of a cerebral AVM; however, measures may be instituted to decrease the likelihood of hemorrhage or subsequent hemorrhage. It is vital that pediatric patients with cerebral AVMs undergo treatment to obliterate the lesion, or are very closely monitored, as they have a high risk of hemorrhage during their lifetime. Monitoring for seizure activity, headaches, or subtle changes in mental status may assist in detecting changes in the size of the AVM or possible hemorrhage. Follow-up MRI/MRA and angiograms should be performed as indicated by the vascular neurosurgery team.

BRAIN DEATH AND ORGAN DONATION

Christine A. Zawistowski

BRAIN DEATH

Pathophysiology

Brain death has the potential to occur from any injury that interrupts blood flow to the brain. In this situation, cell death occurs within a matter of minutes. The cell death leads to tissue edema, which increases the mass of brain tissue in the intracranial vault; this phenomenon is referred to as the "mass effect." The Monro-Kellie hypothesis describes the intracranial vault as a noncompliant fixed space with a fixed volume, in which any increase requires a compensatory decrease in volume or else an increase in pressure will result. Once an increase in intracranial pressure occurs, arterial inflow is impaired; if left untreated, this condition results in cerebral circulatory arrest with ensuing cell damage and death. A compensatory response to the rising pressure in the intracranial vault is for the brain to herniate through the path of least resistance—a downward descent of the brain stem and cerebellum through the foramen magnum, with resulting ischemia and neuronal death. This process depends on the rate of edema and the increase in ICP, which may occur either immediately (e.g., after trauma or a sudden intracranial hemorrhage) or over a period of several days (e.g., after a hypoxic-ischemic insult).

Epidemiology and etiology

Brain death, also known as death by neurologic criteria, is a clinical diagnosis. It is recognized nationally and internationally as a way to declare an individual legally dead.

The United States has adopted the whole-brain formulation of brain death, which is characterized by irreversible loss of function of both cerebral hemispheres and the brain stem. Brain death may occur with any of the following disorders:

- Submersion injuries
- Traumatic brain injury—the most common preceding event
- Smoke inhalation
- Intracranial hemorrhage
- Hypoxic-ischemic insult
- Profound hypotension

The true incidence of brain death in pediatric patients is unknown due to the lack of mandatory reporting. It is believed to account for 1% to 2% of admissions to pediatric intensive care units (PICU) and 11% to 33% of patient deaths in the PICU (Todres, 2006).

Presentation

Brain death may not be immediately apparent upon patient presentation due to the timing of cerebral edema and increased ICP. The patient history should assess for causes of disruption to blood flow and cerebral perfusion. The initial physical examination of brain death will demonstrate the following findings:

- Coma
- Absence of spontaneous movement
- Absence of brain stem function
  - Pupillary light reflex
  - Corneal reflex
  - Oculocephalic/vestibulo-ocular reflex
  - Oropharyngeal reflex
  - Apnea, using an accepted testing procedure

Differential diagnosis

Two major types of insults may be confused with brain death—reversible causes of coma and conditions that involve major impairment of the central nervous system. To diagnose a patient as brain dead, the HCP must determine the cause of coma and ascertain that it is irreversible. Reversible causes of coma include the following:

- Clinically significant drug intoxications with agents such as alcohol, barbiturates, sedatives, or hypnotics
- Therapeutic levels or dosing of anticonvulsants or sedatives
- Neuromuscular blocking agents
- Metabolic and endocrine disorders such as severe electrolyte disturbances or severe hypoglycemia or hyperglycemia
- Uncontrolled hypotension and unresuscitated shock
- Hypothermia

Conditions that involve *major impairment* of the nervous system include the following:

- Persistent vegetative states
- Locked-in syndrome
- Severe peripheral nerve or muscle dysfunction that can cause the patient to be unresponsive

Plan of Care

Once a patient has been identified as potentially being brain dead, formal clinical evaluation begins. The specifics of this evaluation vary from state to state, but most often require documentation of two physical examinations, by more than one physician, and separated by a predetermined time interval depending on the etiology of the brain injury and the age of the patient (Ashwal, 2001). There must be a recognized cause of coma, and all potentially reversible causes of coma must be excluded. Higher brain function must be absent; this outcome is assessed by applying a standardized painful stimulus, such as pressing on the supraorbital nerve, temporomandibular joint, or nail bed of a finger and documenting the following findings:

- Lack of consciousness
- Lack of voluntary movement or responsiveness except for spinal reflexes
- No decorticate or decerebrate posturing
- No convulsions

Spinal reflexes are motor responses confined to a spinal distribution and range from subtle twitches to the *Lazarus sign*, in which both arms are raised up and dropped across the chest. These signs may be seen in some patients and need to be anticipated and explained to inexperienced HCPs and families.

Brain stem function must also be absent to diagnose brain death. Evaluation of the brain stem includes the following findings:

- Absence of sympathetic and parasympathetic regulation of the pupils
  - Pupils in midposition and dilated
  - No direct or indirect response to light
- Disruption of the pathways in the brain stem controlling eye movement
  - Absence of spontaneous eye movement
  - Negative vestibulo-ocular reflex
  - Negative oculocephalic reflex
- Disruption of the afferent trigeminal and efferent facial nerve pathways
  - Absent corneal reflex
- Disruption of afferent and efferent pathways of cranial nerves IX and X
  - Absence of gag reflex and cough
- Absence of vagal efferent activity

- No significant increase in heart rate upon administration of intravenous atropine or negative oculocardiac reflex
- Disruption of the medullary respiratory control centers
  - No respiratory movement at a $PaCO_2$ higher than a set limit during apnea testing

Persistent apnea is a fundamental part of the clinical criteria for the diagnosis of brain death. It is tested by documenting a lack of respiratory effort in response to acute hypercarbic stimulation. In the United States, guidelines recommend an apneic threshold $PaCO_2$ of 60 mmHg or greater and an increase of 20 mmHg above baseline. Apnea testing is optimally performed by pre-oxygenating the patient, followed by delivery of 100% oxygen to the trachea upon disconnection from mechanical ventilation. The certifying HCP must continuously observe the patient for respiratory effort during the duration of the test. The rate of rise of $PaCO_2$ is nonlinear and often requires the patient to spend 10 to 20 minutes off mechanical ventilation. During this period, the patient must remain hemodynamically stable and normally oxygenated.

When all minimum clinical criteria for brain death have been met, there is generally no need to consider confirmatory testing. Nevertheless, indications for confirmatory testing vary by jurisdiction and age of the patient. Such testing should also be done when there is an inability to complete any part of the minimum clinical criteria, when confounding conditions exist, when there is uncertainty or disagreement among certifying HCPs, or to help the family understand the concept of brain death. These tests include the following measures:

- Electroencephalograph
- Tests of intracerebral blood flow: four vessel angiography or radionuclide imaging
- Transcranial Doppler sonography
- Brain stem auditory evoked potentials
- Magnetic resonance angiography with magnetic resonance imaging

Goals of therapy during the assessment period are the same as for any critically ill patient. Normal oxygenation and ventilation that is appropriate for the patient's pulmonary pathology should be maintained. Blood pressure should be kept at the normal mean arterial pressure for age and adjustments made to maintain electrolytes and hematologic indices within normal limits as appropriate.

The patient's family needs to be educated about brain death and supported during this difficult time. Once the determination of brain death has been made, standard end-of-life care should be instituted, including offering the option of organ and tissue donation for eligible patients.

Disposition

During the evaluation for brain death, the patient should be assessed to establish his or her eligibility for organ donation.

This is done by contacting the local organ procurement organization (OPO). For patients who are deemed eligible to donate, the family will be approached for consent/permission. If the family elects to proceed with donation, the OPO often assumes management of the patient once brain death has been determined. For patients who do not become organ donors, standard end-of-life care continues. At this point, the patient is legally dead and the medications and equipment artificially maintaining respirations and blood pressure should be removed in a manner that is sensitive to the family's needs. Bereavement follow-up should be done with the family and community resources for support offered as needed.

ORGAN DONATION

The option to donate organs and tissues is part of end-of-life care in the PICU. The demand for organs continues to outpace the supply. In 2007, slightly more than 27,000 solid-organ transplants were performed in the United States, and 97,000 individuals were on waiting lists for organ transplantation.

In 1968, an ad hoc committee at Harvard Medical School proposed a brain-based definition of death. The Harvard committee met, in part, to develop criteria to pronounce individuals dead who had suffered irreversible, devastating brain injury but continued to have a heartbeat. After the Harvard criteria were developed, a new source of potential organ donors was defined.

As the field of organ transplantation flourished, a large discrepancy developed between supply and demand. Using a definition of death based on cardiopulmonary criteria was seen as a potential way to increase organ donors and to provide the option of donation for patients with devastating neurologic injury who did not meet criteria for brain death. In the 1990s, this process was known as "nonheartbeating organ donation" and today has been retermed "donation after cardiac death" (DCD).

Briefly, DCD is suitable for any patient whose life-sustaining treatment is under consideration for withdrawal and who will likely die soon after the withdrawal of the treatment. In controlled DCD, the patient is taken to the operating room, where a physician removes all life-sustaining treatment, documents asystole, waits a minimum defined period (usually between 2 and 5 minutes), and then declares the patient dead. The organ procurement team then enters the operating room and begins organ recovery. If the patient does not die within 60 minutes of withdrawal of life-sustaining treatment, the organs are no longer suitable for transplantation and the patient is taken back to the intensive care unit for end-of-life care. There continues to be debate about the ethics of this practice (Steinbrook, 2007).

Pathophysiology death by neurologic criteria

The period between declaration of brain death and procurement of organs and tissues is marked by physiologic instability of the donor. The cardiovascular system is especially susceptible to derangement during this period. Cerebral herniation leads to brain stem ischemia, which proceeds in a rostral to caudal fashion. Parasympathetic activation occurs as a result of midbrain ischemia, manifested as apnea, bradycardia, hypotension, and a resultant drop in cardiac output (CO). As ischemia moves to the pons, sympathetic stimulation is superimposed, causing tachycardia and hypertension. Further ischemic extension into the medulla blocks vagal stimulation, causing further sympathetic surge; this adds to the hypertension, causes an elevation of CO, and leads to the potential for arrhythmias ("autonomic storming"). The myocardium itself also becomes neurogenically stunned; catecholamine surge leads to an increase in peripheral vascular resistance that increases myocardial work and oxygen consumption. This effect can result in myocardial ischemia or infarction.

The two other systems most affected by death of the brain are the pulmonary and endocrine systems. Neurogenic pulmonary edema can occur as a result of unopposed sympathetic stimulation. Hyperglycemia occurs secondary to end-organ insulin resistance, physical stress, increases in counterregulatory hormones, and changes in carbohydrate metabolism. Diabetes insipidus and resulting hypernatremia arise from dysfunction of the posterior pituitary when the blood flow to the cells arising in the deep supraventricular and paraventricular nuclei of the hypothalamus is compromised. Hypothyroidism can occur with compromised blood flow to the anterior pituitary; this effect often causes further derangements in cardiovascular function.

In addition to specific organ dysfunction, brain death causes generalized systemic derangements. It leads to a pro-inflammatory state in the whole body. Upregulation of transcriptional levels of TNF- and IL-6 causes an upregulation and induction of the inflammatory response in all organs, which produces further compromise of vital organs.

Epidemiology and etiology

There are no statistics regarding how many potential organ donors exist in the pediatric population. A potential organ donor is defined by the presence of brain death or a catastrophic injury to the brain. According to data collected by the Organ Procurement and Transplant Network, there were 879 pediatric organ donors ages less than 1 year to 17 years of age in 2008; these data were not divided into those declared dead by brain criteria and those declared by cardiorespiratory criteria.

Plan of care

The United Network for Organ Sharing (UNOS) recommends that the following diagnostic studies be performed when a patient is deemed eligible for organ and tissue donation and the family has provided consent/permission:

- Serum chemistry
- Complete blood count with differential
- Urinalysis and urine culture
- Prothrombin time and partial thromboplastin time
- ABO blood typing and A subtyping
- Two blood cultures taken 15 minutes to 1 hour apart from different sites
- Sputum sample for Gram stain and culture
- Liver function tests
- Type and cross-match
- Chest radiograph
- Arterial blood gases (ABG)
- Electrocardiograph
- Echocardiograph
- Bedside diagnostic/therapeutic bronchoscopy
- Serology
- Serial troponins if the patient is a potential heart donor
- Monitor vital signs and urine output

The goal of therapy for the period prior to organ recovery is to maintain stability of the potential donor. This is accomplished by standardized treatments and algorithms, and has proven to be beneficial in minimizing loss of donors, recovering organs initially assessed to be medically unsuitable, and increasing the number of organs procured and transplanted with good outcomes.

Management of respiratory function in the potential donor aims to minimize damage to the lungs and maintain normal oxygenation and ventilation. To assess for lung placement, an oxygen challenge test is performed: Positive end-expiratory pressure (PEEP) is set at 5 mmHg, the fraction of inspired oxygen is set at 1.0 for 20 minutes, and an gasbag analysis is then performed. If the partial pressure of arterial oxygen is greater than 300 mmHg, the lungs are deemed suitable for donation pending evaluation by bronchoscopy.

Ventilator settings should be optimized to achieve an oxygen saturation of more than 95%. Generous tidal volumes of 8 to 10 mL/kg are delivered to prevent atelectasis, although peak airway pressures should be maintained at less than 30 mmHg. Pulmonary toilet and ABGs are performed as needed with the goal of achieving mild respiratory alkalosis.

The hemodynamic performance of the donor may be tenuous. Goals of management include achieving or maintaining normovolemia, maintaining normal blood pressure for age, and optimizing cardiac output. These goals promote adequate perfusion pressure to maintain organ function. Mean arterial pressure should be normal for age and central venous pressure should be 12 mmHg or less. Vasoactive medications should be administered only when the body cannot meet these criteria.

Potential donors may have metabolic derangements that need to be corrected. Hypernatremia adversely affects organ function in the recipient; serum sodium levels should be maintained between 140 and 150 mEq/dL. Cardiac arrhythmias are common, and serum potassium should be kept at a level greater than 4.0 mEq/dL. Acidosis should be corrected by administration of sodium bicarbonate. Glucose levels are frequently elevated and are a risk factor for pancreatic graft dysfunction in the organ recipient; therefore, insulin therapy should administered to maintain blood glucose levels in the range of 120 to 180 mg/dL.

Destruction of the hypothalamus and pituitary gland during cerebral herniation can cause dysregulation of several endocrine functions. If diabetes insipidus develops, arginine vasopressin therapy can reestablish water homeostasis and stabilize serum sodium levels. For patients with severe cardiovascular instability and high vasoactive therapy requirements, replacement with triiodothyronine or thyroxine and/or methylprednisolone can decrease those requirements. Hormone replacement therapy can also eliminate the need for vasoactive therapy altogether in certain patients.

Disorders of blood coagulation are a common consequence of the release of mediators from traumatized or necrotic brain tissue. Blood product replacement should be directed at correcting this coagulopathy and providing adequate oxygen delivery to tissues and organs. An International Normalized Ratio (INR) of less than 2.0, a platelet count greater than 80,000 cells/μL, and hematocrit greater than 30% should be maintained. To minimize the potential for sensitization, cytomegalovirus-seronegative blood and leukocyte filters should be used when transfusing blood products.

While overwhelming infection generally precludes organ donation, bacteremia or fungemia are not absolute contraindications to donation. As such, appropriate anti-infective coverage should be instituted for presumed or proven infections. Donors are often poikilothermic secondary to loss of hypothalamic thermoregulation and the inability to shiver or vasoconstrict. Hypothermia can cause cardiac dysfunction, arrhythmias, coagulopathy, a left shift of the oxygen dissociation curve, and cold-induced diuresis. The patient's core temperature should be maintained between 36.5°C and 38°C (97.7–100.4°F) to prevent these complications. Eye care in the form of lubricants and taping eyelids shut when necessary will maintain these organs and tissues for donation.

Disposition

During the maintenance phase of a potential organ donor, the OPO will be involved in the management and will require notification of any changes in the donor's condition. The agency coordinates the notification of other centers for the distribution of organs. The operating room and personnel need notification of a pending organ recovery. When all supplies and personnel are assembled, the patient is transported to the operating room for organ procurement. The donor's family will have been supported throughout this entire process and will receive follow-up from the OPO to learn the final disposition of their loved one's organs.

Follow-up and support from the health care team is also provided.

CEREBRAL PALSY

Sherri L. Adams and Sanjay Mahant

PATHOPHYSIOLOGY

Cerebral palsy (CP) is a broad term used to describe a group of persistent motor impairments diagnosed in childhood by the age of 3 years. It is defined as a "group of disorders of the development of movement and posture causing activity limitations that are attributed to nonprogressive disturbances that occurred in the developing fetal or infant brain" (Bax et al., 2005, p. 571). Changes in the brain may vary based on the timing and nature (e.g., ischemia) of the insult. The area of brain injury determines the clinical presentation. Some children may have only injury to areas affecting motor control and not have cognitive delay.

EPIDEMIOLOGY AND ETIOLOGY

The description of CP in the literature dates back more than 100 years. The prevalence of this condition, which is estimated at 2 to 2.5 patients per 1,000 live births (Stanley et al., 2000), has not changed in recent decades (Nelson, 2003). CP is the most common physical disability in children (O'Shea, 2008; Rosenbaum, 2003). Its incidence is higher in children born prematurely and children with very low birth weights. Incidence decreases with increasing gestational age (Stanley et al., 2000; Wilson et al., 2007a, 2007b).

The etiology of CP is multifactorial and in many cases is unknown. A central nervous system insult may occur in the prenatal, perinatal, or postnatal period (Wilson et al., 2007a, 2007b). Varying causes such as prenatal infection, prematurity, multiple births, perinatal asphyxia, and intrauterine inflammation have all been implicated in CP. Recent reports suggest that perinatal asphyxia has been overstated in the past as a cause (Wilson et al., 2007a, 2007b). Ischemic changes secondary to vascular insufficiency that are implicated in CP include neuronal migration deficits, periventricular leukomalacia (PVL), and multifocal cerebral injury.

Classification

Classification of CP is based on three criteria:

- Identification of the part of the child's body that is affected (monoplegia, hemiplegia, diplegia, triplegia, or quadriplegia).

- Identification of the motor disorder (spastic, ataxic, dyskinetic, dystonic, choreathetoid), a combination of movement disorders (spasticity and dystonia), and rigidity (rare in children) (Table 33-9).
- Identification of the gross motor function using the Gross Motor Function Classification System (GMFCS), which has five levels of gross motor function and can be helpful in prognosticating future outcomes (Palisano et al., 1997). These scales are age based.

PRESENTATION

Cerebral palsy is diagnosed when the patient is between 12 and 18 months of age, as the child fails to meet gross and/or fine motor developmental milestones (Rosenbaum, 2003). Neurologic findings on physical examination may include persistence of primitive reflexes and a lack of protective reflexes, increased deep tendon reflexes, peripheral hypertonia, and weakness, which may vary between upper and lower extremities or between the right and left sides of the body. Children with CP may also have a generalized hypotonia that progresses to hypertonia. In addition, some children have cognitive impairment.

DIFFERENTIAL DIAGNOSIS

Cerebral palsy is nonprogressive; thus any history of loss of previous skills, developmental slowing or regression, or signs of a lower motor neurologic disorder (myelodysplasia, spinal muscle atrophy, or poliomyelitis) should raise the suspicion of an alternative diagnosis. Other causes of motor impairment such as metabolic or neurodegenerative disorder, neoplasm, or neuromuscular disorder should be considered.

PLAN OF CARE

CP is a clinical diagnosis; thus its diagnosis is based mostly on physical examination findings over time. Neuroimaging may be helpful in determining the cause, time, and extent of the underlying neurologic insult. MRI is recommended over CT scan for evaluating the neural axis (American Academy of Neurology [AAN], 2009). It is not recommended, however, to classify children based on radiologic findings alone; instead, clinical presentation must also be considered when making such determination (Bax et al., 2005). Investigation for a coagulation disorder may be indicated if cerebral infarct is found on MRI; however, the evidence is unclear regarding which investigations are indicated (AAN, 2009). MRI findings are related to the underlying cause of the brain injury. In one recent population-based study of CP, white matter injury related to PVL was the most common finding (43%), followed by basal ganglia lesions (13%), cortical and subcortical lesions (9%), malformations (9%), focal infarcts (7%), and miscellaneous lesions (7%); 11% of patients had normal MRI findings (Bax et al., 2006). Additional investigations, such as metabolic and genetic evaluation, are not diagnostic for CP; thus they should be completed only if the HCP is evaluating these issues as part of the differential diagnosis.

Children with CP may have health issues secondary to their neurological injury, including intellectual impairment, seizure disorder, skin breakdown, visual and hearing impairment, swallowing and feeding problems, respiratory tract infections, osteoporosis, hip subluxation,

TABLE 33-9

Motor/Movement Disorders		
Motor Disorder	**Definition**	**Etiology**
Ataxia	Poor coordination; low muscle tone and poor coordination	Cerebellum
Athetosis	Involuntary, hyperkinetic disorder manifested in writhing movements of the face, trunk, and extremities	Kernicterus
Chorea	Brief, irregular sudden muscle contractions, especially at rest	Caudate nucleus
Dyskinesia	Spastic or repetitive involuntary movements or lack of coordination	Dopaminergic neurons of the substantia nigra pars compacta
Dystonia	Involuntary fluctuating muscle contractions that cause twisting and repetitive movements, abnormal postures, or both	Basal ganglia
Hypotonia	Low muscle tone associated with decreased resistance of muscles to passive stretching	Various etiologies
Rigidity	Joint/muscle inflexibility/stiffness and inflexibility to passive range of motion; rare in children	
Spasticity	Involuntary, velocity-dependent, increased muscular resistance to stretch	Upper motor neuron

scoliosis, and spasticity (Wilson et al., 2007a, 2007b). Consequently, therapeutic management may include care for these disorders and specialty consultation. Optimally an interprofessional team of HCPs should care for the patient to ensure best practice and patient outcomes. For example, physical therapists and occupational therapists may provide interventions for spasticity; orthopedic surgeons may evaluate and treat scoliosis; gastroenterologists, nutritionists, and speech therapists may provide therapies for oral motor dysfunction and gastroesophageal reflux; neurologists may treat seizure disorders; and social workers may provide emotional support and work to secure financial support for equipment and nutritional needs. Developmental and orthotic specialists promote functional capacity in the child with CP.

Spasticity management includes nonoperative interventions such as range of motion exercises, strengthening, and, if the patient is ambulatory, gait training. Positioning, bracing, and casting are also implemented with the goals of appropriate alignment, comfort, and prevention of joint contractures. Medications enlisted in the management of spasticity may be administered via different routes, including the enteral route, injections in the muscle/nerves, and the intrathecal route. Oral medications to reduce spasticity include baclofen, a GABA agonist; dantrolene, which inhibits release of calcium in the sarcoplasmic reticulum; diazepam, which is GABA mediated and has an inhibitor effect; and clonidine and tizanidine, both of which are α_2-adrenergic agonists. Injectable medications include botulinum toxin A, a neuromuscular blocking agent, and phenol, which demyelinates gamma fibers. Systematic review has not revealed strong controlled evidence to support or refute the use of botulinum toxin A for the treatment of spasticity in the lower extremities due to CP (Ade-Hall & Moore, 2009). Conversely, systematic review found high-level evidence supporting the use of botulinum toxin A as an adjunct to managing the upper limbs in children with spastic CP (Hoare et al., 2008). Positioning, splinting/bracing, and therapy should accompany botulinum toxin A administration.

Baclofen may also be administered into the spinal canal, via an intrathecal baclofen pump (ITB). This route allows for direct administration of the medication into the intrathecal space, which circumvents its first-pass metabolism through the liver. Intrathecal baclofen administration is more effective and requires approximately 1,000 times less dosing compared to oral administration. ITBs may be programmed to administer various amounts of baclofen throughout a 24-hour period. These infusion rates may be increased immediately prior to an operation in an attempt to decrease postoperative spasms and acute postoperative pain. HCPs should be aware that baclofen withdrawal can be life-threatening, so symptoms such as hallucinations, increased hypertonia, confusion, agitation,

and hyperthermia must be monitored for very closely. Treatment of these conditions includes administration of baclofen and symptom management. Baclofen is not available in intravenous form. If this medication is to be discontinued, it is recommended that patients be weaned from it slowly.

The five most common surgeries performed in children with CP include gastrostomy tube placement, soft-tissue musculoskeletal procedures, fundoplications, spinal fusions, and bony hip surgeries (Murphy et al., 2006). The most common orthopedic procedures are soft-tissue releases, tendon/muscle transfers, and corrective osteotomies to correct lever-arm dysfunction, where muscle and ground reaction forces are inappropriate or inadequate. Lever-arm dysfunction includes bony malrotation, loss of a stable fulcrum, loss of bony rigidity, and short lever arms (Gage et al., 2009). Children with spastic quadriplegia CP are at high risk for progressive neuromuscular scoliosis, and approximately 60% to 75% of these children will require spinal fusion surgery (Thomson & Banta, 2001).

DISPOSITION AND DISCHARGE PLANNING

Cerebral palsy is a lifelong nonprogressive condition; thus care focus on maximizing quality of life rather than effecting a cure. Early in the diagnosis, families often have questions about how their child will function in society as the individual grows older. Will the child walk, talk, ride a bike, or go to school? Depending on the severity and nature of the causative insult, the answers to these questions may be apparent, but in many instances they become evident only with time. The GMFCS may help the HCP provide more accurate information to families (Rosenbaum et al., 2002). Although many children with CP now live into adulthood, mean life expectancy depends on the severity of the disorder. As many as 50% of children with severe CP survive until they are older than 20 years of age, and almost 100% of those with few functional limitation lives past 20 years of age (Hutton et al., 1998; Strauss et al., 2008). Open and honest answers are best so that families can have a realistic approach to the care of their child and understand what kind of care may be required as the child moves through childhood into adulthood.

The child with CP usually has complex health care needs that are best coordinated by the primary care provider (PCP) through a medical home model (Homer et al., 2008). Routine follow-up at a pediatric treatment or rehabilitation center is invaluable. While CP is often described as a static condition, this label refers only to the cerebral insult. Physical changes such as spasticity, scoliosis, and feeding problems may be progressive and will affect prognosis. Ongoing management by an interprofessional team is essential to prevent and manage problems.

CEREBRAL VASCULAR ACCIDENTS

Michele Grimason, Mark S. Wainwright, and Valerie Eichler

PATHOPHYSIOLOGY

The causes of stroke in children differ substantially from those in adults. A cerebral vascular accident (CVA)—more commonly known as "stroke"—is the result of a sudden interruption of blood flow to a focal region of the brain. Strokes can be further subdivided into two major categories: occlusive and hemorrhagic. Occlusive strokes are the result of hypercoagulable states. Brain ischemia results, but if the blood flow is rapidly reestablished, complete or near-complete resolution occurs. The reverse is seen if localized flow is not reestablished: The brain cells infarct and die. In hemorrhagic stroke, a vessel or aneurysm ruptures and leaks blood into the surrounding tissue and cells (Pappachan & Kirkham, 2008). A small population of children experience strokes with a watershed effect. Hypoperfusion is responsible for the global injury in such patients.

CVAs decrease the circulating blood volume, such that the neurons and brain cells become starved for oxygen and nutrients. Starvation of the cells results in a shift in brain osmolality and stimulates the movement of sodium and water into the astrocytes and other surrounding tissues. The brain cells become edematous, rupture, and ultimately die, with no possibility of their regeneration. In addition, the osmotic changes within the cells cause the release of inflammatory mediators such as tumor necrosing factor, interleukins, and toll receptors (Kochanek et al., 2008). This inflammatory process results in further tissue swelling and edema, further compromising blood flow. If this process is not arrested, the resulting increased intracranial pressure will be so great that the brain will herniate and ultimately the patient will experience brain death.

EPIDEMIOLOGY AND ETIOLOGY

The annual incidence of stroke in children younger than 14 years of age is 2.5 to 3.3 events per 100,000 population (deVeber et al., 2000). The incidence of neonatal strokes has been reported as high as 24.7 events per 100,000 population in infants older than 31 weeks of age (Lynch et al., 2002). Strokes occur more frequently in boys, and are most common in the first year of life (Golomb et al., 2009). Stroke in children is a life-threatening event, associated with a 10% mortality rate, 20% risk of recurrence, and 70% long-term neurologic morbidity in survivors (deVeber et al., 2000; Ganesan et al., 2000). Eighty percent of strokes in pediatric patients are ischemic, while the remainder are hemorrhagic or due to a cerebral sinus venous thrombosis.

Atherosclerosis of large arteries and small-vessel occlusive disease are common causative factors for CVA in adults, but are rarely a source of cerebral vascular disease in pediatric patients (deVeber, 2002; Lynch et al., 2002). The most common risk factors for arterial ischemic stroke (AIS) in children of all ages are congenital or acquired heart disease, arteriopathies (arterial dissection, Moyamoya syndrome, vasculitis), and, less frequently, sickle cell disease (Ganesan et al., 2003; Lynch et al.; Nowak-Gottl et al., 2003). In addition, a number of coagulation abnormalities have been implicated as increasing the risk of stroke in children, such as protein C, protein S, and antithrombin III deficiency; activated protein C resistance; factor V Leiden mutation; prothrombin gene mutation (G20210A); methylenetetrahydrofolate reductase TT677 (MTHFR) mutation; and antiphospholipid antibody syndrome (Lynch et al.). Risk factors for neonatal strokes include cardiac disorders, hypercoagulable conditions, infections, trauma, medications, maternal disorders, and perinatal asphyxia (Sebire et al., 2005; Wu et al., 2002).

PRESENTATION

In the neonate, stroke may present as decreased responsiveness, seizures, or focal weakness. Children are more likely to present with focal neurologic deficits such as hemiparesis, aphasia, visual disturbances, and headache. Occasionally, neck pain or Horner's sign may be noted; these findings are more commonly associated with carotid dissection and ischemic stroke (deVeber, 2003). Risk factors for pediatric AIS are summarized in Table 33-10.

Hemorrhagic strokes may present with headache, vomiting, or both; they are a result of increased intracranial pressure and bleeding. Other presenting signs may include irritability, seizures, and hemiparesis (Al-Jarallah et al., 2000). Patients with hemorrhagic strokes are often healthy individuals prior to the initial symptoms, but have undiagnosed vascular malformations, aneurysms, or brain tumors (Al-Jarallah et al.). Other risk factors for hemorrhagic stroke include underlying hematologic abnormalities and coagulopathies (Table 33-11).

Strokes may also result from cerebral venous occlusion. In neonates and children, seizures are the most common presenting sign of sinus venous thrombosis (SVT) (deVeber et al., 2001). Neonates may also present with hypotonia and irritability, whereas older children may complain of headaches and motor deficits. SVT is most common in the neonatal period, with more than one-half of children with this condition presenting in the first 6 months of life. Dehydration, infection, and maternal risk factors have been associated with the increased frequency of SVT in neonates (Wassey et al., 2008).

TABLE 33-10

Risk Factors for Arterial Ischemic Stroke				
Cardiac	**Hematologic**	**Vasculopathy**	**Infection**	**Genetic/Metabolic**
Congenital heart disease	Hypercoagulable states	Arterial dissection	Meningitis	Mitochondrial disease
Arrhythmia	Sickle cell disease	Moyamoya disease	Varicella	Connective tissue disorders
Cardiomyopathy		Fibromuscular dysplasia	Tuberculosis	Neurofibromatosis type I
Cardiac surgery		Transient cerebral		Fabry disease
Kawasaki disease (KD)		arteriopathy (TCA)		CADASIL
Endocarditis		Vasculitis		Homocysteinuria
		Radiation arteriopathy		

Note: Cerebral autosomal dominant arteriopathy with subcortical infarcts and leukoencephalopathy (CADASIL).

TABLE 33-11

Risk Factors for Hemorrhagic Stroke

Vascular

• Vascular malformations

• Cavernous malformations

• Aneurysms

Brain tumor

Hematologic

• Sickle cell anemia

• Thrombocytopenia

Coagulopathy

Spontaneous dissection

DIFFERENTIAL DIAGNOSIS

The signs and symptoms associated with AIS or hemorrhagic stroke may mimic those of many other disorders such as meningitis, trauma, or tumor. Stroke requires prompt evaluation and intervention, so it should be included high on the differential list when symptoms of headache, seizures, or focal weakness are noted.

PLAN OF CARE

National stroke guidelines are available from the American Heart Association (AHA) and outline the approach to diagnostic study and therapeutic management (Roach et al., 2008). CT scan, or MRI with diffusion-weighted imaging (DWI), is recommended to identify the presence of hemorrhage and extent of infarct. Initial CT (hours) after an ischemic insult may be negative; thus serial evaluation may be required to identify ischemic brain regions. If carotid or vertebral dissection or SVT is a consideration, CT or MRA (CTA/MRA), or venogram, should be performed. Magnetic resonance spectroscopy is useful to evaluate for metabolic (mitochondrial) causes of stroke. A conventional angiogram may be indicated if the CTA or MRA results are normal and dissection, small-vessel vasculitis, arteriovenous malformation, aneurysm, or Moyamoya disease is suspected. A cerebral arteriogram may be ordered to evaluate for thrombosis and vascular anomalies, and an electroencephalograph may indicate subclinical seizure activity. The source of cardioembolic events may be investigated via echocardiograph with bubble contrast or a transesophageal study.

Laboratory studies should include measures of coagulation, platelets, homocysteine, fasting cholesterol, and triglycerides. The HCP should measure the patient's hemoglobin level as well. In small infants with nonfused fontanels, a significant loss of circulating volume to the expandable cranial vault may occur, resulting in a drop in hemoglobin. Testing for protein C, protein S, or antithrombin III deficiency, and for anticardiolipin and antiphospholipid antibodies, allows for evaluation of possible inflammatory processes. Genetic testing may be performed, though its results will not alter the patient's acute management; such testing should include factor V Leiden mutation, prothrombin gene mutation (G20210A), and methylenetetrahydrofolate reductase TT677 mutation (Lynch et al., 2002; Nowak-Gottl et al., 2003). Diagnostic studies for toxins and autoimmune, connective tissue, metabolic, or infectious diseases are guided by the risk factors for the particular child (Ganesan et al., 2003).

Strokes in children with sickle cell disease may be due to arterial ischemia, subarachnoid or intracerebral hemorrhage, aneurysm rupture, dissection, Moyamoya syndrome, or SVT (Kirkham, 2007; Strouse et al., 2006). Imaging studies will identify all of these potential pathologies. If imaging studies do not identify stroke, consider seizures as an etiology.

The average time from initial symptoms to diagnosis of stroke is 35 hours (Gabis et al., 2002). Consequently, the patient may have experienced significant ischemia or cell death by the time of diagnosis.

Management of neonatal strokes is primarily supportive (Roach et al., 2008). AHA Class I recommendations include the following measures:

- Supplementing coagulation factors in coagulation disorders
- Replacing platelets in those with intracranial hemorrhage
- Ventricular drainage for those patients who develop hydrocephalus

AHA Class II recommendations include treating dehydration and anemia, utilizing rehabilitation sources, giving folate or vitamin B in those patients with an MTHFR mutation and an abnormal homocysteine level, and evacuating a hematoma that elevates intracranial pressure.

Approaches to the acute management of AIS due to hematologic, cardiac, or vascular disorders and venous thrombosis are summarized in Table 33-12 and are based on the AHA stroke guidelines (Roach et al., 2008). Heparin—either unfractionated (UFH) or low molecular weight (LMWH)—may be given as long as 1 week after AIS. Tissue plasminogen activator (tPA) is not yet recommended in children outside of clinical trial (Roach et al.).

Although data are limited, acute management of pediatric patients with stroke should also include prevention of fever, maintenance of normoglycemia, and normovolemia to maintain adequate substrate delivery to injured cells (Amlie-Lefond et al., 2008; Roach et al., 2008).

For prevention of recurrent stroke, acetylsalicylic acid (aspirin) is commonly used at a dose of 3 to 5 mg/kg/day, and has proven as effective as warfarin in children. Aspirin increases the risk for Reye's syndrome in children following varicella and other viral infections, so the risks and benefits of this regimen must be considered prior to its administration. For arteriopathy, idiopathic stroke, or Moyamoya disease, aspirin is considered the first choice for stroke prophylaxis (Bernard et al., 2008; Roach et al., 2008). For extracranial dissection or cardioembolic stroke, longer-term treatment should begin with anticoagulants such as warfarin or LMWH.

Regardless of stroke etiology, the patient's clinical presentation dictates the initial therapy. Airway, breathing, and circulation support (ABCs), following standard guidelines, precedes imaging and coagulation. An interprofessional team of specialists should work together to implement AHA stroke guidelines, evaluate care, and provide ongoing consultation. Neurosurgical intervention may be required for either hematoma drainage or cerebral pressure monitoring. Neurology and hematology specialists should work together to implement anticoagulation therapy. Infectious diseases specialists may guide antimicrobial or infectious therapies. Cardiology specialists may be consulted for cardioembolic events and therapy. As previously described, many infants and children with stroke will have neurologic deficits if they

TABLE 33-12

Recommendations for Acute Management of Pediatric Stroke			
Hematologic (*Class, Level*)	**Vasculopathy (*Class, Level*)**	**Cardiac (*Class, Level*)**	**Venous Thrombosis (*Class, Level*)**
Sickle Cell Disease	**Moyamoya Disease**	**Cardioembolic**	**Pediatrics**
Transfusion (ages 2–16 years) with abnormal TCD to reduce SS Hgb (*I.A*) Hydration (*I.C*) Correct hypoxemia (*I.C*) Correct hypotension (*I.C*)	Revascularization (*I.B*) Anticoagulants not recommended except for cases with frequent TIAs or infarcts despite aspirin (*III.C*)	UFH or LMWH prior to warfarin (for non-PFO cases) if risk of recurrence is high (*II.a.B*) Aspirin if risk of recurrence is low (non-PFO cases) (*II.a.C*)	Hydration, control of seizures, treatment of intracranial hypertension (*I.C*) Consider ICP monitoring (*II.b.C*) UFH or LMWH whether or not hemorrhage is present (*II.a.C*) Thrombolysis in selected cases (*II.b.C*)
For acute infarct, exchange transfuse to reduce sickle Hgb to < 30% (*II.a.C*)	**Arterial Dissection**		**Neonates**
Hypercoagulable Disorders	For extracranial dissection, UFH or LMWH as a bridge to oral anticoagulation (*II.a.C*).		Anticoagulation is not appropriate (*III.C*) except in cases of severe prothrombotic disorders, multiple emboli, or propagation despite supportive therapy
Risk of stroke from thrombotic disorders is low but increases in the presence of other risk factors Reasonable to stop oral contraceptives after AIS or cerebral venous thrombosis (*II.a.C*)	Antiplatelet agent, LMWH or warfarin for 3–6 months (*III.C*) Anticoagulation not recommended for intracranial dissection (*III.C*)		

Note: Unfractionated heparin (UFH), low-molecular-weight heparin (LMWH), increased intracranial pressure (ICP), hemoglobin (Hgb), acute ischemic stroke (AIS), transient ischemic attack (TIA), patent foramen ovale (PFO).

survive the event; thus rehabilitation medicine should be consulted early in the hospitalization to assist with goals of care and discharge planning.

The family and the patient (if the clinical condition allows) require information as to the diagnosis, prognosis, risk of recurrence (20%), and therapeutic options (Fullerton et al., 2007). Goals of care are then determined in conjunction with the family. Patients with stroke are managed by a large, interprofessional team; consequently, it is easy for their families to receive fragmented communication. Efforts must be made to coordinate communication through one leading specialty service, such as critical care, to reduce confusion and fragmentation.

DISPOSITION AND DISCHARGE PLANNING

The assessment of longer-term rehabilitation needs, with evaluation by physical, occupational, and speech therapists, should be performed early in the patient's hospital stay (Bernard et al., 2008). Depending on the region of the brain that is affected by the stroke, the recovery phase may by prolonged, with the child experiencing significant residual motor loss. Families and patients should be counseled to anticipate a prolonged (weeks to months) period of recovery. Most patients will require some period of physical and occupational therapy.

Once the decision has been made by the primary medical team that the patient is ready for discharge either to an inpatient rehabilitation facility or to home, discharge planning or social services should plan for and obtain any necessary durable medical equipment (DME). If the patient is discharged to home, a home health medical team will also be in contact with the family. The caregivers and any other family who will be providing care should take a class on basic cardiopulmonary resuscitation training prior to the child being discharged home. Consultation and transfer to an inpatient rehabilitation program may be considered as a bridge to home discharge.

ENCEPHALOPATHY

Gina M. Sanchez

PATHOPHYSIOLOGY

Encephalopathy is a broad term used to define global brain dysfunction that includes a wide range of syndromes and diseases leading to an altered mental state (National Institutes of Health [NIH], 2007). The brain requires a delicate balance of neurotransmitters, substrates, water, and electrolytes to function correctly, as well as adequate perfusion, acid–base balance, and appropriate temperature. Derangement in this delicate milieu, which is essential for optimal neurological function, can cause injury to brain cells, disruption of neurotransmitter signals, and disturbances of electrical impulses within the brain (Parke, 2006).

Cytotoxic injury leading to encephalopathy is a result of an energy crisis—that is, decreased availability of the vital substrates glucose and oxygen and/or inadequate blood flow. The lack of energy leads to anaerobic metabolism and accumulation of lactic acid and other potent neurotoxins and free radicals; such as excess extracellular calcium, glutamate, and neuronal and vascular nitric oxide. These factors, in turn, contribute to further pathological cascades, resulting in impaired—and sometimes permanent—cerebral dysfunction (Volpe, 2001). Even with recovery of perfusion and oxygenation, some neurons will still progress to cellular death, as a result of necrosis or apoptosis (Liou et al., 2003). This may explain the irreversible, static encephalopathy induced by some neurological insults. Furthermore, poor blood flow allows for insufficient removal of toxins and poor delivery of vital substrates. The lack of oxygen and perfusion, combined with the accumulation of carbon dioxide and lactic acid lead, leads to acidosis, osmotic pressure changes, and cytotoxic edema, further exacerbating cerebral ischemia.

Electrolyte derangements can lead to abnormal action potentials and change neuronal membrane excitability (Plum & Posner, 1982). Additionally, toxins, either exogenous or endogenous, disrupt the normal balance of neurotransmitters such as dopamine, GABA, acetylcholine, and serotonin, thereby altering the mental state of the pediatric patient.

EPIDEMIOLOGY AND ETIOLOGY

Acute toxic/metabolic encephalopathies

Acute toxic/metabolic encephalopathy *excludes* the possibility of primary structural brain disease, traumatic brain injury (i.e., brain tumor or hemorrhage), or infection (i.e., meningitis or encephalitis). Instead, it is defined as a condition of acute global cerebral dysfunction resulting in altered consciousness, behavior changes, and/or seizures (Parke, 2006). In general, the pathophysiology of this category of encephalopathy is a result of cytotoxic injury and neurotransmitter disruption as previously described.

Hypoxic-ischemic encephalopathy (HIE) is an important type of toxic/metabolic encephalopathy that occurs after an event deprives the brain of adequate perfusion or oxygenation, resulting in cerebral ischemia and hypoxia due to delivery of insufficient supplies of oxygen to sustain cellular viability. The event can occur before, during, and after birth as a result of trauma, asphyxiation, congenital abnormality, stroke, medications, and prematurity. In older pediatric patients, it can also result from asphyxiation, airway obstruction with foreign body or airway edema, submersion injury, severe asthma, sepsis, low cardiac output states, chronic hypoxia from pulmonary disease, respiratory and circulatory arrest, systemic hemorrhage, carbon monoxide poisoning, and cardiac arrhythmias.

Many factors influence the severity of neurological sequelae associated with HIE, such as the duration of hypoxia and hypotension (Jacinto et al., 2001). It remains difficult to prognosticate the long-term outcome of HIE; factors such as historical features of events leading to injury, physical examination findings, neuroradiological imaging, and neurophysiological data aid in predicting outcomes (Abend & Licht, 2008).

Other etiologies of acute toxic/metabolic encephalopathy are listed in Table 33-13.

Other acute encephalopathies

Infections are a prominent cause of encephalopathy within the pediatric population. Such disease may be a result of direct pathogen insult to brain tissue, systemic inflammatory response, or immune response to infectious agents. Examples of infections associated with encephalopathy include sepsis, viral and bacterial meningitis and encephalitis, fungal meningitis, tuberculosis meningitis, and parasitic infection. AIDS encephalopathy is a complication for many patients with congenital HIV infection. Para-infectious encephalopathy can develop from both active and postinfectious causes such as acute disseminated encephalomyelitis (ADEM), in which lymphocytes attack the myelin sheath (Parke, 2006).

Vasculature disorders can contribute to alterations is cerebral functioning. Severe hypertension, hemorrhage and stroke, and autoimmune disease can result in changes to cerebral vasculature leading to encephalopathy. Hypertensive encephalopathy is a reversible medical emergency in which the systemic blood pressure exceeds the ability of the cerebral vessels to autoregulate it, leading to damaged cerebral arterioles. Posterior reversible encephalopathy syndrome (PRES) is associated with kidney disease; the overall clinical outcome with this type of encephalopathy is good if the patient is treated promptly (Hu et al., 2008). Cerebrovascular hemorrhage may occur with arteriovenous malformations. Bleeding into the parenchyma, subarachnoid, subdural, or epidural spaces can cause marked mental status changes and intracranial pressure changes. Occlusive vascular disease such as thrombi or emboli, although rare in children, can occur, leading to ischemia and infarct. In children, the majority of strokes are ischemic rather than hemorrhagic (Roach et al., 2008). Congenital heart disease, Moyamoya disease, infection, and dehydration are disorders that leave children vulnerable to hemorrhagic infarcts. Traumatic brain injury (TBI) may result in cerebral contusion or intracranial hemorrhage, as well as permitting secondary injury to occur from sequelae such as hypoxia and seizures.

TABLE 33-13

Etiologies for Acute Toxic/Metabolic Encephalopathies
Hypoglycemia
• Ketotic hypoglycemia
• Over-administration of insulin
• Hyperinsulinism
Hyperglycemia
• Diabetic ketoacidosis
• Non-ketotic hyperosmolar hyperglycemia (NKHH)
Electrolyte Imbalances
• Hyponatremia
• Hypernatremia
• Hypercalcemia
• Hypermagnesemia
Organ Dysfunction
• Liver
• Kidney
• Pancreatic
• Adrenal
Medication and Environment
• Ethanol
• Sedative medications
• Salicylates
• Anticholinergic medications
• Chemotherapeutic agents
• Hydrocarbons
• Carbon monoxide
• Lead
• Organophosphates
Inborn Errors of Metabolism
• Hypoglycemia
• Hyperammoninemia
• Lactic acidosis

Intracranial hypertension is the result of an increase in the volume of matter within the skull cavity. The skull becomes rigid after the fusion of the fontanels. Accumulation of blood, CSF, edema, and brain neoplasm in this space will, therefore, raise the intracranial pressure and may lead to cerebral hypoperfusion, edema, and encephalopathy.

Status epilepticus (prolonged), with associated blood pressure instability, hypercarbia, and hypoxia, can precipitate permanent neuronal damage.

Static encephalopathy

Static encephalopathy is a type of cerebral dysfunction this is permanent and nonprogressive. Patients may have abnormal motor function; mental retardation; sensory deficits such as blindness, deafness, and/or inability to communicate; and seizures. Identification of this form of encephalopathy is a diagnosis of exclusion. Cerebral palsy is often considered a manifestation of static encephalopathy, although is not synonymous with it.

Great care must be taken to differentiate progressive disorders from true static encephalopathy. The types of static encephalopathy correlate with the area of the brain affected. Causes of neurological insult in such patients include prematurity, infections, ischemia, asphyxia, ischemia, and kernicterus.

Progressive encephalopathies

Neurodegenerative disorders account for a large portion of progressive encephalopathies. These disorders present as a progressive deterioration of neurological function, sometimes in a previously well child, and are a result of specific biochemical or genetic defects, infections, or other unknown causes. The age of onset varies, as does the rate of progression. The number of disorders is vast and overlaps with many inborn errors of metabolism. Among the more well-known disorders are Tay-Sachs disease, mucopolysaccharidosis types I and II, adrenoleukodystrophy, mitochondrial encephalopathies such as MELAS, and spinocerebellar ataxia.

PRESENTATION

The mental status changes associated with encephalopathy are often initially subtle, yet eventually prompt caregivers to seek medical attention for their child. The report may be of irritability, poor feeding, or lethargy in the infant, or personality or cognitive changes, such as an inability to concentrate, in the older child. In addition, more severe symptoms may be present, such as perceptual deficits, seizures, decreased level of consciousness, or coma.

Physical examination findings also vary along a spectrum from mild to severe. The child may be awake but disoriented, seizing, or unarousable. Deep tendon reflexes may be abnormal. Pupillary response may be absent, pinpoint, or sluggish; nystagmus may be noted. Motor symptoms may be present, such as tremor, asymmetry, asterixis, hemiparesis, myoclonic jerks, hypotonia, hypertonia, and decerebrate or decorticate posturing. The respiratory pattern may be unremarkable; alternatively, the child may demonstrate apnea. The cardiovascular examination may reveal heart murmurs, irregular rhythm, or poor perfusion.

DIFFERENTIAL DIAGNOSIS

The differential diagnosis is based on whether the encephalopathy is acute or progressive and age of presentation. Table 33-14 provides a list of potential diagnoses for consideration.

PLAN OF CARE

Complete blood count with differential, comprehensive metabolic panel, liver function tests that include bilirubin and ammonia levels, coagulation studies, blood gases, and toxicology screens provide an initial basis from which to determine the etiology of the encephalopathy. The CBC

TABLE 33-14

Differential Diagnoses for Encephalopathy
• Abusive head trauma
• Acute disseminated encephalomyelitis
• Anorexia or bulimia
• Arrhythmia
• Asphyxia
• Arteriovenous malformation
• Cardiomyopathy
• Cerebral vascular accident
• Congenital adrenal hyperplasia
• Congenital heart disease
• Diabetic ketoacidosis
• Electrolyte imbalance
• Encephalitis
• Hepatic failure
• Hepatitis
• Hypoglycemia
• Inborn error of metabolism
• Intoxication/overdose
• Intracranial hemorrhage
• Intracranial tumor
• Kernicterus
• Kidney failure
• Mad cow disease (Crutzfeldt-Jakob disease)
• Meningitis
• Neurodegenerative disease
• Psychosis
• Reye's syndrome
• Seizure disorder
• Submersion injury
• Syndrome of inappropriate antidiuretic hormone

is useful in evaluating for inflammation or infection, anemia, and immune function. The metabolic panel will identify electrolyte imbalances, kidney function, hydration status, and serum glucose levels. Liver function tests provide information regarding enzyme activity and accumulation of toxic metabolites such as bilirubin or ammonia. Coagulation panels may reveal coagulopathy or hypercoagulable states, as well as liver function. Arterial blood gases provide information on acid–base and oxygenation/ventilation balance. The carboxyhemoglobin level may be evaluated on the blood gas if the suspected source of the child's illness is a fire or gas heater dysfunction. Toxicology screens are important in every age group.

Other tests that can be used to evaluate for infection are blood, urine, and CSF cultures, as well as viral studies with polymerase chain reaction (PCR). If there is clinical suspicion for inborn errors of metabolism, then serum amino acid panels and urine organic acid panels should be ordered. Thyroid function studies and cortisol levels are useful when an endocrine etiology is suspected.

Neuroimaging is essential for identifying acute causes of encephalopathy, which may be reversible if identified and treated early. The CT scan is usually the first diagnostic study to consider in patients who are encephalopathic. This rapid, noninvasive test yields valuable information when trauma, stroke, neoplasm, and raised ICP are suspected. CT scan is considered the modality of choice to identify acute hemorrhage and calcifications. Depending on the level of density and relation to the brain, it may also identify inflammation, edema, necrosis, infarct, and neoplasms. Neurodegenerative diseases may be identified by changes in the white and gray matter. Contrast-enhanced CT is useful for identification of neoplasm, arteriovenous malformation, and infections such as empyema and abscess.

Magnetic resonance imaging is more sensitive than CT and avoids radiation exposure, but is often less practical. Vascular and hemorrhagic disease is more readily identifiable with MRI, and even more so with newer MRA technology.

Electroencephalography is valuable for identifying seizures, particularly subclinical events. EEG may also allow for confirmation of global dysfunction.

The initial management for a child with encephalopathy is always based on the severity of symptoms and follows the standard resuscitation guidelines for airway, breathing, and circulation (ABCs). In the case of neurological instability, pediatric patients may lose important pharyngeal reflexes, which protect the airway and lungs from aspiration (i.e., gag and cough reflexes). A depressed sensorium may lead to an inadequate respiratory drive, hypoventilation, and respiratory arrest. Neuromuscular weakness or seizures may compromise the patient's airway, oxygenation, and ventilation (Adelson et al., 2003).

Endotracheal intubation in the encephalopathic child is particularly dangerous if increased ICP is suspected;

therefore, proper cerebroprotective technique is necessary to decrease the body's response to laryngoscopy and intubation. Circulatory management in the encephalopathic patient depends on physical examination findings. Patients in shock states should be resuscitated with appropriate isotonic fluids, and vasoactive and inotropic pharmacological agents should be administered if indicated. Vasodilating agents may be necessary for patients in hypertensive states, especially if increased ICP and coagulopathy are present. The patient's glucose level should be checked and therapy directed by these results. Mild hypothermia to improve clinical outcomes in non-neonates is under study (Kochanek et al., 2009).

All medications should be evaluated for their contribution to the patient's encephalopathic state. Complete removal or sudden discontinuation of a medication is not always in the patient's best interest, as additional effects such as withdrawal or seizures may occur; thus a reduced dose or change to another medication may be warranted. Electrolyte and glucose imbalances should be corrected with care to avoid both hypo-osmolar and hyperosmolar states. Antiviral, antifungal, and antimicrobial agents to treat infection should be administered early in the course of disease, if indicated. Medications to treat seizures should be given promptly. For the more static and progressive encephalopathies, spasticity medications can greatly improve the discomfort of children with neuromuscular manifestations.

Early consultation with specialists is important. Depending on the etiology, specialists from critical care, neurosurgery, neurology, nephrology, cardiology, endocrinology, rheumatology, pulmonology, genetics, and rehabilitation medicine are useful in providing direction to diagnostic evaluation and management. Additional consultation with child life specialists, social services, spiritual advisors, and physical and occupational therapists should be considered.

DISPOSITION AND DISCHARGE PLANNING

Intensive care is indicated for patients with severe encephalopathy who require airway and ventilation management, patients who are in shock, those with a rapidly deteriorating neurological status, or those requiring emergency surgery. Hospitalizations can be long and recovery slow. Rehabilitation needs should be identified early in the diagnosis, so as to optimize the physical and cognitive outcomes. Interprofessional coordination is necessary after the acute phase passes, as long-term medications and therapy may be necessary. For those patients with permanent neurological conditions, tracheostomy, home ventilation, and gastrostomy feeding may be required. These technologies require intensive service coordination by the hospital so that families can successfully care for their family member at home.

HOSPITAL PSYCHOSIS AND DEPRESSION

Christopher C. Rich

PATHOPHYSIOLOGY

The exact causes of psychosis and other mental illnesses, such as schizophrenia, generalized anxiety disorder, or major depressive disorder, are not specifically known, but are part of a multifactorial process that contributes to the overall presentation a HCP may encounter with a mentally ill pediatric patient. Neurotransmitters such as dopamine, norepinephrine, and serotonin appear to play vital roles in the intricate balance of chemical reactions in the central nervous system that help regulate an individual's mood and ability to think rationally and clearly. Medications used to treat mood disorders and psychoses often target these neurotransmitters, even though the exact cause of these disorders remains unknown. For the purpose of this section, psychosis will be defined as specified by the American Academy of Child and Adolescent Psychiatry (AACAP): "Psychotic disorders include severe mental disorders which are characterized by extreme impairment of a person's ability to think clearly, respond emotionally, communicate effectively, understand reality, and behave appropriately" (AACAP, 2009b).

EPIDEMIOLOGY AND ETIOLOGY

The evidence supporting diagnosis of pediatric-onset psychosis is rare, particularly in children younger than the age of 11; prevalence in this age group is 0.01 to 0.05 per 1,000 population (Joshi & Towbin, 2002). Five percent of adults who have schizophrenia report that their symptoms began before the age of 15 years (Imran & Clark, 2008). The overall prevalence of psychosis increases dramatically during the adolescent years. The male-to-female ratio is 2:1 in childhood, but is balanced in adulthood (McClellan & Werry, 2001). There is also a suspected correlation between early-onset psychosis with pediatric patients who have impaired cognition and lower intelligence quotients (IQs) (Joshi & Towbin).

Pediatric bipolar disorder was once thought to be quite rare in children and adolescents, but estimates of its prevalence have increased since changes were made in how the disorder is diagnosed in pediatrics. The estimated lifetime prevalence is approximately 1%, with a significant number of adult bipolar patients admitting their symptoms (usually depressive symptoms) originated during their childhood years. Currently, debate focuses on the exact definition of bipolar disorder in pediatric patients and the appropriateness of using adult criteria in this population (American Psychiatric Association [APA], 2000). Manic symptoms in pediatric patients are generally seen as "atypical," most likely due to developmental differences in children and adolescents (McClellan et al., 2007). Interestingly, one-half of bipolar patients are originally diagnosed with schizophrenia (McClellan & Werry, 2001).

Pediatric depression can be fairly common among children and adolescents. The point prevalence is 1% to 2% for prepubertal children and 3% to 8% for adolescents. The lifetime prevalence is 20% by the end of adolescence. The female-to-male ratio of pediatric depression in childhood is 1:1, but in adolescence it changes to 2:1. Notably, there is a twofold to fourfold increase in a child's risk of developing this condition when a first-degree relative has been diagnosed with pediatric depression (Zalsman et al., 2006).

Pediatric anxiety disorders represent one of the most common forms of childhood mental illness. Previous epidemiological studies indicated that the prevalence of having at least one pediatric anxiety disorder ranges from 6% to 20%, with children often having other comorbid anxiety or depressive disorders. Children with anxiety disorders can also be at risk for developing substance abuse disorders (Connolly & Bernstein, 2007). Specifically, pediatric patients with social anxiety disorder have a greater risk of developing both cannabis and alcohol dependence compared to their peers with other anxiety disorders. A recent study found that there was a greater than 6.5 likelihood of cannabis dependence and 4.5 likelihood of alcohol dependence in such patients (Buchner et al., 2008).

Having a chronic medical illness can be very challenging for a pediatric patient, both physically and emotionally. Some evidence suggests that physical illness in childhood can cause psychological stress, which may then lead to anxiety and mood fluctuations. The amount of stress is affected by how long the illness lasts, what the development stage of the child is, whether the illness is life-threatening, and how much support the pediatric patient receives from family and friends. The coexistence of other psychological factors, such as an underlying mood or psychotic disorder, will also affect the overall level of stress (Krener & Wasserman, 1994). This interface between the physical and psychological aspects of a pediatric patient's disease is extremely important. Patients with CNS illnesses, such as tumors or seizures, and those with multiple physical problems have an increased risk of developing psychiatric disorders, such as anxiety and depressive disorders (DeMaso et al., 2009). Influences related to development, cognition, and the pediatric patient's biological, psychological, environmental, and social factors all play vital roles in determining the individual's mental health and overall emotional stability.

PRESENTATION

When assessing a pediatric patient's mental illness, HCPs are encouraged to use the biopsychosocial model to focus on all aspects of the patient's care. Oftentimes, HCPs fail to recognize the multifaceted issues influencing a patient's physical and emotional stability, as the presentation of depression or psychosis in an already medically ill child can be both varied and unique.

The most important factor in determining the proper diagnosis when a pediatric patient presents with acute-onset mental status changes is a detailed and thorough history, including a timeline leading up to the moment the symptoms began. It is vital to ask about family history of medical and psychiatric disorders, the patient's developmental history, past medical and psychiatric treatments, and any previous hospitalizations and medications. Common medications used in pediatric populations can cause adverse side effects consistent with psychotic symptoms—in particular, steroids, prescribed medications, and over-the-counter (OTC) cough medicines, stimulants, diet pills, and consumption of energy drinks. As many as 50% of patients who have been diagnosed with a psychiatric illness also have a diagnosable substance abuse issue. A thorough medical and neurological examination is also imperative.

A pediatric patient who has just recently been diagnosed with type 1 diabetes mellitus, for example, may present with typical depressive symptoms—sad, withdrawn mood; inability to fall asleep; poor self-esteem; low motivation; decreased energy; poor concentration; and even suicidal thinking. These new symptoms may be temporary or last for several weeks. Under these circumstances, the HCP would consider diagnosis of a major depressive disorder, as the patient is having a difficult time adjusting to the news that he or she has a lifelong illness. This same diabetic patient may later present with an altered mental status, fluctuating mood symptoms, and variable energy states; in this setting, the HCP might consider hypoglycemia or hyperglycemia as a reason for the acute mental status change. In each case, the patient exhibits a change in his or her mental state, but the root cause is very different—and the treatment approach will be different as well.

To make a diagnosis of a psychotic disorder, the same *Diagnostic and Statistical Manual of Mental Disorders*, fourth edition (*DSM-IV-TR*) criteria are used for both pediatric and adult patients (APA, 2000). Children often present with visual and auditory hallucinations. Other features of pediatric illness may include the following conditions:

- Disorganized speech and behaviors
- Low motivation
- Poor maintenance of activities of daily living, such as grooming and hygiene
- Paucity of spontaneous speech
- Restricted range of facial expressions or moods
- Significant disturbance in overall social, family, and school functioning
- Disturbance that lasts at least 6 months

- Other disorders, such as substance abuse, a general medical condition, or a mood disorder with psychotic features, have been sufficiently ruled out

Pediatric bipolar disorder can often be a confusing and difficult diagnosis to make in a developing child or adolescent; as with schizophrenia, the same *DSM-IV-TR* criteria are used for both adult and pediatric patients. Pediatric bipolar disorder is characterized by a distinct period of abnormally or persistently elevated, expansive, or irritable mood, lasting at least 1 week or for any duration if the child is hospitalized for the disorder. During the period of mood disturbance, the child will often present with the following symptoms:

- Inflated self-esteem or grandiose mood states
- Decreased need for sleep
- Flight of ideas or a subjective feeling that thoughts are racing
- Pressured speech or more talkative than usual
- Distractibility and an increase in goal-directed activities
- Involvement in risky behaviors that have the possibility of painful consequences

Pediatric bipolar disorder can also present with primarily depressive symptoms, mixed symptoms (where criteria are met for both a manic episode and a depressive episode), or psychotic symptoms in the context of the acute mood disturbance. Some patients may present with catatonic symptoms, such as stiffness, motoric immobility, mutism, peculiar voluntary movements, posturing, and extreme negativism. Catatonic symptoms in a child or adolescent are quite rare, but can be a medical emergency and require swift diagnosis and treatment. In each case, the mood disturbance is not due to a general medical condition such as hyperthyroidism or the direct physiological effects of a substance such as cocaine or methamphetamine (APA, 2000).

DIFFERENTIAL DIAGNOSIS

When a pediatric patient has symptoms of a physical illness and presents with symptoms of a mental illness, the differential diagnosis list lengthens. Other factors take on an important role, such as a patient's genetic history, personality, psychological factors, and social environment. It is vital to determine if the presentation is occurring secondary to a *DSM-IV-TR* psychiatric disorder, such as major depression or schizophrenia, or if the presentation is occurring secondary to an underlying medical issue. Oftentimes HCPs will use the term "functional" versus "organic" when making this distinction. Differentiating between the two is very important for developing an appropriate therapeutic plan.

The differential diagnoses for a *functional psychosis* are substantial and can come from different categories in the *DSM-IV-TR*. Patients who present with psychotic symptoms are simply termed "schizophrenic"; however, the following distinctions should be recognized:

- Brief psychotic disorder (fewer than 30 days of psychotic behavior)
- Schizophreniform disorder (more than 30 days but fewer than 6 months of psychotic behavior)
- Schizoaffective disorder (a combination of both mood and psychotic symptoms, independent of each other)

Pediatric patients who have bipolar disorder can present in a manic, psychotic state and appear as if they have paranoid schizophrenia. Patients who have major depression can also present with derogatory, mood-congruent auditory hallucinations that appear to be due to a primary psychotic illness. As the mood symptoms improve, however, the psychotic symptoms usually subside. If they do not, and if the patient continues to display psychotic symptoms in the context of a normal mood, the patient would likely be diagnosed with schizoaffective disorder as previously described. If a patient presents with catatonic symptoms, it is vital to evaluate him or her for a medical cause such as neuroleptic malignant or serotonin syndromes, as these conditions, if left untreated, can lead to death.

Anxiety disorders can also present with acute mental status changes. When a pediatric patient has experienced a trauma such as physical injury or recent sexual abuse, he or she may present with an altered mental state and dissociative features of post-traumatic stress disorder (PTSD). Children who have an acute streptococcal infection may develop pediatric autoimmune neuropsychiatric disorder associated with *Streptococcus* (PANDA). With this disease, the patient's own immune system attacks parts of the brain that are associated with repetitive movements. Affected patients may present with symptoms suggestive of obsessive–compulsive disorder, tic disorder, and Tourette's syndrome. In particular, the pediatric patient may present with repetitive movements, throat clearing, grunting, and obsessive behaviors. A pediatric patient who is stressed and anxious due to a medical illness or a deceased family member may experience a brief reactive psychosis that should subside as the stress of the event diminishes.

Pediatric patients who have developmental delay, cognitive disorders, or mental retardation may appear to have disorganized thoughts, detachment from reality, and abnormal behaviors, which are attributed to the patient's limited mental capacity. Patients who have pervasive developmental disorders such as autism or Asperger's disorder may display impairment in social interactions, communication irregularities, and repetitive, stereotyped behaviors, which may appear unusual and be confused with psychosis. It should be noted that autistic children do not normally present with hallucinations or delusions (APA, 2000).

At times pediatric patients will present with conversion disorder, which is characterized by confusing neurological signs and symptoms or deficits affecting their motor or sensory function. After a thorough medical work-up for neurological deficit, if no medical condition is found, psychological factors are considered to be the major reason for the dysfunction. Such a disturbance causes significant distress and impairment in overall functioning. Conversion disorder is classified as one of the somatoform disorders, which also include somatization disorder, undifferentiated somatoform disorder, pain disorder, hypochondriasis, and body dysmorphic disorder. It is important to recognize that the pediatric patient with conversion disorder is *not* malingering (i.e., intentionally producing symptoms for external motives, such as avoiding school or criminal consequences) or purposely playing the "sick role" to get more attention from caregivers, as seen in factitious disorder (APA, 2000).

The differential diagnosis list for *organic psychosis* can be as substantial and varied as functional psychosis. When a pediatric patient presents with an acute-onset mental status change, he or she should always have a thorough medical examination and neurological evaluation. The list of potential organic causes is long and includes the following:

- CNS disorders such as seizures (temporal lobe epilepsy), lipid storage disorders, Huntington's chorea, brain tumor, and traumatic brain injury
- Delirium, which can occur secondary to many different medical disorders
- Metabolic disorders, such as endocrine disorders, Wilson's disease, electrolyte disturbances, and blood sugar abnormalities
- Developmental disorders such as velocardiofacial syndrome
- Toxic disorders such as CNS infections, fever, and ingestion of heavy metals; substances such as cocaine, amphetamines, phencyclidine (PCP), alcohol, and OTC cold medicines; or medications such as stimulants, steroids, and anticholinergic agents
- Infectious diseases such as meningitis, encephalitis, and HIV

PLAN OF CARE

The initial therapeutic plan for a pediatric patient who presents with acute onset of mental status change includes ruling out organic causes. For example, a pediatric patient who appears depressed and lethargic may have hypothyroidism; a pediatric patient presenting with euphoria, decreased need for sleep, and paranoia may have used a psychoactive drug such as methamphetamine. In both cases, diagnostic studies could identify the underlying etiology and lead to proper therapeutic management. Laboratory studies include complete metabolic panel, which should include kidney function and liver enzymes; CBC; thyroid-stimulating hormone (TSH); rapid plasma reagin (RPR), and HIV tests for sexually active patients. Additionally, a toxicology screen for drugs of abuse and measurement of therapeutic drug levels for prescribed patient medications, such as valproic acid or lithium, are suggested.

Imaging studies are not traditionally used when assessing patients with acute-onset psychiatric symptoms, but are important in diagnosing CNS infections and lesions. Lumbar puncture, brain MRI, or CT scan may be indicated in these circumstances. An EEG should be considered to evaluate the patient for underlying seizure activity (temporal lobe epilepsy). At times, overt seizure may not be evident and the behavioral disturbances are the only symptomology.

The primary goal in therapeutic management of a pediatric patient who presents with signs of acute mental status changes is to ensure the safety of the patient. It is also important to protect the safety of the family, HCPs, and other hospital staff if the patient is agitated or shows symptoms of aggression or violence. The HCP must evaluate the patient for current suicidal or homicidal ideation, previous suicide attempts, and past episodes of violent or aggressive behaviors. Past episodes of suicidal, violent, or aggressive behavior are the best predictor of future behaviors that might put the patient or other HCPs at risk for harm.

Approaching the patient's management from the biopsychosocial perspective emphasizes biological and psychosocial interventions and focuses the care provided by interprofessional team. The HCP must determine whether the pediatric patient is at risk of harming self or someone else. If the patient is unable to be adequately maintained in the current setting, brief hospitalization on an inpatient psychiatric unit may be indicated. The decision to place the patient in this unit should be made in concert with social services professionals and the psychiatric consultation-liaison team.

If the patient's underlying illness is primarily organic in nature, providing the appropriate therapeutic management will usually address the mental status changes. In contrast, those patients with mental status changes due functional causes such as anxiety, depression, or psychotic illnesses will require ongoing evaluation. If, for example, a pediatric patient's acute-onset racing thoughts, pressured speech, expansive moods, and impulsivity are the result of a manic episode, treating the patient with a mood stabilizer such as lithium or valproic acid is indicated. In any event, it is important to review the specific *DSM-IV-TR* criteria to make the correct diagnosis and then formulate a therapeutic management plan based on the biopsychosocial model.

Medications may be indicated to treat underlying mental status change. This section is not designed to give a comprehensive overview of all drugs used to treat psychiatric illnesses, but will address the most common medications. In general, the following classes of medications are used to treat various illnesses:

- Selective serotonin reuptake inhibitors (SSRIs—fluoxetine, sertraline) are used for depressive and anxiety disorders.

- Mood stabilizers (lithium, valproic acid, carbamazepine, other anticonvulsants) are used to treat unstable moods such as bipolar disorder.
- Antipsychotic medications (haloperidol, clozapine, risperidone, olanzapine, quetiapine, ziprasidone, aripiprazole) are used for a variety of disorders, such as aggression and irritability seen with autism, mood instability, psychosis, tic disorders, and anxiety disorders.

Very few medications have been approved by the U.S. Food and Drug Administration (FDA) to treat pediatric psychiatric disorders. However, in recent years, with the support of research, the list of approved medications has increased (Table 33-15).

TABLE 33-15

FDA-Approved Medications for the Treatment of Children with Mental Health Disorders

Selective Serotonin Reuptake Inhibitors

- Fluoxetine for major depressive disorder (ages 8–18) and obsessive–compulsive disorder (ages 7–17)
- Fluvoxamine for obsessive–compulsive disorder (ages 8–17)
- Sertraline for obsessive–compulsive disorder (ages 6–17)
- Escitalopram for major depressive disorder (ages 12–17)

Tricyclic Antidepressants

- Clomipramine for obsessive–compulsive disorder (ages > 10)

Mood Stabilizers

- Lithium for bipolar disorder (ages 2–18)

Antipsychotic Medications

- Chlorpromazine for severe behavioral disorders (ages 6 months–5 years)
- Prochlorperazine maleate for schizophrenia (ages 2–5)
- Haloperidol for psychosis (ages 3–18), Tourette's syndrome (ages 3–18), and severe behavioral disorders and agitation (ages 3–18)
- Aripiprazole for schizophrenia (ages 13–17); bipolar disorder, manic/mixed (ages 10–17); and autism-related irritability (ages 6–17)
- Risperidone for schizophrenia (ages 13–17); bipolar disorder, manic/mixed (ages 10–17); and autism-related irritability (ages 5–16)

Benzodiazepines

- Lorazepam for pediatric anxiety (age unspecified)
- Diazepam for pediatric anxiety (ages > 6 months)
- Chlordiazepoxide for pediatric anxiety (ages > 6 months)

Source: Adapted from Epocrates Online (http://online.epocrates.com).

One of the many benefits of working with pediatric patients is that they generally improve; there is a resiliency in children that one may not appreciate with adult patients. Abusive parents, broken homes, school problems, peer relationships, physical illness, and mental illness affect pediatric patients differently; children who are resilient are able to overcome these difficulties and move forward with their lives. HCPs and the adults who care for these patients can undoubtedly assist in this process, as pediatric patients require hope, love, and stable, supportive relationships to be successful. These staples promote self-esteem, build confidence, and support the patient's ability to overcome trials and tribulations, which in turn leads to an increased resiliency.

A pediatric psychiatrist, and optimally an interprofessional psychiatric team, is essential in the diagnostic and supportive care of a patient presenting with psychosis or depression. In addition, it may be beneficial to consult a neuropsychologist to consider neuropsychological testing to assess the patient's overall cognitive and adaptive functioning. This assessment may identify the patient's strengths and weaknesses and assist the family in planning for additional social and academic support. Child life specialists are helpful in reducing the effects of hospitalization. Coordinating with the patient's school HCP and counselor ensures academic support for the patient when he or she returns to school. A request for an individual educational plan (IEP) for the patient may also be developed as part of the hospital discharge plan. Awareness of available therapies in the community allows the family to better plan for their child's care.

To ensure appropriate therapeutic management and prevent subsequent acute phases of the illness, the family needs to be educated about the cause of the illness, the significance of regular follow-up care, and the importance of adhering to prescribed medications. Stressing the importance of adherence to medication regimens and outpatient follow-up appointments also reiterates the diagnosis and its need for continued management.

DISPOSITION AND DISCHARGE PLANNING

One of the most important aspects of treatment planning for children with mental health issues is appropriate disposition and coordination of discharge plans with the patient and caregivers. A continuum of care may be accessed to aid in stabilizing the patient, such as group homes, residential treatment centers, inpatient psychiatric units, day treatment programs, intensive outpatient programs, traditional outpatient therapy, and medication management. Group homes and residential treatment centers are indicated when long-term issues are being addressed and the patient has been stabilized following the acute phase of the illness. Inpatient treatment is necessary for patients who cannot be safely maintained in an outpatient setting and require 24-hour nursing care to help stabilize and monitor the acute phase of their illness.

Unfortunately, limited information exists as to the efficacy of inpatient hospitalization when compared to day treatment settings. Oftentimes, inpatient hospitalization is a necessary care strategy when preparing the patient for enrollment in a day treatment program or outpatient care. A study from the *Journal of the American Academy of Child and Adolescent Psychiatry* demonstrated the effectiveness of adolescent day treatment programs. These researchers found that such treatment programs were more cost-efficient and less disruptive for the patient and family than inpatient hospitalization. Notably, however, the programs did not provide the same level of support, structure, and stabilization as are available in a hospital setting (Milin et al., 2000).

The AACAP developed the Child and Adolescent Service Intensity Instrument (CASII) as a scale to help determine the appropriate level of care for a pediatric patient, regardless of setting or diagnosis. This tool is able to integrate three distinct types of disorders: psychiatric disorders, substance abuse disorders, and developmental disorders (including autism and mental retardation). The scores are then combined and the information is assimilated to generate a recommended level of care. The scale ranges from 0 (basic services) to 7 (24-hour care; admission to a locked psychiatric or residential unit). AACAP provides 1- and 2-day courses on the scale's utilization and encourages the use of this tool when determining patient disposition (AACAP, 2009a).

The prognosis for pediatric patients with acute-onset mental status changes varies according to the underlying cause of the illness. A good prognosis is indicated when the pediatric patient has no evident family psychiatric history, good premorbid functioning with no previous psychiatric diagnosis, and an illness that is acute with a relatively short duration. Other positive indicators include a patient who has good insight into the illness and strong social and family support. A poor prognosis is associated with a family history of schizophrenia, impaired premorbid functioning, inadequate social support, and an illness that is insidious and presents over a longer time period.

Regular follow-up appointments with mental health professionals should be established prior to discharge to monitor medications and frequently assess the patient's mental status. If the patient has an underlying medical illness, he or she should have consistent contact with the PCP.

HYDROCEPHALUS AND INTRACRANIAL SHUNT DISORDERS

Judie Holleman, Amanda Johnson, and Paula Zakrzewski

PATHOPHYSIOLOGY

Cerebrospinal fluid (CSF) is primarily produced by the choroid plexus and is deposited within the ventricular system, where it provides nutrients, proteins, and a protective cushion for the brain and spinal cord. The CSF flows through the ventricular system and central spinal canal through a series of channels and then exits. This arrangement allows the subarachnoid spaces and the venous sinuses to reabsorb CSF, which returns the volume to the systemic venous circulation (Rekate, 2008).

Obstruction or malformation of various components of the CSF pathway may cause the accumulation of fluid within one or more of the compartments of the ventricular system (Figure 33-13). Hydrocephalus is the pathologic accumulation of fluid resulting from overproduction of CSF, obstructed channels or aqueducts, or impaired absorption (Rekate, 2008) (Figure 33-14). It is associated with multifaceted congenital abnormalities, complications of prematurity, and other acquired diseases.

Congenital hydrocephalus is frequently obstructive, often within the aqueduct of Sylvius or arachnoid cysts. *Acquired* hydrocephalus is the result of trauma, hemorrhage, or a tumor; it is nonabsorptive in nature. *Iatrogenic* hydrocephalus is a result of inadequate CSF drainage because of a shunting device failure or ventriculostomy closure.

Shunting systems

Prior to the 1950s, the limited array of treatments for hydrocephalus posed great risk of disability and death. Modern treatment options have ensured that affected children have an opportunity for a comparatively normal life. The valve-regulated shunt has become the mainstay of treatment.

Such shunts represent life-saving technology for children and adults, who experience improved and prolonged life expectancy after their placement. However, the challenge of keeping shunts working without complication is difficult. Placing a shunt in an infant or child requires a lifetime of specialized care, including transitioning care delivery from a pediatric-focused HCP to an adult-focused HCP (Rekate, 2008).

Valved shunting systems rely on open communication among the various CSF compartments. Devices commonly used for this purpose include ventricular and lumbar shunts. Ventricular proximal catheters are placed within the lateral ventricles, with the flexible distal catheter being placed with the peritoneum, the pleural cavity, the right atrium, or another absorptive surface area compartment. Lumbar proximal catheters are placed within the lumbar subarachnoid space, with the distal catheter being placed in the same compartment as the ventricular proximal catheter.

Valve options include differential pressure valves and programmable valves. Differential pressure valves open when the intraventricular pressure exceeds a predetermined threshold, thereby allowing CSF to flow (i.e., at low, medium, or high pressure). Programmable valves (e.g., Codman, Strata, Sophie) have the capability to adjust the opening pressure threshold through use of an external magnetic device. In addition, a siphon-resisting device or an antigravity device may be added to mimic physiologic influences of gravity and position on CSF flow.

The introduction of ventricular endoscopy has provided the option of ventricular fenestration for CSF outflow. Endoscopic third ventriculostomy (ETV) offers a key advantage—freedom from shunting devices, thereby eliminating the lifetime risks of infection and device malfunction. The disadvantage of ETV is its moderately high

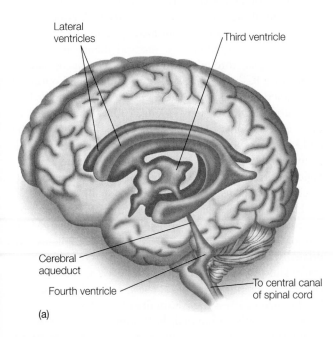

FIGURE 33-13

Ventricles.

Source: Chiras, D. (2008). *Human Biology, 6th Ed.* Sudbury, MA: Jones & Bartlett.

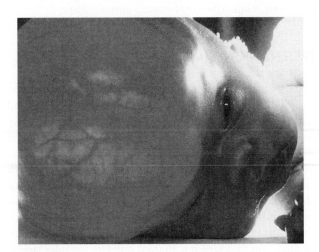

FIGURE 33-14

Hydrocephalus.
Source: © SIU/Visuals Unlimited.

closure or failure rate in the developing infant, which necessitates consideration of further shunting options.

EPIDEMIOLOGY AND ETIOLOGY

The incidence of congenital hydrocephalus is estimated at 1 patient per 1,000 live births. Nevertheless, because hydrocephalus has a high association with myelomengiocele, Chiari II malformation, and other conditions, its true incidence is difficult to determine (Cartwright, 2004; Rekate, 2008). Acquired hydrocephalus can occur after intracerebral hemorrhage, brain tumor, meningitis, or head injury.

According to the Hydrocephalus Association (2009), 40,000 shunt-related operations occur annually in the United States. Potential shunt complications include malfunction, infection, intracranial hypertension or hemorrhage, and disproportionate drainage. A shunt may malfunction from obstruction, catheter misplacement, or disconnection. Obstruction can occur from protein particles occluding either the proximal or distal shunt catheter. Shunts are also associated with infection, which occurs in 5% to 10% of patients after shunt placement (Cartwright, 2004). Intracranial hemorrhage can occur during the placement or removal of the ventricular catheter. In addition, patients are at risk of bowel perforation during the placement of the distal catheter; development of abdominal pseudocysts; and migration of the catheter, which may then erode tissues within the peritoneum.

Insufficient drainage will allow symptomatic hydrocephalus to continue; conversely, over-drainage may cause subdural hemorrhage. Lifelong shunting alters the brain compliance and may lead to slit ventricle syndrome and pseudotumor cerebrii. Other complications of shunt placement include developmental delays, prolonged and frequent hospitalizations, limitations of sport participation, and being stigmatized for having a chronic disease.

PRESENTATION

Symptoms of untreated hydrocephalus can present at any age. During pregnancy, hydrocephalus may be detected with routine prenatal ultrasound. Affected newborns may have irritability, poor oral intake, vomiting not associated with feeding, or simply an enlarging head circumference. Young or school-age pediatric patients may present with chronic headaches, vomiting, visual disturbances, behavior changes, or diminished school capabilities. Mature pediatric or adult patients may also present with memory difficulties or urinary incontinence. In any age group, a symptom of moderate to severe intracranial pressure includes sleepiness and lethargy. Congenital, acquired, or iatrogenic (shunt malfunction) hydrocephalus present with similar symptoms. Caregivers of patients who experience frequent shunt obstruction are often very cognizant of the subtle symptoms of accumulating CSF in their children. Careful attention to their concerns often allows for early detection of shunt malfunctions.

Upon examination, the HCP may note changes in the level of consciousness, ranging from alert and oriented to comatose. An infant may demonstrate prominent scalp veins; a full, tense, or bulging fontanel; or an enlarged anterior or posterior fontanel with split sutures. Pupillary examination may reveal photophobia or sluggish, dilated pupils. Extraocular movement may reveal difficulty with an upward gaze, nystagmus, or "sun setting." Speech may be slurred, and gait may be ataxic.

DIFFERENTIAL DIAGNOSIS

Differential diagnoses for hydrocephalus include gastroenteritis, constipation, migraines, upper respiratory infection, and fever. Hydrocephalus does not cause diarrhea. Ventriculomegaly due to atrophy of surrounding brain tissue can occur after hemorrhage, severe traumatic brain injury, and infection. Differentiation of these diagnoses may be achieved with a detailed history and neurological examination, further radiographic and laboratory studies, or consult with experienced providers.

PLAN OF CARE

Patients with hydrocephalus should be evaluated by the neurosurgical service. These specialists will evaluate the patient's stability, assess the immediate concerns, and plan for further radiographic and medical management. The treatment goal, through shunting and subsequent care, is to decrease ICP, diminish neurologic injury, and optimize CSF function through a system designed to minimize lifelong surgical intervention (Rekate, 2008). The decision to place a shunt must be made judiciously. The younger the child at the time of shunt placement, the higher the risk of infection, which may potentially result in severe neurologic deficits. Shunt placement can increase the already high death risk associated with congenital anomalies (Rekate).

Diagnostic radiographic studies include ultrasound (infants with open fontanels), CT scan, and MRI. Radiographic markers suggestive of hydrocephalus are dilated frontal or temporal horns, an enlarged third ventricle, and periventricular interstitial edema. Anterior and lateral radiographs of the head, chest, and abdomen should be obtained to assess the continuity of the shunt.

A CBC with differential, ESR, and CRP values, along with respiratory, stool, or urinary cultures, may identify an infectious or viral process. A serum metabolic panel (BMP) and antiepileptic drug levels may assist in identifying the etiology of seizures.

An assessment of the shunt should be performed by providers who are knowledgeable about shunts and hydrocephalus. The valve reservoir should be palpated for recoil tension and tubing integrity. Consider a lumbar puncture or consult with the neurosurgery service for a shunt tap to evaluate ICP and obtain a CSF sample for cell count, glucose and protein measurements, and culture.

A patient with acute hydrocephalus with acute neurological decline needs immediate medical management and surgical intervention. Medical management for intracranial hypertension includes the use of osmotic agents (hypertonic saline, mannitol) or diuretics (acetazolamide, furosemide), plus glucocorticoids (dexamethasone) if a space-occupying lesion is present. Surgical intervention may entail the placement of an external ventricular device (EVD) or an emergent shunt placement or revision. The goal is acute CSF diversion. Without diversion, brain herniation and, subsequently, death may result.

DISPOSITION AND DISCHARGE PLANNING

Children with hydrocephalus usually recover quickly from a shunt placement or revision, which typically requires a few days' stay in the hospital. The goals at discharge are threefold: (1) resume regular diet or source of nutrition, (2) return to baseline level of activity and communication, and (3) develop a pain management strategy for home. Most children can resume their normal daily routine, including school attendance, within a few days or weeks.

Within 1 to 3 weeks after hospital discharge, pediatric patients usually have a follow-up visit with the neurosurgeon or PCP to assess their postoperative status and discuss ongoing care. After their initial follow-up visit, they will continue to see the neurosurgeon annually. They should see their PCP, and any other specialists, for regularly scheduled checks.

Long-term outcomes for children with hydrocephalus correlate with the etiology, and reflect the presence of any complications from shunting. The prognosis for patients with hydrocephalus has generally improved with the introduction of modern shunting, although premature infants with hydrocephalus may have poorer outcomes. Notably, members of the latter group may have complex learning disorders, behavior disorders, and cognitive deficits. Children with brain tumors and hydrocephalus often must undergo chemotherapy and/or radiation therapy, which can also affect their cognitive development.

Families and patients need to appreciate that hydrocephalus and shunting are lifelong concerns. Hydrocephalus is not curable, but rather manageable. Educational needs include ensuring that the family and patient have a comprehensive understanding of the signs and symptoms of a shunt malfunction. It is important to incorporate the family and primary caregivers into the plan of care and empower them to recognize and report subtle changes or developments in the patient.

HYPOTONIA IN THE INFANT

Peter Heydemann

PATHOPHYSIOLOGY

Hypotonia is described as decreased resistance to passive motion, where muscle tone is diminished, but strength may be appropriate. It is considered to be a symptom that results from a motor dysfunction, rather than a disorder itself. The dysfunction may occur at different levels of the central nervous system, thereby affecting the musculature. A neuromuscular disorder may be caused by dysfunction at the anterior horn cell or cranial motornuclei, neuromuscular junction, peripheral nerve, or muscle.

EPIDEMIOLOGY AND ETIOLOGY

Hypotonia with onset in the first month of life was the presenting diagnosis in 4% of nonpremature infants at one French university hospital in a study by Laugel and associates (2008). In two-thirds of these infants, the hypotonia was traced to a cerebral etiology. Central (cerebral) hypotonia was more than four times as common as peripheral neuromuscular causes, with hypoxic ischemic encephalopathy (HIE) and hemorrhagic lesions being the most common single diagnosis, found in 42% of the affected children. Metabolic etiologies were present in 6%, and neuromuscular disorders in 14%. Of the various syndromic disorders leading to hypotonia, Down syndrome was the most common (found in 12% of infants with hypotonia), followed by Prader-Willi syndrome (3%) and other syndromes. With peripheral diagnoses, congenital myopathy or dystrophy accounted for 10% of the total number of infants with hypotonia, with more than one-third of these children's conditions found to be due to myotonic dystrophy. Neuronal disorders accounted for 5% of affected infants, nearly all due to spinal muscle atrophy (SMA); there were no neuromuscular junction disorders. Table 33-16 lists common etiologies of hypotonia.

PRESENTATION

In mothers whose infants have hypotonia, intrauterine symptoms during pregnancy are commonly reported upon retrospection. The HCP should inquire about fetal movement, pregnancy and labor problems, APGAR scores, umbilical cord blood gas, feeding patterns, alertness, and movement patterns after birth. Acquisition of a family history for

TABLE 33-16

Localization and Etiology of Hypotonia in the Infant	
Neuro-Axis Site	**Disease**
Brain	Hypoxic ischemic encephalopathy, brain malformation, Down syndrome, Smith-Lemli-Opitz syndrome, other syndromes, metabolic diseases
Spinal cord	Ischemic or traumatic myelopathy
Anterior horn cell	Spinal muscular atrophy
Peripheral nerve	Dejerine-Sotas syndrome, congenital hypomyelinating neuropathy
Neuromuscular junction	Congenital myasthenia, transient neonatal myasthenia, infant botulism
Muscle	Congenital muscular dystrophies (e.g., merosin deficiency; Walker-Warburg syndrome), congenital myopathies
Mixed sites	Myotonic dystrophy, Pompe disease, mitochondrial disorders

neuromuscular disease is essential, especially for maternal myasthenia gravis (MG) and myotonic dystrophy.

Upon physical examination, the child with hypotonia may be noted to have abducted hips, low shoulder and trunk tone, floppy neck, poor suck, facial diplegia, ptosis, absence of deep tendon reflexes (DTRs), and contractures. The neonatal neurologic exam is demonstrated well at http://library.med.utah.edu/pedineurologicexam/html/newborn_ab.html.

Contractures are a feature of low in utero movements. Poor ventilatory effort in the face of hypoxia or hypercarbia is a feature of severe weakness. In the general examination, it is important to evaluate the child for hepatomegaly, retinal disease, cataracts, and myocardial failure, all of which suggest the presence of systemic or metabolic disorders.

DIFFERENTIAL DIAGNOSIS

Cerebral hypotonia is suspected in the presence of dysmorphic features, encephalopathy, low alertness, severe metabolic acidosis (umbilical cord blood), multisystem disease, or sepsis. In severe HIE or traumatic breech delivery, the cervical spinal cord may be injured. Spinal muscular atrophy commonly presents within the first few months of life with hypotonia, low extremity movements, low DTRs, and poor feeding; it is diagnosed by blood deletion analysis of the survival motor neuron (SMN) gene. Neuromuscular junction disorders are commonly characterized by worsening of sucking strength, facial movement, and muscle tone as feeding progresses. Peripheral nerve and muscle diseases often lead the child to have very weak antigravity movements, low DTRs, and sometimes contractures. Increased

DTRs, poor alertness, and dysmorphism suggest cerebral disease. Contractures, absent DTRs, good alertness, and lack of antigravity movements are suggestive of peripheral neuromuscular disease (Vasta et al., 2005). A very low APGAR score with preserved heart rate, in the absence of umbilical cord metabolic acidosis, is also suggestive of peripheral motor disorders.

PLAN OF CARE

Diagnostic studies are prioritized based on the initial presentation as well as evolution of the findings over days to weeks, which is important when hypotonia is due to acute injury such as HIE. The approach in the newborn is generally to obtain brain imaging, EEG, creatine kinase (CK, also known as creatine phosphokinase), and metabolic studies; in dysmorphism, the HCP should also obtain a chromosomal analysis. If hypotonic symptoms persist late in the first week after birth without explanation, then gene studies and repeat CK should be obtained. If hypotonia fluctuates, then a neostigmine test is warranted.

In infancy after the newborn period, some diagnoses become more likely, such as Pompe disease, botulism, and SMA. Head ultrasound is the easiest brain image to obtain, but MRI yields sufficient details for specific diagnoses and may be a secondary test. CK elevation may be transient due to labor trauma; conversely, some myopathies are characterized by normal CK levels. EEG is adjunctive for suspicion of encephalopathy. High-yield gene tests include blood DNA analysis for SMN, myotonic dystrophy, and Prader-Willi syndrome. Metabolic studies include a complete chemistry panel, thyroid studies, blood lactate, ammonia, amino acids, carnitine level, acylcarnitine profile, urine organic acids, and very-long-chain fatty acids. Patients with cardio-hepatomegaly should have blood for alpha-glucosidase level obtained to evaluate for Pompe disease. A diagnostic neostigmine injection may indicate myasthenia. Nerve conduction velocity (NCV) is essential to diagnose neuropathies, and repetitive stimulation is helpful for identifying MG.

Muscle biopsy can be performed in the neonate, but is often deferred until the infant reaches 6 months of age, when muscle cells are closer to the adult size. An ophthalmologic examination may demonstrate retinal anomalies, as seen in some congenital muscular dystrophies.

Symptomatic management of respiratory insufficiency, excessive secretions, and inadequate intake should by managed by oxygen, intubation, mechanical ventilation, suction, and nasogastric or gastrostomy tube feeding as dictated by clinical severity and course. Physical, occupational, and feeding therapists may be needed while the child remains an inpatient. Fractures may occur, so extra-gentle handling is recommended. Dislocated hips, contractures, or fractures require orthopedic consultation. Genetic and neurologic consultations are helpful for the diagnostic evaluation.

Family education is essential to comprehensive care of the infant with hypotonia. Families will be exposed to multiple tests, often requiring many months for results to come back from national and international testing facilities, and will see many specialists as part of the interprofessional team. This ongoing interaction allows for symbiotic communication about goals of care, diagnostic studies and their findings, and prognosis. If the diagnosis is unknown, then plans of care should address quality of life for the patient and family Education may also include the use of home care equipment and devices. Outpatient physical and rehabilitative therapies may be required, as well as supportive splinting adjuncts. Providing good skin care, maintaining a normothermic environment, avoiding ill contacts, and providing adequate nutrition are paramount to preventing infection. Diet counseling, enteral feeding, and nutrition studies may be indicated periodically.

DISPOSITION AND DISCHARGE PLANNING

The specific diagnosis is critical to determine the child's long-term prognosis. Most patients are weaned from intensive support, but some patients (e.g., those with SMA) will require such care on a long-term basis.

Without a specific etiology, counseling is symptomatic and relies on the "wait and see" model. For patients with hereditary disorders, genetic counseling is essential. Involvement in early child development programs is important, as is continued follow-up with specialists as indicated by symptom management. Follow-up with the PCP will support child health maintenance and ensure optimal growth and development. Home care and home medical equipment may be required. Case managers and social workers may facilitate the development and maintenance of home care nursing and support systems. Follow-up with specialists and nutritionists is essential to promote best care and continued evaluation of outcomes of therapeutic strategies.

MENINGITIS AND ENCEPHALITIS

Anne Lam

PATHOPHYSIOLOGY

Meningitis is an inflammation of the leptomeninges—that is, the tissues surrounding the brain and spinal cord. Encephalitis indicates brain parenchymal involvement. As these anatomic boundaries are often not distinct, many patients have evidence of both meningeal and parenchymal involvement and should be considered to have meningoencephalitis (Prober, 2007). A variety of infectious agents may cause meningitis and encephalitis. Suspected bacterial meningitis is a medical emergency and requires immediate

intervention, as the mortality rate of untreated bacterial meningitis approaches 100%.

Bacteria infect the central nervous system by entry from a distant source into the bloodstream or by spreading directly from contiguous infection. In infants and children, bacterial colonization from the upper respiratory tract is usually the source of infection. After bacteremia, meningeal seeding follows. Inflammation persists after bacteria are destroyed by host defenses and antimicrobial therapies (Feigin, 2006).

Cerebral edema results from vasogenic, interstitial, and cytotoxic processes that lead to increased intracranial pressure, coma, and herniation, ultimately resulting in death. In vasogenic edema, increased permeability of the blood–brain barrier allows proteins and fluid to invade the brain parenchyma's extracellular space. This process occurs over a period of hours to days. Interstitial edema is similar to vasogenic edema, in that there is a breakdown in the blood–brain barrier; however, mostly CSF crosses over into the parenchymal extracellular space. Cytotoxic edema results from host and bacterial toxic factors or hypoxia; these conditions decrease the effectiveness of the membrane pump, resulting in increased intracellular sodium. Water then flows into the cells. This process proceeds rapidly following insult (Feigin, 2006). Increased ICP secondary to cerebral edema may lead to hypoxemia, ischemia, and herniation. Cerebral vasculitis, venous sinus occlusion, or subarachnoid hemorrhage may occur from necrotizing arteritis.

EPIDEMIOLOGY AND ETIOLOGY

A variety of infectious agents can cause meningitis. In the developed world, *Streptococcus pneumoniae* and *Neisseria meningitidis* cause 95% of cases of acute bacterial meningitis in children older than 2 months of age (Feigin, 2009). In neonates, group B *Streptococcus* is the most common cause of meningitis, with the maternal genital tract being the source of both early- and late-onset disease (Mann, 2008). Although this etiology is less common, *Escherichia coli* from the maternal genitourinary tract and transplacental transmission and *Listeria monocytogenes* continue to be important agents in neonatal meningitis (Feigin, 2006). Before the introduction of the conjugate *Haemophilus influenzae* type B (Hib) vaccine, Hib was the causative agent in 65% of U.S. bacterial meningitis cases (Feigin, 2006). *H. influenzae* type B must still be considered as possible infectious agent in incompletely vaccinated children and those from low- and middle-income countries.

The most common cause of bacterial meningitis in children 2 to 23 months is *S. pneumoniae*, followed by *N. meningitidis*. Group B *Streptococcus* is responsible for a relatively small number of meningitis cases in this group. In children aged 2 to 29 years, *N. meningitidis* is responsible for the majority of bacterial meningitis cases (Prober, 2007).

Enteroviruses are the most common cause of viral meningoencephalitis, with more than 80 serotypes of these viruses having been identified to date (Prober, 2007). Infection may be mild and self-limiting, or it may range in severity up to severe encephalitis resulting in death. Arboviruses are responsible for some cases of meningoencephalitis in the summer months. The most common pathogens infecting these patients are West Nile, St. Louis, and equine viruses. Severe encephalitis with diffuse brain involvement may be caused by herpes simplex virus type 2 (HSV) in neonates who contract the virus from their mothers at birth. Varicella-zoster virus may cause CNS symptoms; this infection has a close relationship to chickenpox.

PRESENTATION

Meningitis may occur slowly over the course of days or over several hours. The clinical presentation of bacterial meningitis depends on the age of the patient. Fever and meningeal inflammation occur in 85% of patients (Feigin, 2009). Signs and symptoms of meningeal inflammation include headache, irritability, nuchal rigidity, confusion, photophobia, and back pain. Kernig sign—flexion of the hip to 90 degrees with subsequent pain on extension of the leg—and Brudzinski sign—involuntary flexion of the knees and hips after passive flexion of the neck while supine—are present in only 50% of patients. Malaise, restlessness, lethargy, ataxia, anorexia, myalgia, or arthralgia may also be present. Cranial nerve palsies may be present secondary to inflammation or necrosis. Seizures occur in 30% of patients, with 20% occurring prior to the child's admission to the hospital (Feigin, 2006).

Infants may have a late sign of bulging fontanel. Poor feeding, jaundice, or decreased muscle tone may also be present in infants.

Respiratory distress secondary to upper respiratory illness or shock may be observed. Older children may have signs of altered mental status, hypertension, and bradycardia with increased ICP. Patients may exhibit petechiae or purpura, which may be either limited or diffuse.

Exanthems may precede CNS symptoms in infants and children with viral meningitis or encephalitis. A triad of fever, headache, and altered level of consciousness is the clinical hallmark of viral encephalitis in older patients without nuchal rigidity or other focal neurologic symptoms (Whitley & Gnann, 2002).

Some patients will develop shock with profound hypotension. Disseminated intravascular coagulation (DIC) may follow, and death may occur within hours despite adequate therapies.

DIFFERENTIAL DIAGNOSIS

In addition to the bacteria previously listed, many other microorganisms can cause generalized CNS infection with similar clinical presentations. *Mycobacterium tuberculosis*, *Treponema pallidum* (syphilis), and *Borrelia burgdorferi* (Lyme disease) are less typical bacteria that produce signs and symptoms mimicking those of meningitis. Fungi endemic to specific geographic areas and those responsible for infections in compromised hosts, such as *Candida*, *Cryptococcus*, and *Aspergillus*, and parasites such as *Toxoplasma gondii* and those that cause cysticercosis may cause similar symptoms as well.

CNS abscess, subdural empyema, cranial and spinal epidural abscess, and intracranial hemorrhage may also be confused with meningitis. Noninfectious illnesses such as malignancy, collagen vascular syndromes, and exposure to toxins can cause generalized inflammation of the CNS. Bacterial endocarditis with embolism, allergic or demyelinating encephalitis, and vasculitis are other causative agents of signs and symptoms similar to those observed with meningitis.

PLAN OF CARE

Lumbar puncture for CSF analysis and culture is the definitive diagnostic study for meningitis. Contraindications to performing an LP include cardiopulmonary compromise, signs of increased ICP, and focal neurologic signs. When an LP is performed, CSF pressure should be measured. The opening pressure is generally in the range of 200 to 500 cmH$_2$O, but may be lower in infants and children (Tunkel, 2004). Although the yield of CSF cultures and Gram stain may be lowered by antibiotics given prior to LP, CSF findings such as low glucose, high protein, and high white blood cell count will provide evidence for the diagnosis of bacterial meningitis (Tunkel). In children older than 12 months, the normal CSF leukocyte count should be fewer than 6 cells per mm^3.

Polymerase chain reaction (PCR) is a valuable laboratory study for HSV and enteroviral meningitis. McGrath et al. (1997) reported that CSF results in individuals with HSV infection included elevated protein, lymphocytic pleiocytosis, and an increased number of erythrocytes in 84% of patients. While not normally found in CSF, red blood cells (RBCs) may be noted and signal a traumatic tap, possible subarachnoid hemorrhage, or a cerebral vascular event. White cells may enter the CSF in response to local inflammation, bleeding, or infection. The ratio of RBCs and WBCs in the CSF can be compared to the ratio in the serum to help determine the etiology of the presence of RBCs, although many sources question the validity of this process.

Time to identification is shortened from weeks to hours or days with the use of PCR when compared to viral culture results and should be utilized if viral meningitis is suspected (Tunkel, 2004). CSF studies should be repeated if there is no improvement in the patient's clinical status after

48 hours of appropriate antimicrobial therapy in bacterial meningitis (Tunkel, 2004).

Cranial CT scan has limited use in diagnosis of acute bacterial meningitis. In children with suspected increased ICP or altered mental status, an emergent CT scan should be done prior to LP. This imaging may highlight signs of cerebral edema, including slit-like ventricles, areas of low attenuation, and absence of basilar and suprachiasmatic cisterns (El Bashir, 2003). LP should be delayed if the CT findings are consistent with increased ICP.

Patients suspected of having HSV meningitis should have an MRI to evaluate for temporal lobe abnormalities, which have been reported in 90% of patients with HSV-associated encephalitis. Electroencephalography may also be of use, as 80% of patients have generalized slowing or focal slowing with occasional lateralized epileptiform discharges (Rose et al., 1992; Tyler, 2004).

In a child with suspected meningitis, urgent hospital admission with microbiological investigation and antibiotic treatment are the cornerstones of management. If an LP cannot be performed immediately, blood cultures must be obtained, and then antimicrobial therapy initiated. Once Gram stain results are available, targeted antimicrobial therapy should be initiated. In children older than 1 month of age, empirical broad-spectrum antimicrobial coverage with vancomycin and either cefotaxime or ceftriaxone should be started (Tunkel, 2004). Acyclovir should be initiated for all infants and children with suspected HSV-associated encephalitis. Review the discussion of fever in a neonate in Chapter 30 for more information about therapy in this age group.

Animal models have shown decreased inflammation, reduced cerebral edema, decreased ICP, and lessened brain damage with dexamethasone administration (Chavez-Bueno & McCracken, 2005). Adjuvant dexamethasone (0.15 mg/kg every 6 hours, for 2 to 4 days) should be given prior to or concomitant with antibiotic therapy in children with suspected Hib meningitis. Dexamethasone therapy in children who have already received antimicrobial therapy should not be used, as this regimen has not been shown to improve outcomes (Tunkel, 2004). Experts vary in recommending corticosteroid use in infants and children with non-Hib infections, such as pneumococcal meningitis. For infants and children 6 weeks of age or older, dexamethasone may be considered after weighing the potential risks and benefits of its use (American Academy of Pediatrics [AAP], 2006a, 2006b).

Maintaining adequate cerebral perfusion and management of increased ICP are crucial to prevent life-threatening complications of meningitis. Vasoactive agents may be required to maintain adequate blood pressure. Head of bed elevation of 30 degrees, antipyretic administration, hyperventilation, administration of mannitol, and sedation may be necessary as components of increased ICP management in critically ill patients. ICP monitoring or ventricular drainage may also be necessary. Seizure control should be managed with benzodiazepines and anticonvulsant medications as indicated. Subdural effusions occur in one-third of patients with bacterial meningitis, and even more commonly in patients with Hib-associated and pneumococcal meningitis. These individuals are usually asymptomatic and their disease typically resolves spontaneously. Subdural empyema is an uncommon complication that should be suspected with prolonged fever and irritability; patients who develop this condition require surgical drainage with antibiotic therapy (Chavez-Bueno & McCracken, 2005). Encephalopathy may also occur with viral encephalitis.

DISPOSITION AND DISCHARGE PLANNING

The routine use of conjugated Hib vaccines in children has reduced by more than 99% the incidence of invasive disease in children younger than 5 years of age (AAP, 2006a). Two pneumococcal vaccines are available for use in children: PCV13 (Prevnar), which includes coverage for 13 serotypes, and PPV 23 (Pneumovax), the 23-valent pneumococcal vaccine. At the time of PCV7 licensing in 2000, the 7 serotypes of PCV7 accounted for 82% of cases of bacterial meningitis in U.S. children younger than 6 years of age (AAP, 2006b). Use of these conjugate vaccines has been crucial in preventing bacterial meningitis. Meningococcal vaccine is recommended only for children who are older than 2 years of age and in high-risk categories.

Serious complications in patients with bacterial meningitis usually occur within the first 2 to 3 days of treatment, but rarely after 3 or 4 days of appropriate therapy. Between 5% and 10% of patients with bacterial meningitis die. Sequelae are most common in children with pneumococcal meningitis, and include intellectual deficits, hydrocephalus, spasticity, blindness, and severe hearing loss (Mann, 2008). Hearing loss—either unilateral or bilateral—occurs in approximately 30% of patients with bacterial meningitis (Mann). Patients with bacterial meningitis usually remain hospitalized for the duration of intravenous antibiotic therapy. Once therapy is completed, all children with CNS infection should have evaluation for neurologic sequelae.

MUSCULAR DYSTROPHIES

Peter Heydemann

PATHOPHYSIOLOGY

The muscular dystrophies are genetic disorders presenting with progressive muscle weakness. Most dystrophies are due to disorders involving structural proteins in or near the cell membrane. Duchenne muscular dystrophy (DMD) is due to a defective gene for dystrophin, which connects the contractile protein actin to the cell membrane.

EPIDEMIOLOGY AND ETIOLOGY

DMD occurs in 1 in every 3,500 boys and is by far the most common childhood muscular dystrophy. Other muscular dystrophies include various limb girdle dystrophies, some of which are DMD phenocopies, and congenital muscular dystrophies, which may present before the infant reaches 1 year of age. The congenital dystrophies may even present at birth with signs of hypotonia, or prenatally with decreased intrauterine movement. Most childhood dystrophy presents in the first decade of life. DMD is an X-linked recessive defect; thus it affects primarily males. Females are carriers and are usually asymptomatic or exhibit only mild symptoms.

PRESENTATION

Muscular dystrophies commonly present with a gait disturbance due to hip girdle weakness. In DMD, caregivers typically note a child who was late to learn to walk, at age 13 to 15 months or later; moves more slowly than other toddlers; and may display toe walking, rolling gait or waddle, large calves (pseudohypertrophy), or a Gower sign (pushing off the thighs when arising from the ground). Other findings may include language or developmental delay, autistic symptoms, or muscle aching after walking. Weakness is progressive, starting with the voluntary muscles and those of the hips and pelvic girdle.

The diagnostic history should cover activities that display weakness, proximal versus distal weakness, fluctuation in symptoms, nonmuscular symptoms, age, and subtlety of presentation, and family history. Often there is no prior family history; mutations are common in affected children.

DIFFERENTIAL DIAGNOSIS

The differential diagnosis of DMD includes other limb girdle muscular dystrophies and alternative diseases, some of which have specific treatments. Polymyositis/dermatomyositis is treatable by steroids and other immunosuppressants. Pompe disease is a glycogen storage disease, which recently became treatable by monthly infusions of alpha glucosidase. Spinal muscular atrophy (type 3, which occurs after the ability to walk) and the primary muscle disorders, such as limb girdle dystrophies, should be considered, as well as late-presenting congenital myopathies—for example, central core disease. Other chronic childhood diseases

of progressive weakness include neuropathies, such as Charcot-Marie-Tooth disease, and chronic immune demyelinating polyneuropathy. Congenital myopathies may have similarity to DMD, but creatine phosphokinase (CPK) is generally normal, or minimally elevated, and biopsies are non-dystrophic.

PLAN OF CARE

Typical diagnostic testing includes serum CPK and a gene test to confirm the specific type of muscular dystrophy. CPK is elevated, with levels reaching as high as 10,000 U/L, as damaged and inflamed muscle leaks the enzyme. Muscle biopsy—a diagnostic step—is not required when gene testing is positive; if undertaken, it will show dystrophic features including pyknotic and ballooned myocytes, plus fatty and fibrous replacement of muscle tissue. Myotonic dystrophy is the major exception to this biopsy pattern, having a distinctly different pathophysiology and disease pattern compared to the majority of dystrophies. Occasionally electromyography and nerve conduction velocity testing are needed.

Children with muscular dystrophy have progressive problems of movement involving first the leg muscles, with loss of ambulation; then the arms and hands; and then spinal support and respiratory function. Children reach a plateau of ability in mid-childhood, before the start of a decline marked by the eventual loss of ambulation. By later childhood, most patients require a wheelchair for mobility. Optimally, wheelchairs should be equipped with molded seating, spine support, and a tilt-in-space feature.

Corticosteroids are recommended to slow the rate of decline. Due to the well-described risks of steroid therapy, it is recommended that these medications not be started at diagnosis (when some motor strength is still developing), but rather that they be initiated during the plateau phase of the disease. Continuing steroid use into the decline phase will enable the patient to maintain as much function as possible for the longest time. For example, even if ambulation is lost, decline in upper arm strength may be slowed. Prednisone is recommended at a dose of 0.75 mg/kg/day (Bushby et al., 2010a, 2010b). During this phase, the child's functional status needs frequent broad reassessment and supportive care must be modulated to the child's abilities.

By the age of 6 years, the patient should be evaluated by cardiology specialists and have his or her first echocardiograph. Cardiac muscle is involved in all cases of DMD, but children generally remain asymptomatic in their first decade of life. Arrhythmias and cardiomyopathy from myocyte hypertrophy, atrophy, and fibrosis become more common as the disease progresses (Bushby et al., 2010a, 2010b). Cardiac afterload reduction with angiotensin-converting enzyme inhibitiors such as perindopril or enalopril results in more years of normal ejection fraction and asymptomatic cardiac decline. Corticosteroids have a similar and probably additive effect. Digoxin, furosemide, and other cardiac medications may be required in the later stages of the disease.

Progressive spinal muscle weakness leads to profound thoracic cage deformities and impaired ventilatory excursion. As muscle weakness progresses, even the ability to cough and clear secretions is impaired. Restrictive lung disease eventually emerges in all patients due to progressive weakness of the diaphragm and chest wall muscles. The severity of scoliosis has lessened—from a frequent severe complication requiring spinal surgery, to a much less frequent complication of minor severity—with the use of steroids.

The age at which ventilation becomes significantly impaired is increasing, also due to the use of steroids. Even so, many patients need supportive devices such as cough assist, chest vest, home oximetry, noninvasive ventilation, or tracheostomy and mechanical ventilation. Today, portable ventilation is easily possible with laptop-size ventilators.

As the child moves out of the plateau phase, consultation with pulmonology services should be arranged.

Cognitive and executive function impairments are often present due to the abnormal level of dystrophin in the child's brain. This component of muscular dystrophy should be addressed with cognitive testing and special education. Medications for attention-deficit/hyperactivity disorder (ADHD) may be helpful.

Common reasons for emergency department visits by patients with DMD include respiratory insufficiency, often triggered by an upper or lower respiratory infection; fractures due to osteopenia; arrhythmias; and heart failure. Caution must be observed in treatment of pain with narcotics due to the respiratory depression present in a child with a fragile ventilatory system. The incidence of malignant hyperthermia is higher in those patients with DMD and other muscle disorders; consequently, this information should be readily available on a medical alert bracelet so that anesthesiologists are notified of the high risk should a historian be unavailable in an emergency.

DMD has multiple complications besides skeletal muscle weakness, and a detailed plan of care for this disorder is available from the DMD Care Consideration Group (Bushby et al., 2010a, 2010b). Dystrophin is present in smooth muscle, and late complications are common, including constipation, gastroesophageal reflux, and gastroparesis. Good bowel habits should be taught to the presymptomatic child. Over time, chewing becomes weak and jaw excursion may become limited; thus gastrostomy feeding is often required. Pressure ulcers may occur in late adolescence with immobility; the tilt-in-space chair feature is helpful for preventing this complication. Bone density is low in diseases of weakness, especially when individuals are treated with steroids, so good attention to calcium and vitamin D intake is important, including vitamin D levels. Bisphosphonates may be considered.

Psychological support is often necessary given the breadth of problems facing these children, including coping skills, depression, and the knowledge that they will have a shortened life span. Caregivers need their own support, which is partly obtained from local support groups and through websites operated by the Muscular Dystrophy Association (www.mda.org), Parent Project Muscular Dystrophy (www.parentprojectmd.org), and European Neuromuscular Network (www.treat-nmd.eu).

Multiple specialists are needed for complete care of children with DMD and other muscular dystrophies. The interprofessional team may include a neurologist for diagnosis, a cardiologist, a pulmonologist, a physiatrist, an orthopedist, a gastroenterologist, an orthopedist, a rehabilitation team, orthotics specialists, social workers, and wheel chair design and maintenance technicians.

Soon after a diagnosis of DMD or other dystrophy, families must learn about the disease's natural history, the treatments available, and current research. The neuromuscular specialist can be thorough about details, but a less specialized physician needs to give the basic explanation and referral. Genetic counseling is essential to allow family planning decisions.

DISPOSITION AND DISCHARGE PLANNING

The natural history of DMD has changed, and the course is often many years to decades longer than in the past. Factors increasing the life span for affected individuals include corticosteroid usage, aggressive pulmonary and cardiac management, lack of comorbid conditions such as diabetes and cachexia, and the option for tracheostomy with portable ventilator (Moxley et al., 2005).

New treatments are currently in clinical trials, including a medication known as PTC 124; this drug allows translation of the dystrophin protein despite a "stop codon" mutation in the dystrophin gene that causes 10% of DMD. Another clinical trial is exploring the use of "exon skipping," which inserts an antisense oligonucleotide at the site of a deletion mutation in dystrophin RNA and allows continued translation of the dystrophin protein beyond the deletion. Families are anxiously awaiting the results of these trials, which may bring specific treatments those with DMD.

For many families, these new therapies will not come soon enough, and a shortened life span for their child is to be expected. Discussions regarding palliative care and goals of care should start early and often so that life quality is optimized.

NEUROCUTANEOUS DISORDERS

Lisa Milonovich

NEUROFIBROMATOSIS

Pathophysiology

Neurofibromatosis is one of the most common autosomal dominant neurocutaneous disorders. The disorder is further classified into neurofibromatosis type I (NF1) and type II (NF2). NF1 results from a genetic mutation of chromosome 17q11.2, whereas NF2 is caused by a mutation of chromosome 22q1.11. These are two distinct disorders, although they share some overlapping features and are often confused. Both disorders have a high rate of spontaneous mutation, with approximately 50% of the cases arising from de novo mutations (Yohay, 2006). Mutations in the NF1 gene result in loss of function of neurofibromin, which regulates cell growth, particularly of neurocutaneous tissues (Williams et al., 2009; Yohay). The NF2 gene encodes merlin, which is believed to act as a regulator of cellular growth, motility, and remodeling (Yohay).

Epidemiology and etiology

NF1 is a common disorder, affecting approximately 1 in every 2,500 to 3,000 individuals (Williams et al., 2009). NF2 is much less common, with an incidence of only 1 in 40,000 persons. These disorders do not seem to possess a gender or racial predominance, and they demonstrate wide phenotypical variability (Yohay, 2006). Approximately one-third of individuals with NF1 will have serious medical and cosmetic complications, while the other two-thirds will have only minor to moderate manifestations.

Presentation

Patients with *neurofibromatosis type I* usually present in the first few years of life. NF1 is a progressive disorder, so providers must be able to identify the evolving features of the disorder to make the appropriate diagnosis. The National Institutes of Health (NIH) Consensus Development Conference defines NF1 as being present in a patient who displays two or more of the following clinical features:

- Café-au-lait macules
- Freckling in skin folds
- Lisch nodules
- Neurofibromas
- Optic pathway gliomas
- Distinctive bony lesions
- A first degree relative with the disease

Table 33-17 summarizes the diagnostic criteria for NF1 (NIH, 1987).

Neurofibromatosis type II usually does not present until late adolescence or young adulthood. Patients generally experience hearing loss due to the development of vestibular schwannomas (VS) or other symptoms that result from the development of meningiomas or spinal schwannomas. A patient is diagnosed with NF2 if he or she exhibits either bilateral or unilateral VS, meningiomas, glioma, and schwannomas, and has a first-degree relative with the disease (Table 33-18) (NIH, 1987). The average age of symptom onset in patients with NF2 is typically at 20 years; however, diagnosis may be delayed for several years. The presence of café-au-lait spots in patients with NF2 is not necessarily useful, as their incidence in the NF2 population is likely not greater than their incidence in the general population.

Cutaneous manifestations of NF1 include café-au-lait spots, axillary or inguinal freckling, Lisch nodules, and neurofibromas. Café-au-lait spots are often the first clinical

TABLE 33-17

NIH Diagnostic Criteria for Neurofibromatosis Type I

NF1 is present in a person who has two or more of the following criteria:

- Six or more café-au-lait macules larger than 5 mm in the greatest diameter in prepubertal individuals or larger than 15 mm in greatest diameter after puberty
- Two or more neurofibromas of any type or one or more plexiform neurofibromas
- Freckling in the axial or inguinal region
- Tumor of the optic pathway
- Two or more Lisch nodules
- A distinctive osseous lesion
- A first-degree relative with NF1

Source: Adapted from NIH, 1987.

TABLE 33-18

NIH Diagnostic Criteria for Neurofibromatosis Type II

NF2 is present in a person who meets either of the following criteria:

- Bilateral cranial nerve VIII masses on MRI or CT scan
- A first-degree relative with NF2 and with unilateral cranial nerve VIII mass or two of the following:
  - Glioma
  - Meningioma
  - Schwannoma
  - Neurofibromas
  - Juvenile posterior subcapsular lenticular opacity

Source: Adapted from NIH, 1987.

manifestation of NF1 in infants and young children and are present in more than 90% of all NF1 patients (Crawford & Schorry, 2006). These hyperpigmented macules are generally oval-shaped lesions with clearly defined edges. Freckling in the inguinal and axillary areas as well as in other skin folds is another common feature of NF1. Lisch nodules—that is, hamartomas of the iris—do not affect vision and are pathognomonic for NF1. They typically present in patients between 5 and 10 years of age.

Neurofibromas are benign Schwann cell tumors that arise from fibrous tissue surrounding peripheral nerve sheaths (Williams et al., 2009). They can be further classified as cutaneous, subcutaneous, nodular or diffuse plexiform, or spinal. The location, number, and complexity of these fibromas vary from patient to patient. Cutaneous lesions usually present in late childhood or early adolescence; they are rarely associated with pain or neurological deficits. By comparison, subcutaneous and spinal neurofibromas are more likely to be associated with sensory or motor neurological deficits.

Plexiform neurofibromas arise from multiple nerve fascicles and grow along the length of a nerve. These lesions occur in approximately one-third of all patients with NF1 and are usually present at birth. They may continue to appear into adolescence and early adulthood. Plexiform neurofibromas demonstrate erratic growth patterns and often extend into surrounding tissue such as skin, muscle, bone, and internal organs, resulting in pain.

Skeletal abnormalities are a common finding in patients with NF1. Scoliosis is the most common osseous disorder in patients with NF1, though it varies in severity. Although its exact etiology is unclear, scoliosis affects 10% to 30% of patients with NF1 (Crawford & Schorry, 2006). The majority of patients with NF1 have nondystrophic scoliosis. Those with dystrophic scoliosis—the more severe of the two forms—often have rapid progression of their deformity, requiring early intervention and fusion to prevent spinal cord compression. Other, less commonly seen osseous lesions in NF1 include congenital tibial dysplasia, short stature, and sphenoid wing dysplasia.

Optic pathway gliomas are seen in approximately 15% of patients with NF1 and usually appear in the first decade of life. These lesions are generally pilocytic astrocytomas; however, unlike sporadically occurring pilocytic astrocytomas, the lesions in NF1 patients occur along the optic nerve. Most patients are asymptomatic; however, those who are symptomatic may develop proptosis, visual acuity loss, or precocious puberty due to impingement of these masses on the hypothalamus. Unlike sporadically occurring tumors, the presenting symptom of NF-associated optic pathway gliomas is most often precocious puberty. Patients younger than 6 years of age seem to be at the highest risk for development of symptomatic optic pathway gliomas (Listernick et al., 2004). Gliomas also occur in other areas of the brain in as many as 3.5% of patients with NF1

(Williams et al., 2009). When compared with other brain stem gliomas, however, lesions in the NF1 population are often much slower growing and may spontaneously regress.

Cardiac manifestations in patients with NF1 I include vasculopathies such as stenosis, aneurysms, arteriovenous malformations, congenital heart disease, and hypertension. These vasculopathies generally affect the arterial system, with renal artery stenosis being the most common finding and the etiology of hypertension in the pediatric patient with NF1. Cerebral vascular disease may also develop secondary to vascular stenosis or occlusion. Hypertension has been associated with significant morbidity in this population.

Other manifestations of NF1 include neurocognitive disorders and malignancies outside the nervous system. Learning deficits affect approximately one-half of NF1 patients and include verbal and nonverbal language deficits as well as gross and fine motor abnormalities. Attention-deficit/hyperactivity disorder, autism spectrum disorders, and behavioral abnormalities also occur at a higher incidence in children with NF1. The presence of unidentified bright objects (UBO) on T2-weighted MRI of children with NF1 is often associated with these behavioral and cognitive disorders. NF1 patients are also at greater risk than the general population for malignancies such as pheochromocytomas and chronic myeloid leukemia.

Differential diagnosis

A number of possible diseases and disorders may present with similar findings to neurofibromatosis, including multiple endocrine neoplasia type I, abdominal neurofibromatosis, neurofibromatosis type I with Noonan's syndrome, neurofibromatosis type II, and segmental neurofibromatosis.

Plan of care

There is no specific therapeutic management plan for neurofibromatosis. The disease is highly variable in presentation; thus management is tailored to the individual patient, his or her symptoms, and any complications experienced. Given the need for evaluation and management by many-specialty services, patients are often best served at a center that specializes in neurofibromatosis. This practice ensures that neurology, ophthalmology, neurosurgery, dermatology, cardiology, orthopedics, plastic surgery, and other necessary services are coordinated in a comprehensive approach.

It is recommended that patients with NF1 undergo biannual physical examinations during childhood and yearly thereafter (Yohay, 2006). Patients with NF1 should undergo yearly neurological and ophthalmologic examinations. Radiographic testing and EEG should be limited to those patients with NF1 who show a deficit on examination or provide a symptomatic history. Formal behavior and developmental evaluation is also important given the high incidence of development delay and ADHD in patients with NF1. In patients with NF2, neurological and ophthalmologic examinations should be performed yearly, along with audiologic testing and a brain MRI.

Family education and genetic counseling are important when the diagnosis is initially made and throughout the patient's life. The patient's and family's ability to cope with this diagnosis and its associated complications will vary not only based on family dynamics and education, but also based on the patient's developmental age and symptomology at any given time.

Disposition and discharge planning

Similar to the plan of care developed for the patient with neurofibromatosis, the discharge needs and long-term prognosis will depend on the severity of the disease. Genetic counseling is important not only to parents, but also to teenagers and young adult patients as they plan for their future. It is important to advise patients and families of what to expect at each developmental stage, including physical findings, signs of disease progression, and appropriate developmental milestones. Patients with NF1 may face both physical and cognitive challenges, and parents are much better able to address these needs if they are aware and educated on what to expect.

Like NF1 patients, individuals with NF2 have a varying prognosis depending on their clinical symptoms and presentation. As a general rule, those patients with earlier age of symptom onset, higher number of meningiomas, and truncating genetic mutations have a worse prognosis (Evans, 2009).

TUBEROUS SCLEROSIS

Pathophysiology

Tuberous sclerosis complex (TSC) is an autosomal dominant neurocutaneous disorder that is characterized by the development of harmartomas in essentially any organ system. The brain, skin, and kidneys are most often affected. In more than three-fourths of all patients with TSC, a disease-producing mutation can be found in either the TSC-1 gene, present on chromosome 9q34, or the TSC-2 gene, present on chromosome 16p13.3. Both of these genes function as tumor suppressor genes, and a mutation allows for hamartoma development. Genetic products such as hamartin and tuberin function as a complex to modulate cell signaling pathways that are important for regulation of cell growth, migration, and proliferation (Au et al., 2008). Variability in disease expression has been linked to further mosaicism, "second hits," and genetic modifiers.

Epidemiology and etiology

The incidence of TSC is approximately 1 patient per 6,000 to 7,000 population, with approximately two-thirds of all cases representing new mutations. Approximately 1 million individuals are affected worldwide (Krueger & Franz, 2008). The disease affects all racial and ethnic groups. Classically, TSC causes mental retardation, intractable seizures, and angioma formation; however, fewer than 40% of patients exhibit the full complex. The most common morbidity in TSC is intractable seizures, which affect as many as 90% of patients.

Presentation

Historically, the average age for diagnosis of TSC has been reported at approximately 5 years. However, due to the development of diagnostic criteria in recent years, better neuroimaging techniques, and genetic testing, diagnosis can now often be made at an earlier age, potentially antenatally. Definitive diagnosis prior to age 2 years remains a challenge, as the stigmata varies from one individual to another. Patients who present in infancy with TSC often demonstrate seizures or infantile spasms, hypomelanotic skin lesions ("ash leaf spots"), or cardiac rhabdomyomas. When an international consensus conference published the revised diagnostic criteria for tuberous sclerosis in 1998, the most significant change was that experts agreed that there are no pathognomonic clinical signs of TSC (Table 33-19).

TABLE 33-19

Diagnostic Criteria for Tuberous Sclerosis
Major Features

- Facial angiofibromas or forehead plaque pits in dental enamel
- Nontraumatic ungula or periungual fibromas
- Hypomelanotic macules (three or more)
- Shagreen patch (connective tissue nevus) migration line
- Multiple retinal nodular hamartomas
- Cortical tuber
- Subependymal nodule
- Subependymal giant-cell astrocytomas
- Cardiac rhabdomyoma, single or multiple
- Lymphagniomyomatosis, renal angiomyolipoma, or both

Minor Features

- Multiple, randomly distributed
- Harmartomatous rectal polyps
- Bone cysts
- Cerebral white matter radial
- Gingival fibromas
- Nonrenal harmartoma
- Retinal achromic patch
- Confetti-like skin lesions
- Multiple renal cysts

Source: Roach et al., 1998.

Differential diagnosis

The differential diagnosis for TSC includes the following conditions:

- Isolated cardiac rhabdomyomas
- Hypopigmentation
  - Vitiligo
  - Nevus pigmentus
  - Piebaldism
- Ungual fibromas from traumatic injury
- Renal angiomyolipomas

Plan of care

Evaluation of a patient with suspected TSC usually begins with evaluation of the initial symptoms at presentation and then encompasses testing to confirm the diagnosis. The majority of patients with TSC have some type of neurological deficits, either seizures or infantile spasms, developmental delay, or autistic tendencies; thus most patients undergo CT scan or MRI of the brain as part of their initial work-up. EEG is indicated in patients who exhibit seizure activity, but not is necessary in those who are seizure free.

Renal ultrasonography should be performed in all patients at the time of diagnosis. Routine follow-up should be done every few years, as renal angiomyolipomas are most likely to develop in adolescents and adults, although pediatric patients will occasionally develop renal tumors.

ECG is recommended for all patients at the time of diagnosis as well as prior to any surgical procedure. Patients with TSC are likely to exhibit arrhythmias even without the presence of cardiac rhabdomyomas. Wolff-Parkinson-White syndrome is the most commonly reported arrhythmia. Echocardiograph is recommended only for patients who present with symptoms of cardiac rhabdomyomas. This finding is very common in the neonates presenting with TSC, but becomes less likely later in life.

Ophthalmologic examination should be performed at the time of diagnosis, with follow-up exams continuing as clinically indicated. Dermatologic exam may be helpful in confirming TSC in a patient with an atypical presentation of skin lesions. The majority of patients with TSC are at risk for neurodevelopmental and behavioral impairment, which may be exacerbated by lack of seizure control. Formal age-appropriate testing should be done at the time of diagnosis, and again at school entry. Ongoing testing will depend on the patient's age at presentation and degree of disability (Roach & Sparagana, 2004).

Long-term management is directed at treatment and monitoring of the patient's clinical manifestations and complications and screening for potential future lesions. The most common issue facing patients with TSC—and a significant cause of morbidity—is intractable seizures. Many patients have seizures that are refractory to multiple antiepileptic agents. Recent development of imaging techniques to localize the epileptogenic focus, and therefore allow for surgical resection of these foci, has resulted in decrease or cessation of seizures in more than 50% of patients with TSC and drug-resistant seizures (Curatola et al., 2008).

Family education and genetic counseling are other important aspects of the treatment plan. Genetic counseling may be helpful in confirming the diagnosis of TSC, verifying the effected gene, determining the expected clinical course, and planning for future children. Education should be aimed at symptom recognition and the importance of surveillance examinations.

Disposition and discharge planning

As previously noted, patients with TSC have a variable expression of symptoms; consequently, they have a variable long-term prognosis. Recent discovery of the mTOR pathway upregulation in TSC-associated lesions has resulted in animal and clinical trials of rapamycin, an immunosuppressant, as a nonsurgical treatment for TSC-associated tumors. Rapamycin has been shown to induce regression of brain astrocytomas associated with TSC (Schwartz et al., 2007). Other clinical implications of its use are also being investigated.

Discharge planning should focus on symptom management and long-term surveillance for future manifestations of the disease. Patients with TSC require interprofessional evaluation and follow-up. For this reason, management at a center where all necessary specialists (neurology, genetics, neurosurgery) are available is helpful to families as they attempt to coordinate care.

NEUROPATHY

Michele Grimason, Mark S. Wainwright, and Valerie Eichler

PATHOPHYSIOLOGY

Neuropathies may be categorized as nerve disorders, neuromuscular junction disorders, or muscle disorders. Thus they are characterized by either a dysfunction of the nerve signal, destruction of the actual neuron itself or its inflammation, or destruction of the myelin sheath. Neuropathies may be of a congenital nature, such as spinal muscular atrophy (SMA); of an autoimmune nature, such as myasthenia gravis (MG); or an acquired form, such as postinfectious transverse myelitis or Guillain-Barré syndrome (GBS).

SMA is a degenerative disease in which patients experience progressive denervation of muscle. The motor units are reinervated from other close-by units, but in the process the muscle fibers begin to atrophy, eventually leading to neuronal cell death. This process is observed primarily because infants with SMA have a defective or mutated survival motor neuron (SMN) gene located on chromosome 5. This gene is responsible for arresting programmed cell death. In its defective state, it is unable to fulfill this function, leading to continued apoptosis.

MG, interpreted as "grave muscle weakness," is a disorder in which autoimmune destruction of the acetylcholine receptor disrupts normal neuromuscular transmission, leading to profound skeletal muscle weakness. The trigger for MG is unknown, but infection has been implicated. Some sources suggest that the thymus gland has a role in causing MG.

The acquired forms of neuropathy are thought to be triggered by a preceding infection. As many as 70% of patients report experiencing an acute infection within 1 month prior to the onset of their neurologic symptoms. The preceding infection likely activates T and B cells, which in turn trigger macrophage and complement activation, which directly damages the myelin sheath. This macrophage penetration of the sheath appears to strip away the myelin sheath, exposing the axon. As more axons are exposed, the patient develops a progressive, ascending peripheral-to-central weakness that will eventually lead to respiratory insufficiency and possibly respiratory failure (Gillis & Ryan, 2008; Sarnat, 2007; Singhi et al., 2008).

EPIDEMIOLOGY AND ETIOLOGY

In the United States, GBS has emerged as the most common cause of nontraumatic acquired paralysis. The incidence of GBS is approximately 1 to 2 patients per 100,000 patients; in children younger than 18 years of age, however, the incidence is lower—0.5 to 1.5 patients per 100,000 population. In the latter group, the average age of presentation is between 4 and 8 years, with males affected slightly more often than females.

The incidence of MG is approximately 4 to 6 patients per 1 million population, with females affected slightly more often than males. MG is a rare occurrence in childhood, as its onset by the age of 20 years occurs in only 10% to 15% of patients (Singhi et al., 2008). The incidence of SMA is 1 in 5,000 births (Gillis & Ryan, 2008).

Neuropathies in children may be caused by hereditary disorders involving the axon (e.g., Friedreich's ataxia, mitochondrial disorders, SMA, ataxia–telangiectasia) or myelin (Krabbe's syndrome, Nieman-Pick syndrome, congenital muscular dystrophy), immune disorders (GBS), toxins such as heavy metals or botulism, or systemic illnesses such as diabetes.

PRESENTATION

The cardinal signs of neuropathy on the physical examination are the reduction or absence of reflexes. In patients with polyneuropathies, this effect typically begins in the distal portions of the lower extremities (ankle jerks).

In contrast, weakness in patients with myopathies is typically most severe in proximal muscles and has a symmetric distribution. Early in myopathic disease, reflexes are preserved. Decreased or absent reflexes, therefore, suggest a neuropathy.

The presence of pain may indicate either a neuropathic or a myopathic process. If the pain follows a radicular distribution, spinal cord injury or nerve root compression must be considered. The differential diagnosis for myopathic pain includes inflammation (connective tissue disease, or myositis), rhabdomyolysis (metabolic disorders), or muscle pain without myopathy (cramps, ischemia, drug toxicity). Typically, myopathic pain is associated with an elevated level of creatine kinase (also known as creatine phosphokinase); therefore, this study should be obtained first.

If the weakness begins with or involves the cranial nerves, a disorder of the neuromuscular junction (myasthenia gravis, botulism) or GBS should be considered. A pattern of weakness that is diffuse rather than proximal also suggests the presence of a neuromuscular disorder.

Consider spinal cord injury in the differential diagnosis of patients with suspected neuropathy. The presence of back pain, alteration in bowel or bladder function, involvement of more than one limb, or a radicular pattern of pain in a patient who initially presented with weakness should prompt emergent evaluation for spinal cord pathology. As a consequence, the initial examination of the patient with neuropathy or myopathy should carefully investigate the presence of a sensory level. This can be accomplished using a sharp or cold (tuning fork) object and asking the patient to identify where the sensation on the limb or torso changes.

Weakness in patients admitted to the pediatric intensive care unit may be due to critical care illness polyneuropathy or myopathy. These patients are weak (they may first present with difficulty weaning from the ventilator), less often demonstrate muscle atrophy, and commonly have reduced or absent reflexes (Williams et al., 2007). Risk factors for neuropathy in this patient population include prolonged admission to the intensive care unit, sepsis, systemic inflammatory response syndrome, pancreatitis, hyperosmolarity, parenteral nutrition, use of neuromuscular blocking agents, and steroids.

DIFFERENTIAL DIAGNOSIS

Guillain-Barré syndrome is an acute immune-mediated polyradiculoneuropathy. It typically presents with symmetric ascending weakness and diminished or lost reflexes, progressing within 6 weeks of an infection, vaccine administration, trauma, or tick/mosquito bite. Other associated symptoms may include meningismus, vomiting, headache, encephalopathy, ataxia, and ophthalmoplegia (Miller-Fisher syndrome).

In children, the presenting symptoms of transverse myelitis include loss of sensation, weakness, urinary dysfunction, and pain (Pidcock et al., 2007). Symptoms are typically preceded by an infection (averaging 11 days before presentation), immunization (within 30 days of presentation), or trauma (averaging 8 days before presentation). Transverse myelitis is an inflammatory disorder of the spinal cord, which may present with an explosive onset of weakness, loss of sensation, and sphincter disturbance, with permanent deficits occurring in as many as 60% of patients (Defresne et al., 2001).

Differential diagnoses for childhood neuropathies are provided in Table 33-20.

PLAN OF CARE

Diagnostic studies are guided by the differential diagnoses established from the history and physical examination. Emergent imaging of the spine and neurosurgical consultation are indicated in any patient presenting with symptoms of spinal cord dysfunction. In the absence of CNS infection, an intensity in T2 signaling on a contrast-enhanced MRI of the spine, along with cord expansion, assists in confirming the diagnosis of transverse myelitis. Spine MRI in GBS may demonstrate nerve root enhancement, although this finding is not required to establish the diagnosis.

If GBS or transverse myelitis is suspected, spinal fluid should be obtained. The presence of an elevated protein level with a normal cell count helps confirm the diagnosis of GBS. However, caution should be exercised in interpreting a normal protein level as a negative study. In the early stages of GBS (1 to 3 days of symptoms), the protein levels may be normal. In transverse myelitis, demonstration of the absence of CNS infection is a criterion for diagnosis. If the white cell count in the CSF is elevated, an alternative diagnosis (e.g., Lyme disease) should be considered.

Elevation in creatine kinase is a simple first screen study to distinguish between neuropathy and myopathy. If an autoimmune disorder (GBS, Miller-Fisher disease) is suspected, testing for antibodies to GM1, GQ1b, or GalNAc-GD1a ganglioside may be obtained. Electrolytes (sodium, calcium, magnesium) are measured to evaluate reversible causes of neuropathy or weakness. Other studies for metabolic disorders, vitamin deficiency (A, B_1, B_2, B_{12}, D, E), toxins, or drugs associated with neuropathy must be guided by each patient's presentation.

If the patient has fatigueable weakness with preserved reflexes, myasthenia gravis is the leading diagnosis in childhood. Acetylcholine receptor antibodies, Tensilon testing, and single-fiber electromyography (EMG) may be used to confirm the diagnosis.

If the patient is weak, possibly with constipation and ophthalmoplegia with dilated pupils, botulism should be considered. Stool for botulinum toxin testing should be sent.

If myasthenia gravis is suspected in a patient with ptosis, the application of an ice pack to the affected eye for 2 minutes may show resolution of ptosis. Alternatively, 1 mg of Tensilon can be administered parenterally (with atropine readily available for treatment of bradycardia). Cardiorespiratory monitoring is required. If a significant improvement in strength occurs within 1 minute, followed by recurrence of weakness, it strongly supports the diagnosis of MG.

In the acute setting, EMG, nerve conduction studies (NCS), and biopsies are rarely available; therefore, these tests should not be relied up to guide management decisions in the initial evaluation. The technical challenges involved in EMG and NCS require an examiner who is experienced in the performance of these studies in children if the results are to be useful. Testing can localize the pathology to the nerve, neuromuscular junction, or muscle, and distinguish between a demyelinating or axonal pathology. In the case of myasthenia, single-fiber EMG with repetitive nerve stimulation may be needed to confirm the diagnosis if antibody studies are negative. The yield from nerve biopsy is higher when there is greater functional impairment of the affected limb with sensory loss or weakness.

The approach to the acute treatment of children with neuromuscular disease begins by attending to the potential for weakness—particularly with GBS, MG, and botulism—to compromise respiratory function. These patients require frequent assessment of respiration and ability to protect their airway. Treatment of children with GBS

TABLE 33-20

Differential Diagnoses for Neuropathies in Childhood	
Mechanism	**Example and Risk Factors**
Medications	Chemotherapy
Undiagnosed neuromuscular disease	Myotonic dystrophy
Autoimmune disease	Guillain-Barré syndrome, chronic inflammatory demyelinating polyneuropathy
Spinal cord	Spinal cord injury, spinal cord injury without radiological abnormality, transverse myelitis
Critical illness polyneuropathy	Prolonged ventilation, use of steroids during critical illness
Loss of muscle mass	Rhabdomyolysis
Electrolyte imbalance	K^+, Na^+, Ca^{++} imbalance; hypermagnesemia; hypophosphatemia
Systemic illness	Toxin exposure (heavy metals), uremia, HIV or other infection
Vitamin deficiency	B_1, B_6, B_{12}, E; niacin; celiac disease
Genetic	Charcot-Marie-Tooth disease, Friedreich's ataxia, mitochondrial disease

is described in Chapter 35. Limited data are available on the treatment of transverse myelitis. Treatment with methyl-prednisolone at 1 gm/1.72 m²/day for 3 to 5 days, followed by prednisone (1 mg/kg/day for 1 to 2 weeks), has been shown to shorten recovery time. Treatment for myasthenic crisis should be managed in an intensive care unit, with early intubation of the patient occurring, before respiratory compromise becomes evident (Defresne et al., 2001). The mainstay of therapy is pyridostigmine, either 1 mg/kg by mouth every 4 to 6 hours or intravenously given at 1/30th of the oral dose. This medication may also be combined with either plasmapheresis or intravenous immunoglobulin. For critical illness polyneuropathy (Williams et al., 2007), treatment is supportive, but it is recommended that the combination of neuromuscular blockade and corticosteroid therapy be avoided (Mook & Hulsewe-Ewers, 2002). A wide range of pharmacologic options have been tried for management of neuropathic pain (Eisenberg et al., 2007). For acute management of pediatric patients, gabapentin (100 to 1,000 mg/day) is a common choice, as it offers a good side-effect profile.

Regardless of the etiology of the neuropathy, mild to profound weakness and respiratory failure require admission of the patient to an intensive care unit until he or she is stabilized. Neuropathies may follow a long, protracted course; therefore, specialists in neurology, pulmonology, and rehabilitation medicine should be consulted early to assist with their management. For diagnoses of SMA and GBS, the affected infant or child may require long-term mechanical ventilatory management. Early consultation with pulmonary specialists is necessary to assist with both inpatient and outpatient management.

Depending on the outcome and final diagnosis, families and patients must be educated on their particular condition, including what to look for, when to bring them in for evaluation, and which restrictions to either diet or activity are required. A list of basic signs and symptoms of the particular disease should be given to the parents, as well as a list of medications and the rationale for their use.

DISPOSITION AND DISCHARGE PLANNING

Most neuropathies require a long recovery period, and many patients may not fully regain their strength, sensation, or reflexes. Most patients will require some period of physical therapy, plus management of neuropathic pain with opiates, nonsteroidal anti-inflammatory drugs, and gabapentin or equivalent agents.

Once the decision has been made by the primary medical team that the patient is ready for discharge either to an inpatient rehabilitation facility or to home, the case worker should be involved to plan for and obtain any necessary durable medical equipment that the child will need in the home setting. If the patient is discharged to home, a home

health medical team will also be in contact with the family. The number of hours per day allotted for in-home care depends on the complexity of care for the child.

Occasionally, in the event of a prolonged hospital course where the child requires long-term mechanical ventilatory support, a tracheotomy is performed and a tracheostomy placed to allow for a more stable airway and to assist in weaning of support. In this circumstance, the family will require additional instruction on artificial airways, suctioning of the airway, home ventilator management, or any other mode of oxygen delivery that may be used. The caregivers and any other family members who will be providing care should take a class on basic cardiopulmonary resuscitation prior to the child being discharged home. Consultation and transfer to an inpatient ventilator rehabilitation program may be considered as a bridge to home discharge.

SEIZURES

Melissa Reider-Demer and Lisa Milonovich

PATHOPHYSIOLOGY

A seizure is a transient disturbance of brain function that is caused by paroxysmal discharges within the neuronal network. Hypersynchronous discharges originating within the cortex and several key subcortical structures combine with high-frequency bursts of the action potentials to generate a seizure. Seizures typically present with a sudden surge of electrical activity that usually affects motor control, sensory perception, or autonomic functions.

The brain develops rapidly during childhood and adolescence, with development then declining slowly in early adulthood. This pattern of growth may relate to certain types of seizures manifested during childhood.

EPIDEMIOLOGY AND ETIOLOGY

Common causes of seizures include brain malformations, stroke, fever, toxin, infections, and tumor. Approximately 30% to 35% of seizures are associated with genetic abnormalities; another 30% to 35% are related to structural lesions; an unknown etiology accounts for the remaining 30% to 35% (McBride, 1995). Seizures can be categorized as (1) symptomatic (known cause); (2) cryptogenic (causation not defined); or (3) idiopathic (unknown cause). They are among the most common pediatric neurological disorders. The overall prevalence of epilepsy is approximately 1%; as many as 5% of all children experience fever-induced seizures (febrile seizures) before 6 years of age (Philippe & Thiele, 2007). In the United States, an estimated 25,000 to 40,000 children experience their first nonfebrile seizure every year (Hirtz, 2000).

Provoked seizures often result from an acute condition such as hypoglycemia, toxic ingestion, intracranial infection, trauma, or other precipitating factor. *Unprovoked* seizures occur in the absence of such precipitating factors.

Epilepsy is classically defined as the occurrence of two or more unprovoked seizures. Several familial forms of epilepsy have been identified, such as myoclonic epilepsy and progressive myoclonic epilepsy. Approximately 20% of individuals with epilepsy have a genetic predisposition toward their disease (Blosser & Reider-Demer, 2009).

Seizures can also be categorized based on their manifestations and EEG signatures. The EEG displays spontaneous brain activity as a continuous graph of voltage waves over time. Based on the pattern of cerebral involvement, seizures are typically divided into two categories: (1) generalized—derived from both sides of the brain so that the patient is unconscious throughout the seizure, and (2) partial/focal—limited to one side or region of the brain. Focal seizures can be further subdivided into simple or complex (Table 33-21).

TABLE 33-21

International Classification of Epileptic Seizures

I. Partial Seizures (Focal, Localized)

A. Simple partial seizures
   a. With motor signs
   b. With somatosensory or special sensory systems
   c. With autonomic symptoms and signs
   d. With psychic symptoms
B. Complex partial seizures
   a. Simple partial onset followed by impairment of consciousness
   b. With impairment of consciousness at onset
C. Partial seizures evolving to secondarily generalized seizures
   a. Simple partial seizures evolving to generalized seizures
   b. Complex partial seizures evolving to generalized seizures

II. Generalized Seizures (Convulsive or Nonconvulsive)

A. Absence seizures
   a. Typical absences
   b. Atypical absences
B. Myoclonic seizures
C. Clonic seizures
D. Tonic seizures
E. Tonic–clonic seizures
F. Atonic seizures

III. Unclassified Epileptic Seizures

Source: Adapted from Commission on Classification and Terminology of the International League Against Epilepsy. (1981). Proposal for revised clinical and electroencephalographic classification of epileptic seizures. *Epilepsia, 22,* 489–501.

DIFFERENTIAL DIAGNOSIS

Epilepsy differential diagnoses are extensive and often obtuse. Some of the most common diagnoses include sleep disorders, nonepileptic seizures (pseudoseizures), movement disorders, syncope, complicated migraines or migraine variants, and gastroesophageal reflux.

PRESENTATION

A careful history and physical examination may lead to a diagnosis without the need for further diagnostic study (Table 33-22). Some seizures may be less overt and be described as a sensation of "pins and needles" lasting a few seconds. Other seizures may lead to unconsciousness, followed by collapse and a description of violent "jerking" movements lasting several minutes. Still other seizures simply present with strange feelings or sensations, causing the individual to "blank out" for a few seconds or "jerk" an extremity. The HCP may categorize the seizure according to caregiver or patient descriptions, or based on HCP observation.

Generalized seizures

Generalized seizures may be described as tonic, clonic, tonic–clonic, absence, atonic, or myoclonic (Table 33-21). *Tonic* seizures are marked by a sudden onset of sustained extension or flexion of the head, trunk, or extremities. Such seizures commonly occur in clusters, typically during sleep or drowsy states. Several EEG patterns are associated with tonic seizures, such as fast rhythmic activity (spike/multispike) and slow-wave discharges.

Clonic seizures present as rhythmic, repetitive "jerking" movements of the head, trunk, or extremities. The associated EEG correlation tends to demonstrate a spike/multispike pattern and slow-wave discharges at the same frequency as clonic activity.

TABLE 33-22

Obtaining a Seizure History

- Is or was the event a seizure?
- What was the context in which the seizure occurred?
- Did the seizure stop spontaneously?
- Did the patient return to baseline after the seizure?
- Has this ever happened before?
- Did the patient have a fever?
- Was the seizure precipitated by a trauma?
- Did the patient ingest a toxin?
- Did the patient experience a recent hypoxic event?
- Is the patient developmentally normal?
- Was there hypoxia at birth?
- Is there a family history of seizures?

Tonic–clonic seizures involve a combination of tonic and clonic movements. They are characterized by several types of motor behaviors, including generalized tonic extension of extremities, clonic movements, and postictal (period after seizure) confusion and tiredness.

Typical absence seizures present as brief periods of impaired consciousness or confusion often with an associated aura; they usually last no longer than 15 to 20 seconds. Facial automatisms are common, as are repetitive behaviors. Hyperventilation often provokes this type of seizure. The typical EEG finding is 3 to 5 Hz, general slow-wave complexes.

Myoclonic seizures present as brief motor movements lasting less than 1 second. EEGs typically show polyspike or slow-wave complexes that differentiate this type of seizure from the normal sleep pattern. Myoclonic seizures may also have an electro-decrement characteristic.

Atonic seizures can present as slumping to the ground caused by a sudden loss of muscle tone. This brief loss of muscle tone often results in falls and injuries (International League Against Epilepsy, 1981). The ictal EEGs are similar to those for tonic seizures and are clinically correlated with neurological abnormalities.

Partial/focal seizures

Partial seizures can be classified as either simple or complex (Table 33-21). *Simple partial* seizures account for approximately 10% of childhood epilepsy (Pellock, 2005). Intact recall of the event assists with diagnosing this type of seizure, as consciousness is not lost during the episode. Simple partial seizures result when the ictal discharge occurs in a limited area of the cortex—a "focal focus." Aura sensations that occur with the seizure may include visual changes, parenthesis, olfactory hallucination, and temperature disturbances. The precise presentation depends on the locus in the brain. On EEG, bilateral complex, spike, or polyspike, slow waves are prominent, with increased amplitude noted in the frontal regions.

Complex partial seizures are defined by impaired consciousness and imply bilateral spread of the seizure discharge. In addition to impairment or loss of consciousness, patients with such seizures usually present with automatisms such as lip smacking, repeat swallowing, and clumsy motor movements. Postictal confusion and irritation is common. Complex partial seizures usually arise from the temporal or occipital lobes.

Status epilepticus

Status epilepticus is defined as a single seizure lasting longer than 30 minutes or two or more consecutive seizures without return to baseline level of consciousness (Statler & Van Orman, 2008). The most common causes of status epilepticus are febrile illness and abrupt discontinuation of anticonvulsant medication. Approximately 20% of patients who present with status epilepticus have known underlying seizure disorders; however, in as many as 50%, the cause is unknown. Other potential etiologies of status epilepticus include metabolic disorders, infectious encephalopathies, toxic ingestions, and traumatic brain injury (TBI).

Refractory status epilepticus

The diagnosis of "refractory" status epilepticus is considered whenever the patient fails to cease seizure activity after the administration of two appropriately dosed anticonvulsant medications (Statler & Van Orman, 2008). Refractory status epilepticus has been reported in 10% to 25% of pediatric patients, with an associated mortality rate of 20% to 30%, and with neurologic sequelae in more than 50% of patients (Statler & Van Orman).

PLAN OF CARE

Often with a first seizure, several diagnostic studies such as CBC, serum electrolytes, blood urea nitrogen, creatinine, glucose, calcium, and magnesium are performed. However, in one study of 507 children with both febrile and nonfebrile seizures, laboratory studies did not contribute to either diagnosis or management (Hirtz, 2000). Seizures that recur require prompt diagnostic evaluation and a comprehensive therapeutic plan.

The American Academy of Neurology (AAN) recommends that for nonfebrile seizures, laboratory tests should be ordered based on individual circumstances, including suggestive historic or clinical findings such as vomiting, diarrhea, dehydration, or a failure to return to baseline alertness. If drug exposure is in question, a toxicology screen should be performed (Hirtz, 2003). EEG should be ordered selectively, not routinely, after the first unprovoked seizure in a pediatric patient and may be useful for future comparison (Gilbert, 2000).

Diagnostic imaging should be performed if a patient exhibits a postictal focal deficit (Todds paresis), the seizure does not resolve quickly, or the patient has not returned to baseline within several hours of the seizure. MRI is the preferred neuroimaging study (Hirtz, 2000). Lumber puncture is frequently performed when fever is associated with a seizure to evaluate for CNS infection.

The decision to institute antiepileptic drug (AED) therapy should be based on a thoughtful and informed analysis of the variables involved. Almost 30% of medication therapies have significant associated risk of adverse side effects (Carl, 2007). Most adverse effects are mild and dose related. These side effects often include sedation, mental dulling, impaired memory and concentration, dizziness, gastrointestinal upset, rash, and behavioral issues. Idiosyncratic side effects might include aplastic anemia (common with felbamate) and liver toxicity. Thus antiepileptic medications should be prescribed only when the potential benefits of treatment clearly outweigh the potential adverse effects of therapy. In pediatric patients, there is an additional concern that medication therapy may have long-term side effects on brain development, behavior, and learning.

Isolated infrequent seizures, whether convulsive or non-convulsive, pose few medical risks to otherwise healthy individuals. The likelihood of seizure recurrence varies among patients and depends on the seizure type and associated neurological and medical comorbidities. Twenty-five percent of pediatric patients who experience a first unprovoked seizure (usually tonic–clonic) will demonstrate a normal neurological exam and have few or no recurrent seizures (Hirtz, 2003). However, minor seizures that are associated with loss or altered consciousness may have psychosocial and safety ramifications. For pediatric patients, no distinct evidence-based guidelines exist as to the best therapeutic approach following the first unprovoked seizure (Hirtz).

Valproate is the medication of choice for generalized seizures. Lamotrigine and topiramate are suitable alternatives if valproate is ineffective; levitiracetam and zonisamide may also prove to be effective and require further study. Topiramate is widely used for myoclonic seizures. Carbamazipine and lamotrigine can induce myoclonic seizures and should be prescribed only with insight into the patient's seizure history. Ethosuximide is recommended for treatment of absence seizures (Hadjiloizou, 2005). Felbamate is used for those patients whose seizures remain uncontrolled on the previously discussed medications (French, 1999); however, this medication requires a rigorous regimen of monitoring for liver failure, aplastic anemia, or serious rash throughout its administration (Table 33-23).

TABLE 33-23

Antiepileptic Medications				
Name/Use	Class	Pediatric Dose	Side Effects	Notes
Gabapentin Partial seizures	Amino Acid	30–60 mg/kg/day divided TID	Sleepiness	Not a very good AED; good choice for neuropathic pain T½ = 5–7 hours
Phenobarbital Broad-spectrum AED	Barbiturate	3–7 mg/kg/day QD or divided BID	Sleepiness, liver toxicity, inducer of P450 activity	Use in status epilepticus, especially in children younger than 6 months of age T½ = 36–220 hours
Clonazepam Broad-spectrum AED	Benzodiazepine	0.01–0.2 mg/kg/day divided BID to TID	Sleepiness, liver effects with long-term use	Good choice as a bridge medication for lamotrigine; treats hyperekerplexia T½ I = 8–50 hours
Phenytoin Broad-spectrum AED	Hydantoin	5–10 mg/kg/day divided BID to TID	Liver toxicity, blood effects, teratogen, hirsutism, gingival hyperplasia, bone effects, cerebellar atrophy with long-term use	Zero-order kinetics T½ = approximately 20 hours
Ethosuccimide Absence seizures	Succinimide	150 mg/day and increase up to 1,200 mg/day to effect, divided QD to BID	Liver effects, sedation	T½ = 15–45 hours
Carbamezapine Partial epilepsies	Other	10–35 mg/kg/day divided BID to TID	Liver effects, sleepiness, rash, leucopenia and thrombocytopenia	Can worsen a generalized epilepsy T½ = 12–65 hours
Felbamate Broad-spectrum AED, particularly useful for MAE and LGS	Other	15–45 mg/kg/day divided TID to QID	Insomnia, irritability, liver effects, renal effects, rare aplastic anemia*	Important to take scheduled doses; skipping doses can result in status epilepticus T½ = 14–23 hours
Lamotrigine (Lamictal) Broad-spectrum AED	Other	Usual 1–5 mg/kg/day divided BID to TID; usual maintenance is 3 mg/kg/day, but can go up to 7 mg/kg/day	Rash; most concerning is Stevens-Johnson reaction, particularly when lamotrigine is used in combination with VPA	Titrate up slowly; need a bridging medication while titrating upward, such as Klonopin or dilantin
Levetiracetam (Keppra) Partial seizures	Other	10–15 mg/kg/day divided BID up to 50 mg/kg/day	Renal effects, behavior effects, clumsiness or incoordination	T½ = 6–8 hours

(Continued)

TABLE 33-23

Antiepileptic Medications *(Continued)*				
Name/Use	**Class**	**Pediatric Dose**	**Side Effects**	**Notes**
Oxcarbamezepine (Trileptal) Partial seizures	Other	8–10 mg/kg/day divided BID to TID	Rash, liver effects, hyponatremia	May worsen a generalized epilepsy $T\frac{1}{2}$ = 8–10 hours
Topiramate (Topomax) Broad-spectrum AED	Other	1–3 mg/kg/day divided BID initially; may need doses as high as 9 mg/kg/day or higher especially in babies	Behavioral side effects, liver effects, decreased appetite, weight loss, and cognitive effects Need to keep well hydrated because of potential for formation of renal stones and patients can overheat	$T\frac{1}{2}$ = 18–30 hours
Vigabatrin (Sabril)	GABA agonist	2–4 gm QD	Visual loss, somnolence	For infantile spasms or intractable epilepsy Requires ophthalmic monitoring
Rufinamide (Banzel)	Other	10–40 mg/kg divided BID	QT-interval shortening, suicidal ideation, nausea, vomiting, fatigue, rash	ECG required at baseline Used for LGS
Valproic acid† Broad-spectrum AED	Other; fatty acid	15–60 mg/kg/day divided BID to TID	Weight gain, liver effects (hyperammonemia), pancreatitis, blood effects, alopecia, tremor Use with caution especially when changing to lamotrigine	Fulminant hepatic failure more common in patients younger than 2 years of age; need metabolic testing to make sure there is no fatty acid oxidation deficiency; need acylcarnitine and carnitine levels before starting in a patient younger than 2 years of age $T\frac{1}{2}$ = 9–20 hours if monotherapy, longer if polytherapy
Zonisamide (Zonegran) Partial seizures, myoclonic seizures	Other Sulfa	2–4 mg/kg/day divided BID initially; can go as high as 10 mg/kg/day	Sleepiness, behavior changes, renal effects, liver effects Need to keep patient well hydrated because of the potential for formation of renal stones and patients can overheat	Can be used with ACTH in the treatment of IS $T\frac{1}{2}$ = 50–70 hours
Diastat (rectal diazepam) Status epilepticus	Benzodiazepine	In patients younger than age 2 years: 0.5 mg/kg/dose In patients older than age 2 years: 0.3 mg/kg/dose	Sleepiness, respiratory compromise, hypotension	Use for seizures lasting more than 5 minutes and for clustering of seizures greater than two in 1 hour $T\frac{1}{2}$ = 4–6 hours

* There has not been any reported case of aplastic anemia in any child younger than 12 years of age on felbamate. The patients in the pediatric population who tend to get into trouble with felbamate are adolescent girls with autoimmune disease. They have a sevenfold increased risk of developing aplastic anemia while taking felbamate.

† Valproic acid can falsely elevate the thyroid-stimulating hormone (TSH) level. If this occurs, repeat thyroid function tests (TFTs), including a free T4 (usually done by equilibrium dialysis) to test true thyroid function. In complicated cases (such as in patients with septo-optic dysplasias), endocrine specialists may need to be involved. The risk of fulminant liver failure in patients younger than 2 years of age who are developmentally delayed and are on other AEDs is 1:500.

Note: Therapeutic half-life ($T\frac{1}{2}$), every day (QD), twice daily (BID), three times daily (TID), antiepileptic drug (AED), electrocardiograph (ECG), benzodiazepine, adrenocorticotropic hormone (ACTH), Lennox-Gastaut syndrome (LGS), myoclonic-astatic epilepsy (MAE), infantile spasms (IS).

Source: Adapted from Blosser & Reider-Demer, 2009.

Drugs such as carbamazepine, phenytoin, primidone, and phenobarbital are equally effective in controlling complex partial seizures and secondary seizures. Carbamazepine is more effective in treating complex partial seizures compared to valproic acid. Other reasonable alternatives are lamotrigine, topiramate, oxcarbazine, and phenytoin (Table 33-23).

Diastat (rectal diazepam) may be prescribed for rescue therapy. When a patient experiences a seizure that last for 5 minutes or longer, the medication is administered rectally (Table 33-23). Diastat is intended for emergency use only; it may not be prescribed for daily use. This agent may be used in the home, by emergency medical personnel, or in the acute care setting. Caregivers should immediately contact emergency medical services anytime their child or adolescent experiences respiratory distress or an unrelenting seizure at home.

A nonpharmacologic strategy for seizure management is the ketogenic diet. This intervention may be considered in patients who have refractory seizures or who experience problematic adverse effects from AED therapy. The ketogenic diet is consists of high fat, adequate protein, and very low carbohydrate levels, thereby mimicking aspects of starvation by demanding that the body burn fats instead of carbohydrates for energy. When carbohydrate intake is extremely low, the liver converts fats into fatty acids and ketone bodies, which pass into the brain and replace glucose as an energy source. Ketosis has been shown to reduce the frequency of seizures in some patients. The classic 4:1 ratio refers to the total grams of daily fat intake in comparison to total daily grams of protein and carbohydrate intake combined (Fenton, 2009). Unfortunately, compliance with the ketogenic diet is extremely difficult to maintain for families, and its use requires support from neurology and nutrition specialists who are well versed in its implementation and ongoing monitoring. Patient who are placed on a ketogenic diet require hospitalization to safely reach a state of ketosis, followed by frequent outpatient monitoring.

Critical care and seizure management

For those patients who experience status epilepticus, management may be more complex and require intensive care. The goals of patient management in these circumstances include preservation of cardiopulmonary function, cessation of seizure activity, and identification and treatment of the underlying cause, if possible. Patients with prolonged seizure activity may require positioning to maintain a patent airway, supplemental oxygen, or endotracheal intubation and mechanical ventilation. Intravenous access should be obtained, if possible, to allow for management of the seizures with antiepileptic medications. Lorazepam is the first-line therapy for seizure management outside the neonatal period. It has a rapid onset and in most patients stops seizure activity in 2 to 5 minutes (Shields, 1989). If seizure

activity persists, the patient may require additional AEDs, such as phenobarbital or fosphenytoin to stop seizure activity. In addition and if possible, the underlying cause of the seizure activity should be identified. Patients whose seizures occur secondary to a metabolic derangement such as hypoglycemia or hyponatremia must have these derangements treated to stop the seizure activity.

In patients whose seizures are refractory to standard management, the inducement of a drug-induced coma may be necessary. This is usually accomplished by continuous infusion of barbiturates, either pentobarbital or thiopental. Other agents, such as high-dose benzodiazepines and anesthetic agents, have also been used for this purpose. The goal of therapy in these patients is either burst suppression or electrocerebral silence. Patients require both continuous monitoring of electroencephalographic activity and hemodynamic monitoring available only in an intensive care unit.

Complications of status epilepticus in the intensive care environment include rhabdomyolysis, hyperthermia, and cerebral edema. These sequelae should be treated aggressively to minimize further brain injury.

Management of refractory seizures

Surgical intervention may be considered when seizures remain uncontrolled by optimal medical management and diminish an individual's quality of life. Patients with refractory seizures often continue to have uncontrolled seizures after two trials of high-dose monotherapy using two different and appropriate drugs, and one trial of combination therapy.

Focal brain resection is the most common type of epilepsy surgery. Resection may be appropriate when seizures begin in a restricted cortical area and will not impair neurological function. Most commonly, seizure foci originate in the temporal lobe (Carl, 2007).

Corpus callostomy may be recommended for patients with atonic seizures. This surgery involves dividing the corpus callosum and disconnecting the two hemispheres of the brain. Hemispherectomy is the removal of the large cortical areas from one side of the brain when the seizures are derived from almost the entire hemisphere, such as in patients with Rasmussen syndrome.

A vagal nerve stimulator (VNS) is typically recommended for refractory partial seizures in patients who are not considered surgical candidates. The VNS is a palliative device that stimulates the vagus nerve; it is implanted in the upper left chest, similar to a pacemaker. The device provides intermittent stimulation of the left vagus nerve within the neck (Fisher, 1999). Although the exact mechanism underlying its effectiveness is unclear, the VNS appears to reorganize neural electrical firing and avoids unequal surging that may elicit a seizure. Recent studies have shown that metabolic activation of certain thalamic, brain stem, and limbic structures may be important in mediating the effect of VNS. The improvement in seizure control derived from use of VNS is similar to that of new AEDs.

Patients presenting with either first-time or chronic seizure history may require consultation with a number of specialties, including neurology, critical care, metabolic, and infectious diseases. Nutritional consultation optimizes energy demands and ketogenic diet success. If the seizures are refractory and the patient requires surgical intervention, consultation with neurosurgery and/or general surgery may be required. Long-term hospitalization secondary to refractory seizures warrants involvement of the rehabilitative team, child life, and social and spiritual services in the patient's and family's care. Sequelae associated with AEDs may also require the involvement of the gastroenterology/hepatology and hematology services.

Caregiver education involves discussion of hospital admission and goals of therapy, which include cardiopulmonary support and cessation of seizure activity. Families should also be prepared for the diagnostic studies to be performed and contact with specialty consultants as a part of the therapeutic plan. Depending on the patient's response to therapy, families may face a brief acute hospital admission or may need to be prepared for an extensive hospitalization.

DISPOSITION AND DISCHARGE PLANNING

One-third of children with febrile seizures will have more than one episode; however, those with isolated febrile seizures have about the same chance as the general population for developing epilepsy. Approximately one-third of children with unprovoked seizures will also have a recurrence (Scotoni et al., 2004). Long-term prognosis is highly variable and depends on the underlying pathology, adequate seizure control, and the effects of seizure activity and AEDs on quality of life.

Discharge instructions include seizure recognition, maintaining the AED regimen as prescribed, not altering prescription drugs from the prescribed and dispensed medication, and approaches to keeping the patient safe when discharged. Caregiver instructions specific to a seizure include the following guidelines:

- Do not attempt to hold the child.
- Do not try to stop any movements.
- Do not place anything in the child's mouth.
- Clear all items around the child, place something soft under the head, and turn the child to the left side if possible.
- Loosen anything around the child's neck.
- Keep track of how long the seizure lasts with a watch and what the seizure looked like.
- Try to remain calm (Epilepsy Foundation, n.d.).

Medical attention should be sought if it is a first seizure, if the seizure lasts for more than 5 minutes, if the child has high fever or diabetes, if there is a risk for head injury, or if the child's respiratory or cardiac function is compromised.

SUBMERSION INJURIES

Nicole Fortier O'Brien

PATHOPHYSIOLOGY

After submersion, most individuals undergo a period of struggle, that includes breath holding or accidental intake of water into the oropharynx and larynx with resultant laryngospasm. Either effect may result in progressive hypoxia and eventual loss of consciousness. Most victims then experience a loss of protective reflexes with subsequent aspiration of water. In addition, large quantities of water may be swallowed and vomited with aspiration of gastric contents. Aspiration of material into the lungs is known as "wet drowning." In approximately 10% to 20% of victims of submersion injury, severe laryngospasm persists even after loss of consciousness and aspiration into the lungs is prevented (Levine & Morris, 1993; Zuckerman & Conway, 2000); this phenomenon is known as "dry drowning." Unless rescue from the submersion occurs, continued asphyxia and hypoxia will ultimately lead to cardiorespiratory failure and death.

After rescue from submersion, some degree of pulmonary dysfunction is not uncommon in pediatric patients. Aspiration of freshwater results in the denaturing of surfactant, with subsequent alveolar collapse, intrapulmonary shunting, and hypoxia. Saltwater aspiration results in a large osmotic gradient with transudation of fluid from the pulmonary vasculature into the alveoli. This increased intra-alveolar fluid results in surfactant dilution and washout with alveolar collapse, shunting, and hypoxia. In addition, regardless of the type of fluid aspirated, pronounced injury to pulmonary capillaries can occur, leading to increased membrane permeability, exudation of proteinaceous material into alveoli, pulmonary edema, and decreased lung compliance (Sarnaik & Leih-Lai, 2006).

EPIDEMIOLOGY AND ETIOLOGY

Traditionally, drowning has been defined as death from asphyxia within 24 hours of submersion in water. Near drowning has typically been referred to as survival beyond 24 hours after the episode of submersion, even if survival is temporary. In 2002, at the World Congress on Drowning, these definitions were revised. Drowning is now defined as respiratory impairment from submersion in a liquid; its outcome may be death, morbidity, or no morbidity (Bierens, 2006).

According to the Centers for Disease Control and Prevention (CDC, 2008), more than 3,500 fatal drownings occur each year in the United States, with more than 800 of these victims being children younger the age of 14 years. For each fatality, at least another 4 children receive emergency care for nonfatal submersion injuries. Due to underreporting, the frequency of nonfatal drowning is probably much higher than published.

Males are four times more likely than females to suffer a submersion injury. Minority children are also at increased risk of drowning. Alaskan Natives and American Indians experience a drowning rate that is 2.4 times that of Caucasians, and for African Americans the risk is 3.2 times that of Caucasians (CDC, 2008). There is also a bimodal age distribution for submersion injuries, with the first peak in children younger than 4 years of age. Infants younger than the age of 1 year are susceptible to drowning in bathtubs, buckets, or toilets. Toddlers aged 1 to 4 years most often experience submersion injury in residential swimming pools. Lack of appropriate barriers and inadequate supervision are major risk factors for submersion injuries in such young children. Adolescence represents the second peak in age distribution for drowning when such injuries are most often associated with alcohol or drug use and risk-taking behavior (Brenner et al., 2001; Kallas & O'Rourke, 1993).

PRESENTATION

There is a wide spectrum of presentation for pediatric patients suffering a drowning episode. Some patients may be completely asymptomatic. Other patients may have evidence of mild to severe organ dysfunction or present in full cardiopulmonary arrest.

Pulmonary effects

Children rescued after a brief episode of submersion will often have hypoxia limited to the duration of apnea, with resolution occurring during the initial resuscitative efforts. These patients often present with no or few respiratory complaints. Children who experience longer episodes of submersion or who aspirate large quantities of water often have continued hypoxia even after initial resuscitation is complete; they may present to a treatment center with mild to severe respiratory distress or respiratory failure. Progression to acute respiratory distress syndrome is not an infrequent complication of a submersion injury. Aspiration of stomach contents, debris, and bacteria may also result in a secondary pneumonia and contribute to respiratory dysfunction. Initial chest radiographs can be normal, show patchy infiltrates (most commonly in the periphery or bibasilar regions), or show frank pulmonary edema.

Cardiovascular effects

Cardiovascular instability is also often encountered following a submersion injury. Hypoxemia and acidosis can result in life-threatening arrhythmias such as ventricular tachycardia or asystole. Prolonged hypoxia also results in myocardial damage characterized by decreased cardiac output and cardiogenic shock. Hypoxia and inflammatory mediators can also cause pulmonary vasoconstriction, which, if severe enough, results in decreased right ventricular stroke volume, decreased left ventricular preload, and worsened cardiac output (Biagas, 2009).

Neurologic effects

Nonfatal drownings can result in hypoxic-ischemic damage to the brain. Conn et al. (1980) developed a classification scheme that estimates the magnitude of hypoxic insult among submersion victims based on neurologic function on arrival to a treating center. Patients in category A are awake, alert, and have minimal brain injury. Patients in category B have more serious asphyxial injury, show a blunted to stuporous affect, but have normal pupillary reactions and purposeful responses to pain. Patients in category C have experienced more severe brain injury and are comatose, have an abnormal respiratory pattern, and have abnormal motor responses to pain. Patients in category C can be further subdivided based on motor response to pain: C1—decorticate movements, C2—decerebrate movements, and C3—flaccid (Table 33-24).

Effects on other organ systems

Multiple organ dysfunction due to prolonged hypoxemia may complicate the clinical course of pediatric patients suffering an episode of drowning. Renal dysfunction (acute tubular necrosis), hepatic and gastrointestinal dysfunction,

TABLE 33-24

Postsubmersion Neurological Classification	
Category	**Description**
A	Alert, fully conscious
B	Obtunded, stuporous but arousable; purposeful response to pain; normal respiration
C	Comatose, not arousable; abnormal response to pain; abnormal respirations
C1	Flexor response to pain; Cheyne-Stokes respiration
C2	Extensor response to pain; central hyperventilation
C3	Flaccid; apneic

disseminated intravascular coagulation, and profound metabolic acidosis are frequently encountered. Of note, most patients who have suffered a submersion injury do not develop blood volume alterations or electrolyte abnormalities. While most victims aspirate an average of 3 mL/kg, aspiration of more than 11 mL/kg is required for blood volume alterations and aspiration of more than 22 mL/kg is required for electrolyte alterations (Modell & Davis, 1969; Modell & Moya, 1966, 1967).

DIFFERENTIAL DIAGNOSIS

In most instances, the history and physical examination confirm the diagnosis of drowning. The possibility of non-accidental injury should be considered in very young children, and the possibility of suicide should be considered in adolescents. Seizures may also lead to a drowning episode. If the history or physical examination is suspicious, further evaluation should be undertaken. Coexistent spinal cord injury should be considered in all pediatric patients whose submersion event followed a diving incident or was unwitnessed.

PLAN OF CARE

The management of a pediatric patient suffering significant submersion injury with respiratory or hemodynamic compromise starts with CPR in the field. The main goal is to improve oxygenation and ventilation as rapidly as possible so as to improve the neurologic outcome. Immobilization of the patient's neck should be implemented if a spinal cord injury is suspected.

On arrival to the emergency department, the patient's airway, respirations, and peripheral perfusion should be evaluated. Pediatric patients who are asymptomatic following a submersion injury often require no specific interventions; observation alone is sufficient in these situations. Patients with mild to moderate hypoxia can receive supplemental oxygen via nasal cannula or face mask.

Some patients will also require bilevel or continuous positive airway pressure (BiPAP or CPAP, respectively). Positive airway pressure increases functional residual capacity and lung compliance, decreases atelectasis and pulmonary edema, reduces intrapulmonary shunting, and can be effective in reversing hypoxemia (Sarnaik & Leih-Lai, 2006). Patients will often require supplemental oxygen or positive-pressure ventilation for 48 to 72 hours, which is the time it takes for pulmonary surfactant to be regenerated (Burford et al., 2005).

Patients with significant respiratory distress, poor respiratory effort, significant hypoxia, or altered mental status and an inability to protect their airway require intubation and mechanical ventilation. Pediatric patients who progress to acute lung injury and acute respiratory distress syndrome (ARDS) should undergo mechanical ventilation with ventilatory strategies aimed at minimizing barotrauma and volutrauma. Refractory hypoxemia has been treated with extracorporeal membrane oxygenation (ECMO) with some degree of success (Thalmann et al., 2001).

The use of routine antibiotics in victims of submersion injury is not indicated unless the patient becomes febrile, has increasing leukocytosis, has worsening infiltrates on chest radiograph, or develops hemodynamic instability (Miller, 2004). Empiric steroids should also not be administered, as outcomes are not improved and infection rates may be increased with these medications (Salomez & Vincent, 2004). Pulmonary edema is frequently encountered following submersion injury; although patients may require diuretic therapy to counteract this effect, close attention to overall fluid status must be paid prior to administration of these agents.

Arrhythmias such as ventricular tachycardia and asystole are frequently encountered early in resuscitation. Correction of hypoxemia and acidosis and standard CPR techniques with appropriate medication administration should be performed. Hypovolemia should be corrected with isotonic crystalloids or colloids (10 to 20 mL/kg). Inotropic support with dopamine, dobutamine, or epinephrine may be required if hypotension or poor perfusion persists.

Once the ABCs are addressed, neurologic evaluation should be undertaken and a secondary survey with exclusion of other injuries should be performed. Asymptomatic patients require no laboratory or radiologic studies. Initial laboratory evaluation for symptomatic patients should include an arterial blood gas and chest radiograph. A CBC, coagulation studies, and electrolyte panel should also be considered in symptomatic patients.

The degree of CNS injury is now the major determinant of morbidity and survival in pediatric drowning. Historical factors that may correlate with poor neurologic outcome after submersion injury include duration of submersion lasting more than 4 to 5 minutes (Orlowski, 1979; Quan & Kinder, 1992), warm water temperature (Biggart & Bohn, 1990; Kram & Kizer, 1984; Kyriacou et al., 1994), need for CPR in the field (Jacobsen et al., 1983; O'Rourke, 1986), and continued apnea, systole, and coma after arrival to the emergency department (Habib et al., 1996). Once resuscitation is complete, further evaluation of the patient's neurologic status should be undertaken with serial physical exams, labs, and a head CT scan. Laboratory variables such as a pH less than 7.1 and elevated serum glucose have been found to correlate with worse neurologic outcome (Ashwal et al., 1990; Habib et al., 1996). Rafaat et al. (2008) showed that all pediatric patients with an initial abnormal CT scan (loss of gray white, low-density lesions in basal ganglia and thalami, effacement of cisterns) following submersion injury died. Of patients who had an initially normal CT but an abnormal second CT, 54% died, 42% entered into a persistent vegetative state, and only 4% had a good outcome at 6 months after the submersion event. Various neurocritical care therapies such as hyperventilation, osmolar therapy, barbiturate therapy, hypothermia, and intracranial pressure monitoring have not been shown to improve morbidity or mortality in children suffering a hypoxic-ischemic insult, and they should not be used routinely (Bohn et al., 1986; Frewen et al., 1985; Nussbaum & Maggi, 1988; Spack et al., 1997).

Close communication with family members regarding the overall management plan of the pediatric patient suffering submersion injury is imperative. Of particular importance is relaying detailed information about the patient's neurologic exam and findings on head CT scan. This information will help family members make informed decisions about continuing or discontinuing life support.

DISPOSITION AND DISCHARGE PLANNING

Nearly all patients who demonstrate significant problems in gas exchange will do so by 4 to 6 hours after the submersion incident. Therefore, patients who can be observed for this duration of time and who meet the category A criteria from a neurologic perspective can be discharged from the emergency department. Any victim with respiratory symptoms, an abnormal chest radiograph, abnormal blood gas measurements, or an abnormal neurologic exam should be admitted to the hospital for continued observation until these abnormalities have resolved (Mason, 2005). Provided the patient has returned to his or her baseline, routine follow-up with a PCP is appropriate for these children. Children with prolonged hospitalization or neurologic injury may require occupational and physical therapy and rehabilitation evaluation and treatment.

REFERENCES

1. Abend, N., & Licht, D. (2008). Predicting outcome in children with hypoxic ischemic encephalopathy. *Pediatric Critical Care Medicine*, 9(1), 32–39.

2. Ade-Hall, R., & Moore, P. (2009, October 17). Botuliumum toxin type A in the treatment of lower limb spasticity in cerebral palsy [Cochrane Review]. *Cochrane Database of Systematic Reviews, Ovid Evidence Based Medicine Reviews*.

3. Adelson, P., Bratton, S., Carney, N., Chestnut, R., duCoudray, H., Goldstein, B., et al. (2003). Guidelines for the acute medical management of severe traumatic brain injury in infants, children, and adolescents. *Pediatric Critical Care Medicine, 4*, 34–37.

4. Al-Jarallah, A., Al-Rifai, M., Riela, A. R., & Roach, S. (2000). Nontraumatic brain hemorrhage in children: Etiology and presentation. *Journal of Child Neurology, 15*, 284–289.

5. American Academy of Child and Adolescent Psychiatry (AACAP). (2009a). Child and Adolescent Service Intensity Instrument. Retrieved from www.aacap.org/cs/root/member_information/practice_information/casii

6. American Academy of Child and Adolescent Psychiatry (AACAP). (2009b). Glossary of symptoms and illnesses: Psychosis. Retrieved from www.aacap.org/cs/root/resources_for_families/glossary_of_symptoms_and_illnesses/psychosis

7. American Academy of Neurology (AAN). (2009). Practice parameter: Diagnostic assessment of the child with cerebral palsy. Retrieved from http://www.aan.com/globals/axon/assets/2601.pdf

8. American Academy of Pediatrics (AAP). Report of the Committee on Infectious Diseases. (2006a). *Haemophilus influenzae* infections. In *2006 AAP red book*. Elk Grove Village, IL: Author.

9. American Academy of Pediatrics (AAP). Report of the Committee on Infectious Diseases. (2006b). Pnuemococcal infections. In *2006 AAP red book*. Elk Grove Village, IL: Author.

10. American Psychiatric Association (APA). (2000). *Diagnostic and statistical manual of mental disorders* (4th ed., text revision). Washington, DC: American Psychiatric Press.

11. Amlie-Lefond, C., Sebire, G., & Fullerton, H. (2008). Recent developments in childhood arterial ischaemic stroke. *Lancet Neurology, 7*, 425–435.

12. Ashwal, S. (2001). Clinical diagnosis and confirmatory testing of brain death in children. In E. Wijdicks, *Brain death*. Philadelphia: Lippincott Williams & Wilkins.

13. Ashwal, S., Schneider, S., Tomasi, L., & Thompson, J. (1990). Prognostic implications of hyperglycemia and reduced cerebral blood flow in childhood near-drowning. *Neurology, 40*(5), 820–823.

14. Au, K. S., Ward, C. H., & Northrup, H. (2008). Tuberous sclerosis complex: Disease modifiers and treatments. *Current Opinion in Pediatrics, 20*, 628–633.

15. Avner, J. (2006). Altered states of Consciousness. *Pediatrics in Review, 27*, 331–338.

16. Bax, M., Goldstein, M., Rosenbaum, P., Leviton, A., Paneth, N., et al. (2005). Proposed definition and classification of cerebral palsy. *Developmental Medicine and Child Neurology, 47*(8), 571–576.

17. Bax. M., Tydeman, C., & Flodmark, O. (2006). Clinical and MRI correlates of cerebral palsy: The European cerebral palsy study. *Journal of the American Medical Association, 296*(13), 1602–1608.

18. Bernard, T., Goldenberg, N., Armstrong-Wells, J., Amlie-Lefond, C., & Fullerton, H. (2008). Treatment of childhood arterial ischemic stroke. *Ann Neurol, 63*, 679–696.

19. Biagas, K. (2009). Drowning and near drowning: Submersion injuries. In M. Helfaer & D. Nichols (Eds.)., *Rogers handbook of pediatric intensive care* (4th ed., pp. 55–59). Philadelphia: Lippincott, Williams & Wilkins.

20. Bierens, J. (2006). *Handbook on drowning*. New York: Springer Science.

21. Biggart, M. J., & Bohn, D. J. (1990). Effect of hypothermia and cardiac arrest on outcome of near-drowning accidents in children. *Journal of Pediatrics, 117*(2), 179–183.

22. Blosser, C., & Reider-Demer, M. (2009). Neurologic disorders. In C. Burns, A. Dunn, M. Brady, N. Starr, & C. Blosser (Eds.)., *Pediatric primary care* (4th ed., pp. 634–672). St. Louis: Saunders Elsevier.

23. Bohn, D. J., Biggar, W., Smith, C., Conn, A., & Barker, G. (1986). Influence of hypothermia, barbiturate therapy, and intracranial pressure monitoring on morbidity and mortality after near-drowning. *Critical Care Medicine, 14*(6), 529–532.

24. Brenner, R. A., Trumble, A., Smith, G., Kessler, E., & Overpeck, M. (2001). Where children drown, United States. *Pediatrics, 108*(1), 85–89.

25. Bruce, D. (1985). Cerebrovascular dynamics. In H. James, N. Anas, & R. Perkins (Eds.)., *Brain insults in children*. Orlando, FL: Grune & Stratton.

26. Buchner, J., Schmidt, N., Lang, A., Small, J., Schlauch, R., & Lewinsohn, P. (2008). Specificity of social anxiety disorders as a risk factor for alcohol and cannabis dependence. *Journal of Psychiatric Research, 42*(3), 230–239.

27. Burford, A., Ryan, L., Stone, B., Hirshon, J., & Klein, B. (2005). Drowning and near-drowning in children and adolescents. *Pediatric Emergency Care, 21*(9), 610–619.

28. Bushby, K., Finkel, R., Birnkrant, D., Case, L., Clemens, P., Cripe, L., et al. (2010a). Diagnosis and management of Duchenne muscular dystrophy, part 1: Diagnosis, and pharmacological and psychosocial managemement. *Lancet Neurology, 9*(1), 77–93. Retrieved from www.thelancet.com/neurology

29. Bushby, K., Finkel, R., Birnkrant, D., Case, L., Clemens, P., Cripe, L., et al. (2010b). Diagnosis and management of Duchenne muscular dystrophy, part 2: Implementation of multidisciplinary care. *Lancet Neurology, 9*(2), 177–189. Retrieved from www.thelancet.com/neurology

30. Carl, W. B. (2007). Many options for epilepsy: Comparisons of the first and second generation AED. *Lancet, 369*, 1000–1015.

31. Cartwright, C. (2004). Pediatric and developmental anomalies. In M. K. Bader & L. Littlejohns (eEs.)., *AACN core curriculum: Neuroscience nursing* (4th ed., pp. 853–899). St. Louis: Saunders.

32. Centers for Disease Control and Prevention (CDC), National Center for Injury Prevention and Control. (2008). Water-related injuries. Retrieved from http://www.cdc.gov/ncipc/wisqars

33. Chavez-Bueno, S., & McCracken, G. (2005). Bacterial meningitis in children. *Pediatric Clinics of North America, 52*(3), 795–810.

34. Cohen-Gadol, A., & Pollack, B. (2006). Radiosurgery for arteriovenous malformations in children. *Journal of Neurosurgery, 104*, 388–391.

35. Conn, A. W., Montes, J. E., & Baker, G. A. (1980). Cerebral salvage in near-drowning following neurologic classification by triage. *Canadian Anesthetic Society Journal, 27*(3), 201.

36. Connolly, S., & Bernstein, G. (2007). Practice parameters for the assessment and treatment of children and adolescents with anxiety disorders. *Journal of the American Academy of Child and Adolescent Psychiatry, 46*(2), 267–283.

37. Crawford, A. H., & Schorry, E. K. (2006). Neurofibromatosis update. *Journal of Pediatric Orthopedics, 26*(3), 413–423.

38. Curatolo, P., Bombardieri, R., & Sergiusz, J. (2008). Tuberous sclerosis. *Lancet, 372*, 657–668.

39. Davis, R., et al. (1987). Head and spinal cord injury. In M. Rogers (Ed.)., *Textbook of pediatric intensive care*. Baltimore: Williams & Wilkins.

40. Defresne, P., Meyer, L., Tardieu, M., Scalais, E., Nuttin, C., DeBont, B., et al. (2001). Efficacy of high dose steroid therapy in children with severe acute transverse myelitis. *Journal of Neurology, Neurosurgery, and Psychiatry, 71*, 272–274.

41. DeMaso, D., Martini, R., & Cahen, L. (2009). Practice parameters for the psychiatric assessment and management of physically ill children and adolescents. *Journal of the American Academy of Child and Adolescent Psychiatry, 48*(2), 213–233.

42. deVeber, G. (2002). Stroke and the child's brain: An overview of the epidemiology, syndromes and risk factors. *Current Opinion in Neurology, 15*, 133–138.

43. deVeber, G. (2003). Arterial ischemic strokes in infants and children: An overview of current approaches. *Seminars in Thrombosis and Hemostasis, 29*, 567–573.

44. deVeber, G., Andrew, M., Adams, C., Bjornson, B., Booth, F., Buckley, D., et al. (2001). For the Canadian Pediatric Ischemic Stroke Group: Cerebral sinovenous thrombosis in children. *New England Journal of Medicine, 345*, 417–423.

45. deVeber, G., MacGregor, D., Curtis, R., & Mayank, S. (2000). Neurologic outcome in survivors of childhood arterial ischemic stroke and sinovenous thrombosis. *Journal of Child Neurology, 15*, 316–324.

46. DiRocco, C., Tamburrini, G., & Rollo, M. (2000). Cerebral arteriovenous malformations in children. *Acta Neurochirurgica, 142*, 145–158.

47. Dorfer, C., Czech, T., Bavinski, G., Kitz, K., Mert, A., Knosp, E., et al. (2009). Multimodality treatment of cerebral AVMs in children: A single-centre 20 years experience. *Child's Nervous System*. doi: 10.1007/s00381-009-1039-8

48. Eisenberg, E., River, Y., Shifrin, A., & Krivoy, N. (2007). Antiepileptic drugs in the treatment of neuropathic pain. *Drugs, 67*, 1265–1289.

49. El Bashir, H. (2003). Diagnosis and treatment of bacterial meningitis. *Archives of Diseases of Childhood, 88*, 615–620.

50. Epilepsy Foundation. (n.d.). Retrieved from www.epilepsyfoundation.org

51. Evans, D. G. R. (2009). Neurofibromatosis type 2 (NF2): A clinical and molecular review. *Orphanet Journal of Rare Diseases, 4*(16), 1–11.

52. Feigin, R. (2006). Bacterial meningitis beyond the newborn period. In J. Mcmillan, *Oski's pediatrics* (4th ed., pp. 924–934). Philadelphia: Lippincott, Williams & Wilkins.

53. Feigin, R. (2009). Bacterial meningitis beyond the neonatal period. In R. Feigin, J. Cherry, G. Demmler-Harriosn, & S. Kaplan (Eds.)., *Textbook of pediatric infectious diseases* (pp. 443–474). Philadelphia: Saunders Elsevier.

54. Fenton, C. (2009). Manipulation of the types of fats and cholesterol intake can successfully improve the lipid profile while maintaining the efficacy of the ketogenic diet. *Infant, Child and Adolescent Nutrition, 1*(6), 338–341.

55. Fisher, R. (1999). Reassessment of vagus nerve stimulator for epilepsy: A report of the Therapeutic and Technological Assessment Subcommittee of the American Academy of Neurology. *Neurology, 53*, 666.

56. French, J. (1999). Practice advisory: The use of felbamate in the treatment of patients with inactive epilepsy: Report of Quality Standards Subcommittee of the American Academy Epilepsy Society. *Neurology, 52*, 1540.

57. Frewen, T. C., Sumabat, W., Han, V., Amacher, A., Del Maestro, R., & Bibbald, W. (1985). Cerebral resuscitation therapy in pediatric near-drowning. *Journal of Pediatrics, 106*(4), 615.

58. Fullerton, H., Achrol, A., Johnston, S., McCulloch, C., Higashida, R., Lawton, M., et al. (2005). Long-term hemorrhage risk in children versus adults with brain arteriovenous malformations. *Stroke, 36*, 2099–2104.

59. Fullerton, H., Wu, Y., Sidney, S., & Claiborne, J. (2007). Risk of recurrent childhood arterial ischemic stroke in a population-based cohort: The importance of cerbrovascular imaging. *Pediatrics, 119*, 495–501.

60. Gabis, L., Ravi, Y., & Lenn, N. (2002). Time lag to diagnosis of stroke in children. *Pediatrics, 110*, 924–928.

61. Gage, J. R., Schwartz, M. H., Koop, S. E., & Novacheck, T. F. (Eds.). (2009). *The identification and treatment of gait problems in cerebral palsy*. London: Mac Keith Press.

62. Ganesan, V., Hogan, A., Shack, N., Gordon, A., Isaacs, E., & Kirkham, F. (2000). Outcome after ischaemic stroke in childhood. *Developmental Medicine and Child Neurology, 42*, 455–461.

63. Ganesan, V., Prengler, M., McShane, M., Wade, A., & Kirkham, F. (2003). Investigation of risk factors in children with arterial ischemic stroke. *Annals of Neurology, 53*, 167–173.

64. Gilbert, D. (2000). An EEG should not be obtained routinely after first unprovoked seizure in childhood. *Neurology, 54*, 635.

65. Gillis, J., & Ryan, M. (2008). Chronic neuromuscular diseases. In D. Nichols (Ed.)., *Rogers' textbook of pediatric intensive care* (4th ed., pp. 800–809). Philadelphia: Lippincott.

66. Gilman, S. (1998a). Imaging the brain: First of two parts. *New England Journal of Medicine, 338*, 812–820.

67. Gilman, S. (1998b). Imaging the brain: Second of two parts. *New England Journal of Medicine, 338*, 889–896.

68. Goldstein, B., Aboy, M., & Graham, A. (2007). Neurologic monitoring. In D. Nichols (Ed.)., *Rogers' textbook of pediatric intensive care* (4th ed., pp. 862–871). Baltimore: Lippincott, Williams & Wilkins.

69. Golomb, M. R., Fullerton, H. J., Nowak-Gottl, U., & deVeber, G. (2009). Male predominance in childhood ischemic stroke: Findings from the international Pediatric Stroke Study. *Stroke, 40*, 52–57.

70. Habib, D. M., Tecklenburg, F., Webb, S., Anas, N., & Perkin, R. (1996). Prediction of childhood drowning and near-drowning morbidity and mortality. *Pediatric Emergency Care, 12*(4), 255–258.

71. Hadjiloizou, S. (2005). Generalized seizures. In M. Bernard, *Current management of child neurology* (3rd ed., pp. 117–128). Shelton, CT: People's Medical Publishing House.

72. Haslam, R. (2008). Neurologic evaluation. In R. Kliegman, R. Behrman, H. Jenson, & B. Stanton (Eds.), *Nelson's textbook of pediatrics* (18th ed.). Amsterdam: Saunders.

73. Hickey, J. (2003). Diagnostic procedures and laboratory testing for neuroscience patients. In J. Hickey (Ed.), *The clinical practice of neurological and neurosurgical nursing* (5th ed.). New York: Lippincott, Williams & Wilkins.

74. Hirtz, D. (2000). Practice parameter: Evaluation a first non-febrile seizure in children. *Neurology, 55*, 616–623.

75. Hirtz, D. (2003). Practice parameter: Treatment of the child with a first unprovoked seizure: Report of the Quality Standards Subcommittee of the American Academy of Neurology and Practice Committee of the Child Neurology Society. *Neurology, 60*, 166–175.

76. Hoare, B. J., Wallen, M. A., Imms, C., Villanueva, E., Rawicki, H. B., & Carey, L. (2008, August 17). Botulinum toxin A as an adjunct to treatment in the management of the upper limb in children with spastic cerebral palsy [Cochrane Review]. *Cochrane Database of Systematic Reviews, Ovid Evidence Based Medicine Reviews.*

77. Hoh, B., Ogilvy, C., Butler, W., Loeffler, J., Putnam, C., & Chapman, P. (2000). Multimodality treatment of nongalenic arteriovenous malformations in pediatric patients. *Neurosurgery Online, 47*(2), 346–358.

78. Homer, C. J., Klatka, K., Romm, D., Kuhlthau, K., Bloom, S., Newacheck, P., et al. (2008). A review of the evidence for the medical home for children with special health care needs. *Pediatrics, 122*, e922–e937.

79. Hu, M., Wang, H., Lin, K., Huang, J., Hsia S., Chou, M., Chou, M., et al. (2008). Clinical experience of childhood hypertensive encephalopathy over an eight year period. *Chang Gung Medical Journal, 31*(2), 153–158.

80. Hutton, J., Cooke, T., & Pharoah, P. (1998). Life expectancy in children with cerebral palsy. *British Medical Journal, 309*, 431–435.

81. Hydrocephalus Association. (2009). Treatment of hydrocephalus. Retrieved from http://www.hydroasso.org

82. Imran, H., & Clark, A. (2008). Adolescent psychosis: A practical guide to assessment and management. *Psychiatric Times, 25*(10). Retrieved June 10, 2009, from www.psychiatrictimes.com

83. International League Against Epilepsy. (1981). Revised terminology and concepts for organization of the epilepsies: Report of the Commission on Classification and Terminology-Status 2008. Retrieved from www.ilae-epilepsy.org

84. International RadioSurgery Association (IRSA). (2009). Radiosurgery practice guideline initiative: Stereotactic radiosurgery for patients with intracranial arteriovenous malformations (AVM). Radiosurgery Practice Guideline Report #2-03. Retrieved from http://www.irsa.org/AVM%20Guideline.pdf

85. Jacinto, S., Gieron-Korthals, M., & Ferreira, J. (2001). Predicting outcome in hypoxic-ischemic brain injury. *Pediatric Clinics of North America, 48*(3), 647–660.

86. Jacobsen, W. K., Mason, L. J., Briggs, B. A., Schneider, S., & Thompson, J. C. (1983). Correlation of spontaneous respiration and neurologic damage in near-drowning. *Critical Care Medicine, 11*(4), 487–489.

87. James, H., Anas, N., & Perkin, R. (1985). *Brain insults in infants and children.* New York: Grune & Stratton.

88. Jenkins, L., & Kochanek, P. (2007). Developmental neurobiology, neurophysiology, and the PICU. In D. Nichols (Ed.), *Rogers' textbook of pediatric intensive care* (4th ed., pp. 810–825). Baltimore: Lippincott, Williams & Wilkins.

89. Johnston, M. (2006). Development, structure, and function of the brain and neuromuscular systems. In B. Fuhrman & J. Zimmerman (Eds.), *Pediatric critical care* (3rd ed., pp. 767–779). Philadelphia: Mosby.

90. Joshi, P. T., & Towbin, K. E. (2002). Psychosis in childhood and its management. In K. L. Davis, D. Charney, J. T. Coyle, & C. Nemeroff (Eds.), *Neuropsychopharmacology: The fifth generation of progress* (5th ed., pp. 613–623). American College of Neuropsychopharmacology. Philadelphia: Lippincott Williams & Wilkins.

91. Kallas, H. J., & O'Rourke, P. P. (1993). Drowning and immersion injuries in children. *Current Opinion in Pediatrics, 5*(7), 295–302.

92. Kirkham, F. (2007). Therapy insight: Stroke risk and its management in patients with sickle cell disease. *Nature Clin Practice Neurology, 3*, 254–278.

93. Klimo, P., Rao, G., & Brockmeyer, D. (2007). Pediatric arteriovenous malformations: A 15-year experience with an emphasis on residual and recurrent lesions. *Child's Nervous System, 23*, 31–37.

94. Kochanek, P., Bayir, H., Jenkins, L., & Clark, R. (2008). Molecular biology of brain injury. In D. Nichols (Ed.), *Rogers' textbook of pediatric intensive care* (4th ed., pp. 826–845). Philadelphia: Lippincott.

95. Kochanek, P., Fink, E., Bell, M., Bayir, H., & Clark, R. (2009). Therapeutic hypothermia: Applications in pediatric cardiac arrest. *Journal of Neurotrauma, 26*(3), 421–427.

96. Kondziolka, D., Humphreys, R., Hoffman, H., Hendrick, B., & Drake, J. (1992). Arteriovenous malformation of the brain in children: A forty-year experience. *Canadian Journal of Neurologic Science, 19*, 40–45.

97. Kram, J. A., & Kizer, K. W. (1984). Submersion injury. *Emergency Medicine Clinics of North America, 2*(3), 545–552.

98. Krener, P., & Wasserman, A. (1994). Diagnostic dilemmas in pediatric consultation. In M. Lewis & R. King (Eds.), *Child and adolescent psychiatric clinics of North America: Consultation–liaison in pediatrics* (Vol. 3[3], pp. 485–512). Philadelphia: W. B. Saunders.

99. Krueger, D. A., & Franz, D. N. (2008). Current management of tuberous sclerosis complex. *Pediatric Drugs, 10*(5), 299–313.

100. Kyriacou, D. N., Arcinue, E. L., Peek, C., & Kraus, J. F. (1994). Effect of immediate resuscitation on children with submersion injury. *Pediatrics, 94*(2), 137–142.

101. Laugel, V., Cossee, M., Matis, J., de Saint-Martin, A., Echaniz-Laguna, A., Mandel, J., et al. (2008). Diagnostic approach to neonatal hypotonia: Retrospective study on 144 neonates. *European Journal of Pediatrics, 167*, 517–523.

102. Lehman, R., & Mink, J. (2008). Altered mental status. *Clinical Pediatric Emergency Medicine, 9*(2), 68–75.

103. Levine, D. L., & Morris, F. C. (1993). Drowning and near-drowning. *Pediatric Clinics of North America, 40*(2), 321–336.

104. Liou, A., Clark, R., Henshall, D., Yin, X., & CHen, J. (2003). To die or not to die for neurons in ischemia, traumatic brain injury and epilepsy: A review on the stress-activated signaling pathways and apoptotic pathways. *Progress in Neurobiology, 69*(2), 103–142.

105. Listernick, R., Ferner, R., Piersall, L., Sharif, S., Gutmann, D., & Charrow, J. (2004). Late-onset optic pathway tumors in children with neurofibromatosis 1. *Neurology, 63*(10), 1944–1946.

106. Lynch, J., Hirtz, D., deVeber, G., & Nelson, K. (2002). Report of the National Institute of Neurological Disorders and Stroke workshop on perinatal and childhood stroke. *Pediatrics, 109*, 116–123.

107. Mann, K. (2008). Meningitis. *Pediatrics in Review, 29*, 417–430.

108. Mason, R. J. (2005). Near drowning. In R. Mason & J. Murray (Eds.), *Murray & Nadel's Textbook of Respiratory Medicine* (4th ed.). Philadelphia: Mosby Elsevier.

109. McBride, M. (1995). Consultation with the specialist: Status epilepticus. *Pediatrics in Review, 16*, 386–389.

110. McClellan, J., Kowatch, R., & Findling, R. (2007). Practice parameters for the assessment and treatment of children and adolescents with bipolar disorder. *Journal of American Academy of Child and Adolescent Psychiatry, 46*(1), 107–125.

111. McClellan, J., & Werry, J. (2001). Practice parameters for the assessment and treatment of children and adolescents with schizophrenia. *Journal of American Academy of Child and Adolescent Psychiatry, 40*(7 suppl), 4S–23S.

112. McGrath, N., Anderson, N., Croxson, M., & Powell, K. (1997). Herpes simplex encephalitis treated with acyclovir: Diagnosis and long term outcome. *Journal of Neurology, Neurosurgery & Psychiatry, 63*, 321–326.

113. Michelson, D., & Ashwal, S. (2007). Neurologic imaging. In D. Nichols (Ed.),. *Rogers' textbook of pediatric intensive care* (4th ed., pp. 872–886). Baltimore: Lippincott, Williams & Wilkins.

114. Milin, R., Coupland, K., Walker, S., & Fisher-Bloom, E. (2000). Outcome and follow-up study of an adolescent psychiatric day treatment school. *Journal of the American Academy of Child and Adolescent Psychiatry, 39*(3), 320–328.

115. Miller, A. (2004). Infections associated with near drowning. In J. Cohen & W. Powderly (Eds.), *Cohen & Powderly: Infectious diseases* (2nd ed.). Philadelphia: Mosby Elsevier.

116. Modell, J. H., & Davis, J. H. (1969). Electrolyte changes in human drowning victims. *Anesthesiology, 30*(4), 414.

117. Modell, J. H., & Moya, F. (1966). Effects of volume of aspirated fluid during chlorinated fresh water drowning. *Anesthesiology, 27*(5), 662.

118. Modell, J. H., & Moya, F. (1967). The effects of fluid volume in seawater drowning. *Annals of Internal Medicine, 67*(1), 68.

119. Mook, W. V., & Hulsewe-Ewers, R. (2002). Critical illness polyneuropathy. *Current Opinion in Critical Care, 8*, 302–310.

120. Morray, J., Tyler, D., Jones, T., Suntz, J., & Lemire, R. (1984). Coma scale for use in brain-injured children. *Critical Care Medicine, 12*, 1018.

121. Moxley, R., Ashwal, S., Pandya, S., Connolly, A., Florence, J., Mathews, K., et al. (2005). Practice parameter: Corticosteroid treatment of Duchenne dystrophy: Report of the Quality Standards Subcommittee of the American Academy of Neurology and the Practice Committee of the Child Neurology Society. *Neurology, 64*, 13–20.

122. Murphy, N. A., Hoff, C., Jorgensen, T., Norlin, C., & Young, P. C. (2006). Costs and complications of hospitalizations for children with cerebral palsy. *Pediatric Rehabilitation, 9*, 47–52.

123. National Institutes of Health (NIH). (1987, July 13–15). Neurofibromatosis. *NIH Consensus Statement Online, 6*(12), 1–19.

124. National Institutes of Health (NIH). (2007). National Institute of Neurological Disorders and Stroke: Encephalopathy. Retrieved from http://www.ninds.nih.gov/disorders/encephalopathy/encephalopathy.htm

125. Nelson, K. (2003). Can we prevent cerebral palsy? *New England Journal of Medicine, 349*, 1765–1769.

126. Nowak-Gottl, U., Gunther, G., Kurnik, K., Strater, R., & Kirkham, F. (2003). Arterial ischemic stroke in neonates, infants and children: An overview of underlying conditions, imaging methods, and treatment modalities. *Seminars in Thrombosis and Hemostasis, 29*, 405–414.

127. Nussbaum, E., & Maggi, J. C. (1988). Pentobarbital therapy does not improve neurologic outcome in nearly-drowned, flaccid-comatose children. *Pediatrics, 81*(5), 630–634.

128. Ogilvy, C., Stieg, P., Awad, I., Brown, R., Kondziolka, D., Rosenwasser, R., et al. (2001). Recommendations for the management of intracranial arteriovenous malformations: A statement for healthcare professionals from a special writing group of the Stroke Council, American Stroke Council. *Stroke, 32*, 1458–1471.

129. Orlowski, J. P. (1979). Prognostic factors in pediatric cases of drowning and near-drowning. *Journal of the American College of Emergency Physicians, 8*(5), 176–179.

130. O'Rourke, P. P. (1986). Outcome of children who are apneic and pulseless in the emergency room. *Critical Care Medicine, 14*(5), 466–468.

131. O'Shea, T. (2008). Diagnosis, treatment, and prevention of cerebral palsy. *Clinical Obstetrics and Gynecology, 51*(4), 816–828.

132. Palisano, R., Rosenbaum, P., Walter, S., Russell, D., Wood, E., & Galuppi, B. (1997). Development and reliability of a system to classify gross motor function in children with cerebral palsy. *Developmental Medicine and Child Neurology, 39*, 221–222.

133. Pappachan, J., & Kirkham, F. (2008). Cerebrovascular disease and stroke. In D. Nichols (Ed.), *Rogers' textbook of pediatric intensive care* (4th ed., pp. 929–953). Philadelphia: Lippincott.

134. Parke, J. (2006). Acute encephalopathies. In J. McMillan, R. Feigin, C. DeAngelis, & M. Jones (Eds.), *Oski's pediatrics: Principles and practice* (4th ed., p. 2258). Philadelphia: Lippincott, Williams & Wilkins.

135. Pellock, J. (2005). First choice antiepileptic drugs. In M. Bernard, *Current management of child neurology* (3rd ed., pp. 117–128). Shelton, CT: People's Medical Publishing House.

136. Philippe, M., & Thiele, E. (2007). Seizures in children: Determining the variation. *Pediatrics in Review, 28*, 363–371.

137. Pidcock, F., Krishan, C., Crawford, T., Salorio, C., Trovato, M., & Kerr, D. (2007). Acute transverse myelitis of childhood. *Neurology, 68*, 1474–1480.

138. Plum, F., & Posner, J. B. (1982). *The diagnosis of stupor and coma.* Philadelphia: F. A. Davis.

139. Prober, C. (2007). Central nervous system infections. In R. Kliegman, R. Behrman, H. Jenson, & B. Stanton (Eds.), *Nelson's textbook of pediatrics.* Philadelphia: Saunders.

140. Quan, L., & Kinder, D. (1992). Pediatric submersions: Prehospital predictors of outcome. *Pediatrics, 90*(6), 909–913.

141. Rafaat, K. T., Spear, R. M., Parsapour, K., & Peterson, B. (2008). Cranial computed tomographic findings in a large group of children with drowning: Diagnostic, prognostic, and forensic implications. *Pediatric Critical Care Medicine, 9*(6), 567–572.

142. Reilly, P., Simpson, D., Sprod, R., & Thomas, L. (1988). Assessing the conscious level in infants and young children: A paediatric version of the Glasgow Coma Scale. *Child's Nervous System, 4*, 30–33.

143. Rekate, H. (2008). Treatment of hydrocephalus. In A. L. Albright, I. Pollack, & D. Adelson (Eds.), *Principles and practice of pediatric neurosurgery* (2nd ed., pp. 94–108). New York: Thieme Medical Publishers.

144. Roach, E., Golomb, M., Adams, R., Biller, J., Daniels, S., deVeber, G., et al. (2008). Management of stroke in infants and children: A scientific statement from a special writing group of the American Heart Association Stroke Council and the Council on Cardiovascular Disease in the Young. *Stroke, 39*, 2644–2691.

145. Roach, E. S., & Sparagana, S. P. (2004). Diagnosis of tuberous sclerosis complex. *Journal of Child Neurology, 19*(9), 643–649.

146. Rose, J., Stroop, W., Matsuo, F., & Herkel, J. (1992). Atypical herpes simplex encephalitis: Clinical, virologic, and neuropathologic evaluation. *Neurology, 42*, 1809–1812.

147. Rosenbaum, P. (2003). Cerebral palsy: What parents and doctors want to know. *British Medical Journal, 326*, 970–974.

148. Rosenbaum, P., Walter, S., Hanna, S., Palisano, R., Russel, D., Raina, P., et al. (2002). *Cerebral palsies: Epidemiology and causal pathways.* London: Mac Keith.

149. Salomez, F., & Vincent, J. L. (2004). Drowning: A review of epidemiology, pathophysiology, treatment and prevention. *Resuscitation, 63*(3), 266–268.

150. Sarnaik, A., & Leih-Lai, M.(2006). Near-drowning. In B. Fuhrman & J. Zimmerman (Eds.), *Pediatric critical care* (3rd ed., pp. 1556–1563). Philadelphia: Mosby Elsevier.

151. Sarnat, H. (2007). Neuromuscular disorders. In R. Kliegman, R. Behrman, H. Jenson, & B. Stanton (Eds.), *Nelson's textbook of pediatrics* (18th ed.). Philadelphia: Saunders Elsevier.

152. Schwartz, R. A., Fernandez, G., Kotulska, K., & Jozwiak, S. (2007). Tuberous sclerosis complex: Advances in diagnosis, genetics, and management. *Journal of the American Academy of Dermatology, 57*, 189–202.

153. Scotoni, A., Manreza, M., & Guerreiro, M. (2004). Recurrence after a first unprovoked cryptogenic/idiopathic seizure in children: A prospective study from Sao Paolo, Brazil. *Epilepsia, 45*(2), 166–170.

154. Sebire, G., Tabarki, B., Saunders, D., Leroy, I., Liesner, R., Saint-Martin, C., et al. (2005). Cerebral venous sinus thrombosis in children: Risk factors, presentation, diagnosis and outcome. *Brain, 128,* 477–489.

155. Shields, W. (1989). Status epilepticus. *Pediatric Clinics of North America, 36,* 383.

156. Singhi, S., Khadwal, A., & Bansal, A. (2008). Acute neuromuscular diseases. In D. Nichols (Ed.), *Rogers' textbook of pediatric intensive care* (4th ed., pp. 778–797). Philadelphia: Lippincott.

157. Spack, L., Gedeit, R., Splaingard, M., & Havens, P. (1997). Failure of aggressive therapy to alter outcome in pediatric near-drowning. *Pediatric Emergency Care, 13*(2), 98–102.

158. Spetzler, R., & Martin, N. (1986). A proposed grading system for arteriovenous malformations. *Journal of Neurosurgery, 65*(4), 476–483.

159. Stanley, F., Blair, F., & Alberman, E. (2000). *Cerebral palsies: Epidemiology and casual pathways.* London: Mac Keith Press.

160. Statler, K., & Van Orman, C. (2008). Status epilepticus. In D. Nichols (Ed.), *Rogers' textbook of pediatric intensive care* (4th ed., pp. 912–928). Philadelphia: Lippincott, William, & Wilkins.

161. Steinbrook, R. (2007). Organ donation after cardiac death. *New England Journal of Medicine, 357*(3), 209–213.

162. Strauss, D., Brooks, J., Rosenbloom, L., & Shavelle, R. (2008). Life expectancy in cerebral palsy: An update. *Developmental Medicine and Child Neurology, 50,* 487–493.

163. Strouse, J., Hulbert, M., DeBaun, M., Jordan, L., & Casella, J. F. (2006). Primary hemorrhagic stroke in children with sickle cell disease is associated with recent transfusion and use of corticosteroids. *Pediatrics, 118,* 1916–1924.

164. Teasdale, G., & Jennett, B. (1974). Assessment of coma and impaired consciousness: A practical scale. *Lancet, 2,* 81–84.

165. Thalmann, M., Trampitsch, E., Haberfellner, N., Eisendle, E., Kraschl, E., & Kobinia, G. (2001). Resuscitation in near-drowning with extracorporeal membrane oxygenation. *Annals of Thoracic Surgery, 72*(2), 607–608.

166. Thomson, J., & Banta, J. V. (2001). Scoliosis in cerebral palsy: An overview and recent results. *Journal of Pediatric Orthopaedics, Part B, 10,* 6–9.

167. Todres, I. (2006). Brain death. In A. Slonim & M. Pollack (Eds.), *Pediatric critical care medicine* (pp. 790–795). Philadelphia: Lippincott, Williams & Wilkins.

168. Tunkel, A. (2004). Practice guidelines for the mangament of bacterial menigitis. *Clinical Infectious Disease, 39,* 1267–1284.

169. Tyler, K. (2004). Herpes simplex virus infections of the central nervous system: Encephalitis and meningitis, including Mollaret's. *Herpes, 11,* 57A–64A.

170. Vasta, I., Kinali, M., Messina, S., Guzzetta, A., Kapellou, O., Manzur, A., et al. (2005). Can clinical signs identify newborns with neuromuscular disorders? *Journal of Pediatrics, 146,* 73–79.

171. Volpe, J. (2001). Perinatal brain injury: From pathogenesis to neuroprotection. *Mental Retardation and Developmental Disability, 7*(1), 56–64.

172. Wassey, M., Dai, A., Mohsin, A., Shaikh, Z., & Roach, E. S. (2008). Cerebral venous thrombosis in children: A multicenter cohort from the United States. *Journal of Child Neurology, 23,* 26–31.

173. Whitley, R., & Gnann, J. (2002). Viral encephalitis: Familiar infections and emerging pathogens. *Lancet, 359,* 507–513.

174. Williams, S., Horrocks, I., Ouvrier, R., Gillis, J., & Ryan, M. (2007). Critical illness polyneuropathy and myopathy in pediatric intensive care: A review. *Pediatric Critical Care Medicine, 8,* 1–5.

175. Williams, V. C., Lucas, J., Babcock, M. A., Gutmann, D. H., Korf, B., & Maria, B. L. (2009). Neurofibromatosis type 1 revisited. *Pediatrics, 123,* 124–133.

176. Wilson, M., Morgan, E., Shelton, J., & Thorogood, C. (2007a). Cerebral palsy: Introduction and diagnosis (part I). *Journal of Pediatric Health Care, 21*(3), 146–152.

177. Wilson, M., Morgan, E., Shelton, J., & Thorogood, C. (2007b). Primary care of cerebral palsy: A review of systems (part II). *Journal of Pediatric Health Care, 21*(4), 226–237.

178. Wu, Y., Miller, S., Chin, K., Collins, A., Lomeli, S., Chuang, N., et al. (2002). Multiple risk factors in neonatal sinovenous thrombosis. *Neurology, 59*(3), 438–440.

179. Yohay, K. (2006). Neurofibromatosis type 1 and 2. *Neurologist, 12*(2), 86–93.

180. Zalsman, G., Brent, D., & Weersing, R. (2006). Depressive disorders in childhood and adolescence: An overview. In G. Zalsman & D. Brent (Eds.), *Child and adolescent psychiatric clinics of North America: Depression* (Vol. 15[4], pp. 827–841). Philadelphia: W. B. Saunders.

181. Zuckerman, G. B., & Conway, E. E. (2000). Drowning and near drowning: A pediatric epidemic. *Pediatric Annals, 29*(6), 360–366.

Orofacial Disorders

ANATOMY

Samuel M. Maurice, Adam B. Smith, and John W. Polley

The appearance of the human face varies across races, genders, ethnicities, and ages (Farkas et al., 2005). Differences in facial appearance are easily discernable, even among genetically related individuals. Whereas small differences or asymmetries are easily recognized by the naked eye, basic units of facial structure remain relatively constant except in individuals with pathological states. The interplay of the underlying facial skeleton with the overlying soft tissues is responsible for an individual's unique appearance. Facial form is intimately associated with function. The face is ingeniously designed for sight, mastication, respiration, hearing, speech, and expression of emotion.

CRANIAL AND FACIAL SKELETON

The frontal bone overlies the frontal lobes of the brain and makes up the skeleton of the forehead. Prior to suture fusion, the frontal bone is divided sagitally in the midline by the *metopic suture*. The frontal bone articulates with the paired parietal bones posteriorly at the *coronal sutures*. The paired parietal bones meet in the midline at the *sagittal suture*. The paired parietal bones articulate posteriorly with the occipital bone at the *lambdoidal sutures*. The *squamosal suture* separates the parietal bone from the temporal and sphenoid bones laterally (Figure 34-1, Figure 34-2, and Figure 34-3). The metopic, sagittal, coronal, and lambdoidal sutures generally fuse by the time an individuals reaches 2, 22, 24, and 26 years, respectively (Kokich, 1986).

Craniosynostosis refers to premature sutural fusion. Premature fusion of the metopic suture leads to *trigonocephaly*, which is characterized by a pointed, triangle-appearing skull. Premature fusion of bilateral coronal sutures leads to *brachycephaly*, which is characterized by temporal widening and a short anterior–posterior diameter. Premature fusion of the sagittal suture leads to *scaphalocephaly*, which is characterized by temporal narrowing and a long anterior–posterior diameter. Fusion of a unilateral coronal or lambdoid suture leads to *plagiocephally*, or a "twisted skull" appearance.

The *orbit* is composed of seven bones: frontal, lacrimal, ethmoid, maxillary, sphenoid, zygomatic, and palatine. The *maxilla* supports the dentition of the upper jaw, houses the maxillary sinuses, makes up the bony lateral border of the nose (*pyriform aperature*), and is responsible for most of the height of the midface. The maxilla articulates laterally

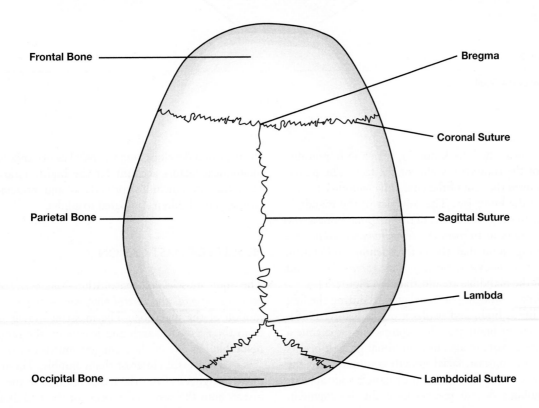

FIGURE 34-1

Superior Aspect of the Cranium.

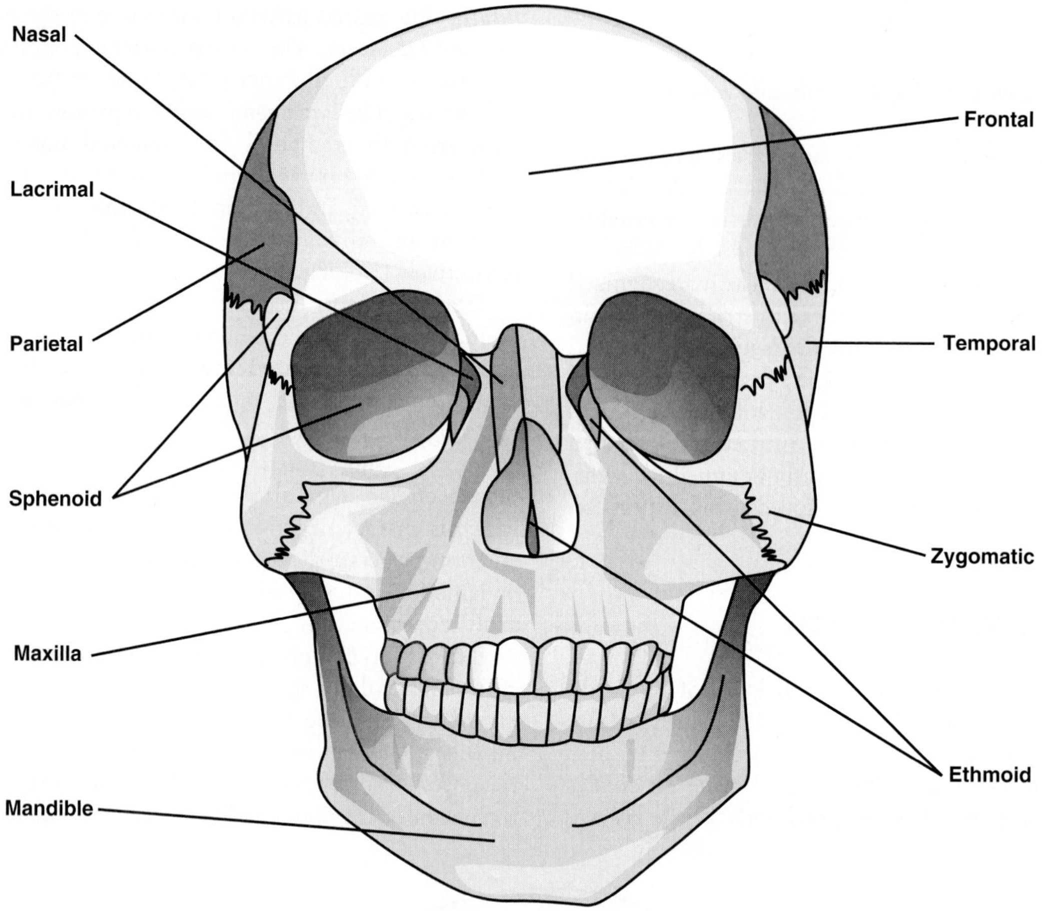

FIGURE 34-2

Frontal View of the Skull.

with the *zygoma* (the "cheek bone"), which is responsible for much of the transverse width of the face. The paired *nasal bones* form the root of the nose. The *mandible* houses the teeth of the lower jaw. The condyles of the mandible articulate with the glenoid fossa of the temporal bone at the base of the cranium to form the *temporomandibular joint* (TMJ), a hinge joint that allows for opening and closing of the jaw. The *condyle, coronoid process, ramus, body,* and *symphysis* of the mandible are illustrated in Figure 34-4.

The primary influence on facial growth during the first 7 years of life is brain and ocular growth (Ranly, 1988). Eighty percent of brain growth is complete by the time a child reaches 2 years of age; only minimal growth occurs after age 7. In contrast, facial growth continues into the second decade of life. The face of the infant is wide appearing and bulbous due to precocious brain development. The ratio of the size of the cranium to the size of the face is 8:1 at birth, but decreases to 2:1 in the adult (Singh & Bartlett, 2004). The paranasal sinuses are poorly developed in children. The face lengthens as the sinuses pneumatize,

the dentition develops, and the nasal cavity enlarges. These anatomical factors account for the higher ratio of upper facial fractures, including orbital roof and intracranial injuries, seen in children compared to adults.

MUSCLES OF MASTICATION

The four muscles of mastication—*masseter, temporalis, medial pterygoid,* and *lateral pterygoid*—are responsible for motion of the mandible. The masseter muscle originates from the zygomatic arch and inserts on the ramus of the mandible. As one of the strongest muscles in the body, it acts as a powerful closer of the mandible. The temporalis muscle originates from the temporal fossa of the skull and inserts onto the coronoid process of the mandible; it acts as a rotator and closer of the mandible. The medial and lateral ptyergoid muscles both originate from the lateral pterygoid plate of the sphenoid bone. The medial ptery-goid muscle inserts onto the medial and inferior border of

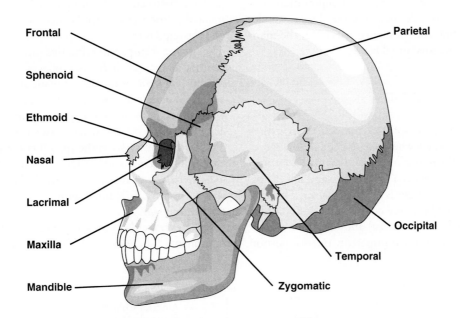

FIGURE 34-3

Lateral View of the Skull.

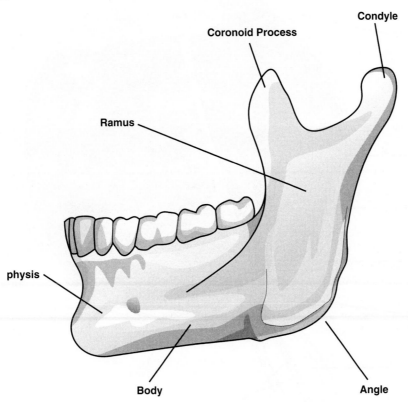

FIGURE 34-4

Lateral View of the Mandible.

Source: Modified from Gray, H. (1918). *Anatomy of the human body.* New York: Lea & Febiger.

the mandibular ramus and acts to close the mandible. The lateral pterygoid muscle inserts onto the temporomandibular joint and acts to protrude the mandible. These muscles are all supplied by branches of cranial nerve V3, the mandibular division of the trigeminal nerve.

EYE AND ORBITAL CONTENTS

The bony orbit and eyelids protect the ocular structures (Figure 34-5). The corners where the upper and lower eyelids meet are called the *medial and lateral canthi*. The *palpebral fissure* is the space between open upper and lower lids. The white outer layer of the eye is called the *sclera*. The conjunctiva is a thin vascular tissue covering the inner aspect of the eyelids (*palpebral conjunctiva*) and the sclera (*bulbar conjunctiva*). The *cornea* is the transparent, anterior portion of the eye responsible for light refraction. The *limbus* is the junction between the cornea and sclera. The *iris* is the pigmented portion of the eye located posterior to the cornea, and the pupil is the circular opening in the center of the iris. The *lens* is a transparent refractive surface lying posterior to the iris and pupil; it focuses images posteriorly onto the retina. The *retina* is the neural tissue at the posterior aspect of the globe that converts visual images into neural signals, which it relays to the brain via the *optic nerve*. The *anterior chamber* represents the space between the cornea and iris. The *posterior chamber* is the space between the iris and the lens. The anterior and posterior chambers are filled with *aqueous humour*. The *vitreous cavity* is the space between the lens and retina. It is filled with a jelly-like material called *vitreous humour*.

Six extraocular muscles are responsible for eye movements. The *medial and lateral rectus muscles* move the

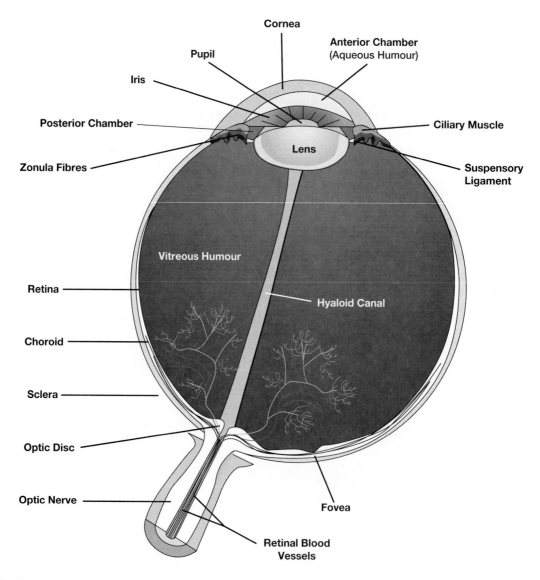

FIGURE 34-5

Ocular Anatomy.

globe medially and laterally, respectively. The *superior and inferior rectus muscles* move the globe superiorly and inferiorly, respectively. The *superior oblique muscle* moves the globe inferiorly and laterally. The *inferior oblique muscle* moves the globe superiorly and medially. These muscles are supplied by three cranial nerves: Cranial nerve IV innervates the superior oblique, cranial nerve VI innervates the lateral rectus, and cranial nerve III innervates the remainder of the extraocular muscles.

Tears are produced by the paired lacrimal glands, which lie beneath the lateral orbital roofs. Tears are directed across the globe and enter small openings at the medial aspects of the upper and lower eyelids, known as the *lacrimal punetum*. Tears travel from the punctum to the *superior and inferior canniliculus* and then onward to the *lacrimal sac* and *nasolacrimal duct*, which empties into the nose via an opening beneath the inferior turbinate.

EAR ANATOMY

The *auricle* or external ear is composed of cartilage and skin. It directs sound waves through the *external acoustic meatus* to the *tympanic membrane* (eardrum). The tympanic membrane, in turn, transmits information to the *auditory ossicles* (bones) of the middle ear—the *malleus, incus,* and *stapes.* The ossicles then transmit these signals to the inner ear structures.

The structures of the middle ear are located in the temporal bone (Figure 34-6). The middle ear is connected to the nasopharynx via the *auditory tube* and to the *mastoid cells* through the *mastoid antrum.* The mucous membrane lining of the mastoid cells and mastoid antrum, which is continuous with that of the middle ear, represents a pathway for the spread of infection from the middle ear (otitis media) to the mastoid cells leading to mastoiditis. The facial nerve courses through the temporal bone before becoming extracranial. Iatrogenic injury to the facial nerve is a potential complication during operations for mastoiditis (Moore & Agur, 1995).

The structures of the external ear are also illustrated in Figure 34-6. Sensation to the external ear is provided by five nerves (Allison, 1978; Boutros & Thorne, 2009). The *great auricular nerve* (C2-3) provides sensation to the medial and lateral sides of the lower half of the ear. The *lesser occipital nerve* (C2-3) supplies the upper posterior portion of the ear. The *auriculotemporal nerve,* a branch of cranial nerve V2, supplies the tragus and root of the helix. The conchal bowl is supplied by *Arnold's nerve,* a branch of cranial nerve X. The external ear canal is supplied by *Jacobson's nerve,* a branch of cranial nerve IX. The ear has a rich blood supply, with contributions from the superficial temporal artery, posterior auricular artery, and occipital artery.

NASAL ANATOMY

Skin, subcutaneous tissue, and muscle make up the outer layer of the nose. The skin of the nasal dorsum and columella is thinner than the more sebaceous skin over the nasal tip and ala (Figure 34-7). The paired *nasal bones, upper lateral cartilages, lower lateral cartilages,* and *septum* make up the supporting structures of the nose (Figure 34-8). The septum is composed of the *perpendicular plate of the ethmoid bone* superiorly, the *vomer* inferiorly, and the *septal cartilage* anteriorly (Figure 34-9). The nares open into the nasal cavity. The nasal mucosa makes up the inner lining of the nasal cavity. The medial wall of the nasal cavity is formed by the nasal septum. The contour of the lateral wall is irregular due to the presence of three *conchae* (turbinates)—the superior, medial, and inferior conchae.

LIP ANATOMY

The topographic anatomy of the lip is illustrated in Figure 34-10. The upper and lower lips are supplied by the *superior and inferior labial arteries,* respectively. The *orbicularis oris muscle* acts as a sphincter, bringing the upper and lower lips together (Figure 34-11); its function is important for oral competence and articulation. The principal elevator muscles of the upper lip include the *levator labii superioris, zygomaticus major and minor,* and *levator angularis oris.* The *depressor angularis oris, depressor labii inferioris,* and *platysma* are the primary lower lip depressors. In repair of lip lacerations, alignment of the *white roll* is of utmost importance. A 1-mm discrepancy in the white roll is visible at a distance of 3 feet (Zide, 1990).

ORAL AND DENTAL ANATOMY

Primary (pediatric/deciduous) dentition is characterized by 20 teeth. Each quadrant consists of a medial incisor, lateral incisor, canine, first molar, and second molar. Primary dentition is conventionally referenced with letters beginning with the upper right second molar to upper left second molar (A–J) and continuing with the lower left second molar to lower right second molar (K–T). Table 34-1 describes the sequence of eruption and shedding of the primary teeth.

The permanent (secondary/adult) dentition is characterized by 32 teeth. Each quadrant contains a medial incisor, lateral incisor, canine, first premolar, second premolar, first molar, second molar, and third molar. Permanent dentition is numbered from 1 to 16 beginning from the right upper third molar to the left upper third molar, and from 17 to 32 beginning from the left lower third molar to the right lower third molar. Table 34-2 describes the sequence of eruption of permanent teeth.

Each tooth consists of three portions: the crown, the root, and the neck. The *crown* is the portion of the tooth that is visible in the oral cavity. It is covered with enamel.

The *root* is the portion of the tooth that is embedded in the bony socket or *alveolus*. It is covered by cementum (a substance that is similar to, but softer than, enamel), and is anchored to the alveolus by a *periodontal ligament*. The *neck* is the portion between the crown and the root. The surfaces of the teeth are made up of "hills" (*cusps*) and "valleys" (*grooves*).

In dental terminology, position is often described in relationship to the midline. "Mesial" denotes being toward the midline, whereas "distad" refers to being away from the midline. "Labial," "buccal," "lingual," and "palatal" refer to a position toward the lip, cheek, tongue, and palate, respectively.

Occlusion refers to the relationship of teeth to one another. Normal occlusion is based on the relationship of the maxillary first molar, in that the mesiobuccal cusp of the maxillary first molar lies in the buccal groove of the mandibular first molar. Three classes of malocclusion were

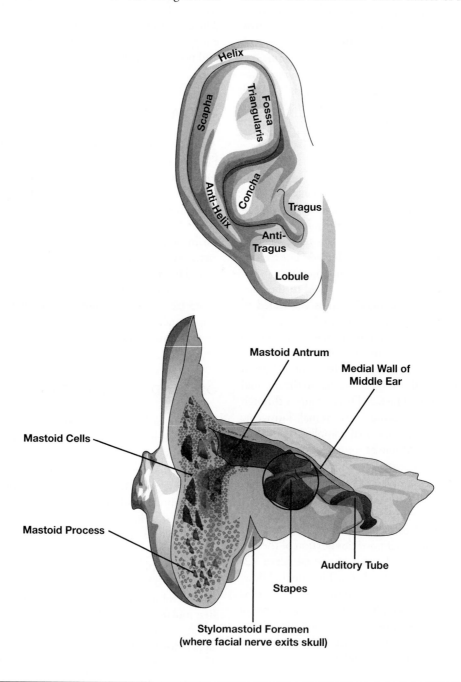

FIGURE 34-6

Anatomy of the Ear.

Note: Middle ear and temporal bone structures (1), external ear (2).
Source: Modified from Gray, H. (1918). *Anatomy of the human body.* New York: Lea & Febiger.

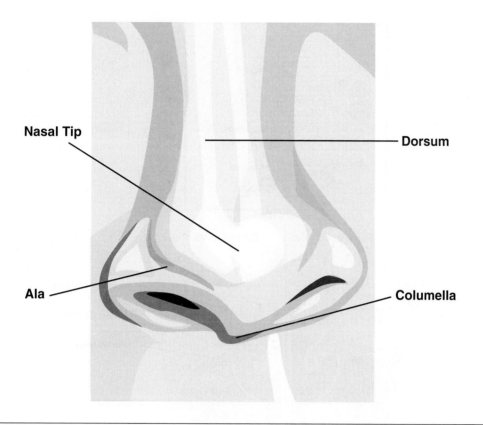

FIGURE 34-7

External Nasal Anatomy.

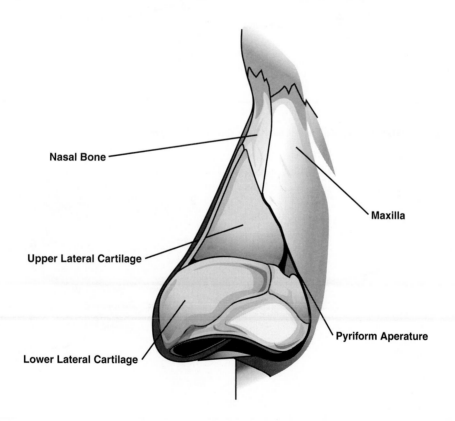

FIGURE 34-8

Anatomy of the Nose.

Source: Modified from Gray, H. (1918). *Anatomy of the human body.* New York: Lea & Febiger.

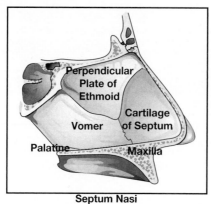

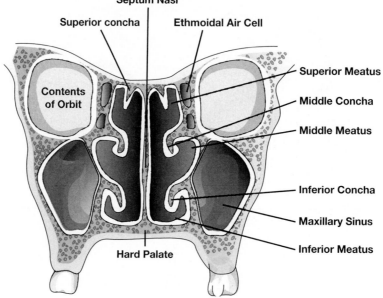

FIGURE 34-9

Internal Nasal Anatomy.

Source: Modified from Gray, H. (1918). *Anatomy of the human body*. New York: Lea & Febiger.

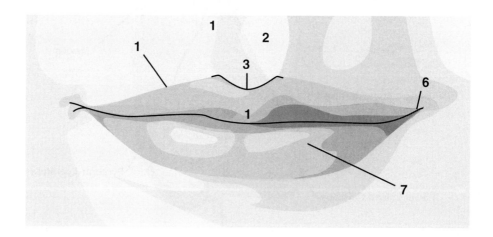

FIGURE 34-10

Topographic Anatomy of the Lip.

Note: Philtral column (1), philtral dimple (2), Cupid's bow (3), white roll (4), tubercle (5), commisure (6), vermillion (7).

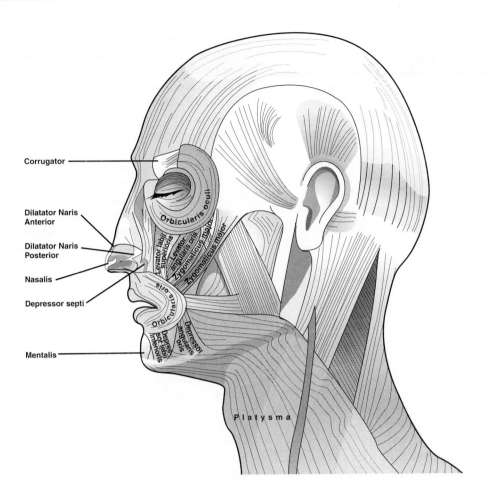

FIGURE 34-11

Facial Musculature.

TABLE 34-1

Primary Dentition Eruption and Shedding		
	Erupt	**Shed**
Upper Teeth		
Central incisor	8–12 months	6–7 years
Lateral incisor	9–13 months	7–8 years
Canine (cuspid)	16–22 months	10–12 years
First molar	13–19 months	9–11 years
Second molar	25–33 months	10–12 years
Lower Teeth		
Central incisor	6–10 months	6–7 years
Lateral incisor	10–16 months	7–8 years
Canine (cuspid)	17–23 months	9–12 years
First molar	14–18 months	9–11 years
Second molar	23–31 months	10–12 years

Source: American Dental Association, 2005.

described by Angle. In Class I malocclusion, the normal relationship is seen, but the teeth are malpositioned or malrotated. In Class II malocclusion, the mandibular molar is distally positioned relative to the maxillary molar. In class III malocclusion, the mandibular molar is mesially positioned relative to the maxillary molar (Proffit et al., 1980).

The tongue is composed of both intrinsic and extrinsic muscles. The intrinsic muscles—including the superior and inferior longitudinal muscles, transverses, and verticalis—are responsible for changing the shape of the tongue. The extrinsic muscles—genioglossus, hypoglossus, styloglossus, and palatoglossus—are responsible for gross tongue movements. Injury to the hypoglossal nerve (CN XII) causes the tongue to deviate to the side of the injured nerve.

SALIVARY GLANDS

Three main paired salivary glands are present (Figure 34-12). The *submandibular* glands lie along the body of the mandible, whereas the *sublingual glands* lie

TABLE 34-2

Permanent Dentition Eruption	
	Erupt
Upper Teeth	
Central incisor	7–8 years
Lateral incisor	8–9 years
Canine (cuspid)	11–12 years
First premolar (first bicuspid)	10–11 years
Second premolar (second bicuspid)	10–12 years
First molar	6–7 years
Second molar	12–13 years
Third molar (wisdom tooth)	17–21 years
Lower Teeth	
Central incisor	6–7 years
Lateral incisor	7–8 years
Canine (cuspid)	9–10 years
First premolar (first bicuspid)	10–12 years
Second premolar (second bicuspid)	11–12 years
First molar	6–7 years
Second molar	11–13 years
Third molar (wisdom tooth)	17–21 years

Source: American Dental Association, 2006.

along the floor of the mouth. The submandibular glands empty into the mouth via *Wharton's ducts*, in close proximity to the lingual frenulum. The sublingual glands empty into the mouth via numerous small ducts located along the floor of the mouth.

The parotid gland, the largest salivary gland, lies over the cheek and anterior to the mandibular ramus. Its duct, known as *Stensen's duct*, travels over the masseter muscle before piercing the buccinator muscle and the buccal mucosa, thereby entering the oral cavity at the level of the maxillary second permanent molar. A Stensen's duct injury should be considered when evaluating patients with lacerations of the anterior cheek. Exploration with cannulation of the duct intraorally may be necessary to confirm the status of the duct.

FACIAL BLOOD SUPPLY

The face is mostly supplied by branches of the external carotid artery. The *facial artery* provides the main blood supply to the face. After branching off the external carotid artery, it travels along the lower mandibular border and then anterior to the masseter muscle. It sends branches to the upper lip (*superior labial artery*), lower lip (*inferior labial artery*), and lateral nose (*lateral nasal artery*). It terminates as the *angular artery*, which supplies the mid- to upper lateral nose and medial corner of the eye (Figure 34-13).

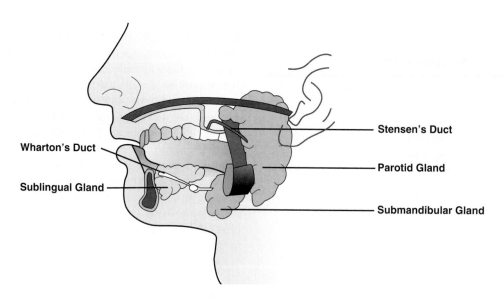

FIGURE 34-12

Salivary Glands.

Source: Modified from Gray, H. (1918). *Anatomy of the human body.* New York: Lea & Febiger.

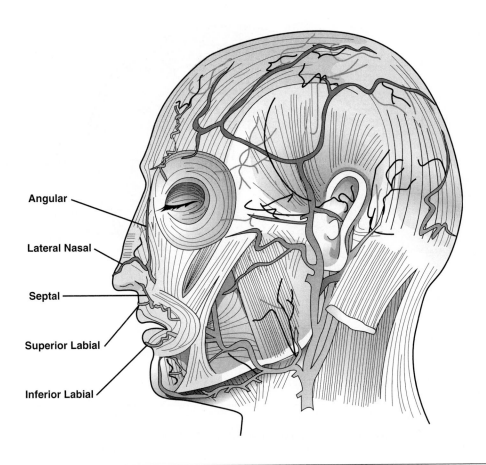

Angular

Lateral Nasal

Septal

Superior Labial

Inferior Labial

FIGURE 34-13

Facial Blood Supply.

Source: Modified from Gray, H. (1918). *Anatomy of the human body.* New York: Lea & Febiger.

The scalp receives its vascular supply from both the external and internal carotid systems. The ophthalmic artery, which is a portion of the internal carotid artery, not only supplies the retina, but also branches off to supply muscles and skin of the forehead via the *supraorbital and supratrochlear arteries.* The *superficial temporal artery* is the smaller terminal branch of the external carotid artery. It passes anterior to the tragus of the ear before bifurcating into a frontal branch and a parietal branch, which supply the lateral scalp and forehead. The *occipital and posterior auricular arteries* also branch off the external carotid artery; they supply the posterior scalp.

Venous drainage of the face parallels the arterial supply. The *facial vein* provides the major route of venous drainage to the face. It begins at the medial canthus of the eye as the *angular vein,* then travels posteriorly to the facial artery, and ultimately drains into the *internal jugular vein.* The angular vein communicates with the *orbital vein.* The orbital vein, in turn, communicates with the *cavernous sinus,* the venous drainage system of the brain. This communication provides a potential route of spread of upper facial infections intracranially (Moore & Agur, 1995).

FACIAL SENSATION

The face and scalp are supplied by branches of the cervical plexus and by branches of the *trigeminal nerve* (CN V). The great auricular nerve (C2-3) extends over the ear lobule and parotid region of the face. The lesser occipital nerve (C2-3) innervates the upper third of the ear and mastoid region. The greater occipital nerve (C2) innervates the posterior scalp.

The trigeminal nerve is the main sensory nerve of the face. Before exiting the cranium, it divides into three main branches: the ophthalmic (V1), maxillary (V2), and mandibular (V3) nerves. The sensory distributions of these branches are illustrated in Figure 34-14.

The *ophthalmic division* (V1) exits the cranium through the superior orbital fissure. There are three major branches of the ophthalmic division: frontal, lacrimal, and naso-ciliary. The frontal branch divides into the *supratrochlear nerve,* which supplies the upper eyelid, conjunctiva, and medial forehead, and the *supraorbital nerve,* which supplies the forehead and anterior scalp. The supraorbital nerve passes beneath the supraorbital rim at the midpupillary

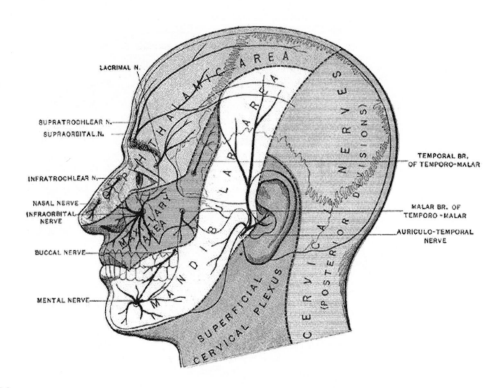

FIGURE 34-14

Sensory Innervation of the Face.

Source: Modified from Gray, H. (1918). *Anatomy of the human body.* New York: Lea & Febiger.

line through either a well-defined foramen or notch. The supratroclear nerve travels freely under the supraorbital rim medial to the supraorbital nerve uncontained in a foramen or notch. The *lacrimal nerve* carries sensation from the conjunctiva and upper eyelid. The *nasocilary nerve* provides sensation to the sclera, cornea, and nose. Its nasal branch carries sensation from the lateral nose, nasal ala, nasal septum, and nasal vestibule.

The *maxillary division* (V2) exits the cranium through the foramen rotundum and then courses anteriorly through the inferior orbital fissure. It then runs along the orbital floor before exiting the infraorbital foramen as the infraorbital nerve. In its course from the foramen rotundum to the infraorbital foramen, V2 gives rises to multiple branches, which supply the palate, tonsils, and maxillary teeth. The zygomaticotemporal and zygomaticofacial nerve branches carry sensation from the skin over the zygoma and temple. Orbital floor fractures often cause numbness to the cheek, lower eyelid, lateral nose, and upper lip due to injury or stretch of the infraorbital nerve as it passes along the floor of the orbit.

The *mandibular division* (V3) exits the cranium thought the foramen ovale. This nerve carries sensory information from the lower jaw and chin, and also provides the motor supply to the muscles of mastication. The major sensory branches of V3 are the auriculotemporal, buccal, lingual, and mental nerves. The buccal branch supplies the buccal mucosa and lower gums. The auriculotemporal nerve is responsible for sensation to the temporal region of the face, lateral scalp, temporomandibular joint, and much of the anterior surface of the ear and external auditory meatus. The lingual nerve supplies sensation to the anterior two-thirds of the tongue and the floor of the mouth. It also receives taste and parasympathetic nerve fibers from the facial nerve (CN VII) via a nerve branch, the *chorda tympani*, to supply taste sensation to the anterior two-thirds of the tongue and autonomic control of the sublingual and submandibular salivary glands, respectively. The *mental nerve* exits the mandible at the mental foramen and innervates the skin of the chin and lower lip.

FACIAL MUSCLES AND THE FACIAL NERVE

Twenty-three paired muscles and one unpaired muscle are responsible for facial expression (Figure 34-11), all of which are innervated by the *facial nerve* (CN VII). The facial nerve exits the cranium through the stylomastoid foramen, a small opening in the temporal bone of the skull. It passes through the parotid gland where it divides into five main branches: *frontal/temporal, zygomatic, buccal, marginal mandibular,* and *cervical.* Table 34-3 summarizes the main facial muscles, their nerve supply, and their function.

TABLE 34-3

Major Facial Muscles		
Muscle	**Branch of Facial Nerve Supplied by**	**Function**
Frontalis	Temporal	Raises forehead and eyebrows
Orbicularis oculi	Temporal and zygomatic	Closes eyelids
Levator labii superioris	Buccal	Elevates upper lip
Zygomaticus major and minor	Zygomatic and buccal	Responsible for smiling and grimacing
Orbicularis oris	Buccal	Purses and protrudes lips
Depressor anguli oris	Buccal and marginal mandibular	Depresses corners of mouth
Depressor labii inferioris	Marginal mandibular	Depresses lower lip
Platysma	Cervical	Depresses mandible and tenses lower facial and neck skin
Mentalis	Marginal mandibular	Protrudes and elevates lower lip
Buccinator	Buccal	Compresses cheek

Source: Modified from Moore, K. & Agur, A. (1995). Essential Clinical Anatomy. Philadelphia: William & Wilkins.

Lacerations over the cheek or temple should raise suspicion of a possible facial nerve injury. Nerve lacerations medial to the lateral canthus of the eye generally do not require nerve repair, as these small zygomatic and buccal branches have multiple interconnections (Anderson, 2006). In the newborn, the facial nerve is vulnerable to injury as it exits the temporal bone of the skull; its location is just deep to the skin. From ages 2 to 4 years, as the temporal bone and mastoid process develop, the facial nerve assumes a more protected course inferior and medial to these bony structures (Kullman et al., 1971). Embryologic development of the facial nerve is both spatially and temporally associated with development of the external and middle ears. Malformations of the external or middle ear should alert the health care practitioner (HCP) to a possible anomaly of the facial nerve (Sataloff, 1990). Hemifacial microsomia, Goldenhar's syndrome, and Möbius syndrome are three syndromes sometimes associated with cases of congenital facial paralysis.

DENTAL ABSCESS AND TRAUMA

Pamela Bourg and Abigail Blackmore

PATHOPHYSIOLOGY

The crown of the tooth is the portion of the tooth that is visible above the gingiva. It has an outer layer that is made up of hard enamel. Found inside the crown is the soft yellow dentin, which contains the pulp chamber, blood vessels, and nerves. The root of the tooth is located in the bone socket and attached to the socket by ligaments (Halpern & Bernardo, 2002).

Dental abscesses are common in children and adolescents due to the morphologic characteristics of the primary tooth and immature permanent tooth. They usually originate from bacterial infections or untreated dental caries. Dental abscesses may also result from a cracked tooth secondary to trauma. They form when pus becomes enclosed in the tissues of the mandible at the tip of an infected tooth. Dentoalveolar abscesses may be classified into three types: gingival, periapical, and periodontal (Nelson & Shusterman, 2000) (Table 34-4).

When children present after dental trauma, the injuries may also be classified as one of three types: avulsion, subluxation, or fracture. A tooth *avulsion* occurs when a tooth comes out of its bone socket. A tooth *subluxation* occurs when the tooth is still in the socket, but is malpositioned. A tooth *fracture* occurs when the tooth is broken, but is still held within the socket. These injuries have the highest prevalence in children 8 to 9 years of age (Halpern & Bernardo, 2002).

EPIDEMIOLOGY AND ETIOLOGY

Dental injuries may occur from unintentional trauma such as sports activities, playground injuries, and bicycle crashes. According Gassner et al. (2004), each year 5% of all younger children experience dentoalveolar trauma; there is no gender prevalence noted with such injuries.

PRESENTATION

A comprehensive history should be elicited in patients who present with dental abscess or trauma. Overt infections,

TABLE 34-4

Abscess Types	
Abscess Type	**Description**
Gingival	Redness and swelling that involves only the gum tissue
Periapical	Originates in the dental pulp Sensitive to heat and cold Pain on percussion
Periodontal	Begins in supporting bone or tissue structures Tooth mobility Dull, throbbing, constant ache

TABLE 34-5

Clinical Presentation of Dentoalveolar Abscess	
Pain	The tooth may be painful to percussion or exhibit spontaneous painful episodes
Mobility	Greater than the normal degree of movement in the socket
Swelling	The soft tissues around the tooth may be edematous and erythematous
	In severe cases, this can extend to the jaw and face
Fever	The child may be febrile (temperature greater than 37.5°C [99.5°F])
	May be paired with general malaise and poor appetite
Breath odor	Children or caregivers may note foul odor on the breath
	Children may complain of a bitter taste in the mouth
Lymphadenopathy	Swollen lymph glands

sequelae, and therapies already administered should be explored. Routine dental care and review of systems apply, as dental abscess may become serious in patients with chronic illness or comorbidities. In children, the missing tooth is often found in the patient's mouth, clothing, or surrounding area.

The primary symptom of dental abscess is pain, although some children may also complain of a bad or bitter taste in their mouth. Foul breath odor may be noted by family members and caregivers. In severe cases, the soft tissues of the tooth and even the face may be affected, resulting in edema or cellulitis (Table 34-5). For patients with concurrent cellulitis of the floor of the mouth, Ludwig's angina may be noted, evidenced by a gagging or strangling sensation. The examination should not be limited to the head and neck; rather, a complete evaluation of the patient is indicated. In the case of trauma, the patient should be evaluated based on trauma protocol. If child maltreatment or violence is suspected, then an evaluation by child maltreatment specialist is warranted.

DIFFERENTIAL DIAGNOSIS

The following diagnoses may present with similar finding as a dental abscess: gingivitis, parotiditis, incomplete dental eruption, buccal cyst, granuloma, cellulitis, neoplasm, and Langerhans cell histiocytosis. Patients presenting with trauma may be victims of child maltreatment.

PLAN OF CARE

The basic principles of treatment for abscess are antimicrobial therapy and drainage. In most patients, the antibiotic of choice is penicillin. Treatment is aggressive, even for a primary tooth abscess, as infection may affect the developing unerupted tooth bud. If the infection involves a vital area, such as the submandibular space, it may develop into Ludwig's angina or a cavernous sinus thrombosis. If it invades the periorbital space, it may involve the orbital structures. In such cases,

parenteral antibiotics are required (Nelson & Shusterman, 2000). To enhance the patient's comfort, extraoral heat can be applied to the affected area. Mild analgesic therapy with acetaminophen or ibuprofen is often sufficient to control pain. Consultation with oral surgery, dentistry, or plastic surgery may be necessary to plan for drainage.

Tooth subluxation is the least problematic of the traumatic injuries. This condition usually requires little or no intervention. For avulsed teeth, therapeutic management differs based on whether primary or permanent dentition is involved. Avulsed primary dentition is not replanted; instead, the area is cleansed and investigated for foreign bodies or fractured roots. Avulsed permanent teeth are cleansed and replanted with splinting. If the avulsed tooth can be replanted into the alveolar bone within the hour, prognosis is good (Halpurn & Barnardo, 2002).

Care should be taken to touch the tooth only on the hard outer enamel surface. It should not be rinsed with water, unless soiled, and then only briefly until clean. Avoid scrubbing or placing the root surface tooth in restrictive materials for transport, as the integrity of the cells within the root surface may be destroyed by such contact. Ideally, the tooth should be placed in a solution of normal saline for transport to treatment. If no commercial saline products are available, milk may be used.

If extensive oral infection or trauma occurs, oral feeding may be difficult. Inpatient care with nutritional support may be necessary.

Dental consultation should be obtained if tooth extraction becomes necessary or if a tooth must be replanted. Consultation with an infectious diseases specialist is warranted if patients with abscess do not improve with therapy or are moderately or severely ill.

Patient and family education involves discussion of plan, diet, and dental hygiene and follow-up. Activities may be restricted with splinted teeth.

DISPOSITION AND DISCHARGE PLANNING

Children and their families should be directed to appropriate follow-up appointments. Follow-up with a dentist is essential for management of long-term complications, such as pulpal necrosis, ankylosis, and displacement of the permanent tooth successors (Rodriguez & Sarlani, 2005).

Prevention of abscess and trauma starts with patient and family education. Good oral hygiene and nutrition reduces the incidence of abscess from dental caries. In addition, use of mouth guards may reduce the incidence of dental injury during sport activities. For example, it is estimated that 200,000 injuries to the mouth and face are prevented each year among high school and college football players who use mouth guards (Halpern & Bernardo, 2002).

MASTOIDITIS

Thomas H. Rand

PATHOPHYSIOLOGY

Mastoid air cells, similar to the paranasal sinuses, are a honeycomb of airspaces within bony septations of the temporal bone. These cells communicate with the middle ear space via the aditus ad antrum. The middle ear space is located behind the tympanic membrane and is ventilated to the pharynx by the Eustachian tube. The mastoid is in close proximity to the inner ear apparatus (cochlea) and the sigmoid venous sinus within the intracranial fossa. Mastoiditis is an infectious complication of the otitis media.

EPIDEMIOLOGY AND ETIOLOGY

During the second half of the twentieth century (the antibiotic era), the incidence of acute mastoiditis dropped dramatically; during the past decade, however, this rate has started to rise (Bahadori et al., 2000). Some have attributed the increased incidence to the development of drug-resistant strains of *Streptococcus pneumoniae*; however, not all experts agree that such a temporal trend has occurred. Other organisms noted to cause mastoiditis include *Streptococcus pyogenes, Pseudomonas aeruginosa*, and *Staphylococcus aureus* (including methicillin-resistant strains).

Surgical management of mastoiditis was developed during the pre-antibiotic era and remains an important part of therapy today when periosteal abscess is present or for other specified complications. Many pediatric patients with chronic otitis media also demonstrate mastoid filling on computed tomography (CT) scan; chronic otomastoid conditions are beyond the scope of this section.

PRESENTATION

The ages at which individuals are typically affected by acute mastoiditis parallel the age-specific frequency of acute otitis media. Most patients with acute mastoiditis have no underlying medical problem.

The pediatric patient with acute mastoiditis has findings of acute otitis media plus tenderness and swelling of the mastoid process. Whereas postauricular swelling pushes the ear pinna up and out in children older than 18 months of age, infants may have the appearance of the ear being pushed down by postauricular swelling due to more limited development of mastoid air cells in the mastoid process. Sagging of the posterior wall of the external ear canal is present in all cases. Most patients have fever. Involvement of the sixth (abducens), seventh (facial), or eighth (vestibular or acoustic) cranial nerves may be noted as well. Gradenigo's triad—consisting of abducens nerve palsy, pain in the trigeminal nerve distribution, and drainage from the ear canal—is attributable to petrositis, but has been seldom seen in the post-antibiotic era. Rupturing of the mastoid abscess into the digastric groove and the sternocleidomastoid space is rare and is referred to as a Bezold's abscess (Gaffney et al., 1991).

DIFFERENTIAL DIAGNOSIS

The physical findings with mastoiditis should be distinguished from those associated with parotitis or postauricular lymphadenitis. Each of these conditions is characterized by a tender mass behind the ear pinna. Parotitis always extends anterior to the margin of the mandible and to the preauricular region. Lymphadenitis is initially separate from the mastoid process of the temporal bone. Mastoiditis is always accompanied by findings of otitis media.

Occasionally, otitis externa may mimic acute mastoiditis. In otitis externa the ear pinna is not pushed forward and outward, the swelling is centered on the ear canal, and movement of the tragus elicits greatest tenderness.

PLAN OF CARE

Blood cultures should be drawn before antibiotic administration in febrile children with serious infections. Occipital pain may prevent exclusion of meningitis by physical examination alone, and a lumbar puncture is necessary. Acute mastoiditis is also often accompanied by pleocytosis of the cerebrospinal fluid (CSF); this response is associated with a parameningeal focus of infection, which results in sterile CSF cultures and likely aseptic meningitis.

If clinical assessment is not adequate to determine the extent of the infection, then CT is the first choice of imaging study to confirm mastoid filling, presence of periosteal abscess, or destruction of bony septations of the mastoid (termed coalescent mastoiditis) (Bluestone, 1998). Intracranial complications such as dural venous sinus thrombosis or epidural abscess are the most clearly defined on magnetic resonance imaging (MRI); hence, MRI should be ordered to evaluate the patient with signs of increased intracranial pressure.

Choice of antibiotics for acute mastoiditis follows the same principles as choice of antibiotic therapy of acute otitis media. Outpatient management with oral antibiotics is a reasonable choice in the infrequent situation of a pediatric patient who appears well enough and does not appear to have a periosteal abscess. However, the majority of patients diagnosed with mastoiditis will have recently taken antibiotics for otitis media without resolution of illness; as such, they will require parenteral therapy to cover Gram-positive and Gram-negative organisms. Outpatient management of *S. pneumoniae* infection is usually accomplished with high-dose amoxicillin (75–90 mg/kg/day) given orally or with ceftriaxone (50–100 mg/kg/day) given intramuscularly or intravenously. Among oral agents, high-dose amoxicillin remains the best choice for infections with *S. pneumoniae* and drug-resistant *S. pneumoniae*.

For inpatients, any of the empiric parenteral regimens for young children with bacterial complications of respiratory tract infections are appropriate. Therapy may be modified for cultures that grow susceptible *S. aureus* (nafcillin or oxacillin), methicillin-resistant *S. aureus* (vancomycin), or oral anerobes such as *Fusobacterium* and *Prevotella* (ampicillin with sulbactam).

Duration of therapy for mastoiditis is longer than the length of therapy for acute otitis media and is individualized based on the patient's clinical signs of recovery. Principles of therapy for osteomyelitis may be applied to management of mastoiditis, including transition from intravenous to high-dose oral antibiotics with signs of improvement and surgery when abscess is present.

Periosteal abscess requires drainage in the operating room. An experienced otorhinolaryngologist may proceed to irrigation and drainage without performing CT imaging prior to surgery. Nevertheless, CT with intravenous contrast provides valuable information regarding bony destruction of the mastoid air cells or other complications. Cultures are obtained from the patient's middle ear fluid and periosteal abscess at the time of surgery to guide further therapy. A tympanostomy tube is placed for continued middle ear drainage. Complicated mastoiditis with destruction of bony septations (coalescent mastoiditis) is an indication for mastoidectomy (Bluestone, 1998).

Early contact with an otorhinolaryngologist is important. Additional specialty consultation (e.g., neurosurgery, critical care, infectious diseases, hematology) may be indicated if extension of infection or central nervous system complications occur.

It is difficult to meet the rigorous demands of prolonged antibiotic therapy in an outpatient setting in young children. Caregivers need to understand the importance of compliance with the plan. If they are unable to meet these demands, then inpatient therapy may be required to ensure adequate antibiotic serum levels. As part of the education plan, the HCP should review the symptoms of recurrence or infection extension and explain when to return to the HCP for evaluation.

DISPOSITION AND DISCHARGE PLANNING

Prognosis is good with early treatment of mastoiditis, and most children recover without sequelae. In contrast, antibiotic penetrance is poor, and extension of the infection is not uncommon. There is also a risk for recurrence with mastoiditis.

An important intracranial complication of acute mastoiditis is thrombosis of the lateral or sigmoid venous sinus. A high index of suspicion for this complication should be maintained in the pediatric patient who remains acutely ill despite treatment with appropriate antibiotics, has an elevated opening pressure on lumbar puncture, or who has mental status changes or sixth or seventh cranial nerve palsy. Pain of the jugular vein and papilledema may be noted. Either CT with intravenous contrast or MRI with vascular phase studies (magnetic resonance venography [MRV]) may detect venous sinus thrombosis. Management of mastoiditis complicated by intracranial venous sinus thrombosis includes mastoidectomy followed by anticoagulation therapy and is best accomplished at a pediatric referral center.

Other potential complications include labyrinthitis, osteomyelitis, and central nervous system conditions such as epidural or subdural empyema, abscess, or meningitis. Both conductive and sensorineural hearing loss may accompany mastoiditis; thus an evaluation with audiology should be considered after the patient's discharge.

Most cases of acute mastoiditis may be avoided with prompt and effective treatment of acute otitis media.

ORBITAL AND PRESEPTAL (PERIORBITAL) CELLULITIS

Amy Babiuch and David Mittleman

ORBITAL CELLULITIS

Pathophysiology

Orbital cellulitis is an acute infectious inflammatory process involving the tissues posterior to the orbital septum. Typically, marked erythema and edema of the eyelid and surrounding skin are present. Orbital cellulitis most commonly results from direct extension of paranasal sinus infection (e.g., ethmoiditis). The infection spreads readily through the thin medial wall of the orbit, known as the lamina papyracea.

Epidemiology and etiology

Orbital cellulitis is much less common than preseptal (periorbital) cellulitis. In a retrospective case series of 315 children admitted to the hospital with preseptal or orbital cellulitis, 18 of the 315 patients (6%) were diagnosed with orbital cellulitis (Ambati et al., 2000). The median age of children hospitalized with orbital cellulitis is 7½ years (Nageswaran et al., 2006). An increased incidence of orbital cellulitis is seen in winter, presumably because of the increased prevalence of sinusitis in the community.

Sinusitis is the most common risk factor for orbital cellulitis in both the pediatric and adult age groups (Mills & Kartush, 1985). Orbital cellulitis can also result from localized periorbital infection, such as dacryocystitis, dacryoadenitis, preseptal cellulitis, or dental infection. Other causes include complications of orbital trauma (especially those involving foreign bodies), complications arising from orbital or paranasal sinus surgery, or vascular seeding of endogenous infection. The most common causative organisms include *Staphylococcus aureus*, *Streptococcus*, and non-spore-forming anaerobes. Although *Haemophilus influenzae* is no longer the leading cause in young children, this pathogen should be considered in non-immunized patients.

Presentation

Signs and symptoms or a diagnosis of sinusitis may be present prior to the development of orbital cellulitis. Symptoms include tenderness, redness, and swelling involving the eyelid and periorbital region (Figure 34-15). The conjunctiva is typically red and chemotic. Systemic symptoms include headache, fever, and lethargy. Proptosis is observed, along with limited extraocular motility, often associated with pain. In patients with advanced disease, optic nerve edema and an abnormal pupillary response, such as an afferent pupillary defect (APD), may be noted (Table 34-6). The infection is often localized to the subperiosteal space of the medial wall of the orbit adjacent to the ethmoid sinus, frequently resulting in abscess formation at that location.

Differential diagnosis

Inflammatory pseudotumor in adolescents and young adults may mimic the appearance of orbital cellulitis. Thyroid orbitopathy is common in older adults, but can also occur in children and should be considered in the differential diagnosis. Orbital tumors—in particular, rhabdomyosarcoma—occur in the same age group as orbital cellulitis and may exhibit rapid growth masquerading as a cellulitis.

Plan of care

Immediate hospitalization is required. CT scan of the orbits and paranasal sinuses with both axial and coronal views, ideally with contrast, should be performed. Blood cultures and a complete blood count (CBC) with differential should be obtained. The white blood cell count often exceeds 15,000 cells/mm^3 with a corresponding neutrophilia that supports the diagnosis of a bacterial infection. A Gram stain and culture of any purulent material from the nose may be helpful in isolating the causative organism. Lumbar puncture should be considered if central nervous system dysfunction or meningeal signs are present.

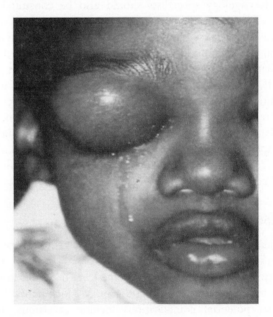

FIGURE 34-15

Orbital Cellulitis.

Source: Courtesy of Amy Babiuch and David Mittleman.

TABLE 34-6

Afferent Pupillary Defect (APD)

A difference in the pupillary reaction of one eye relative to the contralateral eye's pupillary reaction to light. This can be identified by performing the swinging flash light test where the light is swung back and forth from one pupil to the other. Normally, when the light is shined into one eye, both eyes will react with equal constriction of the pupils. If the contralateral pupil dilates upon swinging the light to that eye, an APD is present.

Patients with orbital cellulitis are generally treated with high-dose intravenous antibiotics, such as second- or third-generation cephalosporins. Antibiotic choice may be adjusted based on culture results. Intravenous antibiotics should be continued until the pediatric patient is afebrile and the skin changes begin to resolve (typically 3 to 5 days). A comparable oral antibiotic should then be continued for 2 to 3 weeks.

An ophthalmologic examination should be performed on a daily basis, or more frequently in patients with severe infections, to evaluate for increased proptosis, reduced ocular motility, elevated intraocular pressure, and optic neuropathy. If vision decreases, extraocular motility becomes more limited, or pupillary reaction changes, then a repeat orbital CT scan should be performed immediately. If a subperiosteal abscess of the medial wall is present or develops and does not respond to medical therapy within a few days, surgical drainage is indicated (Greenberg & Pollard, 1998). Abscesses in other locations within the orbit should be drained promptly.

Ophthalmology services should be consulted immediately for examination and therapeutic management. Otolaryngology specialists should also be consulted, as sinusitis is the most common source of infection. Infectious diseases specialists should be consulted if the causative organism is found to be an uncommon pathogen or if the pediatric patient is immunocompromised.

Patients should remain on intravenous antibiotics until definite signs of resolution appear—specifically, decreasing redness, swelling, and tenderness. Upon resolution, the pediatric patient may be discharged from the hospital to complete a long outpatient course of comparable oral antibiotics. It is imperative that the pediatric patient finish the full course of such therapy.

Disposition and discharge planning

Patients with adequately treated orbital cellulitis have a guarded prognosis. Studies of orbital cellulitis report mortality rates of 1% to 2% and some level of vision loss in 3% to 11% of patients (Osguthorpe & Hochman, 1993). Other potential complications include cavernous sinus thrombosis, subdural abscess, brain abscess, and meningitis. Regular follow-up appointments with the otolaryngologist and ophthalmologist will be required.

Parents need instruction regarding recurrence of disease. If increased redness, pain, or swelling occur or the patient experiences a decrease in vision, the caregivers should be instructed to bring the pediatric patient in for reevaluation immediately.

Future episodes of sinusitis should be treated promptly, as rapid evaluation for and treatment of sinusitis can prevent the development of orbital cellulitis. If the patient experiences recurrent bouts of sinusitis (more than three episodes in one year), he or she should be evaluated by an otolaryngologist. Superficial eyelid wounds should be cleansed adequately and observed closely for development of infection.

PRESEPTAL (PERIORBITAL) CELLULITIS

Pathophysiology

Preseptal (periorbital) cellulitis is an acute infectious inflammatory process of the eyelid and surrounding skin, producing marked erythema and edema in the involved tissues. The inflammation is confined to the structures anterior to the orbital septum. The orbital septum is a layer of connective tissue extending vertically from the periosteum of the orbital rim to the levator aponeurosis in the upper eyelid and to the inferior border of the tarsal plate in the lower eyelid; it forms a barrier that prevents infection from extending into the orbit.

Epidemiology and etiology

Preseptal cellulitis is much more common than orbital cellulitis. In a retrospective case series of 315 children admitted to the hospital with preseptal or orbital cellulitis, preseptal cellulitis accounted for 297 of 315 of the diagnosed patients (94%) (Ambati et al., 2000). Preseptal orbital cellulitis commonly affects young children, often prior to the age of five years.

This infection may occur following trauma, puncture wound, laceration of the eyelid, or insect bite. It may also arise secondary to an adjacent skin infection, such as impetigo, herpes zoster, hordeolum, or dacryocystitis. Finally, preseptal cellulitis may result from an upper respiratory infection or sinusitis. *Staphylococcus aureus*, *Streptococcus pneumoniae*, and *Streptococcus pyogenes* are the bacteria most commonly responsible for this infection. *Haemophilus influenzae*, once a common cause in young children, should be considered as a potential pathogen in non-immunized patients.

Presentation

Pediatric patients may have prior symptoms of sinusitis or have a history of a violation of the superficial dermal structures. Symptoms of preseptal cellulitis—tenderness, redness, and swelling involving the eyelid and periorbital region—develop acutely and may evolve into the full presentation within 24 hours. Patients may also have an accompanying low-grade fever. On physical examination, the HCP will note erythema, tense edema, and tenderness of the eyelids and periorbita. The edema may be so severe that the patient is unable to open the eye, and eyelid retractors may be necessary to ensure adequate evaluation of the globe (Figure 34-16). However, there is no proptosis, pain with eye movement, or limitation of ocular motility. Pupillary responses are brisk and equal.

Differential diagnosis

The most important entity to differentiate from preseptal cellulitis is true orbital cellulitis—that is, extension of the infection behind the orbital septum. Eyelid allergy may mimic preseptal orbital cellulitis. A chalazion or hordeolum may produce noninfectious lid swelling.

Plan of care

A CT scan of the orbit should be performed to evaluate for extension of the infection into the orbit. This imaging study may also reveal the presence of a subperiosteal abscess, paranasal sinusitis, or an orbital foreign body. Additional lab tests routinely performed include a CBC with differential, blood cultures, and Gram stain and culture of any purulent material obtained from the nose.

Mild cases in children older than one year of age may be treated on an outpatient basis with broad-spectrum oral antibiotics such as amoxicillin/clavulanate or a cephalosporin for a 10-day course. Infants (younger than one year) and patients with more severe presentations, such as those associated with high fever or other signs of systemic disease, should be hospitalized to receive intravenous antibiotic therapy. Once the fever has resolved and signs of

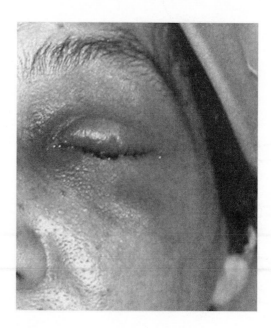

FIGURE 34-16

Preseptal (Periorbital) Cellulitis.

Source: Courtesy of Amy Babiuch and David Mittleman.

recovery—decreased redness, swelling, and tenderness—are present, patients may be discharged to complete a 10- to 14-day course of comparable oral antibiotics. The average length of hospitalization for pediatric patients with complicated preseptal cellulitis is 4 days (Uzcategui et al., 1998). Ophthalmology, otolaryngology, and infectious diseases specialists should be consulted for patients with preseptal cellulitis. Symptoms should abate with treatment. Lid swelling and erythema will decrease with antibiotic therapy, and the patient's normal appearance should be restored. Application of warm compresses can be soothing during the acute process. Clinical improvement should begin to be seen within 24 hours. However, preseptal cellulitis can evolve into the more severe condition of orbital cellulitis despite antibiotic therapy. If the child develops diplopia, fever, worsening of vision, or worsening of symptoms, he or she should be re-evaluated immediately.

Disposition and discharge planning

Patients should be seen daily by an ophthalmologist until there are definite signs of resolution. If vision decreases, extraocular motility becomes limited, or a definite change in pupillary reaction occurs, then a repeat CT scan should be performed immediately. Patients with uncomplicated, treated preseptal cellulitis have a good prognosis. Healing is typically quick, within one to two weeks' time, and visual acuity should remain unaffected. Recurrent preseptal cellulitis is uncommon.

Prompt treatment and evaluation of sinusitis can prevent the development of preseptal cellulitis. Recurrent bouts of sinusitis (more than three episodes in one year) should be evaluated by an otolaryngologist. Superficial eyelid wounds should be cleansed adequately and observed closely for development of infection.

OROFACIAL DEVICES AND SURGICAL REPAIRS

Adam B. Smith, Samuel M. Maurice, and John W. Polley

Craniofacial surgery and orthognathic surgery have continued to advance rapidly and efficiently in both their availability and scope over the past several decades. Many defects that were once considered challenging to repair without severe disfigurement or permanent prosthetics are now repaired successfully with respect to both function and aesthetics. The management of these patients is typically complex, requires a dedicated team approach, and possible requires care at specialty centers to ensure optimal health outcomes (Munro, 1975).

Orofacial devices are used for two broad categories of malformations: traumatic/soft tissue or congenital. Traumatic fractures and soft-tissue defects typically affect patients with otherwise normal anatomy. The therapeutic goals in this situation are to return the patient to as close to the pretraumatic anatomic and functional status as possible. To a lesser extent, issues such as deformational plagiocephaly may be considered to represent a prolonged low-impact trauma to the cranial vault (Teichgraeber et al., 2002).

The most common congenital malformations are premature fusion of normally open osseous interfaces and nonunion of normally fused facial structures (Millard, 1976). Examples include synostosis of the cranial bones and orofacial clefting, respectively. The other commonly encountered congenital abnormalities involve hypoplasia of facial structures or, conversely, hyperplasia manifesting as an imbalance to the surrounding facial anatomy. Micrognathia and maxillary hypoplasia result from these processes.

SURGICAL ACCESS

Access to the orofacial structures (Figure 34-17) presents more of a challenge than access to other areas of the body for obvious reasons. The facial aesthetic appearance is intimately associated with a patient's psyche, and scarring in this region is not as easily concealed as it is in other areas of the body. In addition, a poor choice of access may result in functional deficits that are difficult to correct secondarily, such as lagophthalmos (deSousa et al., 2007). Consequently, particular attention must be made to the extent of the exposure necessary to complete the repair successfully versus the morbidity associated with the access route. Incisions used to access the craniofacial skeleton are divided into four regions (Table 34-7).

Superior orbital and cranial bone incisions

The coronal incision is made well within the hairline at the level of the posterior external auditory meatus in a

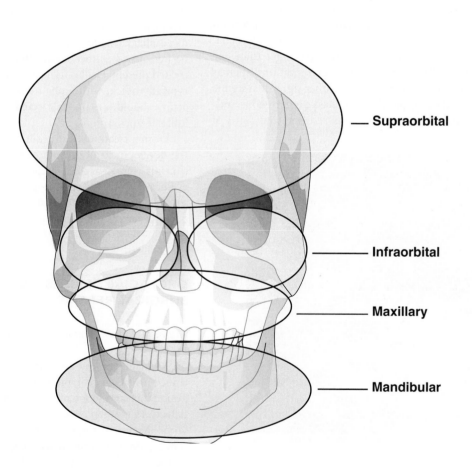

FIGURE 34-17

Access Zones of the Facial Structures.

TABLE 34-7

Access to Traumatic Zones	
Facial Zone	**Common Fractures in the Associated Zone**
Supraorbital, crania	Frontal sinus, superior orbital, naso-ethmoid-orbital, temporal bone
Infraorbital, periorbital	Inferior/lateral orbital, orbital blowout, zygomatic arch, lateral pyriform aperture
Maxillary/midface	Maxillary sinus, Le Fort I, inferior pyriform aperture, tripod/tetrapod
Mandible	Mandibular

retro-auricular fashion (Polley & Cohen, 1992). The cosmetic appearance of the incision as well as limitations of the functional contracture may be minimized via utilization of multiple W-plastys on the lateral portions—a strategy known as the "stealth" approach. More limited access may be obtained via incisions directly at the hairline/forehead interface.

Inferior/lateral periorbital and temporal bone incisions

Access to the periorbital regions both inferiorly and laterally are accomplished via transconjunctival incisions that are well hidden beneath the eyelid. Special attention must be paid postoperatively to ensure the patient does not develop lagophthalmos; should this complication occur, consultation with an ophthamologic specialist should be sought. For a more extensive exposure, subcilliary incisions may be used, with or without extension, toward the lateral canthus. They carry the same risk as transconjunctival incisions and produce an external scar. For zygomatic repairs, a Gillies incision may be placed within the hairline in the temporal region; its width varies depending on the exposure required.

Maxillae and inferior pyriform aperture incisions

Upper buccal sulcus incisions are used to access the midfacial structures (Luce, 1992). These types of incisions are extremely versatile and provide adequate exposure to the maxilla superiorly to the inferior orbits and laterally to the lateral maxillary buttress as well as the base of the pyriform aperture. No external scarring is apparent, and the functional risk is minimal. Closure is typically performed with interrupted absorbable sutures, and care must be taken to

provide adequate oral care in the postoperative period to prevent the accumulation of food and debris in the recesses on these sutures.

Mandible incisions

Inferior labial sulcus incisions are preferred if the exposure will be adequate for the repair, as this type of incision mirrors the upper buccal sulcus incision in both appearance and function. External incisions slightly below the angle of the mandible (Ridson incisions) can afford access in cases of plating or distraction needs that cannot be accomplished via intraoral approach. These obviate an external scar on the lower face.

METHODS OF FIXATION

The methods of fixation are as diverse as the methods of approach just described. The goal of therapy is minimal aesthetic disturbance for maximal functional restoration. Common fractures of the face and their reconstructive options are summarized in Table 34-8.

Rigid fixation is a method commonly used to treat traumatic defects. Titanium plating systems may be used (0.5- to 3.0-mm plates) in a virtually limitless assortment of designs and configurability. Titanium mesh, with subsequent fixation, may be used in very thin bony areas that would otherwise not accept classic anchors (orbit/maxilla). Rigid fixation may also be accomplished via approximation of bony fragments with 23- to 26-gauge wire.

Several absorbable fixation devices have also been introduced. These are used mainly for children, in whom rigid plate fixation might impair future growth of the facial skeleton.

For more complex defects, such as difficult orbital blowout fractures or correction of enophthalmos, split-thickness calvarial bone grafts may be required. For extensive reconstruction procedures, bone grafts from other areas of the body such as the rib or fibula have been harvested.

All of these plating systems and bone grafts have the potential to be palpable by the patient later in life as well as to become infected; in either situation, the fixation may require removal. For these reasons, families should receive information that another surgery may be required in the future to alleviate these problems.

For the fixation of mandibular and maxillary fractures, a popular approach is maxillo-mandibular fixation (MMF). This technique allows rigid fixation of the bony structures in occlusion so that when the native bone has healed, there is a greatly reduced chance of cross-bite or malocclusion. The classic method of MMF is to place

990 PART III Selected Disorders and Their Management

TABLE 34-8

Fracture Reconstruction Options	
Fracture	**Reconstruction Options**
Frontal sinus	ORIF with plating or wire, intracranialization
Superior orbital	Simple reduction, ORIF with 1- to 1.5 mm plating
Naso-ethmoid-orbital	ORIF with 1- to 1.5 mm plating, intercanthal wire to prevent telecanthus
Inferior orbital/orbital blowout	ORIF with 1- to 1.5 mm plating, titanium mesh repair, split-thickness cranial bone grafting
Zygomatic arch	Simple reduction, ORIF with 1.5- to 2 mm plating
Lateral pyriform aperture	ORIF with wire, ORIF with 1-mm plating
Le Fort I	ORIF with 2 mm plating
Maxillary sinus	ORIF with 1- to 2 mm plating, ORIF with wire, simple reduction
Inferior pyriform aperture	ORIF with 1- to 1.5 mm plating, simple reduction
Tripod/tetrapod	ORIF with 1.5- to 2 mm plating multiple fixation points
Mandibular	Maxillo-mandibular fixation, ORIF with 2- to 2.5 mm plating, interdental wires

Note: Open reduction internal fixation (ORIF).

circumdental wires to a preformed semirigid bar on both the upper and lower dentition. These upper and lower bars are then wired together in fixed position, thereby stabilizing both the occlusion and the interdental distances until healing can take place. This strategy, which is known as placing arch bars, is useful even in multiple comminuted mandible fractures. In the event that maximal stabilization does not need to occur or the patient is adentulous, specialized screws may be placed into the upper and lower alveolar cortical bone to provide wire attachment points. These MMF screws offer the benefit of being quicker and easier to remove for the patient, but come at the cost of placement of an invasive screw into the bone that can serve as an infection nydus or potentially damage the tooth roots.

Postoperative management

The postoperative management of a patient with a wired jaw is paramount to his or her care, and is perhaps even more crucial to the overall success of the procedure than the corrective surgery itself (Dethero, 1995). The most important concept with a wired jaw is ensuring the patency of the patient's airway. Every member of the team must be aware of the risk of aspiration and inadvertent asphyxiation in a patient with a wired jaw. Because the patient cannot open his or her jaw to expel emesis, the perceived entrapment of the tongue coupled with anxiety can provoke life-threatening airway obstruction. Patients must wear a wire-cutter on their person at all times when up and out of bed; this device may be secured to the head of the bed when the patient is at rest. The wire-cutter must also accompany the patient when he or she is transported between health care settings. If an emergency situation arises, the wires are to be cut immediately and the airway cleared. Every HCP who cares for the patient must be familiar with this simple but crucial procedure, because there may be no time for intervention by another member of the team.

Dietary consultation is helpful to patients and their families to educate them about the dietary modifications necessary with a wired jaw. Cleaning and dental care while the jaw is wired in occlusion should be performed. The sensation of not being able to open one's jaw after surgery is very anxiety provoking in some individuals; frequent reassurance is invaluable.

NONSURGICAL THERAPY

Deformational plagiocephaly is the malpositioning of an infant's cranial bones. It usually occurs secondary to prolonged exposure to low-impact force over a prolonged period (Teichgraeber et al., 2002). In the newborn, the cranial sutures are particularly malleable, as they must be able to deform to accommodate the neonate's passage through the birthing canal. This malleability persists for several years after birth as the cranial vault gradually becomes less moldable. During this period, prolonged sleeping or positioning on the back, or other positioning issues such as torticollis, can cause a flattening of the cranium in the area of force exertion (Persing et al., 2003). These deformational plagiocephalies can be identified through either physical examination of the sutures and the alignment of the other craniofacial structures, cephalometric analysis, or CT scan.

Once a deformational plagiocephaly is diagnosed, the mainstay of treatment is to eliminate the offending force. In patients with mild deformities, the process will reverse itself quite effectively. In contrast, in moderate to severe defects, molding helmets may be required. A number of manufacturers produce and fit such helmets, which must be adjusted and worn until the desired cranial molding has been achieved (Bruner et al., 2004). For maximal benefit, the caregivers of the child must be instructed as to the daily wearing of the helmet, the procedure for checking points of pressure, and appropriate padding lest pressure ulcers result. The length of treatment depends of the severity of the deformity and the age of the patient.

OROFACIAL SURGERY

Congenital orofacial abnormalities may in some instances require more extensive and invasive devices to obtain a satisfactory reconstruction. The most common craniofacial abnormality is clefting of the lip, the palate, or both (Millard, 1976). The importance of the team approach again cannot be overemphasized in the care of these patients and their families (Munro, 1975).

Mild defects may benefit from minimally invasive procedures, such as lip taping, to bring the final repair under the least tension possible. Children with cleft palates may benefit from having custom-molded palatal plates which may help to minimize nasal reflux of oral contents prior to repair. These devices should be worn at mealtimes and cleaned to prevent bacterial accumulation from attached food particles. Also useful is a specially designed nipple and bottle (Haberman Feeder or Mead Johnson Cleft Lip/Palate Nurser) for ease of feeding. These specially designed bottles may be helpful whether or not a patient has a plate.

For patients with more extensive clefting, nasoavleolar molding (NAM) can greatly assist in the patient's future reconstruction (Figure 34-18 and Figure 34-19) (Kirbschus et al., 2006). In particular, patients with bilateral clefts extending into the alveolus, by definition, have a nontethered premaxillary segment. With NAM, progressive molds made specifically for the patient are constructed to take advantage of the relative pliability of an infant's alveolar bone and circulating maternal estrogens making the soft tissue and cartilage more moldable to bring the premaxillary segment, palate and soft tissue into a more anatomical alignment. This treatment has multifactorial benefits: It

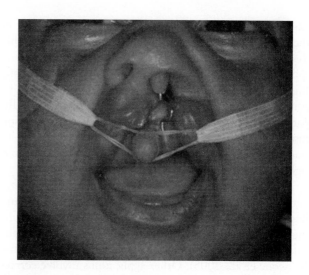

FIGURE 34-19

Nasoalveolar Molding: Internal View.

Source: Courtesy of Dr. Drew Schnitt, MD, Craniofacial Surgeon and Jose Larumber, DDS, Pediatric Dentist.

reduces tension on both the lip repair and the nasal tip flare endemic to these patients. The NAM device may decrease the temptation of osteotomizing the premaxillary segment to set it back and, thereby, may also reduce the need for future Le Fort I orthognathic repositioning (Aburezq et al., 2006). The parents should be counseled by the cleft team that the patient must wear the NAM device consistently and have a routine follow-up schedule with the dentist or orthodontist for adjustments and monitoring.

Orthognathic surgery in the care of the cleft patient, and even in noncleft patients, brings together several principles previously described. Maxillary hypoplasia is quite common in a patient who has had a cleft lip or palate. Micrognathia, retrognathia, and maxillary hyperplasia may all result in class II or III malocclusions that are not amenable to orthodontic correction. Patients may have to undergo correction when they have reached skeletal maturity. For maxillary movement, the Le Fort I osteotomy is a very versatile operation. In an approach typically performed through the upper buccal sulcus incision, the osteotomy is made and secured via rigid internal plate fixation and placement of mandibulomaxillary fixation intraoperatively. For mandibular advancements or setbacks, sagittal splits osteotomies or inverted "L" osteotomies are performed via inferior buccal sulcus incisions and rigidly fixed with mandibular screws and or plates. If the jaw is wired, the same precautions apply as previously described. The importance of airway monitoring in these patients cannot be overemphasized.

Even in the event that MMF is not required, the patient will likely need to wear elastics and have a splint in place to

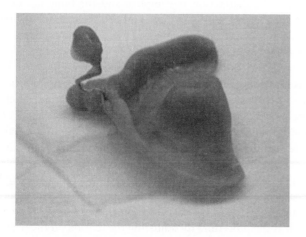

FIGURE 34-18

Nasoalveolar Molding: External View.

Source: Courtesy of Dr. Drew Schnitt, MD, Craniofacial Surgeon and Jose Larumber, DDS, Pediatric Dentist.

ensure satisfactory occlusal reconstitution. Proper wear of the elastics and duration of therapy should be thoroughly discussed with the patient prior to discharge. Intraoral splinting requires special attention to be paid to oral care. Light brushing of the area with mild toothpaste should be performed several times a day or after every meal. Typically, patients are advised not to use a forceful swish-and-spit mouthwash for several days after the surgery, lest the solution find its way through the suture line prior to its watertight seal.

Internal distraction can be used as a nonsurgical therapeutic technique in several areas of the facial skeleton and has also found its way into other areas of the body. The most common application of internal distraction is for the early correction of micrognathia with airway compromise (Cascone et al., 2005). Other applications involve correction of complete midface hypoplasia, such as that associated with Apert's or Crouzon's syndromes. Le Fort III osteotomy, with osteogenic distraction, may greatly reduce or eliminate the need for interposition bone grafting and internal plating (Denny et al., 2003). Osteogenic distraction is based on the principle of active osteoblast activity in response to tension on a bone. As such, new bone can be rapidly laid down and then be held in place until it has ossified into a self-supporting structure.

Internal distractors are composed of three main units: the distal and proximal fixation plates, the extensive mechanism, and the activation arm. All except the activation arm are by necessity in close proximity to the bone. The activation arm extends through the skin to allow for external manipulation of the internal distraction. In a mandibular distraction, external incisions are made directly inferior to the border of the body of the mandible, an osteotomy is performed, the distractor is placed, and the activation arm is situated dorsal to the angle of the mandible and inferior to the lobule of the ear (Cascone et al., 2005). With a Le Fort III distraction, the activation arms are typically hidden in the hairline near the coronal incision.

Proper functioning of the internal distractor and care are based on two central concepts: meticulous care to the armature exit sites and methodical daily distraction. The family of the patient should be instructed in the proper turning of the activator on a once- or twice-daily basis until adequate distraction has been achieved. Should this distraction be interrupted, the bone could ossify prematurely, necessitating a second osteotomy. As the armature is in direct continuity with healing bone and an internal plating system, cleaning and monitoring of the exit site are vital. This area should be cleaned a minimum of twice daily and watched for signs of infection such as erythema or purulent exudate. The vast majority of internal distraction devices must be removed at a second operation, so the family should be prepared for this procedure to occur in several weeks to months. During the hospital stay, the HCP should reinforce these principles to the patient and family as well as educate and inquire about them on follow-up to ensure the best possible outcome.

External distractors are some of the largest and most complex orofacial devices. Their complexity belies their utility: With external distraction, truly majestic transformations are possible. External distractors may be used in conjunction with a halo (an example being the rigid external distractor [RED] device) or in a similar fashion to internal distractors with an activation mechanism and rigid screw fixation to the underlying bone (Polley & Figueroa, 1998). Monobloc advancements, Le Fort III osteotomy, Le Fort I osteotomy, micrognathia corrections, and cranial vault enlargements are all examples of procedures that utilize external distraction (Polley & Figueroa, 1997).

Mobile armature-based distraction relies on several long pins being placed percutaneously into the bones on either side of the osteotomy, followed by daily activation to keep a constant tension on the bone. When the distraction is complete, the external fixator is removed, leaving only the exposing incision and the percutaneous pin holes. Care must be given to the pin holes in much the same way as the armatures of an internal distractor, as they are direct conduits into healing bone from the skin.

Halo-based devices such as the RED rely on rigid halo fixation to the skull and the attachment of skeletal drop wires to the underlying mobile segment of bone. A drop bar with activator is secured to the halo, with the wires then being secured to the activator. Movement of the bone can be controlled in virtually any vector by applying constant tension to the drop wires coming from the mobile segment. When the distraction is complete and the bone has ossified adequately, both the halo and the skeletal drop wires are removed. Minimal evidence of the distraction save the access incision remains.

As with any form of distraction, attention must be given to the maintenance of consistent constant tension across the osseous defect and the underlying bony attachment of the halo. A key concern with halo-based devices is maintenance of the fit. The tension of the cranium-to-halo screws must be checked regularly to ensure that they have not loosened. If this occurs, the halo may become malpositioned, potentially causing harm to the soft tissues and decreasing the tension on the transport segment of bone. Caregivers should be instructed on the care of the halo as well as the procedure for adjusting the tension on the wires. In addition, the halo produces unique challenges in sleeping arrangements. Likewise, with playtime activities, care must be taken to ensure that the halo does not become dislodged or impinge unnecessarily on daily life.

Orofacial devices are diverse in their spectrum and use. They extend from simple plating systems in minimally displaced areas, to external rigid distraction that can lead to large facial modifications. The basic tenet underlying orofacial surgery is to provide the maximal functional outcome while simultaneously preserving the best aesthetic relationships. Of all of the HCP's responsibilities, perhaps the most important is knowledge of airway difficulties in these specialized patients and the ability to deal with them. The team approach is absolutely essential to ensure superb results anatomically, physiologically, and socially in the entire spectrum of the orofacial patient population.

REFERENCES

1. Aburezq, H., Daskalogiannakis, J., & Forrest, C. (2006). Management of the prominent premaxilla in bilateral cleft lip and palate. *Cleft Palate–Craniofacial Journal, 43*(1), 92–95.

2. Allison, G. (1978). Anatomy of the external ear. *Clinics in Plastic Surgery, 5*(3), 419–422.

3. Ambati, B. K., Ambati, J., Azar, N., Stratton, L., & Schmidt, E. V. (2000). Periorbital and orbital cellulitis before and after the advent of *Haemophilus influenzae* type B vaccination. *Ophthalmology, 107*(8), 1450–1453.

4. American Dental Association. (2005). Tooth eruption: The primary teeth. *Journal of the American Dental Association, 137*, 127.

5. American Dental Association. (2006). Tooth eruption: The permanent teeth. *Journal of the American Dental Association, 136*, 1619.

6. Anderson, R. (2006). Facial nerve disorders and surgery. *Selected Readings in Plastic Surgery, 10*(14), 1–41.

7. Bahadori, R., Schwartz, R., & Ziai, M. (2000). Acute mastoiditis in children: An increase in northern Virginia. *Pediatric Infectious Diseases Journal, 19*, 212–215.

8. Bluestone, C. (1998). Acute and chronic mastoiditis and chronic suppurative otitis media. *Seminars in Pediatric Infectious Diseases, 9*, 12–26.

9. Boutros, S., & Thorne, C. (2009). Reconstruction of acquired ear defects. In B. Guyuron, E. Eriksson, & J. Persong (Eds.). *Plastic surgery: Indications and practice* (pp. 717–726). Philadelphia, PA: Saunders Elsevier.

10. Bruner, T., David, L., Gage, H. D., & Argenta, L. C. (2004). Objective outcome analysis of soft shell helmet therapy in the treatment of deformational plagiocephaly. *Journal of Craniofacial Surgery, 15*(4), 643–650.

11. Cascone, P., Gennaro, P., Spuntarelli, G., & Iannetti, G. (2005). Mandibular distraction: Evolution of treatment protocols in hemifacial microsomy. *Journal of Craniofacial Surgery, 16*(4), 563–571.

12. Denny, A., Kalantarian, B., & Hanson, P. R. (2003). Rotation advancement of the midface by distraction osteogenesis. *Plastic and Reconstructive Surgery, 111*(6), 1789–1799; discussion 1800–1783.

13. deSousa, J., Leibovitch, I., Malhotra, R., O'Donnell, B., Sullivan, T., & Selva, D. (2007). Techniques and outcomes of total upper and lower eyelid reconstruction. *Archives of Ophthalmology, 125*(12), 1601–1609.

14. Dethero, B. (1995). A patient education guide for wired jaws. *Plastic Surgery Nursing, 15*(4), 207–210.

15. Farkas, L., Katic, M., & Forrest, C. (2005). International anthropometric study of facial morphology in various ethnic groups/races. *Journal of Craniofacial Surgery, 16*(4), 615–646.

16. Gaffney, R., O'Dwyer, T., & Maguire, A. (1991). Bezold's abscess. *Journal of Laryngology and Otolaryngology, 105*, 765–766.

17. Gassner, R., Tarkan, T., Hachl, O., Moreira, R., & Ulmer, H. (2004). Craniomaxillofacial trauma in children: A review of 3,385 cases with 6,060 injuries in 10 years. *Journal of Oral and Maxillofacial Surgery, 62*, 399–407.

18. Greenberg, M. F., & Pollard, Z. F. (1998). Medical treatment of pediatric subperiosteal orbital abscess secondary to sinusitis. *Journal of AAPOS, 2*(6), 351–355.

19. Halpern, J., & Bernardo, L. (2002). Pediatric trauma emergency treatment for dental injuries. *International Journal of Trauma Nursing, 8*(1), 15–17.

20. Kirbschus, A., Gesch, D., Heinrich, A., & Gedrange, T. (2006). Presurgical nasoalveolar molding in patients with unilateral clefts of lip, alveolus and palate: Case study and review of the literature. *Journal of Craniomaxillofacial Surgery, 34*(suppl 2), 45–48.

21. Kokich, V. (1986). The biology of sutures. In M. Cohen (Ed.). *Craniosynostosis: Diagnosis, evaluation and management* (pp. 81–103). New York: Raven Press.

22. Kullman, G., Dyck, P., & Cody, D. (1971). Anatomy of the mastoid portion of the facial nerve. *Archives of Otolaryngology, 93*(1), 29–33.

23. Luce, E. (1992). Developing concepts and treatment of complex maxillary fractures. *Clinics in Plastic Surgery, 19*(1), 125–131.

24. Millard, D. (1976). *Cleft craft: The evolution of its surgery.* Boston: Little, Brown.

25. Mills, R. P., & Kartush, J. M. (1985). Orbital wall thickness and the spread of infection from the paranasal sinuses. *Clinical Otolaryngology and Allied Sciences, 10*(4), 209–216.

26. Moore, K., & Agur, A. (1995). *Essential clinical anatomy.* Philadelphia: Williams & Wilkins.

27. Munro, I. (1975). Orbito-cranio-facial surgery: The team approach. *Plastic and Reconstructive Surgery, 55*(2), 170–176.

28. Nageswaran, S., Woods, C. R., Benjamin, D. K. Jr., Givner, L. B., & Shetty, A. K. (2006). Orbital cellulitis in children. *Pediatric Infectious Disease Journal, 25*(8), 695–699.

29. Nelson, L., & Shusterman, S. (2000). Dental emergencies. In G. Fleisher & S. Ludwig (Eds.). *Textbook of pediatric emergency medicine* (4th ed., pp. 1613–1615). Philadelphia: Lippincott, Williams & Wilkins.

30. Osguthorpe, J. D., & Hochman, M. (1993). Inflammatory sinus diseases affecting the orbit. *Otolaryngologic Clinics of North America, 26*(4), 657–671.

31. Persing, J., James, H., Swanson, J., Kattwinkel, J., Committee on Practice and Ambulatory Medicine, Section on Plastic Surgery, et al. (2003). Prevention and management of positional skull deformities in infants. American Academy of Pediatrics Committee on Practice and Ambulatory Medicine, Section on Plastic Surgery and Section on Neurological Surgery. *Pediatrics, 112*(1 Pt 1), 199–202.

32. Polley, J., & Cohen, M. (1992). The retroauricular coronal incision. *Scandinavian Journal of Plastic and Reconstructive Surgery and Hand Surgery, 26*(1), 79–81.

33. Polley, J., & Figueroa, A. (1997). Distraction osteogenesis: Its application in severe mandibular deformities in hemifacial microsomia. *Journal of Craniofacial Surgery, 8*(5), 422–430.

34. Polley, J., & Figueroa, A. (1998). Rigid external distraction: Its application in cleft maxillary deformities. *Plastic and Reconstructive Surgery, 102*(5), 1360–1372; discussion 1373–1364.

35. Proffit, W., Epker, B., & Ackerman, J. (1980). Systematic description of dentofacial deformities: The data base. In W. Bell, W. Proffit, & R. White (Eds.). *Surgical correction of dentofacial deformities* (pp. 105–154). Philadelphia: W. B. Saunders.

36. Ranly, D. (1988). *A synopsis of craniofacial growth.* New York: Appleton-Century-Crofts.

37. Rodriguez, D., & Salarni, E. (2005). Decision making for the patient who presents with acute dental pain. *AACN Clinical Issues, 16*(3), 359–372.

38. Sataloff, R. (1990). Embryology of the facial nerve and its clinical applications. *Laryngoscope, 100*(9), 969–984.

39. Singh, D., & Bartlett, S. (2004). Pediatric craniofacial fractures: Long-term consequences. *Clinics in Plastic Surgery, 31*(3), 499–518.

40. Teichgraeber, J., Ault, J., Baumgartner, J. Waller, A., Messersmith, M., Gateno, J., et al. (2002). Deformational posterior plagiocephaly: Diagnosis and treatment. *Cleft Palate–Craniofacial Journal, 39*(6), 582–586.

41. Uzcategui, N., Warman, R., Smith, A., & Howard, C. W. (1998). Clinical practice guidelines for the management of orbital cellulitis. *Journal of Pediatric Ophthalmology and Strabismus, 35*(2), 73–79; quiz 110–111.

42. Zide, B. (1990). Deformities of the lips and cheeks. In J. McCarthy (Ed.). *Plastic surgery* (pp. 2009–2056). Philadelphia: W. B. Saunders.

Pulmonary Disorders

PHYSIOLOGY AND DIAGNOSTICS

Edmundo Cortez and Rani Ganesan

ANATOMY

Children and adults differ in airway anatomy and physiology. It is not until the individual reaches approximately 8 years of age that the pediatric airway anatomy and physiology are similar to that of an adult. The relatively small size of airway and respiratory structures in children play a role in their ability to handle respiratory problems.

Extrathoracic airway

The extrathoracic structures of the pediatric airway are found above the sternal notch. These structures work in concert to prepare inspired air prior to delivery into the intrathoracic structures, primarily the lungs. The nose, paranasal sinuses, pharynx, and larynx warm, humidify, and decontaminate inspired air.

Head. Anatomically, in infants and young children, the occiput is much larger in proportion to the rest of the skull and more protuberant than that in the adult. When the child is in a supine position, there is more neck flexion and the potential for airway obstruction.

Nasal cavity. The nasal cavity plays the major role in humidification and warming of the inspired air to body temperature. Each nasal passage consists of a roof, floor (hard palate), medial wall (nasal septum), and lateral wall (which includes the nasal turbinates). The nose provides the major resistance to air flow in the extrathoracic airway system. This function is demonstrated in infants, who are primarily nasal breathers. These children, with their smaller nasal openings, show significant work of breathing with increased secretions, edema, or blood in their nasal passages.

Sinuses. The ethmoid and maxillary sinuses are usually present at birth. By the time a child reaches 5 to 7 years of age, the frontal sinuses have developed so that they can be radiographically demonstrated. The sinuses insulate the cranial vault, promote phonation and resonation of voice, and produce secretions that aid in trapping foreign material during inspiration. Inflammatory and infectious processes of the sinuses (e.g., sinusitis) may cause significant upper airway difficulty for children. Increased secretions drain into the pharynx and then may be aspirated into the respiratory tract. Locally, sinusitis may lead to cellulitis of the overlying dermal layers or abscess formation within the sinus or its surrounding tissues.

Pharynx. The pharynx consists of the nasopharynx and oropharynx. The nasopharynx is found posterior to the nasal cavity and above the soft palate. The Eustachian tubes, adenoids, and tonsils are located within the nasopharynx. The openings of the Eustachian (pharyngotympanic) tubes lie on the lateral walls of the nasopharynx. Inflammation or obstruction of the nasopharynx often leads to the inability to drain an effusion process from the Eustachian tubes. This problem, in turn, may promote an infectious otitis media process.

The adenoids (nasopharyngeal tonsils) are located on the roof and posterior wall of the nasopharynx. These structures are commonly enlarged during childhood and can lead to obstructive nasal breathing. Because infants are primarily obligate nose breathers, significant nasopharyngeal obstruction often presents as feeding difficulties, increased work of breathing, or obstructive apnea breathing patterns.

Oropharynx. The oropharynx stretches from the soft palate to the tip of the epiglottis. The tongue is attached to the anterior oropharynx by the glossoepiglottic folds. The vallecular space—the area in between these folds—is the landmark into which the tip of a curved McIntosh laryngoscope blade is inserted during an intubation attempt. The lingual tonsil at the base of the tongue and the bilateral palatine tonsils are found at the entrance of the oropharynx. Inflammation of these tonsils may also contribute to an obstructive breathing pattern.

In proportion to the area of the oral cavity, the tongue is relatively large in children. In supine infants or children with decreased muscle tone, the tongue can easily cause airway obstruction by falling and lying flat against the soft palate. The jaw-thrust maneuver, which is taught during advance life support courses, will often improve obstructive breathing by pulling the tongue away from the palate and opening the oropharynx.

Larynx. The larynx is the area of the upper airway located between the pharynx and the trachea. The anatomical borders are the base of the tongue proximally and the trachea distally. The major structures found within the trachea include the thyroid cartilage, cricoid cartilage, bilateral arytenoids cartilage, epiglottis, and vocal cords. The various laryngeal structures contribute to phonation and protect the lower airway system during swallowing and coughing.

The thyroid cartilage is the largest cartilaginous structure of the larynx. It is open posteriorly but is best demonstrated by its anterior prominence (the "Adam's apple"). The cricoid cartilage is a complete ring of cartilage located just below the thyroid cartilage. Due to its small size, and because of its status as the only complete cartilaginous ring in the airway, the cricoid cartilage represents the narrowest point in the pediatric airway proximal to the carina. Its presence explains the recommendations for use of non-cuffed endotracheal tubes in pediatric patients younger than 7 years of age and is associated with a risk of acquired subglottic stenosis at this level following prolonged or multiple tracheal intubation. The bilateral arytenoid cartilages are attached to the posterior and superior borders of the thyroid cartilage. The vocal ligaments are attached to the anterior portion of the arytenoids.

The position of the pediatric larynx is more superior and anterior than that of an adult larynx. The cricoid cartilage of the newborn is approximately at the level of the C4 vertebra. By age 7 years, it is approximately at the level of the C5 cervical vertebra. By adult age, the cricoid cartilage is at the level of the C6 vertebra. These anatomical variances in the pediatric patient create a more acute angle between the base of the tongue and the larynx, which in turn may make it difficult to visualize the larynx during a direct laryngoscopy procedure. Mild extension of the pediatric patient's neck by placement of a roll under the neck and shoulders will relieve the angle and improve visualization.

Epiglottis.   The epiglottis is a leaf-shaped structure found at the posterior border of the thyroid cartilage. In an adult, the epiglottis is firm in shape. In infants, however, this structure is less rigid (floppy) and omega shaped. During tracheal intubation in younger children, visualization of the vocal cords is best facilitated by using the tip of a straight Miller laryngoscope blade to directly lift the epiglottis.

Intrathoracic anatomy

The intrathoracic structures of the pediatric airway are anatomically found below the sternal notch. The trachea, larger bronchi, and smaller bronchioles form the continued conducting airway system that delivers inspired air to the distal alveoli. The alveoli, along with their surrounding connective tissues and pulmonary capillary network, form the components of air exchange within the airway system. The chest wall is made up of cartilage, bone, and muscle that provide outright protection for the lung and heart from direct injury and facilitate the appropriate mechanics necessary to promote air flow in and out of the airway.

Trachea.   The trachea extends from the cricoid cartilage to the carina, where it bifurcates into the left and right mainstem bronchi. As an anatomical landmark, the carina is at approximately the level of the second rib anteriorly. The right mainstem bronchus is larger and bifurcates in a less sharp angle than the left mainstem bronchus—a factor that explains the propensity for aspirated material or objects to enter the right mainstem bronchus more than the left. Incomplete cartilaginous rings that are connected posteriorly by fibrous connective tissue maintain the patency of the trachea and bronchi.

The small diameter of the airway, along with the weaker cartilage found in infants and young children, accounts for the increased resistance and collapse of these airways during high active expiratory flow. This process is commonly demonstrated during crying or in bronchiolitis. Poiseuille's law of resistance states that resistance in a tube is inversely proportional to the radius to the fourth power; it is demonstrated clinically when processes such as edema or secretions reduce the airway size in children and respiratory distress occurs.

Lungs.   The right lung consists of three lobes (upper, middle, and lower), whereas the left lung has two lobes (upper and lower). Each of these lobes has a main lobar bronchus that branches into segmental bronchi deeper within each lobe. At birth, the infant lung usually has 10 right and 9 left segmental bronchi and approximately 50 million alveoli. Embryologically, pulmonary system development starts at approximately 5 to 6 weeks of gestation with the formation of a laryngotracheal groove in the fetus. Even at birth, pulmonary development is incomplete; thus this process continues into adolescence and beyond. The normal adult lung will eventually have 25 segmental bronchi and approximately 500 million alveolar units.

The lung has a dual blood supply coming from both right and left ventricular output. The pulmonary arteries coming from the right ventricle eventually branch into and form the pulmonary capillary system that completely meshes with the alveolar units. This system is the largest capillary bed in the human body. The pulmonary capillary system's main role occurs in gas exchange of O_2 and CO_2. Arteries that carry blood coming from the left ventricle follow and branch with the bronchial tree, respectively. This system's main role is to provide oxygen and nourishment to the bronchi, bronchioles, lymphatic system, and visceral pleura.

Thorax.   As with other parts of the airway system, the chest wall under goes structural changes and reformation with normal growth of the child. In an infant, the ribs of the chest wall are significantly less ossified than those in an adult and are usually articulated in a horizontal plane from the spine. With normal growth and development, the ribs achieve a downward orientation like that of an adult just prior to adolescence. Complete ossification of the ribs may not occur until adulthood. Notably, due to the cartilaginous nature of the pediatric rib cage and the smaller amount of muscle and fatty tissue mass, chest wall compliance is markedly higher in children than in adults. This factor accounts for the significant intercostal and subcostal retractions that are often seen in pediatric patients during respiratory distress.

RESPIRATORY PHYSIOLOGY

Mechanism of breathing

Normal breathing is divided into two cycles—inspiration and expiration. The inspiratory phase of the respiratory cycle is always active. Expiration is passive at rest and active during periods of respiratory distress and exercise.

The inspiratory phase of the respiratory cycle starts with contraction of the diaphragm, accessory muscles, and external intercostal muscles, which leads to an increase in intrathoracic volume. The resulting increase in negative intrathoracic pressure leads to movement of air from the atmosphere into the lungs.

The initiation of normal inspiration is centrally and peripherally controlled. Centrally acting receptors are located in the brain stem and the floor of the fourth ventricle; peripheral receptors are located in the carotid and aortic bodies. Control of breathing occurs mostly in the chemoreceptors located in the medulla. These receptors are very sensitive to changes in extracellular pH, which is directly related to serum $PaCO_2$ levels. The initiation of a breath occurs with a decrease in extracellular pH, which occurs with the elevation of $PaCO_2$. Peripherally located chemoreceptors also mediate the initiation of normal respiratory cycles. These chemoreceptors, which are also located in the carotid and aortic bodies, are typically sensitive only during periods of profound hypoxemia ($PaO_2 < 60$ mmHg). Episodes of profound hypoxemia may occur at higher altitudes, during periods of exercise, or with significant ventilation/perfusion mismatch.

The activation of the centrally and/or peripherally located respiratory centers leads to a contraction of the diaphragm, accessory muscles, and external intercostal muscles. As the diaphragm contracts, it moves downward, producing an increase in vertical lung capacity and lower air pressure in the lungs. When the external intercostal muscles contract, the upward and outward movement of the ribs also increases the lung capacity and lowers the air pressure in the lungs. The resulting pressure drop in the alveoli to less than (more negative than) atmospheric pressure leads to air movement into the lungs.

Expiration may be either a passive or an active process. In exhalation, expiration is passive and depends on the elastic recoil of lung tissue. Active exhalation occurs during exercise or respiratory distress. The introduction of positive abdominal pressure or negative pressure to the upper airway facilitates active exhalation. During normal exhalation, the diaphragm and external intercostal muscles relax, resulting in smaller lung volumes and subsequently intrathoracic pressure that are higher than atmospheric pressure. This pressure change causes air to move out of the lungs.

Alveolar ventilation and oxygenation

The primary physiologic goal of the lung is to provide adequate CO_2 elimination and O_2 uptake during the entire respiratory cycle. Gas exchange occurs anywhere that the respiratory tree interfaces with the pulmonary vasculature. With each breath of inspired gas, a variable amount is wasted and never reaches the gas-exchanging units of

the lung. This gas is lost to regions of the respiratory tree referred to as areas of "dead space" ventilation. Dead space ventilation is divided into two types—anatomic and physiologic. Anatomic dead space refers to large conduction airways. Alveolar dead space refers to alveoli that are unable to participate in gas exchange for any of a number of reasons. To achieve maximum absorption of oxygen and elimination of carbon dioxide, pulmonary blood flow to gas exchanging units of the lung is optimized.

In this text, respiratory physiologic principles refer to CO_2 and O_2 in units of partial pressure (1 mmHg = 1 torr or 1 kPa = 7.5 mmHg) and concentration (1 mL/dL = volume % = 0.45 mmol/L). Partial pressure of a dry gas in the environment is defined as its fraction of total barometric pressure. For example:

$$P_x = F_x (P_{atmospheric\ pressure})$$
$$PO_2 \text{ in atmosphere} = 0.21 \times 760 \text{ mmHg} = 160 \text{ mmHg}$$

The partial pressure of a dry gas in the environment is different from the partial pressure of the same dry gas in the airway. The airway has water vapor pressure, which reduces the overall presence of dry gas.

$$P_x = F_x (P_{atmospheric\ pressure} - P_{water\ vapor\ pressure})$$
$$PO_2 \text{ in airways}(P_iO_2) = 0.21 \times (760 \text{ mmHg} - 47 \text{ mmHg})$$
$$= 150 \text{ mmHg}$$

Effective alveolar ventilation, or alveolar minute ventilation, is the most important factor in determining P_AO_2 at any given P_IO_2 and oxygen consumption in the healthy lung. Total ventilation is directly proportion to a person's respiratory rate and the tidal volume of each breath:

$$\text{Total ventilation} = \text{Respiratory rate} \times \text{Tidal volume}$$

A portion of total ventilation is lost to the anatomic dead space of the conduction zones in the airways. Alveolar minute ventilation, or effective minute ventilation, is the difference between total ventilation and dead space ventilation. Typically, dead space ventilation in the normal adult lung is 1 mL/1 lb of body weight. In diseased lungs, effective minute ventilation is further influenced by physiologic dead space, which includes diseased alveoli that cannot participate in effective gas exchange. Alveolar ventilation in the healthy lung can also be calculated using a variation of Fick's principle, which states that the difference between the amount of gas that enters the organ and the amount of gas that leaves the organ is equal to the amount of gas the organ consumed or produced. For example:

$$CO_2 \text{ elimination } (V_{CO_2}) =$$
$$CO_2 \text{ exhaled } (V_A \times F_{ACO_2}) - CO_2 \text{ inhaled } (V_I \times F_{ICO_2})$$

where V_A represents alveolar ventilation and F_{ICO_2} is zero. The equation may be rearranged and simplified to the alveolar ventilation equation as follows:

$$V_A = V_{CO_2}/F_{ACO_2}$$

where the fraction of alveolar CO_2 is described in terms of a constant K (0.863) and P_{ACO_2}:

$$V_A = (V_{CO_2}/P_{ACO_2}) \times K$$

Note that V_A and P_{ACO_2} are inversely proportional, meaning that, with decreased alveolar ventilation, P_{ACO_2} and, subsequently, P_{aCO_2} levels rise. Upper case "A" represents alveolar and lower case "a" is the designation for arterial.

The alveolar ventilation equation may aid calculation of partial pressure of alveolar oxygen (P_AO_2) in the healthy lung where the partial pressure of inspired CO_2 is zero:

$$P_{AO_2} = P_{IO_2} - (P_{ACO_2}/R) + F$$

where P_{IO_2} refers to F_{IO_2} (atmospheric pressure − water vapor pressure); P_{ACO_2} is P_{aCO_2} in the healthy lung; R (RQ) reflects CO_2 production/O_2 consumption; and F is a negligible constant under normal conditions. The respiratory quotient represents the ratio of carbon dioxide production to oxygen consumption. The typical RQ of a healthy adult is 0.8, which demonstrates that oxygen consumption is higher than carbon dioxide production at normal physiologic states. In hypermetabolic/hyperventilation states of exercise, carbon dioxide production increases significantly due to the higher levels of bicarbonate in the blood and tissues, which result in an increase in RQ to greater than 1. Respiratory quotients are also affected by the proportions of protein, carbohydrate, and fat within the diet. Carbohydrate is metabolized to carbon dioxide, for example; thus an increase in intake of carbohydrate leads to higher carbon dioxide production and a higher RQ.

Normal gas exchange

Just as the delivery of air to zones of ventilation in the respiratory tree is essential in gas exchange, so the diffusion properties of carbon dioxide and oxygen across the alveolar–capillary membrane are equally important in gas exchange. Principles of gas exchange in the lung assume a steady state and are based on conservation of mass. Gas exchange in the lungs occurs through simple diffusion. The partial pressure of a gas drives its diffusive gas transport. Simple diffusion is defined as the net movement of a substance from a region of higher concentration to one of lower concentration. Ideally, diffusion across the blood–gas barrier results in complete equilibrium between the alveoli and the pulmonary arterial blood. In reality, however, a small difference exists. With any disease that affects the blood–gas barrier results in diffusion limitations (or gas exchange limitations), this difference becomes even greater. Diffusion limitations that result in minimal alveolar–arterial PO_2 differences generally do not cause much compromise to overall oxygen delivery or oxygen consumption.

Oxygen. Due to the many chemical reactions that oxygen undergoes in blood, its concentration does not reflect solely its partial pressure and constant solubility. Oxygen exists in bound form with hemoglobin. Hemoglobin is a protein that is composed of four subunits, which are made up of two alpha and two beta chains. This molecule binds with oxygen and the ferrous (Fe^{2+}) form of iron. The concentration of oxygen in blood is the sum of dissolved and bound oxygen. In equation form:

$$C_aO_2 = \text{Dissolved oxygen} + \text{Bound oxygen}$$
$$C_aO_2 = (P_aO_2 \times 0.002) + (1.34 \times Hgb \times O_2 \text{ sat})$$

Note that dissolved oxygen adds only a small portion to the total concentration of oxygen in blood with normal hemoglobin and oxygen saturation. The bound concentration of oxygen adds to the bulk of its content in blood.

The relationship between P_aO_2 and the oxygen saturation of hemoglobin is delicately balanced based on serum pH, temperature, hemoglobin type, 2,3-DPG, pCO_2, and pCO. This relationship is illustrated by the oxygen dissociation curve (Figure 35-1). The oxygen dissociation curve is sigmoidal (or S) in shape, reflecting the three-dimensional shape of hemoglobin. With changes in the previously mentioned factors, the oxygen dissociation curve may shift vertically, may shift horizontally, or may change its shape.

A vertical shift in the curve indicates a change in oxygen capacity. An increased height of the curve occurs when the hemoglobin load increases from the normal level.

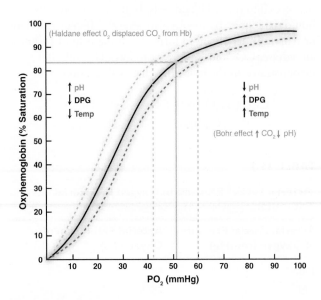

FIGURE 35-1

Oxyhemoglobin Dissociation Curve.

A horizontal deviation (or shift of P_{50}) from baseline indicates a change in the oxygen's affinity to hemoglobin. A leftward shift represents a higher Hgb-O_2 affinity (more efficient loading and less efficient unloading of oxygen molecules), whereas a rightward shift represents a lower Hgb-O_2 affinity (less efficient loading and more efficient unloading of oxygen molecules). Hgb-O_2 affinity is largely determined by serum pH, pCO_2, and temperature.

A change in actual morphology of the curve may indicate a change in the chemical reactions between oxygen and hemoglobin. Because the relationship between oxygen and hemoglobin is complex, remembering four key points of the normal adult curve will allow for a clinician to understand and possibly solve many common problems of oxygen transport that lead to poor tissue perfusion (Table 35-1).

Optimal diffusion of oxygen across the alveolar–arterial wall and efficient oxygen loading to and unloading off hemoglobin molecules are critical processes in oxygen delivery to tissues. In a healthy lung, the alveolar partial pressure of oxygen will be the same as the arterial partial pressured of oxygen. The alveolar–arterial (A-a) gradient in the normal lung ranges from 5 to 15 mmHg. Changes in the diffusion properties of the alveolar–capillary wall, or mismatching of pulmonary blood flow to ventilated lung units, causes increases in alveolar–arterial PO_2 gradients.

Carbon dioxide. Carbon dioxide exists in the human body as dissolved CO_2 (bicarbonate) and as a form bound to deoxygenated hemoglobin (carbamino-hemoglobin). Like oxygen, dissolved CO_2 follows the principles of Henry's law, which states that the partial pressure of CO_2 is directly proportional to its solubility constant and its concentration at a given temperature. At the tissue level, carbon dioxide moves from the interstitium to the serum and eventually dissolves into the red blood cells. In the red blood cells, carbon dioxide may be involved in several different reactions or remain in its dissolved form. With the help of carbonic anhydrase, CO_2 and H_2O react to form H^+ and HCO_3^- as demonstrated in the following chemical reaction:

$$CO_2 + H_2O \leftrightarrow H_2CO_3 \leftrightarrow H^+ + HCO_3^-$$

TABLE 35-1

Arterial Partial Pressure of Oxygen to Arterial Saturation	
Arterial Partial Pressure of Oxygen (mmHg)	**Arterial Saturation of Oxygen (%)**
100	98
40	75
26	50
0	0

When the intracellular concentration of HCO_3^- increases, this ion leaves the cell and Cl^- enters the cell, as the cell seeks to maintain its electrical neutrality. This exchange is known as the chloride shift. H^+ molecules that have stayed within the red blood cell reduce HbO_2 to HHb and O_2:

$$H + HbO_2 \leftrightarrow HHb + O_2$$

The resulting deoxygenated hemoglobin molecule, which has a higher affinity for CO_2 than for O_2, forms carbamino-hemoglobin with carbon dioxide. As the intracellular concentration of free oxygen increases, oxygen molecules move along their concentration gradient into tissue. The unloading of oxygen molecules resulting from the hemoglobin–carbon dioxide bond is known as the Haldane effect.

As red blood cells move to the pulmonary capillary bed, the intracellular concentration of carbon dioxide exceeds that of the serum, which favors movement of dissolved carbon dioxide from the red cells to the alveoli. Concomitantly, chloride shifts back to the extracellular space in exchange for HCO_3^- into the cell. As the concentration of intracellular oxygen increases, the oxygen binds with hemoglobin and hydrogen protons are donated. With the help of carbonic anhydrase, HCO_3^- and H^+ form CO_2 and water. The continued increase in the amount of dissolved carbon dioxide favors movement of this molecule out of the cell. Carbon dioxide and oxygen are in a constant state of movement that favors optimal oxygen delivery to the body's tissues and removal of carbon dioxide to the alveoli.

In the normal lung, the alveolar partial pressure of carbon dioxide is equal to the partial pressure of carbon dioxide in the pulmonary arterial blood. In diseased lung units where the diffusion properties of the alveolar–capillary wall change, alveolar partial pressure of carbon dioxide in the alveoli will generally be lower than that in the arterial blood.

Movement of gas and fluid within the lung

To understand the basic principles of lung function, it is important to understand how fluid shifts within the lung affect the alveolar–capillary gas exchange process. Normally, fluid moves from the pulmonary vasculature to the interstitium, and then drains into the pulmonary lymphatic system, while the alveoli remain relatively dry. The amount of fluid that shifts from the capillary bed to the interstitium is quantified by the Starling equation:

$$J_v = K_f([P_c - P_i] - \sigma[\pi_c - \pi_i])$$

In this expression, J_v quantifies net fluid movement; K_f is the permeability coefficient of the membrane, which depends on the ease of fluid movement across a given surface area; and σ is the reflection coefficient. The reflection coefficient (range: 0–1) indicates the ease of transvascular plasma protein movement. A reflection coefficient of 0 indicates no restriction of plasma protein movement, whereas a value of

1 indicates complete restriction of plasma protein movement. Typically, the reflection coefficient in the normal lung is 0.65, which primarily restricts transvasculature plasma protein movement. Also in the equation, $P_c - P_i$ is the difference between intravascular hydrostatic pressure (P_c) and interstitial hydrostatic pressure (P_i), while ($\pi_c - \pi_i$) is the difference between intravascular oncotic pressure (π_c) and interstitial oncotic pressure (π_i).

Because the permeability coefficient and reflection coefficient favor restriction of protein plasma movement, overall net fluid movement depends on the difference between the hydrostatic and protein osmotic pressures. The hydrostatic pressure in the lung's microvasculature is higher than that of the interstitium, so net fluid movement favors flux into the interstitium. In the normal adult lung, fluid in the interstitium is cleared by the lymphatics at a rate of 10 to 20 mL/hr. In the case of left heart failure, the hydrostatic pressure in the microvasculature becomes higher, which causes more fluid to move toward the interstitium at a rate faster than it can be drained by the lymphatics. This phenomenon is often referred to as "high-pressure" pulmonary edema. If the interstitium and pulmonary lymphatics become overwhelmed with fluid, interventions to lower left atrial pressures or to lower left ventricular preload may improve the patient's pulmonary fluid status. If the lymphatics and interstitium continue to be exposed to a high fluid load, the edema may eventually break through the alveolar wall and cause alveolar edema. At this stage, lung compliance is affected and hypoxemia results.

In the case of an infection or sepsis, the permeability of the pulmonary microvasculature wall is compromised. Such a defect results in leakage of both fluid and protein into the interstitium. As there is no intervention available to directly repair the capillary wall, the goal of therapy in these patients is to treat the underlying disease process.

Diffusion. Normal movement of carbon dioxide and oxygen across the alveolar–capillary membrane depends greatly on the diffusion properties of the membrane itself. It is important to remember that the blood leaving the pulmonary capillaries is in equilibrium with alveolar gas in the healthy lung. The small differences in P_AO_2 and P_aO_2 are not due to diffusion limitations, but rather are due to normal ventilation/perfusion (V/Q) mismatch. Fick's law is applied again when quantifying the amount of oxygen that diffuses across the alveolar–capillary membrane:

$$V_{O_2} = \Delta P_{O_2} \times D_{O_2}$$

where ΔP_{O_2} reflects the gradient of PO_2 between alveoli and pulmonary capillary blood, and D_{O_2} implies diffusing capacity. The diffusing capacity of a molecule is directly proportional to its solubility properties and the surface area of the membrane being crossed; it is inversely proportional

to its molecular weight and the thickness of the membrane being cross. In equation form, this relationship can be summarized as follows:

$$D_{O_2} = (\text{Solubility/Molecular weight}) \times (\text{Area/Thickness})$$

Along with diffusion properties, capillary blood transit time at the alveolar–capillary interface influences oxygen diffusion. In the normal adult lung, the transit time of a single red blood cell along the alveolar–capillary membrane is, on average, 0.75 second, where alveolar and arterial oxygen pressures equilibrate at approximately 0.25 second. During times of extreme exercise, athletes have very high oxygen consumption and elevated cardiac output. This increase in cardiac output shortens the transit time of red blood cells at the alveolar–capillary interface, which decreases the amount of time allowed for complete oxygen equilibration across the membrane. Similarly, diffusion of oxygen is limited at high altitudes, where transit time is faster and P_AO_2 levels are lower. Diffusion limitations in the healthy lung also differ from those of diseased lungs. Diffusion limitations in diseased lungs typically arise when disease at the alveolar–capillary interface causes an increase in membrane thickness.

The movement of all gases across the alveolar–capillary membrane is specific to the properties of each gas and not limited solely on the diffusion properties of the membrane. For instance, nitrous oxide (along with other inert gases) does not chemically react with red blood cells; thus nitrous oxide remains completely dissolved in serum. Nitrous oxide and other inert gases that do not react chemically with red blood cells are considered perfusion-limited gases. In contrast, carbon monoxide reacts very strongly with red blood cells. Because carbon monoxide quickly binds to hemoglobin as it moves across the alveolar–capillary membrane, the partial pressure of dissolved carbon monoxide remains very low, thereby maintaining the alveolar–capillary gradient. This gradient continues to favor movement across the membrane. The movement of carbon monoxide from the alveoli into pulmonary capillary blood is, therefore, limited by the diffusion properties of the membrane: Carbon monoxide is a diffusion-limited gas.

Alveolar ventilation and pulmonary blood flow relationships. Pulmonary blood flow within the lung depends on many factors, including pulmonary vasculature pressure gradients, resistances, and gravity. Normal distribution of pulmonary blood flow in the upright adult lung is described as a series of zones by West (2008). Pulmonary blood flow reflects the difference between hydrostatic pulmonary arterial (P_a) and venous (P_v) capillary pressures and its relationship to alveolar pressure (P_A), as evidenced by pulmonary blood flow that is relatively low to segments of the lung above the heart when compared to those segments that are below the heart. *Zone 1* represents the apex of the lung where alveolar pressure exceeds that of both venous and alveolar hydrostatic pressures. These segments are adequately ventilated, but are normally poorly perfused. In *Zone 2*, pulmonary blood flow depends on the difference between the arterial hydrostatic pressure and the alveolar pressure. Because venous and arterial hydrostatic pressures are greater than alveolar pressure, pulmonary blood flow is completely dependent on pressure gradients with the pulmonary vasculature in *Zone 3* (or lung bases). Lung expansion in this zone is relatively poor, resulting in proportionally lower available gas-exchanging units (V) to perfusion (Q) ratio (Table 35-2). Increases in alveolar–arterial oxygen gradients in different parts of the lung may be caused by mismatching of pulmonary blood flow to ventilated lung units (V/Q).

Lung volumes

Lung volume and lung capacity are often used to describe pulmonary physiology and pathophysiology. It is important to recognize that volume and capacity are not interchangeable and that they reference different physiologic principles. Lung capacity refers to the amount of air that *can* occupy space in the lung, whereas volume describes the amount of air that *does* occupy space in the lung. The lung volumes and capacities that are used to describe the lung's physiologic state are fractions of a person's total lung capacity (TLC). TLC is defined as the maximum amount of air the lung can hold after a maximal inspiration.

TLC is the sum of vital capacity (VC) and residual volume (RV), where VC describes the maximal amount of air forcefully expired after a maximal inspiration and RV is defined as the residual volume present in the lung after the completion of a forced expiration. Vital capacity decreases with increases in residual volume, as in the case in obstructive airway diseases including asthma and emphysema. Vital capacity may also decrease in the case of both pulmonary and extrapulmonary diseases. Interestingly, overall alveolar ventilation may not be adversely affected in the cases of lung disease, because all of the lung's vital capacity is not used during breathing.

Tidal volume (TV) is defined as the amount of air inspired and expired during normal expiration. Functional residual capacity (FRC) describes the lung's remaining volume at the end of normal expiration. TV affects effective alveolar ventilation and oxygenation, whereas FRC represents the balance of static and passive forces between the lung and chest wall.

TABLE 35-2

West Zones	
Zone 1	$P_A > P_a > P_v$
Zone 2	$P_a > P_A > P_v$
Zone 3	$P_a > P_v > P_A$

Lung compliance and elastance

Elastic recoil pressure is defined as an opposing force that resists deformative changes so as to maintain a system in its relaxed state. In the respiratory system, elastance is defined as follows:

$$P_{elas}/\text{Volume}$$

where P_{elas} is the elastic recoil pressure. Elastic recoil pressure is important in understanding the flow dynamics of air as it moves in and out of the lung. The total amount of pressure required to generate flow of air into the lungs is equal to the sum of the respiratory system's elastic recoil, frictional, and inertial pressures, where inertial pressure is negligible.

Compliance is defined as the degree to which a closed compartment will expand when pressure is applied. For example, a thin-walled balloon is highly compliant, as a small amount of pressure application results in significant expansion. In respiratory physiology, the following expression is used to describe compliance:

$$C = \Delta\text{Volume}/\Delta\text{Pressure}$$

where ΔPressure represents the change in lung elastic recoil pressure and ΔVolume is equal to the change in lung volume. With parenchymal lung disease or increased airway resistance, the overall compliance of the respiratory system decreases as the amount of pressure required to change a given total lung volume increases. Changes in lung compliance may also be physiologically normal, as it is in the developing lung. These variations in lung compliance depend on the actual number of expanding air spaces and their different geometric shapes and sizes.

DIAGNOSTICS

As with any pathophysiologic processes of other body systems, observation of the clinical status and direct physical examination remain the primary way to diagnose specific pathology and location within the pediatric airway. Inspiratory sounds (e.g., stridor or stertor) are the usual physical examination hallmark findings for upper airway pathology. Expiratory sounds (e.g., wheezing) usually indicate an intrathoracic process.

A more detailed evaluation of the airway is often required to adequately assess the functionality and anatomic status of the airway. The health care professional's (HCP's) armamentarium of diagnostic studies of the pediatric airway is broad. Radiologic studies include plain radiograph, barium esophagrams, ultrasonography, computed tomography (CT) scans, and magnetic resonance imaging (MRI). Nonradiologic studies may be divided into invasive procedures (rigid and flexible endoscopy) and noninvasive procedures (sleep studies and pulmonary function testing [PFT]).

Radiologic studies

Plain radiographs remain a commonly used and easy-to-perform diagnostic image to evaluate the airway. Lateral and anterior–posterior (AP) films of the neck are useful in the evaluation of nasopharyngeal, oropharyngeal, and laryngeal pathology. Chest radiographs (CXR) in a lateral or AP position aid in delineating tracheal and intrathoracic pathology. A common pathophysiologic issue for young children is foreign body ingestion and aspiration. Almost one-third of the objects in these patients are radiolucent. When such objects are aspirated into the trachea or bronchial tree, inspiratory and expiratory AP CXR (for cooperative patients) or lateral decubitus CXR (for younger or uncooperative children) may help identify the aspiration of a radiolucent object. When inspiratory and expiratory radiographs are obtained, the inspiratory CXR will show normal bilateral lung aeration. The expiratory CXR will show normal aeration on the ipsilateral side and diminished aeration on the contralateral side to the aspirated object.

Normally, aeration is diminished when the lung is placed in the decubitus position. When foreign body is suspected, the side with the foreign body demonstrates normal aeration when placed in the decubitus position.

Barium esophagrams

Barium esophagrams are useful adjuncts if tracheal compression is suspected via physical examination or endoscopy. Vascular anomalies such as an aberrant left pulmonary, vascular ring, or double aortic arch may be present with esophageal compression. If these processes are suspected, further radiologic imaging such as MRI or angiography is warranted prior to surgical correction.

Ultrasound

Ultrasound remains a useful noninvasive imaging tool in the assessment of soft-tissue structures and pathology of the face and neck (e.g., retropharyngeal or peritonsillar abscesses). Because it is a fast and noninvasive diagnostic modality, this technique is especially useful in patients who are uncooperative or are at risk for clinical compromise during sedation.

Computed tomography and magnetic resonance imaging

CT scans and MRI of the pediatric airway are becoming more accepted as noninvasive imaging and diagnostic modalities to precisely delineate pathology and anatomy, especially before any further invasive testing or surgical correction is performed. For difficulties involving the nasal and paranasal structures (e.g., choanal atresia, sinusitis), CT scans are quite useful and essential. MRI and magnetic resonance angiography (MRA) scans are commonly performed when intrathoracic pathology (e.g., vascular ring, mediastinal tumor) is highly suspected.

Compared to other radiologic modalities, the high yield of information produced by these studies carries higher risk for the pediatric patient. CT scans expose the patient to significant radiation. Both CT scans and MRI frequently require the patient to be sedated to obtain clear images. The airway and cardiovascular status of the patient must be carefully assessed prior to conducting these studies under sedation. Clinical experts (anesthesia or critical care) in pediatric sedation and airway management should be involved with the management of the patient whenever such studies are performed in children.

Rigid and flexible endoscopy

The invasive procedures of rigid and flexible endoscopy remain useful and successful modalities in the diagnosis and treatment of common airway issues. Rigid endoscopy should be performed only by physicians (otolaryngologists) who have received training in its use. This technique has significant advantages over flexible endoscopy in that the endoscope acts to protect the airway during the procedure (air flow in and out of the trachea is not markedly obstructed); it also allows special instrumentations (CO_2 laser and optical forceps) to be used in the treatment of airway lesions (e.g., granulation tissue, foreign body, hardened secretions). The disadvantages of rigid endoscopy include the need for the procedure to be performed in an operating room environment, the requirement for general anesthesia to facilitate the procedure, the inability to evaluate the distal airway, and the risk of trauma to the airway because of the rigidity of the scope.

Flexible endoscopy offers several advantages over rigid bronchoscopy. Notably, it allows evaluation and therapy of distal airway pathology. Use of instrumentation through the flexible endoscope allows for the collection of specimens (tissue biopsy, bronchoalveolar fluid analysis) and removal of foreign bodies. Flexible endoscopy does not necessarily require the patient to be deeply sedated or under general anesthesia, and it can be performed by various types of clinicians (critical care, anesthesiology, general surgery, emergency medicine) who are appropriately trained. Flexible endoscopes of variable sizes (including one as small as 2.7 mm in diameter) may be used in patients with a wide range of airway calibers. In infants or intubated patients, the diameter of the scope itself is usually large enough to significantly obstruct air flow. As with other invasive procedures, close cardiorespiratory monitoring and medically trained personnel who can manage airway issues are essential to patient safety.

Sleep studies

Sleep studies are noninvasive methods to determine the cause (central or obstructive) and severity of obstructive breathing patterns in patients. The complexity of the study can range from simple end-tidal CO_2 capnography with chest wall plethysmography, to multichannel sleep monitoring that includes electrocardiograph (ECG) and electroencephalograph (EEG).

Pulmonary function tests

Pulmonary function testing (PFT) has been used in both younger and older pediatric patients. By visualizing flow-volume loops of the patient, either variable or fixed, and the intrathoracic or extrathoracic airway, obstructive processes are commonly identified. Ideally, cooperative patients can best utilize an active breathing apparatus for PFT measurements. In younger and uncooperative patients, passive breathing measurements are evaluated (e.g., partial expiratory flow-volume loop).

ACUTE RESPIRATORY DISTRESS SYNDROME

Mark Riccioni

PATHOPHYSIOLOGY

Acute respiratory distress syndrome (ARDS) is a result of direct or indirect lung injury, specifically to the alveolar capillary barrier that involves both the alveolar epithelium and the capillary endothelium. The alveolar capillary barrier is important in maintaining lung fluid balance, and the loss of this barrier is a key contributor to the development of ARDS (Ware, 2006).

ARDS proceeds through three phases. The first phase is the *acute/exudative phase*, during which several physiologic events occur. Initial injury to the alveolar–capillary interface leads to disruption of epithelial fluid transport and reduced removal of fluid from the alveolar space. As a result, capillary permeability increases and pulmonary edema occurs (Figure 35-2) (Morrison & Bidani, 2002; Ware & Matthay, 2000). The edema impairs gas exchange by increasing the diffusion barrier. An alteration in the diffusion barrier, in

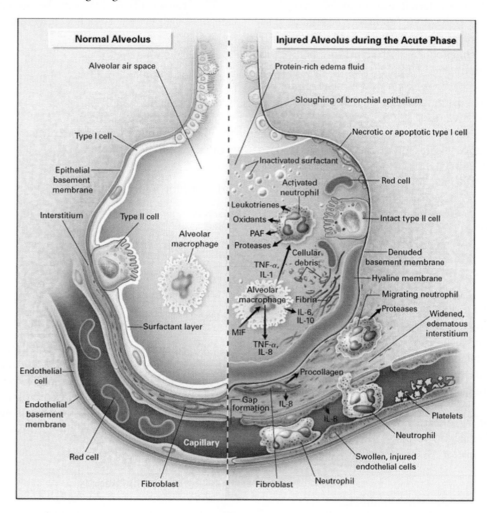

FIGURE 35-2

Acute (exudative) phase of Acute Respiratory Distress Syndrome (ARDS).

Note: In the acute phase of the syndrome (right-hand side), there is sloughing of both the bronchial and alveolar epithelial cells, with the formation of protein-rich hyaline membranes on the denuded basement membrane. Neutrophils are shown adhering to the injured capillary endothelium and marginating through the interstitium into the air space, which is filled with protein-rich edema fluid. In the air space, an alveolar macrophage is secreting cytokines, interleukin-1, 6, 8, and 10, (IL-1, 6, 8, and 10) and tumor necrosis factor (TNF), which act locally to stimulate chemotaxis and activate neutrophils. Macrophages also secrete other cytokines, including interleukin-1, 6, and 10. Interleukin-1 can also stimulate the production of extracellular matrix by fibroblasts. Neutrophils can release oxidants, proteases, leukotrienes, and other proinflammatory molecules, such as platelet-activating factor (PAF). A number of antiinflammatory mediators are also present in the alveolar milieu, including interleukin-1–receptor antagonist, soluble tumor necrosis factor receptor, autoantibodies against interleukin-8, and cytokines such as interleukin-10 and 11 (not shown). The influx of protein-rich edema fluid into the alveolus has led to the inactivation of surfactant. MIF denotes macrophage inhibitory factor.

Source: Used with permission from Ware & Matthay, (2000). The acute respiratory distress syndrome. The New England Journal of Medicine, 342(18), 1334-1349.

turn, may lead to V/Q mismatch and an increase in the A-a gradient, which is followed by an acute inflammatory stage recognized by neutrophil activation. Neutrophils adhere to the injured epithelium and release several injurious metabolites, such as oxidants, proteases, and leukotrines (Ware, 2006). Finally, cytokines are produced in response to inflammation. Examples of pro-inflammatory cytokines include tumor necrosis factor (TNF) and interleukins (IL) 1, 6, and 8. IL-1 and TNF induce release of the chemokine IL-8, which is responsible for pulmonary neutrophil recruitment (Morrison & Bidani, 2002).

In the second phase, referred to as the *proliferative phase*, resolution of ARDS begins. Resolution occurs in part through the actions of the type II cuboidal cells (alveolar epithelium), which produce surfactant, promote fluid transport, and proliferate of injured type I cells. If resolution does not occur, progression to persistent respiratory failure, hypoxemia, decreased lung compliance, and fibrosis will occur (Ware & Matthay, 2000).

The third and final phase is the *chronic/fibrotic phase*. Histologic evidence is present as early as 5 to 7 days from the onset of ARDS. During this phase, mesenchymal cells are formed in the alveolar space with an accumulation of collagen and fibronectin. The fibrosing process is thought to be promoted by IL-1 (Ware & Matthay, 2000).

EPIDEMIOLOGY AND ETIOLOGY

In the past, ARDS was known by several other names, such as shock lung and adult respiratory distress syndrome. In 1994, the American–European Consensus Conference (AECC) recommended both a name change and a standard definition for the disorder as it affected children and adults—hence the name *acute respiratory distress syndrome*. This group also differentiated ARDS from the less severe form of pulmonary disease known as acute lung injury (ALI) (Bernard et al., 1994).

Defining criteria for ARDS are as follows:

- Acute onset
- PaO_2/FiO_2 ratio of less than 200 mmHg
- Evidence of bilateral infiltrates on chest radiograph
- Pulmonary artery wedge press less than 18 mmHg or no clinical evidence of left atrial hypertension

Defining criteria for ALI are as follows:

- Acute onset
- PaO_2/FiO_2 ratio of 200 to 300 mmHg
- Evidence of bilateral infiltrates on chest radiograph
- Pulmonary artery wedge press less than 18 mmHg or no clinical evidence of left atrial hypertension

The AECC definitions have two limitations. First, variability in their sensitivity and specificity arises when they are applied to clinical practice. Second, the interpretation of chest radiographs is subjective (Avecillas et al., 2006).

Estimates of incidence rates for ARDS have varied dramatically, from 1.5 to 78 per 100,000 population. This variation is thought to be due to population size, geographic area, study length, and defining criteria (Avecillas et al., 2006). More recently, the pediatric incidence rate was reported at 12.8 per 100,000 population (Zimmerman et al., 2009).

The causes of ARDS can be grouped into two categories—direct versus indirect lung injury (Frutos-Vivar et al., 2004).

Direct lung injury

- Pneumonia
- Aspiration of gastric contents
- Submersion injury (near-drowning)
- Inhalation injury

Indirect lung injury

- Sepsis
- Thermal injury (burns)
- Pancreatitis
- Trauma
- Transfusion (blood products)

PRESENTATION

ARDS presents with rapid onset of dyspnea leading to hypoxia and respiratory failure. Pulse oximetry values are less than 90% without supplemental oxygen (Ware, 2006; Ware & Matthay, 2000). Auscultation reveals crackles with significant work of breathing. Additional findings are based on the underlying cause and the patient's comorbidities.

DIFFERENTIAL DIAGNOSIS

The differential diagnoses for ARDS include pulmonary hemorrhage, surfactant deficiency, pulmonary malignancies, and congestive heart failure. Pediatric patients with pulmonary hemorrhage will have an acute drop in hemoglobin, which is not routinely seen in ARDS. Those with surfactant deficiency may present with an ARDS-like syndrome of acute-onset respiratory distress and bilateral infiltrates on CXR. Patients with pulmonary malignancies may have lung nodules, and those with congestive heart failure may present with cardiomegaly and hepatomegaly (Morrison & Bidani, 2002).

PLAN OF CARE

The PaO_2/FiO_2 ratio is calculated from arterial blood gas values. A PaO_2/FiO_2 ratio of 200 or less is suggestive of ARDS. Early in the course of the syndrome, respiratory alkalosis may be noted; in later stages, respiratory acidosis is observed. Additional diagnostic studies for ARDS include a basic metabolic panel, complete blood count (CBC) with differential, CXR, echocardiography, and bronchoalveolar lavage (BAL) (Ware & Matthay, 2000). The basic metabolic panel will provide data on kidney function and hydration status. The CBC and differential will provide data on whether a bacterial or viral process is present, as well as allow for ongoing monitoring for anemia.

The hemoglobin level is essential in optimizing arterial oxygen content. The calculation for arterial oxygen content is as follows:

$$(\text{Hgb concentration in gm/dL}) \times 1.36 \text{ mL O}_2/\text{gm}$$
$$\times SaO_2 + 0.003 \times PaO_2$$

Normal values are 18 to 20 mL O_2/dL blood. Normal values will ensure adequate delivery of oxygen to the tissues.

CXR will reveal bilateral infiltrates (Figure 35-3). Echocardiography assists with evaluation of cardiac function.

A pulmonary artery (PA) catheter may be placed for defining criteria. PA wedge pressure of less than 18 mmHg supports the diagnosis of ARDS (Behrman et al., 2004). Fluid obtained from the BAL will be diagnostic for neutrophil activation (Ware & Matthay, 2000).

Management of ARDS focuses on lung-protective strategies. Supplemental oxygen is provided to pediatric patients who show signs of respiratory distress. Noninvasive ventilation (NIV) is considered if little or no improvement occurs with supplemental oxygen support. Examples of NIV include continuous positive airway pressure (CPAP) and bi-level positive airway pressure (BiPAP). NIV may reduce intubation rates and clinical improvement if used early (Yanez et al., 2008).

Intubation and mechanical ventilation are required in those patients who are unable to protect their airway or have impending respiratory or cardiac failure. Three protective lung strategies are employed with patients on mechanical ventilation:

- Lower tidal volumes (7–8 mL/kg) with conventional ventilation (ARDS Network, 2000; Hanson & Flori, 2006)
- Permissive hypercapnea (Laffey et al., 2004; Rogovik & Goldman, 2008; Rotta & Steinhorn, 2006)
- High-frequency oscillatory ventilation (HFOV)

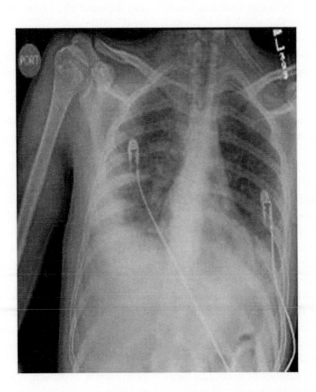

FIGURE 35-3

Bilateral infiltrates in Acute Respiratory Distress Syndrome (ARDS).

Source: Courtesy of Mark Riccioni.

HFOV reduces the risk of ventilator-associated lung injury through the use of smaller tidal volumes, higher mean airway pressures, and limited peak inspiratory pressures (Mehta & Arnold, 2004). Although as many as one-third of pediatric patients requiring mechanical ventilation transition to HFOV, its effectiveness has yet to be determined in reducing long-term morbidity or mortality (Anton et al., 2003; Mehta & Arnold).

Adjunct strategies for management of ARDS include nitric oxide (NO), prone positioning, and administration of exogenous surfactant. Inhaled nitric oxide promotes capillary and pulmonary dilation, thereby improving V/Q matching. It has shown to acutely improve oxygenation in pediatric patients, but has not been proven to reduce the number of ventilator days or the hospital length of stay after 72 hours of administration (Dobyns et al., 1999). The starting dose for nitric oxide is typically 20 parts per million (ppm) but can go as high as 80 ppm. Side effects include hypotension and methemoglobinemia, with the severity of methemoglobinemia increasing with the dose of nitric oxide. Maximum methemoglobin levels are usually reached 8 hours after initiation of inhalation, although levels have been reported to peak as late as 40 hours following initiation of nitric oxide therapy. Following discontinuation or reduction of nitric oxide, the methemoglobin levels usually return to baseline over a period of hours (INO Therapeutics, n.d.).

The prone position is another strategy that has been suggested to improve oxygenation. The physiologic premise underlying prone positioning is to improve V/Q matching by converting the more dependent segments of the lung (lung bases: Zone 3), which are areas where pulmonary perfusion is greater than ventilation, to Zone 2, which includes areas of the lung where ventilation and perfusion are more equal. Note that this strategy has not been proven to reduce the length of hospital stay or the number of ventilator days (Curley et al., 2000).

The third adjunct strategy is supplemental surfactant. Surfactant may prevent atelectasis and improve oxygenation by reducing alveolar surface tension. Patients with ARDS have impaired alveolar epithelium. Dosing is usually 50 to 100 mg/kg, administered one or two times, and within 12 to 48 hours of the initiation of mechanical ventilation (Duffett et al., 2007). Results vary by age for this therapy. In a meta-analysis by Davidson et al. (2006), the use of surfactant in adult patients with ARDS was shown to potentially improve oxygenation, but did not reduce mortality. This analysis lacked sufficient data to evaluate whether surfactant reduced the number of days on mechanical ventilation. In a second meta-analysis of studies in pediatrics by Duffett et al. (2007), mortality, number of ventilator-free days, and days on mechanical ventilation were all significantly reduced with the use of supplemental surfactant.

Conservative fluid management for patients with ARDS is yet another therapeutic modality. Murphy et al. (2009) reported that adult patients with acute lung injury secondary to septic shock who received both adequate initial fluid resuscitation and conservative late fluid management had better outcomes and lower hospital mortality compared to patients who received only conservative late fluid management. Adequate initial fluid resuscitation was defined as an initial fluid bolus of 20 mL/kg and achievement of central venous pressure of 8 mmHg or greater within 6 hours of starting vasopressor therapy. Conservative late fluid management was defined as an even-to-negative fluid balance on at least 2 consecutive days during the first 7 days after the onset of septic shock.

In 2006, the National Heart, Lung, and Blood Institute's Acute Respiratory Distress Syndrome (ARDS) Clinical Trials Network reported conservative (compared to liberal) fluid management in adults improved the oxygen index, lung injury score, and the number of ventilator free days. The patients in the conservative strategy group had a 7-day mean cumulative fluid balance of 136 ± 491 compared to $6,992 \pm 502$ in the liberal strategy group.

Randolph et al. (2005) also analyzed whether cumulative intake versus output affected the duration of weaning from the ventilator, except using a sample of pediatric patients rather than adults. These researchers reported that patients who had a cumulative intake versus output in the highest quartile took longer to wean from the ventilator compared to patients in the other three quartiles. This finding supports the utility of conservative therapy (Randolph et al., 2005).

The nutritional needs of pediatric patients with ARDS remain unknown. In adult patients, researchers have found that providing a diet enriched with eicosapentaenoic acid (EPA), gamma-linolenic acid (LPA), and antioxidants can improve oxygenation and reduce both days on mechanical ventilation and days in the hospital (Singer et al., 2006). EPA and LPA supplementation can also reduce the amount of alveolar inflammatory mediators (Pacht et al., 2003). Enteral nutrition is recommended over parenteral nutrition, as the former approach is associated with fewer infectious complications (Heyland et al., 2003).

As yet, no studies involving pediatric patients have been published that support the use of corticosteroids in ARDS (Randolph, 2009). Use of these medications in adults with ARDS has produced varied results. In one meta-analysis, low-dose corticosteroids were noted to improve mortality and morbidity outcomes without increasing side effects (Peter et al., 2008); however, in another study that was published one year later, they increased the incidence of ARDS in critically ill adults (Tang et al., 2009).

Management of ARDS should incorporate an interprofessional approach. Specialists in critical care medicine, pulmonology, infectious diseases, pharmacy, nutrition, rehabilitation, social work, and child life are just some of the team members who may participate in care. The family is sentinel in care, and family education requires detailed explanation as to the therapies provided because ARDS is a very complex critical illness and often difficult for families to understand. Coordination of communication may be very helpful to promote the parent's understanding and to determine the appropriate goals of care.

DISPOSITION AND DISCHARGE PLANNING

The mortality rate for ARDS remains high—between 20% and 75%—despite the availability of complex therapies to treat this condition. Pediatric patients who have had a prolonged intubation, high PaO_2/FiO_2 ratio, multiple organ dysfunction, immunocompromise, or preexisting condition have the highest rates of death from this condition (Erikson et al., 2007; Flori et al., 2005). Pediatric patients with ARDS may have extended periods of intensive care and may require long-term rehabilitation for chronic lung disease and generalized muscle weakness. In one adult study, neuromyopathy was found in 34% of survivors of prolonged ARDS (Hough et al., 2009).

AIR LEAK SYNDROMES

Elizabeth Elliott

PATHOPHYSIOLOGY

Air leak syndromes include any pathology in which air enters a normally closed space within the thorax. It may develop for two reasons: (1) an acute change in intrapleural pressure, which results in air entry into this space, or (2) a rupture of the alveoli or pericardial sac, which allows air to track into these spaces. A *pneumothorax* is a collection of air in the intrapleural space caused by a rupture in the alveoli or trauma that creates a communication between the outside of the body and the pleural cavity (Figure 35-4). Air leaks may be iatrogenic or spontaneous.

Intrapleural pressure is usually negative compared to atmospheric pressure—a difference that prevents the lungs from collapsing or the chest wall from springing back (Costanzo, 2002). When the negative pressure is disrupted by either a puncture from outside the body or a rupture at the alveolar level, the pressure in the intrapleural space becomes equal to atmospheric pressure, allowing the movement of air into the intrapleural space, and causing collapse of the lung and expansion of the chest wall. A *pneumomediastinum* is a collection of air in the mediastinum due to a communication from the pleural cavity. A *pneumopericardium* is a collection of air in the pericardial space due to a communication from the pleural cavity. In the case of both pneumopericardium and pneumomediastinum, the disruption occurs in either the alveolar or pericardial

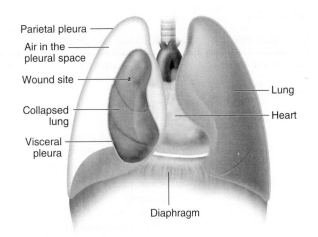

FIGURE 35-4

Pneumothorax.

Source: Pollak, A. (Ed). *Critical Care Transport*. Sudbury, MA: Jones and Bartlett Publishers.

tissue, allowing air to track from the lung tissue along the bronchial tree to the hilum of the lungs, leading to the mediastinum or pericardial sac.

EPIDEMIOLOGY AND ETIOLOGY

Air leak syndromes are uncommon in the general pediatric population. They may be caused by trauma (an open, communicating, or "sucking" chest wound), result from acute changes in lung compliance, rupture of blebs in patients with chronic lung disease (secondary), or may be spontaneous (primary) in certain populations with no underlying lung disease (Taussig & Landau, 1999). Pneumomediastinum and pneumopericardium may result from trauma, rupture of alveoli or bronchi, infection, or fistula formation. The inciting event causing a rupture may be coughing or vomiting, and/or any high inspiratory pressure in a mechanically ventilated patient (Caceres et al., 2008).

PRESENTATION

Given that air leak syndromes are caused by air entry into different parts of the thoracic cavity, the presentation of these syndromes depends on the location of the air. Table 35-3 describes the common presentations and physical examination findings of air leak syndromes. It is also important to note that findings of tracheal deviation to the contralateral side, hypotension, tachycardia, and cyanosis indicate a tension pneumothorax—a *medical emergency* that requires immediate intervention (Robinson et al., 2009).

TABLE 35-3

Common Presentations of Air Leak Syndromes			
Type of Air Leak	**Signs/Symptoms**	**Physical Exam Findings**	**Clinical Findings**
Pneumothorax	• Chest pain • Dyspnea • Tachycardia • Acute change in lung compliance in the mechanically ventilated patient	• Ipsilateral hyperresonance to percussion • Ipsilateral decreased air entry • Ipsilateral decreased vocal fremitus	• Decreased oxygen saturations • Increased peak inspiratory pressures or changes in expired tidal volumes on mechanical ventilator
Pneumomediastinum	• Chest pain • Dyspnea • Neck pain • May be asymptomatic	• Hamman's sign • Subcutaneous emphysema	• Most often none
Pneumopericardium	• Tachycardia • Tachypnea	• Mill wheel murmur • Muffled heart sounds	• Hypotension

DIFFERENTIAL DIAGNOSIS

Due to the potential morbidity and mortality associated with air leak syndromes, it is important to differentiate them from other common conditions that mimic their symptom patterns. In the case of pneumothorax, it can be difficult to differentiate this condition from a large, thin-walled bullae or a skin fold on chest radiograph (Chen et al., 2004). Herniation of the stomach through the diaphragm into the chest wall may also appear similar to a pneumothorax. With pneumomediastinum, it is important to evaluate for the presence of a thoracic or mediastinal mass. Pericarditis can mimic a pneumopericardium on electrocardiograph, but can be differentiated by echocardiograph.

PLAN OF CARE

All air leak syndrome diagnoses are confirmed with diagnostic studies, either radiographic, electrocardiograph, or echocardiograph. Pneumothorax is diagnosed by CXR and is demonstrated by a thin line displaced from the chest wall (Figure 35-5). On one side of the line, there is air-filled lung with appropriate lung vascular markings; on the other side of the line, there is only air without vascular markings (Chen et al., 2004). A tension pneumothorax will also show a shift of the mediastinum to the contralateral side and flattening or inversion of the ipsilateral hemidiaphragm. An arterial blood gas will show impairment of oxygenation and a larger A-a gradient because nonventilated lung is being perfused (Pagana & Pagana, 2002).

Pneumomediastinum is also diagnosed by chest radiograph; on this study, it will appear as radiolucent streaks in the mediastinum (Figure 35-6). Diagnostic studies for pneumopericardium include a CXR, which will show air in the pericardial sac and a "halo" sign (radiolucent band of air partially or completely surrounding the heart) (Figure 35-7). Pneumopericardium may also be demonstrated on echocardiograph, where it is evidenced by global ST-segment elevations and low voltage.

With all air leak syndromes, the goals of therapy are similar: Remove pathologic air from the thoracic cavity and restore normal pressure gradients; relieve tension or pressure in the thoracic cavity; improve oxygenation and ventilation; treat and prevent further cardiovascular collapse; and take measures to prevent recurrence. Global therapies include delivering enough oxygen to ensure adequate oxygenation of the body's tissues and monitoring those patients with risk factors for recurrence closely.

While some pneumothoraces may be treated with close observation, many in the critical care setting will require thoracostomy tube placement to remove air from the intrapleural space (see Chapter 42). In patients with chronic lung disease and recurrent pneumothorax, surgical intervention with thoracoscopy or chemical pleurodesis may be warranted (Robinson et al., 2009). Emergency evacuation of the air-filled space should never wait for radiographic confirmation or thoracostomy tube placement in patients with cardiopulmonary compromise. Needle thoracentesis should be performed to relieve intrathoracic pressure and improve venous return.

Pneumomediastinum rarely causes hemodynamic compromise and is usually a benign condition. Its treatment generally includes observation and treatment of underlying medical conditions (Bullaro & Bartoletti, 2007).

Pneumopericardium is usually self-limited and does not require treatment. The exception is in a patient who experiences circulatory collapse (tension pneumopericardium), in which case the pneumopericardium is drained with either needle aspiration or surgical evacuation. An open thoracotomy may be necessary to close the communicating fistula and point of air entry (Haan & Scalea, 2006).

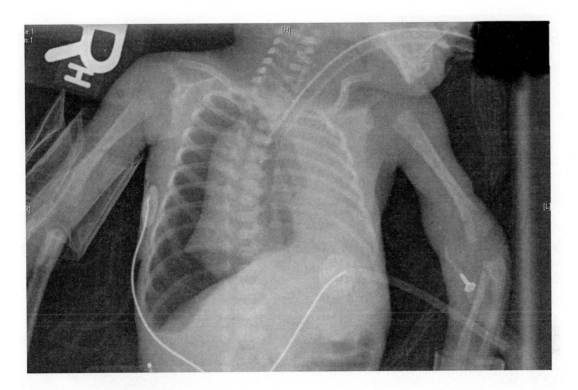

FIGURE 35-5

PA Chest Radiograph of Pneumothorax.

Source: Courtesy of Elizabeth Elliott.

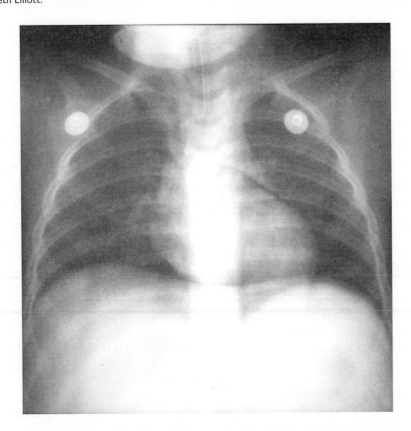

FIGURE 35-6

PA Chest Radiograph of Pneumomediastinum.

Source: Courtesy of Elizabeth Elliott.

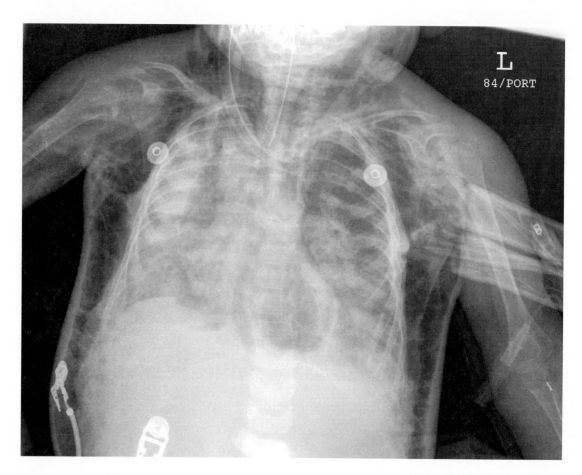

FIGURE 35-7

PA Chest Radiograph of Pneumopericardium with Notable Subcutaneous Air.

Source: Courtesy of Elizabeth Elliott.

Consultation with the critical care team, general surgeon, trauma surgeon, cardiovascular surgeon, or anesthesiologist may be necessary if immediate and emergent airway and ventilation support is required. Pneumopericardium may require a cardiothoracic approach for relief. In patients with chronic lung disease, the pulmonology service may have an established relationship with the patient and family. Patients, depending on their severity of illness or sequelae, may require long-term care and the support of nutrition, rehabilitation team, social work, and child life specialists.

Patient and family education depends on the severity of presentation. Support by social and spiritual advisors is often necessary in the acute life-threatening admission. However, once the patient is stable, education as to the patient's plan of care should be undertaken.

DISPOSITION AND DISCHARGE PLANNING

Because the severity of air leak syndromes varies, not all patients will be quickly discharged from the hospital. Those with underlying disease processes may require prolonged hospital stays. Those being discharged home from the hospital require caregivers who have been taught pain management and vigilance for returning air leaks. Caregivers should also be comfortable with the local wound care of the thoracostomy tube site, bathing, suture care, and recognition of a wound infection. These considerations are especially important in children with chronic lung diseases that predispose them to recurrence. Patients need close follow-up with their primary care provider (PCP). Depending on the cause and treatment of the air leak, they may also require follow-up with a pulmonologist, cardiologist, or surgeon.

APPARENT LIFE-THREATENING EVENTS

Jennifer Chaikin

An apparent life-threatening event (ALTE) is "an episode that is frightening to the observer and that is characterized by some sort of combination of apnea (central or occasionally obstructive), color change (usually cyanotic or pallid, but occasionally erythematous or plethoric), marked change in muscle tone (usually marked limpness), choking, or gagging" (National Institutes of Health, 1987, p. 293).

EPIDEMIOLOGY AND ETIOLOGY

ALTE is the chief complaint in 0.05% to 6% of pediatric emergency visits in the United States. Peak incidence is around 10 weeks of age (Hall & Zalman, 2005; Kiehl-Kohlendorfer et al., 2005). Etiologies are varied; in approximately 50% of patients, the cause remains unknown despite diagnostic study (Figure 35-8) (Davies & Gupta, 2002).

ALTE was previously known as "near-miss sudden infant death syndrome" or "aborted cot death." It remains unclear if the occurrence of an ALTE is a predictor of potential sudden infant death syndrome (SIDS) (Claudius & Keens, 2007). In addition, no studies have shown that SIDS and ALTEs are the result of the same etiology. Fewer than 10% of SIDS victims have a history of a prior ALTE (Brooks, 1996). Most documented cases of ALTE are mild and carry no significant increased risk of death (Smith & Talbot, 2008). However, in those infants with a more severe ALTE, the risk of SIDS increases to as high as 10%, especially when there is ALTE recurrence, the event occurred during sleep, or the infant required CPR (Brooks, 1996).

In 1988, the National Institute of Child Health and Human Development's (NICHD) SIDS cooperative epidemiological study concluded that newborn apnea, or apnea of prematurity, is not a risk factor for SIDS. Studies reviewing monitored infants who died suddenly at home revealed the occurrence of prolonged bradycardia before any prolonged central apnea. The incidence of SIDS has significantly decreased since the practice of placing infants on their backs during sleep was recommended, while the incidence of ALTE has not.

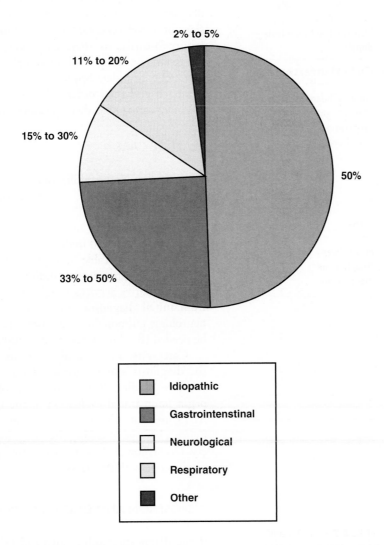

FIGURE 35-8

Etiology of ALTE.

Note: Apparent life-threatening event (ALTE).

DIFFERENTIAL DIAGNOSIS

The differential diagnoses for the symptoms of ALTE are summarized in Table 35-4.

PRESENTATION

Many times the infant reported to have had an ALTE appears normal at the time of evaluation (Kahn, 2004).

TABLE 35-4

Differential Diagnosis of Apparent Life-Threatening Events	
Gastrointestinal	**Metabolic**
Gastroesophageal reflux	Inborn errors of metabolism
Volvulus	Endocrine, electrolyte abnormalities
Intussusception	Urinary tract infection
Swallowing abnormalities	Sepsis
Neurologic	**Child Maltreatment**
Seizure disorder	Abusive head trauma
Febrile seizure	Munchausen-by-proxy syndrome
Intracranial hemorrhage	Smothering
Brain malformations	
Hydrocephalus	
Central nervous system infection	
Malignancy	
Respiratory	**Other**
Infection (respiratory syncytial virus, pertussis, croup, pneumonia)	Food allergy
	Anaphylaxis
	Medication
Obstructive sleep apnea syndrome	
Breath-holding spells	
Laryngotracheomalacia	
Foreign body aspiration	
Congenital central hypoventilation syndrome	
Vascular	
Arrhythmia (prolonged QT, Wolff-Parkinson-White syndrome)	
Congenital heart lesion	
Myocarditis	
Cardiomyopathy	

Source: Used with permission from Hall, K., & Zalman, B. (2005). Evaluation and management of apparent life-threatening events in children. *American Family Physician, 71,* 2301–2308. Copyright © American Academy of Family Physicians. All rights reserved.

The presumption is always that the child did have an apparent life-threatening event regardless of his or her present state. Caregivers should never be made to feel that the event did not happen or that they over-reacted. By definition, the event leads to feelings that their child will die if there is no intervention.

Because the etiological options are many, a complete history is warranted to determine the cause. Table 35-5 provides specific questions useful for completing the history. Of the many questions on this list, a history of prematurity is highly significant. Prematurity, coupled with male gender, respiratory syncytial virus (RSV) infection, or a history of general anesthesia increases the risk for ALTE (Hall & Zalman, 2005). Approximately 1% of all ALTE episodes are related to child maltreatment; consequently, the HCP should consider this possibility in the interview and be observant for cues (Bonkowsky & Tieder, 2009).

Physical examination must be comprehensive and detailed. Pay close attention to any delay in progression of developmental stages, dysmorphic features, or failure-to-thrive, as these conditions may indicate child maltreatment, congenital abnormality, malabsorption, or metabolic disorder. Specific attention to the symptoms exhibited and their order is important. For example, did the bradycardia precede the cyanosis or follow it?

PLAN OF CARE

Resuscitation and stabilization should be provided, as needed, following the ABCs: airway, breathing, and circulation.

Diagnostic studies are based on the patient's symptoms during the ALTE and findings from the history and physical examination. Table 35-6 provides suggestions to consider when selecting initial studies.

Consultative services should be contacted as findings from initial diagnostic study warrant. Specialty care by neurology, pulmonology, or gastroenterology services may be needed (Bonkowsky & Tieder, 2009).

Caregivers are typically anxious and fearful about the diagnosis and prognosis of their infant's condition (Ball & Bindler, 2008). Education of the family should begin upon initial evaluation of the infant. Infants with ALTE are routinely admitted to a monitored unit and experience a barrage of testing that often increases family anxiety. Discussion of the extensive testing plan often helps the family cope with the stress.

DISPOSITION AND DISCHARGE PLANNING

If the diagnostic studies fail to identify a cause and the infant has a history of prematurity, continuation of presenting symptoms, sequelae following the event, or anxious

TABLE 35-5

Historical Inquiry Following Apparent Life-Threatening Events

Caregiver Description of Event

- Was the child awake or asleep?
- What was the position and location of the child (prone versus supine, crib versus bed)?
- Was there any activity at the time of the event (feeding, coughing, gagging)?
- How was the child breathing?
- What was the child's color?
- How was the child's movement and tone?
- How long was the event?

Interventions by the Caregiver

- None? Mouth-to-mouth breathing?
- Gentle stimulation? Vigorous stimulation?
- Blowing air in the face?
- CPR?

History of the Present Illness

- None? Contact with someone who has been ill?
- Any symptoms of illness?
- Fever?
- Poor feeding? Weight loss?
- Rash?
- Irritability, lethargy?
- Currently taking any medications? Immunizations up-to-date?

Previous Medical History

- Prenatal history: birth history?
- Prematurity? Small for gestational age?
- Feeding history: any gagging, coughing episodes?
- Meeting developmental milestones?
- Previous hospitalizations? Prior ALTE?
- Accidents?

Family History

- Congenital, neurological conditions?
- Previous infant/child deaths? Sudden infant death syndrome?
- Smoking in the home?

TABLE 35-6

Diagnostic Studies for Infants with Apparent Life-Threatening Events

Suggested Minimal Evaluation	Expanded Evaluation
Chest radiograph (infection, cardiomegaly)	Arterial blood gas (hypoxia, acidosis)
Complete blood count and differential (infection, anemia)	Blood culture (infection)
Electrocardiograph (arrhythmia, long QT syndrome)	Brain imaging (trauma, malignancy)
Serum electrolytes (metabolic abnormalities, dehydration)	Electroencephalograph (seizures, brain abnormalities)
Serum bicarbonate and lactate (acidosis, hypoxia, toxins, enzyme defects)	Liver function tests (hepatic dysfunction)
Urinalysis (infection)	Lumbar puncture (cerebrospinal culture, infection)
	Nasal swab for respiratory syncytial virus (infection)
	Radioisotope milk scan/ esophageal pH probe (gastroesophageal reflux)
	Echocardiograph (cardiac abnormalities)

Source: Used with permission from Hall, K., & Zalman, B. (2005). Evaluation and management of apparent life-threatening events in children. *American Family Physician, 71,* 2301–2308. Copyright © American Academy of Family Physicians. All rights reserved.

parents, home cardiorespiratory monitoring with recording capability may be considered. Most home monitors can record changes in heart rate and rhythm, transcutaneous carbon dioxide levels, oxygen saturation, and respirations.

Caregiver teaching should include the reason for the monitor and its function. Families should be instructed in proper lead placement, alarm volumes, skin evaluation, and troubleshooting. Emergency agencies should be prenotified of the infant who is at home with a monitor and at risk for ALTE. Emergency numbers should be posted in the home, and a plan for power failure should be established.

Caregivers should be instructed to eliminate all tobacco smoke exposure in the home, as even second-hand smoke may precipitate bronchospasm in young infants. Training in cardiopulmonary resuscitation (CPR) is also required for caregivers.

The duration of home monitoring depends on the frequency and severity of ALTE. If during the time that the home monitor is used the infant does not have any ALTE or significant event recorded, the monitoring may be discontinued. If a significant event is recorded during the home monitoring, the monitoring should continue and further evaluation for the underlying cause should be pursued.

If during an admission the infant has no recurrence of symptoms, no history of prematurity, and no caregiver anxiety, discharge without home monitoring may be considered. Family teaching remains important, however. Smoking and second-hand smoke should be eliminated and CPR training recommended. Follow-up takes place with the PCP or consulting specialty physician. Infants who have had an ALTE usually have no obvious sequelae (Rudolph et al., 2003).

In patients for whom an ALTE etiology is identified, the prognosis is determined by the type and extent of the diagnosis and subsequent treatment. The mortality rate for infants with ALTE is reported at 0 to 4% (Brooks, 1996). Most deaths are associated with serious neurological disorders (especially those with apnea risk) and infants with idiopathic, recurrent ALTE (Hall & Zalman, 2005).

An ALTE may not be preventable. Some experts suggest that prevention of infection and proper nutrition may decrease the likelihood of an infant having an ALTE. Most prevention guidelines are specific to SIDS rather than to ALTE, however. The most significant and consistent advice is to ensure that babies sleep on their backs. If back sleeping causes fussiness for the infant, caregivers can purchase special sleeping wedges that help maintain the side-lying position for the baby during sleep. Infants should not sleep with bumper pads, pillows, large heavy blankets, or stuffed animals, as these items can cause obstruction of the mouth and nasal airways and hindering ventilation. The following preventive measures should be included in caregiver education:

- Ensure that the infant resides in smoke-free surroundings.
- Provide a firm mattress for sleeping.
- Breastfeed the infant, if possible.
- If "blue spells" are noticed in the infant, seek prompt medical advice.
- Avoid overheating; do not over-swaddle the infant.
- Never permit bed linens to cover the infant's face.

ASTHMA

Mary Astor Gomez and Ann Marie Felauer

PATHOPHYSIOLOGY

Asthma is a disease of chronic inflammation that affects primarily the large airways of the lungs. This complex cascade of symptoms results in inflammation, hyperresponsiveness, and airway obstruction, usually following a trigger or stimulus (Murugan et al., 2009).

In the *initial phase*, mast cells, eosinophils, T lymphocytes, macrophages, neutrophils, and epithelial cells combine to start the inflammatory process (National Heart, Lung, and Blood Institute [NHLBI], 2007a). Histamine release from the mast cells results in mucosal edema, excess mucus production, mucus plugs, and bronchospasm.

The *late phase* takes longer to appear and may last 24 hours or longer before subsiding. The inflammatory response combined with eosinophils and platelets results in infiltration and congestion with further airway obstruction and varying degrees of respiratory insufficiency that may progress to respiratory failure (Linzer, 2007). Following an exacerbation, alterations in the epithelium, submucosa, smooth muscles, and bronchial blood vessels lead to airway remodeling (Wilson & Hii, 2006). These structural

changes occur in both proximal and distal airways and can lead to overall changes in an individual's functional residual capacity (FRC) (Sung et al., 2007).

EPIDEMIOLOGY AND ETIOLOGY

The National Interview Health Survey Data (CDC, 2006b) reports that 6.7 million children younger than 18 years of age have asthma; 20% of these patients are younger than 4 years of age. Three million children younger than 15 years of age have had an asthma episode in the past year. Among children who had asthma at 5 years of age, 30% had symptoms of wheezing by 1 year of age and approximately 70% had symptoms by 3 years of years. Males are more likely to have been diagnosed with asthma than females. There is a notable racial discrepancy, in that one-half of all children with asthma in the United States are either Hispanic or African American. Children in lower-socioeconomic households are more commonly afflicted. Asthma accounts for 14 million missed school days each year. Mortality from asthma is highest among African American children (Akinbami, 2006; Amado & Portnoy, 2006; Bloom & Cohen, 2007; Centers for Disease Control and Prevention [CDC], 2006b; Mannino et al., 2002).

Asthma may be caused by a complex interaction of environmental factors such as airborne allergens, viral respiratory infections, and genetics (Bradding & Green, 2010; Hayden & Le Souef, 2007). Studies have found that children with a family history of asthma are at greater risk for developing asthma if they have a lower respiratory tract infection caused by a rhinovirus accompanied by wheezing than if they have lower respiratory tract infection caused by respiratory syncytial virus (RSV) with wheezing (Bartlett et al., 2009). It is still unclear if the viral illness causes asthma in some young infants and children or just exacerbates or reveals an underlying disorder (Bartlett et al.).

Table 35-7 lists common triggers of first-time events or exacerbations of asthma. Response to medications can differ depending on the allergen or trigger. Studies have shown that exposure to cigarette smoke can inhibit the response to steroids while at the same time enhancing the leukotriene modifiers that are commonly used as controller medications (Farber, 2010). Obesity has been linked to increased severity of asthma exacerbations. The predisposition to asthma associated with obesity can be related to overall reduced vital capacity, obstructive sleep apnea, and increased levels of inflammatory cytokines—all of which are more common in obese children when compared to their non-obese counterparts (Farber; Forno & Celedon, 2009; Schramm & Carroll, 2009).

It is important to note distinctions of asthma severity and control. Asthma severity is defined as the intrinsic intensity of the disease to quality of life. According to the National Asthma Education and Prevention Program's (NAEPP) *Expert Panel Report III: Guidelines for the*

TABLE 35-7

Common Triggers for Asthma Events or Exacerbations

- Viral infections and lower respiratory infections
- Cold air or weather fluctuations
- Environmental irritants such as exposure to smoke, chemicals, vapors, and dust
- Allergens including household dust mites, animal dander, molds, cockroaches, pollen, and mold
- Exercise
- Emotions and stress
- Medications such as aspirin or beta blockers
- Foods
- Family history of atopy
- Medical conditions such as gastroesophageal reflux disease (GERD), sinusitis, or rhinitis

Source: NHLBI, 2007b.

Diagnosis and Management of Asthma (EPR III; NHLBI, 2007a), *asthma severity* is classified into four categories based on symptoms:

- Intermittent
- Mild persistent
- Moderate persistent
- Severe persistent

In contrast, *asthma control* is the degree to which manifestations of asthma are minimized and influenced by factors such as the following: if appropriate medication has been prescribed, if there has been adherence to a therapeutic regimen, and to what extent recommended measures have been avoided for clinically applicable aeroallergens or triggers (Lang, 2008).

The EPR III also identifies two domains for asthma: impairment and risk. These domains evaluate factors necessary to address the comprehensive impact of asthma. *Impairment* focuses on current status, assessing symptom frequency and intensity, functional limitations, lung function, and patient compliance. *Risk* evaluation focuses on the future goal of preventing exacerbations, minimizing emergency department (ED) visits and hospitalizations, reducing the tendency for progressive decline in lung function, and providing minimal drug treatment to maintain control and minimize adverse effects from medications (Lang, 2008; NHLBI, 2007a).

Identification and avoidance of triggers and risks is an important, continuous process, as each exacerbation causes additional airway remodeling. Fatal and near-fatal asthma events may involve either a sudden, acute exacerbation or a slow, gradual deterioration over several days or more of poorly controlled asthma. The gradual asthma event accounts for 80% to 85% of all asthma fatalities. Near-fatal asthma is associated with hypoxemia, hypercapnia, lactic acidosis, and dynamic hyperinflation; the slow response to treatment differentiates this form from other severe asthma events. Many

fatal and near-fatal events may be prevented if trigger exposure is reduced. Table 35-8 summarizes the factors related to an increased risk of death from an asthma event or exacerbation (Marshall et al., 2009; Restrepo & Peters, 2008).

PRESENTATION

The common presenting symptoms of the patient with an acute asthma event are wheezing; cough, often at night or after exercise; chest and/or abdominal pain or tightness; shortness of breath; and fatigue with exertion.

The history begins with elicitation of prior exacerbations, including precipitating and aggravating factors; an accounting of medications used daily, including last use of systemic steroids; and any previous hospitalizations, including intubations or intensive care unit admissions for asthma. For some patients, the visit may represent an exacerbation of previously diagnosed disease; for others, it will be their first event. The pediatric patient's history should also include information related to the time of onset of symptoms, medications administered since that time, and indications of whether they provided any symptomatic relief. Accompanying symptoms such as fevers, malaise, or signs of viral illness may help determine if a specific trigger

TABLE 35-8

Risk Factors for Death from Asthma

Asthma History

- Previous severe exacerbation (e.g., intubation or intensive care unit admission for asthma)
- Two or more hospitalizations for asthma in the past year
- Three or more emergency department visits for asthma in the past year
- Hospitalization or emergency department visit for asthma in the past month
- Using more than two canisters of SABA per month
- Difficulty perceiving asthma symptoms or severity of exacerbations
- Other risk factors: lack of written asthma action plan, sensitivity to *Alternaria*

Social History

- Low socioeconomic status or inner-city residence
- Illicit drug use
- Major psychosocial problems

Comorbitities

- Cardiovascular disease
- Other chronic lung disease
- Chronic psychiatric disease

Note: Short-acting beta$_2$ agonist (SABA).
Source: NHLBI, 2007b.

initiated the event. In addition, knowledge of the patient's past medical history such as prematurity, preexisting lung disorders or disease, gastroesophageal reflux, or developmental delays is important to obtain from caregivers, as these factors can contribute to an asthma exacerbation or confound the diagnosis of asthma (Bartlett et al., 2009; Bloomberg, 2010; Camargo et al., 2009; Martinez, 2009; NHLBI, 2007a).

A family history may identify the development of an immunoglobulin E (IgE)–mediated response to allergens such as asthma, allergy, or atopic dermatitis in immediate family members. A family history of atopy is a strong predictor for developing asthma. A complete social history will evaluate the pediatric patient's exposure to triggers and risk factors such as cigarette smoke, low socioeconomic status or inner-city residence, illicit drug use, or other psychosocial problems that may impair compliance to good asthma control (NHLBI, 2007a).

The physical examination should include an evaluation of work of breathing—specifically, the presence of cough, dyspnea, degree and location of accessory muscle use, presence of nasal flaring, respiratory rate, and the child's ability to communicate. Defining criteria used by the World Health Organization (www.who.int) for tachypnea are as follows:

- More than 50 breaths per minute (bpm) for infants 2 to 12 months of age
- More than 40 bpm for those 1 to 5 years of age
- More than 30 bpm for children 5 years of age or older

In a severe event, patients may be able to speak in only short phrases, one- to three-word sentences, or not at all. In addition, the patient's position of comfort or degree of agitation should be noted; sitting upright and being unable to lie down is indicative of severe distress (Restrepo & Peters, 2008). Indications of respiratory failure include agitation with dyspnea or decreasing level of consciousness, inability to speak, central cyanosis, diaphoresis, and inability to lie down (Mannix & Bachur, 2007). The presence of air movement and wheezing, both inspiratory and expiratory, should be evaluated through auscultation. Absence of breath sounds or wheezing is disturbing, as it indicates that air flow is so diminished that it cannot even cause wheezing. Absence of wheezing that is accompanied by evidence of confusion or drowsiness should be considered a medical emergency and quick intervention should occur as respiratory arrest may be imminent (Mannix & Bachur; NHLBI, 2007a; Restrepo & Peters, 2008).

Pulsus paradoxus may be observed during moderate to severe asthma events due to changes in intrathoracic pressures with inspiration. Blood pressures changes of more than 12 mmHg are considered significant, and blood pressure changes of more than 25 mmHg are indicative of severe impairment to cardiac output. Patients with severe

distress may be hypovolemic due to reduced oral intake and increased insensible losses; this condition may result in even greater impairment of cardiac output secondary to decreased venous return (Marshall et al., 2009; NHLBI, 2007a; Restrepo & Peters, 2008).

The clinical examination should also include assessment for potential air leak complications such as pneumothorax, pneumomediastinum, and pneumopericardium. While rare, they are potentially life-threatening conditions for the patient experiencing a moderate or severe event. The use of positive pressure or mechanical ventilation increases the risk for these complications (Marshall et al., 2009).

DIFFERENTIAL DIAGNOSIS

Many disorders of the upper or lower airways may mimic asthma (Camargo et al., 2009) (Table 35-9). Disorders of

TABLE 35-9

Differential Diagnosis for Asthma

Infants and Children

Upper Airway Disease

- Allergic rhinitis and sinusitis

Obstructions Involving Large Airways

- Foreign body in trachea or bronchus
- Vocal cord dysfunction
- Vascular rings or laryngeal webs
- Laryngotracheolmalacia, tracheal stenosis, or bronchostenosis
- Enlarged lymph nodes or tumor

Obstructions Involving Small Airways

- Viral bronchiolitis or obliterative bronchiolitis
- Cystic fibrosis
- Bronchopulmonary dysplasia
- Heart disease

Other Causes

- Recurrent cough not due to asthma
- Aspiration from swallowing mechanism dysfunction or gastroesophageal reflux

Adults

- COPD (e.g., chronic bronchitis or emphysema)
- Congestive heart failure
- Pulmonary embolism
- Mechanical obstruction of the airways (benign or malignant tumors)
- Pulmonary infiltration with eosinophilia
- Cough secondary to drugs (e.g., angiotensin-converting enzyme inhibitors)
- Vocal cord dysfunction

Source: NHLBI, 2007b.

the upper airway may be accompanied by stridor and usually do not respond to short-acting beta$_2$ agonists (SABA) therapy. If at least come degree of malacia is present, symptoms may worsen with the administration of SABAs. Disorders of the lower airway are often associated with asthma-like symptoms such as wheezing, but treatment of the underlying problem is necessary to control the wheezing, airway obstruction, and inflammation that may be present. It is important to evaluate whether the onset of symptoms was abrupt versus insidious (i.e., occurring gradually over time). Evaluation of the wheezing—unilateral versus bilateral, inspiratory versus expiratory, and if accompanied by stridor or hypoxia—can help sort through various other disorders that mimic asthma (NHLBI, 2007a).

Serial spirometric measurements of lung function—either FEV$_1$ (forced expiratory volume in 1 second) or peak expiratory flow (PEF)—may be useful to assess severity of the event or exacerbation and differentiate the diagnosis of asthma. Note that such studies are *not* recommended in a severe or life-threatening asthma event (NHLBI, 2007a).

PLAN OF CARE

Treatment of the pediatric patient with an acute asthma event is based on an initial assessment of the severity of the exacerbation or event, with the goal being to establish control of the asthma and create a plan for follow-up in the future. Criteria for categorizing the severity of asthma events are described in the Table 35-10. *Status asthmaticus* is the global term used when initial therapies do not result in symptom improvement. According to the EPR III guidelines, a patient with a *mild* event can be discharged after observation for 60 minutes following the last SABA treatment if the patient remains symptom free, maintains oxygenation in room air, and is able to eat and drink without difficulty, and the FEV$_1$ or PEF is 70% or more of the predicted value (NHLBI, 2007a). The patient should be admitted to an inpatient unit if he or she continues to have symptoms, has an oxygen requirement, requires SABA therapy more often than every 2 to 3 hours, or has a prior history of asthma-related intensive care admission.

TABLE 35-10

Criteria for Asthma Event or Exacerbation Severity in the Urgent or Emergency Care Setting			
	Mild	**Moderate**	**Severe**	**Subset: Respiratory Arrest Imminent**
Symptoms				
Breathlessness	While walking Can lie down	While at rest (infant—softer, shorter cry; difficulty feeding) Prefers sitting	While at rest (infant—stops feeding) Sits upright	
Talks in	Sentences	Phrases	Words	
Alertness	May be agitated	Usually agitated	Usually agitated	Drowsy or confused
Signs				
Respiratory rate	Increased above normal	Increased above normal	Increased above normal	
Use of accessory muscles; suprasternal retractions	Usually not	Common	Usually	Paradoxical thoracoabdominal movement
Wheeze	Moderate; often only end-expiratory	Loud; throughout exhalation	Usually loud; throughout inhalation and exhalation	Absence of wheeze
Pulse/minute	< 100	100–120	> 120	Bradycardia
Pulsus paradoxus	Absent; pressure < 10 mmHg	May be present; pressure of 10–25 mmHg	Often present; pressure of 20–40 mmHg in a child or > 25 mmHg in an adult	Absence suggests respiratory muscle fatigue
Functional Assessment				
PEF, percent predicted or personal best	≥ 70%	Approximately 40%–69% or response lasts < 2 hours	< 40 %	< 25%, (PEF testing may not be needed in severe attacks)

(Continued)

TABLE 35-10

Criteria for Asthma Event or Exacerbation Severity in the Urgent or Emergency Care Setting *(Continued)*			
	Mild	**Moderate**	**Severe**	**Subset: Respiratory Arrest Imminent**
Functional Assessment				
PaO_2 (on air)	Normal	$\geq$ 60 mmHg	< 60 mmHg: possible cyanosis	
PCO_2	< 42 mmHg	< 42 mmHg	$\geq$ 42 mmHg: possible repiratory fatigue	Hypercapnia/ hypoventilation develops more readily in young children than in adults/ adolescents
SaO_2 percent (on air)	> 95%	90%–95%	< 90%	
Clinical Course				
	• Usually cared for at home • Prompt relief with inhaled SABA • Possible short course of oral systemic corticosteroid	• Usually requires office or emergency department visit • Relief from frequent inhaled SABA • Oral systemic corticosteroid; some symptoms last for 1–2 days after treatment is begun	• Usually requires emergency department visit and likely hospitalization • Partial relief from fequent inhaled SABA • Oral systemic corticosteroids; some symptoms last for > 3 days after treatment is begun • Adjunctive therapies are helpful	• Requires emergency department/ hospitalization; possible intensive care unit • Minimal or no relief from frequent SABA • Intravenous corticosteroids • Adjunctive therapies are helpful

Note: Peak expiratory flow (PEF).
Source: NHLBI, 2007b. www.nhlbi.nih.gov/guidelines/asthma/

Admission to the intensive care unit (ICU) is warranted if the initial presentation is classified as a *severe* exacerbation, a sudden respiratory deterioration occurs, and the child requires close airway monitoring and support. Figure 35-9 reviews the acute management of asthma events. Medication therapy is reviewed later in this section.

The need for diagnostic studies, such as a CXR, vary and are based on the need to differentiate the etiology of the distress, identify comorbidities (e.g., pneumonia), or identify air leak syndromes (NHLBI, 2007a). CXR findings, in the absence of fever or symptoms suggestive of an air leak disorder, are often not clinically significant, and such studies are rarely needed to direct care. They are most valuable for excluding other conditions (Mannix & Bachur, 2007; Matthews et al., 2009; Sung et al., 2007). The CXR findings common to asthma may include hyperinflation with flattening of the diaphragm, subsegmental atelectasis, peribronchial thickening, and a narrowed cardiac silhouette depending on the severity of the exacerbation. If a severe exacerbation is difficult to control, or if a patient has a near-fatal event, then CT scans may be valuable to provide in-depth analysis of both the large and small airways (Sung et al.).

Laboratory studies are not routinely obtained for patients with asthma, but instead are selected based on the severity of the event, comorbidities, and medications administered. Obtaining a blood gas analysis in a patient who experiences a mild or mild-moderate event may not be useful, as mild carbon dioxide retention is expected given the decreased ventilation and airway narrowing; however, serial measurement of blood gas values for those patients who experience moderate-severe or severe events may prove useful for evaluating the need for additional therapy. Patients with this degree of impairment commonly experience some anxiety and agitation given the respiratory acidosis and hypoxia; however, if they progress to lethargy and confusion accompanied by carbon dioxide retention and metabolic acidosis, respiratory arrest may be imminent (Mannix & Bachur, 2007; Marshall et al., 2009; Meert et al., 2007; Restrepo & Peters, 2008). Lactic acid levels may also be elevated when there is significant use of accessory muscles, intrathoracic pressure, and hypoperfusion of skeletal muscles. Consequently, some HCPs find monitoring this value, in addition to blood gasses, useful for patients experiencing a severe event (Meert et al.).

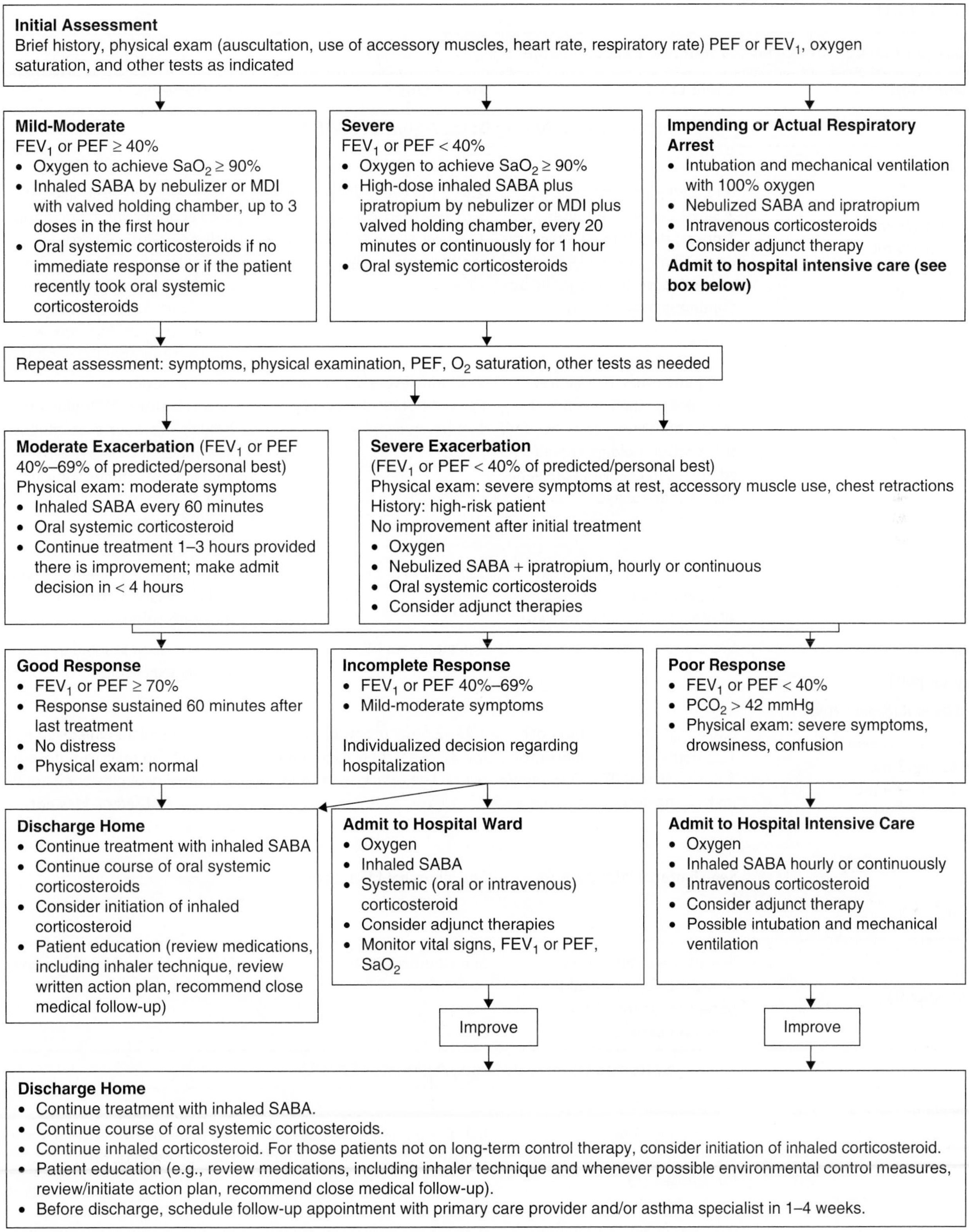

Initial Assessment

Brief history, physical exam (auscultation, use of accessory muscles, heart rate, respiratory rate) PEF or FEV_1, oxygen saturation, and other tests as indicated

Mild-Moderate

FEV_1 or PEF $\geq$ 40%
- Oxygen to achieve $SaO_2 \geq$ 90%
- Inhaled SABA by nebulizer or MDI with valved holding chamber, up to 3 doses in the first hour
- Oral systemic corticosteroids if no immediate response or if the patient recently took oral systemic corticosteroids

Severe

FEV_1 or PEF < 40%
- Oxygen to achieve $SaO_2 \geq$ 90%
- High-dose inhaled SABA plus ipratropium by nebulizer or MDI plus valved holding chamber, every 20 minutes or continuously for 1 hour
- Oral systemic corticosteroids

Impending or Actual Respiratory Arrest
- Intubation and mechanical ventilation with 100% oxygen
- Nebulized SABA and ipratropium
- Intravenous corticosteroids
- Consider adjunct therapy
Admit to hospital intensive care (see box below)

Repeat assessment: symptoms, physical examination, PEF, O_2 saturation, other tests as needed

Moderate Exacerbation (FEV_1 or PEF 40%–69% of predicted/personal best)
Physical exam: moderate symptoms
- Inhaled SABA every 60 minutes
- Oral systemic corticosteroid
- Continue treatment 1–3 hours provided there is improvement; make admit decision in < 4 hours

Severe Exacerbation
(FEV_1 or PEF < 40% of predicted/personal best)
Physical exam: severe symptoms at rest, accessory muscle use, chest retractions
History: high-risk patient
No improvement after initial treatment
- Oxygen
- Nebulized SABA + ipratropium, hourly or continuous
- Oral systemic corticosteroids
- Consider adjunct therapies

Good Response
- FEV_1 or PEF $\geq$ 70%
- Response sustained 60 minutes after last treatment
- No distress
- Physical exam: normal

Incomplete Response
- FEV_1 or PEF 40%–69%
- Mild-moderate symptoms

Individualized decision regarding hospitalization

Poor Response
- FEV_1 or PEF < 40%
- PCO_2 > 42 mmHg
- Physical exam: severe symptoms, drowsiness, confusion

Discharge Home
- Continue treatment with inhaled SABA
- Continue course of oral systemic corticosteroids
- Consider initiation of inhaled corticosteroid
- Patient education (review medications, including inhaler technique, review written action plan, recommend close medical follow-up)

Admit to Hospital Ward
- Oxygen
- Inhaled SABA
- Systemic (oral or intravenous) corticosteroid
- Consider adjunct therapies
- Monitor vital signs, FEV_1 or PEF, SaO_2

Admit to Hospital Intensive Care
- Oxygen
- Inhaled SABA hourly or continuously
- Intravenous corticosteroid
- Consider adjunct therapy
- Possible intubation and mechanical ventilation

Improve

Improve

Discharge Home
- Continue treatment with inhaled SABA.
- Continue course of oral systemic corticosteroids.
- Continue inhaled corticosteroid. For those patients not on long-term control therapy, consider initiation of inhaled corticosteroid.
- Patient education (e.g., review medications, including inhaler technique and whenever possible environmental control measures, review/initiate action plan, recommend close medical follow-up).
- Before discharge, schedule follow-up appointment with primary care provider and/or asthma specialist in 1–4 weeks.

FIGURE 35-9

Management of Asthma Events or Exacerbations: Emergency Department and Hospital-Based Care.

Note: Peak expiratory flow (PEF), forced expiratory volume (FEV), short-acting beta$_2$ agonists (SABA), metered dose inhaler (MDI), short-acting beta$_2$ agonists (SABA).
Source: NHLBI, 2007b. www.nhlbi.nih.gov/guidelines/asthma/

TABLE 35-11

Dosage of Drugs for Asthma Events or Exacerbations

Medication	Child Dose	Adult Dose	Comments
Inhaled Short-Acting Beta$_2$ Agonists (SABA)			
Albuterol Nebulizer solution • 0.63 mg/3 mL • 1.25 mg/3 mL • 2.5 mg/3 mL • 5 mg/3 mL	0.15 mg/kg (minimum dose, 2.5 mg) every 20 minutes for 3 doses, then 0.15–0.3 mg/kg up to 10 mg every 1–4 hours as needed, or 0.5 mg/kg/hr by continous nebulization	2.5–5 mg every 20 minutes for 3 doses, then 2.5–10 mg every 1–4 hours as needed or 10–15 mg/hr continously	Only selective beta$_2$ agonists are recommended. For optimal delivery, dilute aerosol to minimum of 3 mL at gas flow of 6–8 L/min. Use large-volume nebulizers for continous administration. May mix with ipratropium nebulizer solution.
MDI (90 µg/puff)	4–8 puffs every 20 minutes for 3 doses, then 1–4 hours inhalation maneuver as needed, using valved holding chamber; add mask in children younger than 4 years of age	4–8 puffs every 20 minutes up to 4 hours; then every 1–4 hours as needed	In mild-moderate exacerbations, MDI plus valved holding chamber is as effective as nebulized therapy, with appropriate administration technique and coaching by trained personnel.
Bitolterol Nebulizer solution (2 mg/mL)	See albuterol dose; thought to be one-half as potent as albuterol on a milligram basis	See albuterol dose	Has not been studied in severe asthma exacerbations. Do not mix with other drugs.
MDI (370 µg/puff)	See albuterol MDI dose	See albuterol MDI dose	Has not been studied in severe asthma exacerbations.
Levalbuterol (R-albuterol) Nebulizer solution • 0.63 mg/3 mL • 1.25 mg/0.5 mL • 1.25 mg/3 mL	0.075 mg/kg (minumum dose 1.25 mg) every 20 minutes for 3 doses, then 0.075–0.15 mg/kg up to 5 mg every 1–4 hours as needed	1.25–2.5 mg every 20 minute for 3 doses, then 1.25–5 mg every 1–4 hours as needed.	Levalbuterol administered in one-half the milligram dose of albuterol provides comparable efficacy and safety. Has not been evaluated by continous nebulization.
MDI (45 µg/puff)	See albuterol MDI dose	See albuterol MDI dose	
Pirbuterol MDI (200 µg/puff)	See albtuerol MDI dose; thought to be one-half as potent as albuterol on a milligram basis	See albuterol MDI dose	Has not been studied in severe asthma exacerbations.
Systemic (Injected) Beta$_2$ Agonists (SABA)			
Epinephrine 1:1,000 (1 mg/mL)	0.01 mg/kg up to 0.3–0.5 mg every 20 minutes for 3 doses SQ	0.3–0.5 mg every 20 doses for 3 doses SQ	No proven advantage of systemic therapy over aerosol.
Terbutaline (1 m.g/mL)	0.01 mg/kg every 20 minutes for 3 doses, then 2–6 hours as needed SQ	0.25 mg every 20 minutes for 3 doses SQ	No proven advantage of systemic therapy over aerosol.

(Continued)

TABLE 35-11

Dosage of Drugs for Asthma Events or Exacerbations *(Continued)*			
Medication	**Child Dose**	**Adult Dose**	**Comments**
Anticholinergics			
Ipratropium bromide Nebulizer solution (0.25 mg/mL)	0.25–0.5 mg every 20 minutes for 3 doses, then as needed	0.5 mg every 20 minutes for 3 doses, then as needed	May mix in same nebulizer with albuterol. Should not be used as a first-line therapy, but rather should be added to SABA therapy for severe exacerbations. The addition of ipratropium has not been shown to provide further benefit once the patient is hospitalized.
MDI (18 µg/puff)	4–8 puffs every 20 minutes as needed, up to 3 hours	8 puffs every 20 minutes as needed, up to 3 hours	Should use with a valved holding chamber and face mask for children younger than age 4 years. Studies have examined use of an ipratropium bromide MDI for as long as 3 hours.
Ipratropium with albuterol Nebulizer solution (Each 3-mL vial contains 0.5 mg ipratropium bromide and 2.5 mg albuterol)	1.5 mL every 20 minutes for 3 doses, then as needed	3 mL every 20 minutes for 3 doses, then as needed	May be used for as long as 3 hours in the initial management of severe exacerbations. The addition of ipratropium to albuterol has not been shown to provide further benefit once the patient is hospitalized.
MDI (Each puff contains 18 µg ipratropium bromide and 90 µg of albuterol)	4–8 puffs every 20 minutes asneeded, up to 3 hours	8 puffs every 20 minutes as needed, up to 3 hours	Should use with a valved holding chamber and face mask for children younger than 4 years of age.
Systemic Corticosteroids			
Dosing/recommendations apply to all three corticosteroids.			
Prednisone *Methylprednisolone* *Prednisolone*	1–2 mg/kg in 2 divided doses (maximum 60 mg/day) until PEF is 70% of predicted or personal best	40–80 mg/day in 1–2 divided doses until PEF reaches 70% of predicted or personal best	For outpatient "burst," use 40–60 mg in one dose or two divided doses for total of 5–10 days in adults (children: 1–2 mg/kg/day, maximum 60 mg/day, for 3–10 days).

Notes:
- There is no known advantage of using higher doses of corticosteroids in severe asthma exacerbations, nor is there any advantage for intravenous administration over oral therapy provided gastrointestinal transit time or absorption is not impaired.
- The total course of systemic corticosteroids for an asthma exacerbation requiring an emergency department visit or hospitalization may last from 3 to 10 days. For corticosteroid courses of less than 1 week, there is no need to taper the dose. For slightly longer courses (e.g., up to 10 days), there probably is no need to taper the drug, especially if patients are concurrently taking inhaled corticosteroids.
- Inhaled corticosteroids can be started at any point in the treatment of an asthma exacerbation.

Note: Peak expiratory flow (PEF), metered-dose inhaler (MDI).
Source: NHLBI, 2007b. www.nhlbi.nih.gov/guidelines/asthma/

Magnesium levels should be monitored, if magnesium sulfate is administered, to avoid hypermagnesemia. Serum potassium levels should be considered for patients on high-dose albuterol, or continuous albuterol of any dose and non-potassium-sparing diuretics, as intracellular shifts of potassium with activation of the Na^+/K^+ pump may occur. If aminophylline or terbutaline is used as an adjunct therapy, it is vital to follow drug levels given the narrow therapeutic window and subsequent side effects of these medications.

Many therapies for acute asthma events or exacerbations are available, including oxygen, SABA, inhaled ipratropium, and systemic corticosteroids (Table 35-11). The most immediate intervention is to monitor oxygen saturations via pulse oximetry and provide supplemental oxygen via a nonrebreather mask or nasal cannula to achieve a SaO_2 of 90% or greater (NHLBI, 2007a). Most asthmatics are dehydrated on presentation due to poor fluid intake, vomiting (particularly post-tussive), and increased insensible losses from their respiratory tract; therefore, fluid volume or resuscitation may be indicated. The goal of fluid replacement is to establish euvolemia, as over-hydration may lead to pulmonary edema.

Medications

Short-acting beta$_2$ agonists. Short-acting beta$_2$ agonists administered via nebulizer or metered-dose inhaler (MDI) are first-line therapy for symptom relief and bronchodilation (Table 35-11). As many as three doses in the first hour may be administered to relax bronchial smooth muscle, decrease mast cell degranulation, decrease leakage into the airways, and improve mucus clearance (NHLBI, 2007a). For patients with continued symptoms, this medication can be delivered continuously via face mask (Table 35-12). If status improves, the child can be transitioned from continuous albuterol to dosing every 2 or more hours. Tremors, tachycardia, dizziness, or headaches are the most common adverse effects (NHLBI, 2007a; Taketomo et al., 2010).

Ipratropium bromide. Ipratropium bromide is an anticholinergic agent that facilitates smooth-muscle relaxation by inhibition of muscarinic cholinergic receptors. It is used as an inhaled adjunct therapy for its additive effects to SABAs for patients with moderate to severe obstruction (Table 35-11). It is also useful for treating bronchospasm associated with beta blockers. Ipratropium bromide is valuable in averting hospital admission, although its value in shortening length of stay and preventing further deterioration once hospitalized remains unclear (Marshall et al., 2009; Restrepo & Peters, 2008). Adverse effects include dry mouth, papillary dilation, and blurred vision, especially if the face mask delivery device is positioned to direct the inhalation toward the eyes (Linzer, 2007; NHLBI, 2007a; Taketomo et al., 2010).

Corticosteroids. Corticosteroids are used to reduce the inflammation associated with asthma and can be given

in oral, inhaled, or intravenous (IV) form, depending on the severity of the patient's condition. Beta agonists at higher doses can decrease gastrointestinal absorption and cause vomiting; therefore, the IV form is often preferred for its delivery reliability in those patients who are experiencing severe events (Marshall et al., 2009). The standard dose is 1 to 2 mg/kg divided twice daily (NHLBI, 2007a; Taketomo et al., 2010) (Table 35-11). The decision to transition the patient to oral steroids is made at the discretion of the HCP and depends on the patient's ability to tolerate oral intake. The overall length of treatment with steroids can range from 3 to 10 days (average $\approx$ 5 days) depending on the severity of the presentation or until PEF is 70% or more of the expected or personal best (Marshall et al.; NHLBI, 2007a; Restrepo & Peters, 2008; Taketomo et al.). Side effects vary based on dosing and length of therapy. Notably, patients should be monitored for hypertension, hypokalemia, changes in behavior, seizures, and Cushing's syndrome.

Epinephrine. Epinephrine works on alpha$_1$, beta$_1$, and beta$_2$ receptors, resulting in positive inotropy and chronotropy in addition to bronchodilation. The use of epinephrine should be considered cautiously given these additional effects in individuals with a history of cardiovascular disease or arrhythmias (Marshall et al., 2009). The EPR III guidelines recommend the dosing of epinephrine, 0.01 mg/kg, up to a maximum of 0.3 to 0.5 mg every 20 minutes for a total of three doses, subcutaneously, as a possible adjunct therapy (NHLBI, 2007a) (Table 35-11). Many HCPs, however, recommend epinephrine be given intramuscularly rather than subcutaneously, as there is significantly faster absorption by the IM route.

Magnesium. Intravenous magnesium sulfate, 25 to 75 mg/kg/dose, is an adjunct therapy that may provide further smooth-muscle relaxation for patients with severe or life-threatening asthma events. Studies have shown that this medication can improve bronchodilation and potentiate the effects of beta$_2$ agonists (Marshall et al., 2009; NHLBI, 2007a). The main side effect of magnesium sulfate is hypotension (Taketomo et al., 2010).

Terbutaline. There are no statistically significant data supporting the use of intravenous terbutaline for pediatric patients who are nonresponsive to continuous inhaled beta$_2$ agonists; nevertheless, terbutaline infusions are often used in patients with severe or life-threatening exacerbations of asthma (Bogie et al., 2007; Restrepo & Peters 2008). Terbutaline is a beta$_2$ agonist that is thought to provide smooth-muscle relaxation with less tachycardia than commonly noted with mixed alpha$_1$ beta$_{1-2}$ agents such as epinephrine. A loading dose of 2 to 10 μg/kg is usually administered, to be followed by a 0.08 to 0.4 μg/kg/min continuous infusion. Depending on the clinical response, the dosage may be titrated in increments of 0.1 to 0.2 μg/kg/min every 30 minutes. Maximum doses of

10 µg/kg/min have been used successfully (Taketomo et al., 2010). The EPR III guidelines recommend use of subcutaneous terbutaline, 0.01 mg/kg every 20 minutes for three doses, then every 2 to 6 hours as needed (NHLBI, 2007a) (Table 35-11). Side effects include cardiac dysrhythmias, tachycardia, and electrolyte abnormalities (e.g., potassium); therefore, close cardiac monitoring and monitoring of drug levels is warranted (Taketomo et al.).

Methylxanthines. Methylxanthines (aminophylline, theophylline) also relax the smooth muscles of the respiratory tract, which makes them attractive options for use in patients who are nonresponsive to SABAs (Restrepo & Peters, 2008). Current studies have not shown that methylxanthines have any benefit over inhaled SABAs; however, it has been suggested that for those patients who are refractory to continuous administration of albuterol, ipratropium, and magnesium, or in impending respiratory failure, methylxanthines may have some benefit (Marshall et al., 2009; Restrepo & Peters). Side effects include vomiting, tachycardia, agitation, and arrhythmias. In addition, the narrow therapeutic to toxic index of methylxanthines warrants close monitoring and evaluation of drug levels (NHLBI, 2007a; Restrepo & Peters). The EPR III guidelines make no recommendations for use of methylxanthines in asthma treatment.

Antimicrobials. There should be a low threshold to start antimicrobial therapy in patients with moderate to severe asthma events or exacerbations with evidence of pneumonia or a bacterial sinusitis as the trigger (NHLBI, 2007a). Macrolides, which are commonly used for atypical pneumonias in older children, have additional anti-inflammatory effects that may be helpful for the pediatric patient in status asthmaticus; however, studies have not provided any significant data to show any benefit from their empiric use (Marshall et al., 2009). For the infant with acute wheezing and fever, viral infection is the most likely cause; thus antibiotics are not recommended (NHLBI, 2007a).

Ventilation

Heliox. Heliox may be considered for patients who are mildly hypoxemic and demonstrate significant work of breathing due to airway obstruction. Heliox is administered as a gas in concentrations of helium/oxygen ranging from 60/40 to 80/20; the most common mix is 70/30. It is thought to decrease flow turbulence because its density is less than oxygen, resulting in a more laminar flow pattern that delivers nebulized medications to peripheral alveoli more effectively (Marshall et al.; Restrepo & Peters, 2008; Rivera et al., 2006). This mixture may also lower peak airway pressures in intubated patients (Linzer, 2007; Marshall et al.; NHLBI, 2007a). Restrepo and Peters (2008) reported that heliox may reverse airway obstruction in some individuals who do not respond to initial therapies, resulting in improved oxygenation, decreased work of breathing, and enhanced elimination of carbon dioxide.

Noninvasive ventilation. The pediatric patient who presents in respiratory failure may benefit from NIV via CPAP or BiPAP. The goal of NIV is to successfully ventilate the child until the severity of the event or exacerbation has subsided. Not all patients can tolerate the change to positive-pressure ventilation, so NIV should be used judiciously (Restrepo & Peters, 2008). Adult trials of NIV have shown that this treatment leads to improved lung function and gas exchange with a decreased length of stay; results also appear promising in children although more study in this population is needed (Linzer, 2007; Needleman et al., 2004; Nowak, 2009; Schramm & Carroll, 2009). The positive pressure helps to prevent airway collapse and augments tidal volumes, thereby providing support for already fatigued respiratory muscles (Marshall et al., 2009; Schramm & Carroll). An advantage of NIV over mechanical ventilation is that it allows for normal upper airway function and spontaneous cough necessary for airway clearance (Schramm & Carroll).

NIV requires a patient who will cooperate and has been fitted with the appropriate-size mask to ensure adequate delivery of pressure breaths. Sedation may need to be considered to ensure cooperation. In this circumstance, it is important to consider the risks and benefits of using sedatives for patients in respiratory failure prior to use (Schramm & Carroll, 2009).

Mechanical ventilation. Intubation and mechanical ventilation of the pediatric patient with status asthmaticus or near-fatal asthma should be considered only when the benefits versus risks trade-offs have been assessed and respiratory arrest is imminent. Indications for intubation of the patient with severe respiratory failure include hypoxia unresponsive to supplemental oxygen, persistent or increasing hypercapnia, worsening of mental status, and the absence of breath sounds or wheezing (NHLBI, 2007a; Restrepo & Peters, 2008). Other possible indications for mechanical ventilation include pH less than 7.25 or hemodynamic instability (Marshall et al., 2009).

Intubation should occur in a controlled environment. The oral route is recommended because it allows for placement of a larger endotracheal tube, which may help minimize airway resistance and facilitate clearance of secretions (Restrepo & Peters, 2008). Hypotension may occur with intubation due to the immediate reduction in intrathoracic pressure, improved venous return, and generalized hypovolemia; therefore, isotonic fluid boluses and vasopressor agents should be readily available (Marshall et al., 2009). Ketamine may be used prior to intubation as an anesthetic agent, as it carries a lower risk of bronchospasm and hypotension than other commonly used pre-intubation agents (Marshall et al.).

Ventilator management of the asthmatic patient is directed to maintaining adequate oxygenation, minimizing hyperinflation, and avoiding barotrauma; permissive hypercapnia is often necessary (Marshall et al., 2009; NHLBI, 2007a; Restrepo & Peters, 2008).

The mode of ventilation—that is, pressure versus volume—requires careful consideration and evaluation of the patient's minute ventilation, peak inspiratory pressures (PIP), and overall gas exchange, with the goal of minimizing airway pressures so as to avoid barotrauma (Marshall et al.; NHLBI, 2007a; Restrepo & Peters). In pressure ventilation, shifts in mucus plugging, airway obstruction, and the underlying hyperresponsiveness of asthma may contribute to significant variability in minute volumes over time (Marshall et al.). By comparison, volume ventilation may exacerbate already high airway pressures. While experts vary in their recommendations of which mode of ventilation should be used, there is consensus that lower levels of positive end-expiratory pressure (PEEP) are beneficial for asthmatic patients requiring mechanical ventilation; settings of 0 to 4 cm H_2O are common (Marshall et al.; Restrepo & Peters). The inspiratory time (I-time) should be adjusted to account for the prolonged expiratory phase that accompanies status asthmaticus, which may require setting the inspiratory:expiratory (I:E) ratio to 1:2–1:3 or greater (Marshall et al.; Restrepo & Peters).

Sedation may be required to provide comfort to the ventilated patient with asthma. Trials in which ketamine was used for continued sedation while patients were on mechanical ventilation showed no clinical benefits from this regimen (NHLBI, 2007a). In addition to sedation, neuromuscular blockade may be required to provide the ventilator support needed to optimize oxygenation and prevent elevated airway pressures. However, given the risks of profound muscle weakness from concurrent use of systemic steroids and neuromuscular blocking agents, use of these medications should be considered carefully (Marshall et al., 2009). When they are used, vecuronium, rocuronium, cisatricurium, or pancuronium should be considered because they do not induce bronchospasm (Restrepo & Peters, 2008).

Referral to an allergist, pulmonologist, or asthma specialist is recommended for any child with asthma serious enough to require hospital admission (NHLBI, 2007a). These specialists can formulate asthma-oriented plans specifying when to use steroids, SABAs, and other rescue medications. They can also explore trigger identification with the families and determine whether any underlying disorders might be contributing to the asthma.

Patient and family education initially is focused on stabilization and the therapies administered to the patient. New-onset asthma requiring admission to the hospital may be stressful for families who are being newly introduced to the disorder. Daily discussions regarding the plan and titration of therapy will strengthen their ability to support their child or adolescent with asthma. Patients who have frequent reoccurrence of symptoms and hospitalization require involvement by social work to evaluate the family's ability to care for the child.

DISPOSITION AND DISCHARGE PLANNING

Ongoing monitoring after discharge should stress the importance of a follow-up appointment with the PCP within 1 week after discharge. Depending on the severity of the event or exacerbation, weaning from steroids, further medication adjustments, or additional specialty referrals may be necessary. Educational goals for the family are to decrease the child's impairment and reduce the risk of exacerbation. Decreased impairment can occur if symptoms are reduced and pulmonary function improves. Reduced risk will result in fewer exacerbations, emergency department visits, and disease progression. Further evaluation may include CT scan of the chest to evaluate for changes in the proximal and peripheral airways induced by airway obstruction, air-trapping, dynamic hyperinflation, and increased FRC. The inflammation that occurs with even one acute event contributes to irreversible remodeling (Sung et al., 2007).

The patient caregiver should be given an individualized written asthma action plan identifying triggers, strategies for avoidance, recognition of early signs and symptoms, review of medications including inhaler technique, use of control and rescue medications, and pertinent follow-up appointments (NHLBI, 2007b). Asthma action plans (Figure 35-10) may be found at http://www.nhlbi.nih.gov/health/public/lung/asthma/asthma_actplan.pdf. A stepwise approach is employed to use medications most effectively (Camargo et al., 2009; GINA, 2009; NHLBI, 2007a).

BOTULISM AND GUILLAIN-BARRÉ SYNDROME

Vicki L. Craig

PATHOPHYSIOLOGY

Botulism and Guillain-Barré syndrome (GBS) are acute, acquired neuromuscular diseases that cause paralysis, affect pulmonary function, and can cause respiratory failure in the pediatric population. The shared mechanism by which respiratory failure occurs as a consequence of these disease entities involves disruption of the nervous system; however, the specific mechanisms of nervous system involvement are different. Botulism is an infectious disease that affects the neuromuscular junction. GBS is an autoimmune disease that affects the peripheral nervous system.

Botulism

The clinical manifestations of botulism are caused by spore-forming Gram-positive bacilli, *Clostridium botulinum*.

Asthma Action Plan

For:_____   Doctor:_____   Date:_____

Doctor's Phone Number:_____Hospital/Emergency Department Phone Number_____

GREEN ZONE

Doing Well

- No cough, wheeze, chest tightness or shortness of breath during the day or night
- Can do usual activities

And, if a peak flow meter is used,

Peak flow: more than _____
(80 percent or more of my best peak flow)

My best peak flow is: _____.

Take these long-term control medicines each day (include an anti-inflammatory).

Medicine	How much to take	When to take it
_____	_____	_____
_____	_____	_____
_____	_____	_____
_____	_____	_____
_____	_____	_____

Before exercise ☐ _____   ☐ 2 or ☐ 4 puffs _____   5 to 60 minutes before exercise

YELLOW ZONE

Asthma is Getting Worse

- Cough, wheeze, chest tightness, or shortness of breath, or
- Waking at night due to asthma, or
- Can do some, but not all, usual activities

-OR-

Peak flow: _____ to _____
(50 to 79 percent of my best peak flow)

First Add: quick-relief medicine - and keep taking your **GREEN ZONE** medicine.

_____   ☐ 2 or ☐ 4 puffs, every 20 minutes for up to 1 hour
(short-acting beta$_2$-agonist)   ☐ nebulizer, once

Second If your symptoms (and peak flow, if used) return to **GREEN ZONE** after 1 hour of above treatment:

☐ Continue monitoring to be sure you stay in the green zone.

-OR-

If your symptoms (and peak flow, if used) do not return to **GREEN ZONE** after 1 hour of above treatment:

☐ Take: _____ ☐ 2 or ☐ 4 puffs or ☐ Nebulizer
(short-acting beta$_2$-agonist)

☐ Add: _____ mg per day for _____ (3-10) days
(oral steroid)

☐ Call the doctor ☐ before ☐ within _____ hours after taking the oral steroid

RED ZONE

Medical Alert!

- Very short of breath, or
- Quick-relief medicines have not helped, or
- Cannot do usual activities, or
- Symptoms are same or get worse after 24 hours in Yellow Zone

-OR-

Peak flow: less than _____
(50 percent of my best peak flow)

My best peak flow is: _____.

Take this medicine:

☐ _____ ☐ 4 or ☐ 6 puffs, or ☐ Nebulizer
(short-acting beta$_2$-agonist)

☐ _____ mg
(oral steroid)

Then call your doctor NOW. Go to the hospital or call an ambulance if:
- You are still in the red zone after 15 minutes AND
- You have not reached your doctor.

Danger Signs

- **Trouble walking and talking due to shortness of breath**
- **Lips or fingernails are blue**

- Take _____ ☐ 4 or ☐ 6 puffs of your quick-relief medicine AND
- Go to the hospital or call for an ambulance _____ NOW!
  (phone)

FIGURE 35-10

Asthma Action Plan.

Source: National Heart, Lung, Blood Institute. http://www.nhlbi.nih.gov/health/public/lung/asthma/asthma_actplan.pdf

These anaerobic organisms are found commonly in soil and food. Spores or toxin enter the body through open wounds or the gastrointestinal tract. There, the organisms produce neurotoxins that are absorbed into the bloodstream and block the release of acetylcholine from nerve endings, causing paralysis.

Guillain-barré syndrome

GBS can develop after a mild infectious illness, such as common viral respiratory infections or gastroenteritis. An immune response to the infection causes production of antibodies directed against myelin or Schwann cells along peripheral nerves. Demyelination of motor nerves occurs, resulting in paralysis. Motor nerves are most affected in GBS, but sensory and autonomic nerves may be affected as well.

EPIDEMIOLOGY AND ETIOLOGY

Botulism

Three main forms of botulism occur in humans: food-borne, wound, and infant. There is also concern for use of botulinum toxin as a potential biological weapon for terrorists (Arnon et al., 2001). The total number of botulism cases occurring in the United States each year is approximately 110, 70% of which are the infant form (CDC, 2006a). Only infant botulism is described further in this section. Readers interested in food-borne or wound botulism are encouraged to access the CDC's website (www.cdc.gov) for further information.

Infant botulism is a rare disease that affects males and females equally. Ninety-five percent of infections occur before the age of 6 months (Arnon, 2004). In older children and adults, the normal digestive tract flora compete with and prevent *C. botulinum* from colonizing the intestine, averting disease development in these age groups (Sobel, 2005). Unpasteurized honey is a known food reservoir for *C. botulinum* spores and has been definitively linked with infant botulism. Other potential sources of botulinum spores include soil and vacuum cleaner dust (Arnon et al., 1979). In many patients, however, no specific source of *C. botulinum* spores is identified.

Spores may be ingested, inhaled, or ingested. The spores germinate in the intestines. Bacteria then multiply, colonizing the intestine and producing toxin. Toxin is absorbed into the bloodstream, leading to the clinical manifestations of the disease.

Guillain-barré syndrome

GBS is also a rare entity, affecting approximately 1 to 2 persons per 100,000 population worldwide, and is slightly more common in males than females (van Doorn et al., 2008). This disease can occur at any age; however, unlike botulism, GBS is extremely rare in pediatric patients younger than 1 year of age (Evans & Vedanarayanan, 1997).

Typically, an existing history of respiratory or gastrointestinal infection precedes the onset of weakness and other symptoms. Infectious agents that have been associated with development of GBS include *Campylobacter jejuni, Mycoplasma pneumoniae, Haemophilus influenzae,* cytomegalovirus, and Epstein-Barr virus. GBS has also been reported after vaccination, surgery, and other stressful events (van Doorn et al., 2008). It is unclear why some individuals develop an autoimmune response after exposure to infectious agents or other triggers. In GBS, antibodies are produced that attack myelin and peripheral nerves. Recent evidence suggests that antiganglioside antibodies are produced in response to certain triggers and are important in the pathogenesis of GBS (van Doorn et al.).

PRESENTATION

Both infant botulism and GBS present with weakness as a main feature of the illness, which may progress to respiratory failure. If the diagnosis of botulism or GBS is suspected, close observation and monitoring of pediatric patients in a pediatric intensive care unit (PICU) or other closely monitored setting is warranted until a definitive diagnosis and disease course are determined.

Botulism

Although the clinical severity and presentation of infant botulism vary, the typical patient presents with a history that occurs over a few days. Caregivers report constipation, lethargy, poor feeding, and increasing weakness. On physical examination, generalized hypotonia and symmetrical cranial nerve palsies are present. Infants appear to have an "expressionless face," weak cry, ptosis, ophthalmoplegia, sluggish papillary response to light, and poor head control. Gag, suck, and swallow reflexes are diminished or absent. Deep tendon reflexes may be present, but usually will become diminished or absent as the disease progresses. The progression of weakness is descending. Cranial nerve palsies are always present and are part of the definitive diagnosis (Arnon, 2004).

Guillain-barré syndrome

The symptoms of GBS typically present in previously healthy patients, often 4 to 6 weeks following a prior infection. Symptoms begin as progressive and symmetrical weakness in the lower extremities, with ascending paralysis being a cardinal characteristic of this disease. Pain, numbness, and tingling of the extremities are also frequent presenting complaints. Fever is not typically present. In pediatric patients, the combination of weakness, pain, and sensory loss may present as a gait disturbance (Evans & Vedanarayanan, 1997). On physical examination, deep tendon reflexes are absent or diminished. Sensory and vibratory sense may also be diminished. Respiratory muscles and cranial nerves may be affected, causing respiratory insufficiency. Facial weakness, drooling, and ophthalmoplegia (Miller-Fisher syndrome) may be noted as well. Symptoms progress quickly over hours to days, with maximum weakness occurring within 2 to 4 weeks after onset of symptoms (van Doorn et al., 2008).

DIFFERENTIAL DIAGNOSIS

The differential diagnoses for both infant botulism and GBS are vast. A thorough history, physical examination, and appropriate supportive diagnostic study usually leads the HCP to the correct diagnosis without an extensive evaluation.

When considering either infant botulism or GBS as a diagnosis, presenting signs and symptoms that are not typical of these conditions should signal the HCP to consider other diagnoses. In general, infant botulism is considered under the category of evaluation of a "floppy infant." Patients are frequently first admitted to the hospital with diagnoses such as possible sepsis, viral syndrome, dehydration, and failure-to-thrive. Any infant younger than 6 months of age presenting with an acute or subacute onset of hypotonia associated with constipation, listlessness, poor feeding, weak cry, and decreased gag reflex should be suspected of having infant botulism (Francisco & Arnon, 2007). Specifically, other diagnoses that have been originally misdiagnosed as infant botulism and should be considered in the differential diagnosis are spinal muscular atrophy type I (Wernig-Hoffman disease); metabolic disorders; GBS—especially the Miller-Fisher variant in which cranial nerve palsies are presenting signs; and paraneoplastic syndromes (Franciso & Arnon). Differential diagnoses for GBS include bilateral strokes, acute cerebellar ataxia, transverse myelitis, spinal cord tumors, enterovirus, poliomyelitis, toxic neuropathies, tick paralysis, porphyria, botulism, myasthenia gravis, and myopathies (Evans & Vedanarayanan, 1997).

PLAN OF CARE

Botulism

The diagnosis of infant botulism is made by identification of botulinum toxin and *C. botulinum* in the feces of the affected infant. Stool samples may have to be obtained by enema.

Pediatric patients with botulism require supportive care. Notably, cardiopulmonary monitoring throughout the disease course may prevent potentially fatal secondary complications of this disorder and positively affect long-term patient outcomes. The HCP must be alert to the possible need for endotracheal intubation to protect and maintain the airway, and the need for mechanical ventilation to support breathing. Patients require continuous monitoring of respiratory and cardiovascular parameters until it is determined that weakness and paralysis are no longer progressing. Continuous monitoring of vital signs, arterial blood gases, and other noninvasive indicators of oxygenation and ventilation should be documented and followed.

Nutrition is very important, and enteral feeding by nasogastric or nasojejunal tube should be planned. Human milk, if available, or infant formula may be used to feed an infant. Parenteral nutrition poses an increased risk of infection and is not recommended.

The only specific treatment for infant botulism is human botulism immune globulin (BIG-IV), which can be obtained only through the *California Department of Health Infant Botulism Treatment and Prevention Program (IBTPP)*. This therapy is administered as a single dose by intravenous infusion. Information and consultation is available 24 hours a day for suspected cases of infant botulism by telephone at *510-231-7600*. Information on diagnosis and treatment can also be obtained on the IBTPP website: http://www.infantbotulism.org. BIG-IV has been shown in a randomized, double-blind, placebo-controlled trial to significantly decrease the severity of illness and shorten the hospital length of stay of infants with botulism who are treated within 3 days of hospital admission (Arnon et al., 2006).

Consultation with the following specialties are indicated in botulism: critical care, pulmonology, neurology, and infectious diseases. Additional interprofessional care team members may include nutrition, child life, rehabilitative services, social workers, and spiritual support.

Caregiver education includes information about the diagnostic evaluation and results, along with the therapeutic plan of care. Educating the patient and family about the progression of the disease allows them to prepare for interventions. Acute life-threatening presentations require additional support and education as to the immediate and expected therapeutic plan.

Guillain-barré syndrome

The diagnosis of GBS is usually made based on the history and clinical examination findings consistent with GBS. Cerebrospinal fluid (CSF) studies will show elevated protein, normal glucose, and normal cell count. If there are more than 50 white blood cells/mm^3 present in the CSF, other diagnoses should be considered. Lumbar puncture may need to be repeated at a later date if GBS is the leading diagnosis, as the CSF protein may be normal early in the course of the disease. Other tests that may be helpful in supporting the diagnosis of GBS are nerve conduction studies and MRI of the lumbosacral spine using gadolinium contrast.

Approximately 15% of children with GBS will develop respiratory failure and require mechanical ventilation during the disease course (Sladky, 2004). Autonomic dysfunction is the major cause of mortality, and cardiac dysrrhythmias and cardiac arrest may occur. In patients who can cooperate, pulmonary functions such as negative inspiratory force and forced vital capacity can be measured.

In general, antibiotics should be avoided except as specific treatment for complications such as pneumonia and urinary tract infections. The current literature does not support the use of corticosteroids in GBS therapy (Hughes et al., 2006b). Specific treatments that have been shown to shorten the recovery time from GBS and are equally effective are plasma exchange and administration of intravenous immunoglobulin (IVIG) (Hughes et al., 2006a). As there is no greater advantage to plasma exchange, IVIG is most often given, as its administration is less invasive and easier. IVIG is usually given as 0.4 mg/kg/day for 5 days (total of 2 gm/kg).

Consultation with the following specialties are indicated in GBS: critical care, pulmonology, neurology, infectious diseases, and immunology. Additional interprofessional care team members may include nutrition, child life, rehabilitative services, social workers, and spiritual support.

Caregiver education includes information about the diagnostic evaluation and results, along with the therapeutic plan of care. Educating the patient and family about the progression of the disease will allow them to prepare for interventions. Acute life-threatening presentations require additional support and education as to the immediate and expected therapeutic plan.

DISPOSITION AND DISCHARGE PLANNING

Treatment and discharge plans for infant botulism and GBS include physical therapy and transfer to a facility that can provide rehabilitation services. Arrangements for these services should be considered once the patient is recovering and issues that require acute hospital care are resolved.

Full recovery from infant botulism is expected with proper support and care throughout the illness. Prognosis for recovery from GBS is also good, with approximately 80% of patients achieving complete recovery within one year (Evans & Vedanarayanan, 1997).

Most infant botulism follows exposure to unpasteurized honey. An effective prevention strategy, consequently, is to avoid this product in those children who are younger than one year of age.

> **Critical Thinking**
> The progression of weakness is descending in infant botulism and ascending in Guillain-Barré syndrome.

BRONCHIOLITIS

Christine Agee and Samantha Chinderle

PATHOPHYSIOLOGY

Bronchiolitis is an infection of the bronchiolar epithelium characterized by profound submucosal edema, white blood cell peribronchiolar infiltration, increased mucus production, and bronchiolar epithelial cell necrosis (Mandelberg et al., 2003). The viral infection initially occurs in the upper respiratory tract and then spreads to the lower respiratory tract within a few days (Zorc & Hall, 2010). In the lower respiratory tract, the infected respiratory epithelial cells release inflammatory mediators. These mediators augment the immune response, thereby increasing the cellular recruitment to the small, infected airways. This process leads to tissue edema, mucus production, and increased airway resistance; which in turn creates further obstruction of the lumen of the smaller airways.

Bronchioles normally expand on inspiration and constrict on exhalation. In bronchiolitis, the obstructed airways produce a greater resistance in expiratory and inspiratory pathways. The bronchiolar changes obstruct the flow of air, leading to air trapping and hyperinflation. This ball-valve mechanism can result in a mismatch of pulmonary ventilation and perfusion that may lead to hypoxemia (Zorc & Hall, 2010). If the bronchioles become completely obstructed, atelectasis ensues from the absorption of the trapped air (Leung et al., 2005). The increased resistance to air flow leads to an increased respiratory rate and effort as the pediatric patient tries to compensate. This increased work of breathing places the pediatric patient at significant risk for respiratory insufficiency and, ultimately, respiratory failure (Martinón-Torres et al., 2002).

EPIDEMIOLOGY AND ETIOLOGY

Approximately 16% of all pediatric hospitalizations are attributable to bronchiolitis (McBride et al., 2005). Notably, this disease accounts for approximately 80% of lower respiratory infections occurring in the first year of life. Bronchiolitis typically occurs in children younger than 2 years of age, during the winter months, with a peak incidence 2 months of age (Leung et al., 2005). In the United States, bronchiolitis is the leading cause of hospitalization for infants accounting for 100,000 admissions and $700 million in health care costs annually (Cornelli et al., 2007). Despite its high morbidity, bronchiolitis has a relatively low mortality. The pediatric patients at greatest risk for death associated with bronchiolitis are infants younger than 6 months of age, premature infants, and infants with an underlying cardiopulmonary or immunodeficiency disease. Approximately 400 children die from this cause each year (Zorc & Hall, 2010).

Worrall (2008) reported that respiratory syncytial virus (RSV) was detected in 70% of patients with bronchiolitis. In this study, RSV-associated bronchiolitis accounted for approximately three times as many hospitalizations as bronchiolitis caused by other viruses. The enveloped RNA virus, which belongs to the *Paramyxoviridae* family, is a single-stranded genome that has a characteristic syncytial pattern in tissue culture. Due to its delicate nature, the virus is unable to withstand extreme changes in pH or temperature (Leung et al., 2005). Okiro et al. (2010) concluded that viral shedding in nasal secretions had a mean duration of 4.5 days, with an overall range of 1 to 14 days. One of the key findings in their study was a 40% higher rate of recovery from shedding in children who were previously infected. The initial incubation period for RSV varies from 2 to 8 days. RSV is typically present during the months of November through April (Leung et al.).

Several other organisms may also lead to significant bronchiole inflammation (Table 35-12). Molecular diagnostic studies have revealed a 10% to 30% coinfection rate in children with bronchiolitis, signifying that children are often infected with more than one virus (Zorc & Hall, 2010).

Several risk factors for severe disease and complications from bronchiolitis have been identified, including male sex, chronic coexisting medical conditions (chronic pulmonary disease/congenital heart disease), prematurity, low birth weight, immunodeficiency, exposure to cigarette smoke, lower socioeconomic status, lack of breastfeeding, and exposure to crowded environments (daycare programs, siblings) (Hall et al., 2009). Of these risk factors, several have been shown to significantly increase morbidity. For example, prematurity, chronic lung disease, and cyanotic heart disease are correlated with an increased rate of hospitalization as well as an increased length of stay (Figueras-Aloy et al., 2003; Thompson et al., 2004). Genomics is being studied as an etiology of bronchiolitis, with genes linked to innate immunity and vitamin D receptors have been demonstrated to have an association with this disease (Zorc & Hall, 2010).

PRESENTATION

Pediatric patients with bronchiolitis may initially present with mild symptoms of rhinorrhea, congestion, and low-grade fever. After 2 to 5 days, this triad may progress to cough, dyspnea, wheezing, and feeding difficulties. A significant number of patients will experience more debilitating symptoms of respiratory distress, hypoxia, or apnea (Leung et al., 2005). Some infants are at a particularly increased risk of developing apnea—namely, those of younger age, premature birth, with a history of apnea of prematurity, and who initially present with apnea (Willwerth et al., 2006). Of these manifestations, infants who present with respiratory distress, hypoxia, or dehydration are most likely to be hospitalized. Willwerth et al. (2006) found a 2.7% rate of apnea among hospitalized infants with bronchiolitis.

The physical examination of a pediatric patient with bronchiolitis is characteristic for significant respiratory pathology. Most pediatric patients in the early phase of bronchiolitis will have tachypnea, intercostal retractions, expiratory wheezing, and various adventitious sounds (crackles, rhonchi) (Willwerth et al., 2006). These symptoms can progress to a severe form, characterized by respiratory distress with tachypnea, prolonged expiratory phase, nasal flaring, grunting, severe intercostal retractions, tachycardia, irritability, cyanosis, and hypoxemia. Simultaneously, the pediatric patient may show signs of mild conjunctivitis, pharyngitis, otitis media, and dehydration (Leung et al., 2005).

DIFFERENTIAL DIAGNOSIS

Multiple differential diagnoses exist for a pediatric patient with bronchiolitis symptoms. The most frequent differential diagnosis is respiratory distress of similar etiologies, including asthma, pneumonia, and bronchitis (Collins et al., 1996). It can often be difficult to distinguish between these other etiologies (Table 35-13), but it is important to consider them to direct the plan of care appropriately.

PLAN OF CARE

According to the American Academy of Pediatrics (AAP, 2006), HCPs should diagnose bronchiolitis based on history

TABLE 35-12

Viral Etiology of Bronchiolitis by Incidence	
Agent	**% Incidence**
Respiratory syncytial virus	27
Enterovirus	25
Rhinovirus	24
Rhino/enterovirus	16
Parainfluenza virus type 1	3
Parainfluenza virus type 2	0
Parainfluenza virus type 3	2
Parainfluenza virus type 1 or 3	1
Adenovirus	5
Human metapneumovirus	4
Influenza A virus	1
Influenza B virus	1
Coronavirus	1
Mixed viral infection	19

Source: Jartti et al., 2004.

TABLE 35-13

Differential Diagnoses for Wheezing in the Pediatric Patient

- Viral bronchiolitis
- Other pulmonary infections (pneumonia, Mycoplasma, Chlamydia, tuberculosis)
- Laryngotracheomalacia/bronchomalacia
- Foreign body, esophageal or aspiration
- Gastroesophageal reflux
- Congestive heart failure
- Vascular ring
- Allergic reaction
- Cystic fibrosis
- Mediastinal mass
- Bronchogenic cyst
- Tracheoesophageal fistula
- Exacerbation of bronchopulmonary dysplasia
- Pertussis
- Asthma

Source: Leung et al., 2005: Zorc & Hall, 2010.

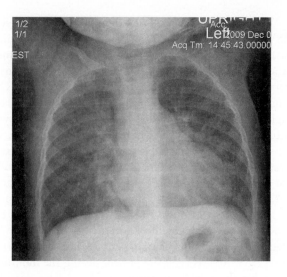

FIGURE 35-11

The pathologic findings of this chest radiograph are consistent with a viral etiology such as bronchiolitis: hyperinflation of the lung fields, diffuse perihilar interstitial bronchial wall thickening, perihilar opacities, and patchy atelectasis.

Source: Courtesy of Christine Agee and Samantha Chinderle.

and physical examination. Only limited evidence supports the use of diagnostic laboratory or radiographic examinations in the typical patient with bronchiolitis (Zorc & Hall, 2010). Nevertheless, some pediatric patients may be more difficult to diagnose, such as patients younger than 2 months of age with fever or those with an unusual clinical course or severe disease. These patients may require a CXR or CBC with differential count (AAP, 2009a). The CXR will typically show hyperexpansion from the increased airway resistance, atelectasis from the airway obstruction, and peribronchiolar thickening (Figure 35-11). It may be difficult to differentiate areas of atelectasis with focal infiltrates associated with pneumonia, as these two processes may look similar on a CXR and may coexist in the patient with bronchiolitis (Leung et al., 2005).

For definitive diagnosis, the study of choice is nasal or throat viral culture. However, these cultures can be expensive and can take anywhere from 3 to 7 days to yield a positive result. Given this limitation, a method used to obtain quicker results—viral genome amplification by polymerase chain reaction (PCR)—may be useful (Leung et al., 2005). Immunologic testing is more convenient as well, as it is rapid and less expensive than PCR (Agency for Healthcare Research and Quality [AHRQ], 2003).

The mainstay of therapeutic management for bronchiolitis is supportive therapy, including oxygen supplementation, intravenous hydration, monitoring of adequate nutrition, various pulmonary regimens, and even corticosteroids (Martinón-Torres et al., 2002). Certain high-risk groups will require hospitalization—for example, premature infants; infants younger than 3 months of age; patients with respiratory rate greater than 70, a pulse oximetry level less than 94%, cardiovascular disease, or

lethargy; and patients with immunodeficiency (Worrall, 2008). There is a strong correlation between a pulse oximetry level of less than 94% and rate of hospitalization, which suggests a relationship between pulse oximetry level and V/Q mismatch (Zorc & Hall, 2010).

Some infants may require CPAP, while approximately 25% of pediatric patients admitted to the intensive care unit require mechanical ventilation (Berner et al., 2008). Conventional ventilation is the most commonly used modality in this population. Once extubated, some patients may require respiratory support with CPAP or supplemental oxygen. The use of chest physiotherapy is not recommended (AAP, 2006).

Heliox, which is composed of helium (an inert gas of low molecular weight) and oxygen, may be used as a temporizing agent until symptoms resolve and is now often considered first-line therapy for pediatric patients with severe infection (Chowdhury et al., 2010). Heliox has a marked reduction in density compared to air; therefore, it is theoretically more apt to reach the lower obstructed airways, leading to decreased airway resistance and improved work of breathing (Martinón-Torres et al., 2002). When given via face mask, it has been reported to shorten length of treatment and duration on CPAP, especially for patients with RSV (Chowdhury et al.).

Nebulized hypertonic saline (3%), has shown some promise, including the ability to produce a 25% decrease in length of stay. The expectation is that this treatment reverses the submucosal and adventitial edema in the bronchiolar lumen, thereby decreasing the thickness and dryness of the mucous plaques. Nebulized hypertonic saline decreases mucosal edema, decreases the concentration of inflammatory mediators, facilitates mechanical removal of thickened mucus, and improves mucociliary transport and function. It may also induce coughing, which helps to maintain airway patency; however, coughing-induced bronchospasm requires immediate cessation of the therapy (Mandelberg et al., 2003; Tomooka et al., 2000; Zhang et al., 2008).

Pharmacologic therapies for bronchiolitis remain controversial. Inhaled therapies such as β_2-adrenergic selective bronchodilators and bronchodilators with an α-adrenergic component (i.e., epinephrine) do not have sufficient evidence to support their use in the treatment of patients with bronchiolitis. Their use may produce a modest short-term benefit, but routine use has not been proven beneficial (Worrall, 2008). The smooth muscle of the respiratory tract seems to play a small role in the pathologic process of bronchiolitis, which may explain the limited value of bronchodilators (Zorc & Hall, 2010).

Early use of high-dose systemic corticosteroids may reduce the length of hospital stay and duration of symptoms in pediatric patients with moderate to severe bronchiolitis (Cornelli et al., 2007; Hall, 2007; Mansbach et al., 2008; Patel et al., 2004). Nevertheless, after reviewing the evidence on the use of corticosteroids, the AAP (2006) concluded that it could not recommend their routine use in the management of bronchiolitis.

Ribavirin, a synthetic analog that acts by suppressing viral RNA polymerase activity and protein inhibition, has not been shown to improve clinical outcomes in bronchiolitis (Leung et al., 2005); consequently, the AAP (2006) does not recommend the routine use of ribavirin in children with bronchiolitis.

Antibiotics are rarely used in this population because bacteremia and bacterial pneumonia are rare coinfections of bronchiolitis. The AAP (2006) recommends that the use of antimicrobials be limited to children with bronchiolitis who have specific indications that suggest the coexistence of a bacterial infection. These agents should not be used as a mainstay of therapy.

If the patient's clinical status is deteriorating and more invasive therapies are required, consultation with the critical care team is recommended for possible admission to the intensive care unit. If the pediatric patient has a prolonged duration of symptoms, abnormal presentation, or possible coinfection, it may be necessary to consult the infectious diseases team for their expertise in reviewing other possible differential diagnoses. Occasionally, bronchiolitis will damage previously healthy lung tissue and require an expert to monitor lung sequelae; this outcome would require a consultation with a pediatric pulmonologist. Pediatric patients who remain in the intensive care unit for a prolonged period of time also usually require a physical medicine and rehabilitation specialist to assist with the restoration of muscle, nerve, and bone function.

Education of the family is an important part of managing the bronchiolitic patient (AAP, 2009a). The entire family needs to learn and practice excellent hand hygiene. In addition, family education centers on delineating to the caregiver the expected clinical course, the process for administering any needed therapies, and prevention of future respiratory infections. Discussions should include encouraging continued lactation support for the breastfeeding mother and restricting ill contacts. Families also need to be able to recognize resurgence of symptoms, such as increased respiratory rate, decreased activity, decreased oral intake, or increased work of breathing.

DISPOSITION AND DISCHARGE PLANNING

While there are no specific criteria for when a patient should be discharged from the emergency department or inpatient unit, patients should have resolution of the symptoms that led to the admission (AAP, 2009a; Tie et al., 2009). Commonly used criteria for discharge include a respiratory rate less than 70 breaths per minute, an oxygen saturation of more than 92% without supplemental oxygen, adequate oral intake, and the ability of the caregiver to clear the airway with bulb suctioning (AAP, 2009a). Pulmonary hygiene can be continued in the home environment if needed for certain patients.

For an uncomplicated course of bronchiolitis, follow-up is with the patient's PCP. The focus of this visit is to ensure that the patient is progressing as expected with no new derangements. For pediatric patients who required hospitalization, follow-up is based on the severity of illness. If the patient developed chronic lung disease, it may be necessary to follow up with a pulmonologist for further management.

Bronchiolitis is a self-limited disease. The prognosis is usually excellent provided there is no lung injury related to mechanical ventilation. Most children recover completely at home within 3 to 5 days (Yarza et al., 2007). Some children will have repeated episodes of wheezing after bronchiolitis, but rarely does this condition persist into asthma beyond adolescence. In conditions where significant lung injury occurs, patients may develop chronic lung disease and associated sequelae.

While there is no definitive treatment for bronchiolitis, a few preventive modalities have some proven efficacy. The primary benefit is the prevention of RSV disease in certain high-risk populations.

The U.S. Food and Drug Administration (FDA) licensed the first preventive therapy, respiratory syncytial virus immune globulin (RSV-IGIV), in January 1996. This preparation of hyperimmune globulin is derived from selected donors with particularly high serum titers of RSV-neutralizing antibody (Meissner et al., 2003). In a large study of at-risk infants, use of RSV-IGIV reduced RSV-related hospitalization rates by 41% (Kimpen, 2002). One advantage of this therapy is that it includes antibodies to a variety of pathogens, not just RSV; however, this preparation is contraindicated in patients with hemodynamically significant congenital heart disease.

A second preventive therapy, palivizumab (Synagis), has been show to be effective as a prophylactic therapy in a variety of pediatric populations (Feltes et al., 2003). This preparation, which was licensed by the FDA in June 1998, is a recombinant humanized murine monoclonal immunoglobulin G anti-F glycoprotein with inhibitory activity against RSV (Leung et al., 2005; Meissner et al., 2003). When Meissner et al. (2003) evaluated the effectiveness of monthly administration of palivizumab during RSV season, their results indicated it achieved a 45% to 55% decrease in the rate of hospitalization. Palivizumab, unlike RSV-IGIV, can be used in patients with hemodynamically significant congenital heart disease (Leung et al.). The recommended dose is 15 mg/kg/dose intramuscular every month during RSV season (Table 35-14).

TABLE 35-14

Recommendations by the American Academy of Pediatrics, Committee on Infectious Diseases, for Use of Palivizumab for Prevention of Respiratory Syncytial Infections	
Eligible Criteria	**Eligible Maximum Number of Doses**
Infants with chronic lung disease	5
Prematurity	5
• Gestational age less than 28 weeks, age less than 12 months at start of RSV season	
• Gestational age of 29 weeks to 32 weeks, age less than 6 months at the start of RSV season	
• Gestational age of 32 weeks 0 days to 34 weeks 6 days, age less than 3 months at the start of RSV season, if one of two risk factors is present:	3
• Daycare program attendance	
• 1 or more siblings younger than 5 years of age in the same household	
Congenital abnormality of airway or neuromuscular disease, age of 12 months or younger at the start of RSV season	5
Hemodynamically significant congenital heart disease, age of 2 years or younger at the start of RSV season:	
• Infants receiving medications to control congestive heart failure	
• Infants with moderate-to-severe pulmonary hypertension	
• Infants with cyanotic heart disease	

Note: Respiratory syncytial virus (RSV).
Source: AAP, 2009b.

Other recommendations recognized as beneficial in preventing and reducing the risk of viral transmission include the following:

• Adequate hand washing
• Avoidance of cigarette smoke
• Breastfeeding—human milk has active immunoglobulins and antibodies, some specific to neutralizing activity against RSV (AAP, 2006)

CHRONIC LUNG DISEASE

Cynthia Etzler Budek and Paula Costanzo

Evolving acute care management over the last 50 years has had a significant impact on the outcome of pediatric patients. The development of critical care units and use of mechanical ventilators in the 1960s resulted in the survival of many patients who would have died from their acute illnesses in earlier eras. Unfortunately, these life-saving treatment modalities often contributed to development of chronic lung disease (CLD) secondary to oxygen toxicity, ventilator barotrauma, and volutrauma. Ongoing advances in treatment modalities, technology, and research have led to a growing and changing population of pediatric patients with varying degrees of CLD.

Many pulmonary and systemic diseases have the potential to progress to CLD or significantly contribute to its development. The most common causes of pediatric CLD are cystic fibrosis (CF), bronchopulmonary dysplasia (BPD), asthma, chronic aspiration pneumonitis due to gastroesophageal reflux disease (GERD), and disorders that lead to bronchiectasis (Rossi & Owens, 2005). This section focuses on general aspects of CLD, with an emphasis on CLD caused by BPD in neonates. Pediatric CLD encompasses a broad spectrum of acuity, ranging from patients with mild lung disease characterized by intermittent acute exacerbations due to respiratory infections, to patients with severe chronic lung injury who require prolonged mechanical ventilatory support.

PATHOPHYSIOLOGY

Acute lung injury due to an underlying disorder, exposure to a toxic substance, or response to treatment modality typically initiates an acute inflammatory response. Cytokines (interleukins 1L-1-beta, IL-6, soluble Inter-Cellular Adhesion Molecule 1 [ICAM-1]) are present early in the *inflammatory phase* and activate mediators that in turn release pro-inflammatory cells and promote cell-to-cell adhesion. Chemokines are released that activate neutrophils, which in turn mediate endothelial cytotoxicity, inhibit surfactant production, and release elastase. Leukotrienes are released and remain present in high levels for an extended period;

they are responsible for bronchoconstriction, vasoconstriction, edema, neutrophil chemotaxis, and mucus production (Kinsella et al., 2006). Overall, the acute inflammatory phase is characterized by airway and parenchymal inflammation with airway hyperreactivity, production of exudate, and mucus plugging of airways.

Resolution of acute inflammation is marked by fibroproliferation of interstitial and perialveolar tissue. During the *fibroproliferative phase,* alveoli septal walls thicken and a heterogeneous pattern develops in which emphysema is interspersed with atelectasis. Diffuse areas of atelectasis cause V/Q mismatch due to the absence of ventilation within perfused small airways, which leads to subsequent hypercarbia and/or hypoxemia.

The fibroproliferative phase is followed by the *lung repair phase,* which is characterized by remodeling of lung parenchyma and airways. The fourth phase is *subsequent lung growth and development,* as the patient continues to grow and mature (Kotecha, 2008). This recovery process from acute lung injury can become complicated by overlapping phases of acute injury and chronic recovery, which leads to progressive CLD, if the underlying disease process or acute illnesses causes repetitive injury to the lung.

Over time, structural changes in parenchyma and small airways alter the structure of pulmonary microcirculation. Pulmonary vessels can become narrowed and torturous with thickened vessel walls—a development that decreases vascular compliance and increases vascular resistance. If significant, these changes in pulmonary vasculature can cause pulmonary hypertension. Systemic-to-pulmonary collateral blood vessels can develop that typically are small; if they are large, however, they can cause significant left-to-right shunting into the pulmonary vasculature bed, ultimately resulting in pulmonary edema and hypoxemia (Kotecha, 2008).

Infants with classic BPD tend to have a late inflammatory response, severe airway damage, and heterogeneity of alveolar damage and fibrosis. As a result, they are more prone to extrapulmonary air leakage and emphysema (American Thoracic Society [ATS], 2003). Very low birth weight (VLBW is defined as a birth weight of less than 1,250 grams) and very premature (24 to 25 weeks' gestational age) neonates have a different pathologic process from classic BPD, commonly referred to as "new" BPD. This unique presentation is likely due to their lung immaturity and stage of lung development as well as their use of exogenous surfactant.

Lung injury in the "new" BPD population results in less fibroproliferation and greater dysregulation of alveolar and capillary growth and development. Pathologic changes consist of alveolar simplification and enlargement, with decreased acinar complexity, fewer and dysmorphic vessels, more uniform inflation with less fibrosis of lungs, and variable airway smooth-muscle hyperplasia. VLBW and very premature infants also have an immature antioxidant system that is charged with handling cytotoxic oxygen free radicals; thus they are more likely to sustain injury to the pulmonary vasculature. Smooth-muscle cell proliferation within pulmonary arteries can lead to increased vasoreactivity and pulmonary artery resistance, making them more susceptible to developing pulmonary hypertension (PH) (Kinsella et al., 2006).

Table 35-15 compares the pathologic changes noted in classic presurfactant BPD and "new" postsurfactant BPD.

EPIDEMIOLOGY AND ETIOLOGY

CLD incidence is difficult to determine from the existing data due to variance in the CLD definitions used in studies, the multifactorial etiologies of CLD, and the wide variability in outcomes from acute lung disease between medical centers. The difficulty in defining CLD is well illustrated by examining the evolving change in BPD definition over the past 40 years.

Northway and his colleagues first described BPD in 1967 as a constellation of clinical features, radiographic findings, and oxygen requirement found in premature neonates at 36 weeks' postmenstrual age (gestational age plus chronologic age). These infants previously required high levels of oxygen therapy and mechanical ventilation for management of respiratory distress syndrome. Classic BPD was later defined in the 1970s as oxygen dependency with specific clinical and radiologic findings at 28 days' chronologic age (Bancalari et al., 1979).

As acute care management of the premature neonate improved and antenatal administration of exogenous surfactant became common practice, younger and lower-birth-weight infants began to survive the neonatal period. As a consequence, most premature infants were still oxygen dependent at 28 days of life and the observed pathologic

TABLE 35-15

Differences in Pathological Features of "Classic/Old" and "New" Bronchopulmonary Dysplasia	
Presurfactant ("Old")	**Postsurfactant ("New")**
Alternating atelectasis with hyperinflation	Less regional heterogeneity of lung disease
Severe airway epithelial lesions (e.g., hyperplasia, squamous metaplasia)	Rare airway epithelial lesions Mild airway smooth muscle thickening
Marked airway smooth muscle hyperplasia	Rare fibroproliferative changes
Extensive, diffuse fibroproliferation	Fewer arteries but "dysmorphic"
Hypertensive remodeling of pulmonary arteries	Fewer, larger and simplified alveoli
Decreased alveolarization and surface area	

Source: Used with permission from Kinsella et al., 2006, p. 1422.

changes of BPD changed. Additional criteria were required for "new" BPD to distinguish those infants who required oxygen because of immature lungs from those infants who required oxygen for CLD.

A revised definition of BPD was proposed in 2001 by the National Institutes of Health consensus conference that described the severity of BPD based on the degree of respiratory support required when infant was closer to full-term age (Jobe & Bancalari, 2001). The new criteria applied to infants who required oxygen for at least the first 28 days of life. Infants less than 32 weeks' gestational age were categorized as having mild, moderate, or severe BPD based on their need for oxygen or positive-pressure ventilatory support at 36 weeks' postmenstrual age or at time of discharge, whichever came first. Infants of 32 weeks' or more gestational age were evaluated at 56 days' chronologic age or at discharge. Categories were defined as follows: patients with mild BPD had no oxygen requirement, those with moderate BPD required less than 30% oxygen, and those with severe BPD required 30% or more oxygen and/or positive-pressure ventilation or nasal CPAP (Jobe & Bancalari).

In 2003, the American Thoracic Society developed a description of chronic lung disease of infancy (CLDI) as the common endpoint of BPD as well as other, less frequently encountered pulmonary conditions: "pneumonia/sepsis, meconium aspiration pneumonia, pulmonary hyperplasia, persistent pulmonary hypertension, apnea, tracheoesophageal fistula, congenital diaphragmatic hernia, congenital heart disease, and congenital neuromuscular disorders" (ATS, 2003, pp. 356–357).

A clinical classification system for PH, which is often associated with severe CLD, was initially developed in 1998 at the Second World Symposium on PH held in Evian, France, and was subsequently referred to as the Evian classification. This classification system was reviewed and revisions made to subclassifications at the 2003 Third World Symposium on PH held in Venice, Italy. The five classifications for PH are pulmonary arterial hypertension, PH with left heart disease, PH associated with lung diseases and/or hypoxemia, PH due to chronic thrombotic and/or embolic disease, and miscellaneous. PH associated with lung diseases is typically associated with a modest increase in pulmonary artery pressure (less than 35 mmHg), and morbidity depends more on the severity of lung disease than on the PH (Simonneau et al., 2004).

As a result of variable terminology as well as the diagnostic overlap of classic and "new" BPD and CLDI, it is difficult to determine the incidence of the differing forms of CLD. Walsh and colleagues (2006) reported a 97% incidence of BPD in VLBW infants. An inverse relationship in frequency of BPD compared to birth weight has been observed, such that increased incidence of BPD is associated with decreased birth weight. One study reported the incidence of BPD based on birth weight (BW) as follows: 42% when BW is 501 to 750 grams, 25% when BW is 751 to 1,000 grams, and 5% when BW is 1,251 to 1,500 grams

(Fanaroff et al., 2007). Another study examined the trends in severity of BPD between 1994 and 2002 and found that the overall incidence of BPD remained unchanged, while the incidence of severe BPD decreased an average of 11% annually (Smith et al., 2005).

The etiology of CLD is multifactorial. An underlying pulmonary or systemic disease may be identified as the primary cause of CLD, but often multiple other factors contribute significantly to the degree of chronic disease (Table 35-16).

TABLE 35-16

Etiology of Pediatric Chronic Lung Disease

Pulmonary Diseases

Cystic fibrosis
Asthma
Bronchopulmonary dysplasia (BPD)
Acute respiratory distress syndrome (ARDS)
Bronchiectasis
Pulmonary hemorrhage disorders
Primary ciliary dyskinesia
Alveolar proteinosis
Children's interstitial lung disease (ChILD)

Congenital Defects

Diaphragmatic hernia
Pulmonary hypoplasia
Tracheoesophageal fistula
Esophageal atresia
Complete tracheal rings
Chest wall deformities
Congenital heart disease with pulmonary vasculature overload

Cardiac Diseases

Patent ductus arteriosus
Left ventricular heart failure

Systemic Diseases

Collagen vascular diseases
Juvenile rheumatoid arthritis
Systemic lupus erythematosus
Vasculitis
Sarcoidosis
Storage and metabolic diseases
Immune deficiency diseases

Neuromuscular Diseases

Spinal muscular atrophy

Infections: Viral, Bacterial, Fungal, Parasitic

Pneumonia
Bronchiolitis
Sepsis
Lung abscess or empyema

TABLE 35-16

Etiology of Pediatric Chronic Lung Disease *(Continued)*

Lung Injuries

Chronic aspiration pneumonitis
Gastroesophageal reflux (GERD)
Swallow dysfunction
Oxygen toxicity
Ventilator-induced lung disease
Inhalation

Thermal

Smoke
Toxic chemical
Exposure
Therapeutic drug
Radiation

For pediatric patients with acute lung disease, therapeutic measures required to support their respiratory needs—such as high oxygen levels, intubation, and aggressive ventilation—often in turn cause additional lung injury and may increase the risk of developing CLD. High levels of oxygen are well known to cause acute lung injury, and younger patients are more susceptible to this complication than older patients. Ventilator barotrauma (trauma due to high peak airway pressures) and volutrauma (trauma due to high tidal volume) may cause over-distention of the alveoli with an ensuing disruption in epithelial cells, protein leakage, and activation of acute inflammatory response. This is particularly true in the neonatal population, in whom oxygen toxicity and ventilator barotrauma/volutrauma are known to be causative factors of BPD. VLBW and very premature infants are particularly susceptible due to their stage of lung development and can develop lung injury after receiving even minimal levels of oxygen and ventilatory support in the antenatal period (Kinsella et al., 2006).

Additional risk factors for BPD have been identified. For example, several studies have suggested a genetic link related to the risk of developing BPD, although none has been confirmed as yet due to problems in replicating the studies. In addition, research is under way to identify biomarkers as early predictors of which infants likely to develop BPD (Bhandari & Bhandari, 2009). Maternal chorioamnionitis not only precipitates premature birth, but also is associated with a higher incidence of BPD in the infant, perhaps due to activation of the acute inflammatory process in the neonatal lung by the infection.

PRESENTATION

Birth history is essential information to elicit for a patient with history of CLDI, beginning with gestational age and birth weight. If the patient was a preterm infant, determine whether antenatal exogeous surfactant was administered. In addition, the degree of respiratory support in the neonatal period should be determined. Specific history to elicit includes neonatal intensive care (NICU) admission, intubation, nasal CPAP versus high-flow oxygen via nasal cannula, and mechanical ventilator support with conventional versus high-frequency oscillatory ventilation. A history of emphysematous cysts, pneumothorax, or pneumomediastinum suggests barotrauma/volutrauma and the possibility of classic BPD. If the patient has a history of PH, information about previous administration of inhaled nitric oxide and either parenteral or oral pulmonary vasodilators will assist in determining the severity of the pulmonary vascular disease. Lastly, it is important to determine if the patient required oxygen during the first 28 days of life. If so, determine if patient still required oxygen or ventilatory support at 36 weeks' postmenstrual age or at the time of discharge to establish the severity of BPD.

If a patient developed CLD in the postneonatal period, it is important to determine whether the lung disease is due to an acute lung injury or a chronic underlying disorder. Elicit history regarding the course of chronic lung disease progression. Note any history of acute exacerbations of CLD, the frequency and nature of hospital and critical care admissions, and the need for intubation and ventilatory support, including noninvasive bilevel positive airway pressure support versus invasive mechanical ventilation.

Lastly, an understanding of the patient's current pulmonary baseline is very important to elicit. Obtain the patient's or caregiver's description of respiratory effort during rest and play/exercise, episodes of cyanotic spells or respiratory distress, precipitating factors for these episodes, typical oxygen saturation levels, oxygen use, sleep pattern, nutritional intake, and pattern of linear growth and weight gain. Current medications should be reviewed, and the frequency of administration of bronchodilator, steroid, diuretic, and pulmonary vasodilator medications noted. Use and effectiveness of airway clearance techniques and devices should be explored as well, including chest physical therapy (CPT) with postural drainage and use of a high-frequency chest compression vest/wrap, oscillating positive expiratory pressure (also called "flutter" therapy), or cough assist device.

Information about any artificial airway and use of a ventilatory support device is a critical element of the current pulmonary baseline. Tracheostomy tubes are surgically placed in those patients who have significant airway pathology that compromises breathing, such as subglottic stenosis or severe tracheomalacia; they are also placed in patients who require long-term use of mechanical ventilation. Note the type and size of the tracheostomy tube, the amount of cuff inflation if the tube has a cuff, and the length of the tube (standard versus customized). Patients with airway concerns such as severe tracheomalacia or recurrent tracheal granulation tissue may have a tracheostomy tube placed with customized, longer length to stent open the airway or bypass the problematic area.

Patients who require ventilatory support may use noninvasive versus invasive (conventional ventilator) devices. If the patient uses a noninvasive bilevel pressure device for ventilatory support, determine its current settings, the method of patient interface with the device (mask versus nasal pillows), the frequency of use, and the patient's tolerance of the device. If the patient uses a mechanical ventilator, determine the current ventilator settings, including the mode of ventilation (assist control versus synchronized intermittent mandatory ventilation [SIMV] mode, pressure versus volume mode), breathing rate versus pressure support alone, inspiratory time, and set pressures (pressure control, pressure support, PEEP). Also elicit details of the patient's use of the ventilator, such as specific hours per day, only while asleep versus around-the-clock, tolerance of the ventilator, and response to transitions on and off the ventilator. Although uncommon, some patients continue to use other noninvasive devices, such as the rocking bed, chest cuirasse, and iron lung for ventilatory support, particularly if they have CLD with an underlying neuromuscular disease; any history related to these devices should not be overlooked.

Pediatric patients can present with a broad spectrum of clinical features depending on the underlying disorder that progressed to CLD, the incidence of repeat acute injury to the lung, the severity of pulmonary disease, and presentation at clinical baseline versus an acute exacerbation of CLD. Tachypnea, a common finding, may sometimes be the only indication on examination of underlying CLD. Breathing may be shallow. Subcostal, substernal, or suprasternal retractions may be present as well as activation of accessory muscles and nasal flaring depending on the degree of increased work of breathing. Expiratory grunting, associated with exhalation against a partially closed glottis, may be heard. Observance of retractions and accessory muscle use may be less than expected given the patient's degree of pulmonary compromise if an underlying neuromuscular weakness is present. Paradoxical breathing—pronounced rising of the abdomen and collapse of the chest wall on inspiration—may be observed; this finding is often observed in infants with airway obstruction or severe malacia, and in patients with neuromuscular disease.

Pediatric patients with history of lung hyperinflation, as in classic BPD, may present with a barrel-shaped thoracic cavity due to an increased ratio of anterioposterior-to-lateral diameter, and the edge of the liver may be palpated well below the right lower costal margin. Other patients may present with a bell-shaped thoracic cavity, especially if they had chronic paradoxical breathing as infants when chest wall was still very compliant. During this developmental period, increased use of the diaphragm due to ineffective intercostal muscles along with very compliant rib cage leads to a narrowing of the upper rib cage and flaring out of the lower rib cage.

Auscultation of lungs may reveal clear breath sounds with good air entry. However, it is not uncommon to auscultate diffuse adventitious sounds. Breath sounds may be diminished over areas of consolidation due to chronic atelectasis. If the patient has a history of airway hyperreactivity, intermittent or pronounced wheezing may be present as well as prolonged exhalation.

PH may be difficult to assess on physical examination due to lung hyperinflation and abnormal breath sounds in the pediatric patient with CLD. Palpation of right ventricular heave or auscultation of accentuated P_2, tricuspid regurgitation murmur, or pulmonary regurgitation murmur suggests the presence of PH (ATS, 2003).

DIFFERENTIAL DIAGNOSIS

Other pulmonary and cardiac conditions should be included in the differential diagnosis when evaluating a pediatric patient with apparent CLD. In the infant population, congenital defects may present along a spectrum ranging from acute respiratory failure in the antenatal period to progression of generalized symptoms of irritability, poor feeding, and mild respiratory distress. Congenital defects to consider include heart defects with pulmonary vasculature overload, diaphragmatic hernia, hypoplastic or agenesis of lung, complete tracheal rings, tracheoesophageal fistula, or esophageal atresia. Structural defects that cause compression of the airway, such as a pulmonary artery sling or innominate artery, or dynamic airway dysfunction, such as severe tracheal or bronchial malacia, can also mimic the signs and symptoms of lung disease. In the general pediatric population, congestive heart failure and underlying systemic diseases such as neuromuscular, metabolic and storage, collagen vascular, and immunodeficiency diseases may present with a chronic respiratory component and should be considered depending on the history and clinical presentation. Swallow dysfunction and GERD should be considered in patients with recurrent aspiration pneumonia. Many of these disorders will contribute to development of CLD if they are not recognized and managed appropriately.

PLAN OF CARE

Chest radiograph is the primary imaging study used to diagnose acute lung processes such as pneumonia and atelectasis as well as monitor progression and response to treatment of CLD. The findings will vary depending on the underlying pathologic process and the stage of lung injury and repair. For example, CXR of patients recovering from acute lung injury may show diffuse opacification. Heterogeneous areas of reticular strands, atelectasis, and consolidation interspersed with emphysematous cysts may be visible depending on the degree of acute lung injury and barotrauma/volutrauma from ventilation. Findings of lung hyperinflation, cystic and atelectatic changes, and scarring may persist in patients with severe CLD. Infants with history of "new" BPD typically have CXR findings of small, gray lungs (Kotecha, 2008).

Pneumothorax or pneumomediastinum may be found if the patient has poor lung compliance and acutely decompensates, especially if the patient requires high-pressure ventilation or increased ventilatory support. The presence of a mediastinal shift may also indicate acute pneumothorax or may be a chronic finding if the patient has history of unilateral lung hypoplasia, which can occur in patients following repair of congenital diaphragmatic hernia.

It is important to compare previous CXR with current images to differentiate findings due to an acute disease process from chronic changes related to CLD. CXR images of CLD may improve over time, with potential resolution of chronic findings occurring as long as the pediatric patient does not have repetitive acute lung injury or progressive underlying disease affecting the lung.

Monitoring of oxygen and carbon dioxide levels is another key diagnostic tool in CLD. Arterial blood gases are utilized during acute stages of illness to evaluate for hypercarbia, hypoxemia, and acidosis, and to guide adjustments in acute care management. Continuous pulse oximetry monitoring of oxygen saturation and end-tidal monitoring of exhaled carbon dioxide (CO_2) are essential during the acute phase of lung injury and subsequent period of stabilization and lung healing. Both modes of monitoring permit rapid recognition of acute changes in the patient's pulmonary status as well as ongoing assessment of oxygenation and ventilation trends, clinical stability, and readiness for oxygen/ventilator weaning during the chronic phase. Pulse oximetry and end-tidal CO_2 monitoring are also important tools utilized in home care for continuous or intermittent monitoring of oxygen saturation and CO_2 levels. The frequency of monitoring reflects the severity of the CLD, the stability of the child's pulmonary status, and the current level of oxygen and ventilator support. Serum bicarbonate, venous or capillary blood gases, and CO_2 transcutaneous monitoring $tcPO_2$ levels are additional monitoring modalities that are useful for intermittent evaluation and monitoring of ventilatory trends, although their utilization is usually limited to hospital or clinic settings.

If the patient is receiving diuretic therapy, serum electrolytes should be checked periodically to evaluate for hypokalemia, hyponatremia, and hypochloremia. Hemoglobin, hematocrit, and red blood cell indices are also evaluated periodically to assure adequate oxygen-carrying capacity. Elevated hemoglobin (Hgb) and hematocrit (Hct) levels may be indicators of chronic hypoxemia, in which case current management of CLD may need to be modified.

Periodically, additional diagnostic studies are indicated to determine the degree of lung injury and either progression or resolution of CLD. Chest high-resolution computed tomography (HRCT) is useful in obtaining additional information about structural abnormalities of the lungs, airway, and pulmonary vasculature. For patients with classic BPD, HRCT typically yields findings of multifocal, asymmetrical areas of hyperinflation as well as linear opacities radiating from the lung periphery to hilum. Chronic GERD with pulmonary fibrosis is often associated with findings of honeycombing, traction bronchiectasis, and "ground glass" opacity. HRCT combined with spiral CT creates a three-dimensional image of the airways, which is especially useful in diagnosing airway abnormalities such as tracheal and bronchial malacia and stenosis (Rossi & Owens, 2005). Serial studies will document changes in CLD and can be utilized to assess the indication for or response to surgical intervention, such as determining the need for surgical resection of a large pneumatocele. HRCT is highly sensitive to chronic lung changes, so it may continue to reveal abnormal findings long after the CXR has indicated improvement in the patient's condition.

Information about pulmonary and cardiac function can be obtained from magnetic resonance angiography (MRA) of the lungs and heart. This technique has an advantage over HRCT, in that it does not require any radiation exposure. Administration of intravenous gadolinium (a contrast medium) permits visualization of pulmonary vasculature and perfusion, which is useful in evaluating patients with PH (Rossi & Owens, 2005). MRA may provide enough detail to direct treatment without requiring invasive cardiac catheterization.

For pediatric patients with PH associated with CLD, serial echocardiographs are often performed to assess the degree of PH and evaluate the response to medical treatment. These studies have the advantage of being readily accessible and noninvasive. The echocardiograph has limited reliability when utilized to diagnose the severity of PH compared to cardiac catheterization, the study of choice. In one study of 25 children, echocardiograph studies correctly diagnosed the presence or absence of PH based on estimated pulmonary artery systolic pressure in 79% of the patients when compared to cardiac catheterization measurements. By comparison, correct diagnosis of severity of PH occurred in only 47% of the echocardiograph studies (Mourani et al., 2008). For patients with PH, cardiac catheterization may be indicated to determine the severity of hypertension, appropriate treatment options, and possible indication for surgical intervention.

Serial B-type natriuretic peptide (BNP) serum levels can be useful for monitoring PH trends. BNP is an endogenous peptide hormone that is released by the right atrium when atrial distention increases the stretch of myocardial fibers. Chronically increased levels of circulating BNP are reflective of increased right-sided heart dilation associated with PH (ATS, 2003). Downward trending of BNP levels can be used as an indirect measure of treatment effectiveness in controlling PH.

Lastly, serial pulmonary function tests (PFTs) are a useful measure of changes in CLD, particularly in relation to lung volume and airway hyperreactivity. While PFTs are technically difficult to obtain and interpret in infants, the studies can be useful in children and adolescents for measuring lung volume, airway hyperreactivity, and responsiveness to bronchodilator therapy. One key limitation is that PFTs cannot be performed in those patients with tracheostomies.

Management of CLD focuses on maintaining the child's clinical stability, promoting optimal growth and development, and minimizing additional acute insult to the pulmonary system, with the hope that pulmonary function may improve and even normalize over time, particularly in patients who have CLD secondary to BPD or ARDS. Pediatric patients have the potential to grow and develop new healthy lung tissue under proper medical management if an underlying medical condition is not causing progressive lung disease or repeat injury to the lungs.

A primary tenet of CLD management is provision of appropriate oxygenation and ventilation when indicated. Oxygenation at rest and during feeding, increased activity, and sleep is assessed over time, so that oxygen flow may be maintained at a level that ensures appropriate oxygenation during all routine activities. Although the optimal oxygen saturation is unknown, it is likely greater than 90%. Ideally, adequate oxygen should be provided to prevent brief changes in saturation to less than 90% and to allow for the fluctuations in saturation observed during daily activities and sleep (Kotecha, 2008).

Once a pediatric patient ventilated for acute respiratory failure has failed multiple weaning attempts or is determined to not be a candidate for weaning because of progressive lung disease, the decision is made to chronically ventilate the child. A tracheostomy tube should be surgically placed as soon as the likelihood of prolonged ventilatory support is recognized to reduce the incidence of airway injury from intubation. Heated humidification of the ventilator circuit is essential in preserving airway integrity. At this point, the focus of management changes from acute ventilator weaning to preparing the patient and his or her caregivers for the patient's discharge to home on chronic ventilation. The patient should be transitioned to a portable ventilator appropriate for home use; currently, many options are available for this transition (International Ventilator Users Network, 2010).

When a pediatric patient has been ventilated for a prolonged period of time, weaning off ventilator support is a gradual process that entails ongoing assessment of weaning tolerance. This weaning process may begin in the hospital setting and continue in the outpatient setting after home discharge on a ventilator. The weaning should begin by slowly decreasing ventilator rate and volume/pressure to levels considered to be developmentally appropriate respiratory parameters for the patient. If the patient is on elevated PEEP to stent open airways due to a history of significant tracheal or bronchial malacia, consider direct visualization of the airway while the patient is awake to assess functional airway dynamics prior to slowly weaning the patient from PEEP. Direct visualization of the airway is obtained by inserting a flexible bronchoscope through the tracheostomy tube—a step that is typically performed by an otolaryngologist or pulmonologist.

Airway dynamics during the various phases of the respiratory cycle are observed while the patient remains on the ventilator, noting the presence and degree of tracheal or bronchial collapse on exhalation during rest and with increased effort (cough or cry) on varying levels of PEEP. This qualitative evaluation of functional airway dynamics provides valuable information about whether significant airway malacia is present, and if so, ideal PEEP levels for stenting the airway open and minimizing its collapse. If airway malacia has resolved, the patient on PEEP can be slowly weaned to normal levels of approximately 5 cm H_2O.

Once ventilator settings are weaned to developmentally appropriate respiratory parameters, the ventilator weaning proceeds by having the patient spend brief periods off the ventilator. While off the ventilator, the patient is closely monitored for tachypnea, increased work of breathing, tachycardia, irritability, signs of anxiety, and oxygen desaturation. Continuous $tcPO_2$ is also a useful noninvasive tool for monitoring for hypercapnia. Tolerance of ventilator weaning is determined not only by monitoring the patient's immediate physiologic response during the period off the ventilator, but also by monitoring for subtle changes in overall behavior, sleep patterns, and weight gain over time. Patients who are not tolerating ventilator weaning may become more irritable or lethargic due to fatigue, may sleep for longer periods or require naps, or may lose weight due to increased breathing effort.

If initial weaning episodes are well tolerated, the intervals of time spent off the ventilator are gradually lengthened until the patient is completely off the ventilator while awake. Ventilator weaning proceeds with brief periods off the ventilator during sleep, starting with the beginning of the sleep cycle—most ventilatory problems associated with sleep are likely to occur late in the sleep cycle. A polysomnograph study should be considered if concerns arise that an underlying sleep disorder is affecting ventilation.

For nonventilated children with CLD who have an acute pulmonary exacerbation, noninvasive CPAP or BiPAP may be used as an interim bridge for ventilatory support if support is anticipated to last for only a brief period of time. Noninvasive ventilation avoids the airway complications due to intubation, yet provides support until pulmonary function improves. Noninvasive ventilatory support may be delivered via mask or nasal cannula/pillow depending on the patient's age, comfort, and ability to form an adequate seal for ventilation.

Diuretic therapy is often initiated in the acute phase of lung disease for treatment of fluid overload or pulmonary edema, and has been shown to improve pulmonary mechanics and decrease pulmonary vascular resistance. Furosemide and bumetanide are commonly used diuretics during the acute phase of CLD, but their chronic use may result in electrolyte imbalances, nephrocalcinosis, or ototoxicity. These diuretics are typically replaced by spironolactone and thiazides, which are used in combination as a safer alternative that is associated with fewer side effects. Fluid restriction is often used in combination with diuretic therapy in the initial acute lung injury phase, and fluids are gradually liberalized as lung disease stabilizes and improves.

Pediatric patients may continue to experience hyperreactivity of the airways following acute lung injury, and some require ongoing bronchodilator therapy for relaxation of airway smooth muscle and subsequent decreased airway resistance. Bronchodilators are weaned as tolerated and administered as needed for exacerbation of reactive airway disease, which is usually associated with upper respiratory viral infections. Patients who require ongoing bronchodilator therapy should be placed on inhaled corticosteroids to prevent exacerbations of their disease. If the child remains on systemic corticosteroids that were previously required for management of acute inflammatory lung injury, these agents are slowly tapered while closely monitoring the patient for pulmonary exacerbations.

The increased energy expenditure associated with increased work of breathing necessitates higher caloric consumption in pediatric patients with CLD. Infants may need as much as 150 kcal/kg/day to maintain adequate growth. Respiratory fatigue and oromotor dysfunction due to prolonged intubation may further impede the patient's ability to achieve oral intake adequate to meet his or her caloric requirements.

Supplemental tube feedings may be required temporarily until the patient's pulmonary and oromotor function improves. If the patient requires continued fluid restriction, the formula should be concentrated to provide the maximum calories in the minimal volume. Additives such as medium-chain triglyceride oil may be used for this purpose. Regular dietary assessment is essential to assure that the child is receiving an appropriate balance of protein, carbohydrates, fat, and vitamins. Notably, excess amounts of carbohydrate can increase the carbon dioxide load on ventilation and further compromise a pediatric patient with CLD.

Dysphagia and gastroesophageal reflux should be evaluated if the initial feeding difficulties do not resolve. Evaluation and treatment of these conditions are critical in reducing the risks of aspiration and further lung damage.

Unfortunately, silent aspiration with absence of gag or cough is all too common in this population. Speech therapy should be involved early to evaluate the patient's swallow function, and any concern about the patient's ability to adequately protect the airway should be further evaluated with a fluoroscopic swallow study. If the patient is unable to swallow adequate volumes to perform this study, a radionucleotide salivagram study can be performed to evaluate swallowing of oral secretions. The latter study may be a particularly useful diagnostic tool in the patient with CLD associated with progressive neuromuscular disease who appears to be chronically aspirating oral secretions, has a tracheostomy, and is nonverbal due to developmental limitations. In this scenario, the patient may be a candidate for surgical laryngotracheal separation to protect the lungs from further injury due to aspiration. Placement of a gastrostomy tube should be considered as soon as the HCP recognizes that a patient is at risk for aspiration of oral feeds due oromotor dysfunction and will require long-term enteral tube feedings.

Gastroesophageal reflux is a common finding in infants, but typically improves over time. Nevertheless, the increased work of breathing observed in patients with CLD and the positive-pressure ventilation to treat them can exacerbate symptoms of reflux, enabling this condition to progress to GERD in both the infant and general pediatric populations. GERD should be suspected in pediatric patients with gagging, emesis, and irritability associated with feedings as well as intermittent desaturation episodes without a precipitating respiratory event. In addition, bronchoscopic findings of upper airway erythema and edema may be suggestive of chronic reflux aspiration.

Measures to control reflux should be initiated early in patients with CLD and suspected GERD to protect the lungs from acid reflux aspiration. In patients with clinical or documented GERD that is unresponsive to therapy, placement of a nasojejunal or gastrojejunal feeding tube and/or Nissen fundoplication may be considered.

Pediatric patients with acute lung disease and severe PH are frequently treated with potent pulmonary vasodilators, such as inhaled nitric oxide and parenteral prostacyclins, in the critical care setting. If the child has underlying parenchymal disease with significant V/Q mismatch, prostacyclin can worsen the V/Q mismatch. Oral vasodilators—sildenafil and bosentan—have been used successfully in treatment of PH associated with CLD that is unresponsive to traditional management. In one study involving six pediatric patients with significant CLD and severe PH, the patients showed significant clinical improvement on sildenafil and/or bosentan as measured by resolution of cardiac failure and successful weaning off oxygen (Krishnan et al., 2008). Response to oral vasodilator therapy is monitored with serial echocardiographs and BNP levels, and vasodilators are slowly tapered once PH is well controlled.

Some infants have severe PH that is refractory to bosentan and sildenafil. These children require continuous parenteral infusion of a potent prostaglandin, epoprostenol, to adequately control their PH. While some of these infants have been discharged home on parenteral epoprostenol administered via central venous catheter, there is risk of possible hypertensive crisis should they lose intravenous access due to the very short (15 minutes) drug half-life (Zaidi et al., 2005). A new parenteral prostacyclin, treprostinil, has the potential for safer home management of severe PH due to its much longer drug half-life.

Patients with CLD who have poor airway clearance of mucus and chronic atelectasis or emphysematous disease are more susceptible to viral and bacterial pulmonary infections. A tracheostomy tube also puts them at greater risk for infection due to the presence of this foreign body in the airway and the inevitable bacterial colonization of the airway. Patients with acute respiratory infection may present with fever, cough, increased tracheal secretions or sputum production, tachypnea, increased work of breathing, cyanotic episodes, and oxygen desaturation. Diffuse rhonchi, crackles, wheezing, and prolonged exhalation may be noted on auscultation. In this scenario, consider obtaining a CXR to evaluate for acute changes in the patient's condition. Sputum or tracheal aspirate may be sent for bacterial culture and Gram stain. Nasal aspirate may be sent for respiratory viral studies, including influenza, respiratory syncytial virus (RSV), parainfluenza, and adenovirus if the patient presents with symptoms consistent with viral respiratory illness.

Symptomatic management should be provided for patients with CLD who are subsequently diagnosed with viral respiratory illness. Appropriate antibiotic therapy should be provided for respiratory bacterial infections, and guided by sputum or tracheal aspirate cultures as needed. If patient has been ill with viral illness and fails to improve with symptomatic management, secondary bacterial infection should be considered and treated with appropriate antibiotic therapy.

Patients with CLD, especially those with tracheostomy tubes who experience recurrent bouts of tracheitis, may benefit from prophylactic antibiotic therapy. Those patients with tracheostomies may develop fewer acute respiratory infections if placed on cycles of inhaled nebulized tobramycin. With these children, the risk of recurrent acute infection and progression of CLD must be balanced against the risk of developing bacterial resistance due to prolonged antibiotic exposure.

In general, pediatric patients with significant or progressive CLD, those with PH, and those requiring mechanical ventilatory support should be followed by a pulmonologist. The pulmonologist is responsible for collaborating with the PCP in the management of the patient's CLD to ensure that pulmonary care is evidence based, is individualized to the patient's unique needs, and optimizes outcomes.

Pulmonary services should also be consulted if assistance is needed with the diagnostic evaluation of patients with suspected CLD or CLD due to unknown etiology, management of acute CLD exacerbation, and atypical, severe, or progressive CLD.

The pulmonologist may perform flexible bronchoscopy, if necessary, to visualize the airway for structural abnormalities such as stenosis, dynamic functional abnormalities such as tracheal or bronchial malacia, and chronic airway changes such as bronchiectasis. The bronchoscopy can be turned into a therapeutic procedure if visualized purulent secretions or mucus plugs causing airway obstruction are removed via saline lavage and suctioning. Bronchoalveolar lavage fluid is typically cultured and can facilitate diagnosis of an infectious process. In addition, determination of ideal PEEP for management of significant malacia is possible, as previously described.

Medical management of pediatric patients with CLD often requires the expertise of other specialty services to optimize treatment and outcomes. Cardiology is often a key specialty in CLD due to the tight interplay of physiology between cardiac and pulmonary function.

A cardiologist is consulted when congenital heart defects or cardiac and/or vascular disease are suspected as an underlying disorder or factor contributing to CLD. The cardiologist can determine the appropriate type of diagnostic evaluation of cardiac structure and function, including echocardiograph versus MRA or cardiac catheterization. In addition, the cardiologist can assist with pharmacologic management of congestive heart failure, pulmonary hypertension, and systemic hypertension, and can advise the HCP about any indication for interventional cardiac catheterization or cardiac surgery.

Other specialty services are consulted as specific patient needs are identified. An ear, nose, and throat (ENT) specialist is typically consulted for the management of the patient who has airway anomalies or disease, or when surgical placement of tracheostomy tube or laryngotracheal separation is indicated. Pediatric patients with suspected obstructive sleep apnea syndrome or central alveolar hypoventilation disorder should be evaluated by a sleep medicine specialist, and a polysomnograph study obtained if necessary. Gastroenterology specialists may be needed for those patients with GERD who are not responding to traditional management.

Therapists are integral members of the interprofessional team, and are typically involved with pediatric patients with CLD, particularly if developmental delay due to prolonged hospitalization or acute illness becomes an issue. Speech therapists are consulted to evaluate the patient's ability to swallow either clinically at the bedside or diagnostically through a fluoroscopic swallow study.

Ongoing oromotor therapy by speech therapists to reestablish a safe swallow in the child with CLD is key. Physical and occupational therapists are consulted to build patient strength and endurance and to improve mobility—important considerations when preparing patient for ventilator weaning. Respiratory therapists are essential in administering inhaled medications, airway clearance methods, and ventilator monitoring and adjustment as necessary. Both respiratory therapists and nurses are important sources of information when evaluating patient response to treatment and readiness for or tolerance to ventilator weaning.

Family involvement in patient care is encouraged throughout the child's hospitalization. Pediatric patient self-care is also encouraged when appropriate and is based on the patient's developmental level. Family caregiver education should include information about the patient's disease process, treatment plan, respiratory equipment, medications, and feeding regimen so that all caregivers understand the rationale and expected outcomes of care. Education should occur at the bedside so that caregivers can first observe care provided by the nursing and respiratory staff, practice their skills under guidance of the staff, and then perform care independently. Basic physical assessment skills should be integrated into the caregiver education, with emphasis on recognizing patient changes from clinical baseline and knowing when and whom to contact with medical concerns.

When they observe that fluctuations in monitor readings may occur without dire clinical events, this learning helps reinforce to caregivers that it is always important to evaluate the child first and not intervene based on the monitor alarms alone. Caregivers should be able to demonstrate competency in providing for the patient's basic care needs, such as bathing, feeding, and medication administration, as well as more complex skills such as providing gastrostomy tube care, administering oxygen therapy, troubleshooting medical equipment such as pulse oximetry monitors, administering inhalation therapy, and performing airway clearance techniques. Instruction in basic cardiopulmonary resuscitation should be considered for caregivers of patients at risk for apneic or cyanotic episodes, and is mandatory for caregivers of patients with tracheostomy tubes, as they are always at risk for acute airway obstruction.

The caregiver education process is more involved and time consuming if the patient has a tracheostomy and requires a ventilator. A requirement that at least two family caregivers be trained to tend to the patient's needs provides for a greater safety net in the home if private nursing care is not available. If the patient has a tracheostomy tube, the caregiver should be able to demonstrate the correct technique in suctioning the tube, independently change the tracheostomy tube while maintaining sterile technique, and respond appropriately in an emergency situation should the artificial airway become obstructed. Ventilator education typically requires multiple teaching sessions with the caregivers due to the technical nature of the instruction. Caregivers should be able to demonstrate competency in performance of ventilator checks to verify settings; maintenance of the ventilator, circuit, and heated humidification system; troubleshooting of ventilator alarms; and adapting the ventilator and circuit for portability away from the bedside.

Finally, education should include discussion of various emergency scenarios throughout the training period to reinforce the appropriate caregiver response in a patient emergency. One option for verifying caregiver competency is to require a 24-hour period during which the caregivers independently provide all aspects of patient care while being monitored by hospital staff. Once caregivers have successfully demonstrated their competency, they should continue to perform patient care and be encouraged to independently take patient off the inpatient unit if feasible to maintain skills and build confidence prior to discharge.

DISPOSITION AND DISCHARGE PLANNING

Limited data have been published regarding CLD outcomes and prognosis due to the complex and multifactorial nature of the problem. One study reported that VLBW and moderately LBW infants had increased hospitalizations for asthma, respiratory infections, and respiratory failure as young adults (Walter et al., 2009). In general, pediatric patients with significant CLD are likely to have some pulmonary dysfunction as adults in the form of hyperinflation, airway obstruction, and hyperreactive airways. Pulmonary function, however, tends to improve with age (Kotecha, 2008). The degree of long-term lung disease is likely related to gestational age, birth weight, presence of pediatric acute and chronic lung disease, and secondary lung injury from respiratory infections, especially infections occurring in infancy.

Discharge planning should be initiated shortly after admission, and becomes fully activated once the patient's medical requirements are understood and goals for discharge clarified. Prior to discharge, the patient should be medically stable on oxygen and a portable ventilator if indicated, should tolerate enteral feeds, and should demonstrate consistent weight gain. Significant caregiver intervention and adjustment in the treatment plan should not be required to maintain medical stability. The goal for the vast majority of pediatric patients is home discharge—even for those patients with severe CLD who require maximum support in the form of a tracheostomy, mechanical ventilator, enteral tube feedings, and continuous parenteral infusions.

Discharge planning for the pediatric patient with CLD typically includes arrangements for home medical equipment and supplies. A durable medical equipment (DME) vendor is identified to supply and maintain the equipment. Patients discharged home on oxygen will require both stationary and portable oxygen sources, as well as a pulse oximetry monitor to assess oxygen saturation levels and response to changes. A portable end-tidal CO_2 monitor may be considered for those patients who are actively weaning from ventilation. Other necessary medical supplies include tracheostomy tubes, suction catheters and machines, enteral feeding tubes and feeding pumps, and nursing supplies and dressings.

For the patient on a ventilator, home equipment needs include the portable ventilator with an appropriate circuit, and a heated humidification system. If the patient is dependent on the ventilator 24 hours per day, a second ventilator should be provided in the home as a backup in the event of mechanical failure of the primary ventilator. Ideally, home ventilators should be used on a trial basis in the hospital setting prior to the patient's discharge to assure the equipment is functioning properly and the patient is tolerating the ventilator.

Private home care nursing services may be available for those patients with significant CLD, especially for those requiring home tracheostomy and ventilator support. Patient eligibility for home nursing depends on medical criteria established by private insurance companies and state public aid agencies, which varies considerably among insurance providers and by state, respectively. Some home nursing is highly recommended, and is even a requirement in some states for pediatric patients on home ventilation due to the need for medically complex care around the clock.

The single most effective method in preventing CLD due to BPD is reduction of premature births. Recent data regarding premature births appear promising. For the first time in 30 years, there was a decrease in the premature birth rate in the United States from 2006 to 2008, when the rate declined from 12.8% to 12.3% of live births (Martin et al., 2010). While this recent trend is certainly encouraging, many preterm infants continue to be born every year who are at high risk for developing CLD. Prevention efforts to address the social and educational factors that lead to premature births should continue.

Research continues to explore factors in the antenatal period that may decrease both the incidence and the severity of BPD. Antenatal maternal administration of antibiotics when intra-amniotic infection is suspected has not decreased the incidence of BPD. Likewise, use of maternal systemic steroids to accelerate fetal lung maturation in the antenatal period has shown no or minimal effect on the incidence of BPD (Bhandari & Bhandari, 2009).

Other preventive measures focus on clinical management of BPD, particularly because of the causative relationship between oxygen toxicity and ventilator barotrauma/volutrauma and development of BPD. A meta-analysis of volume-targeted ventilation compared to pressure-limited ventilation showed no difference between methods of ventilation in terms of the severity of BPD (McCallion et al., 2005). Research efforts continue to explore various ventilation strategies, use of noninvasive ventilation, optimal targets for oxygen saturation, and use of pharmacologic agents such as systemic steroids in an attempt to reduce the incidence of BPD as well as CLD in general. The challenges of research in this area continue to be the multifactorial causes and medical complexity of CLD.

Another aspect of CLD prevention focuses on reducing the risk of additional lung injury secondary to pulmonary infection. Pediatric patients with CLD should be strongly encouraged to receive their routine childhood vaccinations as recommended by the American Academy of Pediatrics, especially pneumococcal, seasonal influenza, and H1N1 influenza vaccines. Palivizumab should be administered to CLD patients who are younger than 2 years of age during the RSV season to decrease the risk and severity of RSV bronchiolitis. Patients and caregivers should be advised to avoid direct contact with ill individuals, and use of good hand washing techniques should be emphasized. Prompt evaluation and treatment of acute respiratory illnesses is imperative.

CONGENITAL CENTRAL HYPOVENTILATION SYNDROME

Daniel J. Lesser

PATHOPHYSIOLOGY

Congenital central hypoventilation syndrome (CCHS), previously known as "Ondine's curse," is characterized by inadequate respiration secondary to a defect of central nervous system (CNS) control of breathing. This disease is now more accurately considered a generalized disorder of the autonomic nervous system (Weese-Mayer et al., 2009). Studies of respiratory control suggest that the *PHOX2B* gene defect causes an abnormality of integration of the chemoreceptors responsible for automatic control of breathing, ultimately leading to abnormal function of ventilatory muscles and inadequate ventilation (Paton et al., 1989). Individuals with CCHS do not respond to elevated levels of carbon dioxide or decreased levels of oxygen; consequently. they cannot be trusted to breathe on their own.

EPIDEMIOLOGY AND ETIOLOGY

CCHS is caused by a defect in the *PHOX2B* homeobox gene (Amiel et al., 2003). Although the mutation usually occurs spontaneously, siblings with CCHS and children of CCHS parents have been described (Silvestri et al., 2002; Sritippayawan et al., 2002; Weese-Mayer et al., 2003). The inheritance pattern of CCHS is autosomal dominant (Silvestri et al.; Sritippayawan et al.).

Although its exact incidence is not known, CCHS is rare. In addition to disordered respiration, this disease is associated with increased incidence of Hirschsprung's disease, tumors of neural crest origin, ophthalmologic dysfunction, and cardiac conduction system abnormalities (Weese-Mayer et al., 1999).

PRESENTATION

Pediatric patients with CCHS often present with respiratory symptoms in the newborn period (Marcus et al., 1991). Some infants may fail to breathe at birth, while others may present in the first several months of life with severe apnea, respiratory arrest, an apparent life-threatening event (ALTE), or cor pulmonale (Marcus et al., 1991). Common physical examination findings include cyanosis, tachycardia, diaphoresis, lethargy, and apnea. Respiratory findings associated with CCHS worsen with sleep. Furthermore, children with CCHS do not show classic signs of respiratory distress (tachypnea, chest wall retractions) when faced with a challenge to the respiratory system.

DIFFERENTIAL DIAGNOSIS

If a child is suspected of having CCHS, alternative diagnoses such as congenital cardiac disease, primary pulmonary disease, metabolic disease, and intracranial pathology should also be considered (Chen & Keens, 2004). Infants with a finding of severe hypoxemia should first be evaluated for pulmonary or cardiac disease, as these entities occur more commonly than CCHS. In addition, metabolic disease and structural pathology of the CNS may first present with hypoventilation and should be considered when evaluating a child with elevated levels of carbon dioxide.

PLAN OF CARE

Gene testing for mutation in the *PHOX2B* gene is available for individuals suspected of having CCHS. The majority of children with CCHS have the abnormal gene *PHOX2B*; thus this test is considered by many to be diagnostic. While gene testing is pending, the following diagnostic studies should be completed: echocardiograph, CXR, MRI of the brain, and further evaluation for metabolic disease (Chen & Keens, 2004). Polysomnography reveals hypoventilation, hypoxemia, frequent arousal, and decreased minute ventilation (Huang et al., 2008).

Therapeutic management of CCHS aims to normalize ventilation during the time when patients are not able to achieve adequate gas exchange (Weese-Mayer et al., 1999). Individuals with CCHS do not breathe adequately on their own, so they require some form of assisted ventilation for at least part of a 24-hour day (Weese-Mayer et al., 1999). Supplemental oxygen alone is not adequate for the treatment of CCHS—this therapy will improve oxygen levels but will not correct hypoventilation. A variety of methods of assisted ventilation have been used in pediatric patients, including positive-pressure ventilation via tracheostomy, noninvasive positive airway pressure ventilation via nasal or face mask, negative-pressure ventilation, and diaphragmatic pacing (Marcus et al., 1991). When choosing a mode of assisted ventilation, the advantages and disadvantages of each type are weighed carefully against the individual needs of the patient and family.

Specialists in pediatric respiratory medicine often manage assisted ventilation in CCHS. In addition, pediatric patients with CCHS may receive care from pediatric neurologists, cardiologists, gastroenterologists, and ophthalmologists. Finally, respiratory therapists, nurses with expertise in home mechanical ventilation and tracheostomy care, and nutritionists contribute substantially to the care of pediatric patients with this disorder.

CCHS profoundly impacts the lives of affected children and their families. Families should be made aware that children with CCHS can manifest rapid cardiopulmonary decompensation when assisted ventilation is not used as prescribed. Pediatric patients with CCHS are especially vulnerable during sleep, episodic illnesses, and exposure to anesthetics. Caregivers should be taught to be vigilant about providing appropriate assisted ventilation and monitoring, as recommended by their HCP (Grigg-Damberger & Wells, 2009).

DISPOSITION AND DISCHARGE PLANNING

Chronic hypoxia can lead to long-term neurologic sequelae. Thus early diagnosis and treatment of CCHS are likely to improve the patient's long-term outcome. Patients who do not receive assisted ventilation continue to hypoventilate and eventually develop cor pulmonale due to chronic hypercapnia. Pediatric patients with CCHS who are adequately ventilated can grow and develop normally, although a significant number manifest learning disabilities (Silvestri et al., 1992).

CCHS is a lifelong disorder for which there is no cure at this time. Pediatric patients with CCHS require chronic ventilatory support, as the respiratory abnormalities associated with this disorder do not improve (Paton et al., 1989). Substantial medical and psychosocial complexities are associated with this disease (Vanderlaan et al., 2004). Despite the challenges of the disorder, however, patients with CCHS can fully develop to lead fulfilling lives.

It is recommended that children with CCHS be followed closely, especially during infancy and early childhood. Those who require assisted ventilation in the home will need coordinated care by multiple HCPs, including physicians, therapists, nurses, and social workers.

Critical Thinking

Pediatric patients with CCHS presenting with seizure or severe lethargy should be considered to have hypoventilation. They should be hyperventilated with supplemental oxygen until the source of the problem can be identified.

FOREIGN BODY ASPIRATION

Minnette Markus-Rodden

PATHOPHYSIOLOGY

A complete or near complete obstruction of the larynx or trachea will cause immediate asphyxia and death. Objects aspirated that are able to pass further along the airway and pass the level of the carina will come to rest at a location dependent upon the age and position of the patient and the characteristics of the object itself. The characteristics of the foreign body aspiration (FBA) and its anatomical location may contribute to further airway obstruction by causing local inflammation, edema, and the formation of granulation tissue.

The types of foreign bodies aspirated vary internationally depending on the individual customs and diets (Tan et al., 2000). Nonfood items are more commonly aspirated in older pediatric patients, but aspiration of food items is common to all age groups. High-risk objects such as nuts, raw vegetables and fruits, and beans can rapidly expand as they absorb moisture, leading to further obstruction (Delghani & Ludemann, 2008).

EPIDEMIOLOGY AND ETIOLOGY

Foreign body aspiration in the pediatric population is a common occurrence. In the United States, more than 17,000 emergency department (ED) visits for aspiration were made by patients 14 years of age or younger in 2000; of those children, 160 died (Schroeder et al., 2002). Pediatric patients aged 9 to 30 months have a decreased ability to protect their airways as compared to adults. They are prone to FBA as a result of their immature neuromuscular swallowing mechanisms, lack of molar teeth, new mobility, and oral orientation (Hill & Voight, 2000). Individuals with underlying neurological disorders or under the influence of drugs or alcohol are also at an increased risk of foreign body aspiration.

PRESENTATION

Prompt diagnosis and management of foreign body aspiration is essential. A detailed history and physical examination, particularly inquiring about any past episodes of violent paroxysmal coughing, must be performed on every patient presenting with possible foreign body aspiration. Most patients will present with coughing/gagging/choking, wheezing, respiratory distress, and fever (Schmidt & Manegold, 2000). Patients may die as a result of a foreign body aspiration while being asymptomatic; therefore, a lack of symptoms should not be viewed as ruling

out the possibility of foreign body aspiration (Schmidt & Manegold).

With the exception to complete airway obstruction, FBA proceeds through three stages of symptoms: the initial event, an asymptomatic period, and symptoms of ensuing complications (Tan et al., 2000). It is common for caregivers to believe the item has been successfully coughed up after the coughing subsides (Schmidt & Manegold, 2000).

DIFFERENTIAL DIAGNOSIS

The differential diagnosis primarily depends on the location of the foreign body and the characteristics of the object. Delay in diagnosis is not uncommon. Most often this problem is due to misdiagnosis by the HCP who relies on negative radiographic studies or a negative history. The caregiver may minimize a history of a coughing or choking episode so that the significance of the event is forgotten. Many of the symptoms of aspiration, such as coughing, wheezing, and decreased breath sounds, are similar to other common childhood illnesses. Differential diagnoses, therefore, include asthma, upper respiratory illness, and pneumonia.

PLAN OF CARE

Several diagnostic studies may aid in the diagnosis of foreign body. A CXR that includes the following positions is most helpful: posterior–anterior views, lateral decubitus views, and inspiration/expiration. On CXR, tracheal foreign bodies typically position themselves in the vertical plane. Inspiratory and expiratory CXRs are helpful in the cooperative pediatric patient, to assess for unilateral air trapping. If it is impossible to obtain these films, then bilateral decubitus CXR obtained during inspiration may allow for evaluation of exhalation and lung deflation (Schunk, 2006). Typically, when the patient is in the decubitus position, the dependent lung will deflate. If the foreign body is located within the bronchial tree, the affected side may have diminished or absent deflation.

Additional imaging studies that prove to be more definitive when CXRs are limited included chest fluoroscopy, CT scan, and bronchoscopy.

In the prehospital setting, acute life-threatening events as a result of foreign body aspiration are treated with back blows and chest compressions in infants, and abdominal thrusts in the older child. If these methods are not successful in removing the foreign body, immediate direct visualization and manual removal is required. Foreign bodies in the lower respiratory tract require removal by rigid bronchoscopy or flexible endocscopy under general anesthesia. Rarely a thoracotomy is necessary (Schunk, 2006). The value of rapid diagnosis and treatment cannot be underestimated as a means to avoid complications associated with anoxia.

Primary management of foreign body aspiration is determined by the condition of the patient as well as by individual hospital policy. Typically, pediatric general surgeons or pediatric otolaryngologists will provide diagnostic and therapeutic interventions. If the patient presents in extremis and the airway is difficult to maintain, however, a consult with the critical care team or anesthesiologist may be required.

The pediatric patient with no postoperative complications or with minimal postoperative risk factors is typically discharged to home within 24 hours. Specific instructions should be provided regarding appropriate food choices, product safety labeling of toys, and child-proofing the environment based on the age of the pediatric patient. Caregivers should also be offered training in how to provide first aid and choking rescue procedures.

DISPOSITION AND DISCHARGE PLANNING

Pediatric patients who have undergone bronchoscopic or endoscopic removal of aspirated foreign bodies and have no operative complications and minimal postoperative risk factors are typically discharged home within 24 hours. Complications of FBA and patient comorbidities may require further medical management within the hospital setting. Admission and discharge criteria should be based on individual risk factors and presentation.

LUNG TRANSPLANTATION

Samuel B. Goldfarb

Bilateral lung transplantation is considered when all other therapies for advanced lung disease have been exhausted. Lung transplantation is an elective procedure that is not indicated for all patients with this type of disease. The most common indication for bilateral lung transplant in the pediatric (0 to 18 years of age) population is cystic fibrosis; the second most common condition is pulmonary hypertension (PH). Other indications are retransplant for bronchiolitis obliterans and congenital heart disease (Aurora et al., 2009).

INDICATIONS

The indication for bilateral lung transplantation in candidates depends largely on the underlying diagnosis. In patients with CF, the trajectory of illness that, despite optimal medical therapy, puts the individual at risk of dying without a lung transplant is the indication for transplant.

Factors that would contribute to the timing of listing for lung transplantation include a baseline FEV_1 that is less than 30% of the predicted value, hypoxemia at rest ($PaO_2 <$ 55 mmHg), worsening severity of hypercapnia, a female or pediatric patient with rapid clinical decline in lung function, and frequent pulmonary exacerbations requiring IV antibiotic therapy with no improvement or worsening of lung function. In patients with PH, indications include New York Heart Association/World Health Organization (WHO) functional class III or IV, rapidly progressive disease, elevated right atrial pressures exceeding 15 mmHg, a cardiac index of less than 2 L/min/m², or failing medical therapy (Oren et al., 2006).

Prior to May 2005, a patient's chance to receive a lung transplantation was based on time accrued on a waiting list and patient/donor blood type; the likelihood of surviving to transplantation was not considered in determining the listing order. Recognizing that many patients died waiting for a suitable donor, investigators have tried to develop methods that predict when the topic of lung transplantation should be discussed with patients and when in the disease course patients should be placed on the transplant list.

Since May 2005, the process of prioritizing patients for lung transplantation has been based on a scoring system known as the Lung Allocation Score (LAS). Transplant candidates who are 12 years of age or older are listed according to the new system. Patients younger than 12 years receive organs based on time accrued on a waiting list. The LAS is calculated from estimates of survival probability while on the lung transplant waiting list and following transplantation. It reflects a comprehensive evaluation that takes into account age and diagnosis as well as several indicators of disease severity, such as FEV_1, body mass index (BMI), serum creatinine, presence of diabetes, 6-minute walk test score, increases in supplemental oxygen need, serum carbon dioxide levels (PCO_2), need for assisted ventilation, functional status, and presence of PH (Egan et al., 2006; Oren et al., 2006; United Network for Organ Sharing [UNOS], n.d.). The referral process to a transplant center should be initiated when a patient's FEV_1 is less than 30% of the predicted value, or sooner if there has been a rapid decline in pulmonary function for patients with primary lung disease. Beginning this process, however, does not imply that the patient will be immediately listed. Other considerations for referral include recurrent hemoptysis that is not controlled by embolization or other means, recurrent or refractory pneumothorax, and frequent respiratory exacerbations requiring antibiotic therapy (Kreider & Kotloff, 2009; Oren et al., 2006). Education of potential candidates regarding bilateral lung transplantation as a future treatment modality can occur as a patient's lung disease worsens. For patients with PH, referral is made when the individual experiences worsening cardiac function or a decline in the effectiveness of pharmacological treatment.

Any patient considered for transplantation must have an adequate social support system and must be able to follow the prescribed medical regimen after transplant. Bilateral lung transplant is an elective procedure; therefore, potential recipients and their families must demonstrate willingness and an ability to adhere to the rigorous therapy, daily monitoring, and reevaluation schedule after transplant (Faro et al., 2007).

CONTRAINDICATIONS

Several absolute contraindications for bilateral lung transplant exist. These conditions include malignancy within the last two years (some centers recommend a five-year disease-free period); infections that include sepsis, active tuberculosis, acquired immunodeficiency syndrome, or hepatitis B or C with histological liver disease; multiple organ dysfunction. severe neuromuscular disease; and documented refractory nonadherence to a medical regimen (Faro et al., 2007; Oren et al., 2006).

Relative contraindications to bilateral lung transplant occur include kidney insufficiency, markedly abnormal BMI, osteoporosis, poorly controlled diabetes mellitus (DM), and colonization with resistant organisms (Faro et al., 2007). Significant kidney dysfunction prior to transplantation can disqualify a patient from the procedure because of the risk of worsening renal function in the post-transplant period. Notably, the use of aminoglycosides in patients with CF is associated with a decline in kidney function (Al-Aloul et al., 2005). Moreover, following transplant there is an increased incidence of chronic kidney insufficiency from use of immunosuppressive medications. One study demonstrated that in the first 3 months post transplant, patients had a 33% decline in glomerular filtration rate (Benden et al., 2009). These findings were in accord with International Society of Heart and Lung Transplantation (ISHLT) registry data that reported a prevalence of hypertension at one year post transplant of 39% and a prevalence of renal dysfunction, as measured by changes in serum creatinine, during the same time frame of roughly 9% (Boucek et al., 2007). Thus judicious use of antibiotics in the pretransplant period to spare kidney function is very important.

Nutritional status affects both pre- and post-transplant mortality. Wasting, defined as a weight less than 85% of the ideal body weight, has been shown to be a predictor of mortality in the pretransplant CF patient independent of lung function, arterial blood oxygen, or carbon dioxide levels (Sharma et al., 2001). In addition, when evaluating all subjects awaiting transplantation, lean body mass depletion has been associated with more severe hypoxemia, reduced 6-minute walking distance, and a higher mortality; even in the setting of a normal BMI (Schwebel et al., 2000). In contrast, in both CF and non-CF transplant candidates, severe obesity is a significant indicator of post-transplant

mortality. A BMI exceeding 27 kg/m^2 was the greatest indicator of mortality in the first 90 days post transplant, whereas in those with a BMI of less than 17 kg/m^2, only a statistically nonsignificant trend was demonstrated toward increased mortality (Madill et al., 2001).

The degree of preexisting bone demineralization represents a major risk factor for severe osteoporosis following lung transplantation (Aris et al., 1996). Corticosteroids, which are used as part of the immunosuppression regimen following transplant, contribute to bone disease by hastening bone resorption and inhibiting bone formation. Ideally, steroid dosing will be gradually reduced to minimize the complications of long-term use (Knoop et al., 2004). The use of antiresorptive therapy to improve bone mineral density has expanded to include lung transplant recipients. While the use of biphosphonates in adults with bone disease shows promise, the long-term efficacy and safety of biphosphonate use in children and adolescents requires further investigation.

In the post-transplant period, there is an increased association of drug-related new-onset DM in the pediatric lung and heart/lung transplant population when compared to either pediatric heart transplant recipients or adult lung transplant recipients (Alvarez et al., 2005; Bradbury et al., 2008; Wagner et al., 1997). Twenty-five percent of all transplanted patients develop DM within the first year following a lung transplant (Aurora et al., 2007). CF patients with cystic fibrosis–related diabetes (CFRD) prior to transplant have more complication-related admissions to hospital post transplant and a higher mortality rate than those without CFRD who undergo transplant (Bradbury et al.). These findings underscore the importance of both pre- and post-transplant management of DM.

TRANSPLANT

Double-lung bilateral sequential transplantation is the procedure of choice in the pediatric population. The survival rate of children undergoing single-lung transplantation was significantly lower than the survival of children receiving bilateral transplants, so the former procedure has been abandoned in this population (Aurora et al., 2008). Organs are matched by height, weight, and blood type. HLA antibody screening is performed, and specific antibodies can be avoided if the recipient has elevated levels.

IMMUNOSUPPRESSIVE THERAPY

Most centers have adopted the immunosuppression protocol set forth by the International Pediatric Lung Transplant Consortium. Triple therapy with or without induction therapy has become standard practice. Roughly 40% of the pediatric centers reporting to the ISHLT use induction

TABLE 35-17

Complications of Lung Transplantation	
Early	**Late**
Hyperacute rejection	Acute rejection
Acute rejection	Chronic rejection/bronchiolitis
Demyelinating disease (due to	obliterans
tacrolimus or cyclosporine)	Bronchiolitis obliterans
Seizure disorder	syndrome
Ectopic atrial tachycardia (EAT)	Infection
Infection	EBV
Bacterial (including atypical	CMV
mycobacterium)	HHV6
Viral (CMV, adenovirus, RSV)	Diabetes
Fungal (*Aspergillus*)	Hypertension
Other (PCP)	Kidney insufficiency/failure
Anastomosis dehiscence	Post-transplant
	lymphoproliferative disease
	Osteoporosis

Note: Cytomegalovirus (CMV), respiratory syncytial virus (RSV), *Pneumocystis jirovecii* pneumonia (PCP), Epstein-Barr virus (EBV), human herpes virus 6 (HHV6).

therapy in the post-transplant period. The majority of patients are given tacrolimus along with either azathioprine or mycophenolate. All centers, at 1 and 5 years post transplant, report the use of oral steroids as part of immunosuppressive therapy (Aurora et al., 2008, 2009).

COMPLICATIONS

Complications from lung transplantation are divided into early and late issues (Table 35-17). Several that warrant special notice are reviewed in the remainder of this section.

Acute rejection

The risk of acute cellular rejection (ACR) is highest in the first few weeks following transplantation. The incidence of ACR ranges from 18% to 50% among those who undergo induction therapy and from 50% to 55% among those who do not (Brock et al., 2001; Knoop et al., 2004; Palmer et al., 1999). Acute rejection is an infrequent problem beyond 1 year post transplant. Notably, infants tend to have a lower frequency of acute rejection than do older children. Risk factors for ACR include HLA mismatching, community-acquired viral infection, and the immunosuppressive regimen (Martinu et al., 2009).

Although acute rejection is often asymptomatic, fever, dyspnea, and hypoxemia can be present. Common findings on chest radiograph include parenchymal densities and bilateral pleural effusions. The FEV_1 and FVC can be diminished.

Distinguishing between rejection and infection on clinical grounds alone is often difficult. Therefore, appropriate evaluation includes bronchoscopy with bronchoalveolar lavage and transbronchial biopsy.

Acute rejection is graded from A0 (none) to A4 (severe); grade A2 acute rejection and higher grades are treated with augmented immunosuppression. The initial therapy is usually pulsed steroids. The few patients in whom acute rejection persists usually respond favorably to additional augmented immunosuppression, usually consisting of a monoclonal or polyclonal T-cell antibody.

Infection

As many as 60% to 90% of lung transplant recipients experience at least one episode of infection after undergoing the procedure (Kanj et al., 1997; Kramer et al., 1993). The risk for serious infection starts in the perioperative period, and infection is the major cause of morbidity and mortality during the first 6 months after transplant surgery. For this reason, prophylactic antimicrobial agents against bacteria, viruses, and fungi are used in most transplant programs. Antimicrobial treatments should be given perioperatively based on donor cultures and the most common hospital pathogens. In the CF population, antibiotic therapy is directed by bacterial sputum colonization and the antibiogram. *Pneumocystis jirovecii* prophylaxis is routine in almost all postoperative lung transplant regimens.

The severity of respiratory viral infections can range from relatively mild to life-threatening in transplant recipients. Respiratory syncytial virus (RSV), influenza, human herpes viruses (particularly HHV6), Epstein-Barr virus, and adenovirus cause significant morbidity and mortality in this population. Cytomegalovirus (CMV) remains the most commonly encountered serious viral infection. The onset of CMV pneumonitis after lung transplant is reported to have a strong correlation with subsequent development of bronchiolitis obliterans, which in turn leads to graft dysfunction and death (Metras et al., 1999). The highest risk for CMV pneumonia is in seronegative patients who receive lungs from seropositive donors. This increased risk persists even when these patients receive aggressive antiviral prophylaxis (Metras et al.). In the pediatric population, respiratory viral infections are associated with an increased mortality at 1 year post transplant (Liu et al., 2009). In this population, an etiology of underlying disease other than CF, younger age, and absence of induction therapy are independently associated with risk of respiratory viral infections (Liu et al.).

While colonization with *Aspergillus* can be as high as 50% in post-transplant patients, invasive disease occurs in only 3% and only in patients colonized with *A. fumigatus* within the first 6 months post transplant (Cahill et al., 1997). Antifungal therapy before and after transplant is, therefore, an important component of care. Risk factors for pulmonary fungal infections in children include grade A2 rejection, repeated acute rejection, a CMV-positive donor, a tacrolimus-based regimen, and pretransplant *Aspergillus* colonization (Danziger-Isakov et al., 2008).

Bronchiolitis obliterans

Bronchiolitis obliterans (BO) is the histopathological correlate of chronic organ dysfunction. It is the leading cause of morbidity and late mortality 1 year after lung or heart–lung transplantation. This inflammatory process ultimately leads to occlusion of small airways by fibromyxoid tissue (Boehler & Estenne, 2003). Both BO and bronchiolitis obliterans syndrome (BOS), the clinical correlate of OB, are manifestations of chronic lung allograft rejection. BOS describes the otherwise unexplained development of an obstructive decrease in pulmonary function. The cardinal clinical feature of BOS is a reduction in FEV_1 or the midexpiratory flow rate (FEF_{25-75}), which does not respond to bronchodilators (Estenne et al., 2002). Roughly one-half of all lung transplant recipients are diagnosed with BO by 5 years after transplant. More than 40% of deaths occurring beyond 1 year post transplant are a direct or indirect result of BO (Aurora et al., 2008).

The etiology of BO remains elusive despite a growing body of basic science and clinical research. Gastroesophageal reflux (GER) has been shown to have an increased association with BO. Furthermore, surgical correction of GER has, in some patients, either stopped or improved the decline in lung function (Davis et al., 2003; O'Halloran et al., 2004; Palmer et al., 2000).

There is no consistently effective treatment strategy for BO. Augmentation of immunosuppression is usually the initial intervention. Options include antithymocyte preparations, cyclophosphamide, methotrexate, photopheresis, and total lymphoid irradiation. All have shown benefit in some patients, but none has proven to be uniformly beneficial (Estenne & Hertz, 2002). Aerosolized cyclosporine is an investigational agent with substantial promise that may provide a survival advantage to lung transplant recipients (Iacono et al., 2004). The use of tacrolimus as a "rescue" therapy in patients who were originally treated with cyclosporine may stabilize the decline in FEV_1 (Sarahrudi et al., 2004). Sirolimus has also been used as a "rescue" agent in BO with some success (Hernandez et al., 2005; Snell & Westall, 2007). Several studies focusing on azithromycin administration, for its anti-inflammatory effect, have shown either improvement or stabilization of lung function (Gottlieb et al., 2008; Shitrit et al., 2005; Verleden & Dupont, 2004). A retrospective study of patients prescribed statins for hypercholesterolemia found a lower incidence of BO and a better long-term survival. Retransplantation may be an option in some individuals.

LIFE EXPECTANCY

Outcomes for bilateral lung transplantation have improved since the early 1990s, when the procedure was first introduced. Survival is the chief indicator of success for this procedure. Survival of pediatric patients is similar to that of adults, with a median survival of 4.3 years being reported over the period 1990–2006. The major cause of death continues to be BO.

There is a survival advantage to children with lung disease of all causes who are transplanted while they are from 1 to 10 years of age when compared to adolescents (Magee et al., 2008). Several hypotheses have been proposed to explain this survival difference. For example, one factor may be that younger patients have fewer episodes of acute rejection and a lower incidence of BO (Ibrahim et al., 2002). Alternatively, this advantage may arise because the adolescent population predominately consists of patients with CF. Studies have also raised concerns that the adolescent age group is more prone to decreased adherence to medical regimens, which in turn may affect long-term survival (De Geest et al., 2005; White et al., 2009; Wray et al., 2006). The risk of early death (within the first 30 days following transplant) attributed to infection is elevated only in patients colonized with *Burkholderia cepacia* complex, whereas no other organisms conferred a survival disadvantage (Meachery et al., 2008).

OBSTRUCTIVE SLEEP APNEA *SYNDROME*

Daniel J. Lesser

PATHOPHYSIOLOGY

Obstructive sleep apnea syndrome (OSAS) occurs commonly in pediatric patients and is associated with severe complications when left untreated (American Academy of Pediatrics [AAP], 2002). The key component of OSAS relates to intermittent obstruction of the upper airway during sleep, resulting in sleep fragmentation and oxygen desaturation (American Thoracic Society [ATS], 1996). Airway obstruction occurs secondary to an anatomically narrow upper airway and/or abnormal upper airway neuromotor tone. An episode of complete or even partial upper airway obstruction may lead to inadequate gas exchange, characterized by hypoxemia and hypercapnia. Eventually, an apnea episode is terminated by the central nervous system with arousal, and respiration is restored (Ward & Marcus, 1996).

EPIDEMIOLOGY AND ETIOLOGY

Although snoring has been estimated to occur in 12% to 20% of school-aged children, OSAS has a prevalence closer to 2% to 3% (Halbower et al., 2007). The peak prevalence of OSAS occurs in children 2 to 8 years of age, usually due to enlargement of the tonsils and adenoids relative to airway size (Marcus, 2001). Nasal obstruction, craniofacial abnormalities, fat deposition in the pharynx, and altered neuromotor tone may also contribute to the etiology of OSAS. Children with craniofacial anomalies, genetic disorders, obesity, cerebral palsy, and neuromuscular disease have an increased incidence of OSAS.

PRESENTATION

Presenting signs and symptoms of OSAS vary with age. Most pediatric patients come to medical attention due to loud snoring, gasping, and labored breathing during sleep (Ward & Marcus, 1996). Toddlers and preschool-aged children may display agitated sleep in addition to noisy breathing and snoring. During wakefulness, younger children with OSAS may also show signs of aggressive behavior, hyperactivity, and inattention. In school-aged children, complaints of agitated sleep, difficulty waking up in the morning, daytime fatigue, and learning difficulties should raise concern for the presence of OSAS (Guilleminault et al., 2005).

DIFFERENTIAL DIAGNOSIS

OSAS must be differentiated from primary snoring, which is defined as snoring without obstructive apnea, frequent arousals from sleep, or gas exchange abnormalities (AAP, 2002). In addition to OSAS, a complaint of daytime sleepiness may be explained by a number of other sleep-related disorders that can occur in pediatric patients, including inadequate total sleep time, delayed sleep phase syndrome, central sleep apnea, and restless leg syndrome. Finally, OSAS should be considered in the differential diagnosis of the child who presents with symptoms of attention-deficit/hyperactivity disorder.

PLAN OF CARE

History and physical examination alone are unreliable when used to distinguish children with primary snoring from those with OSAS (Carroll et al., 1995). Thus polysomnography (sleep study) is the recommended diagnostic test to evaluate children with sleep-related complaints (AAP, 2002). Polysomnography may be used to evaluate the severity of OSAS by quantifying the number of airway obstructions that occur during sleep, assessing for the presence and degree of hypoxemia or hypoventilation, and identifying sleep fragmentation. Other diagnostic tests useful in the work-up of suspected OSAS include blood gas analysis to screen for hypoventilation, echocardiograph to evaluate for pulmonary hypertension, and lateral radiograph of the neck.

Most children with OSAS should be evaluated by an otolaryngologist for consideration of removal of the tonsils and adenoids (AAP, 2002). Children with severe OSAS

undergoing tonsillectomy/adenoidectomy require careful postoperative monitoring and may need to be observed in the hospital after surgery (Ward & Marcus, 1996). In addition, children undergoing the procedure who are very young (younger than 3 years) should be closely monitored. Postoperative respiratory complications of adenotonsillectomy may include hypoxemia, persistent oxygen requirement, and postobstructive pulmonary edema. Children with preexisting OSAS who are undergoing surgical procedures for other medical problems are also at increased risk for postoperative respiratory complications and require careful monitoring. Treatment of preexisting OSAS before elective surgery should be considered.

When used for treatment of OSAS, noninvasive positive-pressure ventilation may often be accomplished through the use of CPAP. A mask interface is attached to the nose and/or mouth and connected to a ventilator that delivers positive pressure to maintain airway patency during sleep. Titration of CPAP settings should occur during polysomnography (Kushida et al., 2008). During CPAP titration in a sleep laboratory, pressures on the CPAP machine are adjusted to alleviate obstructive apnea, markers of sleep fragmentation, and snoring (Kushida et al.). Ideal CPAP settings vary among individuals, and there are no recommended settings based on age or weight. It is currently recommended that pediatric patients requiring CPAP for OSAS be started on a pressure of 4 cm H_2O in a sleep laboratory with further titration to relieve signs of OSAS.

If a child with OSAS is judged to have enlarged tonsils or adenoids, referral to an otolaryngologist is recommended. Neurologic disease or behavior disorders sometimes present with sleep complaints, and consultation with a pediatric neurologist or pediatric sleep behavior disorders specialist may be indicated. If OSAS is refractory to surgery or surgery is not indicated, referral to a pediatric pulmonologist with experience in NIV should be pursued.

After treatment, families are counseled to monitor for return or persistence of symptoms. Ideally, nutritional intervention regarding weight loss and prevention of excessive weight gain will decrease the risk of recurrence of OSAS in obese pediatric patients.

When NV is indicated, a detailed description of the mask interface before it is actually introduced during sleep may increase adherence. If the actual mask is not readily available, then handouts containing descriptions and pictures of the device may be given to families. It is often helpful to remind families that when NIV is used to treat OSAS, it will be used only during sleep—not when the child is engaging in his or her daily activities. After NIV is initiated, families should be counseled regarding possible side effects of wearing the mask, such as skin breakdown and drying of the eyes. Prompt response by HCPs to concerns regarding NIV should improve adherence to the use of the device.

DISPOSITION AND DISCHARGE PLANNING

Although many children improve in terms of their OSAS after adenotonsillectomy, obesity is a risk factor for recurrence (Tauman et al., 2006). In the long term, untreated OSAS in pediatric patients has been linked to neurocognitive impairment, behavioral problems, failure-to-thrive, and cor pulmonale (heart failure secondary to pulmonary hypertension) (Ward & Marcus, 1996). Furthermore, children with undiagnosed OSAS who undergo anesthesia are at increased risk for complications.

Some children may have persistence of snoring post adenotonsillectomy related to postoperative swelling of the upper airway. Thus careful follow-up to monitor for resolution of symptoms is recommended. Polysomnography after surgical treatment of OSAS is recommended in children with persistent symptoms and those with additional risk factors, such as Down syndrome, morbid obesity, or craniofacial syndromes (Marcus, 2001). If OSAS persists post adenotonsillectomy or a child is not a candidate for this operation, then NIV may be indicated (AAP, 2002).

Pediatric OSAS is a relatively prevalent disease process with important implications for long-term cardiovascular and neurocognitive health. Considering the recent increase in pediatric obesity, children with OSAS will be cared for with increased frequency in a number of health care settings. Familiarity with the diagnostic evaluation, complications, and treatment options of OSAS will optimize the care of affected children.

Critical Thinking

Children with risk factors for OSAS should be carefully screened for the presence of obstructive sleep apnea before undergoing elective surgical procedures.

PERTUSSIS

Christine Agee and Jon Meliones

PATHOPHYSIOLOGY

Pertussis is more commonly known as "whooping cough" due to the typical whooping sound that occurs during inspiration of air after the cough. The causative agent in this infection is *Bordetella pertussis,* an aerobic, nonmotile, Gram-negative coccobacillus. Transmission occurs on a human-to-human basis by aerosol droplets. The bacteria multiply on the respiratory epithelium first in the nasopharynx, and then progress to the bronchi and bronchioles. The resultant mucopurulosanguineous exudate compromises small airways and may lead to respiratory failure. Progression of the disease is directly related to the development of marked airway obstruction due to thickened secretions, alveolar atelectasis due to loss of surfactant, and pulmonary hypertension secondary to the hypoxia.

EPIDEMIOLOGY AND ETIOLOGY

Pertussis is the most common vaccine-preventable disease in children younger than 5 years of age (CDC, 2006c)—and its incidence is rising. In 2007, more than 10,000 children in the United States (3.6 per 100,000 population) were reported to have this infection (CDC, 2009). More than 70% of infections occur in children younger than 5 years of age, and 10% to 15% occurs in infants younger than 6 months of age. The most severe cases occur in infants younger than 1 year of age.

Pertussis is highly contagious, with 80% to 90% of those exposed developing the disease (He et al., 1998). Infection typically occurs in late summer and early fall and is endemic every 3 to 5 years. Adults and adolescents are the primary reservoir, and transmission risk increases as their immunity wanes. Individuals are most contagious during the catarrhal stage (Table 35-18); however, because symptoms are nonspecific during this phase, pertussis is usually not diagnosed. It is not until the appearance of the characteristic cough of the paroxysmal stage that diagnosis occurs, when widespread transmission has already occurred. *Bordetella parapertussis* is clinically indistinguishable from *Bordetella pertussis,* but the clinical course of *B. parapertussis* infection is usually milder than that of *B. pertussis* infection (Bortolussi et al., 1995).

Infants can easily become fatigued with the incessant coughing and post-tussive emesis, leading to inadequate oral intake, dehydration, or respiratory failure. Intermittent apnea may also occur in infants and is often associated with paroxysmal coughing; it may occur spontaneously as well, and may be related to vagal stimulation (He et al., 1998). Pneumonia can be a primary manifestation or due to a secondary bacterial infection. Seizures occur in 1% to 2% of infants younger than 6 months of age with pertussis. With severe disease, encephalopathy may develop. The cause of the encephalopathy is unknown but may be related to hypoxia associated with cough, lymphocyte plugging, or intracerebral hemorrhage; this complication is rare, occurring in fewer than 0.4% of patients. Death occurs in fewer than 1% of patients with pertussis, although this risk increases in those younger than 2 months of age, with leukocytosis, or with pneumonia (Mikelova et al., 2003; Southall et al., 1988; Von Konig, 2005).

PRESENTATION

Historical questions to help differentiate pertussis from other respiratory conditions include the immunization status of the patient and his or her caregivers and exposure to an adult with a cough, especially one that is more intense at night.

The characteristic presentation of pertussis occurs in three main stages: catarrhal, paroxysmal, and convalescent (Table 35-18). An incubation period of 7 to 14 days precedes these phases. During this time the patient is asymptomatic (CDC, 2005).

The catarrhal stage begins insidiously, with symptoms similar to those of an upper respiratory infection. On occasion, the catarrhal stage is short or absent (He et al., 1998).

The paroxysmal phase follows and is delineated by an increase in severity and frequency in the cough, with rapidly consecutive forceful coughs in single expiration being followed by a "whoop" (hurried, deep inspiration). Copious viscid mucus and post-tussive vomiting are characteristic of this phase. Choking spells in infants with or without cyanosis may present as opposed to whoops. Evaluation of hydration status is important, especially in young infants. Respiratory distress may progress to respiratory failure in fatigued infants and those with pneumonia. Hypoxia and lung injury may lead to pulmonary hypertension. The resultant pulmonary hypertension may be severe and cause right ventricular failure and intracardiac shunting through a patent foremen ovale or atrial septal defect (Southall et al., 1988).

Older children and adolescents my develop sequelae secondary to forceful coughing, such as chest or abdominal pain, rib fractures, and even air leak syndromes. Facial petechiae are common in all age groups from coughing and post-tussive emesis.

The last stage is the convalescent phase. During this period, symptoms slowly diminish, but the cough recurs easily with common triggers such as cigarette smoke, reactive airway exacerbations, or upper respiratory infections.

Vaccinated children may present with a wide variety of illness severity depending on their level of serologic protection. In older children and adolescents, infection is usually characterized by persistent paroxysmal cough often with post-tussive emesis that is worst at night and that may last as long as 4 to 6 weeks (He et al., 1998).

DIFFERENTIAL DIAGNOSIS

The list of differential diagnoses for pertussis is extensive and based on the presenting symptoms. Diagnoses to consider include infectious diseases, gastrointestinal concerns, and neurological disorders (Table 35-19).

PLAN OF CARE

White blood count may be normal; however, lymphocytosis (absolute lymphocyte count greater than 10,000 cells/μL) can occur and should suggest the diagnosis of pertussis. Higher counts are often associated with more severe disease (Pierce et al., 2000). Other diagnostic studies include bacterial culture, polymerase chain reaction (PCR), direct fluorescent antibody (DFA) testing, and serology. Only the bacterial culture and PCR meet the criteria for laboratory confirmation for national reporting. PCR may be associated with false-positive results and should always be accompanied by culture. Culture is obtained by nasopharyngeal aspirate with a Dacron swab held against the posterior pharynx for at least 10 seconds. Specimens should be split for direct culture and PCR in the laboratory. Best practice for detection methods is evolving, and the CDC (www.cdc.gov) provides up-to-date recommendations. All confirmed infections are to be reported to local health departments (CDC, 2000; Cherry & Heininger, 2004).

Radiographic findings for most patients with pertussis are unremarkable. When present, abnormalities may be subtle, such as peribronchial cuffing, perihilar infiltrates, or atelectasis; consolidations; or, in severe cases, bilateral infiltrates indicative of acute respiratory distress syndrome (Cherry & Heininger, 2004; He et al., 1998).

Therapeutic management often includes hospitalization for young infants due to the severity of illness in this age population; however, patients of any age with moderate to severe respiratory distress, dehydration, or evidence

TABLE 35-18

Phases of Pertussis		
Phase	**Symptoms**	**Duration**
Catarrhal	Symptoms consistent with an upper respiratory infection, such as sneezing, mild cough, rhinorrhea, injected conjunctiva, low-grade fever, malaise, and anorexia	7–10 days Range: 4–21 days
Paroxysmal	Increase in severity and frequency in the cough; rapidly consecutive forceful coughs in a single expiration followed by a "whoop" (hurried, deep inspiration); copious viscid mucus and post-tussive vomiting; choking spells in infants with or without cyanosis may present as opposed to whoops	1–6 weeks Peaks in first weeks
Convalescent	Progressive resolution of cough	2–6 weeks May last up to 3 months

Source: CDC, 2000.

TABLE 35-19

Differential Diagnoses for Pertussis

Foreign body

Bronchiolitis

Aspiration

Viral infections: RSV, adenovirus, influenza A and B, parainfluenza, coronavirus, rhinovirus

Bacteria infections: *Bordetella parapertussis, Bordetella bronchiseptica, Chlamydophila pneumoniae, Mycoplasma pneumoniae,* tuberculosis

Acute exacerbations of chronic bronchitis

Asthma

Postnasal drip

Gastroesophageal reflux

Malignancy

Tuberculosis

Meningitis

Increased intracranial pressure

of encephalopathy must also be admitted. Serial examinations are the best way to measure disease progression. Monitoring infants' oral intake ensures adequate hydration and nutrition. Isolate patients using standard and droplet precautions.

Laboratory confirmation of *B. pertussis* can take days to weeks; therefore, patients with suspected pertussis should begin antimicrobial therapy upon presentation. The antimicrobial approach differs based on the age group. Those patients presenting after 3 weeks of cough may have limited benefit from antimicrobial therapy except in high-risk cases (CDC, 2005). Infants are considered to be at high risk for the first 6 weeks of cough and should be treated. Erythromycin is the medication of choice for both treatment and contact chemoprophylaxis; however, in neonates, it has been associated with infantile hypertrophic pyloric stenosis (IHPS) and should be avoided. Some patients will also not be able to tolerate the adverse gastrointestinal effects of erythromycin. Table 35-20 lists suggested antimicrobial therapies and duration of treatment.

Consultation with the infectious diseases and pulmonology specialists may be indicated if the patient requires additional evaluation or responds poorly to therapy. Because pulmonary hypertension may be associated with pertussis, involving the critical care team and/or cardiology service may be required.

Families often have concerns not only for their ill child, but for other family members and contacts. Review with the family the course of the disease, its means of spread, chemoprophylaxis, and vaccine use for prevention. In China, pertussis is referred to as the "cough of 100 days" (Jenkinson, 2005). This term may be useful when discussing the course with the families, as it will help them

TABLE 35-20

Therapeutic Agent	Duration of Therapy
Erythromycin	
• Treatment of choice	14 days
• May be used for symptomatic patients or nonsymptomatic contacts for prophylaxis	
• Most effective when used early in the disease course	
• Recommended dose in children is 40 to 50 mg/kg/day and in adults is 1 to 2 gm/day, orally in 4 divided doses (maximum 2 gm/day)	
• Infantile hypertrophic pyloric stenosis has been reported in neonates	
Trimethoprim–Sulfamethoxazole	
• Recommended for those who cannot tolerate erythromycin	14 days
• Recommended dose in children is trimethoprim 8 mg/kg/day and sulfamethoxazole 40 mg/kg/day in two divided doses; recommended dose in adults is trimethoprim 320 mg/day and sulfamethoxazole 1,600 mg/day in two divided doses	
• Not recommended for infants younger than 2 months of age	
Clarithromycin	
• Also likely to be effective	10–14 days
• Recommended dose in children is 15 to 20 mg/kg/day orally in two divided doses; maximum = 1 gm/day	
Azithromycin	
• Also likely to be effective	5–7 days
• Recommended dose in children is 10 to 12 mg/kg/day orally in one dose; maximum = 500 mg/day	

Source: CDC, 2000, 2005.

understand the protracted nature of the illness and how long they will need to watch for sequelae of cough such as decreased oral intake and dehydration. Vaccine use for prevention is especially important for adult contacts whose serologic status may no longer be adequate for protection from *B. pertussis.* Families may not be aware of the need for booster dosing for adults.

DISPOSITION AND DISCHARGE PLANNING

Those patients with pertussis who are treated as outpatients can be followed at intervals determined by their symptoms. Children must be excluded from school or daycare programs until completion of 5 days of effective therapy, or if not treated, a minimum of 21 days after onset of cough.

Chemoprophylaxis is recommended for all close contacts, even those who are vaccinated, within the first 3 weeks of exposure. Chemoprophylaxis for 3 weeks or longer after exposure is of lesser benefit except in infants who should receive treatment up to 6 weeks after exposure (CDC, 2000). The routine childhood immunization schedule should be completed regardless of the existence of a documented pertussis infection, as the duration of protection from the disease is unknown. If the infection was diagnosed by a specimen culture, or by contact of a culture-positive patient, then a diphtheria/tetanus (DT) vaccine may be considered instead of the diphtheria, tetanus, and acellular pertussis (DTaP) vaccine (CDC, 2005). HCPs who have appropriately followed standard and droplet precautions during close contact with an infected patient do not require prophylaxis (CDC, 2005).

While the number of deaths from pertussis in the United States has decreased dramatically, mortality from this disease persists, with 10 deaths from this cause being reported in 2007 (CDC, 2009). The most common cause of death is primary or secondary bacterial infection (CDC, 2000).

PNEUMONIA AND PARAPNEUMONIC EFFUSIONS

Jason M. Kane and Jamie Tumulty

PATHOPHYSIOLOGY

Pneumonia is defined as infection and inflammation of the lower respiratory tract in association with detectable radiographic changes of the lung parenchyma. Although the upper airways are colonized with a number of potentially pathologic organisms, microbes that migrate into the lower airways do not lead to pneumonia because of the presence of an intact host defense system. When pneumonia does occur, it is usually the result of a particularly virulent organism, an unusually large innoculum, or impaired host immunity. In an otherwise healthy patient, pathologic organisms can seed the lungs by a number of mechanisms, including inhalation, hematogenous spread, direct inoculation from contiguous areas such as the pleura, or aspiration from the upper airways. Finally, pneumonia can occur when latent disease such as tuberculosis is reactivated in the lung after previously functional host immunity becomes impaired.

Once pathogens reach the lower airways, a number of specific and nonspecific defense mechanisms are triggered. Physical barriers such as cough, reflex bronchoconstriction, surfactant, and mucociliary clearance provide the first line of defense against microorganism invasion. Interaction between toll-like receptors and antigens of the invading organism causes a cascade of biochemical activity that ultimately leads to the activation and production of pro-inflammatory cytokines. Several specific immune defenses—including cellular phagocytosis by macrophages and polymorphonuclear neutrophils, antibody production, and cell-mediated immunity by T lymphocytes—play a role in mitigating infection. Once produced, inflammatory mediators and cytokines cause local tissue edema and increase cellular permeability. Along with fluid that accrues from capillary leak, cellular debris accumulates at the site of infection and surrounding tissue. When fluid collects in the alveolar spaces and alveolar wall edema increases, gas exchange in the affected portion of the lung becomes impaired. Hypoxia and hypercarbia may develop when the remaining unaffected alveoli are too few in number to maintain adequate gas exchange. Clinical symptoms are generally proportional to the extent of progression of illness.

EPIDEMIOLOGY AND ETIOLOGY

Worldwide, childhood pneumonia is the leading cause of mortality in children younger than 5 years of age, accounting for nearly 19% of all deaths in this age group (Rudan et al., 2008). One-half of these deaths are considered vaccine preventable. Even in developed nations, pneumonia has a significant burden of illness, affecting more than 4 million children annually. Although death from childhood pneumonia in industrialized nations is rare, the emergence of drug-resistant organisms has resulted in the increased incidence of more complicated pneumonias.

A number of host risk factors may predispose children to developing pneumonia. The very young and those who are immunocompromised are especially vulnerable to developing pneumonia. Premature infants are at particular risk due to their underdeveloped lungs and exposure to health care-associated organisms as a result of prolonged hospital stays or mechanical ventilation. Individuals with neurologic disease may be at risk for aspiration pneumonia as a result of weak muscle control and poor cough or gag reflexes. Children with musculoskeletal abnormalities, such as severe scoliosis, may not be able to generate strong enough coughs to maintain adequate bronchial clearance and are at risk for retained secretions. Children who are malnourished represent a large percentage of patients who develop pneumonia. Finally, children with chronic lung disease and those living with caregivers who smoke are likely to have cilial motion abnormalities that may contribute to poor airway clearance as well as immune dysfunction.

Infectious pneumonias may be caused by a variety of organisms, including bacteria, viruses, fungi, and parasites. Determining the specific microbiological cause of pneumonia in children is often difficult; however, the patient's age, clinical history, and presenting symptoms can often provide insight into the most likely etiology (Juven et al., 2000; McIntosh, 2002) (Table 35-21).

Before vaccines were readily available, *Streptococcus pneumoniae* and *Haemophilus influenzae* type b were the main bacterial causes of pneumonia worldwide. In the modern era, these organisms remain problematic in developing nations due to lower vaccination rates. The HIB vaccine has all but eliminated *H. influenzae* type b pneumonia from the developed world; however, non-typable *H. influenzae* has emerged as an important pathogen in childhood pneumonia (Heath et al., 2001).

S. pneumoniae remains the most commonly identified bacterial etiology of pneumonia outside of the neonatal period. Less common bacterial etiologies include *H.*

TABLE 35-21

Common Infectious Causes of Community-Acquired Pneumonia by Age		
Age	**Common Cause**	**Other Causes**
Neonates younger than 30 days	Bacteria • *Escherichia coli* • Group B *Streptococcus* • *Listeria monocytogenes*	Bacteria • Group D *Streptococcus* • *Haemophilus influenzae* • *Streptococcus pneumoniae* • *Ureaplasma urealyticum* • *Bordetella pertussis* Viruses • Herpes simplex virus • Cytomegalovirus
1 to 3 months	Bacteria • *Streptococcus pneumoniae* • *Chlamydia trachomatis* • *Bordetella pertussis* Viruses • Respiratory syncytial virus • Influenza virus • Parainfluenza virus • Adenovirus	Bacteria • Haemophilus influenzae • Moraxella catarrhalis • Staphylococcus aureus • Ureaplasma urealyticum Viruses • Cytomegalovirus • Metapneumovirus
3 months to 5 years	Bacteria • *Mycoplasma pneumoniae* • *Chlamydia trachomatis* • *Streptococcus pneumoniae* Viruses • Respiratory syncytial virus • Influenza virus • Parainfluenza virus • Adenovirus • Rhinovirus	Bacteria • *Haemophilus influenzae* • *Moraxella catarrhalis* • *Staphylococcus aureus* • *Neisseria meningitis* • *Mycobacterium tuberculosis* Virus • Varicella-zoster virus

TABLE 35-21

Common Infectious Causes of Community-Acquired Pneumonia by Age *(Continued)*		
Age	**Common Cause**	**Other Causes**
5 years to adolescence	Bacteria • *Mycoplasma pneumoniae* • *Chlamydia trachomatis* • *Streptococcus pneumoniae*	Bacteria • *Haemophilus influenzae* • *Legionella* species • *Mycobacterium tuberculosis* • *Staphylococcus aureus* Viruses • Adenovirus • Epstein-Barr virus • Influenza virus • Parainfluenza virus • Rhinovirus • Respiratory syncytial virus • Varicella-zoster virus

influenzae (non-typable and type b), *Moraxella catarrhalis*, and *Staphylococcus aureus*. From a public health perspective, it is important to note that the incidence of methicillin-resistant *S. aureus* (MRSA) is rising. Originally observed among frequently hospitalized patients and individuals in long-term care, MRSA has emerged as a pathogen now common in the general population; it is often associated with the development of more complicated disease (Buckingham et al., 2003).

Although vaccination has decreased the prevalence of *Bordetella pertussis*, patients with delayed vaccinations and unvaccinated vulnerable infants are at particular risk for developing pertussis pneumonia. Reported cases of pertussis among adolescents and adults have increased since the 1980s despite increasingly high rates of vaccination among infants and children. However, severe pertussis morbidity and mortality occur primarily among infants (Tanaka et al., 2003). In school-aged children and adolescents, *Mycoplasma pneumoniae* and *Chlamydia pneumoniae* are frequently causative agents in community-acquired pneumonia. In addition, *Mycobacterium tuberculosis* should be considered in patients with specific risk factors. Viral pathogens are known to affect children across all age groups, with the most common including respiratory syncytial virus (RSV), influenza A and B, parainfluenza, adenovirus, and metapneumovirus.

Patients who develop pneumonia while hospitalized incur additional morbidity and mortality. Although beyond the scope of this section, clinicians should be familiar with the diagnosis and management of ventilator-associated pneumonias as well as therapy for infections from specific healthcare–associated organisms

(Bigham et al., 2009). Although fungal pneumonia predominantly affects immunocompromised children, outbreaks of certain fungal pathogens—including *Coccidiodes immitis, Histoplasma capsulatum,* and *Blastomyces dermatitidis*—have been known to infect otherwise healthy children living in endemic areas. Parasitic pneumonias are rare and generally result from specific environmental exposures incurred during travel to high-risk areas.

Community-acquired pneumonia may be complicated by the development of parapneumonic effusions or empyemas. Although often associated with severe bacterial pneumonia from *Staphylococcus* or *Streptococcus*, the presence of effusion alone does not necessarily indicate a bacterial etiology. Differentiation between effusion types may be helpful in targeting therapy; however, differentiating among the causes of bacterial pneumonia can be done only with positive microbiological cultures. The first stage of a parapneumonic effusion is the *exudative* phase, in which pleural fluid is free flowing; has a low cell count; and has normal pH, glucose, and protein levels. The second stage is the *fibrinopurulent* phase, which is characterized by bacterial invasion, followed by large numbers of polymorphonucleated white blood cells. Fibrin is deposited on pleural surfaces, where it forms strands, resulting in loculation. The final stage is the *organized*, in which fibroblasts form a membrane on pleural surfaces that restricts lung expansion.

PRESENTATION

In general, pediatric patients with community-acquired pneumonia will present with fever in addition to respiratory symptoms. Tachypnea, cough, nasal flaring, retractions, crackles, and focal findings on auscultation have been shown to be predictors of pneumonia in children (Mahabee-Gittens et al., 2005). Bacterial pneumonia should be strongly suspected in patients younger than 2 years of age who present with tachypnea and fever higher than 38°C (100.4°F) (Table 35-22).

TABLE 35-22

Suggested Age-Specific Criteria for Tachypnea	
Age	**Breaths per Minute**
2 to 12 months	> 50
1 to 5 years	> 40
≥ 5 years	> 30

Source: World Health Organization, www.who.int

Unfortunately, the initial presentation for many children with pneumonia, especially infants, may be nonspecific. Symptoms also will vary based on the patient's underlying health status and the presence of any chronic medical condition. In young infants, along with fever, there may be vague complaints of decreased interest in feeding. Older children may demonstrate fever, cough, dyspnea, abdominal pain or chest pain, or lethargy. Some children appear well, while others may appear toxic. Universally, however, patients with pneumonia will have fever and some respiratory signs.

Distressed infants may present with tachypnea, intercostal retractions, hypoxia, or cyanosis. Breath sounds are easily referred, especially in the smallest infants; thus they are less reliable indicators of focal pulmonary abnormalities in this age group. Grunting can be appreciated in both infants and older children in an attempt to stent open the occluded alveoli. In small infants, this sound is less of a grunt and more of a moan or small cry and, therefore, may be under appreciated. In older cooperative children, the HCP may appreciate focally diminished breath sounds, or crackles. It is important to note that dehydrated children may not demonstrate accessory breath sounds until adequate hydration has occurred. A pleural friction rub may be heard as the result of inflamed pleura, but it may not be audible if a large pleural effusion is present. Tactile fremitus and whispered pectoriloquy tend not to be helpful in the evaluation of children. Cyanosis, when present, is ominous and a late sign of impending respiratory failure.

DIFFERENTIAL DIAGNOSIS

Pneumonia is unlikely without fever and at least one respiratory sign. The best negative predictor of pneumonia in children is the absence of tachypnea alone or other signs of respiratory illness (Margolis & Gadomski, 1998). In patients who do have respiratory signs but no fever, other disorders should be considered as part of the differential diagnosis. Tachypnea and respiratory distress are relatively nonspecific signs that may reflect either pulmonary or systemic disease. Pathologic processes that interfere with oxygen delivery can cause patients to become tachypneic and hypoxic. Hemoglobinopathies, including carbon monoxide poisoning, methemoglobinemia, and severe anemia, can all present with tachypnea and respiratory distress but are unlikely to have coexistent fever. Patients with metabolic acidosis or diabetic ketoacidosis may present with tachypnea or respiratory distress as a compensatory mechanism to normalize pH. Other noninfectious causes of respiratory distress that may mimic pneumonia include foreign body aspiration, reactive airway disease, metastatic malignancy involving the lungs, and congestive heart failure.

Pleural effusions may also present independent of primary pneumonia and are frequently associated with noninfectious disease processes. Differentiation between transudative and exudative effusions may narrow the

TABLE 35-23

Transudative Versus Exudative Pleural Effusions	
Transudative	**Exudative**
Congestive heart failure	Infectious
Pericarditis	Chylothorax
Hypoalbuminemia	Neoplastic disease
Superior vena cava syndrome	Connective tissue disease
Nephrotic syndrome	Iatrogenic: central venous catheter migration or misplacement
Peritoneal dialysis	Immunodeficiency
Atelectasis	Chest trauma

differential diagnosis (Table 35-23). *Transudative* effusions occur when increased hydrostatic pressure in the veins and capillaries forces fluid across a vascular membrane, resulting in a watery, acellular fluid collection. *Exudative* pleural effusions are produced when protein and cells leak out of vascular structures as a result of the inflammatory cascade. The diagnostic and therapeutic approaches to these types of effusions can be quite different.

PLAN OF CARE

Diagnosis of community-acquired pneumonia can often be made clinically in the outpatient setting. In rare circumstances, supportive laboratory examinations may be utilized to guide therapy; however, pneumonia is generally considered a clinical diagnosis and most laboratory evaluations are not necessary prior to the initiation of empiric therapy. Although positive findings on radiographic studies may rule in the diagnosis, a negative chest radiograph (CXR) does not rule out pneumonia, as radiographic findings often lag behind clinical findings.

Clinical history can play an important role in establishing the etiology of community-acquired pneumonia, particularly in older children. A comprehensive history should include an evaluation for exposure to known community pathogens or other sick contacts. Immunization history is critical, with particular attention being paid to seasonal immunizations including influenza and the influenza A subtype H1N1 (H1N1) vaccine. Additional history pertaining to risk factors for tuberculosis should be elucidated in high-risk patients, including travel to endemic areas, residence in homeless shelters, family member incarceration, underlying infection with human immunodeficiency virus (HIV), or known exposure to tuberculosis. Also, depending on the geography, recent exposures may aid in diagnosis. For example, exposure to pigeons, housing construction, or other soil-disrupting activities may suggest histoplasmosis

in certain endemic regions of the United States (Chamany et al., 2004).

Some pathogens are more predominant at various times of year, such as RSV in the fall through spring and influenza during the winter. Patients with simultaneous upper respiratory tract infection symptoms such as rhinorrhea are much more likely to have a viral etiology as opposed to a bacterial etiology; thus a comprehensive review of systems can also aid in diagnosis. Although not pathopneumonic, certain characteristic symptoms may suggest specific etiologies, such as the "staccato" cough of *Chlamydia* pneumonia and the paroxysmal coughing associated with pertussis.

Based on the severity of the patient's illness and underlying comorbidities, selective laboratory tests may be considered. In neonatal patients, regardless of symptoms, the standard of care for the evaluation of fever includes a complete blood count with differential, as well as blood, urine, and cerebrospinal fluid cultures. As patients move beyond the neonatal period, the evaluation for etiology of fever relies more on history and physical examination, and less on laboratory examinations. In older children, routine laboratory tests are indicated only if additional comorbidities warrant evaluation or specific complications are suspected.

In patients for whom laboratory investigations are indicated, there are a limited number of useful tests, most of which have no true diagnostic role in the evaluation of community-acquired pneumonia. These tests include the white blood cell count and differential, sputum culture and Gram stain, blood culture, C-reactive protein, and erythrocyte sedimentation rate. When available, rapid immunoassays for specific seasonal viral antigens may be used to identify certain viral etiologies, but these tests have not been shown to alter initial management decisions. Nevertheless, some authorities recommend rapid viral antigen testing in infants younger than 18 months of age (BTS, 2002).

Laboratory studies may be useful in the moderately ill pediatric patient or in the patient who requires hospitalization. Concerning findings include leukocytosis with left shift or increased neutrophils, and thrombocytosis. Blood cultures are often obtained; however, the utility of blood cultures in the diagnosis and management of pneumonia is minimal. When pneumonia is diagnosed in an outpatient setting, the likelihood of positive blood culture is less than 3%; thus routine use of blood cultures is generally unhelpful and is not recommended (Hickey et al., 1996). In patients who develop complicated pneumonia, pleural fluid can be sent for analysis to aid in diagnosis and guide duration of therapy (Table 35-24). Microbiological studies on pleural fluid may reveal an etiology, although antibiotic treatment prior to obtaining a culture specimen may cause a negative culture result (Gates et al., 2004). Patients who develop empyema will require longer duration of antibiotic therapy compared to those with transudative or reactive effusions.

Routine CXRs are indicated when clinical findings are ambiguous, pleural effusion is suspected, or pneumonia

TABLE 35-24

Pleural Fluid Analysis		
Parameter	Transudate	Exudate
Protein (gm/dL)	< 3.0	> 3.0
Fluid: serum protein	< 0.5	> 0.5
LDH	< 200	> 200
Fluid: serum LDH	< 0.6	> 0.6
WBCs/mm³	< 1,000	> 1,000
RBCs	< 10,000	> 10,000
Glucose	Same as serum	Less than serum
pH	7.4–7.5	< 7.4
Culture	Negative	+/–

Note: Lactate dehydrogenase (LDH), white blood cell count (WBC), red blood cell count (RBC).
Source: Ampofo & Byington, 2007.

has been prolonged or unresponsive to antibiotic therapy. Posterior/anterior and lateral radiographs are useful for localization of pneumonia; however, CXRs have not consistently altered management decisions or improved clinical outcomes (Swingler et al., 1998). Also, routine radiographs have not been shown to differentiate viral from bacterial etiologies (Virkki et al., 2002).

When pleural effusion is suspected, decubitus chest radiographs may provide visualization of a fluid level (Figure 35-12); however, when loculated, this fluid level may be less apparent. Chest ultrasound and chest CT scan (Figure 35-13) have been shown to be similar in their ability to detect loculated effusion and lung necrosis or abscess resulting from complicated pneumonia. Chest CT scan does not provide any additional clinically useful information over chest ultrasound (Kurian et al., 2009), but it can be used for particularly difficult effusions where ultrasound is technically limited or discrepant with the clinical findings. Advantages of ultrasound relative to CT scan include its low cost, ease of use, general availability, radiation free, and lower need for sedation (Calder & Owens, 2009). Ultrasound may also be used to guide the placement of a thoracostomy tube or thoracentesis needle.

Bronchoscopy can be used as both a diagnostic and therapeutic procedure in severe cases of pneumonia or in patients who are refractory to therapy. Bronchial alveolar lavage can be used to collect sputum samples from deep within the lungs to help identify a causative organism. In general, there is no role for routine bronchoscopy in mild cases of community-acquired pneumonia.

The therapeutic management of pneumonia depends on the severity of the infection and associated sequelae, but always includes antibiotic therapy. If the disease is complicated by parapneumonic effusion or abscess, management may include thoracentesis, thoracostomy tube placement, fibrinolytic therapy, video-assisted thoracoscopic surgery (VATS), or thoracotomy. Ideal antibiotic therapy requires isolation of an organism from blood, pleural fluid,

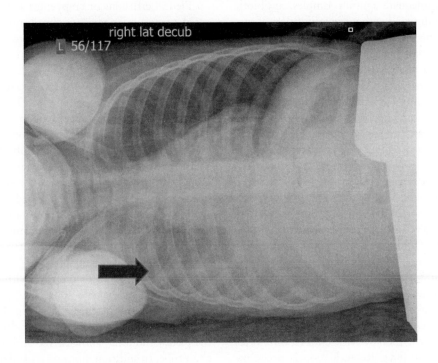

FIGURE 35-12

Decubitus Radiograph of Pneumonia with Pleural Effusion.
Source: Courtesy of Jason M. Kane and Jamie Tumulty.

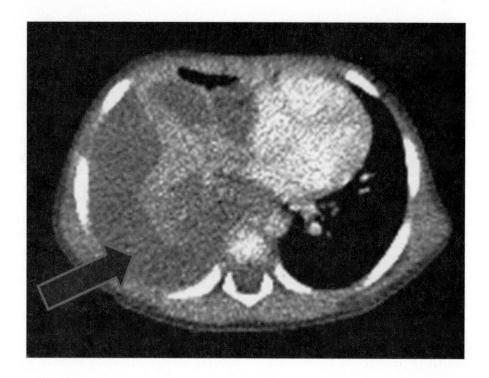

FIGURE 35-13

Computed Tomography of Pneumonia with Pleural Effusion.

Source: Courtesy of Jason M. Kane and Jamie Tumulty.

or sputum. However, because of the low recovery of organisms in routine blood cultures and the inability of younger children to produce adequate sputum samples, antibiotic therapy is frequently initiated without identification of specific microbiological pathogens (McCracken, 2000).

Empiric therapy should be initiated based on patient age and severity of symptoms (Grant et al., 2009; McIntosh, 2002). Neonates with fever should be admitted to the hospital and started on empiric parenteral antibiotics, including ampicillin and gentamycin (or cefotaxime). In older infants with mild cases of pneumonia, enteral amoxicillin is the first-line therapy of choice. Given the concern for penicillin-resistant *S. pneumoniae*, high-dose amoxicillin (80 to 90 mg/kg/day) is recommended. For children who are allergic to penicillin, a macrolide or cephalosporin may be considered; however, 15% of *S. pneumoniae* infections have been shown to be resistant to macrolides (Hyde et al., 2001). In older children, in whom *Mycoplasma* and *Chlamydia* infections are more common, a macrolide is the first-line therapy for treating mild community-acquired pneumonia. In more severe cases, a combination of both a macrolide and a beta-lactam agent should be considered (Table 35-25).

In general, outpatient therapy with enteral antibiotics is prescribed for 7 to 10 days. Re-evaluation is necessary in children who continue to have unresolved symptoms or fever following 48 hours of antibiotic therapy. If patients continue to have fevers and a bacterial etiology is suspected,

HCPs should consider the possibility of treatment failure, resistant organism, empyema, or abscess.

Pleural effusions or empyemas associated with complicated pneumonias may require drainage. Small effusions that are free flowing are unlikely to be complicated and may be able to be managed with antibiotic therapy alone. Patients with large pleural effusions should be referred to pediatric surgeons for consideration of a VATS procedure or thoracostomy tube placement. Drainage options range from simple thoracentesis to open thoracotomy. Simple thoracentesis allows the HCP to analyze the pleural fluid and potentially to narrow the antibiotic therapy on this basis. Thoracostomy tube placement is indicated for all large transudative effusions and the early exudative phase of parapneumonic effusions. The addition of fibrinolytics such as alteplase (tPA), urokinase, and streptokinase may improve drainage during the fibrinopurulent stage and avoid the need for further surgical interventions (Ampofo & Byington, 2007; Gates et al., 2004).

Children who fail to improve with conventional chest tube therapy may benefit from VATS procedure, especially if the procedure is performed early in the course of the disease. VATS offers the advantage of direct visualization of the pleura and lung, allowing for optimal placement of the chest tube. In addition, fibrinolysis and decortication can be performed during the VATS procedure. Studies have suggested that VATS is superior to fibrinolytic therapy alone with respect to hospital length of stay, duration of chest

TABLE 35-25

Empiric Antimicrobial Therapy for Community-Acquired Pneumonia by Age

Age	First-Line Therapies	Additional Considerations
Birth to 1 month	Parenteral ampicillin and gentamicin	Consider cefotaxime in addition to or in lieu of gentamicin
1 month to 3 months (well appearing)	Amoxicillin (high dose)	Alternative agents: sulfamethoxazole–trimethoprim, amoxicillin–clavulanic acid, or macrolide. May also use parenteral ceftriaxone for first dose, then change to oral amoxicillin
1 month to 3 months (ill appearing)	Parenteral cefotaxime or cefuroxime	Consider addition of macrolide if concerns for pertussis or *Chlamydia* infection
4 months to 5 years	Amoxicillin (high dose)	Alternative agents: sulfamethoxazole–trimethoprim, amoxicillin–clavulanic acid, or macrolide
Older than 5 years to adolescence	Macrolide alone if there is low suspicion of *S. pneumoniae*	If symptoms persist or there is concern for *S. pneumoniae*, add a beta lactam antibiotic, including amoxicillin or cephalosporin

tube drainage, narcotic analgesia use, additional radiologic tests, and total fibrinolysis (Kurt et al., 2006).

Patients who have recurrent pneumonia, significant comorbidities, or culture-positive confirmation of rare microbiological organisms should be referred to a pediatric infectious diseases specialist for additional consultation. Immunocompromised patients, including those with HIV or neoplastic diseases, may benefit from early consultation with an infectious diseases specialist to help guide antimicrobial management. Poor growth or recurrent bacterial infections with *S. aureus* or *Pseudomonas aeruginosa* should prompt referral to an immunologist or pulmonologist for evaluation of undiagnosed immunodeficiency or cystic fibrosis. Additional consultation with a pediatric pulmonologist should be considered if patients have a history of prematurity, chronic lung disease, or other pulmonary conditions that warrant longitudinal follow-up and long-term medical management.

Patients who present to outpatient settings with cyanosis or significant respiratory distress should be referred to the emergency department for immediate respiratory stabilization. These individuals should be transported by emergency medical services to the nearest medical facility that can provide advanced airway maneuvers or interventions, as patients with respiratory distress may deteriorate rapidly en route and progress to respiratory failure. Indications for admission to the hospital include a requirement for oxygen to maintain oxygen saturation at a level greater than 91%, severe dehydration, inability to maintain oral hydration, moderate to severe respiratory distress, outpatient enteral antibiotic failure, or insufficient social support structure to facilitate adequate therapy and follow-up.

Patients with severe disease may require admission to the intensive care unit for noninvasive ventilatory support, or endotracheal intubation and mechanical ventilation. In the extreme case of oxygenation or ventilation failure refractory to intubation and mechanical ventilation, extracorporeal membrane oxygenation (ECMO) may be employed as a life-saving rescue therapy. Given that not all pediatric centers are equipped to perform ECMO, early consultation with an ECMO center is recommended for patients who are demonstrating failure to respond to escalation in conventional mechanical ventilation.

Families should be instructed to return to their PCP if the child's symptoms do not begin resolving after 48 hours of antibiotic therapy. If symptoms have not resolved after appropriate antibiotic course, alternative diagnoses or treatment failure should be considered. If the patient has fully recovered with normal physical examination following completion of therapy, no further evaluation is necessary. Repeat CXRs are not indicated after the first case of uncomplicated pneumonia where recovery is complete. If the initial chest radiographs show focal abnormalities, however, a repeat study should be performed after all symptoms have resolved to confirm resolution of the pneumonia. Families should also be instructed to ensure that the patient completes the full course of antibiotics, even after resolution of clinical symptoms.

Immunization status should be reviewed with each family on initial presentation of a child with pneumonia. Patients who experience a delay in vaccination should be given the appropriate vaccines when they become clinically well. Seasonal influenza vaccine should be administered to all children older than 6 months of age. In addition, heptavalent conjugated pneumococcal vaccine should be administered to this population, as this vaccine is effective in preventing invasive pneumococcal disease, radiographic-defined pneumonia, and clinical pneumonia (Lucero et al., 2009). Finally, certain high-risk pediatric patients, including those with congenital cardiac defects or chronic lung disease, should receive immunoprophylaxis against RSV during the winter months.

If at any point signs of respiratory distress such as cyanosis, retractions, audible stridor, or dyspnea are noted, families should be instructed to utilize emergency medical services and request assessment in the nearest emergency department.

DISPOSITION AND DISCHARGE PLANNING

Patients with mild pneumonia treated in the outpatient setting should complete a full course of antibiotics and should expect no residual complications following their illness. Routine follow-up, including maintaining scheduled vaccinations, is recommended. For patients with complicated pneumonia who required surgical drainage, follow-up should be scheduled to occur 1 to 2 weeks after hospital discharge with their PCP. Complete recovery from complicated pneumonia is achieved by the majority of children despite marked abnormalities at presentation and variable approaches to therapy.

Even after significant clinical improvement, CXRs may remain abnormal for children with pneumonia. Chest radiographs should be followed 1 to 2 months following discharge, and repeated every 1 to 2 months until resolution has been achieved.

PULMONARY EDEMA

Elizabeth Elliott

PATHOPHYSIOLOGY

Pulmonary edema is caused by any disruption in the Starling forces favoring increased filtration or decreased absorption of fluid in the pulmonary capillaries. The Starling equation explains these forces:

$$J_v = K_f \left[(P_c - P_i) - (\pi_c - \pi_i) \right]$$

where J_v is the net fluid movement (mL/min) across a capillary wall and is the sum of the hydrostatic and oncotic pressures (Costanzo, 2002). The net fluid movement depends on water permeability (K_f), capillary hydrostatic pressure (P_c), capillary oncotic pressure (π_c), interstitial hydrostatic pressure (P_i), and interstitial oncotic pressure (π_i).

The forces that favor filtration, or the movement of fluid out of the capillary into the interstitial space, are the interstitial oncotic pressure (π_i) and the capillary hydrostatic pressure (P_c). In contrast, the forces that favor absorption, or the movement of fluid from the interstitial space into the capillary, are the interstitial hydrostatic pressure (P_i) and the capillary oncotic pressure (π_c) (Costanzo, 2002). Therefore, any decrease in capillary oncotic pressure or interstitial hydrostatic pressure, and any increase in capillary hydrostatic pressure or interstitial oncotic pressure, will cause pulmonary edema. In addition, any changes in pulmonary capillary permeability will cause pulmonary edema. Abnormalities in lymphatic drainage and surfactant can also contribute to pulmonary edema, especially in congenital pulmonary disease (Taussig & Landau, 1999).

EPIDEMIOLOGY AND ETIOLOGY

Pulmonary edema is not a disease itself, but rather a condition that results from one of many disease processes. Its causes are divided into two categories: cardiogenic and noncardiogenic. Cardiogenic pulmonary edema is most commonly caused by left-sided heart failure. It may result from any mechanism that leads to depressed left ventricular function, including valvular disorders, damage to the myocytes from infectious processes or cardiomyopathies, congenital heart disease, hypertension, or any entity that causes increased peripheral vascular resistance. Because the heart is unable to pump blood efficiently to the body, blood flow will significantly slow and "back up" into the pulmonary circulation, thereby causing a disruption in the Starling forces of the pulmonary capillaries (Brashers, 2002).

Noncardiogenic causes of pulmonary edema are further classified into three categories: pulmonary (intrinsic), neurogenic, and other causes. Intrinsic causes of pulmonary edema include infectious processes such as pneumonia, acute respiratory distress syndrome (ARDS), and pulmonary embolism. In ARDS and infectious processes, the alveolar–capillary membrane becomes damaged and leaky, promoting movement of fluids into the interstitial space. With pulmonary embolism (PE), elevated hydrostatic pressure occurs proximal to the obstruction, promoting filtration (Taussig & Landau, 1999).

Neurogenic pulmonary edema may arise following almost any type of central nervous system insult, including surgery, trauma, or seizures (Fontes et al., 2003). While the mechanism underlying this phenomenon is not completely understood, one of the most commonly cited theories is that pulmonary blood flow increases as a result of catecholamine release from the central nervous system (CNS), leading to an acute elevation of pulmonary capillary pressures due to vasoconstriction (Fontes et al.).

Noncardiogenic pulmonary edema may also occur in cases where pulmonary circulation is relatively increased, such as following transfusion of blood products or at high altitude. The incidence and mechanism of pulmonary edema following acute airway obstruction are unknown, but this condition is well documented in the literature (Uejima, 2001). Other causes may include medication ingestion (salicylates, narcotics), exaggerated immune responses, or administration of some chemotherapeutic agents (Raab et al., 2008; Rogers & Helafaer, 1999).

PRESENTATION

The signs and symptoms of pulmonary edema are similar irrespective of the etiology. Depending on the cause, the patient's past medical history may include congenital heart disease, seizures, or foreign body aspiration (Uejima, 2001). Physical symptoms reported may include shortness of breath, tachypnea, tachycardia, hypoxia, weakness, cough with frothy sputum, diaphoresis, orthopnea, or paroxysmal nocturnal dyspnea.

On physical examination, pediatric patients may exhibit dyspnea, cyanosis, hypoxemia, subcostal retractions, and crackles on auscultation of the lungs. Patients with cardiogenic pulmonary edema may have a third heart sound (S_3). In addition, pink frothy sputum on suctioning of the airway, increased pulmonary capillary wedge pressure, and increasing peak PEEP and oxygen demands may indicate pulmonary edema in the mechanically ventilated patient.

DIFFERENTIAL DIAGNOSIS

The list of differential diagnoses for pulmonary edema is exhaustive and cannot be adequately addressed in the scope of this section. Because pulmonary edema is the result of a disease process, rather than a primary disease, an accurate history and physical examination will support the likely diagnosis.

PLAN OF CARE

Pulmonary edema is often a clinical diagnosis, but it may be supported by diagnostic studies. Chest radiograph will show peribronchial cuffing and perihilar haziness, and at times an enlarged cardiac silhouette (Figure 35-14). There may also be evidence of pleural effusions (Chen et al., 2004). Oxygen saturations are often low. An arterial blood gas will likely show a lower PaO_2 and an increased A-a gradient. Brain natriuretic peptide (BNP) is released, and its level will become elevated when ventricular diastolic pressure rises (Pagana & Pagana, 2002). Pulmonary capillary wedge pressure will also be elevated (greater than 20 mmHg).

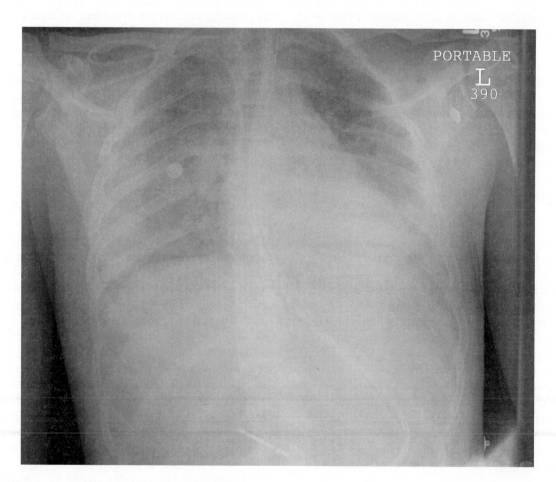

FIGURE 35-14

PA Chest Radiograph of Pulmonary Edema.
Bilateral fluffy alveolar opacifications and congestion.
Source: Courtesy of Elizabeth Elliott.

The goals of therapy in a patient with pulmonary edema are multiple. First, determining the cause allows for development of a tailored therapeutic plan. Second, restoring euvolemic body fluid balance improves oxygenation and relieves dyspnea. Third, the plan should include elements to reverse the disease process, such as medication or procedural therapies. Airway management decisions and timing will depend on the severity of the patient's presentation and the primary cause of the pulmonary edema. Some patients' symptoms will be so severe that they will require immediate noninvasive or invasive ventilation. A thorough assessment of airway, breathing, and circulation are required to stabilize the patient.

The primary therapy for pulmonary edema is supplemental oxygen (Raab et al., 2008; Rogers & Helafaer, 1999) and diuretics (Taussig & Landau, 1999). Some patients may require small amount of oxygen, whereas others will require immediate intubation and mechanical ventilation. Noninvasive ventilation, such as CPAP or BiPAP, has been shown to significantly reduce the need for intubation and reduce hospital mortality in adult patients (Vital et al., 2008). With both noninvasive and invasive means of ventilation, patients with pulmonary edema typically require higher levels of PEEP and oxygen to maintain adequate saturation levels (Uejima, 2001).

Other therapies include elevating the head of the patient's bed to promote pulmonary drainage and use of pharmacologic agents that specifically treat causes of pulmonary edema and promote the movement of fluid back into the intravascular space. In the case of heart failure, the following medication classes are indicated for medical management (Ueijma, 2001)

- Loop diuretics (furosemide, ethacrynic acid): decrease pulmonary microvascular pressure; inhibit the reabsorption of sodium and chloride in the ascending loop of Henle, thereby promoting the increased excretion of water, sodium, and chloride
- Potassium-sparing diuretics (spirinolactone): competitive agonists with aldosterone in the distal renal tubules, causing increase excretion of sodium, water, and chloride
- Thiazide diuretics (chlorothiazide): inhibit sodium and chloride reabsorption in the distal tubules, promoting increased excretion of sodium, water, and chloride
- Angiotensin-converting enzyme inhibitors (enalapril): decrease afterload
- Ionotropes (dobutamine, milrinone): improve contractility of the heart

Ultimately, the therapeutic approach to pulmonary edema is to reverse the cause, by removing the airway obstruction, fixing the failing heart, or reversing lung damage or disease.

An interprofessional team should follow pediatric patients with acute pulmonary edema and those who are at risk for chronic pulmonary over-circulation. If the patient has acute or chronic heart failure, it is important to utilize the expertise of a cardiologist and/or cardiovascular surgeon. Patients with acute pulmonary edema will likely require close monitoring in the PICU by the critical care team. In the case of neurogenic pulmonary edema, a neurosurgeon may help manage a postoperative patient, or the neurology team may help manage a patient who is experiencing seizures. In the case of intrinsic lung disease, a pulmonologist may be of assistance. If the edema is the result of induced airway obstruction (i.e., jaw wired shut), then the orofacial surgeon will be directing care through an arrangement with the critical care team. In addition, infectious diseases or allergy and immunology teams may support plans of care in suspected immune- or infectious-mediated causes of pulmonary edema.

For those patients who will be discharged from the hospital, it is important to start caregiver education early, as pediatric patients are dependent on their caregivers to recognize warning signs and symptoms and administer medications. The HCP should teach caregivers to look for signs of dyspnea, cough with frothy sputum, and fatigue, especially in a patient with a chronic condition whose pulmonary edema is likely to recur. Some patients will require fluid or diet restrictions. As with any disease process, caregivers should be comfortable administering all of the patient's medications prior to discharge home from the hospital.

DISPOSITION AND DISCHARGE PLANNING

The presentation and causes of pulmonary edema vary, as do the rates of morbidity and mortality. Patients with neurogenic pulmonary edema have a rapid onset of symptoms (less than 4 hours in 71.4% of cases) and a rapid recovery (52.4% in less than 72 hours), therefore discharge planning should begin early in the hospitalization (Fontes et al., 2003). It is difficult to stipulate the recovery rates for other causes of pulmonary edema, as they rely on the resolution of the underlying condition. If patients are started on diuretic medications that will continue after discharge, they may require electrolyte monitoring at their follow-up visits, especially monitoring of potassium and chloride levels. Some may even require additional supplementation of these electrolytes in their diets while on diuretic therapy.

A follow-up appointment should be scheduled soon after discharge with the patient's PCP. Additional follow-up appointments may be required with the pulmonologist or cardiologist, depending on the cause of pulmonary edema and the sequelae of the disease process.

SMOKE INHALATION

Mark Riccioni

PATHOPHYSIOLOGY

Lung injury from smoke inhalation is a result of edema, de-epitheliazation of the tracheobronchial region, airway obstruction, and decreased pulmonary compliance (Mlcak et al., 2007). Supraglottic airway edema results from intense heat from a fire or inhalation of steam, whereas lower airway edema occurs due to increased pulmonary capillary permeability. When the tracheobronchial region loses the epithelial layer, psuedomembranous casts are formed. Fibrin is also deposited in the airways. This formation of casts and fibrin can lead to partial obstruction of the airways (Lee & Mellins, 2006; Mlcak et al, 2007). Loss of surfactant leads to atelectasis, and cytokines are released in response to inflammation.

Nitric oxide (NO) has an important role in the pathogenesis of smoke inhalation injury (Enkhbaatar et al., 2009). When NO is formed in the lungs, it leads to a loss of hypoxic vasoconstriction (HPV). HPV helps shunt blood from nonventilated alveoli to ventilated alveoli; thus the loss of HPV causes vasodilation of nonventilated areas of the lung, leading to ventilation/perfusion mismatching (Enkhbaatar et al.). In addition, NO can combine with O_2 and form $2NO_2$, which may further damage the alveolar–capillary membrane (Enkhbaatar et al.). Severe inhalation injuries may lead to acute respiratory ARDS.

EPIDEMIOLOGY AND ETIOLOGY

Lung injury from smoke inhalation occurs secondary to the damage caused by products of combustion such as aldehydes, sulfur oxides, hydrochloric acid, carbon monoxide, chlorine, and cyanide, flame, or airway obstruction from superheated air (Mlcak et al., 2007). Materials such as wool, nylon, polyacrylonitrile, urea-formaldehyde, and melamine-formaldehyde contain nitrogen; burning these materials produces hydrogen cyanide. Polytetrafluorethylene, polyvinyl chlorine (PVC), neoprenes, polyvinyl fluoride, and brominated flame-retardant materials contain substances that, when burned, produce hydrogen chloride, hydrogen fluoride, and hydrogen bromide (Alarie, 2002).

The severity of injury with smoke inhalation depends on which of the aforementioned products of combustion is inhaled, whether the fire occurs in an open versus closed space, and how long the patient is exposed to the products of combustion or superheated air. In 2006, a death from smoke inhalation occurred on average every 162 minutes, leading to more than 2,580 deaths in the United States from this cause. Children ages 0 to 4 years are at greater risk. Fires and burns are the fifth leading cause of unintentional injury deaths in the United States (CDC, 2008), and causes of smoke inhalation include overused electrical outlets, inappropriately used space heaters, unattended candles, cigarette smoking, and children playing with fire materials.

PRESENTATION

The history for a patient suspected of smoke inhalation starts with the type of fire and material burned. Burning of chemicals and plastics may cause more significant injury than burning of wood products. Next, the length of exposure and the location where the patient was found in the structure should be determined. Risk for injury is greater with greater exposure. Young children often hide from the fire in areas of the dwelling that they feel protect them, thereby risking prolonged exposure.

Pediatric patients who present with smoke inhalation often show signs of respiratory distress, hypoxemia, upper airway edema, and wheezing/rhonchi. Edema of the upper airways can lead to stridor and obstruction, which can lead to difficulty in performing intubation. Because symptoms may progress over time, serial evaluations are important. Singed nasal hairs are not a good predictor of exposure in young children who do not yet have these hairs. Soot around the nose and mouth, however, indicates likely inhalation. *If the patient smells like smoke, he or she probably inhaled it.* A thorough secondary survey should follow any resuscitative therapies.

DIFFERENTIAL DIAGNOSIS

The differential diagnosis for smoke inhalation is focused on determining to which of the following the patient was exposed: Toxic products of combustion, flame, and/or superheated air.

PLAN OF CARE

Diagnostic studies include pulse oximetry, CXR, carbon monoxide (CO) and cyanide levels, and direct bronchoscopy. Pulse oximetry measurement may be misleading in patients with smoke inhalation, as carbon monoxide has a 200 times higher affinity for hemoglobin than oxygen, thereby providing falsely high oximetry readings (Dorman-Rosenthal, 2006). Initial CXRs are usually unremarkable but may be useful for baseline study for serial evaluations. Serum carboxyhemaglobin (COHb) levels measure the exposure to carbon monoxide. Levels greater than 2% for nonsmokers or greater than 9% for smokers are indicative of carbon monoxide poisoning (Hampson & Hauff, 2008). Signs of carbon monoxide poisoning vary depending on the level of toxicity. Mild intoxication with a COHb level of less than 20% is evidenced by signs of headache and mild respiratory distress. Irritability, nausea, fatigue, decreased vision, and altered mental status may be seen with levels greater than 40%. Death is associated with COHb levels greater than 60% (Lee & Mellins, 2006).

The results of cyanide levels may not be available for days or weeks depending on the institutional availability for testing (Hall et al., 2007). Direct bronchoscopy is the diagnostic study of choice for suspected inhalation injury (Mlcak et al., 2007).

The therapeutic management approach for smoke inhalation follows the airway, breathing, and circulation (ABCs) resuscitation model. First, establish a patent airway and provide oxygen. Early bronchoscopy and intubation are often considered for those patients at high risk for lung injury, prior to the development of significant respiratory distress or failure. This practice allows for controlled management of the airway before significant tissue swelling develops. Noninvasive mechanical ventilation may be used if significant swelling is not present, if the pediatric patient is able to protect his or her airway, and if there is not an impressive history of inhalation.

Increased secretions can hinder effective ventilation. For this reason, it is important to initiate an airway clearance protocol such as chest physiotherapy, CPAP, or vest therapy (Mlcak et al., 2007).

Several pharmacological agents have been reported to be effective in treating smoke inhalation. β_2-Agonists are used to control bronchoconstriction (Palmieri, 2009). Nebulized heparin combats the obstructive effects of fibrin deposition in the airways (Enkhbaatar et al., 2009). Corticosteroids are effective in reducing inflammation. The risks versus benefits of using inhaled corticosteroids should be considered, however, as these agents' side effects include increased potential for infection, suppression of the hypothalamic–pituitary axis, growth suppression, and reduced bone mineral density (Greenhalgh, 2009).

Hyperbaric oxygen therapy (HBOT) is recommended for patients with severe symptoms, regardless of COHb levels or for those with COHb levels greater than 25%. The main purpose of HBOT is to reduce the neurologic sequelae caused by CO poisoning, such as headache, dizziness, confusion, and seizures. Weaver et al. (2002) found that in adults, three hyperbaric oxygen treatments within a 24-hour period reduced the rate of cognitive sequelae at 6 and 12 months post exposure.

Patients who present with smoke inhalation may benefit from consultation with the following specialists: pulmonology, dermatology or a burn treatment team, critical care, and nutrition. Depending on the extent of injury or sequelae, prolonged hospital stays may be necessary. In this situation, patients and families may require extensive social and spiritual support, child life services, and assistance from the rehabilitation team.

Caregivers should be educated on the sources of carbon monoxide poisoning, such as furnaces, portable gas heaters, and vehicle exhaust. Additional inpatient education may involve long-term pulmonary care, medications, home adjuncts and equipment, dermal care for burns/skin grafts, and return to daily living activities.

DISPOSITION AND DISCHARGE PLANNING

Prognosis and outcomes for pediatric patients with smoke inhalation depend on the severity of the inhalation injury and degree of burns. Late complications of inhalation injury include tracheal stenosis and obstructive/restrictive lung disease (Mlcak et al., 2007). Once discharged, the patient will require follow-up with his or her PCP. Additional services are dependent on the extent of injury, but may include the pulmonary service (if pulmonary function is not back to the patient's baseline), burn team or plastic surgery for extensive burn care, or physical and occupational therapy for continued rehabilitation.

VENTILATION SUPPORT

Andrea Kline and Jason Kane

INDICATIONS FOR MECHANICAL VENTILATION

Mechanical ventilation is indicated when inadequate oxygenation or ventilation is present. A disruption to the pulmonary system can result in hypoxemia, hypercarbia, or both. Respiratory distress and respiratory failure are characterized by the inability to provide adequate gas exchange and occur as a response to various disease processes.

Respiratory distress is characterized by the obvious use of compensatory mechanisms in an attempt to maintain adequate gas exchange. Signs of respiratory distress include tachypnea and increased work of breathing demonstrated by retractions, accessory muscle use, grunting, and/or nasal flaring. Mechanisms to preserve gas exchange and oxygen delivery result in hypoxemia and/or hypercarbia when compensation is no longer possible.

Respiratory failure is described as a progression of signs and symptoms of respiratory distress or respiratory depression accompanied by arterial blood gas values demonstrating a partial pressure of oxygen in arterial blood (PaO_2) of less than 60 mmHg and/or partial pressure of carbon dioxide in the arterial blood ($PaCO_2$) of more than 50 mmHg. Often, blood gas values are not required to determine presence of respiratory failure and need for mechanical ventilation.

Patients with parenchymal lung disease, upper airway abnormalities, chest wall abnormalities, or central nervous system disorders or failure, and patients undergoing operative procedures requiring anesthesia are at risk of requiring mechanical ventilation (Table 35-26).

PHYSIOLOGIC PRINCIPLES

Mechanical ventilation refers to the use of life support technology that assists with the work of breathing for patients who are unable to effectively to do on their own. In pediatric patients, the ultimate goal is to maintain adequate oxygenation and ventilation until the underlying pathologic process resolves.

A number of nonpulmonary indications for mechanical ventilation exist. With respect to respiratory failure, however, there are two broad indications for intubation and mechanical ventilation: (1) failure of oxygenation and (2) failure of ventilation. Although not mutually exclusive, the management of these two conditions requires a comprehensive understanding of the mechanics of artificial ventilation as well as the underlying pathophysiology of the patient.

The failure of adequate oxygenation or ventilation can occur as a result of lung disease, cardiac dysfunction, neurologic abnormalities, or multiple organ dysfunction. Examples of lung disease that often cause patients to be admitted to the ICU include pneumonia, inhalation injury, chest trauma, submersion injury, hydrocarbon aspiration, pulmonary hemorrhage, chronic lung disease or bronchopulmonary dysplasia, chemotherapy-induced pulmonary fibrosis, congenital central hypoventilation syndrome

(CCHS), and asthma. Pediatric patients with congenital cardiac disease may require mechanical ventilation as a strategy to reduce overall metabolic demand and improve the balance between oxygen delivery and oxygen demands, thereby enabling them to avoid anaerobic metabolism and lactic acid production. Patients with neurologic injury may require airway protection or forced hyperventilation as a protective strategy to minimize the risk of cerebral herniation. Thus the overall goals of mechanical ventilation must be to optimize gas exchange, minimize patient work of breathing, and limit additional lung damage from positive pressure or excess volume as a result of mechanical ventilation.

Lung volumes

The total lung capacity (TLC) is the total amount of air in the lungs after a maximal inspiration. The TLC varies with age and height, as well as chest wall anatomy. The vital capacity (VC) is the maximum amount of air that a patient can exhale after a maximal inhalation. The volume of air left in the lungs after maximal exhalation is the residual volume (RV); it is approximately 25% of the TLC. The sum of the VC and RV, therefore, equals the TLC. Because healthy patients do not breathe with maximal inhalation or exhalation, the quantity of air in the lungs and airways at the end of a normal spontaneous exhalation is a practical metric known as the functional residual capacity (FRC). The FRC represents the resting volume of air in the lungs after a spontaneous breath. At FRC, the tendency of the lungs to collapse is exactly balanced by the tendency of the chest wall to expand.

In severe airway *obstruction*, the alveoli may not empty completely due to early airway closure. In addition, expiratory flow may be so limited that insufficient time is available to allow complete emptying of alveoli. This condition gives rise to a higher end-expiratory volume, which increases to the point where a new dynamic equilibrium is reached between inspiratory and expiratory tidal volume. It follows that severe airway obstruction is associated with an increase in FRC (hyperinflation). This development can be particularly problematic in patients with reactive airway disease in whom mechanical ventilation rates do not allow enough time for complete exhalation, such that breath stacking occurs.

In contrast to obstructive pathology, *restrictive* lung disease results in an abnormally low FRC. The FRC also declines when the individual is supine, as the abdominal contents push the diaphragm upward. This phenomenon is most pronounced with space-occupying intra-abdominal processes such as hepatosplenomegaly, abdominal distention, and ascites. Alterations in chest wall compliance or chest anatomy can also negatively impact FRC.

TABLE 35-26

Risks for Respiratory Distress		
Infectious Lung Disease	**Noninfectious Lung Disease**	**Central Nervous System**
Pneumonias: • Bacterial • Viral • Fungal • Atypical • Empyemas	Acute respiratory distress syndrome Foreign body aspiration Smoke inhalation Acute chest syndrome Asthma	Altered mental status Seizures Muscular dystrophy Guillain-Barré syndrome Myasthenia gravis Botulism Congenital central hypoventilation syndrome
Upper Airway	**Chest Wall Abnormalities**	**Operative Procedures**
Laryngomalasia Croup Tracheitis Choanal atresia	Pectus excavatum Pleural effusions Pneumothorax Scoliosis	General anesthesia Moderate sedation Lung transplant

Compliance

Lung compliance is the ability of the lungs to stretch and change in volume relative to a change in pressure. Compliance is greatest at moderate lung volumes, but is much lower at volumes that are either very low or very high. Low compliance implies a "stiff" lung, in which circumstance extra work is required to transport in a normal volume of air. This situation occurs if the lungs become fibrotic and lose their distensibility. When alveoli collapse, increased force is required to reopen them, so overall compliance is decreased. With respect to mechanical ventilation, compliant lungs require lower total pressure to maintain adequate expansion, whereas poorly compliant lungs require higher pressures. Thus poorly compliant lungs are at risk of significant barotrauma when excessive pressures are used to maintain adequate alveolar ventilation. Likewise, very complaint lungs are at risk of trauma from excessive stretch in spite of low pressures when tidal volumes become superphysiologic.

The total compliance of the respiratory system includes compliance of the lungs and resistance to expansion exerted on the lungs by the chest wall (chest wall compliance). Changes in either pulmonary compliance or chest wall compliance can alter the total compliance of the entire respiratory system. For this reason, sedation or neuromuscular blockade may be used to increase total respiratory compliance by limiting the contribution of chest wall rigidity or muscle tone on lung expansion for a given inspiratory pressure. In addition, increased total respiratory compliance is noted in patients with severe body wall edema. These patients may have an increase in total respiratory compliance due to the chest wall edema; however, lung compliance may be normal.

Mean airway pressure

Systemic arterial oxygenation results from interactions between metabolic oxygen demands, cardiopulmonary interactions, and gas exchange across the alveoli. Reducing the metabolic demand or improving cardiac performance may, in and of itself, improve the balance between oxygen delivery and consumption. When needed, mechanical ventilation can improve oxygen delivery by increasing the efficiency of gas exchange.

Oxygenation is a function of mean alveolar pressure. Because alveolar pressure cannot be directly measured, under passive conditions, mean airway pressure (MAP) is reflected by the mean alveolar pressure. This pressure is the average pressure that distends the alveolus and chest wall; it correlates with the alveolar size and recruitment as well as with the intrapleural pressure. With respect to invasive mechanical ventilation, the MAP can be manipulated by changing the minute ventilation, PEEP, inspiratory time fraction (I-time), or tidal volume. A higher MAP results in improved oxygenation. It is essential to monitor for excessive MAP to avoid lung damage from barotrauma or excessive alveolar stretch.

Oxygenation

Knowledge of the concentration of alveolar oxygen can facilitate an understanding of the efficiency of gas exchange across the alveolar membrane. The oxygen tension in the alveoli is computed using the alveolar gas equation:

$$PAO_2 = PIO_2 - (PaCO_2/R) + [(PaCO_2 \times FiO_2 \times (1 - R)/R)]$$

The partial pressure of inspired oxygen (PIO_2) is a function of barometric pressure and the fraction of inspired oxygen and is calculated as follows:

$$PIO_2 = (Barometric\ pressure - 47) \times FiO_2$$

Under steady-state conditions, R (the respiratory quotient) is a function of CO_2 production and varies with the source of metabolic fuel, and PIO_2 represents the inspired oxygen tension adjusted for FiO_2 and water vapor pressure at body temperature. In patients who are receiving dextrose IV fluids as the primary source of carbohydrate, the respiratory quotient is 1. Therefore, for a patient who is in room air ($FiO_2 = 21\%$), at sea level (barometric pressure = 760 mmHg), with a body temperature of 37°C (98.6°F), the formula can be simplified as follows:

$$PAO_2 = (760 - 47) \times 0.21 - PaCO_2/R$$

The difference between the alveolar and arterial oxygen tension can be followed as a marker of oxygen diffusion across the alveolar membranes. A low alveolar–arterial gradient (A-a gradient) indicates free diffusion, whereas a large gradient indicates that oxygen diffusion is impaired. The A-a oxygen gradient is determined by using the results of the previous calculations and measuring the oxygen tension in the arterial blood (PaO_2):

$$A\text{-}a = Alveolar\ O_2 - arterial\ O_2 = [(760 - 47) \times FiO_2 - PaCO_2/R] - PaO_2$$

In healthy children breathing room air at sea level, the A-a gradient is 5 to 15 mmHg. When the gradient between oxygen in the alveoli and the arterial blood increases, it means that less oxygen is diffusing across the alveolar membranes and entering into the systemic circulation. This trend may indicate worsening lung disease. The converse situation, in which the A-a gradient is decreasing, indicates improved oxygen diffusion and, therefore, improvement in overall pulmonary status. The A-a gradient has been used to predict overall outcomes in pediatric respiratory failure (Tamburro et al., 1991).

Alveolar ventilation

Carbon dioxide (CO_2) production varies with the body's metabolic rate. Patients who are mechanically ventilated can experience dramatic fluctuations in their CO_2 levels if the metabolic rate and the ventilatory support are not well matched. Ventilation refers to the clearance of CO_2 from the body. The exchange of CO_2 from the bloodstream to the lungs occurs in the alveoli, and the rate of gas exchange is a function of both the concentration gradient and the alveolar membrane diffusion. *Alveolar ventilation,* in essence, refers to the volume of gas actually exchanged across the alveolar membrane. The clearance of CO_2 from the alveoli is a function of minute ventilation, or the mathematical product of respiratory rate and tidal volume. Thus, if CO_2 production is relatively constant, manipulating the minute ventilation will have a predictable effect on the concentration of CO_2 and rate of elimination. Given that a linear relationship exists between CO_2 concentration and minute ventilation, HCPs can "dial in" the concentration of arteriolar CO_2.

Dead space ventilation

Although alveoli are the site of actual gas exchange, a certain portion of any given breath fills large airways in which no gas exchange occurs. The total volume of airspace that does not participate in gas exchange is referred to as dead space. The *physiologic dead space* is the fraction of the entire breath that does not participate in CO_2 exchange. A breath can fail to result in CO_2 elimination due to either lack of fresh gas delivered to the alveoli (anatomic dead space) or lack of diffusion across the alveolar membrane into the systemic circulation (alveolar dead space). Thus the total physiologic dead space may be thought of as the sum of the anatomic dead space and the alveolar dead space. The physiologic dead space for patients with healthy lungs, then, is primarily a function of anatomy. Patients with significant lung disease, however, will have an increase in total physiologic dead space due to alterations in alveolar gas exchange and increased alveolar dead space.

The dead space fraction—that is, the ratio of the volume of dead space ventilation to the total tidal volume—can be estimated and followed as a function of alveolar ventilation:

$$(Vd/Vt) = (PaCO_2 - PeCO_2)/PaCO_2$$

where $PeCO_2$ is the CO_2 concentration in mixed expired gas and can be measured by end-tidal CO_2 detection (Lum et al., 1998). In healthy patients, the Vd/Vt ratio during spontaneous breathing varies from 0.35 to 0.15 depending on the factors that influence alveolar ventilation. In patients with significant lung disease, the dead space fraction can increase dramatically.

Mechanical ventilation can also contribute to dead space ventilation. The additional volume of tubing associated with this treatment, including the endotracheal tube and the plastic tubing that connects the patient to the ventilator, increases "anatomic" dead space. Excessive alveolar distention from excessively high levels of PEEP or airway pressures can result in compression of pulmonary vasculature, such that there is decreased perfusion to well-ventilated alveoli and an increase in alveolar dead space.

CONVENTIONAL MECHANICAL VENTILATION

While there are no absolute guidelines for which mode of ventilation to select when initiating or adjusting mechanical ventilation, some important considerations must be taken into account when making this decision. Each mode has both advantages and disadvantages. Knowledge of each mode is imperative when making informed decisions regarding optimal ventilation strategies give each pediatric patient's underlying pathology.

Modes of ventilation

Volume-regulated ventilation. Volume-regulated ventilation delivers a set tidal volume to the patient during a preset inspiratory time. The gas is delivered in a continuous-flow manner in this mode of ventilation. Continuous gas flow delivers a high initial pressure that is maintained during inspiration and then abruptly terminated at the end of inspiration. The peak pressure that is reached in the lungs during delivery of the set tidal volume is variable and depends on the patient's underlying pulmonary mechanics/compliance and patient synchrony with mechanical ventilation.

Advantages of this mode include a reduced risk of volutrauma due to the preset tidal volumes and better control over minute ventilation and carbon dioxide clearance. Disadvantages include the need to deliver higher peak pressures to achieve the goal tidal volume or minute ventilation, and the risk of not meeting patient demands for oxygenation due to the continuous-flow pattern gas delivery (Heulit et al., 2008). Volume ventilation modes are clinically useful when lung compliance is relatively static, as this approach reduces the likelihood that excessive pressure will be generated during the mandatory volume delivery should compliance abruptly decrease.

Pressure-regulated ventilation. Pressure-regulated ventilation delivers a pressure-limited breath during a predetermined inspiratory time in conjunction with a preset ventilator rate. The tidal volume that is generated during inspiration is determined by the underlying compliance and resistance in the pulmonary system. Compliant lungs require less pressure to generate greater tidal volumes, whereas stiff lungs require higher pressures to deliver the same amount of tidal volume. Pressure-regulated ventilation always delivers gas flow in a decelerating pattern. In a decelerating gas flow pattern, the gas is moved rapidly from a high initial flow to baseline set pressure for the preset amount of time.

Advantages of pressure-regulated modes include better ventilation of patients with stiff lungs due to the decelerating flow pattern, an overall lower peak pressure needed to achieve the same tidal volume (as compared to volume-regulated modes), and a more even distribution of gas flow. Patients with heterogeneous lung disease benefit from decelerating gas flow due to the initial high level of delivered pressure, which can open alveoli, and the constant pressure, which allows gas to flow from areas that are well aerated to areas with less aeration. Disadvantages of pressure-regulated ventilation include a varying tidal volume delivery based on the patient's underlying pulmonary mechanics (changes in lung compliance) and the lack of guaranteed minute ventilation.

Clinically, pressure-regulated modes are useful in patients who have poor compliance and are at risk for barotrauma when a volume-limited mode is used. With pressure-limited ventilation, the risk of barotrauma is decreased because the HCP can set the peak pressure. However, this mode requires monitoring of tidal volume delivery to minimize the risk of volutrauma as lung compliance changes (Heulit et al., 2008).

Combined: pressure-regulated volume control. Pressure-regulated volume control (PRVC) mode is an assist control mode in which the ventilator breath is delivered as a set tidal volume, as with all volume control modes; however, the ventilator will compute the average pressure required to achieve that volume and adjust the flow accordingly. PRVC is a form of assist-control ventilation. A constant pressure is applied throughout inspiration, regardless of whether the breath is a control breath or an assist breath. This approach may result in improved oxygenation due to the decelerating inspiratory flow pattern (consequence of constant pressure). Unlike traditional volume control, in PRVC the ventilator adjusts the inspiratory pressure from breath to breath, as the patient's airway resistance and respiratory system compliance changes, to deliver the set tidal volume. The ventilator monitors each breath and compares the delivered tidal volume with the set tidal volume. If the delivered volume is too low, it increases the inspiratory pressure on the next breath. If it is too high, it decreases the pressure (Marraro, 2003). Pure PRVC modes are used for assist control and, therefore, are not appropriate for weaning.

Modes of support

Support modes of ventilation can be used in isolation, particularly for weaning from the ventilator, or as an adjunct to other modes of ventilation in which the patient is able to initiate spontaneous respirations. Two forms of support are available: pressure and volume. Usually, the support modes are set to provide assistance when spontaneous breaths are initiated, but generally do not provide a full ventilator breath.

Pressure support. Pressure support ventilation supports spontaneous respirations with a set pressure that is delivered during the inspiratory phase. A second pressure, PEEP, is the amount of pressure that is delivered to the pediatric patient during exhalation and in between respirations. No set rate is delivered in this mode; thus there is no protection from apnea. Pressure support ventilation is primarily used in the weaning phase of ventilation, where it may be useful to promote respiratory muscle training and to compensate for the high resistance of the endotracheal tube during spontaneous respiration.

If the pressure support parameter is set too high, the patient's respiratory rate may decline, as a lower respiratory rate with larger tidal volumes will maintain minute ventilation. Conversely, if the pressure support ventilation is set too low, the respiratory rate will often increase to achieve adequate minute ventilation (Marraro, 2003). If the patient is not able to increase his or her minute ventilation in cases of low pressure support ventilation settings, the child is at risk for developing hypoventilation and atelectasis. Therefore, it is essential to monitor the rate and tidal volume in this mode of ventilation.

Volume support. Volume support ventilation is an alternative strategy to pressure support ventilation when assisting spontaneous respirations. No rate is set in this mode, which is generally used only in the weaning phase of ventilation. In this setting, it may be useful to promote respiratory muscle retraining and compensation for the high resistance of the endotracheal tube during spontaneous respiration.

Values for expected minute ventilation and tidal volume are set in this mode, and the lowest possible pressure is used to deliver the set tidal volume. This volume is delivered when inspiration is sensed and PEEP is delivered at end exhalation and in between breaths. Peak pressure and respiratory rate monitoring are required in this mode of ventilation. Again, patients who do not have adequate ventilatory drive are at risk for apnea when this mode of ventilation is used.

Noninvasive ventilation

Initially developed for use with chronic respiratory insufficiency, noninvasive ventilation (NIV) has become more popular for management of acute and chronic respiratory failure in all pediatric age groups over the last decade (Javouhey et al., 2008) (Table 35-27). NIV is the technique of delivering positive pressure via a noninvasive

TABLE 35-27

Indications for Noninvasive Ventilation	
Acute	**Chronic**
Pneumonia	Chronic lung disease
Bronchiolitis	Cystic fibrosis
Asthma	Neuromuscular disease
Upper airway obstruction	Obstructive sleep apnea
Pulmonary edema	syndrome
End-of-life palliation	

Source: Adapted from Kornecki & Kavanaugh, 2007.

interface such as a full face mask, nasal mask, nasal pillows, or helmet. Contraindications to this mode of ventilation include conditions that impair airway protective reflexes or invoke reduced respiratory drive and frank respiratory failure (Kornecki & Kavanaugh, 2007).

Due to their smaller size, finding an interface (mask, nasal pillows) with the appropriate "fit" for pediatric patients can be challenging. When an appropriate noninvasive interface fit is found, pressure points of skin contact with the device must be monitored for skin breakdown. In some cases, skin barrier devices can be applied between the skin and the interface. A long-term challenge with chronic NIV is the risk for midface hypoplasia.

NIV may spare the pediatric patients from risks associated with invasive ventilation. Benefits of managing patients with NIV include elimination of the risk of upper airway trauma and ventilator-associated pneumonia, reduced or eliminated requirement for anxiolysis and analgesia, ongoing use and exercise of underlying respiratory muscles, reduced cost, and less complex technology (Javouhey et al., 2008).

Continuous positive airway pressure. One form of NIV is continuous positive airway pressure (CPAP), a mode that provides one set level of positive pressure throughout the respiratory cycle. Whether in inspiration, in expiration, or in between breaths, the same pressure level is delivered to the patient through the noninvasive ventilation device. Given that this technology is an assistive ventilation mode, the child must have a consistent respiratory drive to permit its use. CPAP helps prevent alveolar atelectasis, increases FRC, and may provide distending pressure to overcome upper airway obstruction. Monitoring the work of breathing, oxygen saturation, and carbon dioxide levels will provide information on the success of the CPAP trial. Typical levels of CPAP are between 5 to 10 cmH$_2$O.

Bilevel positive airway pressure. Unlike CPAP, bilevel positive airway pressure (BiPAP) provides two levels of pressure during the respiratory cycle—the inspiratory positive airway pressure (IPAP) and the expiratory positive

airway pressure (EPAP), both of which are preset on the device. The BiPAP device is triggered when it senses the pediatric patient's inspiratory effort, at which point it delivers the preset IPAP. When the device senses the end of inspiration, the pressure level drops down to the preset EPAP level. This pressure is then administered until the device again senses that the child is initiating an inspiratory effort. The IPAP pressure is always set higher than the EPAP level.

The bilevel support offered with BiPAP exceeds the level of support available from CPAP alone. Most bilevel devices have spontaneous timed modes. Spontaneous modes do not have a backup rate, whereas spontaneous timed modes have a set backup rate on the device. This approach ensures that the patient is receiving some larger breaths with IPAP. In the event that the pediatric patient is breathing faster than the preset backup rate, the machine will not deliver additional breaths to the patient (the minimum rate preset on the device is met by the patient's own intrinsic rate). BiPAP is useful in many clinical conditions in acute and chronically ill children, and it can be useful in both intrinsic lung disease and upper airway obstruction.

The key to successful noninvasive ventilation with CPAP or BiPAP is a calm and cooperative pediatric patient. In some children, this may require desensitization to the mask and pressure being delivered, as well as slow titration of settings. Desensitization strategies are generally not possible in cases of acute illness. In those situations, the administration of a small dose of an anxiolytic may be required. Often, as patients recognize that they are breathing easier on the device, they become more cooperative with the therapy.

In addition to posing challenges with skin breakdown, use of CPAP and BiPAP may lead to other pressure-related problems. Eye irritation and dryness are not uncommon due to the escaping pressure around the mask, although using eye lubricants and ensuring a proper mask fit can alleviate these symptoms. Abdominal distention has also been reported due to the positive pressure escaping down the esophagus and into the stomach. In most cases, this condition is clinically insignificant; however, if there is concern for gastroesophageal reflux and aspiration associated with abdominal distention, a gastric tube can be placed to decompress the stomach (Kornecki & Kavanaugh, 2007).

High-flow nasal cannula. High-flow nasal cannula (HFNC) is an additional modality offering noninvasive respiratory support. With this approach, gas is delivered—near body temperature and highly saturated with water vapor—through a nasal cannula, making the high flow rate more comfortable for the patient. The gas is delivered to the nasopharynx and can escape through an open mouth, so these considerations must be addressed when selecting candidates for this therapy.

Generally flow rates are set at 1 to 8 L/min for infants and young children, although flow rates can be as high as 40 L/min in older children and adults. Oxygen can also be blended for delivery through the HFNC circuit. Some devices have an internal oxygen blender, whereas others require an external oxygen blender.

In addition to providing heated and humidified gas, some sources have postulated that the rate of flow may deliver a level of positive pressure similar to CPAP. Studies have supported this concept in very small neonates (Kubicka et al., 2008). Some pediatric studies have demonstrated that the application of noninvasive ventilation may avoid or delay the requirement for intubation and mechanical ventilation (Turner & Arnold, 2007).

Alternative ventilation strategies

Airway pressure release ventilation. Airway pressure release ventilation (APRV) is a time-triggered, pressure-limited, time-cycled mode of ventilation that allows unrestricted spontaneous breathing throughout the entire breath cycle. It has been described as continuous positive airway pressure with regular brief intermittent releases in airway pressure. The release phase results in alveolar ventilation and removal of CO_2. Unlike CPAP, however, APRV facilitates both oxygenation and ventilation. The breath begins from an elevated baseline (P-high or measured high pressure) and achieves tidal ventilation with a brief release of the P-high. This brief release allows for CO_2 removal through passive exhalation secondary to elastic recoil. The exhalation time (T-low) is shortened to usually less than one second to prevent alveolar derecruitment and collapse: It is essentially CPAP with a brief release.

APRV was designed to oxygenate and augment ventilation for patients with acute lung injury or low-compliance lung disease. In patients with severe lung disease, APRV may result in significantly lower peak airway pressure compared to conventional ventilator pressures (Garner et al., 1988). Also, lower minute ventilation can be achieved, suggesting that less dead space ventilation occurs. Because APRV is a pressure-targeted mode of ventilation, changes in lung compliance can lead to over-distention or hypoventilation with this mode, mandating monitoring of patients for changes in tidal volume. Also, because APRV is time cycled, there is no synchronization of a patient's spontaneous breathing pattern, which may result in discomfort or patient–ventilator asynchrony. Finally, limited information exists regarding the use of APRV in pediatric patients (Schultz et al., 2001).

High-frequency oscillatory ventilation. High-frequency oscillatory ventilation (HFOV) is characterized by high respiratory rates up to 15 hertz (900 breaths per minute). The rates used vary widely depending on the type of patient and his or her disease condition.

In HFOV, the pressure oscillates in the region of the constant distending pressure (mean airway pressure). Thus gas is forced into the lung during inspiration. Unlike conventional ventilation, in which exhalation is passive, HFOV actively removes air during expiration. This mode generates very low tidal volumes that are generally less than the dead space of the lung. Tidal volume is dependent on endotracheal tube size, amplitude, and hertz.

In HFOV, a diaphragm drives the pressure wave, similar to the system used in a loudspeaker. The pressure wave that is generated at the ventilator is markedly attenuated by passage down the endotracheal tube and the major conducting airways. This helps protect the alveoli from the volutrauma that can potentially occur with traditional positive-pressure ventilation. Although the alveoli are kept at a relatively constant volume, other mechanisms of gas exchange allow ventilation to occur without tidal volume exchange.

Ventilation in HFOV is a function of the frequency, amplitude, and inspiratory–expiratory (I:E) ratio. Amplitude is analogous to tidal volume in conventional ventilation, in which larger amplitudes remove more CO_2. In a seemingly paradoxical twist, lower frequencies remove more CO_2 in HFOV. As frequency decreases, there is less attenuation of the pressure wave transmitted to the alveoli. This results in increased mixing of gas and, therefore, ventilation. The I-time is set as a percentage of total time (usually 33%). The amplitude (ΔP) is a function of power and is subject to variability due to changes in compliance or resistance. As a consequence, power requirements may vary significantly during treatment and from patient to patient. In HFOV, mean airway pressure is the primary determinant of oxygenation and is delivered via a continuous flow through the patient circuit. The MAP in HFOV functions similarly to PEEP in conventional ventilation, in that it provides the pressure for alveolar recruitment.

High-frequency jet ventilation. Compared to conventional ventilation, the major advantages of high-frequency jet ventilation (HFJV) are its improvement of the mucociliary transport system, the recruitment of atelectatic areas, and the improvement of oxygenation while maintaining very low tidal volumes so as to avoid lung barotrauma. Combined HFJV is a technique that requires a conventional ventilator and a HFJV (Brichant et al., 1986). The conventional ventilator is a time-regulated, pressure-controlled ventilation technique. During HFJV, gas is propelled into the lungs at a very high velocity. The incoming gas is forced to stream into the airways in a long spike. The abundant energy of this "jet stream" causes the gas to form a spiral flow, which easily splits into two streams at every bifurcation. Thus fresh gas penetrates through the anatomic dead space, leaving much of the CO_2 in the dead space compressed against the airway walls.

With HFJV, as with conventional mechanical ventilation, inhalation is active or forced, and exhalation is passive. Two factors allow exhalation to occur: (1) The size of each breath (1 to 3 mL/kg) is much smaller than usual and (2) the natural or resonant frequency of the lungs is close to the frequency range being used by HFJV. Thus the lungs recoil readily during HFJV under almost all conditions. The role of conventional ventilation during HFJV is limited to oxygenation. Conventional ventilators can deliver oxygenated gas directly to the alveolar level. They achieve this feat by using relatively long inspiratory times and large tidal volumes, and they have the capability of controlling end-expiratory pressure. These are the factors that most readily control PO_2. Unfortunately, they are also the factors most closely associated with barotrauma. Thus it is useful to minimize these factors by running the conventional ventilator at a low rate (1 to 3 breaths per minute) while the HFJV is providing the majority of the ventilation. Using the conventional ventilator to gradually recruit collapsed alveoli allows the HFJV to achieve the best possible oxygenation and ventilation with the lowest possible airway pressures.

INHALED NITRIC OXIDE

Inhaled nitric oxide (iNO) has been rapidly embraced by critical care HCPs as a means to treat hypoxemic lung diseases such as acute respiratory distress syndrome (ARDS) and, perhaps more rationally, persistent pulmonary hypertension in newborn infants. Its vasodilatory properties can reduce pulmonary artery pressures. As a treatment for hypoxemia in patients with ARDS, inhaled NO is recognized for its ability to selectively increase perfusion to portions of the lung receiving ventilation. Randomized clinical trials have reported temporary improvements in arterial oxygenation but no significant differences in outcomes with this treatment (Dobyns et al., 1999; Finer & Barrington, 2001). NO has been proven effective in decreasing the need for extracorporeal membrane oxygenation (ECMO) in infants with persistent pulmonary hypertension, in whom it has been found to improve systemic oxygenation, and in older children with hypoxic respiratory failure (Hoffman et al., 1997).

SURFACTANT THERAPY

Alterations in endogenous surfactant play a role in the pathogenesis of many causes of acute lung injury and ARDS. Surfactant dysfunction, destruction, and inactivation have also been demonstrated in pediatric patients with acute respiratory insufficiency from certain viral infections. The administration of exogenous surfactant may reduce the need for mechanical ventilation and its associated sequelae by restoring surfactant levels and function. When surfactant is used in patients with acute respiratory failure, studies have shown that patients tend to have more ventilator-free days and decreased duration of ventilation.

Surfactant therapy is well tolerated, with transient hypoxia and hypotension being reported as the most common side effects during administration. To date, there is no apparent consensus as to the optimal dose, timing of administration, and ideal patient population for use of this therapy (Duffett et al., 2007; Willson et al., 2005).

MONITORING DEVICES

Arterial blood gases

Traditionally, arterial blood gases (ABGs) monitoring has been used for evaluation of oxygenation and ventilation. Data obtained from ABG measurements may guide overall ventilator management and can be used to calculate oxygen delivery metrics. Overall metabolic status is reflected in the serum pH, and the coupling of oxygen supply and demand can be reflected by the base excess. When oxygenation monitoring is desired, ABGs are superior methods to capillary blood gases (CBGs), as CBG results poorly correlate with PO_2.

Samples for ABGs should be obtained from a free-flowing arterial source and should be free of air bubbles. Air bubble PO_2 is 158 mmHg. If the sample that is drawn has a PO_2 less than 158 mmHg, then the reading will equilibrate in the sample, resulting in a falsely elevated PO_2. Conversely, if the ABG sample has a PO_2 higher than 158 mmHg, the result will be falsely low on the arterial blood gas (Marcum & Newth, 2007).

The time from obtaining the arterial sample until processing of the results should be minimized due to ongoing consumption of oxygen by the red blood cells in the collected sample. Delayed processing of the sample can affect the accuracy of PaO_2 measurement.

Patient temperature can also affect ABG results. While more recently introduced devices will factor in the patient's temperature, older models do not have this capability.

Pulse oximetry

Pulse oximetry is a noninvasive monitoring modality that is considered the standard of care in inpatient settings due to its continuous and relatively accurate monitoring capabilities. With this technology, two light-emitting diodes and a photodetector emitting light through the capillary bed are used to quantify the fraction of hemoglobin oxygen saturation. Pulse oximetry devices are unable to distinguish between oxyhemoglobin, methemoglobin, and carboxyhemoglobin, so they have limitations in clinical scenarios where these levels may be falsely high or low (Marcum & Newth, 2007). Motion artifact and hypoperfusion states are common causes of inaccurate pulse oximetry readings. Despite these challenges, pulse oximetry is an invaluable tool when monitoring acute and critically ill pediatric patients.

Transcutaneous carbon dioxide

When arterial samples are difficult to obtain, transcutaneous carbon dioxide ($tcPCO_2$) monitoring can be used to assist with assessment of adequacy of ventilation. This method heats the skin surface, causing vasodilation and bringing carbon dioxide to the skin surface. The CO_2 then diffuses across the probe membrane, which enables electrochemical detection of the gas. The best readings are obtained by placing the probe over nonbony, well-perfused surfaces. Limitations of this modality include the results' poor correlation with PO_2, the requirement for frequent device recalibration, and the risk for skin irritation at the probe site. This technology may also yield inaccurate readings in individuals with increased skin thickness, such as in older children and adults (Marcum & Newth, 2007). Nevertheless, $tcPCO_2$ is a useful noninvasive monitoring tool for nonintubated patients or in patients in whom end-tidal CO_2 monitoring is not possible (HFOV).

End-tidal carbon dioxide

Another form of noninvasive CO_2 monitoring is end-tidal carbon dioxide ($ETCO_2$) monitoring. Disposable colorimetric capnometry is a qualitative measure of CO_2 in exhaled gases, displaying a color change upon exposure to exhaled CO_2. Continuous, quantitative, real-time measurement of end-tidal CO_2 concentration is now considered the standard of care for monitoring intubated patients.

CO_2 is systemically delivered to the lungs; thus low cardiac output states can be reflected by low exhaled CO_2 readings in the capnometer. End-tidal CO_2 monitoring is, in essence, a means of monitoring ventilation and measuring cardiac output. A capnograph provides a visual waveform depiction of variations in CO_2 during the respiratory cycle and displays the highest value recorded. Exhaled CO_2 is determined by an infrared light source, an exhalation gas chamber, and a light detector (Marcum & Newth, 2007).

In addition to providing information on ventilation and cardiac output, $ETCO_2$ can be useful in identifying obstructive airway disease. In this case, the display will be sloped rather than square.

While this device is most commonly used in intubated patients, side-stream exhaled CO_2 detectors are available for uses in nonintubated patients. The side-stream device continually withdraws a sample of exhaled gas through a nasal cannula adaptor. Side-stream CO_2 measurement can be a useful adjunct when monitoring acutely ill pediatric patients who are not yet intubated or who have received procedural or conscious sedation.

Volume loops

Many mechanical ventilators have the capability to show flow-volume and pressure-volume loops. These graphical displays of volume, pressure, and flow provide information about the patient's lung physiology and pathology with respect to their response to specific ventilator parameters. Such waveforms can be helpful in monitoring patient–ventilator synchrony, including spontaneous breaths and breaths generated by the mechanical ventilator. The interpretation of volume-flow loops help determine the level of auto-PEEP, and it aids in the evaluation of lung compliance and resistance. When studying waveforms, care must be taken to evaluate their accuracy. In particular, the HCP should recognize that waveform artifacts can occur from condensation or secretion accumulation in the ventilator circuit or air leaks in the system (Burns, 2006).

Pressure-volume loops display the pressure on the horizontal axis and the volume on the vertical axis (Figure 35-15). A pressure-volume loop displaying higher pressures at the first portion of the inspiratory curve results in generation of lower volumes (low compliance). The graphical point where a rapid increase in the curve upslope appears is called the lower inflection point. The lower inflection point represents the time at which alveoli are suddenly opening, allowing for more movement of gas. At the end of inspiration, a sharp angle in the loop marks the beginning of exhalation. The exhalation phase of the loop is notable for a significant reduction pressure associated with a smaller decrease in volume. When over-distention occurs in the lungs, "beaking" of the loop can be observed. Beaking of the graph occurs because there is no longer an increase in tidal volume from additional application in pressure; thus the volume component of the graph remains flat as pressure

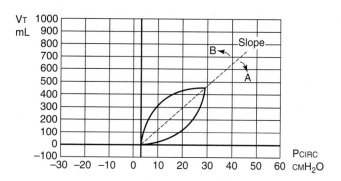

Pressure-volume loop: assessing compliance. The slope (or steepness) of the loop reflects the relationship of volume and pressure. A change in the slope of the loop indicates changes in compliance (A and B). When the slope moves toward A there is a decrease in compliance, while a move of the slope towards B indicates improved compliance.

FIGURE 35-15

Pressure-Volume Loop.

Source: Burns, S. (2006). *Noninvasive Monitoring.* Sudbury, MA: Jones and Bartlett Publishing.

continues to rise. In these cases, no additional tidal volume is achieved in spite of the application of additional ventilator pressure.

In flow-volume loops, the flow is represented on the vertical axis and the volume is represented on the horizontal axis (Figure 35-16). Inspiration is depicted on the upper portion of the slope, and exhalation is depicted on the lower portion of the loop. With increases in flow, the inspiratory volume increases. Exhalation begins when there is cessation in flow. Flow-volume loops can assist in evaluating for upper or lower airway obstruction. For example, a scooped-out appearance of the loop on exhalation demonstrates an obstructive pattern. A response to bronchodilator administration would result in a less scooped-out loop pattern during the exhalation phase (Cheifetz et al., 2008).

PULMONARY HYGIENE

Mucociliary clearance is the primary method of clearing foreign material, bacteria, viruses, and particulate materials from the airway. When mucociliary clearance is dysfunctional or overwhelmed, the cough reflex is crucial in secretion removal. Many conditions in acute illness (bronchiolitis, pneumonia, status asthmaticus) and chronic illness (cystic fibrosis exacerbation, neuromuscular disease) can stimulate excess mucus production, causing the mucociliary system to become overwhelmed. This process may lead to thickening of secretions and atelectasis (Panitch, 2006). In these clinical conditions, assistance with secretion removal, or pulmonary hygiene, is indicated to optimize respiratory status. Several techniques to improve airway clearance are reviewed in this section.

Airway clearance techniques

Conventional chest physiotherapy. Conventional chest physiotherapy (CPT) is a technique for promotion of secretion mobilization that has long been a staple of pulmonary hygiene for acute and chronic illnesses. In this method of airway clearance, external vibration and/or percussion is applied externally to the pediatric patient's chest and/or back to theoretically mobilize secretions. A manual cupping device or electric percussor, or vibrator, may be used. The device used is based on the patient's condition, comfort, and size. This technique is frequently used in conjunction with positioning to facilitate secretion removal from different portions of the lung via gravity. If the pediatric patient is unable to expectorate, this treatment is commonly followed by suctioning of the oropharynx or endotracheal tube.

Inexsufflator (cough-assist device). The inexsufflator device delivers an inspiratory assistance breath to stimulate a cough, which is followed immediately by exsufflation. Exsufflation is performed by a negative-pressure device that enhances the expiratory flow and cough effectiveness. This technique is sometimes coupled with a manual expiratory abdominal thrust to prevent airway collapse and to enhance the peak cough flow (Panitch, 2006). A cough-assist device is often used in pediatric patients with underlying weakness due to prolonged mechanical ventilation and those with chronic respiratory failure (cystic fibrosis, neuromuscular disease), but can be used in most patients requiring assistance with generating an effective cough.

Intermittent positive-pressure breathing. Intermittent positive-pressure breathing (IPPB) uses a noninvasive mask or mouthpiece interface to deliver positive-pressure breaths to spontaneously breathing patients. This therapy is usually delivered in 10 to 15-minute increments several times throughout the day. The goal of IPPB is to enhance the pediatric patient's spontaneous tidal volume, ultimately providing more complete inflation of the lungs while decreasing the occurrence of atelectasis. The positive pressure can be delivered through a standard ventilator circuit or through a noninvasive ventilation machine.

Vest therapy. Vest therapy, also called high-frequency chest wall oscillation, causes gas to move in and out of the lungs at a high velocity for a short period of time. This noninvasive inflatable vest is attached to a high-frequency generator via hoses. Vest therapy facilitates secretion removal by using the high gas flow to shear mucus off the

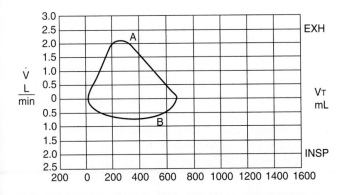

Flow-volume loop. In flow-volume loops, peak expiratory flow rate is noted at A. Peak inspiratory flow rate is noted at B. Flow-volume loops are plotted similarly to pulmonary function tests in which exhalation is plotted first followed by the next inspiration.

FIGURE 35-16

Flow-Volume Loop.

Source: Burns, S. (2006). *Noninvasive Monitoring.* Sudbury, MA: Jones and Bartlett Publishing.

walls of the pulmonary tract; it also decreases the viscosity of the secretions. This technique can be used in acute or chronically ill pediatric patients. It has been well studied in patients with cystic fibrosis, but is frequently used in other patient populations with tenacious secretions or with ineffective cough mechanisms (Panitch, 2006).

Intrapulmonary percussive ventilation. Intrapulmonary percussive ventilation (IPV) delivers low-volume, high-flow "mini-bursts" of positive pressure to the airway using frequencies of 100 to 300 cycles/min, with peak pressures ranging from 10 to 40 cmH_2O. IPV causes vibration, lung expansion, and enlargement of the airways, ultimately facilitating gas exchange in the distal airways. This treatment is often used in conjunction with administration of a bronchodilator and can be used in pediatric patients with a natural or artificial airway. Once the gas has moved past the secretions in the airway, exhalation assists the mucus in returning to the central airway for easier expectoration. This technique has been demonstrated to be effective in managing atelectasis and can be used in patients with acute or chronic respiratory problems (Panitch, 2006). As compared to conventional CPT, IPV is more effective in improving atelectasis and can be safely used in pediatric patients with artificial airways (Deakins & Chatburn, 2002).

Aerosol therapy

Atelectasis is commonly caused by sputum blocking the airway. A variety of aerosol therapies have been used in the treatment of atelectasis. For example, inhaled beta agonists and nebulized saline are often used to treat this problem, although data supporting their use in this indication are lacking. Theoretically, these treatments have mucolytic properties that may help loosen and remove the sections associated with atelectasis.

Recombinant human DNase has been proven to be effective for treating patients with cystic fibrosis, but has not been evaluated extensively in children who have not been diagnosed with the disease (Harms et al., 1998; Quan et al., 2001). DNase has been shown to result in clinical and radiographic improvements in non-CF children with infection-associated atelectasis, however (Hendricks et al., 2005). This effect is presumably due to the infectious sputum, which contains a significant amount of extracellular DNA derived from degenerating leukocytes and epithelial debris. This thick sputum can be broken down by DNase, leading to less viscous sections and easier removal of pulmonary secretions.

VENTILATOR WEANING STRATEGIES

Weaning

The time from intubation until resolution of the acute illness is followed by the weaning phase. As yet, no standard for weaning patients from mechanical ventilation has been developed. Instead, the duration of the weaning phase depends on factors such as patient strength, level of sedation, and fluid status.

Most commonly, gradual reduction in ventilator support is used when weaning pediatric patients from mechanical ventilation. The set ventilator rate is reduced in a stepwise fashion. Some HCPs favor the use of pressure support or volume support during the weaning phase; others prefer to employ moderate amounts of ventilatory support coupled with daily extubation readiness tests (ERT). In these cases, mechanical ventilation is discontinued if the patient passes the ERT. This method has been used more frequently with adult patients than pediatric patients.

Yet another method of weaning from mechanical ventilation uses a "sprinting" technique. With this approach, complete ventilatory support is alternated with periods of assisted spontaneous breathing (Newth et al., 2009).

Weaning protocols have become common in the adult population, but have not yet been well studied in pediatric patients.

Spontaneous breathing test

Some HCPs use spontaneous breathing tests (SBTs) as indicators of extubation readiness. While the technique employed may vary slightly, these trials generally are initiated when the HCP deems the pediatric patient to be nearly ready for extubation. Spontaneous breathing tests are a subjective determination of whether the underlying disease process requiring mechanical ventilation has been resolved sufficiently for the patient to achieve adequate gas exchange and oxygenation with spontaneous breathing (Newth et al., 2009).

Indications of extubation readiness

Evaluation for extubation readiness is especially important in the pediatric population due to these patients' small airway diameter and concerns about the duration of mechanical ventilation in children. Extubation failure rates have been cited as ranging from 4% to 19% in pediatric studies (Turner & Arnold, 2007). Readiness for extubation implies that the weaning is complete and that the patient is sufficiently awake with intact airway reflexes, has manageable secretions, and is hemodynamically stable. Extubation readiness tests are sometimes employed to evaluate for this readiness. The patient is generally evaluated for two hours on CPAP, pressure support, or "T" piece (a simple valveless circuit). Failure criteria include diaphoresis, nasal flaring, increased respiratory effort, apnea, hypotension, cardiac arrhythmias, increased CO_2, and decreased pH. Other data that are commonly acquired to assess extubation readiness include a leak check and assessment of muscle strength with a negative inspiratory force

(NIF) test (Newth et al., 2009). If the pediatric patient does not fully meet the criteria for extubation and spontaneous, unsupported breathing, the HCP may consider extubation to a noninvasive ventilatory support device.

Airway leak test

One method frequently used in an attempt to predict risk for extubation failure is the airway leak test. Some pediatric data suggest that the absence of a leak around the endotracheal tube at a pressure of 30 cm H_2O or greater increases the risk of postextubation stridor and extubation failure. Several pediatric studies have demonstrated a trend of reduced postextubation stridor and reintubation rates when periextubation systemic steroids are administered (Cheng et al., 2006; Lukkassen et al., 2006; Markovitz & Randolph, 2002; Turner & Arnold, 2007).

COMPLICATIONS FROM INTUBATION AND MECHANICAL VENTILATION

While they are certainly life-saving modalities, intubation and mechanical ventilation are not without risk of complication. Complications can occur either during the ventilation course or following extubation (or both). Some complications are short term, while others are more serious and have long-term implications (Table 35-28).

TRACHEOSTOMY

Indications

Many indications for tracheostomy in pediatric patients exist; however, the decision to perform a tracheostomy includes

TABLE 35-28

Complications of Intubation and Mechanical Ventilation
Upper Airway Trauma
• Subglottic stenosis
• Laryngeal trauma (vocal cord paralysis)
• Postextubation airway edema
Lower Airway
• Air leak (pneumomediastinum, pneumothorax)
• Atelectasis
• Ventilator-associated lung disease (volutrauma, barotrauma)
• Ventilator-associated pneumonia
Cardiovascular
• Decreased venous return

Source: Adapted from Kornecki & Kavanaugh, 2007.

consideration of the severity of airway obstruction or respiratory insufficiency and the pediatric patient's overall medical condition (Table 35-29). Currently, the most common indication for pediatric tracheostomy is prolonged mechanical ventilation due to neuromuscular or respiratory insufficiency (Fraga et al., 2009). Benefits of tracheostomy include securement of an airway, facilitation of pulmonary hygiene, and ability to provide positive-pressure ventilation, if needed.

Contraindications

There are no absolute contraindications to tracheostomy. However, a strong relative contraindication is consideration of end-of-life issues in some clinical situations. While the tracheostomy is reversible, the presence of a tracheostomy can imply a desire for further mechanization of the pediatric patient's care.

Tracheostomy (Procedure)

With the exception of emergency situations, tracheotomy is performed in the operating room using general anesthesia

TABLE 35-29

Indications for Pediatric Tracheostomy	
Category	**Examples**
Congenital	Vocal cord paralysis, vascular rings, subglottic stenosis, bronchopulmonary dysplasia, congenital central hypoventilation syndrome, Pierre-Robin sequence, laryngeal web/cysts, pulmonary hypoplasia, craniofacial abnormalities, achondroplasia
Traumatic	Orofacial injury, burns, laryngeal edema, foreign body
Infectious	Epiglottitis, meningitis, tetanus, rabies, botulism
Degenerative disease	Neuromuscular disease, myasthenia gravis
Prophylactic	Head/neck surgery, neurosurgery
Neoplastic	Tumors of the brain, larynx, trachea, pharynx, or tongue; hemangioma; lymphangioma
Allergic	Angioedema, anaphylactic shock
Other	Administration of long-term mechanical ventilation, secretion management/pulmonary hygiene

Source: Adapted from Fraga et al., 2009.

while the patient is intubated. A rigid bronchoscopy should be available throughout the procedure in the event the airway requires manipulation. The patient is placed in the supine position, with a roll under the shoulders to extend and expose the neck. A horizontal skin incision is used, followed by a vertical incision at the level of the third and fourth tracheal rings. The tracheostomy tube is placed through the surgical incision and is often secured using stay sutures (Fraga et al., 2009).

Size and position considerations

Tracheostomy size reflects the underlying etiology necessitating the tracheostomy and the size of the patient's airway. The tube should be small enough to permit vocalization, yet large enough that a leak does not lead to hypoventilation, especially with sleep or mechanical ventilation. It is generally best to use the smallest tracheostomy diameter that allows the pediatric patient to maintain oxygenation and ventilation.

Length of the cannula is another important consideration, as a cannula that is too short may result in inadvertent decannulation or false airway creation. Conversely, a cannula that is too long may result in damage to the carina, stimulation of a vagal response, or intubation of the right or left bronchi (Fraga et al., 2009). Some pediatric patients require customized tracheostomy tube lengths to overcome tracheal abnormalities.

Complications

Most pediatric patients do well with tracheostomy tubes, yet vigilant awareness for risk of complications is required. Pediatric patients are two to three times more likely than adults to suffer complications associated with tracheostomy, largely due to their small size. The incidence of complications has been described as varying between 5% and 49% (Carter & Benjamin, 1983; Fraga et al., 2009; Kremer et al., 2002).

Short-term complications may include bleeding, pneumothorax, pneumomediastinum, subcutaneous emphysema, tracheoesophageal fistula, and infection. Intermediate- and long-term complications may include mucosal injury or ischemia of the tracheal wall, fibrotic changes, and stenosis of the trachea (Fraga et al., 2009). If the tracheostomy tube is cuffed, care must be taken to limit the insufflation of the cuff, as cuff over-distention may also cause ischemic injury and tracheal stenosis.

Tracheal plugging can occur anytime during the presence of an artificial airway. Any acute onset of respiratory distress or inability to ventilate should alert the HCP to consider tracheal plugging or dislodgement as possible etiologies.

Long-term complications of tracheostomy tube presence include granulomatous tissue formation, tracheal stenosis, fusion of the vocal cords, infection, and erosion into the innominate artery. The last complication typically manifests with severe, life-threatening tracheal bleeding (Fraga et al., 2009).

Postoperative care of patients with new tracheostomy tubes

Typically, it takes approximately 7 days after surgery for the tracheostomy track to mature and become established. Often, the surgeon will perform the first tracheostomy change at 5 to 7 days after the procedure. This may be done at the bedside or in the operating room, depending on the size and condition of the pediatric patient.

Many surgeons will leave "stay sutures" in place until the first tracheostomy tube change. Stay sutures are placed directly into the tracheal tissue, allowing tension to be placed on the sutures, by gently lifting the sutures up and away from the neck, in an inadvertent decannulation. This allows the trachea to be pulled up toward the stoma and skin surface, allowing for better visualization of the tract during replacement of the tracheostomy tube (Fraga et al., 2009).

If stay sutures are not present, or if a false passage is created during attempted tracheostomy tube replacement, the patient can be endotracheally intubated from above the site to secure the airway. Patients who have undergone a laryngotracheal separation procedure are *not* candidates for endotracheal intubation from above the tracheostomy site. In these pediatric patients, the larynx and esophagus have been surgically separated and an intubation from above would result in an esophageal intubation.

Until the first tracheostomy change has been performed, gentle cleansing around the site several times per day, and as needed, is indicated. Routine suctioning using an appropriate-size suction catheter may be performed. Monitoring of the site for frank bleeding, purulent drainage, and foul odor is also indicated.

Tracheostomy care and bedside requirements

Once the stoma has been established, stoma site cleansing and monitoring along with routine tracheostomy tube changes are the mainstay of care. Bedside requirements for those with tracheostomies include spare clean tracheostomy tubes in the same size and one size smaller than the tube that is currently in place, appropriate-sized suction catheters or inline suctioning device, cleaning supplies, and clean tracheostomy ties. Established tracheostomy tubes are frequently changed on a weekly basis. Some clinical conditions may require more frequent tracheostomy tube changes.

LONG-TERM MECHANICAL VENTILATION

Indications

The point at which pediatric patients are considered to have chronic respiratory insufficiency is difficult to ascertain. Chronic respiratory insufficiency is generally recognized when a chronic and perhaps irreversible level of respiratory insufficiency leads to hypoxia and/or hypoventilation. Patients with this condition may be identified after repeated unsuccessful attempts at weaning from mechanical ventilation (often over weeks to a month) or when they are no longer afflicted with a superimposed acute respiratory disease. Chronic respiratory failure may be identified in those patients who have no prospect of weaning from mechanical ventilation—for example, because of progressive neuromuscular disease or high spinal cord injury (Keens et al., 2008). A pediatric patient suffering from chronic respiratory failure requires reworking of the therapeutic plan to include chronic ventilatory support, family education, and readying of the home for the necessary technology.

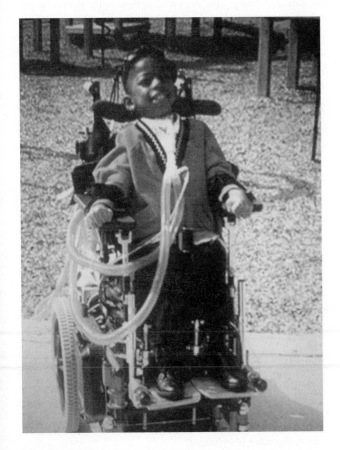

FIGURE 35-17

Home Ventilator.

Source: Courtesy of the National EMSC Resource Alliance.

Home ventilators

Upon determining the presence of chronic respiratory failure and placement of a tracheostomy, the pediatric patient can be placed on a portable positive-pressure ventilator in preparation for hospital discharge (Figure 35–17). Home ventilators are battery powered and relatively portable and mobile. Although advances in these devices have certainly been made, they remain less powerful and technologically advanced as hospital ventilators. For this reason, patients with intercurrent respiratory infection may require hospitalization for transition to a more sophisticated ventilator and ongoing support.

Long-term considerations

When approaching long-term ventilation, the best interests of the family and patient must be considered. Discussions surrounding the pediatric patient's long-term prognosis and quality of life may be indicated prior to instituting long-term mechanical ventilation. Frank discussions should include the caregivers, family, and child (if appropriate) regarding the required level of care, presence of nursing care in the home, and changes in lifestyle. These discussions are required to ensure a successful transition of care for a mechanically ventilated family member, and should occur prior to the implementation of long-term ventilation support. Some families wishing to pursue long-term mechanical ventilation for their child are unable to provide these services within the home. In these cases, a long-term care facility may be a better alternative.

Preparation for discharge

The pediatric patient must be stable on the home ventilator for at least 1 to 2 weeks prior to hospital discharge, allowing time for the child to demonstrate a period of stability on the home settings. This trial period is especially important because home mechanical ventilators do not provide the same level of support as hospital ventilators at the same settings. Frequently, when transitioning from a hospital ventilator to a home mechanical ventilator, the settings will need to be increased to achieve the same level of mechanical ventilation. For this reason, it is important to monitor the patient in the hospital on the *actual ventilator and circuit* that will be used in the home. Patients will tolerate a $PaCO_2$ slightly lower than physiologic, so determining an appropriate range is often the goal when adjusting long-term mechanical ventilation so as to provide a margin of safety within the home (Keens et al., 2008).

Home ventilation strategies

The patient's underlying indication for mechanical ventilation and clinical status will determine how many hours per day the child will require mechanical ventilation. Many pediatric patients are on 24-hour-per-day mechanical ventilation at home. Those demonstrating readiness for weaning may be ready to tolerate trials of "sprinting," or time off the ventilator on a humidified tracheostomy collar. These sprints are initiated only while the patient is awake. They usually begin with trials off the ventilator of only a few minutes, with the time off mechanical ventilation gradually being increased as tolerated. $ETCO_2$, pulse oximetry, and physical examination can be useful to assess the adequacy of ventilation and oxygenation during times off mechanical ventilation. As the duration of time off increases, a polysomnogram may be performed to more formally evaluate adequacy of oxygenation and ventilation, especially during nap and night time.

Complications

Complications of long-term mechanical ventilation include all of the complications that can be encountered in a patient with a tracheostomy in addition to complications specific to mechanical ventilation. Whenever a piece of technology is used, there is a risk of mechanical failure—and this is true for all forms of mechanical ventilation. Abrupt or more insidious mechanical failures, however, can also occur with home ventilators. In this circumstance, the caregiver must be able to recognize the malfunction and begin hand ventilation while preparing a change to the backup ventilator. Ventilator circuits can become either too warm or cool, which can affect the moisture level in the circuit and potentially lead to increased mucus plug formation. Infection remains a risk at all times and can be further exacerbated when ventilator circuits are not maintained in the recommended fashion.

Even pediatric patients who are well managed on long-term home mechanical ventilation will experience times when the ventilator is not fully meeting their respiratory needs, exposing them to periods of alveolar hypoxia and hypoventilation. These events can place the child at risk for developing pulmonary hypertension and cor pulmonale. If this complication is suspected, an echocardiograph may be used to evaluate right-sided heart function. If evidence of pulmonary hypertension or cor pulmonale is found, it may be assumed that the current ventilator settings are inadequate and the pediatric patient should be hospitalized to re-evaluate optimal ventilator settings (Keens et al., 2008). Follow-up echocardiographs will then be required to monitor right-sided heart function.

Chronically ventilated children are at increased risk for more severe courses of common childhood illnesses, in part due to the loss or impairment of some of their normal host defenses. For example, patients with tracheostomy tubes bypass the usual humidifying and filtering functions of the upper airway, which can lead to thicker tracheal secretions and development of tracheobronchitis. In addition,

if the child has an ineffective cough reflex, it can lead to an impaired ability to clear sections, mucus plugging, and atelectasis.

Patient and family education

A significant amount of education is required of the family prior to patient discharge (Table 35-30). Caregivers must be proficient in tracheostomy care, suctioning, and tracheostomy changing. Education must also be provided on the mechanical ventilator, any medications, pulmonary hygiene techniques, safe transport of the patient on mechanical ventilation, emergency procedures, and cardiopulmonary resuscitation. Institutions should have standardized home ventilation protocols for caregiver education prior to discharge. Such guidelines often include a 12- or 24-hour stay at the hospital managing all aspects of the patient's care.

Disposition and discharge planning

The pediatric patient is determined to be ready for discharge when the caregivers have completed their education, the home is ready, and the child is medically stable. While the child remains an outpatient, routine evaluation of the ventilator settings and the patient's overall status should be performed to ensure that the ventilator settings are continuing to meet the needs of the growing child.

TABLE 35-30

Essential Equipment for Home Mechanical Ventilation

- Portable home ventilator
- Home ventilator accessories
  - Ventilator circuits
  - Humidifier
  - Heater and water trap
  - Automobile charging adapter, if available for ventilator model
- Back-up ventilator (essential if the ventilator is used for 20 or more hours per day)
- Battery and battery charger (unless built into the ventilator)
- Supplemental oxygen, if necessary
- E-cylinder of oxygen with regulator, for emergency use
- Aerosol delivery system
- Portable suction
- Suction catheters
- Spare tracheostomy tubes
- Tracheostomy care supplies
- Resuscitation bag
- Pulse oximeter, pulse oximeter probes
- Speaking valve (if indicated)
- Artificial nose
- Bacterial filter for the ventilator circuit

Source: Adapted from Keens et al., 2008.

First-floor residences are often preferred to facilitate transporting the pediatric patient in and out of the home. In some cases, the residence may require an electrical upgrade to support the technology that will be brought into the home. Local utility and phone companies should be notified in writing about the patient's status and ventilator dependence, so that in the event of a power or phone outage, the child's home is on a priority list for reinstitution of service (Keens et al., 2008).

Prior to discharge, the patient and family should be closely linked with a medical center that is capable of caring for the child in case of illness or emergency, and a pediatric care provider with experience in managing special needs health care children should be contacted to handle the patient's primary care needs. The local paramedics and emergency department should be familiar with the child and be able to provide emergency care and transport to the local medical center in case of emergency.

There is no consensus on the frequency with which health care visits to the home should be made. Nevertheless, younger pediatric patients may require more frequent visits, while older, more stable patients may be able to be managed with annual visits. Patients should have scheduled follow-up appointments with all subspecialties necessary, including pulmonary and/or rehabilitation services, prior to discharge. Home care nursing visits should also be arranged to ensure a smooth transition from hospital to home.

VENTILATOR-INDUCED LUNG INJURY

Bradley Tilford

Ventilator-induced lung injury (VILI) is lung injury that develops as a consequence of mechanical ventilation. It most commonly occurs during ventilation for acute lung injury (ALI) or acute respiratory distress syndrome (ARDS), but may occur in other disease states. ALI and ARDS represent points along the same disease spectrum but differ in severity; thus they are often referred to collectively as ALI/ARDS. In the clinical setting, it may be impossible to distinguish whether worsening hypoxia and infiltrates are due to VILI or the underlying disease process.

PATHOPHYSIOLOGY

Alveolar over-distention (volutrauma) and cyclic atelectasis (atelectrauma) are thought to be the primary causes of lung injury during mechanical ventilation. Volutrauma may occur without large tidal volumes. The lungs of mechanically ventilated patients often contain a heterogeneous mix of normal lung and consolidated/collapsed lung that is more difficult to ventilate. The normal lung receives a disproportionate amount of the ventilated breath, so that

the healthy alveoli are over-distended. In contrast, atelectrauma is caused by repetitive expansion and collapse of the mechanically ventilated alveoli, which creates shear forces resulting in distention and injury to the adjacent alveoli.

Both volutrauma and atelectrauma may cause alveolar and interstitial edema, alveolar hemorrhage, surfactant loss, hyaline membrane formation, and alveolar collapse. They also result in an increase in pro-inflammatory cells and cytokines with both local and systemic effects (MacIntyre, 2005).

EPIDEMIOLOGY AND ETIOLOGY

Patients with ALI/ARDS are at the highest risk for developing VILI. The incidence of VILI is difficult to determine due to its similarities to progressive ARDS. Approximately 25% of patients ventilated for reasons other than ALI/ARDS will develop ALI if ventilated for 48 hours or longer. Risk factors for lung injury in these patients include delivery of a large tidal volume on the first day of ventilation, blood transfusion in the first 48 hours of ventilation, acidosis, and restrictive lung disease (Gagic et al., 2004).

PRESENTATION

VILI is difficult to distinguish from progressive ALI/ARDS. Patients typically have increased oxygen requirements and demonstrate worsening infiltrates on CXR. They may have more tachypnea and tachycardia and may develop multiple organ dysfunction syndrome.

DIFFERENTIAL DIAGNOSIS

Many problems may worsen the respiratory condition of mechanically ventilated patients; thus it may be difficult to differentiate between VILI and other causes. Volume overload may result in pulmonary edema and hypoxia, but should improve with diuretic therapy. Ventilator-associated pneumonia often presents with fever and a change in endotracheal tube secretions. Pulmonary embolus may present with hypoxia and tachycardia, but may not be associated with changes on the CXR. Pneumothorax may cause acute hypoxia and hemodynamic instability, but should be readily apparent from the physical examination and CXR. In practice, evaluation and treatment for several potential diagnoses will proceed simultaneously in a deteriorating patient.

PLAN OF CARE

Diagnostic imaging studies include serial CXRs. In some instances, a CT scan of the chest may be indicated.

Although it may provide valuable information, MRI of the chest is often difficult to perform in patients with increasing ventilation demands.

The management of VILI is the same as that for ALI/ARDS. Ventilation strategies should be employed to reduce volutrauma and atelectrauma in all mechanically ventilated patients. Tidal volumes of 6 mL/kg ideal body weight or less are optimal for patients with ALI/ARDS. A tidal volume of 8 mL/kg ideal body weight or less is reasonable for patients without preceding ALI. Maintaining plateau pressures at 30 cmH$_2$O or less will lower the risk of alveolar over-distention. The optimal PEEP needed to prevent cyclic atelectasis is not known, but should be titrated to allow reduction of FiO$_2$ to nontoxic levels. Open lung ventilation strategies, such as high-frequency oscillation, may be useful in reducing both volutrauma and atelectrauma if hemodynamic instability does not preclude the use of a higher mean airway pressure (Yumiko & Slutsky, 2005).

Consultation with radiology and pulmonology specialists may be indicated as the clinical presentation of the patient and CXR worsen. Patients who have increasing ventilator requirements should also be followed by nutrition, occupational and physical therapy, and social work specialists. Discussion with caregivers should include the change in lung pathology and possible long-term sequelae. An interprofessional plan of care should be in place to promote the best outcomes.

DISPOSITION AND DISCHARGE PLANNING

Patients with VILI are at risk for multiple organ dysfunction and may require prolonged mechanical ventilation, vasopressor or inotropic support, and dialysis, among other interventions. Weaning from mechanical ventilation may be slow, and the patient may require a tracheostomy and chronic ventilation. With any pediatric patient with severe illness who requires intensive care, evaluation by the rehabilitation team should be considered.

REFERENCES

1. Acute Respiratory Distress Syndrome Network. (2000). Ventilation with lower tidal volumes as compared with traditional tidal volumes for acute lung injury and the acute respiratory distress syndrome. *New England Journal of Medicine, 342*(18), 1301–1308.
2. Agency for Healthcare Research and Quality (AHRQ). (2003). *Management of bronchiolitis in infants and children.* Evidence Report/Technology Assessment No. 69. Rockville, MD: Author. Retrieved from www.ahrq.gov/clinic/epcsums/broncsum.htm
3. Akinbami, L. (2006). *The state of childhood asthma, United States, 1980–2005.* Advance data from Vital and Health Statistics, No. 381. Hyattsville, MD: National Center for Health Statistics.
4. Al-Aloul, M., Miller, H., Alapati, S., Stockton, P. A., Ledson, M. J., & Walshaw, M. J. (2005). Renal impairment in cystic fibrosis patients due to repeated intravenous aminoglycoside use. *Pediatric Pulmonology, 39*(1), 15–20.
5. Alarie, Y. (2002). Toxicity of fire smoke. *Critical Reviews in Toxicology, 32*(4), 259–289.
6. Alvarez, A., Algar, F. J., Santos, F., Lama, R., Baamonde, C., Cerezo, F., et al. (2005). Pediatric lung transplantation. *Transplant Proceedings, 37*(3), 1519–1522.
7. Amado, M., & Portnoy, J. (2006). Diagnosing asthma in young children. *Current Opinion in Allergy and Clinical Immunology, 6,* 101–105.
8. American Academy of Pediatrics (AAP). (2002). Clinical practice guidelines: Diagnosis and management of childhood obstructive sleep. *Pediatrics, 109*(4), 704–712.
9. American Academy of Pediatrics (AAP), Committee on Infectious Diseases. (2009a). Respiratory syncytial virus. In L. Pickering (Ed.), *2009 red book: Report of the Committee on Infectious Diseases.* Elk Grove Village, IL: Author.
10. American Academy of Pediatrics (AAP), Committee on Infectious Diseases. (2009b). Modified recommendations for use of palivizumab for prevention of respiratory syncytial infections. *Pediatrics, 124*(6), 1694–1701.
11. American Academy of Pediatrics (AAP), Subcommittee on Diagnosis and Management of Bronchiolitis. (2006). Diagnosis and management of bronchiolitis. *Pediatrics, 118*(4), 1774–1793.
12. American Thoracic Society (ATS). (1996). Standards and indications for cardiopulmonary sleep studies in children. *American Journal of Respiratory and Critical Care Medicine, 153*(2), 866–878.
13. American Thoracic Society (ATS). (2003). Statement on the care of the child with chronic lung disease of infancy and childhood. *American Journal of Respiratory and Critical Care Medicine, 168*(3), 356–396.
14. Amiel., J., Laudier, B., Attié-Bitach, T., Trang, H., de Pontual, L., Gener, B., et al. (2003). Polyalanine expansion and frameshift mutations of the paired-like homeobox gene *PHOX2B* in congenital central hypoventilation syndrome. *Nature Genetics, 33*(4), 459–461.
15. Ampofo, K., & Byington, C. (2007). Management of parapneumonic empyema. *Pediatric Infectious Disease Journal, 26,* 445–446.
16. Anton, N., Joffe, K., & Jofee, A. (2003). Inability to predict outcome of acute respiratory distress syndrome in children when using high frequency oscillation. *Intensive Care Medicine, 29*(10), 1763–1769.
17. Aris, R., Neuringer, I. B., Weiner, M. A., Egan, T. M., & Ontjes, D. (1996). Severe osteoporosis before and after lung transplantation. *Chest, 109*(5), 1176–1183.
18. Arnon, S. (2004). Infant botulism. In R. Feigen, J. Cherry, G. Demmler, & S. Kaplan (Eds.). *Textbook of pediatric infectious diseases* (pp. 1758–1766). Philadelphia: Saunders.
19. Arnon, S., Midura, T., Damas, K., Thompson, B., Wood, R., & Chin, J. (1979). Honey and other environmental risk factors for infant botulism. *Journal of Pediatrics, 94*(2), 331–336.
20. Arnon, S., Schechter, R., Inglesby, T., Henderson, D., Bartlett, J., Ascher, M., et al. (2001). Botulinum toxin as a biological weapon: Medical and public health management. *Journal of the American Medical Association, 285*(8), 1059–1070.
21. Arnon, S., Schechter, R., Maslanka, S., Jewell, N., & Hatheway, C. (2006). Human botulism immune globulin for the treatment of infant botulism. *New England Journal of Medicine, 354*(5), 445–447.
22. Aurora, P., Boucek, M. M., Christie, J., Dobbels, F., Edwards, L. B., Keck, B. M., et al. (2007). Registry of the International Society for Heart and Lung Transplantation: Tenth official pediatric lung and heart/lung transplantation report—2007. *Journal of Heart and Lung Transplantation, 26*(12), 1223–1228.
23. Aurora, P., Edwards, L. B., Christie, J., Dobbels, F., Kirk, R., Kucheryavaya, A. Y., et al. (2008). Registry of the International Society for Heart and Lung Transplantation: Eleventh official pediatric lung and heart/lung transplantation report—2008. *Journal of Heart and Lung Transplantation, 27*(9), 978–983.
24. Aurora, P., Edwards, L. B., Christie, J. D., Dobbels, F., Kirk, R., Rahmel, A. O., et al. (2009). Registry of the International Society for Heart and Lung Transplantation: Twelfth official pediatric lung and

heart/lung transplantation report—2009. *Journal of Heart and Lung Transplantation, 28*(10), 1023–1030.

25. Avecillas, J., Freire, A., & Arroliga, A. (2006). Clinical epidemiology of acute lung injury and acute respiratory distress syndrome: Incidence, diagnosis, and outcomes. *Clinical Chest Medicine, 27*(4), 549–557.

26. Ball, J., & Bindler, R. (2008). *Pediatric nursing: Caring for children* (4th ed.). Upper Saddle Ridge, NJ: Pearson.

27. Bancalari, E., Abdenour, G., Feller, R., & Gannon, J. (1979). Bronchopulmonary dysplasia clinical presentation. *Journal of Pediatrics, 95*(5), 819–823.

28. Bartlett, N., McLean, G., Chang, Y., & Johnston, S. (2009). Genetics and epidemiology: Asthma and infection. *Current Opinion in Allergy and Clinical Immunology, 9*, 395–400.

29. Behrman, R., Kliegman, R., & Jenson, H. (2004). *Nelson textbook of pediatrics* (17th ed.). Philadelphia, PA: Elsevier.

30. Benden, C., Kansra, S., Ridout, D. A., Shaw, N. L. Aurora, P., Elliott, M. J., et al. (2009). Chronic kidney disease in children following lung and heart–lung transplantation. *Pediatric Transplantation, 13*(1), 104–110.

31. Bernard, G., Artigas, A., Brigham, K. L., Carlet, J., Falke, K., Hudson, L., et al. (1994). The American–European Consensus Conference on ARDS: Definitions, mechanisms, relevant outcomes, and clinical trial coordination. *American Journal pf Respiratory and Critical Care Medicine, 149*(3), 818–824.

32. Berner, M., Hanquist, S., & Rimensberger, P. (2008). High frequency oscillatory ventilation for respiratory failure due to RSV bronchiolitis. *Intensive Care Medicine, 34*(9), 1698–1702.

33. Bhandari, A., & Bhandari, V. (2009). Pitfalls, problems, and progress in bronchopulmonary dysplasia. *Pediatrics, 123*(6), 1562–1573.

34. Bigham, M., Amato, R., Bondurrant, P., Fridriksson, J., Krawczeski, C. D., Raake, J., et al. (2009). Ventilator-associated pneumonia in the pediatric intensive care unit: Characterizing the problem and implementing a sustainable solution. *Journal of Pediatrics, 154*(4), 582–587.

35. Bloom, B., & Cohen, R. (2007). Summary health statistics for U.S. children: National Health Interview Survey, 2006. National Center for Health Statistics. *Vital Health Statistics, 10*, 234.

36. Bloomberg, G. (2010). The exacerbation component of impairment and risk in pediatric asthma. *Current Opinion in Allergy and Clinical Immunology, 10*, 155–160.

37. Boehler, A., & Estenne, M. (2003). Post-transplant bronchiolitis obliterans. *European Respiratory Journal, 22*(6), 1007–1018.

38. Bogie, A., Towne, D., Luckett, P., Abramo, T., & Wiebe, R. (2007). Comparison of intravenous terbutaline versus normal saline in pediatric patients on continuous high-dose nebulized albuterol for status asthmaticus. *Pediatric Emergency Care, 23*(6), 355–361.

39. Bonkowsky, J., & Tieder, J. (2009). A pragmatic approach to ALTEs. *Contemporary Pediatrics, 26*(11), 54–63.

40. Bortolussi, R., Miller, B., Ledwith, M., & Halperin, S. (1995). Clinical course of pertussis in immunized children. *Pediatric Infectious Disease Journal, 14*, 870.

41. Boucek, M., Aurora, P., Edwards, L. B., Taylor, D. O., Trulock, E. P., Christie, J., et al. (2007). Registry of the International Society for Heart and Lung Transplantation: Tenth official pediatric heart transplantation report—2007. *Journal of Heart and Lung Transplantation, 26*(8), 796–807.

42. Bradbury, R., Shirkhedkar, D., Glanville, A. R., & Campbell, L. A. (2008). Prior diabetes mellitus is associated with increased morbidity in cystic fibrosis patients undergoing bilateral lung transplantation: An "orphan" area? *Internal Medicine Journal, 152*, 540–545.

43. Bradding, P., & Green, R. (2010). Subclinical phenotypes of asthma. *Current Opinion in Allergy and Clinical Immunology, 10*, 54–59.

44. Brashers, V. (2002). Alterations of pulmonary function. In K. McCance & S. Heuther (Eds.). *Pathophysiology: The biologic basis for disease in adults and children* (3rd ed., pp. 1110–1111). St. Louis, MO: Mosby.

45. Brichant, J., Rouby, J., & Viars, P. (1986). Intermittent positive pressure ventilation with either positive end-expiratory pressure or high frequency jet ventilation (HFJV), or HFJV alone in human acute respiratory failure. *Anesthesia and Analgesia, 65*, 1135–1142.

46. British Thoracic Society (BTS), Standards of Care Committee. (2002). British Thoracic Society guidelines for the management of community acquired pneumonia in childhood. *Thorax, 57*(suppl 1), 1–24.

47. Brock, M., Borja, M. C., Ferber, L., Orens, J. B., Anzcek, R. A., Krishnan, J., et al. (2001). Induction therapy in lung transplantation: A prospective, controlled clinical trial comparing OKT3, anti-thymocyte globulin, and daclizumab. *Journal of Heart and Lung Transplantation, 20*(12), 1282–1290.

48. Brooks, J. (1996). Consultation with the specialist: Apparent life-threatening events. *Pediatrics in Review, 17*, 257–259.

49. Buckingham, S., King, M., & Miller, M. (2003). Incidence and etiologies of complicated parapneumonic effusions in children, 1996 to 2001. *Pediatric Infectious Disease Journal, 22*, 499–503.

50. Bullaro, F., & Bartoletti, S. (2007). Spontaneous pneumomediastinum in children: A literature review. *Pediatric Emergency Care, 23*(1), 28–30. doi: 10.1097/01.pec.0000248686.88809.fd

51. Burns, S. (2006). Respiratory waveforms monitoring. In *AACN protocols for practice: noninvasive monitoring* (2nd ed.). Sudbury, MA: Jones and Bartlett.

52. Caceres, M., Syed, Z., Braud, R., Weiman, D., & Garretm, H. E. (2008). Spontaneous pneumomediastinum: A comparative study and review of the literature. *Annals of Thoracic Surgery, 86*, 962–966. doi: 10.1016/j.athoracsur.2008.04.067

53. Cahill, B., Hibbs, J. R., Savik, K., Juni, B. A., Dosland, B. M., Edin-Stibbe, C., et al. (1997). *Aspergillus* airway colonization and invasive disease after lung transplantation. *Chest, 112*(5), 1160–1164.

54. Calder, A., & Owens, C. (2009). Imaging of parapneumonic pleural effusions and empyema in children. *Pediatric Radiology, 36*(6), 527–537.

55. Camargo, C., Rachelefsky, G., & Schatz, M. (2009). Managing asthma exacerbations in the emergency department: Summary of the National Asthma Education and Prevention Program Expert Panel Report 3 guidelines for the management of asthma exacerbation. *Proceedings of the American Thoracic Society, 6*, 357–366.

56. Carroll, J., McColley, S., Marcus, C., Curtis, S., & Loughlin, G. (1995). Inability of clinical history to distinguish primary snoring from obstructive sleep apnea syndrome in children. *Chest, 108*(3), 610–618.

57. Carter, P., & Benjamin, B. (1983). Ten-year review of pediatric trachestomy. *Annals of Otology, Rhinology, and Laryngology, 92*, 398–400.

58. Centers for Disease Control and Prevention (CDC). (2000). *Guidelines for the control of pertussis outbreaks.* Atlanta, GA: Author. Retrieved from http://www.cdc.gov/vaccines/pubs/pertussis-guide/guide.htm

59. Centers for Disease Control and Prevention (CDC). (2005). *Guidelines for the control of pertussis outbreaks.* Atlanta, GA: Author. Retrieved from http://www.cdc.gov/vaccines/pubs/pertussis-guide/guide.htm

60. Centers for Disease Control and Prevention (CDC). (2006a). Botulism: Epidemiological overview for clinicians. Retrieved from http://www.bt.cdc.gov/agent/botulism/clinicians/epidemiology.asp

61. Centers for Disease Control and Prevention (CDC). (2006b). National Health Interview Survey. Retrieved from http://www.cdc.gov/nchs/FASTATS/asthma.htm

62. Centers for Disease Control and Prevention (CDC). (2006c). Vaccine preventable deaths and the Global Immunization Vision and Strategy, 2006–2015. *Morbidity and Mortality Weekly Report, 55*(18), 511–515.

63. Centers for Disease Control and Prevention (CDC). (2008). Fire deaths and injuries: Prevention tips. Retrieved from http://www.cdc.gov/HomeandRecreationalSafety/Fire-Prevention/fireprevention.htm

64. Centers for Disease Control and Prevention (CDC). (2009). *Pertussis.* Atlanta, GA: Author.

65. Chamany, S., Mirza, S., Fleming, J., Howell, J. F., Lenhart, S. W., Mortimer, V. D., et al. (2004). A large histoplasmosis outbreak among high school students in Indiana, 2001. *Pediatric Infectious Disease Journal, 23*(10), 909–914.

66. Cheifetz, I. M., Venkataraman, S. T., & Hamel, D. S. (2008). *Respiratory monitoring.* In D. G. Nichols (Ed.). *Rogers' textbook of pediatric intensive care* (4th ed., pp. 662–685). Philadelphia: Wolters Klowers.

67. Chen, M. L., & Keens, T. G. (2004). Congenital central hypoventilation syndrome: Not just another rare disorder. *Paediatric Respiratory Reviews, 5*(3), 182–189.

68. Chen, M., Pope, T., & Ott, D. (Eds.). (2004). *Basic radiology.* New York: McGraw-Hill.

69. Cheng, K., Hou, C. C., Huang, H. C., Lin, S. C., & Zhang, H. (2006). Intravenous injection of methylprednisolone reduces the incidence of postextubation stridor in intensive care unit patients. *Critical Care Medicine, 34,* 1345–1350.

70. Cherry, J., & Heininger, U. (2004). Pertussis and other *Bordetella* infections. In R. Feigin, G. Demmler, J. Cherry, & S. Kaplan (Eds.). *Textbook of pediatric infectious diseases* (5th ed., Vol 1., pp. 1588–1608). Philadelphia: W. B. Saunders.

71. Chowdhury, M., Pao, C., Pearson, C., Shah, A., Reus, E., Devlin-Jolliffe, A., et al. (2010). Helium–oxygen gas mixtures in infants with acute bronchiolitis: Results of a phase III double-blind, multicentre RCT. *American Journal of Respiratory and Critical Care Medicine, 181,* A2281.

72. Claudius, I., & Keens, T. (2007). Do all infants with apparent life-threatening events need to be admitted? *Pediatrics, 119*(4), 679–683.

73. Collins, P., McIntosh, K., & Chanock, R. (1996). Respiratory syncytial virus. In *Fields' virology* (3rd ed., pp. 1313–1351). New York: Lippincott, Williams & Wilkins.

74. Cornelli, H., Zorc, J., Mahajan, P., Shaw, K., Holubkov, R., Reeves, S., et al. (2007). A multicenter, randomized, controlled trial of dexametha-sone for bronchiolitis. *New England Journal of Medicine, 357*(4), 331–339.

75. Costanzo, L. (2002). *Physiology* (2nd ed.). Philadelphia, PA: Saunders.

76. Curley, M., Thompson, J., & Arnold, J. (2000). The effects of early and repeated prone positioning in pediatric patients with acute lung injury. *Chest, 118*(1), 156–163.

77. Danziger-Isakov, L., Worley, S., Arrigain, S., Aurora, P., Ballmann, M., Boyer, D., et al. (2008). Increased mortality after pulmonary fungal infection within the first year after pediatric lung transplantation. *Journal of Heart and Lung Transplantation, 27*(6), 655–661.

78. Davidson, W., Dorscheid, D., Spragg, R., Schulzer, M., Mak, E., & Ayas, N. (2006). Exogenous pulmonary surfactant for the treatment of adult patients with acute respiratory distress syndrome: Results of a meta-analysis. *Critical Care, 10*(2), R41.

79. Davies, F., & Gupta, R. (2002). Apparent life threatening events in infants presenting to an emergency department. *Emergency Medical Journal, 19,* 11–16.

80. Davis, R., Lau, C. L., Eubanks, S., Messier, R. H., Hadjiliadis, D., Steele, M. P., et al. (2003). Improved lung allograft function after fun-doplication in patients with gastroesophageal reflux disease undergoing lung transplantation. *Journal of Thoracic and Cardiovascular Surgery, 125*(3), 533–542.

81. Deakins, K., & Chatburn, R. (2002). A comparison of intrapulmonary percussive ventilation and conventional chest physiotherapy for the treatment of atelectasis in the pediatric patient. *Respiratory Care, 47*(10), 1162–1167.

82. De Geest, S., Dobbels, F., Fluri, C., Paris, W., & Troosters, T. (2005). Adherence to the therapeutic regimen in heart, lung, and heart–lung transplant recipients. *Journal of Cardiovascular Nursing, 20*(5 suppl), S88–S98.

83. Delghani, N., & Ludemann, J. (2008). Aspirated foreign bodies in children: BC Children's Hospital emergency room protocol. *British Columbia Medical Journal, 50*(5), 252–256.

84. Dobyns, E., Cornfield, D. N., Anas, N. G., Fortenberry, J. D., Tasker, R. C., Lynch, A., et al. (1999). Multicenter randomized controlled trial of the effects of inhaled nitric oxide therapy on gas exchange in children with acute hypoxemic respiratory failure. *Journal of Pediatrics, 134*(4), 406–412.

85. Dorman-Rosenthal, L. (2006). Carbon monoxide poisoning: Immediate diagnosis and treatment are crucial to avoid complications. *American Journal of Nursing, 106*(3), 40–46.

86. Duffett, M., Choong, K., Ng, V., Randolph, A., & Cook, D. (2007). Surfactant therapy for acute respiratory failure in children: A systematic review and meta-analysis. *Critical Care, 11*(3), R66.

87. Egan, T., Murray, S., Bustami, R. T., Shearon, T. H., McCullough, K. P., Edwards, L. B., et al. (2006). Development of the new lung allocation system in the United States. *American Journal of Transplantation, 6*(5 Pt 2), 1212–1227.

88. Enkhbaatar, P., Herndon, D., & Traber, D. (2009). Use of nebulized heparin in the treatment of smoke inhalation injury. *Journal of Burn Care and Research, 30*(1), 159–162.

89. Erickson, S., Schibler, A., Numa, A., Nuthall, G., Yung, M., Pascoe, E., et al. (2007). Acute lung injury in pediatric intensive care in Australia and New Zealand: A prospective, multicenter, observational study. *Pediatric Critical Care Medicine, 8*(4), 317–323.

90. Estenne, M., & Hertz, M. (2002). Bronchiolitis obliterans after human lung transplantation. *American Journal of Respiratory and Critical Care Medicine, 166*(4), 440–444.

91. Estenne, M., Maurer, J., Boehler, A., Egan, J. J., Frost, A., Hertz, M., et al. (2002). Bronchiolitis obliterans syndrome 2001: An update of the diagnostic criteria. *Journal of Heart and Lung Transplantation, 21*(3), 297–310.

92. Evans, O., & Vedanarayanan, V. (1997). Guillain-Barré syndrome. *Pediatrics in Review, 18*(1), 10–16.

93. Fanaroff, A., Stoll, B., Wright, L., Carlo, W., Ehrenkranz, R., Stark, A., et al. (2007). Trends in neonatal morbidity and mortality for very low birthweight infants. *American Journal of Obstetrics and Gynecology, 196*(2), 147.e1–e8.

94. Farber, H. (2010). Optimizing maintenance therapy in pediatric asthma. *Current Opinion in Pulmonary Medicine, 16,* 25–30.

95. Faro, A., Mallory, G. B., Visner, G. A., Elidemir, O., Mogayzel, P. J. Jr., Danziger-Isakov, L., et al. (2007). American Society of Transplantation executive summary on pediatric lung transplantation. *American Journal of Transplantation, 7*(2), 285–292.

96. Feltes, T., Cabalka, A., Meissner, H., Piazza, F., Carlin, D., Top, F., et al. (2003). Palivizumab prophylaxis reduces hospitalization due to respiratory syncytial virus in young children with hemodynamically significant congenital heart disease. *Journal of Pediatrics, 143*(4), 532–540.

97. Figueras-Aloy, J., Carbonell-Estrany, X., & Quero, J. (2004). Case-control study of the risk factors linked to respiratory syncytial virus infection requiring hospitalization in premature infants born at a gestational age of 33–35 weeks in Spain. *Pediatric Infectious Diseases, 23*(9), 815–820.

98. Finer, N., & Barrington, K. (2001). Nitric oxide for respiratory failure in infants born at or near term. *Cochrane Database of Systematic Reviews, 2,* CD000399.

99. Flori, H., Glidden, D., Rutherford, G., & Matthay, M. (2005). Pediatric acute lung injury: Prospective evaluation of risk factors associated with mortality. *American Journal of Respiratory and Critical Care Medicine, 171,* 995–1001.

100. Fontes, R., Aguilar, P., Zanetti, M., Andrade, M., & Teixeira, M. (2003). Acute neurogenic pulmonary edema: Case reports and literature review. *Journal of Neurosurgical Anesthesiology, 15*(2), 144–150. Retrieved from http://www.ncbi.nlm.nih.gov.ezproxyhost.library.tmc.edu/sites/entrez?otool=hamtmc

101. Forno, E., & Celedon, J. C. (2009). Asthma and ethnic minorities: Socioeconomic status and beyond. *Current Opinion in Allergy and Clinical Immunology, 9,* 154–160.

102. Fraga, J., deSouza, J., & Kruel, J. (2009). Pediatric tracheostomy. *Journal of Pediatrics, 85*(2), 97–103.

103. Francisco, A., & Arnon, S. (2007). Clinical mimics of infant botulism. *Pediatrics, 119*(4), 826–828.

104. Frutos-Vivar, F., Nin, N., & Esteban, A. (2004). Epidemiology of acute lung injury and acute respiratory distress syndrome. *Current Opinion in Critical Care, 10*(1), 1–6.

105. Gagic, O., Dara, S., Mendez, J., Adesanya, A., Festic, E., Caples, S. M., et al. (2004). Ventilator-associated lung injury in patients without acute lung injury at the onset of mechanical ventilation. *Critical Care Medicine, 32*, 1817–1824.

106. Garner, W., Downs, J., Stock, M., & Räsänen, J. (1988). Airway pressure release ventilation (APRV): A human trial. *Chest, 94*, 779–781.

107. Gates, R., Hogan, M., Weinstein, S., & Arca, M. J. (2004). Drainage, fibrinolytics, or surgery: A comparison of treatment options in pediatric empyema. *Journal of Pediatric Surgery, 39*, 1639–1642.

108. Global Initiative for Asthma (GINA). (2009). *Global Strategy for Asthma Management and Prevention in Children 5 Years and Younger.* Retrieved from http://www.ginasthma.org

109. Gottlieb, J., Szangolies, J., Koehnlein, T., Golpon, H., Simon, A., & Welte, T. (2008). Long-term azithromycin for bronchiolitis obliterans syndrome after lung transplantation. *Transplantation, 85*(1), 36–41.

110. Grant, G., Campbell, H., Dowell, S., Graham, S. M., Klugman, K. P., Mulholland, E. K., et al. (2009). Recommendations for treatment of childhood non-severe pneumonia. *Lancet Infectious Diseases, 9,* 185–196.

111. Greenhalgh, D. (2009). Steroids in the treatment of smoke inhalation injury. *Journal of Burn Care and Research, 30*(1), 165–169.

112. Grigg-Damberger, M., & Wells, A. (2009). Central congenital hypoventilation syndrome: Changing face of a less mysterious but more complex genetic disorder. *Seminars in Respiratory and Critical Care Medicine, 30*(3), 262–274.

113. Guilleminault, C., Lee, J., & Chan, A. (2005). Pediatric obstructive sleep apnea syndrome. *Archives of Pediatrics and Adolescent Medicine, 159*(8), 775–785.

114. Haan, J., & Scalea, T. (2006). Tension pneumopericardium: A case report and a review of the literature. *American Surgeon, 72*(4), 330–331. Retrieved from http://www.ncbi.nlm.nih.gov.ezproxyhost.library.tmc.edu/sites/entrez?otool=hamtmc

115. Halbower, A., Ishman, S., & McGinley, B. (2007). Childhood obstructive sleep-disordered breathing: A clinical update and discussion of technological innovations and challenges. *Chest, 132*(6), 2030–2040.

116. Hall, A., Dart, R., & Bogdan, G. (2007). Sodium thiosulfate or hydroxocobalamin for the empiric treatment of cyanide poisoning? *Annals of Emergency Medicine, 29*(6), 806–813.

117. Hall, C. (2007). Therapy for bronchiolitis: When some become none. *New England Journal of Medicine, 357*(4), 402–404.

118. Hall, C., Weinberg, G., Iwane, M., Blumkin, A., Edwards, K., & Staat, M. (2009). The burden of respiratory syncytial virus infection in young children. *New England Journal of Medicine, 360*(6), 588–598.

119. Hall, K., & Zalman, B. (2005). Evaluation and management of apparent life threatening events in children. *American Family Physician, 71*(12), 2301–2308.

120. Hampson, N., & Hauff, N. (2008). Carboxyhemoglobin levels in carbon monoxide poisoning: Do they correlate with the clinical picture? *American Journal of Emergency Medicine, 26*(6), 665–669.

121. Hanson, J., & Flori, H. (2006). Applications of the Acute Respiratory Distress Syndrome Network low-tidal volume strategy to pediatric acute lung injury. *Respiratory Care Clinics of North America, 12*(3), 349–357.

122. Harms, H., Matouk, E., Tourmier, G., von der Hardt, H., Weller, P. H., Romano, L., et al. (1998). Multi-center open-label study of recombinant human DNase in cystic fibrosis with moderate lung disease. International Study Group. *Pediatric Pulmonology, 26*, 155–161.

123. Hayden, C., & Le Souef, P. (2007). The genetics of asthma. *Clinical Pulmonary Medicine, 14*(5), 249–257.

124. He, Q., Viljanen, M., Arvilommi, H., Aittanen, B., & Mertsola, J. (1998). Whooping cough caused by *Bordetella pertussis* and *Bordetella parapertussis* in an immunized population. *Journal of the American Medical Association, 280*(7), 635–637.

125. Heath, P., Booy, R., Azzopardi, H., Slack, M. P. Fogarty, J., Molony, A. C., et al. (2001). Non-type b *Haemophilus influenzae* disease: Clinical and epidemiologic characteristics in the *Haemophilus influenzae* type b vaccine era. *Pediatric Infectious Disease Journal, 20,* 300–305.

126. Hendricks, T., de Hoog, M., Lequin, M., Devos, A., & Merkus, P. (2005). DNase and atelectasis in non-cystic fibrosis pediatric patients. *Critical Care, 9,* R351R359.

127. Hernandez, R., Gil, P. U., Gallo, C. G., de Pable Gafas, A., Hernandez, M. C., & Alvarez, M. J. et al. (2005). Rapamycin in lung transplantation. *Transplantation Proceedings, 37*(9), 3999–4000.

128. Heulit, M., Wolf, G., & Arnold, J. (2008). Mechanical ventilation. In G. H. Nichols & A. D. Ackerman (Eds.). *Rogers' textbook of pediatric intensive care.* Philadelphia: Lippincott, Williams & Wilkins.

129. Heyland, D., Dhaliwal, R., Drover, J., Gramlich, L., & Dodek, P. (2003). Canadian clinical practice guidelines for nutrition support in mechanically ventilated, critically ill adult patients. *Journal of Parenteral and Enteral Nutrition, 27*(5), 355–373.

130. Hickey, R., Bowman, M., & Smith, G. (1996). Utility of blood cultures in pediatric patients found to have pneumonia in the emergency department. *Annals of Emergency Medicine, 27*(6), 721–725.

131. Hill, J., & Voight, R. (2000). Foreign bodies. In K. Ashcroft, J. P. Murphy, R. J. Sharp, D. L. Sigalet, & C. L. Snyder (Eds.). *Pediatric surgery* (3rd ed., pp. 146–151). Philadelphia: W. B. Saunders.

132. Hoffman, G., Ross, G. A., Day, S. E., Rice, T. B., & Neling, L. D. (1997). Inhaled nitric oxide reduces the utilization of extracorporeal membrane oxygenation in persistent pulmonary hypertension of the newborn. *Critical Care Medicine, 25*(2), 352–359

133. Hough, C., Steinberg, K., Thompson, T., Rubenfeld, G., & Hudson, L. (2009). Intensive care unit–acquired neuromyopathy and corticosteroids in survivors of persistent ARDS. *Intensive Care Medicine, 35,* 63–68.

134. Huang, J., Colrain, I. M., Panitch, H. B., Tapia, I. E., Schwartz, M. S., Samuel, J., et al. (2008). Effect of sleep stage on breathing in children with central hypoventilation. *Journal of Applied Physiology, 105*(1), 44–53.

135. Hughes, R., Raphael, J., Swan, A., & van Doorn, P. (2006a). Intravenous immunoglobulin for Guillain-Barré syndrome. *Cochrane Database of Systematic Reviews, 1,* CD002063.

136. Hughes, R., Swan, A., van Koningsveld, R., & van Doorn, P. (2006b). Corticosteroids for Guillain-Barré syndrome. *Cochrane Database of Systematic Reviews, 2,* CD001446.

137. Hyde, T., Gay, K., Stephens, D., Vugia, D. J., Pass, M., Johnson, S., et al. (2001). Macrolide resistance among invasive *Streptococcus pneumoniae* isolates. *Journal of the American Medical Association, 286,* 1857–1862.

138. Iacono, A., Corcoran, T. E., Griffith, B. P.,Grgurich, W. F., Smith, D. A., Zeevi, A. et al. (2004). Aerosol cyclosporin therapy in lung transplant recipients with bronchiolitis obliterans. *European Respiratory Journal, 23*(3), 384–390.

139. Ibrahim, J. E., Sweet, S. C.,Flipping, M., Dent, C., Mendelhoff, E., Huddlesron, C. B., et al. (2002). Rejection is reduced in thoracic organ recipients when transplanted in the first year of life. *Journal of Heart and Lung Transplantation, 21*(3), 311–318.

140. Infant Botulism Treatment and Prevention Program (IBTPP). (2004). Retrieved from http://www.infantbotulism.org

141. INO Therapeutics. (n.d.). Nitric oxide prescribing monograph. Retrieved February 13, 2009, from http://www.medicos.md/monograph/view/did/3946#S1.1

142. International Ventilator Users Network, affiliate of Post-Polio Health International. (2010). Home ventilator guide. Retrieved from http://www.post-polio.org/ivun/index.html

143. Jartti, T., Lehtinen, P., Vuorinen, T., Osterback, R., van den Hoogen, B., Osterhaus, A., et al. (2004). Respiratory picornaviruses and respiratory syncytial virus as causative agents of acute

expiratory wheezing in children. *Emerging Infectious Diseases, 10*(6), 1095–1101.

144. Javouhey, E., Barats, A., Stamm, R., & Floret, D. (2008). Noninvasive ventilation as primary ventilatory support for infants with severe bronchiolitis. *Intensive Care Med, 34*(9), 1560–1561.

145. Jenkinson, D. (2005). Whooping cough information. Retrieved from http://www.whoopingcough.net/index.htm

146. Jobe, A., & Bancalari, E. (2001). NICHD/NHLBI/ORD workshop summary: Bronchopulmonary dysplasia. *American Journal of Respiratory and Critical Care Medicine, 163*(7), 1723–729.

147. Juven, T., Mertsola, J., Waris, M., Leinonen, M., Meurman, O., Roivainen, M., et al. (2000). Etiology of community-acquired pneumonia in 254 hospitalized children. *Pediatric Infectious Disease Journal, 19*, 293–298.

148. Kahn, A. (2004). Recommended clinical evaluation of infants with an apparent life-threatening event: Consensus document of the European Society for the Study and Prevention of Infant Death, 2003. *European Journal of Pediatrics, 163*, 108–115.

149. Kanj, S., Tapson, V., Davis, R. D. Madden, J., & Browning, I. (1997). Infections in patients with cystic fibrosis following lung transplantation. *Chest, 112*(4), 924–930.

150. Keens, T., Kun, S., & Davidson Ward, S. (2008). Chronic respiratory failure. In G. H. Nichols & A. D. Ackerman (Eds.). *Rogers' textbook of pediatric intensive care.* Philadelphia: Lippincott, Williams & Wilkins.

151. Kiehl-Kohlendorfer, U., Hof, D., Pegalow, P., Traweger-Ravanelli, B., & Keichl, S. (2005). Epidemiology of apparent life threatening events. *Archives of Disease in Childhood, 90*(3), 297–300.

152. Kimpen, J. (2002). Prevention and treatment of respiratory syncytial virus bronchiolitis and postbronchiolitic wheezing. *Respiratory Research, 3*(suppl 1), S40–S45.

153. Kinsella, J., Greenough, A., & Abman, S. (2006). Bronchopulmonary dysplasia. *Lancet, 367*(9520), 1421–1431.

154. Knoop, C., Haverich, A., & Fischer, S. (2004). Immunosuppressive therapy after human lung transplantation. *European Respiratory Journal, 23*(1), 159–171.

155. Kornecki, A. & Kavanaugh, B. (2007). Mechanical ventilation. In: D. Wheeler, H. Wong, & T. Shanley (Eds.). Pediatric Critical Care Medicine. New York: Springer. page 414.

156. Kotecha, S. (2008). Chronic respiratory complications of prematurity. In L. Taussig & L. Landau (Eds.). *Pediatric respiratory medicine* (2nd ed., pp. 387–411). Philadelphia: Sanders/Elsevier.

157. Kramer, M., Marshall, S. E., Starnes, V. A., Gamberg, P., Amitai, Z., & Theodore, J. (1993). Infectious complications in heart–lung transplantation: Analysis of 200 episodes. *Archives of Internal Medicine, 153*(17), 2010–2016.

158. Kreider, M., & Kotloff, R. (2009). Selection of candidates for lung transplantation. *Proceedings of the American Thoracic Society, 6*(1), 20–27.

159. Kremer, B., Botos-Kremer, A., Eckel, H., & Schlondorff, G. (2002). Indications, complications, and surgical techniques for pediatric tracheotomies: An update. *Journal of Pediatric Surgery, 37*, 1556–1562.

160. Krishnan, U., Krishnan, S., & Gewitz, M. (2008). Treatment of pulmonary hypertension in children with chronic lung disease with newer oral therapies. *Pediatric Cardiology, 29*, 1082–1086.

161. Kubicka, Z., Limauro, J., & Darnall, R. (2008). Heated, humidified high-flow nasal cannula therapy: Yet another way to deliver continuous positive airway pressure? *Pediatrics, 121*(1), 82–88.

162. Kurian, J., Levin, T., Han, B., Taragin, B., & Weinstein, S. (2009). Comparison of ultrasound and CT in the evaluation of pneumonia complicated by parapneumonic effusion in Children. *American Journal of Roentgenology, 193*, 1648–1654.

163. Kurt, B., Winterhalter, K., Connors, R., Betz, B. W., & Winters, J. W. (2006). Therapy of parapneumonic effusions in children: Video-assisted thoracoscopic surgery versus conventional thoracostomy drainage. *Pediatrics, 118*, 547–553.

164. Kushida, C., Chediak, A., Berry, R., Brown, L., Gozal, D., Iber, C., et al. (2008). Clinical guidelines for the manual titration of positive airway pressure in patients with obstructive sleep apnea. *Journal of Clinical Sleep Medicine, 4*(2), 157–171.

165. Laffey, J., O'Croinin, D., McLoughlin, P., & Kavanagh, B. (2004). Permissive hypercapnia: Role in protective lung ventilator strategies, *Intensive Care Medicine, 30*(3), 347–356.

166. Lang, D. (2008). New asthma guidelines emphasize control, regular monitoring. *Cleveland Clinic Journal of Medicine, 75*(9), 641–653.

167. Lee, A., & Mellins, R. (2006). Lung injury from smoke inhalation. *Paediatric Respiratory Reviews, 7*(2), 123–128.

168. Leung, A., Kellner, J., & Davies, H. (2005). Respiratory syncytial virus bronchiolitis. *Journal of the National Medical Association, 97*(12), 1708–1713.

169. Linzer, J. (2007). Review of asthma: Pathophysiology and current treatment options. *Clinical Pediatric Emergency Medicine, 8*(2), 87–95.

170. Liu, M., Worley, S., Arrigain, S., Aurora, P., Ballmann, M., Boyer, D., et al. (2009). Respiratory viral infections within one year after pediatric lung transplant. *Transplantat Infectious Disease, 11*(4), 304–312.

171. Lucero, M., Dulalia, V., Nillos, L., Williams, G., Parreno, R. A., Nohynek, H., et al. (2009). Pneumococcal conjugate vaccines for preventing vaccine-type invasive pneumococcal disease and X-ray defined pneumonia in children less than two years of age. *Cochrane Database of Systematic Reviews, 4*, CD004977.

172. Lukkassen, I., Hassing, M., & Markhorst, D. (2006). Dexamethasone reduces reintubation rate due to postextubation stidor in high risk paediatric population. *Acta Paediatrica, 95*, 74–76.

173. Lum, L., Saville, A., & Venkataraman, S. T. (1998). Accuracy of physiologic deadspace measurement in intubated pediatric patients using a metabolic monitor: Comparison with the Douglas bag method. *Critical Care Medicine, 26*(4), 760–764.

174. MacIntyre, N. (2005). Current issues in mechanical ventilation for respiratory failure. *Chest, 128,* 561S–567S.

175. Madill, J., Gutierrez, C., Grossman, J., Allard, J., Chan, C., Hutcheon, M., et al. (2001). Nutritional assessment of the lung transplant patient: Body mass index as a predictor of 90-day mortality following transplantation. *Journal of Heart and Lung Transplantation, 20*(3), 288–296.

176. Magee, J., Krishnan, S. M., Benfield, M. R., Hsu, D. T., & Shneider, B. L. (2008). Pediatric transplantation in the United States, 1997–2006. *American Journal of Transplantation, 8*(4 Pt 2), 935–945.

177. Mahabee-Gittens, E., Grupp-Phelan, J., Brody, A., Donnelly, L. F., Bracey, S. E., Duma, E. M., et al. (2005). Identifying children with pneumonia in the emergency department. *Clinics in Pediatrics, 44*, 427–435

178. Mandelberg A., Tal, G., Witzling, M., Someck, E., Houri, S., Balin, A., et al. (2003). Nebulized 3% hypertonic saline solution treatment in hospitalized infants with viral bronchiolitis. *Chest, 123*(2), 481–487.

179. Mannino, D., Homa, D. M., Akinbami, L. J., Moorman, J. E., Gwynn, C., & Redd, S. C. (2002). Surveillance for asthma summary. *Morbidity and Mortality Weekly Report, 51*(SS-1), 1–13.

180. Mannix, R., & Bachur, R. (2007). Status asthmaticus in children. *Current Opinion in Pediatrics, 19*, 281–287.

181. Mansbach, J., Clark, S., Christopher, N., LoVecchio, F., Kunz, S., & Acholonu, U. (2008). Prospective multicenter study of bronchiolitis: Predicting safe discharges from the emergency department. *Pediatrics, 121*(4), 680–688.

182. Marcum, J., & Newth, C. (2007). Respiratory monitoring. In D. S. Wheeler, H. R. Wong, & T. P. Shanley (Eds.). *Pediatric critical care medicine.* London: Springer:

183. Marcus, C. (2001). Sleep-disordered breathing in children. *American Journal of Respiratory and Critical Care Medicine, 164*(1), 16–30.

184. Marcus, C. L., Jansen, M. T., Poulsen, M. K., Keens, S. E., Nield, T. A., Lipsker, L. E., et al. (1991). Medical and psychosocial

outcome of children with congenital central hypoventilation syndrome. *Journal of Pediatrics, 119*(6), 888–895.

185. Margolis, P., & Gadomski, A. (1998). The national clinical examination: Does this infant have pneumonia. *Journal of the American Medical Association, 279*(4), 308–313.

186. Markovitz, B., & Randolph, A. (2002). Corticosteroids for the prevention of reintubation and postextubation stidor in pediatric patients: A meta analysis. *Pediatric Critical Care Medicine, 3*, 223–226.

187. Marraro, G. (2003). Innovative practices of ventilatory support in pediatric patients. *Pediatric Critical Care Medicine, 4*(1), 8–21.

188. Marshall, P., Possick, J., & Chupp, G. (2009). Intensive care management of status asthmaticus. *Clinical Pulmonary Medicine, 16*(6), 293–301.

189. Martin, J., Oserman, M., & Sutton, P. (2010). Are preterm births on the decline in the United States? NCHS Data Brief 39. Retrieved from http://www.cdc.gov/nchs/data/databriefs/db39.htm

190. Martinez, F. (2009). Managing childhood asthma: Challenge of preventing exacerbations. *Pediatrics, 123*, S146–S150.

191. Martinón-Torres, F., Rodríguez-Núñez, A., & Martinón-Sánchez, J. (2002). Heliox therapy in infants with acute bronchiolitis, *Pediatrics, 109*(1), 68–73.

192. Martinu, T., Chen, D., & Palmer, S. (2009). Acute rejection and humoral sensitization in lung transplant recipients. *Proceedings of the American Thoracic Society, 6*(1), 54–65.

193. Matthews, B., Shah, S., Cleveland, R., Lee, E., Bachur, R., & Neuman, M. (2009). Clinical predictors of pneumonia among children with wheezing, *Pediatrics, 124*, e29–e36.

194. McBride, S., Chiang, V., Goldmann, D., & Landrigan, C. (2005). Preventable adverse events in infants hospitalized with bronchiolitis. *Pediatrics, 116*(3), 603–608.

195. McCallion, N., Davis, P., & Morley, C. (2005). Volume-targeted versus pressure-limited ventilation in the neonate. *Cochrane Database of Systematic Reviews, 3*, CD003666.

196. McCracken, G. (2000). Diagnosis and management of pneumonia in children. *Pediatric Infectious Disease Journal, 29*, 924–928.

197. McIntosh, K. (2002). Community-acquired pneumonia in children. *New England Journal of Medicine, 346*, 429–437.

198. Meachery, G., De Soyza, A., Nicholson, A., Parry, G., Hasan, A., Tocewicz, K., et al. (2008). Outcomes of lung transplantation for cystic fibrosis in a large UK cohort. *Thorax, 63*(8), 725–731.

199. Meert, K., Clarck, J., & Sarnaik, A. (2007). Metabolic acidosis as an underlying mechanism of respiratory distress in children with severe acute asthma. *Pediatric Critical Care Medicine, 8*(6), 519–523.

200. Mehta, N., & Arnold, J. (2004). Mechanical ventilation in children with acute respiratory failure. *Current Opinion in Critical Care, 10*(1), 7–12.

201. Meissner, H., Long, S., & Committee on Infectious Diseases and Committee on Fetus and Newborn. (2003). Revised indications for the use of palivizumab and respiratory syncytial virus immune globulin intravenous for prevention of respiratory syncytial virus infections. *Pediatrics, 112*(6), 1447–1452.

202. Metras, D., Viard, L., Kreitmann, B., Riberi, A., Pannetier-Miller, A., Garbi, O., et al. (1999). Lung infections in pediatric lung transplantation: Experience in 49 cases. *European Journal of Cardiothoracic Surgery, 15*(4), 490–494; discussion 495.

203. Mikelova, L., Halperin, S., Scheifele, D., Smith, B., Ford-Jones, E., Vaudry, W., et al. (2003). Predictors of death in infants hospitalized with pertussis: A case-control study of 16 pertussis deaths in Canada. *Journal of Pediatrics, 143*(5), 576–581.

204. Mlcak, R., Suman, O., & Herndon, D. (2007). Respiratory management of inhalation injury. *Burns, 33*(1), 2–13.

205. Morrison, R., & Bidani, A. (2002). Acute respiratory distress syndrome: Epidemiology and pathophysiology. *Chest Surgery Clinics of North America, 12*, 301–323.

206. Mourani, P., Sontag, M., Younoszai, A., Dunbar Ivy, D., & Abman, S. (2008). Clinical utility of echocardiography for the diagnosis and management of pulmonary vascular disease in young children with chronic lung disease. *Pediatrics, 121*(2), 317–325.

207. Murphy, C., Schramm, G. E., Doherty, J. A., Reichley, R. M., Gajic, O., Afessa, B., et al. (2009). The importance of fluid management in acute lung injury secondary to septic shock. *Chest, 136*(1), 102–109.

208. Murugan, A., Prys-Picard, C., & Calhoun, W. (2009). Biomarkers in asthma. *Current Opinion in Pulmonary Medicine, 15*, 12–18.

209. National Heart, Lung, and Blood Institute (NHLBI). (2007a). National Asthma Education and Prevention Program, Expert panel report III: Guidelines for the diagnosis and management of asthma (NIH publication no. 08-4051). Retrieved from www.nhlbi.nih.gov/guidelines/asthma/

210. National Heart, Lung, and Blood Institute (NHLBI). (2007b). Asthma action plan. Retrieved from http://www.nhlbi.nih.gov/health/public/lung/asthma/asthma_actplan.pdf

211. National Heart, Lung, and Blood Institute (NHLBI), Acute Respiratory Distress Syndrome (ARDS) Clinical Trials Network. (2006). Comparison of two fluid-management strategies in acute lung injury. *New England Journal of Medicine, 353*(24), 2564–2575.

212. National Institutes of Health (NIH). (1987). National Institutes of Health consensus development conference on infantile apnea and home monitoring. *Pediatrics, 79*(2), 292–299.

213. Needleman, J., Sykes, J. A., Schroeder, S. A., & Singer, L. P. (2004). Noninvasive positive pressure ventilation in the treatment of pediatric status asthmaticus. *Pediatric Asthma, Allergy & Immunology, 17*(4), 272–277.

214. Newth, J., Venkataraman, S., Willson, D. F., Meert, K. L., Harrison, R., Dean, J. M., et al. (2009). Weaning and readiness for extubation in pediatric patients. *Pediatric Critical Care Medicine, 10*(1), 1–11.

215. Northway, W., Rosan, R., & Porter, D. (1967). Pulmonary disease following respirator therapy of hyaline membrane disease. *New England Journal of Medicine, 276*(7), 357–368.

216. Nowak, R., Corbridge, T., & Brenner, B. (2009). Noninvasive ventilation. *American Thoracic Society, 6*, 367–370.

217. O'Halloran, E., Reynolds, J. D., Lau, C. L., Manson, R. J., Davis, R. D., Palmer, S. M., et al. (2004). Laparoscopic Nissen fundoplication for treating reflux in lung transplant recipients. *Journal of Gastrointestinal Surgery, 8*(1), 132–137.

218. Okiro, E., White, L., Ngama, M., Cane, P., Medley, G., & Nokes, D. (2010). Duration shedding of respiratory syncytial virus in a community study of Kenyan children. *BioMed Central Infectious Diseases, 10*(15), 1–7.

219. Oren, J., Estenne, M., Arcasoy, S., Conte, J. V., Corris, P., Egan, J. J., et al. (2006). International guidelines for the selection of lung transplant candidates: 2006 update. A consensus report from the Pulmonary Scientific Council of the International Society for Heart and Lung Transplantation. *Journal of Heart and Lung Transplantation, 25*(7), 745–755.

220. Pacht, E., DeMichele, S., Nelson, J., Hart, J., Wennberg, A., & Gadek, J. (2003). Enteral nutrition with eicosapentaenoic acid, [gamma]-linolenic acid, and antioxidants reduces alveolar inflammatory mediators and protein influx in patients with acute respiratory distress syndrome. *Critical Care Medicine, 31*(2), 491–500.

221. Pagana, K., & Pagana, T. (2002). *Mosby's manual of diagnostic and laboratory tests* (2nd ed.). St. Louis, MO: Mosby.

222. Palmer, S. M., Miralles, A. P., Lawrence, C. M., Gaynor, J. W., Davis, R. D., & Tapson, V. F. (1999). Rabbit antithymocyte globulin decreases acute rejection after lung transplantation: Results of a randomized, prospective study. *Chest, 116*(1), 127–133.

223. Palmer, S., Miralles, A. P., Howell, D. N., Brazer, S. R., Tapson, V. F., & Davis, R. D. (2000). Gastroesophageal reflux as a reversible cause of allograft dysfunction after lung transplantation. *Chest, 118*(4), 1214–1217.

224. Palmieri, T. (2009). Use of β-agonists in inhalation therapy. *Journal of Burn Care and Research, 30*(1), 156–159.

225. Panitch, H. (2006). Airway clearance in children with neuromuscular disease. *Current Opinion in Pediatrics, 18,* 277–281.

226. Patel, H., Platt, R., Lozano, J., & Wang, E. (2004). Glucocorticosteroids for acute viral bronchiolitis in infants and young children. *Cochrane Database of Systematic Reviews, 3,* CD004878.

227. Paton, J. Y., Swaminathan, S., Sargent, C. W., & Keens, T. G. (1989). Hypoxic and hypercapneic ventilatory responses in awake children with congenital central hypoventilation syndrome. *American Review of Respiratory Disease, 140*(2), 368–372.

228. Peter, J., John, P., Graham, P., Moran, J., George, I., & Bersten, A. (2008). Corticosteroids in the prevention and treatment of acute respiratory distress syndrome (ARDS) in adults: meta-analysis. *BMJ, 336,* 1006–1009.

229. Pierce, C., Klein, N., & Peters, M. (2000). Is leukocytosis a predictor of mortality in severe pertussis infection? *Intensive Care Medicine, 159,* 898–900.

230. Quan, J., Tiddens, H., Sy, J., McKenzie, S., Montgomery, M., Robinson, P., et al. (2001). Pulmozyme early intervention trial study group: A two year randomized placebo controlled trial of dornase alpha in young patients with cystic fibrosis with mild lung function abnormalities. *Journal of Pediatrics, 139,* 813–820.

231. Raab, E., et al. (2008). Pulmonary edema. In D. Nichols (Ed.). *Rogers' textbook of pediatric intensive care* (4th ed., pp. 710–711). Philadelphia: Lippincott, Williams & Wilkins.

232. Randolph, A. (2009). Management of acute lung injury and acute respiratory distress syndrome in children. *Critical Care Medicine, 37*(8), 2448–2454.

233. Randolph, A., Forbes, P. W., Gredeit, R. G., Arnold, J. H., Wetzel, R. C., Luckett, P. M., et al. (2005). Cumulative fluid intake minus output is not associated with ventilator weaning during or extubation outcomes in children. *Pediatric Critical Care Medicine, 6*(6), 642–647.

234. Restrepo, R., & Peters, J. (2008). Near-fatal asthma: Recognition and management. *Current Opinion in Pulmonary Medicine, 14,* 13–23.

235. Rivera, M., Kim, T., Stewart, G., Minasyan, L., & Brown, L. (2006). Albuterol nebulized in heliox in the initial ED treatment of pediatric asthma: A blinded, randomized controlled trial. *American Journal of Emergency Medicine, 24,* 38–42.

236. Robinson, P., Cooper, P., & Ranganathan, S. (2009). Evidence-based management of paediatric primary spontaneous pneumothorax. *Paediatric Respiratory Reviews, 10,* 110–117. doi: 10.1016/j.prrv.2008.12.003

237. Rogers, M., & Helafaer, M. (Eds.). (1999). *Handbook of pediatric intensive care.* Baltimore, MD: Williams & Wilkins.

238. Rogovik, A., & Goldman, R. (2008). Permissive hypercapnea. *Emergency Medicine Clinics of North America, 26*(4), 941–952.

239. Rossi, U., & Owens, C. (2005). The radiology of chronic lung disease in children. *Archives of Diseases in Childhood, 90*(6), 601–607.

240. Rotta, A., & Steinhorn, D. (2006). Is permissive hypercapnea a beneficial strategy for pediatric acute lung injury? *Respiratory Care Clinics of North America, 12*(3), 371–387.

241. Rudan, I., Boschi-Pinto, C., Biloglav, Z., Mulholland, K., & Campbell, H. (2008). Epidemiology and etiology of childhood pneumonia. *Bulletin of the World Health Organization, 86,* 408–416.

242. Rudolph, C., Rudolph, A., Hostetter, M., Lister, G., & Seigel, N. (2003). *Rudoph's pediatrics* (21st ed.). New York: McGraw-Hill.

243. Sarahrudi, K., Estenne, M., Corris, P., Niedermayer, J., Knoop, C., Glanville, A., et al. (2004). International experience with conversion from cyclosporine to tacrolimus for acute and chronic lung allograft rejection. *Journal of Thoracic and Cardiovascular Surgery, 127*(4), 1126–1132.

244. Schmidt, H., & Manegold, B. (2000). Foreign body aspiration in children. *Surgical Endoscopy, 14,* 644–648.

245. Schramm, C., & Carroll, C. (2009). Advances in treating acute asthma exacerbations in children. *Current Opinions in Pediatrics, 21,* 326–332.

246. Schroeder, T., Downs, C., & McDonald, A. (2002, October 25). Nonfatal choking-related episodes among children—United States, 2001. *Morbidity and Mortality Weekly Report, 51*(42), 945–948. Retrieved from http://www.cdc.gov/mmmr/preview

247. Schultz, T., Costarino, A. T., Durning, S. M., Napoli, L. A., Schears, G., Godinez, R. I., et al. (2001). Airway pressure release ventilation in pediatrics. *Pediatric Critical Care Medicine, 2*(3), 243–246.

248. Schunk, J. (2006). Foreign body-ingestion/aspiration. In G. Fleisher, S. Ludwig, & F. Henretig (Eds.). *Textbook of pediatric emergency medicine* (5th ed., pp. 307–314). Philadelphia: Lippincott, Williams & Wilkins.

249. Schwebel, C., Pin, I., Barnoud, D., Devouassoux, G., Brichon, P. Y., Chaffanjon, P., et al. (2000). Prevalence and consequences of nutritional depletion in lung transplant candidates. *European Respiratory Journal, 16*(6), 1050–1055.

250. Sharma, R., Florea, V. G., Bolger, A. P., Doehner, W., Florea, N. D., Coats, A. J., et al. (2001). Wasting as an independent predictor of mortality in patients with cystic fibrosis. *Thorax, 56*(10), 746–750.

251. Shitrit, D., Bendayan, D., Gidon, S., Saute, M., Bakal, I., & Kramer, M. R. (2005). Long-term azithromycin use for treatment of bronchiolitis obliterans syndrome in lung transplant recipients. *Journal of Heart and Lung Transplantation, 24*(9), 1440–1443.

252. Silvestri, J. M., Chen, M. L., Weese-Mayer, D. E., McQuitty, J. M., Carveth, H. J., Nielson, D. W., et al. (2002). Idiopathic congenital central hypoventilation syndrome: The next generation. *American Journal of Medical Genetics Part A, 112*(1), 46–50.

253. Silvestri, J. M., Weese-Mayer, D. E., & Nelson, M. N. (1992). Neuropsychologic abnormalities in children with congenital central hypoventilation syndrome. *Journal of Pediatrics, 120*(3), 388–393.

254. Simonneau, G., Galie, N., Rubin, L., Langleben, D., Seeger, W., Dominighetti, G., et al. (2004). Clinical classification of pulmonary hypertension. *Journal of the American College of Cardiology, 43*(12), 5S–12S.

255. Singer, P., Theilla, M., Fisher, H., Gibstein, L., Grozovski, E., & Cohen, J. (2006). Benefit of enteral diet enriched with eicosapentaenoic acid and gamma-linolenic acid in ventilated patients with acute lung injury. *Critical Care Medicine, 43*(4), 1033–1038.

256. Sladky, J. (2004). Guillian-Barré syndrome in children. *Journal of Child Neurology, 19*(3), 191–200.

257. Smith, M., & Talbot, A. (2008). Management of apparent life-threatening events. *Paediatrics and Child Health, 19*(3), 114–120.

258. Smith, V., Zupancic, J., McCormick, M., Croen, L., Greene, J., Escobar, G., et al. (2005). Trends in severe bronchopulmonary dysplasia rates between 1994 and 2002. *Journal of Pediatrics, 146*(4), 469–473.

259. Snell, G., & Westall, G. (2007). Immunosuppression for lung transplantation: Evidence to date. *Drugs, 67*(11), 1531–1539.

260. Sobel, J. (2005). Botulism. *Clinical Infectious Disease, 41*(8), 1167–1173.

261. Southall, D., Thomas, M., & Lambert, H. (1988). Severe hypoxaemia in pertussis. *Archives of Disease in Childhood, 63*(6), 598–605.

262. Sritippayawan, S., Hamutcu, R., Kun, S. S., Ner, Z., Ponce, M., & Keens, T. G. (2002). Mother–daughter transmission of congenital central hypoventilation syndrome. *American Journal of Respiratory and Critical Care Medicine, 166*(3), 367–369.

263. Sung, A., Naidich, D., Belinskaya, I., & Raoof, S. (2007). The role of chest radiography and computed tomography in the diagnosis and management of asthma. *Current Opinion in Pulmonary Medicine, 13,* 31–36.

264. Swingler, G., Hussey, G., & Zwarenstein, M. (1998). Randomised controlled trial of clinical outcome after chest radiograph in ambulatory acute lower-respiratory infection in children. *Lancet, 351,* 404–408.

265. Taketomo, C., Hodding, J., & Kraus, D. (2010). *Pediatric dosage handbook.* Hudson, OH: Lexi-Comp.

266. Tamburro, R., Bugnitz, M., & Stidham, G. (1991). Alveolar–arterial oxygen gradient as a predictor of outcome in patients with nonneonatal pediatric respiratory failure. *Journal of Pediatrics, 119*(6), 935–938.

267. Tan, H., Brown, K., McGill, T., Kenna, M., Lund, D., & Healy, G. (2000). Airway foreign bodies (FB): A 10-year review. *International Journal of Pediatric Otorhinolaryngology, 56,* 91–99.

268. Tanaka, M., Vitek, C., Pascual, F., Bisgard, K., Tate, J., & Murphy, T. (2003). Trends in pertussis among infants in the United States, 1980–1999. *Journal of the American Medical Association, 290,* 2968–2975.

269. Tang, B., Craig, J., Eslick, G., Seppelt, I., & McLean, A. (2009). Use of corticosteroids in acute lung injury and acute respiratory distress syndrome: A systematic review and meta-analysis. *Critical Care Medicine, 37*(5), 1594–1603.

270. Tauman, R., Gulliver, T., Krishna, J., Montgomery-Downs, H., O'Brien, L., Ivanenko, A., et al. (2006). Persistence of obstructive sleep apnea syndrome in children after adenotonsillectomy. *Journal of Pediatrics, 149*(6), 803–808.

271. Taussig, L., & Landau, L. (Eds.). (1999). *Pediatric respiratory medicine.* St. Louis, MO: Mosby.

272. Thompson, W., Shay, D., Weintraub, E., Brammer, L., Cox, N., Anderson, L., et al. (2003). Mortality associated with influenza and respiratory syncytial virus in the United States. *Journal of the American Medical Association, 289*(2), 179–186.

273. Tie, S., Hall, G., Peter, S., Vine, J., Verheggen, M., Pascoe, E., et al. (2009). Home oxygen for children with acute bronchiolitis. *Archives of Disease in Childhood, 94*(8), 641–643.

274. Tomooka, L., Murphy, C., & Davidson, T. (2000). Clinical study and literature review of nasal irrigation. *Laryngoscope, 110*(7), 1189–1193.

275. Turner, D., & Arnold, J. (2007). Insights in pediatric ventilation: Timing of intubation, ventilatory strategies, and weaning. *Current Opinion in Critical Care, 13,* 57–63.

276. Uejima, T. (2001). General pediatric emergencies: Acute pulmonary edema. *Anesthesiology Clinics of North America, 19*(2), 383–389. Retrieved from http://www.ncbi.nlm.nih.gov.ezproxyhost.library.tmc.edu/sites/entrez?otool=hamtmc

277. United Network for Organ Sharing (UNOS). (n.d.). Retrieved from http://www.unos.org/

278. Vanderlaan, M., Holbrook, C. R., Wang, M., Tuell, A., & Gozal, D. (2004). Epidemiologic survey of 196 patients with congenital central hypoventilation syndrome. *Pediatric Pulmonology, 37*(3), 217–229.

279. van Doorn, P., Ruts, L., & Jacobs, B. (2008). Clinical features, pathogenesis, and treatment of Guillain-Barré syndrome. *Lancet Neurology, 7*(10), 939–950.

280. Verleden, G., & Dupont, L. (2004). Azithromycin therapy for patients with bronchiolitis obliterans syndrome after lung transplantation. *Transplantation, 77*(9), 1465–1467.

281. Virkki, R., Juven, T., Rikalainen, H., Svedstrom, E., Mertsola, J., & Ruuskanen, O. (2002). Differentiation of bacterial and viral pneumonia in children. *Thorax, 57,* 38–41.

282. Vital, F., Saconato, H., Ladeira, M., Sen, A., Hawkes, C., Soares, B., et al. (2008). Non-invasive positive pressure ventilation (CPAP or bilevel NPPV) for cardiogenic pulmonary edema [Review]. *Cochrane Database of Systematic Reviews 2008, 3,* CD005351. doi: 10.1002/14651858.CD005351.pub2

283. Von Konig, C. (2005). Use of antibiotics in the prevention and treatment of pertussis. *Pediatric Infectious Disease Journal, 24,* S66.

284. Wagner, K., Webber, S. A., Kurland, G., Boyle, G. J., Miller, S. P., Cipriani, L., et al. (1997). New-onset diabetes mellitus in pediatric thoracic organ recipients receiving tacrolimus-based immunosuppression. *Journal of Heart and Lung Transplantation, 16*(3), 275–282.

285. Walsh, M., Szefler, S., Davis, J., Allen, M., Van Marter, L., Abman, S., et al. (2006). Summary proceedings from the bronchopulmonary dysplasia group. *Pediatrics, 117*(S52–56, 3), 552–556.

286. Walter, E., Ehlenbach, W., Hotchkin, D., Chien, J., & Koepsell, T. (2009). Low birth weight and respiratory disease in adulthood: A population-based case-control study. *American Journal of Respiratory and Critical Care Medicine, 180,* 176–180.

287. Ward, S., & Marcus, C. (1996). Obstructive sleep apnea in infants and young children. *Journal of Clinical Neurophysiology, 13*(3), 198–207.

288. Ware, L. (2006). Pathophysiology of acute lung injury and the acute respiratory distress syndrome. *Seminars in Respiratory and Critical Care Medicine, 27*(4), 337–349.

289. Ware, M., & Matthay, M. (2000). The acute respiratory distress syndrome. *New England Journal of Medicine, 342*(18), 1334–1349.

290. Weaver, L., Hopkins, R., Chan, K., & Churchill, S. (2002). Hyperbaric oxygen for acute carbon monoxide poisoning. *New England Journal of Medicine, 347*(14), 1057–1067.

291. Weese-Mayer, D. E., Berry-Kravis, E. M., Zhou, L., Maher, B. S., Silvestri, J. M., Curran, M. E., et al. (2003). Idiopathic congenital central hypoventilation syndrome: Analysis of genes pertinent to early autonomic nervous system embryologic development and identification of mutations in *PHOX2B. American Journal of Medical Genetics Part A, 123A*(3), 267–278.

292. Weese-Mayer, D. E., Rand, C. M., Berry-Kravis, E. M., Jennings, L. J., Loghmanee, D. A., Patwari, P. P., et al. (2009). Congenital central hypoventilation syndrome from past to future: model for translational and transitional autonomic medicine. *Pediatric Pulmonology, 44*(6), 521–535.

293. Weese-Mayer, D. E., Shannon, D. C., Keens, T. G., & Silvestri, J. M. (1999). Idiopathic congenital central hypoventilation syndrome: Diagnosis and management. *American Journal of Respiratory and Critical Care Medicine, 160*(1), 368–373.

294. West, J. (2008). *Respiratory physiology: The essentials* (4th ed.). Philadelphia: Lippincott, Williams & Wilkins.

295. White, T., Miller, J., Smith, G. L., & McMahon, W. M. (2009). Adherence and psychopathology in children and adolescents with cystic fibrosis. *European Journal of Child and Adolescent Psychiatry, 18*(2), 96–104.

296. Willson, D., Thomas, N. J., Markovitz, B. P., Bauman, L. A., DiCarlo, J. V., Pon, S., et al. (2005). Effect of exogenous surfactant (Calfactant) in pediatric acute lung injury. *Journal of the American Medical Association, 293,* 470–476.

297. Willwerth, B., Harper, M., & Greenes, D. (2006). Identifying hospitalized infants who have bronchiolitis and are at high risk for apnea. *Annals of Emergency Medicine, 48*(4), 441–447.

298. Wilson, J., & Hii, S. (2006). The importance of the airway microvasculature in asthma. *Current Opinion in Allergy and Clinical Immunology, 6,* 51–56.

299. Worrall, G. (2008). Bronchiolitis. *Canadian Family Physician, 54*(5), 742–743.

300. Wray, J., Waters, S., Radley-Smith, R., & Sensky, T. (2006). Adherence in adolescents and young adults following heart or heart–lung transplantation. *Pediatric Transplantation, 10*(6), 694–700.

301. Yanez, L., Yunge, M., Emilfork, M., Lapadula, M., Alcantara, A., Fernandez, C., et al. (2008). A prospective, randomized, controlled trial of noninvasive ventilation in pediatric acute respiratory failure. *Pediatric Critical Care Medicine, 9*(5), 484–489.

302. Yarza, E., Moreno, A., Lazaro, P., Mejias, A., & Ramilo, O. (2007). The association between respiratory syncytial virus infection and the development of childhood asthma: A systematic review of the literature. *Pediatric Infectious Disease Journal, 26*(8), 733–739.

303. Yumiko, I., & Slutsky, A. (2005). High-frequency oscillatory ventilation and ventilator-induced lung injury. *Critical Care Medicine, 32,* S129–S134.

304. Zaidi, A., Dettorre, M., Ceneviva, G., & Thomas, N. (2005). Epoprostenol and home mechanical ventilation for pulmonary hypertension associated with chronic lung disease. *Pediatric Pulmonology, 40,* 265–269.

305. Zhang, L., Mendoza-Sassi, R., Wainwright, C., & Klassen, T. (2008). Nebulized hypertonic saline solution for acute bronchiolitis in infants. *Cochrane Database of Systematic Reviews, 4,* 1–22.

306. Zimmerman, J., Akhtar, S., Caldwell, E., & Rubenfoeld, G. (2009). Incidence and outcomes of pediatric acute lung injury. *Pediatrics, 124*(1), 87–95.

307. Zorc, J., & Hall, C. (2010). Bronchiolitis: Recent evidence on diagnosis and management. *Pediatrics, 125*(2), 342–349.

Child Maltreatment

EPIDEMIOLOGY

Pamela Herendeen

The definition of child maltreatment includes many forms of neglect, physical abuse, sexual abuse, emotional abuse, and threats of harm. The Child Abuse Prevention and Treatment Act (CAPTA) defines child maltreatment as "any recent act or failure to act on the part of a caretaker which results in death, serious physical or emotional harm, sexual abuse or exploitation; or an act or failure to act which presents an imminent risk of serious harm" (U.S. Department of Health and Human Services [HHS], 2010). In 2008, an estimated 3.3 million reports of child maltreatment were investigated. In nearly 24% of these cases, some form of maltreatment was identified. The forms of maltreatment included the following:

- Neglect: 71.1%
- Physical abuse: 16.1%
- Sexual abuse: 9.1%
- Emotional or psychological maltreatment: 7.3%
- Medical neglect: 2.2%
- Other forms of abuse (e.g., abandonment): 9%

Thirty-three percent of victims were younger than 4 years of age; the majority of those victimized were younger than 1 year. Approximately 24% were 4 to 7 years of age. Slightly more females were victimized (51.3%) than males (48.3%). Victimization occurred in all racial pediatric groups, with the breakdown as follows: 45.1% Caucasian, 16.6% African American, and 20.8% Hispanic (HHS, 2010). Fifteen percent of those abused were reported to have a disability—either medical, physical, psychological, or behavioral.

In 2008, child fatalities were estimated at 1,740 victims, with 79.8% of these deaths occurring in children younger than age 4 years. The majority of the fatalities (71.9%) were inflicted by the child's caregivers. The death was attributed to the mother acting alone in 26.6% of cases. Of the total number of fatalities, 39.7% resulted from multiple forms of maltreatment, 31.9% from neglect, 22.9% from physical abuse, and 1.5% from medical neglect. Child abuse reports made by health care professionals (HCPs) accounted for the vast majority (92.7%) of all reports made (HHS, 2010).

Interpretation of child maltreatment incidence and prevalence should include consideration of different methodologies and definitions used to identify and classify the population. Differences among state reporting and investigation practices and problems using hospital discharge diagnoses can affect estimations. Children are often affected by more than one type of maltreatment, and they may suffer multiple incidents over time. In general, it is presumed that current statistics underestimate the true scope of child maltreatment (Keenan & Leventhal, 2009). These data highlight the importance of

considering maltreatment in a patient from any demographic population and the increased vulnerability of the youngest patients—those unable to speak for, or defend, themselves. Subsequent sections in this chapter review specific types of child maltreatment.

APPROACH TO THE MALTREATED PEDIATRIC PATIENT

Sandra L. Elvik

The child or adolescent who presents to an acute care setting for a concern of maltreatment can pose a challenge to the HCP. Historical information is often misleading, and physical injuries can be either life-threatening or occult. In addition, caring for abused and neglected patients can introduce the HCP into a legal setting, which is often unfamiliar territory for such caregivers. HCPs who work with these children can better serve both themselves and their patients by knowing what their responsibilities and resources are within the legal framework of their state.

MANDATED REPORTING LAWS

In 1974, the U.S. federal legislation known as the Child Abuse Prevention and Treatment Act (CAPTA) resulted in all 50 states enacting mandated reporting laws for cases of child abuse/neglect. While state laws are not identical, most share common threads:

- The "mandated reporter" is defined; all states include the HCP in that definition.
- All states provide a "hotline" for reporting child maltreatment.
- Immunity from prosecution is provided if a case is reported in "good faith."
- Punishments from failing to report are delineated; they usually involve monetary fines and/or jail time.

Numerous publications detail the penal codes of each state. In addition, information regarding mandated reporting laws can be accessed from the Internet (Smith, 2007), from state HCP licensing organizations, or from health care agencies.

Despite clearly defined legal statutes, studies have shown that some mandated reporters fail to follow these standards. Reasons for not reporting have included the provider's relationship to the caregivers, a past negative experience with Child Protective Services, and the lack of certainty that the child was maltreated (Flaherty et al., 2008). However, most state laws mandate that the HCP report *suspicion* of child maltreatment, based on the history obtained from the patient or physical manifestations observed during the examination. HCPs are not responsible for proving whether abuse occurred; this task is given to professionals in law enforcement and state child protection agencies.

GENERAL APPROACH TO THE MALTREATED CHILD AND ADOLESCENT

In cases of child maltreatment, the emergency department (ED) is often used as the gateway to health care services. Delivery of initial care in this setting may be a necessary step because of the child's or adolescent's injuries (Canter et al., 2008). A pediatric patient may present with a history of physical or sexual abuse, but may appear otherwise normal. In this situation, Child Protection Teams (CPTs), also referred to as Suspected Child Abuse and Neglect (SCAN) teams, are utilized throughout the country. These teams may include expert interviewers and medical examiners trained specifically in the forensic and medical aspects of child maltreatment. Acute care facilities may have a CPT on their campus or have the ability to refer the child to such a team after acute medical and safety issues have been addressed. Some children, however, present with severe, life-threatening injuries that require stabilization by ED personnel or the critical care team.

The approach to maltreated children in acute care settings is similar to that used with all presenting patients. Life-threatening conditions are identified and treated first. A careful history is then obtained from the caregiver and from the pediatric patient, separately if possible, to discover any possible inconsistencies between the historians. A complete, head-to-toe examination is performed and photographs obtained to identify and document suspicious lesions or traumatic injuries, and to assess the patient's overall health status.

A challenge for the HCP is to assess the consistency of the history and clinical presentation. When the history itself is concerning for maltreatment, or when the history does not explain the clinical presentation, suspicion of maltreatment may be raised and should be reported to the state child protection authorities for investigation. Careful attention should be taken when documenting statements made to the HCP and members of the interprofessional health care team. With inflicted trauma, crucial information regarding the mechanism of injury often changes over time or between historians. In addition, physical injuries can vary over the first few days, so all findings require meticulous documentation of serial examinations. Photographs and diagrams can assist this effort.

THE ROLE OF THE HEALTH CARE PROFESSIONAL IN COURT

HCPs are often intimidated by the prospect of having to testify in a court of law. While there is a possibility that the HCP will be subpoenaed to appear in court, more cases are settled before a witness is ever called. Palusci et al., (2001) noted that in 260 cases of maltreatment involving 455 subpoenas, the pediatrician appeared as a witness less than 5% of the time.

There are different expectations of the HCP witness compared to other types of witnesses. Any person involved with a care of a child maltreatment victim may be called into court to testify to a child's statements, physical injuries, or condition during the patient's time in the acute care setting. Generally, this kind of testimony is referred to as being a *fact* or material witness. Based on the HCP's training, education, and experience, he or she may also be qualified by the court to be an *expert* witness. An expert witness may give a scientific or other specialized opinion about the evidence presented in court (Garner, 2004). For example, the expert witness may be asked to render an opinion as to whether abuse occurred. The HCP who has clearly documented the history and physical examination findings and can explain them in court serves to educate the legal professionals and the jury about medical issues. Testimony from the HCP may protect a child from being returned to an abusive environment.

EMOTIONAL OR PSYCHOLOGICAL MALTREATMENT

Pamela Herendeen

Emotional maltreatment, also described as psychological abuse, occurs when caregivers fail to adequately provide children with affection, love, or nurturance. Emotional maltreatment is difficult to separate out from child neglect, as it is inclusive of educational, medical, and mental health neglect (Dubowitz & Black, 2009). The child may be humiliated, terrorized, isolated, and ridiculed. Other forms of emotional maltreatment include rejection of the child, exposure to violence, deprivation of basic necessities, and confinement. When the caregiver is emotionally absent or inconsistent, the infant may not feel safe, which will affect the child's ability to form normal attachments and experience normal emotions and intellectual curiosity. The infant may respond by becoming more demanding or challenging, leading the caregiver to becoming even more emotionally detached (American Academy of Pediatrics [AAP], 2008; Brady & Dunn, 2009; Dubowitz & Black, 2009; Dubowitz & Finkel, 2009; Kairys et al., 2002).

EPIDEMIOLOGY AND ETIOLOGY

Emotional maltreatment is difficult to measure; it often goes unreported, and it may be difficult to elicit a response from Child Protective Services (CPS) when it is the only allegation. Although psychological maltreatment is a frequent outcome of physical and sexual abuse, it may also exist as a separate indication. It is estimated that emotional maltreatment accounts for 7.3% of all maltreatment (HHS, 2010).

Myriad risk factors may contribute to emotional maltreatment. Indeed, as with child maltreatment in general, it can rarely be attributed to a single causal factor. Mental illness, substance abuse, high stress levels, caregiver developmental delay, and poverty may all affect the caregivers' ability to provide appropriate parenting. Caregivers may have a personal history of emotional abuse, giving them little opportunity to learn appropriate parenting roles. Children and adolescents with a chronic illness may be perceived as different from other children, placing them in a vulnerable position (Brady & Dunn, 2009; Dubowitz & Black, 2009).

PRESENTATION

Pediatric primary care providers (PCPs) are in a pivotal position to recognize emotional maltreatment; they are often the only profession that maintains an ongoing relationship with the family prior to school (Kairys et al., 2002). Behavioral indicators of emotional maltreatment can be identified by a careful history and physical examination. Indicators gathered from the history may include poor compliance with medical recommendations and immunization delay. There may be evidence that the caregiver is socially isolated, overwhelmed, frustrated, depressed, or otherwise experiencing negative feelings toward the child (Brady & Dunn, 2009; Dubowitz & Black, 2009; Kairys et al., 2002). The child may demonstrate significant behavioral problems both at home and in school. In addition, the child may either act out during the visit or remain visibly withdrawn. The interaction between the caregiver and the child should be noted, especially when the caregiver is openly demeaning or hostile (Brady & Dunn, 2009; Kairys et al., 2002).

Physical findings may include a poor growth pattern, untreated medical conditions, failure-to-thrive, altered appetite, poor hygiene, untreated rashes, inappropriate clothing, flattened occiput, or dental decay (Brady & Dunn, 2009; Kairys et al., 2002). Direct observation of the interaction between the child and the caregiver may help elucidate the problem and provide an opportunity to intervene.

DIFFERENTIAL DIAGNOSIS

The differential diagnosis for emotional maltreatment should include organic causes of failure-to-thrive, intentional injury, poor parenting, family social isolation, and mental illness or cognitive delay in the child or parent (Brady & Dunn, 2009).

PLAN OF CARE

No one diagnostic study will lead to the diagnosis of emotional or psychological maltreatment. The provided history and an observed pattern of behavior that is well documented over time will support the diagnosis. Appropriate diagnostic studies aimed at evaluating the patient for an associated or underlying medical condition may be needed, such as a complete blood count, electrolytes, lead screen, urinalysis, and human immunodeficiency virus (HIV) screen in the evaluation of a child with failure-to-thrive (Brady & Dunn, 2009; Dubowitz & Black, 2009). Often a home assessment by a community agency can provide additional information. A mental health evaluation of the child and the caregiver may be necessary.

DISPOSITION AND DISCHARGE PLANNING

It is essential that the appropriate mental health therapies and social support be initiated for the family. Close follow-up from the HCP should be arranged. Any underlying clinical conditions must be treated appropriately, and a safe disposition assured for the child. As always, when there is a concern for maltreatment, a report to the state child protection agency should be initiated.

MUNCHAUSEN SYNDROME-BY-PROXY

Pamela Herendeen

Munchausen syndrome-by-proxy (MSBP) is an atypical form of child abuse that involves the methodical fabrication of an illness in a dependent by the caregiver. First described in 1977, this complex diagnosis is burdened with diagnostic challenges and multiple legal issues. The patient's symptoms typically seem credible and may be consistent with a concerning illness. The caregiver generally appears thoughtful and anxious, leading the HCP down a convoluted path of deception resulting in multiple unnecessary diagnostic and therapeutic interventions for the child (Rosenberg, 2009). The caregiver may accomplish the abuse by fabricating, imagining, exaggerating, or inducing even inducing an illness or its signs and symptoms (Stirling & Committee on Child Abuse and Neglect, 2007) with the goal of meeting his or her own emotional needs (Ayoub et al., 2002).

Other terminology has been used more recently to describe this clinical entity. In an effort to separate the patient's diagnosis from that of the perpetrator, the terms "pediatric condition falsification" (PCF—a diagnosis for the child) and "factitious disorder-by-proxy" (FDP—a diagnosis in the caregiver) have been introduced in the *Diagnostic and Statistical Manual of Mental Disorders,* fourth edition (*DSM-IV*). One could also apply the general term "child abuse, which happens to occur in a medical setting" in an effort to diagnose the child independently of the motivations or diagnosis in the caregiver (Stirling & Committee on Child Abuse and Neglect, 2007).

EPIDEMIOLOGY AND ETIOLOGY

Ayoub et al. (2002) estimate that there are approximately 600 new cases of MSBP in the United States each year; however, most cases likely go unreported due to the persuasive skills of the perpetrators. Victimization is almost always by the child's mother and usually begins in the infant or toddler years. Incidence is equally distributed between male and female children. The abuse often lasts for years due to an inherent delay in diagnosis. The most common causes of death are suffocation and poisoning (Rosenberg, 2009).

PRESENTATION

The symptoms and laboratory findings vary widely; however, the most common presentation is apnea. Other frequent symptoms noted are seizures, bleeding, pain, vomiting and diarrhea, fever, and rash. While the presentation is variable, several common elements can be useful in detecting the problem. Caregivers often seek medical attention from multiple subspecialists or institutions. There may be continued assertions that "something is wrong" despite the absence of objective findings to support a medical condition or reported symptoms. The HCP may evaluate the patient based primarily on the caregiver's history rather than on objective indicators of a medical diagnosis (Rosenberg, 2009; Stirling & Committee on Child Abuse and Neglect, 2007).

DIFFERENTIAL DIAGNOSIS

The differential diagnosis is expansive and depends on the presenting symptoms. HCPs should include MSBP in the differential diagnosis when the source of the patient's problems remains elusive despite careful testing. One must also consider true medical or psychiatric symptoms in the patient and the caregiver who may be contributing to the patient's presentation (Rosenberg, 2009).

PLAN OF CARE

If suspected, confirmation or elimination of a diagnosis of MSBP must be pursued while eliminating other plausible explanations for illness. This complex process often involves an interprofessional team including the HCP, child maltreatment experts, legal consultants, and other family members. Laboratory and imaging studies will be necessary to eliminate the possibility of a medical cause for the patient's reported symptoms and may provide evidence of induced illness. More often, the diagnosis relies on establishing a pattern of behavior in the caregiver that has resulted in unnecessary and potentially harmful medical interventions in the child. This task may be accomplished through careful observation of the child's symptoms, with and without the caregiver present. All medical records should be carefully reviewed and history should be obtained from other HCPs (Rosenberg, 2009).

The use of video monitoring requires collaboration with the hospital's legal team. If it is considered, HCPs must assure a system of continuous supervision and an immediate, preplanned response, or safety plan are available to prevent further injury to the patient (Stirling & Committee on Child Abuse and Neglect, 2007).

DISPOSITION AND DISCHARGE PLANNING

Suspicion of MSBP requires a report to the state child protection agency and close follow-up. Without recognition and intervention of MSBP, a healthy child may experience significant trauma or even death. Requests for further medical interventions should be funneled through the primary HCP. In many instances, a period of removal from the abuser is necessary. The perpetrator should undergo a mental health assessment with the goal of acknowledging the harmful behavior and its effects on the child (Rosenberg, 2009; Stirling & Committee on Child Abuse and Neglect, 2007).

NEGLECT

Pamela Herendeen

Child neglect is defined as the parental omission of care that may result in actual or potential harm to the child (Dubowitz et al., 2000; Schapiro, 2008). There may be an omission in supervision, health care, education, environmental safety, clothing, food, or psychological support. Neglect may have either subtle or severe sequelae (Brady & Dunn, 2009), including long-term effects on the child's mental and physical health and psychosocial development (Dubowitz, 2009). It may be intentional, or it may reflect an inability to meet the child's needs secondary to poverty, the caregiver's mental illness, developmental delays, or physical handicaps (Hymel, 2006). Risk factors for child neglect include poverty, single parenting, and young maternal age; in contrast, family support, accessible community resources, and fiscal solidity are often protective factors

(Schapiro, 2008). Children with special health care needs are also at increased risk due to their extensive care needs not only physically, but also emotionally and financially.

EPIDEMIOLOGY AND ETIOLOGY

Child neglect is the most common form of child maltreatment (Dubowitz et al., 2000; Schapiro, 2008). In 2008, 71% of all child abuse reports, and 32% of all fatalities, were attributed to neglect. This represents a general neglect victimization rate of 7% of all children (HHS, 2010). Given that neglect may be overlooked and is often not reported, the official statistics likely underestimate the true prevalence of the problem (Dubowitz, 2009).

PRESENTATION

The HCP may find the child who is experiencing neglect to have poor hygiene, improper clothing, hunger, fatigue, failure-to-thrive, developmental delay, or emotional and behavior concerns. There may be evidence of inadequate medical and dental care. The school-aged child may have an excessive number of absences from classes. The home may demonstrate unsafe conditions such as fire hazards, poor heating, lack of food, unsanitary conditions, and lack of appropriate supervision. In many instances, the child may experience multiple physical injuries secondary to poor supervision. Children with special health care needs may have missed medications, skin care, or medical appointments (Dubowitz et al., 2000; Dubowitz & Black, 2009; Hymel, 2006).

DIFFERENTIAL DIAGNOSIS

The HCP should attempt to distinguish between purposeful neglect and neglect secondary to the caregivers' inability to care for the child, as the first is reported to the legal system and the latter is referred to support services that can provide assistance or education. Gather data about the family's adherence with agreed-upon medical appointments and prescribed therapies. Determine the knowledge level and understanding that the caregiver has regarding the child's needs, as occasionally a deficit in either may be the cause of the neglect. Medical conditions that cause symptoms shared with those of neglect should also be considered, such as skin disorders, mental health disorders, and failure-to-thrive or developmental delay of organic origin. Finally, the HCP should consider the concept of societal neglect, in which the child's needs are not being met due to inadequate services, policies, and programs available to the family. An example would be children who are not receiving medical, dental, or mental health care because there are no providers available to service them or accommodate their public aid program (Dubowitz, 2009).

PLAN OF CARE

Therapeutic management for the child experiencing neglect is based on the intent and the severity of the effect. Physical needs and life-threatening medical problems must be cared for first. Resources available to the family and the likelihood of behavior change in response to the support should be considered. Some needs may be overwhelming even for well-intentioned families. The help of a community agency, such as home nursing, may be elicited to visit the home and identify any risk factors amenable to change (Brady & Dunn, 2009). Education of the family regarding the needs of children and close medical follow-up are important to evaluate the effect of services.

DISPOSITION AND DISCHARGE PLANNING

Referral to community social service agencies that can provide appropriate resources is recommended. In some instances identified as neglect, the caregiver may have underestimated the level of supervision necessary to prevent injury. In these situations, preventive counseling may be the most appropriate initial intervention (Hymel, 2006). Building on family strengths and establishing the use of both informal and community resources may provide the extra support needed. Collaboration among an interprofessional team of HCPs, social workers, nutritionists, community agencies, and schools may provide the at-risk family with appropriate support in an outpatient setting. If the HCP suspects that the caregivers' pattern of concerning behaviors is placing the child at risk for actual or potential physical or psychological harm, then it is imperative that Child Protective Services be notified (Hymel, 2006).

PHYSICAL ABUSE

Emily Siffermann

Physical abuse is any action that inflicts injury on a child. It may take the form of skin injuries, musculoskeletal injuries, visceral injuries, or head injuries. The most recent national data indicate that physical abuse accounts for 16.1% of the approximately 772,000 substantiated cases of child maltreatment that occur in the United States each year (HHS, 2010).

Child physical maltreatment can occur in any racial group or socioeconomic class. Risk factors for maltreatment have been identified and can be classified into parental, child, or societal characteristics. Parental or household risk factors include substance use, mental illness, domestic violence, single parenting, and a nonrelated adult living in the home. Risk characteristics in a child include younger age, prematurity, low birth weight, and developmental or physical disability. Societal factors include poverty, increased family size, and social isolation (Cooperman & Merten, 2009; Kellogg & Committee on Child Abuse and Neglect, AAP, 2007; Schnitzer & Ewigman, 2005).

CUTANEOUS MANIFESTATIONS: BRUISING, LACERATIONS, AND ABRASIONS

Pathophysiology

Injury to the skin results when a force is applied that exceeds the strength of the skin or its underlying structure. A force applied parallel to the skin may result in an abrasion. A blunt force may stretch the skin past its point of failure, leading to a laceration; contact with a sharp object may create an incision-type laceration. Crushing forces may damage layers of the skin and vasculature, causing

bruises as vessels of varying size and depth rupture. For example, when an implement strikes the skin, its outline may be evident on the skin due to vessel rupture and blood extravasation (Figure 36-1) (Jenny & Reese, 2009).

How quickly a skin injury heals depends on many factors, including the size, depth, amount of associated bleeding, location on the body, and strength of the injured tissue. A variety of host factors including perfusion, tissue oxygenation, medication exposure, nutrition, and individual clotting characteristics, can influence healing and the appearance of an injury over time (Jenny & Reese, 2009). As a result, it is *not* prudent for the HCP to provide a specific timing for an injury. *Efforts to date bruising based on color are not supported by the literature* (Bariciak et al., 2003; Maguire et al., 2005b).

Epidemiology and etiology

Skin injuries are reported in nearly half of all physical abuse cases, either as the only type of injury or in conjunction with other abuse-type injuries. Skin findings are the most common presentation of physical maltreatment. Therefore, a complete skin examination should be performed every time a pediatric patient presents for medical care (Jenny & Reese, 2009).

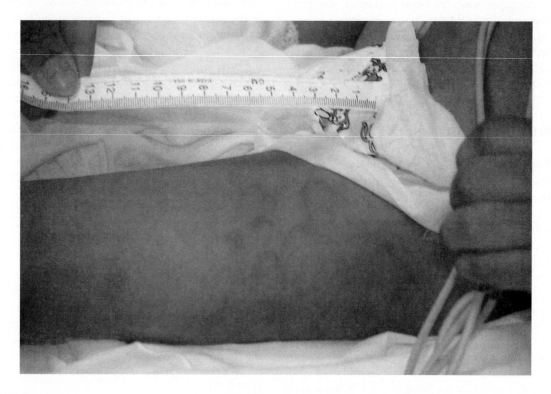

FIGURE 36-1

Pattern Injury.

Source: Courtesy of Emily Siffermann.

Presentation

As with all types of physical maltreatment, the history reported for the cutaneous injury is often lacking or inconsistent with the physical findings. The HCP should consider the history, age, and developmental capabilities of the pediatric patient as well as the extent, distribution, and pattern of the injury when assessing a patient for the possibility of abuse. Accidental skin injuries are common in ambulatory children and typically present over bony prominences such as the forehead, knees, shins, and elbows. Bruising over soft tissues or on protected surfaces of the body is unusual. Examples of these locations include the face, trunk, buttocks, genitals, neck, hands, and feet. In addition, any bruise in an infant or nonambulatory child is cause for concern. In a study of bruising patterns in children presenting for routine health maintenance, the number of bruises increased proportional to age. In infants not yet able to cruise, bruising was found only 2.2% of the time (Pierce et al., 2010; Sugar et al., 1999).

Certain patterns of skin injury provide clues about the mechanism of injury. Loop or parallel linear injuries suggest being struck with an object such as a cord or belt. Multiple skin injuries of uniform shape are suggestive of abuse. The HCP may appreciate the outline of fingers, hands, rings, or any other object that contacted the body (Figure 36-2 and Figure 36-3).

A pattern of injury in which multiple planes of the body are affected, or where injuries are in multiple stages of healing, may refute a provided false history (Maguire et al., 2005a).

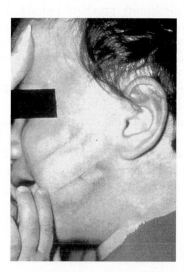

FIGURE 36-2

Pattern Injury.

Source: Courtesy of the National EMSC Resource Alliance.

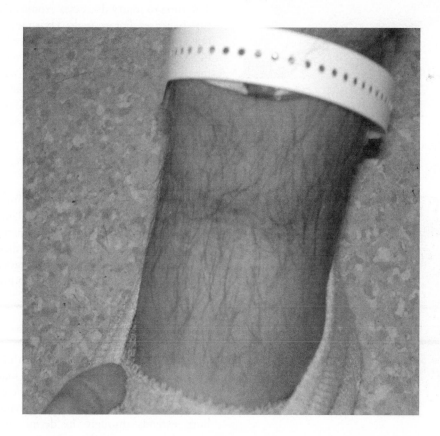

FIGURE 36-3

Ligature Mark on the Ankle.

Source: Courtesy of Emily Siffermann.

Differential diagnosis

The most common differential diagnosis of inflicted skin injuries is accidental injury, which can be readily identified by the history provided and the distribution of injury. Rarely other medical conditions can complicate the diagnosis. An underlying bleeding disorder, for example, can cause bruising disproportionate to the force of injury. In these patients, the distribution is consistent with that usually seen in accidental injury. Various birth marks (Figure 36-4), vasculitides, meningococcal or ricketsial disease, and coagulopathies may present with skin findings that are initially mistaken for abuse. Cultural practices such as coining and cupping used to treat illness may produce petechiae, bruising, abrasions,

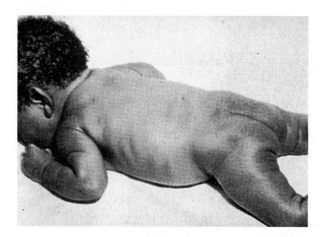

FIGURE 36-4

Mongolian Spots.

Source: Courtesy of the National EMSC Resource Alliance.

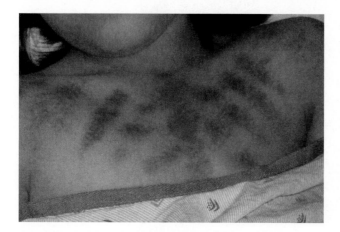

FIGURE 36-5

Coining in Patient with Appendicitis.

Source: Courtesy of the National EMSC Resource Alliance.

and thermal injuries, which often appear in a symmetric pattern (Figure 36-5). Phytophotodermatitis, a condition resulting from a combination of skin exposure to ultraviolet light and to psoralens found in certain plant products, can resemble a bruise or a burn. The unusual distribution of skin affected and the common lack of spontaneous history complicate an accurate diagnosis of phytophotodermatitis (Jenny & Reese, 2009).

CUTANEOUS MANIFESTATIONS: BURNS

Pathophysiology

Thermal burns occur when heat causes damage to tissue proteins, including those making up cell membranes. The depth of the burn depends on the temperature and duration of exposure as well as the thickness of the skin exposed. Blood flow, moisture, and clothing exposure may all affect burn depth. Burn injury renders the body susceptible to excess fluid loss, electrolyte imbalance, hypothermia, and infection.

The time needed to result in a burn depends on the temperature of the exposure. In general, infants and toddlers have thinner skin than adults, which means that they will experience injury more quickly at any given temperature. The time to injury decreases exponentially as the temperature increases. For example, a burn injury can occur within one second at 140°F (60°C) as opposed to minutes at 120°F (49°C) (Jenny & Reese, 2009). This relationship is the basis for the recommendation that home water heaters be set to 120° F (49°C) or less, as it would take 5 minutes to sustain a serious burn at this temperature (Gardner & Committee of Injury Violence and Poison Prevention, AAP, 2007).

Epidemiology and etiology

Hot water scalds are the most common etiology of both inflicted and accidental burns in the United States (Maguire et al., 2008). The peak age of injury is between 9 and 24 months (Agran et al., 2003). Inflicted burns are more severe, resulting in longer hospital stays and increased mortality when compared to accidental burns (Thombs, 2008).

Presentation

In general, burns are extremely painful. A superficial burn involves the epidermis only and manifests as redness. A partial-thickness burn involves the epidermis and some of the dermis resulting in blister formation. A full-thickness burn extends through the dermis and affects the skin appendages; it results in a white-appearing, painless injury.

Most pediatric burns in the United States are accidental scald burns involving hot liquids in the kitchen.

These injuries generally present with burns to an anterior surface of the body, including the face, chest, arms, and hands. Typically, the margins of the burn are irregular, and multiple planes of the body may be involved (Figure 36-6). The burn is deepest and has the widest margin where the liquid initially hits the body. More superficial cascade and splash marks may be seen in the direction of flow, depending on the temperature of the liquid and the clothing worn by the patient.

In contrast, an immersion burn is an inflicted scald burn that occurs when a child is forcefully held in hot liquid. The pattern of these burns is characteristic: The burns tend to be circumferential, demonstrate uniform thickness, and have a clear line of demarcation between injured and uninvolved skin. When the limbs are affected, this pattern is described as a "stocking" or "glove" distribution (Figure 36-7). A burn injury may spare the flexor creases or surfaces in contact with a cooler surface (bathtub, sink). Areas that have thicker skin may have a more superficial depth of injury (Figure 36-8). Restraint injuries or bruising at areas used to immobilize the child during an immersion event may also be found. A trigger event of soiling, enuresis, or other minor misbehavior may be a component of the presenting history (Maguire et al., 2008).

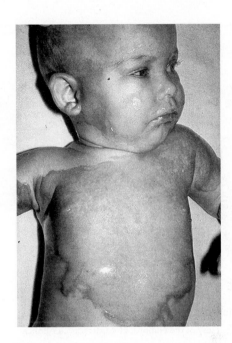

FIGURE 36-6

Accidental Scald Burn.

Source: Courtesy of Amy Melton-Terreros.

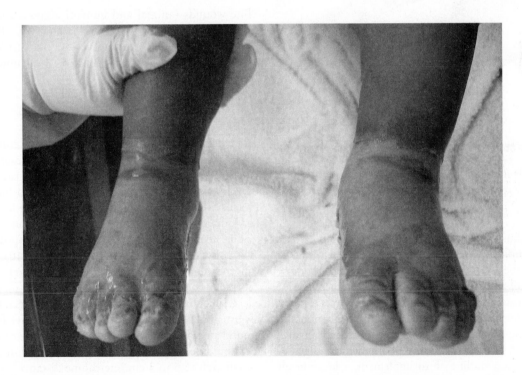

FIGURE 36-7

"Stocking" Distribution Immersion Burn.

Source: Courtesy of the National EMSC Resource Alliance.

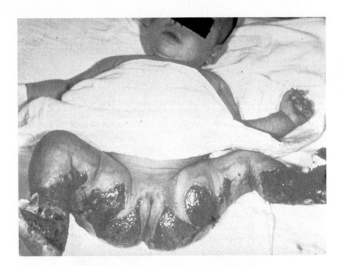

FIGURE 36-8a

Bathtub Immersion Burns.

Source: Courtesy of the National EMSC Resource Alliance.

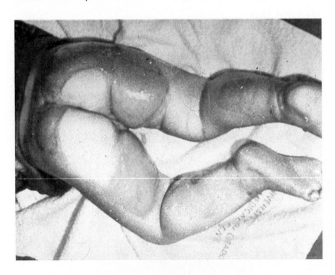

FIGURE 36-8b

Bathtub Immersion Burns.

Source: Courtesy of the National EMSC Resource Alliance.

Contact burns occur when the skin comes into contact with a hot surface. Whether a contact burn is accidental or inflicted may be determined by assessing the pattern of injury, the location of the injury, and the developmental abilities of the child. An accidental contact burn usually affects exposed areas of skin on body parts used to explore or that commonly run into things. Such injuries are more superficial, involve one surface of the body, and have poorly defined edges. A burn with a clear outline of an implement, a location on a protected area of the body, or on multiple surfaces of the body raises concern for inflicted injury (Figure 36-9).

Differential diagnosis

Chemical, flame, electrical, and radiation burns are other types of burns seen in settings of accidents, abuse, or neglect. The history and pattern of injury will help distinguish the mechanism of injury in patients with these burns. Cupping and moxibustion are cultural practices that may lead to these types of burn injuries. A number of other clinical entities may have the appearance of a burn; examples include phyto-photodermatitis, *Staphylococcus* scalded skin syndrome, toxic epidermal necrolysis, impetigo, contact dermatitis, and traumatic or pressure blisters (Jenny & Reese, 2009). Chemical burns in a diaper distribution from senna exposure have been reported as well (Leventhal et al., 2001).

CUTANEOUS MANIFESTATIONS: BITES

Pathophysiology

The injury from a human bite may take the form of a laceration, abrasion, or bruising. The contact from the teeth themselves may cause injury, but there may also be a component of crush or suction injury. As the skin and underlying bruising resolves, it may become more difficult to identify individual teeth imprints.

Epidemiology and etiology

Bite wounds (animal and human) account for 1% of all pediatric emergency room visits; however, the majority (80%) of these injuries involve dog bites (AAP, 2009a). Human bites are most often located on the upper extremities (Jenny & Reese, 2009).

Presentation

A pediatric patient may present with a chief complaint of a bite, or the pattern of a bite mark may be observed during physical examination for another reason. It can be helpful to know the characteristics of a bite from a human adult versus a bite from a child. The human bite leaves a series of individual bruises, abrasions, or lacerations (from individual teeth) arranged in an arch or two opposing arches, with or without central bruising (Figure 36-10). Bites from another child are often multiple, more likely to involve abrasions, and are more commonly located on exposed or accessible surfaces. The arch measured between the canines is usually less than 2 cm. An adult or abusive bite may be found anywhere and often has a larger intercanine distance. It should be noted, however, that a small adult may have a small arch (2.5 to 3 cm intercanine distance) and that the size of a bite mark may be affected by the body surface and type of tissue affected (Jenny & Reese, 2009).

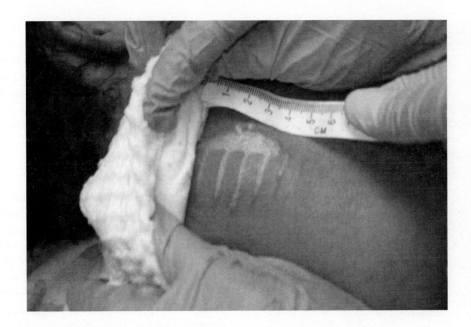

FIGURE 36-9

Contact Burn.

Source: Courtesy of the National EMSC Resource Alliance.

Differential diagnosis

Dog and cat bites are relatively common but their pattern is very different than that of a human bite. Dog bites typically create tears in the skin and cat bites often result in puncture wounds (see Chapter 23).

SKELETAL INJURY

Pathophysiology

Skull fractures occur from blunt trauma or crush forces to the head, either as an object strikes the head or as the head strikes a surface. Short vertical falls rarely result in significant injury; however, falls from somewhat greater heights may result in a simple linear skull fracture (a nondisplaced, single fracture line confined to one calvarial bone). Skull fractures that are depressed, diastatic, or stellate or that extend across a suture line are considered complex and require more force (Cooperman & Merten, 2009).

Long bone fractures of different morphologies can occur depending on the mechanism of force. A direct blow or bending of the bone may result in a transverse, oblique, or incomplete greenstick-type fracture. If the force has a torsional component, it may result in a spiral fracture. Axial loading produces a buckle or torus fracture, usually at the distal third of the long bone. Classic metaphyseal lesions (CML), also known as "bucket handle" or "corner" fractures, may occur from traction or acceleration–deceleration forces.

A CML is a planar fracture through an immature portion of the developing long bone; it is considered highly specific for abuse. Subperiosteal new bone formation (SPNBF) is a radiologic sequela of subperiosteal hemorrhage that may result from trauma. An underlying fracture may or may not be associated with SPNBF (Pierce et al., 2004).

Rib fractures, especially the posterior type, are another injury highly specific for abuse. Posterior rib fractures result from articulation of the rib head and neck over the vertebra during forceful anterior to posterior compression of the chest (Figure 36-11). This mechanism of injury can also lead to anterior or lateral rib fractures. Blunt trauma must also be considered as a cause of anterior or lateral rib fractures (Kleinman, 1998).

Epidemiology and etiology

The most important risk factor for skeletal trauma due to abuse is age, as 55% to 70% of abusive skeletal injuries are identified in infants younger than the age of 1 year. The same age group accounts for less than 2% of accidental skeletal trauma. It is estimated that as many as 43% of these skeletal injuries are clinically occult (Cooperman & Merten, 2009).

Presentation

Any skeletal injury that occurs in a nonambulatory child is highly concerning for physical maltreatment. An infant with a skeletal injury may have no symptoms at all or may

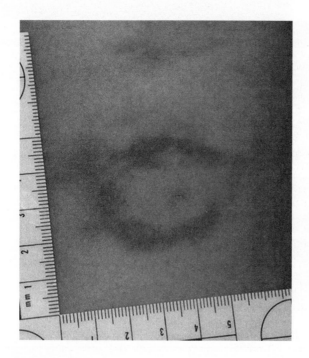

FIGURE 36-10

Bite Mark.

Source: Courtesy of Emily Siffermann.

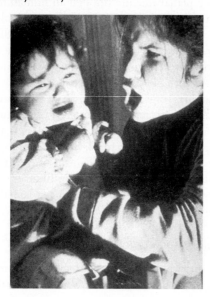

FIGURE 36-11

Forceful Anterior-Posterior Compression of the Chest.

Source: Courtesy of the National EMSC Resource Alliance.

present with a vague complaint such as fussiness or crying. A history of trauma may be absent or minimized, resulting in a clinical history that does not correspond with the forces required to produce the injury.

Fractures have different specificities for abuse. The most specific are fractures of the scapula, spinous process,

sternum and ribs, and the CML. The fractures most specific for abuse are those most likely to be clinically silent; thus they may be found only when radiographs are performed for another reason or when an evaluation for occult injury is actively pursued. Some fractures can be dated within a range of days depending on the amount of healing and calus formation evident on radiography (Kleinman, 1998).

Differential diagnosis

Accidental fractures are very common and expected in the older, ambulatory child. In such patients, a detailed explanatory history should be readily available. In some patients, a few conditions associated with bone fragility should be considered in the setting of pediatric fracture. These conditions include rickets due to vitamin D deficiency or other metabolic disease, osteogenesis imperfecta, osteopenia of prematurity, osteomyelitis, copper deficiency, demineralization from paralysis and immobility, and chronic exposure to certain medications (prostaglandin, glucocorticoid, methotrexate). Other rare conditions that may lead to bone abnormalities include Menkes syndrome, scurvy, congenital syphilis, leukemia, and vitamin A toxicity. These potential diagnoses should be readily suspected during any complete evaluation for physical maltreatment, which would include a detailed past medical, family, diet, and medication history as well as a physical examination, laboratory evaluation, and radiographs (Jenny, 2006).

ABUSIVE HEAD TRAUMA

Pathophysiology

Abusive head trauma (AHT) can result from either blunt trauma or rotational forces (acceleration, deceleration) applied to the head, such as when an infant is vigorously shaken. Injuries such as laceration, scalp hematoma, skull fractures, intracranial hemorrhage, and brain parenchymal contusions may result from contact forces. In contrast, subdural hematoma, cerebral contusions, parenchymal lacerations, axonal injury, brain stem injury, and swelling may result from noncontact or rotational forces applied to the head and brain. Additionally, when it is subjected to rotational forces, the brain moves within the cranial vault, leading to stress and tearing of the bridging veins traversing the subdural space. This effect can lead to subdural and subarachnoid hemorrhage (Rorke-Adams et al., 2009).

Epidemiology and etiology

AHT has the highest mortality rate of all the various forms of physical maltreatment of children. Male caregivers are at greater risk than females for inflicting these injuries. The most frequent perpetrators, in decreasing order, are father, male caregiver, female caregiver, and mother (Starling et al.,

1995). It is estimated that of patients who suffer abusive head trauma, one-third die, one-third survive with persistent neurologic sequelae, and one-third fully recover (Case, 2008).

Presentation

The clinical presentation of AHT varies. Some patients may present with profound signs and symptoms such as obvious mental status change, respiratory failure, or death. Other presentations may suggest brain pathology, such as seizures or apneic episodes. Often the presentation is more subtle, consisting of fussiness, crying, lethargy, vomiting, breathing problems, or increasing head circumference (Rorke-Adams et al., 2009). One study reported that approximately 30% of children who were ultimately diagnosed with AHT were initially misdiagnosed. Of these children, another 30% went on to suffer further injury (Jenny et al., 1999). These data highlight the need to keep AHT in the differential diagnosis of pediatric patients with subtle symptoms. Patients presenting acutely with AHT are at risk for significant complications such as increased intracranial pressure and disseminated intravascular coagulation (DIC). Hymel et al. (1997) reported that in those patients with AHT, prothrombin time (PT) prolongation and activated coagulation are common findings.

Retinal hemorrhages (RH), rib fractures, and CML are other injuries associated with abusive head trauma. They may be more obvious and identified prior to the ultimate diagnosis of AHT; thus, when cranial trauma is evident, associated injuries should be considered.

Retinal hemorrhages are found in 65% to 80% of patients with AHT. While they may occur for other reasons, the findings in patients with AHT are unique—the hemorrhages are bilateral and involve all layers and zones of the retina (Figure 36-12). An indirect ophthalmic examination is necessary to properly evaluate for the presence and extent of RH (Rorke-Adams et al., 2009).

Differential diagnosis

When a pediatric patient presents with a head injury as a result of an accident, there is usually a readily available history to explain the findings. Short vertical falls and falls down stairs, for example, are common histories for both accidental and inflicted trauma. These mechanisms of injury have not been found to cause severe brain injuries. A cutaneous injury to the leading body part or a simple linear skull fracture may be attributed to a short vertical fall. In contrast, more severe injuries should have a corresponding, more severe mechanism of injury.

Several underlying conditions should be considered when evaluating a child with intracranial hemorrhage, including birth trauma, genetic disorders such as glutaric aciduria type I, congenital malformations, infectious disease, and

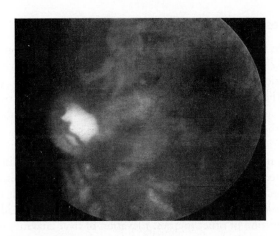

FIGURE 36-12

Retinal Hemorrhages.

Source: Courtesy of Emily Siffermann.

malignancies. Details of the clinical presentation, history, and diagnostic studies should distinguish such processes (Rorke-Adams et al., 2009).

Bleeding disorders should be considered based on the patient and family history. When interpreting coagulation studies in the setting of trauma, damage to the brain parenchyma can lead to activation of the coagulation cascade (Hymel et al., 1997).

VISCERAL INJURY

Pathophysiology

Visceral injuries usually result from forceful blunt trauma to the abdomen or chest. Therefore, in the absence of a clear history of major trauma such as a motor vehicle collision (MVC) or fall from several stories, physical maltreatment should be suspected. Liver lacerations are commonly identified injuries, but other solid-organ tears and contusions may also occur. Hematoma or rupture of hollow viscera and even rupture of the thoracic duct may result from physical maltreatment. Crushing of an organ between the object delivering the force and the spine can contribute to abdominal injuries. Injuries to the mesentery may result from acceleration and deceleration forces. The injuries result in dysfunction of the affected organs, internal bleeding and infection (Nance & Cooper, 2009).

Epidemiology and etiology

Abdominal trauma is a relatively rare presentation of child maltreatment. With a high mortality rate of 45% to 50%, however, it is second only to head trauma as a cause of death from child physical maltreatment. The pediatric patient with inflicted abdominal injuries is more often found to have severe or multiple injuries than the patient with an accidental mechanism of injury (Wood et al., 2005).

Presentation

The clinical presentation of visceral injury is often nonspecific and delayed. This is particularly true in the nonverbal patient who cannot provide a history or localize pain. The difficulty in diagnosing visceral trauma is exacerbated by the usual absence of forthcoming history in cases of abuse. Although outward signs of injury are often lacking, any bruising to the abdomen should prompt further evaluation for internal abdominal injuries. Patients may escape clinical detection until becoming symptomatic with shock or infection. Sometimes injuries are detected only as a result of a clinical evaluation for occult injury prompted by the identification of other injuries. Elevation of liver enzymes may be the only presenting sign of a liver laceration (Lindberg et al., 2009; Nance & Cooper, 2009).

Differential diagnosis

Accidental trauma should be readily identified via history. Other pathologic processes should be apparent on diagnostic study evaluation.

PHYSICAL MALTREATMENT PLAN

The assessment of the pediatric patient starts with the primary survey. The HCP must first address any immediate needs to resuscitate and stabilize the patient. Next comes the secondary survey and identification and management of any serious injuries; Chapter 38 provides a more detailed explanation of trauma management. After the initial steps have been accomplished, a detailed history and physical examination specific for suspected abuse or neglect can take place.

A detailed history should include separate interviews with each caregiver and the pediatric patient when possible. Details about the mechanism of injury, the events leading up to the incident, and caregiver involvement should be elicited. The onset and progression of symptoms in the patient should be obtained. It can be very helpful to find out when the pediatric patient last appeared normal. A developmental history is important to establish the likelihood of the proposed mechanism of injury. A complete social history should be collected to identify and address family risk factors. A past medical, family, diet, and medication history will enable the HCP to screen for genetic conditions or underlying medical problems that may help explain or provide a contextual frame for the injury. Table 36-1 summarizes pertinent history. Characteristics of the history that should alert the clinician to maltreatment are summarized in Table 36-2.

As with a history, the physical examination needs to be complete and well documented. A general assessment of the patient's mental status, affect, nutritional status, and observed developmental abilities is paramount. The HCP should take note of the interaction between the patient and caregivers. Each injury should be described, measured, and

TABLE 36-1

Components of a Comprehensive History

Mechanism of Injury

Time
Position (start, middle, and end of event)
Characteristics of surfaces involved
Surroundings of pediatric patient
Clothing worn by pediatric patient

Caregivers

Location at time of injury
Witnesses to injury

Birth History

Vaginal delivery or cesarean section
Instrumentation
Birth weight
Location of birth (home or hospital)
Vitamin K exposure
Newborn screening results

Past Medical History

Hospitalizations and visits to the primary care provider
Medications
Previous apparently life-threatening event (ALTE)
Vomiting
Apnea
Seizures
Previous injuries or accidents

Family History

Siblings with sudden death, sudden infant death syndrome (SIDS), or ALTE
Sibling with previous injuries or accidents
Bone disease or bone problems
Hearing loss
Dental abnormalities
Diagnosed bleeding disorder
History of easy bruising or excessive bleeding with menses or procedures
Genetic or metabolic disorder

Developmental History

Developmental milestones achieved
Delay suspected by caregiver, health care professional, or teacher
Caregiver's expectation of behavior and development
Caregiver's assessment of pediatric patient's disposition

TABLE 36-1

Components of a Comprehensive History (Continued)

Nutrition History

History of malabsorption symptoms
Total parenteral nutrition
Vitamin D exposure
Failure-to-thrive
Breastfeeding
Access to formula and method of preparation

Social History

Household members and caregivers
Domestic or interpersonal violence
Substance abuse
Mental illness
Social support system
Previous involvement with Child Protective Services

TABLE 36-2

Historical Features Seen in Abusive Injury

No history of trauma
History of minor trauma out of proportion to injury severity
Multiple histories of injury
Evolving history over time
Discrepant history from the same caregiver or between caregivers
History inconsistent with the injury's timing, severity, or pattern
Injury inconsistent with the developmental abilities of the pediatric patient
Injury attributed to a sibling or pet
Delayed presentation for medical care

TABLE 36-3

Tools to Consider in the Evaluation of Suspected Physical Maltreatment

Evaluation of Occult Trauma

Complete blood count (CBC) with platelets
Prothrombin time (PT) and partial thromboplastin time (PTT)
Creatine kinase (CK)
Liver function profile
Amylase and lipase
Urinalysis
Skeletal survey
Cranial imaging (noncontrast computed tomography [CT])

Expanded Evaluation of Trauma

Multiple and/or coned down views of suspected injury
Oblique chest films
Magnetic resonance imaging (MRI) of the brain
Repeat skeletal survey in 2 weeks (without skull views)
Abdominal or chest imaging
Ophthalmologic exam

Tests to Consider as Part of the Differential Diagnosis

Calcium
Phosphorus
Vitamin D levels
Parathyroid hormone
Alkaline phosphatase
Copper or ceruloplasmin
Factor levels
Von Willebrand panel
Disseminated intravascular coagulation (DIC) panel
Erythrocyte sedimentation rate (ESR) and C-reactive protein (CRP)
Urine organic acids (glutaric aciduria type I)
Skin biopsy
Blood or wound cultures

Collaboration with Investigators

Photographs or description of the scene
Relevant measurements (distances or water temperatures)
Histories from witnesses not available to the health care professional
Forensic sample collection

documented with the use of a body chart and photographs. Sequential skin examinations can be useful, as bruises may take time to appear. Skin findings such as birth marks will remain stable, unlike bruising. Every surface should be examined, including often-missed areas such as the scalp, posterior ears, frenulum, hands, feet, genitalia, and anus.

Diagnostic studies can help to evaluate for occult injury and elucidate alternative diagnoses. Table 36-3 summarizes laboratory and imaging studies to consider when physical abuse is suspected. The precise evaluation undertaken depends on the results of the detailed history and physical examination. Consider obtaining a complete blood count (CBC), urinalysis, liver function profile, and creatine kinase to evaluate for acute blood loss, solid-organ injury, or excessive soft-tissue injury. Coagulation studies, including a prothrombin time (PT), activated partial thromboplastin time (aPTT), CBC, and platelet count, can reveal most bleeding diatheses that might potentially confuse the diagnosis. As previously described, abnormal coagulation studies may occur as a result of brain injury alone. Conversely, normal coagulation tests can be present in the face of a true coagulopathy. Consultation from a pediatric hematologist or geneticist can be helpful when questions of an underlying bleeding, metabolic, or bone disorder are raised.

When physical maltreatment is suspected, injury to the skeleton should always be considered. In an older verbal pediatric patient, the radiological evaluation can be tailored to the results of the history and physical examination.

However, it is important to investigate younger and nonverbal patients further because the skeletal injuries specific for abuse can be clinically silent in this population. If a child younger than 2 years of age presents with possible physical maltreatment, a skeletal survey should be completed. This imaging includes dedicated views of the anterior/posterior (AP) and lateral skull, axial skeleton, and each long bone, hand, and foot. A skeletal survey is notably different from the commonly performed "babygram," in which the entire skeleton is viewed in one or two radiographs. Any suspected injury should be further studied with multiple views of that region. Oblique views of the chest may assist in discovering posterior rib fractures.

Skeletal injuries specific to abuse can be difficult to see in radiologic films obtained shortly after the incident. They often appear more readily after healing and new bone formation have begun. For this reason, a repeat skeletal survey without skull views can be obtained 2 weeks after the incident to evaluate for rib fractures, CML, and periosteal elevation.

A bone scan is sometimes performed to detect areas of possible injury; however, its utility is limited by the need to move the patient to the nuclear medicine suite and administer sedation. This technique also has a low sensitivity for skull and metaphyseal injuries (AAP, 2009b).

Imaging of the brain in an infant with suspected abuse is also recommended to evaluate for intracranial hemorrhage and cerebral injury or edema. Both head computed tomography (CT) and magnetic resonance imaging (MRI) can be used to identify injury and can be chosen depending on the clinical setting. When an abnormality is found on the head CT, or if clinical suspicion is high in the face of a normal CT, then an MRI should be obtained. The benefits of CT include its wide availability and brief study time, both of which are attractive qualities for rapid diagnosis in a critically ill pediatric patient. MRI offers less radiation exposure and more specific assessment of injury in the subacute or chronic stage, albeit at the expense of a longer study time usually requiring sedation (AAP, 2009b).

Consulting specialists are determined based on the presenting or suspected injuries and may include:

- Child Protective Services
- Critical care
- Neurosurgery
- Neurology
- Developmental medicine
- Plastic surgery
- Dentistry
- Pediatric surgery
- Gastroenterology
- Orthopedic surgery
- Ophthalmology
- Hematology

- Genetics
- Radiology
- Child life therapists
- Habilitation and rehabilitation

DISPOSITION AND DISCHARGE PLANNING

The goal of early diagnosis of child maltreatment is primarily to keep the patient safe from ongoing abuse that might escalate, leading to further injury or even death. Early intervention can also interrupt exposure to an environment that is not meeting the pediatric patient's emotional and developmental needs. As a HCP, any suspicion of child maltreatment needs to be promptly reported to the state's Child Protective Services. If concern for the patient's safety is an issue, the HCP can hospitalize the patient until state officials can address the safety concerns (AAP, 1998). The HCP can also assist the state with the legal case for abuse by explaining the medical diagnoses and concerns. The medical subspecialty of child abuse pediatrics was recently approved by the American Board of Pediatrics. It is recommended that HCPs seek consultation from professionals with this training, experience, and certification if they have questions regarding the diagnosis and management of child maltreatment.

SEXUAL ABUSE

Gail Hornor

EPIDEMIOLOGY AND ETIOLOGY

Child sexual abuse is defined as engaging a child in sexual activity that the child cannot understand, for which the child is developmentally unprepared and cannot give informed consent, or that violates societal taboos (Leder et al., 2001). Sexual abuse includes both touching and noncontact behaviors. Touching behaviors range from fondling of the breasts, genitalia, or buttocks to oral, genital, or anal penetration. Noncontact behaviors include exposure to pornography, exposure to adults engaging in sexual behavior, or taking pornographic photos of a child.

More than 70,000 children were documented victims of sexual abuse in 2008 (HHS, 2010). This number likely represents only a small fraction of those children who actually experience sexual abuse; in a retrospective study of adults, only approximately 1 in 20 cases of sexual abuse was reported or investigated (Kellogg, 2005). The prevalence of child sexual abuse is estimated to be 1 in 4 for females and 1 in 6 for males (Finkel, 2009).

Sexual abuse may occur in association with other types of maltreatment; that is, the sexually abused child is at risk for other adverse childhood experiences. Dong et al. (2003)

found that child sexual abuse victimization was frequently associated with emotional and physical abuse, and neglect. Sexual abuse is also associated with a home environment affected by interpersonal violence, substance abuse, mental illness, parental mental retardation, separation or divorce, and criminal activity.

Certain characteristics place children at increased risk for sexual abuse, including sex, age, and disability. Females are 2.5 to 3 times more likely to experience sexual abuse than males (Putnam, 2003). However, males may be less likely to disclose abuse when it occurs.

Sexual abuse risk increases with age. According to the HHS (2010), 35% of the children who were sexually abused in 2008 were between 12 and 15 years of age; 23.7% in the age group of 8 to 11 years; 22.4% were between 4 and 7 years; and only 6.5% were younger than 4 years of age. Usually younger children lack the developmental skills to understand and communicate their experiences to the adults in their lives.

Children with disabilities are at increased risk of victimization. Dependency, need for institutional care, and communication difficulties contribute to this risk. Some disabilities render the child vulnerable to being perceived as a noncredible source of information, such as mental retardation, mental illness, and developmental disorders (Putnam, 2003).

PRESENTATION

Children may present with a chief complaint of sexual abuse; at other times, the abuse is not the stated chief complaint and must be identified by the HCP. Common chief complaints that may raise the concern of possible sexual abuse include anogenital trauma, discharge, bleeding, pain, or lesions. Sometimes the sequelae of sexual abuse manifest themselves before children make an outcry about their abuse. Familiarity with these consequences of sexual maltreatment can assist the HCP both in recognizing abuse and understanding children's experience and reaction.

Children experience sexual abuse differently; likewise, the development of medical and mental health consequences from such abuse may vary. However, children who are initially asymptomatic may become symptomatic over time. Sexual abuse may create feelings of powerlessness within the child, leaving the child with a perception of having little control over the event. This leads to stress, which may affect the neurodevelopment of the sexual abuse victim (Dube et al., 2005). Males and females tend to respond differently to the stressor of sexual abuse. Females tend to exhibit internalizing behaviors, such as depression and eating disorders (anorexia, bulimia, obesity); males are more likely to exhibit externalizing behaviors such as delinquency and heavy drinking (Putnam, 2003). An understanding of the underlying feelings of powerlessness and loss of control may aid the HCP in evaluating the behaviors exhibited by some sexual abuse victims.

Sexualized behaviors

Many sexualized behaviors exhibited by children are part of normal development, such as touching or looking at their own or peers' genitalia. Sexual abuse or exposure to sexual behavior (pornography or adults engaging in sexual activity) should be considered when a child exhibits concerning sexual behaviors. Kellogg (2009) states that sexual behaviors that are persistent (with the child becoming angry at distraction attempts), coercive, abusive, developmentally abnormal, or involving children who are four or more years apart in age are concerning. Other factors may contribute to sexual behavior problems in children, such as physical abuse and neglect; however, sexual abuse is the most common contributing factor (Kellogg, 2009).

Mental health sequelae

Other problematic behaviors can develop following child sexual abuse. Sexual abuse victims may exhibit symptoms of attention-deficit/hyperactivity disorder (ADHD) (Mullers & Dowling, 2008). They may be misdiagnosed as having ADHD when the symptoms are actually the result of sexual abuse trauma and should more accurately be diagnosed as post-traumatic stress disorder (PTSD) or anxiety.

Sexual abuse has been linked with a variety of psychiatric disorders in childhood that continue into adulthood. The lifetime incidence of psychiatric diagnoses for those with a history of maltreatment is 56% for women and 47% for men. These rates compare to the much lower (32% to 34%) lifetime incidence of psychiatric disorders in women and men who deny a history of sexual abuse (Martin et al., 2004). The psychiatric disorder most commonly noted in victims of sexual abuse is PTSD. PTSD symptoms may either develop immediately following the event or become apparent months or even years later (Cohen et al., 2004). Other psychiatric disorders that can develop following sexual abuse include depression, suicide, substance abuse, borderline personality disorder, dissociative identity disorder, and eating disorders (Putnam, 2003).

Revictimization

A history of child sexual abuse also places individuals—especially females—at increased risk for sexual revictimization in older adolescence and adulthood (Dubowitz et al., 2001). Filipas and Ullman (2006) found adult sexual abuse to be almost four times more likely in individuals who suffered sexual abuse as a child. Adult revictimization often triggers the emergence of symptoms such as maladaptive coping, self-blame, and PTSD.

Effects on parenting

Given the number of behavioral and psychiatric disorders that can develop following sexual abuse, it might be expected that an individual's history of child sexual abuse would affect his or her ability to parent. Children born to mothers who were sexually abused are more likely to be born preterm, have a teenage mother, and be involved with Child Protective Services (Noll et al., 2008). They are also at increased risk for other types of maltreatment. While mothers with a history of child sexual abuse rarely commit sexual abuse, they are at risk for making poor parenting choices that place their children at risk for sexual abuse by others (Dubowitz et al., 2001). This same population of parents may demonstrate the opposite behavior of hypervigilance, which in turn may affect the parent–child relationship and lead to unnecessary abuse investigation and physical examinations. Parental history of sexual abuse, however, may have the positive effect of making that parent more empathetic to the child if the child is sexually abused.

DIFFERENTIAL DIAGNOSIS

Other life events may lead to mental health and psychosocial sequelae similar to those associated with sexual abuse and should be considered in the evaluation. For instance, many anogenital findings or symptoms may mimic sexual abuse, including chemical, infectious, and irritant causes of vulvovaginitis, and discharge or labial adhesions. Urethral prolapse, urethritis, hematuria, vaginal foreign bodies, torn labial adhesions, and menstruation may lead to bleeding that is mistaken for a sign of sexual abuse. Lichen sclerosis is a dermatological condition resulting in hypopigmented, friable skin in the genital area of preubertal girls and has been erroneously identified as a finding of sexual abuse. Normal prepubertal vascularity and normal anatomic variations can be mistaken for signs of trauma. Infections that are not sexually transmitted can result in discharge and genital vesicles or ulcerations. Consideration should be given to systemic illnesses that can manifest with genital findings, including inflammatory bowel disease.

The pattern of a straddle injury is easily distinguished from penetrative trauma. An accidental straddle injury is usually accompanied by an explanatory history and the injury is often lateral and superficial to the hymenal tissue (Kellogg & Frasier, 2009).

PLAN OF CARE

Triage is the first step in the medical assessment for sexual abuse. Children who present with complaints of anogenital symptoms (bleeding, pain, discharge, or itching) or who present acutely (within 72 hours of the latest incident of sexual abuse) need to be evaluated as soon as possible that same day. Children presenting nonacutely (more than 72 hours since the last incident of sexual abuse and no complaints of anogenital symptoms) do not require an immediate medical assessment. Depending on the institutional protocol and resources, the nonacutely presenting patient may be referred to a child advocacy center or child abuse specialist for evaluation at a later date. Referral to the state's Child Protective Services agency and local law enforcement should be made immediately to assure the child's safety.

The medical assessment for both acute and nonacute sexual abuse is twofold. Like all other conditions, the concern of sexual maltreatment requires obtaining a complete history and a physical examination (Adams et al., 2007). The information gathered needs to include the history of the sexual abuse, a psychosocial history, and a medical history containing inquiry about physical and behavioral signs of abuse. The physical examination should include a complete inspection and detailed documentation of the anus and genitalia.

Interprofessional teamwork is optimal when assessing suspected sexual abuse. The HCP with the most training in sexual abuse assessments should proceed with the evaluation. Depending on the institutional resources available, a pediatric sexual assault nurse examiner may be employed to perform the history and physical examination. A social worker trained in interviewing children may conduct a forensic interview. The HCP must obtain history from the caregiver and pediatric patient separately. Table 36-4 and Table 36-5 identify pertinent information to gather in the suspected sexual abuse history.

When interviewing a child victim, questions should be asked in an open-ended, nonleading, and developmentally appropriate manner. The nature and timing of the abuse as well as the relationship of the alleged perpetrator should be ascertained. Any statements made by the patient regarding his or her sexual abuse must be clearly documented, using quotations when possible. Careful documentation of the pediatric patient's statements may eliminate the need for subsequent interviews. This information is necessary for medical assessment and diagnosis; in addition, many courts have allowed HCPs to testify regarding specific details of a pediatric patient's statements obtained when gathering a medical history (Kellogg, 2005). Information gathered from law enforcement and CPS investigators should be collected in one place to assist in the medical evaluation and minimize repeat interviews.

Anogenital examination

The physical examination for suspected sexual abuse should occur in the context of a complete head-to-toe physical assessment. Any nongenital injuries should be identified and documented in both written and photographic form.

The anogenital examination of all ages and sexes begins with a thorough inspection of the external anogenital anatomy for signs of acute or chronic trauma, lesions, or discharge. Sexual maturity should be assessed and documented. Sexually transmitted infection (STI) testing may be indicated depending on the nature of the sexual abuse disclosure and the presence of any physical findings or complaints (Table 36-6).

Prepubertal female anogenital examination

The examiner must be familiar with normal prepubertal female anogenital anatomy (Figure 36-13). It is not recommended to use a speculum unless unexplained vaginal bleeding is present; in that situation, the examination is performed under general anesthesia (Adams et al., 2007). The prepubertal hymen is sensitive; thus touching it should be avoided. An adequate light for visualization is needed, such as an otoscope. Colposcopy, which provides a source of light and magnification, can assist the examiner with visualization and the ability to photographically document the examination.

The pediatric patient can lie supine in the frog-leg position, possibly in the caregiver's lap, or stirrups and

TABLE 36-4

Psychosocial History

Family Tree

Maternal name and age
Paternal name and age
Children together
Children from previous and/or subsequent relationships
Individuals living in the home with the pediatric patient and where pediatric patient visits

Parental Information

Marital status
Current employment
Educational level
Drug/alcohol concerns
Domestic violence
Mental health concerns
Mental retardation
Involvement with law enforcement
Childhood history of maltreatment: sexual, physical, or neglect

Child/Familial Information

Previous involvement with Child Protective Services
History of placement in foster care or with relatives
Previous child maltreatment concern: sexual, physical, or neglect

Source: Adapted from Hornor, 2005.

TABLE 36-5

Medical History

Injury or surgery involving the genital or anal tissue
Past sexual or physical abuse
Anogenital pain
Anogenital bleeding, itching, or discharge
Dysuria
Pain with bowel movements
Constipation
Recent medical treatment of anogenital conditions

Adolescents

Past consensual or forced sexual intercourse
Timing of past intercourse
Use of birth control and safe sex practices

Source: Adapted from Adams et al., 2007.

TABLE 36-6

Sexual Transmitted Infection Testing

Indications for Children and Adolescents

Signs/symptoms of STI (anogenital discharge, pain, erythema, bleeding, and/or pruritus; lower abdominal pain)
Disclosure of genital–genital contact, genital–anal contact, or oral–genital/anal contact
Anogenital injury without consistent history
Perpetrator known to have an STI

Laboratory Tests

Testing of orifices depends on the sexual abuse history given and the presence of any anogenital or oral symptoms.
Serologies should be completed with a history of anogenital or genital–genital contact.
Gonorrhea: oral, anal, and/or genital culture
Chlamydia: anal and/or genital culture
  • If a nonculture or nucleic acid amplification test (NAAT) method is used to test for gonorrhea/*Chlamydia* and yields a positive result, a culture should be obtained prior to treatment.
Trichomonas: wet mount or culture
Syphilis: rapid plasma regain (RPR)
Hepatitis B: hepatitis B surface antigen
Human immunodeficiency virus: HIV antibody
Vesicular lesions concerning for herpes: viral culture and polymerase chain reaction

Screening for All Adolescents

Urine pregnancy test (females)
Urine NAAT for gonorrhea/*Chlamydia*

Note: Sexually transmitted infection (STI); human immunodeficiency virus (HIV).
Source: Adapted from Leder et al., 2001.

the lithotomy position may be utilized. The prone knee-chest position may facilitate visualization of the hymen and should always be used when there is a suspected abnormal finding noted in the supine position. Proper traction technique, when pulling the labia majora apart, is crucial to visualization of genital anatomy (Figure 36-14). Normal saline or water can be flushed in the vestibule to facilitate visualization of the hymenal opening and rim. Normal prepubertal hymenal configurations are *crescentic* (Figure 36-15), *annular* (Figure 36-16), or *fimbriated* (Figure 36-17). Imagine the hymen as the face of a clock. Attention should be focused on the posterior rim between 3 and 9 o'clock, as this is where abnormalities from sexual abuse generally occur (Pilani, 2008).

Adolescent female anogenital examination

Note the differences in the adolescent hymen (Figure 36-18). Estrogen causes the hymen to hypertrophy and creates redundancy and elasticity in the tissue. The hymenal rim can easily be explored with a swab to check for transactions or notches without resulting in discomfort. As with the prepubertal examination, the inferior portion of the hymen between 3 and 9 o'clock is where findings consistent with previous injury may be discovered. A speculum can be used and a pelvic examination completed if there is unexplained vaginal bleeding, concerns of pelvic inflammatory disease, or a need to perform a Papanicolaou smear.

Male anogenital examination

Inspect the penis, scrotum, and anus for signs of acute or chronic trauma as well as lesions or discharge. If the penis is uncircumcised, retract the foreskin to visualize the urethra. Palpate the scrotum to note the presence of either testes or masses. Note anal folds and the presence of fissures or lacerations. The supine knee chest and lateral decubitus positions are helpful in accomplishing this examination.

Acute presentation

Collection of forensic evidence should be considered for pediatric patients who present acutely (less than 72 hours after the incident) and give a history of orogenital, anogenital, genital–genital, or digital–genital contact, or who present with an acute anogenital injury without a consistent history of how the injury occurred. A forensic evidence kit should be collected for subsequent forensic analysis.

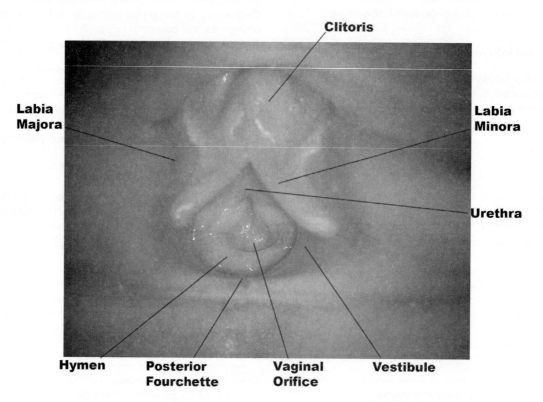

FIGURE 36-13

Normal Prepubertal Female Genital Anatomy.

Source: Courtesy of Gail Hornor.

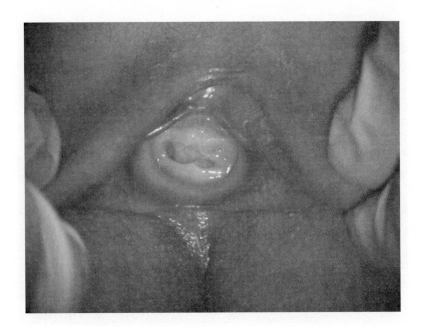

FIGURE 36-14

Traction and Separation for Female Genital Exam.

Source: Courtesy of Gail Hornor.

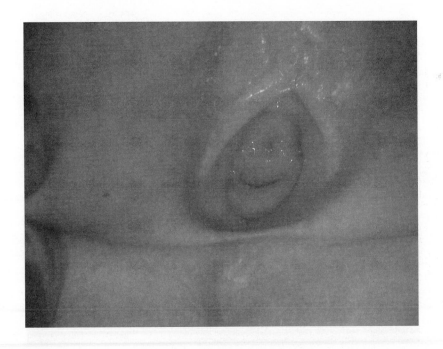

FIGURE 36-15

Prepubertal Crescentic Hymen.

Source: Courtesy of Gail Hornor.

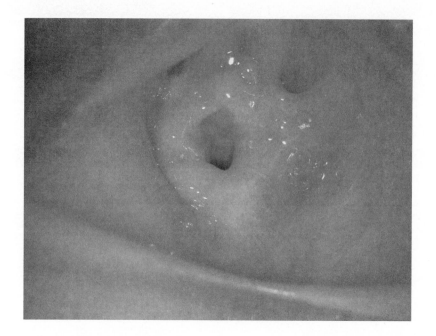

FIGURE 36-16

Prepubertal Annular Hymen.

Source: Courtesy of Gail Hornor.

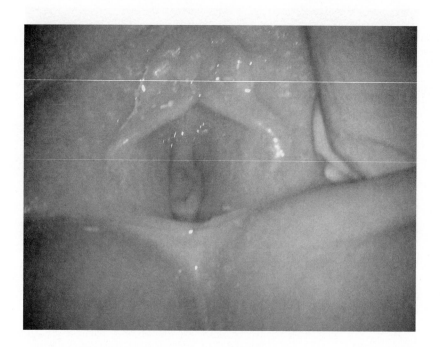

FIGURE 36-17

Prepubertal Fimbriated Hymen.

Source: Courtesy of Gail Hornor.

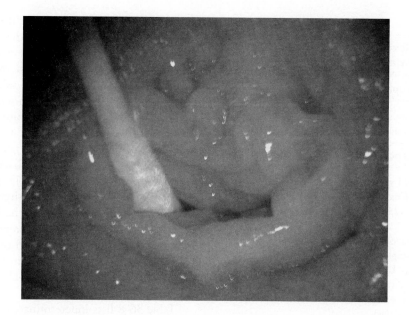

FIGURE 36-18

Normal Pubertal Female Genital Anatomy.

Source: Courtesy of Gail Hornor.

Sexually transmitted infections and pregnancy prophylaxis should be considered for adolescents. Prophylactic treatment for STIs in the prepubertal pediatric population is not routinely recommended when follow-up can be assured, due to the low incidence of STIs in children following sexual abuse. Prepubertal girls are at lower risk for ascending infection than adolescent or adult females (Workowski & Berman, 2006). However, if the child or caregiver is concerned about the possibility of an STI, prophylaxis can be started after all specimens for diagnostic studies have been obtained. Table 36-7 identifies indications and medications for STI and pregnancy prophylaxis.

Interpretation of anogenital findings

Genital or anal physical findings diagnostic of sexual abuse are rare. Fewer than 5% of children who report a history of sexual abuse have a physical finding upon exam (Heger et al., 2002). Explanations for this phenomenon include the nature of the sexual abuse behavior (nontouching, fondling, orogenital contact); elasticity of the hymen or anus, which allows for penetration without tearing or injury; healing of anogenital injuries with little to no residual scarring; delayed disclosure of abuse; and sensitivity of the prepubertal hymen to touch (Adams, 2008). The ultimate goal of the physical examination for suspected sexual abuse

TABLE 36-7

Acute Presentation Sexually Transmitted Infection and Pregnancy Prophylaxis

Indications for STI Prophylaxis

Perpetrator is known to have an STI
Adolescent gives a history of oral–genital, anal–genital, or genital–genital contact
Patient is symptomatic: genital/anal discharge, pain, itching, or bleeding; dysuria; urinary urgency; or lesions
Sexual abuse/assault by multiple perpetrators
Sibling is known to have an STI
Unknown perpetrator
Caregiver or patient request

Indications for Pregnancy Prophylaxis

Pubertal female with history of genital–genital contact
Caregiver/patient request

Indications for HIV Prophylaxis

Perpetrator known to be positive or at high risk for HIV (IV drug user; male who has sex with males; prison) with sexual abuse/assault history involving anal–genital or genital–genital contact
Unknown perpetrator with acute anogenital injury with sexual abuse or assault history involving anal–genital or genital-genital contact

(Continued)

TABLE 36-7

Acute Presentation Sexually Transmitted Infection and Pregnancy Prophylaxis (Continued)

Indications for HIV Prophylaxis

Unknown perpetrator with sexual abuse or assault history involving anal–genital or genital–genital contact

Medications (Adolescent Doses)

Chlamydia: Azithromycin 1 gm orally × 1 or Doxycycline 100 mg orally 2 times per day × 7 days
Gonorrhea: Ceftriaxone 125 mg IM × 1 or Cefixime 400 mg orally × 1
Trichimoniasis: Metronidazole 2 gm orally × 1
Pregnancy: Plan B One-Step (levonorgestrel) orally × 1
HIV (three-drug regimen): Use of this regimen should be discussed with infectious diseases professionals who can assist the patient with education on adherence and follow-up.
 • Kaletra (lopinavir/ritonavir)
 • Combivir (ZDV with lamivudine)

Note: Sexually transmitted infection (STI), human immunodeficiency virus (HIV), intravenous (IV), intramuscular (IM).
Source: Adapted from Smith & Grohskopf, 2005; Workowski & Berman, 2006.

is to ensure positive outcomes for the pediatric patient and family by providing reassurance that despite what has happened, the child's body is normal or will heal.

Anogenital findings are most frequently noted when children are examined acutely following sexual abuse. Approximately 20% of children will have an anogenital finding concerning for sexual abuse (Pilani, 2008). Acute findings include ecchymosis, edema, petechiae, bleeding, abrasions, or transections or tears of the hymen or other anogenital structures (Figure 36-19 and Figure 36-20). Chronic findings (Figure 36-21) are more difficult to detect, but may include healed hymenal transections in the posterior rim extending to the base of the hymen or to the vaginal wall, missing hymenal tissue in the posterior rim, scarring of the posterior fourchette, or perianal scarring (Adams, 2007). Chronic findings should be confirmed in supine and knee-chest position whenever possible.

Table 36-8 lists indeterminate and diagnostic findings associated with sexual abuse. An indeterminate finding may support a child's disclosure of sexual abuse but must be interpreted with caution if the child gives no history of abuse. A diagnostic finding is highly suggestive of sexual abuse even if no disclosure is given unless an explanatory

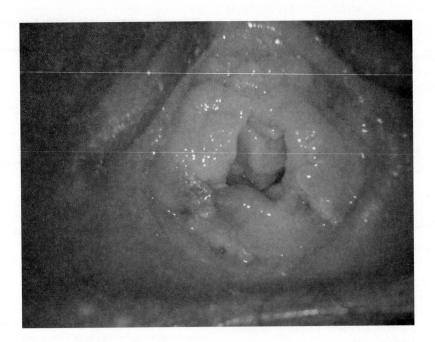

FIGURE 36-19

Acute Anogenital Injury.
Source: Courtesy of Gail Hornor.

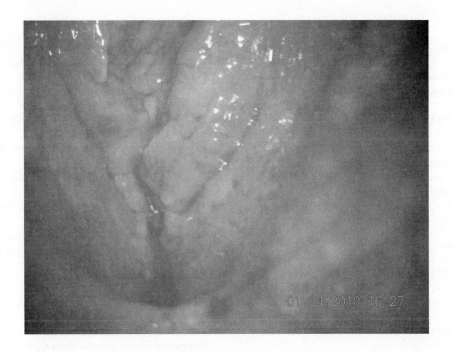

FIGURE 36-20

Acute Anogenital Injury.

Source: Courtesy of Gail Hornor.

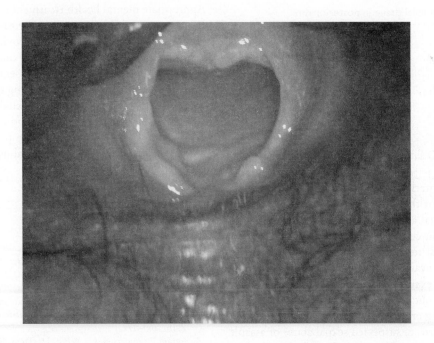

FIGURE 36-21

Chronic Anogenital Injury.

Source: Courtesy of Gail Hornor.

TABLE 36-8

Interpretation of Physical Findings in Suspected Sexual Abuse

Indeterminate Findings

Deep notches or clefts (not transactions) in the posterior hymenal rim between 3 (1500) and 9 (2100) o'clock

Smooth, noninterrupted, narrow hymenal rim between 4 (1600) and 8 (2000) o'clock (appears to be less than 1 mm wide) when the patient is in the knee-chest position or the supine position when floating the hymenal rim with water

Marked, immediate dilatation of the anus to diameter of 2 cm or more, in the absence of other predisposing factors

Diagnostic Findings

Acute lacerations or bruising of labia, penis, scrotum, perianal tissues, or perineum

Fresh laceration of the posterior fourchette, not involving the hymen

Perianal scar, in the absence of predisposing factors

Scar of posterior fourchette or fossa

Hymenal laceration (tear—partial or complete), acute

Bruising/petechiae on the hymen

Perianal lacerations extending deep to the external anal sphincter

Healed hymenal transaction between 4 (1600) and 8 (2000) o'clock

Missing segment of hymenal tissue in posterior rim

Source: Adams, 2008.

history of accidental injury consistent with the injury is provided. The diagnosis of certain STIs raises the concern of sexual abuse (Table 36-9).

DISPOSITION AND DISCHARGE PLANNING

Child advocacy centers (CAC) and child abuse specialists are a resource for the HCP when performing medical assessments for sexual abuse; you should become familiar with your local resources. Consider referral to a CAC or a child abuse specialist for the medical assessment for child sexual abuse if it is available in a timely manner. Second-opinion anogenital exams by a skilled child sexual abuse examiner should be obtained whenever the HCP questions an anogenital finding or an STI.

Reporting concerns of suspected sexual abuse or assault is a moral, ethical, and legal responsibility of all HCPs. All HCPs are mandated reporters and are responsible for understanding the reporting laws of the state in which they practice. Reports of suspected sexual abuse or assault should be made to Child Protective Services and law enforcement.

The HCP examining the child for a sexual abuse concern must ensure that the child's medical needs are met. To do so, referral to other medical specialists may be necessary.

TABLE 36-9

Interpretation of STI Testing

Diagnostic Findings

Report to Child Protective Services:
- Positive oral, anal, or genital GC culture in a child older than the neonate stage
- Positive anal or genital *Chlamydia* culture in a child older than 3 years of age
- Positive RPR or VDRL (syphilis) if perinatal transmission is ruled out
- Positive *Trichomonas vaginalis* culture or wet mount in a child older than 1 year of age
- Positive HIV test if perinatal transmission, contact with contaminated needles, or blood products are ruled out

Indeterminate Findings

Report to Child Protective Services unless vertical or horizontal transmission is likely:
- Anogenital warts (*Condyloma accuminata*)
- Anogenital herpes simplex virus type 1 or type 2

Note: Sexually transmitted infection (STI), *Gonococcus* (GC), rapid plasma regain (RPR), venereal disease research laboratory (VDRL), human immunodeficiency virus (HIV).
Source: Adapted from Adams et al., 2007.

Appropriate mental health treatment is essential in decreasing trauma to child victims and their families. Referral to a mental health specialist skilled in providing trauma-focused cognitive behavioral therapy for sexual abuse victims and nonoffending family members is essential.

Prompt recognition and reporting of child sexual abuse by the HCP can prevent further sexual abuse—not only of the pediatric patient currently receiving treatment, but also of other potential victims. Educate pediatric patients and caregivers regarding child sexual abuse. Be a resource to other HCPs and the community.

REFERENCES

1. Adams, J. (2008). Guidelines for medical care of children evaluated for suspected sexual abuse: An update for 2008. *Current Opinion in Obstetrics and Gynecology, 20*(5), 435–441.
2. Adams, J., Kaplan, R., Starling, S., Mehta, N., Finkel, M., Botash, A., et al. (2007). Guidelines for medical care of children who may have been sexually abused. *Journal of Pediatric & Adolescent Gynecology, 20*(3), 163–172.
3. Agran, P., Anderson, C., Winn, D., Trent, R., Walton-Haynes, L., & Thayer, S. (2003). Rates of pediatric injuries by 3-month intervals for children 0–3 years of age. *Pediatrics, 111*, 683–692.
4. American Academy of Pediatrics (AAP), Committee on Hospital Care and Committee on Child Abuse and Neglect. (1998). Medical necessity for the hospitalization of the abused and neglected child. *Pediatrics, 101*(4), 715–716.
5. American Academy of Pediatrics (AAP), Clinical Report. (2008). Understanding the behavioral and emotional consequences of child abuse. *Pediatrics, 122*(3), 667–673.

6. American Academy of Pediatrics (AAP). (2009a). Bite wounds. In L. Pickering, C. Baker, D. Kimberlin, & S. Long (Eds.). *Red book: 2009 report of the Committee on Infectious Diseases*. (28th ed., pp. 187–191). Elk Grove Village, IL: Author.

7. American Academy of Pediatrics (AAP), Section on Radiology. (2009b). Policy statement: Diagnostic imaging of child abuse. *Pediatrics, 123*(5), 1430–1435.

8. Ayoub, C., Alexander, R., Beck, D., Bursch, B., Feldman, K., Libow, J., et al. (2002). Position paper: Definitional issues in Munchausen by proxy. *Child Maltreatment, 7*(2), 105–111.

9. Bariciak, E., Plint, A., Baoury, I., & Bennett, S. (2003). Dating of bruises in children: An assessment of physician accuracy. *Pediatrics, 112*(4), 804–807.

10. Brady, M., & Dunn, A. (2009). Role relationships. In C. Burns, A. Dunn, M. Brady, C. Blosser, & N. Starr (Eds.). (2009). *Pediatric primary care* (4th ed.). St. Louis, MO: Saunders.

11. Canter, J., Hoffman Rosenfeld, J., Butt, N., & Botash, A. (2008). Physical and sexual abuse of children. In F. Gallahue & L. Melville (Eds.). *Emergency Care of the Abused*. New York: Cambridge University Press.

12. Case, M. (2008). Inflicted traumatic brain injury in infants and young children. *Brain Pathology, 18*, 571–582.

13. Cohen, J., Deblinger, E., Mannarion, A., & Steer, R. (2004). A multi-site, randomized controlled trial for children with sexual abuse–related PTSD. *Adolescent Psychiatry, 43*(4), 393–402.

14. Cooperman, D., & Merten, D. (2009). Skeletal manifestations of child abuse. In R. M. Reese & C. W. Christian (Eds.). *Child abuse medical diagnosis and management* (3rd ed., pp. 122–165). Elk Grove Village, IL: American Academy of Pediatrics.

15. Dong, M., Anda, R., Dube, S., Giles, W., & Felitti, V. (2003). The relationship of exposure to childhood sexual abuse to other forms of abuse, neglect, and household dysfunction during childhood. *Child Abuse & Neglect, 27*(6), 625–639.

16. Dube, S., Anda, R., Whitfield, C., Brown, D., Felitti, V., Dong, M., & Giles, W. (2005). Long-term consequences of childhood sexual abuse by gender of victim. *American Journal of Preventive Medicine, 28*(5), 430–438.

17. Dubowitz, H. (2009). Tackling child neglect: A role for pediatricians. In A. Sirotnak (Ed.). *Child abuse and neglect: Advancements and challenges in the 21st century* (pp. 363–378). Philadelphia: W. B. Saunders.

18. Dubowitz, H., & Black, M. (2009). Child neglect. In R. Reece & C. Christian (Eds.). *Child abuse: Medical diagnosis & management* (3rd ed.). Elk Grove Village, IL: American Academy of Pediatrics.

19. Dubowitz, H., Black, M., Kerr, M., Hussey, J., Morrel, T., Everson, M., & Starr, R. (2001). Type and timing of mothers' victimization: Effects on mother and children. *Pediatrics, 107*(4), 728–735.

20. Dubowitz, H., & Finkel, M. (2009). Child physical abuse and neglect. In T. MacInerny, H. Adam, D. Campbell, D. Kamat, & K. Kelleher (Eds.). *AAP textbook of pediatric care*. Elk Grove Village, IL: American Academy of Pediatrics.

21. Dubowitz, H., Giardino, A., & Gustavson, E. (2000). Child neglect: Guidance for pediatricians. *Pediatrics in Review, 21*(4), 111–116.

22. Filipas, H., & Ullman, S. (2006). Child sexual abuse, coping responses, self-blame, post-traumatic stress disorder and adult sexual revictimization. *Journal of Interpersonal Violence, 21*(5), 652–672.

23. Finkel, M. (2009). Medical aspects of prepubertal sexual abuse. In R. Reese & C. Christian (Eds.). *Child abuse medical diagnosis and management* (3rd ed., pp. 269–320). Elk Grove Village, IL: American Academy of Pediatrics.

24. Flaherty, E., Sege, R., Griffith, J., Price, L., Wasserman, R., Slora, E., et al. (2008). From suspicion of physical child abuse to reporting: Primary care clinician decision-making. *Pediatrics, 122*, 611–619.

25. Gardner, H., & Committee of Injury Violence and Poison Prevention, American Academy of Pediatrics (AAP). (2007). Clinical report: Office based counseling for unintentional injury prevention. *Pediatrics, 119*(1), 202–206.

26. Garner, B. (Ed.). (2004). *Black's law dictionary* (8th ed.). St. Paul, MN: West.

27. Heger, A., Ticson, L., Velasquez, O., & Bernier, R. (2002). Children referred for possible sexual abuse: Medical findings in 2384 children. *Child Abuse & Neglect, 26*(6), 645–659.

28. Hornor, G. (2005). Domestic violence and children. *Journal of Pediatric Health Care, 19*(4), 206–212.

29. Hymel, K. (2006). When is lack of supervision neglect? *Pediatrics, 118*(3), 1296–1298.

30. Hymel, K., Abshire, T., Luckey, D., & Jenny, C. (1997). Coagulopathy in pediatric abusive head trauma. *Pediatrics, 99*, 371–375.

31. Jenny, C., for Committee on Child Abuse and Neglect, American Academy of Pediatrics (AAP). (2006). Clinical report: Evaluating infants and young children with multiple fractures. *Pediatrics, 118*(3), 1299–1303.

32. Jenny, C., Hymel, K., Ritzen, A., Reinsert, S., & Hay, T. (1999). Analysis of missed cases of abusive head trauma. *Journal of the American Medical Association, 281*, 621–626.

33. Jenny, C., & Reese, R. (2009). Cutaneous manifestations of child abuse. In R. Reese & C. Christian (Eds.). *Child abuse medical diagnosis and management* (3rd ed., pp. 19–51). Elk Grove Village, IL: American Academy of Pediatrics.

34. Kairys, S., Johnson, C., & Committee on Child Abuse & Neglect. (2002). The psychological maltreatment of children. *Pediatrics, 109*(4), 1–3.

35. Keenan, H., & Leventhal, J. (2009). The evolution of child abuse research. In R. Reese & C. Christian (Eds.). *Child abuse medical diagnosis and management* (3rd ed., pp. 1–18). Elk Grove Village, IL: American Academy of Pediatrics.

36. Kellogg, N. (2005). The evaluation of sexual abuse in children. *Pediatrics, 116*(2), 506–512.

37. Kellogg, N. (2009). Clinical report the evaluation of sexual behaviors in children. *Pediatrics, 124*(3), 992–998.

38. Kellogg, N., & Committee on Child Abuse and Neglect, American Academy of Pediatrics (AAP). (2007). Clinical report: Evaluation of suspected child physical abuse. *Pediatrics, 119*(6), 1232–1241.

39. Kellogg, N., & Frasier, L. (2009). Conditions mistaken for child sexual abuse. In R. M. Reese & C. W. Christian (Eds.). *Child abuse medical diagnosis and management* (3rd ed., pp. 389–425). Elk Grove Village, IL: American Academy of Pediatrics.

40. Kleinman, P. (Ed.). (1998). *Diagnostic imaging of child abuse* (2nd ed.). St. Louis, MO: Mosby.

41. Leder, M., Knight, J., & Emans, S. (2001). Sexual abuse: When to suspect it, how to assess for it. *Contemporary Pediatrics, 18*(5), 59–92.

42. Leventhal, J., Starling, S., Christian, C., & Kutz, T. (2001). Experience and reason: Laxative-induced dermatitis of the buttocks incorrectly suspected to be abusive burns. *Pediatrics, 107*(1), 178–180.

43. Lindberg, D., Makoroff, K., Harper, N., Laskey, A., Bechtel, K., Deye, K., et al. (2009). Utility of hepatic transaminases to recognize abuse in children. *Pediatrics, 124*, 509–516.

44. Maguire, S., Mann, M., Sibert, J., & Kemp, A. (2005a). Are there patterns of bruising in childhood which are diagnostic or suggestive of abuse? A systematic review. *Archives of Disease in Childhood, 90*, 182–186.

45. Maguire, S., Mann, M., Sibert, J., & Kemp, A. (2005b). Can you age bruises accurately in children? A systematic review. *Archives of Disease in Childhood, 90*, 187–189.

46. Maguire, S., Moynihan, S., Mann, M., Ptotkar, T., & Kemp, A. (2008). A systematic review of the features that indicate intentional scalds in children. *Burns, 34*, 1072–1081.

47. Martin, G., Bergen, H., & Richardson, A. (2004). Sexual abuse and suicidality: Gender differences in a large community sample of adolescents. *Child Abuse & Neglect, 28*(5), 491–503.

48. Mullers, E., & Dowling, M. (2008). Mental health consequences of child sexual abuse. *British Journal of Nursing, 17*(22), 1428–1433.

49. Nance, M., & Cooper, A. (2009). Visceral manifestations of child physical abuse. In R. M. Reese & C. W. Christian (Eds.). *Child abuse medical diagnosis and management* (3rd ed., pp. 167–187). Elk Grove Village, IL: American Academy of Pediatrics.

50. Noll, J., Trickett, P., Harris, W., & Putnam, F. (2008). The cumulative burden borne by offspring whose mothers were sexually abused as children. *Journal of Interpersonal Violence, 10*(3), 1–26.

51. Palusci, V., Hicks, R., & Vandervort, F. (2001). "You are hereby commanded to appear": Pediatrician subpoena and court appearance in child maltreatment. *Pediatrics, 107*, 1427–1430.

52. Pierce, M., Bertocci, G., Vogeley, E., & Moreland, M. (2004). Evaluating long bone fractures in children: A biomechanical approach with illustrative cases. *Child Abuse & Neglect, 28*, 505–524.

53. Pierce, M., Kaczor, K., Aldridge, S., O'Flynn, J., & Lorenz, D. (2010). Bruising characteristics discrimination physical child abuse from accidental trauma. *Pediatrics, 125*, 67–74.

54. Pilani, M. (2008). Genital findings in prepubertal girls: What can be concluded from an examination? *Journal of Pediatric and Adolescent Gynecology, 21*(4), 177–185.

55. Putnam, F. (2003). Ten-year research update review: Child sexual abuse. *Journal of the American Academy of Child and Adolescent Psychiatry, 42*(3), 269–278.

56. Rorke-Adams, L., Duhaime, C., Jenny, C., & Smith, W. (2009). Head trauma. In R. Reese & C. Christian (Eds.). *Child abuse medical diagnosis and management* (3rd ed., pp. 153–119). Elk Grove Village, IL: American Academy of Pediatrics.

57. Rosenberg, D. (2009). Munchausen syndrome by proxy. In R. Reese & C. Christian (Eds.). *Child abuse medical diagnosis and management* (3rd ed., pp. 19–51). Elk Grove Village, IL: American Academy of Pediatrics.

58. Schapiro, N. (2008). Medical neglect of children. *Journal for Nurse Practitioners, 4*(7), 531–533.

59. Schnitzner, P., & Ewigman, B. (2005). Child deaths resulting from inflicted injuries: Household risk factors and perpetrator characteristics. *Pediatrics, 116*, e687–e693.

60. Smith, D., & Grohskopf, L. (2005, January 21). Antiretroviral postexposure prophylaxis after sexual, injection-drug use, or other nonoccupational exposure to HIV in the United States. *Morbidity and Mortality Weekly Report, 54*(RR02), 1–20.

61. Smith, S. (2007). Mandatory reporting of child abuse and neglect. Retrieved from http://www.smith-lawfirm.com

62. Starling, S., Holden, J., & Jenny, C. (1995). Abusive head trauma: The relationship of perpetrators to their victims. *Pediatrics, 95*(2), 259–262.

63. Stirling, S., & Committee on Child Abuse and Neglect. (2007) Clinical report: Behind Munchausen syndrome by proxy: Identification and treatment of child abuse in a medical setting. *Pediatrics, 119*(5), 1026–1030.

64. Sugar, N., Taylor, J., Feldman, K., & Puget Sound Pediatric Research Network. (1999). Bruises in infants and toddlers: Those who don't cruise rarely bruise. *Archives of Pediatric and Adolescent Medicine, 153*, 399–403.

65. Thombs, B. (2008). Patient and injury characteristics, mortality risk and length of stay related to child abuse by burning: Evidence from a national sample of 15,802 pediatric admissions. *Annals of Surgery, 247*(3), 519–523.

66. U.S. Department of Health and Human Services (HHS). (2010). Child maltreatment 2008. Retrieved from http://www.acf.hhs.gov/programs/cb/stats_research/index.htm#can

67. Wood, J., Rubin, D., Nance, M., & Christian, C. (2005). Distinguishing inflicted versus accidental abdominal injuries in young children. *Journal of Trauma, 59*, 1203–1208.

68. Workowski, K., & Berman, S. (2006, August 4). STD treatment guidelines. *Morbidity and Mortality Weekly Report, 55*(RR11), 1–94.

Anthony M. Burda, Arthur Kubic, and Michael Wahl

Toxicologic Exposures

- Poison Control Centers
- General Principles
- Gastrointestinal Decontamination

- Selected Pediatric Poisoning Management
- References

The National Center for Health Statistics (NCHS) defines poisoning as an event resulting from ingestion of, or contact with, harmful substances including overdose or incorrect use of any drug or medication. The most comprehensive statistical data regarding poisoning are available through the National Poison Data System (NPDS) database compiled by the American Association of Poison Control Centers (AAPCC). In 2008, the NPDS reported data on 2,491,049 human exposures. Children younger than 3 years were involved in 46.2% of exposures, and 51.9% of these incidents occurred in children younger than 6 years. A male predominance was found among recorded cases involving children younger than 13 years. In adolescents and adults, the relationship was reversed. Although children younger than 6 years were involved in the majority of exposures, they accounted for just 2% of the 1,315 verified fatalities in the poison center database.

Not surprisingly, more than 90% of all poisoning exposures occurred in the residence. In 79.3% of reports, the route of exposure was ingestion, and approximately 25% of cases were referred to a health care facility for further treatment or evaluation (Bronstein et al., 2009). As a result of the creation of the poison control center system, improved critical care therapies, toxicology training for clinicians, reformulation of very toxic household products, and use of child-resistant packaging, the childhood poisoning fatality rate has fallen to fewer than 50 deaths per year. Prior to the implementation of these safeguards, in the 1940s alone it had been estimated that 400 to 500 children died each year from accidental poisoning.

POISON CONTROL CENTERS

In 2002, the AAPCC established a national toll-free poison help hotline (**1-800-222-1222**), which allows any caller to access his or her designated poison control center from anywhere in the United States. AAPCC member poison centers are staffed around the clock by pharmacists, nurses, physicians, and poison information providers. Consultation is free and available to health care professionals (HCPs) as well as to the general public.

Poison center staff offer assistance with a variety of toxic concerns, such as drug overdose; ocular, dermal, and inhalation exposures; medication errors; envenomations; hazardous material incidences; and foodborne illnesses. As the majority of callers from the general public are managed at the origin of the call, most callers are not referred to a health care facility and substantial cost savings are realized. Additionally, most poison control centers employ public education professionals to conduct poison prevention education and activities.

GENERAL PRINCIPLES

As stated previously, the vast majority of poisoning exposures, especially in the pediatric population, do not require medical intervention in a health care facility. Two reasons explain this observation. First, many pediatric ingestions involve substances that are inherently nontoxic, such that they require no intervention other than simple observation of the patient and calm reassurance to the parent or caregiver (Table 37-1). Second, many ingestions involve only "taste" amounts of substances that are potentially toxic but at such small volume are unlikely to result in significant toxicity. A large percentage of pediatric poisonings reported annually in NPDS result in outcomes of no effect or minor effects.

The three categories of products most commonly involved in pediatric exposures to potentially harmful substances are cleaning products, analgesics, and cosmetics/personal care products. These findings are not unexpected, as pediatric patients have easy access to cleaners stored at floor level under sinks and in vanities, and children's analgesics are available in a variety of pleasantly flavored chewable tablets and liquids. Cosmetics, which are frequently attractively scented and marketed in eye-catching packaging, are often easily accessible to children in purses and medicine cabinets (Table 37-2).

Although most pediatric exposures are of little consequence, it is important for HCPs to be vigilant and recognize those poisons and drugs that can pose a significant risk of injury or death from very small quantities. A number of these substances, which may cause toxicity in a toddler following ingestion of one tablet or 5 mL of a liquid, have been identified (Table 37-3). For example, a teaspoonful (5 mL) of concentrated oil of wintergreen (methylsalicylate) can result in significant salicylate poisoning. One tablet of a sulfonylurea (e.g., glipizide) may cause profound hypoglycemia.

TABLE 37-1

Substances Generally Agreed to be Nontoxic in Common Pediatric Exploratory Ingestions		
Ballpoint pen ink	Bath soap/bubble bath	Antacids
Magic Markers	Makeup/lipstick	Candles
Crayons	Solid deodorants	Play Doh
Pencils	Silica gel packets	Potting soil
Jade plant	Spider plant	Tempra paint

TABLE 37-2

Top Ten Substances Involved in Pediatric Poisoning Reported for Children Five Years of Age or Younger		
Substance	**Total Number of Exposures**	**Percentage of Total Reported Exposures**
Cosmetics/personal care products	172,541	10.7
Household cleaning substances	122,832	7.6
Analgesics	115,059	7.2
Foreign bodies/toys/miscellaneous	95,754	6.0
Topical preparations	86,804	5.4
Cold and cough preparations	65,044	4.0
Vitamins	49,440	3.1
Pesticides	44,644	2.8
Plants	41,752	2.6
Antihistamines	39,686	2.5

Source: Bronstein et al., 2008.

When pediatric patients are treated in an emergency department for poisoning, most are managed with only conservative symptomatic and supportive measures, with or without some form of gastrointestinal decontamination (Table 37-4). Although use of specific poison antidotes are uncommon, their use in selected intoxications may be beneficial and life saving.

TABLE 37-3

Examples of Highly Toxic Substances in One Tablet or One Teaspoonful Dose		
Beta blockers	Calcium-channel blockers	Camphor
Cloroquine	Diphenoxylate-atropine	Ethylene glycol
Hydrocarbon (aspiration)	Methadone	Methanol
Methyl salicylate	Sulfonylureas	Tricyclic antidepressants

TABLE 37-4

Methods of GI Decontamination		
Procedure (where still available)	**Adult**	**Children**
Syrup of ipecac	15 to 30 mL followed by 8 oz (240 mL) of water. May be repeated in 20–30 minutes if no initial effect.	6–12 Months: 5–10 mL followed by 4–8 oz (120–240 mL) of water. 1–12 years: 15 mL followed by 4–8 oz (120–240 mL) of water. May be repeated in 20–30 minutes if no initial effect. *Not recommended for use in children.*
Gastric lavage	Place patient in left lateral/head down position. Administer 200–300 mL aliquots of warm water or 0.9% normal saline through a 36–40 French tube until recovered lavage solution is clear of particulate matter.	Place patient in left lateral/head down position. Administer 10 mL/kg of 0.9% normal saline *only* through a 24–28 French tube until recovered lavage solution is clear of particulate matter.
Activated charcoal	Single dose: 50–100 gm. Multiple doses: 1 gm/kg initially, followed by 25–50 gm every 2–4 hours. Cathartics may be administered with first dose only. Do not administer cathartics with repeat doses.	Single dose: 1 gm/kg. Multiple doses: 1 gm/kg initially, followed by 0.5 gm/kg every 2–4 hours. Cathartics may be administered with first dose only. Do not administer cathartics with repeat doses.
Cathartics	Sorbitol 70%: 1–2 mL/kg. Magnesium citrate: 250–300 mL.	Sorbitol 35%: 4 mL/kg. Magnesium citrate: 4 mL/kg.
Whole-bowel irrigation	Patient should be seated with the head of the bed elevated at least 45 degrees. Administer PEG-ES solution through a nasogastric tube at a rate of 1,500–2,000 mL/hr until rectal effluent is clear.	Patient should be seated with the head of the bed elevated at least 45 degrees. Administer PEG-ES solution through a nasogastric tube at the following rates until rectal effluent is clear: • 9 months to 6 years: 500 mL/hr • 6–12 years: 1,000 mL/hr

GASTROINTESTINAL DECONTAMINATION

GENERAL CONSIDERATIONS

Five procedures have traditionally been employed in the gastrointestinal (GI) decontamination of the poisoned patient: administration of an emetic (syrup of ipecac), activated charcoal, gastric lavage, cathartics, and whole-bowel irrigation. For many years, controversy existed regarding the benefits and risks of each procedure. Considerations in making a decision for their use include the toxicity of the poison/drug, the quantity ingested, the amount of time since ingestion, and the clinical status of the patient.

GI decontamination is unwarranted if a child ingests a nontoxic substance or minimal quantities of potentially toxic substances. For example, making a child vomit to "teach him a lesson" should never be done. GI decontamination should be considered in recent ingestions of potentially toxic substances, in patients demonstrating signs and symptoms of poisoning, or in patients who have ingested poisons/drugs that may demonstrate a delay in onset of symptoms.

Similar to the case for many other medical procedures and medications, research concerning GI decontamination methods in the pediatric population is sparse. This fact, together with the knowledge that a vast majority of unintentional pediatric ingestions are managed without GI decontamination, requires judicious selection of those patients who may benefit from these interventions. Consultation with the regional poison control center may assist in making these determinations.

SYRUP OF IPECAC

For many decades, poison centers, physicians, and pharmacists have advocated the purchase of a 1 fluid ounce (30 mL) bottle of syrup of ipecac (SOI), an over-the-counter emetic, that can be used in the home or the emergency department setting. The pharmacological action of SOI is attributed to two alkaloids found in this medication, emetine and cephaeline. These alkaloids irritate the GI tract and stimulate the chemoreceptor trigger zone, the area responsible for inducing vomiting in the brain.

Due to various concerns—such as the lack of improvement in patient outcome, inability to evacuate the majority of GI contents, potential for adverse outcomes (pulmonary aspiration), and inappropriate usage for contraindicated substances (caustics, hydrocarbons)—administration of this product has dramatically declined in recent years. Another disadvantage associated with SOI-induced emesis is that administration of this product may cause prolonged vomiting, which may then delay administration of other oral treatments such as activated charcoal or *N*-acetylcystine. Additionally, studies in adult volunteers have demonstrated

that SOI administration is inferior to activated charcoal in decreasing the absorption of drugs after 30 to 60 minutes post ingestion. Chronic misuse of SOI by adolescents with eating disorders has resulted in extreme muscle weakness, congestive cardiomyopathy, and death. Lastly, several cases of serious toxicity in children have resulted from Munchausen syndrome by proxy (Manoguerra, Cobaugh, & Members of the Guidelines for the Management of Poisonings Consensus Panel et al., 2005a).

Contraindications to SOI use include age younger than 6 months, an impaired gag reflex, impending coma or seizures, hydrocarbon ingestion, caustics (acid, alkalis) ingestion, and ingestion of sharp foreign bodies. Although generally considered safe, the intense projectile vomiting produced by SOI has caused complications such as dehydration, pulmonary aspiration, Mallory-Weiss tears of the esophagus, and rupture of the diaphragm or stomach. Common minor side effects are drowsiness, protracted vomiting, and diarrhea.

According to the AAPCC, in 1985 usage of SOI reached its peak, being used in 15% of human poisonings of all ages (10.6% of children). In 2007, SOI usage had fallen to 0.1% of human exposures of all ages (0% of children). As a result of the many potential drawbacks associated with SOI use, the American Academy of Pediatrics (AAP) in 2003 *recommended against the usage and home stocking of SOI.*

The AAPCC has taken the position that SOI may be useful in a few rare circumstances: when there is no contraindication to SOI, when no effective alternative therapy is available, when there is a delay of one hour before the patient arrives at the emergency facility, and when administration of SOI will not affect more definitive therapy. However, the availability of SOI is limited, and will become more so, as the only pharmaceutical company making the product has stopped production. Home stocking of SOI and activated charcoal may be considered (if still available) for caregivers who live in remote areas and have limited access to health care facilities. Home use of SOI should be performed only under the direction of the poison control center and should generally be considered under rare circumstances.

GASTRIC LAVAGE

According to the American Academy of Clinical Toxicology, two conditions must be met to warrant use of orogastric lavage following toxicologic exposure: (1) the patient has ingested a potentially life-threatening poison and (2) the procedure is done within one hour after ingestion. In the pediatric population, orogastric lavage is rarely performed for several reasons. Notably, there are no studies evaluating the efficacy and safety of this procedure in this age group. Also, depending on patient age, the size of the lavage tube used ranges from 24 to 40 Fr (7.8 to 13.3 mm external diameter), and this diameter may not allow passage of solid materials such as tablet fragments. At best, orogastric lavage removes 40% of stomach contents, but may simultaneously force gastric contents into the small intestine, where more rapid absorption of the toxin may occur.

Potential complications of gastric lavage include aspiration pneumonia, laryngospasm, tension pneumothorax, tachycardia, atrial and ventricular ectopy, mechanical injury to the gastrointestinal tract, hypernatremia, hyponatremia, and hypothermia. This procedure is contraindicated following ingestion of caustics; following ingestion of hydrocarbons with a high aspiration potential; and in patients with an unprotected airway, instability, or at risk of a GI bleed (American Academy of Clinical Toxicology & European Association of Poisons Centres and Clinical Toxicologists, 2004). Patients should not be intubated merely to facilitate orogastric lavage, as the medical risks associated with intubation may exceed the limited benefits of lavage.

ACTIVATED CHARCOAL

Activated charcoal (AC) is a tasteless, odorless, fine black powder consisting of specially treated charcoal particles that yield a very large surface area (up to 3,000 m^2 per gram). This very large surface area with microscopic pores allows AC to adsorb a very wide variety of drugs and poisons. Theoretically, the optimal dose of AC for a poisoned patient is a ratio of 10:1 AC to ingested agent. A short list of substances not adsorbed well by AC includes alcohols, acids and alkali, hydrocarbons, iron, potassium, magnesium, sodium, and lithium salts.

Human volunteer studies using nontoxic markers suggest that administration of AC alone may be as effective, or even more effective, than combination procedures such as lavage followed by AC. Of the five methods of GI decontamination, administration of AC is considered the most effective and is the most frequently used. The indication for use of AC is the ingestion of poisons or drugs known to be absorbed by AC. This procedure is most effective when AC is given within 1 hour of the exposure, as its efficacy decreases over time. AC should not be given routinely to asymptomatic patients who present many hours after ingestion, as they are unlikely to benefit from this therapy.

Many pediatric patients find the AC slurry to be unpalatable due to its grittiness and black appearance. Tips on improving compliance include placing the slurry in an opaque cup with a lip and using a straw, adding a flavoring agent such as chocolate or cherry syrup, and allowing family members to administer the AC to an apprehensive child. During those incidences when the pediatric patient is unable or unwilling to consume the AC, administration may be facilitated via placement of a nasogastric tube. HCPs in the emergency department should be aware that AC is extremely difficult to remove from clothing, and appropriate protective barriers are recommended when this treatment is used.

Although the incidence of adverse reactions from AC in children is low, rare cases of vomiting, constipation, obstruction, and aspiration have been reported. Contraindications for this procedure include an unprotected airway, hydrocarbon ingestion, caustic ingestion, and a nonintact (anatomically) gastrointestinal tract. AC should not be given to patients who have significant altered mental status, cardiovascular instability, or a high risk of seizures, or for whom intubation is imminent, as the risk of aspiration and its life-threatening complications exceed the benefits of charcoal administration.

Multiple-dose activated charcoal (MDAC) is sometimes employed to enhance total body clearance of several drugs already absorbed in the body. This form of "gastrointestinal dialysis" is theoretically accomplished by interrupting the enterohepatic recirculation of drugs and their metabolites. MDAC is indicated for significant poisonings involving carbamazapine, dapsone, phenobarbital, quinine, theophylline, and possibly some other agents. Contraindications to MDAC include an unprotected airway, vomiting, decreased bowel sounds or signs of bowel obstruction, a combative patient, corrosive ingestion, hydrocarbon ingestion, and whole-bowel irrigation. Do not use any cathartic with repeated doses of AC due to the risk of dehydration and electrolyte imbalances.

CATHARTICS

Cathartics are strong laxatives which theoretically decrease GI transit time of ingested drugs and poisons. The most commonly used agents are sorbitol, magnesium citrate, and magnesium sulfate, all of which act via osmotic action. There are, however, no evidence-based indications for the routine use of cathartics in the poisoned patient.

Although a cathartic such as sorbitol is often administered together with activated charcoal, no data have been published demonstrating improved outcomes with the combination therapy compared to administration of activated charcoal alone. Even though the combination of sorbitol with activated charcoal may increase the overall palatability of the slurry for the pediatric patient, this approach has some problematic disadvantages—namely, nausea, vomiting, abdominal cramps, and transient hypotension. Reported complications in the pediatric population include hypermagnesemia, severe dehydration, and electrolyte imbalances, especially when multiple doses have been given.

Contraindications for the use of cathartics include absent bowel sounds, recent abdominal trauma, recent bowel surgery, intestinal obstruction, intestinal perforation, volume depletion, hypotension, significant electrolyte imbalance, renal failure, and heart block. Cathartics should be avoided in infants younger than 12 months of age.

WHOLE-BOWEL IRRIGATION

Whole-bowel irrigation (WBI) is a form of GI decontamination that utilizes an osmotically balanced polyethylene glycol electrolyte solution (PEG-ES) to rapidly evacuate the contents of the GI tract within 2 to 6 hours. More commonly known for its use as a preoperative bowel preparation, PEG-ES is isotonic and nonabsorbable and does not create the fluid/electrolyte disturbances associated with cathartics.

Based on published anecdotal case reports, this technique has been successfully employed in both children and adults. Indications for WBI include ingestion of adult iron tablets, heavy metals such as lead paint chips or pellets, lithium, and sustained-release drug formulations; it may also be used in body packers (persons who swallow packets of illicit drugs). Because many of these substances are radiopaque, abdominal radiographs may be performed serially to assess the success of this procedure. WBI should not be performed if the poison or drug is adsorbed by activated charcoal because PEG-ES may interfere with the adsorptive capacity of the charcoal.

Contraindications for WBI include an unprotected airway, hemodynamic instability, ileus, bowel obstruction or perforation, intractable vomiting, and GI hemorrhage. Potential adverse effects include nausea, bloating, regurgitation, and pulmonary aspiration. Slowing down the rate of PEG-ES administration or giving a nonsedating antiemetic may be used to control vomiting. Stop WBI if serious ileus or hypotension is noted.

SELECTED PEDIATRIC POISONING MANAGEMENT

The following poisonings were selected based on their inclusion in one of two categories: (1) common household ingestions based on prevalence and identification as one of the most common pediatric ingestions (ethanol in perfumes, hand sanitizers, iron in multivitamins, ibuprofen and acetaminophen in children's analgesic preparations) or (2) "deadly in one dose" status, where exposure is likely to result in severe toxicity (tricyclic antidepressants, methanol, organophosphate pesticides).

ACETAMINOPHEN

Pathophysiology and clinical manifestations

The primary target organ of acetaminophen—also known as *N*-acetyl-*p*-aminophenol (APAP)—toxicity is the liver. Hepatotoxicity may occur from either an acute overdose or chronic supratherapeutic administration. At recommended doses, more than 90% of acetaminophen is metabolized in the liver to glucoronide and sulfate conjugates. Approximately 2% to 5% of APAP is eliminated unchanged in the urine, while 5% is metabolized by the cytochrome p450 subsystem to *N*-acetyl-para-benzoquinoneimine (NAPQI), which is rapidly bound by body stores of glutathione and detoxified. When acetaminophen is ingested in toxic amounts, glucoronide and sulfation conjugation systems become overwhelmed, shifting the route of metabolism to the p450 system. As larger amounts of NAPQI are formed, the glutathione stores used to detoxify this metabolite become depleted. Once glutathione stores drop to less than 30% of normal (typically within 8 hours post ingestion of a toxic dose), free NAPQI begins to directly bind to critical cellular structures within hepatocytes, and cellular injury and death occur.

The clinical course of acetaminophen overdose is characterized by a delayed onset and slow progression over several days. Initial symptoms may be nonspecific and include nausea, vomiting, malaise, and sweating. Within 24 to 36 hours post ingestion, elevations of the hepatic enzymes aspartate aminotransferase (AST) and alanine aminotransferase (ALT) begin to occur. Peak hepatotoxicity develops between 72 and 96 hours post ingestion, possibly accompanied by signs of fulminant hepatic failure, renal failure, coma, encephalopathy, and coagulopathy. At this point patients may begin to recover, require a liver transplant, or die. In the majority of cases, if recovery occurs, it is complete within 5 to 7 days.

Toxic dose and disposition

Following an acute APAP overdose, patients should be referred to the emergency department if the ingested amount is greater than or equal to 200 mg/kg in pediatric patients younger than 6 years of age, or 200 mg/kg or 10 gm (whichever is less) in adults. AAPCC evidence-based clinical guidelines for chronic or supratherapeutic ingestions state that patients should be referred for emergent evaluation if pediatric patients younger than 6 years of age ingest the following doses:

- More than 200 mg/kg in a 24-hour period
- More than 150 mg/kg per 24-hour period for the preceding 48 hours
- More than 100 mg/kg per 24-hour period for 72 hours or longer

Adults should be referred for emergent evaluation if they have a chronic or supratherapeutic ingestion of more than 10 gm or 200 mg/kg (whichever is less) per 24 hours, or more than 6 gm or 150 mg/kg (whichever is less) per 24-hour period for 48 hours or longer (Dart et al., 2006).

Management and antidote

The mainstay of therapy for APAP poisoning is the antidote *N*-acetylcysteine (NAC). In the United States, both an intravenous preparation (Acetadote) and an oral preparation (Mucomyst) are available. The latter is a sterile product originally indicated for nebulization as a mucolytic agent. NAC is the most frequently prescribed poison antidote, according to NPDS.

The mechanism by which NAC counteracts APAP overdose is complex but can be summarized as follows. First, NAC acts as a glutathione substitute in the detoxification of NAPQI. Second, some NAC is converted to glutathione. Third, NAC demonstrates hepatoprotective properties by acting as an antioxidant and free-radical scavenger, thereby improving blood microcirculation.

Two broad indications for use of NAC are presentation with a known or suspected toxic blood level of APAP and evidence of hepatotoxicity. To determine if an APAP blood level requires NAC therapy, a blood level versus time graph (Rumack-Matthew nomogram) is employed. This nomogram, which is included in the NAC product package insert, is also available on online databases and pocket references. It depicts two downward-sloping lines beginning at 4 hours post ingestion: The upper line represents probable toxicity, while the lower line depicts possible hepatotoxicity. In the United States, any APAP blood level plotted above the lower treatment line is an indication for NAC therapy.

NAC therapy is most effective when initiated within 8 hours post ingestion, but is effective at any time after a significant overdose. Treatment need not be delayed in the absence of rapid blood APAP quantification. NAC should be initiated in any pediatric patient demonstrating abnormal liver function tests thought to be caused by APAP toxicity, even if APAP is not detected in the blood.

The Rumack-Matthew nomogram applies only to single acute ingestions, so it is not applicable to instances of chronic supratherapeutic use. In these situations, NAC should be initiated immediately if any APAP is detectable on assay or if elevation of hepatic transaminases is seen.

The U.S. Food and Drug Administration (FDA) has approved two NAC treatment regimens: a 72-hour oral course and a 21-hour IV course. Various studies also have demonstrated the efficacy and safety of shorter oral courses (24 to 36 hours), and individual regional poison control centers have developed guidelines utilizing these strategies. The IV route is preferred in situations where the patient is unable or unwilling to take NAC orally, or in cases where GI bleeding or obstruction is suspected, APAP toxicity presents as encephalopathy, neonatal APAP toxicity from a maternal overdose occurs, or the patient is undergoing decontamination with multidose activated charcoal or whole-bowel irrigation.

Oral NAC is generally considered safe and produces only minor gastrointestinal disturbances during therapy, such as vomiting or diarrhea. Intravenous NAC, by comparison, carries a greater risk of hypersensitivity reactions such as pruritis and urticaria, which have an incidence of 4% to 7% in pediatric patients (Acetadote, 2009). Because the NAC solution has an unpleasant sulfur or "rotten egg" taste and odor, some tips on administration include making sure that NAC is diluted to a concentration of 5%, mixing NAC with any soft drink or juice that the patient would prefer, serving it over ice, and serving it in a covered container. Any oral dose vomited within 1 hour of administration should be repeated.

Criteria for liver transplantation in the setting of APAP have been developed by King's College. They include acidosis, defined as arterial pH of less than 7.3 after adequate fluid resuscitation; coagulopathy, defined as a PT greater than 40 seconds at 40 hours, PT greater than 100 seconds at any time, or rapidly rising PT or INR greater than 6.5; creatinine greater than 3.3 mg/dL; or grade III or IV hepatic encephalopathy. In these patients, IV NAC is administered continually at the rate of 100 mg/kg for 16 hours until the patient improves, undergoes transplant surgery, or fails to survive.

ALCOHOLS: ETHANOL

Pathophysiology and clinical manifestations

Ethyl alcohol (ethanol) is a type of alcohol found in alcoholic beverages and a myriad of household items, including mouthwashes, colognes and aftershaves, hairsprays, some rubbing alcohols, and hand sanitizers. Some of these products, which are not intended for human consumption, include special denatured alcohol (SD alcohol); this type of alcohol contains additives that render the products unpalatable, thereby limiting the potential for ingestion of a large quantity. The major toxicity of ethanol is nonspecific central nervous system (CNS) depression. Clinical manifestations in intoxicated individuals include initial stimulation and loss of inhibitions followed by lethargy, slurred speech, ataxia, stupor, and coma. Pediatric patients may experience facial flushing, vomiting, sweaty skin, respiratory depression, seizures, hypotension, hypothermia, and hypoglycemia.

Ethanol is metabolized primarily in the liver, where alcohol dehydrogenase converts ethanol to acetaldehyde, which is then further degraded by aldehyde dehydrogenase to acetate. Alcohol-naive individuals such as children may metabolize ethanol at a rate of 10 to 25 mg/dL/hr, whereas chronic alcoholics may achieve an elimination rate of 30 mg/dL/hr or more. Profound hypoglycemia, due to impaired hepatic gluconeogenesis that does not correlate with blood alcohol levels, is a greater risk in the pediatric patient. The appearance of this hypoglycemia may be delayed for as long as 6 hours after ingestion.

Toxic dose and disposition

Any symptomatic pediatric patient should be referred to the emergency department for evaluation. Alternatively, a child with an estimated ingestion of more than 0.5 mL/kg of 100% ethanol, which approximates a blood alcohol level of 50 to 75 mg/dL, may be referred to a health care facility. Although there is wide variability in the patient response to alcohol, it has been estimated that the potentially lethal dose of ethanol in a pediatric patient is 3.8 mL/kg of 100% ethanol (Klasco, 2009).

Management and antidote

Regional poison control centers manage many pediatric exposures to "mouthful" or "taste" ingestions of ethanol with home observation and telephone follow-up. In cases of more serious ethanol ingestion, no gastrointestinal decontamination is warranted unless coingestants are suspected. Conservative observation, respiratory and cardiovascular support, and blood sugar and electrolyte monitoring are all that is necessary for patients who present to the emergency department. Hypoglycemia should be corrected with appropriate administration of intravenous dextrose with the addition of oral caloric intake in an awake and alert patient. Hemodialysis is indicated rarely in patients with very high blood alcohol levels who do not respond to standard supportive measures. Hospital admission is advised for any pediatric patient demonstrating significant toxicity, such as marked CNS depression, hypoglycemia, seizures, or fluid/electrolyte abnormalities.

ALCOHOLS: ETHYLENE GLYCOL

Pathophysiology and clinical manifestations

Ethylene glycol is a solvent that is a primary component of automobile radiator antifreeze. This chemical poses a particular hazard to children, as it often has an attractive color and sweet taste. Ethylene glycol is metabolized via the same enzymatic pathway as ethanol; however, its end products are more toxic than the parent compound. These metabolites (oxalic acid, glycolic acid) are responsible for the major toxicities of ethylene glycol: delayed wide anion gap metabolic acidosis, renal tubular injury, and hypocalcemia. Characteristically, patients who ingest large amounts of ethylene glycol will exhibit initial ethanol-like symptoms of inebriation and lethargy, followed 6 to 12 hours later by tachypnea, coma, pulmonary edema, acidosis, and renal failure. Laboratory evidence that may raise the level

of suspicion for ingestion of a toxic alcohol such as ethylene glycol or methanol includes the presence of a wide osmolal gap, wide anion gap, low serum calcium, and calcium oxalate crystals in the urinalysis. The osmolal gap may be calculated using the equation of measured osmolality minus calculated osmolality, where the calculated osmolality is determined by the following equation:

$$\text{Serum Na (mEq/L)} \times 2 + \text{BUN (mg/dL)}/2.8$$
$$+ \text{glucose (mg/dL)}/18 + \text{ethanol (mg/dL)}/4.6$$

The normal osmolal gap ranges from −14 to +10. An osmolal gap greater than 10 should raise the HCP's suspicion that a toxic alcohol such as ethylene glycol, methanol, or isopropyl alcohol may have been ingested.

Regular antifreeze also often contains a fluorescent dye. Thus a Woods lamp may be used on the vomitus or urine of the patient, with evidence of fluorescence raising the suspicion of ethylene glycol poisoning.

Toxic dose and disposition

Children should be referred for emergent evaluation for anything other than witnessed taste or lick ingestion of concentrated (more than 20%) ethylene glycol solutions. Admit any patient who is symptomatic or requires antidotal therapy. The estimated fatal dose of ethylene glycol is 1.4 mL/kg.

Management and antidote

Two major approaches are used in the management of a patient with ethylene glycol poisoning: Inhibiting the enzyme alcohol dehydrogenase terminates the formation of the toxic metabolites of ethylene glycol, while hemodialysis enhances total body clearance of ethylene glycol and its toxic metabolites.

Inhibition of alcohol dehydrogenase is accomplished by either IV administration of fomepizol, also known as 4-methylpyrizol (4-MP), or by oral or IV administration of ethanol. This therapy has several inherent disadvantages, including the need for frequent blood alcohol determinations, wide swings in blood alcohol concentrations, hyponatremia, hypoglycemia, fluid overload, and vein irritation. Commercial preparations of injectable alcohol solutions are no longer available. The therapeutic blood alcohol level is in the range of 100 to 130 mg %. Fomepizol has the advantage of providing 12 hours of alcohol dehydrogenase inhibition with a single dose; it also produces minimal adverse reactions, such as headache, dizziness, and nausea. Indications for administration of 4-MP or alcohol include blood ethylene glycol levels of 20 mg/dL or greater, and suspicion of toxicity based on wide osmolal gap or wide anion gap acidosis.

Hemodialysis is indicated for ethylene glycol levels of 50 mg/dL or greater, and for symptomatic patients with refractory acidosis, pulmonary edema, or renal failure. Because hemodialysis also removes fomepizol and ethanol, adjustments in their dosing must be made during dialysis. Consult a regional poison control center for guidance in this situation.

ALCOHOLS: ISOPROPYL

Pathophysiology and clinical manifestations

Isopropanol, also known as isopropyl alcohol (IPA), is commonly found in rubbing alcohol, dermal astringent and other topical products, and deicing solutions. It is metabolized by alcohol dehydrogenase to form acetone. The clinical manifestations of isopropyl poisoning are similar to those of ethanol poisoning; however, isopropyl's effects are more potent. These effects include CNS depression, gastritis, hypotension, and respiratory depression accompanied by a non-acidotic ketosis. A wide osmolal gap and ketonuria may be present. Similar to ethanol, IPA may cause hypoglycemia when ingested, particularly in pediatric patients. Toxicity has been known to occur following dermal applications of rubbing alcohol as a method of reducing fever in pediatric patients; as a consequence, this practice is discouraged (Klasco, 2009).

Toxic dose and disposition

The estimated toxic dose of IPA is in the range of 0.5 to 1 mL/kg of 70% rubbing alcohol. Due to its unpalatability, pediatric patients who merely taste rubbing alcohol may be observed at home, with telephone follow-up to ensure there are no symptoms from the ingestion. Ingestions of more than a mouthful and symptomatic patients require referral to an emergency department for evaluation. Admit any patient with persistent symptoms for monitoring.

Management and antidote

Management of IPA intoxication consists of supportive care, such as ventilatory support, fluids and vasopressors for hypotension, and blood glucose monitoring. No specific antidote (e.g., fomepizol or ethanol) is indicated. Although hemodialysis removes IPA and acetone, this procedure is generally reserved for seriously poisoned patients who develop coma with hypotension or very high IPA blood levels exceeding 500 mg/dL.

ALCOHOLS: METHANOL

Pathophysiology and clinical manifestations

Methanol, also known as methyl alcohol, is commonly found in automobile gas-line antifreeze, windshield washer solvent, paint strippers, and sterno liquid fuel. Similar to ethanol and ethylene glycol, it is metabolized by alcohol dehydrogenase and aldehyde dehydrogenase to form formaldehyde and formic acid, respectively. These end products are more toxic than the parent compound and are responsible for methanol's major toxicities: wide anion gap metabolic acidosis and optic nerve injury that may result in blindness. Symptoms begin with an ethanol-like intoxication, which is followed hours later by headache, nausea, vomiting, blurred or "snowfield" vision, hypokalemia, tachypnea, acidosis, and death. An early, widened osmolal gap may be noted.

Toxic dose and disposition

Because the estimated toxic dose of 100% methanol is very low (0.25 mL/kg or one-half teaspoonful [2.5 mL] in a 10-kg child), all patients with a known or suspected ingestion of this alcohol should be referred to the emergency department for evaluation. The fatal dose is estimated to be approximately 0.5 mL/kg of 100% methanol (Klasco, 2009).

Management and antidote

Management of methanol intoxication parallels that of ethylene glycol. Fomepizol or ethanol is indicated in any patient with known or suspected methanol poisoning as demonstrated by a blood level of 20 mg/dL or greater, or a wide osmolal gap with or without a wide anion gap metabolic acidosis. Hemodialysis is indicated for blood levels of 50 mg/dL or greater or any symptomatic patient (Klasco, 2009).

IRON

Pathophysiology and clinical manifestations

Iron supplements are available in a variety of adult and pediatric preparations, including women's prenatal vitamin/mineral preparations, high-potency hematinics, and pediatric chewable tablets and liquids. The toxicity in iron poisoning is due to the effects of elemental iron, the concentration of which varies according to the salt form. For example, ferrous sulfate is 20% elemental iron, whereas ferrous fumarate is 33% elemental iron. Thus a ferrous sulfate 325-mg tablet contains 65 mg of elemental iron, while a ferrous fumarate 200-mg tablet contains 66 mg of elemental iron. The toxicity of iron is mediated by the corrosive effect of ferrous (2+) iron on the gastrointestinal tract and multiorgan cellular injury.

Early signs and symptoms of iron toxicity, occurring within 4 to 6 hours of ingestion, include nausea, vomiting, and diarrhea (which may be bloody). They may be followed by a period of apparent improvement or stability; later, however, patients may progress to more serious complications, including metabolic acidosis, coma, hypotension, shock, hepatic failure, coagulopathy, seizures, and death. Hyperglycemia and leukocytosis may be observed. Late complications may include bowel obstruction or stricture.

Toxic dose and disposition

It is important to differentiate among the various types of iron formulations ingested. AAPCC evidence-based clinical guidelines recommend referral to the emergency department for ingestions greater than 40 mg/kg of elemental iron in the form of adult ferrous salt formulations. Toxicity is likely at greater than 60 mg/kg doses. Patients who ingest children's chewable multivitamins containing iron, carbonyl iron formulations, or polysaccharide iron complexes may be observed at home, regardless of the amount ingested (Manoguerraet al., 2005b)

Management and antidote

Orogastric lavage may be considered in life-threatening iron ingestions if it can be performed within one hour; however, iron-containing tablets may be large and form concretions, making passage through the lavage tube difficult. Activated charcoal does not adsorb iron and should not be administered for this indication. Iron tablets are radiopaque and may be visualized with abdominal radiography. If discrete tablets are seen, whole-bowel irrigation may be considered. Supportive measures such as crystalloid fluids and vasopressors for hypotension, intravenous sodium bicarbonate for metabolic acidosis, and benzodiazipines for seizures should be instituted.

Deferoxamine methylate (DFO) is a specific antidote for iron poisoning. DFO acts as a chelating agent, which binds to free iron and forms ferrioxamine, a water-soluble complex that is excreted by the kidneys. This complex may impart a "vin rose" or reddish brown color to the urine. DFO, which is delivered, at a maximum dose, as a 15 mg/kg/hr IV infusion, is indicated for patients with severe iron intoxication, shock, severe acidosis, or serum iron levels greater than 500 µg/dL. The endpoint of therapy is resolution of symptoms. Complications associated with prolonged DFO therapy include acute respiratory distress syndrome (ARDS) and *Yersinia* sepsis.

OPIOIDS

Pathophysiology and clinical manifestations

Opioids are a class of natural and synthetic compounds that were originally derived from the opium poppy, *Papaver somniferum*. These agents are primarily used as antitussives, analgesics, antidiarrheals, and anesthetics. Examples of opioids include naturally derived opiates such as morphine and codeine; semisynthetic agents such as heroin, hydrocodone, and oxycodone; and synthetic agents such as methadone, propoxyphene, and fentanyl.

Opioids' mechanism of action is via stimulation of receptor sites innervated by naturally occurring endorphins. Symptoms of mild intoxication of opioids include euphoria, sedation, miosis, reduced gastrointestinal motility, and a histamine-release mediated skin flush and bronchospasm; some of these effects are responsible for these drugs' potential for addiction. More serious or potentially life-threatening overdoses are evidenced by coma, respiratory depression, bradycardia, hypotension, and possibly acute lung injury (pulmonary edema). Some opioids display unique toxicities. For instance, propoxyphene may produce cardiac conduction disturbances resulting from its quinidine-like fast sodium-channel blockade. Propoxyphene and tramadol may precipitate seizures when taken in overdose amounts. Mepiridine may cause anticholinergic toxicity, and its metabolite normepiridine may cause seizures. Methadone, as a consequence of its long half-life, may cause prolonged symptoms (coma) of 24 hours or more in pediatric patients.

Withdrawal syndrome following opioid addiction is generally uncomfortable and non-life-threatening. Symptoms may include drug craving, nausea, vomiting, diarrhea, diaphoresis, anxiety, myalgia, and mild increase in pulse and blood pressure. Neonates born to opioid-dependent mothers, in contrast, may demonstrate more serious withdrawal symptoms including fever, myoclonus, and seizures.

Toxic dose and disposition

The extent of toxicity seen in a pediatric patient will necessarily depend on the specific opioid taken, the route of administration, the dose, and the existence of any previous tolerance to that agent. In cases where caregivers call poison control centers and give accurate histories of opioid-naive pediatric ingestions of codeine of 2 mg/kg or less, patients may be observed at home, with telephone follow-up, for mild symptoms. Ingestions exceeding this threshold dose should be promptly referred to the nearest emergency department.

Respiratory arrest in a pediatric patient may result from an ingestion of 5 mg/kg of codeine. Toxicity of propxyphene hydrochloride may occur with a dose as small as 10 mg/kg, and may be potentially fatal at a dose greater than 20 mg/kg. Doses of methadone as low as 10 mg have been lethal in pediatric patients. Ingestions of new or used fentanyl patches may also be potentially lethal, as even used patches contain a significant amount of drug in the patch matrix. Ingestion of as few as 6 tablets of diphenoxalate 2.5 mg/atropine 0.025mg (Lomotil) may result in coma and respiratory depression (Klasco, 2009).

Management and antidote

An opioid overdose should be suspected whenever a patient presents with the following triad of symptoms: CNS depression, respiratory depression, and miosis. Monitor the patient's vital signs carefully. Frequent assessments of oxygen saturation, arterial blood gases, and chest radiographs (for developing pulmonary edema) are recommended. Rapid qualitative toxicology screening tests typically will be positive for opiates such as heroin, morphine, and codeine; however, they may not detect semisynthetic or synthetic opioids such as oxycodone, fentanyl, or methadone.

A pure opioid antagonist such as naloxone (Narcan), given in sufficient doses, may reverse nearly all neurologic and respiratory symptoms of opioid overdose, thereby avoiding the need for endotracheal intubation and mechanical ventilation. This agent is readily accessible in emergency departments, anesthesia suites, and emergency medical service vehicles. Naloxone may be administered intravenously, intramuscularly, subcutaneously, intranasally, intralingually, endotracheally, or even nebulized. Due to its extensive first-pass metabolism in the liver, naloxone is not bioavailable orally.

Initial intravenous naloxone doses are 0.4 to 2 mg in children and adults. If no response is observed, doses may be repeated every 1 to 2 minutes. If a total dose of 10 mg has been given without noticeable response, the diagnosis of opioid toxicity should be questioned. Smaller incremental doses, approximately 0.1 to 0.2 mg, should be administered to chronically habituated or opioid-dependent patients to lessen the potential for an acute withdrawal response. In the youngest patients (neonates at birth to age 5 years), an intravenous dose of 0.1 mg/kg (in patients weighing less than 20 kg) is recommended. It is important to note that the duration of effect of naloxone is approximately 20 to 60 minutes, which may be much shorter than the duration of the opioid; thus close monitoring is required, and frequent redosing may be necessary as symptoms recur. Alternatively, an infusion of naloxone in 5% dextrose or normal saline may be started at a rate of two-thirds of the initial reversal dose per hour. Caution should be exercised when discontinuing the naloxone infusion. Patients should remain symptom free for 4 hours before discharge.

Another option that may be considered in opioid-naive patients is administration of a longer-acting opioid antagonist such as nalmefene. Doses of 0.5 to 2 mg may provide reversal of the opioid effects for as long as 8 hours. These products should be avoided in opioid-dependent patients, however, as prolonged withdrawal syndromes may be experienced. Close observation is warranted when using this agent, particularly when patients were exposed to long-acting agents such as methadone.

Seizures associated with opioid overdose (e.g., propoxyphene) should be treated with a benzodiazepine, followed by a barbiturate to treat refractory seizures. Propoxyphene-induced cardiac conduction disturbances, as evidenced by a widened QRS interval, may be treated with IV sodium bicarbonate, in a similar fashion to the treatment for tricyclic antidepressant overdose. Acute lung injury may require supportive care with mechanical ventilation and oxygenation as necessary. A variety of treatment modalities to manage opioid addiction in adolescents and adults exist using maintenance regimens of methadone, oral or transdermal clonodine, naltrexone, or buprenorphine/naloxone.

ORGANOPHOSPHATES

Pathophysiology and clinical manifestations

Organophosphate insecticides (OPI) are pesticides commonly used in and around the home, by professional pest control operators, and agriculturally. Some examples include chlorpyrifos, diazinone, malathion, and parathion. Nerve agents, such as sarin or soman, represent highly toxic organophosphates that are used in chemical warfare.

OPIs exert their toxicity by means of inhibition of acetylcholinesterase and plasma cholinesterase enzymes. This process results in a myriad of clinical manifestations, which can be grouped as muscarinic effects, nicotinic effects, and CNS effects. The muscarinic symptoms are characterized by a cholinergic syndrome that can be remembered by the acronym DUMBELS:

- **D**iarrhea, **D**iaphoresis
- **U**rination
- **M**iosis
- **B**radycardia, **B**ronchorrhea, **B**ronchospasm
- **E**mesis
- **L**acrimation
- **S**alivation

The nicotinic symptoms may be recalled by the "days of the week" (MTWTF):

- **M**ydriasis
- **T**achycardia
- **W**eakness
- hyper**T**ension
- **F**asciculations

Neurologic toxicity is evidenced by agitation, seizures, and coma. Seizures and CNS depression are reported to be more common in pediatric patients than in adults. It is important to note that pediatric patients may demonstrate different presenting clinical manifestations in comparison to adults. In one study, the predominating effects in children were CNS depression, stupor, flaccidity, dyspnea, and coma (Klasco, 2009).

Serious toxicity may result from all routes of exposure to OPIs: ingestion, dermal, or inhalation. Care must be exercised in managing pesticide exposures, because the labeled "inert ingredients" (e.g., hydrocarbon solvent) may also pose a toxicity hazard. All OPI-poisoned patients should be thoroughly decontaminated via removal of clothing and multiple soap-and-water washings. First responders and emergency department staff should wear chemical-protective clothing and gloves to avoid being exposed by these toxic agents.

Toxic dose and disposition

The potential severity of an OPI exposure depends on multiple factors, such as the inherent potency of the agent, the concentration of the active ingredient in the product, the route of exposure, and the duration of exposure. All patients suspected of significant OPI exposure should be referred to the emergency department for treatment. After patient recovery with judicious use of antidotes, patients should be monitored for several days for the delayed onset of an intermediate syndrome characterized by muscle weakness, respiratory paralysis, and cranial nerve palsies, which may persist for 1 to 2 weeks.

Management and antidote

Airway management and respiratory support are priority considerations in the treatment approach to the OPI-poisoned patient. Excessive bronchial secretions should be suctioned, while mechanical ventilation may be necessary in patients who develop respiratory paralysis. Hydrocarbon pneumonitis secondary to aspiration of hydrocarbon solvents should be evaluated by obtaining a chest radiograph.

Three pharmacological agents are employed as antidotal therapy in the setting of OPI poisoning. Atropine sulfate is an anticholinergic agent that reverses muscarinic and CNS symptoms, but not nicotinic effects. Doses of this agent much higher than those commonly used for other indications are necessary to achieve desired effects (Table 37-5). The endpoint of therapy is atropinization, which is demonstrated by dry mucous membranes and lungs clear of wheezes. Tachycardia is not a contraindication to atropine administration.

Pralidoxime chloride, also known as 2-PAM, is a cholinesterase regenerator that can improve muscarinic, CNS, and nicotinic signs and symptoms. It may be administered either in IV bolus doses or as a continuous infusion. 2-PAM should be administered as soon as possible to moderately to severely symptomatic patients before "aging" renders the cholinesterase–phosphate bond irreversible. Continue 2-PAM administration 24 hours after the patient is symptom free.

Parenteral administration of diazepam is indicated for OPI-induced seizure activity. Paralytics such as succinylcholine and mivacurium should not be used in OPI-poisoned patients because their duration of action will be markedly prolonged due to the impaired metabolic degradation by cholinesterase enzymes.

SALICYLATES

Pathophysiology and clinical manifestations

The salicylates encompass a variety of prescription and nonprescription agents, of which aspirin—also known as acetylsalicylic acid (ASA)—is the most widely recognized. Other examples include methyl salicylate (oil of wintergreen) and trolamine salicylate, which are found in muscle rubs; bismuth subsalicylate, which is found in gastrointestinal preparations; salicylic acid, which is found in acne preparations and corn, callous, and wart removers; and magnesium salicylate, which is found in backache and pain relief medications. Salicylates may be found either as single-ingredient products or in combination with other cold, flu, or analgesic remedies.

Salicylate toxicity may occur as a result of an acute overdose or chronic supratherapeutic administration. The mechanism by which salicylates exert their toxicity is complex and involves nearly all organ systems. Multiple metabolic derangements occur—most notably, a significant wide anion gap metabolic acidosis. Acidemia results from Krebs cycle inhibition, uncoupling of oxidative phosphorylation, and increased tissue glycolysis. A respiratory alkalosis, due to direct stimulation of the respiratory center, may precede the metabolic acidosis in adults, but does not always occur in children. A direct irritant effect of the gastrointestinal mucosa accounts for emesis, which may be bloody. Hypoglycemia, particularly in children, may occur due to increased cellular oxygen consumption and impaired gluconeogenesis. Hypokalemia results from increased renal excretion of potassium.

Following an acute salicylate poisoning, a patient may present with nausea, vomiting, hematemesis, gastric pain, tinnitus or impaired hearing, tachypnea, tachycardia, dehydration, and fever. Serious toxicity is evidenced by delirium, seizures, coma, metabolic acidosis, rhabdomyolysis, noncardiogenic pulmonary edema, increased cranial pressure, arrhythmias, and asystole.

Chronic salicylate toxicity may masquerade as other medical conditions and may be misdiagnosed as septicemia, dementia, or encephalopathy. Chronic administration of aspirin during viral illnesses in children has been associated with the development of Reye's syndrome. Symptoms of Reye's syndrome include vomiting, hypoglycemia, hepatic dysfunction, and encephalophy, and may mimic chronic salicylate intoxication.

TABLE 37-5

Selected Antidotes Used in Pediatric Poisoning

Antidote	Indication	Pediatric Dose	Comments
n-Acetylcysteine (NAC): 7-hour oral protocol	Acetaminophen	**PO:** 140 mg/kg then 70 mg/kg every 4 hrs × 17 doses	Unpleasant odor, nausea, and/or vomiting may occur. Shorter courses may be recommended by poison control centers.
n-Acetylcysteine (NAC): 21-hour IV protocol	Acetaminophen	**IV:** 150 mg/kg in 200 mL D_5W over 1 hr, then 50 mg/kg in 500 mL D_5W over 4 hrs, then 100 mg/kg in 1,000 mL D_5W over 16 hrs	Possible anaphylactoid reactions, including rash, urticaria, vasodilation, or hypotension.
Atropine sulfate	Drug-induced bradycardia; organophosphates and nerve agents	**Cardiotoxic drugs:** IV 0.02 mg/kg with a minimum of 0.1 mg **Organophosphates:** IV 0.05 mg/kg, doubling the dose every 5–10 min	Very large repeated doses may be needed in organophosphate poisoning. The endpoint is clearing of secretions. In these patients, tachycardia is not a contraindication for use.
Benzodiazepine	Agitation, seizures, drug-induced tachycardia	**Midazolam/diazepam:** IV/IM 0.1 mg/kg **Lorazepam:** IV/IM 0.04 mg/kg	Can cause CNS or respiratory depression.
Bicarbonate, sodium	Acidosis, serum alkalinization (for wide QRS), urinary alkalinization (aspirin)	**Serum alkalinization:** IV: 1–2 mEq/kg bolus **Urinary alkalinization:** 150 mEq with 20–40 mEq KCl in 1,000 mL D_5W run at twice maintenance to a goal of urine pH of 7.5–8	**Serum alkalinization:** Goal serum pH 7.45–7.55 **Urinary alkalinization:** Monitor potassium frequently
Deferoxamine mesylate	Iron	**IV:** Initial dosing 15 mg/kg/hr	Prolonged administration associated with ARDS and *Yersinia* sepsis. May cause hypotension.
Digoxin immune Fab	Digoxin	**Number of vials:** Digoxin level (ng/mL) × weight (kg)/100	May be useful for other cardiac glycosides. May cause hypocalcemia.
Ethanol	Methanol or ethylene glycol if fomepizole is not available	**IV:** 10% alcohol in D_5W; 10 mL/kg loading dose, then 12 mL/kg/hr maintenance dose **PO:** 40% solution; 2.5 mL/kg loading dose, then 0.3–0.5 mL/kg/hr maintenance dose mixed with juice	Warning: can produce hypoglycemia, hyponatremia, and CNS or respiratory depression. Goal is blood alcohol level of 100–130 mg %. Commercially prepared solutions are no longer available, so ethanol preparations must be compounded by the pharmacy.
Fomepizol (4-MP)	Methanol or ethylene glycol poisoning	**IV:** Loading dose 15 mg/kg, then 10 mg/kg every 12 hours × 4 doses, then 15 mg/kg every 12 hrs	Nausea, dizziness, and headache are possible. Dosage must be increased during dialysis; consult the poison control center.
Glucagon	Beta blockers, calcium-channel blockers	**IV:** 0.05–0.1 mg/kg bolus with a maximum of 5 mg; may be followed by an ongoing IV infusion of response dose over 1 hr	Improves bradycardia and hypotension via non-adrenergic pathway. May cause vomiting and hypokalemia.
Hydroxocobalamin	Cyanide, smoke inhalation	**IV:** 70 mg/kg (up to 5 gm) administered over 15 min to 2 hrs	May cause red discoloration of body fluids. Does not cause hypotension or methemoglobinemia, as does the nitrate/thiosulfate cyanide kit.

(Continued)

TABLE 37-5

Selected Antidotes Used in Pediatric Poisoning (*Continued*)			
Antidote	**Indication**	**Pediatric Dose**	**Comments**
Methylene Blue	Methemoglobinemia	**IV:** 1–2 mg/kg (0.1–0.2 mL/kg) as a 1% solution	Do not exceed 4 mg/kg. Avoid in G-6-PD deficient patients.
Naloxone hydrochloride	Opioids	**IV:** In patients younger than 5 years, give 0.1 mg/kg up to 2 mg, or empirically 0.4–2 mg; may repeat every 1–2 min up to 10 mg total	May precipitate withdrawal in habituated patients; duration of effect is less than 60 minutes; may consider infusion in D_5W or normal saline equal to two-thirds of the patient response dose per hour in long-acting opioid overdoses.
Octreotide acetate	Sulfonylureas	**SQ:** (preferred) 1.25 µg/kg (up to 50 µg) every 6 hr **IV:** (in D_5W or 0.9% NS over 15–30 min) same dosing, increase frequency to every 4 hrs	Rapidly and safely corrects hypoglycemia associated with sulfonylurea exposure.
Pralidoxime chloride (2-PAM)	Organophosphates, nerve agents	**IV bolus:** As a 5% solution in normal saline, 25–40 mg/kg up to 1 gm over 30 min **Infusion:** As a 5% solution in normal saline, 10–20 mg/kg/hr	The endpoint is resolution of symptoms. Administer as soon as possible and continue for 24 hours after the patient is symptom free. Side effects may include hypertension, tachycardia, nausea, and dizziness.
Pyridoxine hydrochloride	Isoniazid (INH)	**IV:** 70 mg/kg; if no response, repeat dose	Effectively corrects coma, acidosis, and seizures associated with INH overdose.

Note: Central nervous system (CNS), acute respiratory distress syndrome (ARDS), intravenous (IV), subcutaneous (SQ).

Toxic dose and disposition

AAPCC evidence-based clinical guidelines recommend referral to the emergency department for acute ingestions of salicylates at a dose exceeding 150 mg/kg or 6.5 gm of aspirin equivalent. Ingestions of 300 to 500 mg/kg or more are associated with serious toxicity. Chronic doses of more than 100 mg/kg per day for 2 days or more may also produce toxicity (Chyka et al., 2007).

Management and antidote

Because salicylate intoxication has the potential to create severe morbidity and mortality, it is important to consider multiple approaches to treatment, such as thorough gastrointestinal decontamination, correction of fluid/electrolyte and acid–base imbalances, and enhancement of elimination. Large ingestions of salicylates—especially those with enteric coatings—may cause slowly dissolving concretions or "bezoars"; thus multiple doses of activated charcoal without a cathartic are indicated to counteract them. Salicylate blood levels should be obtained every 2 hours until a peak is determined, with blood levels than being obtained every 4 hours thereafter.

Salicylate-intoxicated patients are often dehydrated and require intravenous fluid hydration. Wide anion gap metabolic acidosis should be corrected with administration of IV sodium bicarbonate at 1 to 2 mEq/kg per dose. Correct hypoglycemia with administration of IV dextrose. Seizures should be managed with IV benzodiazepines. Obtain a chest radiograph and monitor for noncardiogenic pulmonary edema. If the patient requires mechanical ventilation, it is critical to ensure the patient is hyperventilated to maintain a high arterial pH, thereby preventing salicylates, which are weakly acidic, from crossing the blood–brain barrier.

Because weakly acidic salicylates become more ionized as the urine pH rises, enhanced urinary excretion of salicylates may be achieved via alkalinization of the urine to a target pH of 7.5 to 8. This concept, which is known as "ion trapping," may be accomplished by IV administration of a solution of 5% dextrose in water with 150 mEq of sodium bicarbonate and 20 to 40 mEq of potassium chloride at a rate that is twice the maintenance level; the goal for urine production of 1 to 2 mL/kg/hr. Additional potassium supplementation may be required to maintain a serum potassium of 4 mEq/L, as urine alkalinization is difficult to achieve in the presence of hypokalemia. Obtain arterial blood gases, electrolytes, and urine pH frequently (every 4 to 6 hours), using the results to guide therapy. Urine alkalinization may be terminated when salicylate levels fall below 30 mg/dL.

Emergent hemodialysis may be necessary to enhance elimination of high salicylate blood levels and correct fluid/electrolyte and acid–base abnormalities. Indications for hemodialysis include salicylate levels approaching 100 mg/dL in acute ingestions or 40 to 60 mg/dL in chronic supratherapeutic ingestions, pulmonary edema, renal failure, congestive heart failure or cardiovascular instability, seizures, altered mental status, intractable acidosis, or electrolyte abnormalities.

TRICYCLIC ANTIDEPRESSANTS

Pathophysiology and clinical manifestations

Tricyclic antidepressants (TCAs) are a group of medications named for the triple cyclic ring structure common to all agents in the class. Examples include amitriptyline, clomipramine, desipramine, doxepin, imipramine, and nortriptylene. The pharmacology of TCAs is multifactorial and complex, but can be summarized by emphasizing a few key points.

First, TCAs are potent CNS and respiratory depressants. Rapid coma and respiratory failure may occur following large overdose.

Second, TCAs have extensive anticholinergic activity. This effect can manifest as dry mucous membranes, mydriasis, tachycardia, agitation, delirium, hyperthermia, and decreased gastrointestinal motility.

Third, TCAs possess alpha-adrenergic blockade properties. These characteristics account for their profound hypotensive effect in overdose.

Finally, due to blockade of sodium channels in the myocardium, TCAs may produce marked cardiac conduction abnormalities, which are most notably demonstrated by a widened QRS complex and prolongation of the QT interval on the electrocardiogram (ECG). Life-threatening dysrhythmias including ventricular tachycardia or fibrillation and cardiac arrest are possible. Seizures are also frequently seen, although their cause appears to be multifactorial and is not completely understood.

Toxic dose and disposition

Evidence-based guidelines developed by the AAPCC indicate that ingestion of amounts greater than 5 mg/kg for all TCAs except desipramine, nortriptylene, trimipramine, and protriptylene necessitate referral to an emergency department. Pediatric patients who ingest more than 2.5 mg/kg of desipramine, nortriptylene, or trimipramine, or more than 1 mg/kg of protriptylene, should be referred for evaluation. TCA ingestions in the range of 10 to 20 mg/kg in pediatric patients pose a serious risk of neurologic and cardiovascular toxicity. Admission to a pediatric intensive care unit is advised for any patient demonstrating altered mental status

or cardiovascular toxicity until symptoms have resolved (Woolf et al., 2007).

Management and antidote

Management of TCA overdose consists of appropriate GI decontamination and supportive measures. Patients experiencing rapid obtundation, loss of protective airway reflexes, or coma require rapid endotracheal intubation and ventilatory support. Seizures may be managed through the administration of benzodiazipines (lorazepam) and barbiturates for refractory seizures.

Cardiac conduction defects evidenced by a widened QRS complex of more than 110 to 120 milliseconds may respond to administration of sodium bicarbonate and serum alkalinization. Thus IV sodium bicarbonate at 1 to 2 mEq/kg/dose and hyperventilation in intubated patients with a goal of achieving an arterial pH of 7.45 to 7.55 may correct many of the wide complex tachydysrhythmias associated with TCA overdose. Hypotension may be managed through the administration of IV bolus doses of sodium bicarbonate, crystalloid fluids, and administration of vasopressive agents.

Agents with primarily direct alpha-adrenergic activity (norepinephrine) may offer a theoretical advantage over indirect-acting agents such as dopamine in treatment of TCA overdose. Several important contraindicated therapies should be noted. Although physostigmine salicylate is a short-acting cholinesterase inhibitor used in the management of anticholinergic poisonings, it has been associated with seizures, asystole, and death in the setting of TCA overdose. Consequently, it should never be used in this setting. Class 1-A and 1-C antidysrhythmics (e.g., quinidine, procainamide, disopyramide, flecanide) may worsen cardiac conduction and should be avoided. Although beta blockers (propranolol) may correct tachycardia, their use has been linked to severe hypotension and cardiac arrest and should also be avoided.

REFERENCES

1. Acetadote. (2009). Injection package insert. Retrieved from http://acetadote.com/AcetadotePI_rDec08.pdf
2. American Academy of Clinical Toxicology & European Association of Poisons Centres and Clinical Toxicologists. (2004). Position paper: Gastric lavage. *Clinical Toxicology, 42*, 933–943.
3. American Academy of Pediatrics (AAP). (2003). Ipecac. Retrieved from www.aap.org
4. Bronstein, A., Spyker, D. A., Cantilena, L. R., Jr., Green, J. L., Rumack, B. H, Heard, S. E., et al. (2008). 2007 annual report of the American Association of Poison Control Centers' National Poison Data System (NPDS): 25th annual report. *Clinical Toxicology, 46*(10), 927–1057.
5. Bronstein, A., Spyker, D., Cantilena, J., Louis, R., Green, J., Rumack, B., et al. (2009). 2008 annual report of the American Association of Poison

Control Centers' National Poison Data System (NPDS): 26th annual report. *Clinical Toxicology, 47,* 911–1084.

6. Chyka, P., Erdman, A. R., Christianson, G., Wax, P., Booze, L., Manoguerra, A., et al. (2007). Salicylate poisoning: An evidence based consensus guideline for out of hospital management. *Clinical Toxicology, 45,* 95–131.

7. Dart, R., Erdman, A., Olson, K., Christianson, G., Manoguerra, A., Chyka, P., et al. (2006). Acetaminophen poisoning: An evidence based consensus guideline for out of hospital management. *Clinical Toxicology, 44,* 1–18.

8. Klasco, R. K. (Ed.). (2009, December). *POISINDEX system.* Greenwood Village, CO: Thomson Reuters.

9. Manoguerra, A., Cobaugh, D., & Members of the Guidelines for the Management of Poisonings Consensus Panel. (2005a). Guideline on the use of ipecac syrup in the out of hospital management of ingested poisons. *Clinical Toxicology, 1,* 1–10.

10. Manoguerra, A., Erdman, A., Booze, L., Christianson, G., Wax, P., Scharman, E., et al. (2005b). Iron ingestion: An evidence based consensus guideline for out of hospital management. *Clinical Toxicology, 43,* 553–570.

11. Woolf, A., Erdman, A., Nelson, L., Caravati, E., Cobaugh, D., Booze, L., et al. (2007). Tricyclic antidepressant poisoning: An evidence based consensus guideline for out of hospital management. *Clinical Toxicology, 45,* 203–233.

Traumatic Injuries

EPIDEMIOLOGY

Ruth Bush and Kathleen Corcoran

STATISTICS

Childhood injury statistics are generally reported as intentional or unintentional. Intentional injuries include homicide, suicide, and assault. Unintentional injuries are those caused by road traffic/transportation, fall, fire or burn, drowning, suffocation, and poison. An estimated 9.2 million children (ages 0 to 19 years) visit an emergency department (ED) annually for an unintentional injury (Borse et al., 2008). This number suggests that 25% of individuals younger than the age of 19 years sustain an unintentional injury that requires medical care (American Academy of Pediatrics [AAP] et al., 2008). Children in families with lower socioeconomic status, low maternal education, young maternal age, or caregiver substance abuse; who grow up in a single-parent household; or who are part of a large family with several children are at highest risk for injury (Fallat et al., 2006).

The specialized diagnostic studies and therapeutic management necessary to care for physical wounds, such as those caused by force or the impact of a fall or motor vehicle collision (MVC), distinguishes a traumatic injury from the general care received in a hospital ED (Institute of Medicine [IOM], 2007). The study of pediatric trauma incorporates considerations for a pediatric patient's skeletal size, smaller body surface area, physiologic and immunologic immaturity,

and developmental status in its training and treatment approach (Gausche-Hill, 2009). Unintentional injury, much of which overlaps with the definition of trauma, is the leading cause of morbidity and mortality among children in the United States and is an indication not only of pediatric trauma's substantial, daily impact on the U.S. health care system, but also the far-reaching, long-term economic and societal implications (Borse et al., 2008).

The American College of Surgeons (ACS) uses a two-part criterion to define trauma for data capture. First, a trauma injury must meet the criteria for at least one International Classification of Diseases, Ninth Revision, Clinical Modification (ICD-9-CM) diagnostic code from the injury range 800 to 959.9, excluding the codes for the late effects of injury; superficial injuries (blisters, contusions, abrasions, insect bites); and injuries that result from foreign bodies. Second, a trauma patient must have been admitted to the hospital, transferred via emergency medical services (EMS) from one hospital to another, or died as the result of a traumatic injury independent of hospital admission or hospital transfer status (ACS, 2008). Thus pediatric trauma rates differ from childhood injury rates in that they usually do not include drowning, suffocation, or poisoning incidents, all which are outside of the ICD-9-CM injury code range.

Compared with adults, any given force is more widely distributed through the child's body, making multiple injuries significantly more likely to occur. Injuries patterns range by age (Figure 38-1), and children of all ages are subject to the sequelae of child maltreatment. Of significant injuries, head trauma—that is, traumatic brain injury (TBI)—is the

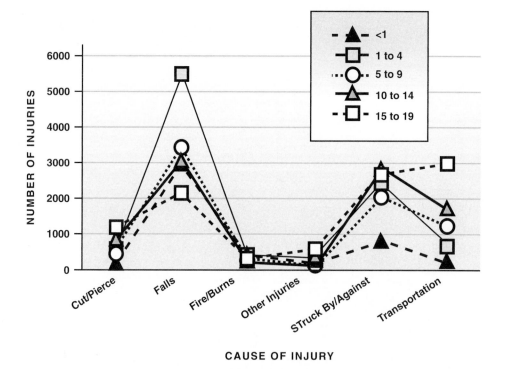

FIGURE 38-1

Nonfatal Unintentional Injury Rates Among Children 0–19 Years of Age.

Source: CDC Childhood Injury Report: Patterns of Unintentional Injuries among 0 -19 Year Olds in the United States, 2000–2006.

most common, followed by thoracic and abdominal injuries. The latter are a common cause of unrecognized fatal injury in children. Blunt trauma related to MVC causes more than 50% of the abdominal injuries and is the most lethal. Lap belt injury, including small bowel injury and Chance fracture, occurs in approximately 5% to 10% of restrained children in MVCs. Bicycle handlebar- and sports-related injuries may also result in abdominal trauma (Avarello & Cantor, 2007).

Falls are the leading cause of nonfatal injury among children younger than 9 years of age, resulting in almost 3 million initial ED visits. The incidence of falls is particularly high among young children, accounting for more than one-half of all ED visits made by members of this age group. In a related and overlapping mechanism of injury, more than 200,000 children ages 14 years and younger are treated in EDs annually for injuries resulting from playground-related activities. After falls, being struck by or against an object, cuts/piercing, and bicycle crashes are predominant injuries within the age 5–14 years group. Animal bites and insect stings, which are unlikely to meet trauma criteria, are also frequently noted in this population. Burns are of particular concern among young males. U.S. EDs treat an average of 121,000 pediatric burn patients per year, with children younger than 6 years old (58%) and males (59%)

being disproportionately represented. Traumatic brain injuries result in an estimated 475,000 hospital visits, 37,000 hospitalizations, and nearly 3,000 deaths each year among children aged 0 to 14 years (Figure 38-2) (Borse et al., 2008; Centers for Disease Control and Prevention [CDC], n.d., a, c, d; D'Souza et al., in press; Langlois et al., 2006; National Center for Injury Prevention and Control [NCIPC], n.d.).

Child maltreatment is an interrelated aspect of pediatric trauma that is defined as any act or series of acts of commission or omission by a parent or caregiver that results in harm, potential for harm, or threat of harm to a child. Suspicion for child maltreatment should be high when treating children with injuries.

Generally, the mortality rate for children seen in the ED after injury is low—approximately 1%. Most pediatric fatalities occur in the field before the patient's arrival at a health care facility. The pattern of pediatric trauma-related deaths is roughly "U" shaped, with the very young (beginning around 1 year of age, when a child begins to walk) and adolescents more likely to die from their injuries (Figure 38-3). Overall, the most common mechanism of traumatic death is transportation related (28%). The most common single-organ system injury is head trauma or TBI, although the mechanism and accident locations vary by age (Figure 38-4) (ACS, 2008; Avarello & Cantor, 2007).

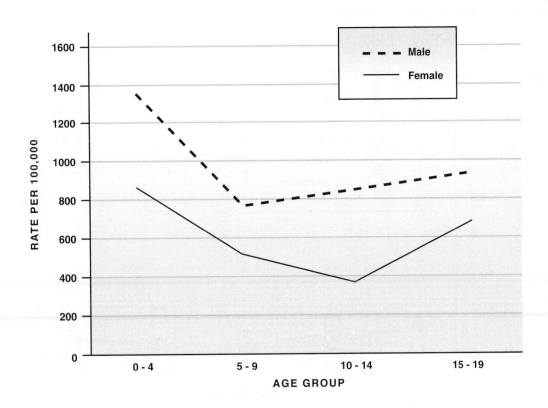

FIGURE 38-2

Average Annual Traumatic Brain Injury-Related Rates for Emergency Department Visits, Hospitalizations, and Deaths, by Age Group and Sex, United States, 1995–2001.

Source: Traumatic Brain Injury in the United States (2006).

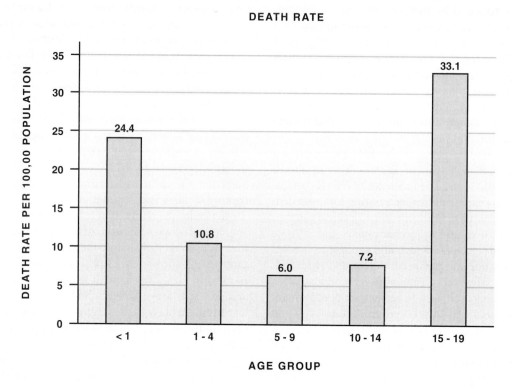

FIGURE 38-3

Unintentional Injury Death Rates among Children 0 to 19 Years of Age, by Age Group, United States, 2000–2005.

Source: CDC Childhood Injury Report: Patterns of Unintentional Injuries among 0 -19 Year Olds in the United States, 2000–2006.

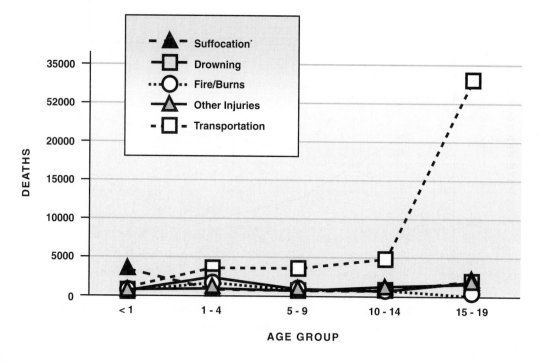

FIGURE 38-4

Leading Causes of Unintentional Injury Death Among Children 0–19 Years of Age.

Source: CDC Childhood Injury Report: Patterns of Unintentional Injuries among 0–19 Year Olds in the United States, 2000–2006.

There is tremendous variability in both pediatric death and injury rates according to race, sex, and location of residence. For example, the overall unintentional injury death rate among children in the United States during the period 2000–2005 was 15.0 per 100,000, but was much higher in American Indian or Alaska Native males. Among all age groups, males have almost twice the injury/death rate of females; after age 1 year, males are also more likely than females to have a nonfatal injury (Figure 38-5) (Borse et al., 2008).

States in the Northeast have the lowest injury death rates. Fire and burn death rates are highest in the South. The death rate from transportation-related injuries is highest in the South and the Upper Plains, while the lowest rates occur in the Northeast, presumably because fewer people drive and more take public transportation in this region. The most frequent sites of fatal accidents are the street (34%) and the home (28%) (ACS, 2008; Borse et al., 2008).

The length of hospital stay for the pediatric trauma patient is generally brief, with a median two-day stay for most mechanisms of injury and a median one-day stay for falls (ACS, 2008). Following triage and treatment in an ED, 41% of pediatric trauma patients are admitted to a general admission/nonspecialty unit bed, 17% to an intensive care unit, and 14% directly to the operating room (with subsequent admission to a floor or specialty bed); 12% are discharged to home without further services; and 5% are transferred to another hospital. The remaining 10% are discharged to a variety of other subcategories (ACS, 2008).

While many of the same limitations that affect calculation of pediatric trauma injury rates extend to and make estimating financial costs difficult, even a rough analysis indicates that trauma care costs are both substantial and increasing. Using estimated 1996 and 2000 figures, the associated annual costs of child and adolescent injuries (ages 0 to 14) range from $50 billion to $80 billion, including current and future medical expenses, other resource costs (such as caregivers), and present and future work losses (AAP et al., 2008; NCIPC, n.d.). Whether through direct association or because of the shared societal costs, pediatric trauma is having an increasingly costly impact on society. Trauma care is an acute, specialized medical discipline requiring highly trained practitioners, special instruments, powerful diagnostic tools such as computed tomography (CT) and magnetic resonance imaging (MRI), and appropriate pharmaceuticals. For the more severely injured patients, intensive care, long hospital stays, and rehabilitation also contribute to the cost of care. While trauma results in disability in people of all ages, issues of disability are more costly among pediatric patients because, theoretically, they still have many future years of life ahead.

It is helpful to examine some of the stratified cost estimates to understand the variation among age groups. Injuries among 5- to 14-year-olds are estimated to cost $34.6 billion annually, of which almost one-third is attributed to fall-related injuries. Among children 4 years of age or younger, colliding with objects (walls, trees) and objects colliding with children (balls, hands) result in the greatest total lifetime costs, estimated at more than $2.2 billion.

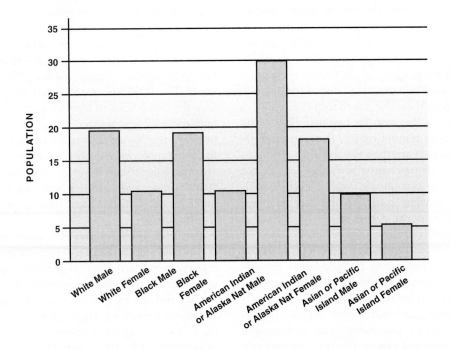

FIGURE 38-5

Unintentional Injury Death Rates among Children 0 to 19 Years, by Race and Sex, United States, 2000–2005.

Source: CDC Childhood Injury Report: Patterns of Unintentional Injuries among 0 -19 Year Olds in the United States, 2000–2006.

Among the very youngest patients, loss of productivity (rather than medical bills) accounts for the greatest costs. Violence has a tremendous impact on older children. Although the available data include individuals beyond the age group of interest, the fact that the direct and indirect costs of youth violence (10- to 24-year-olds)—including medical costs, lost productivity, and lesser quality of life—exceed $158 billion per year gives some sense of violence's impact on pediatric trauma (NCIPC, n.d.).

Another economic consideration is the impact on the regional trauma center host that must treat pediatric trauma patients. Many trauma centers are located in urban inner-city environments and care for a large proportion of public aid and uninsured patients. While research provides compelling evidence that trauma and EMS systems are effective in reducing mortality, morbidity, and lost productivity from traumatic injuries (National Trauma Data Standards [NTDS], 2009), they are also very expensive to operate. In a sophisticated cost–benefit analysis the costs associated with initiating and maintaining a level I adult trauma center were compared with lives saved; the monetary cost was estimated at almost $100,000 per person (Rotondo et al., 2009). The significance of the costs associated with the process will undoubtedly continue to be evaluated within the overarching awareness of health care reform and optimal utilization of resources.

TRAUMA SYSTEMS AND CENTERS

The ACS Trauma Center Designations were designed to establish and to ensure that the infrastructure needed for best practices (and improved outcomes) is present in centers that care for both pediatric and adult patients. The ACS conducts a voluntary program through which trauma centers can complete an in-depth application and then undergo an evaluation site visit, during which time ACS members confirm the presence of the resources outlined in the ACS's *Resources for Optimal Care of the Injured Patient*. Those trauma centers that satisfactorily demonstrate compliance are then classified according to four levels; a level I trauma center is able to provide the highest level of trauma care on-site, while a level IV facility is designed to provide initial trauma care, stabilize the patient, and transfer the patient to a higher level of trauma care if needed (CDC, n.d., b).

To meet the pediatric designation criteria, a pediatric trauma center (PTC) must meet the additional requirements of a certain minimum volume of pediatric patients; availability of specialized medical and support staff; emergency, intensive, acute, and tertiary care; ongoing pediatric-care education, injury prevention, and performance improvement programs; and a trauma registrar for data collection. The ACS guidelines further recommend that pediatric trauma patients be cared for by pediatric surgeons, by pediatric anesthesiologists, and in a pediatric intensive care

unit when necessary. PTCs are designed specifically to care for injured children; thus it is not surprising that several studies have demonstrated that younger and more seriously injured children have improved mortality rates at PTCs or integrative adult-pediatric center (AAP et al., 2008; Ochoa et al., 2007). While there has been some criticism of the use of retrospective methodology and the focus on mortality rather than outcomes in these studies, they remain foundational to evidence-based practice and support the recently published guidelines suggesting that children should be transferred to a facility with specialized pediatric services when appropriate (AAP et al., 2009).

Today's emergency and trauma care systems are treating more patients, with fewer resources, in an environment with tenuous coordination among prehospital EMS, hospital services, and public health providers. To meet this challenge, the Emergency Medical Services for Children (EMSC) program, administered by the U.S. Department of Health and Human Services' Health Resources and Services Administration's Maternal and Child Health Bureau, was designed to develop and evaluate improved procedures and protocols for treating ill or injured children (Junkins et al., 2006). In spite of the implementation of this national program, studies suggest that the majority of injured children continue to be treated in adult facilities (Ochoa et al., 2007). The relatively infrequent exposure of hospital-based emergency care professionals at adult facilities to seriously ill or injured children represents a substantial barrier to the maintenance of essential skills and clinical competency. In its 2007 report titled *Emergency Care for Children: Growing Pains*, the IOM states that pediatric treatment varies widely among emergency care providers, that many of these providers do not properly stabilize seriously ill or injured children, that many under-treat children in comparison to adults, and that many health care professionals (HCPs) fail to recognize injuries resulting from child maltreatment. The IOM also reports that of those hospitals that lack the capabilities to care for pediatric trauma patients, only one-half have written transfer agreements with other hospitals that would facilitate transfer of pediatric patients to a more appropriate facility when needed. These problems are often exacerbated in rural areas where specialized pediatric training and resources may not be available, resulting in increased distance and time for prehospital transport (IOM, 2007).

In 2008, the AAP and Pediatric Orthopaedic Society of North America issued a statement on pediatric trauma management, clarifying that pediatric trauma patients have unique needs that must be considered and integrated into trauma systems as well as state and regional emergency and disaster planning. Highlights of this statement include the following recommendations: Pediatric specialists need to be involved in all planning levels; appropriate pediatric facilities must be identified; potential providers need to have basic pediatric triage skills; and pediatric emergency competency training needs to be disseminated. Research needed to support evidence-based protocols should be supported. Integrated systems of injury management and prevention should also be provided (AAP et al., 2008).

In response to many of the previously described concerns regarding treatment of pediatric patients in EDs, the AAP Committee on Pediatric Emergency Medicine, the American College of Emergency Physicians Pediatric Committee, and the Emergency Nurses Association Pediatric Committee developed a joint policy statement known as *Guidelines for Care of Children in the Emergency Department* (2009). These guidelines address a range of areas, including administration and coordination of pediatric care in the ED; targeted pediatric-specific HCP training; quality and performance improvement; pediatric-specific policies and procedures for triage, analgesia, and consent/permission; support services; and appropriate medication and/or dosing. They also make recommendations for maintaining the equipment and supplies for use with pediatric patients. Through varied strategies, these guidelines, the ACS pediatric trauma center system, and the efforts of the EMSC, hospital EDs are expected to become better prepared to receive, accurately assess, and at a minimum stabilize (and safely transfer if necessary) acutely ill or injured children.

PREVENTION

In 1985, the National Research Council published *Injury in America: A Continuing Public Health Problem*. The message of this report was that injury events are not "accidental acts of fate," but rather are predictable—and, therefore, preventable—phenomena (Hirsch & DeRoss, 2009). Injury prevention has since been recognized as a public health priority. The CDC's Injury Center conducts surveillance, injury risk and protective factor research, and intervention and adoption research designed to determine effective public health practice (CDC, n.d., a; NCIPC, n.d.). The ACS also includes a requirement for all level I and II trauma centers to establish injury prevention as part of their trauma care mission (Hirsch & DeRoss, 2009). Community groups such as the National Safe Kids Campaign and the Injury Free Coalition for Kids have also developed successful injury prevention programs that are geared toward identifying at-risk groups, providing education, and advocating for legislation pertinent to child safety. In New York City, for example, the Injury Free Coalition for Kids created a comprehensive injury surveillance program that has been expanded nationally and employs a five-stage approach: (2) analyze the data, (2) build a coalition, (3) communicate the problem, (4) develop the interventions, and (5) evaluate the program (Hirsch & DeRoss, 2009).

Injury prevention programs appear to be making a difference. Data from the National Vital Statistics System (1987–2004), demonstrate that there has a 43% decrease in the raw, or unadjusted, number of unintentional injury deaths in recent years (Safe Kids Worldwide [SKW], 2007). Motor vehicle fatalities, bicycle injuries, pedestrian injuries, fire and/or burns, unintentional firearm injuries, and falls all declined during this time period. Most dramatically, deaths due to fire and/or burn have been reduced by 58%—a decrease largely attributed to national and regional bodies' adoption of plumbing code language to require antiscald technology and a standard water heater temperature of 120°F (48.9°C) in all newly constructed units (SKW, 2007). Other examples of effective injury prevention programs include the community-wide program in Seattle to promote bicycle helmet usage, which led to an 85% risk reduction for bicycle-related head injuries with the use of helmets, and the CDC initiative to provide smoke alarm installation and fire safety education programs in high-risk communities, which has saved an estimated 1,053 lives (of all ages) (Hirsch & DeRoss, 2009; NCIPC, n.d.).

All 50 states and the District of Columbia now have basic child restraint laws, and 38 states and the District of Columbia have upgraded their child restraint laws to require children as old as 9 years of age to use booster seats or other appropriate restraint devices. The use of restraints in combination with mandatory air bags in newer cars and improved automobile safety are all factors contributing to the 32% decrease in pediatric MVC-related deaths since 1987. Some of these reductions are even more notable because the denominator (i.e., the number of children) has actually increased during this time period, which suggests that the impact is even greater than the raw numbers would suggest.

To evaluate the success of injury prevention programs, as well as to undertake trauma care review, a comprehensive trauma registry system is needed. Trauma registries and other research projects have provided the necessary data to examine pediatric trauma trends, suggest behavior modifications, and evaluate the results of those modifications (AAP et al., 2008). Unfortunately, the actual data points contained in independent hospital registries are often so different in content and structure that making comparisons across registries is extremely difficult (NTDS, 2009). Consequently, the ACS subcommittee on Trauma Registry Programs, supported by the U.S. Health Resources and Services Administration, has created a uniform set of trauma registry variables and variable definitions designed to maximize participation by all state, regional, and local trauma registries. These guidelines are expected to result in a new National Trauma Data Bank that should improve the ability to monitor trends, identify new prevention targets, and evaluate interventions (NTDS, 2009).

Traumatic injuries continue to have significant impact on morbidity, disability, and mortality within the pediatric population. Interventions such as improved motor vehicle restraint systems as well as prevention programs, however, have demonstrated that it is possible to reduce the injury burden from this source.

APPROACH TO THE PEDIATRIC TRAUMA PATIENT

Gerald J. Gracia, Corey Fritz, and Sarah Wilson

Comprehensive and effective evaluation and management of the pediatric trauma patient is based on knowledge of the unique anatomic and pathophysiologic differences in children. The special considerations, unique needs, and characteristics of the injured pediatric patient are the focus of this section.

The initial evaluation of the injured child begins with the across-the-room assessment using the *Pediatric Assessment Triangle*. This global view of the patient's status offers the first cue to resuscitative needs (Figure 38-6). The approach to the patient is then divided into two distinct phases: the primary survey and the secondary survey. The *primary survey*, or initial phase of resuscitation, addresses life-threatening injuries that compromise oxygenation, ventilation, and circulation—also referred to as airway, breathing, and circulation (ABCs). The *secondary survey* is a head-to-toe evaluation of the patient that seeks to identify further injury. High-functioning trauma teams perform many tasks simultaneously; however, for purposes of a written text, the survey is described here as a step-by-step process.

WEIGHT-BASED DETERMINATION FOR RESUSCITATION

Resuscitation in pediatrics is weight-based; thus tools that quickly estimate weight in settings when direct measurement cannot be performed are valuable. Several methods are used for estimating the weight of a pediatric patient, including the Broselow Color-Coded Pediatric Emergency Tape, the Leffler formula, and the Theron formula.

The most commonly used method is the Broselow Tape. To use this device, the HCP places the tape alongside the patient's body and determines, based on the length, the patient's approximate weight and a color code assignment. Each color bar on the tape has information regarding equipment sizes and medication doses for the approximated

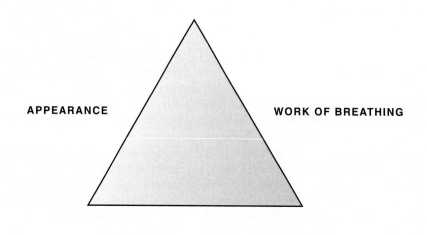

APPEARANCE   WORK OF BREATHING

CIRCULATION TO SKIN

Airway

Breathing

Circulation

Disability/Neurologic Evaluation

Exposure

FIGURE 38-6

Pediatric Assessment Triangle.

weight. The predictive accuracy of these methods for weight estimates were evaluated by So et al. (2009). Their results demonstrated that the Broselow Tape is accurate for weight estimation in children weighing 25 kg or less, but that the Theron formula performs better with patients weighing more than 40 kg. The estimation of weight is performed at the beginning of the primary survey so that size-based information is available as interventions are needed.

Leffler formula:

- Weight in kilograms = (age in months/2) + 4 for children younger than 1 year of age
- Weight in kilograms = (2 × age in years) + 10 for children 1 to 10 years of age

Theron formula: Weight in kilograms =
exp [(0.175571 × age in years) + 2.197099]

PRIMARY SURVEY

The primary survey follows the ABCs of resuscitation (Figure 38-6), starting with *airway* control. Early airway control is paramount. Unlike in adults, the cause of pediatric cardiac arrest is often an initial respiratory arrest. The young child's airway is anatomically different from that of an adult. A young child has a larger occiput, shorter neck, smaller and anterior larynx, "U"-shaped epiglottis, short trachea, and large tongue. During the primary survey, the airway is assessed for signs of obstruction such as foreign bodies or dental, facial, mandibular, tracheal, or laryngeal fractures. The crying child attests to a patent airway. Nonetheless, supplemental oxygen should be applied to all patients, even in the presence of a spontaneously, well-maintained airway. For optimal airway patency, the child's airway must be maintained in the sniffing position (Cooper, 2005).

Several additional maneuvers may be useful for patients with airway obstruction. The initial maneuver is a chin lift or jaw thrust. The chin-lift maneuver is indicated in children who have a depressed level of consciousness with concomitant upper airway obstruction and who are not victims of trauma. The jaw-thrust maneuver is indicated when the movement of the patient's neck is either not possible or not prudent. These maneuvers are potentially helpful in relieving upper airway obstruction.

Nasopharyngeal and oropharyngeal airways are simple adjuncts used for maintaining airway patency in those patients with good respiratory effort. If oral intubation is indicated, use of the jaw-thrust maneuver to improve airway patency during the procedure is often helpful. The cervical spine must be protected during all maneuvers. Do not hyperextend, hyperflex, or rotate the cervical spine. Assume that all pediatric trauma patients have a cervical spine injury until proven otherwise (ACS, 1997).

Should intubation be required to protect the airway, selection of the appropriate endotracheal tube size may be accomplished by direct comparison to the child's fifth digit or by the formula (age + 16)/4 (AAP & American College of Emergency Physicians, 1998). Endotracheal tube position must be evaluated after insertion by the following: Auscultation of bilateral breath sounds and no epigastric sounds; visible mist in the endotracheal tube on exhalation, capnography and bedside $EtCO_2$, and chest radiograph. Traditionally cuffed endotracheal tubes were not used for children less than 8 years of age; however, more recent recommendations support cuffed endotracheal tubes in children beyond the newborn period provided cuff pressure is less than 20 cmH_2O so as to minimize tracheal trauma (American Heart Association, 2006). The narrowest portion of the pediatric airway is the subglottic trachea (cricoid cartilage), which provides a somewhat "physiologic cuff." In rare circumstances, it may be necessary to perform a cricothyrotomy if oral intubation is either contraindicated or too difficult. A cricothyrotomy is a method of last resort, however; it should be reserved until all other means have been exhausted, as it is associated with a significant risk for developing subglottic stenosis. An orogastric or nasogastric tube should be placed shortly after intubation to evacuate gastric contents (reduce aspiration risk) and reduce gastric distention (which may impede diaphragmatic excursion).

Once a patent airway is established, the next step is assessing the child's *breathing*. Infants and small children are primarily diaphragmatic breathers, as their ribs lack the rigidity, muscle maturity, and configuration present in adults. As a result, any compromise of diaphragmatic excursion significantly limits the child's ability to ventilate. Direct injury to the diaphragm, disruption and herniation of intra-abdominal contents, or gastric distention (aerophagia) can severely compromise the pediatric patient's ability to breathe. The mediastinum of a child is very mobile; therefore, mediastinal structures can shift into the contralateral hemithorax as a result of a simple pneumothorax, hemothorax, or tension pneumothorax. Recognition of these emergencies requires immediate intervention. In addition to having a mobile mediastinum, pediatric patients have a thin chest wall, allowing for resonation of sounds to transmit to the other side of the chest (referred breath sounds).

Inspection, auscultation, palpation, and percussion are the key elements to the respiratory assessment. For the awake patient, "look first and touch last" during the assessment to reduce patient anxiety. Observe the following elements:

- Respiratory effort
- Mechanics of breathing
- Air entry

- Jugular vein distention
- Abdominal contour
- Skin color

If ventilatory attempts are present, the rate should be noted. Special attention to the mechanics of breathing will assist in evaluating how much effort is required to adequately ventilate and oxygenate the child. Retractions, grunting, tracheal tugging, accessory muscle use, nasal flaring, and head bobbing are all signs of increased work of breathing. Distended jugular veins require immediate evaluation for potential life-threatening conditions, such as a tension pneumothorax or pericardial tamponade.

The position of the trachea (e.g. midline or shifted) should be noted. The presence of tenderness, instability, or crepitus may suggest underlying lung parenchymal injury or compromise of the pleural space. Chest wall excursion or expansion should also be evaluated. Auscultation of the lung fields is performed immediately if the patient appears to be in distress. Assess whether breath sounds are present, diminished, or absent; compare equality of sounds, and note any adventitious breath sounds. The breath sounds from one lung field may resonate throughout the entire chest cavity of a child; thus the presence of breath sounds alone does not negate an injury or impaired function. Several life-threatening injuries should be identifiable during this step of the evaluation, including flail chest, tension pneumothorax, and open pneumothorax.

Once the airway is secured and adequate ventilation/oxygenation is confirmed, the *circulatory* status of the patient should be addressed. The ability to recognize hypovolemic shock in pediatric trauma patients is essential to obtaining a positive patient outcome. The earliest measured sign of hypovolemia is tachycardia. Unlike in the adult population, the heart rates and blood pressures found in the pediatric population vary significantly based on age (Table 38-1).

Other clinical signs of shock include mental status changes, respiratory compromise, weak or absent peripheral pulses, delayed capillary refill, skin pallor, and hypothermia. Pediatric patients have an impressive cardiovascular reserve, so initial vital signs that are within the age-range norms may not accurately convey the status of the child's circulating volume. Obvious signs of shock, such as a decrease in urine output or hypotension, may not be apparent in early stages (Cooper, 2005) (Table 38-2).

The most common etiology of shock in the pediatric trauma patient is hemorrhagic shock, although concomitant cardiogenic (e.g., cardiac tamponade), obstructive (e.g., tension pneumothorax), and neurogenic (e.g., spinal shock) shock may also exist. The increased reserve of the pediatric cardiovascular system allows children to compensate and maintain normal blood pressures despite even moderate degrees of hemorrhagic shock. Children may maintain a normal systolic blood pressure for age until they have lost as much as 30% of their circulating blood volume (ACS, 1997) (Table 38-3).

The circulating blood volume of a child is 70 to 80 mL/kg, as compared to the typical adult circulating blood volume of 60 mL/kg. A normal systolic blood pressure (SBP) for a child can be calculated using this formula: (age in years × 2) + 90 mmHg. The corresponding expected diastolic blood pressure should be ⅔ × SBP. The initial compensatory mechanism that the HCP should look for during the early stages of hemorrhagic shock is tachycardia. The other compensatory mechanism that occurs as the child's body attempts to maintain normal perfusion and blood pressure is an increase in the systemic vascular resistance,

TABLE 38-1

Age-Based Estimates for Vital Signs and Weight (Blood Pressure Mean ± 2 Standard Deviations)					
AGE	**Weight (kg)**	**Heart rate**	**Resp rate**	**Systolic BP**	**Diastolic BP**
Premature	1	145/min	~40	42 + 10	21 + 8
Premature	1–2	135	~40	50 + 10	28 + 8
Newborn	2–3	125	~40	60 + 10	37 + 8
1 month	4	120	24–35	80 + 16	46 + 16
6 month	7	130	24–35	89 + 29	60 + 10
1 year	10	120	20–30	96 + 30	66 + 25
2–3 years	12–14	115	20–30	99 + 25	64 + 25
4–5 years	16–18	100	20–30	99 + 20	65 + 20
6–8 years	20–26	100	12–25	100 + 15	60 + 10
10–12 years	32–42	75	12–25	110 + 17	60 + 10
>14 years	>50	70	12–18	118 + 20	60 + 10

Source: Data from Thompson, M. et al (2009). Deriving temperature and age appropriate heart rate centiles for children with acute infections. *Archives of Disease in Childhood* 94, 361–365.

TABLE 38-2

Approximate Blood Volumes			
Age	Total Blood Volume (mL/kg)	Age	Total Blood Volume (mL/kg)
Preterm infants	90–105	4–6 years	80–86
Term newborns	78–86	7–8 years	83–90
1–12 months	73–78	Adults	68–88
1–3 years	74–82		

Source: Nathan & Oski, 1998.

TABLE 38-3

Classification of Blood Loss				
	Class I	Class II	Class III	Class IV
Blood loss (%)	> 15%	15–25%	26–39%	> 40%
Cardiovascular	Normal to ↑ heart rate (HR)	↑HR Normal blood pressure ↓ Pulses	↑↑ HR Hypotension Thready pulses	↑↑↑ HR Profound hypotension Absent pulses
Respiratory	Normal rate	Tachypnea	Moderate tachypnea	Severe tachypnea
Central nervous system	Slightly anxious	Irritable, confused, combative	↓ Response to pain	Coma
Skin	Warm, pink Normal capillary refill	Cool extremities Mottling Delayed capillary refill	Cool extremities Mottling pallor Prolonged capillary refill	Cold extremities Pallor Cyanosis
Kidneys	Normal urine output	Oliguria Increased specific gravity	Oliguria Increased blood urea nitrogen (BUN)	Anuria
Acid–base	Normal pH	Normal pH	Metabolic acidosis	Metabolic acidosis

Source: Adapted from Committee on Trauma of the American College of Surgeons, 1993.

which is manifested clinically by mottled/cool extremities, weak/thready distal pulses, delayed capillary refill time, and a narrowed pulse pressure. If the early clinical signs of hemorrhagic shock are not identified and corrected, the child may progress to a preterminal stage of decompensated shock, which is defined as hypotension for age. Hypotension in children may be defined using the following formula: (age in years × 2) + 70 mmHg. The minimum systolic blood pressures for age are listed in (Table 38-1).

Immediate institution of appropriate vascular access and control of external blood loss are the principal elements of treatment during the initial assessment and resuscitation phase of management of the injured child. Typically, vascular access has been obtained in the field, but this issue may need the HCP's immediate attention if two large-bore venous access sites are not present. The locations of the injuries should be considered prior to placing any intravenous access, so as to prevent extravasation of resuscitative fluids. In the event obtaining venous access is futile, an intraosseous line placement may be placed.

Ongoing hemorrhage via open lacerations should be managed initially by direct manual pressure on the wound. Scalp lacerations are managed with compressive dressings or rapid hemostatic maneuvers such as a figure-of-eight suture closure, prior to leaving the resuscitation area. Emergent imaging studies should not be delayed while definitive wound closures are performed. To identify other sources of bleeding, CT is used for patients of all ages, and focal abdominal sonography for trauma (FAST) scans are used for older adolescents and adults as necessary. Blood loss can be intracranial, intra-abdominal, or in an extremity such as a thigh. Intracavitary hemorrhaging is more difficult to manage in the initial assessment phase. Medical anti-shock trousers (MAST) have few or no indications in the pediatric trauma population. Upon securing appropriate venous access, immediate resuscitation with crystalloid solutions should be implemented. In general, 20 mL/kg of a crystalloid solution is the initial step in fluid resuscitation.

Once the airway has been secured, breathing is adequate (ventilation and oxygenation), and the circulatory system has been addressed, a rapid initial evaluation of the neurologic *disability* of the patient is completed. The standard tool for such evaluation is the pediatric version of the Glasgow Coma Scale (GCS). Historically, the neurologic status was determined during the secondary survey; however, current opinions suggest that the GCS score for the child be determined during the primary survey and the assessment then be repeated throughout the resuscitation period. Using the

GCS instrument, patients are scored from 3 (indicating deep unconsciousness) to 15 (alert and neurologically intact). Patients with a GCS score of 8 or less require immediate intervention to secure their airway (Table 38-4).

An alternative method, known as the AVPU, is also commonly used as a fast initial assessment of the injured child. This acronym has the following meaning:

- **A:** alert
- **V:** responds to verbal stimuli
- **P:** responds to painful stimuli
- **U:** unresponsive

TABLE 38-4

Modified Glasgow Coma Scale and Glasgow Coma Scale Modified for Infants and Children

Clinical Parameter	Adult	Infants (Ages 0–12 Months)	Children (Ages 1–5 Years)	Score*
Eye Opening	Open spontaneously	Open spontaneously	Open spontaneously	4
	Open in response to verbal stimuli	Open in response to verbal stimuli	Open in response to verbal stimuli	3
	Open in response to pain only	Open in response to pain only	Open in response to pain only	2
	No response	No response	No response	1
Best Verbal Response	Oriented	Coos and babbles	Oriented, appropriate	5
	Confused	Irritable cries	Confused	4
	Inappropriate words	Cries in response to pain	Inappropriate words	3
	Incomprehensible words or nonspecific sounds	Moans in response to pain	Incomprehensible words or nonspecific sounds	2
	No response	No response	No response	1
Best Motor Response†	Obeys	Moves spontaneously and purposefully	Obeys commands	6
	Localizes	Withdraws to touch	Localizes painful stimulus	5
	Withdraws	Withdraws in response to pain	Withdraws in response to pain	4
	Abnormal flexion	Responds to pain with decorticate posturing (abnormal flexion)	Responds to pain with decorticate posturing (abnormal flexion)	3
	Extensor response	Responds to pain with decerebrate posturing (abnormal extension)	Responds to pain with decerebrate posturing (abnormal extension)	2
	No response	No response	No response	1

*Score ≤ 12 suggests a severe head injury. Score < 8 suggests need for endotracheal intubation and mechanical ventilation. Score ≤ 6 suggests need for intracranial pressure monitoring.

†If the patient is intubated, unconscious, or preverbal, the most important part of this scale is motor response. This section should be carefully evaluated.

Source: Adapted from Davis, R., et al. (1987). Head and spinal cord injury. In M. Rogers (Ed.), Textbook of pediatric intensive care. Baltimore, MD: Williams & Wilkins.

James, H., Anas, N., & Perkin, R. (1985). *Brain insults in infants and children.* New York: Grune & Stratton.

Morray, J., et al. (1984). Coma scale for use in brain-injured children. *Critical Care Medicine, 12,* 1018.

Teasdale, G., & Jennett, B. (1974). Assessment of coma and impaired consciousness: A practical scale. *Lancet, 2,* 81–84.

Reilly, P., Simpson, D., et al. (1988). Assessing the conscious level in infants and young children: A paediatric version of the Glasgow Coma Scale. *Child's Nervous System, 4,* 30–33.

Pupils should be examined individually for position, size, equality, and reactivity (e.g., left 3 → 2 brisk/right 4→ 2 sluggish). The acronym PERLA (pupils, equal round and react to light, accommodation) is an imprecise term and description and should not be used in documentation of an injured patient (Teasdale & Jennett, 1974). It is important to reassess pupils if any neurological changes are noted. Also, note that changes in the size and reactivity of the pupils may be influenced by medications administered during the resuscitation effort.

Alteration in the level of consciousness should prompt an immediate reevaluation of oxygenation, ventilation, and circulation. If these are adequate, assume that the trauma is the cause of the decrease in the level of consciousness. Alcohol and drugs may also reduce the level of consciousness, but they are a diagnosis of exclusion in a person with trauma. Emergent radiographic evaluation may be required in children with altered mental status and head injuries. It is important to reiterate that these imaging modalities should be performed without significant delay.

The final assessment in the primary survey is the complete *exposure* of the patient to briefly look for key injuries missed during attention to the ABCs. It is of utmost importance that in-line stability of the vertebral column is maintained during this portion of the assessment. Once the child has been disrobed completely, a log-roll maneuver can be completed to briefly assess the posterior side of the patient to identify life threats.

Hypothermia must be prevented during the examination, as it may potentiate deleterious physiologic changes. Children are notably more susceptible to hypothermia than adults (Inaba & Seward, 1991). Physiologically, children have larger body surfaces in proportion to their body mass; as a consequence, they lose heat through surface evaporation at a faster rate than adults. In addition, children typically have less body fat to serve as insulation when compared to adults; consequently, they lose heat more rapidly than adults. Moreover, children's heads are large in proportion to their bodies and represent an additional significant source of heat loss that is not typically a concern in adults (Inaba & Seward, 1991). To combat hypothermia in the pediatric trauma patient, create a warm, ambient air environment of 82°F (28°C). This can be accomplished by applying temperature-regulating blankets, placing radiant heaters over the child, and using insulating devices such as blankets, stockinettes, or other materials to maintain the patient's temperature. Additional strategies may include using warmed crystalloid solutions. Blood, blood products, and irrigation fluids may also be warmed.

SECONDARY SURVEY

After the initial assessment (primary survey), the HCP should obtain a full set of vital signs (if not previously recorded), obtain historical information, conduct a thorough, head-to-toe examination, and order additional diagnostic studies as determined. This phase of evaluation is known as the *secondary* survey. If at any time during the secondary survey the patient's condition deteriorates, another primary survey is warranted to evaluate the child for potential life threats.

The full set of vital signs includes blood pressure, heart rate, respiratory rate, oxygen saturation with pulse oximetry, and temperature. These vital signs should be repeated frequently during the secondary survey to monitor the effects of resuscitation. If chest trauma is suspected, auscultatation or pneumatic evaluation of the blood pressure should be obtained in both arms.

An indwelling urinary catheter may be inserted to monitor urine output. Any child demonstrating signs of shock should have an indwelling catheter. If an injury to the urethra is suspected, placement of a urinary drainage catheter is contraindicated. A urethral injury should be suspected if blood is present at the meatus or scrotum, or if an anterior pelvic fracture is suspected.

If indicated, and not previously placed, a gastric tube is inserted at this point in the assessment. If the patient has facial fractures or head injury, insert the gastric tube orally. Gastric decompression and emptying of the gastric contents will help reduce the risk of aspiration, respiratory compromise, vagal stimulation, and bradycardia. Maintaining cervical spine stabilization remains of vital importance through this phase of care.

Obtain information from prehospital providers, when present, to provide perspective on the child's injuries. The mnemonic MIVT (**M**echanism of injury, **I**njuries sustained, **V**ital signs, and **T**reatment) can be used to format the information from prehospital personnel. Knowledge of the mechanism of injury may help to predict injury patterns (Table 38-5). Gather as much information from the patient or family members as possible regarding patient age, preexisting medical conditions, current medications, allergies, tetanus immunization history, previous hospitalizations and surgeries, recent use of drugs or alcohol, and sexual activity and last menstrual period (pregnancy assessment).

The head-to-toe assessment is performed via inspection, auscultation, and palpation. A systematic examination, moving from cephalad to caudad, starts on the anterior side of the body and inspects the patient for lacerations, abrasions, avulsions, contusions, puncture wounds, impaled objects, deformities, ecchymosis, and edema. Once the anterior surface has been evaluated, inspect the posterior surface, including the vertebral column and the rectal tone. It is crucial to maintain cervical spine stabilization and to support extremities with suspected injuries while log-rolling the patient.

TABLE 38-5

Common Injury Mechanisms and Corresponding Injury Patterns in Childhood Trauma		
Injury Mechanism		**Injury Pattern**
Motor vehicle collision: occupant	Unrestrained	Head/neck injuries Scalp/facial lacerations
	Restrained	Internal abdominal injuries Lower spine fractures
Motor vehicle collision: pedestrian	Single	Lower extremity fractures
	Multiple	Head/neck injuries Internal chest/abdomen injuries Lower extremity fractures
Fall from a height	Low	Upper extremity fractures
	Medium	Head/neck injuries Scalp/facial lacerations Upper extremity fractures
	High	Head/neck injuries Scalp/facial lacerations Internal chest/abdomen injuries Upper/lower extremity fractures
Fall from a bicycle	Unhelmeted	Head/neck injuries Scalp/facial lacerations Upper extremity fractures
	Helmeted	Upper extremity fractures
	Handlebar	Internal abdomen injuries

Source: Adapted from ACS (2004).

DIAGNOSTIC STUDIES

Once the primary and secondary trauma surveys are completed and life-threatening injuries are identified and addressed, diagnostic studies may be ordered. Blood typing is the highest priority, which may also include screening and cross-matching. Standard trauma lab tests include complete blood count (CBC), blood urea nitrogen (BUN), creatinine, urinalysis, prothrombin (PT), and partial thromboplastin time (PTT). If abdominal trauma is suspected, additional abdominal laboratory studies may include alanine transaminase (ALT), aspartate transaminase (AST), amylase, and lipase. Specialized trauma centers vary in their selection of "trauma labs." If a female child is older than 10 years of age, consider sending a beta human chorionic gonadotropin or urine pregnancy test. Detailed insight into the diagnostic studies specific to injury is provided in injury-specific sections of this text.

OTHER ASPECTS OF THE PLAN OF CARE

Facilitate the presence of family in the treatment room and involve them in the plan of care. According to the Emergence Nurses Association (ENA, 2005), "It is in the best interest of the patient and family to offer the option for

a family member to be present during invasive procedures and resuscitation situations" (p. 1). The American Academy of Pediatrics concurs with this position: "The option of family member presence should be encouraged for all aspects of ED care" (O'Malley et al., 2008, p. e514). It is important to utilize resources to support the emotional and spiritual needs of the family with child life specialists, spiritual advisors, and social workers.

Providing comfort measures to the pediatric trauma patient includes additional measures along with pharmacologic analgesia. Various pain scales are used to determine pain severity in the injured child. Alternative pain-controlling measures include positioning of the child, distraction and relaxation techniques, soft and calming communication, and use of ancillary services such as social work and child life specialists.

Photographs may need to be taken for documentation purposes. Referrals are made to consulting services based on the injuries identified in the assessment process, such as with orthopedics, neurosurgery, plastic surgery, otolaryngology, or Child Protective Services. If consulting services are not available, transfer of the patient to a trauma center is warranted.

If the patient is stable enough for discharge to home, follow-up appointments should be made with the consulting services as recommended. If no consulting service follow-up is necessary, a follow-up with the primary care provider in 1 to 2 weeks is appropriate.

ABDOMINAL TRAUMA

Emily Hopper and Jodie Roth

PATHOPHYSIOLOGY

In abdominal trauma, the extent of injury is related to body motion, body mass, type of force applied, and density of the underlying structures. Mechanical energy is the most frequent type of force involved in abdominal trauma, and motor vehicle collisions (MVCs), bicycle accidents, and gunshots are all common sources of such forces. These sources produce different responses within the body depending on the type of tissue or structure that receives the energy load. Body mass and velocity both contribute to the amount of force produced and the extent of the subsequent injury (ENA, 2007).

Acceleration and deceleration are two forms of *external force* that may affect the body. *Acceleration* is a force that results in increasing speed of an object. For instance, if a motor vehicle strikes a pedestrian standing on the street corner, the force of energy from the motor vehicle is applied to the pedestrian and results in the acceleration of the pedestrian. Conversely, *deceleration* is a force that results in decreasing velocity. If that same person now hits a curb, the force of energy applied results in deceleration. Falls are an important example of both acceleration and deceleration. Other examples of objects that create energy when in motion are baseball bats, sharp objects, and ammunition. Internal acceleration and deceleration can also occur. For example, organs (e.g., the descending aorta, duodenum) may move independent of other internal structures, due to their fixation points, leading to further injury (ENA, 2007).

When an external force is applied to the body, it produces stress within the body, causing tissue deformation from *internal forces*. The resistance of the tissues to the energy load is a determinant of the degree of force and tissue injury. The internal stressors that result from the external force can be of several types—compressive, shearing, tensile, or overpressure:

- *Compressive stress* occurs from direct application of force to the body.
- *Shearing stress* results from a tangential force in opposite directions.
- *Tensile stress* occurs as opposing forces are applied to the same region resulting in strain. The tensile force pulls tissues and cells apart.
- The stress of *overpressure* directly affects the hollow viscus structures by producing compression. This

compressive force may create too much pressure for the viscus wall, leading to its rupture (Feliciano et al., 2008).

The last form of mechanical energy transfer is blunt versus penetrating injury. In *blunt injury,* the skin remains intact; in *penetrating injury,* the skin is disrupted. Blunt injury can be a result of mechanisms such as MVC, fall, or assault. During this type of event, the energy is dispersed throughout a larger surface area when compared to penetrating trauma, which in turn increases the potential for multisystem involvement. Penetrating injury can be a result of firearms, sharp objects, or machinery. During this type of event, injury occurs via entry through the skin into the underlying structures. All tissues and structures in the trajectory of the offending object are at risk for injury (ENA, 2007; Feliciano et al., 2008).

EPIDEMIOLOGY AND ETIOLOGY

More than 312 million patients worldwide sought medical care for an unintentional injury in 1990. This type of injury is the leading cause of death in people from ages 1 to 44 years; its risk does not show any differentiation based on race, sex, age, or socioeconomic status. Trauma accounts for more than $400 billion annually in lost wages, property damage, medical expenses, and insurance costs in the United States (ACS, 2008), and it places a significant burden on society, the health care system, and individuals (ENA, 2007).

Abdominal trauma is the leading cause of morbidity and mortality in injured children. Pediatric patients may be difficult to assess for abdominal trauma in the acute phase of injury, however, due to their stage of language or cognitive development and level of consciousness. Thorough initial assessment of the pediatric patient with abdominal trauma is essential to prevent complications associated with missed injuries and to reduce death and disability from this cause (Holmes et al., 2002b; Wegner et al., 2006).

The majority of pediatric trauma is a result of blunt injury. Abdominal injuries related to this type of force predominantly affect intra-abdominal solid organs, resulting from a variety of mechanisms including MVCs, falls, bicycle accidents, sports injuries, or all-terrain vehicle (ATV) crashes (Stafford et al., 2002). Only 1% to 10% of admissions to a pediatric trauma center are related to penetrating injury from firearm use, stabbings, or object impalement (Feliciano et al., 2008).

The management of pediatric trauma patients has changed in numerous ways over the last two decades. For example, ultrasound has been introduced as a primary screening tool for abdominal injury in both stable and unstable patients. Focused abdominal sonography for trauma (FAST) ultrasound is gradually replacing diagnostic peritoneal lavage (DPL) in hemodynamically unstable patients as a means of determining the need for emergency laparotomy. The introduction of the 64-slice CT scanner has also improved the diagnosis of intra-abdominal injury. CT scan is more widely used in hemodynamically stable patients with potential abdominal injury and is the primary imaging study used to grade solid-organ injury. Nonoperative management of solid-organ injury is based on clinical response to injury and CT grading of injury; when these assessments are combined, the result is highly predictive of successful management. Patients with pelvic fractures and higher-grade solid-organ injuries may now be managed with angiography to control excessive hemorrhage without having to undergo an operative procedure (Isenhour & Marx, 2007; Schuster-Bruce & Nolan, 1999; Siplovich & Kawar, 1997).

PRESENTATION

The approach to the pediatric trauma patient was described earlier in this chapter. Note that the abdominal assessment is not part of the primary survey and should not be performed until the primary survey is completed and the patient responds appropriately to resuscitative efforts. Information about the events, environment, and mechanism of injury related to the incident, such as restraint status, fall height, and gunshot range, is important in predicting patterns of damage (Feliciano et al., 2008). This history surrounding the event may not always be available due to the pediatric patient's condition or the absence of a family historian.

The abdominal examination should be conducted in a systematic fashion using the following sequence: inspection, auscultation, percussion, and palpation. In abdominal trauma, however, auscultation and percussion often have limited value. Documentation of positive and negative findings on physical examination is crucial.

A benign abdominal exam is characterized by the following findings:

- No outward signs of trauma to the abdomen
- Soft, nontender, nondistended abdomen
- FAST exam that shows no free intraperitoneal fluid (may be used with older adolescents and adults)

A positive exam may be associated with these findings:

- Abdominal tenderness
- Abdominal wall contusion, abrasions, or ecchymosis ("seat-belt sign")
- Abdominal distention
- Signs of peritonitis (e.g., guarding, rebound tenderness, abdominal wall rigidity)
- Referred pain or tenderness
- Blood at the urethral meatus

- Pelvic instability
- Gross blood on rectal exam
- Positive FAST exam with the presence of free intraperitoneal fluid (used with older adolescents and adults)

The reliability of the physical examination may be affected by altered mental status, the patient's age, or the presence of distracting injuries. In the event of a pregnant pediatric patient, the severity of injury and adequacy of resuscitation will affect both maternal and fetal outcomes. The mother must be treated to treat the fetus; therefore, radiographic studies are not withheld (ACS, 2008; Eastern Association of the Surgery of Trauma, 2001; Lutz et al., 2004; Moss & Musemeche, 1996).

DIFFERENTIAL DIAGNOSIS

The following differential diagnoses should be considered when evaluating the pediatric trauma patient for abdominal injury:

- Child maltreatment
- Injuries to solid and/or hollow organs
- Mesenteric laceration
- Diaphragmatic injury
- Pregnancy
- Coagulopathy
- Vascular injury
- Pelvic fracture
- Abdominal wall contusion (Feliciano et al., 2008; Moore et al., 2003)

PLAN OF CARE

The standardized trauma laboratory panels can help provide a structured approach for rapid assessment of the pediatric trauma patient. In the hemodynamically unstable patient, waiting for laboratory results may be detrimental. In contrast, in the stable patient, screening laboratory evaluation may provide helpful supplementary information to the physical examination findings and prevent exposure to unnecessary radiographic studies (Isaacman et al., 1993; Keller et al., 2004).

The abdominal trauma laboratory panel may or may not include the following tests:

- Arterial blood gas (ABG)/venous blood gas (VBG)
- Urinalysis (UA)
- Urine pregnancy test (HCG)
- Aspartate aminotransferase (AST)/alanine aminotransferase (ALT)
- Amylase/lipase
- Complete blood count (CBC)

- Prothrombin time (PT)/partial thromboplastin time (PTT)/International Normalized Ratio (INR)
- Type and cross-match

ABG/VBG is recommended for rapid screening in the hemodynamically unstable patient. The important values that can be obtained from this test include the base deficit, electrolytes, hematocrit (Hct), and hemoglobin (Hgb). These values help estimate the degree of shock, acidosis, need for blood product transfusion, and the efficacy of resuscitation (ACS, 2008).

UA has a high sensitivity for detecting intra-abdominal injury but is nonspecific for type or degree of injury. Microscopic hematurias containing more than 5 red blood cells (RBCs) per high-power field (HPF) indicate the need for further evaluation of the abdomen (Brown et al., 2001; Cotton et al., 2004). *Urine HCG should be obtained in all female patients of childbearing age (10 years of age or older).* Ideally, this test should be done before any radiographic studies are completed.

With the AST/ALT tests, elevated enzymes may suggest the presence of liver injury. A finding of abnormally elevated AST (more than 450 IU/L) or ALT (more than 250 IU/L) indicates the need for CT scan to further evaluate the degree of injury; however, the degree of enzyme elevation does not correlate with the degree of injury or the need for operative intervention (Hennes et al., 1990; Puranik et al., 2002).

Amylase and lipase are not good predictors of pancreatic injury during the initial evaluation. The presence of abdominal pain and elevated amylase and lipase 24 hours after injury or upwardly trending values have greater predictive values for pancreatic trauma (Feliciano et al., 2008).

CBC is useful for trending Hgb and Hct in the setting of solid-organ injury. The CBC results help guide the decision-making process related to transfusion or operative management. The PT/PTT/INR tests are baseline coagulation studies that are important to obtain in those patients with known blood dyscrasias or those who are taking anticoagulant therapy.

Blood type and cross-match are performed on all patients who are suspected of having blunt abdominal trauma. Having type and screen results readily available decreases the amount of time required to further cross-match blood. All patients who have suffered penetrating injury or who are hemodynamically unstable require a type and cross-match to be drawn during the initial screening lab work. O-negative blood can be used in an emergent situation until the final cross-match data are obtained (ACS, 2008).

Chest and abdominal radiographs are often performed as screening films in a patient who has experienced multisystem trauma. Pelvic radiographs may be performed to determine the presence of fractures, as these injuries are often the source of significant blood loss. Flat lateral or upright radiographs may be used in hemodynamically stable patients to visualize free air, diagnose diaphragmatic injury, and visualize foreign bodies when CT is unavailable. These radiographs are useful in patients who have suffered penetrating trauma to detect the presence of retroperitoneal air or to determine the path of the missile (ACS, 2008; ENA, 2007).

The CT scan is the preferred diagnostic modality for detecting intra-abdominal injury in children. It can be used to identify hematomas, free fluid or air, and retroperitoneal, pelvic, or solid-organ injury. The data obtained via CT scan can also be used to grade solid-organ injuries, thereby guiding nonoperative management. These scans must be performed using intravenous contrast to identify active bleeding or "blush" from the vascular structures (ENA, 2007). Not all injuries are immediately identifiable on CT. For example, diaphragmatic, bowel, and pancreatic injuries are often not detected via initial CT scan. In the absence of a solid-organ injury, the presence of a significant volume of free fluid in the abdomen is associated with hollow viscus or mesenteric injury in 30% to 94% of patients (Feliciano et al., 2008). CT scan has questionable utility in individuals with penetrating injuries; instead, patients with apparent peritoneal damage from penetrating trauma are often taken to the operating room for emergent abdominal exploration. The CT scan is indicated for hemodynamically stable patients only (ENA, 2007).

FAST is a tool that is used in the evaluation of possible intra-abdominal injury for older adolescent and adult patients; it is rarely used in children. The primary goal with this type of ultrasound is to identify free intraperitoneal fluid. This rapid, noninvasive technique can be used for serial examinations. The sensitivity of the test depends on the operator's skill level and the volume of free fluid in the peritoneal cavity. Although FAST can detect as little as 100 mL of fluid, the results are not considered to be a positive exam unless at least 200 to 500 mL of fluid is detected. FAST is indicated for both hemodynamically stable and unstable patients (ENA, 2007). The four areas of the abdomen that are examined with this technique are the hepatorenal fossa (Morrison's pouch), splenorenal fossa, pericardial sac, and pelvis (pouch of Douglas) (ACS, 2008). The key limitation of FAST is its inability to diagnose hollow viscus or retroperitoneal injuries (ENA, 2007).

A diagnostic peritoneal lavage is a rapidly performed invasive procedure for identifying intraperitoneal blood. The popularity of this technique has decreased in the past several years as high-speed CT scanners have become more widely available; it is rarely used in children. In the peritoneal lavage procedure, a small incision or puncture is made below the umbilicus through the fascia and into the peritoneal cavity. A catheter is introduced; if gross blood (more than 10 mL) or gastrointestinal contents are withdrawn, it is considered a positive finding. If the initial aspiration does not show gross blood, then warmed isotonic solution

(10 mL/kg in a pediatric patient or 1 L in an adult) is infused rapidly through the catheter. Once the bag of fluid has infused, the fluid is allowed to drain by gravity. This fluid will then be analyzed for the presence of red or white cells (RBC or WBC), amylase, bile, feces, and food fiber (ENA, 2007). A positive test is confirmed by the presence of more than 100,000 RBC/mm³, more than 500 WBC/mm³, or positive Gram stain for bacteria. This technique can be used in both hemodynamically stable and unstable patients (Feliciano et al., 2008).

ORGAN-SPECIFIC INJURIES

Spleen

The spleen is the organ that is most commonly injured in abdominal trauma. Recent changes in management encourage nonoperative or operative preservation (splenic salvage) of this vital organ rather than its removal.

Presentation. Physical examination findings for splenic injuries are nonspecific:

- Left-sided rib pain or tenderness
- Presence of Kehr's sign (pain in the left shoulder secondary to pathology below the left diaphragm, referred pain as a result of diaphragmatic irritation by subphrenic blood)
- Localized tenderness in the left upper quadrant or generalized tenderness

- Ecchymosis or abrasions to the left upper quadrant
- Penetrating wound to left torso
- Hypotension and tachycardia
- Associated pelvic fracture, rib fractures, or diaphragmatic rupture (Feliciano et al., 2008; Moore et al., 2003)

Plan of care. CT of the abdomen with IV contrast is the modality of choice for the diagnosis of injury to the spleen. Oral contrast does not increase the sensitivity of this method for identifying injury. Small injuries that do not result in a hemoperitoneum may be missed by ultrasonography, whereas CT is useful in grading of splenic injury.

The presence of "blush" or extravasation of contrast may represent ongoing bleeding or the likelihood of arterial injury. Patients with this finding may need further evaluation via serial CT scanning, angiography, or surgery (Feliciano et al., 2008). One of the difficulties in using CT when evaluating patients for a splenic injury is the risk that fluid in the peritoneal cavity or pelvis may be falsely attributed to the spleen when there is actually a concurrent mesenteric or bowel injury.

Grading systems for splenic injuries may be based on either CT appearance or intraoperative appearance of the spleen. These systems describe the degree of parenchymal damage, capsular disruption, and vascular disruption of the splenic structures. Table 38-6 summarizes the grading system developed by the American Association for the Surgery of Trauma (AAST) (Feliciano et al., 2008; Moore et al., 2003).

The spleen performs a number of immunologic functions, such as removal of nonopsonized bacteria,

TABLE 38-6

American Association for the Surgery of Trauma Spleen Injury Scale		
Grade	**Type of Injury**	**Description of Injury**
I	Hematoma	Subcapsular, nonexpanding, less than 10% surface area
	Laceration	Capsular tear, nonbleeding, less than 1 cm parenchymal depth
II	Hematoma	Subcapsular, nonexpanding, 10% to 50% surface area; intraparenchymal, nonexpanding, less than 5 cm in diameter
	Laceration	Capsular tear, active bleeding; 1–3 cm of parenchymal depth that does not involve trabecular vessel
III	Hematoma	Subcapsular, more than 50% surface area of expanding; rupture subcapsular hematoma with active bleeding; intraparynchymal hematoma more than 5 cm or expanding
	Laceration	More than 3 cm parenchymal depth or involving trabecular vessels
IV	Hematoma	Ruptured intraparynchymal hematoma with active bleeding
	Laceration	Involving segmental or hilar vessels producing devascularization (more than 25% of spleen)
V	Hematoma	Hilar vascular injury that devascularizes the spleen
	Laceration	Completely shattered spleen

Note: Advance one grade for multiple injuries up to grade III.
Source: Adapted with permission from Moore, et al. (1995). Organ Injury Scaling: Spleen and Liver (1994 Revision). J Trauma, 2(3), 323–324.

synthesis of immunoglobulin M antibody, opsonins tuft-sin, and properdin synthesis. Blunt abdominal trauma is the most common indication for splenectomy. The risk of *overwhelming postsplenectomy infection* (OPSI) in the pediatric patient is significant and is associated with a 50% mortality rate. This risk increases with younger patient age at the time of splenectomy and is highest in the first two years following surgery (Cadili & de Gara, 2008). Asplenic patients are at risk for infections from the encapsulated organisms *Streptococcus pneumoniae, Haemophilus influenzae,* and *Meningococcus,* as well as *Escherichia coli* and *Staphylococcus aureus.*

The nonoperative approach (splenic salvage) is the preferred method for managing patients who are hemodynamically stable due to the risks associated with asplenia. It avoids the morbidity associated with operative intervention and helps preserve immune function. Nonoperative management involves bed rest, nothing-by-mouth (NPO) status, close hemodynamic monitoring for 24 to 48 hours, serial abdominal examinations, serial Hgb and Hct measurements (every 4 to 6 hours within the first 24 hours), blood product transfusions when indicated, and maintenance IV fluids. Fluid administration should be titrated to limit blood loss and prevent hemodilution, while tissue perfusion is maintained (Hatoum et al., 2002). When the patient has remained hemodynamically stable after a period of observation, activity and diet can slowly be advanced. The observation period depends on the grade of the injury and hemodynamic stability (Moore et al., 2003). The time frame has been traditionally calculated by grade of injury +1 day; however, the most recent data support management consisting of overnight bed rest for grade II and II injuries and two nights of observation for higher-grade injuries (St. Peter et al., 2008). The literature also supports the practice of monitoring hemodynamically stable pediatric patients on surgical rather than intensive care units (Mehall et al., 2001). Use of adjunctive splenic artery embolization in patients with "blush" on CT scan or ongoing splenic bleeding increases the success rate of nonoperative management (Davis et al., 1998).

Patients who are hemodynamically unstable are not suitable candidates for nonoperative management. Operative management may include repair, partial splenectomy, or total splenectomy. Different risks are associated with each approach, such as rebleeding, pseudoaneurysms, abscess formation, pneumonia, atelectasis, iatrogenic splenic injury, and need for splenectomy (Moore et al., 2003).

Consultations may include a number of subspecialty services depending on the degree of injury, such as trauma surgery, infectious diseases, interventional radiology, critical care, and rehabilitation medicine. If additional traumatic injuries exist, then consultations may include many other subspecialty services.

Patient and family instructions should include anticipatory guidance on returning to contact sports and other activities where there is risk for a blow to the torso. The length of time for which activity is restricted often depends on provider preference and the degree of injury, but may be in the range of 2 to 6 months). The importance of seeking medical evaluation for any febrile illness must be stressed, especially in patients with potentially compromised splenic function. Prophylactic antibiotics during febrile illness may be considered (Stylianos & APSA Liver/Spleen Trauma Study Group, 2002; Wegner et al., 2006).

Disposition and discharge planning. Outcomes worsen as the injury grade increases. The majority of pediatric patients with a splenic injury will heal without operative intervention with little consequence. The nonoperative success rate in children exceeds 90%. Failure of nonoperative management is associated with blush seen on CT, concurrent injury, and higher grade of injury. The use of angiography has reduced the risk of failure when the choice is made to manage patients nonoperatively (Schuster-Bruce & Nolan, 1999). Asplenic patients have a lifelong risk for serious or potentially fatal infections. The risk of OPSI is higher for younger patients; there is a direct correlation between age and OPSI (Cadili & de Gara, 2008). Improvements in immunologic therapy may lead to new therapies for the asplenic patient. Pseudoaneurysms may develop following the injury and are reported be to more common now that patients are often managed nonoperatively.

The pediatric patient with a splenic injury who was treated nonoperatively will need postdischarge follow-up in the clinic per the trauma clinician's discretion. The patient who underwent surgery will be followed routinely per the surgeon's judgment. Follow-up CT scans in patients managed nonoperatively are controversial, as management is rarely altered with the additional information made available through such imaging (Feliciano et al., 2008). Postsplenectomy vaccination with pneumococcal, *Haemophilus influenzae,* and meningococcal vaccines should be considered at 14 days, although the timing of such vaccination remains controversial. Daily penicillin prophylaxis is recommended for all pediatric patients who have undergone splenectomy before 5 years of age and prior to any future surgical or dental procedures. Consider consulting infectious diseases specialists for decisions regarding antibiotic prophylaxis (Feliciano et al., 2008; Moore et al., 2003).

Liver

While statistically the spleen is the most often injured solid organ, the liver has the highest risk for injury in blunt trauma due to its large size and partially exposed anatomic location. Nonoperative approaches to management of such injuries are common, with success rates in the range of 95% to 97% (Feliciano et al., 2008; Moore et al., 2003).

Presentation. Physical examination findings for liver injuries are nonspecific:

- Diffuse abdominal tenderness due to hemoperitoneum
- Localized tenderness seen in the right upper quadrant (RUQ)
- Occasional referred right shoulder pain
- Ecchymosis or abrasions to the RUQ
- Penetrating wound to the right torso
- Right-sided rib pain or tenderness
- Hypotension and tachycardia
- Associated pelvic or rib fractures (Fleisher et al., 2006)

Plan of care. Ultrasound and CT scanning are the primary diagnostic modalities for hemodynamically stable pediatric patients with blunt abdominal trauma (Stylianos, 2005). The FAST exam has a high sensitivity for hemoperitoneum in grade III liver injury or higher. Because diagnosis of the anatomic location of injury is difficult, however, CT is the diagnostic modality of choice. CT scanning of the abdomen and pelvis with IV contrast is used to evaluate for contrast extravasation, hemoperitoneum, evidence for associated nonhepatic injury, grading of injury, and occurrence of pseudoaneurysm (a late finding).

Grading systems are based on both the intraoperative and CT appearance of the liver. The scoring system evaluates the presence and degree of subcapsular or intrahepatic contusion, biliary disruption, and vascular injury.

Table 38-7 summarizes the grading system developed by the AAST (Moore et al., 2003).

Nonoperative management is the most common approach to liver injury. Criteria for nonoperative management include appropriate grading of the injury by CT scan and the AAST grading scale, hemodynamic stability, no evidence of peritonitis, minimal transfusion requirement related to the injury, and no associated intra-abdominal or retroperitoneal injuries requiring operative management. Nonoperative management consists of bed rest, NPO status, close hemodynamic monitoring for 24 to 48 hours, serial Hgb and Hct (every 4 to 6 hours for the first 24 hours), blood products when indicated, maintenance IV fluids, and serial abdominal examinations. Fluid administration should be titrated to limit blood loss and prevent hemodilution, while tissue perfusion is maintained (Hatoum et al., 2002). The observation period depends on the grade of the injury and the patient's hemodynamic stability (Moore et al., 2003). The time frame has been traditionally calculated as the grade of injury plus one day; however, new data support overnight bed rest for patients with grades II and II injuries and two-night observation for patients with higher-grade injuries (St. Peter et al., 2008). Evidence also supports the practice of monitoring hemodynamically stable pediatric patients on surgical rather than intensive care units (Mehall et al., 2001).

There is a higher risk for nonoperative failure in patients with large hemoperitoneum, contrast extravasation, pseudoaneurysm, and high-grade injury. Even so, these conditions are not contraindications for nonoperative management. Use of adjunctive hepatic artery embolization in patients

TABLE 38-7

American Association for the Surgery of Trauma Liver Injury Scale		
Grade	Type of Injury	Description of Injury
I	Hematoma	Subcapsular, less than 10% surface area
	Laceration	Capsular tear, less than 1 cm parenchymal depth
II	Hematoma	Subcapsular, 10% to 50% surface area: intraparenchymal less than 10 cm in diameter
	Laceration	Capsular tear, 1–3 cm parenchymal depth, less than 10 cm in length
III	Hematoma	Subcapsular, greater than 50% surface area of ruptured subcapsular or parenchymal hematoma; intraparenchymal hematoma, greater than 10 cm or expanding
	Laceration	3 cm parenchymal depth
IV	Laceration	Parenchymal disruption involving 25% to 75% hepatic lobe or 1–3 Couinaud's segments within a single lobe
V	Laceration	Parenchymal disruption involving greater than 75% of the hepatic lobe or more than 3 Couinaud's segments within a single lobe
	Vascular	Juxtahepatic venous injuries (retrohepatic vena cava/central major hepatic veins)
VI	Vascular	Hepatic avulsion

Note: Advance one grade for multiple injuries, up to grade III.
Source: Adapted with permission from Moore, et al. (1995). Organ Injury Scaling: Spleen and Liver (1994 Revision). J Trauma, 2(3), 323–324.

with "blush" or extravasation on CT scan increases the success rate of nonoperative management (Feliciano et al., 2008; Moore et al., 2003; Wegner et al., 2006).

Patients who are hemodyamically unstable with massive liver disruption and intractable bleeding, despite blood and fluid administration, need emergent surgical consultation and possible exploratory laparotomy. There is an associated high risk for massive intraoperative hemorrhage secondary to manipulation of venous injuries, which often results in patient death (Feliciano et al., 2008; Wegner et al., 2006).

Consultations may include a number of specialty services depending on the extent of the injury, such as trauma surgery, infectious diseases, interventional radiology, critical care, hepatology (in case of severe injury), and rehabilitative medicine. If additional traumatic injuries exist, then consultations may include many other specialty services.

Patient and family instructions should include anticipatory guidance on returning to contact sports and other activities where there is a risk for a blow to the torso. The length of time for which activity is restricted often depends on provider preference and the degree of injury, but is usually in the range of 2 to 6 months (Stylianos & APSA Liver/Spleen Trauma Study Group, 2002; Wegner et al., 2006).

Disposition and discharge planning.

Patients have a higher chance of survival with nonoperative management. Success rates of nonoperative management range from 85% to 90% (Wegner et al., 2006). Post injury complications potentially include recurrent bleeding, hemobilia (upper gastrointestinal bleeding from the biliary tract), biliary fistula, and intra-abdominal abscess. Poorer outcomes have been reported with surgical management and in those patients with associated injuries (Feliciano et al., 2008; Sikhondze et al., 2006).

The pediatric patient with a liver injury who was treated nonoperatively will require postdischarge follow-up in the clinic as per the trauma clinician's discretion. The patient who underwent surgery will be followed routinely as per the surgeon's judgment. Follow-up CT scans in patients managed nonoperatively are controversial, as management is rarely altered with the additional information made available through such imaging (Feliciano et al., 2008).

Pancreas

Pancreatic injuries are associated with a high morbidity and mortality, frequently as a result of delays in diagnosis and missed injury. The retroperitoneal location of the pancreas makes noninvasive diagnostic modalities less reliable. In addition, the diagnosis of pancreatic injury is difficult because it frequently requires an invasive procedure to determine the integrity of the duct (Feliciano et al., 2008; Keller et al., 1997).

Presentation. Pancreatic injuries are uncommon, as this organ is well protected from outside forces. When a pancreatic injury is found, it is often associated with trauma to the intestine (duodenum) and liver.

Early findings on physical examination include the following:

- Soft-tissue contusion in the upper abdomen
- Handlebar marking
- Tenderness to the lower ribs and costal cartilage
- Epigastric tenderness out of proportion to the finding of the abdominal examination
- Concomitant lower thoracic spine fracture
- Signs of peritonitis such as rebound tenderness, guarding, or abdominal wall rigidity
- Hypotension and tachycardia due to blood loss
- Presence of vomiting

Late findings on physical examination include the classic triad of persistent abdominal pain, palpable abdominal mass, and persistently elevated amylase levels (Fleisher et al., 2006; Moore et al., 2003).

Plan of care. CT evaluation of the pancreas may fail to identify pancreatic injury in the acute post injury period. This tendency does not reflect inaccuracies of this diagnostic method, but rather the evolving nature of the pancreatic injury. The sensitivity of CT in identifying pancreatic injury is much greater several hours after the injury; therefore, CT scan should be repeated in the pediatric trauma patient with persistent abdominal pain, elevated amylase, or fever. Repeat scanning with both IV and oral contrast should be completed to maximize the ability to accurately define the anatomy.

Serum amylase is often obtained on admission as part of the initial trauma panel. A normal serum amylase does not exclude major pancreatic trauma; the sensitivity and specificity of an early amylase level are low with this type of injury. By comparison, repeat serum amylase levels (more than 3 hours post injury) or those that are trending higher over time have greater diagnostic accuracy for pancreatic injury, especially when imaging studies are inconclusive (ACS, 2008; Feliciano et al., 2008; Jobst et al., 1999). Serum amylase may also be elevated as a result of facial trauma (Greenlee et al., 1984).

Grading of pancreatic injuries is based on the integrity of the pancreatic duct. Ductal integrity can be determined via the following modalities: magnetic resonance cholangiopancreatography (MRCP), endoscopic retrograde cholangiopancreatography (ERCP), abdominal CT with fine cuts of the pancreas, and operative exploration. Absolute serum amylase values do not correlate with the degree of injury (Table 38-8) (Moore et al., 2003).

TABLE 38-8

American Association for the Surgery of Trauma Pancreatic Injury Scale

Grade	Type of Injury	Description of Injury
I	Hematoma	Minor contusion without duct injury
	Laceration	Superficial laceration without duct injury
II	Hematoma	Major contusion without duct injury or tissue loss
	Laceration	Major laceration without duct injury or tissue loss
III	Laceration	Distal transection or parenchymal injury with duct
IV	Laceration	Proximal (to right of superior mesenteric vein) transection or parenchymal injury
V		Massive disruption of pancreatic head

Source: Adapted with permission from Moore, et al. (1995). Organ Injury Scaling: Spleen and Liver (1994 Revision). J Trauma, 2(3), 323–324.

Nonoperative management is appropriate in pediatric patients with grade I or II pancreatic injuries. Nonoperative strategies may include bed rest, bowel/pancreatic rest, nasogastric decompression, parenteral nutrition (PN), enteral feedings with elemental formula, or octreotide-therapy. Disruption of the duct may necessitate surgery or endoscopic stent placement (Keller et al., 1997; Wales et al., 2001).

Early operative management is recommended for those patients with higher-grade injury (grade III or V) to reduce the incidence of pseudocyst formation and prolonged hospitalization. Operative procedures may include urgent laparotomy, closed section drainage, distal pancreatectomy with splenic preservation, oversewing the proximal duct with drainage reconstruction of the distal pancreas, damage control surgery, or the Whipple procedure (pancreaticoduodenectomy) (Feliciano et al., 2008; Keller et al., 1997; Wales et al., 2001).

Consultations may include a number of specialty services depending on the extent of injury, such as trauma surgery, infectious diseases, interventional radiology for drain placement, critical care, gastroeneterology, endocrinology, and rehabilitative medicine. If additional traumatic injuries exist, then consultations may include many other subspecialty services.

Patient and family instructions should include anticipatory guidance on returning to contact sports and other activities where there is risk for a blow to the torso. The length of time in which activity is restricted often depends on provider preference and the degree of injury. The importance of seeking medical evaluation for any febrile illness must be stressed. Early satiety and colicky abdominal pain many be indicative of pancreatitis or pseudocyst formation (Stylianos & APSA Liver/Spleen Trauma Study Group, 2002; Wegner et al., 2006).

Disposition and Discharge Planning.   To minimize postoperative complications and preserve endocrine function, efforts should be made operatively to preserve at least 20% of the pancreatic tissue. Fistula, abscess, pancreatitis, and pseudocyst formation are complications that may potentially be seen in the pediatric patient with pancreatic injury.

Pseudocysts often form in patients who are managed nonoperatively. The outcome in this circumstance is determined by the status of the pancreatic duct. Percutaneous drainage may be effective if the pancreatic duct is intact. Percutaneous drainage should, therefore, be preceded by ERCP to determine duct integrity. If duct stenosis or injury is noted, operative management may be indicated (Moore et al., 2003).

The pediatric patient with a pancreatic injury who was managed nonoperatively will require postdischarge follow-up in the clinic as per the trauma clinician's discretion. The patient who underwent surgery will be followed routinely as per the surgeon's judgment.

Kidney

The pediatric patient is at higher risk for kidney trauma than the adult. This risk is increased due to the high incidence of preexisting kidney abnormalities, larger size of kidneys relative to patient size, and a deficiency of perinephric fat in the pediatric patient (Feliciano et al., 2008).

Presentation.
- Contusion, hematoma, or ecchymosis to the back or flank
- Abdominal or flank tenderness
- Hematuria (gross or microscopic)
- Palpable flank mass
- Tenderness in the flank, costovertebral angle
- Stab wounds posterior to the anterior axillary line (Feliciano et al., 2008; Moore et al., 2003)

Plan of care.   The most common sign of kidney trauma is hematuria, although the degree of hematuria does not correlate with the degree of injury. Those patients with microscopic hematuria of more than 50 RBCs per HPF, gross hematuria, penetrating abdominal injury, or multisystem trauma should undergo abdominal CT with IV contrast (Stylianos, 2005).

Intravenous pyelogram (IVP) may be used in the intraoperative setting to evaluate kidney function. Although IVP detects injury, it does not allow for precise grading of the injury. In pediatric patients with radiographic evidence of vascular injury or unilateral renal nonfunction, a renal arteriogram may be warranted.

The AAST grading of kidney injury is based on abdominal CT findings. This scale, which is summarized in Table 38-9, is predictive of morbidity and mortality in blunt and penetrating kidney trauma (Feliciano et al., 2008).

Approximately 95% of pediatric patients can be managed nonoperatively. Nonoperative management consists of bed rest for 24 to 72 hours or until gross hematuria resolves, IV hydration, serial Hct and Hgb, and blood pressure monitoring. Broad-spectrum antibiotics should be considered as well (Stylianos, 2005). In grade III or IV lacerations, follow-up imaging is recommended within 24 to 48 hours of injury to evaluate the amount of extravasation, kidney perfusion, and hematoma size.

Complications associated with nonoperative high-grade injuries can be managed with nonsurgical techniques such as stenting, percutaneous drainage, and angiographic embolization. Outcomes are improved when renal exploration is avoided. Patients are observed for stability of blood pressure, Hgb, Hct, and resolution of gross hematuria before discharge (ACS, 2008; Moore et al., 2003).

Surgical intervention for the injured kidney is indicated in patients with hemodynamic instability and penetrating injuries, rather than based on the injury grade. Bleeding that is not controlled by angiographic embolization requires operative management. Ultimately, 90% to 100% of grade V injuries require nephrectomy (Feliciano et al., 2008; Moore et al., 2003).

Consultations may include a number of specialty services depending on the extent of injury, such as trauma surgery, infectious diseases, interventional radiology, critical care, urology, nephrology, and rehabilitative medicine. If additional traumatic injuries exist, then consultations may include many other specialty services.

Patients and families should receive instructions that limited activty is allowed for 2 to 4 weeks after *gross* hematuria resolves. Patients may resume normal activity when *microscopic* hematuria has completely resolved. Although hypertension is rare in the post-trauma period, it may develop in the following months and require medical management. Delayed hemorrhage is a significant risk in the first weeks after injury. Medical evaluation should be sought with febrile illness (Stylianos, 2005; Stylianos & APSA Liver/Spleen Trauma Study Group, 2002).

Disposition and discharge planning. Mild kidney injuries usually resolve without complications. Nonoperative management of the pediatric patient with moderate to severe blunt injury and hemodynamic stability leads to long-term renal salvage and function. In devascularized injuries, kidney function may be altered secondary to scarring and parenchymal volume loss (Stylianos, 2005).

Blood pressure should be monitored over the first few months following the kidney injury to observe for hypertension. Urinalysis should also be monitored for resolution of hematuria. Follow-up CT scans or ultrasounds will be done at the clinician's discretion to evaluate for hematoma resolution (Stylianos, 2005).

TABLE 38-9

American Association for the Surgery of Trauma Renal Injury Scale		
Grade	**Type of Injury**	**Description of Injury**
I	Contusion	Microscopic or gross hematuria; urologic studies normal
	Hematoma	Subcapsular, nonexpanding without parenchymal laceration
II	Hematoma	Nonexpanding perirenal hematoma confined to the renal retroperitoneum
	Laceration	Less than 1 cm parenchmyal depth of renal cortex without urinary extravasation
III	Laceration	Greater than 1 cm parenchymal depth of renal cortex without collecting-system rupture or urinary extravasation
IV	Laceration	Parenchymal laceration extending through the renal cortex, medulla, and collecting system
	Vascular	Main renal artery or vein injury with contained hemorrhage
V	Laceration	Completely shattered kidney
	Vascular	Avulsion of renal hylum that devascularizes the kidney

Source: Adapted with permission from Moore, et al. (1995). Organ Injury Scaling: Spleen and Liver (1994 Revision). J Trauma, 2(3), 323–324.

Hollow viscus injury

A high incidence of hollow viscus injury accompanies penetrating trauma. Notably, any penetrating injury in which the peritoneum is breached increases the risk for small bowel perforation. The risk following blunt trauma increases proportionately to the number of solid organs that are injured. Intestinal injuries have been reported in fewer than 5% of pediatric patients who have experienced blunt abdominal trauma (Feliciano et al., 2008).

Presentation
- Abdominal wall ecchymosis or abrasion
- Abdominal tenderness
- Seat-belt sign
- Associated injuries such as lumbar distraction fracture (Chance fracture—a distraction fracture usually at the T12–L2 level) and solid-organ injury
- Signs of peritonitis such as rebound tenderness, guarding, or abdominal wall tenderness
- Handlebar marks (ACS, 2008; Cotton et al., 2004; Feliciano et al., 2008)

Plan of care. Mesenteric and small bowel injuries from blunt trauma are often delayed findings. Their diagnosis is usually based on clinical suspicion and physical examination. Frequent evaluation of the abdomen is the most important tool for early diagnosis and management. Although the WBC, Hct, and serum amylase are not good early indicators of injury, they are often useful when following trends.

Ultrasonography is a valuable screening tool for detecting abdominal injury. While it is unreliable for detection of bowel injury, it remains highly sensitive and specific for detecting hemoperitoneum (Feliciano et al., 2008; Kurkchubasche et al., 1997). The use of diagnostic peritoneal lavage is no longer common; however, when this procedure is performed, its results may show gross blood indicating bowel, mesenteric, or solid-organ injury. A cell count ratio of 1 or greater has a high specificity and 100% sensitivity for such injury (Fang et al., 1998). When hollow viscus injury is present, CT findings may include free fluid, thickened bowel, extraluminal air, mesenteric fat streaking, mesenteric hematoma, and vascular or luminal extravasation of contrast (Frick et al., 1999; Kurkchubasche et al., 1997).

The AAST grading of hollow viscus injury is based on intraoperative findings, with the exception of the duodenal or mesenteric injury, which can be evaluated by CT, ultrasound, or upper GI study. Definitive repair is relatively straightforward and is based on the grade of injury (Feliciano et al., 2008).

Children with duodenal and mesenteric hematomas may be managed nonoperatively. In contrast, large expanding or pulsatile hematomas must be explored.

Nonoperative management for a duodenal hematoma may consist of nasogastric decompression, parenteral nutrition, or nasojejunal enteral feeding beyond the hematoma (Clendenon et al., 2004; Moore et al., 2003; Shilyansky et al., 1997).

After their initial resuscitation, patients with bowel injury should undergo an exploratory laparotomy. These injuries are then addressed according to their potential for mortality. Injuries to large blood vessels and hemorrhage from solid-organ injuries are a priority for intervention. After hemorrhage is controlled, the gastrointestinal tract is explored and any identified injuries are repaired.

The routine use of postoperative nasogastric tubes is controversial in trauma patients, as prospective, controlled, randomized trials have found no advantage with their use in nontrauma patients undergoing similar procedures (Feliciano et al., 2008). Postoperative antibiotics are often administered for 24 hours following a gastric or small bowel injury. Parenteral nutrition is not usually required; early enteral nutrition is preferred whenever possible.

Abdominal compartment syndrome

Abdominal compartment syndrome (ACS) is a life-threatening complication of pediatric abdominal trauma. Most often occurring after laparotomy, it results in coagulopathy, acidosis, hypothermia, and bowel edema. Intra-abdominal packing may also contribute to the increased intra-abdominal pressure. Intra-abdominal pressure is monitored indirectly by monitoring urinary bladder pressure; ACS is present when the pressure is approximately 15 to 35 mmHg. Immediate decompression of the abdomen is necessary in this circumstance to maintain cardiopulmonary, bowel, and kidney function (Feliciano et al., 2008; Perks & Grewal, 2005)

Consultations may include a number of specialty services depending on the extent of injury, such as trauma surgery, infectious diseases, interventional radiology, critical care, and rehabilitative medicine. If additional traumatic injuries exist, then consultations may include many other specialty services.

Patient and family instruction includes discussion of postoperative activity limitations. The family should evaluate wounds daily for signs of wound infection. Medical evaluation should be sought for any patient with febrile illness, worsening abdominal pain, or bilious vomiting (Feliciano et al., 2008).

Disposition and discharge planning. Postoperative complications may include small bowel obstruction, malabsorption from small bowel resection (intestinal failure), abscess formation, or wound infection. Many pediatric patients with hollow viscus injury make a full recovery without complication (Feliciano et al., 2008; Moore et al., 2003).

The pediatric patient with a duodenal or mesenteric injury who was managed nonoperatively will require post-discharge follow-up in the clinic as per the trauma surgeon's discretion. The patient who underwent surgery will be followed routinely as per the surgeon's judgment.

Diaphragm injury

Diaphragmatic injury in the pediatric trauma patient is rare. If not recognized early, this injury may lead to incarceration or obstruction of the intestine, sepsis, and death. In addition, injuries to the diaphragm are a predictor of associated injuries and a marker of severity. The left hemidiaphragm is the most commonly injured (Ramos et al., 2000). These injuries can be asymptomatic, thereby delaying their diagnosis.

Presentation
- Dyspnea
- Orthopnea
- Chest pain (pleuritic)
- Referred scapular pain
- Decreased breath sounds
- Flail chest
- Localized or diffuse severe abdominal tenderness
- Guarding
- Rebound tenderness
- Progressive abdominal distention
- Anxiety
- Increased oxygen demand
- Tachycardia (ACS, 2008; Moore et al., 2003)

Plan of care. Diagnosis of diaphragmatic injuries can be difficult. Mechanisms such as direct injury to thoracoabdominal area, fall from high elevation, or history of a crush injury often coincide with diaphragm injury.

The initial CXR is normal in 50% of patients. Some patients may demonstrate evidence of small pneumothorax, small hemothorax, elevated diaphragm or "blurring" of the hemidiaphragm, an abnormal gas shadow obscuring the hemidiaphragm, abnormal air–fluid levels, nasogastric tube seen in the left thoracic cavity, fractured ribs with or without displacement, sternal fractures, or flail chest. Rarely, the liver can be seen in the right hemithoracic cavity. If a diaphragmatic injury is suspected, the need for a chest tube has to be carefully assessed prior to placement to prevent injury to herniated organs.

With diaphragmatic injury, the stomach may be visualized within the left hemithoracic cavity on an upper GI; also, barium enema may reveal a herniated colon within the thoracic cavity. On occasion, ultrasound may show evidence of a diaphragmatic rupture. Diagnostic peritoneal lavage is not clinically useful for evaluation of diaphragmatic rupture; rather, exploratory laparotomy or thoracoscopy are required for definitive diagnosis.

Diaphragmatic injuries are classified according to the AAST organ injury scale for diaphragmatic injuries. This scale allows for standardization of description of injury (Feliciano et al., 2008).

Patients with suspected or confirmed diaphragmatic injury need immediate operative exploration via laparotomy or thoracotomy. Nasogastric tubes should be inserted with care and not forced. Priorities of operative management include control of hemorrhage and gastrointestinal spillage. All herniated viscera are carefully reduced before the injury is repaired (Feliciano et al., 2008; Moore et al., 2003).

Consultations may include a number of specialty services depending on the extent of injury, such as trauma surgery, critical care, cardiothoracic surgery, pulmonology, plastic surgery, gastroenterology, and rehabilitative medicine. If additional traumatic injuries exist, then consultations may include many other specialty services.

Patient and families should receive instructions regarding limited activity and avoidance of contact sports. Aggressive mobility and pulmonary therapies are encouraged to prevent postoperative pneumonis; these measures include chest physical therapy, blowing bubbles, and incentive spirometry (Feliciano et al., 2008; Moore et al., 2003).

Disposition and discharge planning. Complications may include suture line dehiscence, hemidiaphragmatic paralysis/eventration secondary to phrenic nerve injury, empyema, subphrenic abscess, respiratory insufficiency, strangulation or perforation of abdominal viscera, recurrent bowel obstruction, sepsis, or pneumonia. Postoperative follow-up is mandatory to minimize sequelae. Medical evaluation should be sought for any patient who develops febrile illness, chest or abdominal pain, and dyspnea.

Spine injury

Seat-belt compression with hyperflexion and distraction from deceleration in a motor vehicle collision is a common mechanism of spine injury in children. The pediatric patient's anatomy differs from an adult, in that the iliac crests are not fully developed enough to secure the seat belt, thereby allowing the belt to position itself over the abdomen. Moreover, the child's intra-abdominal organs are less protected by the pelvis and thorax compared to the adult's organs. These anatomic differences increase children's risk for lumber spine fractures, dislocation, and paraplegia. In evaluating the pediatric patient with a "seat-belt sign" or intra-abdominal injury, it is important to assume the child has an associated spinal injury until proven otherwise

(Santschi et al., 2005); cervical spinal cord injuries are reviewed later in this chapter.

Pelvic fractures

Pelvic fractures are not common injuries in children. When present, they are associated with high-energy trauma to the lower torso. Unlike adults, children have lower mortality from pelvic trauma and are more likely to have associated injuries including abdominal and spinal cord (Holden et al., 2007; Nabaweesi et al., 2008).

Presentation
- Ecchymosis over iliac wings, pubis, labia, or scrotum
- Deformity
- Abnormal movement
- Pain on palpation of pelvic ring
- Hematoma to scrotum or vulva
- Lacerations on rectal or vaginal exam
- High-riding prostate or blood at the urinary meatus
- Abnormal peripheral pulses
- Leg-length discrepancy
- Asymmetry in rotation of the hips (ACS, 2008; Moore et al., 2003)

Plan of care. Physical examination assessing for pelvic stability should be completed prior to undertaking any diagnostic studies. Pushing both sides of the pelvis carefully toward midline with the HCP's hands on the anterior superior iliac spine, along with gently externally rotating the pelvis, assesses for stability. Pelvic bleeding may be exacerbated by excessive rocking of the pelvis.

An anterior–posterior (AP) pelvic radiograph is often performed as a screening film for patients who have suffered abdominal trauma, as it useful in identifying the presence (or absence) of pelvic fracture in conjunction with the physical examination. If a fracture is identified, additional views are often helpful in determining its extent. Inlet/outlet radiographs are completed at a 45-degree angle to the patient; inlet views may show AP displacement of the injury, while outlet views may show vertical displacement.

Computed tomography is slowly becoming a routine part of the diagnostic evaluation in patients with suspected pelvic fracture. This imaging modality is useful in determining occult fractures that are not found by physical examination or radiographs. It is also helpful in determining the integrity of the sacroiliac (SI) joint complex (Feliciano et al., 2008; Moore et al., 2003).

In evaluating pelvic injury, the HCP should take note of the three major mechanisms that cause disruption of the pelvic ring. The most common mechanism is lateral compression, often found after MVCs in which the car has been broadsided. The second most frequent mechanism is AP compression (also known as an "open book" fracture);

and the third mechanism is the vertical shear often seen after a fall from height.

Pelvic fractures are classified according to the degree of displacement or ligamentous instability. This classification system is helpful in assessing the risk of vascular injury and predicting fracture-associated pelvic hemorrhage and other injuries. A number of other classification systems are also available, but these should be used only as a general guide for treatment. The Torode and Zieg pelvic (1985) classification system is frequently used in pediatric patients (Signorino et al., 2005).

Pelvic fractures can produce significant hemorrhage even with minimal radiographic abnormality; thus initial management focuses on hemorrhage control and fluid resuscitation. Four temporary external compression methods may be used to assist with control of bleeding: pelvic binder (bedsheet or commercially available product), MAST, pelvic clamps, and external fixation (used in definitive treatment).

Angiography can be diagnostic and/or therapeutic in the pediatric patient with a hemorrhaging pelvic fracture. Indications for this procedure include presence of contrast blush on CT, pelvic or retroperitoneal hematoma, and hemodynamic instability (ACS, 2008; Feliciano et al., 2008; Moore et al., 2003).

Closed, nonhemorrhagic, noncomplex pelvic fractures may be managed with analgesia, bed rest, and limited or non-weight-bearing status depending on the injury. Urologic service consultation should be considered in any patient with confirmed or suspected injury to the urethra or bladder (Tolo, 2000).

The treatment of unstable fractures in the pediatric trauma patient is not the same as that in the adult. Patients with an immature pelvis are unlikely to require operative intervention for control of bleeding, as excessive hemorrhage is rare. Instead, operative intervention, including internal or external fixation, is used only when conservative interventions fail. The thick pelvic periosteum in the pediatric patient typically helps to stabilize the fracture, and significant bone remodeling occurs in skeletally immature patients.

Treatment of unstable fractures in the pediatric patient with an immature pelvis, and in adolescents with a mature pelvis, should follow the adult guidelines for operative management. Likewise, malaligned and acetabular fractures may require operative intervention. The benefits of operative management in open fractures include hemorrhage control, wound therapy, deformity prevention, improved mobility, and decreased risk of growth disruption (Beaty & Kasser, 2005).

Consultations may include a number of specialty services depending on the extent of injury, such as trauma surgery, critical care, orthopedic surgery, urology, and rehabilitative medicine. If additional traumatic injuries exist, then consultations may include many other specialty services.

Patients and family education should include the need for protected weight-bearing status, with a gradual return to activity being expected. An average of 4 to 6 weeks is needed for healing, as children's bones heal relatively quickly. Moderate assistance is needed at discharge for mobility and self-care. Average functional outcomes at 6 months are normal (Beaty & Kasser, 2005, Signorino et al., 2005).

Disposition and discharge planning.   Potential complications of pelvic fractures may include deep vein thrombosis, limb discrepancy, neurologic deficits, acetabular growth disturbance, hip subluxation, urologic disorders, and sexual dysfunction. Long-term morbidity in the pediatric patient is rare (Beaty & Kasser, 2005; Feliciano et al., 2008). Follow-up care depends on the clinician's preference. Repeat radiographs are usually obtained one week post injury to evaluate for bone regrowth. Physical therapy should start early and continue until mobility is restored.

Penetrating abdominal injury

Any wound from the nipple line to the gluteal crease has the potential to disrupt the peritoneal or retroperitoneal cavities (Moore et al., 2003). Although penetrating trauma is often categorized as stabbing or gunshot wounds, almost any object has the potential to penetrate the abdomen if used with enough force (ENA, 2007).

Stab wounds.   Approximately one-third of stab wounds are associated with significant harm (Moore et al., 2003). Intra-abdominal organs commonly injured from stab wounds include the small bowel, colon, diaphragm, and liver. Not all stab wounds penetrate the peritoneum, however (ENA, 2007). Management is based predominantly on serial physical examinations. Laparotomy should be considered when the patient exhibits omental evisceration, peritoneal penetration, free air on abdominal radiograph, or blood on DPL. The use of diagnostic studies in abdominal stab wounds is patient specific (Feliciano et al., 2008).

Gunshot wounds.   Gunshot wounds may be caused by either low- or high-velocity weapons. Lower-velocity plains cause cutting and lacerating types of injury, whereas higher-velocity weapons transfer kinetic energy directly to the viscera (ACS, 2008). In addition, plains have the potential to ricochet off of bony structures and fragment into secondary missiles. Approximately 80% of gunshot wounds are associated with significant injury. Gunshot wounds often involve the small bowel, colon, liver, and vascular structures (ACS, 2008).

Physical examination is less reliable with peritoneal penetration; thus routine laparotomy is a common practice for gunshot wounds at many trauma centers. Plain radiographs of the abdomen may be helpful in patients with a retained plain. CT of the abdomen or pelvis may be helpful in visualizing the plain's trajectory (Feliciano et al., 2008).

Damage control surgery is a limited operative procedure performed to control injuries that are life-threatening. Indications include hypothermia, acidemia, and coagulopathy. Damage control is considered in three stages: limited procedure for hemorrhage control and contamination control, resuscitation in the intensive care setting, and reoperation (Feliciano et al., 2008; Moore et al., 2003).

CARDIOTHORACIC TRAUMA

Justin T. Hamrick and Jennifer L. Fuller

Despite safety campaigns and federal legislation, trauma remains the greatest cause of morbidity and mortality among pediatric patients aged 1 to 14 years in the United States (Bliss & Silen, 2002; Ceran et al., 2002). Although thoracic trauma accounts for only 10% of all pediatric trauma, it carries increased morbidity and mortality and may be a marker for significant injury (Peclet et al., 1990). While the overall mortality of pediatric trauma is 3%, thoracic injury has an overall mortality rate of 12% (Fuhrman & Zimmerman, 2006). Most thoracic trauma presents as a part of multisystem trauma; it occurs in isolation in fewer than 1% of pediatric trauma patients. When this condition presents with concomitant head injury, the mortality increases even further (Peclet et al., 1990). The majority of cardiothoracic trauma in the pediatric population is to due blunt injury (60% to 92%), with MVC-related events accounting for almost 75% of all injuries (Ceran et al., 2002; Smyth, 1979; Tovar, 2008). The most common thoracic injuries are pulmonary contusion, pneumothorax, and rib fractures (Nakayama et al., 1989).

Due to the high morbidity and mortality associated with thoracic injuries in children, it is important to establish an accurate diagnosis and therapeutic plan as outlined in pediatric advanced life support (PALS) and advanced trauma life support (ATLS) protocols (American Heart Association [AHA], 2006; Kortbeek et al., 2008). Therefore, management of thoracic trauma requires stabilization and resuscitation as detailed by these guidelines (AHA, 2006; Kortbeek et al., 2008). A recent study demonstrated that predictors of significant thoracic trauma in pediatrics include increased respiratory rate, low systolic blood pressure, femur fractures, Glasgow Coma Scale score of less than 15, or abnormal chest examination (Holmes et al., 2002a). A focused physical examination followed by plain CXR, and high-resolution CT, are often indicated when thoracic injury is suspected.

As compared to adults, pediatric patients are at increased risk of morbidity and mortality from thoracic injuries for several reasons. Notably, the pediatric population has a higher oxygen consumption per body weight, a smaller lung functional residual capacity, and a higher airway closing capacity, thus elevating children's risk for atelectasis and significant hypoxia (Woosley & Mayes, 2008). Young pediatric patients, with their weak intercostal musculature and increased chest wall compliance, will typically demonstrate tachypnea and hypoxia in the face of thoracic trauma (Bliss & Silen, 2002). These physiologic features allow for significant forces to be transferred to the thoracic structures without overt evidence of external injury or rib fractures. The pediatric thoracic cavity is smaller and transmits sounds more easily than the same structure in adults, making the physical examination extremely difficult and unreliable.

CARDIAC TRAUMA

Cardiac trauma is a rare occurrence in pediatrics and is usually secondary to blunt trauma with an overall incidence of cardiac injuries being less than 3% (Hehir et al., 1990; Pitetti & Walker, 2005). The rarity of this condition may be due to the mobility of the mediastinal structures, which allow greater amounts of energy to be delivered to the underlying contents without disruption. Although occurrence rates are low, children who experience cardiac trauma may have profound hemodynamic sequelae and instability, thereby making the diagnosis and prompt interventions essential.

As with other types of pediatric trauma, the mechanism of action and the pediatric patient's anatomy lead to unique patterns of injury. Because the cardiac structures lie in an anterior location in the pediatric chest, approximately 40% of pediatric patients with a cardiac injury will have involvement of the right ventricle. The left ventricle is equally affected in 40% of patients, while the right and left atria are affected only 24% and 3% of patients, respectively. Mortality increases dramatically when more than one chamber is involved (Roddy et al., 2005).

Cardiac injury may result in functional defects (conduction abnormalities, decreased cardiac output), histologic changes (hemorrhage, infarction), or damage to vascular structures (Eshel et al., 1987). The initial cardiac evaluation in the pediatric trauma patient may be difficult. For instance, an elevated heart rate may occur secondary to trauma and agitation, but may also be an early indicator of impending circulatory collapse. Noninvasive blood pressure values may also be difficult to interpret in the agitated patient. Cardiac output, therefore, is best monitored by skin temperature and color, capillary refill, pulse quality, and heart rate.

Myocardial contusion

Cardiac contusion is the most frequent cardiac injury and commonly occurs with multisystem trauma (Kulshrestha et al., 1990). Associated injuries may include pulmonary contusions and rib fractures (Fuhrman & Zimmerman, 2006; Ildstad et al., 1990).

Myocardial contusion consists of an area of focal tissue injury that is histologically similar to infarction and may clinically present as a low cardiac output state manifested as unexplained hypotension and inadequate oxygen delivery combined with multiple arrhythmias (Ildstad et al., 1990; Pitetti & Walker, 2005; Roddy et al., 2005). Symptoms include chest pain, respiratory distress, and tachypnea. Physical examination may reveal an irregular rhythm, gallop rhythm, and rales. Diagnosis is usually made based on elevations in cardiac enzymes—specifically, troponin I (Hirsch et al., 1997). Elevations in cardiac troponin I can be diagnostic, whereas abnormalities of creatinine kinase are usually nonspecific (Biffl et al., 1994; Dowd & Krug, 1996; Pitetti & Walker, 2005). Studies have shown that severity of injury does not correlate with the amount of enzyme elevation (Langer et al., 1989).

Supportive information may be obtained through echocardiography, radionucleotide studies, and an electrocardiograph (ECG). An echocardiograph may show focal wall motion abnormalities, while a radionucleotide study may demonstrate focal areas of decreased perfusion. ECG provides rapid screening for suspected contusion, and may reveal ST-segment or T-wave changes, premature beats, and atrial or ventricular arrhythmias. A normal ECG does not rule out a suspected contusion, however, as ECG abnormalities may not appear until 12 to 48 hours after the injury. Most cardiac contusions have little clinical significance (Fuhrman & Zimmerman, 2006).

Treatment is generally supportive. Initial hemodynamic instability is rare and usually a result of persistent arrhythmias (Pitetti & Walker, 2005). Consequently, children with suspected myocardial contusions require cardiac monitoring. Although symptoms may not be present for as long as 48 hours post injury, most cardiac sequelae present within the first 12 hours (Grisoni & Volsko, 2001). Severe sequelae include ventricular wall rupture, aneurysm formation, cardiac tamponade, and necrosis resulting in cardiac failure (Roddy et al., 2005)

Commotio cordis

Cardiac concussion (commotio cordis) is usually the result of a low-impact, low-velocity blow to the chest, which may interrupt repolarization of the myocardium. This injury is primarily associated with athletic participation and is a leading cause of sudden death (Koehler et al., 2004; Maron et al., 2002). Therapeutic management is directed at arrhythmia recognition and treatment.

Valvular injury

Valvular insufficiency may be the result of direct blunt or penetrating trauma or rupture of retaining or surrounding structures (papillary muscles, chordae tendineae). Direct forces increase the chamber pressures against closed valves, thereby damaging the valves and supporting structures (Kleikamp et al., 1992). Diagnosis usually relies on clinical suspicion, physical examination, and diagnostic echocardiography. The presence of additional injuries (pneumothorax, hemothorax) may make transthoracic echocardiography (TTE) difficult; as a consequence, transesophageal echocardiography (TEE) is often the study of choice when valvular injury is suspected (Pathi et al., 1996).

Some valvular injuries may go undiagnosed for extended periods of time. Their ongoing presence may lead to ventricular overload and subsequent failure, pulmonary hypertension, or significant arrhythmias (Kleikamp et al., 1992). The aortic valve is the most commonly affected in this type of injury, followed by the mitral and tricuspid valves (Pathi et al., 1996).

Aortic insufficiency is usually more severe than other valvular abnormalities. Increasing left ventricular end diastolic volume may increase ventricular load and dilatation beyond the point of effectively increasing cardiac output, as demonstrated by the Frank-Starling curve. Over time, these effects may lead to left ventricular overload and failure. Physical examination demonstrates a midsystolic murmur heard best at the right lower sternal border. Therapeutic management is directed at maintaining forward flow across the aortic valve; this goal is accomplished by maintaining euvolemia and arterial pressures, optimizing cardiac contractility, and avoiding vasoconstriction.

Mitral valve insufficiency usually results from a more significant force due to this valve's posterior anatomic location (Roddy et al., 2005). Physical examination may identify a holosystolic murmur best heard at the cardiac apex. In addition, rales maybe auscultated as a result of increasing pulmonary pressures and pulmonary edema. A central venous pressure tracing may show prominent V waves. Therapeutic management is directed at decreasing afterload while maintaining cardiac output with volume resuscitation (Roddy et al., 2005). Surgical repair or valvular replacement is usually needed in the first week after the injury (Pathi et al., 1996).

Isolated tricuspid insufficiency is extremely rare and usually clinically insignificant. If associated with other injuries, however, it may lead to significant decreases in cardiac output. Therapeutic management is directed at increasing preload with fluid resuscitation while maintaining cardiac output and right ventricular contractility. In severe injuries, surgical correction maybe required (Kleikamp et al., 1992).

Septal injuries

First described by Hewett in 1847 in a 5-year-old child run over by a cart, septal defects (either atrial or ventricular) may occur as the direct or indirect result of trauma (Dunseth & Ferguson, 1965). Traumatic compression of the cardiac chambers during ventricular systole may injure the myocardial wall (Dunseth & Ferguson, 1965). This presentation may include arrhythmias, decreased cardiac output, or complete cardiovascular collapse. A triad of chest trauma, cardiac murmur, and conduction abnormality is highly suspicious for septal injury (Dunseth & Ferguson, 1965). For instance, a newly detected holosystolic murmur best heard at the lower sternal border may indicate the existence of a traumatic ventricular septal defect (VSD). Diagnosis is usually made by echocardiography. The therapeutic plan seeks to reduce afterload, maintain cardiac output, and decrease left-to-right shunting until definitive surgical correction can be performed.

Coronary artery injuries

Coronary arteries may be injured as the result of blunt or penetrating trauma. Dissections or fistulas may form between the coronary arteries and the cardiac chambers, leading to a coronary steal phenomenon and myocardial ischemia. Those patients with complete lacerations of the coronary arteries are unlikely to survive. Physical examination may include a continuous murmur heard best over the lower sternal border, which increases with inspiration (Roddy et al., 2005). ECG may demonstrate patterns characteristic of myocardial ischemia, and an echocardiograph will likely reveal fistula formation. Surgical intervention is usually required to correct this type of injury (Sato et al., 2007).

Pericardial injuries

Accumulation of pericardial air or fluid in an intact pericardium will increase pericardial pressures and result in tamponade, thus making pericardial injuries a life-threatening situation. *Hemopericardium* derives from a tear of the myocardium, or laceration of parietal pericardium or epicardial surfaces, whereas *pneumopericardium* results from fistula formation in either the esophagus or the bronchial tree. Hemopericardium is most often associated with right ventricular injury due to the thinness of the ventricular wall (Eshel et al., 1987). Rapid accumulation of air or fluid may cause the classic signs and symptoms of cardiac tamponade. Slow accumulation from a small injury may go unrecognized and result in chronic hemopericardium and pericarditis. Complaints may include chest pain, dyspnea, or a feeling of fullness in the chest.

Physical examination findings include Beck's triad, pericardial rub, pulsus paradoxus, cyanosis or hypoxia, and tachypnea. *Beck's triad* (jugular vein distention, distant or muffled heart sounds, and hypotension) is less reliable in the young pediatric patient. The most accurate diagnostic study for pericardial tamponade is echocardiography

(Milner et al., 2003). A CXR may reveal cardiomegaly, although normal findings do not rule out cardiac tamponade. The therapeutic plan includes intravenous fluid resuscitation to maintain cardiac output in the face of elevated pericardial pressures and pericardiocentesis. Definitive surgical correction entails creation of a pericardial window or repair of the causative injury (Woosley & Mayes, 2008).

Great vessel injuries

Injuries to the aorta and great vessels are uncommon in pediatric patients, having a less than 1% incidence following blunt trauma (Sartorelli & Vane, 2004; Trachiotis et al., 1996). More than 75% of patients die prior to arrival at the hospital (Peclet et al., 1990).

Physical examination findings may include significant differences between upper and lower extremity blood pressures, paraplegia, and fractures of the first rib and sternum. Diagnostic studies include CXR, chest CT, aortic angiography, and echocardiography (Sivit, 2002). Aggressive perioperative blood pressure and heart rate control will lessen the stress on the aortic wall and prevent free rupture while preparing for surgical repair (Sartorelli & Vane, 2004; Woosley & Mayes, 2008).

THORACIC TRAUMA

Compared to adults, children have a more compliant chest wall with more elastic ribs and a mediastinum with more mobile structures (Tovar, 2008). These anatomical differences make the pattern of pediatric thoracic injury different from that seen in adult patients. Notably, children may have significant thoracic trauma in the absence of rib fractures.

Rib fractures

Rib fractures may occur in as many as 25% to 30% of all blunt chest traumas in pediatric patients (Balci et al., 2004; Garcia et al., 1990). Although less common in young children, these injuries may occur more frequently in adolescents and serve as a marker for significant injury (Bliss & Silen, 2002; Garcia et al., 1990). Most fractures are diagnosed by CXR. Posterior rib fractures may be more difficult to detect via CXR, with oblique views being required to identify them. Posterior rib fractures should also alert the HCP to the possibility of physical abuse. Fractures of the first rib may be associated with nerve or vascular injury. Flail chest is extremely uncommon in the pediatric population but may be the cause of significant respiratory compromise when present (Figure 38-7). Therapeutic management is supportive, including adequate pain control and prevention of pneumonia, atelectasis, and hypoxia.

Pulmonary contusions

Pulmonary contusions are the most common thoracic injury in the pediatric population (Cooper et al., 1994; Haxhija et al., 2004; Nakayama et al., 1989; Smyth, 1979). At least one other organ system is involved in as many as 80% of children (Bonadio & Hellmich, 1989). This kind of injury may result from direct compression, shearing forces, or laceration from fractured ribs (Balci et al., 2004). More than 70% of pulmonary contusions occur without evidence of injury to the bony thorax (Bonadio & Hellmich, 1989). Absence of external signs of trauma and lack of respiratory compromise, therefore, are not unusual. Upon patients' admission, 90% of lung injuries are evident on CXR as focal consolidation, although some contusions may not be visible on CXR until 24 hours after the initial insult (Bonadio & Hellmich, 1989; Smyth, 1979) (Figure 38-8). At the tissue level, findings include alveolar hemorrhage, atelectasis, and edema (Bliss & Silen, 2002; Lichtmann, 1970). Exchange of gases is impaired, with alterations of the capillary alveolar membrane and alveolar fluid accumulation being noted (Tovar, 2008).

Clinical manifestations of pulmonary contusions include hypoxia, hypoventilation, decreased pulmonary compliance, and ventilation–perfusion mismatch (Allen & Cox, 1998; Bliss & Silen, 2002). Hypoxia that is resistant to oxygen therapy may be observed. Diagnosis is made by auscultation of the affected area, focal tenderness, or hemoptysis (Bonadio & Hellmich, 1989). Some milder contusions may be missed by CXR and physical examination, yet be found with the use of more sensitive studies such as chest CT (Woosley & Mayes, 2008).

Therapeutic management includes supplemental oxygen, fluid restriction, incentive spirometry, and early

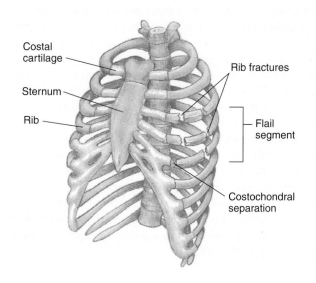

FIGURE 38-7

Flail Chest.

Source: Pollak, A. (Ed). *Critical Care Transport.* Sudbury, MA: Jones & Bartlett Publishers.

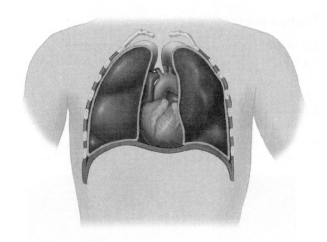

FIGURE 38-8

Left Pulmonary Contusion.

Source: Pollak, A. (Ed). *Critical Care Transport.* Sudbury, MA: Jones & Bartlett Publishers.

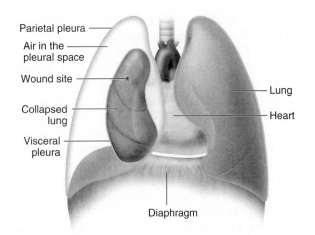

FIGURE 38-9

Pneumothorax.

Source: Pollak, A. (Ed). *Critical Care Transport.* Sudbury, MA: Jones & Bartlett Publishers.

mobilization. The severity of most contusions peaks at 2 to 3 days post injury, with the injury generally resolving within 1 week (Bonadio & Hellmich, 1989). Occasionally, if extensive lung tissue is involved, then mechanical ventilation and positive end-expiratory pressure are needed (Bliss & Silen, 2002). Secondary complications may include pneumonia, pneumatoceles, and acute respiratory distress syndrome (ARDS).

Pneumothorax and hemothorax

Injury to the lung parenchyma, thoracic structures, or vasculature may result in air or blood accumulation in the pleural space. A *pneumothorax* may result from closure of glottic structures at the time of direct thoracic compression or rupture of smaller airways after lung parenchymal laceration (Figure 38-9). This type of injury may also occur after tracheal, bronchial, or esophageal rupture (Sivit, 2002). A pneumothorax has the lowest mortality rate among the various thoracic injuries (Peclet et al., 1990). A small pneumothorax causes only mild symptoms but may quickly worsen in a patient receiving positive-pressure ventilation; by comparison, a large tension pneumothorax may quickly compromise cardiac output (Figure 38-10 and Figure 38-11).

Symptoms of pneumothorax may include tachypnea, hypoxia, and, increased work of breathing. Physical examination may reveal hypotension, a distended hemithorax with hyperresonance, and absent breath sounds—although all of these findings can be difficult to assess in children in the trauma bay. Contralateral shift of the mediastinal and neck structures is highly suggestive of tension pneumothorax. CXR may often be deferred if the physical examination indicates the existence of a tension pneumothorax. In such circumstances, performance of an immediate needle thoracentesis should be followed by chest tube placement.

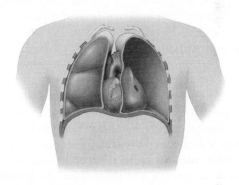

FIGURE 38-10

Tension Pneumothorax.

Source: Pollak, A. (Ed). *Critical Care Transport.* Sudbury, MA: Jones & Bartlett Publishers.

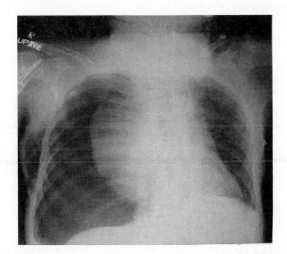

FIGURE 38-11

Right-sided Tension Pneumothorax.

Source: Courtesy of Justin T. Hamrick and Jennifer L. Fuller.

Stabilization of the airway and ventilation along with cardiovascular support may be required.

A *hemothorax* is usually the result of a rupture of low-pressure pulmonary vessels but may also occur following a great vessel injury. This condition has a high mortality rate (Peclet et al., 1990). Cardiac output may be compromised from direct cardiac compression or decreased venous return. Hemothorax may be more difficult to detect if mild, or it may present with complete cardiac collapse. Physical examination may reveal decreased or absent breath sounds with hyporesonance and shift of the mediastinal and neck structures to the contralateral side of the chest (Figure 38-12).

CXR is most often the definitive diagnostic study for hemothorax. It is followed by immediate therapeutic management that involves blood transfusion (only if the hemothorax is large volume and causing hemodynamic instability) and placement of a chest tube to allow for drainage (see Chapter 42). The placement of a chest tube may be diagnostic, prognostic, and therapeutic. The character of the drainage from the tube is important. If the drainage is sanguineous, the chance that a surgical intervention will be required is much higher if the blood is bright red (arterial) rather than dark red (venous). Drainage of intestinal contents implies that the patient has either an esophageal injury or a bowel injury with associated diaphragmatic rupture. A persistent air leak implies an underlying lung laceration, and large leaks may indicate total bronchial disruption (Mattox & Allen, 1986), requiring surgical intervention and cardiopulmonary support. While there is no absolute amount of drainage that by itself prompts surgical intervention, a persistent drainage of more than 10 mL/kg/hr increases the likelihood of surgical intervention. Chest tubes are generally removed when drainage is less than 2 to 3 mL/kg/hr and there is no persistent air bubbling in the drainage chamber off of wall suction.

Tracheal and bronchial disruption

Although they are less common in pediatric patients, tracheal and bronchial disruptions have a high mortality rate if undetected. Depending on the location of the disruption, the patient may present with neck distention, pneumomediastinum, extensive subcutaneous emphysema, or bilateral or unilateral pneumothoraces (Figure 38-13 and Figure 38-14). These injuries may rapidly progress to

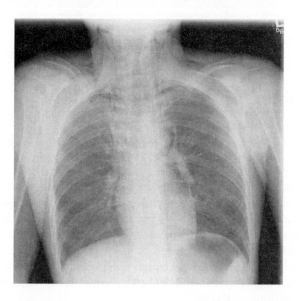

FIGURE 38-13

Plain radiograph demonstrating bronchial disruption with pneumomediastinum and extensive subcutaneous emphysema.

Source: Courtesy of Justin T. Hamrick and Jennifer L. Fuller.

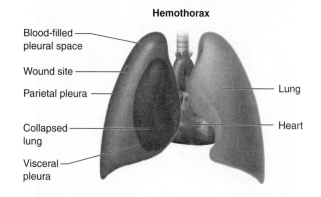

FIGURE 38-12

Hemothorax.

Source: Pollak, A. (Ed). *Critical Care Transport.* Sudbury, MA: Jones & Bartlett Publishers.

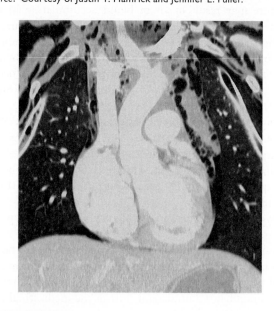

FIGURE 38-14

Computed tomography bronchial disruption with pneumomediastinum and extensive subcutaneous emphysema.

Source: Courtesy of Justin T. Hamrick and Jennifer L. Fuller.

cardiac collapse as the intrathoracic pressure increases and cardiac output and venous return are compromised (Tovar, 2008). Diagnosis is usually made by CXR or chest CT. but may require direct fiber-optic bronchoscopy to determine the extent of the injury. Large airway injury should be suspected if airway continuity appears disrupted or if a large, continuous air leak is present (Sivit, 2002). Therapeutic management options range from supportive care to surgical intervention.

Superior vena cava syndrome

Superior vena cava (SVC) syndrome, also known as superior mediastinal syndrome, is a condition that involves compression of the superior mediastinal structures, which ultimately compromises venous return to the heart. In traumatic injuries, it may also be a result of abscess or hematoma formation. SVC syndrome may occur in tandem with increased intracranial pressure (ICP), decreased cardiac output, or complete cardiac collapse. It also has some nontraumatic etiologies, such as a result of malignant masses and following surgery for congenital heart disease (Issa et al., 1983). Physical examination findings include distended neck veins, facial edema, upper thoracic edema, subcutaneous air, tachypnea, hypoxia, increased work of breathing, and signs of decreased cardiac output. CXR may reveal a widened mediastinum and subcutaneous air, whereas chest CT scan may reveal a mass with direct compression of mediastinal structures. Thoracotomy may be required to treat this condition.

Esophageal disruption

Esophageal injury, although rare (occurring in fewer than 0.2% of all blunt thoracic trauma patients), may result from direct penetrating injury or from blunt force trauma. It has a high incidence of co-injury; thus esophageal disruption should be suspected in patients with pneumomediastinum, hemomedistinum, or hemothorax. Diagnosis is confirmed by a contrast esophageal study. Therapeutic management involves surgical exploration and repair (Glatterer et al., 1985). Patients must be monitored for complications such as mediastinitis and abscess formation (Sivit, 2002).

Diaphragmatic injury

Diaphragmatic herniation or rupture may occur as the result of blunt or penetrating thoracoabdominal trauma. Although seen in fewer than 1% of pediatric trauma patients, it is usually the result of high-energy force to the thoracoabdominal area and may be a marker for additional significant injuries (Barsness et al., 2004). Physical examination reveals decreased breath sounds on the side of the injury, and possible transmission of bowel sounds within the thoracic cavity.

Diagnosis of traumatic diaphragmatic rupture may be delayed by several days, years, or even decades. Presentations include nausea, vomiting, chest pain, shoulder pain, and dyspnea, although some patients remain asymptomatic at the time of diagnosis. One proposed reason for the delay in diagnosis may be the presence of omentum, which seals the diaphragmatic defect during the initial presentation; symptomatic herniation may then occur months to years later. Traumatic diaphragmatic herniation should be considered in any patient with a history of chest or abdominal trauma who is presenting with signs of acute bowel obstruction (Kulstad, 2003). Diagnosis may be made by CXR, which reveals an elevation of the hemithorax and presence of intrathoracic bowel loops. CXR is more sensitive to left-sided injury, whereas chest CT has a higher rate of diagnosis when a bilateral injury is present (Sivit, 2002). Rupture is most likely to occur on the left hemithorax. Therapeutic management involves immediate gastric decompression and surgical repair (see page 1159).

EXTREMITY FRACTURES

Summer Watkins and Prasad Gourineni

PATHOPHYSIOLOGY

Fracture healing occurs in three stages—inflammation, reparative, and remodeling—all of which are necessary for proper bone formation. The healing time is faster in children than in adults, and is indirectly associated with age; this outcome reflects children's growth potential and thicker, more active periosteum (Kliegman et al., 2007).

The *inflammation* stage begins within the first 24 hours after injury. A hematoma forms within, and around, the fracture. The intracellular components migrate to this site to aid in the formation of first cartilage and then bone. Because pediatric bone is much more vascular than adult bone, the response in children is greater than that seen in adults. Notably, the inflammation created can cause fevers within the first 5 days after injury. Peptide-signaling proteins (TGF-β, fibroblast growth factor [FGF], PDGF, and BMPs) and immunoregulatory cytokines (IL-1, IL-6) are the key cellular components in fracture healing (Green & Swiontkowski, 2008).

During the *reparative* stage, cartilage and new blood vessels are formed and the fracture union is completed. Complications during this stage may include nonunion or malunion. In nonunion, the bone heals in two separate pieces instead of one. Although the resulting bone may be strong enough for basic use, it is at higher risk for refracture. Consequently, patients are advised to avoid strenuous use of the bone during the reparative stage. In malunion, the fracture heals out of alignment. For small children, there is a higher chance that the deformity will resolve within 6 to 12 months due to rapid remodeling. However, surgical correction may be indicated for severe cases or if the deformity causes an alteration in function.

During the *remodeling* stage, the new bone is molded into shape. Normal day-to-day forces placed upon the old fracture site give the bone strength. The old bone is reabsorbed and the new bone is formed. This process commonly occurs more quickly in the child than in the adolescent.

EPIDEMIOLOGY AND ETIOLOGY

Fractures of the skeletal system are a frequent occurrence in the pediatric population due to their underdeveloped bones and high activity levels. Developing bone is easier to break because of its incomplete ossification. A child is more likely to break a bone than to injure a tendon or ligament due to the presence of open growth plates and unossified cartilage.

The most common fracture types differ by age group. An infant may present with a clavicular fracture from birth trauma. In active, walking children, accidental fractures are more common. As the child reaches school age, distal radial, supracondylar (Figure 38-15), and tibial fractures are more prevalent. Such injuries can result from a fall with an outstretched hand or a trip and fall. As the growth plates close in adolescence, fracture patterns come to resemble those in adults.

Physeal or growth plate injuries are a special concern for the growing child. The location of a fracture relative to the growth plate has implications for permanent sequelae such as growth disturbances and osteoarthritis (Laine et al., 2010). Common fracture sites that result in such complications include the distal radius, distal femur, and distal tibia. Physeal injuries account for 30% of all pediatric fractures and occur twice as often in the upper extremities as compared to the lower extremities (Canale & Beaty, 2007). Orthopedic observation after these fractures is very important to address any growth disturbances or angulation problems that may arise. Growth plate fractures are classified by the Salter-Harris grading system (Table 38-10). Five types of fractures are distinguished depending on the location around the growth plate. Each type poses its own risk factor for growth disturbance and often determines whether surgical intervention will be necessary (Figure 38-16).

Fractures that extend into the joints space are also a concern in the pediatric population. Intra-articular injury can lead to the development of osteoarthritis (Laine et al., 2010). Identifying whether the fracture involves this critical space is important for determining long-term prognosis.

Long bone fractures are also classified by type. There are several common fractures that are typical in the pediatric population. These include buckle (Figure 38-17), complete, greenstick, and plastic deformation. Within the complete fracture group, the pattern of the fracture is also described—for example, oblique, spiral, transverse, or displaced. The two components of displacement include translation and angulation (Figure 38-18).

PRESENTATION

Any child who presents with an injury must be evaluated for a fracture. An infant or toddler with a fracture may be fussy and refuse to move the affected extremity and have pain with palpation. An older child or adolescent may be able to explain what happened and localize pain to the affected site. Referred pain may radiate from the hip to the knee or ankle. Neurological disability may sometimes hinder the child's ability to locate the injury. For example, numbness, tingling, or other variations of altered sensation may indicate nerve or vascular injury. Palpation over the affected site will usually elicit a pain response. The observer may feel crepitus, bone movement, or an uneven bony surface. Breaks in the skin and dark oozing blood may be indicative of an open fracture.

DIFFERENTIAL DIAGNOSIS

Trauma can cause tissue injury, pain, localized swelling, and lack of use without evidence of fracture. Ligament or tendon injuries are more common in the adolescent/teenage group. Infection in the form of osteomylitis or synovitis may mimic a fracture. In addition, underlying pathology may sometimes result in fracture. For example, malignancy, cyst, or osteopenia from immobility or chronic kidney disease may result in pathologic fracture.

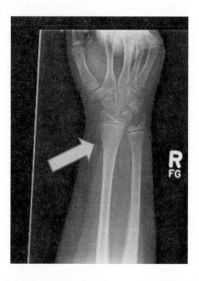

FIGURE 38-15

Distal humerus supracondylar fracture.

Source: Courtesy of Summer Watkins and Prasad Gourineni.

TABLE 38-10

Salter-Harris Fracture Classification

FRACTURE TYPE	DESCRIPTION	EXAMPLE
I	Fracture through growth plate	
II	Fracture through growth plate and metaphysis	
III	Fracture through growth plate and epiphysis	
IV	Fracture throgh growth plate, metaphysis, and epiphysis	
IV	Crushing of the growth plate	

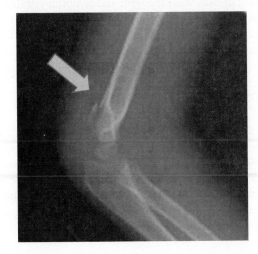

FIGURE 38-16

Salter III fracture of lateral distal tibial epiphysis.

Source: Courtesy of Summer Watkins and Prasad Gourineni.

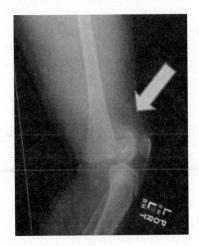

FIGURE 38-17

Distal radius buckle fracture.

Source: Courtesy of Summer Watkins and Prasad Gourineni.

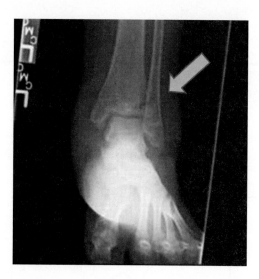

FIGURE 38-18

Acute comminuted and displaced fracture of the distal femur involving the growth plate.

Source: Courtesy of Summer Watkins and Prasad Gourineni.

PLAN OF CARE

Radiographs are important in fracture identification; both anterior–posterior and lateral views may be needed to determine the existence and extent of such injury. CT, bone scan, or MRI can also be used to further aid in diagnosis. The HCP should attempt to localize the area of injury prior to obtaining radiographical data. The least amount of radiation exposure should be of high importance in all circumstances, with the exception of child maltreatment. When this kind of abuse is suspected, a skeletal survey should be performed to evaluate for both old and new fractures.

When a fracture is suspected, immobilization, diagnostics, and pain control are important. Many fractures can be managed minimally with simple immobilization. By comparison, more complex fractures may require orthopedic surgery or traction for realignment or stabilization. Stable, nondisplaced, closed fractures in children are usually immobilized in a well-padded splint (posterior mold) until an evaluation by an orthopedic surgeon can be performed. The fracture will then be placed in a cast. Avoiding use of the affected extremity will promote healing and bone formation. The cast or splint should be kept clean and dry, and nothing should be placed in it—abrasions and foreign body entrapment can lead to a serious infection. More complicated fractures, such as displaced or open fractures, may require manipulation with sedation or open reduction with internal fixation with general anesthesia. Intramedullary rods, pins, or plates can be placed to stabilize long bone fractures. This hardware is generally removed once the bone is healed to allow for proper growth in the skeletally immature child. For large fractures, such as a femur fracture, there is a risk for fat embolism and severe bleeding.

Hemodynamic monitoring is usually required for the first 24 to 48 hours.

Open fractures are of special concern due to the possibility of osteomyelitis, cellulitis, or improper healing. A grading system is used to describe the severity of the open fracture. Grade I fractures are smaller, usually less than 1 cm in length, with little soft-tissue injury. Grade II fractures are more extensive, with greater soft-tissue damage and wounds greater than 1 cm in length. Grade III open fractures have extensive soft-tissue and osseous damage, often with significant wound contamination. These wounds have the highest risk for infection and improper healing. Grade I fractures associated with lacerations longer than 1 cm are no longer considered emergent; these injuries may only need to be irrigated, debrided, splinted, and treated with oral antibiotics for 24 to 72 hours. A first-generation cephalosporin antibiotic is generally used for this purpose (Skaggs et al., 2005). With higher-grade fractures, surgical exploration, debridement, and bone stabilization may be required. Antibiotic therapy for Gram negative coverage is typically added. Special consideration is given to wounds that were exposed to grass or a farm yard. For these wounds, a third antibiotic is added for anaerobic coverage.

While caring for the child with a fracture, pain control is of critical importance. Sedation or a hematoma block is generally used for fracture reduction and alignment. Intravenous narcotics should be administered for larger fractures such as those involving the humerus, femur, and tibia, which typically cause severe pain. Oral narcotics can be given once the patient is tolerating a general diet. Consider a stool softener if the patient is expected to use these medications for more than a few days. Once the patient reports pain to be mild to moderate, he or she can be transitioned to acetaminophen.

Patient and family education focuses on how to maintain the splint or cast, what the signs and symptoms of infection and compartment syndrome are, who to call or when to go to the emergency department should they occur, and how to manage the child's pain.

DISPOSITION AND DISCHARGE PLANNING

Some patients will require physical or occupational therapy to recover functional mobility after initial therapy. Follow-up with orthopedic surgery or the primary care provider depends on the type of fracture and the severity of the injury. For instance, children with growth plate injuries will need to be closely followed by their primary care provider for signs of impaired growth.

> **Critical Thinking**
> If a fracture involves a physis (growth plate), the family should be informed of the possibility of growth disturbance.

FACIAL TRAUMA

Pamela Bourg and Abigail Blackmore

PATHOPHYSIOLOGY

Facial trauma may be blunt or penetrating in nature, disrupting soft tissue, facial musculature, blood vessels, and the facial skeleton. Young children are especially susceptible to craniofacial trauma due to their greater cranial mass-to-body ratio.

The face is divided into three functional divisions. The upper third of the face comprises the lower portion of the frontal bone, the supraorbital ridge, and the frontal sinuses. The midface consists of the orbits, maxillary sinus, and nasal bones. The lower third of the face is made up of the teeth-bearing bones of the maxilla and mandible.

The facial muscles covering the bones are responsible for facial movements; for example, mandibular muscles open and close the jaw. Cranial nerve innervation in the face allows for many everyday facial functions. Certain cranial nerve functions may be affected by ocular, maxillofacial, and neck trauma.

EPIDEMIOLOGY AND ETIOLOGY

Although trauma is the most common cause of death in children, facial trauma is relatively uncommon in the pediatric population. A pediatric patient's facial proportions change as the face grows from infancy through young adulthood. In the very young child, the large cranium and prominent forehead generally protect the face from injury. Falls, sport-related injuries, and motor vehicle collisions are the most common causes of facial fractures (Meier & Tollefson, 2008). Although isolated abrasions, contusions, and lacerations may occur with any of the previously mentioned mechanisms of injury, the most extensive and devastating soft-tissue injuries occur from animal (especially dog) bites.

The gender distribution of facial fractures remains relatively equal until children reach school age, when injuries to boys predominate. This sex-related difference in fracture incidence is often attributed to boys having more frequent involvement in contact sports, physical activity, and dangerous peer behavior (Hatef et al., 2009).

PRESENTATION

A full description of the event and mechanism of injury should be obtained as part of the injury, and any wound contamination should be determined. Definitive complaints, such as pain or malocclusion, may be difficult for pediatric patients to express. Therefore, a comprehensive health history should be obtained from parents or caregivers (Wilson, 1999). If recent preinjury photographs (school pictures) are available, they also may be beneficial in determining the extent of the injury (Paige et al., 2000).

Special consideration should be made when performing physical assessment in the very young pediatric patient. The apprehension that results from the HCP approaching and manipulating a young child's face may be significant.

Initial evaluation of injuries to the facial skeleton should begin with close observation. Start with a full anterior view of the face and a "bird's-eye" view from the top of the head with attention to possible asymmetry. Next, systematically palpate the face to avoid errors of omission (Paige et al., 2000). The increased subcutaneous facial fat in the pediatric patient, the tendency for minimal fracture displacement, and poor compliance may also limit the ability to make an accurate diagnosis.

The orbital assessment should include an evaluation of visual acuity, pupillary size and response, visual fields, diplopia, and extraocular muscle function. Concurrent injuries are common with facial injuries. Close observation for subconjunctival hemorrhage or hyphema (blood in the anterior chamber of the eye) may require urgent ophthalmologic consultation.

The midface exam starts with the nose and includes inspection for facial symmetry and nasal obstruction (Figure 38-19). Fractures of the zygomatic arch may result in significant facial asymmetry. Malocclusion of the jaw may result from mandibular fractures, and close intraoral inspection may provide further evidence of jaw fracture. High-energy injuries to the craniofacial skeleton may result in Le Fort–type fractures (Table 38-11). The fractures in prepubescent children, however, often have a more oblique pattern due to the lack of paranasal sinus development and the presence of undescended secondary dentition that reinforces the midface (Paige et al., 2000).

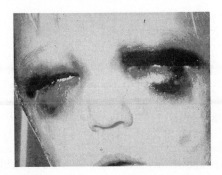

FIGURE 38-19

Facial Trauma.

Source: Courtesy of the National EMSC Resource Alliance.

TABLE 38-11

Le Fort Fractures

FRACTURE TYPE	DESCRIPTION	
LE FORT I	A transverse maxillary fracture through the lower maxilla including the maxillary aleolar process, portion of the maxillary sinus, the hard palate, and the lower aspect of the pterygoid plates. Teeth are usually contained in the detached portion of the maxilla.	
LE FORT II	A pyramidal fracture that passes through the nasal bone; lacrimal bone; floor of the orbit; infraorbital margin; across the upper portion of the zygomatic-maxillary suture line, maxillary sinus, and pterygoid plate; along the lateral wall of the maxilla; and into the pterygopalatine fossa. *This facture results in a floating maxilla and nose with possible cribiform plate fracture.*	Le Fort III Le Fort II Le Fort I
LE FORT III	This fracture is a complete separation of the facial bones from their cranial attachments (craniofacial dysjunction). The facture passes through the nasofrontal suture, the junction of the ethmoid and frontal bone, the superior orbital fissure, lateral wall of the orbit, zygomaticofrontal and temporal suture, with a high fracture of the pterygoid producing a *dishface* deformity.	

DIFFERENTIAL DIAGNOSIS

The following differential diagnoses may be considered: soft-tissue damage, head injury (TBI), ophthalmic injuries, and dental injuries and avulsions.

PLAN OF CARE

CT images provide excellent detail of the cranium, midfacial structures, and mandibular condyle. If this modality is unavailable, a panoramic radiography may be valuable in determining the extent of injury (Hatef et al., 2009). Serial Hgb and Hct monitoring enables the HCP to identify ongoing blood loss, which may not be immediately evident.

Mild airway swelling and obstruction may quickly lead to respiratory failure. Nasotracheal intubation may be contraindicated depending on the severity of the maxillofacial trauma; thus endotracheal intubation may be required.

When both endotracheal and nasotracheal intubation are not possible, a tracheotomy may be performed (Mohan et al., 2009).

Soft-tissue lacerations should be repaired within 8 to 12 hours after the injury is sustained. However, if the laceration is clean, its edges may be reapproximated as long as 24 hours post injury. In general, pediatric facial fractures are approached more conservatively than similar injuries in adult patients. For example, mandibular fracture, without displacement or malocclusion, is managed with observation, soft diet, avoidance of physical activity, and analgesics.

Pediatric patients have enormous potential for restitutional and regenerative remodeling (Hatef et al., 2009). This accelerated rate of healing may be both beneficial and problematic. Fracture reduction becomes more difficult if care is delayed due to early bone healing. Consequently, fracture reduction and fixation should be performed as soon as possible (Meier & Tollefson, 2008). When severe displacement or malocclusion is present, surgical intervention with fixation may be required (see the review of orofacial devices and surgical repairs in Chapter 34).

Depending on the site of and severity of injury, the patient may have other concurrent injuries. Thus consultations with other services may include neurosurgery, plastic surgery, ophthalmology, otolargyngology, and dentistry.

Instructions for parents or caregivers regarding activity restrictions, dietary restrictions, signs and symptoms of infection, and appropriate dosing of antibiotics and analgesic medications are appropriate. For wound care, the patient's parent or caregiver should be instructed to wash the hands with soap and water prior to undertaking any wound care or dressing changes. Generally, facial bandages may be unwieldy and difficult to keep in place, especially on children. Even so, some HCPs may ask that a wound remain covered for 24 to 48 hours. When removing a bandage, peel carefully toward the center of the wound, not away from it. Should resistance be felt, or the bandage sticks to the wound, use warm water on the bandage and lift it away slowly. Most wounds may be kept clean with a mild soap and water, followed by carefully patting them dry with a clean towel. Caregivers should also be instructed on the application of antibiotic ointment to the wounds, as appropriate.

If a child has a wound on the lip or mouth, encourage the patient to rinse the mouth after eating or drinking. The caregivers' education should recommend a soft-foods diet and avoidance of foods that may burn or sting, such as orange juice or hot, spicy foods.

DISPOSITION AND DISCHARGE PLANNING

If the patient is discharged with sutures in place, caregivers should be informed of when and where to follow up for their removal. Sutures may need to remain in place for a period ranging from 5 days to 2 weeks. Some sutures are absorbable and do not need to be removed. Follow-up appointments with the primary care provider and any necessary specialists should be arranged before the patient's discharge from the emergency department or hospital unit.

Every year, more than 12,000 children between the ages 0 and 19 years die from unintentional injury; approximately 33 children dies form this cause every day, Thus age-appropriate injury prevention should be discussed at every health care visit. For example, teaching families about proper car seat installation and seat-belt use in children has reduced injuries. Inappropriately restrained patients are at greater risk of significant facial injury than those appropriately restrained for their age (Arbogast et al., 2002).

The potential for disfigurement associated with facial fractures may resonate strongly with caregivers, and provide motivation for proper restraint—in particular, booster seats and rear seat location. Other safety devices that warrant discussion include proper use of helmets and bite blocks during contact activities.

OPHTHALMIC TRAUMA

Amy Babiuch and David Mittleman

An estimated 2.4 million eye injuries occur in the United States every year, 35% of which affect persons aged 17 or younger (Prevent Blindness America, 2008). Eye injuries are the leading cause of monocular visual disability and noncongenital unilateral blindness in children. As many as 59% of pediatric eye injuries occur during sport and recreational activities (Jandeck et al., 2000). Additionally, data from the 2000 Kids' Inpatient Database (KID) indicate that superficial wounds of the eye and adnexa account for 7.1% of hospitalizations for pediatric ocular injury (Brophy et al., 2006). Evaluation of the child with trauma to the eye should also include basic trauma evaluation if orbital blowout or blunt force trauma is present. Conversely, any patient involved in a motor vehicle collision should be evaluated for ophthalmic trauma.

Corneal abrasion

Pathophysiology. A corneal abrasion occurs when there is a breach in the corneal epithelium. The area devoid of epithelium will be visible with a blue light filter after staining with fluorescein. If an abrasion occurs over the pupillary area, vision may be severely impaired (Kanski, 2003).

Epidemiology and etiology. Corneal abrasions are likely under-reported ocular injuries, as they usually do not require hospitalization. Abrasions commonly occur from fingernail scratches, contact lenses, foreign bodies, and debris.

Presentation. Symptoms include pain, redness, tearing, photosensitivity, blurred vision, and foreign body sensation. These symptoms occur upon injury and last through healing. On physical examination, the cornea will stain positively with fluorescein dye under a blue light. In the anterior chamber (the area between the cornea and the iris), a cellular reaction may be present. If a surrounding area of corneal whitening is present, suspect a corneal ulcer. If the shape of the abrasion is vertically oriented, then a foreign body may be embedded under the upper eyelid. Young children and individuals with special health care needs may not be able to provide a description of having pain in their eye or a history of when or how it started. Consider a corneal abrasion in such pediatric patients with blepharospasm, tearing, or photosensitivity.

Differential diagnosis. The differential diagnoses to consider in a corneal abrasion include corneal ulcer, severe dry eye syndrome, vernal keratoconjunctivitis, and corneal foreign body.

Plan of care. No diagnostic testing is necessary beyond physical examination. Therapeutic management includes application of a fourth-generation fluoroquinolone or ciprofloxacin four times daily to the affected eye until healed. As the systemic absorption of these drugs is minimal, they are used routinely by pediatric ophthalmologists. Steroid eye drops or steroid/antibiotic combination eye drops should *never* be prescribed in the setting of a corneal abrasion as these medications increase the rate of infection. The eye should *not* be patched, as this practice may also increase the incidence of infection and formation of a corneal ulcer.

An ophthalmologic consultation is not necessary in the setting of an acute corneal abrasion, as patients may be readily diagnosed by an emergency department HCP. However, some patients may benefit from an ophthalmologic evaluation.

Patient and families should receive education that a foreign body sensation, blurred vision, pain, and photosensitivity are all common symptoms associated with corneal abrasion. These symptoms will abate as the abrasion heals; healing may take as long as 1 week. Pain medication will not be helpful in the setting of a corneal abrasion. If symptoms worsen, the pediatric patient should be reevaluated promptly.

Disposition and discharge planning. Although complete healing is generally expected within 1 week, large abrasions may take as long as 2 weeks to heal. Unfortunately, development of an infection within the structures of the affected eye sets the stage for a less than optimal prognosis. Additionally, a deep central abrasion could cause scar formation, which is associated with a guarded prognosis. Scars can lead to a decrease in visual acuity potential, and resultant amblyopia. In most patients, however, the overall prognosis is good.

The patient should follow up within 2 days to be evaluated for healing and presence of developing infection. If evidence of infection, such as corneal whitening, is identified, the patient should be evaluated by an ophthalmologist within 1 day. If the abrasion does not heal within 1 week, the patient should be referred to an ophthalmologist for further evaluation. If the pediatric patient experiences

worsening of symptoms or decreasing vision, he or she should be seen sooner.

Wearing protective goggles during contact sports activities decreases the risk of eye trauma. Activities that may reinjure the affected eye should be avoided until the patient is cleared by a HCP. Providing preventive and developmental education regarding pediatric patients running, jumping, or playing with objects that may cause serious eye injuries is recommended. Contact lenses should not be worn in the setting of an acute abrasion.

Corneal and conjunctival foreign body

Pathophysiology. A corneal or conjunctival foreign body involves the embedding of a foreign body within the cornea or conjunctiva. A foreign body in the cornea can be at any level of the cornea—that is, involving only a superficial epithelial breach or representing a full-thickness stromal penetration, leaving Descemet's membrane intact. While most conjunctival foreign bodies are usually embedded within the conjunctival stroma, it is imperative to confirm that the foreign body does not involve the underlying sclera (Kanski, 2003).

Epidemiology and etiology. Corneal and conjunctival foreign bodies are likely under reported ocular injuries as many do not require hospitalization. Foreign bodies commonly occur from playground and household debris.

Presentation. Symptoms include pain, redness, tearing, photosensitivity, blurred vision, and foreign body sensation. On physical examination, a foreign body will be present. If the foreign body is metallic, a surrounding rust ring may be noted. A corneal infiltrate with an anterior chamber (the area between the cornea and the iris) cellular reaction may be present. The foreign body and surrounding area will stain positively with fluorescein under a blue light. Young children and individuals with special health care needs may not be able to provide a description of having a foreign body in their eye or a history of how and when it occurred. Consider a foreign body in such pediatric patients with blepharospasm, tearing, or photosensitivity.

Differential Diagnosis. The differential diagnosis to consider in a corneal and conjunctival foreign body includes corneal ulcer, severe dry eye syndrome, vernal keratoconjunctivitis, and corneal abrasion.

Plan of care. No further diagnostic testing is necessary unless globe penetration by the foreign body is suspected (e.g., peaked pupil or flat anterior chamber).

In this circumstance, a CT scan should be performed to evaluate the globe shape and form (2-mm axial and coronal cuts). In addition, a Seidel test (Table 38-12) should be completed.

The foreign body should be removed, and corneal burring should be undertaken if a rust ring is present. This procedure can be performed by any trained medical professional depending on the level of comfort and expertise with such injuries as well as the pediatric patient's level of cooperation. Some pediatric patients will require an examination under anesthesia for removal of the foreign body; this step should be performed by an ophthalmologist. Application of a fourth-generation fluoroquinolone or ciprofloxacin four times daily to the affected eye until healed is recommended. The systemic absorption of these drugs is minimal, so these drugs are used routinely by pediatric ophthalmologists. Steroid eye drops or steroid/antibiotic combination eye drops should *never* be prescribed in the setting of a corneal foreign body as these medications increase the risk of infection. The eye should *not* be patched, as this practice also increases the incidence of infection and formation of a corneal ulcer.

The urgency of an ophthalmologic consultation depends on the referring HCP's ability to successfully remove the entire foreign body.

Patient and families should receive education that a foreign body sensation, blurred vision, pain, and photosensitivity are all common symptoms associated with corneal and conjunctival foreign bodies before and *after* removal. These symptoms will abate as the underlying abrasion from the foreign body heals, but may take as long as 1 week. Pain medication will not be helpful in this setting. If symptoms worsen, the pediatric patient should be re-evaluated promptly.

Disposition and discharge planning. Complete healing is expected within 1 week, although large abrasions associated with foreign bodies may take as long as 2 weeks to heal. Scarring can occur with deep foreign body penetration or as a result of rust rings. Scars may, in turn, lead to a decrease in visual acuity potential, with resultant amblyopia.

TABLE 38-12

Seidel Test
• Use a fluorescein strip to apply fluorescein dye to the area of the suspected open ocular wound.
• Use a blue light filter to observe the area in question.
• Fluid leaking from the anterior chamber will appear green under the light—this is a positive test.

The prognosis is guarded depending on the size, depth, and location of the foreign body.

If the foreign body was removed successfully, the patient should follow up with an ophthalmologist within 2 to 3 days. If the foreign body was not removed, the patient should see an ophthalmologist that day or the next day for evaluation and removal. In the setting of foreign body removal and evidence of infection, such as corneal whitening, or the presence of a rust ring from a metallic foreign body, the patient should be evaluated by an ophthalmologist within 1 day. If healing does not occur within 1 week, the patient should be referred to an ophthalmologist for further evaluation. If the pediatric patient experiences worsening of symptoms or decreasing vision, he or she should be seen sooner.

Wearing protective goggles during contact sports activities decreases the risk of eye trauma. Activities that may reinjure the affected eye should be avoided until the patient is cleared by a HCP. Providing preventive and developmental education regarding pediatric patients running, jumping, or playing with objects that may cause serious eye injuries is recommended.

Traumatic iritis

Pathophysiology. Traumatic iritis commonly occurs following blunt trauma from anteroposterior compression with expansion along the equatorial plane of the eye. This compression causes a transient increase in the intraocular pressure. The extent of the damage depends on the severity of the blow. Blunt trauma also commonly causes an inflammatory reaction that leads to chemotaxis of leukocytes and leakage of proteins into the anterior chamber—the condition known as iritis (Kanski, 2003).

Epidemiology and etiology. The most common causes of contusions are being struck by or against an object (44.3%), motor vehicle collisions (MVC) (26.6%), and falls (11.0%) (Brophy et al., 2006). Other frequent causes of blunt trauma include assault, domestic accidents, sports injuries (elbows, balls), elastic luggage straps, and champagne corks.

Presentation. Symptoms of traumatic iritis include pain, redness, photosensitivity, tearing, blurred vision, and a history positive for blunt trauma within the last 72 hours. On physical examination, conjunctival hyperemia may be present, along with a constricted and poorly reactive pupil. On slit lamp examination (see Chapter 50), an anterior chamber cellular reaction will be present.

Differential diagnosis. Differential diagnoses to consider in blunt trauma include corneal abrasion, uveitis, microhyphema, and intraocular tumor.

Plan of care. Diagnostic study is not required. If the symptoms do not resolve, an ophthalmologist will perform a more in-depth work-up to evaluate for the differential diagnoses listed previously. Therapeutic management should include cycloplegia with cyclopentolate 1% three times daily.

An immediate referral is not necessary. If child maltreatment is suspected, then the Child Protective Services team should be contacted.

Patient and families should receive education that complete healing is expected within 1 to 2 weeks. Symptoms should decrease in intensity over this period of time. If symptoms worsen or vision decreases, the pediatric patient should be reevaluated promptly.

Disposition and discharge planning. No long-term effect on visual function from traumatic iritis is expected, and the prognosis is good. There is no risk of recurrence unless the patient is exposed to additional trauma.

Arrange an appointment for the pediatric patient to follow up with an ophthalmologist within 3 to 5 days. If the pediatric patient experiences worsening of symptoms or decreasing vision, he or she should be evaluated sooner. Long-term follow-up is usually not required.

Wearing protective goggles during contact sports activities decreases the risk of an eye trauma. Activities that may reinjure the affected eye should be avoided until the patient is cleared by a HCP. Providing preventive and developmental education regarding the use of a helmet during appropriate sports activities can help the child avoid blunt trauma to the face and eye areas.

Traumatic hyphema

Pathophysiology. Hyphema typically occurs secondary to blunt trauma from anteroposterior compression with expansion along the equatorial plane of the eye. This compression causes a transient increase in the intraocular pressure. The extent of the damage depends on the severity of the blow. When blunt trauma disrupts the vessels of the major arterial circle of the iris, or when disruption of ciliary bodies causes hemorrhage into the anterior chamber, the condition is called a hyphema (Kanski, 2003).

Epidemiology and etiology. Hyphemas, like other contusions of the eye, are most commonly caused by being struck by or against an object (44.3%), motor vehicle collisions (MVC) (26.6%), and falls (11.0%) (Brophy et al., 2006). Other causes of such blunt trauma include assault, domestic accidents, sports injuries (elbows, balls), elastic luggage straps, and champagne corks.

Presentation. Symptoms of traumatic hyphema include pain, redness, blurred vision, and a recent history of blunt trauma to the ocular area. On physical examination, layered blood is visible in the anterior chamber when the patient is sitting up (Figure 38-20). This layered blood may fill the entire chamber and can be red or black in color. It will not appear layered if the patient is supine; instead, it will cover the entire chamber and obscure the pupil when the patient is in this position. Hyphema is easier to visualize in patients with a light-colored iris. Blood that fills the entire anterior chamber and is black is called an "eight ball hyphema"; it suggests that the blood has become deoxygenized. These patients should be seen immediately by an ophthalmologist, and there should be a high suspicion for a ruptured globe. Patients with hyphema may also have other signs of trauma in the surrounding structures, such as ecchymosis, subconjunctival hemorrhage, and eyelid or facial lacerations.

Differential diagnosis. The differential diagnosis for traumatic hyphema is limited, as there are very few entities that may be confused clinically with this injury. The only masquerading syndrome to consider in this clinical scenario is an intraocular tumor.

Plan of care. A sickle-cell prep test should be performed on all African American patients. A CT scan should be performed to evaluate for the presence of a foreign body or orbital fracture (2-mm axial and coronal cuts). A Seidel test (Table 38-12) should be performed if an open globe is suspected, such as when the patient has a peaked pupil. The HCP should conduct a visual examination if the pediatric patient is stable and cooperative, as these findings will provide a baseline for subsequent serial evaluations.

Oral prednisone in the form of a multidose pack, or its equivalent, based on the patient's age and weight, should

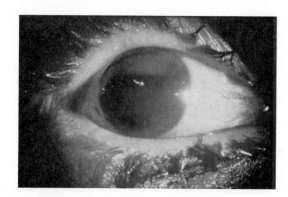

FIGURE 38-20

Hyphema with Patient in the Supine Position.

Source: Walton, W., Von Hagen, S., Grigorian, R., and Zarbin, M. (2002). "Management of TraumaticHyphema," Survey of Ophthalmology 47(4), 297–334. Courtesy of Marco A. Zarbin, MD, PhD.

be started. In addition, prednisolone acetate 1%, atropine 1%, and intraocular pressure lowering drops should be started. Avoid carbonic anhydrase inhibitors in sickle-positive patients, as these agents can increase sickling of the red blood cells and decrease outflow through the trabecular meshwork. The eye should be shielded with a metal eye shield, and the patient should be placed on 24-hour strict bed rest (Kunimoto et al., 2008). It is not necessary to keep the room darkened. The head of the bed can be kept at 30 degrees, although this positioning is not a necessity.

Ophthalmology consultation should be obtained immediately. If child maltreatment is suspected, then the Child Protective Services team should be contacted. If concurrent traumatic wounds are present, then consultation with the appropriate service (e.g., neurosurgery, plastic surgery, dentistry, or orthopedics) is warranted.

Patient and families *must* be educated that strict bed rest is imperative to prevent a rebleed and for healing; emphasize that their adherence to these instructions will promote the best healing. If the pediatric patient's social circumstances do not allow for strict bed rest, then hospitalization is recommended.

Disposition and discharge planning. The immediate risk to the patient with traumatic hyphema is that of secondary hemorrhage, which can occur as long as 1 week following trauma, although its likelihood is greatest in the first 4 days post injury. Most commonly, hyphemas will resolve without surgical intervention. In the setting of high intraocular pressure that cannot be controlled with medication, surgery to "wash out" the anterior chamber is necessary. Prognosis is guarded with this condition. Those patients who present with vision of 20/200 or worse, who have a hyphema affecting more than one-third of the anterior chamber, or who have a delayed presentation to an ophthalmologist are at higher risk of poor outcomes. Even in the setting of uncomplicated small hyphemas, permanent damage to intraocular structures can lead to complications later in life, such as glaucoma.

The pediatric patient should be followed by an ophthalmologist on a daily basis until the hyphema has resolved. Patients who are discharged to home will also be seen on a daily basis. Transportation must be available by way of family members or friends. Long-term ophthalmology follow-up is necessary to observe for complications of hyphema such as glaucoma.

Wearing protective goggles during contact sports activities decreases the risk of an eye trauma. Activities that may reinjure the affected eye should be avoided until the patient is cleared by the ophthalmologist. Providing preventive and developmental education regarding the use of a helmet during appropriate sports activities can help the child avoid blunt trauma to the face and eye areas.

Orbital blow-out fracture

Pathophysiology. A blow-out fracture of the orbital floor occurs when a large object strikes the orbit, causing a sudden increase in the orbital pressure. Because the bones of the orbital floor are weaker than those of the roof or lateral wall, they are the most common sites of fracture. The medial orbital wall is also frequently damaged in such events (Kanski, 2003).

Epidemiology and etiology. The most common causes of orbital floor fractures are being struck by or against an object (37.1%), motor vehicle collisions (34.5%), and falls (7.1%) (Brophy et al., 2006). Other causes of blunt trauma include assault, domestic accidents, sports injuries (elbows, balls), elastic luggage straps, and champagne corks.

Presentation. Symptoms include pain, possibly accompanied by diplopia and blurred vision. There is a positive history of blunt trauma to the orbital region. On physical examination, eyelid edema and ecchymosis are typically seen, occasionally with subcutaneous or conjunctival emphysema. Hypoesthesia over the inferior orbital rim can be present if the infraorbital nerve has been involved in the injury. Enophthalmos (sunken globe) may be present. Diplopia with muscle restriction secondary to entrapment may be seen. *Bradycardia that occurs with eye movement secondary to the oculocardiac reflex can be present in the setting of muscle entrapment; patients with this presentation require immediate surgical intervention.* Hyphema may be present.

Differential diagnosis. Differential diagnoses to consider in an orbital blow-out fracture include orbital edema without fracture, tripod fracture, and Le Fort fracture.

Plan of care. CT scan of the orbit (2-mm coronal and axial cuts) through the maxillary sinus should be obtained with bone windows. In addition to reviewing the CT scan for fracture, the globe should be evaluated for rupture and presence of a foreign body. A Seidel test (Table 38-12) should be performed if an open globe is suspected—for example, in a patient with a peaked pupil.

Cephalexin or an equivalent broad-spectrum oral antibiotic should be started. In addition, oral prednisone in the form of a multidose pack, or equivalent, based on the patient's age and weight, should be prescribed. The patient should be instructed to avoid nose blowing. Cold packs can be used to decrease swelling, bruising, and pain.

The urgency of the situation is determined by the presence or absence of extraocular muscle involvement. If muscle entrapment is apparent, referral to or consultation from an ophthalmologist should be obtained immediately for surgical intervention. The plastic surgery service can be consulted if additional facial trauma is present. If child maltreatment is suspected, then the Child Protective Services team should be contacted.

Activity should be restricted until a release is given from an ophthalmologist or plastic surgeon.

Disposition and discharge planning. Only those fractures that result in muscle entrapment or enophthalmos require surgical intervention. Sometimes an implant is necessary to reform the orbital floor. Atrophy of tissue can occur over long periods of time, so that successive surgical procedures may be warranted. Prognosis for visual function is good. If muscle entrapment or enophthalmos occurs, diplopia can ensue if not corrected surgically; uncorrected diplopia can lead to amblyopia.

If no muscle entrapment is present, the patient should follow up with an ophthalmologist within 1 week. Wearing protective goggles during contact sports activities decreases the risk of an eye trauma. Activities that may reinjure the affected eye should be avoided until the patient is cleared by the ophthalmologist. Preventive and developmental education regarding pediatric patients running, jumping, or playing with objects that may cause eye injuries is recommended.

Eyelid laceration

Pathophysiology. Eyelid lacerations occur when there is a disruption of the dermal and vascular structures of the eyelid. Loss of tissue, disruption of the nasolacrimal system, and disruption of the levator aponeurosis can also occur depending on the site, severity, and depth of the laceration (Kanski, 2003).

Epidemiology and etiology. Eyelid lacerations can occur from assault, domestic accidents, sports injuries (elbows, balls), elastic luggage straps, and champagne corks.

Presentation. Symptoms include pain, bleeding, swelling, and bruising. Physical examination reveals a partial- or full-thickness eyelid laceration. Lacerations can also involve the nasolacrimal system or the eyelid levator muscle.

Differential diagnosis. Differential diagnoses to consider in an eyelid laceration include a nasolacrimal duct laceration and an eyelid laceration with underlying ruptured globe injury.

Plan of care. CT scan of the orbit (2 mm coronal and axial cuts) through the maxillary sinus should be obtained with bone windows. The CT scan should be evaluated for the presence of a foreign body, globe rupture, or orbital fracture. A Seidel test (Table 38-12) should be performed if an open globe is suspected—for example, in a patient with a peaked pupil.

Tetanus toxoid should be given. If the wound resulted from an animal bite, the appropriate broad-spectrum oral antibiotic should be prescribed. If possible, the animal should be confined and tested for the rabies virus.

Referral to or consultation with an ophthalmologist or plastic surgeon for wound closure should be obtained immediately. If child maltreatment is suspected, then the Child Protective Services team should be contacted.

Patients and their families should be aware that long-term follow-up may be necessary.

Disposition and discharge planning. Further surgical intervention may be necessary in severe injuries involving tissue loss, disruption of the levator aponeurosis, or disruption of the nasolacrimal system. The severity of the wound and tissue loss will ultimately determine the level of scarring and need for future interventions. Pediatric patients younger than 9 years of age are at risk for development of amblyopia. Prognosis is good for visual function. However, the prognosis is guarded for appearance. Follow-up should be determined by the surgeon who performs the wound closure.

Wearing protective goggles during contact sports activities decreases the risk of an eye trauma. Activities that may reinjure the affected eye should be avoided until the patient is cleared by the ophthalmologist. Providing preventive and developmental education regarding pediatric patients running, jumping, or playing with objects that may cause serious eye injuries is recommended.

Corneal laceration and ruptured globe

Pathophysiology. Severe blunt trauma results in anteroposterior compression with expansion along the equatorial plane of the eye. This compression causes a transient increase in the intraocular pressure. The extent of the damage depends on the severity of the blow. When the eye wall cannot absorb the pressure from compression, a rupture occurs. Typically the rupture occurs in the anterior direction and is accompanied by prolapse of intraocular structures, most commonly the iris (yielding a peaked pupil) (Kanski, 2003).

Penetrating trauma occurs with sharp objects or flying foreign bodies. Outcomes may include either full-thickness (open globe injury) or partial-thickness corneal lacerations. Scleral lacerations are typically full thickness and cause an open globe injury.

Epidemiology and etiology. The most common causes of open wounds of the eyeball are being cut or pierced

(27.4%), struck by or against an object (26.6%), and other nonspecified injuries (18.4%) (Brophy et al., 2006). Other causes of blunt trauma include assault, domestic accidents, sports injuries, elastic luggage straps, and champagne corks (Kanski, 2003).

Presentation. Symptoms include pain, tearing, nausea and vomiting, decreased vision, and a history positive for trauma. On physical examination, a peaked or irregular pupil may be seen. The presence of a 360-degree subconjunctival hemorrhage is highly suspicious for an open globe injury. The globe may appear misshapen, with low or undetectable intraocular pressure being noted. A Seidel test (Table 38-12) will be positive.

Differential diagnosis. The differential diagnosis is limited to either a corneal laceration or a ruptured globe.

Plan of care. CT scan of the orbit (2 mm coronal and axial cuts) through the maxillary sinus should be obtained with bone windows. The CT scan should be evaluated for the presence of a foreign body, globe rupture, or orbital fracture. In addition, blood work or other studies necessary for surgical clearance should be obtained.

The eye should be protected immediately with a metal (fox) shield; if a metal shield is not available, use a cup taped over the eye. Intravenous (IV) access should be obtained, and an antiemetic, broad-spectrum antibiotic, and tetanus toxoid prophylaxis given. The patient should be admitted to the hospital with nothing by mouth (NPO) status and placed on strict bed rest.

Referral to or consultation with an ophthalmologist should be obtained immediately for surgical intervention. If child maltreatment is suspected, then the Child Protective Services team should be contacted.

The pediatric patient and family should be aware that follow-up will be frequent in the postoperative period, and they should have a mode of transportation available to keep those appointments. The patient will need to remain on restricted activity with his or her eye shielded at all times at home in the immediate postoperative period.

Disposition and discharge planning. Pediatric patients younger than 9 years of age are at risk for development of amblyopia in the injured eye, despite the anatomical outcome. Prognosis is guarded. The severity of the injury, the involvement of foreign bodies, infection, and scarring are all factors that may limit the visual prognosis.

The patient should be seen by an ophthalmologist on postoperative day one and then at the discretion of the surgeon. Frequently, patients are discharged following surgery. However, if the pediatric patient has suffered other injuries or has questionable stability postoperatively, it may be necessary for the child to remain in the hospital. The pediatric patient and family should be aware that follow-up will be frequent in the postoperative period. Additionally, the pediatric patient will require long-term follow-up with an ophthalmologist.

Wearing protective goggles during contact sports activities decreases the risk of an eye trauma. Activities that may reinjure the affected eye should be avoided until the patient is cleared by the ophthalmologist. Providing preventive and developmental education regarding pediatric patients running, jumping, or playing with objects that may cause serious eye injuries is recommended.

SPINAL CORD INJURY

Dean Barone

Spinal cord injury (SCI) is described by level and extent of injury using the *International Standards for Neurological and Functional Classification of Spinal Cord Injury* established by the American Spinal Injury Association (ASIA, 2003). Injury severity ranges from temporary to permanent, and may impair motor, sensory, or autonomic function. This type of injury may occur following either a traumatic or nontraumatic event (Table 38-13). *Tetraplegia* (formerly known as quadriplegia) is an injury in one of the eight cervical segments, whereas *paraplegia* is an injury in the thoracic, lumbar, or sacral segments.

TABLE 38-13

Spinal Cord Injury Impairment Scale		
Category	**Scale**	**Defining Characteristics**
A	Complete	No sensory or motor function preserved below S4–S5
B	Incomplete	Sensory function present; no motor function preserved below the neurologic level extending through S4–S5
C	Incomplete	Motor function preserved below the neurologic level with muscle grade less than 3
D	Incomplete	Motor function preserved below the neurologic level with muscle grade of 3 or greater
E	Normal	Sensory and motor function preserved

Source: American Spinal Injury Association, 2003.

PATHOPHYSIOLOGY

Incomplete and complete lesions

Spinal cord injury is divided into incomplete and complete lesions. An *incomplete lesion* leaves residual motor or sensory function more than three segments below the level of injury. In an incomplete lesion, observing the patient for signs of preservation of long tract function is important. Signs of an incomplete lesion include sensation or voluntary movement in the lower extremities, "sacral sparing" (sensation around the anus, voluntary rectal sphincter contractions), and voluntary toe flexion. Long tract signs include clonus, muscle spasticity, or bladder involvement, which usually indicates a lesion in the middle or upper parts of the spinal cord or in the brain (Bondurant & Oro, 1993; Waters et al., 1991).

A *complete lesion* is defined as having no preservation of motor and/or sensory function more than three levels below the level of injury. The persistence of a complete lesion beyond 24 hours may be prognostic, in that the function is unlikely to recover (Greenberg, 2006).

Spinal shock

Spinal shock is a temporary condition that follows some SCIs and results in loss of all sensorimotor function below the level of injury. It can last for several days until reflex arcs recover. Findings include flaccid paralysis and loss of rectal tone and reflexes. This condition can lead to venous pooling and relative hypovolemia.

Neurogenic shock

In neurogenic shock, impairment follows acute SCI of the sympathetic nervous system below the level of injury, leaving the parasympathetic nervous system unopposed and resulting in a triad of vasodilation (hypotension), hypothermia, and bradycardia rather than the tachycardia more commonly noted with hypotension. Neurogenic shock is unlikely to occur with SCI below the level of T6.

Autonomic dysreflexia

With the return of reflex arcs following spinal shock, some patients experience an imbalance of reflex sympathetic discharges from triggers below the level of injury, such as bladder or bowel distention. This effect leads to massive arterial vasoconstriction and reflex hypertension. Some patients experience severe headaches from the vasodilation above the level of injury. Parasympathetic responses produce profound sweating and skin flushing; bradycardia develops in an attempt to control the hypertension.

Spinal cord injury with out radiographic abnormality

Spinal cord injury without radiographic abnormality (SCIWORA) is diagnosed when radiographic studies of the bony and ligamentous structures are free of any overt abnormality despite underlying injury. Radiographic studies used in the setting of SCI have expanded beyond flexion/extension radiographs to now include CT and MRI, however; thus some sources now refer to this condition as *spinal cord injury without neuroimaging abnormality* (Yucesoy & Yuksel, 2008).

It is postulated that SCIWORA results from the normally increased elasticity of the spinous ligamentous and paravertebral soft tissue in younger children (Pang & Wilberger, 1982). The spinal cord injury in this circumstance may be either complete or incomplete. Children with SCIWORA may have a delay between injury and the onset of objective sensorimotor dysfunction, ranging from minutes to days. The age range for children with SCIWORA is 1.5 to 16 years, with a higher incidence being noted in children younger than 9 years. Children with Chiari I malformation or Down syndrome may also be at increased risk for this type of injury (Bondurant & Oro, 1993; Hamilton & Myles, 1992).

EPIDEMIOLOGY AND ETIOLOGY

Spinal cord injury most frequently occurs between the ages of 16 and 30 years; the mode age is 19 years. Nevertheless, nearly 10% of the 11,000 patients who experience SCI each year are children between the ages of 1 and 15 years. Injury to children younger than 5 years of age is rare. In young children, laxity in the ligamentous structures of the spine, a high head-to-body-weight ratio, immaturity of the spinal musculature, and underdeveloped skeletal structures increase the risk for SCI with trauma. More injuries occur at the C1–C2 level. By the age of 8 years, however, pediatric patients more closely approximate their adult counterparts in terms of spinal structure, and impairment more commonly occurs at the C5–C6 level (Figure 38-21). Mortality from SCI is higher in children than adults and is attributed to secondary associated injuries (National Spinal Cord Injury Statistical Center [NSCISC], 2010).

The most common causes of spinal cord injury are motor vehicle collisions (41%), acts of violence (15%), falls (27%), and sports (8%), especially diving. Injuries from penetrating trauma are often worse than those resulting from blunt trauma (NSCISC, 2010; Rhee et al., 2006). Other causes may include birth trauma, malignancy, and spondylosis. Injury may be primary to the spinal cord or secondary, due to such conditions as ischemia or edema.

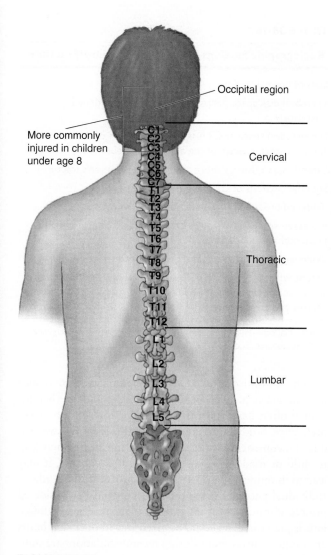

More commonly injured in children under age 8

Occipital region

Cervical

Thoracic

Lumbar

FIGURE 38-21

Spinal Injuries.

PRESENTATION

In the history, a description of the mechanism of injury (if known), concurrent medical problems, timing of onset, progression of symptoms, motor and sensory functional history, and bowel and bladder function should be ascertained. Physical examination requires serial evaluations, as the level of injury may progress depending on the underlying etiology. Motor weakness can be described as summarized in Table 38-14.

Incomplete lesions can be classified into four syndromes based on their clinical presentations: central cord syndrome, Brown-Sequard syndrome, anterior cord syndrome, and posterior cord syndrome.

Central cord syndrome—the most common incomplete spinal cord lesion—occurs from translational movement of spinal vertebrae. The mechanism of injury is often a blow

TABLE 38-14

Muscle Strength Grade	
Scale	**Description**
0	No contraction or movement
1	Slight contraction but no movement
2	Movement but not against gravity
3	Movement against gravity
4	Movement against mild resistance
5	Normal strength

to the upper face and forehead that causes hyperextension of the neck. The patient will present clinically with motor weakness of the upper extremities greater than the lower extremities, decrease in sensation below the level of the injury, and rectal and/or urinary sphincter dysfunction.

Brown-Sequard syndrome is a hemisection of the spinal cord that occurs from penetrating injuries, epidural or subdural hematomas, tumors, or arteriovenous malformations. The patient will present clinically with contralateral findings of dissociated sensory loss—that is, a loss of pain and temperature with preservation of light touch. The ipsilateral findings take the form of loss of proprioception, vibration, and motor paralysis.

Anterior cord syndrome, also known as anterior spinal artery syndrome, results from compression of the anterior spinal cord from bone, soft tissue or a mass, or occlusion of the anterior spinal artery. The patient presents clinically with plegia below the level of injury and a dissociated sensory loss. The sensory dissociation is a loss of pain and temperature sensation with the preservation of position sense, two-point discrimination, and deep pressure sensation.

Posterior cord syndrome, also known as contusion cervicalis posterior, is caused by compression of the posterior portion of the spinal cord from bone, tissue, or a mass. The patient presents clinically with paresthesia and pain in the neck, upper arms, and torso.

DIFFERENTIAL DIAGNOSIS

The following differential diagnoses should be considered for a patient presenting with nontraumatic spinal cord injury:

- Vascular: hematoma, ischemia
- Neoplastic: primary, metastatic
- Inflammatory/infection: abscess, tuberculosis, granuloma, transverse myelitis
- Diseases in the "other" categories: amyotrophic lateralizing sclerosis, Friedreich's ataxia, multiple sclerosis, cerebral palsy, spinal bifida
- Toxins/medications: methotrexate, cytosine arabinoside, radiation

PLAN OF CARE

All trauma patients at risk for SCI should be treated as if they have a spinal cord injury until proven otherwise (Table 38-15). The single most important treatment strategy is initial manual spinal stabilization while simultaneously addressing the patient's need for airway, breathing, and circulatory support (ABCs). The jaw thrust without neck extension is the best maneuver for airway positioning when SCI is suspected; however, if this position is ineffective, then the chin lift or jaw thrust with neck extension may be necessary. Respiratory impairment is directly related to the level of SCI, with patients who are injured at higher levels (C1–C2) having no cough and minimal vital capacity. Intubation of the patient with a suspected or confirmed SCI is often difficult and best performed by a specialist skilled in the procedure (AAP & AHA, 2006).

Diagnostic studies for SCI include radiographs, CT, and MRI. In the immediate post injury setting, cervical radiographs are easy to obtain and useful to evaluate the patient for cervical instability. However, they are not practical for full spinal evaluation, may not identify small fractures, and are inadequate at identifying cord injury. When obtained, these images should include anteroposterior, lateral, and odontoid views and the cervical segments through C7–T1 (Table 38-16). Spiral CT is very sensitive (99.3%) for identifying spinal fractures and may be more convenient if the patient also requires CT of the head (Brown et al., 2005). MRI is highly sensitive for identifying soft-tissue, ligamentous, or nonbony injuries. It is less convenient in the immediate postresuscitation period, but is highly valuable in identifying cord and secondary injury. If a patient complains of neck pain, has impaired sensation or motor function, or is unresponsive, then spinal immobilization should be maintained until diagnostic studies can be completed and evaluated by those who are expert in the interpretation of spinal cord imaging.

Neurogenic shock must first be differentiated from hemorrhagic shock due to a traumatic injury, as hemorrhage is best treated with blood until the bleeding is controlled. Initial management for both conditions, however, consists of isotonic fluid resuscitation.

Table 38-15

Trauma Associated with Risk for Spinal Cord Injury

Head, neck, or spinal trauma

Fall from a height

Motor vehicle collision: passenger or thrown from vehicle

Diving

Contact sports

Abusive head trauma

TABLE 38-16

Radiographic Findings in Spinal Cord Injury/Fracture

Loss of normal lordosis

Vertebral disk space narrowed anteriorly or widened posteriorly

Prevertebral space at C3 less than two-thirds of the anteroposterior width of the adjacent vertebral body

Lateral mass offset by more than 1 mm (Jefferson's fracture)

Spondylolisthesis of C2 (hangman's fracture)

Widened predental space greater than 5 mm

Increased space between the occiput and C1 and/or widened predental space (atlantoaxial dislocation)

Widening of an intervertebral disk space (distraction injury)

Odontoid view remarkable for one lateral mass of C1 forward and closer to the midline while the other lateral mass appears narrow and away from the midline (rotator subluxation)

Source: Gausche-Hill, M., et al. (2007). *APLS: The pediatric emergency medicine resource.* Sudbury, MA: Jones and Bartlett.

The administration of methylprednisolone to reduce inflammation in SCI, once considered standard therapy, is now often based on institutional protocol or physician preference. Studies of outcomes with this therapy have produced inconsistent results; thus, while the therapy may lead to mild or modest improvement in some patients, it may lead to immune impairment or avascular necrosis in others. Individual patient risks and benefits should be considered prior to administration of this agent. When methylprednisolone is prescribed, it should be given within the first 8 hours after injury. Intravenous dosing recommendations are standard at 30 mg/kg over 15 minutes, followed in 45 minutes by infusion at a rate of 5.4 mg/kg/hr. Bracken et al. (1997) recommend that administration last for 24 hours if this therapy is started within 3 hours of injury and continue for 48 hours if started 3 to 8 hours after injury.

Additional therapies include aggressive gastric decompression, as ileus is common in conjunction with SCI and may increase the patient's risk for aspiration if untreated. Once spinal shock has resolved, autonomic dysreflexia may develop. Treatment is to reduce and manage known triggers such as bowel and bladder distention. Short-acting antihypertensives may be considered before undertaking any procedures or tests expected to initiate the dysreflexia. Atropine may be beneficial for bradycardia not associated with respiratory impairment and hypoxia (Abd & Braun, 1989).

Consultation with neurosurgical or orthopedic spine specialists will determine the need for surgical stabilization or other surgery and is based on the mechanism and extent of injury. Other consultative services that may be sought include critical care for respiratory, hemodynamic, and vascular complications associated with spinal cord injury/trauma; gastroenterology for bowel training; urology for bladder training; the pain team for treatment of associated or neuropathic pain; pulmonology for respiratory support; neurology for ongoing care and control of spasticity, psychiatry for grief and/or depression, child life therapy and spiritual support for coping; and rehabilitation therapy for optimization of function.

After the patient has survived the acute phase of the spinal cord injury, the rehabilitative phase begins. The objectives during this phase include maximizing the patient's medical, functional, and psychological outcomes, and educating the patient and family regarding the new care needs. Education should begin at admission so that the family may aid in the prevention of or reduction of secondary complications such as pressure sores and aspiration. Discussion as to the serial diagnostic studies and their findings, the use of multiple therapies, and possible surgical intervention will enable families to engage in sound decision making and optimize outcomes.

DISPOSITION AND DISCHARGE PLANNING

The prognosis for functional recovery is based on the completeness of injury and time. The more complete the spinal cord injury is, especially on initial examination at 72 hours to 1 week following the injury, the less favorable the possibility of neurological recovery (ASIA & International Medical Society of Paraplegia, 2001). Neurological recovery usually peaks at 3 to 6 months post injury, although there have been reports of continued recovery at 1 year. Patients with complete injuries usually recover one level below the lowest motor level observed on the initial evaluation. Except for those in Category D and E, fewer than 1% of those with SCI fully recover. Approximately 50% of all SCIs and 92% of sport SCIs result in tetraplegia. Among those patients with tetraplegia, 17% have complete lesions and 38% have incomplete lesions. Among those with paraplegia, 23% have complete lesions and 22% have incomplete lesions. Lesions above C3 have the highest mortality rate. Survival after 24 hours is highly associated with 10-year survival (85%). Mortality is higher in the first year after injury than for subsequent years. Death after 24 hours is most commonly associated with pneumonia, sepsis, or pulmonary emboli (National Spinal Cord Injury Association [NSCIA], 1998; NSCISC, 2010).

Length of stay in hospital and rehabilitation settings has decreased over the past 30 years. Patients now average 12 days in the hospital and 38 days in the rehabilitation setting—down from 24 days and 98 days, respectively (NSCISC, 2010). During rehabilitation, functional outcome may be predicted and realistic goals established. The Functional Independence Measure (FIM) is a predictive tool often used for this purpose. The FIM is a 7-point scale that measures 18 items in 6 categories: mobility, locomotion, self-care, continence of bowel and bladder, communication, and social cognition. A score of 1 indicates total dependence on a caregiver, whereas a score of 7 reflects complete independence. Additional functional assessment scales that may be employed include the Quadriplegic Index of Function, Modified Barthal Index, Walking Index for SCI, Capabilities for Upper Extremity Instrument, Spinal Cord Independence Measure, and Canadian Occupational Performance Measure.

Critical Thinking

If a patient complains of neck pain, has impaired sensation or motor function, or is unresponsive; spinal immobilization should be maintained until diagnostic studies can be completed and evaluated by those expert in their interpretation.

THERMAL INJURIES

Elaine R. Lamb

BURNS

Pathophysiology

Burn injury in pediatric patients differs greatly from that of their adult counterparts. Injury severity varies based on weight, age, and body habitus. Children are macrocephalic, with greater body surface-to-mass ratios than adults—a factor that makes them prone to additional complications associated with burn injury. The skin of a child is also thinner than that of an adult (Duffy et al., 2006).

The anatomy of the skin plays a significant part in the assessment of burn injury. It is essential in determining severity and depth of the burn, and is used by providers for predicted outcome measurement. The skin consists of three layers: the epidermis, the dermis, and subcutaneous. To understand the depth of burn injury and the significance of this factor in burn injury, one must comprehend the physiology and function of each part (Figure 38-22).

First, the epidermis—the outermost layer of the skin—is the protective layer that provides the control for thermoregulation and protection from foreign objects. The epidermis is made up of cells called keritanocytes. This layer is avascular and, therefore, dependent on the underlying support of the second layer, the dermis, for growth and support. In the process of wound healing, the epidermis undergoes proliferation through the growth of new keritanocytes from newly generated epithelial cells provided by the dermis (Duffy et al., 2006).

The dermal layer—the second layer of the skin—is the most functional portion of the skin anatomy. It contains many of the vital characteristics and components that support the skin's function. Mostly made up of cells called fibroblasts that secrete collagen and elastin to provide the elasticity and strength of the skin, this layer also houses important components such as blood vessels, lymphatic channels, nerves, sweat glands, follicles, cytokines, and

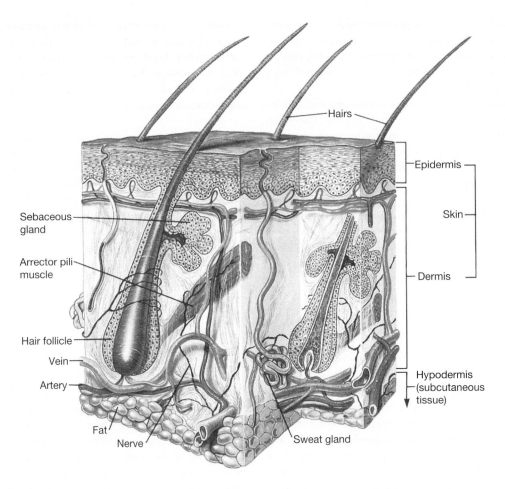

FIGURE 38-22

Anatomy of the Skin.

growth factors (Duffy et al., 2006). The hair follicle perhaps plays the most important role in wound healing in this layer: It is where new epithelial cells are generated, and serves as an excellent marker for clinical assessment of burn wound depth. The absence of the hair follicle indicates dermal damage and raises concern for a deeper injury to the third layer of the skin. In addition, the presence of cytokines in this layer is an important aspect of wound healing. The aggravation of cytokines results in inflammation, edema, and the phenomena commonly referred to in burn wound injury as "third spacing," which is clinically easily identified by diffuse swelling and drainage.

Once injury has occurred to the third layer of skin, the subcutaneous layer, wound healing is at a great deficit. It is generally accepted that in the absence of dermal components, wound healing does not occur.

In all burn injuries, the body mounts both a local and a systemic response to the injury. The local and systemic responses are proportional to the severity of the burn injury, or total body surface area (TBSA) involved. Three zones of local injury constitute the physiologic response to injury: the *zone of coagulation*, the *zone of stasis*, and the *zone of hyperemia* (Table 38-17).

The systemic response is also determined by the TBSA of the burn. Burn injuries extending over more than 15% TBSA are generally associated with a worse systemic response than smaller burns. The body undergoes a fluid shift that generally occurs 12 to 48 hours post injury. During this time frame, protein, electrolytes, and water shift from the microvasculature to the wound. Further injury to the blood vessels in the zone of coagulation and zone of stasis occurs as a result of increased capillary permeability and vasodilation. This process results in diffuse edema and places the patient at risk for compartment syndrome in either the extremity, orbital, or abdominal regions (Saffle, 2007).

In cases of significant systemic response, the patient is at risk for developing "burn shock." This phenomenon is characterized by the depletion of interstitial and intravascular volume, poor venous return, decreased preload, decreased cardiac output, hypotension, inadequate tissue perfusion, organ dysfunction, and circulatory collapse. If not controlled, it can lead to death.

If a patient is progressing toward shock, the renal system becomes highly vulnerable to additional injury. Inadequate resuscitation of the major burn may lead to inadequate kidney perfusion, renal vasoconstriction, decreased kidney

TABLE 38-17

Zones of Local Injury

ZONE OF COAGULATION *(site of injury)*:
cells in this area receive maximum contact with the heat source, necrosis ensues

ZONE OF STASIS *(area extending peripherally from sit of injury)*:
decreased blood supply, high risk for burn wound progression without adequate fluid resuscitation

ZONE OF HYPEREMIA *(located furthest from injury)*:
cells sustain minimal injury, mild inflammation, spontaneously heal in 7-10 days

blood flow, and decreased glomerular filtration. If this state continues to go untreated, or if fluid resuscitation continues to be inadequate, it can lead to kidney failure and acid–base/electrolyte imbalances.

Additionally, in the absence of proper fluid resuscitation or in cases of severe electrical injury, rhabdomyolyis can occur. This condition is characterized by the destruction of muscle cells, which in turn results in circulating myoglobin. The circulating myoglobin can occlude the kidney tubules and lead to subsequent kidney dysfunction.

Unique to burn injury is a state referred to as the hypermetabolic response, which is thought to occur predominantly in the period 24 to 72 hours after burn injury. During this time, the body experiences an increase in resting energy expenditure and cardiac output. It is thought that these demands nearly double in this condition. The body begins to undergo gluconeogenesis, characterized by insulin resistance and increased protein catabolism. Signs and symptoms of this process include weight loss, a negative nitrogen balance, and a decrease in normal energy stores. The risk of infection also increases during this time, as translocation of gastrointestinal flora may occur. Cautious monitoring of body temperature is imperative, as significant heat loss is observed. Overall, the hypermetabolic response produces generalized endocrine disruption, resulting in increased cortisol, glucagons, and catecholamine secretion.

Epidemiology and etiology

The most common mechanism of injury in pediatric patients with burns are scalds, which account for 65% to 80% of all burns in children younger than 14 years of age

(Figure 38-23). Contact burns, from sources such as an iron or other hot surface, account for approximately 20% of all pediatric burns. Electrical injury is rare in the pediatric population. High-voltage injuries are highly unlikely, as children are not generally at risk for occupational exposure, unlike the adult population. Of all electrical injuries in children younger than 12 years of age, nearly two-thirds are associated with low-voltage household current, including electrical cords, extensions, and wall outlets (Figure 38-24). Perhaps of greatest concern is the incidence of child maltreatment associated with burn injury (Figure 38-25 and Figure 38-26), reported in the literature to be as high as 20%.

According to Safe Kids Worldwide, in 2001, 532 children younger than age 14 died due to unintentional fire/burn-related injury. On average, 8 children younger than age 14 die from scald-related injures each year (children younger than age 4 account for nearly all of these deaths). In flame- and fire-related death and injury, nearly all cases of childhood death associated with residential fires are due to children's play (Safe Kids Worldwide, 2009).

The impact of pediatric burn injuries on health care resource utilization is not insignificant. Each year, more than 90,000 children younger than the age of 14 years are treated in U.S. hospital emergency departments for burn-related injuries. Scald injuries in children younger than 14 years of age are estimated to cost payers $2.1 billion annually. The estimated total charges for admission to a pediatric burn center average $22,700 per child (Klein et al., 2008). In addition, a retrospective study of data from the National Burn Repository noted that victims of child maltreatment by burning account for increased severity

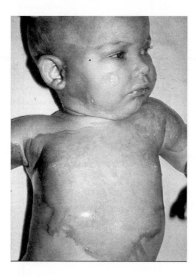

FIGURE 38-23

Scald Burn.

Source: Courtesy of the National EMSC Resource Alliance.

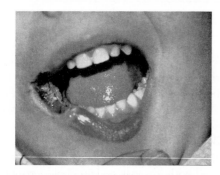

FIGURE 38-24

Electrical Burn.

Source: Courtesy of the National EMSC Resource Alliance.

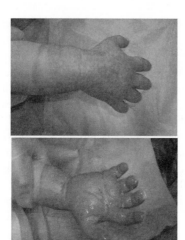

FIGURE 38-25

Child Maltreatment Burn-Glove Pattern.

Source: Courtesy of Elaine R. Lamb.

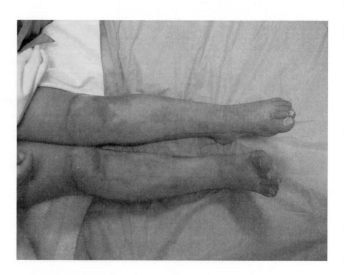

FIGURE 38-26

Child Maltreatment Burn-Stocking Pattern.

Source: Courtesy of Elaine R. Lamb.

of injury, increased hospital length of stay, and increased associated hospital/health care costs (American Burn Association, 2009).

Presentation

The assessment of a pediatric burn victim follows the general approach described for the trauma patient. Unique to burn care, however, is a focus on inhalation injury in the early assessment of the airway. Most early airway emergencies in pediatric burn injury involve the upper airway. In the exposure of the patient, note and account for an estimated TBSA for the burn. Several methods for determining this area are available. In particular, use of an objective software program is simple and may assist in standardizing an otherwise subjective analysis. The Sage Diagram (www. sagediagram.com) is an easily accessible (via the Internet), free-to-use program employed by several pediatric burn centers in the United States. Burn centers also generally accept the Lund and Browder chart as the standard for communication regarding TBSA (Table 38-18). The Rule of Nines, although less commonly used, is also an easy-to-use tool for assessment (Figure 38-27). If an assessment tool is unavailable, or if the HCP is on scene of the incident, a reasonable alternative is to utilize the size of the child's palm as an estimate of 1% TBSA (Figure 38-28).

Part of the exposure of the burned child includes ensuring that the burning process is ceased. If a hot substance is present on the skin, it needs to be addressed at this time. In addition, prompt covering of the patient is essential because the patient will be at greater risk for heat loss due to the loss of integumentary protection.

Pertinent questions to ask in the history regard the mechanism of injury. Is there associated trauma? Is the mechanism described consistent with the pattern witnessed, or is there concern for maltreatment? The agent involved is important as well. Contact, flame, and grease (or other liquids of high consistency) tend to penetrate the dermis and may lead to a burn of greater depth.

In burn care, fluid resuscitation is based on the time of injury, not the time of presentation. Document whether fluids were administered prior to assuming care, as these are considered when ordering subsequent fluid therapy. Verify that immunizations are to up-to-date, particularly tetanus immunization; a tetanus booster is indicated if the child is behind in this schedule.

Burn wound injuries are classified into three categories: superficial, partial thickness, and full thickness. These injuries are categorized based on their depth and the damage to the anatomy of the skin structure.

Superficial injury is restricted to the epidermal layer. The most common example of this type of burn is the simple sunburn (Figure 38-29). The affected area is erythematous, painful, and usually absent of bullae. In this process the keritanocytes slough, but generally regenerate spontaneously within approximately 1 week (Duffy et al., 2006).

Partial-thickness injury extends into the dermal layer of the skin. It is the most frequent burn for which treatment is sought in a health care setting. Partial-thickness injuries can further be classified based on the damage to the dermis as *superficial partial thickness* or *deep partial thickness* (Figure 38-30 and Figure 38-31). Almost all partial-thickness injuries, however, present with bullae, and are generally very painful given the exposure of nerve endings. A superficial

TABLE 38-18

Lund and Browder Chart								
	Age in Years					**Percentage Burned**		
Area	0–1	1–4	5–9	10–15	Adults	Second Degree	Third Degree	Total
Head	19	17	13	10	7			
Neck	2	2	2	2	2			
Anterior trunk	13	13	13	13	13			
Posterior trunk	13	13	13	13	13			
Right buttock	2 ½	2 ½	2 ½	2 ½	2 ½			
Left buttock	2 ½	2 ½	2 ½	2 ½	2 ½			
Genitalia	1	1	1	1	1			
Right upper arm	4	4	4	4	4			
Left upper arm	4	4	4	4	4			
Right lower arm	3	3	3	3	3			
Left lower arm	3	3	3	3	3			
Right hand	2 ½	2 ½	2 ½	2 ½	2 ½			
Left hand	2 ½	2 ½	2 ½	2 ½	2 ½			
Right thigh	5 ½	6 ½	8 ½	8 ½	9 ½			
Left thigh	5 ½	6 ½	8 ½	8 ½	9 ½			
Right leg	5	5	5 ½	6	7			
Left leg	5	5	5 ½	6	7			
Right foot	3 ½	3 ½	3 ½	3 ½	3 ½			
Left foot	3 ½	3 ½	3 ½	3 ½	3 ½			
					Total			

Source: Adapted from Lund, C., & Browder, N. (1944). The estimation of areas of burns. *Surgical Gynecology and Obstetrics, 79,* 352–358.

RULE OF NINES

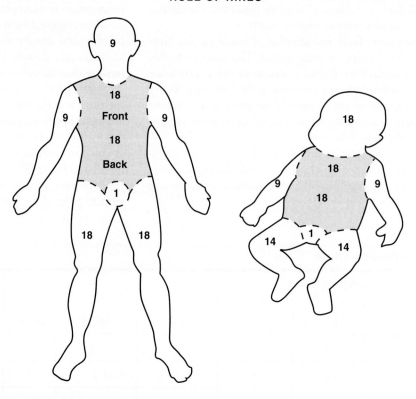

FIGURE 38-27

Rule of Nines.

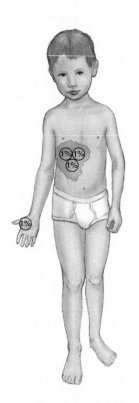

FIGURE 38-28

Child's Palm to Estimate the Burn Surface Area.

Source: Pollak, A. (Ed). (2011). *Critical Care Transport*. Sudbury, MA: Jones & Bartlett.

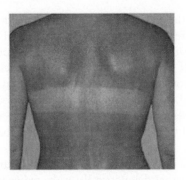

FIGURE 38-29

Superficial Burn.

Source: Courtesy of Elaine R. Lamb.

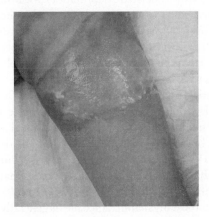

FIGURE 38-30

Superficial Partial Thickness Burn.

Source: Courtesy of Elaine R. Lamb.

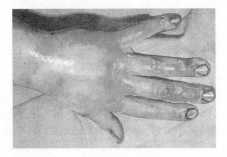

FIGURE 38-31

Deep Partial Thickness Burn.

Source: Courtesy of Elaine R. Lamb.

partial-thickness injury is generally restricted to the upper one-third of the dermal layer and will heal with the assistance of topical antimicrobials in approximately 2 to 3 weeks. Scalds are a mechanism of injury often associated with these burns. In contrast, a deep partial-thickness injury generally has a zone of necrosis that extends to the deep dermal tissue and may require approximately 3 to 6 weeks with the assistance of topical antimicrobials to heal (Duffy et al., 2006). Clinical assessment of these burn injuries involves

inspection for capillary refill, which can easily differentiate such an injury from a full-thickness burn. Mechanisms of injury often associated with deep partial-thickness injury include scalds, flame injuries, grease burns, and mechanical injuries (such as road rash or treadmill injuries).

Full-thickness burns involve penetration of the zone of injury beyond the dermal layer. In this case, the hair follicles are disrupted and not present on clinical evaluation (Figure 38-32). Given their absence, the likelihood of spontaneous healing is minimal. Assess for the presence or absence of capillary refill. The absence of capillary refill—also known as a "nonblanching" wound—is highly suspicious for a full-thickness injury. A common misunderstanding is that these wounds are nonpainful because the nerve endings are theoretically not preserved; however, in most patients there are surrounding or interspersed areas of partial-thickness injury that can cause great discomfort for the patient (Duffy et al., 2006). Mechanisms of injury often associated with full-thickness injury include prolonged contact with hot surfaces (e.g., contact burns or higher-consistency liquids), flame injury, immersion injury (often child maltreatment), and mechanical injury.

Differential diagnosis

The differential diagnoses for burn injury are summarized in Table 38-19.

Plan of care

In most cases of burn injury, there is little need for the involvement of ancillary laboratory or diagnostic studies.

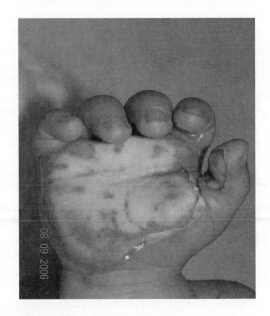

FIGURE 38-32

Full Thickness Burn.

Source: Courtesy of Elaine R. Lamb.

TABLE 38-19

Differential Diagnoses for Burns

- Burn injury
- Toxic epidermal necrolysis
- Purpura fulminans
- Staphylococcal scalded skin syndrome
- Soft-tissue infection
- Epidermis bullosa

Most pediatric burn injuries are associated with TBSA of 15% or less. In the absence of associated traumatic findings, further tertiary examinations are unnecessary.

In contrast, patients with burns covering more than 15% TBSA should have additional studies ordered at baseline, including a basic metabolic panel (serum electrolytes, blood urea nitrogen, creatinine) and a serum prealbumin. Prealbumin is the nutritional marker for the hypermetabolic state and serves as a means to evaluate nutritional efficiency during resuscitation. Hypoalbuminemia is common in patients with extensive burns. Although the baseline prealbumin may be within normal range, this level should be continually monitored every 72 hours, as a drop is anticipated. Members of the burn community well know that blunting the nutritional loss of protein can serve to expeditiously treat the hypermetabolic response, thereby reducing the risk of poor patient outcome. Anticipate a false hypocalcemia level on initial evaluation. When accounting for the associated hypoalbuminemia, calcium levels are usually normal after adjustment. Hyponatremia and hypoglycemia are also not unusual initial findings, particularly in the child weighing less than 30 kg, due to depleted glycogen stores.

In some unique cases of burn injury, additional diagnostic studies are warranted. Smoke inhalation injuries should be further evaluated with a carboxyhemoglobin level. Carboxyhemoglobin binds to heme containing enzymes, including hemoglobin and mitochondrial cytochromes; a level greater than 20% is considered significant for injury. A baseline arterial or venous blood gas is indicated, with repeat evaluation as clinically relevant. Metabolic acidosis is common; however, if the severity of acidosis is greater than would be expected with the associated carbon monoxide level, then cyanide poisoning should also be considered.

Electrical injuries in pediatric patients, as mentioned earlier, are predominantly the result of low-voltage current. Such injuries require little evaluation with diagnostic studies. All patients with electrical injury should have their urine tested at the bedside or via urinalysis to evaluate urine pH for acidosis associated with injury. A goal urine pH is greater than 6. A urine myoglobin level is necessary in patients who have sustained high-voltage electrical injury or have pigmented urine. In addition, all patients should have a baseline ECG to evaluate for ST-segment changes.

A review of the literature suggests that evaluation of cardiac enzymes (Creatinine Kinase-MB or troponin I) is not helpful in the patient who has sustained a low-voltage electrical injury. If patients have a noted ST-segment change, a cardiology consult and admission for telemetry monitoring are indicated. In the absence of loss of consciousness, findings of ST-segment changes, or high-voltage injury, most patients will be able to be discharged from the emergency department.

Any patient noted to have associated traumatic injury should be further diagnostically evaluated as indicated for the problem.

Initial care of the pediatric burn injury is not different from that of any other trauma patient. Directed care to first manage any associated abnormalities with the patient's airway, breathing, or circulation should be the primary concern. Given the overwhelming need for rapid fluid resuscitation in the burned patient, however, it is imperative that during the circulatory assessment, IV access is obtained for all patients with burns covering more than 15% TBSA and in most patients with burns affecting 5% to 10% TBSA.

Burns less than 15% TBSA may not require aggressive IV fluid resuscitation. If the child has sustained a less than 5% TBSA burn and is able to tolerate adequate oral intake, obtaining IV access may not be necessary. For burns of 5% to 10% TBSA, IV resuscitation at the daily maintenance rate is usually sufficient. For burns of 10% to 15% TBSA, 1 to 1½ times the daily maintenance rate is generally accepted as desirable. Burns with 15% or greater TBSA require careful, well-observed, large-volume fluid resuscitation in a critical care setting (Greenhalgh, 2007; Sheridan, 2002).

The Parkland formula is well accepted as a starting point for fluid resuscitation in most major burn centers (Table 38-20 and Table 38-21). Although continuous monitoring for cardiovascular compromise through evaluation of blood pressure, presence of pulses, and perfusion is indicated, urine output remains the standard for the assessment of effective fluid resuscitation in the pediatric burn patient.

Complications of fluid over-resuscitation may be severe and include the potential for compartment syndrome, acute respiratory distress syndrome, increased dependence on mechanical ventilation, and overall increased mortality. In addition, the presence of overwhelming edema can impede capillary perfusion and further progress burn wound depth (Bak et al., 2009). Complications of fluid under-resuscitation are similarly significant, including hypovolemic shock, kidney failure, potential for wound progression (related to inadequate perfusion), and increased mortality.

Constant monitoring of circulatory status is essential, along with frequent neurovascular checks of all involved extremities. Torso burns, particularly circumferential injuries, are at increased risk for decreased chest wall compliance and ventilatory compromise. If compromise of either extremity perfusion or chest wall compliance occurs, an escharotomy may be warranted. To accomplish this

TABLE 38-20

Parkland Formula for Major Burn Fluid Resuscitation (15% or More TBSA)

Intravenous Fluids

4 mL × weight in kg × % TBSA burned = volume of LR to deliver in 24 hours
- Infuse first one-half of fluid over first 8 hours post burn injury
- Infuse second one-half of fluid over next 16 hours post burn injury

Important: Time the fluid delivery from the time of burn injury (not the time of the patient's arrival at the hospital) and deduct any fluids received in transit (see example in Table 38-21).

For patients weighing less than 30 kg, deliver maintenance IVF with dextrose in addition to the Parkland formula fluids.

Urine Output

Goal for patients weighing less than 30 kg: 0.5–1 mL/kg/hr
Goal for patients weighing more than 30 kg: 1–2 mL/kg/hr
If urine output is "too high," titrate LR infusion down by one-third.
If urine output is "too low," titrate LR infusion up by one-third.
Reassess urine output in 2 hours and adjust as needed.

Note: Total body surface area (TBSA), lactated Ringer's solution (LR), intravenous fluids (IVF).

TABLE 38-21

Parkland Formula Example

It is noon in the ED. A 1-year-old, 10-kg male arrives with 20% TBSA burns to his torso and lower extremities from a scald injury that occurred at 10:00 A.M. In transit, the patient received a normal saline bolus of 200 mL by the EMS providers. How would you resuscitate this child?

Parkland formula: 4 mL × weight × % TBSA burned = volume of LR to deliver in 24 hours
4 mL × 10 kg × 20% = 800 mL for 24 hours

Subtract the fluid received in transit:

800 mL – 200 mL (given by EMS as a saline bolus) = 600 mL
600/2 = 300 mL (amount to be given over the first 8 hours post injury and then the following 16 hours)
The time of the burn injury was 10:00 A.M.; it is now noon. Therefore, you have until 6 P.M. to infuse the first 8 hours of fluid. This is 6 hours from now.

Lactated Ringer's solution:

300 mL/6 hrs = 50 mL/hr (to infuse from noon until 6 P.M.)
300 mL/16 hrs = 19 mL/hr (to infuse from 6 P.M. to 10:00 A.M. tomorrow)
Maintenance IVF of D_5LR at 40 mL/hr also needs to be infused because the child weighs less than 30 kg.
At 2 P.M. you evaluate the patient and note urine output to be only 0.2 mL/kg/hr. What do you do next?
Titrate the LR rate up by one-third:
⅓ of 50 mL = 15 mL, 15mL + 50 mL = a new rate of 65 mL/hr of LR
Do not titrate the D_5LR maintenance IVF; its remains at 40 mL/hr regardless of urine output due to depleted glycogen stores and risk of hypoglycemia.

Note: Total body surface area (TBSA), lactated Ringer's solution (LR), intravenous fluids (IVF).

procedure, coagulating electrocautery is used to make incisions through the thick eschar, relieving the pressure in the affected area.

Within the first 24 hours after burn injury, the patient's nutritional status must be addressed to manage the hypermetabolic state. Due to the depletion of nutritional protein as a result of the inflammatory process and gluconeogenesis, high-protein and high-calorie feedings are necessary. Consider placement of a nasogastric tube in the patient with major burns.

Overall, given the critical nature and individualized care necessary for the pediatric burn-injured patient, the American Burn Association (2001) recommends that all children with significant burns be cared for in centers with personnel and equipment specially trained and designed for this vulnerable population. Emergent referral to a facility that does offer this unique care is warranted if unavailable.

Topical antimicrobial coverage is commonly used in the initial management of patients with burns. Systemic antibiotic therapy as prophylaxis is unnecessary, and enteral or parenteral antibiotics should be employed only on a case-by-case basis as necessary given the patient's clinical condition (Patel et al., 2008).

A wide variety of topical antimicrobial agents are available for use in pediatric burn patients. Commonly used creams and ointments include Silvadene, Bacitracin, and Sulfamylon (which provides better penetration to poorly perfused areas such as the cartilage of the ear). Over the last decade, the long-acting silver dressings have become popular for use on partial-thickness burns, as their application allows for fewer dressing changes. Many of these products can be left in place for 5 to 7 days, reducing the pain and anxiety associated with the dressing change procedure. Products available include hydrocolloids, silver foams, and nanocrystalline silver sheets. Unfortunately, these products do not work for all wounds and are occlusive in some cases, prohibiting frequent assessment of the wound. Mechanisms of injury that require special consideration are listed in Table 38-22.

For full-thickness injuries, operative intervention may be necessary. The two most commonly performed procedures are a split-thickness skin graft and full-thickness skin graft. Both procedures involve the transplantation of either epidermis (split-thickness skin graft) or epidermis and dermis (full-thickness skin graft) from the patient to the burned area for definitive treatment.

Care of the burned patient requires the involvement of team members from many different specialties. Nutrition/dietary services, occupational therapy, physical therapy, child life, social work, and the patient's family must all be included in determining the appropriate plan of care.

Disposition and discharge planning

Pediatric burn survivors require frequent care visits upon disposition from the hospital. At a minimum, weekly follow-ups are necessary until epithelialization occurs. Long-term scar management is done in conjunction with

TABLE 38-22

Special Considerations in Pediatric Burns	
Source/Site	**Management Considerations**
Chemical	Cleanse immediately; do not attempt to alkanize; call poison control
Eye	Seek an ophthalmology consult; use an erythromycin ointment
Perineum	Place an urinary drainage catheter (in case of edema, pain, and possible urethral obstruction); use bacitracin

therapy support using silicone pads, compression garments, or scar massage with a thick emollient. The overall desired outcome is the absence of hypertrophy and maintenance of function/mobility. Long-term physical and occupation therapy is often recommended. Frequent monitoring for growth restriction, deformities, and contractures may be necessary depending on the severity of the burn. Use of sunscreen, with sun-protective factor (SPF) greater than 25, is necessary to avoid secondary tissue damage (Kassira & Namias, 2008).

Some children may have prolonged hospitalizations or home stays; they may also be disfigured or traumatized. Peer assimilation and reintegration into school will require a coordinated plan with the school system and caregivers of friends.

HYPERTHERMIA

Pathophysiology

Heat is exchanged through four mechanisms:

- *Conduction* is the process in which there is contact with cooler surfaces.
- *Convection* occurs when heat dissipates as cooler air passes over the body.
- *Radiation* is the direct release of heat into the environment.
- *Evaporation* is heat loss from perspiration or through a fluid medium.

The physiologic response and management of heat exchange is primarily managed by the hypothalamus.

The process of hyperthermia occurs when adaptive mechanisms of heat exchange become overwhelmed. Oxygen consumption and carbon dioxide production increase as the resting energy expenditure and metabolic rate increase. The optimal core body temperature is generally between 36 °C and 37.5°C (96.8°F to 99.5°F). Cellular death occurs more rapidly at higher temperatures as it is accelerated by inflammatory factors and hematologic and endothelial changes. Children are at greater risk than adults for heat-related illness for a multitude of reasons and, therefore, require special consideration (Table 38-23).

Epidemiology and etiology

The occurrence of hyperthermia and heat=related illness is largely affected by geographical location (Balbus & Malina, 2009). Hyperthermia is often associated with tropical and wilderness medicine. However, during summer months, particularly in a heat wave, there is a potential for serious health risk from this cause. From 1999 to 2003, more than 3,400 heat-related deaths occurred in the

TABLE 38-23

Pediatric Considerations and Risk Factors for Hyperthermia

- Greater surface area-to-mass ratio; therefore, increased risk with environmental exposure to heat (radiation)
- Lower blood volume—children younger than 5 years of age fail to increase their cardiac output in significant heat stress
- Lower amount of sweat produced per gland
- The nonambulatory child is unable to escape the heat
- Special concerns—the adolescent athlete (consider hypertrophic cardiomyopathy)
- Obese, sickle cell disease, and cystic fibrosis patients are at greater risk
- Dehydrated patients are at greater risk

United States. Although most occurred in the elderly population, 7% involved children younger than 15 years of age (Grubenhoff et al., 2007).

Presentation

Heat-related illness is classified into three categories based on severity: heat cramps, heat exhaustion, and heat stroke.

Heat cramps. The most minor of all heat-related illnesses is heat cramps. This condition is characterized by muscle cramps, most often in the large muscles of the legs, but occasionally in the abdomen. The discomfort can be spasmodic and generally follows exertional stress. The onset of the muscle cramps is generally during a time of rest after exercise and is believed to result from an electrolyte imbalance. On physical examination, a hard, firm, palpable mass may be noted in the affected muscle during spasm. Core body temperature is often normal.

Heat exhaustion. Heat exhaustion is characterized by vague symptoms related to volume depletion and elevated body temperature:

- Fatigue and weakness
- Nausea and vomiting
- Increased thirst and dehydration
- Headache
- Myalgia or muscle cramps
- Dizziness and irritability
- Orthostatic blood pressure changes
- Tachycardia
- Tachypnea
- Sweating (may or may not be present)

Heat stroke. Heat stroke is the most severe of the heat-related illnesses and is a life-threatening medical emergency due to its concomitant risk of multiple organ dysfunction syndrome and death. Core temperature may be greater than

41°C (105.8°F). Heat stroke is characterized by symptoms of significant central nervous system dysfunction, respiratory distress, and hemodynamic instability:

- Seizures
- Delirium
- Coma
- Hallucinations
- Severe headache
- Cerebellar dysfunction—ataxia

Tachypnea, hyperventilation, and dyspnea typically are noted as the patient attempts to compensate for lactic acidosis and hypoxemia. These effects can progress to acute respiratory distress syndrome (ARDS). Tachycardia, decreased cardiac output, and elevated central venous pressure are common. Patients with heat stroke no longer sweat. Cutaneous dilation, which is necessary to attempt body cooling, requires a significant volume of blood that is taken from central circulation, in turn lowering peripheral vascular resistance. Inadequate fluid intake and increased insensible losses add to the decreased total body volume. Consequently, hypotension ensues and the patient is at risk for both hypovolemic and distributive shock. Hypotension is a late sign, and should alert the HCP to imminent circulatory collapse. Acute kidney failure may develop as a result of inadequate kidney perfusion. As overall failure of the body's systems continues, the patient may progress to disseminated intravascular coagulation (DIC), with associated hematuria, purpura, and melena.

Differential diagnosis

Several heat-related illnesses exist, ranging from minor to critical. Generally, as heat exposure increases, so does the severity of illness. The management of the patient with heat-related illness is dictated by the clinical findings associated with presentation. Table 38-24 outlines the differential diagnoses for consideration when evaluating the patient with a possible heat related illness.

Plan of care

Heat cramps. Diagnostic studies that may be of value in the evaluation of the patient with heat cramps include serum and urine electrolytes. Laboratory data may reveal hyponatremia, hypochloremia, and occasional hypokalemia with a low urine sodium.

Therapeutic management includes replacement of fluid losses. Generally, patients can be sufficiently rehydrated with oral electrolyte solutions. For patients with prolonged muscle cramps, IV hydration starting with a normal saline bolus of 10 to 20 mL/kg may be warranted. Patients should be moved to a cool location as soon as possible. Rest is encouraged.

TABLE 38-24

Differential Diagnoses for Hyperthermia

- Heat cramps
- Heat exhaustion
- Heat stroke
- Dehydration
- Central nervous system infections
- Sepsis
- Status epilepticus
- Intracranial hemorrhage
- Hypothalamic dysfunction
- Drug ingestion: anticholinergic medications, stimulants, salicylates
- Drug withdrawal
- Serotonin syndrome
- Neuroleptic malignant syndrome
- Malignant hyperthermia
- Hemorrhagic shock
- Encephalopathy

Heat Exhaustion. Patients with heat exhaustion may have either hyponatremia or hypernatremia. They are usually dehydrated with an elevated blood urea nitrogen (BUN). The hematocrit may be elevated due to hemoconcentration. If concern arises that the patient may be progressing to heat stroke, then further diagnostic inquiry is warranted, such as an evaluation of respiratory, liver, kidney, and coagulation function.

Primary management of the patient with suspected heat exhaustion is to first move him or her to a cool location. Remove all clothing to improve heat loss through evaporation and convection. Generally, passive cooling is sufficient and can be achieved using cool packs and wet towels. Diuretics, including caffeinated or carbonated beverages, are to be avoided. Hemodynamic instability, emesis, and severe muscle cramps are indications for intravenous fluid administration. Ensure that all laboratory data are obtained prior to the administration of intravenous fluids, so that serial evaluations may be performed as deemed necessary based on the patient response.

Heat stroke. As with other victims of environmental or traumatic injury, it is important to start with evaluation of the ABCs (airway, breathing, and circulation) plus temperature. Core body temperature can reach levels greater than 41°C (105.8°F).

Table 38-25 listed the recommended diagnostic studies in suspected heat stroke. Electrolyte abnormalities are to be expected, including hyponatremia or hypernatremia, hypokalemia, hypoglycemia, and azotemia (a decrease in the glomerular filtration rate and an increase in the BUN and creatinine). Elevated transaminase levels may be observed with associated liver injury. Elevated prothrombin and partial thromboplastin times and a decreased platelet count are suggestive of DIC. In addition, an elevated serum creatinine kinase level and myoglobin may indicate significant muscle breakdown and rhabdomyolysis.

The goal in management of the patient with heat stroke is to lower the core temperature enough to maintain physiologic stability (Grubenhoff et al., 2007). This goal is achieved through rapid IV fluid administration and active cooling. The patient should be moved to a cool location with various cooling therapies considered. Any cooling

TABLE 38-25

Diagnostic Studies for Hyperthermia

Diagnostic Study	Evaluation
Hepatic transaminase levels	Liver damage
Complete blood count (CBC), prothrombin time (PT)/partial thromboplastin time (PTT), fibrinogen, platelets	Disseminated intravascular coagulation (DIC)
Electrolytes	Hyperkalemia, hyponatremia, acid–base imbalances
Glucose	Hypoglycemia and/or liver injury
Creatine kinase (CK)	Rhabdomyolysis
Arterial blood gas (ABG)	Acid–base imbalances
Urinalysis (UA)	Acute kidney failure and rhabdomyolysis
Chest radiograph (CXR)	Acute respiratory distress syndrome (ARDS), pulmonary edema, aspiration pneumonia
Computed tomography (CT) of the brain	Intracranial hemorrhage (ICH) or cerebral edema
Electrocardiograph (ECG)	Myocardial ischemia

therapy should be ceased once the core temperature is less than 39°C (102.2°F) to avoid hypothermia. Elevation of the lower extremities to improve central perfusion may be useful.

Antipyretic therapy may be considered. Anticholinergic drugs should be avoided, however, as they can induce tachycardia, dry flushed skin, dilated pupils, decreased gastrointestinal motility, and urinary retention—all of which can worsen the symptoms associated with heat stroke. Consider benzodiazepines to treat seizures, agitation, or shivering.

Intravenous fluid administration is guided by hypovolemia, dehydration, and laboratory study. Urinary output should be maintained at a rate greater than 1 to 3 mL/kg/hr to promote hydration and prevent dehydration-related kidney failure. It also may be necessary to provide dextrose 25% for treatment of hypoglycemia related to heat stroke.

Rhabdomyolysis develops in 25% to 30% of all patients with heat stroke. The initial therapy for this complication consists of the administration of isotonic IV fluid boluses. It may be necessary to alkalanize the urine with an osmotic diuretic, such as mannitol. Urine should be alkalanized to a pH greater than 7. Loop diuretics, such as furosemide, should be avoided, because these agents promote renal tubular acidosis and myoglobin deposits that may lead to acute tubular necrosis (Wagner & Boyd, 2008).

If all methods of fluid resuscitation are unsuccessful, hemodialysis is a strategy of last resort for management of kidney failure. If rhabdomyolysis ensues, close monitoring for the development of compartment syndrome is warranted.

Disposition and discharge planning

The prognosis associated with heat stroke varies, and is influenced by many factors. Poor prognostic indicators include a core temperature greater than 41°C (105.8°F), sustained temperatures greater than 38.8°C (101.8°F), coma lasting longer than 2 hours, pulmonary edema, sustained or delayed hypotension, acute kidney failure with hyperkalemia, lactic acidosis, and liver transaminase values greater than 1,000.

Heat-related injuries are generally preventable; thus patient education is important. Suggested topics for family education include the following guidelines:

- Avoid leaving children unattended in closed spaces in warm weather.
- Educate coaches and athletes on environmental factors related to heat-induced illness.
- Educate adolescents on the role of alcohol in heat-related illness.
- Encourage the use of sun protection.

HYPOTHERMIA

Pathophysiology

Hypothermia is defined as a body temperature less than 35°C (95°F). Once the body temperature drops to this level, the gas solubility in blood increases. Along with this phenomenon, there is a low partial pressure of carbon dioxide, a low partial pressure of oxygen, and a higher overall pH. Shivering can lead to an increase in oxygen consumption and carbon dioxide production. The oxyhemoglobin dissociation curve shifts left, which leads to respiratory depression and central nervous system alterations. Eventually, the patient may further decompensate with metabolic acidosis and a fall in cardiac output. At 30°C (86°F), the patient's pupils may be fixed, coagulation impaired, and GI motility halted. Hyperglycemia and pancreatitis may also be present.

Local injury occurs as freezing of the tissue leads to formation of extracellular ice crystals. A change in the osmotic gradient also results in intracellular dehydration. Collectively, this progression leads to formation of intracellular ice crystals and eventual cell death. External dermal ischemia is present as well, having an appearance similar to burn injury necrosis.

Epidemiology and etiology

Most dermal cold injury is isolated to the extremities and referred to as frostbite. Diabetes mellitus, artherosclerosis, and smoking may all exacerbate the impact of cold on the extremities. Each year, more than 650 deaths from hypothermia occur in the United States.

Presentation

Hypothermia is classified as mild, moderate, or severe, based on the patient's core temperature (Table 38-26). Physical examination findings vary based on the severity. The effects of hypothermia are usually gradual. Early findings may be subtle and not recognized. Mental awareness or judgment may be impaired. There is usually the feeling of cold progressing to numbness. Shivering is common during mild hypothermia.

TABLE 38-26

Hypothermia		
Category	Temperature (°C)	Temperature (°F)
Mild	34–36	93.2–96.8
Moderate	32–34	89.6–93.2
Severe	< 32	< 89.6

As the core temperature drops, further alterations in metabolic function are noted, including apathy to the environment. This effect becomes even more profound when combined with ingestion of alcohol. Signs of moderate to severe hypothermia are as follows:

- Altered mental status
- Seizures
- Coma
- Tachycardia, followed by bradycardia, followed by asystole
- Constipation
- Oliguria

Frostbite dermal injury

In the initial management of the patient with hypothermia, the HCP must take precautions to handle the patient gently during all transfers and care so as to prevent cold-associated arrhythmias or further tissue damage. Care starts with attention to the airway, breathing, and circulation (ABCs). During the evaluation of circulatory status, ventricular fibrillation or asystole may be noted. Cardiopulmonary resuscitation should be initiated as clinically indicated. Immediate removal of any wet or cold clothing is imperative, and the patient should be placed in a warm environment.

Differential diagnosis

The differential diagnoses for hypothermia and frostbite are listed in Table 38-27.

Plan of care

Relevant diagnostic studies to be considered in the evaluation of the patient with hypothermic injury include the following:

- ABG (adjusted for temperature)
- ECG: expect a progressive bradycardia associated with a fall in cardiac output; associated T-wave inversion; prolonged PR, QRS, and QT intervals; and the presence of J waves

TABLE 38-27

Differential Diagnoses for Hypothermia
- Status epilepticus - Trauma - Cerebral edema - Burn injury - Intracranial hemorrhage

- PT/PTT: coagulopathy frequently occurs despite normal levels
- CBC: platelet number and function decreased
- AST/ALT: elevated and metabolism impaired
- Glucose: Hyperglycemia
- Amylase/lipase: elevated, associated pancreatitis
- Electrolytes
- Radiographs if dermal injury is present; consider angiography if indicated

The management of hypothermia varies based on the severity of injury. For the patient with mild hypothermia, passive external warming is generally sufficient. This care involves the removal of wet clothing, application of warm clothing, and use of a warm covering (Figure 38-33). Active rewarming can be initiated as well via forced-air rewarming. Beware of a phenomenon called "afterdrop"—the continued fall of body temperature during the rewarming process.

In cases of moderate to severe hypothermia, active core rewarming may be initiated. Generally, core rewarming is less prone to the "afterdrop" phenomenon or life-threatening arrhythmias. Core rewarming is achieved through a variety of techniques:

- Humidified heated oxygen
- Warmed IV fluid (isotonic)
- Peritoneal and pleural lavage with warmed isotonic sterile solutions
- Extracorporeal membrane oxygenation (ECMO)

No matter which rewarming technique is used, it is important to continually monitor core temperature and closely monitor for hypoglycemia. Administration of fresh frozen plasma may be necessary if the patient becomes coagulopathic.

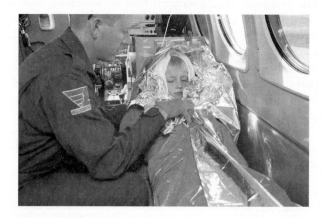

FIGURE 38-33

Hypothermia Management.

Source: © Jones & Bartlett Learning. Courtesy of MIEMSS.

Frostbite. Frostbite, or the dermal injury sustained in hypothermic conditions, is managed similarly to burn wound care. Initial treatment in the prehospital setting should be cautiously monitored to avoid periods of rewarming and refreezing. The provider should be wary of the presence of ice crystals in the intracellular space and the potential for worsening injury with this process. Rubbing of the area is also contraindicated, as it may induce mechanical trauma.

Upon arrival at the hospital, active rewarming is to be initiated. A water bath with an antimicrobial agent (such as chlorhexedine or iodine) should be employed at a temperature of 40ºC (104 ºF). Dry heat use is contraindicated. Pain management with narcotics is necessary, as the rewarming process for frostbite is extremely painful. Once the wound has been immersed in the rewarming solution, it should be permitted to air dry at the conclusion. Do not rub the area. Tetanus administration is recommended in all cases.

Wound management is similar to that for full-thickness burns. Digits should be separated, and the affected extremities should be placed on non-weight-bearing status and elevated. Administration of topical antimicrobials is indicated. If compartment syndrome or severe necrosis ensues, amputation may be necessary (Figure 38-34).

Disposition and discharge planning

Frequent follow-up is required for the management of the patient with frostbite injury; this includes wound care and interprofessional involvement of the rehabilitation team if pertinent given the severity of the injury. Prevention edtucation should be disseminated to all patients and families, including the following guidelines:

• Dress young children and infants in one more layer than adults would wear in the same environment.
• Limit the amount of exposure to the cold.
• Have children come indoors from cold outdoor environments frequently to warm up,
• Stay as dry as possible in winter weather.

TRAUMATIC BRAIN INJURY

Nicole Fortier O'Brien

PATHOPHYSIOLOGY

Morbidity and mortality associated with head trauma occur due to injury suffered in two distinct phases: primary and secondary. The primary phase of injury occurs at the moment of impact, when mechanical forces cause direct disruption of the brain parenchyma. *Primary injuries* can be either focal or diffuse in nature. Types of focal brain injury include intracranial contusion and extra-axial hemorrhage (epidural hematoma, subdural hematoma, subarachnoid hemorrhage). An *epidural hematoma* results from injury to the middle meningeal artery or vein, venous sinuses, or diploic veins (Figure 38-35). A *subdural hematoma* is caused by bridging vein rupture (Figure 38-36 and Figure 38-37). Tearing of small vessels in the pia mater results in *subarachnoid hemorrhage* (Figure 38-38). Diffuse brain injury, commonly called *diffuse axonal injury*, is typically produced by acceleration or deceleration forces that result in shear trauma at the interface of gray and white matter.

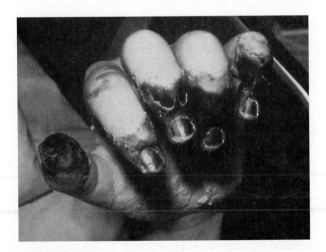

FIGURE 38-34

Frostbite Gangrene.
Source: Courtesy of Dr. Jack Poland/CDC.

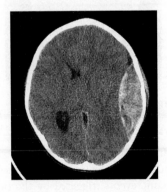

FIGURE 38-35

CT Scan: Epidural Hematoma with Midline Shift.
Source: Courtesy of Nicole Fortier O'Brien.

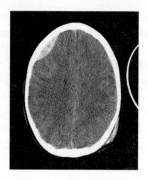

FIGURE 38-36

CT Scan: Subdural Hematoma.

Source: Courtesy of Nicole Fortier O'Brien.

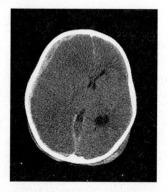

FIGURE 38-37

CT Scan: Subdural Hematoma with Midline Shift.

Source: Courtesy of Nicole Fortier O'Brien.

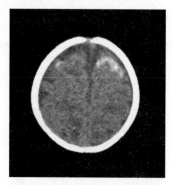

FIGURE 38-38

CT Scan: Subarachnoid Hemorrhage.

Source: Courtesy of Nicole Fortier O'Brien.

The secondary phase of injury comprises sequelae of local and systemic events triggered by the primary injury. Three basic mechanisms leading to secondary brain injury can be defined: Ischemia, energy failure, and excitotoxicity result in cell death and secondary brain injury. Axonal injury and death, cerebral edema, and intracranial pressure abnormalities may also contribute to secondary brain injury (Kochanek, 2006).

Post-traumatic ischemia, energy failure, excitotoxicity, and cell death

Following traumatic brain injury, cerebral blood flow is decreased. Adelson and colleagues (1997) assessed cerebral blood flow in infants and children following brain injury and found that mean cerebral blood flow for these patients on admission was 25.1 mL/100 gm/min. Seventy-seven percent of patients had cerebral blood flow of less than 20 mL/100 gm/min. Contributors to diminished cerebral blood flow following brain injury may include a decreased vasodilatory response to cyclic guanosine monophosphate, cyclic adenosine monophosphate, and prostanoids; loss of endothelial production of nitric oxide; and production of endothelin-1 (Kochanek et al., 2000). In addition, increased release of excitatory neurotransmitters such as glutamate, aspartate, and acetylcholine early after brain injury has been reported (Ruppel et al., 2001). Hypoperfusion in conjunction with increased metabolic demand from excitotoxicity results in neuronal damage and death and secondary brain injury.

Axonal injury

Shearing and rapid deformation of axons during a traumatic event can damage the axonal cytoskeleton, thereby producing impairment of axoplasmic transport. Subsequent axonal swelling occurs in bulb formations that accumulate transported proteins and calcium. Ultimately, damaged axons become disconnected, die, and contribute to secondary brain injury (Povlishock & Christman, 1996).

Cerebral edema and intracranial pressure abnormalities

Intracranial pressure is a function of the volume and compliance of the intracranial compartment. Under normal conditions, the brain parenchyma accounts for 80% of the intracranial volume, blood for 10%, and cerebrospinal fluid (CSF) for 10%. The skull is a fairly rigid, noncompliant structure. Therefore, an increase in the volume of any one of the intracranial components necessitates a decrease in another, or an increase in intracranial pressure (ICP) will occur (the Monro-Kellie doctrine).

Elevations in ICP typically peak 24 to 72 hours following brain injury. Cerebral edema with resultant increased intracranial volume and ICP elevation may be caused by intracellular swelling (cytotoxic edema), capillary endothelial cell dysfunction and increased permeability (vasogenic edema), or increased periventricular fluid (interstitial edema) (Figure 38-39). When Barzo et al. (1997) performed MRI to localize the increase in brain water after traumatic brain injury, they found that cellular

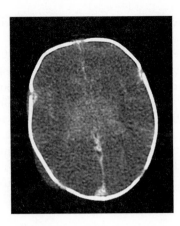

FIGURE 38-39

CT Scan: Severe Cerebral Edema.

Source: Courtesy of Nicole Fortier O'Brien.

swelling is the predominant contributor to cerebral edema in this setting.

After resolution of early post-traumatic hypoperfusion, some pediatric patients develop increased cerebral blood flow greater than that necessary to meet metabolic demands (Kochanek et al., 2000). This loss of autoregulation can lead to excessive blood flow and contribute to elevated ICP. In addition, excessive CSF production can occur in the face of increased blood flow. Diminished absorption of CSF by arachnoid villi also often occurs following subarachnoid hemorrhage. Thus increased CSF volume due to either increased production or decreased absorption can contribute to elevated ICP.

Intracranial hypertension from all of these factors contributes to secondary brain injury by compromising cerebral perfusion. If significant enough, elevations in ICP can produce further injury through herniation syndrome.

EPIDEMIOLOGY AND ETIOLOGY

Traumatic brain injury (TBI) is the leading cause of childhood death and disability in developed nations (Krug et al., 2000). Each year in the United States, 435,000 children visit the emergency department due to head trauma. Of these pediatric patients, 37,000 require hospitalization and 2,685 die as a direct result of their injury (Langlois et al., 2004). An unknown—and likely much larger—number experience minor head injury and do not seek treatment.

Dunning et al. (2004) prospectively described a large cohort of children with head injury in an attempt to further delineate the epidemiology of TBI in this population. Fifty-five percent of the children suffering brain injury were younger than age 5 years, and 28% were younger than 2 years of age. Males were more likely than females to

experience head injury, with males accounting for 65% of the study cohort. In addition, most pediatric patients suffered only mild TBI, with 98% of the children presenting with a Glasgow Coma Scale (GCS) score of 15. Dunning et al. (2004) also described the most common mechanisms of injury in pediatric head trauma patients: 73% had suffered falls, a collision or bicycle crash was experienced by 12% of patients, and a projectile caused injury in 10%.

PRESENTATION

Traumatic brain injury is classified as mild, moderate, or severe based on the results of a neurologic assessment using the GCS. Minor head injury is defined as having a GCS score in the range of 13 to 15 and may be associated with symptoms such as brief loss of consciousness, disorientation, headache, or vomiting. Concussion is a type of minor TBI associated with symptoms but no abnormalities on head CT. Moderate TBI is defined as having a GCS score in the range of 9 to 12, whereas severe TBI is characterized by a GCS score of 8 or less. Moderate and severe head injury are typically associated with more significant symptoms than those seen in mild head injury as well as with abnormal brain imaging.

In another study by Dunning et al. (2006), presenting symptoms of children seeking emergency services following TBI included headache or irritability in 21%, vomiting in 11%, and loss of consciousness in 5%. Post-traumatic seizures occur in 3% to 8% of patients with TBI (Davis et al., 1994; Schunk et al., 1996). In addition, skull fracture and scalp hematoma without other symptoms are not uncommon. Transient defects such as cortical blindness have also been reported in a small percentage of pediatric patients.

DIFFERENTIAL DIAGNOSES

In most instances, history and physical examination are sufficient to confirm the diagnosis of head trauma. The possibility of abuse head trauma should be considered in young children with no history of trauma but the following symptoms:

- Loss of consciousness
- Altered mental status
- Vomiting
- Increasing head circumference

PLAN OF CARE

A goal of initial evaluation is to identify, on clinical grounds, those patients with TBI who require immediate medical or surgical intervention versus those who can be treated with observation alone without intervention. This practice limits exposure to unnecessary radiation. The Children's Head Injury Algorithm for the Prediction of Important Clinical Events (CHALICE) study involved a prospective cohort of 22,772 patients and described patient characteristics that can help predict whether a head CT should be obtained (Table 38-28). Per the CHALICE criteria, if no concerning variable is present, the pediatric patient is at low risk for intracranial pathology and no CT should be performed. The authors reported 98% sensitivity and 87% specificity for prediction of clinically

significant head injury based on these criteria (Dunning et al., 2006).

More recently, the Pediatric Emergency Care Applied Research Network (PECARN) study involved a prospective cohort of 42,412 patients and looked at predictors of clinically important traumatic brain injuries (Table 38-29). The authors reported a 100% negative predictive value and a 100% sensitivity for these predictors in children younger than 2 years of age and a 99.95% negative predictive value and a 96.8% sensitivity in children 2 years of age or older. If no predictor is present

TABLE 38-28

CHALICE Criteria

The CHALICE criteria are used for pediatric patients not likely to have clinically important traumatic brain injury and who may *not* require head CT. If any of these criteria are present or the GCS is less than 14 or 15, a CT scan is required.

Historical Features	Physical Exam Findings	Mechanism of Injury
No loss of consciousness for more than 5 minutes	GCS ≥ 14 in a child older than 1 year of age	Not a high-speed accident
No abnormal drowsiness	GCS ≥ 15 in a child younger than 1 year of age	No fall from a height more than 3 meters
No vomiting more than three times	No suspicion of penetration injury	Injury not due to a fast-moving projectile or object
No suspicion of inflicted head trauma	No suspicion of depressed skull fracture	
No seizures	No suspicion of basilar skull fracture	
	No focal neurologic deficit	
	No swelling or laceration of more than 5 cm in a child younger than 1 year of age	

Note: Children's Head Injury Algorithm for the Prediction of Important Clinical Events (CHALICE), Glasgow Coma Scale (GCS).
Source: Dunning et al., 2006.

TABLE 38-29

PECARN Criteria

These criteria are used for pediatric patients who are not likely to have clinically important traumatic brain injury and who may *not* require head CT. If any of these criteria are present, the GCS is less than 14, or the patient is acting abnormally, a CT scan is required.

Age: Younger Than 2 Years	Age: 2 Years or Older
GCS ≥ 14	GCS ≥ 14
No altered mental status	No altered mental status
No nonfrontal scalp hematoma	No loss of consciousness of any duration
No loss of consciousness for more than 5 seconds	No history of vomiting
No severe injury mechanism	No severe injury mechanism
No palpable skull fracture	No clinical signs of basilar skull fracture
Acting normally according to parents	No severe headache

Note: Pediatric Emergency Care Applied Research Network (PECARN), Glasgow Coma Scale (GCS).
Source: Kupperman et al., 2009.

in a patient, a head CT may be deemed unnecessary (Kupperman et al., 2009).

After assessing the pediatric patient's airway, breathing, and circulation (ABCs), the initial evaluation of a child with TBI should include a physical examination to evaluate for extracranial injury. Chiaretti et al. (2002) noted that multiple trauma is common in patients who have suffered moderate to severe head injury, with 39% of patients having damage to more than one organ system. The physical examination should also evaluate for cervical spine injury.

All children who have suffered TBI require observation. This observation can be done at home after a brief period of observation in the emergency department if the mechanism of injury is associated with a low risk of TBI, there was no loss of consciousness, the child presents with a normal mental status, the child has no headache, the child has experienced no more than one or two episodes of vomiting, and caregivers are reliable. Pediatric patients who experience a brief, immediate post-traumatic seizure with normal head CT do not necessarily require admission unless other concerning findings are present. Observation in the hospital should be carried out if a brain injury is documented by radiographic images, the child has a depressed or basilar skull fracture, the child has persistently altered mental status (even with a normal CT), or the child has continued vomiting. Observation in the hospital should also be arranged if caregivers are unable to return should it become necessary (Schutzman & Greenes, 2001).

Patients who have suffered moderate to severe TBI require admission to the critical care unit for continued observation and care. If these patients have or develop a GCS score of 8 or less, pupillary dysfunction, lateralizing signs, posturing, or systemic hypertension/bradycardia, they are likely to have impending herniation and require immediate intervention. A cerebroprotective rapid-sequence intubation strategy should be used to secure the airway (Figure 38-40). Circulatory stabilization needs to be undertaken, including rapid replacement of vascular volume with isotonic or hypertonic fluids and maintenance of adequate blood pressure with continued fluid resuscitation or vasoactive agents if required. Aggressive treatment to immediately lower ICP, including mild hyperventilation with 100% oxygen and administration of thiopental, mannitol, or hypertonic saline, should be performed. Once stabilization has been achieved, a head CT should be obtained to determine if the child has a space-occupying lesion that requires surgical intervention.

Ongoing therapy in the critical care unit should focus on maintenance of physiologic stability and management of intracranial hypertension. Intracranial pressure should be controlled as outlined by the Society of Critical Care Medicine (2003) guidelines for the acute medical management of severe traumatic brain injury in infants, children, and adolescents (Figure 38-41).

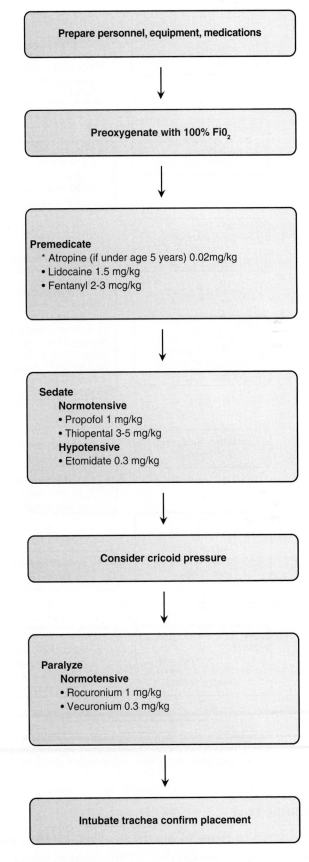

FIGURE 38-40

Cerebroprotective Rapid Sequence Intubation Strategy.

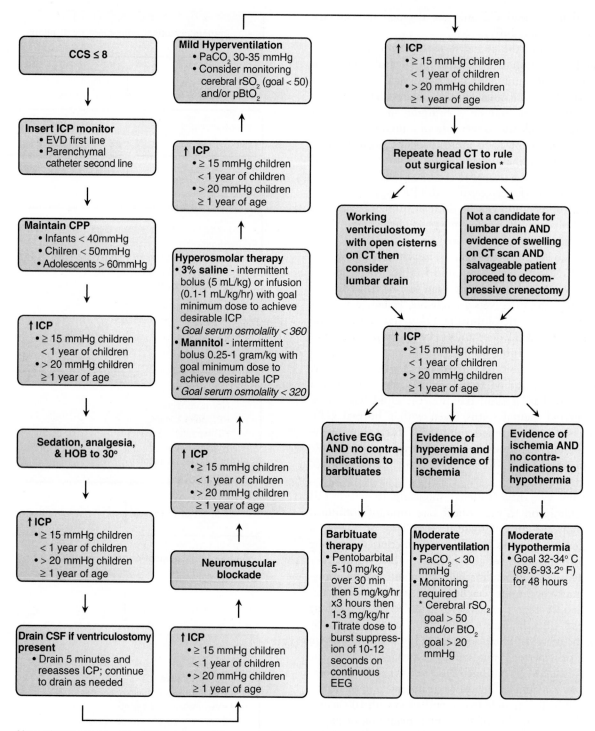

Note: glascow coma score (GCS), intracranial pressure (ICP), external ventricular drain (EVD), cerebral perfusion pressue (CPP), head of bed (HOB), cerebrospinal fluid (CSF), sodium (Na), partial pressure carbon dioxide (PaCO₂), regional oxygen saturation (rSO₂), brain tissue oxygenation (pBtO₂), electroencephalogram 9EEG).

FIGURE 38-41

Critical Pathway for the Treatment of Established Intracranial Hypertension in Pediatric Traumatic Brain Injury.

Source: Society of Critical Care Medicine (2003). Guidelines for the acute medical management of severe traumatic brain injury in infants, children, and adolescents. *Crit Care Med,* 31(6), S407–91.

When indicated and when the patient's ventricles are sufficiently open to make placement technically possible, an external ventricular drain (EVD) should be inserted (review the discussion of intracranial shunt access/installation and ventricular drainage in Chapter 44). The EVD allows for monitoring of the ICP as well as treatment of elevated ICP by intermittent drainage of cerebrospinal fluid. When placement of an EVD is not possible but measuring ICP is indicated, an intraparenchymal monitor ("bolt") should be placed. Intraparenchymal monitors are capable of making continuous measurements of ICP but cannot drain cerebrospinal fluid; as a consequence they are not a treatment modality for elevated ICP.

Several major studies in children with severe TBI report that an ICP greater than 20 mmHg is associated with a poor outcome (Downward et al., 2000; Esparza et al., 1985; Pfenninger et al., 1983; Shapiro & Marmarou, 1982). Thus therapy should be directed to maintain ICP below this level. In infants with open sutures and a lower physiologic mean arterial blood pressure, the goal ICP should possibly even be lower than 20 mmHg. Optimal cerebral perfusion pressure

$$CPP = Mean\ arterial\ pressure - ICP$$

for age should be maintained using intravenous fluid boluses and vasoactive medications if necessary. Common thresholds for CPP are more than 40 to 50 mmHg for infants, more than 50 to 60 mmHg for children, and more than 60 mmHg in adolescents. In addition, aggressive treatment of seizures and control of hyperthermia should be undertaken.

Neurosurgical consultation should be obtained if brain injury is detected on CT or if a depressed, diastatic, or basilar skull fracture is noted. Neurology consultation may be necessary to determine whether seizures associated with TBI require prolonged treatment with antiepileptic drugs. Occupational, physical, and speech therapy consultation is appropriate for most patients following head injury. In addition, an orthopedics consult will often be required to manage coexisting bony injuries.

Close communication with family members regarding the overall management plan for the pediatric patient with TBI is imperative. Of particular importance is relaying detailed information about the patient's neurologic exam, findings on head CT, and expected course of the hospitalization. This information will help family members cope with a stressful situation and make informed decisions throughout the care of the patient.

DISPOSITION AND DISCHARGE PLANNING

Children with mild brain injury discharged to home either directly from the emergency department or after a period of hospital observation do not need to be awakened from sleep for monitoring. If caregivers note a worsening mental status, continued vomiting, worsened headaches, or seizures, medical attention should be sought. Within a few days of initial evaluation, primary care providers should follow up with pediatric patients who have suffered mild brain injury. This evaluation should focus on any persistent concussive symptoms, mental status testing, neurologic testing, and exertional provocative testing. The level of activity that caregivers should allow as well as the appropriateness of return to play for athletes should be determined by the PCP based on this evaluation.

Children who have suffered moderate to severe TBI will often have persistent significant deficits in cognitive and motor function even after discharge from the hospital. In addition to follow-up with their PCP, most will require occupational, physical, and speech therapy and rehabilitation treatment on either an inpatient or outpatient basis. Follow-up with the neurosurgery and neurology services may also be indicated. In addition, home health care and nursing may be required to provide appropriate care to the most significantly head-injured pediatric patients in their homes.

Of all children suffering traumatic brain injury, 95% will survive. However, in children suffering severe TBI, survival is only 65% (Sumich et al., 2007). In addition, long-term difficulties often occur in children who are survivors of TBI. Hawley et al. (2004) reported that behavioral, emotional, memory, and attention problems were present in 10% to 18% of children who suffered mild head injury, in 25% of children with moderate head injury, and in 33% of children suffering severe head injury. Personality change was also noted in 21% of children suffering mild injury, 46% suffering moderate injury, and in 69% suffering severe injury. In children with moderate to severe head trauma, there is also a high incidence of disability in motor function and in performance of activities of daily living (Sesma et al., 2008).

Given the significant morbidity and mortality associated with pediatric TBI, prevention should be one of the primary focuses of child health care. Caregivers, schools, daycare providers, pediatricians, communities, and government bodies all share responsibility for prevention of such injuries. Outside the home, motor vehicle safety, including the appropriate use of car seats, should be undertaken. Additionally, no child younger than the age of 13 years should be allowed to ride in the front seat of a vehicle due to the increased incidence of injury in younger children in MVCs in which airbags deploy. Helmet use while bicycling, skateboarding, and skiing should be encouraged. Inside the home, childproofing, appropriate storage of firearms, and water safety are paramount. Neglect and abuse prevention are difficult; however, caregivers should be educated regarding the dangers of shaking a baby.

POST-TRAUMATIC STRESS DISORDER

Corey Fritz and Sarah Wilson

PATHOPHYSIOLOGY

Post-traumatic stress disorder (PTSD) is an anxiety disorder that occurs after the exposure to one or more traumatic events. This condition is distinguished from an immediate stress reaction by its persistence, with symptoms typically lasting more than 1 month (American Academy of Child and Adolescent Psychiatry [AACAP], 2009). The essential feature of PTSD is the development of characteristic symptoms following a psychologically distressing event that causes intense fear, terror, and feelings of helplessness (AACAP, 2009; American Psychiatric Association [APA], 2000).

The psychologically distressing event is often one that is unusual to the pediatric patient. It may vary from a motor vehicle collision to physical or sexual abuse. It can also encompass a serious threat to the child's life or physical integrity, caregiver or other significant relative., and/or home or community (APA, 2000). Pediatric patients can develop PTSD without being the direct victims of the traumatic event. For example, they may vicariously experience the trauma by witnessing or viewing (television, Internet) other persons being seriously injured or killed (APA, 2000).

PTSD is differentiated into acute distress disorder, PTSD-acute type, or PTSD-chronic type by the length of time that the person exhibits symptoms (Table 38-30).

EPIDEMIOLOGY AND ETIOLOGY

Pediatric patients appear to be more susceptible to developing PTSD than adults. The prevalence of PTSD in adults

TABLE 38-30

Differentiating Stress Disorders	
Diagnosis	**Duration of Symptoms**
Acute stress disorder	Less than 1 month
Post-traumatic stress disorder, acute type	More than 1 month but less than 3 months
Post-traumatic stress disorder, chronic type	3 months or more

Source: APA, 2000.

is 8% to 9%, while the prevalence in children is 13% to 45% (Ziegler et al., 2005). Numerous factors contribute to the probability that a pediatric patient will develop PTSD. This disorder is more common in those from a low-socioeconomic status and living in an area in which violence is endemic (Bassuk et al., 2001). Nevertheless, PTSD has not been reported to have an association with any particular cultural or ethnic group (AACAP, 2009). Females are more likely to be diagnosed with PTSD than males (APA, 2000), and they may also develop more severe and longer-lasting PTSD symptoms when exposed to traumatic events. Males, however, are more likely to be exposed to such events (AACAP, 2009).

PRESENTATION

Characteristic symptoms of PTSD in the pediatric patient include reexperiencing the traumatic event, avoidance of stimuli associated with the event or numbing of general responsiveness, and increased arousal (AACAP, 2009; APA, 2000). These diagnostic criteria were established by the American Psychiatric Association (2000) and are described in the *Diagnostic and Statistical Manual of Mental Disorders,* fourth edition (*DSM-IV-TR*).

Reexperiencing the traumatic event

It is common for the individual affected by the event to have recurrent and intrusive recollections or distressing dreams of the event. In rare instances, patients may exhibit dissociative states where components of the event are relived and the person behaves as though experiencing the event for the first time. This state may last from a few seconds to several hours or days. In addition, intense psychological distress often occurs when the person is exposed to new events that resemble or symbolize the original traumatic event, such as the anniversary of the incident. In a young child, however, this criterion may be difficult to elicit (AACAP, 2009; APA, 2000).

Avoidance of stimuli associated with the event or numbing of general responsiveness

The individual affected by a traumatic event often attempts to avoid activities or situations that may evoke thoughts or memories of the event. This behavior may lead to a decreased interest in usual activities or refusal to discuss the event. In young children, it may be manifested by the loss of previously attained developmental or language milestones.

Increased arousal

In the pediatric patient, symptoms of physiological arousal in conjunction with PTSD are common. These symptoms include sleep disturbances (difficulty falling or staying asleep, recurrent nightmares), an increased startle response, irritability, or outbursts of anger. At school, children and adolescents are frequently reported to have trouble with concentration and task completion, which may result in a decline in grades. Affected youths may be involved in schoolyard fights, and younger children might display oppositional behaviors. Pediatric patients who have PTSD as a result of a sexual abuse may exhibit high-risk sexual behaviors (AACAP, 2009; APA, 2000).

Many of these symptoms may be common among pediatric patients without the diagnosis of PTSD. Their occurrence should prompt the HCP to elicit any traumatic events history and perform a mental health evaluation accordingly (AACAP, 2009).

DIFFERENTIAL DIAGNOSIS

Various disease and disorder states may have attributes or symptoms similar to PTSD. Table 38-31 outlines these conditions.

PLAN OF CARE

Measurement and diagnosis of PTSD in the pediatric patient are evaluated by patient self-report, observations by the caregivers, and psychological symptom analysis. Diagnosis requires that the pediatric patient be able to describe the event. Some patients may be unwilling to discuss the event; in these circumstances, there must be clear evidence of a precipitating event for the diagnosis of PTSD to be considered. Testing for and diagnosis of PTSD are usually accomplished by a mental health professional (MHP). A traumatic experience should not be implicated

as the cause of the pediatric patient's symptomology by the MHP or HCP (AACAP, 2009).

Several tools are available to the MHP when evaluating a pediatric patient for PTSD. Two widely used, and clinically tested, evaluation tools for psychological symptom analysis are the Trauma Symptom Checklist for Children (TSCC) and the Trauma Symptom Checklist for Young Children (TSCYC). The TSCC evaluates six areas of symptomology: anxiety, depression, anger, post-traumatic stress, dissociation, and sexual concerns. It is used in pediatric patients aged 8 to 16 years (Briere, 1996). The TSCYC was developed following the success of the TSCC, and measures symptomology in pediatric patients as young as 3 years of age (Briere et al., 2001).

Therapeutic management reflects the level of functional impairment and is based on a comprehensive care model that includes cognitive-behavioral therapy (CBT), family therapy, psychodynamic psychotherapy, and occasionally pharmacotherapy (AACAP, 2009; Stirling & Amaya-Jackson, 2008). Caregivers, school personnel (with permission), and the primary care provider should be included in the therapy. Deblinger and colleagues (1996) found that when caregivers were included in the CBT, patients experienced a significant improvement in symptoms such as depression and behavioral problems.

Trauma-focused therapies may be the most useful for the pediatric patient with PTSD, because traumatic memories (or avoidance of them) often produce psychological distress. The goal of such therapy is to develop mastery over the memory. Indirect methods of addressing traumatic issues, such as art and play techniques, while important, have not proved superior to directly addressing the child's traumatic experience (AACAP, 2009).

The evidence base for psychopharmacologic approaches to treating pediatric patients who suffer from PTSD is not yet well established, although in adults,

TABLE 38-31

Mental and Physical Conditions That May Mimic Post-traumatic Stress Disorder

• Attention-deficit/hyperactivity disorder (ADHD)	• Hyperthyroidism
• Oppositional defiant disorder (ODD)	• Migraine
	• Asthma
• Panic disorder	• Seizure disorders
• Social anxiety disorder (SAD)	• Catecholamine- or serotonin-secreting tumors
• Obsessive–compulsive disorder (OCD)	• Prescription drugs such as sympathomimetics, steroids, selective serotonin reuptake inhibitors (SSRIs), and antipsychotics
• General anxiety disorder (GAD)	
• Major depressive disorder (MDD), bipolar disorder	• Nonprescription agents such as caffeine, diet pills, antihistamines, and cold medicines
• Primary substance abuse	

Source: AACAP, 2009.

selective serotonin reuptake inhibitors (SSRIs) have been reported to reduce symptoms. Psychopharmacologic intervention, however, should be considered an adjunct to, rather than a substitute for, psychotherapy and should be used with caution (AACAP, 2009; Stirling & Amaya-Jackson, 2008).

Pediatric patients presenting with symptoms associated with PTSD will likely require a number of specialty consultations. These consults will often depend on the presenting symptoms; therefore, MHPs, psychologists, psychiatrists, neurologists, and behavioral medicine specialists are often involved early in the patient's presentation. In addition, personnel from the social work and child life services may become involved if the patient is admitted. It should be noted that pediatric patients who present with physiologic symptoms may also be evaluated by the corresponding subspecialties.

The pediatric patient and caregiver should be educated about PTSD, along with the therapeutic goals and management plan. With caregiver permission, it is also helpful to include the patient's teachers in the education so that they, too, can work on supportive reinforcement of positive behaviors of the child. In therapy with the MHP, the caregivers must explore and address the psychological distress that the traumatic event has had on them, as this understanding will lower their own distress and allow them to be stronger supports for their children.

DISPOSITION AND DISCHARGE PLANNING

The outcomes for children with PTSD vary. Some pediatric patients will improve very slowly over time, with or without treatment. Others will continue to have symptoms of chronic PTSD years later. Some sources suggest that younger pediatric patients may be more vulnerable to permanent effects. It is not yet known if earlier recognition and treatment will change these outcomes (AACAP, 2009).

Accommodation for the child's condition may need to be arranged in the school setting, and is determined by the MHP, caregivers, and school personnel. Reasonable removal or limitations of reminders of the traumatic event may be useful. If functional impairment is significant, removal from the inciting atmosphere may be required (AACAP, 2009).

REFERENCES

1. Abd, A., & Braun, N. (1989). Management of life-threatening bradycardia in spinal cord injury. *Chest, 95*(3), 701–702.

2. Adelson, P., Clyde, B., Kochanek, P., Wisniewski, S., Marion, D., & Yonas, H. (1997). Cerebrovascular response in infants and young children following severe traumatic brain injury: a preliminary report. *Pediatric Neurosurgery, 26*(4), 200–207.

3. Allen, G. S., & Cox, C. S. (1998). Pulmonary contusion in children: Diagnosis and management. *Southern Medical Journal, 91*(12), 1099–1106.

4. American Academy of Child and Adolescent Psychiatry (AACAP). (2009). *Practice parameters for the assessment and treatment of children and adolescents with posttrauma stress disorder.* Washington, DC: Author. Retrieved from http://www.aacap.org/galleries/PracticeParameters/Final%20for%20Web%20December%202009%20PTSD.pdf

5. American Academy of Pediatrics (AAP) Committee on Pediatric Emergency Medicine, American College of Emergency Physicians (ECEP) Pediatric Committee, & Emergency Nurses Association (ENA) Pediatric Committee. (2009). Joint policy statement: Guidelines for care of children in the emergency department. *Pediatrics, 124*(4), 1233–1243.

6. American Academy of Pediatrics (AAP) Section on Orthopaedics, American Academy of Pediatrics (AAP) Committee on Pediatric Emergency Medicine, American Academy of Pediatrics (AAP) Section on Critical Care, American Academy of Pediatrics (AAP) Section on Surgery, American Academy of Pediatrics (AAP) Section on Transport Medicine, American Academy of Pediatrics (AAP) Committee on Pediatric Emergency Medicine, Pediatric Orthopaedic Society of North America, Krug, S., & Tuggle, D. (2008). Management of pediatric trauma. *Pediatrics, 121*(4), 849–854.

7. American Academy of Pediatrics (AAP) & American College of Emergency Physicians (ACEP). (1998). *Advanced pediatric life support instructor manual* (pp. 75–87). Dallas, TX: Author.

8. American Academy of Pediatrics (AAP) & American Heart Association (AHA). (2006). *Pediatric advanced life support.* Dallas, TX: Author.

9. American Burn Association. (2001). *2001 practice guidelines for burn care.* Chicago: Author.

10. American Burn Association. (2009). National Burn Repository 2009 report. Retrieved from http://www.ameriburn.org/2009NBRAnnualReport.pdf

11. American College of Surgeons (ACS). (1997). Pediatric trauma. In *Advanced trauma life support instructor course manual* (6th ed., pp. 353–375). Chicago: First Impression.

12. American College of Surgeons (ACS). (2008). The National Trauma Data Bank 2009 pediatric report. Retrieved from http://www.facs.org/trauma/ntdb/ntdbpediatricreport2009.pdf

13. American College of Surgeons (ACS), Committee on Trauma. (2004). *Advanced trauma life support for doctors: Student manual.* Chicago: Author.

14. American College of Surgeons (ACS), Committee on Trauma. (2008). *Advanced trauma life support for doctors* (8th ed.). Chicago: Author.

15. American Heart Association (AHA). (2006). 2005 American Heart Association (AHA) guidelines for cardiopulmonary resuscitation (CPR) and emergency cardiovascular care (ECC) of pediatric and neonatal patients: Pediatric advanced life support. *Pediatrics, 117*(5), e1005–1028.

16. American Psychiatric Association (APA). (2000). *Diagnostic and statistical manual of mental disorders* (4th ed, Text Revision). Washington, DC: Author.

17. American Spinal Injury Association (ASIA). (2003). *International standards for neurological classification of spinal cord injury.* Chicago: Author.

18. American Spinal Injury Association (ASIA) & International Medical Society of Paraplegia. (2001). *International standards for neurological and functional classification of spinal cord injury patients.* Chicago: ASIA.

19. Arbogast, K., Durbin, D., Kallan, M., Menon, R., Lincoln, A., & Winston, F. (2002). The role of restraint and seat position in pediatric facial fractures. *Journal of Trauma Injury, Infection, and Critical Care, 52*(4), 693–697.

20. Avarello, J., & Cantor, R. (2007). Pediatric major trauma: An approach to evaluation and management. *Emergency Medicine Clinics of North America, 25*, 803–836.

21. Bak, Z., Sjoberg, F., Eriksson, O., Steinrall, I., & Janerot-Sjoberg, B. (2009). Hemodynamic changes during resuscitation after burns using the parkland formula. *Journal of Trauma Injury, Infection, and Critical Care, 66*(2), 329–336.

22. Balbus, J., & Malina, C. (2009). Identifying vulnerable subpopulations for climate change health effects in the United States. *Journal of Occupational and Environmental Medicine, 51*(1), 33–37.

23. Balci, A., Kazez, A., Eren, S., Ayan, E., Ozalp, K., & Eren, M. N. (2004). Blunt thoracic trauma in children: Review of 137 cases. *European Journal of Cardiothoracic Surgery, 26*(2), 387–392.

24. Barsness, K., Bensard, D., Ciesla, D., Partrick, D., Hendrickson, R., & Karrer, F. (2004). Blunt diaphragmatic rupture in children. *Journal of Trauma, 56*(1), 80–82.

25. Barzo, P., Marmarou, A., Fatouros, P., Hayasaki, K., & Corwin, F. (1997). Contribution of vasogenic and cellular edema to traumatic brain swelling measured by diffusion weighted imaging. *Journal of Neurosurgery, 87*(6), 900–907.

26. Bassuk, E., Dawson, R., Perloff, J., & Weinreb, L. F. (2001). Posttraumatic stress disorder in extremely poor women: Implications for health care clinicians. *Journal of the American Medical Women's Association, 56*, 79–85.

27. Beaty, J., & Kasser, J. (2005). *Rockwood and Wilkins' fractures in children* (6th ed.). Philadelphia: Lippincott, Williams, & Wilkins.

28. Biffl, W., Moore, F., Moore, E., Sauaia, A., Read, R., & Burch, J. (1994). Cardiac enzymes are irrelevant in the patient with suspected myocardial contusion. *American Journal of Surgery, 168*(6), 523–527; discussion 527–528.

29. Bliss, D., & Silen, M. (2002). Pediatric thoracic trauma. *Critical Care Medicine, 30*(11 2uppl), S409–415.

30. Bonadio, W., & Hellmich, T. (1989). Post-traumatic pulmonary contusion in children. *Annals of Emergency Medicine, 18*(10), 1050–1052.

31. Bondurant, C., & Oro, J. (1993). Spinal cord injury without radiographic abnormalities and Chiari malformation. *Journal of Neurosurgery, 79*, 833–838.

32. Borse, N., Gilchrist, J., Dellinger, A., Rudd, R., Ballesteros, M., & Sleet, D. (2008). *CDC childhood injury report: Ppatterns of unintentional injuries among 0–19 year olds in the United States, 2000–2006.* Atlanta, GA: Centers for Disease Control and Prevention, National Center for Injury Prevention and Control. Retrieved from http://www.cdc.gov/safechild/images/CDC-childhoodinjury.pdf

33. Bracken, M., Shepard, M., Holford, T., Leo-Summers, L., Aldrich, E., Fazi, M., et al. (1997). Administration of methylprednisolone for 24 or 48 hours or tirilazad mesylate for 48 hours in the treatment of acute spinal cord injury: Results of the Third National Acute Spinal Cord Injury Randomized Controlled Trial. National Acute Spinal Cord Injury Study. *Journal of the American Medical Association, 277*(20), 1597–1604.

34. Briere, J. N. (1996). *Trauma symptom checklist for children (TSCC) professional manual.* Odessa, FL: Psychological Assessment Resources.

35. Briere, J., Johnson, K., Bissada, A., Damon, L., Crouch, J., Gil, E., et al. (2001). The Trauma Symptom Checklist for Young Children (TSCYC): Reliability and association with abuse exposure in a multi-site study. *Child Abuse & Neglect, 25*, 1001–1014.

36. Brophy, M., Sinclair, S. A., Hostetler, S. G., & Xiang, H. (2006). Pediatric eye injury-related hospitalizations in the United States. *Pediatrics, 117*(6), e1263–e1271.

37. Brown, C., Antevil, J., Sise, M., & Sack, D. (2005). Spiral computed tomography for the diagnosis of cervical, thoracic, and lumbar spine fractures: Its time has come. *Journal of Trauma, 58*(5), 890–895.

38. Brown, S., Haas, C., Dinchman, K., Elder, J., & Spirnak, J. (2001). Radiologic evaluation of pediatric blunt renal trauma in patients with microscopic hematuria. *World Journal of Surgery, 25*(12), 1557–1560.

39. Cadili, A., & de Gara, C. (2008). Complications of splenectomy. *American Journal of Medicine, 121*, 371–375.

40. Canale, S., & Beaty, J. (2007). *Campbell's operative orthopaedics* (11th ed.). Philadelphia: Elsevier.

41. Centers for Disease Control and Prevention (CDC). (n.d., a). *The CDC injury research agenda, 2009–2018.* Atlanta, GA: Author. Retrieved from http://www.cdc.gov/injury/ResearchAgenda/CDC_Injury_Research_Agenda-a.pdf

42. Centers for Disease Control and Prevention (CDC). (n.d., b). *CDC trauma care: Aaccess to trauma care. Getting the right care, at the right place, at the right time.* Atlanta, GA: Author. Retrieved from http://www.cdc.gov/TraumaCare/

43. Centers for Disease Control and Prevention (CDC). (n.d., c). *Injuries among children and adolescents.* Atlanta, GA: Author. Retrieved from http://www.cdc.gov/print.do?url=http%3A//www.cdc.gov/ncipc/fact-sheets/children.htm

44. Centers for Disease Control and Prevention (CDC). (n.d., d). Web-based Injury Statistics Query and Reporting System (WISQARS) [online]. Atlanta, GA: Author. Retrieved from www.cdc.gov/ncipc/wisqars

45. Ceran, S., Sunam, G., Aribas, O., Gormus, N., & Solak, H. (2002). Chest trauma in children. *European Journal of Cardiothoracic Surgery, 21*(1), 57–59.

46. Chiaretti, A., Piastra, M., Pulitano, S., Pietrini, D., DeRosa, G., Barbaro, R., et al. (2002). Prognostic factors and outcomes of children with severe head injury: An 8-year experience. *Child's Nervous System, 18*(3), 129–136.

47. Clendenon, J., Meyers, R., Nance, M., & Scaife, E. (2004). Management of duodenal injuries in children. *Journal of Pediatric Surgery, 39*(6), 964–968.

48. Committee on Trauma of the American College of Surgeons. (1993). *Advance Trauma Life Support Course for Physicians* (5th ed.). Chicago: Author.

49. Cooper, A. (2005). Early assessment and management of trauma. In K. Ashcroft, G. Holocomb, & J. Murphy. (Eds.). *Pediatric surgery* (pp. 168–184). Philadelphia: Elsevier Saunders.

50. Cooper, A., Barlow, B., DiScala, C., & String, D. (1994). Mortality and truncal injury: The pediatric perspective. *Journal of Pediatric Surgery, 29*(1), 33–38.

51. Cotton, B., Beckert, B., Smith, M., & Burd, R. (2004). The utility of clinical and laboratory data for predicting intra-abdominal injury among children. *Journal of Trauma: Injury, Infection, and Critical Care, 56*(5), 1068–1075.

52. Davis, K., Fabian, T., Croce, M., Gavant, M., Flick, P., Minard, G., et al. (1998). Improved success in nonoperative management of blunt splenic injuries: Embolization of splenic artery pseudoaneurysms. *Journal of Trauma: Injury, Infection, and Critical Care, 44*(6), 1008–1015.

53. Davis, R., Mullen, N., Malela, M., Taylor, J., Cohen, W., & Rivara, F (1994). Cranial computed tomography scans in children after minimal head injury with loss of consciousness. *Annals of Emergency Medicine, 24*(4), 640–645.

54. Deblinger, E., Lippmann, J., & Steer, R. (1996). Sexually abused children suffering posttraumatic stress symptoms: Initial treatment outcome findings. *Child Maltreatment, 1*(4), 310–321.

55. Dowd, M., & Krug, S. (1996). Pediatric blunt cardiac injury: Epidemiology, clinical features, and diagnosis. Pediatric Emergency Medicine Collaborative Research Committee: Working Group on Blunt Cardiac Injury. *Journal of Trauma, 40*(1), 61–67.

56. Downard, C., Hulka, F., Mullins, R., Piatt, J., Chestnut, R., Quint, P., et al. (2000). Relationship of cerebral perfusion pressure and survival in pediatric brain injured patients. *Journal of Trauma, 49*(4), 654–658.

57. D'Souza, A., Nelson, N., & McKenzie, L. (In press). Pediatric burn injuries treated in US emergency departments between 1990 and 2006. *Pediatrics.*

58. Duffy, B., McLaughlin, P., & Eichelberger, M. (2006). Assessment, triage, and early management of burns in children. *Clinical Pediatric Emergency Medicine, 7*, 82–93.

59. Dunning, J., Daly, J., Malhotra, R., Stratford-Smith, P., Lomas, J., Lecky, F., et al. (2004). The implications of NICE guidelines on the management of children presenting with head injury. *Archives of Disease in Childhood, 89*(8), 763–767.

60. Dunning, J., Daly, J., Lomas, J., Lecky, F., Batchelor, J., Mackway-Jones, K., et al. (2006). Derivation of the children's head injury algorithm for the prediction of important clinical events decision rule for head injury in children. *Archives of Disease in Childhood, 91*(11), 885–891.

61. Dunseth, W., & Ferguson, T. (1965). Acquired cardiac septal defect due to thoracic trauma. *Journal of Trauma, 5*, 142–149.

62. Eastern Association of the Surgery of Trauma. (2001). *Practice management guidelines for the evaluation of blunt abdominal trauma.* Retrieved from http://www.east.org/tpg/bluntabd.pdf

63. Emergency Nurses Association (ENA). (2005). Position statement: Family Presence at the bedside during invasive procedures and cardiopulmonary resuscitation. Retrieved from http://www.ena.org/about/position/position/Pages/Default.aspx

64. Emergency Nurses Association (ENA). (2007). *Trauma nursing core course* (6th ed.). Des Plaines, IL: Author.

65. Eshel, G., Gross, B., Bar-Yochai, A., Azizi, E., & Mundel, G. (1987). Cardiac injuries caused by blunt chest trauma in children. *Pediatric Emergency Care, 3*(2), 96–98.

66. Esparza, J., M-Portillo, J., Sarabia, M., Yuste, J., Roger, R., & Lamas, E. et al. (1985). Outcome in children with severe head injuries. *Child's Nervous System, 1*(2), 109–114.

67. Fallat, M., Costich, J., & Pollack, S. (2006). The impact of disparities in pediatric trauma on injury-prevention initiatives. *Journal of Trauma: Injury, Infection, and Critical Care, 60*(2), 452–454.

68. Fang, J., Chen, R., & Lin, B. (1998). Cell count ratio: New criterion of diagnostic peritoneal lavage for detection of hollow organ perforation. *Journal of Trauma: Injury, Infection, and Critical Care, 45*(3), 540–544.

69. Feliciano, D., Mattox, K., & Moore, E. (2008). *Trauma* (6th ed.). New York: McGraw-Hill.

70. Fleisher, G., Ludwig, S., & Henretig, F. (2006). *Textbook of pediatric emergency medicine* (5th ed.). Philadelphia: Lippincott Williams & Wilkins.

71. Frick, E., Pasquale, M., & Cipolle, M. (1999). Small-bowel and mesentery injuries in blunt trauma. *Journal of Trauma: Injury, Infection, and Critical Care, 46*(5), 920–926.

72. Fuhrman, B., & Zimmerman, J. (2006). *Pediatric critical care* (3rd ed.). Philadelphia: Mosby-Elsevier.

73. Garcia, V., Gotschall, C., Eichelberger, M., & Bowman, L. (1990). Rib fractures in children: A marker of severe trauma. *Journal of Trauma, 30*(6), 695–700.

74. Gausche-Hill, M. (2009). Pediatric disaster preparedness: Are we really prepared? *Journal of Trauma, 67*(suppl), S73–S76.

75. Glatterer, M., Toon, R., Ellestad, C., McFee, A., Rogers, W., Mack, J., et al. (1985). Management of blunt and penetrating external esophageal trauma. *Journal of Trauma, 25*(8), 784–792.

76. Green, N., & Swiontkowski, M. (2008). *Skeletal trauma in children* (4th ed.). Philadelphia: Elsevier.

77. Greenberg, M. (2006). *Handbook of Neurosurgery* (6th ed.). New York: Thieme.

78. Greenhalgh, D. (2007). Burn resuscitation. *Journal of Burn Care and Research, 28*(4), 555–565.

79. Greenlee, T., Murphy, K., & Ramm, M. (1984). Amylase isoenzymes in the evaluation of trauma patients. *American Surgeon, 50*(12), 637–640.

80. Grisoni, E., & Volsko, T. (2001). Thoracic injuries in children. *Respiratory Care Clinics of North America, 7*(1), 25–38.

81. Grubenhoff, J., duFord, K., & Roosevelt, G. (2007). Heat-related illness. *Clinical Pediatric Emergency Medicine, 8*(59), 59–64.

82. Hamilton, M., & Myles, S. (1992). Pediatric spinal injury: Review of 174 hospital admissions. *Journal of Neurosurgery, 77*, 700–704.

83. Hatef, D., Cole, P., & Hollier, L. (2009). Contemporary management of pediatric facial trauma. *Current Opinion in Otolaryngology & Head and Neck Surgery, 17*, 308–314.

84. Hatoum, O. A., Bashenko, Y., Hirsh, M., & Krausz, M. (2002). Continuous fluid resuscitation for treatment of uncontrolled hemorrhagic shock following massive splenic injury in rats. *Shock, 18*(6), 574–579.

85. Hawley, C., Ward, A., Magnay, A., & Long, J. (2004). Outcomes following childhood head injury: A population study. *Journal of Neurology, Neurosurgery, and Psychiatry, 75*(5), 737–742.

86. Haxhija, E., Nores, H., Schober, P., & Hollwarth, M. (2004). Lung contusion–lacerations after blunt thoracic trauma in children. *Pediatric Surgery International, 20*(6), 412–414.

87. Hehir, M., Hollands, M., & Deane, S. (1990). The accuracy of the first chest x-ray in the trauma patient. *Australia and New Zealand Journal of Surgery, 60*(7), 529–532.

88. Hennes, H., Smith, D., Schneider, K., Hegenbarth, M., Duma, M., & Jona, J. (1990). Elevated liver transaminase levels in children with blunt abdominal trauma: A predictor of liver injury. *Pediatrics, 86*(1), 87–90.

89. Hirsch, M., & DeRoss, A. (2009). Injury prevention and the national agenda: Can we make America injury free? *Journal of Trauma, 67*(suppl), S91–S93.

90. Hirsch, R., Landt, Y., Porter, S., Canter, C., Jaffe, A., Ladenson, J., et al. (1997). Cardiac troponin I in pediatrics: Normal values and potential use in the assessment of cardiac injury. *Journal of Pediatrics, 130*(6), 872–877.

91. Holden, C., Holman, J., & Herman, M. (2007). Pediatric pelvic fractures. *Journal of the American Academy of Orthopaedic Surgeons, 15*(3), 172–177.

92. Holmes, J., Sokolove, P., Brant, W., & Kuppermann, N. (2002a). A clinical decision rule for identifying children with thoracic injuries after blunt torso trauma. *Annals of Emergency Medicine, 39*(5), 492–499.

93. Holmes, J., Sokolove, P., Brant, W., Palchak, M., Vance, C., Owings, J., et al. (2002b). Identification of children with intra-abdominal injuries after blunt trauma. *Annals of Emergency Medicine, 39*(5), 500–509.

94. Ildstad, S., Tollerud, D., Weiss, R., Cox, J., & Martin, L. (1990). Cardiac contusion in pediatric patients with blunt thoracic trauma. *Journal of Pediatric Surgery, 25*(3), 287–289.

95. Inaba, A., & Seward, P. (1991). An approach to pediatric trauma: Unique anatomic and pathophysiologic aspects of the pediatric patient. *Emergency Medicine Clinics of North America, 9*(3), 523–548.

96. Institute of Medicine, Committee of the Future of Emergency Care in the U.S. Health System. (2007). Emergency care for children: Growing pains. Retrieved from http://books.nap.edu/openbook.php?record_id=11655

97. Isaacman, D., Scarfonw, R., Kost, S., Gochman, R., Davis, H., Bernado, L., et al. (1993). Utility of routine laboratory testing for detecting intra-abdominal injury in the pediatric trauma patient. *Pediatrics, 92*(5), 691–694.

98. Isenhour, J., & Marx, J. (2007). Advances in abdominal trauma. *Emergency Medicine Clinics of North America, 25*, 713–733.

99. Issa, P., Brihi, E., Janin, Y., & Slim, M. (1983). Superior vena cava syndrome in childhood: Report of ten cases and review of the literature. *Pediatrics, 71*(3), 337–341.

100. Jandeck, C., Kellner, U., Bornfeld, N., & Forester, M. H. (2000) Open globe injuries in children. *Graefe's Archive for Clinical and Experimental Ophthalmology, 238*(5), 420–426.

101. Jobst, M., Canty, T., & Lynch, F. (1999). Management of pancreatic injury in pediatric blunt abdominal trauma. *Journal of Pediatric Surgery, 34*(5), 818–824.

102. Junkins, E., O'Connell, K., & Mann, N. (2006). Pediatric trauma systems in the United States: Do they make a difference? *Clinical Pediatric Emergency Medicine, 7*, 76–81.

103. Kanski, J. (2003). *Clinical ophthalmology: A systematic approach* (5th ed.). New York: Butterworth-Heinemann Elsevier Science.

104. Kassira, W., & Namias, N. (2008). Outpatient management of pediatric burns. *Journal of Craniofacial Surgery, 19*(4), 1007–1009.

105. Keller, M., Coln, C., Trimble, J., Green, M., & Weber, T. (2004). The utility of routine trauma laboratories in pediatric trauma resuscitations. *American Journal of Surgery, 188*, 671–678.

106. Keller, M., Stafford, P., & Vane, D. (1997). Conservative management of pancreatic trauma in children. *Journal of Trauma: Injury, Infection, and Critical Care, 42*(6), 1097–1100.

107. Kleikamp, G., Schnepper, U., Kortke, H., Breymann, T., & Korfer, R. (1992). Tricuspid valve regurgitation following blunt thoracic trauma. *Chest, 102*(4), 1294–1296.

108. Kliegman, R., Behrman, R., Jenson, H., & Stanton, B. (2007). *Nelson textbook of pediatrics* (18th ed.). Philadelphia: W. B. Saunders.

109. Klein, M., Hollingworth, W., Rivara, F., Krmer, C., Askay, S., Heimbach, D., et al. (2008). Hospital costs associated with pediatric burn injury. *Journal of Burn Care and Research, 29*(4), 632–637.

110. Kochanek, P. (2006). Severe traumatic brain injury in infants and children. In B. Fuhrman & J. Zimmerman (Eds.), *Pediatric critical care* (3rd ed., pp.1595–1617). Philadelphia: Mosby Elsevier.

111. Kochanek, P., Clark, R. S., Ruppel, R. A., Adelson, P. D., Bell, M. J., Whalen, M. J., et al. (2000). Biochemical, cellular, and molecular mechanisms in the evolution of secondary brain damage after severe traumatic brain injury in infants and children: Lessons learned from the bedside. *Pediatric Critical Care Medicine, 1*(1), 4–19.

112. Koehler, S., Shakir, A., Ladham, S., Rozin, L., Omalu, B., Dominick, J., et al. (2004). Cardiac concussion: Definition, differential diagnosis, and cases presentation and the legal ramification of a misdiagnosis. *American Journal of Forensic Medicine and Pathology, 25*(3), 205–208.

113. Kortbeek, J., Al Turki, S., Ali, J., Antoine, J., Bouillon, B., Brasel, K., et al. (2008). Advanced trauma life support, 8th edition, the evidence for change. *Journal of Trauma, 64*(6), 1638–1650.

114. Krug, E., Sharma, G., & Lozano, R. (2000). The global burden of injuries. *American Journal of Public Health, 90*(4), 523–526.

115. Kulshrestha, P., Das, B., Iyer, K., Sampath, K., Sharma, M., Rao, I., et al. (1990). Cardiac injuries: A clinical and autopsy profile. *Journal of Trauma, 30*(2), 203–207.

116. Kulstad, E., Pisano, M., & Shirakbari, A. (2003). Delayed presentation of traumatic diaphragmatic hernia. *Journal of Emergency Medicine, (24)*4, 455–457.

117. Kunimoto, D., Kanitkar, K., & Makar, M. (2008). *The Wills eye manual: Office and emergency room diagnosis and treatment of eye disease* (5th ed.). Philadelphia: Lippincott, Williams & Wilkins.

118. Kupperman, N., Holmes, J., Dayan, P., Hoyle, J., Atabaki, S., Holubkov, B., et al. (2009). Identification of children at very low risk of clinically-important brain injuries after head trauma: A prospective cohort study. *Lancet, 374*(9696), 1160–1170.

119. Kurkchubasche, A., Fendya, D., Tracy, T., Silen, M., & Weber, T. (1997). Blunt intestinal injury in children. *Archives of Surgery, 132,* 652–658.

120. Laine, J., Kaiser, S., & Diab, M. (2010). High-risk pediatric orthopedic pitfalls. *Emergency Medicine Clinics of North America, 28,* 85–102

121. Langer, J., Winthrop, A., Wesson, D., Spence, L., Pearl, R., Hoffman, M., et al. (1989). Diagnosis and incidence of cardiac injury in children with blunt thoracic trauma. *Journal of Pediatric Surgery, 24*(10), 1091–1094.

122. Langlois, J., Rutland-Brown, W., & Thomas, K. (2006). *Traumatic brain injury in the United States: Emergency department visits, hospitalizations, and deaths.* Atlanta, GA: Centers for Disease Control and Prevention, National Center for Injury Prevention and Control. Retrieved from http://www.cdc.gov/ncipc/tbi/TBI_in_US_04/TBI%20in%20the%20US_Jan_2006.pdf

123. Lichtmann, M. (1970). The problem of contused lungs. *Journal of Trauma, 10*(9), 731–739.

124. Lutz, N., Nance, M., Kallan, M., Arbogast, K., Durbin, D., & Winston, F. (2004). Incidence and clinical significance of abdominal wall bruising in restrained children involved in motor vehicle crashes. *Journal of Pediatric Surgery, 39*(6), 972–975.

125. Maron, B., Gohman, T., Kyle, S., Estes, N., & Link, M. (2002). Clinical profile and spectrum of commotio cordis. *Journal of the American Medical Association, 287*(9), 1142–1146.

126. Mattox, K., & Allen, M. (1986). Systematic approach to pneumothorax, haemothorax, pneumomediastinum and subcutaneous emphysema. *Injury, 17,* 309–312.

127. Mehall, J., Ennis, J., Saltzman, D., Chandler, J., Grewal, H., Wagner, C. et al. (2001). Prospective results and standardized algorithm based on hemodynamic status for managing pediatric solid organ injury. *Journal of the American College of Surgeons, 193*(4), 347–353.

128. Meier, J., & Tollefson, T. (2008). Pediatric facial trauma. *Current Opinion in Otolaryngology & Head and Neck Surgery, 16*(6), 555–561.

129. Milner, D., Losek, J., Schiff, J., & Sicoli, R. (2003). Pediatric pericardial tamponade presenting as altered mental status. *Pediatric Emergency Care, 19*(1), 35–37.

130. Mohan, R., Iyer, R., & Thaller, S. (2009). Airway management in patients with facial trauma. *Journal of Craniofacial Surgery, 20*(1), 21–23.

131. Moore, E., Cogbill, T., Jurkovich, G., Shackford, S., Malangoni, M., & Champion, H. (1995). Organ injury scaling: Spleen and liver (1994 revision). *Journal of Trauma: Injury, Infection, and Critical Care, 38*(3), 323–324.

132. Moore, E., Cogbill, T., Malangoni, M., Jurkovich, G., Shackford, S., & Champion, H. (1990). Organ injury scaling: Pancreas, duodenum, small bowel, colon and rectum. *Journal of Trauma: Injury, Infection, and Critical Care, 30*(11), 1427–1429.

133. Moore, E., Mattox, K., & Feliciano, D. (2003). *Trauma manual* (4th ed.). New York: McGraw-Hill.

134. Moore, E., Shackford, S., Pachter, H., McAninch, J., Browner, B., Champion, H., et al. (1989). Organ injury scaling: Spleen, liver and kidney. *Journal of Trauma: Injury, Infection, and Critical Care, 29*(12), 1664–1666.

135. Moss, R., & Musemeche, C. (1996). Clinical judgment is superior to diagnostic tests in the management of pediatric small bowel injury. *Journal of Pediatric Surgery, 31*(8), 1178–1182.

136. Nabaweesi, R., Arnold, M., Chang, D. C., Rossberg, M., Ziegfeld, S., Sawaya, D., et al. (2008). Prehospital predictors of risk for pelvic fractures in pediatric trauma patients. *Pediatric Surgery International, 24,* 1053–1056.

137. Nakayama, D., Ramenofsky, M., & Rowe, M. (1989). Chest injuries in childhood. *Annals of Surgery, 210*(6), 770–775.

138. Nathan, D., & Oski, F. (1998). *Hematology of infancy and childhood.* Philadelphia: W. B. Saunders.

139. National Center for Injury Prevention and Control (NCIPC). (n.d.). *The economic costs of injuries among children and adolescents.* Atlanta, GA: Centers for Disease Control and Prevention, National Center for Injury Prevention and Control. Retrieved from http://www.cdc.gov/print.do?url=http://www.cdc.gov/ncipc/factsheets/CostBook/Cost_of_Injury-Children.htm.

140. National Spinal Cord Injury Association (NSCIA). (1998). Spinal cord statistics. Retrieved from www.makoa.org/nscia/fact02.html

141. National Spinal Cord Injury Statistical Center (NSCISC). (2010). Spinal cord injury facts and figures at a glance. Retrieved from https://www.nscisc.uab.edu/public_content/pdf/Facts%20and%20Figures%20at%20a%20Glance%202010.pdf

142. National Trauma Data Standards (NTDS). (2009). Data dictionary 2010 admissions. Retrieved from http://www.ntdsdictionary.org/dataElements/documents/NationalTraumaDataStandardDictionary2010.doc

143. Ochoa, C., Chokshi, N., Upperman, J., Jurkovich, G., & Ford, H. (2007). Prior studies comparing outcomes from trauma care at children's hospitals versus adult hospitals. *Journal of Trauma, 63*(suppl), S87–S91.

144. O'Malley, P., Brown, K., Krug, S., & Committee on Pediatric Emergency Medicine. (2008). Patient-and family-centered care of children in the emergency department. *Pediatrics, 122*(2), e511–e521.

145. Paige, T., Bartlett, S., & Whitaker, L. (2000). Facial trauma and plastic surgical emergencies. In G. Fleisher & S. Ludwig (Eds.). *Textbook of pediatric emergency medicine* (4th ed., pp. 1383–1395). Philadelphia: Lippincott, Williams, & Wilkins.

146. Pang, D., & Wilberger, J. (1982). Spinal cord injury without radiographic abnormalities in children. *Journal of Neurosurgery, 57,* 114–121.

147. Patel, P., Vasquez, S., Granick, M., & Rhee, S. (2008). Topical antimicrobials in pediatric burn wound management. *Journal of Craniofacial Surgery, 19*(4), 913–922.

148. Pathi, V., Jones, B., & Davidson, K. (1996). Mitral valve disruption following blunt trauma: Case report and review of the literature. *European Journal of Cardiothoracic Surgery, 10*(9), 806–808.

149. Peclet, M., Newman, K., Eichelberger, M., Gotschall, C., Garcia, V., & Bowman, L. (1990). Thoracic trauma in children: An indicator of increased mortality. *Journal of Pediatric Surgery, 25*(9), 961–965; discussion 965–966.

150. Perks, D., & Grewal, H. (2005). Abdominal compartment syndrome in the pediatric patient with blunt trauma. *Journal of Trauma Nursing, 12*(2), 50–54.

151. Pfenninger, J., Kaiser, G., Lutschg, J., & Sutter, M. (1983). Treatment and outcome of the severely head injured child. *Intensive Care Medicine, 9*(1), 13–16.

152. Pitetti, R., & Walker, S. (2005). Life-threatening chest injuries in children. *Clinical Pediatric Emergency Medicine, 6*(1), 16–22.

153. Povlishock, J., & Christman, C. W. (1996). The pathobiology of traumatically induced axonal injury in animals and humans: A review of current thoughts. In F. Bandak, R. Eppinger, & A. Ommaya (Eds.), *Traumatic brain injury: Bioscience and mechanics.* New York: Mary Ann Liebert.

154. Prevent Blindness America. (2008). The scope of the eye injury problem. Retrieved from http://www.preventblindness.org/resources/Non Customizable/NC_FS93_08-083_Scope_Eye_Injury.pdf

155. Puranik, S., Hayes, J., Long, J., & Mata, M. (2002). Liver enzymes as predictors of liver damage due to blunt abdominal trauma in children. *Southern Medical Journal, 95*(2), 203–206.

156. Ramos, C., Koplewitz, B., Babyn, P., Manson, D., & Ein, S. (2000). What have we learned about traumatic diaphragmatic hernias in children? *Journal of Pediatric Surgery, 35*(4), 601–604.

157. Rhee, P., Kuncir, E., Johnson, L., Brown, C., Velmaho, G., Martin, M., et al. (2006). Cervical spine injury is highly dependent on the mechanism of injury following blunt and penetrating assault. *Journal of Trauma, 61*(5), 1166–1170.

158. Roddy, M., Lange, P., & Klein, B. (2005). Cardiac trauma in children. *Clinical Pediatric Emergency Medicine, 6*(4), 234–243.

159. Rothrock, S. (2007). *Tarascon pediatric emergency pocketbook* (5th ed.). Lompac, CA: Tarascon Publishing.

160. Rotondo, M., Bard, M., Sagraves, S., Toschlog, E., Schenarts, P., Goettler, C., et al. (2009). What price commitment: What benefit? The cost of a saved life in a developing level I trauma center. *Journal of Trauma, 67*(5), 915–923.

161. Ruppel, R., Kochanek, P. M., Adelson, P. D., Rose, M. E., Wisniowski, S. R., Bell, M. J., et al. (2001). Excitatory amino acid concentrations in ventricular cerebrospinal fluid after severe traumatic brain injury in infants and children: The role of child abuse. *Journal of Pediatrics, 138*(1), 18–25.

162. Safe Kids Worldwide (SKW). (2007). Trends in unintentional childhood injury deaths. Retrieved from http://www.usa.safekids.org/content_documents/2007_InjuryTrends.doc

163. Safe Kids Worldwide (SKW). (2009). Injury facts: Burn injury. Retrieved from https://www.safekids.org

164. Saffle, J. (2007). The phenomenon of "fluid creep" in acute burn resuscitation. *Journal of Burn Care and Research, 28*(3), 382–395.

165. Santschi, M., Echavé, V., Laflamme, S., McFadden, N., & Cyr, C. (2005). Seat-belt injuries in children involved in motor vehicle crashes. *Canadian Journal of Surgery, 48*(5), 373–376.

166. Sartorelli, K., & Vane, D. (2004). The diagnosis and management of children with blunt injury of the chest. *Seminars in Pediatric Surgery, 13*(2), 98–105.

167. Sato, Y., Matsumoto, N., Komatsu, S., Matsuo, S., Kunimasa, T., Yoda, S., et al. (2007). Coronary artery dissection after blunt chest trauma: Depiction at multidetector-row computed tomography. *International Journal of Cardiology, 118*(1), 108–110.

168. Schunk, J., Rodgerson, J., & Woodward, J. (1996). The utility of head computed tomographic scanning in pediatric patients with normal neurologic examination in the emergency department. *Pediatric Emergency Care, 12*(3), 160–165.

169. Schuster-Bruce, M., & Nolan, J. (1999). Priorities in management of blunt abdominal trauma. *Current Opinion in Critical Care, 5*(6), 500–505.

170. Schutzman, S., & Greenes, D. (2001). Pediatric minor head trauma. *Annals of Emergency Medicine, 37*(1), 65–74.

171. Sesma, H., Slomine, B., Ding, R., & McCarthy, M. (2008). Executive functioning in the first year after pediatric traumatic brain injury. *Pediatrics, 121*(6), 686–1695.

172. Shapiro K., & Marmarou, A. (1982). Clinical applications of the pressure–volume index in treatment of pediatric head injuries. *Journal of Neurosurgery, 56*(6), 819–825.

173. Sheridan, R. (2002). Burns. *Critical Care Medicine, 30*(11), S500–S514.

174. Shilyansky, J., Pearl, R., Kreller, M., Sena, L., & Babyn, P. (1997). Diagnosis and management of duodenal injuries in children. *Journal of Pediatric Surgery, 31*(6), 880–886.

175. Signorino, P., Densmore, J., Werner, M., Winthorp, A., Stylianos, S., Guice, K., et al. (2005). Pediatric pelvic injury: Functional outcome at 6-month follow-up. *Journal of Pediatric Surgery, 40*, 107–113.

176. Siplovich, L., & Kawar, B. (1997). Changes in the management of blunt splenic and hepatic injuries. *Journal of Pediatric Surgery, 32*(10), 1464–1465.

177. Sivit, C. (2002). Pediatric thoracic trauma: Imaging considerations. *Emergency Radiology, 9*(1), 21–25.

178. Sikhondze, W., Madiba, T., Naidoo, N., & Muckart, D. (2006). Predictors of outcome in patients requiring surgery for liver trauma. *Injury, 38*(1), 65–70.

179. Skaggs, D., Friend, L., Alman, B., Chambers, H. G., chmitz, M., Leoke, B., et al. (2005). The effect of surgical delay on acute infection following 554 open fractures in children. *Journal of Bone and Joint Surgery of America, 87*(1), 8–12.

180. Smyth, B. (1979). Chest trauma in children. *Journal of Pediatric Surgery, 14*(1), 41–47.

181. So, T., Farrington, E., & Absher, R. (2009). Evaluation of the accuracy of different methods used to estimate weights in the pediatric population. *Pediatrics, 123*(6), e1045–E1051.

182. Society of Critical Care Medicine. (2003). Guidelines for the acute medical management of severe traumatic brain injury in infants, children, and adolescents. *Critical Care Medicine, 31*(6), S407–S491.

183. St. Peter, S., Keckler, S., Spilde, T., Holcomb, G., & Ostlie, D. (2008). Justification for an abbreviated protocol in the management of blunt spleen and liver injury in children. *Journal of Pediatric Surgery, 43*(1), 191–194.

184. Stafford, P., Blinman, T., & Nance, M. (2002). Practical points in evaluation and resuscitation of the injured child, *Surgical Clinics of North America, 82*(2), 273–301.

185. Stirling, J., & Amaya-Jackson, L. (2008). Clinical report: Understanding the behavioral and emotional consequences of child abuse. *Pediatrics, 122*, 667–673.

186. Stylianos, S. (2005). Outcomes from pediatric solid organ injury: Role of standardized care guidelines. *Current Opinion in Pediatrics, 17*, 402–406.

187. Stylianos, S., & APSA Liver/Spleen Trauma Study Group. (2002). Compliance with evidence-based guidelines in children with isolated spleen or liver injury: A prospective study. *Journal of Pediatric Surgery, 37*(3), 453–456.

188. Sumich, A., Nelson, M., & McDeavitt, J. (2007). TBI: A pediatric perspective. In N. Zasler, D. I. Katz, & R. D. Zafonte (Eds.), *Brain injury medicine: Principles and practice.* New York: Demos.

189. Teasdale, G., & Jennett, B. (1974). Assessment of coma and impaired consciousness: A practical scale. *Lancet, 2*, 81–84.

190. Tolo, V. (2000). Orthopaedic treatment of fractures of the long bones and pelvis in children who have multiple injuries. *Journal of Bone & Joint Surgery, 82*(2), 272–280.

191. Torode, I., & Zeig, D. (1985). Pelvic fractures in children. *Journal of Pediatric Orthopaedics, 5*(1), 76–84.

192. Tovar, J. (2008). The lung and pediatric trauma. *Seminars in Pediatric Surgery, 17*(1), 53–59.

193. Trachiotis, G., Sell, J., Pearson, G., Martin, G., & Midgley, F. (1996). Traumatic thoracic aortic rupture in the pediatric patient. *Annals of Thoracic Surgery, 62*(3), 724–731; discussion 731–722.

194. Wagner, C., & Boyd, K. (2008). Pediatric heatstroke. *Air Medical Journal, 27*(3), 118–122.

195. Wales, P., Shuckett, B., & Kim, P. (2001). Long-term outcome after nonoperative management of complete traumatic pancreatic transaction in children. *Journal of Pediatric Surgery, 36*(5), 823–827.

196. Waters, R., Adkins, R. H., Yakura, J., & Sie, I. (1991). Profiles of spinal cord injury and recovery after gunshot injury. *Clinical Orthopedics, 267*, 14–21.

197. Wegner, S., Colletti, J., & Van Wie, D. (2006). Pediatric blunt abdominal trauma. *Pediatric Clinics of North America, 53*(2), 243–246.

198. Wilson, R. (1999). *Handbook of trauma pitfalls and pearls*. Philadelphia: Lippincott, Williams & Wilkins.

199. Woosley, C., & Mayes, T. (2008). The pediatric patient and thoracic trauma. *Seminars in Thoracic and Cardiovascular Surgery, 20*(1), 58–63.

200. Yucesoy, K., & Yuksel, K. (2008). SCIWORA in MRI era. *Clinical Neurology and Neurosurgery, 110*(5), 429–433.

201. Ziegler, M., Greenwald, M., DeGuzman, M., & Simon, H. (2005). Posttraumatic stress responses in children: Awareness and practice among a sample of pediatric emergency care providers. *Pediatrics, 115*, 1261–1267.

PART IV

Emergency Preparedness

Chapter 39
Principles of Disaster Management and Clinical Practice

Principles of Disaster Management and Clinical Practice

DISASTER MANAGEMENT

Catherine J. Goodhue and Jeffrey S. Upperman

Recent natural and man-made disasters across the globe have highlighted the importance of emergency/disaster planning and preparedness at the individual, hospital, community, state, federal, and global levels. The effects of these disasters are far-reaching, including loss of infrastructure (water, power, sewage, roadways), financial crisis, and loss of the basic needs of individuals and families. Billions of dollars have been spent in the past decade to increase both homeland security and public health preparedness in the United States (Markenson et al., 2006).

Despite these efforts, the Institute of Medicine (IOM, 2007a) reports that emergency departments are unable to provide care for a large influx of victims in the event of a major disaster. While disaster preparedness frameworks exist, pediatric concerns and needs are rarely addressed in disaster planning (Markenson et al., 2006; IOM, 2007b). A recent survey found that only 6% of emergency departments in the United States had all of the recommended equipment and supplies needed to respond appropriately to a disaster scenario (Gausche-Hill et al., 2007). Hospital emergency/disaster planners are obligated to prepare their facilities for an influx of victims of all ages, including children, and for a wide range of disaster situations.

There are four stages of emergency/disaster planning:

- Mitigation
- Preparedness
- Response
- Recovery

During the *mitigation* phase, a yearly hazard vulnerability assessment (HVA) is performed by evaluating the types of potential natural disasters in the region. Since the terrorist attacks in the United States on September 11, 2001, all hospitals have also been forced to consider the possibility of terrorist activities, including chemical, biological, radiological, nuclear, and explosive (CBRNE) attacks. A hospital emergency/disaster plan is then developed based on the types of disasters most likely to occur in that region.

In the *preparedness* phase, hospitals ensure readiness through tabletop discussions and full-scale disaster drills. The Joint Commission (TJC) requires hospitals to conduct two drills each year, which serve to test the operability of the hospital disaster plan. According to Kaji et al. (2008), however, no method has been validated to assess hospital disaster preparedness. Also, a recent regional analysis concluded that facilities rarely drill with mock pediatric victims, with the exception of pediatric hospitals (Ferrer et al., 2009; Ferrer et al., in press). After a drill, the hospital completes an after-action report, which documents performance and outcomes of the drill.

Emergencies can be further classified as "routine" or "crisis." Routine emergencies are those that occur somewhat regularly, such as earthquakes, hurricanes, fires, and traffic accidents, allowing emergency management personnel to prepare specifically for them. Drills for routine types of emergencies are typically scripted, so that a practiced response becomes possible. Crisis emergencies, in contrast, are unlike previously experienced emergencies, as the scripted plans are inadequate to meet the demands imposed by the new situation. Hurricane Katrina in 2005, the 2010 Haiti earthquake, and the 2011 Japan earthquake and tsunami are examples of crisis emergencies, based on the combination of their size, flooding extent, extent of injury, and loss of infrastructure. Improvisation and innovation on the part of the emergency response team become paramount in large-scale disasters (Leonard & Howitt, 2008).

As part of their emergency preparedness activities, hospitals should also take the following steps:

- Encourage individual preparedness
- Provide additional disaster education and training for staff, including specific pediatric content
- Develop relationships with hospitals in the region for transferring patients and pooling resources in the event of a major disaster

It is crucial to develop mutual aid agreements *before* disaster strikes. In addition, hospitals may wish to develop contingency plans to house family members and even pets of their health care staff. When health care professionals (HCPs) feel comfortable about the safety and well-being of their families, they are more likely to be available to care for the community at large (Qureshi et al., 2005).

The *response* stage includes the actions taken immediately following a disaster. The hospital will declare a disaster and commence its disaster operations using the Hospital Emergency Incident Command System (HICS). If there is actual structural damage to the hospital, a decision to evacuate may be made. Otherwise, the hospital will "shelter in place." Hospitals should expect victims to present by various modes of transportation or by emergency medical services (EMS). Victims will vary in severity from the "walking wounded" to those who are critically injured. Noninjured and mentally traumatized individuals may also arrive and will need to be evaluated. Resources, both supplies and personnel, may become scarce depending on the magnitude of the disaster. If a significant number of children are involved, additional supplies may be required, including cribs, diapers, formula, pediatric dosages of medications, and pediatric emergency equipment. Plans should include sheltering of displaced children who may arrive without an accompanying adult. Hospitals should also plan for the identification of children such as taking photographs and marking forearms with names and birth dates when available.

During the *recovery* phase, after the victims have been treated and systems are operational, the hospital resumes its normal operations. In a recent U.S. governmental press release, the Federal Emergency Management Agency (FEMA) and the Department of Health and Human Services' (HHS) Administration on Children and Families announced an agreement establishing a Disaster Case Management Plan to assist families in the aftermath of a disaster (HHS & FEMA, 2009). In the wake of Hurricanes Katrina and Rita, case management will provide direct assistance to families affected by a disaster.

As the hospital engages in normal operations during the emergency situation, any displaced children should be reunited with their families. Psychological support should be provided to hospital staff as needed. After-action reports are completed and the hazard vulnerability assessment is re-evaluated. The hospital emergency/disaster plan should be revised based on lessons learned during the response stage.

TYPES OF MASS-CASUALTY INCIDENTS

Mass-casualty incidents (MCIs) are disasters involving large numbers of victims, which can overwhelm the health care delivery system. Several such events have been directed specifically at children: The Columbine High School shootings in Colorado in 1999 and the school hostage situation in Russia in 2004, for example, received international media coverage. The Oklahoma City bombing in 1995, while not directed at children, injured and killed a number of children housed in the daycare center in the building that was targeted. Recent hurricanes, tsunamis, and earthquakes have affected a large number of children. Disaster planners must include children in their plans and HCPs must be adept at caring for pediatric victims should disaster strike.

Disasters can be classified into *natural* and *man-made* events. Natural disasters commonly occurring in North America include floods, earthquakes, hurricanes, tornados, and wildfires (Foltin et al., 2006). A tsunami, another natural disaster, although not as frequently seen, caused significant loss of life and property in Indonesia and other areas bordering the Indian Ocean in 2004, and northeastern Japan in 2011. Epidemics or pandemics are another type of "natural" disaster. While they lack the immediate impact of other natural disasters due to their insidious onset, they can instill much fear and panic across the globe.

Flooding can cause near-drowning (submersion injury) and a variety of skin disorders related to prolonged contact with water and gastrointestinal problems associated with contaminated drinking water (Foltin et al., 2006). Structural damage to roadways may impede the disaster response.

Earthquakes can cause significant structural damage as well as injury and death. The most prevalent injuries expected are orthopedic and soft-tissue trauma (Ballow et al., 2008). The exact injuries experienced will depend on where the victim was at the time of the quake (e.g., inside a structure that subsequently collapses). Tsunamis, associated with underwater earthquakes, cause enormous waves that flood coastal areas. Structural damage, flooding, and loss of life ensue (Foltin et al., 2006).

Hurricanes cause structural damage not only from the winds but also from the surges of ocean waves. Injuries are caused by flying debris as well as flooding. Tornados also cause structural damage and injuries associated with flying debris (Foltin et al., 2006).

Wildfires mainly cause structural damage, but inhabitants may become overwhelmed by smoke and may suffer a range of thermal burn injuries. Those with underlying pulmonary conditions may experience increased symptoms (Foltin et al., 2006). There is future risk of mudslides in the burned area due to loss of vegetation.

Man-made disasters may be either accidental (industrial explosion or derailment of train cars carrying hazardous chemicals) or intentional (terrorist bomb). Although industrial mitigation plans may curtail these types of accidents, they are nonetheless more unpredictable than natural disasters. Terrorist attacks are the least predictable of disasters, causing not only injury and death, but also public disorder, panic, and anxiety (Foltin et al., 2006).

The injuries associated with an industrial accident depend on the type of substance released. Also, there may be an associated explosion, with the release of chemicals into the atmosphere, soil, and bodies of water. Respiratory symptoms as well as possible thermal burns and blast injuries may occur in victims (Foltin et al., 2006).

Blast injuries can cause a wide range of injuries depending on the type of explosive used, the area in which the detonation occurs (i.e., enclosed space versus open space), and the distance from site of detonation to victim. Primary blast injuries occur directly to the body from the blast wave: blast lung injury, air embolization, intestinal perforation, and auditory injury. Most victims with primary blast injuries die in the field; however, if they do present to the emergency department, the HCP must focus on airway, breathing, and circulation, as with all trauma patients (Foltin et al., 2006).

Secondary blast injuries are the most common type of blast injury. These injuries result from flying shrapnel or debris and may be classified as either penetrating or blunt. Tertiary injuries are the result of the victim being struck by the "blast wind"; penetrating and blunt trauma injuries result. The associated fires and structural collapse can also cause injuries such as thermal burns, smoke inhalation, and crush injuries to victims (Foltin et al., 2006).

The injuries associated with chemical, biological, radiological, and nuclear events depend on the specific agent but can include skin irritation or burns, respiratory impairment, gastrointestinal symptoms, and widespread fear and panic. Surveillance system access is crucial to the response to these potential events (Boyer et al., 2009).

Issues that arise in the aftermath of a disaster will vary depending on the type of catastrophe. Mental health issues, for example, may include acute stress disorder and post-traumatic stress disorder (PTSD). Thus response to mental health issues must addressed in any comprehensive disaster response plan (Gold et al., 2009; American Academy of Pediatrics [AAP], 2000).

Displacement of large numbers of families has occurred in recent history. Shelters may not be prepared to handle such an influx of children, as they may lack basic equipment such as cribs, bottles, formula, and diapers. Crowded conditions in these shelters may give rise to outbreaks of infectious diseases such as norovirus (Rebman et al., 2008). Children may become separated from their families and will require chaperones to ensure their well-being and safety as well as reunification with their families. Children and adults with chronic conditions may experience exacerbations due to loss of routine medications.

In light of recent disasters across the globe, community, state, and federal disaster planners should reevaluate their own response plans and prepare to incorporated lessons learned into current disaster plans.

PEDIATRIC VULNERABILITIES

Children and the elderly are the most vulnerable populations affected by a disaster. Pediatric vulnerabilities and their potential consequences are described in Table 39-1. To protect themselves, families should be encouraged to develop and maintain a home emergency supply kit and emergency plan. Alternative childcare plans should be developed in the event that the child is at school or en route to or from school and the parents are at work when a disaster strikes (Markenson et al., 2006).

One subpopulation of children who merit attention consists of children with special health care needs, whether medical, physical, emotional, or cognitive (McPherson et al., 1998). Some of these children may be dependent on durable medical goods, such as wheelchairs or ventilators; their medical equipment (ventilators) may also require electricity. Other children with emotional or cognitive impairments may need a chaperone continuously. Some medically impaired children may depend on caregivers to maintain their airway (via suctioning) or provide nutrition (physically feeding or via feeding tubes). Families of children with special health care needs will require assistance in (1) identifying the specific needs of their child (2) procuring additional resources, and (3) developing appropriate disaster plans for home and school. Primary care providers (PCPs) need to assist the child and family with disaster planning in the following ways:

- Alerting utility providers to the need for emergency assistance during power outages
- Developing backup power supply plans in the event that utility providers are unable to restore power in a timely manner
- Storing a supply of routine medications and equipment in case interruption in the supply chain occurs in the course of a disaster
- Identifying contingencies for procuring extra medications and equipment during a disaster
- Educating the family to provide care if routine caretakers are unable to do so in the event of a disaster
- Maintaining the child's current medical information (Markenson et al., 2006)

SURGE PLANNING AND STRUCTURAL SUPPORT

In the event of a disaster, the influx of injured victims can overwhelm a health care facility. Resources, including both supplies and personnel, can become depleted, jeopardizing comprehensive care of victims. Hospitals must have plans to deal with a potential "surge" of victims. Currently, many hospitals already operate at "surge" levels (IOM, 2007a), and would be quickly overwhelmed by a disaster surge of patients.

The U.S. Department of Health and Human Services HHS (Barbera & Macintyre, 2007) has defined two components of surge: *capacity*, which is the ability to respond to a significant increase in the number of patients, and *capability*, which is the ability to deal with specialized or unusual needs of victims (e.g., an adult facility with an influx of pediatric victims). A disaster response, although initiated at the local or hospital level, may move to the community, state, and/or federal levels depending on the magnitude of the emergency. Unfortunately, gaps in pediatric surge planning, as in disaster planning in general, have yet been fully addressed. Therefore, children and adolescents must be factored into comprehensive surge plans at all planning levels (National Commission on Children and Disasters, 2010, http://www.ahrq.gov/prep/nccdreport/nccdreport.pdf).

NATIONAL SURGE PLANNING

The primary legislative act that governs the U.S. federal disaster response is the Robert T. Stafford Disaster Relief and Emergency Assistance Act (1988). FEMA is the federal agency whose primary responsibility is disaster response (Moss & Shelhamer, 2007). Following the events of September 11, 2001, the federal government created the U.S. Department of Homeland Security (DHS), which functions

TABLE 39-1

Pediatric Physiologic and Anatomic Differences and Vulnerabilities	
Type of Differences	**Consequences**
Corporeal	
• Smaller in size • Wide range of weight • Larger head size in proportion to body	• Vulnerable to heavier agents that accumulate close to ground • Adult-only providers may have difficulty estimating weight (drug dosages and fluid resuscitation are weight-dependent) • Prone to head injury; also prone to increased heat loss when uncovered
Integumentary System	
• Larger body surface area • Skin thinner and less keratinized	• Toxins more rapidly absorbed • Prone to deeper level burns
Circulatory System	
• Varied compensatory mechanisms in shock • Smaller blood volume • Wide range of heart rate and blood pressure depending on age	• Can maintain heart rate despite blood volume loss; may give a false impression of normalcy to providers unaccustomed to children • More vulnerable to shock and dehydration • Adult-only providers may not recognize normal versus abnormal ranges
Respiratory System	
• Larger tongue in relation to oropharynx • Higher larynx • Smaller lungs • Minute ventilation/kg faster • Wide range of respiratory rate depending on age	• At risk for airway obstruction especially when prone • More difficult to intubate • Prone to barotrauma • Airborne toxins absorbed more rapidly • Adult-only providers may not recognize normal vs. abnormal ranges
Musculoskeletal System	
• More pliable skeleton—more cartilaginous • Epiphyseal plates unfused • Cervical spine more flexible	• At risk for internal injuries without fractures • At risk for growth plate fractures • May sustain spinal cord injury without radiographic changes
Immunologic System	
• "Uneducated" immune system • Herd immunity inexperience	• Increased risk for infection • More susceptible to infectious agents
Metabolic/Endocrine System	
• Higher metabolic rate and limited reserves	• At risk for hypoglycemia • Less able to compensate with prolonged exposure to stressors
Maturational	
• Infants are nonverbal; young children have limited verbal abilities • Depend on adult caregivers for needs • Younger children lack motor skills • Limited cognitive ability related to danger	• Cannot verbalize symptoms • Unable to meet needs if caregiver injured or killed • Unable to flee from danger on own • May move closer to danger rather than flee
Neuropsychological	
• Age-based responses to trauma are varied • Response also based on caregiver's responses to the trauma	• Regression, tantrums, separation anxiety, depression, anger, somatic complaints, increased risk-taking • May increase child's distress

Source: Adapted from Foltin et al., 2006.

to prevent and prepare the country for the possibility of terrorism (Markenson et al., 2006). DHS also reviewed the federal response plan and created the National Response Plan (NRP), which provides an all-hazards, unified structural approach to disaster responses in the United States. This plan describes how various federal departments and agencies will work together and coordinate the activities of local, state, and tribal governments and other private agencies in the event of a disaster (DHS, 2005).

The NRP has 15 emergency support functions (ESF), of which number eight (ESF 8) is for public health and medical services. In addition, a series of Incident-Specific Annexes and Support Annexes sustain the ESFs. Disaster Medical Assistance Teams (DMATS) are one type of response from the federal level. Many state emergency operations plans are based on the NRP and many local emergency operation plans are based on state plans (Markenson et al., 2006).

Mandated by the U.S. Homeland Security Presidential Directive 5 (HSPD-5), the National Incident Management System (NIMS) was released in 2004. NIMS is a framework for governmental agencies (federal, state, local, and tribal), nongovernmental agencies, and the private sector to work together to respond and recover from disasters and to prepare for them (Markenson et al., 2006).

Finally, the U.S. Strategic National Stockpile (SNS) was established to resupply large quantities of medical supplies and medications ("push packs") to states and communities within 12 hours of a federal directive. Unfortunately, the SNS can only stock FDA-licensed pharmaceuticals for only FDA-approved indications. Many of the antidotes and antimicrobials in the SNS do not have pediatric indications. However, the SNS has been improving its pediatric capabilities (Markenson et al., 2006).

COMMUNITY SURGE PLANNING

The initial response to a disaster occurs at the local level. Unfortunately, community planners generally have not considered children when creating their plans. Pediatric HCPs should actively participate in developing these disaster plans to ensure that pediatric considerations are incorporated (Markenson et al., 2006). Community citizens as well as HCPs can take the Community Emergency Response Teams (CERT) training (www.citizencorps.gov/cert), which provides disaster preparedness education and training specific for that community.

Community pediatric HCPs can play an important role in advocating for the inclusion of children in local, state, and national disaster plans. They may function as a resource for the community at large and encourage their patients and families to create family emergency plans for home, school, and work. These community providers must also be alert for suspicious presentations of illnesses. It is important for pediatric HCPs in the community to further

educate themselves in disaster preparedness (Fagbuyi & Upperman, 2009; Markenson et al., 2006).

Pediatric HCPs working in private offices and community clinics can also register as emergency volunteers through their local or regional Emergency System for the Advance Registration of Volunteer Health Professionals (ESAR-VHP) program. This registration process verifies the credentials of an HCP, including education and licensure. In the event of a large-scale local or regional disaster, the individual is notified to report to a specific location to provide care. Providers with credentials and privileges at specific hospitals should assess that facility's disaster plan, as they may formally be incorporated into the plan.

Community-wide drills provide an opportunity for community stakeholders to interact with one another. Stakeholders may include EMS providers, fire department personnel, law enforcement, hospitals, schools, local public health, service groups, and nonsecular organizations (Foltin et al., 2006). Lessons learned from these drills are then integrated into the community disaster plan.

HOSPITAL SURGE PLANNING

The first step in hospital surge planning involves evaluation of the neighborhood in which the hospital resides and identification of facilities with children (schools, daycare centers, playgrounds, gyms) who could potentially flood the health care facility. Advanced technologies such as geographic information systems (GIS) can be utilized to estimate pediatric surge in that facility's area (Mills et al., in press). Community and general hospitals should examine their ability to care for an influx of pediatric patients; conversely, children's hospitals should be prepared to care for adult disaster victims. Each facility must evaluate its pediatric bed surge capacity, including the number of intensive care beds. Memoranda of understanding (MOU) should be developed to facilitate transferring of patients in the event of a disaster. Community and general hospitals should not expect to transfer all pediatric patients to a children's hospital but rather must be prepared to care for potential pediatric victims themselves. In the event of a disaster, hospitals should plan to be self-sufficient for at least 48 to 72 hours (Foltin et al., 2006).

The facility's emergency preparedness manual should incorporate an all-hazards approach and follow the Incident Command System (ICS). This system is used in emergency management and provides a "common language" for all disaster response participants (e.g., hospital, EMS, fire, law enforcement). The ICS can expand depending on the magnitude and needs in a specific event. Five ICS management functions are identified:

- Incident command: Responsible for all aspects of the incident
- Operations: Responsible for determining tactics and directing all resources

- Planning: Responsible for monitoring resources, collecting and analyzing data, and documenting the response
- Logistics: Responsible for procuring resources and services
- Finance/administration: Responsible for monitoring costs associated with the incident

Under these functions are standardized titles including commander, officer, chief, supervisor, director, and leader. The people assigned to specific roles should be easily identifiable and often wear labeled vests indicating their role (Foltin et al., 2006; http://training.fema.gov/IS/crslist.asp).

Health care facilities should identify a rapid pediatric triage tool to be used in a disaster event involving large numbers of children. The JumpSTART algorithm is one of a few pediatric-specific triage tools and is commonly used in prehospital care (Figure 39-1). The Pediatric Visual Assessment Triangle (Dieckmann, 2006), another commonly used pediatric triage tool, is used in the hospital setting following an MCI. Using this tool, responders rapidly assess children for appearance, breathing, and circulation. Staff must be familiar with the tool selected by the facility. Pediatric victims should be reassessed frequently.

In the event of a large-scale disaster, additional health care personnel will be vital to the hospital's ability to care for an influx of victims. Staff are needed to care for the current patients as well as the surge of patients. Up-to-date telephone trees are essential to the disaster response. In addition, personnel are needed not only to respond immediately to the incident, but also to relieve current staff at the end of their shifts. Moreover, personnel are needed to be "on alert" for a possible response (Boyer et al., 2009).

Pediatric-specific equipment, supplies, and pharmaceuticals must be available at all health care facilities in the event of an MCI. Currently, few facilities have all of the recommended supplies and equipment for children (Gausche-Hill et al., 2007). Facilities not usually treating children should consider stocking the Broselow tape, which provides recommendations for color-coded prepackaged medications/supplies based on the child's length. Pediatric supplies should also include items such as cribs, diapers, and formula. Advanced informatics systems, including the Pediatric Emergency Decision Support System (PEDSS), can be utilized by a hospital to develop a pediatric-specific disaster plan. PEDSS incorporates census data and the necessary pediatric supplies, equipment, pharmaceuticals required for a specific disaster (earthquake), and devises a plan specific for that facility (Neches et al., 2009).

Full-scale disaster drills are a valuable training strategy that enable staff to become familiar with procedures and specific supplies, such as decontamination equipment. It is important for facilities to drill with child victims. To this end, members from community organizations can be recruited to participate in drills. Pediatric-specific disaster education classes are also important, and staff should be encouraged to participate in these educational opportunities.

Hospitals should expect to receive unaccompanied minors in the event of a major disaster. Some may not be injured but will still require supervision and a safe place to shelter until reunited with family. Procedures should be in place for identifying and eventually reunifying children with their families. The National Center for Missing and Exploited Children (www.missingkids.com) should be utilized to assist with the reunification of children and their families in large-scale disasters (Blake & Stevenson, 2009).

In the aftermath of a major disaster, hospitals should provide mental health assistance for their personnel (Boyer et al., 2009). Mental health services should also be expanded to provide services for children and their families (Gold et al., 2009).

DECONTAMINATION

Exposure to chemicals (industrial accidents, terrorist weapons), radiological products (nuclear accidents, terrorist "dirty bombs"), and biological agents (anthrax) requires decontamination of the victims prior to therapeutic management. In the past, the decontamination process occurred in the field by hazardous materials (hazmat) teams. The threat of terrorism and the possibility of accidental industrial and nuclear accidents, however, have increased the need for healthcare facilities to prepare for a potential influx of contaminated victims. In the event of exposure to hazardous substances (chemical, biological, radiological), victims require decontamination for three purposes: (1) to prevent or reduce absorption of toxin(s); (2) to prevent and reduce contamination of others (emergency services workers and HCPs); and (3) to prevent contamination of the health care facility (Koenig et al., 2008).

The U.S. Occupational Safety and Health Administration (OSHA, 2005) has developed guidelines for hospital-based health care personnel. Hospital emergency/disaster plans must establish a decontamination area; some facilities utilize outside trailers or shelters/tents, for this purpose, whereas others have a fixed unit for this purpose. Appropriate numbers of staff must be trained on donning personal protective equipment (PPE) and decontamination procedures. Notably, the PPE is bulky and can impede fine motor skills such as starting an intravenous line. A person's voice also becomes muffled when wearing the equipment, and hearing can be diminished. In addition, HCPs can become overheated in the PPE depending on the climate. Personnel should be monitored for heat fatigue, dehydration, and potential effects from the toxin. They should also recognize that young children may be fearful of the fully protected health care worker. Despite the existence of well-developed plans, contaminated victims may

PEDIATRIC MCI TRIAGE

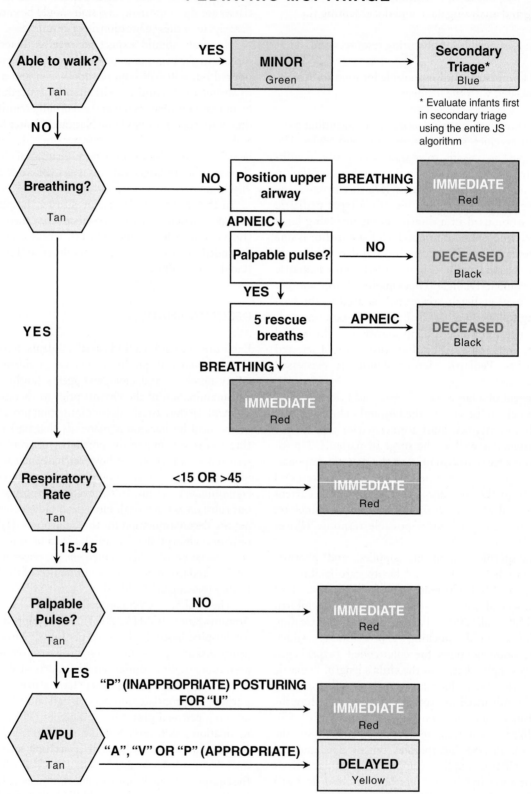

FIGURE 39-1

Color-Coded JumpSTART Pediatric MCI Triage Algorithm. http://www.jumpstarttriage.com/uploads/Simplified_algorithm.gif

Source: Courtesy of Lou Romig, MD.

still present to the emergency department with staff being unaware of the patients' exposure to the toxin. However, once identified, protocols can be implemented to diminish further contamination of the facility (Boyer et al., 2009; Foltin et al., 2006).

The area where contaminated victims are initially contained is considered the "hot zone." The most effective and safest decontamination procedure, which is carried out in this zone, includes undressing and showering with tepid water and using a mild soap. After decontamination, victims enter the "cold zone," where medical evaluation and treatment are performed. Emergency measures can be initiated in the "hot zone" if necessary and if resources are available. It is essential to ensure security and crowd control in these areas (Koenig et al., 2008).

Although the OSHA guidelines do not address the pediatric population, a number of pediatric considerations must be addressed in the facility's own decontamination plan. *Children in Disasters: Hospital Guidelines for Pediatric Preparedness* (2008) provides general guidelines and age-specific recommendations for pediatric decontamination:

- Avoid separation of families
- Assist caregivers with decontamination if needed

- Recognize that older children might be resistant or challenging
- Maintain a water temperature of at least 98°F (37°C)
- Carefully monitor the child's airway
- Incorporate large-volume, low-pressure water delivery systems (child friendly)
- Recognize that smaller children may present a larger problem with regard to any of these points

The age-specific recommendations include three age groups: children younger than 2 years of age; children aged 2 to 8 years; and children aged 8 to 18 years (Table 39-2). It is crucial that health care personnel who may be involved in the decontamination of victims, including children, participate in regular training programs to ensure competency with their facility's protocol.

In part, disaster management requires foresight and proactive planning by a network of local, state, federal, and (at times) global agencies (Table 39-3). As disaster management and preparedness become more sophisticated, the roles of HCPs and health care centers will evolve. Numerous resources are available to individuals and facilities to help them become better equipped to support their communities at times of crisis.

TABLE 39-2

Age-Based Decontamination Recommendations		
Younger Than 2 Years of Age	**2 to 8 Years of Age**	**8 to 18 Years of Age**
• Ambulatory children should be undressed by the caregiver and/or "hot zone" personnel	• Caregiver and/or "hot zone" personnel should assist ambulatory children with undressing	• Ambulatory children can undress themselves when instructed by "hot zone" personnel
• "Hot zone" personnel and/or the caregiver should undress nonambulatory children and place them on a stretcher	• "Hot zone" personnel and/or the caregiver should undress nonambulatory children and place them on a stretcher	• "Hot zone" personnel and/or the caregiver should undress nonambulatory children and place them on a stretcher
• Place clothes/items in containers or bags and label them	• Place clothes/items in containers or bags and label them	• Place clothes/items in containers or bags and label them
• The caregiver and/or "hot zone" personnel must accompany the child in the shower	• The caregiver and/or "hot zone" personnel should accompany both ambulatory and nonambulatory children in the shower	• Ambulatory children can shower themselves; nonambulatory children should be assisted by "hot zone" personnel and/or the caregiver in the shower
• Keep the child on a stretcher, as children become very slippery in the shower		
• Ensure airway maintenance		
• After the shower, the caregiver and/or "cold zone" personnel should dry the child and put a gown on the child	• After the shower, the child should dry off and put on a gown	• After the shower, the child should dry off and put on a gown
• Give the child a unique identification number on a wristband and triage to the appropriate area for evaluation	• Give the child a unique identification number on a wristband and triage to the appropriate area for evaluation	• Give the child a unique identification number on a wristband and triage to the appropriate area for evaluation
• Try not to separate children from their families unless critical medical issues arise	• Try not to separate children from their families unless critical medical issues arise	• Try not to separate children from their families unless critical medical issues arise

Source: Adapted from Centers for Bioterrorism Preparedness Program Pediatric Task Force, NYC DOHMN Pediatric Disaster Advisory Group, NYC DOHMH Healthcare Emergency Preparedness Program (2008). *Children in disasters: Hospital guidelines for pediatric preparedness.*

TABLE 39-3

Abbreviations Related to Disaster Management	
CBRNE	Chemical, Biological, Radiological, Nuclear, Explosive
CERT	Community Emergency Response Teams
DHHS	Department of Health and Human Services
DHS	Department of Homeland Security
DMAT	Disaster Medical Assistance Teams
EMS	Emergency Medical Services
ESAR-VHP	Emergency System for the Advance Registration of Volunteer Health Professionals
ESF	Emergency Support Functions
FDA	Food and Drug Administration
FEMA	Federal Emergency Management Agency
GIS	Geographic Information Systems
HICS	Hospital Emergency Incident Command System
HSPD	Homeland Security Presidential Directive
HVA	Hazard Vulnerability Assessment
ICS	Incident Command System
MCI	Mass-Casualty Incident
MOU	Memoranda of Understanding
NIMS	National Incident Management System
NRP	National Response Plan
OSHA	Occupational Safety and Health Administration
PPE	Personal Protective Equipment
SNS	Strategic National Stockpile
TJC	The Joint Commission

BIOLOGICAL DISASTERS

Asha S. Payne and Daniel B. Fagbuyi

BIOLOGICAL TERRORISM

Definition

Biological terrorism is defined as the use of viruses, bacteria, or other naturally occurring agents as weapons with the intention of causing harm or death to people, animals, or plants. A key component of these agents is the fear they generate and the subtlety with which they are introduced to the general population. It is the job of HCPs to be vigilant in recognizing such potential threats to the population, especially given that the signs and symptoms of the effects from biological terrorism may mimic many common illnesses. Aberrations in location, time of year, or the presence of nonendemic bacteria and viruses should raise suspicion

of biological terrorism, and public health authorities should be notified of a potential threat. Table 39-4 lists questions that HCPs should ask to heighten their awareness of a potential terrorism threat.

The U.S. Centers for Disease Control and Prevention (CDC, 2007) has outlined three categories of biological agents, classified according to their ease of spread and the severity of illness. Category A agents pose the highest risk to the general population, as they are easily spread and have major public health impact, including high death rates, potential for causing mass hysteria, and panic; they are covered in depth here. Category B agents (Table 39-5) are not as easily spread, but do result in moderate illness and panic. Category C agents (Table 39-6) are emerging pathogens that could be engineered for mass destruction; they are readily available, spread, and produced, and have the potential to have a major public health impact.

Category A agents pose the highest risk to the public and national security and, therefore, are of the highest priority. These agents are spread or transmitted easily from person to person, result in high mortality, and may cause public panic and social disruption. In addition, they are easily manufactured and deployed without sophisticated delivery systems, and have the ability to kill or injure hundreds or thousands of people.

A unique and challenging feature that distinguishes a biological exposure from the immediate effects of conventional or nuclear explosives, and chemical exposure, is the delay in the onset of illness (hours to days) associated with biological weapons. This unique feature is key to how illness from biological agents may be unrecognized, present to the "nontraditional" first responder (pediatrician or tertiary facility), and culminate in widespread secondary exposure over large geographic areas (Foltin et al., 2006).

TABLE 39-4

Index of Suspicion of a Possible Bioterrorism Threat
1. Are there large numbers of patients presenting with similar symptoms?
2. Is this diagnosis clinically appropriate for this locale?
3. Is there a cluster of patients from a specific locale presenting with similar symptoms?
4. Are these unusual symptoms for this particular time of year?
5. Is this an endemic disease presenting at a different time of year?
6. Is this a rare disease? (Could this be the index case?)
7. Is there a common geographic factor among the patients presenting with these symptoms?
8. Is there a high case fatality rate or an unusually virulent organism?
9. Is this an uncommon disease with terrorism potential?
10. Is there an increasing disease incidence of a common disease?

TABLE 39-5

Category B Agents			
Disease or Threat	**Organism(s)**	**Source**	**Clinical Presentation**
Brucellosis	*Brucella* spp.	Animal contact (sheep, goats) Consumption of contaminated dairy or undercooked meat Inhalation of aerosol	Nonspecific febrile illness, sweats, headaches, back pain Chronic form possible: recurrent fevers, joint pain, fatigue
Glanders	*Burkholderia mallei*	Prolonged contact with infected animal Laboratory workers	Constitutional symptoms Cutaneous symptoms: abscess-like, can be acute or chronic Mucocutaneous symptoms: increased mucus production Pulmonary: pneumonia, lung abscess, effusions Bacteremia
Melioidosis (Whitmore's disease)	*Burkholderia pseudomallei*	Endemic to Southeast Asia, northern Australia Inhalation of bacteria, through open wounds, ingestion of contaminated water	Acute, localized: nodule in the skin at the pathogen's entry point Constitutional symptoms Pulmonary: fever, myalgia, cough, pneumonia Bacteremia/multifocal abscess formation: seen in immunocompromised individuals Chronic suppurative infections also possible: organs, bone, skin
Psittacosis (orinthosis)	*Chlamydia psittaci*	Inhalation of infected bird droppings	Can be asymptomatic Atypical pneumonia likely Prominent headache
Q fever	*Coxiella burnetii*	People who work with animals (e.g., sheep), inhalation	Atypical pneumonia Mild hepatitis Chronic forms, including chronic endocarditis and chronic fatigue syndromes
Ricin	*Ricinus communis*	Castor beans—limited information on effect on humans Chewing or swallowing beans Inhalation possible from dust from processing beans	Ingestion: nausea, vomiting, abdominal pain, may lead to severe dehydration Inhalation: dyspnea, cough, chest tightness, progressing to pulmonary edema and respiratory failure
Typhus fever	*Rickettsia prowazekii*	Human body louse; head lice and flying squirrels also reservoirs Self-inoculation also possible	Fever Severe headache Maculopapular rash, turns purpuric CNS complications DIC Hypovolemic shock possible
Toxins from common organisms	Epsilon toxin of *Clostridium perfringens* Staphylococcal enterotoxin B	Epsilon toxin: unclear affect on humans Staphylococcal enterotoxin B: ingestion most frequent, inhalational also possible, but less is known	Epsilon toxin: produces neurological complications in animal models Staphylococcal enterotoxin B: self-limited diarrheal illness when ingested, Inhalational: fever, malaise, cough, nausea, vomiting Toxic shock syndrome also possible
Viral encephalitis	Venezuelan equine encephalitis (VEE) Eastern equine encephalitis (EEE)	VEE: seen mostly in horses in Latin America EEE: commonly referred to as "sleeping sickness"; seen in humans; uncommonWEE: seen in humans; uncommon	VEE: self-limited flu-like illness, approximately 1% of patients progress to encephalitis, 20% mortality EEE: self-limited to severe nonspecific viral syndrome similar to VEE, mortality > 50%, neurologic sequelae likely

(Continued)

TABLE 39-5

Category B Agents *(Continued)*			
Disease or Threat	**Organism(s)**	**Source**	**Clinical Presentation**
	Western equine encephalitis (WEE)		WEE: mostly self-limited infection, high rate of severe disease in children, neurological sequelae for children
Food safety threats	*Salmonella* spp.	*Salmonella*: fecal matter from animals contaminate food, including meat products, eggs, vegetables	*Salmonella*: fever, diarrhea, abdominal cramping, all usually self-limited; may lead to bacteremia in older, very young, or immuncompromised populations
	Escherichia coli O157:H7	*E. coli*: unpasteurized dairy, undercooked meat, contaminated fruits and vegetables, those with cattle contact	*E. coli*: bloody diarrhea, severe abdominal pain, and vomiting; diarrhea may lead to hemolytic uremic syndrome in children
	Shigella	*Shigella*: person-to-person and fecal–oral transmission	*Shigella*: bloody diarrhea, fever, abdominal pain; some individuals are asymptomatic carriers
Water Safety Threats			
Cholera	*Vibrio cholerae*	Cholera: contaminated food and drinking water, shellfish, contact with inadequately treated sewage	Cholera: profuse watery diarrhea, vomiting, can rapidly lead to dehydration, shock and death
Cryptosporidium	*Cryptosporidium parvum*	*Cryptosporidium*	*Cryptosporidium*: usually asymptomatic in immunocompetent hosts, immunocompromised hosts

Note: Central nervous system (CNS), disseminated intravascular coagulation (DIC).

TABLE 39-6

Category C Agents		
Disease	**Source/Transmission**	**Clinical Presentation**
Hanta virus, two forms:	Inhalation of stool aerosols of infected rodents	
Hemorrhagic fever with renal syndrome (HFRS)		HFRS: fever, myalgias, malaise thrombocytopenia and DIC develops, diffuse bleeding diathesis; fluid accumulation in retroperitoneal spaces leading to back pain and hypotension, development of oliguric renal failure, hypotension; abnormal renal function leading to polyuria, electrolyte loss
Hantavirus pulmonary syndrome (HPS)		HPS: fever, chills, myalgia, malaise, abdominal symptoms; prolonged PTT, and thrombocytopenia, but no bleeding diathesis; dyspnea and pulmonary edema, hypotension and shock

(Continued)

TABLE 39-6

Category C Agents *(Continued)*		
Disease	**Source/Transmission**	**Clinical Presentation**
Tick-borne hemorrhagic fevers Example: Crimean-Congo hemorrhagic fever	Argasid or ixodid ticks	High fever, myalgias, headache, vomiting, relative bradycardia, then hemorrhage into the skin (causing purple discolorations), saliva, urine; development of hematemesis, epistaxis; all lead to hypovolemia, shock, death
Multidrug-resistant tuberculosis (*Mycobacterim tuberculosis*)	Aerosols Rates of drug resistance greater than 4% in Eastern Europe, Latin America, Africa, Asia (Mushtaq et al., 2006)	Fever, malaise, weight loss, cough; hyponatremia possible
Yellow fever	Mosquitoes: primary vector; transmit the disease between monkeys, but also to humans	Possibly asymptomatic; symptomatic infection includes fever, headache, photophobia, abdominal, back, and joint pain, vomiting; jaundice

Note: Disseminated intravascular coagulation (DIC), partial thromboplastin time (PTT).

In contrast, a biological event would likely result in patients presenting in various locales over time, similar to a natural infectious disease outbreak. Of note, such an intentional epidemic would likely be more compressed in time due to the synchronous exposure of multiple individuals, involve relatively "exotic" diseases uncommon in a given geographic area, and might cause patients to exhibit a particularly high degree of morbidity and mortality. Some of the diseases caused by agents of bioterrorism are highly contagious, and special isolation precautions will be necessary for the safety of EMS personnel.

ANTHRAX

Pathophysiology

Anthrax is caused by *Bacillus anthracis*, an aerobic, Gram-positive rod with spore–forming capability. As a result, it can persist in the environment for as long as several decades, withstanding the effects of air, sunlight, and some disinfectants that might mitigate other biological agents (Moran et al., 2008). Anthrax spores enter the body via a breakdown in the skin, through the gastrointestinal (GI) tract, or through the respiratory system. Regardless of the mode of entry, the spores enter macrophages, germinate, and become vegetative bacteria. The macrophages then migrate to regional lymph nodes, where they break open, releasing bacteria into the lymphatic system, and replicate, eventually leading to a massive bacteremia and sepsis. The bacteria also secrete an exotoxin that produces sepsis and death. Interestingly, presence of the bacteria does not seem to engender an immune response from the body (Dixon et al., 1999).

Epidemiology and etiology

Most cases of anthrax occur related to agricultural settings, as B. *anthracis* is a naturally occurring organism in the environment. Cutaneous anthrax may affect persons who deal directly with animal hides, especially unprocessed or untanned hides; thus this condition is also known as "wool-sorter's disease." Inhalational anthrax, in contrast, is much less common. Humans develop this disease when they are exposed to spore-containing products such as raw animal meat and hides. The last time a person was affected with inhalational anthrax in the United States was in February 2006, after the individual came in contact with animal hides he purchased from the Ivory Coast several months earlier (CDC, 2006b).

Presentation

Anthrax produces three forms of disease: cutaneous, gastrointestinal, and inhalational. As noted earlier, inhalational anthrax is the most severe form of the disease. After exposure to the spores, the clinical presentation in inhalational anthrax occurs in two disease stages. In the first stage, patients present with nonspecific symptoms including fever, cough, dyspnea, vomiting, chills, headache, and abdominal pain. These symptoms last for several hours to several days, and are then followed by a period of apparent recovery. In the second stage, the patient experiences an abrupt return of fever, dyspnea, and diaphoresis. Cyanosis (perhaps from massive lymphadenopathy in the chest), hypotension, and shock develop, leading to death. The second stage is very short, sometimes with death occurring within several hours after the reemergence of symptoms.

Cutaneous anthrax occurs when spores enter broken skin. Spores can enter anywhere, but most commonly invade the body through the face and head or extremities. Approximately 3 days after the person's exposure to this form of anthrax, the spore germinates in the skin, forming a painless, pruritic papule or macule. The lesion then progresses to a large round ulcer. Small vesicles then appear around the periphery of the lesion. Eventually a depressed black eschar forms in the center with a prominent edematous circumference (Figure 39-2). Within 1 to 2 weeks, the eschar dries and falls off. Systemic symptoms, like those noted with inhalational anthrax, may occur, but are rare.

Two forms of the GI disease are possible: upper GI (oropharyngeal) and lower GI. The mechanism that favors one manifestation over the other is unclear. In the oropharyngeal form, ulcers develop in the oral or pharyngeal cavities, leading to lymphadenopathy, edema, and sepsis. The lower GI disease affects the terminal ileum or cecum, causing nausea, vomiting, and malaise. Bloody diarrhea, sepsis, ascites, and an acute abdomen then develop.

Differential diagnosis

Inhalational anthrax, especially given its initial nonspecific, "flu-like" symptoms, can resemble a variety of more benign, less virulent diagnoses, including viral and *Mycoplasma* pneumonia. The mediastinal widening seen on chest radiograph (Figure 39-3) may also resemble that observed with other diagnoses; it may present with acute or chronic mediastinal changes including silicosis, sarcoidosis, and histoplasmosis. Legionnaires' disease, psittacosis, tularemia, and Q fever should also be included in the differential diagnosis.

Cutaneous anthrax can resemble several skin conditions, especially in the early stages of infection when the painless, ulcer is present. It may resemble ulceroglandular

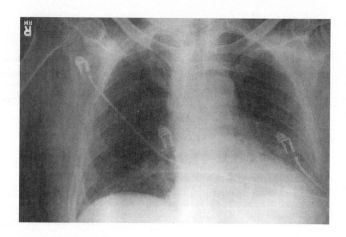

FIGURE 39-3

Inhalational Anthrax.

Source: Reproduced from Jernigan, J. et al., "Bioterrorism-Related Inhalational Anthrax: The First 10 Cases Reported in the United States," Emerging Infectious Diseases 7(6): 2001. Courtesy of CDC.

tularemia, plague, and Glanders. In addition, an ulcer with regional lymphadenopathy may occur in staphylococcal lymphadenitis or cutaneous tuberculosis.

Gastrointestinal anthrax may resemble acute gastroenteritis or ulcers. In addition, the bloody diarrhea may mimic gastroenteritis caused by *Salmonella*, *Shigella*, or *Campylobacter* gastroenteritis and *Clostridium difficile* infection. Irritable bowel diseases should also be a consideration in those patients with abdominal pain and bloody diarrhea. The mouth ulcers seen in GI anthrax may sometimes be confused with viral infections causing mouth sores such as gingivostomatitis or coxsackie virus.

Plan of care

The index of suspicion must be high to diagnose anthrax. If lab personnel are not alerted to the possibility of anthrax, misidentification may occur because of the presence of *Bacillus cerus*, which is often a contaminant. Initial identification of anthrax can be performed in most labs. Additional confirmatory tests (polymerase chain reaction [PCR], immunohistochemical staining) will often need to be sent to special reference labs. Any clinician with a concern for anthrax should promptly alert public health authorities.

Inhalational anthrax is diagnosed after clinical suspicion for the disease is raised. Chest radiograph (CXR) or computed tomography (CT) may show a widened mediastinum, large pleural effusions, or necrotizing pneumonic lesions (Figure 39-3). In addition, blood cultures will be positive within 6 to 24 hours after collection; given the rapidity of clinical deterioration in the second stage of the disease, however, they may not be positive prior to a patient's death. Blood cultures should be obtained prior to administration of antibiotics, because as few as two doses of antimicrobial

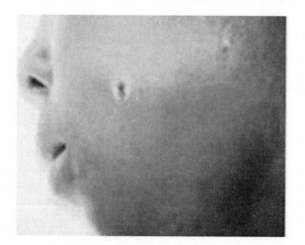

FIGURE 39-2

Cutaneous Anthrax.

Source: Courtesy of Centers for Disease Control and Prevention.

therapy can affect blood culture results (Inglesby et al., 1999). Sputum culture or nasal swabs are not diagnostic.

Although cutaneous anthrax may be diagnosed from the lesion fluid, the HCP should avoid actively trying to express fluid from the wound. Culture from the skin has approximately 60% to 65% positivity, likely due to competition among other local bacteria.

Treatment for all types of anthrax consists of ciprofloxacin or doxycycline for 60 days. Patients should be started on intravenous (IV) therapy with the chosen antibiotic, then transitioned to oral therapy when clinically stable. Although fluoroquinolones are not recommended for pediatric patients younger than the age of 16 years and doxycycline for those younger than age 9, the benefits of treatment outweigh the risk (Inglesby et al., 1999). Inhalational anthrax, once clinically suspected, requires immediate antimicrobial therapy with ciprofloxacin, doxycycline, or penicillin (when susceptabilities are available) and treatment should continue for 60 days.

The length of therapy is prolonged because antimicrobial therapy prevents the development of an immune response (Friedlander et al., 1993). Compliance with this prolonged treatment regimen is paramount to avert any untoward complications and death.

As with any potential exposure to biological threat, local and state health departments will be helpful in guiding overall patient management and resource allocation. Consult infectious disease specialists as necessary.

Many factors will determine which public health message related to anthrax exposure is disseminated and how it is shared with potential patients: how much advanced warning exists prior to anthrax release; the number of individuals affected; the plausible geographic spread of the anthrax spores; the availability of general public vaccine and rapidity of emergency use; and authorization or approval of anthrax vaccine for public use, especially given that the vaccine is not approved for use in pediatric patients. Family and patient messaging will focus on being calm and not giving into panic. Addressing public concerns and providing guidance on prophylaxis, treatment, case definitions, and exposures; defining who is "high risk"; and guiding individuals when to seek medical care are all important steps when anthrax contamination is a threat. Person-to-person spread of anthrax has not been documented. Caregivers and patients should look to the federal agencies such as the CDC, professional organizations such as the American Academy of Pediatrics (AAP), and their individual "medical homes" for further guidance.

Disposition and discharge planning

Death from treated cutaneous anthrax is rare; for untreated cases, mortality is approximately 20%. Inhalational anthrax has a fatality rate in the range of 50% to 70%, even with treatment (AAP, 2006). Postexposure prophylaxis is required only after inhalational exposure. Pediatric patients should take ciprofloxacin or doxycycline for 60 days (Inglesby et al., 1999). The lengthy course of therapy is recommended to account for suspected prolonged exposure to anthrax spores.

A vaccine for anthrax is available, but it is in limited use. The anthrax vaccine adsorbed (AVA, is a six-dose series given to all U.S. active and reserve military personnel. Of note, it is appears to be safe and effective in preventing disease after exposure, but only if appropriate antibiotic therapy is given at the time of anthrax exposure. It is licensed for use only in adults older than 18 years of age.

BOTULISM

Pathophysiology

Clostridium botulinum is an anaerobic, spore-forming, Gram-positive bacillus that occurs naturally in soil. The spores are able to tolerate a wide range of temperatures (Kman & Nelson, 2008). Although seven different antigenic subtypes (A–G) have been identified, all of the toxins affect the body similarly.

Intoxication with botulinum toxin begins with entry of the spores through ingestion or broken skin. After entering the body, the spores germinate into bacteria and produce the toxin, which is readily absorbed through the GI tract. Similarly, the toxin is readily absorbed from the wound or respiratory tract. Irrespective of the entry route, the toxin is taken up by presynaptic neurons, and then cleaves a protein important for fusion of the vesicles to the presynaptic membrane. Thus acetylcholine is not released into the synaptic cleft, resulting in absence of depolarization of the postsynaptic membrane and, subsequently, a flaccid paralysis.

The botulinum toxin is the most poisonous substance known to man. Although the exact lethal dose is not known, one gram of crystalline botulinum toxin could kill more than 1 million people if inhaled (Arnon et al., 2001; Kman & Nelson, 2008; Moran et al., 2008).

Epidemiology and etiology

Botulism is acquired when persons come into contact with the spores directly; human-to-human transmission is not possible. Spores are most commonly encountered from food contaminated with the spores, so that the disease has the potential to affect all age groups. The botulinum toxin is colorless, odorless, and likely tasteless. It is most commonly associated with vegetables such as corn, carrots, and beans, or contaminated condiments such as honey, and foods held at room temperature such as potatoes, condiments, and peanuts (Arnon et al., 2001). Naturally occurring food-borne disease is rare. Approximately 110 cases of botulism are reported to the CDC each year, 70% of which involve infants (CDC, 2006a).

Presentation

Botulism is the clinical syndrome of intoxication with the botulinum toxin. Three types of naturally occurring human botulinum are infantile/intestinal (germinating bacteria elaborates toxin in the gut), food-borne (preformed toxin in food), and wound (rare, but spores infect a wound and release toxin). In contrast, deliberate release of botulinum toxin would likely occur via aerosol or contamination of food or water supplies.

The incubation period for botulism ranges from 6 hours to 10 days, but is usually 1 to 3 days. Pediatric patients may present with profound low muscle tone, weak cry, poor feeding, lethargy, irritability, eyelid lag, and, classically, flaccid, symmetrical, descending, purely motor paralysis that progresses to profound respiratory distress and failure requiring intubation and mechanical ventilation. Although the sensory nervous system remains intact, the patient's level of consciousness may deteriorate as respiratory failure ensues. Of note, the toxin does not enter cerebrospinal fluid (CSF), which means that mental status changes do not occur (Arnon et al., 2001).

The time to onset of symptoms following exposure varies: The larger the burden of exposure, the faster the onset of symptoms. Given that cases of inhaled botulism remain rare, the time for onset of symptoms is not known (Arnon et al., 2001).

Differential diagnosis

Botulism is often confused with Guillain-Barré syndrome or myasthenia gravis. Botulism can be differentiated from these disorders because of the preponderance of cranial nerve symptoms and the absence of sensory nerve damage. In Guillain-Barré syndrome, the patient has a history of recent infection, which is not usually present in botulism. Moreover, in Guillain-Barré syndrome, the paralysis is ascending; in botulism, it is descending. The Miller-Fischer variant of Guillain-Barré syndrome, however, is characterized by bulbar palsy, areflexia, and ataxia. (See the section on neuropathy in Chapter 33 and the section on botulism and Guillain-Barré syndrome in Chapter 35 for more information.) Myasthenia gravis is characterized by recurrent episodes of paralysis, whereas botulism is usually a single episode. Botulism can also be misdiagnosed as ethanol intoxication, tick paralysis (parasthesias and ascending paralysis), and, though rare, poliomyelitis.

Plan of care

The diagnosis of botulism is initially a clinical one. Routine lab tests are often normal. Confirmatory tests require several days to complete and often need to be sent to the CDC or one of several public health laboratories around the United States. Cerebrospinal fluid findings are normal.

Imaging will produce negative results in botulism; thus this tool is useful in excluding other diagnoses. Excretions or skin biopsy can be tested for botulinum toxin at sophisticated laboratories.

Supportive care and passive immunization are the hallmarks of care in affected pediatric patients. An antitoxin is available from the CDC and local health departments; it combats botulinum toxin serotypes A, B, and E. A heptavalent antitoxin vaccine against serotypes A–G is available to the military and high-risk individuals (Smith & Rusnak, 2007); it may be used in pediatric patients. Consultation with public health officials is necessary prior to dosing. The mainstay of therapy consists of supportive care with airway protection and mechanical ventilation. Although costly, administration of human botulinum immune globulin (BIG-IV) in children younger than 1 year of age and of trivalent antitoxin in pediatric patients 1 year of age or older (through adulthood) may shorten illness duration and avert the need for intubation and mechanical ventilation. Antibiotics should not be administered, as they can lead to toxin release through bacterial lysis.

Any cases of botulism—either suspected or proven—should be immediately reported to state and local health departments. The diagnosis of botulism indicates that the patient will have a long-term rehabilitation, potentially including long-term mechanical ventilation, enteric feeds, and home nursing care.

Disposition and discharge planning

The fatality rate from botulism has fallen due to the advent of supportive care, with rates between 3% and 5% observed in patients who receive appropriate medical care (CDC, 2010a). Pediatric patients discharged from the hospital will need continued supportive care. Coordination of care should include the family, HCP, and home health agencies. Prophylaxis with vaccine is futile in the acute setting of exposure, as the protective immune response to the vaccine may take as long as 6 months. Standard precautions should be instituted. Secondary spread from the pediatric patient to a health care worker is unlikely.

SMALLPOX

Pathophysiology

Smallpox (*Poxvirus variolae*) has been used as a biological weapon for centuries. The World Health Organization (WHO) sought to eradicate smallpox on a worldwide level, succeeding in doing so in 1977. Shortly thereafter, routine vaccination stopped in the United States and around the world.

Smallpox is a DNA virus, a member of the orthopoxvirus family. It is a brick-shaped structure and is placed in the same category as monkeypox (a zoonotic disease), cowpox, and vaccinia. All infections with smallpox begin with the virus entering the body via the nose or oropharynx and infecting macrophages. The virus then migrates to the regional lymph nodes, where it multiplies. Asymptomatic viremia then ensues, allowing infection and further replication of the virus in the spleen, bone marrow, and lymph nodes. Virus is then released from these sites, leading to a secondary viremia. Eventually, all organs, including the skin, are infected.

Epidemiology and etiology

Smallpox has the capability of spreading from person to person, usually by droplet or aerosols expressed from the oropharynx of infected persons. Transmission via direct contact, including via linens, can also occur. Affected patients are most infectious during the 7 to 10 days of rash, but may remain infective until the eschars and crusts fall off (Cleri et al., 2006). Animal or insect vectors are not known to carry the disease. As such, the patients most likely to become infected from contact with an index case will be family members or other close contacts. The transmission vector becomes important when discussing vaccination and temporizing measures to isolate the disease.

Presentation

Approximately 8 days after infection with smallpox (a period that includes development of an asymptomatic viremia), the patient develops a secondary viremia, which is followed by a fever and toxemia. Additional symptoms such as malaise, myalgias, and gastrointestinal complaints may be present. The virus is housed in leukocytes, which then localize in dermal and mucosal blood vessels. Two to three days later after this event, lesions on the mouth and oropharynx appear and spread to the face and arms, then eventually to the trunk and legs. Initially, the rash includes a higher number of lesions over bony prominences and areas of high trauma. The rash, which is initially maculopapular, can become vesicular, then pustular, evolving over the course of several days. The lesions are round and firm, sometimes having a central umbilication (Figure 39-4). One well-known characteristic of smallpox is that the lesions are at the same stage of development all over the body. By day 8 or 9, the lesions crust over. As the eschars fall off, they leave a depressed, often hypopigmented scar.

Another form of smallpox is variola minor, which is seen in patients with partial immunity to the smallpox virus. Overall, its symptoms are less severe. The initial fever and constitutional symptoms are mild, and may be confused with an influenza-like illness. The rash goes through a similar evolution of stages as regular smallpox, but it evolves more quickly, and is not as concentrated.

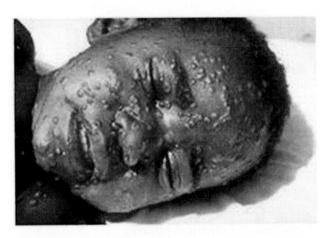

FIGURE 39-4

Smallpox.

Source: Courtesy of Centers for Disease Control and Prevention.

More severe forms of smallpox include malignant and hemorrhagic smallpox. In malignant or "flat" smallpox, the viral prodrome is more severe. It begins as the rash typically seen with smallpox, but never progresses to the pustular stage; instead, the rash persists in the form of soft papules or vesicles. Hemorrhagic smallpox also has a more severe prodrome than typical smallpox. It appears more as a dusky erythematous rash, which then evolves to petechiae and hemorrhage. This form of smallpox may be confused with meningococcemia. In both types, mortality is high.

Differential diagnosis

Clinically, smallpox is most often confused with varicella, especially given the frequency of varicella in pediatric patients. The rash associated with smallpox often features a higher concentration of lesions on the face and upper extremities, whereas a higher predominance of lesions on the trunk is noted with varicella. In addition, varicella is not found on the palms or soles. Finally, in varicella, the lesions are often at different stages of maturation; as noted earlier, smallpox lesions all have the same clinical appearance. Smallpox may also be confused with disseminated herpes, acne, or insect bites.

Plan of care

Given the concern for bioterrorism, any suspicion for smallpox should be immediately reported to local and state public health officials. Suspected patients should be placed in respiratory isolation. Appropriate measures must be taken to ensure the safety of others, including workers in the laboratory. Collection of specimens should be limited to those who are, or recently have been, vaccinated. Similarly, samples should be sent only to laboratories with appropriate containment measures. Fluid from unroofed lesions or eschars can be sent for testing. Identification is performed using electron microscopy.

Definitive testing can be done with viral culture growth, with characterization of specific strains performed via PCR and restriction fragment length polymorphisms (RFLP).

Smallpox is managed with supportive care. No antiviral medications have been proven effective in humans, although cidofovir has shown promising results in animal studies (Cleri et al., 2006). Cidofovir may also be considered for postexposure prophylaxis.

Homes of patients affected with smallpox will require extensive decontamination. Families of affected patients will need support with the diagnosis and managing the home rehabilitation.

Disposition and discharge planning

The overall mortality rate for smallpox is approximately 30%. However, for the hemorrhagic or flat forms of smallpox, fatality rates exceed 95% (Cleri et al., 2006). The main complication from smallpox infection is encephalopathy. Complications may also arise from vaccination for this disease, including encephalitis, necrosis at the site of the vaccination, and eczema vaccinatum (in which the vaccine lesion extends to all eczematous areas in the body). Persons who are vaccinated may also develop a mild, diffuse form of the disease. Pediatric patients affected by smallpox may require additional visits to the dermatologist for consideration of scar modification. Postexposure prophylaxis should be provided. Relative contraindications to postexposure prophylaxis include human immunodeficiency virus (HIV) infection or immunosuppression, eczema, and pregnancy, as well as household contacts with the same contraindications.

Routine vaccination for smallpox was recommended for U.S. pediatric patients until the early 1970s. Since that time, it has not been a routine recommendation. While, in theory, some older members of the population should be protected against smallpox, the duration of immunity has never been established (Henderson et al., 1999). Lifelong immunity from the vaccine is not likely, considering the experience with other vaccines such as for pertussis.

A small reserve supply of the smallpox vaccine is in storage, under the control of the CDC (Henderson et al., 1999). WHO also maintains vaccine reserves. Currently, the vaccine is given to U.S. military personnel prior to deployment. The vaccinia immune globulin (VIG) is also maintained in a small quantity under control of the CDC and should be given to patients with eczema vaccinatum (generalized vaccinia). The dose for VIG is 0.6 mL/kg (Henderson et al., 1999).

TULAREMIA

Pathophysiology

Tularemia is caused by *Francisella tularensis*, a very infective (requiring only a very small innoculum to cause disease), but not particularly virulent bacteria. *F. tularensis* is an intracellular, Gram-negative cocco-bacillus. Infection with this organism occurs when skin or mucous membranes contact the carcass or body fluids of an infected animal. In addition, individuals may become infected when bitten by a tick or deer fly infected with the bacteria—hence the common name of "rabbit fever" given to this disease. In tularemia, the bacteria enter through the skin, mucous membranes, GI tract, or lungs, then spread to regional lymph nodes and multiply in macrophages. Subsequently, infection is disseminated throughout the body.

Infection may occur after inhalation of aerosols or contact with contaminated food and water (Dennis et al., 2001). However, person-to-person transmission has not been documented.

Epidemiology and etiology

F. tularensis is widely found in the North America, with almost all states in the United States having reported cases. Further, it is endemic in Europe and Asia, occurring in mostly rural areas. Rabbits are easily affected during outbreaks. Ticks and deer flies also transmit the disease; thus cases in the United States are most common during the summer months. Nevertheless, infection may occur year-round. One-fourth of cases occur in pediatric patients younger than 14 years of age (AAP, 2009).

Presentation

Seven clinical syndromes of tularemia have been identified:

- Pneumonic
- Typhoidal
- Ulceroglandular (systemic symptoms, ulcerative lesion, lymphadenopathy)
- Glandular (lymphadenopathy, fever)
- Oculoglandular (ocular, lymph node)
- Oropharyngeal (tonsillitis, lymph node)
- Septicemic (sepsis, any of the above)

The clinical presentation depends on the method of exposure. If used as a bioterrorism agent, *F. tularensis* likely will be released as an aerosol and the clinical syndrome of typhoidal tularemia with pneumonia will predominate (Dennis et al., 2001).

Typhoidal tularemia represents systemic illness without a focal lesion. Affected patients exhibit nonspecific constitutional symptoms such as fever, headache, chills, and GI symptoms such as nausea, vomiting, and diarrhea. Cough may also be present. In tularemia pneumonia, patients can develop any combination of pharyngitis, bronchiolotis, hilar lymphadenitis, or pneumonitis.

Ulceroglandular tularemia is the most common form. After contact with an infected animal, an ulcerative skin lesion develops at the site. Simultaneously, a patient develops a fever, chills, and malaise. Initially, the skin lesion is papular; it then becomes pustular, and finally ulcerates and forms a black eschar. Tender lymphadenopathy is frequently present.

Differential diagnosis

The differential diagnosis of tularemia pneumonia includes the more common forms of community-acquired pneumonia, such as those resulting from *Staphylococcus*, *Streptococcus*, or *Mycoplasma* infection. Given the history of contact with animals, Q fever should also be included in the differential diagnosis. Inhalational anthrax and pneumonic plague should be considered. Brucellosis and Q fever, again due to animal exposure, should be considered when evaluating for a diagnosis of typhoid tularemia. Finally, typhoid caused by *Salmonella typhi* should be considered.

Plan of care

Definitive diagnosis is made through culture of *F. tularensis* from sputum, nasal pharyngeal washing, or secretions or exudates from potentially affected patients. Serological testing using enzyme linked immunosorbent assay (ELISA) is also possible. Antibodies against *F. tularensis* can be measured, but such measurements do not become reliable until 2 weeks after the onset of infection. CXR may reveal atypical pneumonia with pleural effusions and enlarged hilar lymph nodes.

Streptomycin 15g/kg intramuscular (IM) twice daily is the drug of choice for treating pediatric patients with tularemia. IV gentamicin 2.5 mg every 8 hours is also a reasonable alternative. Therapy with either of these drugs should be continued for 10 days (Dennis et al., 2001). Amikacin is another alternative (AAP, 2009).

As with other diseases with terrorist implications, state and local public health officials should be consulted whenever tularemia is suspected. Concerned caregivers should seek guidance from the CDC and their HCP.

Disposition and discharge planning

Mortality from treated tularemia is low, less than 2% (Dennis et al., 2001; Moran et al., 2008). Infected individuals will require close follow-up care with their HCP. Postexposure prophylaxis for 14 days consists of either doxycyline or ciprofloxacin. Only those persons with a possible direct exposure to *F. tularensis* should be considered candidates for prophylaxis; such treatment is not necessary for all household contacts of patients.

VIRAL HEMORRHAGIC FEVERS

Pathophysiology

Viral hemorrhagic fevers (VHF) are a group of viruses that cause fever and bleeding diathesis. All belong to one of the four following families of RNA viruses: filoviridae, arenaviridae, bunyaviridae, and flaviviridae. Unfortunately, information on these diseases is limited, as they have a low incidence and often affect a limited population. It is clear that VHFs comprise a diverse group of highly contagious illnesses with high morbidity and mortality. The exact pathophysiology of how these viruses work is largely unknown, although they all affect the vasculoendothelial system. Infection with such viruses leads to fevers and thrombocytopenia, coagulation dysfunction, or hemorrhage through a variety of undetermined mechanisms.

Epidemiology and etiology

Humans are infected with VHF in several ways. Many of the causative viruses are spread via aerosols, but others are spread by tick bite or contact with infected animals, blood, or secretions. Rodent feces are also known harbors of disease. Human-to-human transmission is possible for selected viruses, and has resulted in community and hospital outbreaks (Kman & Nelson, 2008).

Presentation

Signs and symptoms range widely, but most include abrupt onset of fever, body aches, conjunctivitis, facial flushing, myalgia, petechiae, mucosal bleeding, vomiting, and diarrhea. These nonspecific symptoms may last as long as 1 week before the conjunctival or mucosal hemorrhage ensue. Affected patients may also suffer from hematochezia, hematuria, and hematemesis. Filoviruses can cause necrosis of the liver, spleen, and kidneys (Borio et al., 2002). Jaundice may occur in Rift Valley or yellow fevers.

Differential diagnosis

The differential diagnoses for VHFs are broad. Influenza, sepsis, meningiococcemia, dengue fever, shigellosis, and salmonellosis should all be considered. Disseminated intravascular coagulopathy, idiopathic thrombocytopenia purpura, thrombocytopenia purpura, and hemolytic uremic syndrome may all mimic the coagulopathy present in VHFs.

Plan of care

In the setting of a bioterrorist attack, the HCP would likely not be able to elicit a history of travel to an area in Africa, Asia, or South America—an association that would be expected for this infection in its natural setting. Evidence of large numbers of patients with fever and coagulopathy should also alert HCPs to the possibility of a bioterrorism event. Any concern of a VHF, resulting from bioterrorism or another source, should prompt rapid communication with local and state health departments. Appropriate measures must be taken to ensure the safety of others, including personnel in the laboratory. Testing of samples needs to be coordinated through laboratories with Biosafety Level 4 clearance.

The mainstay of treatment for VHFs is supportive care. Intubation and mechanical ventilation may be required given the severe course of disease. Fluid resuscitation and invasive monitoring should be performed, as the ongoing pulmonary capillary leak and bleeding diathesis associated with these infections may worsen pulmonary edema and blood loss. Vasopressors will likely be needed to maintain adequate blood pressure and tissue perfusion. Ribavarin, an antiviral agent, may lower morbidity and mortality, but is not active against filoviruses and flaviviruses. Data are limited regarding ribavirin's use in all of the VHFs.

Given the high morbidity and mortality for VHFs, state and local public health officials should be contacted promptly when this diagnosis is suspected. Family members who were in close proximity to affected patients, especially when the patient was likely infected, should be closely monitored for fever.

Disposition and discharge planning

Mortality for VHFs ranges between 25% and 90%, with the highest mortality noted in conjunction with Ebola virus. The high morbidity associated with VHFs make ongoing medical care likely. Patients should make every attempt to coordinate their care with a primary care provider.

Yellow fever vaccine is the only approved VHF vaccine. Postexposure prophylaxis is not recommended given the limited utility and availability of ribavirin (Borio et al., 2002). Those persons who have been exposed to the bodily fluids of, or have had close contact with, patients suspected of having VHFs should be monitored closely for fever. Respiratory and contact precautions with gloves, gown, mask, and use of N-95 masks with eye protection will reduce the likelihood of transmission. Patients should be placed in respiratory isolation. Decontamination is achieved with hypochlorite disinfectants.

BLAST INJURIES

Phillip Jacobson

In the last decade, considerable attention has been focused on preparation for terrorist incidents. Much of this preparation is designed to address the possibility of chemical, biological, or radiation incidents. In reality, however, the majority of terrorist attacks involve conventional explosive devices (DePalma et al., 2005). Conventional explosives are easy to obtain or produce and can cause much damage; they also spread considerable fear. During terrorist incidents, dual explosions are common. After the initial blast, rescue workers and onlookers gather near the blast sight, upon which a second explosive device is detonated to maximize the number of casualties. Many experts believe that in the future, conventional explosives may also be used as dispersal devices to spread nuclear, chemical, or biological weapons (so-called dirty bombs).

Conventional explosives can cause considerable traumatic injury, and their victims tend to be young. Both pediatric and adult victims of explosions have higher injury severity scores, have more body regions injured, and require more surgeries than victims of conventional trauma. They also have higher in-hospital mortality (Daniel-Aharonson et al., 2003; Kluger et al., 2004; Shamir et al., 2005).

The number of casualties in an explosive incident is influenced by many factors, including the magnitude of the explosion, the number of people in the area, collapse of a building or structure, rescue speed, and medical resource availability. Casualty rates are higher when an explosion takes place in a confined space versus open air. Arnold et al. (2004) reviewed the literature from 29 terrorist bombings and compared morbidity and mortality of victims in the events. Considerable differences were observed depending on whether the explosion occurred with structural collapse, in a confined space, or in open air (Table 39-7). Hospitalization rates were thought to be higher in the confined-space group than the structural-collapse group because more patients suffered immediate death in the latter group (Arnold et al., 2004).

GENERAL PRINCIPLES OF EXPLOSIONS

An explosion is a rapid chemical conversion of a solid or a liquid into a gas with energy release. Either high-order or low-order explosives may be used.

TABLE 39-7

Explosion Site Morbidity and Mortality			
	Immediate Mortality	Hospitalization Rate	Emergency Department Use
Open air	4%	15%	15%
Confined space	8%	36%	36%
Structural collapse	25%	25%	48%

Source: Arnold et al., 2004.

Low-order explosives, also known as propellants, cause a slow release of energy. Energy is released by deflagration, mostly in the form of heat. As a consequence, objects "go up in flames." Examples of low-order explosives include gunpowder and Molotov cocktails (CDC, 2010b).

High-order explosives cause a quick release of energy, otherwise known as detonation. In this type of explosion, much of the energy is released in the form of pressure to the surrounding medium, resulting in a transformation of the physical space around the point of explosion. If the explosion occurs on land, the surrounding air in all directions becomes compressed from the pressure initiated at the point of explosion. The strength of the explosion determines the amount of pressure release and the degree to which the medium is compressed. Pressure waves degrade rapidly degrade, with much of the energy being converted into sound waves. As a blast pressure wave propagates, a vacuum is created in the space previously occupied by molecules of the surrounding medium. In a land explosion, air is then sucked back in to the evacuated space. The negative phase of the Friedlander waveform (Figure 39-5) represents this vacuum (Stuhmiller et al., 1991). A blast pressure wave (Figure 39-6) that occurs in a confined space reflects off walls and reverberates,

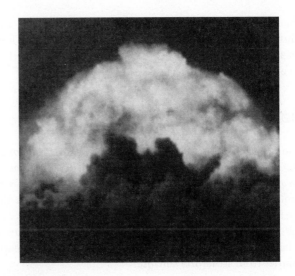

FIGURE 39-6

A large conventional explosion is shown from a distance. Beyond the fireball, the blast wave appears as a sharp line that is caused by refraction of light by the higher-density gas at the shock front.

Source: Courtesy of FEMA News Photo.

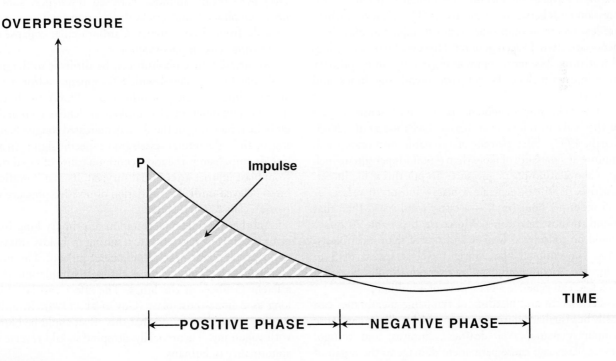

FIGURE 39-5

Friedlander Waveform: Ideal Pressure-Time History of an Air Blast in an Undisturbed, Free-Field Environment. The impulse is the integral of pressure over time. P is the peak overpressure.

Source: Stuhmiller, J., Phillips, Y., & Richmond, D. (1991). *The Physics and Mechanisms of Primary Blast Injury. Conventional Warfare: Ballistic Blast and Burn Injuries* (pp. 243–244). Washington, D.C.: Office of the Surgeon General.

changing the characteristics of the wave considerably, and causes multiple impacts of the wave on the victims. This phenomenon explains why severity of injury is greater when an explosion occurs in a confined space.

BIOLOGICAL AND CLINICAL EFFECTS

Four types of injuries are associated with blasts. *Primary blast injuries* are caused by the pressure of the blast waves. *Secondary injuries* occur when flying objects strike the victim. *Tertiary injuries* occur when victims fly through the air and strike other objects or surfaces. *Quaternary injuries* include various other types of injuries, such as burns, inhalational injuries from toxic gases or dust, and traumatic injuries from structural collapse.

Primary injury

As previously noted, primary blast injuries arise from the pressure blast waves associated with high-order explosions (Wightman & Gladish, 2001). Pressure blast waves can cause tissue detachments (including amputations) from shear forces. They can also cause stress damage to organs with a gas tissue interface. In addition, primary injuries can be sustained during the negative-pressure portion of the blast wave, as the vacuum effect induces different compression rates between air and tissue. These injuries, which are less common than other types of injury in blast incidents, are often delayed in onset. However, they can be life-threatening. The most common organs sustaining primary blast injuries include the tympanic membrane, lungs, and GI tract.

The tympanic membrane is the most sensitive part of the body to injury from blasts (DePalma et al., 2005; Garth, 1997). Fifty percent of tympanic membranes will rupture at a pressure of more than 5 pounds per square inch (psi) above atmospheric pressure. To put this value in perspective, 5 psi can generate a blast wind of 70 m/sec, or 145 miles per hour (mph)—a faster wind speed than that found in most hurricanes. Moreover, 5 psi and 70 m/sec would be considered weaker and slower than most blasts: Most conventional blast waves travel at speeds of 3 to 8 km/sec. A commonly used conventional military explosive, C4, can generate a blast wave of 4 million psi.

Perforation and bleeding of tympanic membranes can easily be visualized during otoscopy. Milder blasts can cause temporary neurapraxia, deafness, tinnitus, and vertigo. Severe blasts can cause permanent damage to the organ of Corti, and can result in permanent hearing loss.

Pulmonary injuries are the second most common primary injury overall, and the most common form of life-threatening primary blast injury. A pressure of approximately 15 psi is required for pulmonary injuries to occur. Pulmonary injuries result more frequently when

blasts occur in closed spaces, and there is an associated increased incidence when burns are present. Three different manifestations of primary blast injuries of the lungs are observed: alveolar damage, blood vessel disruption, and inflammation.

Alveolar damage can result in pneumothorax and/or pulmonary interstitial emphysema. Air that dissects along the bronchovascular sheath can result in air leak syndromes such as subcutaneous emphysema, pneumomediastinum, pneumopericardium, or pneumoperitoneum.

- Blood vessel injury of the lungs can result in pulmonary contusion, hemorrhage, laceration, or hemothorax. If air enters the pulmonary venous system, a systemic arterial air embolism may form; however, damage and ruptured tissues on the venous side of the system may also lead to venous arterial embolism.
- Inflammatory injuries include disseminated intravascular coagulation (DIC) and acute respiratory distress syndrome (ARDS).

Clinical manifestations of primary blast injury to the lung can be nonspecific and include tachypnea, cyanosis, chest pain, dyspnea, and pharyngeal petechiae. Crackles, decreased breath sounds, dullness to percussion, and hemoptysis may be noted with pulmonary contusion. Decreased breath sounds, increased resonance, subcutaneous crepitance, and tracheal deviation may accompany air leaks from alveolar injury. Cardiovascular collapse may result from tension pneumothorax.

An arterial air embolism can be difficult to diagnose. It should be considered with ST-segment and/or T-wave abnormalities on electrocardiograph (ECG) (with coronary air embolus), focal neurological deficits (cerebral air embolus), mottling of the skin, demarcated tongue blanching, or air in the retinal vessels (most specific sign). An arterial air embolism is the most common cause of rapid death from blast injuries after initial survival. Its manifestation is often delayed until after initiation of positive-pressure ventilation (Ho & Ling, 1999).

Another possible manifestation of primary lung injury is a pronounced vagal effect, resulting in bradycardia and hypotension (with normal peripheral pulses). The mechanism of this phenomenon is through stimulation of the afferent C fibers in the lungs. The effect can last for as long as 2 hours post blast (Guy et al., 1998). In animal studies, researchers found that this effect could be blunted with vagotomy. Theoretically, atropine should reverse this abnormality in humans.

The colon is the most common site of injury in the gastrointestinal tract. Stretch and/or ischemia of the bowel wall may cause it to weaken and even rupture—an outcome that may occur either immediately or up to several days after a blast incident (Paran et al., 1996). Hemorrhagic injury of the bowel can also occur, ranging in severity from mild petechiae to large hematomas (Sharpnack et al., 1991). Solid organs of the gut are generally spared from injury due to their homogeneity.

Research has shown that the central nervous system (CNS) is also adversely affected by primary blast injury. In one animal study, rats subjected to blast effects suffered cognitive impairment and biochemical changes to the hippocampus (Cernak et al., 2001). Another study found that animals exposed to a blast developed diffuse axonal injury (Singer et al., 2005). It was previously thought that human victims of blasts had a high incidence of PTSD solely due to a psychological effect. Evidence is accumulating that this outcome is more likely due to a postconcussive syndrome (Cernak et al., 1999). Other authors report electroencephalograph (EEG) abnormalities and attention-deficit disorder may result from primary blast injury (Born, 2005). Autopsies of human victims who sustained only primary blast injuries of the CNS reveal diffuse punctuate hemorrhages and disintegration of Nissl substance (Guy et al., 2000).

The eyes and face can also be injured as a result of primary blast injury. Ruptures of the globe, serous retinitis, hyphema, and implosion of the maxillary sinus have been observed.

Secondary injury

Flying objects from a weapon or other matter may result in secondary blast injuries to any part of the body, although injuries to the eye are common. These injuries can be either blunt or penetrating in nature. Secondary injury is the leading cause of death in blasts.

Tertiary injury

Injuries sustained when victims are thrown through the air, or strike the ground or other surfaces, are known as tertiary blast injuries. Those persons closest to the explosion are at the greatest risk for such damage. Victims tend to be of lighter weight; thus children are more susceptible to tertiary injuries. The heaviest part of a young child is the head; consequently, traumatic brain injury is common in tertiary injury.

Quaternary injury

Crush injuries, burns, and toxic exposures are examples of quaternary injuries, and are especially common in persons trapped by structural collapse. Crush syndrome occurs after prolonged compression and compromised circulation of muscle tissue. Reperfusion results in rhabdomyolysis from muscle breakdown, which in turn leads to electrolyte abnormalities (hyperkalemia, hyperphosphatemia, hyperuricemia, hypocalcemia), acidosis, and release of inflammatory mediators. Kidney failure, cardiac dysrhythmias, compartment syndrome, DIC, ARDS, and shock are clinical manifestations (Gonzalez, 2005).

Carbon monoxide and cyanide gases are commonly released from burning building materials and may pose a threat to nearby victims. Unconventional weapons can also release other toxic chemicals, radiation, or biological agents.

BLAST INJURY MANAGEMENT

Before victims of an explosion arrive at the hospital setting, it is advisable to obtain as much information as possible about the event, including the type and severity of the explosion and the approximate number of casualties. Did the explosion occur in a closed or open space? Was there a structural collapse or fire? If it is apparent that a large number of critically injured patients will be arriving, the possibility of a mass-casualty incident should be contemplated. In a mass casualty, the casualty burden exceeds the capability of onsite resources. If an incident is defined as a mass casualty, specific triage protocols should be followed, and limited resources such as equipment and personnel should be appropriated accordingly.

As with all life-threatening traumatic injuries, blast injury management begins with the initial resuscitation strategies. Additional consideration should be given to the possibility of toxic exposure from the products of combustion of normal structural materials or from a terrorist weapon of mass destruction. Basic decontamination techniques should be performed unless there is a high degree of certainty that no exposure to toxic materials occurred. If chemical eye exposure is a concern, irrigation should be performed for 60 minutes, to ensure toxin clearance.

Endotracheal intubation and positive-pressure mechanical ventilation can be problematic, or even life-threatening due to the possibility of weakened or damaged lung tissue from primary blast injury or superheated air. These measures may lead to, or exacerbate, air leaks, air embolus, or hemorrhage. If positive-pressure ventilation is instituted, a minimum pressure setting is recommended. For larger children and adults, unilateral lung ventilation can be applied by intubating and ventilating the unaffected lung only. Smaller children and infants may be too small for this technique to be feasible. If an arterial air embolus is suspected, 100% supplemental oxygen should be given (it displaces the nitrogen in the embolus) and the patient placed in the left lateral recumbent position to reduce the possibility of coronary air embolus by trapping the embolus in the apex of the right ventricle until dissolution. Hyperbaric oxygen therapy, if available, may be considered to provide recompression, which improves air solubility. Smoke inhalation is also treated with 100% supplemental oxygen.

For those patients with crush injuries, reperfusion of the injury may quickly lead to crush syndrome. Early fluid resuscitation to restore circulating volume and promote kidney excretion of potassium with isotonic saline of

10 to 20 mL/kg/hr and an infusion mix of bicarbonate and mannitol is recommended by Yokata (2005). Initiation of this treatment in the field is considered ideal if practical for rescuers. Bicarbonate may prevent "myoglobin and uric acid deposition in the renal tubules" and improves acidosis and hyperkalemia. Mannitol not only increases extracellular fluid volume by osmotic effect, but also helps protect the kidneys by "enhancement of filtration pressure, increase in tubular flow, and inhibition of damage from reactive oxygen species" (Yokata, 2005, pp. 347–348).

Impaled objects are common with secondary blast injury and should not be removed without the supervision of the surgical team. For purposes of circulatory support, fluids and blood transfusions should be administered, as needed. In a mass-casualty incident, efforts should be made to preserve as much blood in the blood bank as possible; thus auto-transfusion, such as with hemothorax, should be considered (Wightman & Gladish, 2001). When shock is refractory to fluid resuscitation, consider the diagnosis of a spinal cord injury.

After immediately life-threatening injuries are addressed and the patient is stabilized, the care for victims of blast injuries is similar to that for other trauma victims. Additionally, patients with suspected primary blast injury should have serial physical examinations—and, if warranted, diagnostic imaging—of the head, thorax, and abdomen due to the possibility of traumatic brain, pulmonary, or gastrointestinal injury as previously described. Blast injury patients also experience a higher incidence of severe limb injuries, especially those requiring amputation; therefore, they should be monitored for crush and compartment syndromes. For those individuals with crush syndrome, hemodialysis may be required. Compartment syndrome may require fasciotomy.

Ruptured tympanic membranes will generally heal spontaneously. Patients should be advised to avoid swimming until healed. If debris is seen in the ear canal, it should be removed by an otolaryngologist if possible and topical antibiotics should be administered to prevent secondary infection. Prednisone should be prescribed for sensorineural hearing loss.

PSYCHOSOCIAL IMPLICATIONS

Children are particularly at risk during blasts, because they may not have the physical or cognitive ability to recognize danger and run from it. In addition, they may not understand where safety lies or how to reach it. They may hide, thinking this step will be protective; instead, it tends to increase their risk in a building collapse.

Patients may have feelings of anxiety, confusion, and fear immediately after the event, which then persist in a pathologic pattern known as post-traumatic stress disorder. As with other disasters, there is a direct correlation between the psychological effects on the caregivers and those on the

pediatric patients. Pediatric patients should be referred to mental health services when psychological difficulties are observed (AAP, 2006).

CHEMICAL DISASTERS

Asha S. Payne and Daniel B. Fagbuyi

BIOTOXINS

Biotoxins are by-products or extracts of naturally occurring plants or bacteria. They include strychnine, digitalis, brevetoxin, colchichine, and nicotine. In addition, ricin, saxitoxin, tetrodotoxin, and trichothecene are included in this category of agents. Several biotoxic agents are extracted from marine organisms or animals. Tetrodotoxin is the deadly chemical found in pufferfish, for example, while both brevetoxin and saxitoxin are produced by dinoflagellates, leading to neurotoxic shellfish poisoning and paralytic shellfish poisoning, respectively. The remaining agents are chemicals extracted from plants. Trichothecene (T-2) mycotoxin is produced by certain strains of fungi. Abrin, which is similar to ricin, comes from the seeds of the rosary pea; ricin comes from castor beans. Colchicine and digitalis are toxic chemicals from plants, but have approved medical uses. Colchicine is extracted from meadow saffron, but is used to medically treat gout. Digitalis is a toxin from foxglove plants, but also is a chemically important compound in digoxin, a medication used for heart conditions. Finally, strychnine comes from plants. Only strychnine and ricin are described here.

Pathophysiology

Strychnine is a naturally occurring alkaloid obtained from the seeds of the *Strychnos nux-vomica* plant. It can be absorbed through various routes, including the GI tract, intact skin, and respiratory tract (Makarovsky et al., 2008). It functions by inhibiting postsynaptic inhibition in the brain and spinal cord, leading to excessive motor neuron activity, resulting in seizures (Makarovsky et al., 2008).

Ricin is a poison that is exposed when castor bean seeds are either crushed or chewed. Individuals can be exposed to this toxin either through ingestion, inhalation, or injection. Once it enters the cell, ricin inhibits protein synthesis by inactivating ribosomes, eventually leading to cell death (Audi et al., 2005).

Epidemiology and etiology

Various species of *Strychnos* are found throughout the world, including Southeast Asia, South America, and parts of Africa. Over the years, use of strychnine has waned, and the compound is now largely limited to use as a rodenticide; as a consequence, strychnine poisoning is rare. Exposures have been associated with adulterated street drugs and ingestion of rodenticide, either intentionally or accidentally. Strychnine is colorless, odorless, and bitter tasting.

Ricin is present in the mash created during the processing of castor beans into castor oil. This white powder readily dissolves in water, but can also easily travel through the air.

Presentation

Within 30 minutes of exposure to strychnine, prodromal symptoms begin. Affected patients often describe a heightened sensorium, hyperreflexia, muscle twitches, and apprehension. The classic presentation of the syndrome is seizures in an awake, alert patient with an intact sensorium. The seizures last from 30 seconds to 2 minutes, and affect not only major muscle groups, but also smaller ones in the face, diaphragm, and eyes. As a result, an impairment of respiration occurs during these seizures. Each seizure is triggered by very minor sensory stimuli. A potentiation effect is observed, with each seizure being more intense than the prior. There is a period of approximately 10 to 15 minutes between seizure episodes. Due to the prolonged contraction of all muscles, including the diaphragm, patients develop hyperthermia, metabolic acidosis, rhabdomyolysis, and myoglobinuric kidney failure (Makarovsky et al., 2008).

Four to six hours after ingestion of ricin, affected patients may develop nonspecific symptoms such as abdominal pain, vomiting, and diarrhea. Symptoms continue to progress, eventually leading to fluid loss, hypotension, and organ failure. After injection with ricin, patients develop symptoms similar to those associated with sepsis—namely, fever, vomiting, and diarrhea. Death occurs from multisystem organ failure. Inhalation of ricin toxin likely leads to respiratory failure, but limited information is available regarding the actual presentation due to a paucity of cases.

Differential diagnosis

Seizure disorders that cause generalized seizures may mimic strychnine exposure. However, the hallmark of strychnine is the alert sensorium during the seizure. Other conditions in the differential diagnosis for seizures include meningitis and toxin exposure. Tetanus should also be considered when strychnine is suspected.

The profound GI symptoms occurring after ricin ingestion can mimic may other ailments, including *Salmonella* infection, typhoid, cholera, *Campylobacter* infection, *Shigella* infection, or other causes of gastroenteritis.

Plan of care

Strychnine can be detected in the blood and urine, but these levels do not correlate well with the clinical presentation, nor are they useful to guide therapy. Ricin poisoning is also a clinical diagnosis. No tests are commercially available to diagnose ricin poisoning in humans (Audi et al., 2005).

Airway management and seizure control are the cornerstone of therapy in strychnine poisoning. Endotracheal intubation with mechanical ventilation is recommended. Convulsions should be controlled aggressively with benzodiazepines and paralytics as needed. Controlling the seizures will help to limit the sequelae of prolonged hypoxia and muscle breakdown. Patients should have limited stimulation, as even minor stimulation can trigger seizure activity. Gastrointestinal decontamination is not likely to be helpful, as strychnine is rapidly absorbed into the bloodstream.

Supportive care is important in ricin exposure. Aggressive fluid resuscitation and support are needed to combat the fluid losses after ingestion of ricin. For a suspected ingestion, patients should be given activated charcoal, and possibly cathartics, to increase excretion of the ricin toxin. Supportive care is also the mainstay of treatment for inhalational ricin poisoning. Intubation and mechanical ventilation will likely be needed.

Critical care HCPs should provide comprehensive management of patients affected by strychnine or ricin ingestion. Neurologists may be aid in differentiating strychnine ingestion from other acute seizure disorders. As with any potential exposure to chemical threat, local and state health departments will be helpful in guiding overall patient management and resource allocation.

Any family member who may have been affected by exposure to these agents should seek medical attention. Large numbers of patients with similar symptoms should raise suspicions for terror agent use and should be immediately reported to the local state and public health authorities (Table 39-8).

TABLE 39-8

Chemical Disaster Resources

American Academy of Pediatrics, Committee on Environmental Health and Committee on Infectious Diseases. (2000). Chemical–biological terrorism and its impact on children: A subject review. *Pediatrics, 105*(3 Pt 1), 662–670.

Centers for Disease Control and Prevention. (2009). Facts about strychnine. Retrieved from http://emergency.cdc.gov/agent/strychnine/basics/facts.asp

Centers for Disease Control and Prevention. (2009). Facts about sulfur mustard. Retrieved from http://emergency.cdc.gov/agent/sulfurmustard/basics/facts.asp

Centers for Disease Control and Prevention. (2008). Questions and answers about ricin. Retrieved from http://emergency.cdc.gov/agent/ricin/qa.asp

Centers for Disease Control and Prevention. (2008). Toxic syndrome description: Vesicant/blister agent poisoning. Retrieved from http://emergency.cdc.gov/agent/vesicants/tsd.asp

Foltin GL, Schonfeld DJ, Shannon MW (Eds.). (2006). *Pediatric terrorism and disaster preparedness: A resource for pediatricians.* AHRQ Publication No. 06(07)-0056. Rockville, MD: Agency for Healthcare Research and Quality.

Styrchnine. Retrieved from http://toxnet.nlm.nih.gov/cgi-bin/sis/search/r?dbs+hsdb:@term+@rn+57-24-9

Disposition and discharge planning

The majority of the pathogenesis of strychnine poisoning occurs within the first 24 hours after exposure. If patients can survive this time period, their prognosis is favorable. Prognosis is also favorable for ricin exposure once patients survive the acute period, which occurs 48–72 hours after exposure.

Patients affected with either strychnine or ricin poisoning will need to have continued care and follow-up from their primary care provider.

Prevention measures include encouraging individuals to avoid chewing or crushing castor beans to avoid exposure to ricin.

NERVE AGENTS

Pathophysiology

The four best-known nerve agents are sarin, tabun, soman, and VX. Although they have subtle differences in their chemical structures, of these chemicals function as acetylcholinesterase (AChe) inhibitors.

The damage done by these agents is twofold. First, nerve agents lead to an overstimulation of nicotinic and muscarinic receptors. Acetylcholine (ACh) is released by neurons in both the sympathetic and parasympathetic nervous systems, and its release activates both muscarinic and nicotinic receptors. ACh is then broken down by AChe into its constituent parts, acetic acid and choline. In the presence of nerve agents, AChe binds to the nerve agent, preventing it from interacting with ACh, and leading to excess stimulation of the nicotinic and muscarinic receptors.

Second, nerve agents permanently bind AChe. After a period of time, the AChe–nerve agent complex forms a stable bond, preventing it from interacting with ACh. The time course of this process, which is called aging, varies among the nerve agents. It occurs within minutes of soman exposure, for example. AChe must be regenerated, a process that may take several months (Barthold & Scheir, 2005; Holstege et al., 1997; Martin & Lobert, 2003).

Epidemiology and etiology

There is very little information regarding the epidemiology of nerve agents. These chemical weapons are classified as weapons of mass destruction.

Presentation

The clinical presentation of nerve agent exposure will vary depending on the method and route of exposure. Characteristic mnemonics such as *SLUDGE* or *DUMBELLS* are associated with cholinergic toxicity; they summarize the overstimulation of the muscarinic receptors (Barthold

& Schier, 2005). *DDUMBBBELS* is actually a more accurate representation of the full mnemonic of signs and symptoms: *d*iaphoresis, *d*iarrhea, *u*rination, *m*iosis, *b*radycardia, *b*ronchorrhea, *b*ronchospasm, *e*mesis, *l*acrimation, and *s*alivation. Excessive activation of the nicotinic receptors includes symptoms that are somewhat contradictory to muscarinic activation, including mydriasis, fasciculations, muscle cramps, pallor, flaccid paralysis, hypertension, and tachycardia (Holstege et al., 1997; Lee, 2003; Borak & Sidell, 2002).

The respiratory symptoms are the most serious consequences of nerve agent exposures. The combination of bronchospasm and bronchorrhea with muscle fatigue and paralysis can lead to hypoxia and respiratory failure, even in intubated, mechanically ventilated patients (Bogucki & Weir, 2002). Various cardiac manifestations are possible, including bradycardia, tachycardia, and dysrhythmias. Neurological complications include seizures, parathesias, insomnia, and depression; eye-related effects include lacrimation and miosis.

Differential diagnosis

Nerve agents are organophosphates; thus the clinical symptoms may be similar to accidental exposure to organic pesticides. The excessive lacrimation and rhinorrhea seen may also mimic exposure to choking agents such as chlorine gas.

Plan of care

Laboratory studies have limited utility in the diagnosis or management of nerve agent poisoning. Currently, it is not possible to directly measure the concentrations of nerve agents in the urine or serum. Plasma and erythrocyte cholinesterase activity is a surrogate for direct testing. Plasma cholinesterase is also made in the liver and is affected by nerve agents (Holstege et al., 1997). Clinical imaging is not needed for the diagnosis of nerve agent poisoning or exposure, but may be used as an adjunct to supportive care.

Decontamination is the first and most important step after nerve agent exposure, for the benefit of both the patient and the HCP (Barthold & Schier, 2005; Holstege et al., 1997). Extensive decontamination of the body should occur, including immediate removal of clothing and copious water irrigation (Balali-Mood & Balali-Mood, 2008). Eyes should be flushed for at least 10 minutes with water. Soap and dilute bleach solutions may be used to neutralize remaining nerve agents on the body, with their application carefully avoiding the eyes. Harsh substances that may damage the skin should be avoided, as additional absorption of the nerve agent may be possible through damaged tissues.

Proper assessment of airway, breathing, and circulation are the guiding principles of initial management after exposure. Patients with severe respiratory distress and imminent failure should be intubated and placed on mechanical ventilation. Use of succinycholine should be avoided, as it is metabolized by plasma cholinesterase, leading to prolonged neuromuscular blockade.

Frequent administration of atropine will improve bronchorrhea and bronchospasm. Atropine is a muscarinic receptor antagonist whose use leads to reduced secretions. Relief of bronchorrhea and bronchospasm are the therapeutic endpoints for atropine dosing (Holstege et al., 1997, Lawrence & Kirk, 2007). Due to its antimuscarinic effects, this medication is also useful in mitigating the nausea, vomiting, abdominal pain, bradycardia, and sweating associated with nerve agent exposure. However, it has no effect on paralysis, which is mediated by nicotinic receptors.

Pralidoxime is also useful in nerve agent poisoning. Overall, it regenerates AChe by binding the nerve agent, allowing the AChe to be functional in the synaptic cleft. Its effect is most apparent in skeletal muscle (Barthold & Schier, 2005). Diazepam should also be available for the treatment of nerve agent—induced seizures. Midazolam may have a role in the treatment of similar seizures, but remains under investigation for this indication.

State and local health departments should be notified immediately when concerns about nerve agent exposure arise. A mass-casualty event should be anticipated when such agents are used. Experts in emergency and critical care medicine as well as decontamination will be needed (Table 39-8).

Family members who were in contact with patients after exposure should promptly undergo decontamination procedures to mitigate their own exposure. They should be monitored closely for development of symptoms.

Disposition and discharge planning

The prognostic outcome after nerve agent exposure depends on the specific agent and the route of exposure. Atropine, pralidoxime, and diazepam (and midazolam in study) are useful medications in this setting and work on various aspects of the pathophysiology that may improve survival: Atropine reduces secretions, pralidoxime reduces the chance of aging, and diazepam reduces seizures. There is no outcome information on these agents in the setting of chemoterrorism in pediatric patients.

Patients may need to be debriefed by local and federal authorities after exposure to provide assistance in determining assailants, if necessary.

There are no vaccines to prevent clinical symptoms after exposure to nerve agents occurs. Although not studied in pediatric patients, pyridostigmine bromide (PB) tabs have been used in military personnel as pre-exposure prophylaxis, with administration taking place within a week of possible exposure. Other therapies include the dermal application of

SERPACWA (*s*kin *e*xposure *r*eduction *p*aste *a*gainst *c*hemical *w*arfare *a*gents). No pediatric studies on SERPACWA have been reported (Hutchinson & Shahan, 2002).

VESICANTS

Pathophysiology

Overall, the exact mechanism of vesicant pathophysiology is unknown. One leading theory regarding these agents' mode of action suggests that alkylation with the purines of DNA leads to DNA fragmentation, which then activates a polymerase enzyme to repair fragmented DNA. Overstimulation of the repair enzymes depletes the cells of nicotinamide adenine dinucleotide (NAD), thereby preventing glycolysis; this effect shuts off ATP synthesis and ultimately leads to cell death (McManus & Huebner, 2005). Separation of the dermis–epidermis layer is the visual result (Rice, 2003). An alternative theory posits that sulfur mustard interacts and forms intermediaries that react with DNA, RNA, and proteins. Interaction with DNA and RNA leads to altered protein synthesis, and eventual depletion of NAD. Apoptosis then leads to tissue damage and decreased tissue repair.

Epidemiology and etiology

The three major vesicants are sulfur mustard, Lewisite, and phosgene oxime.

Sulfur mustard is a yellow-brown oily liquid that smells like garlic, mustard, or horseradish, although the pure form is clear and does not have a smell. The vapor from sulfur mustard can penetrate through clothing to affect skin. It can slowly penetrate through thicker materials such as leather and wood. Similarly, it can be aerosolized and inhaled, affecting the mucous membranes and gastrointestinal and respiratory systems.

Lewisite is also an oily liquid, but it is colorless. Impure Lewisite preparations can be range from yellow to blue-black. This vesicant is noted to smell like geraniums.

Phosgene oxime is technically considered an urticant owing to the erythema and urticaria it causes. Its effects are not covered in this text.

Overall, vesicants are rarely lethal. They cause blisters that require medical attention, sometimes for prolonged periods of time.

Presentation

After exposure, the eyes, respiratory tract, and skin are the areas most affected by exposure to vesicants. Of note, although the exposure to sulfur mustard may seem more driven by direct contact with the chemical, this agent is very lipophilic; thus it penetrates skin more deeply than the other vesicants, leading to systemic effects (Kehe & Szinicz,

2005). The exact presentation depends on the route of exposure (McManus & Huebner, 2005). However, the greatest effects will be seen in relation to cells that divide rapidly, if not frequently.

Skin affected by sulfur mustard is affected in a different manner than occurs with a thermal, electrical, or corrosive burn (Rice, 2003). Initially the skin is pale and painless; it then turns erythematous and painful within 4 to 8 hours of exposure. Warm, moist areas such as the genitalia, perineum, lower back, and axillae, are most often affected (Rice, 2003; Zilker, 2005). Vesicles and blebs appear the day after exposure. The vesicles vary in size and may coalesce; they are filled with a clear, translucent fluid. Within a week, eschars form. In addition, skin remains very sensitive to the lightest, shearing trauma (Nikolsky's sign). After 4 to 6 days, skin begins to slough off. During this time, the skin remains red and edematous. Two to three weeks after initial exposure, the sloughing finally ends and the skin begins to heal.

The clinical presentation of Lewisite exposure is different than that of sulfur mustard exposure. Pain begins on contact and vesicles develop within minutes, whereas effects from sulfur mustard exposure occur only after a several-hour delay.

Ocular exposure to sulfur mustard results in symptoms at much lower concentrations than needed to injure the airways (Safarinjad et al., 2001; Zilker, 2005). Conjunctivitis, eyelid edema, and blepharospasm can develop as early as 4 to 12 hours after exposure and are related to exposure level (McManus & Huebner, 2005). The corneal epithelium may develop vesicles and slough off. Effects with higher exposure levels include visual disturbances, keratitis, and ulceration. Similar symptoms occur with Lewisite exposure. However, as with Lewisite skin exposure, the pain begins upon contact with the chemical agent.

The respiratory tract is also very sensitive to sulfur mustard. Upper airway symptoms may include hoarseness, sneezing, rhinorrhea, lacrimation, and increased mucus production. The lower airway is also affected, leading to tracheobronchitis, coughing, pseudomembrane formation, pulmonary edema, and ulcerations (McManus & Huebner, 2005, Zilker, 2005). Secondary infection is also possible.

Sulfur mustard can also affect the hematopoietic system, with leucopenia or pancytopenia occurring several days after the exposure. In contrast, Lewisite does not appear to affect the hematopoietic system. Exposure can, however, lead to "Lewisite shock," in which systemic absorption results in capillary damage and loss of vascular oncotic pressure due to the extravasation of proteins and plasma, leading to hypotension.

Differential diagnosis

The differential diagnoses after vesicant exposure constitute a broad list. Infectious causes of blebs and skin sloughing include Stevens-Johnson syndrome, staphyloccocal scalded

skin syndrome, and toxic epidermal necrolysis. In addition, pemphigus vulgaris and bullous pempigoid are noninfectious causes of skin blistering. Finally, chemical burns, such as those from acids or strong bases, should be considered (McManus & Huebner, 2005).

Plan of care

Exposure to sulfur mustard is a diagnosis made based on the patient's history and clinical presentation. Some patients may report the smell of garlic, but it may not be consistently mentioned.

Early decontamination is critical both for the affected patient and for HCPs. Despite not causing immediate symptoms, sulfur mustard bonds to the skin within minutes of exposure; thus clothing should be removed and safely disposed. Skin can be decontaminated with talc or flour (Kehe & Szinicz, 2005). Immediate decontamination is ideal. Because patients rarely have symptoms at the time of exposure, however, decontamination is not usually performed rapidly. Late decontamination should be done to protect HCPs who are treating the patient. Copious rinsing with water should be performed to remove the remaining sulfur mustard. Using limited amounts of water will merely serve to increase the permeability of the skin to the chemical, enhancing its absorption.

Patients with respiratory compromise or definitive large inhalation exposures should be monitored closely. Symptomatic relief with humidified air can be helpful with cough and hoarseness. Early tracheostomy is recommended for patients with persistent stridor and hoarseness, as laryngospasm is a continuing threat (Kehe & Szinicz, 2005). A secondary pneumonia is also possible. Antibiotics should be administered only after presence of a specific organism has been identified. Pseudomembrane formation is a persistent concern, requiring bronchoscopy and debridement for relief.

Supportive burn care will likely be required. Debridement should be performed for larger vesicles. Fluid resuscitation and ongoing management is similar to that for burns, although not as much fluid loss should be expected. Silver sulfadiazine can be applied to the skin once the vesicles have broken to reduce secondary infection; it should be used cautiously in pediatric patients as these lesions can absorb excess amounts of the product. Pain can be treated with mild analgesics, as narcotics are rarely needed. Low-potency topical corticosteroids can be used to treat the topical irritation. Skin grafting is rarely necessary.

Healing takes several weeks. Microscopic analysis of the skin reveals that alkylation extends beyond the initial vesicles. Thus these cells are damaged, and healing (ideally) comes from the outer edges inward. If the cells on the outer edge of the lesion are also damaged, then cell replication will be hampered, further delaying wound healing. Scars formed from sulfur burns are more pliable than thermal burns; thus wound contractures are less concerning, even in the axilla and groin (Rice, 2003).

Eye exposure should prompt irrigation with copious amounts of buffered saline. Contact lenses should be removed. Eye lubricants will be helpful in preventing the eyelids from adhering together. Topical antibiotics prevent infection, and corticosteroids may be helpful.

Severe leukopenia is possible, starting at day 3 and with the nadir being reached 7 to 9 days after exposure (Kehe & Szinicz, 2005). Antibiotics are recommended to protect the body against intestinal flora. Kehe and Szinicz (2005) suggest that granulocyte colony-stimulating factor (GCSF) and granulocyte-macrophage colony-stimulating factor (GM-CSF) be considered.

Experts in burn care may be needed to manage the skin damage and lesions. Critical care physicians should be consulted in the case of respiratory compromise.

Families of affected patients should be prepared for the possible disfigurement associated with skin damage.

Disposition and discharge planning

Despite a prolonged healing course, most skin lesions heal well with supportive care. However, larger, full-thickness burns may require skin grafting. Affected skin may exhibit alternating areas of hypopigmentation and hyperpigmentation. Long-term ocular damage is possible, including late conjunctivitis and corneal opacification (Kehe & Szinicz, 2005). Long-term respiratory symptoms are also possible, including chronic bronchitis, asthma, pulmonary fibrosis, and bronchiectasis. Given that sulfur mustard is a known carcinogen, a long-term concern for lung cancer, skin cancer, and leukemia exists.

Affected patients will need regular visits to specialists from the ophthalmology, pulmonology, and possibly oncology services. Primary care providers should be intimately involved to coordinate care.

There are no preventive measures that can be taken to guard against the effects of sulfur mustard.

CHOKING AGENTS

Choking agents encompass a broad category of chemicals that cause respiratory symptoms. For the purposes of this text, only chlorine gas is reviewed.

Pathophysiology

Chlorine gas is a yellow-green gas with a pungent odor (Warden, 2005). It is intermediately soluble in water; thus it is able to cause damage to both the upper and lower airways. More water-soluble agents react early with tissues, leading to damage of only the upper airways. The reaction of chlorine with water forms both hypochloric and hypochlorus acids. Damage to lung tissue is more than an acidic injury, as toxicity leads to increased vascular permeability at the alveolar–capillary membrane and pulmonary edema (Bogucki & Weir, 2002).

Epidemiology and etiology

Chlorine gas is widely used and transported across the United States every day. It is one of the top 10 chemicals produced by gross weight. Consequently, much of the U.S. population is vulnerable to exposure from this agent (Evans, 2004). Chlorine is used in many industries, including paper making, pharmaceuticals, and plastic production.

Presentation

Patients exposed to chlorine gas will present with signs of lacrimation and irritation on the nasal and oral mucosa. In addition, they may complain of burning in the nose and throat, choking, and chest pain. Affected patients may also develop copious secretions in the nasal and respiratory passages, exertional dyspnea, and laryngospasm. If a large exposure has occurred, patients may develop frank pulmonary edema that can lead to respiratory failure (Bogucki & Weir, 2002).

Differential diagnosis

Patients presenting in respiratory distress should be evaluated for signs of pneumonia, laryngospasm, asthma, or other respiratory distress syndromes.

Plan of care

The diagnosis of chlorine gas exposure is determined by history. Pulmonary function tests are not helpful in diagnosing exposure to chlorine gas, as they may show a restrictive or an obstructive pattern.

Exposure to chlorine gas should prompt immediate decontamination. Clothing and contact lenses should be removed, and patients should be decontaminated with copious amounts of soap and water. Removing any source of residual gas limits the possibility of further exposure.

After decontamination, care is supportive. All exposed patients should be closely monitored. Strict bed rest helps minimize exertional dyspnea—even minimal exertion may shorten the latency periods and hasten clinical worsening (Bogucki & Weir, 2002). Should intubation and mechanical ventilation be required for respiratory reasons, higher positive end-expiratory pressure (PEEP) may be necessary due to the presence of pulmonary edema (Parrish & Bradshaw, 2004). Antibiotics are not needed in the acute setting, but may be required if a secondary pneumonia develops. Diuretics have limited utility.

Critical care HCPs may be needed to manage the respiratory complications of chlorine gas poisoning. As with all exposures to possible chemical terrorism threats, consultation with state and local public health authorities is recommended (Table 39-8).

Family members who were in proximity to the potential exposure site or the affected patient should be monitored closely for development of symptoms.

Disposition and discharge planning

Prognosis for chlorine gas exposure is good with supportive care. Most patients affected recover lung function. Patients will need to follow up with their PCP to coordinate future care, as needed. Lung function may be followed by the pulmonology service. There are no prevention strategies available for chlorine gas exposure.

RADIATION INJURIES

Phillip Jacobson

The events of September 11, 2001, prompted discussion and concern as to how the communities should prepare for future terrorist incidents, especially those involving weapons of mass destruction. Weapons involving the use of radioactive substances are included in this category. The following are examples of some of the worst radiation disasters in history. In 1945, nuclear weapons were detonated over the cities of Hiroshima and Nagasaki in Japan. In these cities, 66,000 and 39,000 people were killed, respectively, and many more people and animals were exposed to toxic levels of radiation (Avalon Project, n.d.). In 1986, a meltdown occurred at a nuclear power plant in Chernobyl, Ukraine, that caused 21,000 square kilometers of land to become contaminated in Ukraine, Belarus, and Russia. Seventeen million people were exposed to excess radiation, and 135,000 people were permanently evacuated from their homes (Likhtarev et al., 2002). Four years later, an excess of thyroid cancer took the lives of many exposed children and adolescents, with the contaminated area remaining uninhabitable. As these examples demonstrate, detonation of a nuclear bomb and a breach of a nuclear reactor have the potential to result in massive devastation.

FUTURE INCIDENTS

National security experts believe that the next most likely terrorist-related radiological incident will not involve the aforementioned concerns, but rather will involve the use of a radiological dispersion device (RDD). Such devices seek to expose the population to a single radiological agent via conventional explosive or nonexplosive means. A primary purpose in the use of a RDD is to spread fear and panic. The exposed area would likely involve a few city blocks; mitigation efforts, though difficult, would be easier than with nuclear detonations or spills (Timins & Lipoti, 2003).

The next most likely potential incident is considered to be either an attack on a nuclear power plant or a planned breach of such a facility. A breach in the reactor core by either means allows for the generation of an atmospheric plume of radioactive gases—most notably, radioactive iodine (^{131}I). People at vast distances would be at risk for exposure in such an event (Mettler & Voelz, 2002).

The least likely potential incident would be another nuclear weapon detonation. Initially, destructive effects would result from intense thermal energy and air blast. Next, ionizing radiation would be released as an intense pulse during the first minute of the explosion and fission, with the formation of activation products following on the heels of these events (residual radiation) (Mettler & Voelz, 2002).

GENERAL PRINCIPLES OF IONIZING RADIATION

Ionizing radiation comprises high-frequency energy emitted from an unstable atom trying to achieve stability. A "binding energy" holds the nucleus of atoms together despite repelling positive forces. When the nucleus becomes unstable, this extraordinarily powerful energy is released. For stability, the proton-to-neutron ratio in the atom should be 1:1.2. Radioactivity occurs when this ratio is imbalanced (Moulder, 2002). When biological organisms are exposed to high doses of ionizing radiation, free radicals are produced, chemical bonds are disrupted, and deoxyribonucleic acid (DNA) is damaged.

Two major categories of ionizing radiation exist: electromagnetic and particulate. *Electromagnetic* radiation consists of gamma rays and x-rays. Gamma rays—high-energy rays with a short wavelength—are highly penetrating. X-rays are lower-energy rays, with a longer wavelength, and are less penetrating.

Particulate radiation consists of alpha particles, beta particles, and neutrons. Neutrons are highly penetrating and damaging; they are emitted only during a nuclear detonation. Beta particles are high-energy electrons emitted from the nucleus; they are also highly penetrating. By comparison, alpha particles are relatively large and cannot penetrate skin or clothes. They are composed of two neutrons and two protons and must be internalized to create physiological effects. In 2006 in Great Britain, the radioactive element polonium was used to poison Alexander Litvinenko, a former Russian KGB agent (McPhee & Leiken, 2009). This element is known to emit alpha particles, which as previously noted, do not pass through clothing. Polonium was, therefore, relatively safe for the perpetrator to carry.

However, once internalized, the victim soon became severely ill; Litvinenko ultimately died.

Radiation cannot be detected by the senses. It cannot be seen, felt, tasted, or smelled. Thus someone can be exposed to a lethal dose of radiation without realizing it, and a radiation incident may not be immediately recognized. In 1987, in Goiania, Brazil, a canister of radioactive cesium (^{137}Cs) was stolen from a hospital and released in the streets, exposing several people to toxic doses of radiation (REAC/TS-CDC, 2006). Ten days elapsed before the radiation poisoning was recognized. Ultimately, 250 people were contaminated, and 4 people died of acute radiation syndrome.

Radiation hazard is related to the exposure and absorption of radioactivity. Exposure and absorption depend on four factors: time, distance, dose, and shielding. *Time* reflects the total amount of time of exposure to the radioactive source. *Distance* to the source is important to the degree of exposure. The inverse square law applies, such that as the distance from a radioactive source doubles, exposure becomes one-fourth of the original exposure. *Dose* is proportional to the strength of the radioactive source, measured by the number of radioactive disintegrations per second, in units of Curies (Ci), or Becquerels (Bq). *Shielding* is the type of barrier that exists between the patient and the radioactive source. Different types of barriers will prevent the penetration of different types of ionizing radiation. For instance, lead is a well-known barrier to Roentgen radiation (x-rays). Breaks in the integumentary barrier, such as occurs with trauma or burns, will diminish the shielding effect of skin and cause an increase in the severity of radiation injury.

The total dose of exposure is measured in a unit called rad (radiation absorbed dose). One rad is equivalent to 0.01 J (joule) of energy per 1 kg of tissue. The amount of tissue damage from radiation is measured in rem (radiation equivalent man). Other measurement units of note include the Gray (Gy) and the Sievert (Sv). One Gy is equal to 100 rad; one Sv is equal to 100 rem (Leikin et al., 2003).

Four important principles are associated with exposure of a victim to ionizing radiation:

- *External exposure* occurs when part or all of the body is exposed to radiation from an external source, but the victim does not harbor any radioactive material with his or her body. The victim is not radioactive and cannot expose others to radiation.
- *External contamination* occurs when radioactive matter lands on victims. These victims can transmit radioactivity to others. Removal of clothing removes 90% of the radioactive material.
- *Internal contamination* occurs when radioactive material is inhaled, ingested, or penetrates the surface of the body through a wound.

- *Incorporation* occurs when specific organs take up radioactive material in a victim who has been internally contaminated. The chemical—and not radiological—behavior of the radioactive material determines the organ(s) of incorporation. For example,[131] I will be incorporated in the thyroid gland, which readily takes up iodine as part of its normal physiology (*Advanced Hazmat Life Support Provider Manual*, 2003).

BIOLOGICAL AND CLINICAL EFFECTS

Chromosomal breaks occur directly from radiation energy. DNA damage from ionizing radiation, however, can occur either directly (20%) or indirectly (80%). Indirect damage is incurred when body water is ionized with H^+ and OH^-. Free radical formation can then lead to a generalized inflammatory response. The biological effects of ionizing radiation at the cellular level can take from seconds to hours to become manifest, whereas the clinical effects can take from hours to years to appear (Figure 39-7) (Zajtchuk et al., 1989).

Radiation disasters associated with blasts or other violent occurrences can lead to further injury from blast pressure effect, flying objects causing blunt or penetrating injuries, or thermal injury. These issues may be life threats that need to be addressed during initial assessment and management of the patient.

Radiation injury can lead to an entity known as the *acute radiation syndrome*. "The acute radiation syndrome is a broad term used to describe a range of signs and symptoms that reflect severe damage to specific organ systems and that can lead to death within hours or up to several months after exposure" (National Council on Radiation Protection [NCRP], 2001, p. 30). Cell death can occur either directly from ionizing radiation or by impairment of cell division. Organ systems with the most rapidly dividing cell lines (i.e., the least differentiated cells), such as the hematopoietic and the gastrointestinal systems, are most easily affected. Consequently, pediatric patients are more susceptible to these effects than adults. Infants and fetuses are the most vulnerable (Figure 39-8). Factors that determine the time of onset of acute radiation syndrome and its severity include the total dose of radiation absorbed, the dose rate, the percentage of body exposure, and the presence of trauma, burns, or other associated medical conditions. A total dose of less than 7 Gy is unlikely to result in acute radiation syndrome, for example; in contrast, a total radiation dose of 2.5 to 4.5 Gy produces a 50% death rate within 60 days. Pediatric patients may have a lower threshold than adults for development of acute radiation syndrome or ensuing death.

The acute radiation syndrome is classified into four phases: prodromal, latent, manifest illness, and death or recovery. The *prodromal* phase can begin within the first 48 hours after radiation exposure. During this time, there is immediate damage to cell membranes associated with release of inflammatory mediators. Nausea or vomiting and low-grade fever can occur during this phase. Onset of these symptoms within 2 hours of exposure is a poor prognostic indicator.

The onset of the *latent* phase usually occurs within 2 to 4 days after exposure, but can occur anytime up to 21 days post exposure. It occurs only with lower doses of exposure such as those in the range of 2 to 3 Gy. During this time, blood cell lines such as lymphocytes and platelets decrease their production of new cells due to the radiation effect on the rapidly dividing cells of the bone marrow.

The onset of the *illness* phase can occur up to 30 days after radiation exposure. Victims are extremely susceptible

to anemia, bleeding, infection, and impaired wound healing. Body systems affected include the hematopoietic, gastrointestinal, central nervous, and integumentary systems. A decrease in lymphocytes, granulocytes, platelets, and reticulocytes is observed. The change in absolute lymphocyte count (ALC) is a sensitive indicator and has been used as a correlate for the radiation dose received.

The epithelial lining of the gastrointestinal tract is one of the most rapidly dividing cell lines of the body; thus it is very susceptible to radiation toxicity. However, it takes larger doses of radiation (8 Gy) than the hematopoietic system to have a clinical effect. During the illness phase of the acute radiation syndrome, severe nausea, vomiting, and diarrhea can develop. Disruption of capillary integrity occurs,

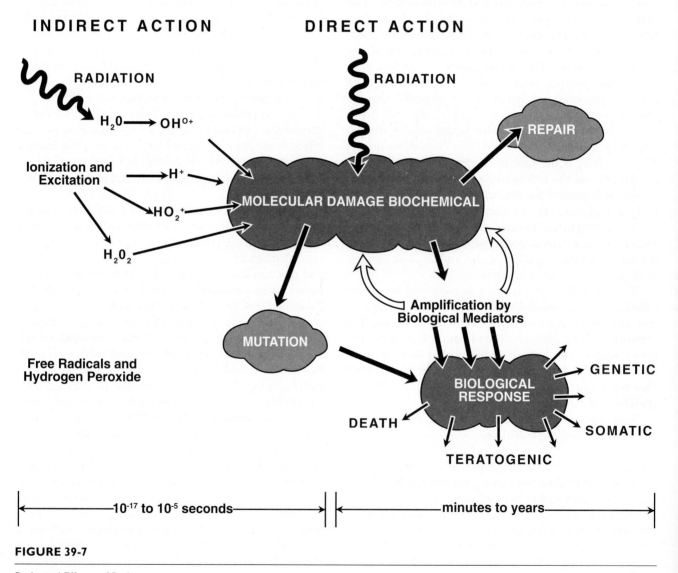

FIGURE 39-7

Biological Effects of Radiation.

Source: Zajtchuk, C. R., Cerveny, T. J., & Walker, R. I. (1989). *Medical Consequences of Nuclear Warfare Textbooks of Military Medicine.* Washington, D.C: Dept. of the Army.

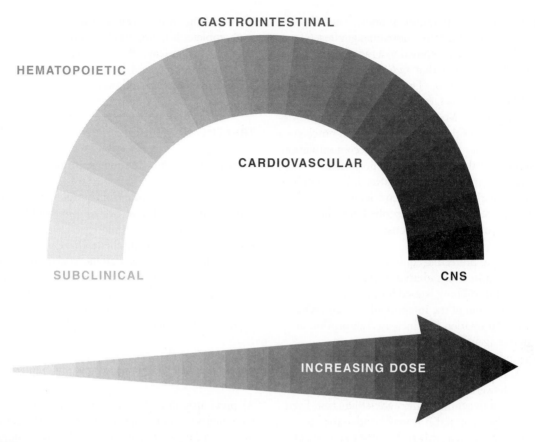

FIGURE 39-8

Organ System Effects of Radiation.

Source: Zajtchuk, C. R., Cerveny, T. J., & Walker, R. I. (1989). *Medical Consequences of Nuclear Warfare Textbooks of Military Medicine.* Washington, D.C: Dept. of the Army.

leading to hypovolemia, electrolyte imbalances, and shock. Translocation of bacteria may also occur, further endangering the patient through opportunistic infection.

The central system is less frequently affected by radiation. Primary central nervous system manifestations of acute radiation syndrome occur only after the person receives a radiation dose of at least 30 Gy. Victims experience cerebral edema associated with disorientation, convulsions, coma, and hyperthermia. A radiation dose of this magnitude, with central nervous system involvement, is universally fatal.

Radiation victims can also have local exposure to radiation, causing lesions on the skin. The type of lesion depends on the dose received. Epilation, erythema, dry desquamation, wet desquamation, and necrosis can all occur, with increasing severity of these manifestations reflecting higher radiation doses. Skin lesions from radiation can be distinguished from thermal and chemical burns, which have a more rapid onset and are more painful early in the course of the disease process. Radiation burns, by comparison, can take several days to weeks to fully develop.

IMMEDIATE CLINICAL MANAGEMENT

In preparation for the arrival of radiation victims, HCPs should divide the emergency department (ED) into "dirty" and "clean" areas to reduce the spread of possible external contamination with radioactive substances. All personnel should wear personal protective equipment, including surgical scrubs and gowns, surgical face shield, caps, and shoe covers. Double gloves are also recommended. The inner set of gloves should be taped to the gown. All HCPs should wear a dosimeter underneath their gown to measure the dose of radiation to which they are exposed while administering care to the exposed patient. The hospital radiation safety officer, or other designate (radiation oncologist), should take a leadership role in decontamination and processing of radioactive materials.

Consultation with the Radiation Emergency Assistance Center (REAC/TS) should then be initiated. The phone number for this agency is 865-576-3131 during business hours, and 865-576-1005 after business hours. The following website may also be useful: http://orise.orau.gov/reacts/.

In caring for the patient exposed to a radiation incident, the HCP should remember that *radiation poisoning is not immediately life-threateningn*. The first priority of treatment should be the ABCs (airway, breathing, circulation) of trauma management. Many centers will remove the victim's clothing as part of the initial resuscitation process—a step that also provides the bulk of the decontamination. Clothing should be double-bagged in polyethylene bags. Decontamination can be completed after initial stabilization. Decontamination procedures are identical to those employed for the chemical events described in earlier in this chapter, with the following exceptions:

- Different personal protective equipment, as described previously, is required for radiation incidents.
- Less rigorous skin rubbing is used for radiation events, to prevent disruption of the integrity of the skin, which can lead to inflammation and increased absorption of the radioactive agents.
- Only soap and water are used for decontaminating victims of radiation events—no bleach or alcohol rubs. Washing or showering for radiation incidents may require less than five minutes per cycle (Radiation Event Medical Management, n.d.). It may be advisable to shampoo the hair first, as this is the most likely site of body contamination (this decontamination procedure may already have taken place in the field before the pediatric patient arrived in the ED).

With the proper precautions, it is safe for HCPs to treat victims of radiation exposure. Lack of knowledge can lead to increased morbidity and mortality for victims of radiation exposure. "No health care provider has ever received a significant dose of radiation from handling, treating, and managing patients with radiation injuries and/or contamination" (REACT/S-CDC, 2006).

A complete blood count (CBC) with differential and absolute lymphocyte count should be performed every 4 to 6 hours. Nasal and throat swabs and 24-hour urine and fecal samples are sent for laboratory analysis to identify and quantify the degree of internal contamination. Wound swabs and irrigation fluid should also be sent for analysis. If the patient is suspected to have received a significant radiation dose, blood should be sent for cytogenetic analysis of lymphocytes, also known as *cytogenetic dosimetry* (REACT/S-CDC, 2006). The details of the event, including the involved radioactive agent(s) and the proximity of the victim to the source, in addition to the diagnostic tests previously described, may provide important information on the degree of exposure and the risk of developing acute radiation syndrome and internal contamination.

After the initial resuscitation and decontamination are complete, it is important to provide supportive care to manage the patient's fluid and electrolyte abnormalities, traumatic injuries, and burns. Rigorous infection control procedures should be followed.

TREATMENT OF ACUTE RADIATION SYNDROME

Treatment of acute radiation syndrome is supportive.

- For excessive vomiting, 5-HT_3 antagonists can be given. Intravenous fluids and electrolytes should be administered as needed.
- For anxiety, administer benzodiazepines.
- For a profound decrease in blood cell lines, the administration of colony-stimulating factors for granulocytes, platelets, or red blood cells should be considered under the supervision of a hematologist. In more severe cases, bone marrow transplants may be required.

TREATMENT OF INTERNAL CONTAMINATION

As previously described, radiation victims may have internal contamination. Routes of entry into the patient include inhalation, ingestion, absorption through wounds or skin, and injection. Once it is determined that a patient has internal contamination with a radioactive agent, it may be necessary to administer antidotes to enhance the elimination of the agent or to block its effects. *Antidotes are administered based on the chemical nature, and not the radiological nature of the inciting agents.* The sooner the treatments are initiated, the less toxic the effect of the radiation. The following strategies are used in antidote administration: chelation, competitive inhibition, enhanced gastrointestinal elimination, and enhanced renal elimination.

Chelation

Chelation with diethylenetriaminepentaacetic acid (DTPA) is therapeutic for internal contamination with heavy metals such as americium, californium, curium, and plutonium. This compound comes in two forms: calcium DTPA (Ca-DTPA) and zinc DTPA (Zn-DTPA). Ca-DTPA is 10 times more effective than Zn-DTPA. For adults and adolescents, administration is as follows:

- 1 gm Ca-DTPA IV initially in the first 24 hours, followed by 1 gm Zn-DTPA IV daily for maintenance.
- For children younger than 12 years of age: 14 mg per kg Ca-DTPA IV initially, followed by 14 mg per kg Zn-DTPA IV daily (NCRP, 2009, pp. 191–193).

Initial administration of DTPA should take place as soon as possible after contamination. Adults and adolescents may receive the initial dose via nebulization if the contamination occurred by inhalation; nebulized DTPA is not approved for pediatric use. BAL (dimercaprol) chelation can be used for polonium toxicity. BAL is a highly toxic drug and should be administered with caution:

- The dosage is 2.5 mg per kg IM four times a day for two days, then twice a day on the third day, and once a day for 5 to 10 days (NCRP, 2009, pp. 189–190).
- Alkalinization of the urine protects the kidneys during BAL administration.

A less toxic alternative to BAL for chelation is dimercaptosuccinic acid (DMSA), otherwise known as Chemet. The dose of DMSA is 10 mg per kg per dose by mouth every 8 hours for 5 days, followed by 10 mg per kg per dose every 12 hours for 14 days (NCRP, 2009, pp. 209–210).

Potassium iodide (KI) is extremely effective in *competitively inhibiting* its radioactive counterpart, ^{131}I, from being taken up by the thyroid gland. This radioisotope is released during the breach of nuclear power plants. KI will block 90% of the uptake of the radioisotope if given within 1 hour of exposure; it will block 50% of the uptake if given within 5 hours of the exposure. Its protective effects last for 24 hours. Thyroid function should be monitored closely during its administration. Table 39-9 provides dosing guidelines (U.S. Food and Drug Administration [FDA], n.d.).

Prussian Blue (ferric ferrocyanide) is an ion exchanger that binds the toxins in the gastrointestinal tract that travel through the enterohepatic cycle. Prussian Blue is not absorbed through the gastrointestinal tract; however, the toxins are excreted in the stool. Its use is an example of *enhanced gastrointestinal elimination*. This approach is highly effective in the treatment of internal contamination with ^{137}Cs or thallium, and was used for patients exposed in Goiania, Brazil. The dosing is as follows:

- For infants: 0.2–0.3 mg per kg orally 3 times a day (not FDA approved)
- For children 2–12 years of age: 1 gm by mouth 3 times a day
- For children older than 12 years of age: 3 gm by mouth 3 times a day

Dosing continues for a minimum of 30 days and can be adjusted based on the degree of internal contamination (NCRP, 2009, pp. 201–209).

Enhanced urinary elimination

Enhanced urinary elimination is another useful tool for certain radioisotopes. Administration of excess fluid helps with the urinary excretion of tritium. Uranium is toxic to the kidneys, and is best eliminated with alkalinization of the urine to a pH of 8–9. In pediatric patients, administration of sodium bicarbonate at a dose of 1 mEq/kg IV every 4 to 6 hours is used to achieve this goal. The dose should be titrated to effect. The doses of bicarbonate for alkalinization of the urine are identical to those used for ingestion of other chemical toxins, such as tricyclic antidepressants. Some patients may need dialysis based on the severity of the kidney injury.

TABLE 39-9

Dosing Guidelines for Potassium Iodide				
	Predicted Thyroid Exposure (Gy)	KI Dose (mg)	Number of 130-mg Tablets	Number of 65-mg Tablets
Adults: > 40 years	≥ 5	130	1	2
Adults: > 18–40 years	≥ 0.1	130	1	2
Pregnant/lactating women	≥ 0.0 5	130	1	2
Adolescents: > 12–18 years*	≥ 0.0 5	65	1/2	1
Children: > 3–12 years	≥ 0.0 5	65	1/2	1
Children: > 1 month–3 years	≥ 0.0 5	32	1/4	1/2
Children: birth–1 month	≥ 0.0 5	16	1/8	1/4

*Treat adolescents weighing 70 kg or more as adults.

Note: Gray (Gy), potassium iodide (KI).
Source: Adapted from U.S. Department of Health and Human Services, Food and Drug Administration, Center for Drug Evaluation and Research. (2001). Potassium iodide as a thyroid blocking agent in radiological emergencies. Retrieved from http://www.fda.gov/downloads/Drugs/GuidanceComplianceRegulatoryInformation/Guidances/ucm080542.pdf

TREATMENT OF LOCAL SKIN CONTAMINATION

Radioactive toxins that come into contact with the skin should be decontaminated using gentle scrubbing with soap and water. Further management is supportive. The contaminated area should be protected after cleaning. Prevention and treatment of infection are important. Good nutrition should be assured to promote positive nitrogen balance and healing. Analgesics should be administered as needed for pain control. Plastic surgery or burn services should be consulted as necessary for ongoing management and follow-up.

PSYCHOSOCIAL IMPLICATIONS

Pediatric patients may suffer from the psychological impact of radiation injury or exposure (AAP, 2003). Problems such as developmental regression, chronic fear and anxiety, nightmares and sleep problems, altered play, and social withdrawal can occur. As with other disasters, there is a direct correlation between the psychological effects on the parents as to that on pediatric patients. Pediatric patients should be referred to mental health services when psychological difficulties are observed.

IMPORTANT PHYSIOLOGICAL CONSIDERATIONS

In radiation disasters, pediatric patients are at higher risk for contamination and toxic effects than adults for the following reasons:

- Children are closer to the ground and can more easily inhale settled radiotoxins.
- Children have a higher minute ventilation, and may inhale radiotoxins more quickly.
- Children have thinner and more delicate skin, and proportionately a greater body surface area, allowing radiotoxins to penetrate their bodies more easily.
- Children have a smaller intravascular volume, causing them to circulate a higher concentration of radiotoxin (Yu, 2003).

LONG-TERM MEDICAL EFFECTS

Long after exposure to radiation, pediatric patients remain more susceptible than adults to malignancy. This greater risk arises because of their higher mitotic index and longer life span in which to develop problems. Higher rates of leukemia, thyroid cancer, and breast cancer have been reported in this population (AAP, 2003).

REFERENCES

1. *Advanced Hazmat Life Support Provider Manual* (3rd ed.). (2003). Tucson, AZ: University of Arizona.
2. American Academy of Pediatrics (AAP), Committee on Environmental Health and Committee on Infectious Diseases. (2000). Chemical–biological terrorism and its impact on children: A subject review. *Pediatrics, 105*(3 Pt 1), 662–670.
3. American Academy of Pediatrics (AAP). (2003). Radiation disasters and children: Committee on Environmental Health. *Journal of the American Academy of Pediatrics, 111*, 1455–1466.
4. American Academy of Pediatrics (AAP). (2006). *Pediatric terrorism and disaster preparedness: A resource for pediatricians.* AHRQ Publication No. 06(07)-0056. Rockville, MD: Agency for Healthcare Research and Quality.
5. American Academy of Pediatrics. (2009) *Red book.* Elk Grove Village, IL: Author.
6. American Academy of Pediatrics (AAP), Markenson, D., Reynolds, S., & Committee on Pediatric Emergency Medicine and Task Force on Terrorism. (2006). The pediatrician and disaster preparedness, *Pediatrics, 117*(2), e340–362. Reaffirmed February 1, 2010.
7. Arnold, J., Halpern, P., Tsai, M-C., & Smithline, H. (2004). Mass casualty terrorist bombings: A comparison of outcomes by bombing type. *Annals of Emergency Medicine, 43,* 263–273.
8. Arnon, S., Schechter, R., Inglesby, T., Henderson, D., Bartlett, J., Ascher, M., et al. (2001). Botulinum toxin as a biological weapon: Medical and public health management. *Journal of the American Medical Association, 285*(8), 1059–1070.
9. Audi, J., Belson, M., Patel, M., Schier, J., & Osterloh, J. (2005). Ricin poisoning: A comprehensive review. *Journal of the American Medical Association, 294*(18), 2342–2351.
10. Avalon Project, Documents in Law, History and Diplomacy. (n.d.). Avalon Project: The atomic bombings of Hiroshima and Nagasaki. Retrieved from http://avalon.law.yale.edu/20th_century/mp10.asp
11. Balali-Mood, M., & Balali-Mood, K. (2008). Neurotoxic disorders of organophosphorus compounds and their managements. *Archives of Iranian Medicine, 11*(1), 65–89.
12. Ballow, S., Behar, S., Claudius, I., Stevenson, K., Neches, R., & Upperman, J. S. (2008). Hospital-based disaster preparedness for pediatric patients: How to design a realistic set of drill victims. *American Journal of Disaster Medicine, 3*(3), 171–180.
13. Barbera, J. A., & Macintyre, A. G. (2007). Medical surge capacity and capability: A management system for integrating medical and health resources during large-scale emergencies. U.S. Department of Health and Human Services. Retrieved from www.hhs.gov/disasters/discussion/planners/mscc/mscc080626.pdf
14. Barthold, C., & Schier, J. (2005). Organic phosphorus compounds: Nerve agents. *Critical Care Clinics, 21*(4), 673–689, v–vi.
15. Blake, N., & Stevenson, K. (2009). Reunification: Keeping families together in crisis. *Journal of Trauma, 67*(2 suppl 2), S147–S151.
16. Bogucki, S., & Weir, S. (2002). Pulmonary manifestations of intentionally released chemical and biological agents. *Clinics in Chest Medicine, 23*(4), 777–794.
17. Borak, J., & Sidell, F. (1992). Agents of chemical warfare: Sulfur mustard. *Annals of Emergency Medicine, 21*(3), 303–308.
18. Borio, L., Inglesby, T., Peters, C., Schmaljohn, A., Hughes, J., Jahrling, P., et al. (2002). Hemorrhagic fever viruses as biological weapons: Medical and public health management. *Journal of the American Medical Association, 287*(18), 2391–2405.
19. Born, C. (2005). Blast trauma: The fourth weapon of mass destruction. *Scandinavian Journal of Surgery, 94,* 279–285.
20. Boyer, E. W., Fitch, J., & Shannon, M. (2009). Pediatric hospital surge capacity in public health emergencies. Agency for Healthcare Research and Quality. Retrieved from http://www.ahrq.gov/prep/pedhospital.pdf

21. Centers for Bioterrorism Preparedness Program Pediatric Task Force, NYC DOHMH Pediatric Disaster Advisory Group, & NYC DOHMN Healthcare Emergency Preparedness Program. (2008). Children in disasters: Hospital guidelines for pediatric preparedness. Retrieved from www.nyc.gov/html/doh/downloads/pdf/bhpp/hepp-peds-childrenindisasters-010709.pdf

22. Centers for Disease Control and Prevention (CDC). (2006a). Botulism: Epidemiological overview for clinicians. Retrieved from http:www.bt.cdc.gov/agent/botulism/clinicians/epidemiology.asp

23. Centers for Disease Control and Prevention (CDC). (2006b, March 3). Inhalation anthrax associated with dried animal hides-Pennsylvania and New York City, 2006. *Morbidity and Mortality Weekly Report, 55*, 280–282.

24. Centers for Disease Control and Prevention (CDC). (2007). Emergency preparedness and response. *Bioterrorism Overview*. Retreived from http://emergency.cdc.gov/bioterrorism/overview.asp

25. Centers for Disease Control and Prevention (CDC). (2010a). Botulism. Retrieved from http://www.cdc.gov/ncphi/disss/nndss/casedef/botulism_current.htm

26. Centers for Disease Control and Prevention (CDC). (2010b, March). Explosions and blast injuries: A primer for clinicians. Retrieved from http://www.bt.cdc.gov/masscasualties/explosions.asp

27. Cernak, I., Savic, J., Ignjatovic, D., & Jevtic, M. (1999). Blast injury from explosive munitions. *Journal of Trauma, 47*, 96–103.

28. Cernak, I., Wang, Z., Jiang, J., Bian, X., & Savic, J. (2001). Ultrastructural and functional characteristics of blast injury-induced neurotrauma. *Journal of Trauma, 50*, 695–706.

29. Cleri, D., Porwancher, R., Ricketti, A., Ramos-Bonner, L., & Vernaleo, J. (2006). Smallpox as a bioterrorist weapon: Myth or menace? *Infectious Disease Clinics of North America, 20*(2), 329–357, ix.

30. Daniel-Aharonson, L., Waisman, Y., Dannon, Y., & Peleg, K. (2003). Epidemiology of terror-related versus non-terror-related traumatic injury in children. *Pediatrics, 112*, e280–e284.

31. Dennis, D., Inglesby, T., Henderson, D., Bartlett, J., Ascher, M., Eitzen, E., et al. (2001). Tularemia as a biological weapon: Medical and public health management. *Journal of the American Medical Association, 285*(21), 2763–2773.

32. DePalma, R., Burris, D., Champion, H., & Hodgson, M. (2005). Blast injuries. *New England Journal of Medicine, 352*, 1335–1342.

33. Dieckmann, R. A. (2006). Pediatric assessment. In *Pediatric education for prehospital professionals: Student manual* (2nd ed.). Elk Grove Village, IL: American Academy of Pediatrics. Retrieved from http://peppsite.com

34. Dixon, T., Meselson, M., Guillemin, J., & Hanna, P. (1999). Anthrax. *New England Journal of Medicine, 341*(11), 815–826.

35. Evans, R. (2005). Chlorine: State of the art. *Lung, 183*(3), 151–167.

36. Fagbuyi, D. B., & Upperman, J. (2009). The role of pediatric health care providers. *Clinical Pediatric Emergency Medicine, 10*(3), 156–158.

37. Ferrer, R. R., Balasuriya, D., Iverson, E., & Upperman, J. S. (In press). Pediatric disaster preparedness of a hospital network in a large metropolitan region. *American Journal of Disaster Medicine.*

38. Ferrer, R. R., Ramirez, M., Sauser, K., Iverson, E., & Upperman, J. (2009). Emergency exercises and drills in healthcare organizations: Assessment of pediatric involvement using after-action reports. *American Journal of Disaster Medicine, 4*(1), 23–32.

39. Foltin, G. L., Schonfeld, D. J., & Shannon, M. W. (Eds.). (2006). Pediatric terrorism and disaster preparedness: A resource for pediatricians. American Academy of Pediatrics. AHRQ Publication No. 06(07)-0056. Retrieved from http:ahrq.gov/RESEARCH/PEDPREP/pedresource.pdf

40. Friedlander, A. M., Welkos, S. L., Pitt, M. L., Ezzell, J. W., Worsham, P. L., Rose, K. J., et al. (1993). Postexposure prophylaxis against experimental inhalation anthrax. *Journal of Infectious Diseases, 167*(5), 1239–1243.

41. Garth, R. (1997). Blast injury of the ear. In G. J. Cooper, H. A. F. Dudley, D. S. Gann, R. A. Little, & R. L. Maynard (Eds.), *Scientific foundations of trauma* (pp. 225–235). Oxford, UK: Butterworth-Heinemann.

42. Gausche-Hill, M., Schmitz, C., & Lewis, R. J. (2007). Pediatric preparedness of U.S. emergency departments: A 2003 survey. *Pediatrics, 120*(6), 1229–1237.

43. Gold, J. I., Montano, Z., Shields, S., Mahrer, N. E., Vibhakar, V., Ybarra, T., et al. (2009). Pediatric disaster preparedness in the medical setting: Integrating mental health. *American Journal of Disaster Medicine, 4*(3), 137–146.

44. Gonzalez, D. (2005). Crush syndrome. *Critical Care Medicine, 33*, S34–S41.

45. Guy, R., Glover, M., & Cripps, N. (2000). Primary blast injury: Pathophysiology and implications for treatment. Part III: Injury to the central nervous system and the limbs. *Journal of the Royal Naval Medical Service, 86*, 27–31.

46. Guy, R., Kirkman, E., Watkins, P., & Cooper, G. (1998). Physiologic responses to primary blast. *Journal of Trauma, 45*, 983–987.

47. Henderson, D., Inglesby, T., Bartlett, J., Ascher, M., Eitzen, E., Jahrling, P., et al. (1999). Smallpox as a biological weapon: medical and public health management. Working Group on Civilian Biodefense. *Journal of the American Medical Association, 281*(22), 2127–2137.

48. Ho, A., & Ling, E. (1999). Systemic air embolism after lung trauma. *Anesthesiology, 90*, 564–575.

49. Holstege, C., Kirk, M., & Sidell, F. (1997). Chemical warfare: Nerve agent poisoning. *Critical Care Clinics, 13*(4), 923–942.

50. Hutchinson, T., & Shahan, D. (Eds.). (2002). Serpacwa. In: *Drugdex System* (Vol. 111). Greenwood Village, CO: Micromedex.

51. Inglesby, T., Henderson, D., Bartlett, J., Ascher, M., Eitzen, E., Friedlander, A., et al. (1999). Anthrax as a biological weapon: Medical and public health management. Working Group on Civilian Biodefense. *Journal of the American Medical Association, 281*(18), 1735–1745.

52. Institute of Medicine (IOM). (2007a). *Hospital-based emergency care: At the breaking point*. Washington, DC: National Academies Press.

53. Institute of Medicine (IOM). (2007b). *Emergency care for children: Growing pains*. Washington, DC: National Academies Press.

54. Kaji, A. H., Langford, V., & Lewis, R. J. (2008). Assessing hospital disaster preparedness: A comparison of an on-site survey, directly observed drill performance, and video analysis of teamwork. *Annals of Emergency Medicine, 52*(3), 195–201.

55. Kehe, K., & Szinicz, L. (2005). Medical aspects of sulphur mustard poisoning. *Toxicology, 214*(3), 198–209.

56. Kluger, Y., Peleg, K., Daniel-Aharonson, L., & Mayo, A. (2004). The special injury pattern in terrorist bombings. *Journal of the American College of Surgeons, 199*, 875–879.

57. Kman, N., & Nelson, R. (2008). Infectious agents of bioterrorism: A review for emergency physicians. *Emergency Medicine Clinics of North America, 26*(2), 517–547, x–xi.

58. Koenig, K. L., Boatright, C. J., Hancock, J. A., Denny, F. J., Teeter, D. S., Kahn, C. A., & Schultz, C. H. (2008). Health care facility-based decontamination of victims exposed to chemical, biological, and radiological materials. *American Journal of Emergency Medicine, 26*(1), 71–80.

59. Lawrence, D., & Kirk, M. (2007). Chemical terrorism attacks: Update on antidotes. *Emergency Medicine Clinics of North America, 25*(2), 567–595; abstract xi.

60. Lee, E. (2003). Clinical manifestations of sarin nerve gas exposure. *Journal of the American Medical Association, 290*(5), 659–662.

61. Leikin, J. B., McFee, R. B., Walter, F. G., & Edsall, K. (2003). A primer for nuclear terrorism. *Disease-a-Month, 49*, 485–516.

62. Leonard, H. B., & Howitt, A. M. (2008). "Routine" or "crisis": The search for excellence. *Crisis Response, 4*(3), 32–35.

63. Likhtarev, I. A., Kovgan, L. N., Jacob, P., & Anspaugh, L. R. (2002). Chernobyl accident: Retrospective and prospective estimates of external dose of the population of Ukraine. *Health Physics, 82*, 290–303.

64. Makarovsky, I., Markel, G., Hoffman, A., Schein, O., Brosh-Nissimov, T., Tashma, Z., et al. (2008). Strychnine: A killer from the past. *Israeli Medical Association Journal, 10*(2), 142–145.

65. Markenson, D., Reynolds, S., & Committee on Pediatric Emergency Medicine and Task Force on Terrorism. (2006). The pediatrician and disaster preparedness. *Pediatrics, 117*(2), e340–e362. Retrieved from http://www.pediatrics.org/cgi/content/full/117/2/e340

66. Martin, T., & Lobert, S. (2003). Chemical warfare: Toxicity of nerve agents. *Critical Care Nurse, 23*(5), 15–20; quiz 21–12.

67. McPhee, R. B., & Leikin, J. B. (2009). Death by polonium-210: Lessons learned from the murder of former Soviet spy Alexander Litvinenko. *Seminars in Diagnostic Pathology, 26*, 61–67.

68. McManus, J., & Huebner, K. (2005). Vesicants. *Critical Care Clinics, 21*(4), 707–718, vi.

69. McPherson, M., Arango, P., Fox, H., Lauver, C., McManus, M., Newacheck, P. W., et al. (1998). A new definition of children with special health care needs. *Pediatrics, 102*(1 Pt 1), 137–40.

70. Mettler, F. A. Jr., & Voelz, G. L. (2002). Major radiation exposure: What to expect and how to respond. *New England Journal of Medicine, 346*(20), 1554–1561.

71. Mills, J. W., Curtis, A., & Upperman, J. S. (In press). Using a geographic information system (GIS) to assess pediatric surge potential after an earthquake. *Disaster Medicine and Public Health Preparedness.*

72. Moran, G., Talan, D., & Abrahamian, F. (2008). Biological terrorism. *Infectious Disease Clinics of North America, 22*(1), 145–187, vii.

73. Moss, M. L., & Shelhamer, C. (2007). The Stafford Act: Priorities for reform. New York University Center for Catastrophe, Preparedness and Response. Retrieved from www.nyu.edu/ccpr/pubs/Report_StaffordActReform_MitchellMoss_10.03.07.pdf

74. Moulder, J. E. (2002). Radiobiology of nuclear terrorism: Report on interagency workshop. *Radiation Research, 158*, 118–124.

75. Mushtaq, A., El-Azizi, M., & Khardori, N. (2006). Category C potential bioterrorism agents and emerging pathogens. *Infectious Disease Clinics of North America, 20*(2), 423–441.

76. National Commission on Children and Disasters. (2010). *2010 Report to the President and Congress.* AHRQ Publication No. 10–M037. Rockville, MD: Agency for Healthcare Research and Quality.

77. National Council on Radiation Protection & Measurements (NCRP). (2001). *Management of terrorist events involving radioactive material.* Report No. 138. Bethesda, MD: Author.

78. National Council on Radiation Protection & Measurements (NCRP). (2009). *Management of persons contaminated with radionuclides: Handbook.* Report No. 161. Bethesda, MD: Author.

79. Neches, R., Ryutov, T., Kichkaylo, T., Burke, R. V., Claudius, I. A., & Upperman, J. S. (2009). Design and evaluation of a disaster preparedness logistics tool. *American Journal of Disaster Medicine, 4*(6), 309–320

80. Paran, H., Neufeld, D., Schwartz, I., Kidron, D., Susmallian, S., Mayo, A., et al. (1996). Perforation of the terminal ileum induced by blast injury: Delayed diagnosis or delayed perforation? *Journal of Trauma, 40*, 472–475.

81. Parrish, J., & Bradshaw, D. (2004). Toxic inhalational injury: Gas, vapor and vesicant exposure. *Respiratory Care Clinics of North America, 10*(1), 43–58.

82. Qureshi, K., Gershon, R. R. M., Sherman, M. F., Straub, T., Gebbie, E., McCollum, M., et al. (2005). Health care workers' ability and willingness to report to duty during catastrophic disasters. *Journal of Urban Health, 82*(3), 378–388.

83. Radiation Event Medical Management (REMM), U.S. Department of Health and Human Services. (n.d.). Decontamination procedures: Radiation event medical management and about decontamination of children video. Retrieved from http://www.remm.nlm.gov/ext_contamination.htm, http://www.remm.nlm.gov/about_decon_video.htm

84. REACT/S-CDC, Radiation Emergency Assistance Center/Training Site (2006, December 5). Emergency management of radiation accident victims. *REAC/TS- CDC Course.* Lecture conducted from Oak Ridge Institute for Science and Education, Oak Ridge, TN.

85. Rebman, T., Carrico, R., & English, J. F. (2008). Lessons public health professionals learned from past disasters. *Public Health Nursing, 25*(4), 344–352.

86. Rice, P. (2003). Sulphur mustard injuries of the skin. Pathophysiology and management. *Toxicology Reviews, 22*(2), 111–118.

87. Safarinejad, M., Moosavi, S., & Montazeri, B. (2001). Ocular injuries caused by mustard gas: Diagnosis, treatment, and medical defense. *Military Medicine, 166*(1), 67–70.

88. Shamir, M. Y., Rivkind, A., Weissman, C., Sprung, C. L., & Weiss, Y. G. (2005). Conventional terrorist bomb incidents and the intensive care unit. *Current Opinion in Critical Care, 11*, 580–584.

89. Sharpnack, D., Johnson, A., & Phillips, Y. (1991). The pathology of primary blast injury. In R. F. Bellamy & R. Zajtchuk (Eds.), *Conventional warfare: Ballistic blast and burn injuries* (pp. 271–294). Washington, DC: Office of the Surgeon General.

90. Sidell, F., & Borak, J. (1992). Chemical warfare agents: II. Nerve agents. *Annals of Emergency Medicine, 21*(7), 865–871.

91. Singer, P., Cohen, J., & Stein, M. (2005). Conventional terrorism and critical care. *Critical Care Medicine, 33*, S61–S65.

92. Smith, L., & Rusnak, J. (2007). Botulinum neurotoxin vaccines: Past, present, and future. *Critical Reviews in Immunology, 27*(4), 303–318.

93. Stuhmiller, J., Phillips, Y., & Richmond, D. (1991). The physics and mechanisms of primary blast injury. In R. F. Bellamy & R. Zajtchuk (Eds.), *Conventional warfare: Ballistic blast and burn injuries* (pp. 243–244). Washington, DC: Office of the Surgeon General.

94. Timins, J. K., & Lipoti, J. A. (2003). Radiological terrorism. *New Jersey Medicine, 100*(6), 14–22.

95. U.S. Department of Health and Human Services (HHS) & Federal Emergency Management Agency (FEMA). (2009). FEMA and Department of Health and Human Services' Administration on Children and Families improve disaster case management through interagency agreement. Retrieved from http://www.fema.gov/news/newsrelease.fema?id=50037.

96. U.S. Department of Homeland Security (DHS). (2005). U.S. Department of Homeland Security fact sheet. Retrieved from www.dhs.gov/xlibrary/assets/NRP_FactSheet_2005.pdf

97. U.S Department of Labor, Occupational Safety and Health Care Administration (OSHA). (2005). OSHA best practices for hospital-based first receivers of victims from mass casualty incidents involving the release of hazardous substances. Retrieved from www.osha.gov/dts/osta/bestpractices/html/hospital_firstreceivers.html

98. U.S. Food and Drug Administration (FDA). (n.d.). Guidance: Potassium iodide as a thyroid blocking agent in radiation emergencies. Retrieved from www.fda.gov/downloads/Drugs/GuidanceComplianceRegulatoryInformation/Guidances/ucm080542.pdf

99. Warden, C. (2005). Respiratory agents: Irritant gases, riot control agents, incapacitants, and caustics. *Critical Care Clinics, 21*(4), 719–737, vi.

100. Wightman, J., & Gladish, S. (2001). Explosions and blast injuries. *Annals of Emergency Medicine, 37*, 664–678.

101. Yokata, J. (2005). Crush syndrome in disaster, *Japanese Medical Association Journal, 48*(7), 341–352.

102. Yu, C. E. (2003). Medical response to radiation-related terrorism. *Pediatric Annals, 32*, 169–176.

103. Zajtchuk, C. R., Cerveny, T. J., & Walker, R. I. (1989). *Medical consequences of nuclear warfare: Textbooks of military medicine.* Washington, DC: Department of the Army.

104. Zilker, T. (2005). Medical management of incidents with chemical warfare agents. *Toxicology, 214*(3), 221–231.

PART V

Procedures

Bonnie J. Stojadinovic

Arterial Catheter Insertion

INDICATIONS

The three main indications for entering a peripheral artery are continuous blood pressure monitoring, titration of vaso-active agents, and blood/laboratory specimen collection.

CONTRAINDICATIONS

Contraindications to arterial catheter insertion are a positive Allen test (Table 40-1), absence of a palpable radial or femoral pulse, cellulitis or other infection near the insertion site, burn injury near the insertion site (relative), coagulation defect (relative), and placement of concomitant central venous catheter in the same lower extremity (relative).

COMPLICATIONS

The most common complications of peripheral artery catheterization are thrombosis or arteriospasm resulting in obstruction to distal perfusion, bleeding, and infection. Careful preparation prior to the procedure, and diligent care after placement are important to minimizing the risks of untoward complications.

EQUIPMENT

Table 40-2 lists the suggested equipment for use during arterial catheterization. Suggestions for catheter sizes by weight are provided.

TABLE 40-1

Allen Test

The Allen test is used to test collateral blood supply to the hand and patency of both the ulnar and radial arteries. It is performed prior to radial arterial blood sampling or cannulation.

- Elevate the forearm and have the patient make a fist for about 30 seconds.
- Apply pressure over the ulnar and radial arteries so as to occlude flow in both.
- With the patient's forearm still elevated, open the hand. It should appear blanched (pallor can be observed at the fingernails).
- Release ulnar pressure. The color should return in less than 7 seconds.

Inference: Ulnar artery supply to the hand is sufficient and it is safe to cannulate the radial artery.

If color does not return or returns after 7 to 10 seconds, then the ulnar artery supply to the hand is not sufficient and the radial artery cannot be safely cannulated.

TABLE 40-2

Equipment for Arterial Catheter Insertion

1. Appropriate-size armboard (optional), tape, and small roll for under wrist (*if inserting a radial arterial line*).
2. Towel or blanket to place under hip (*if inserting a femoral arterial line*).
3. 2% chlorhexidine, 70% alcohol, or 10% povidone-iodine based on patient age and/or institution-specific protocol for site preparation.
4. Sterile gown, sterile gloves, mask, surgical hat, and eye protection.
5. Sterile towels, sterile drape (for femoral placement), and sterile gauze pads.
6. Syringes.
7. 1% lidocaine solution (without epinephrine) based on institution-specific protocol.
8. Appropriate-size safety cannula over needle or procedure tray with appropriate size catheter over guidewire.*
9. Hemodynamic monitoring system.
10. 0.9% saline with heparin 1–3 units/mL per institution-specific protocol; papaverine if ordered.
11. Prethreaded needle and suture (3.0 or 4.0 silk) or other securement device.
12. Scalpel (for cutting sutures thread if being used for securement).
13. Transparent or semipermeable dressing.

Catheter Recommendations		
Size	**Length**	**Access Site**
22–24 gauge	3.5 cm	Radial artery line for patients weighing less than 10 kg
20–22 gauge	3.5 cm	Radial artery line for patients weighing more than 10 kg
2.5 French	2.5–5 cm	Femoral artery line for patients weighing less than 10 kg
3.0 French	5–8 cm	Femoral artery line for patients weighing more than 10 kg

Source: Cook Medical Equipment Insert, August 2007.

* Use the shortest and smallest femoral line possible to avoid occluding blood flow in the artery. The line should always remain below the umbilicus when fully inserted.

PROCEDURE

Although performing an upper and a lower extremity arterial puncture and catheter insertion are similar in many ways, there are slight differences. Care should be taken to follow the variances unique to each site.

UPPER EXTREMITY

Prior to performing an upper extremity arterial puncture and catheter placement, explain the procedure to the patient and family. Obtain informed consent or permission per institution-specific policy, and complete a "time-out" (universal protocol). Perform an Allen test on the identified site. If negative, mark the pulse site. *Never puncture both the radial and ulnar arteries in the same extremity; distal arterial flow obstruction may result.* Assemble the necessary equipment, wash hands, and put on sterile gloves and eye protection.

Next, prepare the chosen site using an armboard (optional), tape, and small role for under the wrist. Cleanse the chosen site with 2% chlorhexidine, 70% alcohol, or 10% povidine-iodine based on the patient's age and/or institution-specific protocol. Chlorhexidine solution is recommended for those patients who are 2 months of age or older. Scrub the site for 30 seconds. Allow the solution to dry completely (30 to 60 seconds).

Anesthetize the site with 1% lidocaine solution, without epinephrine, based on institution-specific protocol. This step is optional, and access should not be delayed to complete it in an emergency.

Using the safety catheter over needle or catheter over guidewire technique, puncture the skin and direct the catheter toward the underlying artery at approximately a 30-degree angle. Watch for flashback of blood while continuously advancing the catheter and needle/guidewire. When flashback occurs, insert the catheter a bit farther before removing the needle/guidewire. If bright red blood returns rapidly, attach a syringe with 0.9% normal saline or with heparin flush solution. The addition of papaverine may (or may not) be required depending on if arteriospasm is anticipated. Aspirate from the catheter; if rapid blood return is still present, advance the catheter while flushing gently. Advance the catheter to its hub to reduce the risk for dislodgement or kinking.

Securely affix the catheter with tape or another securement device. Apply a transparent or semipermeable dressing per institution-specific protocol. Attach the arterial catheter tubing set and transducer for monitoring and waveform assessment.

LOWER EXTREMITY

Preparation is similar to that for the upper extremity, with the exception of the Allen test. Prepare the chosen site using a towel or blanket to place under the patient's hip and drape the area with sterile towels and sterile drape. Mark the pulse site.

Cleanse the chosen site with 2% chlorhexidine, 70% alcohol, or 10% povidine-iodine based on patient age and/or institution-specific protocol. Chlorhexidine solution is recommended for those patients who are 2 months of age or older. Scrub the site for 2 minutes. Allow the solution to dry completely (30 to 60 seconds).

Anesthetize the site with 1% lidocaine solution, without epinephrine, based on institution-specific protocol. This step is optional, and access should not be delayed to complete it in an emergency.

Utilizing the Seldinger technique (see Chapter 41), puncture the skin with the safety catheter over needle or catheter over guidewire, and direct the catheter toward the underlying artery at approximately a 30-degree angle. Watch for flashback of blood while continuously advancing the catheter and needle/guidewire. When flashback occurs, insert the catheter a bit farther before removing the needle/guidewire. If bright red blood returns rapidly, attach a syringe with 0.9% normal saline or with heparin flush solution. The addition of papaverine may (or may not) be necessary depending on if arteriospasm is anticipated. Aspirate the catheter; if rapid blood return is still present, advance the catheter while flushing gently. Advance the catheter to its hub to reduce the risk for dislodgement or kinking.

Secure the catheter to the skin with sutures. Apply a transparent or semipermeable dressing per institution-specific protocol. Attach the arterial catheter tubing set and transducer for monitoring and waveform assessment.

POSTPROCEDURE CARE

After successfully completing the arterial puncture and catheter placement, continuously assess the patient for complications. Check the warmth, color, and pulses in the extremity distal to the catheter placement. Monitor for signs of infection and bleeding, especially around the catheter site or from tubing connections.

PROCEDURE NOTE

An example procedure note for the insertion of a femoral arterial catheter is as follows:

- Date and time.
- Procedure: Arterial catheter placement.
- Indication: Continuous blood pressure monitoring and arterial blood gas sampling.
- Performed by: State names and positions.
- Procedure explained to caregivers, permission/consent obtained.
- "Time-out" taken (universal protocol).
- Sedation/analgesia: Patient was premedicated with midazolam *0.1 mg/kg* intravenous (IV) for sedation and fentanyl *0.1 mg/kg* IV for pain control.

- Site: Right femoral artery.
- Site preparation: The right groin was exposed by elevating the right hip onto a small roll. It was then prepped and draped in sterile fashion and cleansed for 2 minutes using a 2% chlorhexidine scrub. Next, 2 mL of 1% lidocaine was injected into the subcutaneous tissue for topical anesthetic.
- Procedure: Skin puncture was performed with a 22-gauge needle and the needle was advanced into the right femoral artery at a 30-degree angle on the first attempt. A 3-French 5-cm single-lumen catheter was then inserted using the Seldinger technique. Pulsatile blood flow of bright red blood was noted. A syringe with 0.9% normal saline was used to check for patency; it flushed easily with rapid return of bright red blood. Waveform confirmed the arterial location.
- Site at conclusion of procedure: The catheter was sutured in place with 3.0 silk thread and a transparent, occlusive dressing was placed. No bleeding at the site. Blood loss: none.

- Specimens sent: Blood gas.
- Patient condition following procedure: The patient tolerated the procedure without changes in vital signs and has appropriate pain/sedation score post procedure (state specifics). Distal extremity pulses are strong, skin temperature warm, and color pink.
- Signature of health care professional.

BIBLIOGRAPHY

1. American College of Surgeons. (2004). *Advanced trauma life support* (7th ed.). Chicago: Author.
2. Behrman, R., Kliegman, R., & Jenson, H. (Eds.). (2007). *Nelson textbook of pediatrics* (18th ed.). Philadelphia: W. B. Saunders.
3. Dieckman, R. A., Fiser, D. H., & Selbst, S. M. (1997). *Illustrated textbook of emergency and critical care procedures.* St. Louis: Mosby.
4. Fleisher, G. R., & Ludwig, S. (2005). *Textbook of pediatric emergency medicine* (5th ed.). Philadelphia: Lippincott Williams & Wilkins.
5. Verger, J., & Lebet, R. (Eds.). (2008). *AACN procedure manual for pediatric acute and critical care.* Philadelphia: W. B. Saunders.

Central Venous Catheter Insertion and Removal

INSERTION OF A CENTRAL VENOUS CATHETER

INDICATIONS

Central venous catheter (CVC) insertion and removal are essential procedures used in acute and critically ill pediatric patients. The femoral and subclavian vein sites are discussed in this chapter, as they are the most frequently used sites in pediatric patients. The femoral vein site is preferred in children due to its association with fewer complications and greater health care professional (HCP) comfort with this location (Custer, 2008; Kaplan & Brilli, 2007).

General indications for CVC placement include the following:

- Unavailability of venous access at peripheral sites
- Delivery of high-flow fluids or blood products
- Central venous pressure measurement and monitoring
- Blood sampling
- Continuous renal replacement therapy
- Administration of high-concentration/high-osmolality or sclerosing parenteral solutions (Donkin, 2008; Froehlich et al., 2009; Seneff, 2003)

CONTRAINDICATIONS

Several contraindications must be considered before placing a CVC. Infection or vascular compromise over the insertion site or adjacent to the insertion site should cause the HCP to evaluate the availability of another site (Braner et al., 2007; Donkin, 2008). Coagulopathies, high-pressure mechanical ventilation, morbid obesity, and abnormal vascular anatomy are other relative contraindications (Braner et al., 2007; Donkin, 2008; Tsui et al., 2008). Special consideration is required in the coagulopathic patient if selecting the subclavian route—this artery is difficult to compress because as it lies beneath the clavicle, making bleeding difficult to control (Braner et al., 2007). A patient receiving high-pressure ventilation may be more likely to have a pneumothorax on insertion of a subclavian CVC. Morbid obesity and abnormal vascular anatomy may complicate site location and insertion of the CVC (Braner et al., 2007; Donkin, 2008; Tsui et al., 2008).

Certain insertion sites have specific contraindications. The femoral vein should not be used in small neonates, in the presence of abdominal trauma, or in those patients who will undergo cardiac catheterization in the near future (Custer, 2008; Donkin, 2008). The subclavian vein should not be used in small infants or in patients with any of the following conditions: high intrathoracic pressure, presence of a pneumothorax or hemothorax to the contralateral

side of line insertion, or fracture to the ipsilateral clavicle or anterior proximal ribs (Braner et al., 2007; Hijazi et al., 1997).

COMPLICATIONS

General complications for CVC placement can be categorized as infectious, mechanical, and thrombotic. Complications by category and insertion site are listed in Table 41-1.

EQUIPMENT

The equipment to be used for CVC insertion will vary based on institution, but the general considerations are listed in Table 41-2.

TABLE 41-1

Complications of Central Venous Catheter Placement by Category or Insertion Site	
Category or Site	**Complications (listed in order of general prevalence)**
Infectious	1. Bloodstream infection
	2. Local cellulitis
Mechanical	1. Malpositioning or displacement (especially with mobility)
	2. Hematoma
	3. Arterial puncture
	4. Pneumothorax or hemothorax
	5. Nerve injury
	6. Air embolism
	7. Dysrhythmia
	8. Guidewire embolism
Thrombotic	1. Thromboembolism
	2. Thrombophlebitis
Femoral vein	1. Infection (not significant in pediatric patients)
	2. Thromboembolic events
	3. Arterial puncture
Subclavian vein	1. Pneumothorax, hemothorax, and hydrothorax
	2. Arterial puncture (subclavian)
	3. Central venous thrombosis (superior vena cava syndrome)
	4. Malposition
	5. Cardiac tamponade
	6. Cardiac arrhythmias
	7. Infection (not immediate)
	8. Air embolism
	9. Aortic perforation

TABLE 41-2

Equipment for Central Venous Catheter Placement

Sterile barrier materials (sterile gown, cap, gloves, goggles, towels/drapes, mask)
Cleansing solution (e.g., 2% chlorhexidine gluconate)
Tape, dressings, antimicrobial patch
IV tubing—new
IV fluid—new
Central line
Catheter insertion kit
The size and length of the catheter vary depending on the insertion site, number of lumens, and age and size of the patient.
Suture (type dependent on child and HCP preference)
Bath towel or rolled-up sheet
Portable ultrasound machine with sterile covers for probes (if available)
Availability of STAT (immediate) chest radiography or abdominal film (to verify placement)

Insertion Site	Number of lumens	Age	Weight	Minimum Size (French)	Maximum Length (cm)
Femoral	Single	0–6 months	~3–8 kg	3	30
	Single	6 months–2 years	8–13 kg	4	45
	Single	2 years–adult	>13 kg	5	60
	Double	0–6 months	~3–8 kg	4	30
	Double	6 months–2 years	8–13 kg	5	45
	Double	2 years–adult	>13 kg	7*	60
	Triple	6 months–2 years	8–13 kg	5	45
	Triple	2 years–adult	> 13 kg	7	60
Subclavian	Single	0–6 months	~3–8 kg	3	10
	Single	6 months–2 years	8–13 kg	4	15
	Single	2 years–adult	>13 kg	5	20
	Double	0–6 months	~3–8 kg	4	10
	Double	6 months–2 years	8–13 kg	5	15
	Double	2 years–adult	>13 kg	7*	20
	Triple	6 months–2 years	8–13 kg	5	15
	Triple	2 years–adult	> 13 kg	7	20

*There is less complication risk if a catheter smaller than 5 French is used in children younger than 5 years of age.

Source: Donkin, 2008; Hijazi et al., 1997; Janik et al., 2004; Lozon, 2004; Marschall et al., 2008.

PROCEDURE

The general procedure for insertion of a CVC is described in Table 41-3, with the femoral and subclavian vein approaches being shown in Figure 41-1 and Figure 41-2, respectively. The HCP should first assess the patient's clinical status, history of any previous CVC insertions and their locations, and pertinent laboratory values, particularly coagulation studies. Age-appropriate education regarding the CVC procedure should be provided to the pediatric patient and the caregiver(s), including the indications for the CVC, potential complications, general insertion techniques, analgesia and sedation to be used, and postprocedure care.

Caregiver(s) presence during the procedure can be offered at this time as well. The HCP should obtain and document informed consent or permission for the procedure.

As recommended by The Joint Commission, a "time-out" procedure (universal protocol) should be performed with the patient and care team to reassess the need for the CVC procedure, verify the correct patient, and verify and mark the correct and appropriate insertion site for the catheter (Donkin, 2008; Tsui et al., 2008). The HCP should assess the age, size, and insertion site to determine the size and length of the catheter to be used (Table 41-2). A catheter with the minimum number of lumens should be selected to help decrease the risk of infection (O'Grady et al., 2011).

A general method for estimating the length of the catheter required to reach the superior vena atriocaval junction is based on the external distance from the insertion site to the intercostal space between the second and third ribs at the costochondral area (Hijazi et al., 1997).

The pediatric patient should be placed on a cardiorespiratory monitor. Analgesia and sedation medication should be administered to the pediatric patient if indicated. The patient should be positioned and landmarks identified depending on the insertion site to be used (Table 41-3).

TABLE 41-3

Femoral and Subclavian Vein: Positioning, Landmarks, Techniques, and Pearls in the Pediatric Patient

Femoral Vein (FV)

Positioning

Externally rotate, flex, and abduct the patient's legs; "frog leg" positioning is often used. May need to place towel roll under the hip to further expose landmarks.

Landmarks

The femoral vein is located midline from the artery, which lies medial to the genitofemoral nerve. From lateral to medial, the order is nerve→artery→vein. The inguinal ligament is perpendicular to the femoral nerve, artery, and vein.

Technique

Clean the site prior to insertion for 2 minutes. To prevent the needle from puncturing the femoral artery, place the nondominant finger or thumb on the femoral artery while advancing the needle. Insert the needle 2 to 3 cm inferior to the inguinal ligament, at a 30- to 45-degree angle and 0.5 to 0.75 cm (may have to insert farther in large or obese patients) into the groin. Once blood is returned, continue with the Seldinger technique as described in text.

Pearls

1. Insert the needle inferior to the inguinal ligament to minimize the risk of retroperitoneal hematoma.
2. The procedure can be done without general anesthesia in children.
3. It is not associated with an increased risk of infection in pediatric patients
4. The right FV often easier to cannulate than the left due to the more direct path to the inferior vena cava.
5. Direct the needle within the sagittal plane; a common error is to direct the needle toward the umbilicus.

Subclavian Vein (SV): Infraclavicular Approach

Positioning

Place the patient in a supine position with the head of bed lowered by 15 to 30 degrees° (Trendelenburg position). Turn the patient's head away from the insertion site, with arms down. A towel or small blanket placed under the shoulders, between the scapulae, may help isolate landmarks.

Landmarks

Suprasternal notch, junction of middle and medial thirds of clavicle, and pectoral shoulder groove. The SV and subclavian artery are located inferior to the middle third of the clavicle. The SV is fixed just below the clavicle by fibrous attachments and lies on top of the artery, separated from it by the anterior scalenus muscle.

Technique

Clean the site prior to insertion for 30 seconds. Place the nondominant finger in the suprasternal notch. Directing the needle toward the suprasternal notch, with the bevel up, insert the needle 1 to 2 cm below the junction of the middle and medial thirds of the clavicle at a 30-degree angle. The needle should be inserted and advanced parallel to and beneath (posterior to) the clavicle. Once the vein is entered, rotate the bevel of the needle caudally (toward the heart) to ensure the catheter position in the superior vena cava. Venipuncture may require slow withdrawal of the needle (always using negative pressure on the syringe attached to the needle). Once the vein is accessed, proceed with the Seldinger technique as described in text.

Pearls

1. The proper patient position helps with insertion success.
2. The right SV preferred because the top of the lung is higher on the left (increased risk for pneumothorax).
3. Care must be taken with insertion to advance the needle by "marching down" the clavicle (just beneath) to avoid puncturing the subclavian artery or pleura.
4. Auscultate for bilateral breath sounds following insertion.
5. There are generally less infection risk with use of the SV site.
6. It is technically more difficult site and success is dependent on provider experience.
7. The SV is the ideal site in certain conditions: shock/hypovolemia (it is less likely that SV will collapse due to fibrous muscle attachments), obese/edematous patients (the clavicle is more easily identifiable than other sites), or prolonged use (related to less infection and thrombosis complications).

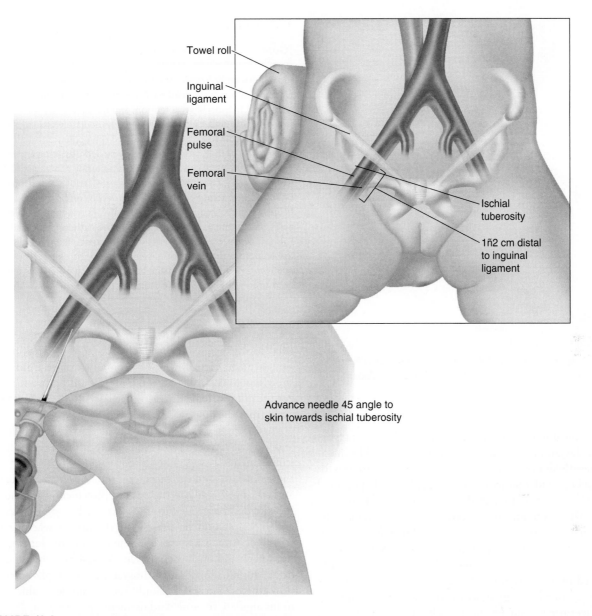

Advance needle 45 angle to
skin towards ischial tuberosity

FIGURE 41-1

Femoral vein approach.

Source: Modified from Henretig FM, King CC, eds. *Textbook of Pediatric Emergency Procedures.* Baltimore, Md: Williams & Wilkins; 1997:269.

The HCP should complete appropriate hand hygiene and put on the maximal sterile barrier equipment (gown, gloves, hat, mask) prior to beginning the procedure (Donkin, 2008; Marschall et al., 2008; O'Grady et al., 2011).

Cleanse the insertion site area with 2% chlorhexidine solution (if the patient is 2 months of age or older), 70% alcohol, or 10% povidine-iodine. Scrub non-groin sites for 30 seconds and groin sites for 2 minutes. Allow the solution to dry completely (30 to 60 seconds) (Garland et al., 2001; Marschall et al., 2008; Miller et al., 2010).

Once the sterile supplies are in place, the catheter hubs and lumens should be flushed with sterile saline or heparinized saline solution. An optional step is to anesthetize the insertion site area with 1% lidocaine without epinephrine; however, this step may obscure the landmarks. To decrease the number of placement attempts and decrease some of the associated complications with insertion, an ultrasound device, if available, is recommended to be used to assist in locating the vein and during the insertion of the needle and the catheter (Froehlich et al., 2009; Milling et al., 2005; National Institute for Clinical Excellence [NICE], 2002; Rothschild, 2001). The ultrasound probes should be covered with a sterile barrier, and an assistant should hold it in place during the procedure.

The *Seldinger* technique is the preferred method for inserting CVCs, particularly for the femoral and subclavian veins (Custer, 2008; Kaplan & Brilli, 2007).

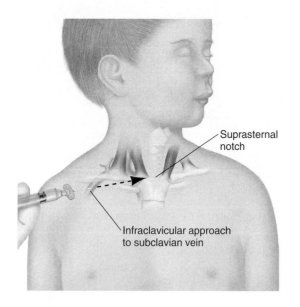

Suprasternal
notch

Infraclavicular approach
to subclavian vein

FIGURE 41-2

Subclavian vein approach.

Source: Modified from Henretig FM, King CC, eds. *Textbook of Pediatric Emergency Procedures.* Baltimore, Md: Williams & Wilkins; 1997:273.

The specific initial insertion techniques for the femoral vein and subclavian vein sites are listed in Table 41-3. The introducer needle should be held at a 30- to 45-degree angle with the bevel up, and a puncture site should be made proximal to the actual vein (Custer, 2008; Donkin, 2008; Tsui et al., 2008). An option during the needle insertion is to have the needle attached to a syringe to apply negative pressure with insertion into the vein (Kaplan & Brilli, 2007; Seneff, 2003; Tsui et al., 2008). The introducer needle should be gently advanced until the vein is entered and flashback of venous blood is confirmed. A guidewire is then placed through the introducer needle and advanced easily. If resistance is met, the guidewire should be pulled back, and advanced again. If resistance continues to be met, the guidewire must be removed and the needle can be adjusted within the vein or removed and another puncture attempted. If ectopic or erratic beats on the cardiorespiratory monitor are noted, the guidewire should be pulled back until the beats disappear (Braner et al., 2007).

Once the guidewire is advanced to the desired length, the introducer needle should be removed over the guidewire. *The end of the guidewire must always be in view and secured by the HCP* (Kaplan & Brilli, 2007; Seneff, 2003)—a technique that helps to prevent the complication of guidewire embolization (Table 41-4). A clamp can be placed on the end of the guidewire or an assistant can hold the wire until its removal. Bleeding at the site often occurs when the guidewire is advanced and the insertion needle is removed. Direct pressure on the insertion site with gauze

TABLE 41-4

Guidewire Embolization

Guidewire embolization is a rare complication in CVC placement, but it can lead to devastating consequences such as stroke, hemorrhage, infection, and death. If guidewire embolization occurs, the HCP must immediately ensure the patient's cardiorespiratory status and then contact radiology to proceed with locating the guidewire and designing a plan for retrieval. Retrieval can be accomplished using snares and often can be done through the puncture site without the need for an introducer sheath. Prevention of guidewire embolization is of utmost importance. The HCP must always maintain visualization and security of the guidewire. When the catheter is placed over the guidewire, the guidewire should protrude from the distal lumen before the catheter is inserted into the skin. Once the guidewire protrudes from the lumen, a clamp or fingers must hold onto the guidewire as the catheter is advanced.

can decrease the bleeding. If the size of the catheter is large (dialysis catheter), an optional 0.25- to 0.5-cm skin incision is made vertically or horizontally from the insertion site (Kaplan & Brilli, 2007). Care should be taken not to cut the guidewire by directing the bevel of the scalpel blade away from the guidewire.

A dilator should then be threaded over the guidewire and advanced with a twisting motion through the skin and subcutaneous tissue. The dilator should be removed over the guidewire, and the catheter inserted over the guidewire and advanced easily to the desired placement as previously measured. The guidewire should then be removed easily, and blood should be present in the lumen where it was removed. Attach a syringe to the hub of this lumen, and draw back and flush each lumen. An assistant should order or call for an immediate radiograph to check placement of the catheter. The HCP should remain sterile, if able, so as to manipulate the line if adjustments are required.

Once the CVC is confirmed to be in the desired location on the radiograph, the HCP should secure the line with sutures or a nonsuture securement device. An antimicrobial dressing, such as one impregnated with chlorhexidine gluconate, may be applied if indicated by hospital policy followed by a sterile occlusive dressing (O'Grady et al., 2011). During the entire procedure, the HCP should continually assess the patient's status and ensure adequate pain and sedation management.

POSTPROCEDURE CARE

Immediately following the procedure, the patient (if awake) and the caregiver(s) should be updated about the outcome of the procedure. The following orders should be recorded in the chart or computerized system: radiograph to check for CVC position, orders to use the CVC, fluids or medications to be initiated or changed to this access device, and specific fluids for central venous pressure (CVP) monitoring. The HCP must also document the procedure.

Care and monitoring of the CVC in the pediatric patient is critical to optimize the catheter's functioning and minimize complications. Signs of bleeding, hematoma, or infection at the site, and vascular changes distal to the site should be monitored by the HCP and/or nurses frequently in the first hours following placement, and then on an ongoing basis as determined by each institution's policies. Other signs of complications, such as decreased aeration of lung fields (potential pneumothorax or hemothorax) or malfunctioning of the CVC, should be reported immediately. The catheter position should be reconfirmed by radiograph on an ongoing basis (at a frequency determined by the patient's status).

CVCs account for the majority of catheter-related bloodstream infections (CRBSIs) (O'Grady et al., 2011). The Center for Disease Control and Prevention (CDC) developed and updated the *Guidelines for the Prevention of Intravascular Catheter-Related Infections* to assist HCPs and caregivers who insert and care for CVCs in pediatric patients (O'Grady et al, 2011). Many of these recommendations for insertion have been incorporated into the procedure technique described in this chapter. In regard to the care of the CVC after insertion, the CDC details specific evidence-based guidelines to prevent CRBSIs (O'Grady et al., 2011). Some of these recommendations are highlighted in Table 41-5.

Suggestions to prevent thrombus formation associated with CVC in the pediatric patient are poorly supported by evidence. The use of intermittent or continuous flushing with saline or an anticoagulant (heparin) has been recommended for lumens not in continuous use. Prophylactic infusion with urokinase once a week has also been recommended, but remains a controversial practice because complications such as bleeding have been reported; this medication is no

longer available in the United States (Lehne et al., 2010). Although the use of heparin-coated CVCs is purported to decrease the risk of thrombus formation, their efficacy has not been thoroughly examined (de Jonge et al., 2005).

PROCEDURE NOTE

An example procedure note for the insertion of a right femoral CVC is as follows:

- Date and time.
- Procedure: CVC insertion.
- Indication: Fluid resuscitation, IV access, CVP monitoring, caustic medication infusions.
- Performed by: State names and positions.
- Procedure explained to patient and caregivers, permission/consent obtained.
- "Time-out" taken (universal protocol).
- Sedation/analgesia: (List medications, dose, and route) prior to the procedure.
- Site: Right femoral vein.
- Site preparation: Patient positioned in a "frog-leg" position and placed on a cardiorespiratory monitor. Area cleansed (state cleansing agent used) for 2 minutes. Solution air-dried for 60 seconds. Maximal sterile barrier precautions employed. Eye-hole dressing and sterile drapes used.
- Procedure: State site of access. Accessed with ultrasound guidance with (state specific device) 21-g needle on first attempt. 4 Fr, triple-lumen, 20-cm Teflon CVC inserted using the Seldinger technique. Blood aspirated from all lumens and flushed easily. Patient remained sedated during procedure.
- Site at conclusion of procedure: No active bleeding or vascular compromise at site or to distal right lower extremity. Blood loss: None. CVC secured in place with nonsuture device and transparent/occlusive dressing.
- Specimens sent: None.
- Patient condition following procedure: Radiograph confirmed placement at (state exact location) and initial CVP reading was (state specifics). Patient tolerated procedure without changes in vital signs or ectopy and has appropriate pain/sedation score postprocedure (state specifics).
- Signature of health care professional.

REMOVAL OF A CENTRAL VENOUS CATHETER

INDICATIONS

The need for a CVC must be evaluated daily following the insertion in the pediatric patient. The complication rate with placement of a CVC increases with the length of

TABLE 41-5

Guidelines to Prevent Catheter-Related Bloodstream Infections

- Remove the CVC when it is no longer needed.
- Replace the CVC dressing in the pediatric patient only when it becomes damp, loosened, or visibly soiled.
- Replacing the CVC dressing in the adolescent patient once weekly.
- Do not use antimicrobial ointments on CVC dressings.
- Do not submerge the catheter or dressing under water.
- Do not replace the CVC on a routine basis.
- Do not replace administration sets (intravenous tubing and add-on devices) more often than every 72 hours.
- Replace tubing for blood products or lipid emulsions within 24 hours of initiating infusion.

Note: Central venous catheter (CVC).

placement, particularly with placements exceeding 5 days. Thus, these devices should remain in place for as brief a period as possible (O'Grady et al., 2011). Indications for early CVC removal include pathogen growth on the line or a systemic bloodstream infection. In particular, if a fungal organism is cultured from a CVC, the line must be removed as soon as possible to prevent systemic infection (Mermel et al., 2001).

CONTRAINDICATIONS AND COMPLICATIONS

The main contraindication to consider before removing a CVC is the coagulation status of the patient. If the patient has a significant bleeding diasthesis, the removal of the CVC may need to be delayed until the problem is treated or resolved. Other complications during removal of a CVC may include the inability to remove the catheter, breakage of a portion of the catheter during removal, or air embolism.

EQUIPMENT

The equipment required for a CVC removal generally includes clean gloves, sterile gauze (2 × 2 cm and 4 × 4 cm), occlusive dressing (petroleum jelly gauze optional), and sterile scissors or suture removal kit (Smith, 2008). Other personal protective equipment may be required by institutional policy. CVCs may be removed by HCPs and registered nurses who have received the appropriate education.

PROCEDURE/POSTPROCEDURE CARE

The CVC removal procedure should be explained to the patient and the caregiver(s), along with the indications for removal. An order to remove the CVC should be written in the patient's medical record. The necessary equipment and personnel should be gathered. A "time-out" (universal protocol) should be taken to ensure that the removal of the CVC is being performed on the correct patient, at the correct site, and that the CVC is no longer indicated or needs to be removed for another reason. All infusions should be discontinued or transferred to another access device. If dextrose concentrations of more than 12.5% are infusing through the line and infusions are to be transferred to a peripheral device, then new therapeutic plans must be written. These higher concentrations are contraindicated for peripheral delivery (Smith, 2008). Proper hand hygiene and aseptic technique prior to beginning and throughout the removal of the catheter must be observed.

Position the patient in such a way as to expose the catheter and insertion site. There is no evidence to support a specific patient position for central line removal. For the removal of a CVC from the femoral vein, the patient should be supine with legs extended.

Put on clean gloves and any other personal protective equipment required by the unit or institution. Remove the dressing carefully, and remove the CVC securement device or sutures using the suture removal kit.

If the patient is able to follow directions, instruct him or her to inhale first and then exhale only with the removal of the CVC. Prepare to remove the CVC on *exhalation* if the patient is on mechanical ventilation or is too young to follow instructions. This technique is based on the concept that negative intrathoracic pressure is generated on inhalation, with this negative pressure drawing air into the vein or CVC tract and resulting in air embolism (McGee & Gould, 2003). Place a sterile gauze over the insertion site and remove the CVC with an assertive and steady movement. Ensure that line is intact and that all parts are removed. If difficulty removing the CVC is encountered, do not force the removal and call for assistance from another HCP.

Firm pressure should be applied to the site for at least 5 minutes or until bleeding has subsided. An occlusive dressing should be applied over the site for 24 hours, and the patient should be required to lie flat for 30 minutes after removal of the catheter to prevent an air embolus while the tract is sealing (Smith, 2008). Petroleum jelly gauze should be placed over the catheter site if the CVC was in place for longer than 2 weeks to ensure that no air will be sucked into the tract, causing an air embolus (Smith, 2008).

Supplies should be disposed of properly and gloves and personal protective equipment removed. Other postprocedure care should include monitoring for bleeding or infection at the site and for signs and symptoms of air embolism.

PROCEDURE NOTE

An example procedure note for the removal of a CVC at the subclavian vein site is provided here:

- Date and time.
- Procedure: CVC removal.
- Indication: CVC no longer needed and peripheral venous access obtained.
- Performed by: State names and positions.
- Procedure explained to patient and caregivers, permission/consent obtained/
- "Time-out" taken (universal protocol).
- Sedation/analgesia: None required.
- Site: State access site.
- Site preparation: Patient positioned in supine position with right subclavian vein areas visible.
- Procedure: CVC dressing and sutures removed. CVC removed easily on exhalation and no ectopic beats noted

on monitor with removal. Pressure with sterile gauze maintained over site for five minutes.

- Site at conclusion of procedure: No active bleeding or vascular compromise at site. Blood loss: None. No signs of infection noted. A petroleum jelly gauze and occlusive dressing applied to site.
- Specimens sent: None.
- Patient condition following procedure: Patient tolerated removal of CVC without changes in vital signs.
- Signature of the HCP.

BIBLIOGRAPHY

1. Bessoud, B. (2003). Experience at a single institution with endovascular treatment of mechanical complications caused by implanted central venous access devices in pediatric and adult patients. *American Journal of Roentgenology, 18*, 527–532.

2. Braner, A. A. V., Lai, S., Eman, S., & Tegtmeyer, K. (2007). Central venous catheterization: Subclavian vein. *New England Journal of Medicine, 357*(24), e26.

3. Custer, J. W. (2008). Procedures. In J. W. Custer & R. Rau (Eds.). *The Johns Hopkins Hospital. Harriet Lane handbook: Manual for pediatric house officers* (18th ed., pp. 69–77). Philadelphia: Mosby.

4. de Jonge, R. C. J., Polderman, K. H., & Gemke, R. J. B. J. (2005). Central venous catheter use in the pediatric patient: Mechanical and infectious complications. *Pediatric Critical Care Medicine, 6*(3), 329–339.

5. Donkin, M. L. (2008). Central venous non-tunneled catheter insertion: perform. In J. T. Verger & R. M. Lebet (Eds.). *AACN procedure manual for pediatric acute & critical care* (pp. 1134–1142). St. Louis: Saunders Elsevier.

6. Froehlich, C. D., Rigby, M. R., Rosenberg, E., S., Li, R., Roerig, P. L., Easley, K. A., et al. (2009). Ultrasound-guided central venous catheter placement decreases complications and decreases placement attempts compared with landmark technique in patients in a pediatric intensive care unit. *Critical Care Medicine, 37*(3), 1090–1096.

7. Garland, J. S., Alex, C. P., Mueller, C. D., Otten, D., Shivpuri, C., Harris, M. C., et al. (2001). A randomized trial comparing povidone-iodine to a chlorhexidine gluconate-impregnated dressing for prevention of central venous catheter infections in neonates. *Pediatrics, 107*(6), 1431–1436.

8. Graham, A. S., Ozment, C., Tegtmeyer, K., Lai, S., & Braner, D. A. V. (2007). Central venous catheterization. *New England Journal of Medicine, 356*, e 21.

9. Hijazi, O. M., Cheyney, J. J., Guzzetta, P. C., & Toro-Figueroa, L. O. (1997). Venous access and catheters. In D. L. Levin & F. C. Morriss (Eds.). *Essentials of pediatric intensive care* (2nd ed., Vol. 2, pp. 1189–1215). New York: Churchill Livingstone.

10. Janik, J. E., Conlon, S. J., & Janik, J. S. (2004). Percutaneous central access in patients younger than 5 years: Size does matter. *Journal of Pediatric Surgery, 39*(8), 1252–1256.

11. Kaplan, J., & Brilli, R. J. (2007). Vascular access. In D. S. Wheeler, H. R. Wong, & T. P. Shanley (Eds.). *Pediatric critical care medicine: Basic science and clinical evidence* (pp. 253–273). London: Springer.

12. Lehne, R. A., Moore, L. A., Crosby, L. J., & Hamilton, D. B. (Eds.). (2010). Anticoagulant, antiplatelet, and thrombolytic drugs (2010). In *Pharmacology for nursing care* (7th ed., Chapter 51, p. 614). St. Louis: Saunders, Elsevier.

13. Lozon, M. M. (2004). Pediatric vascular access and blood sampling techniques. In J. R. Roberts, J. R. Hedges, A. S. Chanmugam, C. R. Chudnofsky, C. B. Custalow, & S. C. Dronen (Eds.). *Clinical procedures in emergency medicine* (4th ed., Chapter 19). Philadelphia: Saunders.

14. Marschall, J., Mermel, L. A., Classen, D., Arias, K. M., Podgorny, K., & Anderson, D. J. (2008). Strategies to prevent central line–associated bloodstream infections in acute care hospitals. *Infection Control and Hospital Epidemiology, 29*(S1), S22–S30.

15. McGee, D. C., & Gould, M. K. (2003). Preventing complications of central venous catheterization. *New England Journal of Medicine, 348*(12), 1123–1133.

16. Mermel, L. A., Farr, B., Sherertz, R., Raad, I., O'Grady, N., Harris, J., et al. (2001). Guidelines for the management of intravascular catheter–related infections. *Clinical Infectious Diseases, 32*(9), 1249–1272.

17. Miller, M., Griswold, M., Harris, J., Yenokyan, G., Huskins, C., Moss, M., et al. (2010). Decreasing PICU catheter-associated bloodstream infections: NACHRI's quality transformation efforts. *Pediatrics, 125*(2), 206–213.

18. Milling, T. J., Rose, J., Briggs, W. M., Birkhahn, R., Gaeta, T. J., Bove, J. J., et al. (2005). Randomized, controlled clinical trial of point-of-care limited ultrasonography assistance of central venous cannulation: The Third Sonography Outcomes Assessment Program (SOAP-3) trial. *Critical Care Medicine, 33*(8), 1875–1877.

19. National Institute for Clinical Excellence (NICE). (2002). Guidance on the use of ultrasound locating devices for placing central venous catheters. Technology Appraisal Guidance No. 49. Retrieved from http://www.nice.org.uk

20. O'Grady, N. P., Alexander, M., Dellinger, E. P., Gerberding, J. L., Heard, S. O., Maki, D. G., et al. (2011). Guidelines for the prevention of intravascular catheter-related infections. Retrieved from http://www.cdc.gov/hicpac/pdf/guidelines/bsi-guidelines-2011.pdf

21. Randolph, A. G., Cook, D. J., Gonzales, C. A., & Prible, C. G. (1996). Ultrasound guidance for placement of central venous catheters: A meta-analysis of the literature. *Critical Care Medicine, 24*, 2053–2058.

22. Rothschild, J. M. (2001). Ultrasound guidance of central vein catheterization: Evidence report/technology assessment. In Agency for Health Care Research and Quality, *Making health care safer: A critical analysis of patient safety practices*, No. 43 (pp. 245–253, AHRQ publication no. 01-E058). Rockville, MD: Author.

23. Seneff, M. G. (2003). Central venous catheters. In R. S. Irwin, J. M. Rippe, F. J. Curley, & S. O. Heard (Eds.). *Procedures and techniques in intensive care medicine* (3rd ed.). Philadelphia: Lippincott, Williams & Wilkins.

24. Smith, L. G. (2008). Central venous non-tunneled catheter: Care and management. In J. T. Verger & R. M. Lebet (Eds.). *AACN procedure manual for pediatric acute and critical care* (pp. 1055–1062). St. Louis: Saunders Elsevier.

25. Tsui, J. Y., Collins, A. B., White, D. W., Lai, J., & Tabas, J. A. (2008). Placement of a femoral venous catheter. *New England Journal of Medicine, 356*(28), e30.

Chest Tube Insertion and Removal

INSERTION OF CHEST TUBE

INDICATIONS

Chest tubes (thoracostomy tubes) are placed to evacuate air, fluid, or blood from intrapleural and mediastinal spaces as well as to assist with lung reexpansion. Indications for the placement of a chest tube include pneumothorax, hemothorax, effusions, and empyemas.

CONTRAINDICATIONS

While there are no absolute contraindications to the placement of a chest tube, the health care professional (HCP) must give special consideration to the risk versus benefit of inserting a chest tube in a pediatric patient who is on anticoagulation medications, is coagulopathic, or has a skin infection at the insertion site of the chest tube.

COMPLICATIONS

Complications associated with chest tube placement may include pneumothorax, hemothorax, bleeding, infection, cardiac dysrhythmias, pulmonary contusion, or lacerations and puncture of liver, spleen, or diaphragm.

EQUIPMENT

Table 42-1 lists equipment needed for performing chest tube insertion.

PROCEDURE

After obtaining informed consent or permission, complete a "time-out" procedure (universal protocol) to reassess the need for the procedure and to verify the correct patient; then administer appropriate analgesia and sedation. Explain the procedure to the patient and the caregiver(s).

Position the child in a supine position or with the affected side up, with the arm raised above the head (Figure 42-1). A chest tube should be placed anteriorly toward the apex of the lung for pneumothorax, and more inferior and posterior for fluid evacuation. Identify the insertion site, which should be one to two intercostal spaces below anticipated entrance of tube into pleural space. Select the appropriate-sized chest tube (Table 42-2). The HCP should don sterile gown, gloves, hat, and mask, and use sterile technique to prep (per institutional policy) and drape the insertion site.

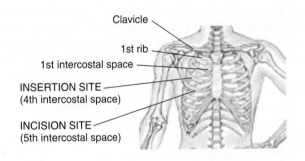

FIGURE 42-1

Chest Tube Placement Location.

Source: Gausche-Hill et al., (Eds.) (2007). *APLS: The Pediatric Emergency Medicine Resource*, 4th ed. Jones and Bartlett Publishers.

TABLE 42-1

Equipment for Chest Tube Insertion	
Sterile prep solution	Kelly clamp
Sterile gloves and towels	Tonsillar clamp
25-gauge needle	Dissecting scissors (straight)
Syringes	Needle holder
1% lidocaine injectable	Hemostats
Pain/sedation medication	Closed drainage system
Sutures 0–2 nonabsorbable polyester	Suction source
Gauze	Sterile dressing material
Scalpel	Chest tube (see Table 42-2)

TABLE 42-2

Guide for Selecting the Appropriate-Size Chest Tube	
Patient Age	Approximate Chest Tube Size (French)
Neonate < 5 kg	8–12
0–1 years (5–10 kg)	10–14
1–2 years (10–15 kg)	14–20
2–5 years (15–20 kg)	20–24
5–10 years (20–30 kg)	20–28
> 10 years (20–50 kg)	28–40
Adult (> 50 kg)	32–40

The chest tube insertion depth may be measured by overlying the tube across the hemithorax to its anticipated final position, noting that all holes of the tube must be through the pleura after placement. Subcutaneous local anesthetic of 1% lidocaine *without* epinephrine should be administered at the anticipated incision site and along the dissection path through the subcutaneous tissues.

Make a sterile incision two to three times the diameter of the tube, located two to three intercostal spaces below the anticipated entry site of the tube. Using a tonsillar clamp or blunt-tipped scissors, open the instrument to spread the subcutaneous tissue, thereby creating a tunnel to the point where the intercostal space will be penetrated by the tube. Using the tonsillar clamp to advance into pleural space, roll the clamp over the superior edge of the rib. Advance the tip of the tonsillar clamp through the pleural space, spreading the clamp to enlarge the hole enough to accommodate the size of the tube. Upon entering the pleural space, a rush of air will be heard or pleural fluid will be returned; do not advance the instrument farther. Remove the clamp, insert an index finger into the newly created incision, and advance the fingertip into the pleural space. Grasp the tube with the hemostat and guide it along the finger into the pleural space; remove the hemostat from the tube and then advance the tube to the premeasured distance. Connect the tube to drainage device and suction as appropriate.

Secure chest tube with heavy polyester suture using either the purse string or mattress suturing technique (see Chapter 52). Apply sterile dressings.

POSTPROCEDURAL CARE

Care following the insertion of a chest tube includes documenting proper positioning of the chest tube with a chest radiograph (CXR) as well as monitoring drainage and tolerance of drainage by the patient, insertion site and dressings, functioning of the chest tube, and resolution of symptoms.

PROCEDURE NOTE

An example procedure note for the insertion of a chest tube for pneumothorax is as follows:

- Date and time.
- Chest tube insertion: State site of access.
- Indication: Pneumothorax.
- Performed by: State names and positions.
- Procedure explained to patient and caregivers, permission/consent obtained.
- "Time-out" taken (universal protocol).

- Sedation/analgesia: 1 mg of morphine was given intravenously for pain.
- Site preparation: Patient was positioned on the left side with the arm above the head. The right chest was prepped (state cleansing agent used) and draped in sterile fashion. 1% lidocaine was used to anesthetize the surrounding skin area.
- Procedure: A 2-cm skin incision was made at the fifth intercostal space in the midaxillary area. A subcutaneous tunnel was created until the pleural space was entered, with a rush of air being noted. A 12 French thoracostomy tube was inserted. The chest tube was attached to 20-cm wall suction and a CXR obtained.
- Site at conclusion of procedure: No active bleeding at site. Blood loss: None. Chest tube sutured to the skin with 2-0 nonabsorbable suture; a sterile dressing was applied.
- Specimens sent: None.
- Patient condition following procedure: Radiograph confirmed placement at (state exact location); report status of pneumothorax. Patient tolerated procedure without changes in vital signs and has an appropriate pain/sedation score post procedure (state specifics).
- Signature of health care professional.

REMOVAL OF CHEST TUBE

INDICATIONS

Chest tube removal is indicated when the reason for its placement has been resolved. These indications may include the absence of pneumothorax, hemothorax, effusion, empyema, or an acceptable decrease in surgical drainage.

CONTRAINDICATIONS

Contraindications to the removal of a chest tube include persistence of the reason the chest tube was placed or an air leak. Special consideration should be made for those patients on anticoagulation therapy or with unresolved coagulopathies.

COMPLICATIONS

Complications that may occur with the removal of a chest tube include pneumothorax, reaccumulation of fluid, infection, air leak, or bleeding.

EQUIPMENT

The following equipment is required for removal of a chest tube:

- Petroleum gauze
- 2 × 2 sterile gauze pad
- Occlusive dressing
- Clamps
- Suture removal kit

Pain medication should be administered prior to chest tube removal.

PROCEDURE

After performing "time-out" (universal protocol), administer pain and sedation medications as needed. Explain the procedure to the patient and the caregiver(s). Remove the dressing from the chest tube site. Cut sutures while holding the tube securely in place. Do not cut purse string sutures; if they are used, they will be tied immediately after tube removal to close the wound. Place a small piece of petroleum gauze onto sterile gauze pad, and place this dressing over the chest tube site. While maintaining constant pressure over the insertion site, instruct the patient to hold his or her breath or, as age appropriate, to exhale and hold his or her breath. Remove the chest tube on exhalation. *Pediatric patients on mechanical ventilation should have chest tubes removed at the end of inspiratory phase of a mechanical breath.* While holding constant pressure over the site, tie the purse sting sutures, if present, and cover the gauze with an occlusive dressing. Immediately auscultate for equal bilateral breath sounds.

POSTPROCEDURAL CARE

Care after the removal of a chest tube includes evaluation and monitoring for respiratory distress and obtaining a CXR to evaluate for pneumothorax or reaccumulation of fluid.

PROCEDURE NOTE

An example procedure note for the removal of a chest tube is as follows:

- Date and time.
- Chest tube removal: State site and type.
- Indication: Resolved pneumothorax.
- Performed by: State names and positions.
- Procedure explained to patient and caregivers.
- "Time-out" taken (universal protocol).
- Sedation/analgesia: Morphine 1 mg given IV for pain was administered prior to the removal of the chest tube.
- Site preparation: After personal protective equipment, the occlusive dressing and sutures were removed.
- Procedure: Petroleum gauze was placed over the insertion site with the chest tube removed upon exhalation. Purse string sutures were tied.
- Site at conclusion of procedure: No ongoing bleeding. Blood loss: None. An occlusive dressing was applied.
- Specimens sent: None.
- Patient condition following procedure: The patient had bilateral equal breath sounds after the tube was removed and tolerated the procedure well without complication. A CXR noted no reaccumulation of pneumothorax.
- Signature of health care professional.

BIBLIOGRAPHY

1. King, C., & Henretig, F. M. (Eds.), & King, B. R., Loiselle, J. M., Ruddy, R. M., & Wiley, J. F. III (ASSOCIATE Eds.). (2008). *Textbook of pediatric emergency procedures*, 2nd ed. Philadelphia: Wolters Kluwer Health/Lippincott Williams & Wilkins.
2. Zeh, H. J. III, & Staveley-O'Carroll, K. F. (2000). Thoracic procedures. In H. Chen & C. J. Sonnenday (Eds.). *Manual of common bedside surgical procedures: By the Halsted residents of the Johns Hopkins Hospital*, 2nd ed. (pp. 111–142). Philadelphia: Lippincott Williams & Wilkins.

Intracardiac Line Removal

INDICATIONS

The removal of intracardiac lines is indicated when there is no longer a need for intracardiac pressure monitoring.

CONTRAINDICATIONS

The contraindications to the removal of an intracardiac line include bleeding, abnormal coagulation studies, clotted chest tubes, lack of intravenous (IV) access, and unavailability of one unit of packed red blood cells (PRBCs) at the bedside. Multiple intracardiac lines should be removed individually, with a minimum of one hour allotted between removals to allow for assessment of possible adverse events.

COMPLICATIONS

Complications associated with the removal of intracardiac lines include bleeding, cardiac tamponade, and hemodynamic instability.

EQUIPMENT

The following equipment should be assembled at the bedside prior to line removal:

- Suture removal kit (scissors, tweezers)
- Gauze
- Occlusive dressing
- Sterile gloves
- One unit PRBCs immediately available at the bedside, per the institution's policy

Consider pain and sedation medications are indicated.

PROCEDURE

Complete a "time-out" procedure (universal protocol) to reassess the need for the procedure and to verify the correct patient and site; then administer appropriate analgesia and sedation. Explain the procedure to the patient and the caregiver(s). Review the chest radiograph (CXR) for abnormal line placement or kinks in the catheter. In addition, the patient's hemoglobin (Hgb), hematocrit (Hct), prothrombin time (PT), partial thromboplastin time (PTT), International Normalized Ratio (INR), and platelet count should be within normal limits. The pediatric patient should also have a patent IV catheter for resuscitation if needed. One unit of PRBCs should be immediately available at bedside when removing intracardiac lines.

Ensure patency of chest tubes by evaluating for drainage and the absence of clots in the tubing. Perform hand hygiene and don sterile gloves. Remove the occlusive dressing and, using sterile tweezers and scissors, cut the suture holding the intracardiac line in place. Slowly withdraw the catheter while holding gauze over the site; stop the removal if any resistance is noted. Maintain pressure and examine the tip of the catheter once removed to ensure entire catheter has been removed.

Cover the site with an occlusive dressing. Evaluate for bleeding at the site or in chest tube(s). Obtain a CXR to evaluate for bleeding or tamponade, and obtain a hematocrit level one hour after line is removed.

POSTPROCEDURAL CARE

Postprocedural care following the removal of intracardiac lines includes monitoring for bleeding and signs and symptoms of cardiac tamponade. Chest tubes should be assessed frequently for patency by assessing tube for clots or a sudden cessation of drainage as well as monitoring for increased bloody drainage within the collection chamber. A hematocrit checked one hour after removal of the intracardiac line should be obtained sooner when signs of bleeding exist.

PROCEDURE NOTE

An example procedure note for the removal of an intracardiac line is as follows:

- Date and time.
- Removal of the left atrial intracardiac line.
- Indication: Completion of intracardiac monitoring.
- Performed by: State names and positions.
- Procedure explained to patient and caregivers.
- "Time-out" taken (universal protocol).
- Sedation/analgesia: (List medications, dose, and route) prior to the procedure.
- Preparation: CXR without evidence of tamponade, left atrial intracardiac line in proper position and no kinking of line noted, Hgb 14, Hct 41, platelets 156, PT 14, PTT 38, INR 1.37. Patent IV and chest tubes were verified and one unit of PRBCs was present at the bedside.
- Procedure: After donning sterile gloves, the occlusive dressing was removed, the site inspected, and the suture removed. The line was removed without resistance or bleeding. The catheter was intact upon removal.
- Site at conclusion of procedure: Occlusive dressing applied. Blood loss: None.
- Specimens sent: None.

- Patient condition following procedure: Chest tubes patent; no evidence of bleeding. CXR without evidence of new fluid accumulation. Patient tolerated the procedure without complication. Will obtain HCT level in one hour and continue to monitor for signs of tamponade and bleeding.
- Signature of healthcare professional.

BIBLIOGRAPHY

1. Verger, J. T., & Lebet, R. M. (Eds.). (2008). *American Association of Critical Care Nurses procedure manual for pediatric acute and critical care.* St. Louis, MO: Saunders Elsevier.

Judie Holleman, Amanda Johnson, and Paula Zakrzewski

Intraventricular Catheter Insertion and Shunt Access

INDICATIONS

The indications for ventricular access are collection of cerebrospinal fluid (CSF) for analysis or fluid reduction and insertion of a catheter for intracranial pressure monitoring. This procedure requires knowledge of neuroanatomy, CSF physiology and flow dynamics, cerebral autoregulation, and management of increased intracranial pressure and cerebral perfusion pressure.

CONTRAINDICATIONS

Contraindications to consider before ventricular access are coagulopathy or a history of bleeding disorders; immunologic compromise or deficiency; and, in some patients, the underlying condition of the ventricles and surrounding brain tissue.

COMPLICATIONS

The highest incidence of a potentially life-threatening intracranial hemorrhage is during the insertion of a ventricular access catheter. Removal of a ventricular catheter also carries a lower risk for intracranial hemorrhage. The removal or drainage of CSF or shift of intracranial contents and pressure can cause intraventricular or subdural hemorrhage. The risk of infection increases anytime the cranial vault is invaded. The risk of infection should also be considered when entering any CSF shunting system.

EQUIPMENT

The equipment necessary for ventricular access is listed in Table 44-1.

PROCEDURE

After obtaining informed consent or permission, complete a "time-out" procedure (universal protocol) to assess the need for the procedure and to verify the correct patient. The site should be marked, just behind the coronal suture and perpendicular to the mid-pupillary line. Shave the site if needed, and drape it. Cleanse the area with povidine-iodine solution for 30 seconds and allow it to air dry for 30 to 60 seconds.

Next, open and assemble the sterile kit and equipment. Using sterile technique, irrigate the collection device with normal saline.

Make a small skin incision and retract to expose the cranium. The hand drill is then held perpendicular to the cranium, and the burr hole is created to the dura. A small

TABLE 44-1

Equipment for Ventricular Access	
Sterile Equipment	**Cranial Access Kit**
Gloves, gowns, suction and suction apparatus, towels, half-sheets and drapes, surgical cap, and masks	A preassembled generic or custom kit that includes:
Anesthetic, local or systemic	• Sutures
Povidone-iodine scrub solution, pads or swabsticks	• Scalpel with no. 11 blade
Bone wax or Gelfoam	• Scalp retractor
Intraventricular catheter for placement	• Forceps
20-gauge angiocatheter/ butterfly needle for a tap	• Sterile scissors
Sterile cerebrospinal fluid collection system or bag	• Needle holder
Proper attachment devices or Luer locks	• Disposable cautery
	• Twist or hand drill with bits
Intracranial Pressure Monitoring Equipment	**Cardiorespiratory Monitoring Equipment**
Transducer cable compatible with bedside monitor	Bedside monitor with pressure transducer capabilities
External gauge transducer	
Pressure tubing	
Three-way stopcock	
0.9% normal Saline without preservative	

slit incision is made in the dura, and the ventricular catheter is inserted at a trajectory to the ipsilateral inner canthus. Vital signs are continuously monitored during catheter passage. Attach the catheter to the drainage device. Allow the CSF to flow and fill the catheter and stopcock. Calibrate the zero marking on the collection device to the patient's designated zero point—that is, the foramen of Monro or the heart. As the CSF fills the manometer column, it levels off. This point can be confirmed by noting a slight variation in the fluid meniscus, fluctuating with the patient's respirations. Document the pressure reading.

A CSF sample should be sent for diagnostic studies such as glucose, protein, cell count, and culture. Secure the catheter, via suturing or tunneling, per institution-specific policy and apply a sterile, occlusive dressing.

The procedure for a ventricular–peritoneal shunt tap is similar. However, instead of a burr hole and ventricular catheter, a 20-gauge angiocatheter or butterfly needle is used to access the shunt reservoir. The catheter or needle tubing can also be attached to a manometer for continued CSF drainage and pressure monitoring. Calibrate the zero of the manometer to the foramen of Monro or tragus for intracranial shunts, and parallel to the lumbar spine for lumbar shunts.

POSTPROCEDURE CARE

Maintenance of ventricular drainage devices is usually dictated by an institution-specific policy. Observe for signs of bleeding from the site and in catheter drainage. Monitor for catheter patency and drainage volume. Regularly document pressure readings. Collect daily CSF samples, and monitor for signs of infection and changes in level of consciousness that may be associated with reaccumulation of CSF or too fast-paced removal of fluid.

PROCEDURE NOTE

An example procedure note for the insertion of a ventricular drainage catheter is as follows:

- Date and time.
- Ventricular drainage catheter insertion.
- Indication: Hydrocephalus.
- Performed by: State names and positions.
- Procedure explained to caregivers, permission/consent obtained.
- "Time-out" taken (universal protocol).
- Sedation/analgesia: 0.5 mg morphine was given intravenously for pain.
- Site preparation: The patient was positioned supine and the insertion site marked, just behind the coronal suture and perpendicular to the mid-pupillary line. The area was shaved and sterile drapes placed. The site was cleansed with povidone-iodine solution for 30 seconds and allowed to dry for 1 minute.
- Procedure: A 0.5-cm skin incision was made and the skin retracted to expose the cranium. A burr hole was made to the dura, which was opened with a small slit incision. The ventricular catheter (state size) was inserted at a trajectory to the ipsilateral inner canthus until free flow of CSF was noted. Vital signs were continuously monitored during catheter passage. Catheter attached to CSF drainage device and clear fluid noted. A sterile occlusive dressing was applied. The drainage device was calibrated at the foramen of Monro. Pressure: State specifics.
- Site at conclusion of procedure: No active bleeding at site. Blood loss: None.
- Specimens sent: Glucose, protein, cell count, and culture.
- Patient condition following procedure: Patient tolerated the procedure without changes in vital signs or level of consciousness and has appropriate pain/sedation score post procedure (state specifics).
- Signature of the healthcare professional.

BIBLIOGRAPHY

1. Cartwright, C. (2004). Pediatric and developmental anomalies. In M. K. Bader & L. Littlejohns (Eds.). *AACN core curriculum: Neuroscience nursing* (4th ed., pp. 853–899). St. Louis: Saunders.
2. Sullivan, J. (2005). Intraventricular catheter insertion (assist), monitoring, care, troubleshooting and removal. In J. Verger & R. Ledbet (Eds.). *AACN procedure manual for pediatric acute and critical care* (pp. 561–569). St. Louis: Saunders.

Lumbar Puncture

- Indications
- Contraindications
- Complications
- Equipment

- Procedure
- Postprocedure Care
- Procedure Note
- Bibliography

INDICATIONS

Indications for performing a lumbar puncture (LP) may be divided into two categories: diagnostic and therapeutic. The major diagnostic indicators for LP involve infectious diseases, inflammatory processes, neurologic conditions, oncologic conditions, metabolic processes, and opening cerebral spinal pressure readings (Custer, 2008; Ellenby et al., 2006; Sorscher, 2008; Weaver et al., 2003). The therapeutic indications for LP in a pediatric patient may include the delivery of anesthetic or chemotherapeutic agents, antimicrobials, and/or to relieve increased intracranial pressure (ICP) through drainage of cerebrospinal fluid (CSF) (Custer, 2008; Ellenby et al., 2006; Sorscher, 2008; Weaver et al., 2003). Specific conditions in which this procedure is indicated are listed in Table 45-1.

TABLE 45-1

Indications for Lumbar Puncture	
Diagnostic	Infectious diseases
	• Meningitis
	• Encephalitis
	Inflammatory processes
	• Transverse myelitis
	• Acute disseminating encephalomyopathy
	Neurologic conditions
	• Multiple sclerosis
	• Guillain-Barré syndrome
	Oncologic conditions
	• Systemic neoplasms (breast cancer, melanoma)
	• Hemapoietic cancers (leukemia, lymphoma)
	• CNS tumors
	Metabolic processes
	Opening pressure reading
	Determination:
	• Hydrocephalus
	• Pseudotumor cerebri
Therapeutic	Delivery of medications
	• Anesthetic agents
	• Antimicrobial agents
	• Chemotherapeutic agents
	Relieve increased intracranial pressure
	• Drainage of CSF

Note: Central nervous system (CNS), cerebrospinal fluid (CSF).

CONTRAINDICATIONS

The *first* major contraindication to performing an LP procedure is increased ICP manifested by focal neurologic findings such as papilledema or retinal hemorrhages,

signs of cerebral herniation, or signs of increased ICP on radiographic imaging (Custer, 2008; Ellenby et al., 2006; Sorscher, 2008; Weaver et al., 2003). When increased ICP exists, an LP decreases the intraspinal pressure by permitting the rapid release of CSF; this rapid decrease in pressure has the potential to lead to cranial vault content shift and herniation (Custer, 2008; Ellenby et al., 2006; Sorscher, 2008). Controversy exists regarding the use of a computed tomography (CT) scan of the head prior to performing all LPs. A negative CT scan, however, does not completely exclude elevated ICP, which further complicates the decision (Custer, 2008). A discussion should occur among the interprofessional team whenever increased ICP, intracranial hemorrhage, focal mass lesions in the brain or spinal cord, or focal neurologic signs are suspected prior to performing a LP (Custer, 2008; Ellenby et al., 2006; Sorscher, 2008).

The *second* most important contraindication to performing an LP is the presence of a coagulation disorder—in particular, a bleeding diasthesis (Custer, 2008; Ellenby et al., 2006; Sorscher, 2008). Prior to this procedure, the pediatric patient's platelet count should be greater than 50,000/mm³ with no signs of active bleeding (Custer, 2008).

A *third* contraindication is cardiorespiratory instability. The healthcare professional (HCP) must assess for cardiorespiratory compromise prior to performing an LP in the pediatric patient. Notably, the positioning required for the performance of an LP will often occlude or decrease the size of the pediatric airway due to the hyperflexion of the neck resulting in obstruction. The flexed position also may diminish the ability of the patient to have full use of the muscles of respiration and aggravate mild respiratory distress, allowing it to progress to respiratory failure (Custer, 2008; Ellenby et al., 2006; Sorscher, 2008).

COMPLICATIONS

The most common complication from the LP procedure is the post lumbar puncture headache (PLPH) or the postdural puncture headache (PDPH), which generally develops within three days following the procedure (Chordas, 2001; Lee et al., 2007; Weaver et al., 2003). The PLPH/PDPH is thought to be caused by CSF leaking into the dura and paraspinous spaces from the hole created by the spinal needle (Chordas, 2001; Lee et al., 2007; Weaver et al., 2003). The leakage results in intracranial hypotension as the pain-sensitive intracerebral veins stretch and expand (Weaver et al., 2003).

Studies conducted in adults and pediatric patients examining prevention and treatment strategies for PLPH/PDPH have yielded varying results. Preventive measures include selecting a small-gauge LP needle (20 gauge or 22 gauge in pediatric patients), inserting the LP needle with the bevel parallel to the longitudinal dural fibers, minimizing CSF volume removal, reinserting the stylet before withdrawing the needle, and allowing the patient free mobility following the procedure (Chordas, 2001; Custer, 2008; Lee et al., 2007; Weaver et al., 2003). The majority of PLPH/PDPHs are treated with conservative management strategies such as bed rest, hydration, and analgesics, although none of these approaches is strongly supported by rigorous evidence (Lee et al., 2007). If these strategies do not resolve the headache, methylxanthines (theophylline, caffeine) or an epidural blood patch maybe considered as therapeutic options (Chordas, 2001; Lee et al., 2007; Weaver et al., 2003).

Additional but less frequently noted complications that may result from the LP procedure include backache or back pain, bleeding into the CSF, nerve palsies, infection, subdural hematoma, herniation, acquired intraspinal epidermoid tumors, and cardiorespiratory compromise (Chordas, 2001; Custer, 2008; Ellenby et al., 2006; Lee et al., 2007; Sorscher, 2008; Weaver et al., 2003). Table 45-2 describes potential complications following the LP procedure, their therapeutic management, and prevention strategies.

EQUIPMENT

The equipment required for the LP procedure is listed in Table 45-3.

PROCEDURE

The HCP should assess the patient's clinical status, history of any previous LP or neurologic procedures, and pertinent laboratory values. Age-appropriate education regarding the LP procedure should be provided to the pediatric patient and the caregiver(s). These instructions include the indications for the LP, potential complications, the general

TABLE 45-2

Complications Following Lumbar Puncture				
Complication	**Etiology/Symptoms**	**Onset**	**Management**	**Prevention Strategies**
Postlumbar puncture headache (PLPH) or postdural puncture headache (PDPH): most common complication	Headache (HA) related to leakage of CSF into paraspinous tissues from the puncture hole	Within 72 hours to 5 days, and may last several days	Bed rest Hydration Analgesia Methylxanthines (caffeine or theophylline) Epidural blood patch	Choose a smaller LP needle gauge Insert the LP needle with the bevel parallel to the longitudinal dural fibers or the spinal column (if patient is in a lateral decubitus position, the bevel is facing toward the ceiling) Minimize CSF volume removal Reinsert the stylet before withdrawing the needle Allow the patient free mobility upon recovery from the procedure
Infection	From introduction of skin flora into subarachnoid spaces	Immediate or several days after LP	Antimicrobials based on cultures	Strict asepsis
Iatrogenic intraspinal epidermoid tumors	Caused by epidermal material entering spinal canal	Following procedure	Advance needle with the stylet in place	Always use a stylet in the LP needle
Dyesthesias	Pain sensations from the spinal needle coming in contact with sensory roots	During LP procedure	Reposition the spinal needle	None

(Continued)

TABLE 45-2

Complications Following Lumbar Puncture *(Continued)*				
Complication	**Etiology/Symptoms**	**Onset**	**Management**	**Prevention Strategies**
Backache	From muscular and ligament relaxation secondary to local trauma	Following procedure; can last several days-months	Symptom management	None
Nerve palsies: visual and auditory disturbances	Traction on cranial nerves due to ↓ CSF volume	Following procedure	Symptom management Generally resolves with time	Careful technique
Herniation	Dislocation of neural elements through cranial compartments related to a large pressure gradient between the cranial and lumbar compartments; can occur after LP if ↑ ICP	Following procedure	Symptom management	Delay procedure if there are signs of ↑ ICP, focal neurologic findings, or head trauma Obtain a head CT scan (does not eliminate all risk)
Traumatic LP	When blood is introduced into CSF from rupture of venous plexuses around the spinal sac	During procedure	None	Careful technique Experience
Subdural hematoma	In patients with bleeding disorders, ↓ CSF volume can place traction on dural vessels causing rupture; symptoms include more severe HA than PLPH/PDPH, persistent vomiting, blurred vision, and disorientation; can lead to irreversible neurologic damage and death	Usually after multiple dura punctures; immediate to delayed diagnosis	Symptom management Repeat LP or laminotomy to drain blood/hematoma	Delay the procedure if a coagulation disorder/bleeding diasthesis is present Administer platelets (if platelet count < 50,000 mm^3) or clotting factors

Note: Cerebrospinal fluid (CSF), intracranial pressure (ICP), computed tomography (CT).

procedure, anesthetic agents, any analgesia and sedation to be used, and postprocedure care. The caregiver(s) can be offered the option of being present during the procedure at this time as well. The HCP should obtain and document informed consent or permission for the procedure.

As recommended by The Joint Commission, a "time-out" procedure (universal protocol) should be performed with the patient and care team to reassess the need for the LP procedure, verify the correct patient, and verify and mark the appropriate site for the LP (Sorscher, 2008). Cardiorespiratory monitoring ensures patient tolerance of the required positioning for the procedure. If a topical anesthetic cream and dressing are to be used, this combination must be placed over the LP site 30 to 60 minutes prior to

the procedure. Analgesia and sedation medication may be administered to the pediatric patient if indicated.

A critical aspect to the LP procedure is the positioning of the patient. The patient should be placed in the sitting or lateral recumbent position (Figure 45-1 and Figure 45-2). If an opening pressure is desired, the lateral recumbent position is required, with the assistant extending the hips of the patient upon initial withdrawal of the CSF specimen (Carlson et al., 2006; Ellenby et al., 2006; Sorscher, 2008; Weaver et al., 2003).

The landmarks for the LP in the pediatric patient are the spinous processes between the superior iliac crests. With the patient in the sitting or lateral recumbent position with the hips aligned evenly, draw an imaginary line

TABLE 45-3

Equipment for Lumbar Puncture Procedure

Sterile barrier materials (sterile gown, cap, gloves, goggles, towels/drapes, mask)
Cleansing solution (e.g., povidone-iodine)
Anesthetic agents (optional)
• 1% lidocaine, 25- or 27-gauge needle, and small syringe **OR**
• Topical anesthetic cream and occlusive dressing
Sterile gauze

Lumbar Puncture Tray		

1. LP/spinal needle with stylet

Age	LP Needle Size (gauge)	LP Needle Length
1 year	22 G	1.5 in. (3.8 cm)
1–12 years	22 G	1.5 or 2.5 in. (3.8 or 6.4 cm)
> 12 years	22 G or 20 G	3.5 in. (8.9 cm)

Type	Brand	Advantage	Disadvantage
tip design	Quincke	Inexpensive	↑ Incidence of PDPH
Pencil point or atraumatic design	Sprotte or Whitacre	↓ Incidence of PDPH	Expensive, ↑ failure rate

2. Syringes (3 mL, 5 mL, and extra as needed)
3. Manometer with 3-way stopcock
4. Collection tubes (at least 4)

Postprocedure bandage or dressing
Bath towel or roll or personnel for position

Note: Postdural puncture headache (PDPH).

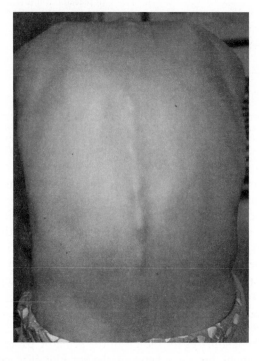

FIGURE 45-1

Sitting Position.
Source: Courtesy of Holly Parker.

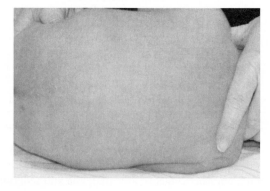

FIGURE 45-2

Lateral Recumbent Position.
Source: Courtesy of Holly Parker.

between the iliac crests and the point of intersection with the spine (Figure 45-3). The intersection is the L4–L5 interspace and is the ideal insertion point for the LP needle. The space above L3–L4 or below L5–S1 may also be used if the HCP is unable to access the CSF at L4–L5 (Carlson et al., 2006; Ellenby et al., 2006; Sorscher, 2008; Weaver et al., 2003). The interspace should be marked

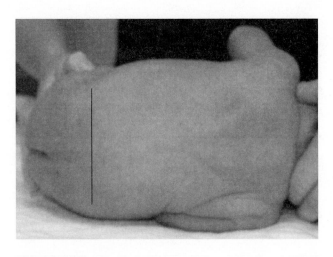

FIGURE 45-3

Lumbar Puncture Landmark.

Source: Courtesy of Holly Parker.

prior to the procedure, as it may become obscured by the administration of subcutaneous injection.

After the patient is properly positioned, any topical anesthetic cream and dressing should be removed and cleaned. A circular area (approximately 10.2 to 15.2 cm [4 to 6 in.] in diameter) around the insertion site should be cleansed with an approved cleansing agent (e.g., povidone iodine). The HCP should complete appropriate hand hygiene and put on the sterile barrier equipment (sterile gloves, hat, mask, gown [optional]) prior to beginning the procedure (Sorscher, 2008). A sterile drape with an eye-hole is placed on the patient's back to allow visualization of the puncture site and the patient. An optional step is to anesthetize the puncture site area (above and below the interspace area) with 1% lidocaine *without* epinephrine; it should be noted that this approach may obscure the landmarks.

The spinal needle should be inserted, with the bevel parallel to the dural fibers ("up" or toward ceiling if the patient is in the lateral recumbent position), into the desired interspace (L4–L5, L3–L4, or L5–S1) at a 15- to 30-degree angle toward the patient's head. This angle is essentially directed toward the umbilicus. As the needle is inserted, it should pass through the skin, subcutaneous tissue, supraspinous ligament, interspinous ligament between spinous processes, ligamentum flavum, epidural space, and subarachnoid space (Ellenby et al., 2006; Weaver et al., 2003). The "popping" sensation or a sensation of less pressure is felt as the needle passes through the ligamentum flavum. The entry through the ligamentum flavum is not always felt in the neonate or young infant (Custer, 2008). If the needle abruptly stops or hits a spinous process (bone), gently pull back on the needle and reangle the needle into the interspace. The total depth of insertion of the needle varies on the patient size and body habitus, and can range from 1 to

8 cm (approximately 0.5 to 4 in,) (Sorscher, 2008; Weaver et al., 2003). Once the needle is in the correct position, the bevel can be rotated toward the head to help assist with CSF flow into the needle (Weaver et al., 2003). Next, the stylet should be withdrawn slowly to assess for CSF return. If no CSF is visualized, return the stylet into the needle and reposition needle or further insert needle slowly.

If an opening pressure is to be obtained, the stopcock and manometer should be attached to the LP needle once CSF is visualized. Again, the patient must be in the lateral recumbent position and the legs must be extended when obtaining the pressure—extreme flexion may cause a false elevation of the pressure measured (Carlson et al., 2006; Ellenby et al., 2006; Sorscher, 2008; Weaver et al., 2003). The pressure measurement is recorded at the level where the CSF in the manometer ceases to rise (Ellenby et al., 2006).

Once the pressure is obtained, the manometer can be removed. The CSF should be allowed to passively flow into the collection tubes. Approximately 1 mL of CSF in each tube is required. If the CSF stops flowing, rotation of the needle slightly within the space may allow for further CSF drainage.

Once the required CSF is obtained, the stylet should be replaced into the needle and the needle withdrawn in one fluid motion. Sterile gauze should be applied with direct pressure over the insertion site, followed by cleansing and bandaging of the site. The collection tubes are labeled appropriately and sent to the lab for analysis (Table 45-4). During the entire procedure, the HCP should assess the patient status and ensure adequate pain and sedation management.

POSTPROCEDURE CARE

Immediately following the procedure, the patient (if awake) and the caregiver(s) should be updated on the outcome of the procedure. Orders should be recorded in the chart or computerized system detailing the specimens to be obtained from each collection tube. The HCP must then document or dictate the procedure.

TABLE 45-4

Cerebrospinal Fluid Specimen Tube Labeling	
Tube 1	Cultures including Gram stain, bacterial, fungal, and viral studies
Tube 2	Biochemistry: glucose and protein; lactate
Tube 3	Hematology: cell count and differential
Tube 4	Additional studies (cytologies or serologies)

Following the LP procedure, the patient's vital signs, neurologic and neurovascular examination, and pain/comfort level should be monitored frequently as determined by the patient's status and protocols. The puncture site should be assessed for CSF or other drainage, redness, or swelling in the first hours after the procedure. The HCP should also follow up on CSF study results.

PROCEDURE NOTE

An example procedure note for the lumbar puncture is as follows:

- Date and time.
- Lumbar puncture.
- Indication: For diagnostic evaluation of CNS infection.
- Performed by HCP and assisted by care nurse.
- Procedure explained to the patient and caregivers, permission/consent obtained.
- "Time-out" taken (universal protocol).
- Site: L4–L5 vertebral space.
- Patient placed on cardiorespiratory monitoring.
- Patient positioned in left lateral recumbent position with head, neck, and hips/knees flexed.
- Site preparation: L4–L5 area cleansed with povidone iodine for 2 minutes. Sterile barrier precautions employed. Eye-hole dressing applied to the back (optional—1% lidocaine administered around the insertion site).
- Analgesia: No systemic sedation/analgesia given.
- Procedure: 20-gauge needle inserted into the L4–L5 space without difficulty and clear, colorless CSF obtained. Opening pressure 15 cmH_2O. 4 mL of CSF collected. Stylet reinserted into needle, and needle removed without incident. Sterile gauze and pressure applied and bandage secured. Patient's vital signs were monitored throughout

procedure. Patient had no cardiorespiratory compromise and tolerated the procedure well.
- Site at conclusion of procedure: No active drainage of clear fluid (CSF). Blood loss: None.
- Specimens sent: Tube 1: culture and Gram stain; Tube 2: glucose and protein; Tube 3: cell count and differential, Tube 4: hold for additional studies.
- Patient condition following procedure: Patient tolerated procedure without changes in vital signs. Neurovascular exam findings in all extremities were appropriate. Patient and caregiver(s) updated about procedure.
- Signature of healthcare professional.

BIBLIOGRAPHY

1. Carlson, D., DiGiulio, G., Givens, T., Gonzalez Del Rey, J., Hodge, D., Jaffe, D., et al. (2006). Illustrated techniques of pediatric emergency procedures. 4.1 Lumbar puncture. In G. Fleisher, S. Ludwig, F. Henretig, R. Ruddy, & B. Silverman (Eds.). *Textbook of pediatric emergency medicine* (5th ed., pp. 1882–1884). Philadelphia: Lippincott Williams & Wilkins.

2. Chordas, C. (2001). Post-dural puncture headache and other complications after lumbar puncture. *Journal of Pediatric Oncology Nursing, 18*(6), 244–259.

3. Custer, J. (2008). Procedures. In J. Custer & R. Rau (Eds.). *The Johns Hopkins Hospital. Harriet Lane handbook: Manual for pediatric house officers* (18th ed., pp. 80–84). Philadelphia: Mosby.

4. Ellenby, M., Tegtmeyer, K., Lai, S., & Braner, D. (2006). Lumbar puncture. *New England Journal of Medicine, 355*, 13.

5. Lee, L., Sennett, M., & Erickson, J. (2007). Prevention and management of post-lumbar puncture headache in pediatric oncology patients. *Journal of Pediatric Oncology Nursing, 24*(4), 200–207.

6. Sorscher, M. (2008). Lumbar puncture: Perform. In J. T. Verger & R. M. Lebet (Eds.). *AACN procedure manual for pediatric acute and critical care* (pp. 623–631). St. Louis: Saunders Elsevier.

7. Weaver, J., Davidson, R., & Tabar, V. (2003). Cerebrospinal fluid aspiration. In R. Irwin, J. Rippe, F. Curley, & S. Heard (Eds.). *Procedures and techniques in intensive care medicine* (3rd ed., pp. 187–195). Philadelphia: Lippincott, Williams & Wilkins.

Tracy Lynne Mackie

Postpyloric Feeding Tubes Insertion

INDICATION

Postpyloric feeding is defined as enteral nutrition delivered past the pyloric sphincter of the stomach. It is often associated with feedings that pass through the duodenum and the ligament of treitz into the jejunum. Most pediatric patients who require postpyloric feeding are acutely ill or have long-term complex medical conditions. Enteral nutrition is preferred for patients who have a functional gastrointestinal (GI) tract yet cannot maintain nutritional requirements through the oral route. Enteral nutrition, as opposed to parenteral nutrition, is commonly considered to be crucial to maintain GI mucosa, to ensure normal permeability of the GI tract, and to prevent bacterial translocation and reduce the risks of sepsis (Jabbar & McClave, 2005; Lee et al., 2006; Niv et al., 2009; Slagt et al., 2004).

General indications for the bedside placement of postpyloric feeding tubes (PPT) are to increase caloric intake; to decrease the risk of aspiration by decreasing the frequency of vomiting or gastroesophageal reflux (GER); and to manage GER due to poor gastric mobility, gastric fullness, or poor sphincter control (Jabbar & McClave, 2005; Singla & Olsson, 2008; Ukleja & Sanchez-Fermin, 2007). Postpyloric feedings are provided as continuous infusions; thus those patients who require a bolus feeding regimen are not candidates for PPT placement. Additional diagnoses that may benefit from a PPT are listed in Table 46-1.

TABLE 46-1

Diagnoses Often Requiring Postpyloric Tube Feeding

- Behavioral problems, delayed self-independence and/or development, delayed skill acquisition, feeding aversion or refusal
- Constipation
- Cystic fibrosis
- Decreased gastric emptying
- Down syndrome
- Dysphagia
- Esophageal atresia
- Failure-to-thrive
- Gastroesophageal reflux
- Intestinal failure
- Intestinal strictures
- Malrotation
- Necrotizing enterocolitis
- Neurologically disabling conditions or developmental delays
- Oral–motor impairment and other swallowing disorders/dysfunction
- Racheoesophageal fistula
- Seizures
- Severe scoliosis
- Spasticity
- Racheoesophageal fistula
- Trauma
- Underlying pulmonary or cardiac disease

Older children may have indications for postpyloric feeding that are similar to those for younger children; however, they may also have etiologies more similar to those of adults. These adult etiologies include gastroparesis not responsive to prokinetics (in the early postoperative period or in critically ill patients), large gastric residual volumes associated with gastric feedings, recurrent aspiration, proximal enteric fistula, gastric outlet obstruction (pyloric or duodenal outlet stenosis in cancer patients), severe pancreatitis, or hyperemesis gravida (Niv et al., 2009).

Bedside PPT placement with insufflation has a very high success rate. It is also associated with fewer and less severe complications than tubes placed in conjunction with imaging or a surgical technique, can be accomplished more quickly, has fewer scheduling demands, and can be completed at a lower cost. Placement accuracy, however, is generally less with bedside placement than with imaging or surgical technique (de Silva et al., 2002; Lee et al., 2006; Niv et al., 2009; Slagt et al., 2004; Spalding et al., 2000).

CONTRAINDICATIONS

The most obvious contraindications to placement of a PPT are acute airway or life-threatening issues. Obstruction or perforation anywhere in the GI tract (i.e., esophagus, gastric outlet, intestine) is also a contraindication.

The procedure duration may be 30 minutes to 1 hour and depends on patient stability and tolerance. Pediatric patients must be able to tolerate a supine or low Fowler's position (semi-upright 45-degree angle with knees bent or straight), and ideally should be able to roll or be positioned to their right side (Niv et al., 2009; Ukleja & Sanchez-Fermin, 2007).

COMPLICATIONS

Common complications with PPT placement include failure of placement, dislodgement, leakage, pain or irritation of nasal or throat passages, infection, clogging, GER (from tube interference in the esophageal sphincters), epistaxis, diarrhea or cramping, dumping (i.e., symptoms of faintness, palpitations, sweating, tachycardia, rebound hypoglycemia, and diarrhea), and metabolic complications (excess free water intake, hyperglycemia, caloric discrepancies) (McCord, 2008; Niv et al., 2009; Singla & Olsson, 2008).

EQUIPMENT

Postpyloric tubes are generally weighted tubes that include a guidewire or stylet. They come in many different materials and lengths. Tube size and length must be appropriate for the age and size of the patient. Other materials needed for bedside placement include a 3-way stopcock, a 60-mL syringe, a 1-mL syringe with normal saline; sterile water or a water-soluble lubricant, a permanent felt-tip marker, pH paper, a stethoscope, a nasogastric tube, tape, a transparent film dressing, and a feeding pump to infuse feeds. Blue dye to check PPT position is optional.

PROCEDURE

After obtaining informed consent or permission, complete a "time-out" procedure (universal protocol) to reassess the need for the procedure and to verify the correct patient. Discussion with the patient and the family covers the indications for PPT use, the procedure, and the need for an abdominal radiograph after the procedure to confirm placement of the tube in the small bowel.

Many health care professionals (HCPs) report that metoclopramide or erythromycin may be useful in the initial placement of a postpyloric tube, as these medications increase gastric motility, thereby promoting tube migration (Niv et al., 2009; Ukleja & Sanchez-Fermin, 2007). A recent Cochrane review, however, found no benefit from metoclopramide in promoting tube progression into the small bowel (Silva et al., 2002). Naloxone given prior to tube placement (via a gastric tube) in patients receiving opioid analgesia has been shown to increase gastric mobility and the subsequent success rate of PPT placement (Ukleja & Sanchez-Fermin, 2007).

After preparing the patient, measure the distance needed to reach the stomach from the point of entry and mark it with a permanent marker. Next, measure the distance needed for the PPT to reach the distal part of the duodenum (ligament of Treitz), and mark it with the permanent marker. Position the patient supine (or in low Fowler's position if unable to tolerate lying flat). Connect a 3-way stopcock, 60-mL empty syringe, and the 1-mL syringe with normal saline to the stopcock.

Lubricate the PPT with the water-soluble lubricant, and first insert the tube as per the usual nasogastric placement procedure. Check for gastric position by injecting air, auscultating for a "pop," withdrawing stomach contents, and checking for gastric pH. Compare measurement of the gastric placement with the duodenal placement marking on the PPT, and then arrange the pediatric patient into the right lateral decubitus position. Inject 10 mL/kg of air via the 60-mL syringe (to a maximum of 500 mL) and advance the tube one-half of the way to the duodenal mark. Inject another 10 mL/kg of air, and then complete the insertion of the tube. If any resistance or change in resistance is noted, the tube may be coiling in the stomach. In this situation, retract the tube to the gastric position, remove residual air from the stomach, and reattempt the insertion/advancement (Table 46-2).

Slagt et al. (2004) suggest insertion of an additional nasogastric tube to decompress the stomach post procedure and the injection of blue dye into the PPT as a placement verification method. If blue dye injected in the PPT fails to be aspirated through the nasogastric tube, then it suggests the PPT is positioned correctly.

When the correct positioning has been achieved, remove the guidewire. Lubricating the guidewire by instilling 1 mL of normal saline into the PPT tube allows for easier removal (Lee et al., 2006). Stabilization and security of the PPT with tape and/or transparent film dressing is paramount (McCord, 2008).

POSTPROCEDURE CARE

Assessment of the patient's comfort and tolerance should be ongoing. Because the diameter of the PPT is smaller than that of a nasogastric tube, flushing the tube every 4 to 6 hours, as well as before and after feeding, helps maintain patency. If tubes become occluded, they may be cleared by flushing warm water or pancreatic enzymes (McCord, 2008; Niv et al., 2009).

TABLE 46-2

Placement Checks for Postpyloric Feeding Tube Insertion		
Placement Check Method	**Desired Findings for Postpyloric Placement**	**Findings for Gastric Placement**
Aspirate air from tube	Minimal air in the duodenum/jejuneum	Tube is likely in the esophagus or stomach if a large volume of air is aspirated
Aspirate secretions from tube	Small volumes of yellowish fluid	Large volumes of bile or stomach contents mean the tube is likely in the stomach
Test pH of secretions	pH of 6–7 in the duodenum/jejuneum	Stomach pH < 5
Inject 10 mL of air and withdraw the air	Resistance is felt and air is not returned	Air return is likely if the tube is coiled in the stomach
Flush 10 mL of normal saline into the tube and aspirate	Less than one-half of the volume is aspirated	Volume is held in the stomach; likely to be able to aspirate the volume back

If a PPT is inserted as an intervention for a long-term complex medical condition, inclusion of the interprofessional care team (nutrition, dental, occupational therapy, speech therapy, child life) in the patient's care promotes its safe and efficacious use (Fayed et al., 2007; Lefton-Greif & Arvedson, 2007).

PROCEDURE NOTE

An example procedure note for the insertion of a PPT is as follows:

- Date and time.
- Postpyloric feeding tube placement with insufflation.
- Indication: Patient no longer able to safely tolerate gastric bolus feeding.
- Performed by: State names and positions.
- Procedure explained to patient and caregivers, permission/consent obtained.
- "Time-out" taken (universal protocol).
- Medications administered: List medications, dose, and route.
- Patient preparation: Discussion with patient and parents about PPT indications, procedure, postprocedure care, radiographs, and future use. Questions answered. Patient positioned as per procedure.
- Procedure: PPT measured for gastric and distal duodenal positions and marked with a permanent marker. PPT lubricated and inserted via left nare on first attempt. Gastric position verified by air "pop," aspiration of stomach contents, and pH of 3. Patient positioned in the right lateral decubitus position, 85 mL of air injected through the PPT, and then the tube advanced to the duodenal marking with no resistance. Abdominal radiograph confirms PPT in duodenum.
- Specimens sent: None.
- Patient condition following procedure: Patient upset immediately following procedure but easily comforted by parents. No abdominal distention noted or discomfort reported.
- Signature of the HCP.

BIBLIOGRAPHY

1. de Silva, P. S. L., Paulo, C. S. T., de Oliveria Iglesias, S. B., de Carvalho, W. B., & Santana e Menses, F. (2002). Bedside transpyloric tube placement in the pediatric intensive care unit: A modified insufflation air technique. *Intensive Care Medicine, 28*, 943–946.

2. Fayed, N., Berall, G., Dix, L., & Judd, P. (2007). A dynamic and comprehensive practice model of paediatric feeding practice. *International Journal of Therapy and Rehabilitation, 14*(1), 7–15.

3. Jabbar, A., & McClave, S. A. (2005). Pre-pyloric versus post-pyloric feeding. *Clinical Nutrition, 24*, 719–726.

4. Larson, P. G. (2008). Technology dependent children: Gastrostomy tube. In R. M. Perkin, J. D. Swift, D. A. Newton, & N. G. Anas (Eds.), *Pediatric hospital medicine textbook of inpatient management* (2nd ed., pp. 723–726). Philadelphia: Lippincott Williams and Wilkins.

5. Lee, A. J., Eve, R., & Bennett, M. J. (2006). Evaluation of a technique for blind placement of post-pyloric feeding tubes in intensive care: Application in patients with gastric ileus. *Intensive Care Medicine, 32*, 553–556.

6. Lefton-Greif, M. A., & Arvedson, J. C. (2007). Pediatric feeding and swallowing disorders: State of health, population trends, and application of the international classification of functioning, disability, and health. *Seminars in Speech and Language, 28*(3), 161–165.

7. McCord, S. S. (2008). Gastrostomy and gastrostomy–jejunostomy tubes: Care and management. In J. T. Verger & R. M. Lebet (Eds.), *AACN procedure manual for pediatric acute and critical care* (pp. 715–724). St. Louis, MO: Saunders.

8. Niv, E., Fireman, Z., & Vaisman, N. (2009). Post pyloric feeding. *World Journal of Gastroenterology, 15*(11), 1281–1288.

9. Silva, C. D., Saconato, H., & Atallah, A. N. (2002). Metoclopramide for migration of naso-enteral tube. *Cochrane Database of Systematic Reviews, 4*, CD003353. doi: 10.1002/14651858.CD003353

10. Singla, S., & Olsson, J. M. (2008). Enteral nutrition. In R. M. Perkin, J. D. Swift, D. A. Newton, & N. G. Anas (Eds.). *Pediatric hospital medicine textbook of inpatient management* (2nd ed., pp. 797–808). Philadelphia: Lippincott Williams and Wilkins.

11. Slagt, C., Innes, R., Bihari, D., Lawrence, J., & Shehabi, Y. (2004). A novel method for insertion of post-pyloric feeding tubes at the bedside without endoscopic or fluoroscopic assistance: A prospective study. *Intensive Care Medicine, 30*, 103–107.

12. Spalding, H. K., Sullivan, K. J., Soremi, O., Gonzalez, F., & Goodwin, S. R. (2000). Bedside placement of transpyloric feeding tubes in the pediatric intensive care unit using gastric insufflation. *Critical Care Medicine, 28*, 2041–2044.

13. Ukleja, A., & Sanchez-Fermin, P. (2007). Gastric versus post-pyloric feeding: Relationship to tolerance, pneumonia risk, and successful delivery of enteral nutrition. *Current Gastroenterology Reports, 9*, 309–316.

Peripherally Inserted Central Catheter Insertion and Removal

INSERTION OF A PERIPHERALLY INSERTED CENTRAL CATHETER

Peripherally inserted central catheters (PICCs) are soft, flexible catheters composed of either silicone or polyurethane. They are inserted via a peripheral vein and advanced until the tip of the catheter terminates within a central vessel such as the superior or inferior vena cava.

Common sites for insertion of a PICC in neonates include the saphenous and scalp veins. The three vessels most often used in the pediatric population for such access are the basilic, median cubital, and cephalic veins. Of these, the basilic vein is the vein of choice for PICC placement, as it is relatively straight and large in diameter. Cephalic veins are considered less desirable secondary to difficulty passing the guidewire or catheter into the subclavian vessel (Mickler, 2008).

PICCs are favored over surgically placed venous catheters for long-term intravascular therapy because they are associated with ease of insertion, low cost, and low complication risk. These catheters are relatively comfortable for patients and allow for an easy transition of therapy from the hospital to the home (Levy et al., 2010; Racadio et al., 2001).

INDICATIONS

- Vascular access (short or long term)
- Blood sampling (in PICCs larger than the 2 Fr size)
- Medication delivery
- Long-term antibiotic therapy
- Parenteral nutrition
- Central venous pressure monitoring (polyurethane catheter only)
- Vesicant or hyperosmolar medications
- Vasoactive medications/infusions
- Limited or inadequate peripheral access

CONTRAINDICATIONS

There are several contraindications that the health care professional (HCP) should consider prior to placement of a PICC. An extremity with a prior history of thrombosis, vascular surgery, peripheral neuropathy, circulatory compromise, burn, radiation, injury, hematoma, or skin condition at the insertion site should not be used for PICC insertion. In addition, an allergy to any components used within the device is an absolute contraindication. PICC placement may be delayed in patients with coagulopathies,

known or suspected infections, and device infections, though these conditions are not absolute contraindications (Mickler, 2008).

COMPLICATIONS

Complications of PICC insertion are generally the same as those associated with other central venous catheter (CVC) placement and can be categorized as infectious, mechanical, or thrombotic. However, the risks of pneumothorax and hemorrhage are considerably less with PICC insertion than with CVC placement, as the insertion sites are in peripheral veins versus large central vessels such as the femoral and subclavian veins. PICCs are also associated with fewer bloodstream infections than surgically placed tunneled catheters (Levy et al., 2010).

In recent years, the addition of ultrasound guidance for PICC insertions has led to lower thrombosis rates. Ultrasound allows for a more direct visualization of the vessel during the insertion process and, therefore, fewer venipunctures and less risk for thrombosis (Stokowski et al., 2009).

Migration, occlusion, and dislodgement are known complications associated with PICCs. The rates of these complications are significantly lower with the use of suture securement versus sutureless securement (Graf et al., 2006).

Complications linked to PICCs and means of preventing them are summarized in Table 47-1.

PATIENT SELECTION

The decision-making process for placement a PICC takes a variety of factors into account. The need for long-term access, the disease process, any comorbidities, and the duration and type of therapy being administered are initial factors in determining the placement of a PICC. Once the decision to place a PICC has been made, the age and size of the patient and the vessel size are assessed. Visualization with ultrasound assists with determination of the vessel location, vessel size, patency, and pathway (Stokowski et al., 2009). Next, the HCP must determine if a single-lumen or multilumen catheter is needed.

If placement of the PICC line requires analgesia and sedation, a second provider will be needed to administer and monitor this medication. Depending on the age of the pediatric patient, a child life specialist may be helpful in preparing and supporting the patient (Mickler, 2008; Moureau, 2008).

TABLE 47-1

PICC Complications and Their Prevention

Complication	Prevention/Resolution
Catheter-related bloodstream infection (CRBSI)	Meticulous site preparation and insertion technique
Bleeding/hematoma	Minimize punctures, apply pressure
Phlebitis/site infection	Meticulous site/dressing care, scrub access ports
Infiltration/extravasation	Low risk with PICCs; monitor the site
Pneumothorax	Low risk with PICCs; use a curved J wire
Venous air embolism	Valsalva maneuver
Catheter fracture/sheering	Low risk with polyurethane; use 5-mL or larger syringes with silicone PICCs
Catheter erosion	Ensure the catheter tip is centrally placed, not placed midline
Thrombosis	Use the appropriate catheter size in relation to the vessel size
Mechanical obstruction	Flush after infusions with heparin
Catheter dislodgement or kinking	Secure with sutures or catheter securement device
Catheter migration	Careful measurement prior to insertion
Leakage	Monitor site and connectors
Inability to pass guidewire or place catheter	Use ultrasound guidance; see the "Clinical PICC Pearls" section
Inexperience personnel	Supervise inexperienced personnel

Note: Peripherally inserted central catheter (PICC).

EQUIPMENT

- Ultrasound with a vascular probe and sterile gel
- Cardiorespiratory monitor
- Soft restraints
- Site antiseptic (e.g., chlorhexidine)
- Local anesthetic (lidocaine, EMLA Cream, Senera Patch)
- Tourniquet
- Sterile gown and sterile gloves
- Hat or cap and mask
- Appropriate-size PICC insertion kit (contents may vary depending on the manufacturer, but should include a needle, scalpel, flexible guidewire, peel away dilator/sheath, and tapered PICC catheter)
- Sterile barriers such as full bed drapes and a sterile ultrasound probe cover
- Sutures or a sutureless securement device
- Extension tubing
- Needle-less injection cap and injector
- Sterile saline flush
- Heparinized saline flush
- Sterile gauze
- Transparent semipermeable dressing
- Measuring tape and surgical skin marker

PROCEDURE

Informed consent or permission should be obtained prior to initiation of the procedure. A "time-out" (universal protocol), confirming the right procedure, the right patient, and the right site, should be performed. The time-out should also include the patient's name and another identifying factor such as the medical record number or birth date.

For placement of the PICC in the basilic, median cubital, and cephalic veins, the HCP places a tourniquet on the patient's upper arm near the axilla. The arm is placed at a 90-degree angle away from the body and rotated to expose the ventral surface of the upper arm. The ultrasound probe is placed on the anticubital fossa, and the median cubital and forearm basilic vessels are identified. The probe is then moved toward the axilla until the median cubital and forearm basilic veins form the upper arm basilic vein. The point immediately above the bifurcation will serve as the insertion site for the catheter; it is marked with a surgical skin marker.

Remove the tourniquet. With the patient's arm still at a 90-degree° angle, apply a tape measure at the insertion site and pull it toward the clavicle to the right of the sternum to the region of the sternocleidomastoid notch.

While holding the tape, turn downward and take the measurement at the first intercostal space or one finger breadth below the head of the right clavicle if the patient is younger than 2 years of age. If the patient is 2 to 4 years of age, use two finger breadths; the patient is older than 4 years of age, use three finger breadths. This location typically lies slightly above the nipple line. If the left arm is used, remember to measure across to the right of the sternum.

The patient should be appropriately anesthetized, the site prepped (e.g., 2% chlorhexidine or 10% povidone-iodine solution) according to institutional protocol, and a tourniquet replaced on the upper portion of the arm. The HCP should don a hat, mask, sterile gown, and gloves. The patient is draped in sterile fashion and all supplies needed for the procedure placed in an orderly fashion near the insertion site. This arrangement allows for the supplies to be readily available without the HCP having to turn or reach out, risking dislodgement of the needle.

The PICC should be trimmed with one clean cut based on the prior determined measurement. Holding a sterile covered vascular ultrasound probe in the nondominant hand, reidentify the basilic vein. Once the vessel has been identified, take the needle in the dominant hand, and while watching on the ultrasound monitor puncture the skin at a 45-degree angle. A small "star or cross" will appear at the tip of the needle on the ultrasound screen. When the vessel has been accessed, blood should flow from the needle.

Once flow is established, lower the angle of the needle, lay the probe aside, stabilize the needle with the nondominant hand, and using the dominant hand, gently thread the guidewire through the needle for a distance of approximately 25 cm. If ectopic beats are noted on the cardiorespiratory monitor during insertion of the guidewire, gently pull back the wire until the ectopic beats have resolved. Holding the guidewire, remove the needle, and with the scalpel perform a dermatotomy at the insertion site (make two small nicks in the skin on the top and side of the guidewire, taking care not to cut the wire or puncture the vessel). *Always* have the proximal end of the guidewire in view and secured by either manually holding or placing a hemostat on the end to prevent migration of the guidewire into the vessel and right atrium (Kaplan & Brilli, 2007; Seneff, 2003). Holding the wire in the nondominant hand, thread the dilator/sheath over the guidewire using a slight twisting motion as it passes through the skin and subcutaneous tissue. If resistance is met, withdraw the dilator/sheath and make the dermatotomy slightly deeper and larger. Pushing against resistance will damage the sheath. Attempt to pass the dilator/sheath the full length.

Remove the guidewire, unscrew the dilator, and remove it from the sheath. Place a thumb over the sheath to minimize blood loss. The tourniquet can be removed at this time.

If the patient is not mechanically ventilated during the procedure, there is an increased risk of air embolism during this portion of the procedure. To decrease this risk, remove the thumb and insert the catheter into the sheath at the end of *end of expiration*. If the patient is awake, have him or her perform the Valsalva maneuver and insert the catheter during this time.

Next, insert the pre-trimmed PICC into the sheath until it stops. Using both hands, break the wings on the sheath downward and then peel the sheath back, exposing the catheter. Pull back and peel the sheath out approximately 1 cm at a time, while simultaneously pushing the catheter in 1 cm. Continue this process until the sheath is removed. Continue to push the catheter in until the tapered area of the catheter is under the skin. This tapered region occludes any oozing at the insertion site.

Ensure that all lumens have blood return and flush with ease. Secure the catheter with either sutures or a catheter securement device, and place a sterile occlusive dressing over the site per institutional protocol (Figure 47-1 and Figure 47-2). Obtain a chest radiograph (CXR) to verify the placement of the catheter. The tip of the catheter should lie within the lower third of the superior vena cava (SVC) near the junction of the right atrium (Figure 47-3). The large amount of blood flow in the SVC allows for dilution of the infusate, and the relatively large size of this vessel allows the catheter tip to float near the center of the vessel, thereby decreasing the risk of contact with, and erosion through, the vessel wall. Lower placement puts the patient at risk for ectopy, whereas higher placement in the SVC or in the subclavian vein (SCV) increases the risk of erosion through the vessel wall (especially as the catheter tip is a blunt cut) and thrombus formation (Racadio et al., 2001).

POSTPROCEDURE CARE AND FAMILY EDUCATION

The catheter, site, and dressing care should be based on individual institutional protocols. The *Guidelines for the Prevention of Intravascular Catheter-Related Infections* document developed by the American Academy of Pediatrics (AAP) serves to assist HCPs in the insertion and care of PICCs. While many of the guidelines are interspersed throughout the description of the procedure in this section, refer to Table 47-2 for detailed recommendations (O'Grady et al., 2002).

The use of a transparent semipermeable dressing allows for visual access to the insertion site. Of importance, no power injectors (such as are used during a radiological procedure) should be used on PICCs, as there is an increased risk of catheter fracture with this intervention, especially with silicone catheters. Ideally, there should be no blood pressures taken, no venipunctures, and no additional intravenous line placements in an extremity with a PICC. If the PICC will be used in a home setting, a home health agency familiar with PICCs should be contacted prior to the patient's discharge to ease the transition to home.

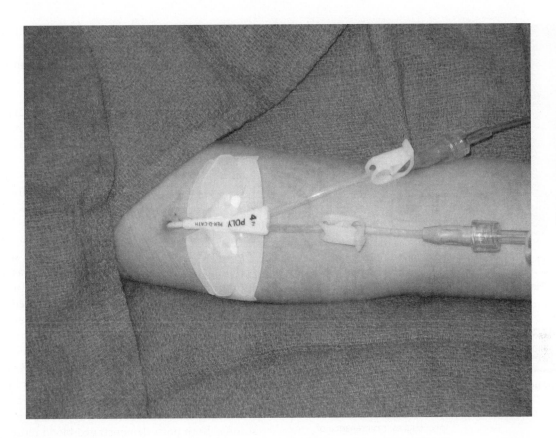

FIGURE 47-1

PICC Line.

Source: Courtesy of Valarie Eichler.

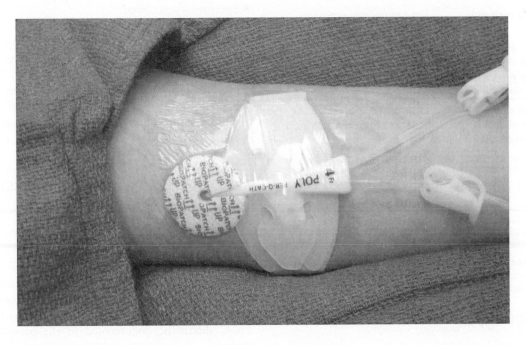

FIGURE 47-2

PICC Line with Securement Device.

Source: Courtesy of Valarie Eichler.

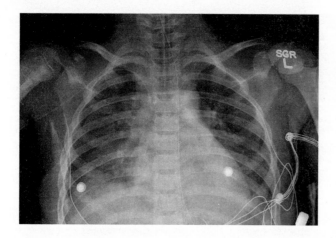

FIGURE 47-3

PICC Tip Placement in Lower Third of Superior Vena Cava.

Source: Courtesy of Valarie Eichler.

TABLE 47-2

CRBSI Prevention Guidelines	
Recommendation	**Rationale**
Education for HCPs	Ensures proper insertion procedures, maintenance of PICCs, and prevention of CRBSIs
Surveillance	Monitor site for signs of infection
Hand hygiene	Ensures proper hand hygiene prior to and after palpating the catheter site
Insertion site prep with chlorhexidine	Ensures uniform site preparation
Aseptic insertion technique, including use of gown, hat, mask, sterile gloves, and maximal sterile barrier	Ensures the proper insertion procedure is followed
Catheter site care; replacement of soiled, damp, or loosened dressings	Ensures proper site care and lessens the risk of CRBSIs
Chlorhexidine sponge dressings	May reduce the incidence of infection; an unresolved issue—no recommendation at present
Sutures and sutureless securement devices	No recommendation at present

Note: Catheter-related bloodstream infection (CRBSI), peripherally inserted central catheter (PICC).
Source: Adapted from O'Grady et al., 2002.

PROCEDURE NOTE

An example procedure note for the insertion of a PICC is as follows:

- Date and time.
- PICC placement: Modified Seldinger technique.
- Indication: Vascular access, parenteral nutrition.
- Performed by: State names and positions.
- Procedure explained to caregivers, permission/consent obtained.
- "Time-out" taken (universal protocol).
- Sedation/analgesia: (list medications, dose, and route) prior to the procedure. The patient was mechanically ventilated during the procedure; no additional medications were administered.
- Site: Right basilica vein.
- Site Preparation: The right upper arm was prepped with 2% chlorhexidine per protocol. Sonosite was utilized for the procedure. The patient and the entire bed were draped in sterile fashion.
- Procedure: Using a modified Seldinger and sterile technique, a 21-gauge Argon steel needle was inserted into the right basilic vein on the first attempt. A 0.018-in 80-cm Cook guidewire was inserted and the needle was removed. A dermatotomy was performed at the insertion site, and a peel-away introducer/sheath was threaded over the wire. The wire was removed intact. After removal of the dilator, a 4 Fr BARD double-lumen PICC trimmed at 21 cm was inserted into the sheath, and the peel-away sheath was removed. The catheter was advanced and secured with 3.0 silk sutures. Both ports demonstrated blood return and flushed with ease.
- Site at conclusion of procedure: No active bleeding or vascular compromise at site or to distal right upper extremity. Blood loss less than 2 mL. A Biopatch and transparent semipermeable dressing placed.
- Specimens sent: None.
- Patient condition following procedure: Stable. Complications: None. CXR revealed the tip in the SVC at the junction of the RA. Catheter is cleared for use as well as blood sampling. Procedure and indications for procedure discussed with the pediatric intensive care unit (PICU) attending physician (state name) who was physically present on the unit during the procedure.
- Signature of HCP.

REMOVAL OF A PERIPHERALLY INSERTED CENTRAL CATHETER

Once therapy has been completed, the PICC should be removed. Maintaining indwelling devices longer than clinically required increases the risk of catheter-related bloodstream infections (CRBSIs). PICCs can be removed by HCPs and registered nurses who have received appropriate training and education. An order to remove the PICC should be documented in the patient's medical record.

Prior to removal of the PICC, the patient's coagulation status should be assessed. Coagulopathy is a consideration during removal, but is not an absolute contraindication, unless there is systemic heparinization. Complications related to PICC removal may include inability to remove the catheter, fracture of the catheter during removal, or air embolism.

The procedure for PICC removal should be explained to both the patient and the family. Keeping the child informed will assist in decreasing his or her anxiety level during the procedure. As with the insertion procedure and depending on the age of the pediatric patient, a child life specialist may be helpful with distraction during the removal process (Mickler, 2008).

A "time-out" (universal protocol) detailing the right procedure, the right patient, and the right site should be performed. The time-out should also include the patient's name and another identifying factor such as the medical record number or birth date.

Wash hands and gather supplies needed for removal (Table 47-3). Determine the length of the PICC at the insertion time. This measurement can be found in the procedure note documented at the time of PICC insertion. The length at removal should then be compared to the length at insertion to ensure that a catheter fracture did not occur during the removal process.

Place the patient in a supine position with the arm extended at a 90-degree angle. With a slow, even motion,

gently pull the hub and catheter as a single unit until the tip is just inside the insertion site. If the patient is able to perform the Valsalva maneuver (having the child hum will produce the same effect as the Valsalva maneuver), he or she should do so at the time the catheter is removed from the skin. At the same time, the HCP places an occlusive dressing such as a petroleum impregnated gauze or a small amount of antibiotic ointment at the site and covers it with a sterile gauze and transparent dressing. This occlusion at the catheter site will prevent air embolism along the catheter tract. A new occlusive dressing should be applied daily until the site has epithelialized.

If the catheter does not come out easily, do not pull against resistance, especially for a silicone PICC. Instead, reposition the extremity and attempt to remove the PICC. If the PICC has been indwelling for a long period of time, placing a warm compress over the insertion site for a few minutes will often loosen the catheter from surrounding tissues. Have a tourniquet immediately available to place on the upper arm if suspicion for catheter fracture arises. In the unfortunate event of fracture or inability to remove the catheter, interventional radiology should be consulted for catheter removal. If catheter fracture or air embolism is suspected, the patient should be turned immediately to a left lateral decubitus position. This position may allow the air or catheter fragment to remain within the right atrium until it can be retrieved (Moureau, 2008).

TABLE 47-3

PICC Removal Equipment

Equipment	Rationale
Gather all needed supplies	Decreases anxiety and facilitates completion of the procedure in a prompt manner
Clean gloves	Prevents exposure to blood-borne pathogens
Alcohol or adhesive removal pads	Releases the adhesive on the dressing and catheter securement device if present
Tourniquet	For application to the upper arm in the event of catheter fracture/ breakage
Sterile gauze	To control bleeding at the insertion site
Petroleum-impregnated gauze or antibiotic ointment	Prevents air from entering the vascular system via the catheter tract
Transparent dressing	Covers the insertion site and gauze, preventing air entry into the vascular system; protects against infection until the site has epithelialized
Sterile scissors or suture removal kit	Removal of sutures

Note: Peripherally inserted central catheter (PICC).
Source: Adapted from Moureau, 2008.

CLINICAL PICC PEARLS

- If resistance is met when threading the guidewire, do not force the wire; instead, pull back and reposition the needle, and then re-attempt the procedure. If resistance is met when the guidewire has been inserted approximately 10 to 15 cm, then try repositioning the patient's arm at a 90-degree angle, lifting the shoulder slightly, as the wire may be pinched between the clavicle and first rib.
- Ensure that the patient is properly sedated and pain control is adequate. Pain leads to anxiety, which in turn causes valves to close off, making it difficult or impossible to pass the guidewire and catheter. A child life specialist can assist with the awake patient.
- To keep the catheter from trailing into the external or internal jugular vein, turn the patient's head toward the arm being accessed. This maneuver momentarily occludes the vessel and decreases the chance of a jugular placed catheter.
- If the catheter is either kinked, curved upon itself, or embedded in the jugular vein, use the jet technique to reposition it. Place the patient in a sitting position or at a 45-degree angle. Using a 10- to 20-mL syringe filled with sterile saline, flush the catheter quickly. The increased flow of saline and the normal blood flow should flip the tip of the PICC into the appropriate

portion of the SVC. Obtain a new CXR to verify tip placement. If the tip has crossed into the left SCV (if placed in the right arm) or into the right SCV (if placed in the left arm), place the patient in a sitting position or at a 45-degree angle, rotate the patient slightly right or left, and use the jet technique as previously described. Gravity and the increased flow should flip the tip of the PICC into place. Obtain another CXR to verify placement.

- If unable to reposition the PICC, then interventional radiology may be consulted and the use of fluoroscopy may be indicated. Sometimes just waiting 24 hours and repeating the CXR may allow for the tip to drop into the appropriate place.

BIBLIOGRAPHY

1. Graf, J., Newman, C., & McPherson, M. (2006). Sutured securement of peripherally inserted central catheters yields fewer complications in pediatric patients. *Journal Journal of Parenteral and Enteral Nutrition, 30*(6), 532–535.
2. Kaplan, J., & Brilli, R. (2007). Vascular access. In D. S. Wheeler, H. R. Wong, & T. P. Shanley (Eds.). *Pediatric critical care medicine: Basic science and clinical evidence* (pp. 253–273). London: Springer.
3. Knue, M., Doellman, D., Rabin, K., & Jacobs, B. (2005). The efficacy and safety of blood sampling through peripherally inserted central catheter devices in children. *Journal of Infusion Nursing, 28*(1), 30–35.
4. Levy, I., Bendet, M., Samra, Z., Shalit, I., & Katz, J. (2010, May). Infectious complications of peripherally inserted central venous catheters in children. *Pediatric Infectious Disease Journal, 29*(5), 426–429.
5. Mickler, P. (2008). Neonatal and pediatric perspectives in PICC placement. *Journal of Infusion Nursing, 31*(5), 282–285.
6. Moureau, N. (2008). Peripherally inserted central venous catheter: Care, management, and removal. In J. T. Verger & R. M. Lebet (Eds.). *AACN procedure manual for pediatric acute & critical care* (pp. 1095–1101). St. Louis: Saunders Elsevier.
7. O'Grady, N., Alexander, M., Dellinger, E., Gerberding, J., Heard, S., Maki, D., et al. (2002). Guidelines for the prevention of intravascular catheter-related infections. *Pediatrics, 110*(5), 1–24.
8. Racadio, M., Doellman,D., Johnson, N., Bean, J., & Jacobs, B. (2001). Pediatric peripherally inserted central catheters: Complication rates related to catheter tip location. *Pediatrics, 107*(2), e28.
9. Seneff, M. (2003). Central venous catheters. In R. S. Irwin, J. M. Rippe, F. J. Curley, & S. O. Heard (Eds.). *Procedures and techniques in intensive care medicine* (3rd ed.). Philadelphia: Lippincott, Williams & Wilkins.
10. Stokowski, G., Steele, D., & Wilson, D. (2009). The use of ultrasound to improve practice and reduce complications rates in peripherally inserted central catheter insertions. *Journal of Infusion Nursing, 32*(3), 145–155.

Tracy Lynne Mackie

Peritoneal Catheter Insertion

INDICATIONS

Peritoneal catheters are placed in the lower abdomen and are used for peritoneal dialysis, paracentesis, or peritoneal lavage. The placement of peritoneal catheters in pediatric patients is important, yet challenging, as many factors influence these devices' insertion and maintenance.

Indications for peritoneal catheter placement include acute or chronic kidney failure, inborn errors of metabolism, dialysis after corrective cardiac surgery for congenital heart lesions, sampling or management of peritoneal fluid through paracentesis or peritoneal lavage due to trauma, internal bleeding, ascites, malignancies, or infection (Brant & Brewer, 2004; Sudel & Li, 2007; Whitehouse & Weigelt, 2009).

CONTRAINDICATIONS

Contraindications for peritoneal catheter placement are commonly divided into relative and absolute contraindications (Sudel & Li, 2007; Whitehouse & Weigelt, 2009). Table 48-1 lists common contraindications, but each clinical situation needs to be considered through the lens of thorough clinical assessment and judgment.

TABLE 48-I

Contraindications to Peritoneal Catheter Placement		
Indication	**Relative Contraindications**	**Absolute Contraindications**
Dialysis	Recent abdominal surgery	Ostomies
	Prior surgeries with resultant scarring	Omphalacele
	Existing peritoneal catheter	Gastroschesis
	Anticipated complications post care	Hernias
		Obesity
Paracentesis	Present infection	Hemodynamic instability
Peritoneal lavage	Coagulopathy	Intestinal perforation
	Thrombocytopenia	Recent surgery
	Recent surgery	
	Cirrhosis	
	Obesity	
	Pelvic fractures	

COMPLICATIONS

The complication risk for peritoneal catheter placement depends on the indications and urgency of placement (Ash & Daugirdas, 2007; Brant & Brewer, 2004;

Sudel & Li, 2007; Whitehouse & Weigelt, 2009). Complications can be classified into categories based on the length of time of placement—that is, short term versus long term (Table 48-2). A peritoneal catheter that is inserted for dialysis purposes may be considered a long-term catheter with a subsequent risk for general systemic complications similar to that of other long-term invasive catheters.

EQUIPMENT

General equipment required for peritoneal catheter insertion includes the following items:

- Nasogastric tube and urinary drainage catheter to decompress the stomach and the bladder, respectively (time permitting)
- Hair clippers
- Cleansing agent (10% povidone-iodine solution, 2% chlorhexidine, or 70% isopropyl alcohol)
- Sterile drapes
- Local anesthetic 1% lidocaine *without* epinephrine
- 16-, 21-, or 23-gauge needles or angiocatheters with syringe (depending on the specific procedure)
- Sterile containers for fluid collection, specimens, culture tubes
- Dialysis tubing setup
- Sterile dressing
- Peritoneal catheter

Medication for pain and sedation may be considered depending on the patient's hemodynamic status and the indication for the peritoneal catheter.

Dialysis catheters may be either straight or curled, and some have a metal stylet or wire to guide their insertion. Longer-term catheters are usually made of silicone or polyurethane and have one or two cuffs that lie under the skin where granulation tissue grows to secure the catheter in place and seal out bacteria from the catheter tract (Ash, 2003; Ash & Daugirdas, 2007; Brant & Brewer, 2004; Veys et al., 2002).

A Tenckhoff catheter is straight or coiled and has two cuffs located 5 to 6 cm apart; these cuffs sit in the rectus muscle of the abdominal wall to secure the catheter. These catheters are placed surgically, blindly at the bedside, or through peritoneoscopy.

A Swan Neck catheter is a U-shaped catheter with a 120-degree arc between the two cuffs so that it fits in the peritoneum pointing toward the pelvis and anchors on the skin without kinking. Presternal Swan Neck catheters are longer and tunnel under the skin up to the sternum for patients who require catheter access at a higher placement. This type of placement may be necessary for patients who bathe in a bathtub or obese patients whose body habitus complicates abdominal catheter placement.

TABLE 48-2

Common Complications of Peritoneal Catheter Placement

Longer-Term Catheter Placement (Peritoneal Dialysis Access)	Shorter-Term Catheter Placement (Paracentesis or Peritoneal Lavage)
• Peritonitis (procedure, exit site, management/use) • Infection of site or tunnel • Pneumoperitoneum • Perforation of internal organs or vessels (commonly bladder, stomach, and iliac veins) • Bleeding • Hypotension (from procedure or fluid loss) • Inadequate patency of tube (poor fluid return) • Misplacement/preperitoneal placement (abdominal wall fluid infusions, pain) • Leaking catheters (exit site, catheter junctions, dialysis setup) • Pain • Hernias (congenital hernias that appear due to increased abdominal pressures, or new hernias) • Leakage around site (of fluid ingoing or outcoming) • Omental attachment • Migration (internal fixation, outflow failure) • Cuff extrusion or erosion	• Peritonitis (procedure, exit site, management/use) • Infection of site or tunnel • Pneumoperitoneum • Perforation of internal organs or vessels (commonly bladder, stomach, and iliac veins) • Bleeding • Hypotension (from procedure or fluid loss) • Inadequate patency of tube (poor fluid return) • Misplacement/preperitoneal placement (no fluid return, bloody fluid returns, pain) • Leaking catheters (exit site, catheter junctions) • Pain • Hernias (congenital hernias that appear due to increased abdominal pressures, or new hernias)

A Toronto-Western catheter is surgically placed with two perpendicular silicone disks that hold the omentum and bowel away from the catheter. It has a modified deep cuff to help position the catheter and secure it in place.

An Advantage (T-fluted) catheter is a specialized catheter designed to lie at right angles next to the parietal peritoneum so that it cannot migrate outward; fluid is distributed along both sides into the peritoneal cavity. This catheter may be placed surgically, blindly at the bedside, or via peritoneoscopy. It tends to have less omental attachment and outflow failure than other tubes.

PROCEDURE

Three methods of peritoneal catheter placement are commonly used: surgical, blind, and blind with mini-trochar/peritoneoscopy. The surgical technique provides direct visualization of catheter placement but requires general anesthetic, a larger incision, and longer recovery. It is also often more difficult to schedule, and has a higher associated cost to the health care system. Whereas a blind technique involves inexpensive equipment, optimal catheter placement is not always achieved with this method, and there is a higher risk of bowel and bladder perforation. Mini-trochar and peritoneoscopy-guided catheter placement allows direct visualization of catheter placement without use of open surgical technique.

When considering placement of a peritoneal catheter, the health care professional (HCP) should think about the timing of catheter placement and the ability of the patient to go without fluids or solids for more than 6 hours. Informed consent or permission for the procedure is per institutional policy, and the procedure must be discussed with the patient and the caregiver. Immediately prior to performing the procedure, perform a "time-out" (universal protocol) to ensure the procedure is still indicated and to verify patient identity.

Consider whether the patient will need general anesthesia or a local anesthetic with sedation. The risks and benefits of each method should be evaluated. Administer intravenous cephalosporin prophylaxis 30 minutes prior to the procedure or, if administering via the oral route, 1 to 2 hours prior to the procedure. Depending on the patient's age, ability, and situation, have the pediatric patient empty the bladder or insert a urinary drainage catheter to decompress the bladder, and consider insertion of a nasogastric tube to decompress the stomach. Monitor cardiorespiratory status and vital signs throughout the procedure. Assess the location and size of the liver, spleen, bladder and other organs via ultrasound if time and availability permit. Clip hair (as needed), and then cleanse the skin with the selected agent. Use sterile technique to drape the abdomen.

If placing the catheter at the bedside, use peritoneoscopy if available. For catheter placement, the landmark for midline or left lateral placement is 2 to 3 cm below the umbilicus or lateral border of the rectus muscle, one-halfway between the umbilicus and the anterior superior iliac spine. The indwelling catheter tip should lie within the pelvis without bending or kinking. The exit site should avoid the diaper or waist line and should be directed downward.

Administer local anesthetic to site, gradually including deeper tissues. Create a 1- to 2-cm incision and dissect the fascia with a blunt hemostat. For paracentesis, use a Z-track technique with a 16-gauge needle or angiocatheter 3 cm into the peritoneal cavity, removing the fluid with a syringe. For an indwelling catheter, insert a 21-gauge needle into the peritoneum and then inject contrast dye if using fluoroscopy to verify catheter placement. Insert a trochar and upsize peritoneal catheters until the size of choice is in situ. The inner cuff of the catheter should be securely attached within the rectus muscle, and the outer cuff should be 1.5 to 2 cm from the exit site, secured within the subcutaneous tissue. Moncrief-Popovich proposed a method of tunneling the external catheter length under the skin to minimize infection risk and ensure security while the catheter site is healing and granulation tissue is forming around the cuffs.

Obtain an abdominal radiograph to confirm catheter tip placement. Flush the catheter with 20 mL of normal saline, and then drain the saline to ensure patency of the catheter and return of clear fluid. As much as 10–20 mL/kg of normal saline may be used per flush if needed (Ash, 2003; Ash & Daugirdas, 2007; Brant & Brewer, 2004; Li et al., 2009; Maya, 2007; Sudel & Li, 2007; Veys et al., 2002; Whitehouse & Weigelt, 2009).

POSTPROCEDURE CARE

If the catheter is not removed during the procedure, dress the catheter site with sterile gauze dressings to secure and immobilize the catheter. Securing the catheter also promotes healing and decreases infection risk. Pediatric patients may shower after a few weeks, after the catheter site is sealed and healed. Patients and caregivers should be taught hand washing techniques, catheter care, and maintenance techniques. They should also be educated on the signs and symptoms to monitor for infection.

PROCEDURE NOTE

An example procedure note for paracentesis is as follows:

- Date and time.
- Paracentesis.
- Indications: Peritonitis; to obtain culture.
- Performed by: State names and positions.
- Procedure explained to patient and caregivers, permission/consent obtained.
- "Time-out" taken (universal protocol).
- Sedation/analgesia: (List medications, dose, and route) prior to the procedure.

- Site preparation: Bladder emptied. NPO for 6 hours. Site cleansed with 10% povidone-iodine. Abdomen draped with sterile towels. Local anesthetic, 1% lidocaine 1 mL, infiltrated subcutaneously at the insertion site. A sterile ultrasound probe used to landmark and assess the liver, spleen, bladder, and other structures near the insertion site. Cardiopulmonary monitoring on.
- Procedure: A 1-cm incision was made 2 cm below the umbilicus, halfway between the umbilicus and the anterior superior iliac spine. The fascia was dissected with a blunt hemostat, and a Z-track technique was used with a 16-gauge needle into the peritoneal cavity. Using a 60-mL syringe, 42 mL of clear, pale, yellow fluid was removed; it was transferred to sterile collection containers, and then sent to the laboratory. The needle was removed.
- Site at conclusion of procedure: The site was dressed with a sterile dressing. Blood loss: None.
- Specimens sent: Peritoneal fluid sent for culture and Gram stain.
- Patient condition following procedure: Patient tolerated procedure well with no significant changes in vital signs. Parents present and have no further questions.
- Signature of health care professional.

BIBLIOGRAPHY

1. Ash, S. R. (2003). Chronic peritoneal dialysis catheters: Overview of design, placement, and removal procedures. *Seminars in Dialysis, 16*(4), 323–334.
2. Ash, S. R., & Daugirdas, J. T. (2007). Peritoneal access devices. In J. T. Daugirdas, P. G. Blake, & T. S. Ing (Eds.). *Handbook of dialysis* (4th ed., pp. 356–375). Philadelphia: Lippincott Williams & Wilkins.
3. Brant, M. L., & Brewer, E. D. (2004). Peritoneal dialysis access in children. In B. A. Warady, F. S. Schaefer, R. N. Fine, & S. R. Alexander (Eds.). *Pediatric dialysis* (pp. 83–89). Dordrecht, Netherlands: Springer.
4. Li, C., Cui, T., Gan, H., Cheung, K., Lio, W., & Kuok, U. (2009). PD in the developing world: A randomized trial comparing conventional Swan-Neck straight-tip catheters to straight-tip catheters with an artificial subcutaneous swan neck. *Peritoneal Dialysis International, 29*, 278–284.
5. Maya, I. D. (2007). Ultrasound/fluoroscopy-assisted placement of peritoneal dialysis catheters. *Seminars in Dialysis, 20*(6), 611–615.
6. Sudel, B., & Li, B. U. K. (2007). Paracentesis/peritoneal lavage. In D. M. Goodman, T. P. Green, S. M. Unti, & E. C. Powell (Eds.). *Current procedures: Pediatrics* (pp. 123–126.) New York: McGraw-Hill.
7. Veys, N., Van Biesen, W., Vanholder, R., & Lameire, N. (2002). Peritoneal dialysis catheters: The beauty of simplicity or the glamour of technicality? Percutaneous vs surgical placement. *Nephrology Dialysis and Transplantation, 17*, 210–212.
8. Whitehouse, J., & Weigelt, J. (2009). Diagnostic peritoneal lavage: A review of indications, technique, and interpretation. *Scandinavian Journal of Trauma, Resuscitation and Emergency Medicine, 17*(13), 1–5.

Bonnie J. Stojadinovic

Rapid-Sequence Intubation

Rapid-sequence intubation (RSI) describes a sequential process of preparation, sedation, and paralysis to facilitate safe, emergent tracheal intubation. RSI is generally the preferred method for airway access in patients who have varying levels of consciousness and are presumed to have a full stomach. Careful preparation (including preoxygenation) and the use of specific techniques, such as applying cricoid pressure and avoiding positive-pressure ventilation, enables the health care professional (HCP) undertaking RSI to minimize the risks of hypoxia and aspiration.

The success of RSI depends on the following factors:

- Sedation and paralysis to eliminate protective airway reflexes and spontaneous respiration. Difficulties with intubation and/or ventilation must be anticipated and a contingency plan put in place.
- Pharmacologic agents for sedation and paralysis. These agents should be selected based on the presence of clinical features such as hypotension or preexisting conditions such as asthma.
- A simple, systematic approach to preparation and execution.

INDICATIONS

RSI is a valuable strategy for airway access in a variety of situations. A few of these indications are listed here:

- PaO_2 less than 60 mmHg with FiO_2 of 0.6 or greater in the absence of cyanotic congenital heart lesions
- $PaCO_2$ greater than 50 mmHg that is acute and unresponsive to other interventions
- Actual or imminent upper airway obstruction
- Neuromuscular weakness with a maximum negative inspiratory pressure less than −20 cmH_2O or vital capacity less than 12 to 15 mL/kg
- Therapeutic hyperventilation such as for intracranial hypertension, pulmonary hypertension, or metabolic acidosis
- Hemodynamic instability
- Significant facial trauma or thermal injury
- Severe brain injury with the need for controlled ventilation
- Any patient in whom a natural airway cannot be maintained or whose protective airway reflexes such as cough or gag are absent
- Any patient who exhibits signs of respiratory exhaustion or impending ventilatory failure

CONTRAINDICATIONS

There are few contraindications to RSI. Relative contraindications include facial or neck injuries that prevent visualization of the airway anatomy and severely increased intracranial pressure. HCPs who are skilled in the maneuver, such as anesthesia specialists, should only intubate patients with epiglottitis. Anatomical features that are suggestive of a difficult airway are listed in Table 49-1. The Mallampati score determines the difficulty of intubating poorly visualized airways (Figure 49-1). Seek anesthesia

TABLE 49-1

Causes for a Difficult Pediatric Airway	
Injuries and Illnesses	**Anatomical Features**

- Trauma to lips, teeth, tongue, and nose
 - Mandibular trauma
 - Avulsion of teeth (potential choking risk)
 - Oral bleeding
 - Severe laryngeal edema
   - Burns or smoke inhalation
   - Repeated intubation attempts
   - Repeated failed extubation
 - Retropharyngeal hematoma
 - Abscess
 - Swollen uvula
 - Tonsillitis
 - Croup
 - Epiglottis (*do not* attempt to intubate)
 - Foreign body aspiration
	- Macroglossia
	 - Micrognathia
	 - Obesity
	 - Occipito-atlantoid instability
	 - Congenital muscular dystrophy
	 - Cervical spine subluxation
	 - Cervical spine fusion/immobilization

Note: This is not an exhaustive list, but rather is meant to highlight those causes most commonly found in pediatric patients. Additional causes exist and must be considered prior to any intubation attempt.
Source: Adapted from American College of Surgeons, 2004.

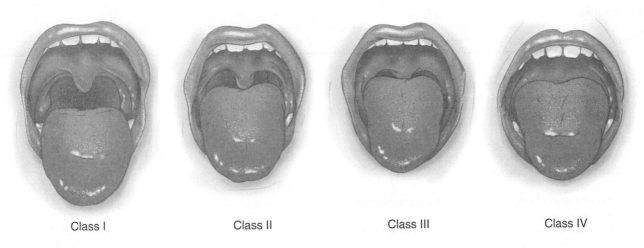

Class I   Class II   Class III   Class IV

FIGURE 49-1

Mallampati Score.

The Mallampati classification is based on the structures visualized with maximal mouth opening and tongue protrusion in the sitting position. Although it was originally described without phonation, some have suggested that the minimum Mallampati score with or without phonation best correlates with intubation difficulty.

Class 1: Full visibility of hard and soft palate, fauces, tonsils, uvula, and pillars.

Class 2: Visibility of hard and soft palate, fauces, upper portion of tonsils, uvula, and pillars.

Class 3: Soft and hard palate and base of uvula are visible.

Class 4: Only hard palate visible.

Source: Pollak, A. (2011). *Critical Care Transport.* Jones and Bartlett Publishers.

consultation for a Class 3 or 4 score, or whenever successful intubation is in doubt.

COMPLICATIONS

Even when the utmost care is used, complications from RSI are possible. The most common of these problems is bronchial intubation—specifically, placement of the tube into the right main stem bronchus. This error may be easily corrected by pulling the endotracheal tube (ETT) back until bilateral breath sounds are reestablished. Other potential complications include esophageal intubation, aspiration of stomach contents, and physical trauma to any part of the airway. Spinal injury can occur in patients with cervical malformations, injury, or tumor. Intubation can lead to hypertension, tachycardia, arrhythmias, and intracranial and intraocular hypertension.

EQUIPMENT

Table 49-2 lists suggested equipment for use during RSI. Equations for determining ETT size and length are provided in the table.

PROCEDURE

Age-appropriate education regarding the procedure should be provided to both the patient and the caregivers. This explanation may need to be brief when RSI is performed emergently. In most settings, informed consent or permission is not required.

As recommended by The Joint Commission, perform a "time-out" procedure (universal protocol) to assess the need for the intubation and to verify the correct patient. Assemble the necessary equipment and use standard precautions. Place the child supine with the head in the sniffing position, the neck slightly flexed at the shoulders, and the head slightly extended at the occipito-atlantoid junction. One HCP should be dedicated to monitoring cardiorespiratory function.

Suction the oropharynx with a large-bore suction catheter. If the child is still breathing spontaneously, consider use of pharmacologic support (Table 49-3). While the medications take effect, maintain support of spontaneous ventilation with 100% oxygen and a self-inflating or flow-inflating resuscitation bag. If the child has risk factors for gastric distention (Table 49-4), the use of cricoid pressure and placement of a nasogastric tube prior to intubation can reduce the risk of vomiting and aspiration of stomach

TABLE 49-2

Rapid-Sequence Intubation Equipment

1. Oxygen source
2. Suction device
   A. Wall or portable vacuum source
   B. Tubing
   C. Suction
3. Equipment for bag-mask ventilation
   A. Oral/nasal airways
   B. Ventilation bags (flow-inflating or self-inflating)
   C. Tubing
   D. Masks (range of sizes appropriate for patient age/size)
   E. Airway pressure manometer
   F. Positive end-expiratory pressure (PEEP) valves or alternative device
4. Equipment for intubation
   A. Laryngoscope handle
   B. Laryngoscope blades (Miller 0, 1, 2; Wis-Hipple 1½; MacIntosh 2, 3)
   C. Working light source with a secured/tightened bulb
   D. Replacement light bulbs for the laryngoscope blade
   E. Endotracheal tubes (ETT): cuffed and uncuffed
   F. Cardiorespiratory monitoring equipment
5. ETT placement
   Colorimetric and digital measurement device for expired carbon dioxide

Guidelines for Determining the Appropriate Size and Length of ETT

$$size = \frac{16 + age\ in\ years}{4}$$

Example: $16 + 8\ (age\ in\ years)/4 = 6.0$ cm ETT
For a cuffed tube, consider using an ETT that is 0.5 cm smaller.

$length = ETT\ size \times 3$

Example: ETT size 4.0 cm $\times$ 3 = 12 cm insertion length

   G. Stylets (small and large)
   H. Medications (optional in emergent scenario)
      1. Anticholinergic agent for secretion control
      2. Benzodiazepine for sedation
      3. Narcotic for pain control
      4. Neuromuscular blocking agent for paralysis

TABLE 49-3

Pharmacologic Support for Rapid-Sequence Intubation

Administer in the following order:
• Anticholinergic agent for secretion control (if used)
• Benzodiazepine for sedative
• Narcotic for pain control
• Neuromuscular blocking agent for paralysis

TABLE 49-4

Risk Factors for Gastric Distention

• Food intake within 4 to 6 hours of intubation
• Bowel obstruction (mechanical or functional)
• Pharyngeal or upper gastrointestinal bleeding
• Tense abdominal distention resulting from any cause
• Trauma or illness onset within a few hours of eating

contents during the procedure. Intubation proceeds when the patient is adequately sedated and paralyzed.

The general procedure for oral intubation is described in Figure 49-2. Give several large breaths with 100% oxygen with a bag-mask device to hyperoxygenate the patient prior to the intubation attempt. In the flaccid patient, the mouth naturally falls open; however, additional visualization can be achieved by using the thumb and index finger of the right hand in a scissors fashion between the teeth. Using the left hand, place the laryngoscope blade into the right corner of the patient's mouth and sweep the blade toward the center and deep into the pharynx, moving the tongue leftward and

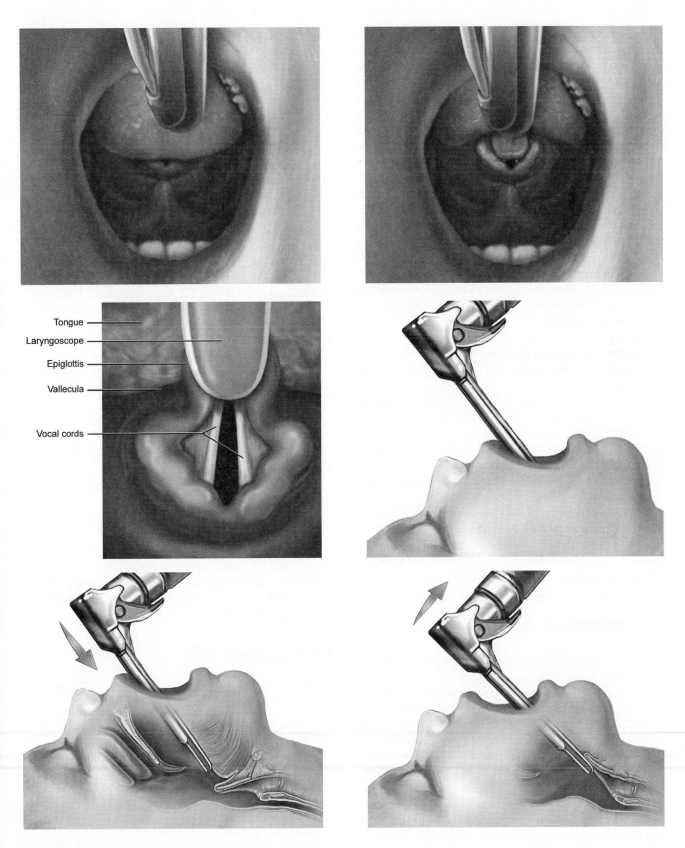

Tongue

Laryngoscope

Epiglottis

Vallecula

Vocal cords

FIGURE 49-2

Rapid-Sequence Intubation Tube Placement.

Source: Copyright © Nucleus Medical Media, All rights reserved.

out of the way. Advance the laryngoscope blade to the base of the tongue. Place the tip of the laryngoscope blade into the vallecula or onto the epiglottis itself, and visualize the larynx by lifting the mandible with pressure on the laryngoscope handle directed toward the ceiling at a 45- to 60-degree angle to the patient's chest. To prevent lip, tooth, or alveolar damage, *do not* use the laryngoscope as a crowbar or rock the laryngoscope blade against the teeth. Visualization of the larynx requires lifting along the line of the laryngoscope handle—*do not* pivot on the fulcrum. Have an assistant apply gentle cricoid pressure to visualize the vocal cords if they are difficult to see. After visualizing the vocal cords, advance the ETT from the right corner of the mouth—not along the laryngoscope blade—into the pharynx and through the vocal cords. Align the appropriate predetermined marking on the tube with the vocal cords (usually a bold or double line, 2 to 5 cm from the tip, depending on the tube size and manufacturer). Repeat the procedure as necessary until placement is obtained.

Do not prolong intubation attempts. Hypoxia may aggravate the underlying illness or injury. If the intubation is not completed successfully after three attempts, consider anesthesia consultation.

No one verification method is reliable for confirming accurate ETT placement. Consequently, several techniques are required to assess placement: Observe for good chest rise and fall, listen for symmetrical breath sounds and absence of epigastric sounds, watch for improving color and oxygen saturation, and use a colorimetric and digital device to measure expired carbon dioxide through the ETT.

After placement is verified, inflate the cuff (if present) with the minimum occlusive volume or minimal leak pressure necessary to prevent tube dislodgement or shifting. Secure the tube with either tape or a commercially manufactured ETT-securing device per institution policy.

POSTPROCEDURE CARE

Once successful placement of the ETT has occurred, and preliminary verification of its position in the trachea is obtained, obtain a chest radiograph to assess the depth of ETT placement. Correct placement comprises an ETT tip located at mid-trachea. This position varies with age, so expect the accurately positioned ETT tip to lie between the patient's clavicles. Adjust the position as necessary. Monitor the patient's expired carbon dioxide with capnography and oxygenation with pulse oximetry. Perform respiratory physical assessment and blood gas monitoring based on institution-specific protocols. Provide ongoing pain medication and sedation medication while the patient is intubated. Consider ongoing paralytic medication based on institution-specific policy and the needs of the patient.

PROCEDURE NOTE

An example procedure note for rapid-sequence intubation is as follows:

- Date and time.
- Oral endotracheal intubation.
- Indication: Respiratory failure secondary to bronchiolitis, thick secretions, and chronic lung disease.
- Performed by: State names and positions.
- Procedure and indication explained to caregivers, who verbalized understanding.
- "Time-out" taken (universal protocol).
- Mallampati score determined to be Class 2.
- Sedation/analgesia: Patient was premedicated with fentanyl 5 μg/kg IV, midazolam 0.1 mg/kg IV, and vecuronium 0.1 mg/kg IV. A neuromuscular blocking agent was administered only after ability to effectively ventilate the patient was established.
- Procedure: Patient was preoxygenated with 100% oxygen, and the oral pharynx was suctioned of a moderate amount of clear secretions. A Miller 1 straight blade was introduced, and direct visualization of the vocal cords was performed. A 3.0 cuffed endotracheal tube was inserted into the oral pharynx and advanced through the vocal cords. Once the cuff was inserted, end-tidal CO_2 was documented. Symmetrical breath sounds were ausculated. The location of the ETT was confirmed with direct visualization of the tube advancing through the cords, end-tidal CO_2, auscultation, and chest radiograph. The tube was secured with silk tape, and its location was recorded as 18 cm at the lip.
- Patient condition following the procedure: Radiograph confirmed ETT placement mid-trachea. Patient tolerated procedure without changes in vital signs and had an appropriate pain/sedation score post procedure (state specifics).
- Signature of HCP.

BIBLIOGRAPHY

1. American College of Surgeons. (2004). *Advanced trauma life support* (7th ed.). Chicago: Author.
2. Dieckman, R., Fiser, D., & Selbst, S. (1997). *Illustrated textbook of emergency and critical care procedures.* St. Louis: Mosby.
3. Fleisher, G., & Ludwig, S. (2005). *Textbook of pediatric emergency medicine* (5th ed.). Philadelphia: Lippincott Williams & Wilkins.
4. Gausche-Hill, M., Henderson, D., & Goodrich, S. (2004). *Pediatric airway management for the prehospital professional.* Sudbury, MA: Jones and Bartlett.
5. Gerardi, M., Sacchetti, A., Cantor, R., Santamaria, J., Gausche, M., Lucid, W., et al. (1996). Rapid-sequence intubation of the pediatric patient. *Annals of Emergency Medicine, 28,* 55–74.
6. Pollak, A. (Ed.). (2011). *Critical care transport.* Sudbury, MA: Jones and Bartlett.
7. Verger, J., & Lebet, R. (Eds.). (2008). *AACN procedure manual for pediatric acute and critical care.* Philadelphia: W. B. Saunders.

Slit Lamp

The slit lamp is a biomicroscope for viewing the *anterior* structures of the eye, eyelids, lashes, conjunctiva, sclerae, cornea, anterior chamber, irides, and lens, and includes fluorescein staining (Fleisher & Ludwig, 2005). Many slit lamps also have an applanation tonometer attached to allow for the measurement of intraocular pressure.

INDICATIONS

The slit lamp examination is used for the following purposes:

- To inspect the anterior segment of the eye (conditions requiring magnification):
  - Lids
  - Lashes
  - Conjunctiva/sclera
  - Cornea
  - Anterior chamber
  - Irides
  - Lens
- For diagnosing eye injuries/conditions:
  - Red eye—blepharitis, conjunctivitis, dacryocystitis
  - Corneal abrasion
  - Foreign body—use an ocular anesthetic agent; examine with fluorescein dye; evert the lid with a cotton swab to explore areas under the upper lid
  - Eyelid lacerations—evaluate for lacrimal duct involvement
  - Fracture—orbital floor fractures may result in entrapment of extraocular muscles with complaints of diplopia
  - Corneal epithelial defect
  - Keratoconjunctivitis
  - Hyphema (layering of blood in the anterior chamber)
  - Hypopyon (layering of white blood cells in the anterior chamber)
  - Lens dislocation
  - Herpetic infections (dendritic lesions)
  - Iritis/uveitis
- To aid in the removal of a corneal foreign body

CONTRAINDICATIONS

Contraindications to a slit lamp examination include the following conditions:

- Inability to be in a seated position (although there are now some hand-held slit lamp devices
- Head injury
- Anatomic disruption (eyelids swollen shut)
- Developmental age and/or disability
- Ruptured globe (open or closed)

If a rupture of the globe is suspected or there is an impaled object, *do not* use fluorescein dye in the eye or remove the object. Instead, follow these guidelines:

- Cover the injured eye with a protective device or shield.
- Consult ophthalmology immediately; consider consulting neurosurgery.
- Do not upset the child, as he or she may inadvertently perform a Valsalva maneuver, resulting in extrusion of intraocular contents.

COMPLICATIONS

There are no complications from using slit lamp.

EQUIPMENT

The following equipment is needed to perform a slit lamp examination:

- Exam gloves
- Anesthetic solution (e.g., 0.5% proparacaine)
- Fluorescein stain strips
- Woods lamp (blue light filter)
- Slit lamp
- Eye wash/irrigation solution

PROCEDURE

First, assess the patient's clinical status, history of any previous eye illnesses, or injuries. Age-appropriate education regarding the Woods lamp/slit lamp procedure should be provided to the pediatric patient and the caregiver(s), including information on the indications, general technique, topical anesthetic agent to be used, and postprocedure care. The caregiver(s) can be offered the opportunity to be present during the procedure at this time as well. The requirement for informed consent or permission for this procedure varies by institution. Perform a "time-out" (universal protocol) to verify the correct patient.

Follow standard precautions. With the patient lying in the supine position, instill one drop of anesthetic solution into the affected eye(s). Ask the patient if there is immediate pain relief with the instillation of the anesthetic drops. Pain relief is usually diagnostic for an anterior eye structure injury or illness. Next, moisten a fluorescein strip with the ophthalmic anesthetic agent and stain the eye.

The patient should be positioned in the upright-seated position. Have the patient rest the forehead firmly against the headrest with the chin in the chin rest. Adjust the slit lamp to accommodate the patient's height. Then, turn off the lights in the examination room and turn on the slit lamp. The light source is mounted on a swinging arm. Knobs are used to change the width and the height of the light beam. In addition, a variety of filters may be used during the examination. Only white and blue filters are used in the acute care settings, however. The vertical alignment is preferred.

For examination of the patient's right eye, the light source should be moved to the patient's left at a 45-degree angle while the biomicroscope is directly in front of the eye. Repeat the procedure if the left eye is to be examined, moving to the patient's right at a 45-degree angle. Using the white light, the slit beam should be set at the maximum height and minimum width. To examine the patient, move the light source across the patient's cornea, by moving the entire base of the slit lamp forward and backward. Then move the entire base of the lamp left and right to scan across the eye. The 45-degree angle between the microscope and the light source should be the "default" position. Do not move the arm of the light source in an arc-shaped fashion.

Examine the eye at the level of the conjunctiva and the cornea at the pupillary margin, and then push the joystick forward to examine the iris. Next, pull back the joystick to focus on the cornea. Move the focus inward, halfway between the iris and the cornea. This maneuver will bring the light to the center of the aqueous humor to allow for visualization of cells if any are present.

The lowest lighting setting is adequate for routine examination, in which the structures of the eye are examined. The slit lamp permits detailed evaluation of external eye injury or illness; thus the health care professional (HCP) should assess the patient for inflammation of lids and lashes (blepharitis) and for "pointing" or inner canthus and lacrimal punctum inflammation (dacryocystitis).

Use a high-intensity setting when examining the anterior chamber with the narrow "slit" beam. Shorten the slit beam to 1 mm, and examine the anterior chamber of the eye for cells (e.g., red and white blood cells) and "flare." Flare is described as "headlights in fog" and may indicate acute injury or acute or chronic iritis/uveitis. It signals an increase in aqueous humor protein content, which is consistent with an inflammatory process in the eye. Observe the patient for blood in the anterior chamber (hyphema) or layered white blood cells (hypopyon). These findings are graded by the percentage of the vertical diameter of the visible iris (Roberts & Hedges, 2004). Last, assess for any corneal abrasion, corneal defects, foreign bodies, or rust rings.

PROCEDURE NOTE

An example procedure note for use of the slit lamp to examine a corneal abrasion is as follows:

- Date and time.
- Slit lamp examination: State which eye.
- Indication: pain, blepharospasm.
- Performed by: State names and positions.
- Procedure explained to patient and caregivers, permission/consent obtained.
- "Time-out" taken (universal protocol).
- Site preparation: With the patient lying in the supine position, the right eye was anesthetized with 1 drop of 0.5% proparacaine. The patient had immediate relief of pain. The patient's right eye was stained with fluorescein.
- Procedure: The room was darkened. Using a Woods/slit lamp, both eyes were examined while in a sitting position. A corneal abrasion was noted in the 6 o'clock position of the right eye. The patient was then positioned in front of a slit lamp for the external exam. A 1-cm circular corneal abrasion of the right eye was confirmed on slit lamp examination in the 6 o'clock position. No foreign body or globe rupture was noted. All other structures appeared intact. The patient's right eye was irrigated with eye wash irrigation solution at the conclusion of the procedure. (In the patient chart, document the injury with a drawing or picture of the injury if possible.)
- Specimens sent: None.
- Patient condition following procedure: The patient tolerated the procedure well and had no adverse reaction to the ophthalmic or eyewash irrigation solutions.
- Signature of health care professional.

BIBLIOGRAPHY

1. Fleisher, G., & Ludwig, S. (2005). *Textbook of pediatric emergency medicine* Philadelphia: Lippincott, Williams and Wilkins.
2. Roberts, J. R., & Hedges, J. R. (2004). *Clinical procedures in emergency medicine* (4th ed.). Philadelphia: Saunders.

Wound Closure

Wound assessment should be made promptly following the injury to promote optimal wound healing, reduce probability of infection, and ensure the desired cosmetic results (Hollander & Singer, 1999). Evaluation of the wound includes assessment of the age of the wound; its size and depth; the mechanism of injury; any corresponding fractures; and exploration of foreign bodies within the wound, visually or by radiograph. Fully appraise the adjacent tissue and structures around the injury, documenting neurovascular integrity or compromise.

A wound may be closed by three intention approaches:

- *Primary:* All tissues, including the skin, are closed with suture material.
- *Secondary:* The wound is left open and closes naturally.
- *Tertiary:* The wound is left open for a number of days and then closed.

Reports in the literature vary regarding when it is reasonable to close a wound by primary intent. The maximum time lapse from injury onset to use of this technique ranges from 6 to 12 hours; the time may be longer for wounds in areas with a rich vascular supply, such as the face and scalp. When developing a plan for wound closure, the patient's underlying health concerns, developmental age, follow-up, and available resources must be considered.

Many wounds require a higher level of specialization for repair and follow-up. Circumstances that would require a consultation or referral include large wounds that may require serial revisions or grafting, inability to achieve or preserve homeostasis or motor/sensory function, open fractures, or concern for poor cosmetic outcomes. Wounds that should be closed by secondary intent (natural healing) include highly contaminated wounds, noncosmetic animal bites, abscess cavities, or wounds greater than 24 hours of age.

Special challenges in wound closure arises with wounds at the vermillion border, tongue, scalp, eyelid margins, and exposed cartilage. Lacerations that cross the vermillion border of the lip are especially challenging to repair due to the increased vascularity at this site, the precision needed to align the two edges, and the inability to infiltrate the site with local anesthesia (because it would disrupt landmarks). Ideally, a nerve block or minimal sedation is used for the repair. The first stitch is most crucial and aligns the edges of the vermillion border; therefore, repair by a plastic surgeon is recommended.

Most tongue lacerations are left to heal by secondary intent. Those that require repair include bisecting or gaping wounds, wounds greater than 1 cm, and avulsions or amputations (Patel, 2008).

Scalp lacerations need to be profusely irrigated and explored, due to the risk of subgaleal infection. Shaving of hair is not recommended, especially on the scalp and eyebrows. A water-based lubricant can be helpful in controlling adjacent hairs, allowing for better visibility during wound repair. Lacerations of most medial and lateral sections of the eyelids, deep lacerations that follow along the facial nerve, and all wounds with exposed cartilage (nose and ears) should be repaired by specialists such as plastic surgery or ophthalmology.

PROCEDURE

Pediatric procedural preparation depends on multiple variables, including the developmental age of the patient, the amount of anxiety and pain the patient is actively experiencing, previous painful experiences, and the support structure present with the patient. Be honest and sensitive. Use simple words and phrases, comparing what is to come to the sights, sounds, smells, and experiences the patient might have previously encountered. Descriptive and familiar words such as "soft," "cold," "hot," "soap," "medicine," "sting," "tug," "string," "opening," and "closing" are all helpful in explaining wound closure to a pediatric patient. Child life specialists, when available, may provide patient and family support before, during, and following the procedure.

Wound preparation begins with adequate local anesthesia. If the situation is nonemergent, a topical agent can be applied to reduce the pain of later injected anesthesia. One frequently used product is a combination of lidocaine 4%, epinephrine 0.1%, and tetracaine 0.5% (LET). LET should not be used on any area that has poor vascular supply due to the vasoconstriction induced by epinephrine. Furthermore, LET should not be used in large wounds, because the amount needed to achieve adequate anesthesia will likely exceed the recommended dose of 4 mg/kg lidocaine (Berede, 1993). Apply the LET solution to a cotton ball, and place it in and over the adjacent wound edges for 30 minutes; the duration of action is 45 to 60 minutes. Next, proceed to infiltrative anesthesia, which is administered via the wound. In this step, injectable lidocaine is routinely used. For the wounds of the face or scalp, lidocaine with epinephrine aids in homeostasis. Maximum dosing is 4.5 mg/kg lidocaine *without* epinephrine, or 7 mg/kg lidocaine *with* epinephrine (Taketomo et al., 2010). The pain of the anesthetic injection may be lessened by using smaller-gauge needles, warming the solution, or buffering the solution with sodium bicarbonate.

Irrigating the wound reduces the bacteria load and is vital to the prevention of wound infection. Normal saline or tap water should be delivered under a pressure of 5 to 8 pounds per square inch (psi) and with a minimum volume of 200 mL per 1 cm of laceration. This irrigation can be accomplished using an 18-gauge catheter and a 35-mL syringe (Singer et al., 1994). Antiseptic solutions should not be used for irrigation, as these products are cytotoxic to the wound bed. Following irrigation, debride the wound and explore for remaining debris and retained foreign bodies as indicated.

Table 51-1 lists the supplies needed to perform simple suturing. When choosing a suture material, nonabsorbable sutures are the best option, as they are associated with less noticeable scarring. Exceptions to this choice might include patients who cannot return for removal and patients with certain types of facial lacerations. Table 51-2 and Table 51-3 summarize suggested recommendations for suture type and size.

When suturing, the needle driver is held in the dominant hand. The thumb and ring finger rest in the rings of the driver, and the index finger is extended along the driver's shaft for stability. The thumb controls the opening and closing of the needle driver's jaw. Load the needle at a 10- to 15-degree angle relative to the needle driver, approximately one-half to one-third of the way from the needle tip, with the needle pointing upward. In the nondominant hand, hold the forceps as if holding a writing utensil, using it to lift the wound edges and to manipulate the needle.

It is best to approximate the middle of the wound first and work in both directions away from the middle. The wound portions yet to be closed can be subsequently divided in halves, thereby resulting in a final even closure. Table 51-4 summarizes suggested recommendations for the length of time nonabsorbable suture should remain in place prior to removal.

TABLE 51-3

Suture Size Recommendations	
Face	5-0 or 6-0
Scalp	4-0 or 5-0
Hands	4-0 or 5-0
Trunk	3-0 or 4-0
Feet	3-0 or 4-0
High-tension areas	3-0 or 4-0

Several basic suturing patterns can be used to accurately appose tissues, distribute wound tension, and evert suture lines.

SIMPLE INTERRUPTED

Simple interrupted suturing is the most basic and most often used pattern. Each "bite" is approached with the needle entering the skin at a 90-degree angle, 1 to 3 mm from the wound edge. This technique fosters optimal wound edge eversion and approximation. The needle then exits the tissue perpendicular to the skin surface, utilizing the forceps or the released needle driver for grasping the needle. Bites of skin should be equal and evenly spaced on both sides of the wound. The width of each suture

TABLE 51-1

Supplies and Equipment for Suturing			
Needle driver	Local anesthetic	Normal saline	4 × 4 gauze
Forceps	3- to 5-mL syringe	Cleansing solution	Topical antibiotic
Scissors	26-gauge needle	Sterile drapes	Dressing
Suture material	19-gauge needle	Sterile gloves	
	35-mL syringe	Sterile basin	

TABLE 51-2

Suture Types		
Absorbable	Plain and chromic guts	Weak; poor knot security; absorbs in 1 week; high tissue reactivity
	Polyglactin (Vicryl)	Long lasting; stiff and difficult to handle
	Polyglycolic acid (Dexon)	Original absorbable; usually preferred
Nonabsorbable	Silk	Soft; easy to work with; good knot security; high tissue reactivity Reserved for mouth, lips, and eyelids.
	Nylon (Ethilon; Dermalon)	Strong; stiff, moderately hard to work with
	Polypropylene (Prolene; Surgilene)	Poorest knot security; most difficult to work with

TABLE 51-4

Suture Removal Recommendations	
Scalp	7–10 days
Face	3–5 days
Trunk	7–14 days
Extremities	7–14 days
Flexor aspect	7–10 days
Extensor aspect	10–14 days

should equal the distance between sutures; sutures closer to the skin edge and closer to one another ensure better healing. The long end of the thread is wrapped around the needle holder twice, which is then used to transfer the loops of suture around the short end. The first double knot is then pulled gently. When using a braided suture (silk), three throws are usually adequate for securing a knot. However, if using a more slippery monofilament material such as nylon, five or six throws may be necessary, in an alternating construction to prevent slippage. Keep all knots on one side of the wound, leaving a 3- to 4-mm tail.

CONTINUOUS/RUNNING

The continuous/running pattern is similar to the simple interrupted pattern, except that there are no individual sutures. Instead, one continuous length of suture is used, similar to stitching on a baseball. The advantage with this technique is its speed; the disadvantage is the greater potential for poor approximation of wound edges.

BURIED SIMPLE

Circular in profile, the buried simple pattern is used to close the deep layers of tissue. The knot should be placed deep; and cut leaving no tail. Absorbable sutures should *always* be used with this technique.

MATTRESS

The mattress technique produces more eversion than a simple suture and provides added strength; it is ideal for palms and soles of feet, or other areas of tissue tension. The *vertical mattress* has a similar approach as a simple suture, yet a second, superficial bite is taken in the same vertical plane. In contrast, the *horizontal mattress* advances the "second bite"

horizontally deep in the tissue rather than superficially. This pattern is specifically useful in wounds that are prone to natural inversion.

SUBCUTICULAR

The subcuticular pattern gives the best cosmetic results, and is simple and quick to place. It entails intradermal horizontal bites, using absorbable suture material. This approach allows the suture to remain in place for a longer period of time without the development of cross-hatch scarring. Once the wound is closed, wound tapes are frequently used for reinforcement.

FLAP/CORNER

The goal with the flap/corner stitch is to spare the vascular supply to a skin tip. A three-point suture is used to bring the wound edges together; it should be the first suture placed in a flap/corner wound.

Wound closure tapes, staples, and tissue adhesive are other closure alternatives. Tissue tape may be used for superficial or partial-thickness lacerations that are subject to considerable tension. This type of tape is also often used in conjunction with other wound closure methods for approximation of edges or wound reinforcement.

Wound staples are frequently used to close lacerations involving the scalp. They offer the advantage of rapid placement, but do not allow for meticulous wound edge approximation.

Tissue adhesives, such as 2-octylcyanoacrylate, are less painful and are quickly applied. They are ideal for small, clean lacerations that are not subject to large degrees of tension or mobility. A topical anesthetic may be used prior to their use. Wound preparation is as previously described. Unlike sutures, tissue adhesives do not require removal at a later date. Site selection is important because the product needs to remain dry for at least five days after application. Tissue adhesives are not intended for use inside of wounds, but rather they form a water-resistant barrier to the outside of the wound. Wound edges are manually approximated and adhesive applied, ideally in three layers. The first layer dries in less than 3 minutes. Excessive adhesive must be removed from surrounding tissues quickly. Extreme caution is warranted when applying such materials near or around the eyes. Infection rates for wounds closed with tissue adhesives are similar or better to those for sutured wounds.

Postprocedural care instructions for the family consist of keeping most wounds clean, dry, and covered for 48 hours. After 48 hours, the wound can be kept open to air, or covered with a simple dressing to keep the wound clean. Tap water and regular bath soap are sufficient for wound cleansing. Patients are told to avoid total submersion, such as in bath tubs and swimming pools. Application of an over-the-counter antibiotic ointment is recommended two to three times per day until sutures are removed, followed by judicious use of sunscreen to sun-exposed sites, for as long as a year following injury. Systemic antibiotics are not routinely recommended in immunocompetent patients, unless the injury involved a bite, intraoral laceration, or open fracture; extended into cartilage, joints, and tendons; or excessively contaminated wounds (Cummings & Del Beccaro, 1995). Confirm that the patient has an up-to-date tetanus vaccination. If this status is unknown, provide the vaccine during the presenting visit.

Potential complications of laceration repair or other wound closure techniques include infection, dehiscence, tissue necrosis, nerve injury, scar formation, skin hypersensitivity, and retained foreign body. Vital and routine aspects of wound closure will aid in limiting these complications. Thoroughly irrigate and explore wounds, evert superficial wound edges, and avoid excessive tension on sutures. In addition, educate the patient and the caregivers on signs and symptoms of infection, wound care, and indications for which to return to the healthcare professional (HCP).

PROCEDURE NOTE

An example procedure note for wound closure is as follows:

- Date and time.
- Laceration repair of left forehead.
- Indication: Wound through dermis.
- Performed by: State names and positions.
- Consent/permission: Obtained in English from both parents; risks and alternatives discussed.
- "Time-out" taken (universal protocol).
- Sedation/analgesia: LET 2 mL placed over the wound 30 minutes prior to the procedure.

- Site preparation: Procedural preparation and distraction were delivered by the child life specialist. The child was placed in a supine position. The 2-cm horizontal laceration was then irrigated with high-pressure normal saline. No foreign body was observed. The area was cleansed (be specific including irrigation solution volume) and draped in the usual sterile fashion. Anesthesia was achieved by infiltrating the wound edges with 3 mL of buffered 1% lidocaine.
- Procedure: Four 5-0 interrupted nylon sutures were placed with good approximation of wound margins. The patient remained pain free during the procedure.
- Site at conclusion of procedure: No active bleeding. Blood loss: None. Topical antibiotic ointment and a dressing were applied.
- Specimens sent: None.
- Patient condition following procedure: Child tolerated the procedure well.
- Signature of health care professional.

BIBLIOGRAPHY

1. Berede, C. (1993). Toxicity of local anesthetics in infants and children. *Journal of Pediatrics, 122,* S14.
2. Bruns, T., & Worthington, J. (2000). Using tissue adhesive for wound repair: A practical guide to Dermabond. *American Family Physician,* 61, 1383–1388.
3. Cummings, P., & Del Beccaro, M. (1995). Antibiotics to prevent infection of simple wounds: A meta-analysis of randomized studies. *American Journal of Emergency Medicine, 13,* 396.
4. Edlich, R., Rodeheaver, G., Morgan, R., et al. (1988). Principles of emergency wound management. *Annals of Emergency Medicine, 17*(12), 1284–1302.
5. Hollander, J., & Singer, A. (1999). Laceration management. *Annals of Emergency Medicine, 34,* 356.
6. Patel, A. (2008). Tongue lacerations. *British Dentistry Journal, 204*(7), 355.
7. Singer, A., Hollander, J., Subramanian, S., Malhotra, A., & Villez, P. (1994). Pressure dynamics of various irrigation techniques commonly used in the emergency department. *Annals of Emergency Medicine, 24*(1), 36–40.
8. Taketomo, C., Hodding, J., & Kraus, D. (2010). *Pediatric dosage handbook.* Hudson, OH: Lexi-Comp.

PART VI

Laboratory Values

Laboratory Values

The reference ranges provided here are general parameters. Consultation with the clinical laboratory is advised.

CHEMISTRIES

Amylase: 30–110 unit/L
Blood urea nitrogen (BUN): 5–20 mg/dL
Calcium: 4.5–5.5 mEq/L **or** 9–11 mg/dL
Carbon dioxide (CO_2): 22–30 mEq/L
Chloride: 95–110 mmol/L
Creatinine:
• < 1 month: 0.2–0.4 mg/dL
• Child: 0.3–0.7 mg/dL
• Adolescent: 0.5–1.0 mg/dL
Glucose: 60–110 gm/dL
Lactate: 2–20 mg/dL
Lipase: 20–140 unit/L
Magnesium: 1.8–2.2 mg/dL
Osmolality:
• Serum: 275–296 mOsm/kg
• Urine: 50–1400 mOsm/kg
Phosphorus: 3.5–6 mg/dL
Potassium: 3.5–5.3 mEq/L
Sodium: 135–146 mEq/L
Uric Acid: 2–7 mg/dL

LIVER FUNCTION STUDIES

Albumin: 3.5–5 gm/dL
Alkaline Phosphatase (ALP): 40–400 IU/L
Ammonia:
• Newborn: 90–150 µg/dL
• > 1 month: 40–120 µg/dL
Bilirubin:
• Total Bilirubin: > 12–15 mg/dL
• Direct Bilirubin:
  • Newborn: > 1.5 mg/dL
  • 1 month: > 0.5 mg/dL
Gamma-Glutamyl Transpeptidase (GGT): 8–78 IU/L
Lactate Dehydrogenase (LDH):
• Newborn: 290–500 unit/L
• > 1 month: 110–145 unit/L
Prealbumin:
• Newborn to 6 months: 7–39 mg/dL
• 7 months to 3 years: 2–36 mg/dL
• > 3 years: 12–40 mg/dL
Serum Glutamate Pyruvate Transaminase (SGPT) **or** Alanine Transaminase (ALT): 7–56 IU/L
Serum Glutamic-Oxaloacetic Transaminase (SGOT) **or** Aspartate Aminotransferase (AST): 5–35 IU/L
Total Protein: 6–8 gm/dL
Triglycerides: < 170 mg/dL

HEMATOLOGY AND MARKERS OF INFLAMMATION

C-reactive Protein (CRP): < 0.8 mg/dL **or** 10 mg/L
Erythrocyte Sedimentation Rate (ESR):
• < 2 months: 1–5 mm/hr
• > 2 months: 1–8 mm/hr
Hematocrit: 30–42%
Hemoglobin: 12–16 gm/dL
Mean Corpuscular Hemoglobin (MCH): > 30 pg/cell
Mean Corpuscular Hemoglobin Concentration (MCHC): 28–33%
Mean Corpuscular Value (MCV):
• Newborn: 95–121 fL
• 6 months to 2 years: 70–86 fL
• 12 to 18 years:
  • Female: 78–102 fL
  • Male: 78–98 fL
• > 18 years: 78–98 fL
Platelet Count: 150–350 ($\times 10^3$/mm^3)
Red Blood Cell (RBC) (million/mm^3):
• < 1 month: 3.6–6.6
• 1 to 6 months: 2.7–5.4
• 6 months to 6 years: 3.7–5.3
• 6 to 12 years: 4.0–5.2
• Female:
  • 12 to 18 years: 4.1–5.1
  • > 18 years: 3.8–5.2
• Male:
  • 12 to 18 years: 4.5–5.3
  • > 18 years: 4.4–5.9
Red blood cell distribution width (RDW):
• Newborn: < 18
• 1 to 6 months: < 16
• > 7 months: < 15
Reticulocyte Count:
• Newborn: 2–6%
• 1 to 6 months: 0–3%
• > 6 months: 0.5–1.5%
White blood cell (WBC): 5–14 ($\times 10^3$/mm^3):
• Segmented neutrophils: 45–65%
• Band neutrophils: 0–5%
• Eosinophils: 15–40%
• Basophils: 0–3%
• Lymphocytes: 15–40%
• Monocytes: 2–8%

COAGULATION STUDIES

D-Dimer: 0–0.5 µg/mL
Fibrinogen: 150–400 mg/dL

International Normalized Ratio (INR): 1.5–2
activated Partial Thromboplastin Time (aPTT): 25–35 sec
Partial Thromboplastin Time (PTT): 20–36 sec
Prothrombin Time (PT): 12–15 sec

THYROID FUNCTION STUDIES

Free Thyroxine Index (FTI):
- Newborn: 7.6–20
- 1 to 4 months: 7.4–17.9
- 4 to 12 months: 5.1–14.5
- > 1 year: 5–14

Thyroid-Stimulating Hormone (TSH):
> 7 days: 0–10 µIU/mL

Thyroxine (T_4):
- Newborn: 9–20 µg/dL
- > 1 month to 1 year: 5.5–16 µg/dL
- > 1 year: 4–12 µg/dL

T_3:
- Newborn: 100–470 ng/dL
- 1 to 5 years: 100–260 ng/dL
- > 5 years: 90–240 ng/dL

T_3 Uptake: 35–45%

CARDIAC ENZYMES

Creatine Kinase (CK) **or** Creatine Phosphokinase (CPK):
- Infant: 20–200 unit/L
- Child: 10–90 unit/L
- CPK Fractionated:CPK1-MB: 0–4%

Troponin: > 0.03 ng/L

COMPLEMENTS

C3: 96–195 mg/dL
C4: 15–20 mg/dL

BLOOD GAS

Measured	Arterial	Capillary	Venous
pH	7.35–7.45	7.35–7.45	7.32–7.42
pCO_2 (mmHg)	35–45	35–45	38–52
pO_2 (mmHg)	70–100	60–80	24–48
HCO_3 (mEq/L)	19–25	19–25	19–25
TCO_2 (mEq/L)	19–29	19–29	23–33
O_2 saturation (%)	90–95	90–95	40–70
Base excess (mEq/L)	5 to +5	5 to +5	5 to +5

CEREBROSPINAL FLUID STUDIES

Cell Count:
- < 1 month: < 22 WBC/mm^3
- > 1 month: < 0.7 cells/mm^3

CSF Glucose/Serum Glucose:
- Newborn: 44–128%
- > 1 month: 50%

Glucose:
- Newborn: 34–119 mg/dL
- > 1 month: 40–80 mg/dL

Protein:
- Newborn: 20–170 mg/dL
- > 1 month:
  - Lumbar: 5–40 mg/dL
  - Ventricular: 5–15 mg/dL

Traumatic tap:

RBCs (CSF)/RBCs (blood) × WBCs (blood) **or**
× protein (blood); subtract value from
obtained value on bloody CSF

WBCs (CSF) or protein (CSF): product
calculated above = true CSF WBC or true CSF protein

BIBLIOGRAPHY

1. Kuhn, M. (2007). *Lab reference pocket guide with drug effects*. Sudbury, MA: Jones and Bartlett.
2. National Institutes of Health Clinical Center. (n.d.). Pediatric laboratory ranges. Retrieved from http://www.cc.nih.gov/ccc/pedweb/pedsstaff/pedlab.html
3. Selected normal pediatric laboratory values. (n.d.). Retrieved from http://wps.prenhall.com/wps/media/objects/354/362846/London%20App.%20B.pdf
4. Taketomo, C., Hodding, J., & Kraus, D. (2010). *Pediatric dosage handbook* (17th ed.). Hudson, OH: Lexi-Comp.

Index